S0-CFU-543

William F. Cleary
11-22-97
Santa Cruz

Strombeck's Small Animal Gastroenterology

Strombeck's Small Animal Gastroenterology

THIRD EDITION

W. Grant Guilford, B.V.Sc., Ph.D., F.A.C.V.Sc.
Senior Lecturer, Small Animal Medicine
Department of Veterinary Clinical Sciences
Massey University
Palmerston North, New Zealand

Sharon A. Center, D.V.M.
Associate Professor
Department of Clinical Sciences
College of Veterinary Medicine
Cornell University
Ithaca, New York

Donald R. Strombeck, D.V.M., Ph.D.
Professor Emeritus
School of Veterinary Medicine
University of California
Davis, California

David A. Williams, M.A., Vet.M.B., Ph.D., M.R.C.V.S.
Chief, Section of Small Animal Medicine
Veterinary Teaching Hospital
Purdue University
West Lafayette, Indiana

Denny J. Meyer, B.S., D.V.M.
Professor, Department of Pathology
Service Chief, Clinical Pathology
College of Veterinary Medicine
Colorado State University
Fort Collins, Colorado

W.B. SAUNDERS COMPANY
A Division of Harcourt Brace & Company
Philadelphia London Toronto Montreal Sydney Tokyo

W.B. SAUNDERS COMPANY

A Division of Harcourt Brace & Company

The Curtis Center
Independence Square West
Philadelphia, PA 19106

Library of Congress Cataloging-in-Publication Data

Strombeck's Small animal gastroenterology.— 3rd ed. / W. Grant Guilford . . . [et al.]

p. cm.

Rev. ed. of: Small animal gastroenterology / Donald R. Strombeck.

Includes bibliographical references and index.

ISBN 0–7216–3760–4

1. Dogs—Diseases. 2. Cats—Diseases. 3. Veterinary gastroenterology. I. Guilford, W. Grant.
   II. Strombeck, Donald R. Small animal gastroenterology.

SF992. G38S77   1996

636.7'089633—dc20   95-22527

STROMBECK'S SMALL ANIMAL GASTROENTEROLOGY   ISBN 0–7216–3760–4

Copyright © 1996, 1990, 1979 by W.B. Saunders Company

All rights reserved. No part of this publication may be reproduced or transmitted in any form or by any means, electronic or mechanical, including photocopy, recording, or any information storage and retrieval system, without permission in writing from the publisher.

Printed in the United States of America.

Last digit is the print number: 9   8   7   6   5   4   3   2   1

Preface

In the six years since the second edition, knowledge of veterinary medicine and veterinary gastroenterology has continued to grow at a rapid rate. To keep pace with this new information, three additional authors have been invited to contribute to *Strombeck's Small Animal Gastroenterology*. Sharon Center, Dave Williams, and Denny Meyer are experts in their fields and have made invaluable contributions to the text.

All chapters of the third edition have been extensively updated. The chapters on the liver, pancreas, malabsorption, and diagnostic techniques have been completely rewritten. Throughout the revision, we have maintained several aims. The first has been to provide the practitioner with a workable guide to the diagnosis and treatment of gastrointestinal disease. The second has been to provide an extensive reference work on the physiology of the canine and feline gastrointestinal system and on the etiopathogenesis and pathophysiology of its diseases for those veterinarians with a penchant for deeper understanding of gastroenterology. To some degree these two aims are contradictory. With exhaustive discussion of pathophysiology we run the risk of obscuring clinical details, much to the frustration of the busy practitioner. To circumvent this problem we have further expanded the chapters on the diagnostic evaluation of common gastrointestinal problems. In addition, we have continued to place a "clinical synopsis" at the beginning of the description of all diseases receiving extensive discussion or that have confusing diagnostic criteria. The "clinical synopsis" represents a collection of prominent clinical features along with a pragmatic suggestion as to therapy. Pragmatism does not sit well with medicine, and so it is our plea that clinicians take these therapeutic recommendations as guides for subsequent modification according to the particular needs of the patient under their care.

The third aim of the present edition is to highlight areas in which knowledge of small animal gastroenterology is lacking in the hope of stimulating research in those areas.

As with the second edition, we hope this book will enable clinicians to have a better understanding of the gastrointestinal problems that constitute an important part of small animal practice. Your critical suggestions are again invited.

W. Grant Guilford

Acknowledgments

First and foremost we wish to thank the veterinary clinicians and researchers whose dedication and hard work have provided the published information that forms the foundation of this book.

Grant Guilford extends personal appreciation to the co-authors of this edition for the long nights and weekends required to condense their knowledge and experience into the chapters of this book. It has been a great pleasure for me to work with colleagues with such dedication to excellence. I also wish to thank the partners and families of my co-authors. I have been demanding of your loved ones' time, and I thank you for your patience. Once again, I thank the veterinarians who have trained, inspired, and encouraged me, most notably Drs. Edward Kirk, Boyd Jones, and Doug and Sandy Cooper of New Zealand; C. B. Chastain, Brent Jones, Dudley McCaw, and Dennis O'Brien of Missouri; and Gerald Ling, Donald Strombeck, and Quinton Rogers of Davis. I also wish to affectionately thank my family, Patricia and Parry, for their constant support, and my wife, Sandra Forsyth, for her care and patience.

Sharon Center extends appreciation to the many residents and faculty members, particularly Drs. John Randolph, William Hornbuckle, and Bud Tennant, who each contributed in special ways, endorsing, supporting, and stimulating my interest in hepatobiliary disease in the dog and cat over the past 15 years at Cornell. I also wish to extend a special recognition to the many referring practitioners, medicine and ICU technicians, and faculty involved in ancillary support services in our teaching hospital, especially Drs. Amy Yeager and Ned Dykes, who made possible the case load, excellent patient care, and diagnostic evaluations that provide much of the case-based information presented in the hepatobiliary chapters of this book. Acknowledgment is also made to Dr. Peter Rowland, who enthusiastically and tirelessly reviewed countless liver biopsies with me while he was at Cornell. My initial interest in liver disease was inspired by one of my professors, Dr. Don Strombeck, while I was a veterinary student at the University of California at Davis. I thank him for his excellent example that a veterinary clinician and educator can advance both scientific knowledge and its practical application in the field of veterinary gastroenterology. Lastly, I especially wish to acknowledge my husband, Kirk Sapa, for his seemingly unlimited patience, good will, sense of humor, encouragement, and willingness to keep our household functional while I was immersed in the chapters I contributed to this text.

Donald R. Strombeck wishes to reiterate the acknowledgments expressed in the preface to the first edition and affectionately acknowledges his wife, Elizabeth Strombeck, for her patience and encouragement.

David Williams gratefully acknowledges the assistance of his wife, Catherine, in the preparation of the manuscripts, as well as her moral support and encouragement. He also wishes to recognize the productive and enjoyable interactions with the numerous veterinarians, veterinary students, and technicians who have worked in his laboratories at the University of Florida, Kansas State University, and Purdue University over the last decade.

Denny Meyer graciously acknowledges (1) the many practitioners that contributed specimens for examination and provided patient follow-up; (2) the interaction with clinicians and pathologists (especially Dr. Bob Shields) at the University of Florida and Drs. Joel Andres, College of Medicine, and Daisy Franzini, Veterans Administration Hospital, for providing an opportunity to study comparative hepatic histopathology, and, most recently, Colorado State University, notably clinical stimulation by Dr. David Cameron Twedt, his residents, and the pathology mentorship of Dr. David Getzy; (3) Bob Zink and the other histotechnicians at Colorado State University for the many, many special stains (no more retic stains, Frank) that were professionally made; and (4) Sterling Winthrop, notably Dr. Harry Olson, for providing a scientific environment and opportunity to complete the manuscripts. Denny warmly dedicates the effort to the three most precious jewels in the crown of his life, Jae, Jen, and Chris. To the former, his delightful wife, there are no words to express the gratitude for understanding, tolerating, and enduring, once again, the solitude of late evenings, most weekends, and holidays while Meyer was at the office. Jae, you are special and wonderful.

The Authors

Contents

Color Plates follow page 642.

Notice

Companion animal practice is an ever-changing field. Standard safety precautions must be followed, but as new research and clinical experience grow, changes in treatment and drug therapy become necessary or appropriate. The authors and editors of this work have carefully checked the generic and trade drug names and verified drug dosages to assure that dosage information is precise and in accord with standards accepted at the time of publication, Readers are advised, however, to check the product information currently provided by the manufacturer of each drug to be administered to be certain that changes have not been made in the recommended dose or in the contraindications for administration. This is of particular importance in regard to new or infrequently used drugs. Recommended dosages for animals are sometimes based on adjustments in the dosage that would be suitable for humans. Some of the drugs mentioned here have been given experimentally by the authors. Others have been used in dosages greater than those recommended by the manufacturer. In these kinds of cases, the authors have reported on their own considerable experience. It is the responsibility of those administering a drug, relying on their professional skill and experience, to determine the dosages, the best treatment for the patient, and whether the benefits of giving a drug justify the attendant risk. The authors and editors cannot be responsible for misuse or misapplication of the material in this work.

The Publisher

1

Integration of Gastrointestinal Functions

DONALD R. STROMBECK

INTRODUCTION

Functions basic to the gastrointestinal tract include those of motility, secretion, and absorption. Each function is regulated so it integrates with a similar function in another part of the gastrointestinal tract; that is, gastric motility is integrated by reflexes or hormones with colonic motility. Function of each type is regulated so it integrates with the other types of functions; that is, gastric secretion is integrated by reflexes or hormones with gastrointestinal motility. Absorption of electrolytes and nutrients, once thought to be unregulated, is influenced by many neural and endocrine/paracrine chemicals.

Functions in the gastrointestinal tract is also integrated with other systems of the body. Gastrointestinal function changes in response to events in other systems, and it is also determined by regulatory mechanisms that are located outside of the system. In the early nineteenth century William Beaumont described changes in gastric function caused by mental or psychologic stimulation. Recent studies show how injection of many peptide hormones and other chemicals into parts of the brain stimulate or inhibit specific gastrointestinal functions. Many of the gastrointestinal peptide hormones are now identified as neurotransmitters in the nervous system (Table 1–1). Function in the gastrointestinal tract also causes changes in other systems. Cause-or-effect alterations in gastrointestinal function are either normal or abnormal. Because abnormal changes are often merely exaggerations of a normally well-regulated process, understanding the normal is important to understanding the pathogenesis of disease.

The gastrointestinal functions that begin in the posterior pharynx with the initiation of swallowing are reflex events, not under voluntary control. From that point on, the only conscious control is over the external anal sphincter. The functions of the pharynx and esophagus are entirely motor, in order to move food to the stomach; the actions are controlled by nerves that have their cell bodies in the brain stem. As food passes from the pharynx to the stomach, sphincters open and close the beginning and end of the esophagus. Nerves also control their function.

The movement of food into the stomach causes relaxation of the region near the entrance, which allows more food to enter without causing a great increase in intragastric pressure. Relaxation is a neurally mediated phenomenon. Motility increases in more caudal parts of the stomach in order to mix and empty its contents. This augmentation of motility,

under the control of events occurring both inside and outside the stomach, is mediated by nerves and hormones. Events occurring in the small intestine influence gastric motility, with the primary objective of inhibiting motility and reducing the amount of chyme entering the small intestine. That prevents overloading of the digestive and absorptive capacities of the intestinal tract.

The stomach responds to a meal by secreting hydrochloric acid and protein-digesting enzymes. The stimuli for secretion are quite specific, amino acids and gastric distention being the most important. The amount of gastric secretion is related directly to the volume of the diet and the amount of protein it contains. A prime mediator of secretion is the hormone gastrin, the release of which is subject to feedback control. Secretion also depends on the parasympathetic nerve supply to the stomach.

Chyme enters the small intestine at a programmed rate so that adjustments in pH can be made before the acidity and pepsin degrade pancreatic enzymes and mucosal cell structures. Chyme can be hyperosmolar, and regulation of its delivery to the intestine prevents excessive amounts from entering and osmotically drawing large amounts of extracellular fluid into the lumen. The stimuli of acidity and hyperosmolality reduce the rate of gastric emptying by reflex pathways that involve neural and endocrine messengers.

The pancreas and intestinal mucosa secrete enzyme and alkaline fluid into the intestine. Specific stimuli of acid pH, amino acids, and fatty acids cause the release of hormonal messengers from the intestinal mucosa, stimulating secretion of an alkaline and enzyme-rich pancreatic juice. The composition of this secretion is variable and reflects a purposeful

Table 1–1

PARACRINE OR HORMONAL MESSENGERS IDENTIFIED IN ENTEROENDOCRINE CELLS

5-hydroxytryptamine	Neurotensin
Glucagon/glicentin	Cholecystokinin
Somatostatin	Motilin
Substance P	Gastrin
Gastric inhibitory peptide	Peptide YY
Secretin	β-endorphin/β-lipotropin
	Pro-γ-melanocyte-stimulating hormone

response to the intestine's immediate needs, which may be either to neutralize acids or to digest proteins. The small intestine contains many different hormones that help integrate all events during digestive periods.

The motility of the resting intestine changes when food enters. That is necessary to delay the food's passage so processing can be complete. The motility change involves an increase in the strength and amplitude of rhythmic segmentation. The stimulus for this change is distention of the intestine by chyme. A neural reflex that is contained entirely within the wall of the intestine mediates the motility response. This motility is augumented by increased activity in parasympathetic fibers coming to the intestine from outside the gut. Some intestinal hormones can also increase motility. Intestinal motility can be inhibited in a few situations, often involving a pathologic process.

Bile is added to chyme in the intestine at a rate determined by neural events in the vagi and by hormones released from the mucosa of the gut. These cause the gall bladder to contract. They also stimulate the liver to secrete bile acids, an important process because the pool of bile acids must circulate through the intestine and back to it via the liver two or three times during every meal.

Digestion of food is a chemical process; the amounts and kinds of both enzyme and substrate in the gut and the conditions under which the reaction must take place determine the rate of digestion. The process progresses to completion unless nutrients are sequestered by fiber, or secretion or motility in the intestine is abnormal. Absorption of nutrients is also an unregulated event, dependent on the surface area of the intestinal mucosa, the integrity of the mucosal epithelial cells, and the absence of disease in the lamina propria and lymphatics. Carbohydrate digestion and absorption depends on normal disaccharidase levels and a normal glucose transport mechanism in the epithelial cell. Lipid absorption requires normal lymphatic drainage and a surface area of the small intestine that has not been appreciably reduced.

The rate of blood flow to secreting organs dictates their rate of secretion because the circulation must provide both fluid and electrolytes, needed to secrete a modified extracellular fluid, and the energy required for its formation. Rate of blood flow is also important in the intestine, where it influences the absorption of nutrients and electrolytes. Both neural events and hormones regulate the rate of splanchnic blood flow in response to a meal.

Hormones have a trophic effect on the mucosa of the alimentary tract; that is, they are required for mucosal growth and maintenance of normal size. These are important in maintaining the mucosa's secretory and absorptive functions.

A vast complicated system of microorganisms lives within the gastrointestinal tract. The host and this system live in harmony, but only as a result of the maintenance of normal functions in the alimentary canal. Overgrowth of the microflora is prevented by acid secretions of the stomach, by normal peristalsis, and by the inherent immune system of the gut. Gastrointestinal function is optimal with the intestinal microflora intact and properly ordered. When the balance within its ecology is upset, major clinical signs of disease appear.

CONTROL OF GASTROINTESTINAL FUNCTION

Gastrointestinal motor function results from control exerted on the muscles by both primitive and sophisticated nervous systems and by the endocrines. Neural and endocrine control also regulate secretory and absorptive functions. Because both of those functions depend on

changes in blood flow to the organ, control of microcirculation to the gut becomes important. Finally, the gross and microscopic structures of the tissues in the gastrointestinal tract depend for both growth and renewal on outside trophic influences.

MOTILITY AND FLUID TRANSPORT IN THE GASTROINTESTINAL TRACT

Basic Factors in Motility[1-5]

Most motility in the gastrointestinal tract is a function of smooth muscle. The only exception is in the esophagus. A combination of myogenic, neural, and hormonal factors regulate smooth muscle motility.

The myogenic factors are fundamental to gastrointestinal function because denervated gut exhibits both localized and propagated contractions. Spontaneous motor activity and autorhythmicity, which are features of myogenic activity, are run by slow waves, pacesetter potentials, basic electrical rhythm or electrical control activity, synonymous terms used to describe the regular periodic depolarizations that can be recorded (Figure 1–1). At the peak of each depolarization there is an increased excitability or an increased probability for a spike discharge, which triggers muscle contraction. The number of spikes that occur during the period of maximum depolarization determines the strength or amplitude of the contraction. Neural and humoral control over the smooth muscle influences the spikes and contractions. The periodicity of the slow wave or electrical control activity determines the rhythmic nature of the muscle contractions. Thus, this myogenic factor sets the basic pattern of the mechanical event.

In the small intestine, slow waves appear to arise in the area between circular and longitudinal muscle, possibly from interstitial cells of Cajal, and activity spreads through the circular muscle, which is the most important muscle for both segmental and peristaltic contractions. Slow waves arise in circular smooth muscle in the colon. Slow waves are generated by changes in ion movements across the membranes of the smooth muscle cell. The nature of the mechanism is far from resolved, although it has been suggested it results from either changes in sodium conductance (permeability changes for the ion) or from the modulating current produced by an oscillating electrogenic ion pump.

The local flow of current from one cell to another propagates slow waves. The factor that determines the amount of propagation is the degree of electrical coupling between muscle cells. Propagation occurs in the longitudinal muscle layer

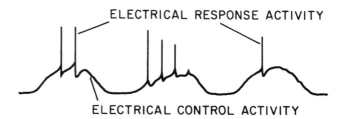

FIGURE 1-1. Schematic of electrical activity of smooth muscle in the gastrointestinal tract. A basic electrical control activity (slow waves) is always present that does not cause muscle contractions. Electrical response activity follows stimulation by a variety of means and results in muscle contractions.

before spreading to the circular layer. The degree of electrical coupling may be influenced by hormones and by mechanical deformation of the muscle. This has an effect on contractile activity.

The rate of depolarization generating slow waves in smooth muscle differs between the parts of the gastrointestinal tract. Slow wave frequency is higher at the beginning of the small intestine than at the end.

By virtue of its myogenic properties, smooth muscle usually responds to being stretched by contracting, but if the muscle is actively contracting when stretched, it can respond by relaxing. Thus, stretch produced by distention can, on one hand, stimulate contractile motility (as in rhythmic segmentation and peristalsis), or, on the other hand, it can cause relaxation (as in the fundus of the stomach or in the colon during filling). This latter phenomenon, called receptive relaxation, assists the stomach and colon in receiving and holding large volumes without developing increased intraluminal pressure.

The contraction of smooth muscles occurs during the most excitable period, which is at the height of slow wave depolarization (Figure 1–1). Each contraction is accompanied by a period of rapid depolarization and repolarization. The electrical activity at this time has been called fast activity, action potentials, and electrical response activity, but is now best known as spike potentials. The most important influences for its activity are neural and hormonal factors.

Basic Factors in Fluid Transport

The secretions produced by various organs in the gastrointestinal tract differ in composition from the extracellular fluid from which they are derived. Energy-dependent transport processes are required to produce different ion concentrations on opposing sides of the membranes. The ion transport mechanisms have neural and humoral regulation.

Neurologic Control of Motility and Fluid Transport

REGULATION BY INTRINSIC NERVOUS SYSTEM.[6–8] Control of motility and fluid transport, which is primarily due to secretion, is accomplished at the most rudimentary level by a primitive self-contained intrinsic nervous system. This system consists of subserous, myenteric, submucosal, and mucosal intrinsic plexuses, including their intercommunications. A simple reflex arc, illustrated in Figure 1–2, consists of (1) a receptor that responds to chemical or mechanical stimuli in the lumen of the gastrointestinal tract; (2) a synapse; and (3) an efferent nerve fiber to a smooth muscle fiber or a secretory cell. Thus, this mechanism allows the gut to respond to events in the immediate vicinity. In general, stimulation of a local reflex arc elicits an excitatory response resulting in secretion or smooth muscle contraction. The neurotransmitter for this pathway is acetylcholine, with a nicotinic receptor at the ganglionic synapse and a muscarinic type at the neuromuscular junction.

The intrinsic nervous system is essential to gastrointestinal function. That is not always true for the extrinsic nerves. For example, a vagotomy changes motility and secretion in the small intestine very little. In other organs the extrinsic nerves are important for function (see later). Without outside assistance, the intrinsic nervous system is unable to maintain an adequate level of function to prevent a loss of homeostasis.

Basic function in the ganglionic synapse can be modified

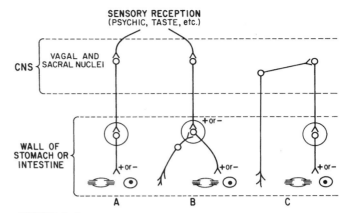

FIGURE 1–2. (A) Schematic showing how control of function in muscle and secretory cells is augmented or inhibited directly by the central nervous system (CNS). (B) Effect of the CNS to influence activity that is stimulated or inhibited by events within the alimentary tract. (C) Events in the gastrointestinal tract regulate function by long pathways that synapse in the CNS.

by gastrointestinal endocrines and norepinephrine, the neurotransmitter for the sympathetic nervous system. Gastrin and cholecystokinin stimulate, and secretin inhibits, the release of acetylcholine and the contraction of smooth muscle in the gastroesophageal sphincter and intestines. Norepinephrine inhibits the release of acetylcholine in the ganglia.

REGULATION BY EXTRINSIC NERVOUS SYSTEM.[6,9,10] The most important way to regulate function in the gastrointestinal tract is by the extrinsic nervous system and by hormones secreted in one part of the tract and acting on another part. The extrinsic nervous system consists of both efferent and afferent fibers in the vagal, sacral, and splanchnic nerves (Figure 1–3). The vagal and sacral nerves contain parasympathetic fibers that are the most important for regulating normal events. The splanchnics contain sympathetics that are less important in that a sympathectomy does not produce visible signs of disrupted function, whereas cutting the parasympathetic results in significant losses of function. In general, reflexes that receive stimuli in a proximal part of the bowel and produce a response in a more distal part are anticipatory: They prepare the distal section for imminent events. For example, during the cephalic phase of gastric secretion, the

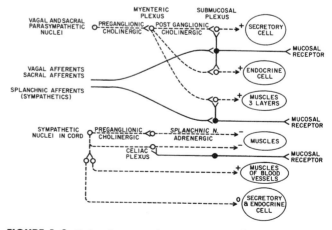

FIGURE 1–3. Role of autonomic nervous system in regulating gastrointestinal function. Parasympathetics are mostly facilitatory, and sympathetics are inhibitory. Role of sympathetics is unimportant in normal function.

stimulus to the animal of the presence of food before it arrives in the stomach results in a vagally mediated secretion of gastric juice that is rich in enzymes. The later presence of food in the stomach stimulates a gastroileal reflex that causes the ileum to evacuate its contents in anticipation of food that will be arriving soon. In contrast, reflexes that receive stimuli in a distal part of the bowel and produce a response in cranial parts are usually inhibitory. For example, chemical or mechanical stimulation of the duodenum causes inhibition of gastric motility by the enterogastric reflex; carbohydrates and fat in the ileum inhibit gastric emptying of solids.

Parasympathetic Control. The efferent fibers in the vagal and sacral nerves are primarily excitatory and function to initiate and reinforce the motility and secretion that are necessary during the digestive period. They are all preganglionic in that they synapse on the ganglia of the intrinsic nervous system and, as shown in Figure 1–2, they can modulate ongoing activity in the reflex arcs of the intrinsic system. The neurotransmitter in these pathways is acetylcholine; chemicals in the area of the synapse can modify its release, as shown in Figure 1–4. The nerves which carry these cholinergic fibers also contain nonadrenergic noncholinergic fibers that cause relaxation of smooth muscle when stimulated.[11] They are responsible for receptive relaxation of the stomach, vagally mediated relaxation of the stomach and gastroesophageal sphincter, descending inhibition of the intestine during peristalsis, and inhibition of the internal anal sphincter. The neurotransmitter is most likely vasoactive intestinal peptide or in some cases adenosine triphosphate. Recent studies show nitric oxide to be an important mediator for nonadrenergic noncholinergic (NANC) neural inhibition of gastrointestinal smooth muscle in a pathway (Figure 1–5). Nitric oxide mediates muscle relaxation by stimulating 5' cyclic guanosine monophosphate (cGMP). Some postganglionic fibers in the colon are adrenergic, causing relaxation of smooth muscle when their parasympathetic innervation is stimulated. Nicotine stimulation of the ganglionic receptors produces relaxation, and this response is blocked by adrenergic antagonists. Thus, parasympathetic stimulation can elicit three types of

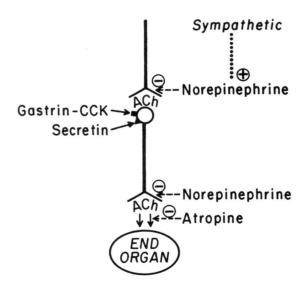

FIGURE 1–4. Diagram of ganglionic synapse and connection between nerve ending and structure innervated. Acetylcholine (Ach) release can be inhibited by norepinephrine, and its binding on receptor sites is blocked by atropine. The gastrin and secretin families of gut hormones possess receptors that can either augment or inhibit neural activity.

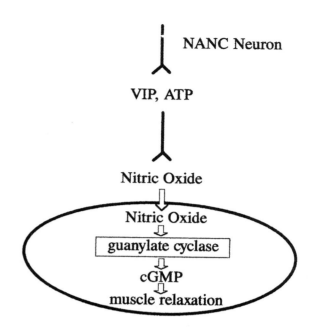

FIGURE 1–5. Schematic of neural pathway that releases nitric oxide as a neurotransmitter.

chemical responses, with the main result being muscle contraction and stimulation of secretion.

Sympathetic Control. Sympathetic nerve fibers leave the spinal cord through the ventral roots. Their preganglionic fibers synapse in the celiac and mesenteric ganglia in regions remote from the walls of the bowel. Postganglionic fibers follow the arterial blood supply to the end organs and terminate on secretory cells, gastrointestinal smooth muscle, and blood vessel smooth muscle. Stimulation of these fibers usually reduces secretion, relaxes gastrointestinal smooth muscle, and causes blood vessel muscles to contract. Sympathetic fibers also terminate on ganglia, where their effect is to inhibit the release of acetylcholine, by this means blocking transmission through an excitatory pathway (Figure 1–4). The postganglionic neurotransmitter for sympathetic fibers is norepinephrine. This amine affects both smooth muscle function and acetylcholine release but does not directly affect secretory function. Norepinephrine reduces rates of fluid secretion, although that response is secondary to the amine's effect in reducing blood flow. In summary, the overall effects of sympathetic activity are to reduce muscle activity and cell secretion, although it is questionable whether those effects are physiologically important in the normal animal. Increased sympathetic activity is important in the pathogenesis of the hypomotility that frequently follows trauma, surgery, and acute stress. In the extreme case, gastric dilatation or paralytic ileus develops.

NEURAL CONTROL OF HORMONE RELEASE.[12] Gastrointestinal hormones act in a complex way in concert with the nervous system to regulate gastrointestinal function. Some of the hormones are released by a stimulus that acts through the nervous system. The best example of this is the vagally induced release of gastrin during feeding. This is a reflex over extrinsic nerves. An example of neurally released hormones over an intrinsic pathway is the release of gastrin from the gastric antrum in response to chemicals on the mucosal surface. Both of these neural pathways are cholinergic.

Chemical transmission in the neural regulation of the gastrointestinal tract occurs via a number of peptides as well as acetylcholine, norepinephrine, and nitric oxide (Table 1–2). All of the enteric neuropeptides are found in neurons elsewhere in the body, notably the brain. The peptides are grouped into families: (1) substance P, (2) vasoactive intestinal peptide, PHI, and secretin, (3) opioids, (4) bombesin, (5) gastrin-cholecystokin (CCK), and (6) pancreatic polypeptide and neuropeptide y (NPY). Somatostatin and neurotensin are other neuropeptides or paracrines.

Substance P is an excitatory transmitter acting within the myenteric plexus on cholinergic neurons and also directly on smooth muscle during the peristaltic reflex. VIP is a neurotransmitter that stimulates pancreatic secretion, intestinal secretion, blood flow, and smooth muscle relaxation. Opioids released on neural stimulation after smooth muscle motility affect the myenteric plexus and the muscle directly; the net effect is to delay transit. Opioid peptides also inhibit intestinal secretion. Bombesin is released during vagal stimulation and is the noncholinergic mediator of gastrin release. The effects of gastrin-CCK, pancreatic polypeptide, and somatostatin are summarized in Table 1–4.

Endocrine Control of Motility and Fluid Transport[7,13–15]

The mediators of gastrointestinal function are chemicals that bind to receptor sites and evoke a response. The chemicals released by neural reflexes are secreted instantly, in exact amounts, and at the point where they act. Endocrines are chemical mediators that are also released in exact amounts but perform their function at a point distant from release, with a physiologic response that is less rapid. The actions of both the neurotransmitters and the endocrines produce specific responses. The gastrointestinal endocrines are produced by peptide-secreting cells, some of which are also amine-precursor-uptake decarboxylase (APUD) cells that originate in the neural crest of the embryo and migrate to sites in the gastric, intestinal, and pancreatic tissues. The hormones these produce are mostly polypeptides, many with structural and functional similarities. Some cells produce biogenic amines such as serotonin, which acts as a chemical messenger. A variety of stimuli, acting locally or remotely, release the hormones; each has receptor sites in all tissues of the gastrointestinal tract. Thus, to a greater or lesser degree, they have effects on all aspects of gastrointestinal function, with their most important effects on secretion. The variety and amounts of hormones described make the gastrointestinal system the largest and probably most complex endocrine organ in the body.

RELEASE OF HORMONES BY INTRALUMINAL EVENTS. Endocrines are released in response to specific chemical stimuli acting on the mucosa of the stomach and intestine. The receptors are highly specific in that they respond well to only certain stimuli. For example, gastrin release is mediated by amino acids of the sarcosine series (glycine, alanine, serine) that bathe the antral mucosa. Cholecystokinin is released by L-isomers only of tryptophan, phenylalanine, and valine, by fatty acids with carbon chains greater than 10, and to a slight extent by acid pH. Secretin is released by acid pH, with a threshold at 4.5, and the degree of acidity below pH 4.5 determines the amount released. Enteroglucagon release is stimulated by monosaccharides in the small intestine, and glucose is more effective than galactose and fructose. Present knowledge indicates the stimuli are chemicals that act directly on the endocrine cell to stimulate hormone release, and the effect is not blocked by any known inhibitors of neural transmission. In general, calcium stimulates endocrine

Table 1–2

NEUROTRANSMITTER OR NEUROMODULATORY SUBSTANCES IN ENTERIC NERVOUS SYSTEM

Acetylcholine	Somatostatin
Norepinephrine	VIP
5-Hydroxytryptamine	Enkephalin
Purine nucleotides	Substance P
Dopamine	Bombesin
Neurotensin	GABA
Cholecystokinin	Gastrin
Glycine	Histamine
Motilin	Thyrotropin-releasing
Angiotensin	hormone
Secretin	Prostaglandins
Galanin	PHI
Neuropeptide y	GRP

release when placed in the lumen of the gut. The mechanisms for release are unknown.

RELEASE OF HORMONES BY HORMONES. The release of endocrines from peptide-secreting cells is not under feedback inhibition by blood levels of the endocrine. Other endocrines, however, stimulate and inhibit their release. Secretin and glucagon inhibit the release of gastrin, and catecholamines stimulate its release. Many of the important endocrines of the gut stimulate the release of insulin.

RELEASE OF HORMONES BY NEURAL REFLEXES. Neural reflexes throughout the gastrointestinal tract release endocrines. This is the most important means of hormone release in the stomach. Elsewhere in the gut, the release of endocrines depends more on intraluminal chemicals. Vagotomy does not significantly alter normal digestive processes in the gastrointestinal tract caudal to the stomach. Gastrin is released from the antrum of the stomach by local neural reflexes in which mechanical distention stimulates a cholinergic pathway. The same mechanical stimulus in the fundus of the stomach triggers a neural reflex with a longer pathway, causing G cells to release gastrin in the antrum. Chemical stimuli in the fundus stimulate gastrin release via the same pathway. Both of the antral and fundic receptors are also a part of long reflex arcs that synapse in the central nervous system and have afferent and efferent fibers in the vagi.

Neural and Endocrine Chemical Effects on Receptor Sites

There are two main families of gut hormones: secretin and those structurally similar, and gastrin and its related peptides. There are separate receptor sites for each family. Every neurally or chemically responsive tissue in the gastrointestinal tract has receptors for these two families of endocrines and for the neurotransmitters. The affinity of a receptor site is greatest for the chemical that produces its principal effect on that tissue. The substance exerting greatest affinity at its preferred site is a full agonist of function in that tissue. Other members of the same family of peptides have the ability to bind to the site, although usually with less affinity for it. Because their binding produces less than normal stimulation of function, they are only partial agonists of function. The number of peptide molecules binding at a receptor site is determined by its affinity for the site and by the number of similar molecules in the vicinity. If a partial agonist is present in high concentrations, the peptide will displace any full agonist present at lower levels, resulting in stimulation that is less than maximum. Affinity for a site is expressed as the rate at which the chemical associates and dissociates with the receptor. The interactions of two members of a peptide family can be illustrated with gastrin and its likeness, cholecystokinin. Gastrin causes maximum gastric acid secretion when it occupies its receptor sites on oxyntic cells. Cholecystokinin binds to the receptor with less affinity than gastrin, but if large amounts of the former are present, it will displace gastrin. In this case the resulting secretion is less than maximum, because cholecystokinin is only a partial agonist of secretion even though it is a stimulator of secretion. As stated earlier, there must also be a receptor for the secretin family of peptides, and when the receptor is occupied by secretin there is an inhibition of acid secretion. Gastric acid secretion requires interaction of activities at receptors for acetylcholine, gastrin, and histamine; these chemicals must interact with their respective sites before the secretion rate is optimum There are also receptor sites that regulate motility in the gastrointestinal tract. An example is shown in Figure 1–4, where the gastrin family of peptides are agonists of intestinal motility and secretin is an inhibitor. The interaction of these chemicals has important effects in the fed animal, which is not to imply they disappear in the fasting state. Basal levels of the chemicals are present at all times. They contribute to a function that continues at low levels during the interdigestive period.

Endocrines Designed to Regulate Gastrointestinal Function

GASTRIN-CHOLOECYSTOKININ FAMILY. The basic gastrin molecule consists of 17 amino acids, and the molecule of cholecystokinin is made up of 33 amino acids. The C-terminal five amino acids are identical in the two hormones (Table 1–3). Thus, that terminal is considered the hormones' active site. The C-terminal tetrapeptide has about one-tenth the molar potency of the complete gastrin molecule in its ability to stimulate gastric acid secretion. Although they vary in potency, all forms of gastrin from the tetrapeptide to the heptadecapeptide are full agonists for gastric secretion. Pentagastrin, a pentapeptide, has considerably more activity. Cholecystokinin stimulates pancreatic enzyme secretion and contraction of the gall bladder. For it to be biologically active, the heptapeptide must possess a sulfated tyrosyl residue, and that is present in the seventh position from the C-terminus. The C-terminal octapeptide is five times as potent as the parent molecule, and the activity of the decapeptide is 10 times as potent. Desulfation of the tyrosyl residue results in a loss of potency. The gastrin heptadecapeptide is found in a sulfated and nonsulfated form in its tyrosyl residue at position 6 from the C-terminus. They are gastrin II and I, respectively. Gastrin differs from cholecystokinin in that sulfation is not necessary for full biologic activity. Moreover, the decapeptide of cholecystokinin becomes a full agonist of gastric acid secretion if its tyrosyl residue is desulfated. The sulfated tyrosyl is not as effective an agonist of gall bladder contraction and pancreatic secretion if it is in the 6-position from the C-terminus. The gastrin-cholecystokinin family contains another member, called caerulein, that is not found in mammals but occurs as a decapeptide in frog skin. The effects of this peptide on gastrointestinal function have revealed many of the function–structure relationships for members of the family.

Gastrin and cholecystokinin, like other gastrointestinal hormones, have receptors on all organs in the system. Thus, excitatory or inhibitory effects have been demonstrated for these hormones infused into experimental animals. The responses are due to the pharmacologic effects of the hor-

Table 1–3

PARTIAL STRUCTURE OF GASTRIN (16 AMINO ACIDS) AND CHOLECYSTOKININ (33 AMINO ACIDS) SHOWING END OF PEPTIDES THAT POSSESS BIOLOGIC ACTIVITY

Gastrin (10 amino acids)	Ala-TyrS-Gly-Trp-Met-Asp-Phe-NH₂
Cholecystokinin (26 amino acids)	TyrS-Met-Gly-Trp-Met-Asp-Phe NH₂

mone, and the question arises as to whether all the described effects are also physiologic; that is, are they the same effects produced by the small amounts of hormones released under physiologic conditions? In the dog and cat, gastrin concentrations increase from about 20 pmol/L to 70 pmol/L after a meal, and the changes in gastrointestinal function produced by those levels of gastrin are considered physiologic (Table 1–4). Those changes in gastrin levels stimulate gastric secretion of acid and enzymes, motility of the antrum, insulin release, and splanchnic blood flow. Gastrin, being structurally similar to cholecystokinin, is a full agonist of pancreatic secretion of enzymes. Because it is less potent than cholecystokinin in stimulating gall bladder contraction and secretion of bile by the liver, however, it is only a partial agonist of those functions. Cholecystokinin's major function is to stimulate pancreatic secretion, gall bladder contraction, and the secretion of bile by the liver. Its functions outside those organs are mainly on the stomach, where cholecystokinin is a partial agonist of acid secretion in the dog and a full agonist of acid secretion in the cat. Cholecystokinin stimulates the release of insulin and glucagon. The major effects of both gastrin and cholecystokinin on gut motility are to delay gastric emptying.

The heptadecapeptide of gastrin has a half-life of 3 minutes. A larger peptide of gastrin, consisting of the 17 residue form joined with another 17 amino acids, has a half-life of 9 minutes. The kidneys and intestines remove gastrin from the circulation. The liver removes fragments of gastrin molecules. The half-life of cholecystokinin is 2.6 minutes, and the kidney plays an important role in its removal and catabolism. With such a short half-life the hormone has to be taken up by other tissues in the body. It was thought the liver is the most important organ in removal of gut endocrines from the portal circulation, but cholecystokinin, like intact gastrin, is not removed and catabolized by the liver. It seems logical that the liver would not remove these hormones because they are secreted into the portal circulation and must make a pass through the circulation before they reach their target organ. If the liver removed them during the initial pass-through, all their effects would be lost. Only if there were a portal type of circulation between the site of hormone release directly to the target organ would hormone inactivation by the liver be unimportant. It has been suggested that a portal system exists between the antrum and fundus of the stomach to transport gastrin directly to its site of action.[16]

SECRETIN-GLUCAGON FAMILY. Secretin is similar in structure to glucagon, gastric inhibitory polypeptide (GIP), and vasoactive intestinal peptide (VIP), all of which are similar in function to varying degrees. The octapeptides at the N-terminus are identical in secretin and glucagon except for one amino acid. A total of 14 amino acids occupy the same positions in both hormones (secretin has 27 amino acids, and glucagon has 29). Secretin requires the complete sequence of the 27 amino acids to be biologically active. Secretin is basic because of its four arginine molecules, a histidine, and sev-

Table 1–4

SUMMARY OF BIOLOGIC ACTIVITIES OF GASTROINTESTINAL HORMONES

	GASTRIN-CHOLE-CYSTOKININ FAMILY		SECRETIN FAMILY				OTHER HORMONES		
	Gastrin	Chole-cystokinin	Secretin	Glucagon	Gastric Inhibitory Peptide	Vasoactive Intestinal Peptide	Somato-statin	Pancreatic Polypeptide	Prosta-glandins
Esophagus									
Gastroesophageal sphincter	ss	|	|	|	|	|			
Stomach									
Acid secretion	S	sS	|	|	|	|	|	sS	|
Pepsin secretion	S	sS	SS	|	|	|	|		
Motility fundus	|	|	|						
Motility antrum	S	S	|	|	|	|		+	|
Emptying	|	|	|	|	|	|	|	+	|
Blood flow	S	S	|	|		S			S
Gastrin release			|	|	|	|	|		
Small intestine									
Fluid secretion	ss	ss	ss	S	S	S	|		S
Fluid absorption		si	si			|	|		|
Motility	ss	S	|	|	|	ss	|	+	S
Blood flow	S	S	|	S		S	|		S
Secretin release	S						|		
Pancreas									
Fluid secretion	ss	ss	S	|	–	sS	|	sS	|
Enzyme secretion	S	S	ss	|		S	|		–
Blood flow	S	S	S	S	–	S			
Liver									
Bile secretion	ss	S	S	S		sS			–
Gall bladder									
Motility	ss	S	ss	|		|	|	|	
Metabolic									
Insulin release	S	s	S	S	S	S	|		
Glycogenolysis				S	–	S		–	
Lipolysis			+	S	|	S			
Glucagon release	–	S	|	–		S		|	

S = full agonist for activity, sS = partial agonist for activity, ss = slight stimulation, \| = inhibits activity, si = slight inhibition, – = no effect on activity. Responses are those seen with physiologic blood levels of hormones.

eral glutamines. Secretin's molecular structure is unique in its unusual tertiary conformation, which must be maintained in order for it to possess biologic activity.

In some respects, secretin has effects opposite to those of the members of the gastrin family, even though the hormone is designed to complement and potentiate the actions of cholecystokinin on pancreatic secretion. Secretin serves to mobilize the alkaline secretion of the pancreas in order to neutralize acid secretions entering the duodenum. Thus, it is not surprising that secretin has properties inhibiting gastric secretion. Another means of reducing the effects of acidity in the small intestine is to inhibit gastric motility, and secretin is capable of delaying gastric emptying. Other physiologic functions of secretin, probably less important, are stimulation of pancreatic trypsin secretion, insulin release, biliary secretion, and inhibition of motility of the small intestine and resting pressure in the gastroesophageal sphincter.

Secretin has a short half-life (2.5 minutes) in dogs. Some can be removed by the liver, and the kidney can play an important role in its rate of disappearance. It is unlike vasoactive intestinal peptide, which the liver rapidly degrades.

Glucagon was first identified as a hormone secreted by the pancreas. Pancreatic glucagon is also produced in the gastric mucosa. Related but different glucagons found in the gastrointestinal mucosa are called enteroglucagons. Pancreatic glucagon is a peptide containing 29 amino acid residues, 14 of which are in the same position as in the secretin molecule. One of the enteroglucagons is the same size as pancreatic glucagon. Because glucagon is quite different from secretin in tertiary structure, there is a major difference in their effects on the primary target organ of secretin, the pancreas. In contrast to secretin, glucagon inhibits pancreatic secretion. The major role of enteroglucagon is not established, but the conditions under which it is released may help in understanding its physiologic significance. Glucose and long-chain triglycerides in the diet stimulate release of the hormone. Its blood level remains elevated for five hours after a meal. This is in contrast to the shorter peak activities of other gut hormones. The peak activity may be long because the highest levels of enteroglucagon occur in the ileum.[5] This is in contrast to gastric inhibitory polypeptide (GIP), found mainly in the cranial small bowel, which inhibits gastric motility. Enteroglucagon's high concentration in the intestine and its ability to inhibit gastric and intestinal motility may serve to delay transit of food in the entire gastrointestinal tract in response to a signal from the caudal small bowel. Enteroglucagon has glycogenolytic effects like those of glucagon. Because glucose stimulates enteroglucagon's release in the intestine, it is paradoxical that a hyperglycemic agent is released with the impending absorption of glucose. Because enteroglucagon is a signal for insulin release, its effect is modified by an antagonist of hyperglycemia. The catabolic sites of enteroglucagon are unknown.

Vasoactive intestinal peptide (VIP) is a hormone produced in the mucosa of the small intestine. It was named for the first properties found for it: production of vasodilation and hypotension. VIP is related structurally most closely to secretin in this group of four hormones. It consists of 28 amino acid residues that form a tertiary structure like that of secretin, consisting of a helix in one part and random coil in the other. The entire sequence is necessary for full biologic activity.

VIP is a neurotransmitter released from nerve endings to a variety of gastrointestinal organs upon stimulation of extrinsic nerves. VIP is not released to the circulation, and its normally low and constant blood levels reflect spillover from synapses where the neurotransmitter is released. Many different stimuli promote VIP release. Some of its physiologic effects are evident on the gastroesophageal and other gastrointestinal sphincters, where VIP release following nerve stimulation results in sphincter relaxation and opening.

Other major effects of VIP are to inhibit motility in the stomach and gall bladder, to stimulate the release of glycogen stores and insulin, and, most importantly, to stimulate the secretion of fluid in the small intestine. This hormone has effects on other systems. In the respiratory system, VIP relaxes bronchi and dilates pulmonary vessels, whereas in the cardiovascular system it produces hypotension by dilating peripheral vessels. VIP is inactivated in the tissues where it is released. Some that escapes to the circulation is inactivated as it passes through the liver.

Gastric inhibitory polypeptide (GIP) is produced in the mucosa of the duodenum and jejunum. It consists of 43 amino acid residues and structurally resembles glucagon more closely than it does secretin and VIP. Because extracts of the small intestine inhibit gastric secretion, resection of a large part of the small intestine results in a hypersecretion of gastric juices. These effects are now known to be due to gastric inhibitory polypeptide.

GIP is released by glucose and fats in the small intestine, and its levels can be measured in the peripheral circulation. Therefore, GIP can affect different parts of the gastrointestinal tract. An important function of GIP is to inhibit the stom-

ach's secretion of acid and pepsin. Secretin, a member of the same family, has these same properties, but GIP is much more potent as an inhibitor. GIP also inhibits gastric motility. *Enterogastrone* is the term used to describe a single humoral agent that affects gastric function in response to fats in the small intestine. It is apparent that enterogastrone is a response mediated by a number of hormones: the members of the secretin-glucagon family of gut hormones. Other major important functions of GIP involve carbohydrate metabolism. GIP is released by intraluminal glucose.

GIP causes a release of insulin. This effect of the hormone is greater than that of hyperglycemia. Thus, GIP may be a primary signal for the pancreas to respond to a glucose load being absorbed from the small intestine. In the same context, it is suggested that cholecystokinin's release of insulin is an advance signal for the absorption of amino acids and fatty acids from the intestine. The catabolic sites of GIP are unknown, but it is apparent the kidney but not the liver is important in removal of GIP from the portal circulation.

Somatostatin is a peptide hormone that was first shown to inhibit the release of growth hormone from the pituitary. The hormone consists of 28 amino acids and is found throughout the gastrointestinal tract, with the largest quantities found in the antrum, duodenum, and pancreas. Somatostatin functions as a paracrine in the gastrointestinal tract. Cells producing somatostatin have long cytoplasmic processes that terminate near gastric mucosal cells secreting hydrochloric acid or gastrin (Figure 1–6). In contrast to endocrine glands that release hormones to produce effects in distant tissues, paracrine cells release hormones for regulation of function in neighboring cells. Somatostatin has a physiologic role in regulating gastric acid secretion and release of insulin and glucagon. Somatostatin levels increase after feeding, especially with high protein and high-fat meals.

Somatostatin inhibits secretion throughout the gastrointestinal tract. It also inhibits the normal occurrence of cyclic interdigestive migrating motility complexes. Somatostatin's major effect is to inhibit the release of most known gastrointestinal hormones. It is a potent inhibitor of secretin and CCK release. It is difficult to evaluate the effects of infusing pharmacologic doses of somatostatin on gastrointestinal function. Because somatostatin is a paracrine, the highest concentration of the hormone is at the target cell where the hormone is released. Circulating blood levels are much lower and do not indicate what concentrations must be released to be effective at the target cell. Somatostatin has a short effect; the hormone has a half-life of 1.8 minutes. Somatostatin is removed by the liver but is also degraded by peptidases near its site of release.

Pancreatic polypeptide consists of 36 amino acids and is produced in the pancreas. Release of the hormone is stimulated by high-protein meals and to a lesser extent by fats in the duodenum. Cholinergic pathways mediate the reflex for pancreatic polypeptide release. Pancreatic polypeptide modulates the pancreatic responses to feeding. Its effects are largely inhibitory, but under some conditions the hormone can stimulate small amounts of secretion.

Neurotensin, a peptide hormone consisting of 39 amino acids, is produced in the ileal mucosa. Fats entering the small intestine stimulate neurotensin release. Pharmacologic levels inhibit gastric secretion and gastric emptying, but physiologic levels have only a slight effect to produce that inhibition. Thus, neurotensin is not likely an enterogastrone whose release is stimulated by fat entering the small intestine. A major function has not been defined for neurotensin.

Motilin is a peptide hormone consisting of 22 amino acids and produced in the cranial small intestine. Plasma motilin

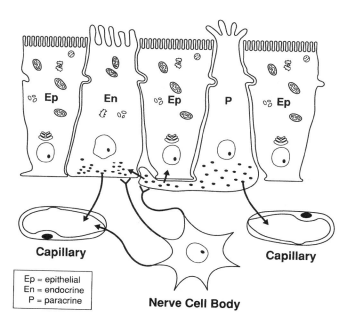

Ep
En
Ep
P
Ep

Capillary

Capillary

Ep = epithelial
En = endocrine
P = paracrine

Nerve Cell Body

FIGURE 1-6. Schematic showing anatomic and functional relations of mucosal epithelial cells, endocrine cells, paracrine cells, neurons of intrinsic nervous system, and mucosal capillaries. Endocrine secretion can be stimulated or inhibited by nerve activity and paracrine secretions. Nerve endings, endocrine, and paracrine cells can all secrete chemical transmitters into capillaries.

concentrations increase during interdigestive periods, and the increases coincide with the activity of the interdigestive myoelectric complex (IMC). Motilin is believed to initiate IMC activity. Other stimulants of motilin release include fats and acid pH in the duodenum. The physiologic importance of stimulation by these conditions is unknown. The major and maybe only significant biologic action of motilin is to increase motility during the intergastric period; the increase appears to be for smooth muscle throughout the gastrointestinal tract. Motilin has a short effect because its half-life is about 4.5 minutes. The kidneys are responsible for its clearance, but peptides with such a short half-life are removed by more than one vascular bed.

Peptide YY consists of 36 amino acids and is produced primarily in the ileum and colon. It is structurally similar to pancreatic polypeptide. Peptide YY inhibits gastrointestinal motility in the unfed state. The hormone inhibits gastric acid and pancreatic bicarbonate secretion; meals, and especially fats in the duodenum, stimulate the release of peptide YY. Release of unusual amounts of peptide YY could be evident in animals with malabsorption, resulting from increased amounts of fats reaching the ileum and colon. The effect would be an inhibition of gastric acid and pancreatic bicarbonate secretions.

PROSTAGLANDINS.[17,18] Prostaglandins are hydroxy-fatty acids with many biologic effects in the gastrointestinal tract. They act as local regulators (secreted at one site and not transported by the circulation to act at another) because they are degraded where they are released and any escaping are almost totally inactivated by a single pass through the liver and lungs. Prostaglandins can be intracellular messengers; they are involved with secretion of fluid in the intestine.

Prostaglandins consist of 20 carbons that are hydroxylated at carbons 11 and 15. The E-type prostaglandins contain a hydroxyl group at carbon 9, and the F-type contain a ketone group at that point. The 20-carbon chain is folded back on

itself, and carbons 8 through 12 form a closed five-member ring (Figure 1–7). Prostaglandins are synthesized from dihomo-gamma-linolenic acid, eicosapentaenoic acid, or arachidonic acid. Prostaglandins that contain an unsaturated bond in the five-carbon ring are designated the A- or B-type, depending on the location of the bond.

Synthesis and storage of prostaglandins take place in the muscle and mucosa of the gastrointestinal tract, the pancreas, and the liver. Release from those tissues has been evoked by feeding, acetylcholine, vagal stimulation, gastrin, histamine, theophylline, and cyclic AMP. The prostaglandins released can be found in gastric juice. Glucagon stimulates the release of prostaglandins from the liver. Release of these fatty acids is reduced by anti-inflammatory drugs such as aspirin and indomethacin. Their action is to inhibit the synthesis of prostaglandins, and the drug's anti-inflammatory and analgesic properties are due to their antiprostaglandin properties. After formation, the prostaglandins are rapidly inactivated in the wall of the gastrointestinal tract, and by the liver, lungs, and blood. Inactivation is accomplished by a dehydrogenase and reductase in the tissues and by an isomerase in the blood. Prostaglandins have a wide range of biologic activity on different tissues and are very potent in minute quantities. If they were not readily inactivated, they would exert their effect on other systems, particularly the cardiovascular.

Effects on Gastrointestinal Motility. Prostaglandins have varied effects on gastrointestinal motility. They stimulate contraction of longitudinal smooth muscle of the small and large intestine, and they can either stimulate or inhibit contractions of circular smooth muscle. The facilitatory response is due to stimulation via the intrinsic plexuses, whereas the inhibiting effect is the result of a direct action of prostaglandins on the muscle. In the dog, prostaglandins of the E-type PGEs inhibit motility in the gastric antrum and jejunum and augment ileal motility. The PGEs increase motility in both the jejunum and ileum. Their effects on large-bowel motility are not clear. Because prostaglandins stimulate secretion of fluid in the small intestine, it is difficult to determine their effects on the transit time of contents moving through the intestine; prostaglandins change the variables of intestinal secretion and motility (both determining transit). Prostaglandins may be involved in local regulation of gastrointestinal motility. A large number of different anti-inflammatory drugs are used in small animal medicine, and those that inhibit prostaglandin synthesis may affect bowel function in some patients.

Effects on Gastrointestinal Secretion. Prostaglandins of the E- and A-type inhibit gastric secretion, a property that makes them a most useful agent in future treatment of ulcers caused by hypersecretion of acid.[18] They are effective when given parenterally or orally, inhibiting the stimulation of acid and pepsin secretion produced by histamine, gastrin, vagal activity, cholinergics, or food. These prostaglandins also prevent ulcer formation as produced experimentally by pylorus ligation, steroid administration, or constant infusion of stimu-

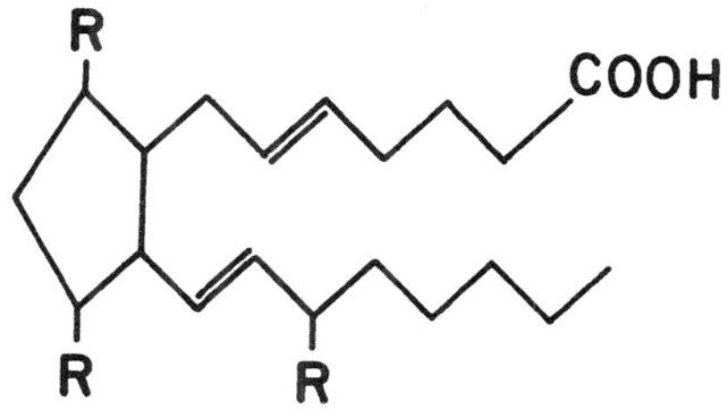

R

COOH

R

R

FIGURE 1-7. Structure of prostaglandins, which consists of a fatty acid chain of 20 carbons folded in the middle. R = oxy or hydroxy groups.

lants to gastric secretion. Methyl analogues have been synthesized that, given orally, effectively inhibit gastric secretion.

Prostaglandins act directly on the oxyntic cell to inhibit acid secretion. They interfere with cyclic AMP's intracellular role of stimulating secretion. Cyclic AMP is the intracellular mediator for histamine's stimulation of acid secretion, and prostaglandins have direct effects on that adenine nucleotide, which is the likely basis for its inhibitory effects. Prostaglandins stimulate gastric bicarbonate and mucus secretion.

A commonly observed effect of prostaglandins is diarrhea. As mentioned earlier, altered intestinal motility may be a factor in its genesis. However, prostaglandins also stimulate secretion of fluid in the intestine. That follows intra-arterial infusion of all types of prostaglandins in the dog. The secretion is the result of profound changes in the circulation and is the direct effect of the prostaglandins on the epithelial cell. Prostaglandins increase mesenteric blood flow, and some of the secretion results from increased filtration of fluid from the capillary bed. They also inhibit sodium absorption and stimulate chloride secretion in isolated preparations of ileal mucosa. It is uncertain which of these factors is the more important in producing the secretion. Prostaglandins are an important cellular mediator in intestinal secretion caused by some enterotoxins. Increased intracellular prostaglandin levels are associated with increases for intracellular cyclic AMP and free calcium. Diarrhea can also be seen during estrus; it may be due to high circulating levels of prostaglandins released. Prostaglandins are also released from injured tissues and have been implicated in the pathogenesis of some chronic bowel diseases. If prostaglandins are the prime mediators of pathology in the intestinal tract, anti-inflammatory drugs to inhibit prostaglandin synthesis should control the clinical signs, but with a few exceptions that are not seen.

Pancreatic secretion of fluid and electrolytes is uninhibited by the E-type prostaglandins. There is no effect on enzyme secretion. These effects are accompanied by a decrease in blood flow.

The prostaglandins are potent vasoactive agents. The E- and A-types are hypotensive because they are vasodilators and cause gastric mucosal blood flow to increase. These effects on increasing blood flow may be the most important cytoprotective attribute of prostaglandins in the gastrointestinal tract. Intestinal blood flow is also augmented by prostaglandins that stimulate intestinal secretion. A physiologic role for prostaglandins on blood flow is difficult to evaluate. Most experimental studies on prostaglandin's effects are based on its intra-arterial infusion. Because prostaglandins are rapidly inactivated by the tissues and blood in which they are released, the concentrations of prostaglandins at the sites where they are released under physiologic conditions are not known.

Prostaglandins also contribute to the integrity of the gastric mucosal barrier. Protection of the barrier is due to prostaglandin's effect of increasing blood flow, inhibiting acid secretion, and stimulating secretion of bicarbonate and mucus. Inhibition of these effects by nonsteroidal inflammatory drugs often results in gastrointestinal erosions or ulcers.

Trophic Action of Gastrointestinal Hormones[19-21]

Gastrointestinal hormones influence the growth of the mucosa of the gut, which has one of the most rapid turnovers of any tissue in the body. These hormones also have trophic effects on the pancreas and liver. Numerous events engaged during the fed state stimulate growth of the gastrointestinal mucosa. Nongastrointestinal factors such as thyroxine and growth hormone also support growth. Animals subjected to starvation lose more than half of their small intestinal weight while losing only one-third of their body weight. Absence of stimuli for hormone secretion results in gastrointestinal atrophy. The physical presence of food in the intestine also promotes growth. Food and intestinal motility combine to cause desquamation of villous cells, the loss of which stimulates proliferation of epithelial cells. Epithelial cells contain chalones that inhibit production of new cells; desquamation of mucosal cells results in loss of the inhibitory chalones, and replication increases to replace lost cells.

The growth-stimulating property of gastrin is the best understood. This hormone stimulates the synthesis of RNA, DNA, and proteins in the oxyntic glands, duodenal mucosa, and pancreatic exocrine tissue. Gastrin stimulates cell division in the stomach and duodenum, but has no trophic effects on the antral mucosa. The trophic effects of gastrin are best illustrated in animals fed by total parenteral nutrition, in which the fasting serum levels of gastrin decrease significantly. Tissues of the gastrointestinal tract and pancreas atrophy, which can be prevented by adding small physiologic amounts of gastrin to the parenteral solutions. The trophic effects of gastrin are inhibited by secretin, but not by the histamine analogues that inhibit gastrin-stimulated secretion. Gastrin may also have a physiologically regulative trophic effect on colonic mucosa.

Cholecystokinin exerts a trophic effect on the pancreas in addition to its well-known ability to stimulate the synthesis of protein enzymes for export. The cholecystokinin effect on the pancreas is reflected by an increase in organ size and in DNA content. Cholecystokinin has no trophic action on gastric or duodenal mucosa. Large amounts of cholecystokinin compete with gastrin for receptor sites in the stomach and competitively inhibit the trophic effects of gastrin.

Secretin stimulates pancreatic growth but less so than CCK. Secretin inhibits gastric mucosal growth. It may act by blocking the action of gastrin.

Enteroglucagen may have a trophic effect on mucosa of the gastric oxyntic mass, small intestine, and colon. A close correlation is reported between hyperproliferation of small intestinal mucosa and enteroglucagon levels in humans with some intestinal diseases. Such a relationship has not been verified with studies showing a trophic effect during infusion of enteroglucagon.

Hormones inhibiting or stimulating release of trophic hormones have indirect trophic effects. Somatostatin inhibits, and bombesin stimulates mucosal growth by their respective effects on gastrin release. Other hormones produced in gastrointestinal mucosa, such as epidermal growth factor, have trophic effects on the mucosa, but it is uncertain whether such hormones have a physiologic role on growth.

The capacity to synthesize gastrointestinal hormones depends on the trophic effects of pituitary hormones. Removal of growth hormone by hypophysectomy decreases antral gastrin levels to one-fourth of normal, and subsequent injection of growth hormone increases this decrement significantly.

Smooth muscle as well as mucosa can be stimulated to grow. Smooth muscle thickness increases in the wall of hollow viscera or tubes in the gastrointestinal tract following chronic distension due to obstruction. Both longitudinal and circular muscles thicken; both hypertrophy and hyperplasia of smooth muscle cells cause the increase in size. Similar changes are seen for the intrinsic nervous sytem in these tissues. Whether any hormones stimulate the trophic changes is unknown. Gastrin can have such an effect on the smooth muscle of the pyloric sphincter. Administration of pentagastrin to pregnant bitches results in 25% to 30% of the pups being born with pyloric hypertrophy.[22] It is uncertain whether the changes are caused by cholecystokinin and secretin, which are released secondarily to the pentagastrin effects. These hormones also cause changes in the intrinsic nerves of the sphincter, which may affect sphincter growth and subsequent function after birth.

Trophic factors are also important for the maintenance of normal liver size and for its regeneration following resection. These factors are discussed in Chapter 3.

BLOOD FLOW AND DIGESTIVE FUNCTIONS[23–27]

Regulation of blood flow is as important to gastrointestinal function as regulation of motility, secretion, and absorption. Increasing blood flow to sustain augmented function is a response to stimulation of the organ's function. Increased blood flow is appropriate because motility and fluid transport functions in the gastrointestinal tract are energy dependent. During the unfed state, total gastrointestinal blood flow is low, and after feeding it increases dramatically. During many physiologic states and in some pathologic ones, blood flow can be reduced to less than normal by shunting flow from the gastrointestinal system to other organs where optimum flow has a higher priority. In some situations blood can be shunted within the organ from one region to another. Thus, total blood flow can be diverted to and from the gastrointestinal tract, and it can be redistributed within an organ in the system. Figure 1–8 is a schematic of the circulation in the gastrointestinal tissues. The total flow of blood has a generally low priority in this system compared with the needs of other systems. Regulation of circulation in the gastrointestinal system is the result of neural and endocrine factors and the basic properties of the microcirculation.

Autoregulation of blood flow occurs in the gastrointestinal tract. This is the phenomenon of the maintenance of normal blood flow through the capillary beds despite wide variations in arterial inflow pressure. The mechanism for this ability to maintain homeostasis is in the inherent property of vascular smooth muscle to respond to pressure changes. The responses cause a constriction of the resistance vessels when the arterial pressure increases and a vasodilation when the pressure decreases. Autoregulation operates over a wide range of arterial pressures from 70 mm Hg to 170 mm Hg to maintain the blood flow constant in gastrointestinal organs. Other inherent mechanisms maintain blood flow to the villi of the small intestine at the expense of the submucosa and muscle layers. Villous blood flow can be maintained at normal rates when arterial pressure falls to as low as 30 mm Hg. Autoregulation also plays an important role in preventing great increases in capillary blood pressure during portal hypertension. The response is a vasoconstriction of the resistance vessels so that arterial inflow is reduced. Autoregulation is an important mechanism that can override outside influences on intestinal blood flow. Neural and endocrine factors can change total blood flow. Most increase blood flow, although a few (mediated by the sympathetics and such hormones as vasopressin) reduce blood flow by their potent vasoconstrictive actions. If these influences prevailed, the intestinal mucosa would be deprived of nutrients that are necessary to maintain its integrity. Autoregulatory escape intervenes, so that adequate blood flow is maintained despite the vasocon-

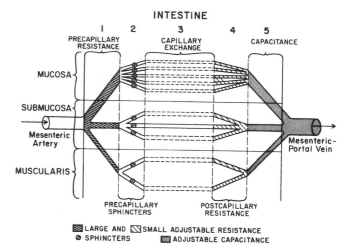

FIGURE 1–8. Schematic of blood flow in intestine. The major blood flow is through the mucosa. Hydrostatic pressure in capillaries is determined by resistance in arterioles and venules and by pressure in mesenteric veins. Hydrostatic pressure determines magnitude and direction of fluxes of fluid in capillaries. Precapillary sphincters determine whether blood flows through a capillary. Blood can be selectively shunted from the muscularis and submucosa into the mucosa at times when splanchnic circulation is reduced. The mucosa has the highest priority for maintenance of circulation. Some large shunt vessels are present whereby blood flow can bypass capillary beds.

strictive influences. Blood flow to structures other than the mucosa is reduced while mucosal flow actually increases. Thus, the overall effect is a redistribution of intestinal blood flow. Autoregulation is thought to be partially controlled by locally produced metabolic products such as carbon dioxide, adenosine compounds, and Krebs cycle intermediates. This metabolic control of blood flow is more important in vascular beds outside the gastrointestinal tract.

The splanchnic bed of the dog contains 21% of the total blood volume. Neural influences are the most important to reduce splanchnic blood flow, and hormones are most important in its augmentation. The venous side of the splanchnic bed contains 14% of the total blood volume. It is a capacitance bed containing venous vessels that are more richly endowed with smooth muscle than are other systemic veins. An increase in the tone of these vessels reduces the capacity of the bed and shunts more blood into the arterial system. A decrease in venous tone results in splanchnic pooling of blood and a corresponding decrease in venous return to the heart, cardiac output, and arterial pressure. Thus, neural and hormonal influences can change the amount of blood in the splanchnic bed without changing its blood flow.

Neural regulation is due to splanchnic sympathetic nerves that cause vasoconstriction in both the arterial and venous vessels of the stomach, intestines, pancreas, and liver. This can reduce an organ's blood content by 40%. Activation of this sympathetic effect is physiologic under some conditions such as exercise, and it is pathologic in conditions such as shock. Stimulation of the parasympathetic system causes vasodilation and increased blood flow, but not directly. There are no known vasodilator fibers in the vagal and sacral efferent fibers. A local vasodilator reflex operates within the wall of the intestine. This neural pathway is noncholinergic and nonadrenergic, and it is suggested that serotonin is either the neurotransmitter or the chemical released to produce vasodilation.[28]

Gastrointestinal blood flow doubles or triples during the functional hyperemia produced during digestive activity. This effect is produced by the gut endocrines gastrin, cholecystokinin, vasoactive intestinal peptide, and glucagon. Histamine is released during gastric secretion and contributes to the augmented blood flow. Crude secretin increases intestinal blood flow, but synthetic secretin has no effect on the circulation, which indicates the crude hormone preparations used in older studies contained other agents with vasoactive properties. Hormones that increase gastrointestinal blood flow also tend to increase oxygen consumption. Acetylcholine also has a vasodilating effect when infused into the mesenteric artery. This effect is blocked by atropine. The vasodilating effects of gastrin and cholecystokinin are also blocked by atropine, which suggests the effects of these hormones are mediated through cholinergic receptors. Glucagon's vasodilating effects are not altered by atropine. Postprandial vasodilation is not readily reduced by normal physiologic events such as exercise, which is able to reduce the augmented gut blood flow by only 10% to 15%. Because blood flow doubles or even triples during digestive events, but infusions of pharmacologic amounts of cholecystokinin or gastrin increase blood flow by only 50%, there must be other means of increasing it. Other gut hormones with vasodilating properties probably participate in functional hyperemia of the gut. Some of the prostaglandins have potent vasodilating effects on the splanchnic microcirculation. Some are more potent than the vasoactive peptides in augmenting blood flow, and they may have a physiologic role in the production of hyperemia. Serotonin may function in a similar manner. Most of the serotonin in the body is found in the gastrointestinal tract, but the reasons are unknown. It has been proposed that it participates in peristalsis and in postprandial hyperemia. It is thought that serotonin's acting as a vasoactive chemical is directly involved both in the previously described reflexly elicited vasodilation and as a neurotransmitter released on blood vessels following nerve stimulation. A number of pharmacologic agents increase splanchnic blood flow. They act on either the alpha adrenergic receptors, blocking transmission so as to produce vasoconstriction, or on the beta receptors to stimulate vasodilation. Epinephrine and isoproterenol are chemicals that act in this manner.

Nitric oxide inhibits vascular smooth muscle and thereby promotes mucosal blood flow. Nitric oxide may be the final vasodilating mediator for neural stimulation and many circulating chemicals that increase mucosal blood flow. Substances such as acetylcholine, bradykinin, and gastrin increase mucosal flow by stimulating nitric oxide synthesis. Nitric oxide also stimulates hepatic blood flow, which helps protect animals with reduced hepatic circulation when caused by problems such as endotoxemia.

A naturally occurring substance, vasopressin, reduces splanchnic blood flow.[29] The effect of this peptide on blood flow has been studied in animals infused with pharmacologic levels of the hormone. For this reason, there is some question whether the amount normally released has a physiologic action in the gastrointestinal tract. Acute stress stimulates the release of vasopressin from the neurohypophysis, and it is generally thought that the amount of hormone released in situations such as hemorrhagic shock is sufficient to play an important role in the marked vasoconstriction of the splanchnic vascular bed that characterizes the shock.

INTEGRATION IN THE FED AND UNFED STATES

In summary, the most important facilitatory influences on gastrointestinal motility are neurally mediated, whereas the major inhibitory factors are mediated by hormones (Table 1–5). Control by extrinsic nerves is indispensible for function

Table 1–5

NEURAL AND ENDOCRINE REGULATION OF NORMAL FUNCTION IN THE GASTROINTESTINAL TRACT

		FACILITATION	INHIBITION
Esophagus	Gastroesophageal sphincter	N	N
Stomach	Acid secretion	N and E	E
	Pepsin secretion	N and E	E
	Motility fundus	N	N
	Motility antrum	N	E
	Emptying	N	E
	Gastrin release	N	E
	Blood flow	E	N
Small intestine	Fluid secretion	E	N
	Fluid absorption	N (?)	E (?)
	Motility	N	E
	Blood flow	E	N
Pancreas	Fluid secretion	E	–
	Enzyme secretion	E	–
	Blood flow	E	N
Liver	Bile secretion	E	N (?)
Gall bladder	Motility	N and E (?)	–

Summary of primary means of stimulating and inhibiting physiologic activity in different parts of the gastrointestinal tract. N = facilitation or inhibition is primarily by neural means. E = effect is primarily by endocrines released from the gut. (?) = a major effect is unknown.

in the esophagus and stomach, whereas most of the remainder of the gastrointestinal tract can function without regulation exercised by the extrinsic nerves. Secretion of gastric juices depends on both extrinsic neural regulation and regulation imposed by endocrines, whereas inhibition of gastric secretion is a function of the endocrine system alone. Facilitation of secretion in other parts of the system is largely mediated by the endocrines, and inhibitory mechanisms appear to play a minor role. Splanchnic blood flow is stimulated primarily by gut hormones and is inhibited under physiologic situations by neural means. The trophic effects on gastrointestinal tissues are secondary to normal neural innervation and endocrine secretion and hence are responses rather than regulated changes.

This simplified overview is not to detract from recent reviews that have described how the gastrointestinal tract is far more complex than previously thought. The small intestine is an exquisitely designed sensory organ for monitoring activity at all levels;[30] that was hardly mentioned in this chapter. Also, ion transport, which has been viewed as largely unregulated, is now known to be affected by the nervous system in a very complex way.[31] The major work yet to be done in gastrointestinal physiology is to show how mechanisms learned from in vitro and unphysiologic studies are integrated and function in the normal animal.

The integration of gastrointestinal function described in this introduction is for animals in the fed state. The gastrointestinal tract also demonstrates important integrated functions in the unfed state, such as a coordinated pattern of motility that acts as an interdigestive housekeeper to clear the gastrointestinal tract of accumulating bacteria and debris.[32] Evidence for such motility was originally gained from electrical recordings showing caudal-moving bands of large-amplitude action potentials starting in the duodenum and moving through the small intestine. The duration of a complex at each level of the bowel is 7.0 to 4.8 minutes. The length of each complex is 25 to 36 cm in the cranial small intestine and 6.0 to 12.0 cm in the caudal part. Two complexes can be in the intestine at any one time; 1.5 to 2.0 hours is required for a complex to travel from the duodenum to the ileum. Similar activity is seen in the gastroesophageal sphincter, stomach, and gall bladder. The cyclic activity in the colon migrates in both the cranial and caudal directions. During the active myoelectric and motor activity, small amounts of secretion are produced by the stomach, pancreas, and biliary system. The fluid produced assists the motility in its housekeeping activity. Enteric neural mechanisms that are modulated by the central nervous system and by circulating hormones regulate the interdigestive motility and secretory activities. The activity ceases with feeding. Loss of the interdigestive housekeeping activity in unfed animals could be a basis for disease.

REFERENCES

1. Bass P. In vivo electrical activity of the small bowel. In: Code CF (ed) Handbook of Physiology, Sec. 6, Vol. 4, Alimentary Canal. American Washington, DC, Physiological Society, 2051–2074, 1968.
2. Bortoff A. Myogenic control of intestinal motility. Physiol Rev 56:418–434, 1976.
3. Duthie HL. Electrical activity of gastrointestinal smooth muscle. Gut 15:669–681, 1974.
4. Szurszewski JH. Electrical basis for gastrointestinal motility. In: Johnson LR ed Physiology of the Gastrointestinal Tract. Raven Press, New York, 383–422, 1987.
5. Makhlouf GM. Isolated smooth muscle cells of the gut. In: Johnson LR (ed) Physiology of the Gastrointestinal Tract. Raven Press, New York, 555–569, 1987.
6. Kosterlitz HW. Intrinsic and extrinsic nervous control of motility. In: Code CF ed Handbook of Physiology, Sec. 6, Vol. 4, Alimentary Canal. Washington, DC, American Physiological Society, 2147–2172, 1968.
7. Makhlouf GM. The neuroendocrine design of the gut. Gastroenterology 67:159–184, 1974.
8. Wood J.D. Physiology of the enteric nervous system. In: Johnson LR (ed) Physiology of the Gastrointestinal Tract. Raven Press, New York, 67–109, 1987.
9. Youmans WB. Innervation of the gastrointestinal tract. In: Code CF (ed) Handbook of Physiology, Sec. 6; Vol. 4, Alimentary Canal. American Physiological Society, Washington, DC, 1655–1664, 1968.
10. Roman C, Gonella J. Extrinsic control of digestive tract motility. In: Johnson LR (ed) Physiology of the Gastrointestinal Tract. Raven Press, New York, 507–533, 1987.
11. Cooke AR. Control of gastric emptying and motility. Gastroenterology 68:804–816, 1975.
12. Dockray GJ. Physiology of enteric neuropeptides. In: Johnson LR (ed) Physiology of the Gastrointestinal Tract. Raven Press, New York, 41–66, 1987.
13. Barrington EJW, Dockray GJ. Gastrointestinal hormones. J Endocr 69:299–325, 1976.
14. Rayford PL, Miller TA, Thompson JC. Secretin, cholecystokinin, and newer gastrointestinal hormones. New Eng J Med 294:1093–1101, 1157–1164, 1976.
15. Walsh JH. Gastrointestinal hormones. In: Johnson LR (ed) Physiology of the Gastrointestinal Tract. Raven Press, New York, 181–253, 1987.
16. Taylor TV, Torrance B. Is there an antral-body portal system in the stomach? Gut 16:781–784, 1975.
17. Waller SL. Prostaglandins and the gastrointestinal tract. Gut 14:402–417, 1973.
18. Whittle BJR, Vane JR. Prostanoids as regulators of gastrointestinal function. In: Johnson LR (ed) Physiology of the Gastrointestinal Tract. Raven Press, New York, 143–180, 1987.
19. Johnson LR. The trophic action of gastrointestinal hormones. Gastroenterology 70:278–288, 1976.
20. Popper H. Implications of portal hepatotrophic factors in hepatology. Gastroenterology 66:1227–1230, 1974.
21. Johnson LR. Regulation of gastrointestinal growth. In: Johnson LR (ed) Physiology of the Gastrointestinal Tract. Raven Press, New York, 301–333, 1987.
22. Dodge JA, Karim AA. Induction of pyloric hypertrophy by pentagastrin. Gut 17:280–284, 1976.
23. Bynum TE, Jacobsen ED. Blood flow and gastrointestinal function. Gastroenterology 60:325–335, 1971.
24. Lundgren O. The circulation of the small bowel mucosa. Gut 15:1005–1013, 1974.
25. Bowen JC, Fang W-F, Pawlik W, et al. Gastrointestinal hormones and blood flow. In: Thompson JC (ed) Gastrointestinal Hormones. University of Texas Press, Austin, 391–393, 1975.
26. Parks DA, Jacobson ED. Mesenteric circulation. In: Johnson LR (ed) Physiology of the Gastrointestinal Tract. Raven Press, New York, 1649–1670, 1987.
27. Granger DN, Kvietys PR, Perry MA, et al. The microcirculation and intestinal transport. In: Johnson LR (ed) Physiology of the Gastrointestinal Tract. Raven Press, New York, 1671–1697, 1987.
28. Biber B: Vasodilator mechanisms in the small intestine. Acta Physiol Scand Suppl 401, 1973.
29. Schapiro H Britt LG. The action of vasopressin on the gastrointestinal tract. Amer J Dig Dis 17:649–667, 1972.
30. Mei N. Intestinal chemosensitivity. Physiol Rev 65:211–237, 1985.
31. Hubel KA. Intestinal nerves and ion transport: Stimuli, reflexes, and responses. Am J Physiol 248:G261–G271, 1985.
32. Sarna SK. Cyclic motor activity; migrating motor complex. Gastroenterology 89:894–913, 1985.

2 Microflora of the Gastrointestinal Tract and Its Symbiotic Relationship with the Host

DONALD R. STROMBECK

INTRODUCTION

The microflora of the gastrointestinal tract consists of hundreds of different species of bacteria. One part of the microflora (that in the colon) is the most complex ecosystem in the body. The numbers of bacteria in this region are 10^{10} to 10^{11} per gram. Bacterial numbers in the stomach and small intestine vary in the normal animal, depending on whether nutrients are present. The numbers and distribution of the intestinal flora are normally stable,[1-3] maintained in a symbiotic relationship with the animal. The vast reservoir of microorganisms in the gut poses a potential threat to the animal if they escape from the alimentary tract and multiply in other parts of the body. Despite a number of physiologic mechanisms to control that threat, alternations can occur, resulting in disease.

The numbers and types of microorganisms vary with each part of the gastrointestinal tract. Each species has its own preferred niche. The numbers are maintained at a low level in the stomach and intestines. Many changes in normal gastrointestinal function cause the number of bacteria to increase in the cranial bowel. Such changes can also cause species of bacteria to colonize sites they do not normally occupy. Disruption of the normal flora permits colonization by foreign bacteria that are ingested. Diarrhea can develop from colonization by foreign microorganisms. Antibacterial agents can influence the number and distribution of bacteria in the intestines, which are determined by the type of diet. Diet and antibiotic therapy are therefore commonly used to control intestinal problems.

The intestinal microflora affects the metabolism of a host's nutrients, digestive enzymes, bile constituents, and steroids. It also has an impact on the structure and function of the intestinal mucosa. Thus, the intestinal microflora has important effects on the health of the host; conversely, the state of function and nutrition in the host determines the population of the microflora.

NORMAL MICROFLORA[3-8]

The numbers of microorganisms vary with each region of the gastrointestinal tract. The oral cavity is considered in this section, because it represents a major source of bacteria that populate the rest of the alimentary tract. The number of bacteria in the mouth is 10^7 per gram, as shown in Figure 2–1. The contents of the fasting stomach are practically sterile, containing only 10^1 to 10^2 organisms per gram of residual secretions. After a meal, the numbers increase to 10^4 to 10^5 per gram. After secretion of hydrochloric acid has reduced the pH to less than 3, the numbers decline to relatively few. Numbers in the empty small intestine are normally 10^1 to 10^2 per gram in the cranial part, increasing to 10^3 to 10^4 in the caudal part. When food is present, these counts increase by 10^2 to 10^3 bacteria per gram of intestinal contents. The number of bacteria in the colon is 10^{10} to 10^{11} per gram, a fairly constant number (as in the mouth). The numbers in each

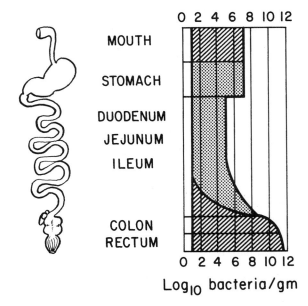

FIGURE 2-1. Numbers of bacteria in the alimentary tract. Diagonal bars indicate regions where bacteria are present at all times. Dotted area in the stomach and small intestine indicates the numbers of bacteria when nutrients are present. When this part of the gastrointestinal tract is empty the numbers of bacteria fall to 10^1 bacteria per gram.

part are controlled by several different factors, discussed later.

The gastrointestinal tract contains a microflora consisting of large numbers of certain species of bacteria that are always found, making them the most important in the makeup of the normal resident population. The normal microflora is also made up of some species of bacteria that are always present, but in smaller numbers. Additionally, the gastrointestinal microflora always contains a small number of contaminants or transients from the mouth and from the diet. Most current knowledge about microflora of the gut is from studies on normal residents and transients that together make up the smallest part of the population; very little is known about the anaerobic organisms that make up the major part of the normal microflora. They exceed the aerobes by 1000 or more to 1. Until recently, it was not possible to study the anaerobes because no techniques were available for isolating, identifying, and quantitating those bacteria and investigating their properties. The great number of different bacteria in the normal microflora adds to the problem of gaining knowledge and an understanding of the entire ecosystem.

An important source of intestinal organisms is swallowed saliva. The predominant organisms in saliva are members of the *Bacteroides, Streptococcus, Lactobacillus,* and *Neisseria* genera (Table 2–1). Also frequently found are *Staphylococcus, Corynebacterium, Spirochaetes, Vibrios,* and yeasts. Bacteria in the stomach are transients deposited by saliva and food. Thus, all the typically oral organisms can be found in gastric contents after a meal. Organisms found in the fasting stomach are mostly acid-resistant species such as clostridia, streptococci, lactobacilli, *Escherichia coli,* and fungi. The cranial small intestine contains mostly gram-positive organisms, mainly clostridia, streptococci, lactobacilli, staphylococci, and fungi. In the middle and caudal regions, the concentration of bacteria increases, and the microflora begins to approach the composition of the flora in the colon. This level of the small intestine contains coliforms at concentrations of 10^5 per gram and enterococci at 10^4 per gram. Bacteroides and bifidobacteria are also found in low numbers throughout the small intestine. Clostridia in the small intestine are found in greater numbers in dogs than in humans.[9] The numbers of bacteria are dramatically increased in the large intestine at a point immediately across the ileocecal sphincter. In summary, all varieties of bacteria found in the mouth can be found in the colon, although their proportions differ. The predominant bacteria in the large intestine are anaerobes, with bacteroides and bifidobacteria found in the highest numbers. Enterobacteria, streptococci, and lactobacilli are found in large numbers. All other organisms exist in low concentrations.

REGULATION OF GASTROINTESTINAL MICROFLORA

The distribution and size of bacterial populations in the gut are determined by normal gastrointestinal function and by environmental factors within the lumen of the tract. The microflora is established shortly after birth[10] and remains rela-

Table 2–1

COMPOSITION OF MICROFLORA OF ALIMENTARY TRACT

FAMILIES	GENERA		MOUTH	STOMACH	SMALL INTESTINE	LARGE INTESTINE
Pseudomonadaceae	Pseudomonas*	AE				+
Enterobacteriaceae	Escherichia coli*	FAN	--	10^1-10^3		10^7-10^8
	Klebsiella*	FAN		10^1-10^2	10^1-10^3	10^7-10^8
	Enterobacter (aerobacer)*	FAN		$10^{1.8}$	$10^{1.6}$	
	Proteus*	FAN				
Bacteroidaceae	Bacteroides*	AN	+	0	10^1	10^8-10^{10}
	Fusobacterium*	AN	+			
Neisseriaceae	Neisseria	FAN	+			+
	Veillonella	AN	+			$10^{5.9}$
Micrococcaceae	Staphylococcus*	FAN	+	$10^{0.4}$	$10^{0.4}$	$10^{4.7}$
Lactobacilliaceae	Streptococcus*	FAN	+	$<10^1$	10^1-10^3	10^8-10^9
	Lactobacillus*	FAN	+	$<10^1$-$10^{1.3}$	10^2	10^8-10^9
	Bifidobacterium*	AN	+		+	$10^{6.6}$
	Ruminococcus					+
Propionobacteriaceae	Eubacterium	AN	--			+
Corynebacteriaceae	Corynebacterium	FAN	+			$10^{8.7}$
Bacillaceae	Bacillus	AN				$10^{5.4}$
	Clostridium*	AN	--	$10^{0.3}$-10^3	$10^{0.1}$-10^4	10^7-$10^{9.1}$
Yeasts						10^5

*Clinically significant microorganisms
AE = Aerobe
FAN = facultative anaerobe

AN = Anaerobe
+ = Present
-- = Absent

Numbers are organisms per gram or milliliter of contents.
Data compiled from references 4–8.

tively constant from then on, unless changes within the host alter normal physiologic function or changes are dictated in the intraluminal environmental factors by changes in the environment in which the host lives. These factors are interactions between members of the resident microflora. Physiologic regulation consists of those functions necessary to maintain each species of bacteria in its own niche and in proper numbers. This maintenance prevents the pathologic effects produced by bacterial overgrowth of a normal resident or colonization of a part of the bowel either by a normal resident that does not belong at that site or by a transient organism that is pathogenic if it is able to colonize.

Physiologic Mechanisms of Regulation by Host

SECRETION OF GASTRIC HYDROCHLORIC ACID.[3,9,11] Normal secretion of hydrochloric acid maintains a relatively sterile environment in the stomach. The bacteria that reach the stomach from the mouth are destroyed by hydrochloric acid. The normal flora of the small intestine, especially the cranial part, consists of transients from the mouth. When gastric secretion of acid is inhibited or reduced, the numbers of bacteria in the small intestine increase. Acid secretion is also important in preventing colonization or invasion by pathogenic bacteria. When secretion of acid is inhibited in the dog, the numbers of *E. coli* and clostridia increase. Thus, the fecal type of flora that prevails in the colon moves cranially in the small intestine from the ileum, where it is normally established at a reduced level. The achlorhydric stomach is usually heavily colonized with bacteria. The animal with gastritis is therefore susceptible to increased numbers of gastric bacteria. This patient is unable to produce a secretion of gastric juices with a pH less than 3 because back diffusion of hydrogen ions is greatly accelerated. Procedures and situations such as feeding that neutralize gastric acid secretion have a similar effect. The use of antacids or drugs such as anticholinergics and H_2 blockers can cause bacterial numbers to increase in the stomach and small intestine. It is questionable whether other secretions in the gastrointestinal tract have a primary function in controlling the total numbers of bacteria.

NORMAL INTESTINAL MOTILITY.[3,12–14] Normal peristalsis is necessary to maintain low concentrations of bacteria in the small intestine. It accomplishes this by moving the contents containing bacteria in an aboral direction, preventing any organisms from multiplying excessively within a given section of the intestine. Such motility provides a housekeeping function by cleaning out bacteria faster than they can multiply. The housekeeping motility is driven by electrical activity called the migrating myoelectrical complex (MMC), which moves slowly through the empty stomach and intestine at regular intervals. When drugs or disease disrupting MMC activity results in a loss of the housekeeping function, numbers of gastrointestinal bacteria can increase.[15] In the absence of normal motility, intestinal microflora increase significantly and fecal organisms will appear in the cranial part of the small intestine.[16,17] Under these circumstances, bacteroides, bifidobacteria, and coliforms predominate. The rate of peristalsis is less in the ileum than in the duodenum and jejunum, probably one of the factors allowing establishment of a partial fecal flora in the ileum. The normal microflora is disrupted by diarrhea and will not return until normal motility is restored.[18]

MUCOSAL BARRIER.[5,19] The mucosal barrier prevents mucosal adherence and invasion by pathogenic bacteria. The barrier is a one-cell-thick epithelial layer with a protective surface coating of mucus, polysaccharides, and immunoglobulins. In addition, a population of nonpathogenic bacteria, normally adhered to the mucosal surface, form an integral part of the barrier because they prevent colonization by pathogenic transient bacteria.

Pathogenicity of some noninvading organisms is related to their ability to attach to a cell's surface and elaborate an enterotoxin. Most of these organisms must penetrate the surface constituents and adhere to the cell surface before they can produce clinical signs of disease. Bacteria adhere to the mucosal surface by fimbriae they possess, by agglutinins they secrete that act as an adhesive, and by adhesive properties of the bacterial capsule. Each of the normal bacteria attached to the intestinal mucosa has a preferred site on either the villus tips or in the crypts. In many cases, it is necessary for the normal flora to be displaced before a pathogen can adhere. Organisms that produce enterotoxins include some of the vibrios,[20] *E. coli*,[20] *Klebsiella*,[21] *Salmonella*,[22] and *Clostridium*.[23] Some of these groups of microorganisms consist of strains that produce specific adherence factors, which is why they are pathogenic.[24] Other strains are incapable of mucosal binding and are therefore nonpathogenic.[25] Enterotoxins must bind to sites on epithelial cells in order to cause diarrhea. It is possible that enterotoxins produced by the nonpathogenic strains are inactivated or destroyed in the lumen of the intestine by inhibitors or intestinal and bacterial proteases[25] and that binding is not possible. Enterotoxins are inhibited by normal contents of the intestine, although they are quite resistant to proteolytic destruction.[26]

The epithelial cell barrier is affected by the presence of normal numbers of bacteria.[27] Germ-free animals have cuboidal rather than columnar mucosal cells; the rate of cell turnover is slower in the germ-free than in the conventional animals. Germ-free animals have few inflammatory cells in their lamina propria. In contrast, when intestinal bacterial numbers are increased over normal the lamina propria can show many inflammatory cells and rapid turnover of epithelial cells that appear damaged. Therefore, the kinds and numbers of bacteria living in the intestinal lumen have profound affects on the mucosal surface and the barrier it provides.

Immunoglobulins synthesized by the host in the lamina propria are also important barriers to disease.[28] This secretory IgA is directed against specific organisms that can be pathogenic. Secretory IgA does not regulate the numbers of bacteria in the lumen of the intestine, nor is it thought to be directed against bacteria normally present on the mucosal surface.[25] The predominant members of the normal flora possess a low degree of immunogenicity.[29] The barrier produced by this local immunity is important primarily when pathogenic transients become a threat because normal physiologic function, for example, peristalsis, is lost or the balance within the normal microflora is disrupted. One mechanism of action by the immune response is IgA's prevention of bacterial adhesion. Another mechanism is antibacterial in that the antibody causes destruction or inhibition of growth of bacteria that come in contact with the mucosal surface. This response depends on viable mucosal cells and is independent of complement.[25] It can be considered a type of cellular immunity.

Environmental Factors That Regulate Microflora

BACTERIAL MICROFLORA INTRAREGULATION.[3] The normal intestinal microflora in an animal is established during the first few weeks of life. Once established, it is difficult to change and impossible to eradicate. There is some daily variation in the microflora of the stomach and intestines because those organs contain a population of transients that can change with eating habits. The population of the microflora is very stable because outsiders have difficulty in colonizing the gut. Stability is also reflected in the near impossibility of changing the microflora intentionally. Even pathogens introduced orally are normally unable to colonize and cause disease.[30–32] Attempts have been made to convert a "putrefactive flora" to a "lactic flora" in patients with chronic diarrhea, but oral administration of large numbers of *Lactobacillus acidophilus* produces no changes in the distribution or number of any members of the normal microflora.[5,33] That has been attempted unsuccessfully also in the treatment of hepatic encephalopathy with the view that non-urease-producing organisms will replace organisms in the intestines that split urea to ammonia.[5] Newly introduced microorganisms are able to colonize with greater ease if they have been cultivated in an environment closely resembling the environment to which they are introduced.[25] In a totally strange environment the lag phase in their growth is prolonged, and they are mechanically eliminated before they can multiply and colonize; adaptation and colonization will require more than the short time taken for the normal passage of intestinal contents. Most human cultures believe the consumption of fermented milk products to be beneficial, attributing the effects to the consumption of lactobacillus organisms. To the contrary, the studies cited here and numerous others show that transient bacteria entering the oral cavity have great difficulty in colonizing. It should be recognized that this is of major importance to the host. A number of environmental factors are responsible for maintaining the size and distribution of the normal flora, and they are more important than local immune mechanisms for the prevention of disease.

The most important factor determining the numbers of any one species of bacteria in the gut is the makeup of the remainder of the population. Bacterial growth of any single species is much slower in the intestine of a conventional animal than in the germ-free intestine. (One study showed that when *E. coli* was the only bacteria present in the intestines of an animal, 95 isolates of anaerobic bacteria had to be added in order to reduce the very high numbers of *E. coli* to the low levels in the normal intestine.[25])

The rate of growth of each species of bacteria is determined, directly or indirectly, by dietary nutrients.[34,35] As an example, consider when one of two organisms is able to digest insoluble polysaccharides and use the soluble carbohydrate products that are formed, and the second organism cannot split the polysaccharide but can use only the soluble products. Thus, both organisms depend on the organism that prepares the nutrients for use. The rate of growth of each, however, is determined by the organism that is able to use the products more readily, and that growth, in turn, affects the growth of the organism preparing the nutrients for use. Some bacteria may be able to use nutrients that others cannot use, which places them in a position where they do not have to compete. The predominating organisms of the large intestine are carbohydrate fermenters, which use ammonia as their major source of nitrogen.[36]

Bacterial growth rates are determined by the amount of available oxygen. Aerobes and facultative anaerobes consume any available oxygen, after which the aerobes are unable to grow, whereas the anaerobic bacteria can. Conditions in the large intestine are essentially anaerobic, and this is partly the reason that anaerobes there outnumber aerobes by 1000 to 1.

The growth of specific bacteria in the intestines is determined indirectly by some of the metabolic products formed. Some volatile fatty acids produced by bacteroides and col-

iforms act to inhibit the growth of other bacteria.[37] That is the basis for the resistance in some species to infection by salmonella and shigella given by mouth. Other bacteria can directly influence the concentrations of different populations in the microflora. The coliforms can release chemicals that kill related bacteria. These substances are called colicines, and when the populations of colicine-producing serotypes is great, there are fewer different strains in the microflora. When more transients are present, fewer colicines are produced and a greater variety of related strains is found.[38]

DIETARY INFLUENCE ON INTESTINAL MICROFLORA.[39] Many of the beneficial effects of "bland" and "hypoallergenic" controlled diets may be due to changing intestinal microflora to populations more favorable to normal physiologic functioning of the alimentary tract. Diet influences the intestinal microflora of animals,[11,33] although more is known about the effects in humans. In general, humans eating a Western type of diet (higher in meat, fat, and protein) have fecal levels of anaerobes that are higher and levels of aerobes that are lower than people on a largely vegetarian diet.[41] Anaerobes can produce carcinogens, and it remains to be seen how strong this relation is.[42] More recent experimental studies show that a high-protein diet causes an increase in numbers of anaerobic bacteroides that persists after return to a conventional diet.[43] Numbers of clostridia are lower on a high-protein diet. A low-protein diet causes coliforms to increase and bacteroides and bifidobacteria to decrease. Fungi increase and staphylococci decrease on a low-protein diet. There is some evidence that the fecal flora is not changed when a human adopts a vegetarian diet as an adult.[44]

A number of studies have produced conflicting reports on the effects of elemental no-residue diets on the composition of the fecal microflora. When nutrients were given that require no digestion and are completely absorbed in the upper small bowel, early reports indicated that fecal bacterial counts dropped precipitously,[45] whereas later studies reported no change in the numbers of most fecal bacteria with this type of diet.[40] Other studies indicate that an elemental diet does produce a decrease in the numbers of some aerobes.[5] The volume of feces is reduced when a no-residue diet is fed, and the feces consist primarily of desquamated epithelial cells, mucus, and microorganisms. The mucosal cells that slough in a normal continuous process provide the supply of nutrients for colonic bacterial growth.

Very few studies have looked at the effect of diet on the normal microflora at different sites in the intestinal tract. There are dietary effects that change both the locations of colonization and the numbers of bacteria. Protein deficiency is associated with tropical sprue, which is characterized by increased total numbers of bacteria in the small intestine and by higher than normal concentrations of coliforms.[46] The diet in this case may cause the changes in the population of microorganisms, which in turn cause the pathology. It is also possible that the overgrowth of the microflora is an event secondary to the malnutrition. Whatever the case, this illustrates that diet has a profound effect, still little understood, on the microflora of the entire intestinal tract. Malnutrition in general has a profound effect on microbial contamination by a wide variety of organisms, which can be a feature of many chronic debilitating diseases. There is an overgrowth of yeast in some cases, and of anaerobes in others. The microflora varies in response to diet probably more in the small intestine than in the large intestine. In general, the specific requirements for the normal bacteria in the colon are for complex polysaccharides.[47] There is a general lack of proteolytic activity by the most predominant members, and they rely on ammonia for their nitrogen needs.

Dietary effects on the intestinal microflora can be demonstrated by different diets changing the fecal activities of bacterial enzymes. These enzymes include beta-glucuronidase, beta-glucosidase, beta-galactosidase, nitroreductase, azoreductase, 7-alpha-dehydroxylase, and cholesterol dehydrogenase.[3,27] Increases in activities of these enzymes can increase the metabolites of nutrients and bile acids. For example, coprostanol and coprostanone, metabolites of cholestrol, can increase. The metabolites of bile acids can damage intestinal epithelial cells; some of the bacterial enzymes may also have that property. The bacterial enzymes can also convert food additives to chemicals capable of damaging the epithelium. Diets formulated from milk proteins and high in fiber produce significant changes in fecal bacterial enzyme activities, and these changes are associated with reduced incidence of some bowel problems.

Endogenous and Exogenous Antibacterial Agents

Most of the luminal factors that regulate the growth of intestinal bacteria are related to the diet or are produced by the bacteria themselves. An additional endogenous substance that regulates their numbers is bile acids, which are inhibitory to many intestinal microorganisms.[48] Bile acids most likely regulate bacterial growth. The level of bile acids in the intestine is determined by the amount of fat in the diet; high-fat diets cause an increase in fecal concentration of bile acids. An increased amount of bile acids in the colon may be significant in causing chronic disease. Bile acids that are not absorbed and reach the region of greater bacterial populations are metabolized to form deconjugated bile acids and hydroxylated forms that interfere with fluid absorption and motility in the small and large intestines.[49] Some of the metabolic products of bile acid degradation by bacteria are carcinogenic.

Antibiotics are the most important agents administered to animals for the purpose of eliminating, suppressing, or drastically altering the microflora.[5] Presurgical use of unabsorbed antibiotics has been advocated to "sterilize" the gastrointestinal tract. Combinations of neomycin or kanamycin with polymyxin or bacitracin have been recommended to minimize postsurgical infection, but controlled trials have shown no benefit over untreated presurgical preparation. More recent recommendations include the use of neomycin and metronidazole combinations. Because no single antibiotic is regularly effective against both aerobes and anaerobes, a combination of several drugs is used to suppress or eradicate both types of organisms. Unfortunately, fecal bacterial counts do not change with erythromycin, chloramphenicol, tetracycline, or probably most other antibiotics. Most bacteria have become resistant to neomycin. It can suppress some normal bacteria that are still sensitive, allowing the remaining flora to overgrow and cause an imbalance. In fact, some studies have shown that effective suppression of anaerobes without any effect on aerobes can cause coliforms to increase in parts of the gut from normal levels of 10^2 to levels of 10,[7] resulting in death. That is an extreme example, but it shows what can happen if antibiotics are used indiscriminately in the alimentary tract.

CONTROL OF THE GASTROINTESTINAL MICROFLORA IN THE GASTROENTEROLOGY PATIENT

Many gastrointestinal tract problems are thought to result from changes in the microflora of the gut. Changes in the intestinal microflora may involve normal flora that become pathogenic, or they may result from transient strains that are ingested with food and are able to colonize. Managing the problems associated with such changes requires an understanding of the fundamental concepts presented in this chapter.

More than 500 different varieties of bacteria are found in the gastrointestinal tract, and as a group they are not sensitive to any single antibacterial agent. Thus, any single antibiotic will suppress the numbers of only part of the microflora. The balance of the entire system is then upset, and other members of the normal flora will multiply and exceed normal numbers. Most antidiarrheal agents are formulated with a single antibacterial agent. The antibiotics used most often are directed against the aerobes, that is, the coliforms, which constitute less than 1 out of every 1000 organisms found in the large intestine. It is therefore important to recognize that treatment directed against such a small part of the microflora has insignificant effects.

Drugs are often used with the idea that they can sterilize the gut, or at least effectively reduce the numbers of bacteria. Antibiotics can reduce the numbers of some microorganisms in the gut, but after a week their numbers return to normal. Many bacteria are able to develop resistance to an antibiotic within 24 hours. Thus, it is important to realize that the very large concentrations of microorganisms in the colon (up to 10^{11} per gram of contents) cannot be suppressed by token amounts of antibacterial agents given orally.

If, indeed, gastrointestinal disease is related to changes in the microflora, it becomes important to consider factors determining the population of the microflora that can be controlled by the clinician and client. These factors have been listed in the preceding sections, and only a few of them can possibly be controlled.

Bacterial interactions have been shown to be important in determining the size and extent of the microflora population. Attempts have been made to put this factor to practical use by administering *Lactobacillus* cultures to patients with chronic bowel disease and hepatic encephalopathy. Unfortunately, cultures of nonpathogenic microorganisms offer little hope in modifying the microflora as it exists.

In addition to internal environmental factors, external ones (such as stress) play a significant role in the development of gastrointestinal disease, which is accompanied by changes in the microflora. It is not known how stress changes the microflora and causes clinical signs to appear. In many cases it may be stress-induced changes in motility of the gut that produce a diarrhea: The changes in motility change the microflora, resulting in clinical signs. The normal population does not return until after normal function is regained.

The microflora of the gut is determined by the type of nutrients the host consumes. The basis for this is just beginning to be understood. The beneficial effects of many different controlled diets in the treatment of chronic disease of the gut has been apparent for centuries. The response to these diets may reside in avoidance of an allergy-stimulating antigen. Controlled diets may also be beneficial because they result in a change in intestinal microflora to a population that is compatible with normal intestinal function.

The basis for chronic gastrointestinal disease will be understood better when more accurate means are developed for evaluating the intestinal microflora. Analyses of fecal samples for total numbers and types of bacteria yield useful information only when known pathogens, such as *Salmonella*, are present. Techniques must be developed to identify and quantitate microorganisms in the stomach and, more important, in the small intestine.

REFERENCES

1. Gorbach SL, Nahas L, Lerner PI, et al. Studies of intestinal microflora. Effects of diet, age and periodic sampling on numbers of fecal microorganisms in man. Gastroenterology 53:845–855, 1967.

2. Zubrzycki L, Spaulding EH. Studies on the stability of normal fecal flora. J Bact 83:968–974, 1962.

3. Simon GL, Gorbach SL. Intestinal flora and gastrointestinal function. In: Johnson LR (ed) Physiology of the Gastrointestinal Tract. Raven Press, New York, 1729–1747, 1987.

4. Broido PW, Gorbach SL, Nyhus LM. Microflora of the gastrointestinal tract and the surgical malabsorption syndromes. Surg Gynecol Obstet 135:449–459, 1972.

5. Drasar BS, Hill MJ. Human Intestinal Flora. Academic Press, London, 1974.

6. Gorbach SL. Intestinal microflora. Gastroenterology 60:1110–1129, 1971.

7. Greenlee HB, Belbart SM, DeOrio AJ, et al. The influence of gastric surgery on the intestinal flora. Amer J Clin Nutr 30:1826–1832, 1977.

8. Mitsuoka T, Kaneuchi C. Ecology of the bifidobacteria. Amer J Clin Nutr 30:1799–1810, 1977.

9. Broido PW, Gorbach SL, Condon RE, et al. Upper intestinal microfloral control. Arch Surg 106:90–93, 1973.

10. Smith WH, Crabb WE. The faecal bacterial flora of animals and man; its development in the young. J Path Bact 82:53–66, 1961.

11. Smith HW. Observations on the flora of the alimentary tract of animals and factors affecting its composition. J Path Bact 89:95–122, 1965.

12. Dixon JMS, Paulley JW. Bacteriological and histological studies of the small intestine of rats treated with mecamylamine. Gut 4:169–173, 1963.

13. Donaldson RM. Role of indigenous enteric bacteria in intestinal function and disease. In: Code CF (ed) Handbook of Physiology, Sec. 6, Vol. 5, Alimentary Canal. American Physiological Society, Washington DC, 2807–2837, 1968.

14. Sumners RW, Kent TH. Effects of altered propulsion on rat small intestinal flora. Gastroenterology 59:740–744, 1970.

15. Scott LD, Cahall DL. Influence of the interdigestive myoelectric complex on enteric flora in the rat. Gastroenterology 82:737–745, 1982.

16. Drasar BS, Shiner M. Studies on the intestinal flora. II. Bacterial flora of the small intestine in patients with gastrointestinal disorders. Gut 10:812–819, 1969.

17. Gorbach SL, Tabaqchali S. Bacteria, bile, and the small bowel. Gut 10:963–972, 1969.

18. Gorbach SL, Neale G, Levitan R, et al. Alterations in intestinal microflora during experimental diarrhea. Gut 11:1–6, 1970.

19. Rowley D. Specific immune antibacterial mechanisms in the intestines of mice. Amer J Clin Nutr 27:1417–1423, 1974.

20. Formal SB, DuPont HL, Hornick RB. Enterotoxic diarrheal syndromes. Ann Rev Med 24:103–110, 1973.

21. Klipstein FA, Engert RF. Purification and properties of Klebsiella pneumoniae heat stable enterotoxin. Infect Immun 13:373–381, 1976.

22. Koupal LR, Deibel RH. Assay, characterization, and localization of an enterotoxin produced by Salmonella. Infect Immun 11:14–22, 1975.

23. McDonel JL, Duncan CL. Histopathological effect of Clostridium perfringens enterotoxin in the rabbit ileum. Infect Immun 12:1214–1218, 1975.

24. Jones GW, Rutter JM. Contribution of the K88 antigen of Escherichia coli to enteropathogenicity; protection against disease by neutralizing the adhesive properties of K88 antigen. Amer J Clin Nutr 27:1441–1449, 1974.

25. Freter R. Interactions between mechanisms controlling the intestinal microflora. Amer J Nutr 27:1409–1416, 1976.

26. Strombeck DR, Harrold D. Comparison of the rate of absorption and proteolysis of (^{14}C) choleragen and (^{14}C) bovine serum albumin in the rat jejunum. Infect Immun 12:1450–1456, 1975.

27. Simon GL, Gorbach SL. Intestinal flora in health and disease. Gastroenterology 86:174–193, 1984.

28. Clancy R, Bienenstock J. Secretory immunoglobulins. Clin Gastroenterol 5:229–249, 1976.

29. Carter PB, Pollard M: Studies with Lactobacillus casei in gnotobiotic mice. In: Heneghan JB (ed) Germ-Free Research. New York, Academic Press, 379–383, 1973.

30. Orcutt R, Schaedler RW. Control of staphylococci in the gut of mice. In: Heneghan JB (ed) Germ-Free Research. New York, Academic Press, 435–440, 1973.

31. Ralovich B, Emody L, Barna K, et al. Excretion of orally administered intestinal bacteria in humans. Abl Bakt Hyg. I. Abt Orig A 226:82–90, 1974.

32. Smith HW: Survival of orally administered E. coli K12 in alimentary tract of man. Nature 255:500–502, 1975.

33. Dubos R. Man Adapting. Yale University Press, New Haven, 1965.

34. Wolin MJ. Metabolic interactions among intestinal microorganisms. Amer J Clin Nutr 27:1320–1328, 1974.

35. Zollner N, Ruckdeschel G, Wolfram, G. Verhalten der darmflora des menschen be formeldiaten mit wechselndem kohlenhydratgehalt. Nutr Metabol 18:127–136, 1975.

36. Bryant MP. Nutritional features and ecology of predominant anaerobic bacteria of the intestinal tract. Amer J Clin Nutr 27:1313–1319, 1974.

37. Meynell GG. Antibacterial mechanisms of the mouse gut. II. The role of Eh and volatile fatty acids in the normal gut. Brit J Exp Path 44:209–210, 1963.

38. Branche WC, Young VM, Robinet HG, et al. Effect of colicine production on Escherichia coli in the normal human intestine. Proc Soc Exp Biol Med 114:198–201, 1963.

39. Hentges DJ: Does diet influence human fecal microflora composition? Nutr Rev 38:329–336, 1980.

40. Finegold SM, Atteberry HR, Sutter VL. Effect of diet on human fecal flora: Comparison of Japanese and American diets. Amer J Clin Nutr 27:1456–1469, 1974.

41. Drasar BS, Hill MJ. Intestinal bacteria and cancer. Amer J Clin Nutr 25:1399–1404, 1972.

42. Hill MJ, Crowther JS, Drasar BS, et al. Bacteria and etiology of cancer of the large bowel. Lancet 1:95–100, 1971.

43. Maier BR, Flynn MA, Burton GC, et al. Effects of a high-beef diet on bowel flora: A preliminary report. Amer J Clin Nutr 27:1470–1474, 1974.

44. Moore WEC, Cato EP, Holdeman LV. Anaerobic bacteria of the gastrointestinal flora and their occurrence in clinical infections. J Infect Dis 119:641–649, 1969.

45. Winitz M, Adams RF, Seedman DA, et al. JA. Studies in metabolic nutrition employing chemically defined diets. Amer J Clin Nutr 23:546–559, 1970.

46. Garcey M, Stone DE. Microbial contamination of the gut: Another feature of malnutrition. Amer J Clin Nutr 26:1170–1174, 1973.

47. Moore WEC, Holdeman LV. Special problems associated with the isolation and identification of intestinal bacteria in fecal flora studies. Amer J Clin Nutr 27:1450–1455, 1974.

48. Floch MH, Binder HJ, Filburn B, et al. The effect of bile acids on intestinal microflora. Amer J Clin Nutr 25:1418–1426, 1972.

49. Midtvedt T. Microbial bile acid transformation. Amer J Clin Nutr 27:1341–1347, 1974.

3

Gastrointestinal Immune System

W. GRANT GUILFORD

INTRODUCTION

The concept of a gastrointestinal immune system functioning independently from the systemic immune system was first proposed in 1919 by Besredka,[1] following his demonstration that rabbits orally immunized with enteropathogenic bacteria were protected against dysentery regardless of the titers of serum antibody. In 1922, Davies[2] was able to demonstrate fecal antibodies against enteropathogenic bacteria before the development of serum antibodies. The significance of this observation was broadened in the 1960s when several laboratories showed that a unique immunoglobulin (IgA), with properties distinct from serum immunoglobulins, was the major gut immunoglobulin.[3] From these beginnings, researchers have gone on to demonstrate that the gut mucosa contains the largest B cell system of the body.[3]

In its broadest sense, the gastrointestinal immune system may be thought to include all the processes, both antigen specific and antigen nonspecific, that protect the body against the deleterious effects of material in the intestinal lumen. The intestinal milieu contains factors that are antigenic or nonantigenic, particulate or soluble, injurious or nutritious, and persistent or transient. This necessitates a particularly versatile immune system that will eliminate injurious agents but be tolerant of persistent harmless antigens. Effective gastrointestinal immunity depends on four interrelated processes (Figure 3–1): exclusion from the mucosa of luminal materials; elimination of, or tolerance to, antigens that reach the mucosa; and regulation of the immune response.

The exclusion of antigenic material from the mucosa is the primary function of mucosal immune systems and the function to which they are best adapted. The processes of exclusion begin in the lumen. Large molecules are rendered nonantigenic by efficient digestion, and bacterial numbers are limited by interactions of flora, bactericidal gastrointestinal secretions, and peristalsis. Exclusion also depends on an effective mucosal barrier.[4] A single layer of epithelial cells separates the body from gastrointestinal content. The quantity and diversity of luminal material demands epithelial "permselectivity," allowing the body to receive adequate nutrition and to "sample" passing gastrointestinal antigens, but to prevent overwhelming exposure to deleterious antigens. Intestinal permeability, the components of the mucosal barrier, and the antigen-nonspecific factors controlling bacterial numbers are discussed in detail in other chapters.

IgA secretion contributes to this mucosal exclusion. IgA secretion is initiated in the gut-associated lymphoid tissue (GALT) and is an antigen-specific method of mucosal exclusion. It is a unique feature of mucosal immune systems (Table 3–1), and is discussed in considerable detail in this chapter.

Once an antigen penetrates the gastrointestinal epithelium, it induces an immune response. Immune responses to food antigens and bowel bacteria are commonplace in healthy animals. The immune response results in either sensitivity or tolerance to the antigen. Another unique feature of the gastrointestinal immune system is its propensity to mount immune responses dominated by T cell suppression that ultimately render the immune system tolerant to ingested antigens and microbial flora. Tolerance to benign, persistent antigens avoids subjecting the mucosa and body to the harmful effects of prolonged, immune-mediated inflammation. Antigen sensitivity results in elimination of pathogenic antigen. Elimination occurs through either antigen-nonspecific or antigen-specific mechanisms. The antigen-nonspecific mechanisms include the elimination of antigen by the mononuclear-phagocytic system, the inflam-

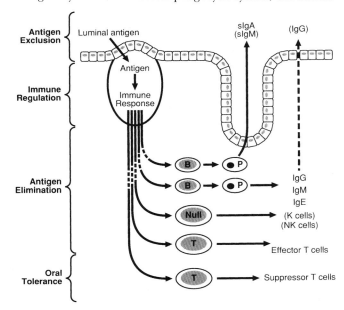

FIGURE 3-1. The gastrointestinal immune system. Effective gastrointestinal immunity depends on four interrelated processes: antigen exclusion, antigen elimination, oral tolerance, and immune regulation (modified from reference 3). By permission of Scandinavian Press.

Table 3–1

DISTINGUISHING FEATURES OF THE GUT-ASSOCIATED LYMPHOID SYSTEM
Preponderance of IgA secretion
Propensity to mount immune responses dominated by T cell suppression
Lymphocyte migration and the mucosal immunologic network

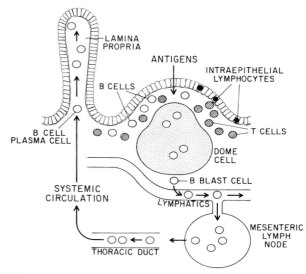

FIGURE 3–2. Diagram of development of local intestinal immunity. Antigens are absorbed by M cells in the epithelium over the Peyer's patches. Antigens interact with antigen-presenting and T helper cells in Peyer's patches resulting in the stimulation of IgA-committed B blast cells. The blast cells migrate through lymphatics to the systemic circulation and "home" to the lamina propria of intestinal mucosa where they mature to IgA-committed B lymphocytes and IgA-secreting plasma cells.

matory response, and the alternate complement cascade. Antigen-specific methods of elimination include secretion of IgG and IgE, and activation of the cell-mediated immune response.

Antigen elimination and tolerance are not just local events. They result in systemic, as well as local, tolerance and mucosal immunity at all mucosal surfaces of the body. These systemic manifestations of the gastrointestinal immune response relate to a third characteristic feature of the gastrointestinal immune system: the tendency of antigen-exposed lymphocytes to migrate from the gut lymphoid tissue and populate other lymphoid tissues and mucosal surfaces. This lymphocyte migration has led to the concept of a mucosal immunologic network (Figure 3–2).[5]

The regulation of the gastrointestinal immune system promotes and integrates mucosal exclusion, antigen elimination, and antigen tolerance into a remarkably effective system of mucosal defense that neatly balances the demands of protection with those of nutrition. Abnormalities in immune regulation are currently thought to contribute to a number of important digestive system diseases, including gluten enteropathy, food allergies, inflammatory bowel disease, lymphocytic cholangitis, and chronic hepatitis.

The majority of this chapter describes the mechanics, function, and consequences of the immune response in GALT. Those aspects of the immune response unique to mucosal immune systems are given greatest emphasis. The mononuclear-phagocytic system, immunity to parasites, passive immunity, and the role of the immune system in producing gastrointestinal disease are also described.

THE MONONUCLEAR-PHAGOCYTIC SYSTEM

The mononuclear-phagocytic system is comprised of macrophages distributed throughout the body. The mononuclear-phagocytic system is distinct from the reticuloendothelial system because it excludes cells that inadvertently take up particulate matter such as epithelial and endothelial cells.[6] All of the cells of the mononuclear-phagocytic system originate from precursors in the bone marrow and reach the tissues in the circulatory system. These circulating juvenile macrophages are called monocytes. Monocytes enter the tissues under the influence of various chemotactants. Some macrophages are found in connective tissues (histiocytes), and large numbers are located in lymph nodes, spleen, bone marrow, and gut-associated and bronchus-associated lymphoid tissue. Macrophages of particular importance to the gastrointestinal immune response are found in association with GALT, in gastrointestinal lymph nodes, or lining the sinusoids of the liver (Kupffer cells). Within GALT, macrophages are found immediately below the specialized epithelium of the lymphoid nodules and sparsely distributed throughout the lamina propria. In lymph nodes, macrophages congregate primarily in the medulla of the

lymph node. Within the liver, macrophages form part of the fenestrated endothelial sheet that lines the sinusoids. The hepatic mononuclear-phagocytic system represents 75% to 80% of the intravascular clearance capacity.[7]

Functions of the Mononuclear-Phagocyte System

ANTIGEN TRAPPING. The functions of the mononuclear-phagocytic system are numerous. Together, the phagocytes of the system represent an efficient and extensive antigen-trapping net. In addition, they are intimately involved in the immune response, and are able to secrete a wide variety of factors important in the mediation of inflammation.

The macrophages of the mononuclear-phagocytic system are ideally situated to trap antigen carried to them in lymph or blood, or passed to them by other cells. Ingestion of antigen by macrophages is a nonspecific process that is facilitated by, but not dependent on, opsonins and antibody. Macrophages can function effectively even on first exposure to an antigen. After the development of antibody, however, the efficiency of phagocytosis is enhanced because macrophages possess receptors for both complement and antibody. In addition, following antibody production antigen trapping by lymph nodes is magnified by the recruitment of dendritic cells. These macrophage-like cells possess numerous long interdigitating cytoplasmic processes that, once coated by antibody, can absorb antigen onto their surface for presentation to lymphocytes. Dendritic cells have been identified in the Peyer's patches and lamina propria of the intestine, where they presumably have a similar role to the dendritic cells of the lymph nodes.[8]

The phagocytic role of the mononuclear-phagocyte system is essential for homeostasis and tissue healing. It is responsible for the clearance from the body of tissue debris, aged or damaged cells, infectious agents, and nonliving antigens such as bacterial endotoxins and immune complexes. Significant differences have been detected in the phagocytic capacity of canine macrophages harvested from different tissues of the body.[9]

ROLE IN THE SPECIFIC IMMUNE RESPONSE. The mononuclear-phagocyte system is involved in the initiation, regulation, and effector arm of the immune response. The immune response is launched largely by the presentation of antigen to lymphocytes by macrophages. Macrophages conserve representative samples of ingested antigen on their cell surface where it is presented, in association with class II major histocompatibility (MHC II) antigens, to lymphocytes. The MHC II antigens are surface glycoproteins usually found on certain lymphocytes and antigen-presenting cells such as macrophages and dendritic cells. The MHC antigens are the product of the major histocompatibility gene complex. Their expression is thus under genetic control, providing a mechanism by which the immune response can be genetically controlled. The process of antigen presentation is fundamental to the immune response.

The release of interleukin 1 and interferon by macrophages plays an important role in immune regulation. Macrophages are important in the destruction of virus-infected and tumor cells. They are particularly effective at cytotoxicity and microbial killing once stimulated by interferons.

ROLE IN THE NONSPECIFIC IMMUNE RESPONSE. Macrophages are important in the initiation, amplification, and regulation of inflammation. The inflammatory response, if restricted in duration, severity, and extent, is a beneficial process and contributes to the repair of injury or elimination of infection. If protracted, flagrant, or extensive, however, the inflammatory response can become detrimental to the host, as is exemplified by the macrophage's role in endotoxic shock and granulomatous enterocolitis. Macrophages influence the inflammatory response by secreting factors such as complement, proteases, platelet activating factor, prostaglandins, leukotrienes, oxygen-derived free radicals, interleukin 1, and cachectin (see Chapter 4). The release of these mediators has a wide range of biologic effects including the production of anorexia, weight loss, fever, leukopoiesis, synthesis of acute-phase proteins, and sequestration of iron (resulting in anemia).

Factors Affecting Function of the Mononuclear-Phagocyte System

Many factors affect the function of the mononuclear-phagocytic system. Its activity depends on an adequate supply of oxygen, glucose, and other sources of energy. Infectious, neoplastic, and autoimmune diseases stimulate the monocyte-macrophage system, as do estrogens, small quantities of endotoxin, and various immunomodulators such as BCG. The activity of the system is enhanced by antibodies, interferons, and opsonins such as fibronectin and C-reactive protein. Fibronectin, a macrophage-produced protein, is an important nonspecific opsonin of particulate matter. If it is depleted, bacterial clearance by the mononuclear-phagocyte system is severely hampered.

The activity of the monocyte-phagocyte system is decreased by inadequate blood flow and by the acute-phase protein serum amyloid A, released by the liver. Uptake of toxic products that damage macrophages, such as asbestos, and the saturation of the system with overwhelming quantities of antigen eventually interfere with function. Shock, trauma, reduced hepatic mass, splenectomy, and corticosteroids also inhibit the

system. It appears that trauma may adversely affect phagocytosis by changing the number or binding affinity of macrophage surface receptors for immunoglobulins, complement fragments, and fibronectin.[7] A similar change has been noticed in hemorrhage. Hepatic vascular shunts markedly decrease phagocytic activity by reducing liver mass and blood flow.

In summary, a number of clinical situations can alter function of the mononuclear-phagocyte system. Depression of activity can be expected during starvation, postsurgical periods, shock, trauma, and any condition reducing hepatic blood flow or delivery of nutrients to the liver. The more pronounced the phagocytic defect, the greater the mortality. In addition, many of the common clinical signs of disease such as anorexia, weight loss, fever, and anemia can result from the secretory products of the activated mononuclear-phagocyte system.

STRUCTURE AND FUNCTION OF THE GASTROINTESTINAL LYMPHOID TISSUES

Components of the Gut-Associated Lymphoid Tissue

The gut-associated lymphoid tissue (GALT) is comprised of aggregated and nonaggregated lymphoid tissue within the gastrointestinal mucosa. The aggregated lymphoid tissues consist of lymphoid nodules and Peyer's patches. The nonaggregated lymphoid tissues includes luminal, intraepithelial, and lamina propria leukocytes. Some authors also include the mesenteric lymph nodes and the lymphoid tissue associated with ductal epithelium (DALT) as part of GALT. These lymphoid aggregates share anatomic proximity and some functions with GALT, but both tissues have important differences in structure and/or immune response compared to GALT. Therefore, for the purposes of this chapter, they are not included as components of GALT.

Lymphoid Nodules

Lymphoid nodules are present throughout the intestine and are the predominant type of aggregated lymphoid tissue in the large bowel of the dog. They are particularly numerous in the rectum.[10] Lymphoid nodules contain a single follicle of lymphoid cells, and range in size from approximately 0.5 to 3 mm. They occupy both the lamina propria and the submucosa.[10] The follicle-associated epithelium of the lymphoid nodules has not been as well studied as that which overlies the Peyer's patches, but the epithelia over both types of lymphoid tissue appear to be similar. M cells (see later) have been identified in the follicle-associated epithelium of lymphoid nodules in the guinea pig and are well described in the Peyer's patches of many species including the dog.[11] The structural organization and function of the isolated follicle in the lymphoid nodules also appears to be similar to that of the aggregated follicles in the Peyer's patches. B and T cells segregate within the nodule to the follicular and parafollicular areas, respectively. Helper cells constitute the major subset of T cells within the nodules.[12]

Peyer's Patches

Peyer's patches are differentiated from isolated lymphoid nodules by their large size. They consist of a collection of lymphoid follicles (5 to 900 in humans) that are located in the lamina propria and submucosa of the small intestine. Peyer's patches are covered by a follicle-associated epithelium, are innervated by peptidergic neurons, and possess efferent but not afferent lymphatics that drain into the mesenteric lymph nodes. They can be recognized grossly in both the cat and the dog, and number approximately 20 in the dog.[13] In dogs they appear as whitish elevations measuring from a few millimeters to 4 cm in their longer diameter. A continuous strip of lymphoid tissue occupies the last 20 to 25 cm of the canine ileum. Occasionally pinpoint-sized collections of lymphoid follicles resembling Peyer's patches are present in the colon and rectum of dogs.[13]

In some species, Peyer's patches are anatomically and perhaps functionally heterogeneous.[6] In the newborn sheep, Peyer's patches containing only B cells have been recognized in the ileocecal area. These Peyer's patches involute in early adulthood, and it has been proposed they are primary lymphoid organs that represent the bursa-equivalent in this, and perhaps other, species. Similarly, ileal Peyer's patches in dogs contain fewer T cells, less IgA-secreting B cells and more IgM-secreting B cells than more proximal Peyer's patches.[14] These findings are compatible with a role for ileal Peyer's patches in the early development of the B cell system of the dog.[14] In contrast to ileal Peyer's patches, the Peyer's patches in the jejunum appear to be secondary lymphoid organs. They persist throughout life and contain up to 30% to 40% T cells. Several days of antigen stimulation are necessary for the expansion and differentiation of jejunal Peyer's patches, but antigen is not required for their initial formation.[16] Newborn animals require several days or weeks of antigen stimulation to produce a fully developed Peyer's patch.

The primary functions of Peyer's patches, in animals other than the neonate, are to sample luminal antigen, present that antigen to subepithelial lymphocytes, initiate and regulate the immune response, and export resultant immunocompetent lymphocytes to the other mucosal lymphoid tissues of the body. Some studies have indicated that Peyer's patches are essential for the development of the mucosal immune response, whereas others have suggested that all components of GALT, including the lymphoid nodules and diffuse lymphoid tissues of the lamina propria, can populate the mucosa with an effective mucosal immune system.[3] The immune response of GALT is discussed in detail later in this chapter.

FOLLICLE-ASSOCIATED EPITHELIUM. The domed surface of Peyer's patches is covered by a specialized epithelium called the follicle-associated epithelium (Figure 3–2). In the duodenum and jejunum of dogs, the follicle-associated epithelium consists predominantly of absorptive epithelial cells with smaller numbers of goblet cells and M cells interspersed between the absorptive cells.[15] In contrast, in the ileum of dogs, M cells are the major cellular component of the dome epithelium.[15] In most species, lymphocytes are commonly observed between the epithelial cells, as is the occasional macrophage. The follicle-associated epithelium is derived from epithelial cell proliferation in the surrounding crypts. Up to 30 crypts may supply a single dome with cells. The number of goblet cells in the follicle-associated epithelium is reduced compared to that in the surrounding nonlymphoid epithelium, and it contains no IgA-transporting capacity.[17] This reduction is thought to create a mucus and IgA "break" that facilitates exposure of luminal antigen to the lymphoepithelium. Species and age differences exist in the percentage of M cells in the follicle-associated epithelium. In laboratory animals, M cells account for 10% to 50% of the follicle-associated epithelium. In newborn ruminants the follicle-associated epithelium has been reported to consist predominantly or

exclusively of M cells.[11] The capillary networks under the dome epithelium generally lack fenestrae, and are less permeable to some macromolecules than most villus capillaries.[18] The reduced permeability may have a protective function given the propensity for uptake of antigen by M cells in the dome epithelium.

M CELLS. M cells are specialized epithelial cells that are present in the follicle-associated epithelium of tonsillar, gut-associated, and bronchus-associated lymphoid tissue (Figure 3–3).[11,19] They can be identified with certainty only by electron microscopy. In light microscopy their presence is suggested by discontinuity of the intestinal brush border[11] especially following staining for brush border alkaline phosphatase.[17]

The term *M cell* has been used synonymously with "lymphoepithelial cell" and "follicle-associated epithelial cell." The name initially derived from the observation that the cells' apical surface contained microfolds rather than microvilli. When microvilli were also observed on the apical surface, the notation M cell was retained. Instead of designating "microfold cell," the term came to designate "membranous epithelial cell." This later term is descriptive of the mature M cell's attenuated rim of apical cytoplasm. This "membranous" cytoplasm surrounds one or more intrusive cells, which are usually lymphocytes, lymphoblasts, or macrophages. These cells indent the M cell cytoplasm to form a central hollow that brings the leukocytes within 0.3 µm of the lumen.

The precursor cell and the site of differentiation of M cells is unresolved. Some of the data suggest that M cells differentiate from mature absorptive cells on the domes of the lymphoid follicles. Other data suggest that at least some of the M cells develop directly from undifferentiated crypt cells and migrate onto the dome as they mature. It has been postulated that the differentiation and function of M cells is influenced by the underlying lymphoid follicle. M cell numbers in specific pathogen-free mice can triple within seven days of exposure to a normal animal housing environment.[20]

It is unlikely that M cells have any digestive or nutrient absorptive function. Instead, it appears that M cells function to take up small quantities of intact luminal antigens by micropinocytosis and transport these antigens in vacuoles to the underlying macrophages and lymphoid tissues for participation in the immune response. M cells represent the pri-

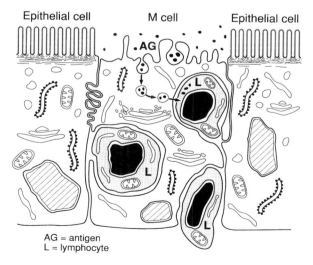

AG = antigen
L = lymphocyte

FIGURE 3–3. Schematic of M cell showing intraepithelial lymphocytes (L) migrating through the cell.

mary physiological route for nonreceptor-mediated transport of macromolecules across the mucosal barrier.[4] The M cells attain this function very early in development and retain their transport capability throughout adulthood. In comparison, the absorptive enterocytes lose much of their ability to transport macromolecules soon after birth.

The material transported by M cells includes particulate matter, proteins, and some microorganisms. The scant glycocalyx of the M cell appears to contain specific receptors for some pathogenic microorganisms. Some pathogens, such as certain types of *Mycobacteria, Salmonella, Yersinia, Campylobacter, E. coli, Chlamydia,* reoviruses, rotaviruses, astroviruses, and coronaviruses, can utilize M cells to access the body.[21] Other bacteria, such as certain strains of *E. coli,* adhere to, but are not endocytosed, by the M cells. This adherence can precede the adherence of the bacterium to the absorptive enterocytes, and it is possible, in such cases, that the M cell plays an important role in the colonization of the bowel by the pathogen. The transport of macromolecules such as proteins by M cells raises the possibility that they may play a role in allergic disease.

M cells may also have the capability to transport material from the lamina propria into the bowel lumen, although the importance of this function is unknown. Lymphocytes from Peyer's patches have been observed to migrate through gaps in the apical cytoplasm of M cells. This may be a major route by which lymphocytes leave the mucosa to enter the bowel lumen.

LYMPHOID TISSUE. The lymphoid tissue of the Peyer's patch consists of three major areas: the follicle, which contains a germinal center; the dome overlying the follicle; and an interfollicular area.[5,19,22] Like the lymphoid nodules, the B and T cells are somewhat compartmentalized within these regions of Peyer's patches. The follicle is composed primarily of B cells with an occasional T helper cell. The dome consists of a mixture of B cells, T cells, and macrophages, and the interfollicular area contains mainly T cells. Many of the B cells in the dome area appear to be of mature memory clones.[23] Some authors recognize a fourth area at the follicular rim composed largely of null cells and T cells with the suppressor/cytotoxic phenotype.[19,22] Overall, the adult Peyer's patch contains 40% to 70% B lymphocytes and 11% to 40% T cells.[19] The majority of B cells in the follicles of the Peyer's patch are precursors of IgA-secreting plasma cells. Precursors of B cells for all immunoglobulin isotypes are, however, present. Postcapillary, high endothelial venules are seen at the interface between the T- and B-dependent areas of the follicles and are the sites for lymphocyte emigration from the vascular bed.[5] The lymphocytes bind to endothelial receptors ("vascular addressins") on the high endothelial venules.[24] The high endothelial venules of Peyer's patches express different addressins than peripheral nodes.[24]

Peyer's patches contain few plasma cells, and do not appear to be important sources of immunoglobulin in vivo, although they can easily be induced to produce antibodies in vitro.[25] Likewise, lymphocytes from Peyer's patches do not seem to undertake antibody-dependent cellular cytotoxicity in the absence of previous sensitization. In contrast, T cells capable of cytotoxicity have been isolated from Peyer's patches.[22]

Luminal Leukocytes

Leukocytes can be found in the gut lumen, closely associated with the mucosa.[26] In the rabbit appendix such cells contain approximately equal numbers of B and T cells along with some null cells and macrophages. Luminal leukocytes appear to migrate from the mucosa driven by luminal antigen. They have not been demonstrated as yet to migrate back into the mucosa.[22] During infectious and inflammatory bowel diseases their numbers are increased and their ranks expanded by polymorphic cells. Luminal lymphocytes increase in number in giardiasis and are often found closely associated with *giardia* trophozoites.[27] The function and importance of these luminal leukocytes is unknown. Their presence in the feces has been utilized as a diagnostic indicator of intestinal inflammation.

Intraepithelial Lymphocytes

Intraepithelial lymphocytes reside between the intestinal epithelial cells. They are probably derived from the lamina propria and are particularly common in the follicle-associated epithelium. In the jejunum of healthy adult dogs, the intraepithelial lymphocytes number approximately 11 to 15 per 100 epithelial cells. Their numbers are somewhat lower in preweaned puppies and in the ileum of adult dogs.[28] Their numbers increase up to fivefold following exposure of the bowel to microbial antigen.[29]

Intraepithelial lymphocytes are a morphologically, phenotypically, and functionally heterogeneous lymphoid cell population.[30] Disagreement exists over the precise subtype classification of intraepithelial lymphocytes, but in general it is considered that the majority are T lymphocytes, and most of these T cells are of the suppressor/cytotoxic phenotype.[5,12,22,24,29] It is still unclear to what extent this phenotypic majority reflects functional predominance,[17] but growing evidence suggests the primary role of the intraepithelial T cell is immunosuppression.[24] Furthermore, this immunosuppressive function may be important in the development of oral tolerance.[24,30]

An important subpopulation of intraepithelial lymphocytes consists of large granular lymphocytes.[29-31] In some species, these may comprise more than 50% of the intraepithelial lymphocytes.[32] There is also evidence for the presence of mast cell precursors in the epithelium,[33] and some investigators have suggested (perhaps incorrectly) that granulated lymphocytes are in fact mast cell precursors.[34] Very few B cells are found in the intraepithelial compartment.[35]

Intraepithelial lymphocytes are known to increase in number in human celiac disease and giardiasis, but their precise role in gastrointestinal disease is unknown. It is thought they can synthesize interferon and may promote expression of MHC II antigens by epithelial cells.[36] In wheat-sensitive enteropathy of Irish Setters, intraepithelial cell numbers increase from approximately 10 lymphocytes per 100 enterocytes to 19 lymphocytes per 100 enterocytes after susceptible dogs are challenged with gluten.[37] This increase in intraepithelial lymphocytes after gluten feeding occurs in all susceptible dogs, but it is only associated with accompanying pathologic changes in villus height, brush border enzyme content, and bowel permeability if the dogs have been *reared* on a cereal-containing diet. Thus, it appears likely that in spite of their increased numbers, intraepithelial lymphocytes do not mediate gluten toxicity in the wheat-sensitive enteropathy of Irish Setter dogs.[38]

Some of the intraepithelial granular lymphocytes have natural killer-like properties and are cytotoxic against enterovirus infected cells. They are effective even in the absence of previous sensitization and may represent an important "front-line" defense.[31] Paradoxically, some coccidia and enterovirus species undergo development in the intraepithelial natural killer-like cells.[32] In addition, it is possible that intraepithelial lymphocytes return to the lamina propria and circulation after antigen priming,[22] thus serving a sentinel role.

Lamina Propria Leukocytes

LAMINA PROPRIA LYMPHOCYTES. The lamina propria contains a wide variety of leukocytes. In dogs, the greatest numbers of immunocytes are found in the duodenum and decrease toward the distal small intestine.[39] In contrast to the intraepithelial compartment, B cells are common in the lamina propria. In the species studied, including cats and dogs, IgA-producing B cells are the predominate B cell subtype.[40,41] The ratio of IgA to IgM to IgG in normal canine mucosa is 2:1:1.[39] In dogs, the greatest numbers of IgA-containing immunocytes are found in the duodenum and become less numerous in more caudal parts, with the exception of a rise in number in the colonic lamina propria adjacent to the submucosa. Using an immunoperoxidase assay, the numbers of IgA-containing cells per counting zone (0.1 mm × 0.5 mm of a 6 μm section) in the dog have been reported to range from 68 ± 3.29 (in the apical lamina propria of the duodenum) to 4.21 ± 1.24 (in the apical lamina propria of the colon).[41,42] In "normal" human mucosa, 70% to 90% of the B cells are IgA-producing cells, including plasma cells and their immediate precursors, compared with less than 5% in peripheral lymph nodes. Smaller numbers of IgG-, IgM-, and IgE-containing lymphocytes have also been identified in normal human mucosa.

T cells with helper, suppressor, and cytotoxic functions are also present in the lamina propria of the species studied. In contrast to the intraepithelial compartment, the majority of the T cells are of the helper subset.[12,25] The presence in the lamina propria of natural killer cells and killer cells capable of antibody-dependent cellular cytotoxicity is debated.[5] However, recent evidence supports the availability of a full complement of cytotoxic cells in the lamina propria.[22,43,44]

The relative numbers of the B and T cell and other leukocytes in the gut differ with antigenic stimulation, the age of the animal, and the sampling site in the intestine (both in luminal versus submucosal and oral versus aboral directions). In human adults, B cells, T cells, and null cells have been reported to make up 25%, 50%, and 25% of the lamina propria lymphoid pool, respectively.[22] In calves, the proportions of lymphoid subsets in the lamina propria is similar, with 28% and 45% expressing B and T cell phenotypes, respectively.[45] In diseased mucosa, the number of leukocytes in the lamina propria increases. The IgA isotype usually remains predominant, but the relative numeric increase is largest for the IgG-secreting cells.[3]

The lamina propria lymphocytes are intimately involved in all aspects of the immune response, including antigen elimination, oral tolerance, and immune regulation. The lamina propria plasma cells are the source of the majority of the IgA for antigen-specific exclusion.

Macrophages, neutrophils, eosinophils, and mast cells are said to comprise less than 1% of lamina propria leukocytes in the normal human.[22] These lamina propria leukocytes are the cellular basis for gastrointestinal inflammation and serve a variety of other functions, including phagocytosis and antibody-dependent cellular cytotoxicity.

GLOBULE LEUKOCYTES. Globule leukocytes have been identified in the gastrointestinal epithelium of a variety of species including dogs.[34,46] Distinctive features of globule leukocytes include an unlobed nucleus and membrane-bound eosinophilic granules.[46] The origin and function of globule leukocytes is uncertain. In dogs they appear closely related to eosinophils, whereas in rats and ruminants morphologic transformation between mast cells and globule leukocytes has been demonstrated.[34,46,47] Globule leukocytes markedly increase in number in parasitized gastrointestinal tracts[34,46] and, in the author's experience, are not infrequently increased in canine inflammatory bowel disease.

LAMINA PROPRIA MAST CELLS. Two types of mast cells have been identified in the gut of rats, mice, sheep, and humans (those species in which suitable histochemical techniques have been applied).[34,48] They have been termed "mucosal" and "connective tissue" mast cells, in recognition of their distinctive distributions. The mucosal mast cells are located primarily in the lamina propria, whereas the connective tissue mast cells are located in connective tissues throughout the body. In the bowel, connective tissue mast cells may be found in the submucosa, muscularis mucosa, and serosa. In rats, connective tissue mast cells predominate in the tongue, esophagus, and nonglandular stomach, whereas mucosal mast cells predominate (up to 90%) in the glandular stomach and intestines.[49] It is likely that mast cell polymorphism also occurs in dogs and cats. Mast cells with properties reminiscent of rat mucosal mast cells have been identified in the gastrointestinal tract of cats.[50]

Mucosal mast cells have been overlooked, until recent years, because of different staining properties to those of the conventional (connective tissue) mast cells. For instance, after standard formalin fixation, mucosal mast cells fail to stain with toluidine blue and other stains that are commonly used to identify connective tissue mast cells.[16,51]

Mucosal and connective tissue mast cells have different ultrastructure, biologic behavior, and perhaps function.[34,51] Connective tissue mast cells are twice as large as mucosal mast cells, possess single-lobed nuclei, are long lived, maintain relatively constant levels in tissues, and elaborate prostaglandins (among other mediators) in response to stimulation. In addition, they have many uniform-sized intracytoplasmic granules, have IgE only on their surfaces, and contain high concentrations of heparin and histamine. In contrast, mucosal mast cells are smaller (10 μm), possess unilobed or bilobed nuclei, are shorter lived, proliferate rapidly in response to interleukin-3, and elaborate leukotrienes to a greater degree after stimulation. Mucosal mast cells have fewer, variable-sized intracytoplasmic granules, have cytoplasmic as well as surface IgE, possess a different type of protease, and contain chondroitin sulfate (not heparin) and only small amounts of histamine.

Rat mucosal mast cells are resistant to certain secretagogues and antiallergic compounds that influence connective tissue mast cells.[49] For instance, significant histamine release from mucosal mast cells will occur following challenge with substance P but not somatostatin, vasoactive intestinal polypeptide, neurotensin, morphine, certain endorphins and bradykinin, all of which can induce connective tissue mast cells to release histamine. No secretory response by either cell type occurs on exposure to acetylcholine, bombesin, motilin, or pentagastrin. Theophylline and sodium cromoglycolate inhibit antigen-induced histamine secretion by connective tissue mast cells. Theophylline, but not cromoglycolate, has the same effect on mucosal mast cells.[52] Corticosteroids inhibit mast cell secretion and can dramatically reduce mast cell numbers in the intestine within 24 hours.[53] Sulfasalazine may also inhibit mast cell secretion.[54] These findings may partly explain the efficacy of these drugs in the therapy of inflammatory bowel disease.

Precursors of mucosal mast cells are present in Peyer's patches and mesenteric lymph nodes. It is probable that early in the immune response Peyer's patches supply the gastrointestinal mucosa with mucosal mast cells in a similar manner to which they supply mucosal T and B cells.[55] It has recently been suggested that both types of mast cell are derived from a common lineage and that the cell's phenotypic expression is controlled by microenvironmental factors.[56]

Mast cell discharge is now known to have many more stimuli than just IgE antibody-antigen complexes. The hormones and neuropeptides mentioned earlier are but some of these stimulating influences. Other known activators include bile, the activated complement fragments C3a, C4a, and C5a, products of macrophages (such as interleukin-1), certain classes of IgG, and a T cell lymphokine.[34,52,54] Whether the mucosal mast cell subtype responds to all of these secretagogues remains to be established.

Vagal stimulation also appears to facilitate histamine secretion. Interestingly, mucosal mast cell secretion can be conditioned to an odor, flashing light, or noise in the same way salivation can be conditioned to bell ringing.[57,58] The nervous pathways involved in the conditioned mast cell response have not been determined, but substance P–containing nerves have been demonstrated closely associated with the intestinal mast cells of rats,[54] and studies of human bowel mucosa have revealed that a high proportion of mucosal mast cells are apposed to nerves.[59] Electron microscopic studies have demonstrated membrane-to-membrane contact between mast cells and axon like processes, providing a microanatomic basis for the phenomenon just described. These observations raise the possibility that the acute diarrhea manifested by many fearful dogs on presentation to veterinary clinics may result from a substance P–mediated, conditioned discharge of the mucosal mast cell.

The functions of mast cells, in general, are complex and considerably more extensive than the mediation of immediate hypersensitivity. They have a role in delayed hypersensitivity, inflammation, immunoregulation, smooth muscle contraction, cytotoxicity, and healing via stimulation of angiogenesis and fibrosis.[34,54] How many of these functions are shared by *mucosal* mast cells, in particular, is largely speculative.

Mast cell functions are initiated by the release of mediators, of which mast cells contain a wide array. Vasodilation, increased vascular permeability, and inflammation result from the release of vasoactive and inflammatory mediators such as histamine, leukotrienes, platelet activating factor, proteases, and kallikreins (see Chapter 4).[6,54] Smooth muscle contraction can be stimulated by leukotrienes (such as leukotriene C4) released by mucosal mast cells. Collectively, the release of these mediators can lead to secretory diarrhea and increased intestinal permeability.[52]

Some mast cell mediators have antinflammatory or healing effects. Thus, proteases released by canine mast cells are capable of degrading vasoactive intestinal peptide and substance P, two substances with potent effects on glandular secretion and smooth muscle tone.[60] Histamine activation of H_2-receptor-bearing suppressor lymphocytes has been widely demonstrated,[54] and may reinforce the suppressor-dominated functions of GALT. Histamine has been shown to induce fibroblast proliferation.[33] Serotonin release by mast cells is known to stimulate jejunal crypt cell renewal.[22]

Mast cells may be involved in the pathogenesis of many gastrointestinal diseases.[52] Increased numbers of mucosal mast cells have been noted in inflammatory bowel disease and celiac disease.[5,51] Mast cell proliferation has also been associated with intestinal fibrosis.[54] Mucosal mast cells appear to be important in the elimination of helminth infections (see

immune response to parasites discussed later), and they have a documented role in the pathogenesis of dietary allergies. In addition, release of chemotactic factors by mast cells may result in the accumulation of eosinophils and neutrophils at sites of inflammation, resulting in the characteristic pathology of such disorders as eosinophilic gastroenteritis.

The recent revelations regarding the many functions of mast cells (in addition to their traditional role in immediate hypersensitivity) and the discovery of mast cell heterogeneity may prove to alter currently accepted roles of the mast cell in the pathogenesis of bowel disorders, and may demand the development of a new range of pharmaceuticals effective in the modulation of mucosal mast cell function.

Duct-Associated Lymphoid Tissue

Duct-associated lymphoid tissue (DALT) is found aggregated about glandular ducts. The secretion of IgA by salivary DALT has been proposed to play an important role in defense of the oral cavity in some species.[61] Migration of IgA-bearing lymphocytes from GALT to salivary tissue has also been demonstrated.[62] In contrast to lymphoid nodules and Peyer's patches, M cells have not been demonstrated in salivary DALT, and antigen is thought to be exposed to the lymphoid tissue by retrograde passage through the salivary ducts.[61] The significance of DALT in the dog and cat is unknown. Both IgA and IgM have been detected in the saliva of these species.[63,64] The parotid salivary glands of the dog appear to secrete saliva particularly rich in IgA (0.52 mg/mL).[63] It is uncertain whether these salivary immunoglobulins are locally produced or derived from serum. The latter process is likely in view of the recent demonstration of selective serum IgA and IgM transport into the saliva of sheep by a process thought to be analogous to the way in which IgA is transported into bile.[65]

Mesenteric Lymph Nodes

Lymph nodes are secondary lymphoid organs whose position and structure are designed to facilitate antigen trapping and immune elimination. They are well-organized tissues with a clearly defined capsule, cortex, medulla, and afferent and efferent lymphatics.[6] B lymphocytes are arranged into nodules in the cortex and are separated from the medulla by a T cell–rich paracortical zone. In contrast to GALT, lymph nodes contain numerous plasma cells. These cells are located in the medulla. Lymph enters through the cortex of the node and is directed to the medulla along lymphatic sinuses. Antigen is trapped by mononuclear-phagocyte cells in the medulla or by dendritic cells in the cortex. The macrophages then migrate to the cortex and present the antigen to B and T cells for initiation of the immune response (see description of the mononuclear-phagocyte system).

The structure and function of the mesenteric lymph nodes is similar to that of the peripheral lymph nodes. They are located in the mesentery close to mesenteric vessels. In dogs, they average 6 × 2 × 0.5 cm in size and vary in number. The mesenteric lymph nodes (inclusive of colic lymph nodes) drain the jejunum, ileum, cecum, and most of the colon. The duodenum and rectum are drained by the celiac and internal iliac lymph nodes, respectively.[10,28] Lymph leaving the mesenteric nodes enters the intestinal lymphatic trunks, the cisterna chyli, the thoracic duct, and ultimately the venous system.

Mesenteric lymph nodes are involved in the circulation of gut-associated lymphocytes. They are the first port of call for these migrant gut-derived lymphocytes and may, in contrast to the Peyer's patch, provide an environment suitable for maturation of precursor IgA-committed B cells into plasma cells. It has also been suggested that the mesenteric nodes amplify the GALT immune response by additional antigen presentation, resulting in further B cell proliferation.[17] Lymphocytes derived from the mesenteric lymph nodes show a tendency to "home" back to the mesenteric lymph nodes and intestinal lamina propria (and to a lesser extent the other mucosal surfaces).[22] Also in contrast to GALT, in response to antigen the mesenteric lymph nodes mount a very vigorous elimination response with little evidence of generation of tolerance. A component of this elimination response is the secretion of immunoglobulins other than IgA. The humoral secretions of the mesenteric lymph nodes contain a much greater proportion of IgG and IgE than do the secretions of GALT. Particularly vigorous immune responses cause hyperplasia of the abdominal lymph nodes (mesenteric lymphadenopathy).

The Liver and Gastrointestinal Immunity

The liver serves an important role in gastrointestinal immunity, by virtue of its vast mononuclear-phagocyte system and by the secretion of IgA into bile. In cats, the liver is a major source of intestinal IgA. IgA is the predominant immunoglobulin in feline bile, followed by IgM, and lastly IgG.[64,66,67] Disagreement exists over the quantity of IgA in canine bile.[6,68]

There are two sources of IgA in bile. The first is an hepatic "IgA pump." A proportion of dimeric IgA produced in the lamina propria of the bowel escapes secretion by the gastrointestinal epithelium and enters the lymphatic, portal, and systemic circulations. This dimeric IgA subsequently binds secretory component present on the surface of the hepatocyte and is transported through the hepatocyte and pumped into the bile.[69] The second source of biliary IgA appears to be local synthesis within the liver.

Biliary IgA may have a role to play in local immunity of the biliary tree. In addition, the hepatic IgA pump is able to remove IgA-antigen complexes, a mechanism that offers a convenient method of ridding the circulation of food and bacterial antigen-antibody complexes generated in the intestine.[69]

IMMUNE RESPONSE OF THE GUT-ASSOCIATED LYMPHOID TISSUE[6]

The antigen-specific immune response of the gastrointestinal tract is initiated and, to some degree, regulated in the aggregated lymphoid tissues of GALT. The first steps in the initiation of the immune response are those of antigen uptake and presentation. Immunoresponsive cells subsequently undergo a closely regulated clonal expansion to produce precursors of antibody-secreting cells, and cells involved in cell-mediated immunity, immune memory, and immunoregulation. A peculiar feature of GALT is its predisposition to produce precursors of IgA-secreting plasma cells. Other characteristic features are its propensity to mount immune responses dominated by T cell suppression, and the rapid migration of immune response cells from aggregated lymphoid tissues to mucosal surfaces and lymphoid tissues throughout the body. In these positions the immune

response cells are responsible for developing local secretory immunity and ultimately rendering the entire immune system tolerant to benign mucosal antigens. This combination of immunity at the mucosal surface and oral tolerance provides effective defense against the complex antigenic environment of the mucosal surfaces.

Antigen Uptake and Presentation in GALT

Luminal antigen reaches GALT either after being sampled by the M cells of the Peyer's patches or lymphoid nodules or following invasion of the mucosal barrier. One consequence of a defective mucosal barrier is an alteration in the predominant route by which an antigen is exposed to the immune system. Antigen penetrating the mucosa through the absorptive epithelium bypasses the Peyer's patch and lymphoid nodules and is transported directly to either the mesenteric nodes via the lymphatics or the liver via the mesenteric portal system. The route of exposure of antigen to the immune system may be important in determining the primacy of local versus systemic immunity or immunologic responsiveness versus tolerance.[4,22]

After penetrating the epithelium, the antigen is trapped by an antigen-presenting cell. In the Peyer's patch and lamina propria the most important antigen-presenting cell is the subepithelial, MHC II positive macrophage (Figures 3–4 and 3–5). Antigen presentation in both the Peyer's patch and lamina propria is supplemented by dendritic cells.[17] On occasion, B cells, endothelial cells, and epithelial cells can act as antigen-presenting cells following the expression of MHC II antigens on their surfaces. MHC II–positive epithelial cells have been identified in intestinal villi and follicle-associated epithelium. It appears that normal enterocytes can express MHC II antigens and present antigen to T cells.[4] In vitro this results in proliferation of T cells of the cytotoxic-suppressor phenotype rather than the helper phenotype. The expression of enterocyte MHC II antigens is increased in a number of gastroenteric diseases,[4] perhaps under the influence of lymphokines from the natural killer-like cells of the intraepithelial compartment[3,17,20] The increased MHC II expression is associated with stimulation of helper T cells, rather than suppressor cells, perhaps leading to further inflammation.[4] Thus, augmented presentation of antigen by epithelial cells may play a role in the pathogenesis of inflammatory gastrointestinal diseases.[17]

Antigen-presenting cells present antigen to B cells and neighboring T cells, which together go on to generate a cell-mediated and humoral response to the antigen.

Cell-Mediated Response of GALT[6]

Effective generation of effector T cells (and antibody) depends on the interaction of a T helper cell with an antigen-MHC II complex on the surface of an antigen-presenting cell. Secretion of interleukin-2 from T helper cells stimulates the clonal expansion of effector T cells primed by binding to an antigen-MHC I complex on the surface of an antigen-presenting cell (Figure 3–4). Several factors limit this proliferation, including the activity of concomitantly generated suppressor T cells. The stimulated T effector cells can differentiate into a number of populations, including memory cells and cytotoxic cells, and can synthesize numerous biologically active factors called lymphokines.

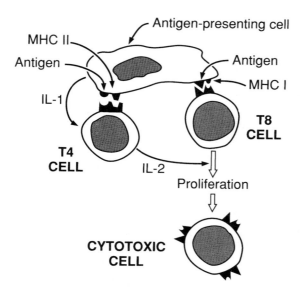

FIGURE 3-4. Schematic illustrating functions of macrophages in cellular and humoral immunity. T4 and T8 cells are helper and cytotoxic cells, respectively (from reference 6, Fig. 7–4).

CELLULAR CYTOTOXICITY. Cytotoxic T cells can kill in a specific or nonspecific manner. In the antigen-specific mechanism, the T cell recognizes the inciting antigen in association with MHC 1 antigens on the target cell, adheres to, and perforates the target's membrane via insertion of a tubular structure that results from the polymerization of cytotoxic proteins called perforins. Stimulated cytotoxic T cells can also disrupt neighboring cells in a nonspecific manner by releasing soluble lymphotoxins into the local environment. The cytotoxicity of T cells is augmented by other types of cellular cytotoxicity. These include antibody-dependent cellular cytotoxicity and cell lysis by natural killer cells and activated macrophages.

Antibody-dependent cellular cytotoxicity is mediated by leukocytes with receptors for immunoglobulin. These cells bind to antibody-coated cells and lyse them. Leukocytes capable of antibody-dependent cellular cytotoxicity include neutrophils, macrophages, eosinophils, and a population of non-B, non-T ("null") lymphocytes called killer cells. Antibody-dependent cellular cytotoxicity can significantly enhance the cytotoxic capability of leukocytes. There is evidence to suggest that IgA is an effective antibody for this process.[17]

Natural killer cells are "null" lymphocytes similar to killer cells but may be functionally differentiated in that they do not require antibody for activity. They do have immunoglobulin receptors, however, and thus can participate in antibody-dependent cellular cytotoxicity. Natural killer cells have cytotoxicity against a wide range of cells including virus-infected, neoplastic, and foreign cells. They are activated by interferon. Natural killer-like cells are a particularly important subpopulation of the bowel epithelium.

Macrophages may become cytotoxic when activated by T cell lymphokines, most notably interferon. They are cytotoxic to microorganisms and tumor cells. The lamina propria contains significant numbers of macrophages.

Cell-mediated cytotoxicity helps eliminate pathogens that penetrate the mucosal barrier and is critical to the destruction of neoplastic and, perhaps, dysplastic cells. Eosinophil-mediated, antibody-dependent cellular cytotoxicity is impor-

tant in the elimination of helminths in the bowel lumen. Lysis of virus-infected cells by natural killer-like cells may be a critical first-line defense of the bowel against enteroviruses.

Cell-mediated cytotoxicity, however, may also be important in the pathogenesis of bowel disorders. Chronic inflammation and persistent delayed hypersensitivity reactions damage tissue by release of inflammatory products and by self-directed cytotoxicity. The self-directed cytotoxicity results from the nonspecific cytotoxicity of soluble mediators released by T cells and macrophages. In addition, on occasion cytotoxic cells will specifically lyse self-tissue. The mechanisms for such autoimmunity are poorly understood but appear to be partly explained by the development of antiepithelial cell antibodies, capable of arming cells for antibody-dependent cellular cytotoxicity, and by alterations of target cell surface glycoproteins during the course of inflammation.[70,71] These specific and nonspecific mechanisms of tissue destruction are known to play an important role in the pathogenesis of inflammatory bowel disease.

LYMPHOKINES. The activated T cell is capable of secreting a large number of lymphokines other than the cytotoxins. These lymphokines have immunoregulatory and inflammatory functions. One group of lymphokines is the interferons, which are responsible for an impressive array of immunoregulatory effects, including the activation of macrophages, the inhibition of macrophage migration, the inhibition of tumor cell growth, and the enhancement of both suppressor and cytotoxic T cell activities. Another important group of lymphokines is the interleukins. Interleukins-1 (a monokine) and 2 are particularly important in the early events of the immune response. Interleukin-3 encourages the maturation of immature T cells and the proliferation of mucosal mast cell populations. T cells regulate B cell immunoglobulin isotype, proliferation and differentiation through the release of isotype switch factor(s), and growth and differentiation factors, all of probable importance to the development of secretory (IgA) immunity.

Activated lymphocytes are responsible for producing a macrophage chemotactic factor, a macrophage fusion factor, and a fibroblast stimulation factor, which contribute to the development of the granulomatous inflammation and fibrosis characteristic of some chronic bowel and liver diseases. T cell lymphokines may be responsible for the villus atrophy and crypt hyperplasia that occurs in many enteropathies. Certainly, in experimental helminthiasis and giardiasis of rodents, and intestinal allograft transplantation in dogs, such pathologic changes appear to be T cell mediated.[72] The increased cellular turnover may help rid the body of pathogens adherent to the epithelium. The shortened villi reduce epithelial absorptive area, a process which, although resulting in nutrient malabsorption, may reduce additional mucosal ingress of pathologic substances.

SUPPRESSOR CELLS. Regulation of the immune response by suppressor cells is an integral part of the immune response. The cells that mediate immunosuppression are poorly defined but probably include suppressor T lymphocytes, macrophages and cells with similarities to natural killer cells. Suppressor B cells have also been detected. To add to the confusion it is possible that suppressor T cells and cytotoxic T cells are different physiologic states of the same T cell.[73]

The activity of suppressor cells is comparable to that of helper cells, but different antigenic epitopes vary in their ability to stimulate suppressor or helper activities. Suppressor T cells inhibit immune responses by releasing soluble suppressor factors. Some of these factors restrain antigen-specific responses, but others are antigen nonspecific. Macrophages may function as suppres-

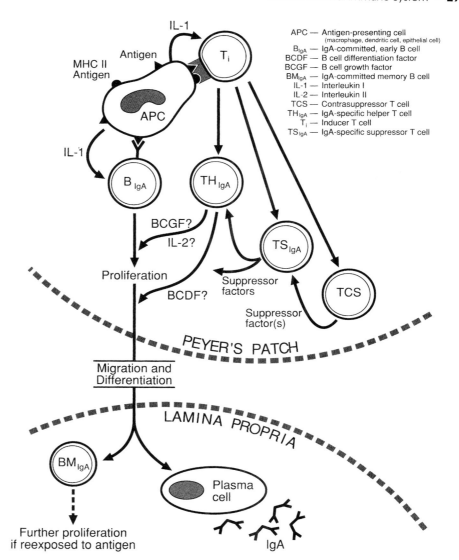

FIGURE 3–5. Schematic diagram of putative features of antigen presentation and generation of the IgA immune response in GALT.

APC — Antigen-presenting cell
　　　　(macrophage, dendritic cell, epithelial cell)
B_{IgA} — IgA-committed, early B cell
BCDF — B cell differentiation factor
BCGF — B cell growth factor
BM_{IgA} — IgA-committed memory B cell
IL-1 — Interleukin I
IL-2 — Interleukin II
TCS — Contrasuppressor T cell
TH_{IgA} — IgA-specific helper T cell
T_i — Inducer T cell
TS_{IgA} — IgA-specific suppressor T cell

sor cells by releasing prostaglandin E_2. This eicosanoid inhibits lymphocyte proliferation and differentiation and restrains the secretion of interleukin-2 and the lymphokines involved in the accumulation and activation of macrophages, thus providing a possible mechanism by which granulomatous inflammation can be self-regulated.

Cellular-dependent immune suppression is an integral part of immunoregulation and an important component of the phenomenon of "oral tolerance." It assumes particular importance in tissues such as the gastrointestinal tract in which the elimination of antigen, an important means of switching off the immune response, is often incomplete. Therefore, it is not surprising that one of the characteristic features of GALT is a predisposition to mount immune responses dominated by T cell suppression rather than T cell help. Recently, this function has been shown to involve the generation of suppressor T cell cascades that are capable of generating cells and factors with widespread suppressive effects on the local and systemic immune systems, but which largely spare the secretion of IgA.[70,74] A failure to suppress adequately GALT's elimination response to luminal antigens is currently thought to be important in the genesis of inflammatory bowel disease, and may play a role in certain dietary

allergies.[70] Defects of cell-mediated immune suppression have also been reported in human chronic active hepatitis and primary biliary cirrhosis.[12]

B Cell Differentiation and Immunoglobulin Isotype Regulation

When antigen is presented to the lymphoid tissues of GALT, the regulatory T cells bind to the MHC II-foreign antigen complex on the surface of the antigen-presenting cell and undergo clonal expansion (Figure 3–5). A helper, suppressor, and contrasuppressor response is generated. Under the influence of interleukin-1 secreted by the antigen-presenting cell, the helper regulatory cells begin secretion of stimulatory lymphokines (presumably interleukin-2 and B cell growth factor). The combined influence of interleukin-1 and the T helper-derived lymphokines encourages the proliferation of an antigen-specific clone of isotype-committed B cells that have been previously primed by binding to the foreign antigen. As the B cells divide, they are thought to be further influenced by other T cell lymphokines (B cell differentiation factors). The result is the terminal differentiation of the isotype-committed B cells into memory cells or plasma cells capable of secreting immunoglobulin specific for the inciting antigen.

In clear contrast to the systemic lymphoid tissues, most of the B cells in GALT bear the IgA immunoglobulin isotype and are committed to differentiate into clones of IgA-secreting plasma cells. This phenomenon appears to be due to the influence of T cells specific for IgA responses that act at multiple levels of B cell differentiation.[75,77]

GALT contains regulatory T cells that induce the majority of the immature IgM-bearing B cells present in the aggregated lymphoid tissues to switch to immature, IgA-bearing, IgA-committed lymphocytes.[75,77] (IgM is the isotype normally present on immature, isotype-uncommitted B cells.) These so-called switch T cells have been demonstrated in Peyer's patches but may also occur in lymphoid nodules and the lamina propria.[17,75] It is speculated that they induce isotype switching by release of a lymphokine (perhaps interleukin-5) that affects the course of DNA recombinations within the B lymphocyte. Recent evidence suggests that some of these switch cells may also contribute to the clonal expansion of IgA-committed B cells.[76] It has been suggested that isotype switching and proliferation of gut B cells is not restricted to the aggregated tissues of GALT but it can also occur in the lamina propria, and contribute to isotype-switching and proliferation of poorly differentiated Peyer's patch–derived B cells.[3,17]

A second proposal, to explain the predominance of IgA-committed B cells in GALT, suggests that the Peyer's patch (or lamina propria) provides a microenvironment in which antigen (such as lipopolysaccharide) can stimulate B cell proliferation but not differentiation. The proliferation leads to conventional, T cell–independent, sequential isotype switching from IgM to IgG to IgA due to repeated recombinations within the B cell genome, which eventually result in a disproportionate expression of the gene coding for IgA.[17,77,78]

Isotype-specific T cells whose primary function is to regulate the response of the *isotype-committed* B cells have also been identified in GALT.[75,77,79] The majority of these isotype-specific regulatory T cells help the continued development of the B cells committed to IgA production.[75,77] A small number of isotype-specific T cells regulate the response of the primitive B cells that either retain their surface IgM or go on to bear IgE or IgG.[5,77] These regulatory cells tend to suppress, rather than encourage, development of IgG-, IgM-, or IgE-committed cells.

Contrasuppressor T cells have been identified in GALT. Although these cells have a role in the immunoregulation of GALT, recent work has shown no evidence of isotype specificity of the contrasuppressor T cells.[75] This finding suggests IgA contrasuppression is not the primary reason for IgA dominance in GALT. Rather, IgA dominance results from both the "switch" cell conversion of early, isotype-uncommitted B cells to IgA-committed B cells, and from preferential help for development of these IgA-committed B cells by IgA-specific regulatory T cells.[75]

The sequence of events just described is not the only pathway for antibody production. For example, a few antigens do not require the cooperation of T cells to achieve humoral immunity. T-independent antigens tend to be large molecules with repeating antigenic determinants. One example, of relevance to the gastrointestinal tract, is lipopolysaccharide. Lipopolysaccharide from the cell wall of *E. coli* can function as a polyclonal activator of B cells. Thus, it can cause nonspecific B cell proliferation (perhaps important for the generation of B cells expressing IgA).

Little IgA secretion occurs in the Peyer's patch itself. Instead, the terminal differentiation of the IgA-committed B cells occurs later, either on route to, or at, distant lymphoid or mucosal sites. Several possibilities have been put forward to explain the lack of IgA secretion in the Peyer's patch. It has been proposed that the IgA-secreting precursors emigrate rapidly from GALT prior to their maturation to IgA-secreting cells.[3,23] An alternative explanation is provided by the discovery in the Peyer's patch of IgA-specific suppressor T cells.[79] Thus, terminal differentiation of IgA-committed B cells may occur only in tissues with an appropriate helper-to-suppressor T cell ratio.[22] It has been proposed, furthermore, that helper T cells responsible for elaboration of B cell differentiation factors are preferentially located in tissues other than GALT, for instance the mesenteric lymph nodes.[80]

Lymphocyte Migration and the Mucosal Immune Network

After interaction with antigen, lymphocytes leave the Peyer's patch and lymphoid nodule and begin a migration that carries them through intestinal lymphatics, mesenteric lymph nodes, spleen, thoracic duct, and blood vasculature and deposits them, three to six days later, in mucosal tissues throughout the body (Figure 3–2). The majority of lymphocytes derived from GALT or mesenteric nodes will return to the lamina propria of the segment of the gut that generated them, but a proportion will localize in respiratory, reproductive, salivary, and lacrimal mucosal tissues.[3,5] Selective localization in mucosal tissues depends in part on lymphocyte receptors expressed on the endothelium of mucosal postcapillary venules.[81]

This migration has led to the concept of a mucosal immunologic network that, through intermucosa transfer of immunologically competent cells and humoral secretions, specifically protects the body surfaces against pathogens.[5] The mucosal tissues probably also receive a minor contribution of cells from peripheral lymph nodes and spleen facilitating integration between the systemic and mucosal immune systems.[3]

It has become apparent that a number of the cellular components of GALT are capable of this migration. The first recognized and best studied migratory cell is the B cell. Other migratory cells are T cells and perhaps mast cells.

B LYMPHOCYTE MIGRATION. The majority of B cells activated by antigen and T cell lymphokines in GALT begin migration as undifferentiated, IgA-committed lymphocytes. A major subpopulation of these lymphocytes undergoes considerable differentiation as it migrates. When the lymphocytes reach the mesenteric lymph nodes, approximately one-half are IgA-containing lymphoblasts. In the thoracic duct, the proportion increases further. The B cells that enter the lamina propria from peripheral blood are dominated by IgA-committed lymphocytes but a variable number of IgM- and IgG-committed lymphocytes are also present.[3,17] Further antigen-driven IgA-B cell proliferation of substantial magnitude, including isotype switching, apparently continues in the lamina propria and eventually leads to a 70% to 90% dominance of lamina propria lymphocytes by IgA-containing lymphoblasts or plasma cells.[3,17] There is evidence for mucosal migration of small numbers of IgM- and IgG-bearing lymphocytes.[5] The extent and significance of this migration is poorly defined.

The stimulus for this mucosal homing is unknown. Suggested factors have included receptor affinities for mucosal endothelial determinants, variations in blood flow, and epithelial chemotactic factors.[17] The role of luminal antigen in lymphocyte homing has not been resolved.[17,82] In humans, lamina propria lymphocytes have been shown to be derived from circulating lymphocytes that lack a specific lymph node homing receptor.[83] It is possible, therefore, that the preferential migration of lymphocytes to the lamina propria might be guided by homing receptors specific to the lamina propria.[83] It is noteworthy that lymphoblasts can distinguish between homing receptors in the colon and jejunum, allowing preferential migration to one or other site.[82]

T Lymphocyte Migration. Accumulating evidence indicates that T lymphocytes migrate in a similar manner to B cells, albeit in smaller numbers. Reinjection of T lymphoblasts derived from mesenteric lymph nodes or thoracic duct results in their selective lodging in the bowel lamina propria and, unlike B cells, bowel epithelium.[5,16] The relative proportions of migrating T suppressor and T helper subtypes is unknown, but members of both subsets appear to migrate. The migration of suppressor cells to lymphoid tissues throughout the body, in addition to mucosal surfaces, is considered important in the development of oral tolerance. The migration of helper subsets may be important for the proliferation and differentiation of B cells in the lamina propria. The homing of T cells to GALT and mesenteric nodes can be reduced by their prior incubation with vasointestinal polypeptide, an observation pertinent to the discussion of the neuroendocrine modulation of the immune system.[84]

Mast Cell Migration. The possibility of analogous mast cell migration has been proposed.[3,5] Some support for this hypothesis is provided by the observation that Peyer's patches, lamina propria, and mesenteric nodes all have significantly greater mucosal mast cell precursor populations than do bone marrow and spleen.[55]

IgA: Properties, Secretion, Assay, and Function[3,6]

IgA Properties and Secretion. IgA is the predominant immunoglobulin in most, but not all, of the body secretions of cats and dogs (Tables 3–2 and 3–3).[63–64] It is the second most abundant immunoglobulin in the serum of cats and the third most abundant in the serum of dogs (most studies).

IgA is a carbohydrate-rich immunoglobulin that is distinguished by its propensity to form dimers and to combine with an epithelial transmembrane protein called "secretory component." The IgA monomer has a structure like that of the other immunoglobulin monomers. It consists of two heavy chains linked together by disulfide bonds and two shorter light chains attached to one end of each heavy chain by disulfide linkages, as shown in Figure 3–6. The molecular weight of the monomer is about 160,000 daltons. Monomeric IgA is found only in small quantities in the serum and is probably derived largely from IgA-secreting cells in the bone marrow.[85] In contrast to that in humans, almost all serum IgA in the dog and cat is dimeric, and most of this is derived from GALT.[40,86]

The major form of IgA produced by intestinal plasma cells is a dimer. It is composed of two immunoglobulin monomers linked by either a single joining (J) chain or perhaps by a J-chain dimer, and it has a molecular weight of approximately 320,000 daltons.[17] The J chain is produced by mucosal immunocytes, regardless of the immunoglobulin class they produce. However, J chain does not combine with IgG and is therefore not secreted by IgG plasma cells but is degraded

Table 3–2

THE IMMUNOGLOBULIN CONCENTRATIONS OF FELINE BODY FLUIDS

SPECIMEN	MEAN VALUES AND RANGE OF IMMUNOGLOBULIN LEVELS (MG/DL)		
	IgG	IgA	IgM
Serum	1894 (1171–2258)	285 (203–582)	247 (60–390)
Colostrum	3570 (2750–4674)	254 (50–488)	110 (31–300)
Milk	189 (95–255)	13 (9–20)	20 (10–40)
Saliva	2 (0–6)	7 (3–20)	3 (0–12)
Nasal secretion	5 (0–39)	7 (3–29)	2 (0–15)
Tracheal fluid	20 (0–146)	42 (0–156)	11 (0–34)
Tears	2 (0–17)	14 (5–33)	4 (0–12)
Bile	11 (3–41)	46 (18–89)	54 (6–96)
Fecal fluid	3 (0–20)	35 (10–84)	34 (0–234)

From reference 64.

intracellularly.[3] It is a 15,000 dalton peptide chain, linked by disulfide bonds to the heavy chains of the IgA dimer. The incorporation of the J chain into the dimer furnishes the binding site for secretory component and is thus an essential prerequisite for secretion.[17]

Plasma cells release the IgA dimer into the interstitium of the lamina propria. A small quantity enters the portal system or intestinal lymphatics, but the majority diffuses to the epithelium and binds to secretory component on the basal and basolateral surface of the epithelial cell (Figure 3–7). Secretory component is an 85,000 to 95,000 dalton glycoprotein that is synthesized by the epithelial cells of the intestine and some other tissues. In human small intestine it is produced primarily by the epithelial cells in the intestinal crypts, whereas in the colon it is generally also present in the surface epithelium.[3] Altered distribution and quantity of secretory component has been observed in a number of diseases in humans, the significance of which is unknown.[3] The synthesis of secretory component is independent of IgA synthesis. Thus, individuals with IgA deficiency can produce secretory component, and people with secretory component deficiency can produce but not secrete IgA.[22] Deficient secretory component secretion has been proposed as a rare cause of failed secretory immunity and severe diarrhea in humans.[3]

Secretory component occupies a transmembrane position and acts as a receptor for the J chain–containing IgA dimer. The binding stimulates pinocytosis by the epithelial cell, and

Table 3–3

THE IMMUNOGLOBULIN CONCENTRATIONS OF CANINE BODY FLUIDS

SPECIMEN	MEAN VALUES AND RANGE OF IMMUNOGLOBULIN LEVELS (MG/DL)		
	IgG	IgA	IgM
Serum	980 (520–1730)	50 (20–120)	170 (70–270)
Colostrum	1200	285	15
Milk	10	130	15
Saliva	2 (0–5)	52 (17–125)	3 (1–7)
Bowel fluid	20	300	60
Tears		25	23

From reference 63. By permission of Blackwell Scientific Publications.

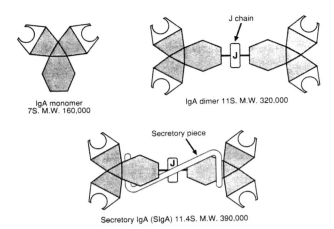

FIGURE 3–6. Structure of IgA monomer and dimer formed by interaction of monomers with J chain. Secretory piece is added before the dimer can attach to mucosal surface (from reference 6, Fig. 12–4).

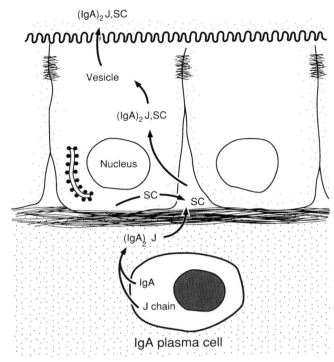

FIGURE 3–7. Schematic of secretion of IgA into the intestinal lumen. IgA = immunoglobulin A; J = joining chain; SC = secretory component.

the IgA-receptor complex is packaged into vesicles for transport to the apical epithelial surface. Here the vesicle fuses with the plasma membrane and the dimeric IgA-secretory-component-complex is released into the bowel lumen. This complex of secretory component, J chain, and dimeric IgA is called secretory IgA (sIgA). It has a molecular weight of approximately 390,000 daltons. Secretory component stabilizes the dimeric IgA within the intestinal lumen. This appears to result from disulfide and noncovalent bridging of the secretory component to the IgA dimer and the resultant protection of the constant region of the IgA molecule from proteolysis by either bacteria or endogenous digestive enzymes.[6,17]

The secretion rate of IgA in humans has been estimated to be 0.78 g/meter of intestine/day. In the fasting dog, a rate of 0.25 g/meter/day has been suggested.[63] The canine vascular IgA pool has a daily turnover of 75%,[68] presumably due to a combination of hepatic catabolism and resecretion into the bowel via the liver and, perhaps, salivary tissue.

REGULATION OF IGA SECRETION. The regulation of IgA secretion by IgA-committed lymphocytes is largely dependent on the properties of the inciting antigen, and the influence of the cell-mediated immune response of GALT. The secretory immune response continues while the antigen remains in the lumen and declines if the antigen is eliminated (plasma cells have life span of three to six days). The local humoral response is much more persistent and vigorous if antigen is presented locally rather than systemically.

Regulation of the secretory immune response also partly depends on nonimmunologic mechanisms.[6,22] These regulatory influences include the genetic makeup of the host and nonspecific immunosuppressive factors such as histamine (via H_2 receptors). The autonomic nervous system seems to facilitate gastrointestinal IgA secretion in coordination with the presence of swallowed antigens. In addition, substance P release has been reported to enhance IgA production by GALT; VIP decreases IgA secretion but increases IgM; somatostatin decreases IgA production;[87,88] and secretin appears to increase the luminal concentrations of both IgA and IgG.[22]

IGA ASSAY. A wide range of serum IgA concentrations in the dog has been reported. These differences result largely from variations in the assay technique used and from discrepancies in the ages of dogs included in the reference popula-

tion. Most laboratories utilize a single radial immunodiffusion technique. Important potential sources of assay-related discrepancy include the use of different forms of IgA as the standards and the utilization of disparate formulas to interpret the precipitation rings.[89] The time at which serum IgA concentrations reach adult levels is poorly defined, but by 12 months of age most dogs appear to have IgA concentrations within or approaching the adult range (Table 3–4).[90] Two recent reports suggest that by 16 to 17 weeks of age there is sufficient IgA in the serum of normal animals to allow differentiation between dogs with normal concentrations of IgA and those that are deficient.[90,91] As well as using age-matched reference ranges, it is important to use the reference range provided by the laboratory running the assay. Most authors consider serum IgA levels less than 20 mg/dl as clearly deficient.

The assay of serum IgA concentration in cats is affected by similar factors as those which affect that of the dog. By 6 to 9 months of age the total serum protein and gamma globulin concentrations of cats rises to adult levels.[40] The environment of the cat has been shown to affect the serum IgA concentration (Table 3–5).[66]

Secretory IgA can be measured in intestinal content. Total immunoglobulin concentration in canine intestinal fluid was found to range from 110 to 810 mg/dl, with a mean of 380 mg/dl. On average, 80% (300 mg/dl) of this immunoglobulin was IgA, 15% (60 mg/dl) was IgM and 5% (20 mg/dl) was IgG. The concentration of IgA in canine feces ranges from 80 to 540 mg/dl with a mean of 300 mg/dl.[92] IgA also has been detected in the feces of cats and it appears that bile may make a significant contribution to intestinal IgA levels in this species.[64] After extraction from feces by centrifugation with an equal weight of PBS, feline fecal fluid had an average IgA concentration of 35 mg/dl with a range of 10 to 84 mg/dl.[64]

It has been assumed that the serum concentrations of IgA

Table 3–4

SERUM IGA CONCENTRATIONS (MG/DL) IN HEALTHY BEAGLES

AGE	MEAN IGA CONCENTRATION	95% CONFIDENCE INTERVAL
4–6 months	36	18–56
12 months	63	24–166
24 months	58	34–147

From reference 90. By permission of Blackwell Scientific Publications.

Table 3–5

SERUM IGA CONCENTRATIONS (MG/DL) IN HEALTHY CATS

AGE	ENVIRONMENT	MEAN	RANGE
Adults	Cattery	285	102–582
Adults	Cattery	175	35–500
Adults	SPF*	277	42–600
0.5–1.5 years	Household	71	25–188
1 year	SPF	33	30–50
14 weeks	SPF	22	12–30
12 weeks	SPF	123	30–254

*SPF = specific pathogen free
From references 64, 66, 120.

in the dog and cat reflect the adequacy of the secretory IgA response. Unfortunately, this does not seem to be the case, because the sIgA level in tears from dogs with low serum IgA concentration is often not different from that in dogs with normal serum IgA concentration.[93] Furthermore, secretory IgA and serum IgA concentrations will be different in the presence of defective intestinal epithelial transport of IgA. Therefore, the measurement of sIgA in tears, saliva, feces, or intestinal secretions may help determine the clinical relevance of suspected IgA deficiency. Another assessment of intestinal sIgA quantity can be made by immunohistochemical demonstration of immunoglobulin-containing cells in the lamina propria. Caution is necessary when interpreting the results of intestinal histochemistry, however, because IgA-bearing cells can be demonstrated in normal numbers in the mucosa of German shepherds with small intestinal bacterial overgrowth and low serum IgA concentration.[94] This implies that any impairment of mucosal IgA secretion in the German shepherd is due to faulty synthesis or secretion of IgA, rather than an absolute deficiency of IgA-committed cells.[94]

IGA FUNCTION AND CONSEQUENCES OF IGA DEFICIENCY. Intestinal sIgA has been likened to an antiabsorptive paint. Its primary function is to facilitate exclusion of specific bacterial, viral, and macromolecular antigens from the mucosa by preventing antigen-mucosal adherence. This blocking of mucosal adherence is not a specific function of IgA molecules, because immunoglobulins of the other classes share the ability. However, these other immunoglobulins, with the exception of secretory IgM (sIGM), cannot function in the intestinal lumen because they are unable to resist proteolytic degradation. Secretory IgA may also augment the nonspecific mechanisms of mucosal defense. It has been established, for example, that proteolysis of intestinal antigens is considerably greater in immunized animals than in nonimmunized controls, and it has been suggested this enhancement results from interaction in the intestinal mucus coat of antigen-antibody complexes with pancreatic enzymes.[95]

Dimeric IgA in the lamina propria contributes to the elimination of mucosal antigen by antibody-dependent macrophage cytotoxicity of bacteria[3,32] and by the rapid hepatic clearance of those IgA-antigen complexes that enter the vasculature and lymphatics.[31] However, IgA, in contrast to IgG, is not efficient at the fixation of complement and its role as an opsonin is controversial.[82] When IgA binds to antigen within the mucosa, it blocks the binding of IgG and therefore inhibits the phlogistic consequences of IgG-antigen complexes and IgG-facilitated phagocytosis.[32] The action of IgA in the mucosa may thus be likened to that of a wet blanket that suppresses the development of excessive gastrointestinal inflammation during mucosal antigen elimination.

Local humoral immunity is of known importance in some coronavirus infections, such as transmissible gastroenteritis of swine, in which serum IgG provides no protection. Some evidence suggests this is also true for canine coronavirus.[96] Local

IgA production has been shown to occur in canine parvovirus infection, and IgA-deficient dogs appear more susceptible to parvovirus infection.[90] Specific IgA synthesized against macromolecules prevents damage by enterotoxins and decreases absorption of dietary antigens. When secretory IgA is deficient, there is an increase in the circulating levels of dietary and bacterial antigens and the appearance of abnormal immune-mediated responses secondary to prolonged activation of the systemic immune system by circulating antigen.

The functions of IgA are further revealed by the diseases commonly suffered by people and animals deficient in IgA, although the accuracy of these conclusions is obscured to some degree by the increase in IgM secretion that commonly accompanies IgA deficiency. Selective IgA deficiency is the most common primary immunodeficiency in humans. Many of these IgA-deficient people are asymptomatic, but predispositions to a number of diseases have been identified. Infectious gastrointestinal disease and malabsorption syndrome occur reasonably frequently,[25,90] and cases of ulcerative colitis and regional enteritis associated with IgA deficiency also have been reported.[97] Disease associations in other body systems include upper respiratory infections, pneumonia, recurrent skin and urinary tract infections, allergies, and autoimmune diseases such as rheumatoid arthritis, SLE, and chronic active hepatitis.[98] In dogs, selective deficiencies of serum IgA levels have been reported in beagles,[90] German shepherds,[89] sharpeis,[91] and a variety of other breeds.[99] Diseases associated with this deficiency are similar to those of humans and include pyoderma, parvovirus, chronic small intestinal disease, atopy, food allergy, respiratory infections, and otitis externa.[89–91,99]

Secretion and Function of Immunoglobulins Other Than IgA

IgG, IgM, and IgE are also present in the lamina propria. Some of this non-IgA immunoglobulin is produced in the lamina propria, although most comes from the plasma. Although quantitatively small compared to the large quantities of IgA produced, these other immunoglobulins are still important in mucosal protection. Rather than a first-line defense directed at antigen exclusion (the major function of IgA), they become important when the epithelial barrier is broached. They defend the body by the processes of opsonization, complement fixation, and encouragement of an inflammatory response, all properties not shared by IgA. They also play an important role in the reaction to helminth parasites.

IMMUNOGLOBULIN M. IgM is a 900,000 dalton pentameric aggregate of the basic Y-shaped immunoglobulin molecule.

The immunoglobulin monomers are bound by disulfide bonds, and two of the subunits are linked by a J chain. IgM is the predominant immunoglobulin produced in the systemic primary immune response, and IgM-bearing cells are the predominant immunocyte in the lamina propria of pups.[39] IgM can bind to secretory component and is excreted through epithelia via the same intracellular route as IgA.[3] IgM is found in large quantities in feline serum, bile, intestinal fluid, colostrum, and milk (Tables 3–2 and 3–3). In the dog, it reaches its highest concentrations in serum and intestinal fluid. In healthy dogs, the mean serum IgM concentration is 187 ± 74.[9] In cats and dogs, IgM is usually the second most abundant immunoglobulin in body secretions.

IgM is highly efficient at complement fixation, virus neutralization, opsonization, and agglutination of particulate antigen. Through these mechanisms it takes part in both antigen elimination and antigen exclusion in the gastrointestinal tract. In comparison to sIgA, however, sIgM is more rapidly degraded in the intestinal lumen.[17]

IMMUNOGLOBULIN G. Immunoglobulin G is a monomeric immunoglobulin. It has a molecular weight of 180,000 daltons. IgG is the predominant immunoglobulin produced in an anamnestic systemic immune response. It does not bind to secretory component and so is not actively extruded into body secretions. However, its small size relative to the other immunoglobulins results in passive extravasation of small quantities of IgG into most of the body secretions (Tables 3–2 and 3–3). This leakage is markedly accelerated if inflammation or hypersensitivity responses increase vascular permeability.

IgG is the dominant antibody in serum and colostrum of both the dog and the cat. It will readily activate complement, facilitate antibody-dependent cellular cytotoxicity, and opsonize and agglutinate particulate antigen. The phlogistic properties of IgG result from the fixation of complement and the facilitation of phagocytosis. The complement cascade spawns a number of complement fragments that attract inflammatory cells and result in mast cell degranulation. Phagocytosis ultimately results in cell death and release of enumerable inflammatory mediators. Together these influences generate inflammation, with all its consequences (see Chapter 4).

It is unlikely that IgG has an important function in the defense of the normal intestine because of low luminal concentrations and rapid degradation. However, IgG may play an important role in diseases characterized by inflammation and increased permeability. Following prolonged gastrointestinal inflammation, IgG-containing cells increase dramatically in the lamina propria, and IgG antibodies to intestinal tissue may be demonstrated.[3,100] Two examples of diseases in which IgG contributes to the disease process are helminthiasis and inflammatory bowel disease.

IMMUNOGLOBULIN E. IgE is a monomeric immunoglobulin with a molecular weight of 196,000 daltons. Its existence in the cat is suspected but not convincingly established.[40,66] IgE possesses a unique ability to bind to mast cells and basophils. It is found in very low concentrations in serum and can be detected in intestinal fluid and feces. It is rapidly degraded in the intestinal lumen.[17]

IgE-containing lymphocytes may be found in skin, mucous membranes, mesenteric nodes, and spleen. Under appropriate stimuli it appears that Peyer's patches generate precursor IgE cells, which migrate to the lymphoid tissues in the bowel.[3] The origin of gastrointestinal mucosal IgE is uncertain. The local synthesis of IgE by plasma cells in the lamina propria may contribute a small quantity of IgE to the mucosa. The possibility that some of the mucosal IgE might also be derived from IgE-containing mucosal mast cells must be considered.[17] It appears, however, that the major site of production of intestinal IgE, at least in the parasite-infected rat, is the mesenteric lymph nodes, which secrete the immunoglobulin into the lymphatics, from where it eventually reaches the mucosa via the bloodstream.[22,101] IgE does not bind to secretory component, and so the small quantities of IgE found in intestinal secretions is presumed to derive from passive exudation from the vasculature and mucosa.

IgE is the antibody responsible for immediate hypersensitivity. Mast cells and basophils are stimulated to degranulate when antigen binds in an appropriate manner to IgE molecules on their surfaces. This results in the release of a large number of inflammatory mediators. Immediate hypersensitivities presumably enhance elimination of the inciting antigen from the mucosa, but the increased permeability that accompanies the response results in the loss of plasma proteins into the gut, and increased absorption of macromolecules from the lumen. IgE is also important in the defense against parasites. Luminal concentrations of IgE are known to increase in both parasitic infections and food allergies.[102]

ORAL TOLERANCE[6,103]

Oral tolerance is the phenomenon whereby prior oral exposure to an antigen induces a specific immunologic unresponsiveness on subsequent systemic (or oral) exposure to the same antigen.[77] Oral tolerance is a specific immune response. It results in a reduced or absent IgG, IgE, or cytotoxic response to the inciting antigen, but the IgA response is preserved.[77,103] Tolerance manifests as nonreactivity, but it is important not to equate this with a total lack of an immune response. On the contrary, tolerance is an active, ongoing arm of the "specific immune response," which instead of resulting in antigen elimination results in its tolerance. Like other forms of the specific immune response, tolerance will decline unless antigen is reexposed.

Oral tolerance has been induced by many materials including food proteins, haptens, bacteria, viruses, cellular antigens, and pollens.[74,77,103] The mechanisms of tolerance to each of these categories of antigen may be slightly different.[103] Without reexposure, oral tolerance to soluble proteins can last from three to four months, whereas tolerance to bacteria may be more shortlived.[103] Tolerance to intestinal bacterial flora also appears to be less complete than tolerance to many other antigens. Both humoral and cell-mediated immune responses to bacteria are dampened, but they are not eliminated. These findings, along with the observation that suppressor cells to bacterial-induced immune responses appear only after relatively vigorous mucosal stimulation by bacterial flora,[77] establish that the tolerogenic response to bacteria allows conservation of some immunoreactivity, perhaps to facilitate mucosal defence.

Oral tolerance to soluble proteins can be induced by either a single large dose or by repeated feeding of smaller doses over several weeks. Small doses given over prolonged periods are usually more effective than the same total dose given once.[103] Intermittent exposure and rapid antigen uptake predisposes to immunoreactivity.[104]

Oral tolerance begins with exclusion of antigen from the lamina propria. As discussed earlier, antigen exclusion has both specific (IgA) and nonspecific aspects.[4] In this regard, effective digestion is particularly important. Digestion can result in macromolecular fragments too small to be antigenic, or it can reduce sensitizing proteins to fragments that, although retaining their antigenicity, induce tolerance rather than sensitization.[95] The secretion of IgA and IgM into the lumen of the gut contributes to tolerance more than immunoreactivity. This results from the effectiveness with which these antibodies prevent antigen from entering the lamina propria. IgA also has a tolerogenic role within the lamina propria, where its function as a blocking antibody results in a wet blanket effect.

The majority of evidence suggests that the profound hyporeactivity of the systemic immune system to noninvasive antigens (that characterizes oral tolerance) is due to an antigen-specific suppressor T cell network. The suppressor T cells are derived from Peyer's patches and/or the intestinal epithelium, and migrate to various lymphoid organs including the mesenteric lymph nodes, spleen, thymus, and peripheral lymph nodes.[24,74,77,103,105] The suppressor T cells release soluble suppressor factors that inhibit the effector T cells of the immune response.[74] In addition to suppressor T cells, tolerance to intestinal bacteria in some species may involve suppressor macrophages.[77] Suppressor B cells may also play a role in the induction of tolerance to some antigens.[77,103] Suppressor B cells have been identified in Peyer's patches and mesenteric lymph nodes within a week of ingestion of haptens. Their production of IgG appears to produce suppression.[103] Antibody exerts a direct negative feedback on the production of more antibody when it binds to immunoglobulin receptors on B and suppressor T cells. In addition, antibody-antiantibody networks that suppress the immune response have been proposed. Circulating immune complexes also exert a negative feedback on the immune response and may contribute to systemic hyporeactivity.[74,103] IgA-antibody-antigen complexes, in particular, have been incriminated.[103]

The liver also plays a role in generating oral tolerance.[106] Oral tolerance can be experimentally generated by exposure of the liver to antigen in the portal blood.[106] There have been reports that portocaval shunting decreases tolerance induction to certain orally administered antigens. The majority of antigen that escapes the lamina propria is removed by the mononuclear-phagocytic system of the liver and mesenteric nodes.[103] It has been postulated that the Kupffer cells of the liver remove sensitizing antigen aggregates and allow tolerogenic protein fragments to reach peripheral tissue.[103] This phagocytic function of the liver is important because exposure of the systemic lymphoid tissues to gut antigens often results in immunoreactivity rather than tolerance.[103]

Oral tolerance is necessary to prevent chronic gastrointestinal inflammation to antigens in the lumen of the gastrointestinal tract, and reduces the likelihood of systemic hypersensitivities to ingested antigens. It is noteworthy from the therapeutic standpoint that short-term feeding of antigen to animals already parenterally sensitized to that antigen does not necessarily induce tolerance. In fact, ingestion of antigen in these circumstances may actually boost IgG and IgE titers.[103]

IMMUNITY TO PARASITES[6,107]

Epidemiological evidence suggests that the gastrointestinal immune response is important in the elimination of many gastrointestinal parasites of the dog and cat. For instance, it is rare to see ascarid infections in animals older than one year; hookworm infections of adult dogs are usually subclinical, whereas those of puppies are often fatal; and coccidial infection rarely causes signs of gastrointestinal disease except in the very young. Unfortunately, however, there is very limited experimental work to examine the extent to which the immune system is involved in these phenomena. Furthermore, the constituents of the immune response to parasites of small animals remain poorly elucidated.

Evidence, largely derived from other species, suggests the immune reaction to parasites is a complex integration of spe-

cific and nonspecific immune responses. The particular facets of the immune response that are important in a particular infection depend on a number of factors, including the host species, the class of parasite, and whether the parasite resides extracellularly, intracellularly, or within the lumen of the bowel. Genetic factors dictate whether an animal is susceptible to a parasitic infection and whether it will mount an immune response to the parasite.[108] As befits a well-adapted parasite, the immune response is often ineffective in eliminating the entire parasitic burden. Parasites have evolved a number of highly successful ways of avoiding the immune response of the host.

NONSPECIFIC RESISTANCE TO PARASITES. Nonimmunologic factors are important in the resistance to parasites. Interspecies and intraspecies competition limits parasite numbers and inhibits development. The specific immune response to parasites often initiates nonspecific mechanisms of elimination. The best example of this interaction is the IgE-dependent mast cell degranulation that results in the so-called self-cure response to helminth parasites. Another example is the T cell–mediated increase in epithelial cell turnover rate, which results in cryptal hyperplasia and villus atrophy in response to parasites such as giardia, hookworm, and roundworm. The villus atrophy and increased epithelial cell loss presumably inhibit attachment of the parasite but are also responsible for many of the clinical signs that accompany such diseases. Furthermore, both of the specific immune responses of T cell lymphokine release and IgE-mediated mast cell discharge stimulate increased mucus secretion. Copious secretion of mucus is reputed to interfere with the ability of parasites to attach to the mucosa.

SELF-CURE PHENOMENON. The self-cure phenomenon (Figure 3–8) to helminths has been best studied in *Haemonchus contortus* infections in sheep and *Nippostrongylus brasiliensis* infections in rats, but similar mechanisms are thought to result in the elimination of other helminth parasites. Helminth parasites secrete antigenic products into the mucosa that, in rodents at least, result in the migration of T cell precursors into the lamina propria, a response which appears essential for expulsion of the parasites. In response to the parasite, mucosal mast cells (and globule leukocytes) increase rapidly in number to peak at about five times the original level.[51] This proliferation is T cell dependent and interleukin-3 induced. Concomitantly, with this mast cell response there is the development of an IgE-dominated humoral response. A prominent source of this IgE is the

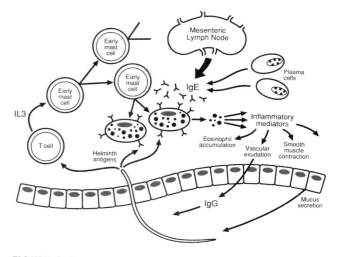

FIGURE 3–8. Schematic representation of the immune responses involved in the self-cure reaction against intestinal helminths.

mesenteric lymph nodes. The IgE enters the lamina propria via the circulatory system and rapidly binds to the mucosal mast cells. Eventually, there is a combination of helminth antigen and mast cell–bound IgE that results in mast cell degranulation and the release of the mediators of goblet cell discharge and immediate hypersensitivity such as histamine and leukotrienes.[109] These compounds promote smooth muscle contraction, increased vascular permeability, and, perhaps, reductions in intestinal fluid and water absorption. The result is vigorous intestinal contractions and profuse fluid and mucus exudation into the intestinal lumen. The exuded fluid is rich in IgG and may contain immunoreactive cells. Morphologically, there is cryptal hyperplasia, edema in the villus tips, and enterocyte detachment.[109] The combination of processes results in dislodgement and expulsion of the majority of the worms.

HUMORAL RESPONSES OTHER THAN THE SELF-CURE RESPONSE. Parasite antigens are very adept at stimulating an IgE-mediated humoral response. However, even though IgE is the most significant humoral response to parasites, IgM, IgG, and IgA isotypes are also produced during parasitism.

In the lumen of the intestine, the immunoglobulin that comes in contact with parasites in the greatest concentration is IgA, but its function against parasites remains uncertain. Animals infected with *Giardia* develop both a systemic IgG and a secretory IgA response against the parasite.[31] Humans with hypogammaglobulinemia (but not selective IgA deficiency) are predisposed to persistent giardiasis.[100] IgA is protective in coccidial infections.[33] A range of cell types, including lymphocytes, neutrophils, and macrophages, have receptors for IgA.[33] Adherence to trophozoites by neutrophils and phagocytosis of trophozoites by macrophages are increased in the presence of IgA and IgG,[107] and it appears that IgA can facilitate cytotoxicity against murine giardiasis.[33] These observations are of particular interest in light of the observation that lymphocytes and macrophages can be found in direct contact with *Giardia* trophozoites where they usually reside, that is, in the intestinal lumen.

Within the tissues, antibodies protect the host by neutralizing proteolytic enzymes secreted by larvae to penetrate tissues, by blocking oral and excretory pores, and by inhibiting development. Probably the most important role of antibody in the tissues, however, is the mediation of antibody-dependent cellular cytotoxicity. This process appears to be of particular importance in the defense against helminth larvae in the tissues.

CELL-MEDIATED RESPONSE TO PARASITES. Sensitized T lymphocytes may successfully attack helminths or their larvae that are within the tissues. The cell-mediated immune response incites a local immune response (granuloma) that inhibits parasitic growth or migration. In addition, cytotoxic T cells may be able to kill some larvae. The blood eosinophilic response to parasites is usually greatest in response to parasites that have migratory forms in the tissues. The eosinophilia may be a result of an eosinophil-stimulating lymphokine released by sensitized T lymphocytes.

EVASION OF THE IMMUNE RESPONSE BY PARASITES. Well-adapted parasites have evolved a number of mechanisms to avoid the host immune response. These include mimicry of host antigens, antigenic variation, shedding of the glycocalyx, and immunosuppression of the host.[6]

NEUROENDOCRINE REGULATION OF THE GASTROINTESTINAL IMMUNE RESPONSE

In recent years, strong evidence has emerged to support neuroendocrine modulation of the immune system. This modulation is readily apparent in the gastrointestinal tract, where leukocytes are exposed to relatively high concentrations of neuropeptides.[87,110] The conditioned response of mast cell secretion, previously cited, is an appropriate example. Another is the ability to condition guinea pigs to develop an exudative peritoneal response to a skin scratch by previously pairing the skin scratch with intraperitoneal injections of a bacterial filtrate.[111]

The anatomic basis for such responses has come with the demonstration of innervation of mast cells and lymphoid tissues, including GALT, and with the discovery of substance P, vasoactive intestinal peptide, and somatostatin receptors on leukocytes.[87,110] Functional studies have also suggested that leukocytes may possess receptors for bombesin, endorphins, enkephalins, and neurotensin.[110] The types of neuropeptide receptors on leukocytes and the origins and functions of the selected neuropeptides found in the gastrointestinal system are shown in Tables 3–6 and 3–7.

It is also apparent that communication between the neuroendocrine system and the immune system is bidirectional.[87] Thus, good evidence suggests that secretory products of the immune system can influence neural activity and many mediators classically thought to have been synthesized by neuroendocrine tissue only are also elaborated by leukocytes. The latter include vasoactive intestinal peptide produced by neutrophils and mast cells, a somatostatinlike peptide secreted by basophils, and ACTH secreted by lymphocytes and macrophages.[87] These observations suggest the immune system may have a sensory role to inform the central nervous system of problems, such as infection, which are not recognized by the classical sensory pathways.[112] However, the neuroendocrine-immune axis provides a mechanism (in addition to the less specific effects of steroid hormones and catecholamines) by which psychosomatic factors such as stress can influence disease processes. It is unlikely that stress initiates inflammation, but clinical observations suggest stress may influence the subsequent course and severity of disease.[87] For instance, the release by neurons and leukocytes of inflammatory neuropeptides, such as substance P, and the influence of this and other neuropeptides on inflammation, mucus secretion, smooth muscle activity, and vascular permeability may be important in the pathogenesis of inflammatory bowel disease.

VACCINATION AGAINST GASTROINTESTINAL DISEASE

The long-lasting immunity produced after recovery from a variety of gastroenteric diseases establishes that prolonged and effective mucosal immunity to enteropathogens can occur. However, it has as yet been difficult to develop success-

Table 3–6

NEUROPEPTIDE RECEPTORS ON IMMUNE EFFECTOR CELLS

NEUROPEPTIDE	RECEPTOR-BEARING IMMUNE CELLS
Bombesin	Phagocytes
Beta-endorphin	Lymphocytes, NK cells
Enkephalin	T lymphocytes, NK cells
Neurotensin	Mast cells, neutrophil
Somatostatin	Lymphocytes, monocytes, mast cells
Substance P	Lymphocytes, mast cells
VIP	Lymphocytes, NK cells

Table 3–7

NEUROPEPTIDES SHARED BY THE GASTROINTESTINAL
AND IMMUNE SYSTEMS

NEUROPEPTIDE	SOURCE	TARGET CELL	EFFECT
Somatostatin	Pancreas	Lymphocyte	Decreased proliferation
	APUD cell	Lymphocyte	Decreased IgA
	Basophil		
Substance P	C, A, fibers	T cell	Increased proliferation
	Intestinal P cell	B cell	Increased IgA
	APUD cell	Monocyte	Chemotaxis
		Neutrophil	Increased phagocytosis
		Mast cell	Secretion
VIP	Cholinergic fibers	T cell	Decreased proliferation
	VIP-ergic fibers	T cell	Altered migration
	APUD cell	NK cell	Altered cytotoxicity
	Neutrophil	B cell	Increased IgM
	Eosinophil	B cell	Decreased IgA

Modified from references 87 and 110.

ful long-lasting vaccines against enteric pathogens unless the pathogenicity of the organism involves an initial period of bacteremia or viremia (e.g., parvovirus).[113] Nevertheless, an apparently effective vaccine against canine coronavirus (a virus that appears to undergo only limited viremia) has been developed, and modest success has been observed with enterotoxigenic *E. coli* fimbrial vaccines in farm animals.[114]

The best recognized means of protecting an animal against infectious disease is by parenteral vaccination. However, parenteral injections do not usually stimulate prolonged secretion of mucosal IgA that will prevent colonization of the gastrointestinal mucosa. Parenteral vaccination will result in the production of circulating IgG antibodies that enter the gut in amounts proportional to the serum IgG level.[115] The amounts of these antibodies secreted into the gut, however, are so small, they are rapidly degraded by proteases and only have a minor influence on colonization.[116] The access of IgG to the gut lumen is greatly increased during gastrointestinal inflammation by the breakdown of the mucosal permeability barrier. Thus, parenteral vaccination against enteric pathogens will limit the severity of disease caused by enteroinvasive organisms, but is less effective at disease prevention.

Prevention of gastroenteric infectious disease relies on an active secretory antibody response. The most effective means of stimulating the synthesis of secretory IgA is by oral administration of antigens.[117] A greater IgA response occurs if an oral priming exposure is followed by an oral boosting exposure. As discussed in the section on oral tolerance, other important factors include the nature of the antigen (soluble vs. insoluble), the dose of antigen, the timing of administration, and the genetic nature of the animal. A major problem experienced in the development of effective oral vaccines is to find methods to preserve the immunogenicity of the antigen while minimizing its pathogenicity. There is a delicate balance between attenuation and immunogenicity.[118] For instance, heat inactivation of cholera enterotoxin causes a loss in its toxicity but changes the toxin from a protease-resistant molecule to one that is protease susceptible.[119] An important area of current research focuses on using oral carrier vaccines. These are usually immunogenic attenuated enteroinvasive microbes (such as adenovirus, *Salmonella*, or *Yersinia*) that have been genetically engineered to carry one or more antigens of another pathogen for which no immunogenic attenuated strain is available.[118] By using these techniques it may be able to create multivalent vaccines based on a single carrier vaccine.[118] Other methods of vaccination for enteric disease that are under examination include intraperitoneal injections, the use of powerful adjuvants, and delivery of the antigen by liposomes.[113]

REFERENCES

1. Besredka A. De la vaccination contre les typhoides par la voie buccale. Ann Inst Pasteur 33:882, 1919.
2. Davies A. An investigation into the serological properties of dysentery stools. Lancet 2:1009, 1922.
3. Brandtzaeg P, Valnes K, Scott H, et al. The human gastrointestinal secretory immune system in health and disease. Scand J Gastroenterol 20 (suppl 114):17–38, 1985.
4. Sanderson IR, Walker WA. Uptake and transport of macromolecules by the intestine: Possible role in clinical disorders (an update). Gastroenterology 104:622–639, 1993.
5. Bienenstock J. The mucosal immunologic network. Ann Allergy 53:535–540, 1984.
6. Tizard I. Veterinary Immunology, 3rd ed. WB Saunders, Philadelphia, 1987.
7. Doran JE, Lundsgaard-Hansen P. Role of the reticuloendothelial system in the pathogenesis of organ damage. Brit J Hosp Med 39:221–225, 1988.
8. Pavli P, Doe WF, Hume DA. Enrichment and characterization of dendritic cells from the lamina propria of murine intestine. Gastroenterology 94:A346, 1988.
9. Portiansky EL, Castellano MC. Normal phagocytic capacity of macrophages isolated from different canine organs. Anat Histol Embryol 18:199–204, 1989.
10. Evans HE, Christensen GC. The alimentary canal. In: Miller's Anatomy of the Dog. WB Saunders, Philadelphia, 455–506, 1979.
11. Egberts HJA, Brinkhoff MGM, Mouwen JMVM, et al. Biology and pathology of the intestinal M cell. A review. Vet Q 7:333–336, 1985.
12. Harty RF, Leibach JR. Immune disorders of the gastrointestinal tract and liver. Med Clin N Am 69:675–745, 1985.
13. Stewart THM, Hetenyi C, Rowsell H, et al. Ulcerative enterocolitis in dogs induced by drugs. J Path 131:363–378, 1980.
14. Hogenesch H, Felsburg PJ. Isolation and phenotypic and functional characterization of cells from Peyer's patches in the dog. Vet Immunol Immunopath 31:1–10, 1992.
15. Hogenesch H, Felsburg PJ. Ultrastructure and alkaline phosphatase activity of the dome epithelium of canine Peyer's patches. Vet Immunol Immunopath 24:177–186, 1990.
16. Bienenstock J, Befus D. Gut- and bronchus-associated lymphoid tissue. Am J Anat 170:437–445, 1984.
17. Brandtzaeg P, Bjerke K, Kett K, et al. Production and secretion of immunoglobulins in the gastrointestinal tract. Ann Allergy 59:21–39, 1987.
18. Allan CH, Trier JS. Structure and permeability differ in subepithelial vil-

lus and Peyer's patch follicle capillaries. Gastroenterology 100:1172–1179, 1991.

19. Wolf JL, Bye WA. The membranous epithelial (M) cell and the mucosal immune system. Ann Rev Med 35:95–112, 1984.

20. Smith MW, James PS, Tivey DR. M cell numbers after transfer of SPF mice to normal animal house environment. Am J Path 128:385–389, 1987.

21. Grutzkau A, Hanski C, Hahn H, et al. Involvement of M cells in the bacterial invasion of Peyer's patches: A common mechanism shared by *Yersinia enterocolitica* and other enteroinvasive bacteria. Gut 31:1011–1015, 1990.

22. Hanauer SB, Kraft SC. Intestinal immunology. In: Berk JE, Haubrich WS, Kalser MH (eds) Gastroenterology. WB Saunders, Philadelphia, 1607–1631, 1985.

23. Bjerke K, Brandtzaeg P. Immunoglobulin- and J chain-producing cells associated with lymphoid follicles in the human appendix, colon and ileum, including Peyer's patches. Clin Exp Immunol 64:432–441, 1986.

24. Brandtzaeg P, Halstensen TS, Kett K, et al. Immunobiology amd immunopathology of human gut mucosa: Humoral immunity and intraepithelial lymphocytes. Gastroenterology 97:1562–1584, 1989.

25. Dobbins WO. Gut immunopathology: A gastroenterologist's view with emphasis on pathophysiology. Am J Physiol 242:G1–8, 1982.

26. Heatley RV, Bienenstock J. Luminal lymphoid cells in the rabbit intestine. Gastroenterology 82:268–275, 1982.

27. Owen RL, Nenamic PC, Stevens DP. Ultrastructural observations on giardiasis in a murine model. Gastroenterology 76:757–769, 1979.

28. Thomas J. Anderson, NV. Interepithelial lymphocytes in the small intestinal mucosa of conventionally reared dogs. Am J Vet Res 42:200–203, 1982.

29. Carman PS, Ernst PB, Rosenthal KL, et al. Intraepithelial leukocytes contain a unique subpopulation of NK-like cytotoxic cells active in the defense of gut epithelium to enteric murine coronaviruses. J Immunol 136:1548–1553, 1986.

30. van Garderen E, van Dijk JE, van den Ingh TS. Intestinal intraepithelial lymphocyte: A review of the literature. Vet Q 13:225–232, 1991.

31. Targan SR, Kagnoff MK, Brogon MD, et al. Immunological mechanisms in intestinal diseases. Ann Int Med 106:853–870, 1987.

32. Befus AD, Bienenstock J. Immunity to infectious agents in the gastrointestinal tract. J Am Vet Med Assoc 181:1066–1068, 1982.

33. Befus D, Lee T. Unique characteristics of local responses in host resistance to mucosal parasitic infections. Vet Parasitol 20:175–194, 1986.

34. Huntley JF. Mast cells and basophils: A review of their heterogeneity and function. J Comp Path 107:349–372, 1992.

35. Van der Heijden PJ, Stok W. Improved procedure for the isolation of functionally active lymphoid cells from the murine intestine. J Immunol Meth 103:161–167, 1987.

36. Cerf-Bensussan N, Quaroni A, Kurnick JT, et al. Intraepithelial lymphocytes modulate Ia expression by intestinal epithelial cells. J Immunol 132:2244–2252, 1984.

37. Hall EJ, Batt RM. Development of wheat-sensitive enteropathy in Irish setters: Morphologic changes. Am J Vet Res 51:978–982, 1990.

38. Hall EJ, Batt RM. Dietary modulation of gluten sensitivity in a naturally occurring enteropathy of Irish setter dogs. Gut 33:198–205, 1992.

39. Hart IR. The distribution of immunoglobulin-containing cells in canine small intestine. Res Vet Sci 27:269–274, 1979.

40. Barlough JE, Jacobson RH, Scott FW. The immunoglobulins of the cat. Cornell Vet 71:397–407, 1981.

41. Willard MD, Williams JF, Stowe HD, et al. Number and distribution of IgM cells and IgA cells in colonic tissue of conditioned sex- and breed-matched dogs. Am J Vet Res 43:688–692, 1982.

42. Willard MD, Leid RW. Nonuniform horizontal and vertical distributions of immunoglobulin A cells in canine intestines. Am J Vet Res 42:1573–1579, 1981.

43. Gibson PR, van de Pol E, Pullman W, et al. The role of mononuclear and LAK cell-mediated cytotoxicity in the pathogenesis of inflammatory bowel disease. Gastroent 94:A146, 1988.

44. Hogan PG, Hapel AJ, Doe WF. Antibody-dependent-cellular-cytotoxicity of intestinal lamina propria mononuclear cells. Gastroent 94:A189, 1988.

45. Nagi AM, Babiuk LA. Bovine gut-associated lymphoid tissue. Morphological and functional studies. J Immunol Meth 105:23–37, 1987.

46. Baldwin F, Becker AB. Bronchoalveolar eosinophilic cells in a canine model of asthma: Two distinctive populations. Vet Pathol 30:97–103, 1993.

47. Huntley JF, McGorum B, Newlands GF, et al. Granulated intraepithelial lymphocytes: Their relationship to mucosal mast cells and globule leucocytes in the rat. Immunol 53:525–535, 1984.

48. Huntley JF, Newlands GFJ, Gibson S, et al. Histochemical demonstration of chymotrypsin-like serine esterases in mucosal mast cells in four species including man. J Clin Pathol 38:375–384, 1985.

49. Atkins FM. Intestinal mucosal mast cells. Ann Allergy 59:44–53, 1987.

50. Schachter M, Longridge DJ, Wheeler GD, et al. Immunocytochemical and enzyme histochemical localization of kallikrein-like enzymes in colon, intestine, and stomach of rat and cat. J Histochem Cytochem 34:927–934, 1986.

51. Jarret EEE, Haig DM. Mucosal mast cells in vivo and in vitro. Immunol Today 5:115–118, 1984.

52. Barrett KE. Mast cells, basophils and immunoglobulin E. In: Metcalfe DD, Sampson HA, Simon RA (eds) Food Allergy, Adverse Reactions to Foods and Food Additives. Blackwell Scientific, Oxford, 13–35, 1991.

53. Soda K, Kawabori S, Perdue MH, et al. Macrophage engulfment of mucosal mast cells in rats treated with dexamethasone. Gastroent 100:929–937, 1991.

54. Befus D, Fujimaki H, et al. Mast cell polymorphisms. Present concepts, future directions. Dig Dis Sci 33 (suppl): 16s–22s, 1988.

55. Kawanishi H, Ihle JM. In vitro induction and characterization of mast cells from murine Peyer's patches. Scand J Immunol 25:109–120, 1987.

56. Kitamura Y, Nakano T, Kanakura Y. Transdifferentiation between mast cell subpopulations. Dev Growth Differ 28:321–325, 1986.

57. Russell M, Dark KA, Cummins RW, et al. Learned histamine release. Science 225:733–734, 1984.

58. MacQueen G, Marshall J, Perdue M, et al. Pavlovian conditioning of rat mucosal mast cells to secrete rat mast cell protease II. Science 243:83–85, 1989.

59. Stead RH, Dixon MF, Bramwell NH, et al. Mast cells are closely apposed to nerves in the human gastrointestinal mucosa. Gastroent 97:575–585, 1989.

60. Caughey GH, Leidig F, Viro NF, et al. Substance P and vasoactive intestinal peptide degradation by mast cell tryptase and chymase. J Pharmacol Exp Ther 244:133–137, 1988.

61. Nair PNR, Schroeder HE. Duct-associated lymphoid tissue (DALT) of minor salivary glands and mucosal immunity. Immunol 57:171–180, 1986.

62. Jackson DE, Lally ET, Nakamura MC, et al. Migration of IgA-bearing lymphocytes into salivary glands. Cell Immunol 63:203, 1981.

63. Heddle RJ, Rowley D. Dog immunoglobulins. I. Immunochemical characterization of dog serum, parotid saliva, colostrum, milk and small bowel fluid. Immunol 29:185–195, 1975.

64. Yamada T, Tomoda I, Usui K. Immunoglobulin compositions of the feline body fluids. Jpn J Vet Sci 46:791–796, 1984.

65. Scicchitano R, Sheldrake RF, Husband AJ. Origin of immunoglobulins in respiratory tract secretion and saliva of sheep. Immunol 58:315–321, 1985.

66. Pedersen NC. Basic and clinical immunology. In: Holzworth J (ed) Diseases of the Cat, Vol. 1. WB Saunders, Philadelphia, 146–181, 1987.

67. Schultz RD, Scott FW, Duncan JR, et al. Feline immunoglobulins. Infect Immun 9:391–393, 1974.

68. Vaerman JP, Heremans JF. The immunoglobulins of the dog. II. The Immunoglobulins of canine secretions. Immunochem 6:779–786, 1969.

69. Hodgson HJF. Gut-liver interactions in the IgA system. Scand J Gastroenterol 20(suppl 114):39–44, 1985.

70. Strober W, James SP. The immunologic basis of inflammatory bowel disease. J Clin Immunol 6:415–432, 1986.

71. Panzini B, Fournier D, Podolsky DK. Emergence of antigenic glycoprotein structures in ulcerative colitis detected through monoclonal antibodies. Abs 902 In: Proc Dig Dis Week, A-226, 1988.

72. Ferguson A, MacDonald TT. Effects of local delayed hypersensitivity on the small intestine. Ciba Found Symp 46:305–319, 1977.

73. Antczak DF, Gorman NT. Cellular interactions in immune responses. In: Halliwell REW, Gorman NT (eds) Veterinary Clinical Immunology. WB Saunders, Philadelphia, 107–134, 1989.

74. Gautam SC, Battisto JR. Orally induced tolerance generates an efferently acting suppressor T cell and an acceptor T cell that together down-regulate contact sensitivity. J Immunol 135:2975–2983, 1985.

75. Kawanishi H, Kiely J. In vitro induction of a contrasuppressor immunoregulatory network by polyclonally activated T cells derived from murine Peyer's patches. Immunol 63:415–421, 1988.

76. Benson EB, Strober W. Regulation of IgA secretion by T cell clones derived from the human gastrointestinal tract. J Immunol 140:1874–1882, 1988.

77. Elson CO. Induction and control of the gastrointestinal immune system. Scand J Gastroentol 20(suppl 114):2–14, 1985.

78. Gearhart PJ, Cebra JJ. Differentiated B lymphocytes. Potential to express particular antibody variable and constant regions depends on site of lymphoid tissue and antigen load. J Exp Med 149:216–227, 1979.

79. Hoover RG, Lynch RG. Isotype-specific suppression of IgA: Suppression of IgA responses in BALB/c mice by T cells. J Immunol 130:521–523, 1983.

80. Kawanishi H, Saltzman LE, Strober W. Mechanisms regulating IgA class-specific immunoglobulin production in murine gut-associated lymphoid tissues. II. Terminal differentiation of postswitch sIgA-bearing Peyer's patch B cells. J Exp Med 158:649–669, 1983.

81. Gallatin WM, Weissman IL, Butcher EC. A cell-surface molecule involved in organ-specific homing of lymphocytes. Nature 304:30–34, 1983.

82. Doe WF. The intestinal immune system. Gut 30:1679–1685, 1989.

83. Berg M. Murakawa Y, Camerini D, et al. Lamina propria lymphocytes are

derived from circulating cells that lack the Leu-8 lymph node homing receptor. Gastroent 101:90–99, 1991.

84. Ottaway CA. In vitro alteration of receptors for vasoactive intestinal peptide changes the in vivo localization of mouse T cells. J Exp Med 160:1054–1069, 1984.

85. Mestecky J, Czerkinsky C, Russell MW, et al. Induction and molecular properties of secretory and serum IgA antibodies specific for environmental antigens. Ann Allergy 59:54–59, 1987.

86. Vaerman JP, Heremans JF. Origin and molecular size of immunoglobulin-A in the mesenteric lymph of the dog. Immunol 18:27–38, 1970.

87. Shanahan F, Anton P. Neuroendocrine modulation of the immune system. Possible implications for inflammatory bowel disease. Dig Dis Sci 33 (March suppl): 41S–49S, 1988.

88. Staniesz AM, Befus D, Bienenstock J. Differential effects of vasoactive intestinal polypeptide, substance P, and somatostatin on immunoglobulin synthesis and proliferations by lymphocytes from Peyer's patches, mesenteric lymph nodes, and spleen. J Immunol 136:152–156, 1986.

89. Whitbread TJ, Batt RM, Garthwaite G. Relative deficiency of serum IgA in the German shepherd dog: A breed abnormality. Res Vet Sci 37:350–352, 1984.

90. Felsburg PJ, Glickman LT, Jezyk PF. Selective IgA deficiency in the dog. Clin Immunol Immunopath 36:297–305, 1985.

91. Moroff SD, Hurvitz AI, Peterson ME, et al. IgA deficiency in sharpei dogs. Vet Immunol Immunopath 13:181–188, 1986.

92. Reynolds HY, Johnson JS. Quantitation of canine immunoglobulins. J Immunol 105:698–703, 1970.

93. Ginel PJ, Novales M, Lozano MD, et al. Local secretory IgA in dogs with low systemic IgA levels. Vet Rec 132:321–323, 1993.

94. Batt RM, Barnes A, Rutgers HC, et al. Relative IgA deficiency and small intestinal bacterial overgrowth in German shepherd dogs. Res Vet Sci 50:106–111, 1991.

95. Walker WA: Pathophysiology of intestinal uptake and absorption of antigens in food allergy. Ann Allergy 59:7–20, 1987.

96. Pollock VH, Zimmer JF. Intestinal immunity. Proc 8th Kal Kan Symp, 81–86, 1984.

97. Ammann AJ, Hong R. Selective IgA deficiency: Presentation of 30 cases and a review of the literature. Medicine 50:223–236, 1971.

98. Guilford WG. Primary immunodeficiency diseases of dogs and cats. Comp Contin Ed Pract Vet 9:641–650, 1987.

99. Campbell KL, Neitzel C, Zuckermann FA. Immunoglobulin A deficiency in the dog. Canine Pract 16:7–11, 1991.

100. Strober W, James SP. The immunopathogenesis of gastrointestinal and hepatobiliary disease. J Am Med Assoc 258:2962–2969, 1987.

101. Mayrhofer G. Sites of synthesis and localization of IgE in rats infested with Nippostrongylus brasiliensis. Ciba Found Symp 46:155–175, 1977.

102. Belut D, Moneret-Vautrin DA, Nicolas JP, et al. IgE levels in intestinal juice. Dig Dis Sci 25:323–332, 1980.

103. Tomasi TB. Oral tolerance. Transplant 29:353–356, 1980.

104. Faria AMC, Garcia G, Rios MJC, et al. Decrease in susceptibility to oral tolerance induction and occurrence of oral immunization to ovalbumin in 20- to 38-week-old mice. The effect of interval between oral exposures and rate of antigen intake in the oral immunization. Immunol 78:147–151, 1993.

105. Mattingly JA, Waksman BH. Immunologic suppression after oral administration of antigen. I. Specific suppressor cells formed in rat's Peyer's patches after oral administration of sheep erythrocytes and their systemic migration. J Immunol 121:1878, 1978.

106. Mowat AM. The regulation of immune responses to dietary protein antigens. Immunol Today 8:93–98, 1987.

107. Zajac AM. The role of gastrointestinal immunity in parasitic infections of small animals. Sem Vet Med Surg 2:274–281, 1987.

108. Gasbarre LC, Leighton EA, Davies CJ. Influence of host genetics upon antibody responses against gastrointestinal nematode infections in cattle. Vet Parasitol 46:1–4, 1993.

109. Perdue MH, Ramage JK, Burget D, et al. Intestinal mucosal injury is associated with mast cell activation and leukotriene generation during Nippostrongylus- induced inflammation in the rat. Dig Dis Sci 34:724–731, 1989.

110. O'Dorisio MS. Neuropeptides and gastrointestinal immunity. Am J Med 81(suppl 6B): 74–79, 1986.

111. Ader R. Psychoneuroimmunology. London, Academic Press, 1981.

112. Blalock JE, Harbour-McMenamine D, Smith EM. Peptide hormones shared by neuroendocrine and immunologic systems. J Immunol 135:858S–861S, 1985.

113. Husband AJ. Novel vaccination strategies for the control of mucosal infection. Vaccine 11:107–112, 1993.

114. Moon HW, Bunn TO. Vaccines for preventing enterotoxigenic Escherichia coli infections in farm animals. Vaccine 11:213–220, 1993.

115. Pierce NF, Reynolds HY. Immunity to experimental cholera. II. Secretory and humoral antitoxin response to local and systemic toxoid administration. J Infect Dis 131:383–389, 1975.

116. Parrott DMV. The gut as a lymphoid organ. Clin Gastroenterol 5:211–228, 1976.

117. Porter P, Kenworthy R, Noakes DE, et al. Intestinal antibody secretion in the young pig in response to oral immunization with Escherichia coli. Immunol 27:841–853, 1975.

118. Morris JG, Tacket CO, Levine MM. Oral carrier vaccines: New tricks in an old trade. Gastroenterology 103:699–701, 1992.

119. Strombeck DR, Harrold D. Comparison of the rate of absorption and proteolysis of (14C) choleragen and (14C) bovine serum albumin in the rat jejunum. Infect Immun 12:1450–1456, 1975.

120. Hiraga C, Kanaki T, Ichikawa Y. Immunobiological characteristics of germ-free and specific pathogen-free cats. Lab An Sci 31-391–396, 1981.

4 Gastrointestinal Inflammation

W. GRANT GUILFORD

INTRODUCTION

Inflammation is the vascular and cellular response of tissue to injury. It is a protective mechanism by which phagocytes, immunoglobulins, complement, and other serum constituents are concentrated at the sites of tissue damage. Inflammation is usually an acute process concluded by elimination of the inciting cause and by tissue repair. If the inflammatory response fails to eliminate the cause, chronic inflammation will ensue and damage to the tissues may result. In this way the inflammation seen in disorders such as inflammatory bowel disease becomes detrimental to the host. Injurious processes that are capable of inciting inflammation include physical damage, infection, ischemia, toxins, neoplasia, and immune reactions (including immediate, cytotoxic, immune complex, and delayed hypersensitivity reactions).

VASCULAR CHANGES DURING INFLAMMATION[1-3]

Vasodilation and increased blood flow to perturbed tissues occur early in the inflammatory process. Increased vascular permeability and exudation of plasma, leukocytes, and red blood cells into the tissues accompany the vasodilation. Later in the inflammatory process blood flow tends to decline, platelets adhere to vessel walls, and intravascular clotting may ensue. Activated Hageman factor, contained in the exuded plasma, initiates the clotting cascade, the fibrinolytic cascade, and kallikrein synthesis. Kinins generated by kallikrein contribute to the vascular dilation and increased permeability. The results of these vascular changes are dilution of toxins by exuded fluid and isolation of microorganisms and damaged tissues by a defensive cordon of accumulated phagocytes, fibrin, and occasionally obstructed vasculature. The vascular changes are a result of various mediators, the most potent of which are the kinins, histamine, certain prostaglandins, and perhaps certain neuropeptides and nitric oxide.

CHEMOTAXIS AND THE CELLULAR CHANGES DURING INFLAMMATION[4]

Chemotaxis is the process by which leukocytes move to damaged tissue along concentration gradients of chemotactic substances. It is at present an important area of research because chemotaxis is an early (perhaps inciting) event in the inflammatory process, and one that determines the accumulating cell types and hence the microscopic classification of the inflammation. The more mobile leukocytes (neutrophils, eosinophils) enter the tissues first, followed later by monocytes. Some chemotactic substances attract most phagocytes, whereas others are specific for neutrophils, monocytes, or eosinophils. In addition to chemoattraction, many of these substances stimulate other biologic functions of the phagocyte, such as degranulation and phagocytosis. Neutrophils are attracted by complement fragments, immune complexes, eicosanoids, soluble bacterial products, oxygen-derived free radicals, kallikrein, certain lymphokines, and various tissue breakdown products including collagen and fibrin fragments. Of these products, leukotriene B_4, 5-HETE, complement fragments C5a and C567, and N-formyl-methionyl-leucyl-phenylalanine (FMLP) are the most potent chemotactic products known. As a result of the wide variety of chemotactic products that attract neutrophils, most types of inflammation have some component of neutrophil infiltration. Eosinophils are attracted by complement fragments, histamine, certain leukotrienes, and the eosinophilic chemotactic factor of anaphylaxis (ECF-A). ECF-A is released by mast cells and basophils and is composed of two polypeptides: alanine-glycine-serine-glutamine and valine-glycine-serine-glutamine. Monocytes are attracted by complement fragments, certain bacterial peptides such as FMLP, some lymphokines, and collagen-breakdown products.

Once present in the tissues, the phagocytes adhere to and ingest foreign antigen and tissue debris. Serum opsonins such as fibronectin, C-reactive protein, antibody, and complement facilitate adherence, as does trapping of the antigen against exuded fibrin.

After ingestion the phagocytosed material in the phagolysosome is exposed to various toxic products and digestive enzymes. These include proteases, toxic proteins, and oxygen-derived free radicals. The latter are produced in great quantity by the respiratory burst of neutrophils.

INFLAMMATORY MEDIATORS

Eicosanoids[5-11]

Eicosanoids are derivatives of 20 carbon fatty acids. The most prevalent eicosanoids in mammalian systems appear to be those

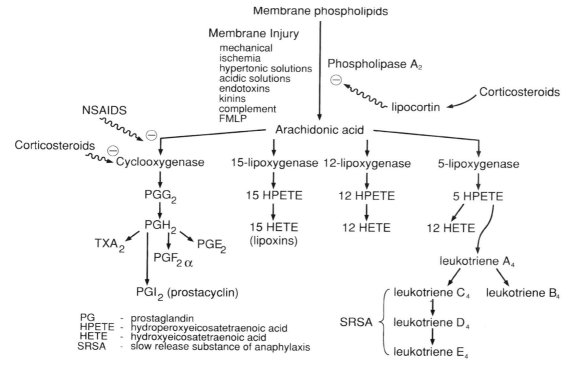

FIGURE 4-1. The arachidonic acid cascade.

formed by the arachidonic acid cascade (Figure 4–1). Cell injury activates membrane phospholipases, in particular phospholipase A_2. The phospholipases initiate the arachidonic acid cascade by releasing arachidonic acid from membrane phospholipids. In the gut, perturbations capable of releasing arachidonic acid include mechanical stimulation, ischemia, and exposure of bowel tissue (including resident leukocytes) to hypertonic solutions, acid or alkali, chyme, bile acids, bacterial endotoxins, FMLP, bradykinin, complement, and coagulation factors. Glucocorticoids inhibit arachidonic acid release by generating a membrane-bound protein called lipocortin. Once released into the cytoplasm, the arachidonic acid may be metabolized by either cyclooxygenases or lipoxygenases to various prostaglandins, hydroxyeicosatetraenoic acids (HETEs), or leukotrienes. Which of these pathways predominates depends on the concentration of these enzymes in the different tissues and the presence or absence of different inhibitors. For instance, most nonsteroidal anti-inflammatory agents inhibit cyclooxygenase but not lipoxygenase channeling eicosanoid synthesis toward leukotrienes.[12] In the bowel, prominent eicosanoid pathways recognized to date appear to be the synthesis of leukotriene B_4, leukotriene D_4, prostaglandin E_2 (PGE$_2$), prostaglandin F$_2$ alpha, prostacyclin, thromboxane B_2, and HETE.[12] The precise cellular origin of gastrointestinal eicosanoids has not been determined. Likely sites are leukocytes, platelets, and endothelial cells in the lamina propria. Their biotransformation is rapid. Half-lives range from seconds to minutes.

Leukotrienes

Leukotrienes are eicosanoids derived from the metabolism of arachidonic acid by lipoxygenases. The quantitatively most important leukotriene pathways in the gastrointestinal tract are those catalyzed by 5-lipoxygenase and 15-lipoxygenase. The principal arachidonic acid–derived product of 15-lipoxygenase is 15-hydroxyeicosatetraenoic acid, which has an important role in the modulation of 5-lipoxygenase. Enzyme activity of 5-lipoxygenase is prominent in leukocytes. The leukotriene products of 5-lipoxygenase (Figure 4–1) have potent inflammatory properties. The leukotriene precursors, 5-hydroperoxyeicosateraenoic acid (5-HEPTE) and hydroxyeicosatetraenoic acid (5-HETE), impair net colonic fluid absorption; 5-HETE is also a chemotactic substance. Leukotriene B_4 attracts neutrophils and to a lesser extent eosinophils and monocytes. It may also increase vascular permeability and stimulate neutrophils to adhere to vascular endothelium. At high concentrations leukotriene B4 stimulates neutrophil degranulation and superoxide generation. Leukotrienes C_4, D_4, and E_4 collectively comprise slow-reacting substance of anaphylaxis. They cause a sustained contraction of certain smooth muscle, including that of the bowel. Leukotrienes C_4, D_4, and E_4 also cause vasodilation and increase vascular permeability of microvasculature. These leukotrienes cause these effects at much lower concentrations than histamine.

Leukotriene B_4, leukotriene D_4, and HETEs are found in high concentrations in rectal mucosal samples taken from humans with ulcerative colitis. The severity of the inflammation positively correlates with the concentration of leukotriene B_4. Inhibitors of leukotriene synthesis (such as 5-lipoxygenase inhibitors and glucocorticoids) have resulted in significant decreases in inflammation and intestinal secretion in ulcerative colitis in humans and in various experimental colitis models.[13] Along with prostaglandins, leukotrienes appear responsible for much of the colonic secretory response in human ulcerative colitis.[12] It is likely these eicosanoids are very important proinflammatory mediators in inflammatory bowel disease, and the advent of 5-lipoxygenase inhibitors, such as zileuton, into the clinical arena is eagerly awaited.

Prostaglandins

Prostaglandins (PG) are eicosanoids derived from the metabolism of arachidonic acid by cyclooxygenase. Further metabolism of prostaglandin intermediates yields the prostacyclin (PGI_2), thromboxane (TxA_2), PGF_2 alpha, PGE_2, and PGD_2 prostaglandin series. In most tissues, prostacyclins are produced predominantly by vascular endothelium, whereas platelets produce the thromboxanes, and most nucleated cells produce the PGE_2, PGF_2 alpha, and PGD_2 series. The prostaglandins have a wide range of biologic activity. Tissue and species differences do occur. The individual prostaglandin series have different and often opposing effects. In vivo, the eicosanoids are released together, and complex interactions between them probably determine the net biologic effect. In general, prostaglandins tend to serve a protective role in the gastrointestinal tract rather than being primary mediators that incite gastrointestinal inflammation. This is particularly clear in the stomach, where prostaglandins, especially PGE_2, have been shown to be "cytoprotective." The cytoprotection probably results from a number of beneficial effects, including inhibition of mast cell mediator release,[14] stimulation of mucus and bicarbonate secretion, enhanced mucosal blood flow, decreased acid secretion, and enhanced epithelial proliferation and repair. Prostaglandins, particularly PGE_2, also appear to be largely protective in the intestine. PGE_2 can stimulate mucus secretion by the bowel, increase bowel mucosal blood flow (as can prostacyclin), maintain or enhance villus height after radiation damage, and protect the bowel against certain perturbations including alcohol-induced colitis, acetic acid–induced colitis, and clindamycin-induced colitis.[5] Furthermore, PGE_2 induces suppressor cell activity in peripheral blood lymphocytes and perhaps in bowel lymphocytes. The exacerbation of colitis that can occur following ingestion of nonsteroidal anti-inflammatory agents provides further, albeit indirect, evidence of prostaglandin-mediated cytoprotection of the bowel.[13]

Although prostaglandins may not incite inflammation in the gastrointestinal tract, it is likely that in some situations they have a mild permissive effect on the inflammatory process and probably mediate some of its consequences, such as pain and diarrhea. Prostacyclin and PGE_2 alone do not increase vascular permeability, but they potentiate the increased macromolecular leakage that occurs due to other mediators. In some situations prostaglandins may induce diarrhea, abdominal cramping, and perhaps nausea. Prostaglandin-mediated diarrhea probably results from increased secretion of fluid and electrolytes, in combination with altered contractility. PGF_2 alpha and thromboxane cause smooth muscle contraction, whereas prostacyclin causes smooth muscle relaxation. PGE_2 causes longitudinal smooth muscle contraction and circular smooth muscle relaxation. It has been suggested that PGE_2 is the mediator responsible for the decreased colonic segmenting contractions noted in humans with ulcerative colitis.[15] PGE_2 stimulates intestinal net secretion of chloride, potassium, sodium, and water. PGF_2 alpha also promotes secretion. Prostacyclin increases secretion of fluid and electrolytes in the large bowel but has variable effects in the small bowel. Increased synthesis of prostaglandins may mediate the intestinal secretion that occurs in a number of diarrheal diseases including certain immune-mediated diseases[16] and those due to enterotoxins from E. coli and Salmonella typhimurium. Increased prostaglandin synthesis may also be involved in diarrhea due to excess thyroxine, excess vasoactive intestinal polypeptide, unconjugated bile acids, celiac disease, mastocytosis, neural crest tumors, and miscellaneous other disorders.[5]

The role of prostaglandins in inflammatory bowel disease is unclear. Synthesis of prostaglandins, in particular PGE, PGF_2 alpha, prostacyclin, and thromboxane, increases during this disorder. This synthesis may alter local blood flow, influence smooth muscle contractility, and contribute to the diarrhea associated with the condition, but, based on the experimental evidence just cited, it is more likely to protect the mucosa than markedly exacerbate the inflammation.

Bacterial N-Formyl-Methionyl Oligopeptides

Bacterial N-formyl-methionyl oligopeptides are proinflammatory chemotactic oligopeptides derived from many species of intestinal bacteria, including E. coli. Bacterial formyl oligopeptides, such as N-formyl-methionyl-leucyl-phenylalanine (FMLP), can cross the undamaged mucosa, but the rate of entry is slow and is controlled by a combination of enzymatic degradation and restricted mucosal permeability.[17,18] The absorption of FMLP-like peptides can be markedly increased by damage to the mucosal barrier.[18] Absorption of FMLP results in increased intestinal vascular permeability, interstitial edema, hyperemia, and increased mucosal permeability.[17] These changes appear to be partly mediated by neutrophil oxidants.[17] Neutrophils possess high- and low-affinity receptors for FMLP. FMLP bound to the high-affinity receptors stimulates migration of the neutrophil. As the neutrophil approaches the area of inflammation, the concentration of the chemoattractant increases, and FMLP eventually binds to its low-affinity receptor. The low-affinity receptor stimulates the neutrophil to phagocytose, degranulate, undergo the respiratory burst, and to elaborate eicosanoids and oxidants.

It is possible that bacterial formyl oligopeptides are the inciting or perpetuating cause of inflammatory bowel disease (Figure 4–2). Neutrophils from human patients with ulcerative colitis have increased responsiveness to FMLP.[19] FMLP may be important in inflammatory disorders of the dog and cat bowel, but it should be noted that, in contrast to other species, one study suggests FMLP is not chemotactic to canine neutrophils.[20]

Histamine

Histamine (beta-imidazolyl-ethylamine) is released by degranulation of mast cells following a variety of stimuli (see Chapter 3 on the gastrointestinal immune system). The importance of histamine as a mediator of inflammation in the digestive system has not been established. Visceral mast cells contain less histamine than connective tissue mast cells. Histamine has a variety of effects on tissues. Some, but not all, of these effects are known to occur in the digestive system. Histamine dilates microvessels, increases vascular permeability, contracts gut smooth muscle, attracts eosinophils, stimulates gastric acid secretion, and contracts the hepatic veins of dogs. Histamine may have immunosuppressive activity, and it can induce fibroblast proliferation.

Serotonin[21]

The majority of serotonin (5-hydroxytryptamine) in the body is found in the enterochromaffin cells of the bowel and in platelets. Serotonin has been identified in the mast cells of

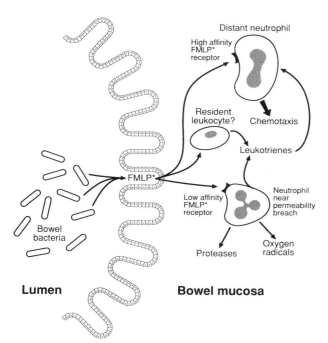

*FMLP — Formyl-Methionyl-Leucyl-Phernylalanine

FIGURE 4–2. Chemotactic peptides and gastrointestinal inflammation.

rodents and cattle, but not of other species. Its importance as an inflammatory mediator is unknown. Release of serotonin from enterochromaffin cells is increased by mechanical stimulation, hypertonicity, acidity, norepinephrine, and vagal influences. Platelets release serotonin following aggregation. The effects of serotonin vary in different tissues and species. In most species studied, serotonin causes splanchnic vasoconstriction, has little influence on capillary permeability (except in rodents), and increases small intestinal motility but decreases gastric and large-bowel motility. In the dog, intravenous infusion of serotonin reduces gastric secretion of pepsin and acid, but increases the secretion of mucus. Serotonin also stimulates secretion of fluid in the intestines. In the rat stomach, some evidence indicates that serotonin may be an important mediator of the phenomenon of adaptive mucosal cytoprotection.[22]

Kallikreins and Kinins[23]

Kinins are short-lived polypeptides derived from the action of kininogenases (serine proteases) on serum globulins called kininogens. Important kininogenases include kallikreins, trypsin, and plasmin. Kallikreins can be secreted by neutrophils, mast cells, basophils, and platelets (Figure 4–3). Kallikrein-like enzymes have been detected in the gastrointestinal mast cells of cats. A tissue kallikrein is found in high concentration in the pancreas, and kallikreins may be detected in salivary, pancreatic, and intestinal secretions. A plasma kallikrein is produced by the action of activated Hageman factor on plasma prekallikrein. Kallikrein, in turn, exerts a positive feedback on its own formation by activating Hageman factor and the coagulation cascade (Figure 4–4). In addition to their role in kinin generation and activation of

coagulation, kallikreins may be involved in the activation of complement and in the physiology of water and electrolyte movement across membranes. Various plasma protease inhibitors, such as C1 esterase inhibitor, alpha-2-macroglobulin, and alpha-1-antitrypsin, inhibit the formation of kinins. The kinins are inactivated by kinases, one of which is otherwise known as angiotensin converting enzyme.

Two important kinins are bradykinin and kallidin. They are potent vasodilators and increase capillary permeability. They contract some bowel smooth muscle preparations and relax others. They stimulate pain responses if injected intraperitoneally or into various viscera. Kinins are chemotactic to leukocytes. Some of their effects may be mediated by kinin-stimulated release of eicosanoids and heparin. Kinins are likely to be important inflammatory mediators in the digestive system. They appear to play an important role in the local and systemic consequences of pancreatic inflammation. In the treatment of pancreatitis, the use of aprotinin (Trasylol), a protease inhibitor that blocks kallikrein and trypsin synthesis, has met with limited success.

Complement Fragments[24]

The complement system may be directly activated by many stimuli of relevance to the digestive system. These include IgG or IgM complexed with antigen, certain bacteria including some strains of *E. coli*, helminth cuticles, fungal cell walls, plasmin, kallikrein, and endotoxin. The consequences of complement activation include lysis of microorganisms and cells, promotion of coagulation, activation of the kinin and eicosanoid cascades, and the release of complement fragments with proinflammatory effects. Complement fragments C5a and C567 are chemotactic. Fragments C3a and C5a increase vessel permeability. Strong evidence indicates that immune complex formation and complement activation contribute to the pathogenesis of inflammatory bowel disease.[25]

Platelet Activating Factor[26]

Platelet activating factor (PAF) is a phospholipid mediator derived from leukocytes, mast cells, platelets, and vascular endothelium. PAF stimulates platelet aggregation and promotes the release by platelets of a large number of mediators including serotonin and thromboxane. At very low concentrations, PAF primes neutrophils to respond to stimuli such as complement and FMLP (see earlier discussion). PAF is chemotactic and stimulates neutrophil adherence to endothelial surfaces, leading to degranulation, vascular damage, and increased vascular permeability. It has been suggested that PAF produced by a mildly injured vascular endothelium may initiate a vicious cycle that leads to further vascular injury mediated by neutrophils, and to microvascular thrombi and ischemia.[13,26] Formation of PAF is increased in some experimental models of colitis.[27] It has been suggested that PAF is an important mediator of endotoxic shock. Infusion of PAF into rats causes gastric damage and hemoconcentration.[28]

Interleukins[13,29]

Interleukin-1 is a polypeptide produced by a variety of cells but in particular activated macrophages. It is an important

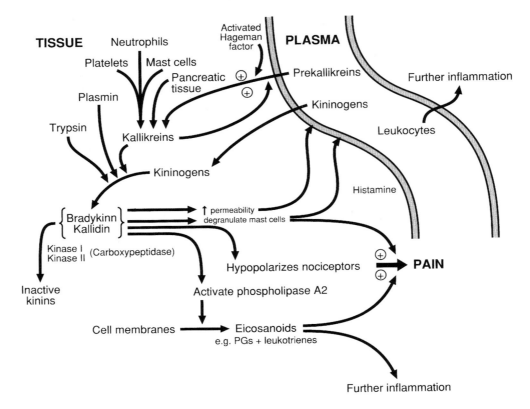

FIGURE 4-3. The kinin system.

mediator of inflammation in many tissues, and has a broad range of proinflammatory effects on the gut immune system (Figure 4–5).[13] Interleukin-1 alters endothelial cell membranes, resulting in adherence of leukocytes, increased procoagulant activity, and the release of platelet activating factor. It decreases plasma iron concentration, a change that may inhibit bacterial growth and free radical generation. Interleukin-1 induces formation of arachidonic acid metabolites and acute-phase proteins, and causes fever, stimulation of lymphocytes, neutrophilia, fibroblast proliferation, and collagen synthesis. The fibrosis that accompanies chronic inflammation may be partly due to interleukin-1, and partly a result of transforming growth factor (beta).

Colonic cells derived from humans and laboratory animals with ulcerative colitis synthesize greatly increased amounts of interleukin-1.[30,31] Interleukin-1 tissue concentrations correlate with the severity of colitis in humans.[32]

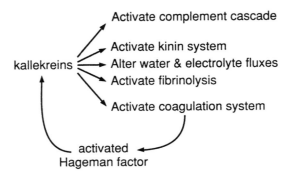

FIGURE 4-4. Consequences of kallikrein activation.

Interleukin-1 receptor antagonist is a specific glycoprotein that competitively binds to interleukin-1 receptors on leukocytes and mesenchymal cells, suppressing the proinflammatory effects of interleukin-1.[13] In a rabbit model of immune-mediated colitis, administration of interleukin-1 receptor antagonist resulted in a dose-dependent reduction in infiltration of the lamina propria by mononuclear cells, production of leukotriene B_4 and prostaglandin E_2, and tissue damage.[13] These observations suggest interleukin-1 receptor antagonists play an important role in controlling gastrointestinal inflammation.

Interleukin-2 is produced mainly by activated lymphocytes and plays an important role in the proliferation and differentiation of lymphocytes. Interleukin-2 levels are increased in the colon tissue of humans with colitis.[13]

Interleukin-6 and interleukin-8 are proinflammatory cytokines that are present in higher levels in inflamed bowel.[13]

Cachectin[29,33]

Otherwise known as tumor necrosis factor, cachectin, a polypeptide, is derived from activated macrophages. It has very similar properties to the interleukins, although it apparently does not share the latter's effects on the immune system. Cachectin induces interleukin. Along with interleukin, cachectin is responsible for the anorexia and fever that accompanies inflammatory disease. Cachectin induces fibroblast proliferation and the vascular changes described for interleukin-1.

Cachectin is induced by endotoxin and may be the prime mediator of endotoxic shock. When infused into mice or rats

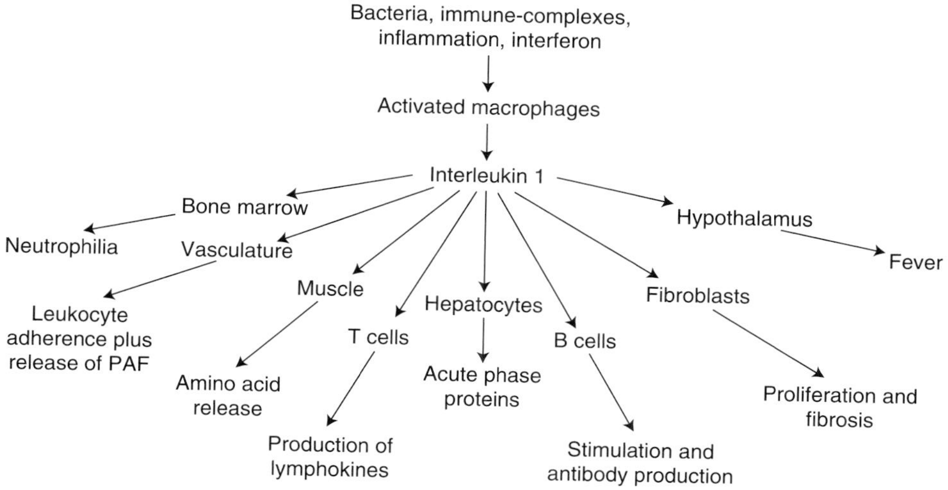

Bacteria, immune-complexes,
inflammation, interferon

Activated macrophages

Interleukin 1

Bone marrow

Neutrophilia

Vasculature

Hypothalamus

Fever

Muscle

Hepatocytes

Fibroblasts

Leukocyte
adherence plus
release of PAF

T cells

B cells

Amino acid
release

Acute phase
proteins

Proliferation and
fibrosis

Production of
lymphokines

Stimulation and
antibody production

FIGURE 4-5. Biologic activities of interleukin-1 (modified from Figure 19-8, reference 1).

in quantities similar to those produced endogenously, cachectin causes diarrhea, shock, and severe organ damage, including ischemic and hemorrhagic lesions of the gastrointestinal tract and pancreas. The hemorrhagic necrosis appears to occur due to vascular events such as procoagulation.

Neuropeptides[34]

The enteric nervous system releases several neuropeptides from unmyelinated afferent nerve endings. In addition to their function in the relay of sensory information and the control of gastrointestinal motility, some of these mediators are capable of causing vasodilation, plasma extravasation, and disordered smooth muscle contraction. Substance P is thought to be one of the most important mediators of this so-called neurogenic inflammation. It is produced by enterochromaffin cells as well as sensory neurons. The secretion of substance P by sensory neurons is magnified by antidromic activation of their axon collaterals ("axon reflexes"). Chemical and physical irritation, including colonic distension,[35] can cause its release. The peptide results in vasodilation, plasma extravasation, pain, and smooth muscle contraction. Some of the vascular effects of substance P may be mediated by histamine. The concentration of substance P in the inflamed mucosa of humans with inflammatory bowel disease is significantly elevated.[36] Recently, substance P and vasoactive intestinal polypeptide (VIP) have been shown to enhance the immunoreactivity of GALT (gut-associated lymphoid tissue).[37,38]

VIP may also contribute to inflammation. By itself, it does not increase vascular permeability, but it does potentiate vascular leakage induced by other mediators.[10] VIP inhibits T cell proliferation but increases natural killer cell cytotoxicity and increases immunoglobulin production from B cells.[13] VIP is a potent vasodilator,[39] and it also stimulates pancreatic, intestinal, and salivary secretions. The excessive release of VIP in VIPomas is associated with watery diarrhea. The tissue levels of VIP tend to decrease in human colitis.[13]

In contrast to VIP and substance P, another peptide hormone, somatostatin, appears to inhibit neurogenic inflammation. Somatostatin inhibits T cell proliferation, decreases immunoglobulin production, and reduces the release of cytokines.[13] Decreased somatostatin-containing cells have been observed in the colonic tissue of humans with inflammatory bowel disease, implying a predisposition to inflammation.[13]

The importance of neurogenic inflammation in the gas-

trointestinal system remains to be established. Species differences appear to exist, and some experimental evidence suggests that neurogenic inflammation may vary in importance in different viscera and different regions of the bowel.

Oxygen-Derived Free Radicals[40-45]

Free radicals are molecules with unpaired electrons in one or more orbitals. They are unstable and highly reactive molecules with the propensity to oxidize other molecules. Oxygen-derived free radicals are radicals derived from the incomplete reduction of oxygen. The univalent reduction of oxygen yields superoxide anion. This reaction is catalyzed by several enzymes found in high concentration in the liver (xanthine oxidase), bowel mucosa (xanthine oxidase, aldehyde oxidase), and phagocytes (NADPH oxidase). The high concentration of radical-generating enzymes in the digestive system and the large numbers of resident phagocytes in the bowel predispose the digestive system to free radical–mediated disease. Superoxide anion may also be generated by nonenzymatic autoxidation reactions, such as those with iron, and with certain flavins and quinones. Superoxide anion is a precursor for other oxygen-derived radicals, such as hydrogen peroxide and hydroxyl radical. Superoxide dismutase enzymes catalyze the dismutation of superoxide anion to hydrogen peroxide. The divalent reduction of oxygen by enzymes such as monoamine or diamine oxidase may also form hydrogen peroxide. In the presence of transition metals such as iron, superoxide anion and hydrogen peroxide can interact to produce the potent oxidizing agent, hydroxyl radical. Hydrogen peroxide in the presence of chloride ion and certain peroxidases, such as neutrophil myeloperoxidase, leads to the production of hypochlorous acid. Hydroxyl radical and halogenated peroxides, such as hypochlorous acid, are thought to be the most toxic of the oxygen-derived free radicals.

Tissues employ a number of defenses against free radical attack. These include antioxidant micronutrients such as vitamin E, vitamin C, selenium, glutathione, and sulfur-containing amino acids. Important micronutrient interactions have been recognized. For instance, high levels of polyunsaturated fatty acids increase the requirements for antioxidants. An adequate level of vitamin C helps prevent depletion of vitamin E. The enzymes superoxide dismutase, catalase, and the selenium-dependent glutathione peroxidase and phospholipid glutathione peroxidase are also important defenses. Ceruloplasmin and ferritin, through copper sequestration and iron sequestration and oxidation also play a protective role. Mucin is known to scavenge hydroxyl radical and may play a role in the defense of the bowel epithelium. The bowel mucosa contains some of the highest concentrations of superoxide dismutase, catalase, glutathione, and vitamin E in the body.

Oxygen-derived free radical formation is only of pathologic consequence if their rate of production exceeds their rate of inactivation. The small quantities of radicals produced during normal oxidative metabolism are easily dealt with by the antioxidant defenses. During inflammation, however, the rate of production of the radicals by phagocytes greatly increases, overwhelming the antioxidant defenses. An excess of free radicals may also result from a depletion of antioxidant protection. Antioxidants may be depleted by chronic inflammation or by absolute or relative dietary deficiencies. Whether derived from increased production or inadequate scavenging, an excess of oxygen-derived free radicals will cause considerable tissue damage, including lipid peroxidation and damage to DNA, carbohydrates, collagen, enzymes, and transport proteins. Lipid peroxidation results in decreased membrane fluidity, altered permeability, and perhaps cell lysis. Damage to DNA carries the attendant likelihood of neoplasia. Free radicals and some of their products (hydroxy-alkenals) are also chemotactic. They enhance eicosanoid production and may stimulate the release of cytokines such as cachectin.[46]

Oxygen radicals may play an important role in the mucosal injury of ulcerative colitis and other inflammatory disorders of the bowel.[13,45] Sulfasalazine, and/or its active metabolite 5-aminosalicylate, is an oxyradical scavenger. This action may partly explain the successful deployment of this drug against ulcerative colitis. Sulfasalazine also inhibits the transformation of LTA_4 to LTB_4, weakly inhibits cyclooxygenase, and impairs binding of interferon to cellular receptors.[8,13] Free radicals may be involved in the pathogenesis of acute gastric mucosal injury from chemicals such as aspirin.[47] Hydroxyl radical degrades mucin, perhaps predisposing the epithelium to injury. Selenium deficiency has been associated with increased risk of esophageal cancer in humans, perhaps because of inadequate antioxidant protection. Radicals may mediate much of the liver damage resultant from certain toxicants such as carbon tetrachloride, acetaminophen, and endotoxin.[43,45,48] They also appear to be involved in the pathogenesis of pancreatitis,[45] and they play an important role in the tissue necrosis and inflammation resulting from gastrointestinal ischemic disorders.

Lactoferrin

Lactoferrin occurs in many gastrointestinal secretions, and is released by degranulating neutrophils. An antibacterial role has been attributed to this protein because of its ability to deprive bacteria of iron. Recent observations have suggested that during inflammation, superoxide anion releases iron from lactoferrin. The increased concentration of iron amplifies the inflammatory process by facilitating the generation of hydroxyl radicals and by enhancing neutrophil adhesion to the endothelium.[26]

Proteases[10]

Phagocytes, in particular neutrophils, release proteolytic enzymes into the tissues. These include kallikreins, plasminogen activator, elastase, collagenases, cathepsins, a serine protease, hyaluronidase, and lysozyme. Substrates of these enzymes include kinins, plasminogen, elastin, collagen, fibrin, proteoglycans, clotting and complement factors, immunoglobulins, and hyaluronic acid. These enzymes are thought to function in tissue defense and repair, but excessive release can damage healthy tissues and may activate the kinin, complement, and coagulation systems. The release of elastase by neutrophils is very destructive to vascular integrity.

CONSEQUENCES OF INFLAMMATION

Elimination of Microorganisms and Foreign Antigen

As an important consequence of the inflammatory process, phagocytes, which have been concentrated at the inflammatory focus by the chemotactic and vascular events described earlier, release a multitude of toxic products and digestive enzymes that eliminate invasive microorganisms and other foreign antigen. As previously mentioned, an important consequence of the exudation of plasma at inflammatory sites is the dilution of toxins and the carriage of protective antibodies into the tissues. Antigen not rapidly eliminated is walled off from the body by intravascular clotting, extravascular fibrin, the physical presence of amassed phagocytes, and ultimately by fibrous tissue.

Tissue Healing

Healing begins with the removal of debris by the processes of liquefaction and phagocytosis. Absorption, sloughing, or drainage remove the debris liquified by enzymatic digestion. Proliferation of fibrous tissue or regeneration then fill tissue defects at the inflammatory site. Macrophages are responsible for eliminating much of the debris from the inflammatory focus. They also stimulate fibrosis. The extent of tissue regeneration depends on both the extent of damage and the type of tissue destroyed. Hepatocytes have a remarkable capacity to regenerate, provided the reticulin framework of the lobule is intact. Bowel epithelium also regenerates readily, provided denudation is not complete. Glandular epithelium, however, has less capacity for regeneration. Massive cellular destruction and chronic irritation result in the formation of considerable amounts of fibrous tissue. Hepatic cirrhosis, chronic pancreatitis, fibrosing gastritis, and fibrosing colitis are examples of such processes.

Tissue Damage

If the inciting cause is not rapidly eliminated, damage to host tissues will occur. The tissue damage results from the chronic secretion of toxic products by phagocytes, and from concurrent elaboration of cytotoxic products by the immune response. The toxic agents most often incriminated in causing nonspecific damage to host tissues are oxygen-derived free radicals, proteases (especially elastase), cytokines, and certain toxic proteins. For instance, major basic protein released from eosinophils is toxic to epithelial surfaces.

Villous atrophy is a common morphologic response to a variety of different pathologic processes, one of which is inflammation. Villous atrophy results from villous contraction after a reduction in the quantity of villous epithelial cells.

Acute inflammatory processes cause epithelial loss through rapid necrosis and/or sloughing of large expanses of epithelium. Chronic inflammation appears to cause epithelial loss by the secretion of T cell–derived lymphokines that cause premature loss of immature enterocytes from the villi. The consequence of villous atrophy is malabsorption. Severe tissue damage in the bowel can result in significant fluid, electrolyte, and protein loss. The consequences of inflammatory damage in the liver are discussed in Chapter 30 on hepatic disease.

Altered Motility[34]

Gastrointestinal inflammation, even if restricted to the mucosa, can result in disordered bowel motility. The pathogenesis of the motility disturbances are not clear but probably result either from a direct effect of mediators, such as PGE_2 or leukotrienes, on smooth muscle function, or from an indirect effect of these mediators on the enteric nervous system. Direct projection of nerves between the mucosa, submucosa, and muscle layers has been demonstrated. Communication from mucosa to muscularis may also occur via spinal reflex arcs.

In ulcerative colitis in humans, there is a tendency for rhythmic segmentation to be reduced, resulting in a flaccid bowel with little resistance to the passage of luminal content and thus diarrhea. Hypermotility accompanies certain parasitic and bacterial disorders of the bowel and may help clear these undesirable agents from the bowel. On occasion, smooth muscle spasms may occur. This results in abdominal pain and may be the forerunner of intussusception. Motility derangements can also result from inflammation in organs other than the bowel. For instance, localized or generalized ileus can develop secondary to pancreatitis or cholecystitis.

Increased Bowel Permeability

Inflammation results in increased bowel permeability. The increased absorption of luminal antigens may perpetuate the inflammatory process by attracting more inflammatory cells and further activating of the immune system. The mechanisms by which inflammation increases permeability are probably multifactorial. Mucosal denudation is an obvious cause. Of interest is an in vitro demonstration that gamma interferon will increase epithelial tight junction permeability.[49] It is probable that many other inflammatory mediators increase bowel permeability. The consequences of increased permeability include fluid, electrolyte, protein, and cell loss, as well as increased absorption of antigenic and toxic materials.

Systemic Consequences

Inflammatory processes in the gastrointestinal system can result in fever, nausea, anorexia, weight loss, and leukocytosis. These signs result from the release of certain mediators, such as interleukin-1 and cachectin, and from the absorption of toxic products. Signs pertaining to fluid, electrolyte, or albumin loss may be noted. Inflammation results in the generation of a number of mediators that can activate the complement cascade, the kinin system, and the coagulation cascade. This interaction becomes important in acute pancreatitis, where local inflammation can take on global consequences through the initiation of disseminated intravascular coagulation. Chronic inflammation is usually accompanied by a significant lymphocytic immune response. Soluble immune complexes derived from the humoral arm of the lymphocytic response may lead to distant manifestations of the inflammatory process. Three well-recognized systemic complications of gastrointestinal immune reactions are uveitis, polyarthritis, and dermatitis. On occasion, chronic inflammation is associated with amyloidosis. So-called reactive amyloidosis appears to result from ineffective degradation of the serum acute-phase proteins that occur in persistently elevated concentration during chronic inflammation. In the digestive system, amyloid is most commonly deposited in the liver of dogs and the pancreas of aged cats, but the intestinal tract is occasionally affected. Renal amyloidosis is occasionally observed in human patients with granulomatous enteritis.

REGULATION OF INFLAMMATION

Digestive system inflammation is prevented by maintaining an effective permeability barrier to luminal antigens. Once initiated, inflammation is largely controlled by eliminating the inciting cause. The predominance of noncomplement mediated (IgA) humoral responses in the bowel further restricts inflammation, as does a variety of other processes. For example, free radical scavengers restrict damage due to release of oxyradicals. Protease inhibitors such as alpha-1-antitrypsin and alpha-2-macroglobulin enter the areas of inflammation through the permeable vessel walls and block the activity of proteases, including those released from neutrophils and those that activate complement. A low molecular weight inhibitor, called antileukoprotease, has also been identified in human mucus and salivary secretions.[10] Proteases released by canine mast cells are capable of degrading vasoactive intestinal peptide and substance P. Proteases released by eosinophils partially reduce mast cell–mediated and basophil-mediated inflammation. Serum amyloid A, an acute-phase protein, dampens the immune response to inflammation.

CATEGORIES OF INFLAMMATION[2,50,51]

Inflammatory processes are usually classified according to their longevity and the predominant exudate or cell type at the inflammatory focus. Two important factors determining the cell types present at the inflammatory site are the particular chemotactic factors produced by the inciting tissue insult and the duration of the inflammation. The categories of inflammation most frequently observed in the gastrointestinal tract are mucoid, fibrinous, hemorrhagic, suppurative, lymphocytic-plasmacytic, eosinophilic, and granulomatous. It is important to note that, like most biologic processes, inflammation defies textbook classification. Intergrades of these classical descriptions are common.

Mucoid Inflammation

Mucoid inflammation is characterized grossly by mucus adherent to feces or mucosa, and microscopically by increased numbers of goblet cells. Mucoid inflammation is caused by chronic mild irritants. These include bacterial and viral infections of low virulence, parasitic disorders, and low-grade immune-mediated processes such as mild chronic colitis.

Fibrinous (Pseudomembranous) Inflammation

Pseudomembranous inflammation is a type of fibrinous inflammation characterized by the formation of a dense white or yellowish plaque on the mucosal surface. On occasion cylindrical fibrinous casts are passed in the feces, giving the initial impression that the patient has sloughed a segment of bowel. Causes of pseudomembranous inflammation include canine and feline parvovirus, *Salmonella, Clostridium difficile,* and perhaps *Bacteroides* and *Fusobacterium* Spp. In the peritoneal cavity, serous and fibrinous inflammation are important manifestations of peritoneal irritation. Feline infectious peritonitis is an important cause of fibrin exudation in cats. Fibrous organization of peritoneal fibrin can lead to abdominal adhesions.

Hemorrhagic Inflammation

Hemorrhagic inflammation can result from diapedesis of red blood cells through highly permeable vasculature, or from hemorrhage through small vessels disrupted by inflammation, trauma, microorganisms, or toxic products. Causes include infection with highly virulent organisms such as *Salmonella, Clostridium perfringens, Neorickettsia helminthoeca,* canine hepatitis virus, Leptospira, and parvovirus. Infection with *Prototheca* can cause a hemorrhagic colitis. Hemorrhagic colitis due to *Candida, Zygomycetes, Aspergillus,* and other opportunists has been reported in cats, most commonly in association with panleukopenia. Other causes include poisoning by heavy metals such as arsenic and thallium, plants such as *Amanita* mushrooms, and various household products. Uremia, ischemic disorders such as shock and organ torsion, and immune-mediated disorders such as chronic colitis, can also cause hemorrhagic inflammation. Severe pancreatic inflammation is commonly hemorrhagic in nature.

Suppurative (Purulent) Inflammation

Suppurative inflammation is characterized grossly by pus and microscopically by marked neutrophil infiltration or accumulation. Causes of suppurative inflammation in the liver include bacteremias and viral diseases such as canine hepatitis. Infections of bowel by bacteria such as *Salmonella,* coliforms, *Yersinia enterocolitica,* and certain anaerobic bacteria can result in suppuration (see Table 24–4). In liver, pancreas, and bowel, disorders resulting in ischemia or necrosis are eventually accompanied by neutrophilic infiltrates. Most suppurative processes are acute in nature.

Lymphocytic-Plasmacytic Inflammation

Lymphocytic-plasmacytic inflammation is said to result from "chronic antigenic stimulation." The inciting antigens, however, are poorly defined. In the bowel, the most important antigens are probably proteinaceous products absorbed from the lumen. On occasion, self-antigens probably initiate the inflammation (autoimmunity). In the liver, the inciting antigens are also unknown.

The gross appearance of tissues affected by lymphocytic-plasmacytic inflammation is often unremarkable, and microscopic diagnosis is not without difficulty. The normal bowel has a small complement of lymphocytes, plasma cells, eosinophils, and histiocytes in the lamina propria (especially along the proprial-submucosal junction). The majority of these lymphocytes and plasma cells are committed to IgA secretion (see Chapter 3). In the inflamed bowel the numbers of lymphocytes and plasma cells increase, and their distribution may widen to include the lamina propria of villi. Furthermore, the proportion of IgG- versus IgA-secreting plasma cells increases. Considerable experience is necessary to differentiate normal bowel from mild lymphocytic-plasmacytic enteritis.

Lymphocytic-plasmacytic inflammation is prominent in the idiopathic disorders of lymphocytic-plasmacytic enteritis, chronic gastritis, chronic colitis, chronic hepatitis, and cholangiohepatitis. Lymphocytic infiltrates are common in gluten enteropathy, *Campylobacter* enterocolitis, and cryptosporidiosis. Bacterial overgrowth, giardiasis, and carcinomas are sometimes associated with mild infiltrations of these cell types (see Table 24–3).

Eosinophilic Inflammation

Small numbers of eosinophils are a normal finding in the lamina propria of the bowel, and mild eosinophilic infiltration is a common component of many inflammatory processes, including inflammation resulting from immune-mediated diseases. Known causes of eosinophilic inflammation are parasitic infections and type 1 hypersensitivity disorders (see Table 24–1). On many occasions, the cause of the eosinophilic infiltration is not apparent. Examples include eosinophilic ulcers and hypereosinophilic syndrome in cats, oral eosinophilic granulomas in Siberian Huskies, and eosinophilic gastroenteritis. The eosinophil's release of proteases, oxyradicals, PAF, leukotrienes, and various toxic proteins has a proinflammatory function. Diamine oxidase released by eosinophils dampens the inflammatory response by degrading histamine.

Granulomatous Inflammation

Granulomatous inflammation is characterized by an accumulation of macrophages, some of which mesh to form multinucleated giant cells, and by the deposition of collagen about the irritant focus. The release of interleukin-1 and fibronectin from macrophages stimulates the collagen deposition. Granulomatous inflammation is a chronic process usually resulting from antigens of a relatively indestructible nature. Causes include phycomycosis, systemic mycoses, mycobacteria, tissue stages of parasites, and imbedded foreign material such as starch (see Table 24–2). In cats granulomatous colitis due to FIP has been recognized. Idiopathic granulomatous inflammation occasionally occurs in the bowel and liver. A granulomatous colitis, characterized by accumulation of macrophages containing PAS-positive granules, has been reported in Boxers and French Bulldogs.

Granulomas on occasion may be dominated by eosinophils rather than macrophages. So-called eosinophilic granulomas have been reported in the oral cavity of dogs and cats and the stomach and intestine of dogs. Their cause is unknown.

THERAPY OF INFLAMMATION

Inflammation is best treated by attention to the primary cause. When the cause of chronic inflammation is not apparent and infective causes are considered unlikely, anti-inflammatory drugs such as prednisone are commonly employed. With the exception of 5-aminosalicylate, nonsteroidal anti-inflammatory drugs (NSAIDS) are *not* recommended for the treatment of gastrointestinal inflammation. Good evidence indicates that most NSAIDS worsen bowel inflammation, possibly by increasing bowel permeability or interfering with suppressor T cell function. Furthermore, they may lead to mucosal ulceration. It is likely that free radical scavengers and specific inhibitors of leukotrienes will eventually find application in the treatment of gastrointestinal inflammation. Therapy of gastrointestinal inflammation is described in more detail during the discussion of specific disorders.

REFERENCES

1. Tizard I. Veterinary Immunology. WB Saunders, Philadelphia, 267–280, 1987.
2. Jones TC, Hunt RD. Veterinary Pathology. Lea & Febiger, Philadelphia, 175–213, 1983.
3. Thompson RG. General Veterinary Pathology. WB Saunders, Philadelphia, 163–229, 1984.
4. Nast CC, LeDuc LE. Chemotactic peptides. Mechanisms, functions, and possible role in inflammatory bowel disease. Dig Dis Sci 33:50S–57S, 1988.
5. Hawkey CJ, Rampton DS. Prostaglandins and the gastrointestinal mucosa: Are they important in its function, disease, or treatment? Gastroenterology 89:1162–1188, 1985.
6. Eva Doran J, Lundsgaard-Hansen P. Role of the reticuloendothelial system in the pathogenesis of organ damage. Br J Hosp Med 39:221–225, 1988.
7. Highland RL, Upson DW. Simplified role of prostaglandins in the gastrointestinal tract. Comp Contin Ed Pract Vet 8:188–194, 1986.
8. Goetzl EJ, Burrall BA, Baud L, et al. Generation and recognition of leukotriene mediators of hypersensitivity and inflammation. Dig Dis Sci 33:36S–40S, 1988.
9. Schumert R, Towner J, Zipser RD. Role of eicosanoids in experimental colitis. Dig Dis Sci 33:58S–64S, 1988.
10. Venge P, Lindbom A. Inflammation. Almqvist & Wiksell International, Stockholm, 1985.
11. Rask-Madsen, J. The role of eicosanoids in the gastrointestinal tract. Scand J Gastroenterol 22:7S–19S, 1987.
12. Wardle TD, Hall L, Turnberg LA. Inter-relationships between inflammatory mediators released from colonic mucosa in ulcerative colitis and their effects on colonic secretion. Gut 34:503–508, 1993.
13. Cominelli F, Kam L. Inflammatory mediators of inflammatory bowel disease. Cur Opin G 9:534–543, 1993.
14. Hogaboam CM, Bissonnette EY, Chin BC, et al. Prostaglandins inhibit inflammatory mediator release from rat mast cells. Gastroenterology 104:122–129, 1993.
15. Snape WJ, Kao HW. Role of inflammatory mediators in colonic smooth muscle function in ulcerative colitis. Dig Dis Sci 33:65S–70S, 1988.
16. Karayalcin SS, Sturbaum CW, Dixon MU, et al. Immune system-stimulated colonic secretion is mediated by the enteric nervous system. Gastroenterology 94:A217, 1988.
17. von Ritter C, Grisham MB, Hollwarth M, et al. Neutrophil-derived oxidants mediate formyl-methionyl-leucyl-phenylalanine-induced increases in mucosal permeability in rats. Gastroenterology 97:778–780, 1989.
18. Ferry DM, Butt TJ, Broom MF, et al. Bacterial chemotactic oligopeptides and the intestinal mucosal barrier. Gastroenterology 97:61–67, 1989.
19. Anton PA, Targan SR, Shanahan F. Neutrophil differences in FMLP-induced chemiluminescence and FMLP receptor number in patients with inflammatory bowel disease. Gastroenterology 94:A9, 1988.
20. Trowald-Wigh G, Thoren-Tolling K. Chemiluminescence and chemotaxis assay of canine granulocytes: A methodological study. Acta Vet Scand 31:79–86, 1990.
21. Douglas WW. Histamine and 5-hydroxytryptamine (serotonin) and their antagonists. In: Goodman Gilman A, Goodman LS, Rall TW (eds) The Pharmacological Basis of Therapeutics. Macmillan, New York, 628–635, 1985.
22. Wallace JL, Gingras GR. Mediation of adaptive cytoprotection by 5-hydroxytryptamine? Gastroenterology 94:A485, 1988.
23. Douglas WW. Polypeptides—angiotensin, plasma kinins, and others. In: Goodman Gilman A, Goodman LS, Rall TW (eds) The Pharmacological Basis of Therapeutics. Macmillan, New York, 653–659, 1985.
24. Tizard I. Veterinary Immunology. WB Saunders, Philadelphia, 115–126, 1987.
25. Jewell DP, Patel C. Immunology of inflammatory bowel disease. Scand J Gastroenterol 20:119S–126S, 1985.
26. Jacob HS, Vercellotti GM. Granulocyte-mediated endothelial injury: Oxidant damage amplified by lactoferrin and platelet activating factor. In: Halliwell B (ed) Oxygen Radicals and Tissue Injury. Upjohn Symposium, Michigan, 57–62, 1987.
27. Boughton-Smith NK, Whittle BJR. Formation of the pro-inflammatory mediatory, PAF-Acether in different models of colitis. Gastroenterology 94:A45, 1988.
28. Wallace JL, MacNaughton WK, Guarner F, et al. Role of leukotrienes as mediators of gastric damage and hemo-concentration induced by platelet-activating factor. Gastroenterology 94:A485, 1988.
29. Dinarello CA. Interleukin-1. Dig Dis Sci 33:25s–35s, 1988.
30. Ligumsky M, Simon PL, Karmeli F, et al. Interleukin-1—possible mediator of the inflammatory response in ulcerative colitis (UC). Gastroenterology 94:A263, 1988.
31. Rachmiliwitz D, Simon PL, Sjogren R, et al. Interleukin-1: A sensitive marker of colonic inflammation. Gastroenterology 94:A363, 1988.
32. Sartor RB, Chapman EJ, Schwab JH. Increased interleukin-1 beta concentrations in resected inflammatory bowel disease (IBD) tissue. Gastroenterology 94:A399, 1988.
33. Beutler B, Cerami A. Cachectin: More than a tumor necrosis factor. New Eng J Med 316:379–385, 1987.
34. Mayer EA, Raybould H, Koelbel C. Neuropeptides, inflammation, and motility. Dig Dis Sci 33:71s–77s, 1988.
35. Stapelfeldt WH, Go VLW, Szurszewski JH. Colonic distension releases substance P in the guinea pig inferior mesenteric ganglion. Gastroenterology 94:A441, 1988.
36. Mazumdar S, Das KM. Immunocytochemical localization of vasoactive intestinal polypeptide and substance P in the colon from normal subjects and patients with inflammatory bowel disease. Am J Gastroenterol 87:176–181, 1992.
37. Croitoru K, Ernst PB, Bienenstock J, et al. The effect of substance P (SP) and vasoactive intestinal polypeptide (VIP) on murine intestinal natural killer activity. Gastroenterology 94:A80, 1988.
38. Hart R, Wagner F, Duncygier H. Substance P enhances immune responses of the gut associated lymphoid tissue. Gastroenterology 94:A174, 1988.
39. Blank MA, Kimura K, Jaffe BM. Vasoactive intestinal polypeptide (VIP) antagonist (N-AC0TYR^1, D-PHE^2)-GRF(1-29)-NH$_2$: An inhibitor of vasodilatation in the feline colon. Gastroenterology 94:A39, 1988.
40. Grisham MB, Granger DN. Neutrophil-mediated mucosal injury. Role of reactive oxygen metabolites. Dig Dis Sci 33:6S–15S, 1988.
41. Hitt ME. Oxygen derived free radicals—their pathophysiology and implications. Comp Contin Ed Pract Vet 10:939–946, 1988.
42. Machlin LJ, Bendich A. Free radical tissue damage: Protective role of antioxidant nutrients. FASEB J 1:441–445, 1987.
43. Cross CE, Halliwell B, Borish ET, et al. Oxygen radicals and human disease. Ann Intern Med 107:526–545, 1987.
44. VanSteenhouse JL. Free radicals: relation to tissue damage—a review. Vet Clin Path 16:29–35, 1987.
45. Parks DA, Bulkley GB, Granger DN. Role of oxygen-derived free radicals in digestive tract diseases. Surgery 94:415–422, 1983.
46. Clark IA, Thumwood CM, Chaudhri G, et al. Tumor necrosis factor and reactive oxygen species. In: Halliwell B (ed) Oxygen Radicals and Tissue Injury. Upjohn Symposium, Michigan, 122–129, 1987.
47. Phian G, Regillo BA, Szabo S. Free radicals and lipid peroxidation in ethanol- or aspirin-induced gastric mucosal injury. Dig Dis Sci 32:1395–1401, 1987.
48. Mitchell JR. Acetaminophen toxicity. New Eng J Med 319:1601–1602, 1988.
49. Madara JL. Gamma-interferon (Gamma-IFN) enhances intestinal epithelial permeability by altering tight junctions. Gastroenterology 94:A276, 1988.
50. Barker IK, Van Dreumel AA. The alimentary system. In: Jubb KVF, Kennedy PC, Palmer N (eds) Pathology of Domestic Animals. Academic Press, Orlando, 1–202, 1985.
51. Van Kruiningen HJ. Gastrointestinal system. In: Thomson RG (ed) Special Veterinary Pathology. BC Decker, Toronto, 133–227, 1988.

5

Approach to Clinical Problems in Gastroenterology

W. GRANT GUILFORD

INTRODUCTION

Diagnosis of medical problems begins with a thorough history and a complete physical examination. If therapy, prognosis, and the likelihood of communicability cannot be determined from the clinical examination, a diagnostic evaluation is advisable. The problem-oriented approach to diagnosis is recommended because it provides a systematic method to approach complex cases (Table 5–1). The diagnostic workup should consist of an orderly series of procedures designed to determine if a particular problem is due to a certain type of disease. The sequence of diagnostic tests that is chosen depends, to a large extent, on logistical concerns such as cost of the procedures and availability of staff and diagnostic equipment. The procedures selected early in the workup are designed to answer more general questions (such as the identity of the organ system(s) involved); they tend to be less invasive, less expensive, and have a higher diagnostic yield than procedures for identifying specific problems or diseases. At times tests designed to detect unlikely, but treatable, diseases are performed early in the workup simply because they diagnose diseases whose outcome the clinician can influence.

Ideally, the workup concludes with an accurate diagnosis. Unfortunately, because of financial constraints, limited knowledge about many canine and feline diseases, and restricted availability of refined diagnostic techniques, the diagnostic workup is often concluded before a specific disease entity is definitively diagnosed. This need not be of concern, provided the diagnostic procedures have sufficiently defined the initial complaint to a point where appropriate therapy, accurate prognosis, and the likelihood of communicability to animals and humans have been determined.

History Taking

The history provides the most rapid and inexpensive progress toward a diagnosis. History taking has been referred to as the greatest of all of the medical arts. Along with the physical examination, it is the foundation on which all future diagnostic procedures are selected. The initial aims of the interview are formulation of a patient profile, definition of the owner's chief complaint, identification of clinical signs of disease, and acquisition of information pertaining to the clinical signs of the present illness (Table 5–2).

A patient profile that includes information about the patient's age, sex, breed, diet, environment, vaccinations, and medical history must be acquired. Breed predispositions to many gastrointestinal diseases have been recognized (Table 5–3). It is extremely important that the history defines the owner's chief complaint. What concerns an owner about a pet may not necessarily be the clinical sign that most concerns the veterinarian. Failure to address the owner's primary concern, while pursuing clinical signs per-

Table 5–1

A PROBLEM-ORIENTED APPROACH TO DIAGNOSIS AND TREATMENT OF GASTROINTESTINAL DISEASES

Step 1 Information gathering (establishing a database)
    A. History
    B. Physical examination
    C. Admission laboratory work
Step 2 Identify and list all problems
Step 3 Establish rule-outs for each problem
Step 4 Design a plan to diagnose each problem
Step 5 Prioritize the workup of each problem and institute diagnostics
    A. Threat to health of patient
    B. Owner's degree of concern
    C. Logistics and expense of workup
Step 6 Update the problem list until a diagnosis is reached or the problem is sufficiently refined
    A. Institute therapy
    B. Advise of prognosis
    C. Educate client about the disease
Step 7 Follow up on each problem
    A. Resolution of signs: end of problem
    B. Unsuccessful therapy: institute further diagnostics

Table 5–2

THE COMPONENTS OF THE MEDICAL INTERVIEW

Patient profile
Owner's primary complaint
Identification of clinical signs of disease
Sequence, frequency, and progression of sign(s)
Character of vomitus or diarrhea
Severity of the signs
Location of site of disease causing the sign(s)
Aggravating or alleviating factors
Review of body systems

50

Table 5–3

SUSPECTED OR CONFIRMED BREED PREDISPOSITIONS TO GASTROINTESTINAL DISEASES

BREED	PREDISPOSITION
Abyssinian	Megaesophagus due to myasthenia gravis
Airedale terrier	Pancreatic carcinoma
Basenji	Lymphocytic/plasmacytic enteritis, hypertrophic gastritis, lymphangiectasia
Beagle	Chronic hepatitis, IgA deficiency
Bedlington terrier	Copper-induced hepatopathy
Belgian shepherds	Gastric carcinoma
Bouviers	Muscular dystrophy and dysphagia
Boston terrier	Vascular compression of the esophagus, constipation
Boxers	Gingival and circumanal neoplasia, mastocytoma, histiocytic colitis
Brachycephalic breeds	Pyloric stenosis
Cairn terriers	Microscopic portovascular dysplasia, portosystemic shunts, congenital bronchoesophageal fistula
Cocker spaniel	Gingival, oropharyngeal, and circumanal neoplasia, chronic hepatitis, portosystemic shunts, cricopharyngeal achalasia
Dachshund	Colonic perforation
Doberman pinscher	Parvovirus, chronic hepatitis
English bulldog	Vascular compression of the esophagus, cleft palate, constipation, fecal incontinence
English springer spaniel	Fucosidosis
Fox terrier	Circumanal neoplasia
German shepherd	Oropharyngeal neoplasia, exocrine pancreatic insufficiency, inflammatory bowel disease, stress-induced diarrhea, megaesophagus, vascular compression of the esophagus, sialocele, hepatic angiosarcoma, perianal fistula, bacterial overgrowth, mesenteric torsion
German short-haired pointer	Oropharyngeal neoplasia
Golden retriever	Oropharyngeal neoplasia
Great Dane	Gastric dilatation-volvulus, megaesophagus
Greyhound	Megaesophagus
Irish setter	Wheat-sensitive enteropathy, megaesophagus, vascular compression of the esophagus, esophageal sarcoma, gastric dilatation-volvulus, perianal fistula
Irish wolfhound	Intrahepatic portosystemic shunts
Jack Russell terrier	Salivary gland necrosis
Labrador	Chronic hepatitis, megaesophagus
Large-breed dogs	Gastric dilatation-volvulus
Lhasa apso	Pyloric stenosis
Lundenhund	Protein-losing enteropathy
Manx cat	Constipation, fecal incontinence
Miniature schnauzer	Hemorrhagic gastroenteritis, hyperlipidemia, pancreatitis, megaesophagus, portosystemic shunts
Newfoundland	Megaesophagus
Pointer	Hepatic angiosarcoma, esophageal sarcoma, cleft palate
Poodle	Sialocele, hemorrhagic gastroenteritis
Rottweiler	Parvovirus, gastric eosinophilic granuloma
Scottish terriers	Chronic hepatitis
Sharpei	IgA deficiency, food intolerances, inflammatory bowel disease, hiatal herniation, megaesophagus
Shih tzu	Cleft palate, pyloric stenosis
Siamese cat	Megaesophagus, gastric retention, intestinal adenocarcinoma
Siberian husky	Oral eosinophilic granuloma
Skye terriers	Chronic hepatitis
Small-breed dogs	Hemorrhagic gastroenteritis, pyloric stenosis
Standard poodles	Lobular dissecting hepatitis
Swiss sheepdog	Cleft palate
Weimaraner	Oropharyngeal neoplasia
West Highland white terrier	Copper-associated hepatopathy, chronic hepatitis
Wirehaired fox terrier	Megaesophagus
Yorkshire terriers	Portosystemic shunts, lymphangiectasia

ceived as more serious by the veterinarian, is an important cause of owner dissatisfaction. The history should begin with general questions pertaining to this complaint and proceed to more specific interrogation as signs of disease are revealed.

Signs of digestive system dysfunction may be classified as primary or secondary signs according to their specificity for gastrointestinal disease (Table 5–4). Primary signs, such as dysphagia, regurgitation, vomition, bloat, borborygmus, diarrhea, dyschezia, melena, tenesmus, abdominal pain, flatulence, icterus, and ascites, strongly suggest digestive system dysfunction is present (either as a result of local or systemic disease). Secondary signs, such as anorexia, fever, depression, dehydration, polyphagia, weight loss, polydypsia, hypersaliva-

tion, shivering, and shock, are not at all specific for gastrointestinal system disease but, collectively, are commonly seen when this system is abnormal. The identification of all primary and secondary signs aids in determining the most likely site of the problem and assessing the severity of the animal's condition.

Historical information to be determined about each clinical sign is depicted in Table 5–2. It is important to determine when a sign was first noticed, and which of a number of signs was seen first. The frequency of occurrence of a given sign must also be noted. Additional information should be collected on the duration of a symptom and the intervals between periods of illness. The character of vomitus and bowel movements often provides useful information for dif-

Table 5-4

CLINICAL SIGNS OF GASTROINTESTINAL DISEASE

PRIMARY SIGNS	SECONDARY SIGNS
Dysphagia	Anorexia
Regurgitation	Fever
Vomition	Depression
Bloat	Cardiovascular signs
Borborygmus	Hypersalivation
Diarrhea	Shivering
Dyschezia	Behavioral changes
Melena	Perineal pruritis
Tenesmus	Polyphagia
Abdominal pain	Dehydration
Flatulence	
Icterus	
Ascites	

ferential diagnosis. The clinician should attempt to determine the anatomic location of the dysfunction. Identification of the site of a problem is of great value in deciding which procedures should be ordered first in a workup of the case. The severity of the sign or the limitation of function imposed by the disease should also be described. The severity of the process determines the necessity of supportive therapy and the appropriate amount of diagnostic effort. The owner should be queried to discover any factors that incite, aggravate, or alleviate the sign. Knowledge of aggravating or alleviating factors will not only help the clinician arrive at a diagnosis but often provide valuable clues toward outlining a successful management program. The history is concluded by screening other systems of the body with appropriate questions. The importance of this systems review cannot be overemphasized. The gastrointestinal system influences, and in turn is influenced by, other body systems. Even when the predominant clinical signs appear to result from gastrointestinal disease, asking questions pertaining only to the gastrointestinal tract ignores the strong likelihood that a disease of another system may be causing secondary gastrointestinal dysfunction. Furthermore, it is not uncommon for animals to have more than one disease process affecting different body systems.

The Physical Examination

The objective of the physical examination is to recognize and describe gross deviations of physical appearance and behavior of the patient from those recognized as normal for the animal's age, sex, and breed. Information gathered from laboratory or radiologic procedures cannot make up for an incompletely conducted physical examination. The discussion here is limited to physical examination features directly pertinent to the gastrointestinal system, but the clinician should examine all body systems when presented with an animal manifesting signs of gastrointestinal disease. Ophthalmic and neurologic examinations should not be forgotten because at times they can provide invaluable clues to the cause of the gastrointestinal dysfunction (for example, FIP; third eyelid prolapse and diarrhea syndrome; cranial nerve abnormalities suggestive of vomiting due to an intracranial mass).

UNRESTRAINED PATIENT. The physical examination should begin by observing the unrestrained patient on the floor. The animal's size, weight, mentation, posture, respiratory rate,

and behavior can be evaluated at this time while it is likely to be less excited. This is also a convenient time to give the patient food or water if swallowing or mastication is to be observed.

OROPHARYNX AND CERVICAL AREA. Physical examination for diagnosis of gastrointestinal signs includes examination of the oral and pharyngeal cavities. Complete examination of these structures often requires the patient to be anesthetized. Particular attention should be paid to the presence of foreign bodies that can become fixed in the oral cavity and pharynx. Examination of the tongue is assisted by dorsally directed digital pressure between the mandibular rami. Failure to recognize a string foreign body about the base of the tongue can seriously delay a diagnosis of obstruction due to a linear foreign body. The cervical region is examined for salivary gland abnormalities, lymphadenopathy, and masses that may be interfering with the movement of a bolus through the esophagus and for evidence of any dilated, flaccid, or air-filled enlargements of the esophagus. In cats, careful palpation of the neck for thyroid nodules is recommended.

ABDOMINAL PALPATION. Abdominal palpation is an important part of the physical examination. Palpation is best accomplished by standing directly behind a patient made to stand on the examining table. Palpation must be systematic, and best sensitivity is afforded by alternating application and release of firm inward pressure on the abdomen by the fingers of both hands laid flat against the patient's abdomen. Raising the front end of the animal facilitates palpation of cranial abdominal organs. Sedation or anesthesia may be necessary for adequate examination. The stomachs of cats and dogs are usually difficult to palpate unless distended by ingesta. The intestines should feel soft, smooth, and should slide freely from between the examiner's hands. The ileocecal area of cats can often be palpated as a firmer knotlike structure in the midcranial abdomen, and should not be confused with an abdominal mass. The colon can usually be defined because of its content of feces. Fecal material will normally indent or fragment when gently squeezed between the fingers, thus differentiating it from abdominal masses. The liver of healthy dogs is usually very difficult to palpate, whereas in healthy cats the liver can usually be felt. When examining tractable animals, standing in front of the patient and hooking the fingers behind the costochondral arch facilitates palpation of the liver. Abdominal fluid may be detected by observation of a fluid wave that radiates from a site of percussion on one side of the abdomen to the other side of the abdomen.

ABDOMINAL AUSCULTATION. Examination of the gastrointestinal tract may include auscultation of the abdomen.[1] Most bowel sounds originate in the stomach; those that originate in the small intestine and colon are briefer. The colon generates sounds of high amplitude, short duration, and low frequency. Air increases the amplitude and frequency of sounds, especially in the stomach. However, fluid in the small intestine increases the number of sounds. Bowel sounds are caused by accumulated fluid and gas moving from one region to another. Peristaltic motility must be reduced for fluid and gas to accumulate. Thus, paradoxically, abnormal increases in bowel sounds are a reflection of a partial loss of intestinal motility rather than an augmentation of motility. Increased bowel sounds will result from agitation of abnormal accumulations of air and liquid in the stomach, as well as from faster movement of fluid and gas through the small intestine and colon as a result of decreased segmental contractility. If sounds are to be heard, sufficient motility must remain to produce movement of the accumulated fluid and gas. Few bowel sounds are heard when motility has disappeared, as in an ileus.[2] In general, auscultation of the abdomen is most useful for the detection of ileus. Failure to detect borborygmus after two to three minutes of auscultation suggests ileus. Auscultation of the abdomen will also occasionally reveal a vascular murmur that is produced by an intra-abdominal circulatory problem such as an arteriovenous shunt.

RECTAL EXAMINATION. Examination of the abdominal cavity is not complete without a digital examination of the rectum. The rectal examination will provide a sample of stool for examination and will reveal abnormalities of the anus, anal glands, rectum, prostate, pelvic diaphragm, and pelvis. The importance of this procedure is obvious when the patient has signs of tenesmus or obstipation but is just as important in evaluating vomiting or diarrhea.

HALITOSIS

Owners frequently complain about halitosis in dogs and less frequently in cats. Common causes of halitosis are listed in Table 5–5. Important medical history includes the nature of the diet and whether the animal practices coprophagia. High-protein diets or diets with poorly digestible protein are sometimes associated with halitosis, perhaps because of the excretion in the breath of odiferous products, such as ammonia, hydrogen sulfide, indoles, and skatoles, derived from the fermentation of incompletely absorbed protein in the large bowel. Remnants of food retained in the oral cavity and degraded by bacteria may also be sufficient to cause disagreeable smells.

Physical examination must include careful inspection of the ears, oral cavity, and lips. It is not uncommon for the smell of otitis externa to be mistaken for halitosis. Similarly, cheilitis is common in certain breeds, such as cocker spaniels, and can result in a surprisingly strong objectionable smell. The most common cause of halitosis is dental disease. Occasionally, other inflammatory or necrotizing oral or pharyngeal lesions such as neoplasia cause halitosis. The odor predominantly

Table 5–5

CAUSES OF HALITOSIS

Dietary associated
  Food remnants
  Highly proteinaceous diets
  Coprophagia
Diseases of the lips
  Chelitis
Oral cavity diseases
  Inflammatory or necrotizing oral lesions
  Foreign bodies
Pharyngeal diseases
  Inflammatory or necrotizing pharyngeal lesions
  Pharyngeal foreign bodies
  Tonsillar crypt foreign bodies
Nasal cavity and sinus disease
  Inflammatory diseases
  Necrotizing diseases
Dental disease
  Periodontitis
  Gingivitis
  Tooth root abscesses
  Tartar
Esophageal diseases
  Megaesophagus
Malassimilation
Systemic diseases
  Uremia
  Liver disease

results from the breakdown of sulfur-containing amino acids derived from oral bacteria or cellular debris. Discharges from nasal lesions that drain caudally into the pharynx can also result in halitosis. Foreign bodies impacted in the nasal cavity, pharynx, oral cavity, or tonsillar crypts can cause halitosis either by inciting inflammation and necrosis or because of their own fermentation, as in the case of food. The fermentation of retained food in a dilated or obstructed esophagus is an occasional cause of halitosis, as are protein malassimilation and systemic diseases such as uremia and liver failure.

Most cases of halitosis can be diagnosed by history and a through physical examination of the mouth, oral cavity, and pharynx. Occasionally, radiographs of the teeth, nasal cavity, pharynx, or esophagus are required. Examination of the nasopharynx with a dental mirror or endoscope and the nasal cavity with a rhinoscope is sometimes helpful. Management of halitosis depends on the primary cause but can include the provision of a highly digestible diet and dental prophylaxis.

DROOLING AND XEROSTOMIA

Drooling can result because of excessive production of saliva (ptyalism, hypersalivation, sialorrhea), or because of failure to swallow saliva produced in normal quantities (pseudoptyalism). Prominent causes of drooling are listed in Table 5–6. Drooling is a common response of the dog to imminent feeding and to high ambient temperature. In the cat drooling often accompanies purring.

Hypersalivation may be seen with inflammatory or painful oropharyngeal lesions. Important examples are foreign bodies and insect bites. Toxins responsible for excess salivation include those that irritate the oral cavity (caustics), thallium, metaldehyde, organophosphates, cresol, the secretions of various toads and newts, and certain plants such as *Amanita* mushrooms, nettles, and dumbcane. Certain medications, especially in cats, can result in copious salivation. Examples include trimethoprim/sulfadiazine, piperazine, metronidazole, cephalexin, and disinfectants. Any disease that results in nausea causes hypersalivation. Ptyalism is a characteristic clinical sign of portosystemic shunts in cats. Drooling has been reported with several diseases of the salivary gland, including infarction of the mandibular salivary gland and parotid salivary gland hyperplasia. Infectious disorders such as rabies, pseudorabies, botulism, and tetanus can result in drooling. Several dogs with gastroesophageal leiomyomas diagnosed at the University of California (UCD) VMTH have been observed to drool. The cause of the hypersalivation was not determined, but the drooling resolved after surgical removal of the leiomyoma.

Pseudoptyalism occurs when an animal is unable or unwilling to swallow saliva. Pseudoptyalism can result from conformational abnormalities of the mouth and lips (Saint Bernards), diseases causing oral deformity, disorders of the lips, or disorders of swallowing.

The diagnostic evaluation of drooling relies heavily on the history and physical examination. Great care is required if rabies is at all suspected. Careful observation of the patient will often differentiate drooling due to nausea or swallowing difficulty from the other causes of hypersalivation. The differentiation of these categories of drooling is important because they have widely disparate diagnostic workups. Animals hypersalivating due to nausea will usually demonstrate other signs of nausea such as depression, lip licking, and retching. The appropriate workup to institute is that described for the evaluation of vomiting. Animals drooling due to swallowing disor-

Table 5–6

CAUSES OF DROOLING: PTYALISM AND
PSEUDOPTYALISM

Physiologic
  Imminent feeding
  Hyperthermia
  Purring
Toxicants/irritants
  Poisons (caustics, metaldehyde, organophosphates, cresol, ivermectin, others)
  Plants (*Amanita* mushrooms, nettles, dumbcane, philodendron, poinsettia, others)
  Insect/spider bites
  Secretions of toads and newts
Medications
  Antibiotics (trimethoprim/sulfadiazine, cephalexin)
  Anthelmintics (piperazine, levamisole, bunamidine)
  Disinfectants
  Others
Oropharyngeal diseases
  Inflammatory lesions
  Neoplasia
  Foreign bodies
Salivary gland diseases
  Parotid salivary gland hyperplasia
  Mandibular salivary gland infarction
Infectious disorders
  Rabies
  Pseudorabies
  Botulism
  Tetanus
Pseudoptyalism
  Conformational or innervation problems of the mouth and lips
  Deforming diseases of the mouth and lips
  Swallowing disorders
  Trigeminal neuritis
Miscellaneous
  Disorders causing nausea
  Hypoparathyroidism
  Portosystemic shunts (cats)
  Gastroesophageal leiomyoma

ders will often show evidence of dysphagia, and should be evaluated as such.

Consequence of persistent drooling include cheilitis and acne. Hypersalivation leads to increased aerophagia. The treatment of hypersalivation is varied because of the wide disparity of causes. Refractory hypersalivation can be treated by extreme measures such as excision of salivary glands or parasympathetic denervation.

Xerostomia, or dryness of the mouth, is uncommon. Panting animals will occasionally have a dry mouth. Xerostomia can be caused by feline and canine dysautonomia. It has also been reported following extensive radiation therapy of the head and neck and as a result of Sjogren syndrome. The latter is an autoimmune disease of the lacrimal and salivary glands.

DYSPHAGIA, REGURGITATION, VOMITING, RETCHING, GAGGING, AND EXPECTORATION

Definitions and Differentiation

Dysphagia, regurgitation, vomiting, retching, and gagging are important clinical signs associated with problems in the pharynx, esophagus, stomach, and small intestine (Table 5–7). In contrast, expectoration is a sign of airway disease or (particularly in cats) accumulation of debris, such as fur, in the laryngopharynx. Dysphagia, gagging, and regurgitation are evaluated differently than vomiting, retching, and expectoration. Failure to differentiate these problems during the clinical examination (Table 5–8) is a major cause of misdiagnosis. It is important to note, however, that patients may present with a mix of these clinical signs. For instance, regurgitation and vomiting are occasionally observed concurrently when chronic vomition leads to an esophagitis.

Dysphagia is defined as difficult or painful swallowing. Dysphagia may be further divided according to the anatomic area in which the swallowing dysfunction originates. Although regurgitation is the most prominent clinical sign of both oropharyngeal dysphagia and esophageal dysphagia, it is usually possible on a clinical basis to separate the two syndromes. Patients affected by oropharyngeal dysphagia make exaggerated swallowing movements and usually food will drop from the mouth within seconds of prehension. In contrast, esophageal dysphagia results in more delayed regurgitation and is usually not associated with exaggerated swallowing movements. More refined definition of dysphagia into disorders of the oral, pharyngeal, cricopharyngeal, esophageal, or gastroesophageal stage of swallowing requires barium swallows and fluoroscopy.

Regurgitation is defined as the retrograde expulsion of ingesta from the esophagus or pharynx. It most often results from esophageal disease. Regurgitation is a passive event with few prodromal signs. There is no abdominal effort and no initiation of reflex neural pathways other than the gag reflex (although some dogs may show a degree of retrograde peristaltic activity similar to vomiting).[3] Food is regurgitated from the esophagus and pharynx primarily under the influence of gravitation. There are usually no prodromal signs of nausea, although drooling because of inability to swallow saliva can on occasion give the impression of hypersalivation due to nausea. Regurgitated food is usually undigested and may take on a tubular shape if originating in the esophagus. The pH should not be acidic unless food has been first refluxed from the stomach. Regurgitated material from the esophagus is rarely bile stained, except for the infrequent occasions when regurgitation is preceded by esophagogastroduodenal reflux. Regurgitation may occur immediately after eating or may be delayed for several hours. Pharyngeal and cranial esophageal problems are typically characterized by immediate regurgitation, whereas esophageal disorders involving the lower cervical or intrathoracic segment are characterized by regurgitation that may be delayed for hours after eating.

Vomiting is the forceful, reflexive ejection of gastric content from the stomach following stimulation of a neural reflex

Table 5–7

CLINICAL SIGNS ASSOCIATED WITH DISORDERED
PHARYNGEAL, ESOPHAGEAL, GASTRIC, AND/OR
SMALL INTESTINAL FUNCTION

Vomiting	Cough
Regurgitation	Abdominal pain
Dysphagia	Bloat
Anorexia	Retching
Polyphagia	Malnutrition
Pica	Shivering
Hypersalivation	Polydipsia
Esophageal colic	Melena
Dyspnea	Dehydration

Table 5–8

DIFFERENTIATION OF OROPHARYNGEAL DYSPHAGIA,
ESOPHAGEAL DYSPHAGIA, AND VOMITING

	OROPHARYNGEAL DYSPHAGIA	ESOPHAGEAL DYSPHAGIA	VOMITING
Abdominal effort	None	None	Marked
Signs of nausea	None	None	None
Time of food ejection	Immediate	Delayed, possibly for hours	Delayed, possibly for hours
Character of food ejected	Undigested	Undigested	Can be partially digested, bile stained, and with acid pH
Number of swallowing attempts with single bolus	Multiple	Usually single	Single
Visible evidence of bolus passing in the cervical esophagus	Not present	Present, maybe prolonged	Present
Ability to drink	Poor	Variable	Normal
Pain on swallowing	Possible	Possible	Absent
Associated signs frequently seen	Dyspnea, cough	Dyspnea, cough	Retching
Aggravating and alleviating factors frequently seen	Food consistency; exercise	Food consistency	None

that has synaptic centers in the brain stem. As described in Chapter 13, vomiting is accomplished by pronounced contraction of the muscles of the diaphragm and abdomen. It is always preceded by signs of nausea such as restlessness, depression, hypersalivation, lip licking, frequent swallowing, and retching. Low pH or presence of bile in the ejected material implies but does not prove vomiting. Material of alkaline pH may be vomit or it may have been regurgitated. Alkaline vomitus is not uncommon and results from reduced gastric acid secretion, gastroduodenal reflux, swallowed saliva, and the buffering of food.

Gagging is a reflexive contraction of the constrictor muscles of the pharynx resulting from stimulation of the pharyngeal mucosa. Retention of food in the pharynx can stimulate the gag reflex, with regurgitation following. *Retching* is an involuntary and ineffectual attempt at vomiting. Retching is produced by contractions of the diaphragm and abdominal muscles, the same motor events that cause vomition. Retching and gagging should be carefully differentiated from expectoration. *Expectoration* refers to the ejection of airway and laryngopharyngeal discharges or debris. It is usually accompanied by the harsh loud sounds of forceful expiration. It is not uncommon for owners to confuse the forceful expectoration of airway fluid, such as commonly occurs with tracheobronchitis, with retching, gagging, or even vomiting. Differentiation is readily made by examination of pharynx and the ejected material, and by the presence or absence of nausea. Dogs with tracheobronchitis expectorate small quantities of white foam and do not show evidence of nausea or pharyngeal diseases that might cause gagging. Cats frequently expectorate and regurgitate to clear accumulated fur and saliva from the laryngopharynx and esophagus. This is often mistaken by owners as "vomiting" due to fur balls.

EATING DIFFICULTY

Eating difficulty may result from disorders of the jaw, oral cavity, tongue, pharynx, or esophagus. Eating difficulty should be differentiated from inappetence, a distinction that may escape the client. The diagnostic procedures employed in the evaluation of a patient experiencing eating difficulty depend on the tenta-tive localization of the site of the disorder. This is determined by history, physical examination, and observation of the patient consuming a meal. Together, these endeavors can usually differentiate disorders of prehension, mastication, and the oropharyngeal or esophageal phase of swallowing.

Disorders of Prehension and Mastication

Animals with disorders of the oral cavity, tongue, or jaws have difficulty grasping and chewing food. The principal causes of prehension and mastication difficulty are listed in Table 5–9. History of importance includes a review of the rabies vaccination record; inquiry as to any consumption of carrion that may result in botulism; and exposure to plants, electrical cord, insects, or caustic products that could produce stomatitis. Generalized weakness in association with the eating difficulty is supportive of diseases such as myasthenia gravis or botulism.

Physical examination may reveal weak, ineffectual, or uncoordinated jaw movements. If the tongue is affected, animals may have difficulty lapping water and soft foods, and the tongue may loll out of the mouth. An affected animal may place its head deeply into its water bowl to allow drinking. On occasion the patient will hold its head to one side to avoid painful lesions on one side of the mouth or jaw. Inability to open the mouth is commonly associated with disorders of the masticatory muscles such as masticatory muscle myositis (trismus), abnormalities of the temporomandibular joints, and retrobulbar abscess. Physical inability to close the mouth is most often due to the coronoid process locking ventrally and laterally to the zygomatic arch, or due to temporomandibular dysplasia. Trigeminal nerve neuritis is characterized by an acute onset of transient, flaccid paralysis of the muscles that close the mouth, resulting in a slack jaw that dangles open. Neurologic examination may reveal evidence of neuropathies of other cranial nerves, or CNS lesions. Oropharyngeal examination may disclose painful oropharyngeal lesions worthy of culture (rarely helpful) or biopsy. Signs of systemic disorders (uremia, sepsis, SLE) may be observed. The diagnostic procedures of utility for the evaluation of these disorders are listed in Table 5–10.

Table 5–9

CAUSES OF DIFFICULT OR PAINFUL PREHENSION AND MASTICATION

Stomatitis/Glossitis/Gingivitis
  Physical agents (electrical cord burns, trauma, insect bites)
  Caustics agents (petroleum products, alkalis, acids, thallium)
  Bacterial infections (*Bacteroides melaninogenicus?*)
  Viral infections (feline rhinotracheitis, calici, FeLV, FIV)
  Fungal infections (Candida)
  Foreign bodies (fiberglass, imbedded plant material)
  Autoimmune diseases (SLE, pemphigus and pemphigoid diseases)
  Immune-mediated disorders (toxic epidermal necrolysis, idiopathic feline glossopharyngitis, eosinophilic granuloma)
  Immunodeficiencies
  Systemic disorders (uremia, sepsis)
Oral/Glossal Neoplasia
  Squamous cell carcinoma
  Fibrosarcoma
  Melanoma
  Rhabdomyosarcoma
Neurologic Disorders
  Rabies
  Trigeminal paralysis
  Polyneuropathies
  Neosporosis
  Neuropathies of cranial nerves VII, IX, X, XII
  CNS lesions (cerebellar disorders, brain stem lesions, hydrocephalus)
Neuromuscular Junction Disorders
  Myasthenia gravis
  Botulism
Musculoskeletal Disorders
  Masticatory myositis (eosinophilic, plasmacytic/lymphocytic)
  Masticatory muscle myopathy
  Temporomandibular joint arthropathy
  Open-mouth jaw locking
  Renal secondary hyperparathyroidism
  Hyperparathyroidism
  Mandible fracture or subluxation
  Craniomandibular osteoarthropathy
Miscellaneous Disorders
  Retrobulbar abscess
  Salivary gland disorders
  Dental disorders (tooth root abscesses, fractured teeth, odontoclastic resorption)

Table 5–10

DIAGNOSTIC PROCEDURES OF VALUE FOR THE DIAGNOSIS OF DIFFICULT OR PAINFUL PREHENSION AND MASTICATION

PROCEDURE	USEFULNESS
Anesthesia Oropharyngeal Examination	Oropharyngeal lesions, foreign bodies
Neurologic Examination	Disorders of cranial nerves V, VII, IX, X, and XII, CNS lesions, polyneuropathies
Admission Laboratory Work	
Blood eosinophil count	Masticatory myositis
BUN level	Uremia
CPK level	Myositis
Calcium/phosphorus levels	Hyperparathyroidism
Serum Tests	
ANA	SLE
Acetylcholine receptor antibody test	Myasthenia gravis
Fine Needle Aspiration	
Temporomandibular joints	Inflammatory/infectious arthritis
Masticatory muscles	Myositis
Mandibular or retropharyngeal lymph nodes	Neoplasia, lymphadenitis
Radiographs	
Teeth	Abscess
Temporomandibular joints	Arthropathy, subluxation
Maxilla and mandible	Osteoporosis, fracture, craniomandibular osteoarthropathy
Ultrasound	
Retropharyngeal area	Lymphadenopathy, foreign body, neoplasia
Biopsy	Oral lesions, myositis, myopathy, salivary gland disorders

Oropharyngeal Dysphagia

Dysphagia may result from dysfunction of the tongue, pharynx, or esophagus. Important causes of dysphagia are listed in Table 5–11. Animals with oropharyngeal dysphagia will usually prehend food readily but are unable to swallow the food normally. If concurrent dysfunction of the tongue is present, prehension and mastication, as well as swallowing, may be compromised. Affected animals may throw their heads back, or conversely ventroflex their necks while swallowing. They may drool persistently because of incomplete swallowing of saliva. Nasal discharge may develop after reflux of food into the nasopharynx and nasal cavity. A cough may be present if food or saliva retained in the pharynx by ineffectual pharyngeal contractions is aspirated into the airway. The gag reflex may be impaired. Useful diagnostic procedures are listed in Table 5–12 and include review of rabies vaccination record; neurologic examination with particular attention to cranial nerves VII, IX, X, and XII; general anesthesia followed by a thorough oropharyngeal examination, including oropharyngeal palpation (use gloves); examination of the tongue, palate, tonsils, and tonsillar crypts, paying particular attention to the presence of masses or foreign bodies; exami-

nation of the nasopharynx with a retroflexed endoscope; pharyngeal radiographs; and fluoroscopic examination of the swallowing of barium liquid and barium-coated food.

Esophageal Dysphagia

Dysphagia due to esophageal disease is usually characterized by the clinical sign of regurgitation. The diagnostic approach to esophageal dysphagia is described under the problem of regurgitation.

REGURGITATION

The differentiation of regurgitation from vomiting has been described. Regurgitation is usually a result of esophageal dysfunction, and less frequently pharyngeal disorders. Causes of regurgitation are listed in Table 5–13. The diagnostic procedures commonly employed for the evaluation of patients with regurgitation are listed in Table 5–12.

History

Rabies vaccination status should be assessed before examining any case of regurgitation. Exaggerated swallowing efforts in association with immediate regurgitation in a pup is indicative of cricopharyngeal achalasia. Regurgitation in young pups is most commonly a result of idiopathic megaesophagus or a vascular anomaly such as persistent right aortic arch. If a dilated esopha-

Table 5–11

CAUSES OF OROPHARYNGEAL DYSPHAGIA

Glossal Disorders
  Glossal neoplasia
  Neuropathies of cranial nerves VII, IX, XII
  Hydrocephalus, brain stem lesions
Pharyngitis/Tonsillitis
  Physical agents (trauma, heat, insect bites)
  Caustics agents (petroleum products, alkalis, acids, thallium)
  Infections (bacteria, infectious canine hepatitis, candida)
  Immune-mediated disorders (idiopathic feline glossopharyngitis,
    eosinophilic granuloma, allergic pharyngitis)
  Immunodeficiencies
  Systemic disorders (uremia, sepsis)
Pharyngeal Neoplasia
  Squamous cell carcinoma, fibrosarcoma, melanoma, tonsillar
    carcinoma, nasopharyngeal polyps
Retropharyngeal Disorders
  Lymphadenopathy, lymphadenitis
  Neoplasia
  Hematoma, abscess
Pharyngeal, Neuromuscular Disorders
  Rabies
  Pseudorabies
  Neuropathies of cranial nerves VII, IX, X
  CNS lesions (cerebellar disorders, brain stem lesions)
  Cricopharyngeal achalasia
  Hypoparathyroidism
  Idiopathic multiple neuromuscular dysfunctions
  Myasthenia gravis
  Muscular dystrophy in Bouviers
  Botulism
Palate Disorders
  Congenitally short or cleft palate
Miscellaneous
  Fractured or dislocated hyoid bones
  Neosporosis
  Pharyngeal foreign bodies
  Salivary gland neoplasia
  Sialocele
  Trigeminal paralysis

Table 5–12

DIAGNOSTIC PROCEDURES OF VALUE FOR THE DIAGNOSIS OF DYSPHAGIA AND REGURGITATION

PROCEDURE	USEFULNESS
CBC	Pneumonia, immune-mediated disease, hypoadrenocorticism, lead toxicosis
Serum chemistry profile	Myositis, hypoadrenocorticism
CPK	Myositis
Urinalysis	Proteinuria supportive of SLE
Fecal	Spirocerca lupi
ANA	SLE
ACTH stimulation test	Hypoadrenocorticism
Distemper titers	Distemper
Acetylcholine receptor antibody test	Acquired myasthenia gravis
Oropharyngeal exam under anesthesia	Foreign body, tonsils, masses
Survey radiographs	Megaesophagus, mediastinitis, peri-esophageal masses, esophageal or pharyngeal foreign bodies, fractured hyoid bones
Swallowing study	Megaesophagus, motility disorders, stricture, fistula, diverticula, hiatal disorders, periesophageal masses, esophageal masses, vascular ring anomalies, reflux esophagitis, cricopharyngeal achalasia
Gastrogram	Gastric disorders, pyloric obstruction
Endoscopic exam of nasopharynx	Pharyngeal masses, foreign bodies.
Esophagoscopy and biopsy	Esophagitis, obstructive diseases
Esophageal manometry	Achalasia, esophageal neuromuscular diseases, gastroesophageal reflux
CSF tap	Brain stem diseases, distemper
Evoked potentials	Brain stem diseases
EEG	Hydrocephalus
CT scan/MRI	Brain stem disease, hydrocephalus
Electromyography	Myopathy, polyneuropathy
Nerve conduction velocities	Polyneuropathy
Repetitive stimulation	Neuromuscular junction diseases
Tensilon test	Myasthenia gravis
Muscle biopsy	Polymyopathy, polymyositis
Nerve biopsy	Polyneuropathy
Toxicology	Plasma cholinesterase, lead, thallium
Exploratory surgery	Periesophageal masses, hiatal disorders

gus is recognized in a pup, and a vascular ring anomaly is ruled out by a barium swallow, the probable diagnosis is idiopathic megaesophagus, and it is rarely justified to proceed with further diagnostics. In older dogs, however, the incidence of regurgitation due to secondary megaesophagus is much higher, and a more indepth workup is justified. A history of acute onset of regurgitation following bone or chew-toy ingestion raises the possibility of esophageal foreign body. Cats frequently regurgitate fur. Regurgitation beginning several weeks after a general anesthetic suggests esophageal stricture following gastroesophageal reflux. Regurgitation of solids but not liquids is suggestive of partial obstruction of the esophagus. The patient's environment determines the likelihood of toxicities causing esophagitis or vagal neuropathy (for example, lead), and dictates the likelihood of access to carrion that may cause botulism. An associated cough may be indicative of concurrent aspiration pneumonia, or rarely, bronchoesophageal fistulation. The history is concluded by screening other systems of the body with appropriate questions to help detect systemic causes of swallowing dysfunction and to identify incidental problems.

Physical Examination

A complete physical examination should be performed. Particular attention is paid to examination of the oropharynx and neck for evidence of oropharyngeal foreign bodies or cervical

masses. In some dogs, a dilated cervical esophagus may be visualized by forcibly compressing the animal's thorax while briefly occluding its nostrils. If there is gas present in a flaccid esophagus, the result will be a ballooning dilation of the cervical part of the esophagus, visible to an observer carefully regarding the animal's left cervical area. Fermentation of food in a dilated esophagus may result in gurgling sounds and halitosis. Other physical examination findings that aid differential diagnosis of regurgitation include evidence of CNS disorders, lower motor neuron dysfunction (polyneuropathy), distemper, muscle weakness (myasthenia gravis, hypoadrenocorticism, botulism), muscle pain (polymyopathy), and skin or mucous membrane lesions (SLE). Dysautonomia, an important cause of regurgitation in the cat, has characteristic clinical signs including dilated pupils and dry mucous membranes.

Admission Laboratory Work

Admission laboratory tests (CBC, serum chemistry profile, urinalysis, fecal flotation) rarely help differentiate the causes of regurgitation. Exceptions include laboratory work suggestive of lead toxicity (basophilic stippling, nucleated RBC);

Table 5–13

CAUSES OF REGURGITATION

PHARYNGEAL DISORDERS
Pharyngeal obstructive disorders
   Foreign bodies
   Pharyngeal tonsillar neoplasia
   Retropharyngeal lymphadenopathy
Pharyngeal neuromuscular disorders
   Rabies
   Botulism
   Neuropathies of cranial nerves IX, X
   CNS lesions (cerebellar disorders, brain stem lesions)
   Cricopharyngeal achalasia
   Myasthenia gravis
Palate disorders
   Congenitally short or cleft palate

ESOPHAGEAL DISORDERS
Esophagitis
Esophageal obstructive disorders
   Foreign bodies
   Stricture
   Neoplasia
   Vascular ring anomalies
   Periesophageal masses
   Granulomas (spirocerca lupi)
Esophageal neuromuscular disorders
   Megaesophagus*
   Motility abnormalities
Esophageal diverticula
Hiatal disorders

MISCELLANEOUS
   Physiologic (lactating bitches)

---

*Megaesophagus has a large number of possible causes. They are listed in Table 11–3.

SLE (anemia, lymphopenia, thrombocytopenia, acanthocytes, proteinuria); hypoadrenocorticism (eosinophilia, lymphocytosis, neutropenia, decreased sodium/potassium ratio); and *Spirocerca lupi* (ova).

Diagnostic Imaging

Survey radiographs of the pharynx, neck, and chest identify most cases of megaesophagus and many cases of pharyngeal and esophageal foreign body. They occasionally reveal a hiatal disorder. The detection of megaesophagus does not obviate the need for further diagnostics because megaesophagus in itself has a variety of possible causes (see Chapter 11). Swallowing studies using liquid barium followed by barium-coated food confirm obstructive disorders such as vascular anomalies, and they may detect esophageal diverticula. Fluoroscopy in association with the barium swallow is required to detect pharyngeal dysfunction, such as cricopharyngeal achalasia, and esophageal motility abnormalities. Ultrasonography is useful for detecting masses causing esophageal compression in the pharynx and neck.

Endoscopy

Endoscopy and endoscopic biopsy may be required for the identification of esophagitis and esophageal neoplasia. Unfortunately, esophageal biopsy is difficult without a suction or speculum forcep biopsy instrument.

Miscellaneous Diagnostic Procedures

Various other diagnostic tests may be required. These include the tensilon test and the acetylcholine receptor antibody test (myasthenia gravis); toxicologic analyses for lead, thallium, and pseudocholinesterase; serum CPK level (polymyositis); electrodiagnostics and nerve or muscle biopsy (neuropathies and myopathies); CSF taps or CT scans (brain stem diseases); and the ACTH test (hypoadrenocorticism). Thoracotomy may be required for the definitive diagnosis of vascular ring anomalies and hiatal disorders.

CHRONIC VOMITING

The differentiation of vomiting from regurgitation was described earlier. The causes of vomiting are listed in Table 5–14. The diagnostic procedures commonly employed for the evaluation of patients with chronic vomiting are listed in Table 5–15.

History

The signalment of the animal helps determine the likelihood of several disorders causing vomiting. For instance, young animals are more likely to ingest foreign bodies, and linear foreign bodies are particularly common in cats. Uncastrated young male dogs are more likely to rove the neighborhood and be traumatized or ingest poisons or garbage. Pancreatitis is common in fat small-breed dogs.

Knowledge of the patient's environment, diet, and any concurrent medication is helpful. Repeated access to trash, organophosphates, cleaners, toxic mushrooms, or ornamental plants may be responsible for chronic vomiting. Aggravation of vomiting by a certain diet raises the possibility of food intolerance or allergy. Almost any drug can cause vomiting as an idiosyncratic reaction.

The frequency and chronicity of the vomiting, the content of the vomitus, the animal's attitude and appetite, and the presence or absence of weight loss help determine the severity of the condition. Digested blood ("coffee grounds") in the vomitus indicates upper gastrointestinal hemorrhage. Fresh blood streaks in the vomitus are of less concern than "coffee grounds," and are usually due to capillary microtrauma from chronic vomiting. Foul-smelling vomitus can be due to stasis of gut content (with associated bacterial overgrowth), mucosal necrosis, or putrefication of food. Persistent vomiting of large volumes of liquid in spite of food restriction is highly suggestive of pyloric or upper intestinal obstruction. Vomiting of food greater than 12 hours after ingestion is pathognomonic for delayed gastric emptying. Causes of delayed gastric emptying are listed in Table 5–16. So-called projectile vomiting is traditionally ascribed to pyloric obstruction, but can occur from virtually any disorder causing violent vomiting. The history is concluded by screening other systems of the body with appropriate questions to help detect systemic causes of vomiting and identify incidental problems.

Physical Examination

A complete physical examination including abdominal palpation and rectal examination should be performed. Particular attention is paid to attitude, hydration, and cardiovascular

Table 5-14

CAUSES OF VOMITING

Adverse Reactions to Food
  Indiscretions
  Intolerances
  Allergies
Gastrointestinal Inflammatory Disorders
  Pharyngitis
  Gastritis (atrophic, hypertrophic, eosinophilic, others)
  Inflammatory bowel disease of small and large intestine
  Infectious enteritis (viral, bacterial, fungal)
  Hemorrhagic gastroenteritis
  Gastrointestinal neoplasia
  Gastric polyps
  Gastroduodenal ulcers
  Lymphangiectasia
Gastrointestinal Obstruction
  Foreign bodies
  Pyloric hypertrophy
  Mural thickenings (neoplasia, granulomas, strictures)
  Extraluminal compression (masses, adhesions)
  Delayed gastric emptying
  Ileus
  Constipation
Gastrointestinal Ischemic Disorders
  Intussusception
  Organ and mesenteric avulsion
  Infarction
  Organ torsions
Parasitism
  Ollulanus tricuspis
  Ascarids
  Physaloptera
  Salmon poisoning
  Heartworm (cats)
Disorders of Other Abdominal Organs
  Hepatobiliary inflammation, hepatic neoplasia, bile duct
    obstruction, cholelithiasis, portosystemic shunts
  Pancreatitis, pancreatic adenocarcinoma
  Kidney failure
  Peritonitis
  Metritis, pyometra
Systemic Diseases
  Uremia
  Hepatic failure
  Sepsis and toxemias
  Congestive heart failure
  Metastatic neoplasia
  Acidosis
  Electrolyte imbalance (hypokalemia, hypocalcemia, hypercalcemia)

Endocrine Diseases
  Adrenocortical insufficiency
  Diabetic ketoacidosis
  Hyperthyroidism
  Hyperparathyroidism
  Hypoparathyroidism
  Gastrinomas
Neurologic Diseases
  Dysautonomia
  Myenteric ganglionitis
  CNS tumors or trauma
  Meningitis
  Encephalitis
  Hydrocephalus
  Vestibular disturbances
  Visceral epilepsy?
Drugs, Poisons, and Chemical Agents
  Apomorphine
  Thiacetarsamide
  Chemotherapeutics
  Narcotics
  Xylazine
  Digitalis
  Anti-inflammatories
  Insecticides
  Copper sulfate
  Lead
  Ethylene glycol
  Mycotoxins (e.g., *Fusarium* spp. and "vomitoxin" on moldy wheat)
  Household plants (e.g., poinsettia)
  Others
Miscellaneous
  Atherosclerosis
  Anaphylaxis
  Diverticular malformations
  Heat stroke
  Motion sickness
  Pain, fear, other psychogenic
  Pregnancy

status. The neurologic examination should not be forgotten because persistent vomiting can result from CNS lesions. The physical examination may reveal the cause of the vomiting (e.g., obstructions) or yield findings that reduce the number of other possibilities (e.g., pain, jaundice, lymphadenopathy). The physical examination contributes to the assessment of the seriousness of the condition and dictates the volume of fluid deficit (if any). Rectal examination may detect melena, and in dogs with an intestinal obstruction it often reveals a dry, tacky mucosa.

Tabletop Assessment

By the conclusion of the clinical examination, the clinician should have been able to differentiate expectoration, gagging, retching, regurgitation, and vomiting. The clinician should also have decided if the vomiting represents a serious departure from normality. Dogs and cats commonly vomit once or twice every few weeks. If the frequency of the vomiting increases beyond that accepted as normal for the particular animal, a significant abnormality is likely. Occasional flecks of fresh blood in vomitus are not of concern whereas "coffee grounds" are. Other warning signs of serious disease include prolonged, frequent vomition; depression; anorexia; weight loss; weakness; dehydration; hyperpnea; pale, congested, or discolored mucous membranes; slow capillary refill; weak rapid pulse; fever; melena; delayed gastric emptying; abdominal organomegaly; pain, masses, or effusions; and continued vomiting while food is being withheld.

If the cause of the vomiting is not apparent following the clinical examination and warning signs of serious disease are present, the clinician is obligated to recommend supportive therapy and a diagnostic workup to determine safe and effective therapy. In the absence of warning signs, therapeu-

Table 5–15

DIAGNOSTIC PROCEDURES OF VALUE FOR THE DIFFERENTIAL DIAGNOSIS OF CHRONIC VOMITING

PROCEDURE	USEFULNESS
Dietary trials	Food intolerance
CBC	Sepsis, toxemia, eosinophilic gastritis, hypoadrenocorticism, lead toxicosis, blood loss, hydration
Serum chemistry profile	Hypoadrenocorticism, ketoacidosis, protein-losing gastropathy, uremia, liver disease, electrolyte levels
Urinalysis	Renal disease, liver disease, hydration, ketoacidosis
Blood gas	Acid-base status
Fecal flotation	Physaloptera, ascarids, Nanophytes
Fecal occult blood	Neoplasia, ulcers
Vomitus microscopic examination	*Ollulanus tricuspis*, neoplasia
ACTH stimulation test	Hypoadrenocorticism
Liver function test	Liver disease
Serum amylase and lipase tests	Pancreatitis
Serum antibody/antigen tests	Heartworm, RMSF, histoplasmosis
Survey radiographs	Obstructions, foreign bodies, liver and kidney size, masses, pancreatitis, peritonitis
Ultrasonography	Masses, metastatic neoplasia, mural thickenings, foreign bodies
Barium suspensions	Gastric disorders, pyloric obstruction, gastric emptying of liquids, intestinal obstruction
Barium-impregnated plastic spheres (BIPs)	Gastric emptying rate of food, ileus, other motility disorders, partial obstructions
Fluoroscopy	Gastrointestinal motility disorders
Enteroclysis	Intestinal motility disorders, partial obstructions
Scintigraphy	Gastric emptying
Endoscopy	Luminal and mucosal gastric, duodenal, and large-bowel disease
CSF tap	Brain stem diseases, increased CSF pressure, meningoencephalitis
Evoked potentials	Brain stem diseases
EEG	Hydrocephalus
CT scan/MRI	Brain stem disease, hydrocephalus
Toxicology	Plasma cholinesterase, lead, serum osmolality (ethylene glycol)
Gastric acid secretory testing	Achlorhydria, hyperacidity
Serum gastrin	Gastrinoma
Phenobarbital trial	Visceral epilepsy?
Exploratory celiotomy	Full thickness biopsy, APUDomas, chronic pancreatitis

Admission Laboratory Data

A laboratory database consisting of a CBC, serum chemistry panel, urinalysis, and fecal flotation should be gathered. Look for evidence in the database of systemic diseases, such as kidney and liver insufficiency, toxemias (e.g., pyometra, peritonitis), diabetes mellitus, hypoadrenocorticism, and lead toxicity. If the database points to any of these disorders, further diagnostic tests such as organ biopsy, liver function tests, ACTH stimulation tests, and lead levels may be required. The data-

base may confirm parasitism (Physaloptera, Salmon poisoning) and aid in the identification of eosinophilic gastritis and protein-losing gastropathies. The detection of metabolic alkalosis and paradoxical aciduria is suggestive of persistent vomiting due to pyloric obstruction but can also occur from other causes of vomiting. Perusal of the PCV, serum albumin, electrolyte panel, and blood gas data helps tailor the fluid (crystaloid, plasma, blood) and electrolytes (Na, K, Cl, HCO_3) administered.

Amylase, Lipase, and Trypsin-like Immunoreactivity

On occasion the history (fat dog, high-fat diet) and the physical examination (anterior abdominal pain) strongly suggest pancreatitis. At other times the diagnosis is less readily apparent. Amylase and lipase tests are commonly used to confirm pancreatitis. Unfortunately, the diagnostic accuracy of lipase and amylase is poor (both sensitivity and specificity), particularly in cats, and in the face of renal disease. Assay of serum trypsinlike immunoreactivity has greater specificity for acute

Table 5–16

CAUSES OF DERANGED GASTRIC EMPTYING

DELAYED GASTRIC EMPTYING
Mechanical obstruction
  Pyloric foreign body
  Gastric neoplasia
  Pyloric hypertrophy
  Antral mucosal hypertrophy
  Antral polyps
  Extrinsic compression of antrum or pylorus
Acid-base and electrolyte imbalances
  Hypokalemia
  Acidosis
Increased sympathetic nervous system activity
  Nervousness
  Stress
  Pain
Decreased parasympathetic nervous system activity
  Feline dysautonomia
  Anticholinergics
  Vagal neuropathy (solids only)
Miscellaneous causes of delayed motility
  Constipation
  Inflammatory or ulcerative stomach or intestinal disease
  Postgastric dilatation-volvulus
  Gastric surgery
  Gastric neoplasia
  Uremia
  Hepatic encephalopathy
  Diabetic gastroparesis
  Acute hyperglycemia
  High-calorie parenteral nutrition
  Tranquilizers
  Idiopathic

ACCELERATED GASTRIC EMPTYING
  Malabsorption syndromes
  Maldigestion syndromes
  Duodenal ulcers
  Gastrinomas
  Myenteric ganglionitis
  Vagal neuropathy (liquids only)
  Pyloroplasty

tic trials, such as controlled diets, are acceptable but, unfortunately, many cases of chronic vomiting are refractory to symptomatic therapy.

pancreatitis than amylase and lipase, but is unlikely to have improved sensitivity.

Survey Abdominal Radiographs[4]

Gastrointestinal tract foreign bodies and intestinal obstruction are common causes of vomiting that can occasionally be diagnosed by survey radiographs. Radiographs also assess gastric size, position, and content; detect gross abnormalities in liver and kidney size; and help detect abdominal fluid, abdominal masses, organ torsions, bowel perforation, peritonitis, and pancreatitis.

Abdominal Ultrasound[5–7]

Abdominal ultrasound and radiographs are complementary examinations. Ultrasound is more sensitive for detecting abdominal masses including intraorgan miliary masses (e.g., metastatic neoplasia), mural thickenings, lymphadenopathy, pancreatitis, and hepatic disorders. In contrast to radiography, the ultrasound image is enhanced by ascitic fluid and compromised by aerophagia.

Dietary Trial

Patients with no warning signs of serious disease (other than their chronic vomiting), whose condition remains undiagnosed after initial laboratory and imaging procedures, should be considered candidates for dietary elimination challenge trials to diagnose food sensitivity. Place the animal on the elimination diet for at least two weeks (see Chapter 23). Use an easily digestible, selected protein diet such as cottage cheese or tofu and boiled white rice. If signs resolve, slowly modify the basic diet until a tolerable balanced diet is determined. If signs do not resolve, more extensive and invasive diagnostic procedures are then justified.

Endoscopy

Endoscopic examination and biopsy of the stomach, duodenum, and colon is the most effective method of diagnosing inflammatory bowel disease, currently considered the most common cause of chronic vomiting in dogs and cats. Endoscopy also facilitates dignosis of many other diseases that cause vomiting, including gastritis, gastroduodenal ulcers, gastric neoplasia, pyloric stenosis, and foreign bodies. Although endoscopy is a high-yield diagnostic procedure, it does have some shortcomings. Endoscopy does not permit the diagnosis of motility disorders or partial obstructions of the jejunum (e.g., from annular adenocarcinoma), and it may miss nonmucosal mural lesions of the stomach or bowel. It was these deficiencies that led to the development of BIPs (see later).

Contrast Radiography with Barium Sulfate Liquid[4]

With the advent of endoscopy, the emphasis of gastrointestinal contrast radiography has moved toward procedures that assess gastrointestinal motility or detect intestinal obstructions rather than detect mucosal abnormalities. However, double-contrast gastrograms allow examination of the gastric mucosa for ulcers (for example) and may be useful if an endoscope is unavailable. Liquid gastrograms may help detect gastric mural lesions such as gastric adenocarcinoma. Administration of barium liquid will also detect gross obstructive disorders of the pylorus or intestine. Barium-coated food gives a crude estimate of gastric emptying time.[8] Gastric emptying usually begins within 30 minutes of ingestion.

Contrast Radiography with Barium-Impregnated Polyethylene Spheres (BIPS)

BIPS (Ken Bowman Assocs, Diamond Bar, CA 91765) are a convenient new radiographic method to detect motility abnormalities and obstructions of the gastrointestinal tract that can cause vomiting (or diarrhea) in dogs and cats. Two sizes of BIPS (5 mm and 1.5 mm diameter) are packaged together in gelatin capsules. The primary function of the large BIPS is detection of obstructions (particularly partial obstructions), whereas the transit of the small BIPS provides an estimate of the gastrointestinal transit time of food. It appears that BIPS have better sensitivity for detecting partial obstructions than barium liquid (especially in the hands of nonradiologists). Furthermore, in contrast to barium liquid they quantitatively assess the transit of food through the gastrointestinal tract, rather than qualitatively assess the transit of liquid.

BIPS are either administered with food or on an empty stomach. Several radiographs are then taken at convenient times over the next 12 to 24 hours and the gastric emptying and intestinal transit rate of the markers compared to normal data. If these rates are normal, gastrointestinal motility abnormalities or physical obstruction are highly unlikely. If emptying or transit times are delayed, the cause might be physical obstructions (e.g., foreign bodies, pyloric stenosis, tumors), functional obstructions (e.g., ileus, gastric dysrhythmias), or both. The decision as to whether an obstruction is functional or physical is made by a combination of history, clinical signs, laboratory findings, radiographic appearance, and the BIPS radiographic pattern (for example, persistent bunching of the BIPS in the small intestine is highly suggestive of physical obstruction of the small bowel).

Miscellaneous Diagnostic Imaging Techniques

Fluoroscopy facilitates diagnosis of gastric and intestinal motility disorders. Enterocylsis, a technique in which large volumes of barium liquid followed by water is directly infused into the small bowel via a duodenal catheter, is a technically difficult but very sensitive technique for diagnosing small-bowel partial obstructions.[9] It also provides information about small-bowel motility and mucosal topography. Scintigraphy provides objective evidence of delayed gastric emptying.

Exploratory Celiotomy[10,11]

Exploratory celiotomy may be required for the diagnosis of mural diseases of the gastrointestinal tract (such as leiomyomas), small-bowel lesions out of reach of the endoscope, gastrinomas, and low-grade diseases of some organs such as chronic pancreatitis. Pyloric hypertrophy and large-mass lesions of the gastric wall may be apparent on endoscopy, but definitive diagnosis may require full thickness biopsy. The complication rate following celiotomy is approximately 30%, with 60% of the complications disease related, and the remainder predominantly surgical or anesthesia related.[11]

Miscellaneous Diagnostic Evaluations

Various other tests may further aid in diagnosing some cases of vomiting. Microscopic examination of the vomitus may reveal *Ollulanus tricuspis* larvae (cats) or cytologic evidence of inflammation, infection, or neoplasia. Unfortunately, cytologic specimens are often distorted by the gastric acidity. CSF taps, CT scans, or magnetic resonance imaging (MRI) may be required to detect animals vomiting because of CNS lesions. The detection of an atropine-responsive bradycardia in a vomiting animal raises the likelihood that the vomiting is due to CNS lesions causing increased intracranial pressure. The entity of visceral epilepsy (vomiting due to a seizure focus in an area of the brain controlling visceral function) is an as yet unproven cause of vomiting. The basis for its diagnosis has been amelioration of the vomiting with phenobarbital, in the absence of demonstrable CNS disease. An ACTH test may be necessary for the diagnosis of hypoadrenocorticism. A small percentage of dogs with spontaneous hypoadrenocorticism and most dogs with iatrogenic hypoadrenocorticism have normal serum sodium and potassium levels, thus making the diagnosis difficult without the ACTH test. Elevated plasma gastrin levels support (but do not confirm) the diagnosis of gastrinoma. Gastric acid secretory testing may be useful for the diagnosis of achlorhydria or gastric hyperacidity syndromes.

CHRONIC DIARRHEA

The primary clinical sign of intestinal disease is diarrhea, but a variety of other clinical signs can also occur (Table 5–17). Diarrhea is often classified as of small-bowel or large-bowel character. *Small-bowel diarrhea* refers to diarrhea as a consequence of small intestine dysfunction. The disordered small intestinal function can result from diseases of the intestine itself, or from diseases of digestive organs such as the pancreas and liver that interfere with the ability of the small intestine to absorb food. The term *large-bowel diarrhea* refers to diarrhea resulting from diseases of the cecum, colon, or rectum.

History

The patient's signalment, vaccination history, and environment should be determined. Young animals are more prone to nutritional, microbial, and parasitic causes of diarrhea. Certain breed predispositions are apparent (Table 5–3). Diarrhea due to parvovirus or distemper is an important consideration in an unvaccinated animal. A free-ranging animal is more likely to develop infectious, toxic, and traumatic disorders.

The animal's diet should be ascertained. Adverse reactions to food are a prominent cause of diarrhea, and the history is a rapid way to identify responsible nutrients. Furthermore, the nature of the diet markedly influences the character of feces. For instance, poorly digestible high-fiber diets produce frequent bulky stools. If the diarrhea ceases when the animal is not fed, but starts again soon after feeding is reinstituted, an osmotic diarrhea is probable. Evaluation of the animal's weight in relation to caloric intake helps identify animals with problems in the absorption of nutrients.

Table 5–17

SMALL AND LARGE INTESTINAL DYSFUNCTION: PRIMARY AND SECONDARY SIGNS	
Primary Sign: Diarrhea	Change in frequency, consistency, or volume of bowel movements
Secondary Signs	Abdominal distention
	Abdominal pain
	Anal pruritus
	Borborygmus
	Dehydration
	Fecal incontinence
	Flatulence
	Halitosis
	Melena
	Polydipsia
	Polyphagia
	Shivering
	Tenesmus
	Vomiting
	Weight loss

The duration of the diarrhea and the frequency of normal and abnormal bowel movements help determine the severity of the condition. However, before relying on the client's testimony the clinician must establish if the client regularly observes the animal's bowel movements. Unobserved bowel movements are usually assumed to be normal. Diarrhea of several days to a week's duration is likely to respond to symptomatic therapy, whereas diarrhea of greater than one to two weeks is likely to respond only once diagnostic effort has identified a cause and specific treatment has been instituted. At times, patients pass a normal bowel movement in the morning, but subsequent bowel movements during the day become soft or watery. This pattern is often due to different levels of physical activity during the day and night. Inactivity promotes increased water resorption from feces, producing normal bowel movements, whereas increased activity encourages transit and exacerbates diarrhea.[12] Alteration in activity is also one reason why some dogs presented with the complaint of diarrhea will have normal stools in the hospital but not at home. The prognosis is poorer for patients that show frequent unrelenting diarrhea than for those with chronic intermittent diarrhea interspersed with periods in which they pass normal stools.

The frequency of bowel movements also assists differentiation of small- and large-bowel diarrhea. In small-bowel diarrhea the frequency is usually two to four times per day, whereas in large-bowel diarrhea the frequency is much higher (often four to ten times per day). Tenesmus and dyschezia (painful defecation) are also hallmarks of large-bowel disease. Fecal incontinence is frequently a result of large-bowel diseases and less frequently of small-bowel disorders. Clients sometimes fail to differentiate between the complaints of fecal incontinence and diarrhea. The clinician should be careful to differentiate the two conditions because they have some different causes and their workups and therapy are widely divergent.

The physical appearance of feces is of important diagnostic value. Fecal consistency can vary from formed feces that are merely soft at one end, as seen in mild diarrhea, to those that are watery and completely without form, as severity increases. Both large- and small-bowel diarrhea can result in unformed feces, but defecation of large volumes of liquid feces is more characteristic of small-bowel diarrhea. Fecal diameter may be reduced as a result of rectal strictures. The presence of excess mucus and fresh blood on the stool is suggestive of large-

Table 5–18†

CAUSES OF STEATORRHEA

MALDIGESTION
Exocrine pancreatic insufficiency
  Pancreatic atrophy
  Chronic pancreatitis
  Pancreatic duct obstruction
Hepatobiliary disease
  Liver failure
  Intrahepatic cholestasis
  Extrahepatic cholestasis

MALABSORPTION
  Inflammatory bowel diseases
  Neoplasia of the small intestine
  Stagnant loop syndrome (bacterial overgrowth)
  Lymphangiectasia

MISCELLANEOUS
  Hyperthyroidism
  Gastrinomas
  Dumping syndromes
  Unaccustomed high-fat diet*

---

*Dogs and cats can consume 40% and 64% fat diets (% dry matter), respectively, without steatorrhea, provided they are given sufficient time to become accustomed to the diet.
†Small-bowel diarrhea of any cause will produce a mild secondary steatorrhea.

bowel disease. The appearance of mucus must be explained to some clients.

Fecal color varies considerably with small-bowel diarrhea. The primary determinate of fecal color is the extent of metabolism of bile pigments in feces. Rapid transit time is associated with the yellow and green colors of incompletely metabolized bilirubin. Melena refers to black tarry feces resulting from upper gastrointestinal blood loss. Normal dogs and cats commonly have black feces, however, and it is important not to assume black feces are due to melena. Increased quantities of fecal fat impart a gray color to the feces. The stool may appear greasy and if wrapped in paper will cause an oily spot. Steatorrhea is an important observation; the abnormality has a number of different causes (Table 5–18). Unfortunately, the diagnostic value of steatorrhea is compromised by the fact that small-bowel diarrhea of any cause will induce mild secondary steatorrhea.[13]

The presence of undigested material in feces should be noted. The discovery of sharp materials, such as bone fragments, raises the possibility that traumatic colitis is the cause of the diarrhea. Foreign material, such as food wrappings, in the feces is suggestive of "garbage can enteritis." The presence of undigested particles of digestible foods in the feces is usually due to pancreatic insufficiency or too rapid intestinal transit.

Fecal odor should be noted. Maldigestion and malabsorption often result in a characteristic sour odor. Steatorrhea can be associated with a rancid smell.

The history is concluded by screening other systems of the body with appropriate questions to help detect systemic causes of diarrhea and identify incidental problems.

Physical Examination

Attitude, behavior, and posture should be examined while the animal is unrestrained. Abnormal posture raises the possibility of painful abdominal diseases. Dogs with painful diseases of the perianal area will sometimes carry their tail away

from their perineum. Cats with hyperthyroidism will often appear hyperactive. Body weight, hydration status, and cardiovascular function should be assessed. Weight loss as a result of malassimilation may be apparent.

Abdominal palpation is an important part of the physical examination. On occasion, loops of bowel filled with fluid and gas can be palpated. Bowel infiltrated by inflammatory or neoplastic cells may feel thickened on palpation. Masses causing partial intestinal obstruction are accessible to palpation in most regions of the intestine but often go undetected because of their small size. Detection of hepatomegaly raises the likelihood of hepatic or cardiac involvement in the diarrheic process. Absence of intestinal sounds following two to three minutes of abdominal auscultation is suggestive of ileus.

The perineal area should be carefully examined for evidence of perianal fistula and perineal hernias, both of which can cause clinical signs suggestive of large-bowel disease. The rectal examination provides fecal material for inspection. Fecal impaction, rectal masses, rectal strictures, rectal foreign bodies, and anal sac diseases, all of which can cause signs suggestive of large-bowel disease, may be discerned.

Tabletop Assessment

At the conclusion of the clinical examination the clinician should be able to differentiate small-bowel from large-bowel diarrhea and to assess the severity of the patient's condition.

DIFFERENTIATION OF SMALL-BOWEL FROM LARGE-BOWEL DIARRHEA. Because the workups of large-bowel and small-bowel diarrhea are different, it expedites diagnosis to tentatively localize the site of the intestinal dysfunction by use of a number of dissimilar, but not mutually exclusive, clinical features of small- and large-bowel diarrhea (Table 5–19). The different manifestations of disease in these two areas of the digestive tract reflect their different positions along the gastrointestinal tract and the different functions of the large and small bowel. The proximity of the large bowel to the formed fecal mass means blood from the large intestinal mucosa is passed as a fresh coating on the feces (hematochezia), whereas blood from the upper gastrointestinal tract is passed digested and admixed with the feces (melena). The large bowel is primarily a storage organ; it contributes little to digestion and absorption of nutrients. Therefore, disordered large-bowel function is associated with frequent defecation and minimal weight loss. In contrast, the primary function of the small bowel is absorption of nutrients. Thus, small intestinal diseases are commonly associated with weight loss and less often with marked increases in fecal frequency.

It is important to note that many animals will have diarrhea that does not fit neatly into a small-bowel or large-bowel classification. Reasons for this include the relatively high prevalence of diseases that can affect small and large bowel simultaneously (e.g., inflammatory bowel disease). Furthermore, chronic small-bowel diarrhea can eventually result in a low-grade colitis, presumably due to exposure of the colon to malabsorbed toxins (such as fatty acids and bile acids) and to other derangements of the colonic microenvironment.

ASSESSMENT OF SEVERITY. Intestinal disease can markedly affect fluid, electrolyte, and nutritional homeostasis. Warning signs of serious disease include prolonged periods of severe diarrhea; depression; anorexia; weight loss; weakness; dehydration; hyperpnea; pale, congested, or discolored mucous membranes; slow capillary refill; weak rapid pulse; fever; melena; and abdominal organomegaly, pain, masses, or effusions.

Table 5-19

DIFFERENTIATION OF LARGE- AND SMALL-BOWEL DIARRHEA: CLINICAL SIGNS

CLINICAL SIGN	SMALL BOWEL	LARGE BOWEL
Limitation of function	Weight loss usual, defecation urgency rare	Weight loss unusual, defecation urgency common
Quality of stool	Loose, no form, watery, possible fat droplets, undigested food, melena, color variable, malodorous	Loose to formed, mucus frequent, sometimes fresh blood, no undigested food, color usually brown
Quantity of stool	Volume is always increased	Volume may be normal or increased
Frequency	Usually increased; 2 to 4 times/day	Invariably increased; 4 to 10 times/day
Exacerbating factors	Diet changes, high-fat diets, poorly digestible diets	Stress and psychologic factors may be important
Associated phenomena	Abdominal distention, flatus, borborygmus, halitosis, melena, polydipsia, polyphagia, vomiting, weight loss	Tenesmus, anal pruritus

If the cause of the diarrhea is not apparent following the clinical examination and warning signs of serious disease are present, the clinician is obligated to recommend supportive therapy and a diagnostic workup to determine safe and effective therapy. In the absence of warning signs, symptomatic therapy and treatment trials are an acceptable approach.

CHRONIC SMALL-BOWEL DIARRHEA

The common causes of chronic small-bowel diarrhea and the diagnostic procedures frequently employed for the evaluation of such patients are listed in Tables 5-20 and 5-21, respectively.

Admission Laboratory Work

For complex or refractory cases of diarrhea the minimum laboratory database should include a complete blood count, a serum chemistry profile with electrolyte levels, a urinalysis, a fecal flotation for parasite ova, and a rectal scrape.

Direct smears of saline-admixed fresh feces for detection of protozoa can be helpful. In the cat, serologic tests for FeLV, feline immunodeficiency virus, FIP, and thyroxine measurement may be warranted. The laboratory database evaluates the patient for systemic diseases, such as infections, hyperthyroidism, and hepatic and renal insufficiency, that may result in signs of gastrointestinal disease. Furthermore, the database identifies incidental problems in other body systems, facilitates choice of fluid therapy, and aids in the identification of gastrointestinal problems, such as parasitism, eosinophilic gastroenteritis, protein-losing enteropathies, and infectious colitis. Eosinophilic gastroenteritis, hypoaderenocorticism, and some parasitic diseses are associated with a peripheral eosinophilia. Panhypoproteinemia characterizes protein-losing enteropathies, and the triad of lymphopenia, hypoalbuminemia, and hypoglobulinemia characterizes lymphangiectasia. The rectal scrape[14] helps identify patients with a large-bowel component to their diarrhea. Patients with small-bowel diarrhea usually do not have high numbers of neutrophils on rectal scrapes.

Tests of Pancreatic Function

Exocrine pancreatic insufficiency (EPI) is a readily treatable cause of chronic diarrhea that should be ruled out early in the diagnostic workup. This is particularly important if the patient has small-bowel diarrhea, gross steatorrhea is observed, or a Sudan stain of fresh feces is strongly positive for undigested fat. The disease is most common in German shepherds but is occasionally diagnosed in other breeds of dogs and in cats. The diagnosis of EPI in dogs is best made by assay of serum trypsin like immunoreactivity (TLI) or by the BT-PABA test. Fecal digestion tests (azocasein) are useful in cats.[15] A less satisfactory approach to confirm the diagnosis is a treatment trial with a pancreatic enzyme supplement. Diarrhea due to many causes will appear to respond, or partially respond, to enzyme supplementation, resulting in overdiagnosis of EPI and at times needless supplementation.

Survey Abdominal Radiographs

Partial obstructions due to foreign bodies, intussusceptions, or masses are occasional causes of diarrhea that in some instances can be diagnosed by survey radiographs. Although not common causes of diarrhea, the serious consequences of misdiagnosing these disorders makes abdominal radiography (especially with BIPs) a recommended part of the early workup of chronic cases. Furthermore, survey radiographs detect gross abnormalities in liver and kidney size and help detect abdominal fluid, abdominal masses, organ torsions, bowel perforation, peritonitis, and pancreatitis.

Abdominal Ultrasound

Abdominal ultrasound and radiographs are complementary examinations. Ultrasound is more sensitive for the detection of abdominal masses, intestinal mural thickenings, intussusceptions, and mesenteric lymphadenopathy.[5] Ultrasound-guided percutaneous biopsy or aspiration of masses or abnormal organs is an effective diagnostic procedure with a low complication rate.[16,17]

Dietary Trial

Animals with no warning signs of serious disease (other than their chronic diarrhea), whose diarrhea remains undiagnosed after the initial laboratory and imaging procedures, should be further investigated with elimination challenge diets for the diagnosis of food sensitivity. As described in

Table 5-20

CAUSES OF SMALL-BOWEL DIARRHEA

Dietary
Food poisoning
Gluttony
Sudden change of diet
Intolerance
Wheat-sensitive enteropathy
Allergy
Stomach
Dumping syndromes
Hyperacidity
Achlorhydria
Small Intestinal Disease
Infectious enteritis (viral, fungal, bacterial enterotoxins and endo-
toxins, invasive bacteria)
Parasites (cryptosporidia, giardia, strongyloides, ascarids, hookworms,
Salmon poisoning)
Inflammatory bowel disease (eosinophilic, plasmacytic/lymphocytic,
other)
Infiltrative neoplasia (lymphosarcoma, mastocytosis)
Other infiltrative disease (fucosidosis, amyloidosis)
Partial intraluminal obstruction (neoplasia, strictures, fungal
granuloma, foreign body, intussusception)
Extraluminal obstructions (hernias, adhesions, masses)
Brush border enzyme defects
Bacterial overgrowth
Ileus (hypokalemia, hypoalbuminemia, enteritis, dysautonomia,
other)
Hypermotility (myenteric ganglionitis)
Ischemic diseases (mesenteric avulsion, infarction, torsions,
strangulations)
Lymphangiectasia
Hemorrhagic gastroenteritis
Pancreatic Disease
Chronic pancreatitis
Pancreatic neoplasia
Juvenile atrophy
Obstruction of pancreatic ducts
Liver Disease
Liver failure
Intrahepatic cholestasis
Bile duct obstruction
Kidney Disease
Uremia
Nephrotic syndrome
Miscellaneous Systemic Disorders
Toxemias (pyometra, abscess, peritonitis)
Septicemias (leptospirosis)
Congestive heart failure
Immunodeficiencies (IgA deficiency)
Autoimmune diseases (SLE)
Hypoadrenocorticism
Hyperthyroidism
APUDomas (gastrinomas, VIPomas, carcinoid syndrome)
Thyroid carcinoma
Metastatic neoplasia
Acrodermatitis
Various toxins and drugs

Table 5-21

DIAGNOSTIC PROCEDURES FOR DIAGNOSING CHRONIC SMALL-BOWEL DIARRHEA

PROCEDURE	USEFULNESS
CBC	Sepsis, toxemia, eosinophilic gastroenteritis, hypoadrenocorticism, lymphangiectasia, PLE, lead toxicosis, hydration
Serum chemistry profile	Hypoadrenocorticism, uremia protein-losing enteropathy, liver disease, electrolyte levels
Urinalysis	Renal disease, liver disease, hydration
Blood gas	Acid-base status
Fecal flotation	Ascarids, nanophytes
Fecal direct smear	Giardiasis
Fecal Sudan stain	Steatorrhea
Fecal occult blood	Neoplasia, ulcers
Fecal digestion tests	Exocrine pancreatic insufficiency
Fecal culture	Bacterial enteritis
Peroral string test	Giardiasis
Trypsinlike immuno-reactivity test	Exocrine pancreatic insufficiency
Serum antibody/antigen tests	FeLV, FIV, histoplasmosis
Serum thyroxine level	Hyperthyroidism
Serum vitamin B_{12}/folate test	Bacterial overgrowth
Breath hydrogen test	Bacterial overgrowth, carbohydrate malabsorption
Xylose absorption	Carbohydrate malabsorption
Fecal total fat excretion	Fat malabsorption
Survey radiographs	Intussusception, foreign bodies, liver and kidney size, masses, pancreatic abscess, peritonitis
Ultrasonography	Masses, metastatic neoplasia, mural thickenings
Dietary trials	Food intolerance
Barium-impregnated plastic spheres (BIPs)	Intestinal partial obstruction, gastric emptying, intestinal motility disorders
Fluoroscopy	Gastrointestinal motility disorders
Enteroclysis	Intestinal motility disorders, partial obstructions
Scintigraphy	Protein-losing enteropathy
Endoscopy	Luminal and mucosal gastroduodenal and large-bowel disease, giardiasis, bacterial overgrowth
Toxicology	Plasma cholinesterase, lead
ACTH stimulation test	Hypoadrenocorticism
Liver function test	Liver disease
Plasma gastrin	Gastrinoma
Percutaneous aspiration of bowel	Neoplasia, eosinophilic enteritis
Exploratory celiotomy	Full thickness biopsy, APUDomas, chronic pancreatitis

Endoscopy

Endoscopic biopsy is an effective technique for diagnosing intestinal mucosal diseases that are associated with morphologic changes. The procedure may identify intestinal inflammation of various causes or intestinal neoplasia. Gastroscopic food sensitivity testing can identify some animals with immediate food sensitivities causing diarrhea. Aspiration of duodenal fluid for cytology can be used to diagnose giardiasis. Aspirated duodenal fluid may also be quantitatively cultured for the definitive diagnosis of small intestinal bacterial overgrowth. Endoscopy, however, does not permit diagnosis of intestinal motility disorders, secretory diarrheas, or brush border enzyme defects, and it is likely to miss lesions in the intestinal submucosa or muscularis. Furthermore, the restricted working length of many endoscopes compromises the ability of the

Chapter 23, use an easily digestible, selected protein diet such as cottage cheese or tofu and rice for at least two weeks. If signs resolve, slowly modify the basic diet until a tolerable balanced diet is determined. If signs do not resolve, more extensive and invasive diagnostic procedures are then justified. Diseases such as food allergy and gluten sensitivity do not have pathognomonic histopathologic changes, and can be diagnosed only by such trials.

endoscope to detect diseases primarily manifested in the jejunum (such as partial obstructions). To be of value, endoscopic examination must be thorough, and multiple biopsies of lesions at standardized areas of the gastrointestinal tract should be performed. If clinical signs suggest the possibility of an enterocolitis, colon biopsy may also be performed.

Tests for Malabsorption

Tests for malabsorption do not give a causal diagnosis, many are time consuming, and they are all plagued to a greater or lesser degree by poor sensitivity and specificity. In the past, one of their major functions has been to provide the clinician with evidence that exploratory surgery and small intestinal biopsy are warranted. With the advent of the endoscope, the decision to biopsy the small intestine is less momentous. For these reasons, and because of the improved sensitivity of endoscopic biopsy (in comparison to malabsorption tests) for the detection of common morphologic mucosal diseases such as inflammatory bowel disease, many clinicians now perform endoscopy prior to instituting screening tests for malabsorption. If the clinician takes this approach, it should not be forgotten that endoscopic examination does not screen for the same spectra of diseases as do malabsorption tests. Endoscopy and endoscopic biopsy only permit diagnosis of intestinal diseases that have abnormal mucosal morphology. In contrast, malabsorption tests evaluate function; they identify abnormal carbohydrate or fat assimilation due to diseases such as motility disorders, bacterial overgrowth, or brush border enzyme deficiencies that need not, or do not, have morphologically recognizable abnormalities on bowel biopsy. Therefore, endoscopy should not be considered a replacement for tests of malabsorption.

Screening tests for malabsorption that have been used in the cat and dog include those that assess the absorption of xylose, fat, glucose, galactose, lactose, cobalamin, folate, vitamin A, and radio-labeled oleic acid. Screening tests of malassimilation include quantitative analysis of fecal fat, Sudan stain for fecal fat, radio-labeled triglyceride (^{131}I-triolein), breath hydrogen analysis, and the assessment of fecal-reducing substances and fecal pH. These tests vary considerably in their simplicity, availability, and reliability. The tests for carbohydrate and fat malassimilation I use most commonly are breath hydrogen analysis and the direct/indirect Sudan stain for fecal fat, respectively. Fecal Sudan stains need to be performed and interpreted carefully because the potential for methodologic errors is high (see Chapter 6). In particular, a consistent diet of moderate fat content needs to be fed prior to the test (e.g.; Prescription Diet c/d), and the feces tested need to be fresh. In my experience the fat absorption/plasma turbidity test is not to be recommended because of frequently misleading results.

Tests for Bacterial Enteritis/Enterocolitis

Infection with bacterial pathogens does not appear to be a common cause of *chronic* small-bowel diarrhea but enteroadherent streptocci and enterotoxigenic *E. coli* may be important in some situations. Unfortunately, these diseases cannot be diagnosed by fecal cultures. However, enteroadherent bacteria can sometimes be detected histologically in small-bowel biopsy specimens, and typing of fecal coliforms to identify pathogenic strains can be performed by some centers. Specific bacterial pathogens, such as *Salmonella* spp., *Campylobacter jejuni* spp., and *Yersinia enterocolitica*, will occasionally be cultured from the feces of animals showing small-bowel diarrhea or, more commonly, large-and small-bowel diarrhea (enterocolitis). It is important to remember, however, that these bacteria can be cultured in small to moderate numbers from many normal animals. Interpretation of culture results is made easier if the laboratory provides a comparative estimate of the number of the bacterial pathogen in relation to other bacterial flora. It is assumed a heavy and relatively pure growth of a known pathogen or a member of the fecal flora is significant, particularly if a rectal scrape shows corresponding suppurative inflammation. In contrast, culture of low numbers of pathogens among healthy mixed flora is more difficult to interpret. Fecal clostridial enterotoxin levels can be performed if clostridial enterocolitis is suspected.

Tests for Small Intestinal Bacterial Overgrowth (SIBO)

Overgrowth of the upper small intestine by normal bacterial flora is probably a more common cause of chronic small-bowel diarrhea than persistent infection by bacterial pathogens. A diagnosis of SIBO cannot be made by fecal culture because very high numbers of bacteria are normally cultured from the feces, and those numbers do not reflect the numbers or composition of bacteria found in the small intestine. A definitive diagnosis of bacterial overgrowth can, however, be made by quantitive anaerobic and aerobic culture of duodenal fluid aspirated by endoscopy, suction capsule biopsy, or by needle at surgery. The breath hydrogen test provides firm supportive evidence for bacterial overgrowth, as does depressed serum vitamin B_{12} in association with an elevated serum folate level.

Whenever possible, antibiotic trials should be avoided for the diagnosis of SIBO or chronic bacterial enteritis. Without attention to the underlying cause of bacterial overgrowth, and because of the rapid acquisition of antibiotic resistance by gastrointestinal bacterial pathogens, these conditions are often only at best temporarily responsive to treatment trials with broad-spectrum antibiotics. In addition, some drugs used for treatment trials, such as metronidazole, have well-recognized effects other than their antibacterial activity that seriously compromise interpretation of results. Once a diagnosis of SIBO has been made, further diagnostic tests to attempt to identify an underlying cause should be considered.

Contrast Radiography

Liquid barium follow-through studies can identify some partial obstructions of the intestine. In general, however, this is a low-yield diagnostic procedure for the diagnosis of chronic diarrhea, especially if already preceded by ultrasonography. BIPs are a new method to detect partial obstructions or motility abnormalities of the stomach or bowel resulting in diarrhea, as discussed earlier. Fluoroscopy assists diagnosis of gastric and intestinal motility disorders. Enteroclysis (see earlier) is a technically difficult but sensitive technique for the diagnosis of small-bowel partial obstructions. It also provides information about mucosal morphology and small-bowel motility.

Exploratory Celiotomy

Exploratory celiotomy allows visual inspection, palpation, and multiple biopsies of the abdominal organs. A major advantage of celiotomy over endoscopy is that it allows full thickness rather than pinch biopsies (see later). Biopsy samples of the intestine should be taken even if the intestine looks and feels normal. Exploratory celiotomy may also be required for the diagnosis of small-bowel lesions out of reach of the endoscope, and some "occult" diseases of other abdominal organs such as low-grade pancreatitis and APUDomas.

Intestinal Biopsies

On most occasions, small intestinal biopsies, whether attained by endoscopy, guided suction biopsy capsules, or celiotomy, yield nonetiologic-specific pathology such as intestinal inflammation, villus atrophy, and cellular infiltration. Sometimes a cause may be apparent, such as when infectious agents, neoplastic cells, or lymphangiectasia are evident. In some cases, such as eosinophilic gastroenteritis, the prominent cell type found suggests an immune-mediated problem. Diagnostic conclusions often depend on the interpretation of the biopsy result in the light of previous diagnostic findings or the response to subsequent therapy. For example, a diagnosis of idiopathic inflammatory bowel disease is made only after a previous workup, including dietary trials, has ruled out obvious causes of intestinal inflammation.

Many intestinal diseases need full thickness biopsy (rather than mucosal pinch biopsies) for diagnosis, either because of location of the disease in the submucosa, myenteric plexus, or muscularis, or because of sparse or patchy incidence in the mucosa. Full thickness biopsy specimens are usually obtained by celiotomy but a laproscopic technique has been described.[18]

Full thickness intestinal biopsy sites are more likely to dehisce than endoscopic biopsy sites. In particular, the biopsy sites of debilitated animals are at increased risk of dehiscence. In such patients, full thickness intestinal biopsy should be performed only after great circumspection and preferably in association with nutritional support. In contrast, recent evidence has suggested that hypoalbuminemia, per se, is not a risk factor for dehiscence of intestinal biopsy sites.[19]

In some institutions, examination of small intestinal biopsy specimens by a dissecting microscope has been found useful to confirm villous atrophy. Furthermore, subcellular fractionation techniques have been utilized with success to detect brush border enzyme deficiencies.

Colon (or rectal) biopsy in animals with small-bowel diarrhea is warranted when enterocolitis is suspected or when biopsy of the small bowel cannot be performed for reasons such as anesthetic risk or expense. Obtaining a sample of large-bowel mucosa is a relatively simple procedure in comparison to biopsying the small bowel. In the anesthetized patient, all it requires is two pairs of rat tooth forceps and a pair of scissors (or a scalpel blade). The first pair of forceps is used to prolapse the rectal mucosa through the anus, and the second pair is used to select and elevate a mucosal fold to be snipped off. If necessary, large-bowel biopsy can be performed without anesthesia by using a suction biopsy instrument. Quite frequently, pathologic processes found in the large bowel biopsy will, to a lesser or greater extent, reflect the histopathologic changes in the small bowel.

Miscellaneous Diagnostic Evaluations

Various other diagnostic procedures may be useful for the diagnosis of some cases of chronic small-bowel diarrhea. Fecal occult blood tests may be required to confirm gastrointestinal blood loss but beware the animal's diet does not contain mutton or beef because false positive tests can result.[20] Measurements of fecal osmolality and fecal electrolyte concentrations have proved useful in human medicine for differentiating secretory and osmotic diarrhea but require more investigation in small animal patients before they can be recommended.

Assays of various hormones or their metabolites may be required to diagnose endocrinopathies such as the APUD tumors. Elevated plasma gastrin level supports (but doesn't confirm) the diagnosis of gastrinoma. In animals with an exposure history, a histoplasmosis titer may be helpful.

Percutaneous fine needle aspiration of thickened bowel loops can provide supportive evidence of inflammatory bowel disease. Diagnosis of protein-losing enteropathy can be assisted by [111]indium-labeled transferrin and [51]chromium-labeled albumin tests. Measurement of fecal alpha-l-antitrypsin may also prove useful.[21] Absorption tests, with substrates such as chromium-labeled EDTA, polyethylene glycol, or lactulose/mannitol, have been used to gauge bowel mucosal permeability. Such tests are tedious to perform but do provide a limited amount of useful clinical information, such as a guide to the mucosal response to therapy.[22]

CHRONIC LARGE-BOWEL DIARRHEA

The prevalent causes of chronic large-bowel diarrhea and the diagnostic procedures commonly employed for the evaluation of such patients are listed in Tables 5–22 and 5–23, respectively.

Admission Laboratory Work

For refractory cases of large-bowel diarrhea, useful diagnostic procedures to complete the database include a complete blood count, a serum chemistry profile with electrolyte levels, a urinalysis, and one or more fecal flotations for parasite ova. Examination of two or three fecal samples for parasites is recommended in all cases. False negative fecal examinations are not uncommon with lowly fecund parasites, such as *Trichuris vulpis*. Direct smears of saline-admixed fresh feces for detection of protozoa such as *Giardia* or *Entamoeba histolytica* can be helpful. Cytologic examination of fecal smears or, preferably, rectal scrapings may reveal protozoa, *Histoplasma* organisms, inflammatory cells suggestive of colitis, or spores of *Clostridium perfringens* supportive of *Clostridium perfringens* enterotoxin-associated diarrhea. The observation of large numbers of neutrophils in rectal scrapings is suggestive of bacterial colitis. In cats, serum tests for FeLV, FIV, and FIP may be appropriate.

The laboratory database allows the clinician to evaluate the patient for systemic diseases, such as uremia, that may result in signs of colitis; identifies any incidental problems in another system of the body; facilitates choice of fluid therapy; and aids in the identification of gastrointestinal problems, such as infectious, parasitic, and eosinophilic colitis.

Treatment Trials

In view of the high prevalence of chronic idiopathic colitis, many clinicians institute treatment for this disorder early in the workup of patients with uncomplicated chronic large-bowel diarrhea. A tentative diagnosis of chronic idiopathic colitis is made following a successful response to a treatment trial with a controlled diet or sulfasalazine. Similarly, in endemic areas, treatment trials

Table 5–22

CAUSES OF LARGE-BOWEL DIARRHEA

Inflammatory Large Intestinal Disease
Acute nonspecific colitis
Chronic colitis (plasmacytic/lymphocytic, eosinophilic, granulomatous, histiocytic, suppurative)
Infectious colitis (FIP, FeLV, histoplasmosis, *Salmonella, Campylobacter, Clostridium perfringens, Clostridium difficile, Prototheca, Yersinia enterocolitica*)
Parasites (trichuris, giardia, hookworms, Salmon poisoning, *Balantidium coli, Entamoeba histolytica,* coccidia)
Pseudomembranous colitis (antibiotic associated)

Obstructive Large-Bowel Disease
Intraluminal obstruction (constipation, megacolon, neoplasia, strictures, foreign body, intussusception)
Extraluminal obstructions (hernias, adhesions, masses)

Ischemic Large-Bowel Disease
Trauma, infarction, torsion, strangulation, ileocolic intussusception, stress?

Neoplastic Large-Bowel Disease
Adenocarcinoma
Benign polyps
Lymphosarcoma
Plasmacytoma
Others

Noninflammatory Large-Bowel Disease
Cecal inversion
Congenital malformations
Diverticular malformations
Exposure to secretagogues (unconjugated bile acids, hydroxylated fatty acids)
Motility abnormalities ("irritable bowel syndrome")

Systemic Disorders
Toxemias (pyometra, abscess, peritonitis)
Uremia
Metastatic neoplasia
Toxicities

Diet Related
Food poisoning
Intolerances or allergy
Foreign material (bones, hair, wrapping material)

Miscellaneous
Acute pancreatitis (segmental colitis)
Secondary to chronic small-bowel diarrhea (malabsorbed bile acids, etc.)

Table 5–23

DIAGNOSTIC PROCEDURES OF VALUE FOR THE DIAGNOSIS OF CHRONIC LARGE-BOWEL DIARRHEA

PROCEDURE	USEFULNESS
CBC	Sepsis, toxemia, eosinophilic colitis, hydration
Serum chemistry profile	Uremia, electrolyte levels
Urinalysis	Renal disease, hydration
Fecal flotation	Trichuris
Fecal direct smear	Giardiasis, Entamoeba, *Balantidium coli*
Fecal cytology/rectal scrape	Bacterial colitis, inflammatory bowel disease, Entamoeba, *Balantidium coli*, clostridial spores, prototheca
Fecal culture	Salmonella, campylobacter enterocolitis, *Clostridium difficile*
Fecal clostridial enterotoxin	Clostridial enteritis
Serum antibody/antigen tests	FeLV, FIV, histoplasmosis, FIP
Survey radiographs	Ieocolic intussusception, foreign bodies, constipation
Barium enemas	Ileocolic intussusceptions, cecal inversion, masses, diverticula
Ultrasonography	Pelvic masses, metastatic neoplasia, mural thickenings, ileocolic intussusceptions
Endoscopy	Colitis, neoplasia, foreign bodies, cecal inversion
Controlled diet trial	Food intolerance, chronic colitis
Fiber trial	"Irritable bowel syndrome," bile acid malabsorption, perturbed flora, perturbed colonic secretion
Sulfasalazine trial	Chronic colitis
Cholestyramine trial (dogs)	Bile acid malabsorption
Stress reduction	"Irritable bowel syndrome"
Manometry?	"Irritable bowel syndrome"
Exploratory celiotomy	Pelvic and pericolonic masses, biopsy

---

against whipworms are often instituted early in the workup, even if fecal flotation does not detect whipworm eggs.

Diagnostic Imaging

Survey abdominal films, barium or air enemas, and ultrasound are only occasionally helpful in the diagnosis of large-bowel diarrhea. They will periodically reveal rectal foreign bodies, bowel thickenings, mesenteric lymphadenopathy, cecal inversion, and ileocolic intussusceptions. In general, these procedures have been superseded by endoscopy, but they are of value if tenesmus (rather than the other signs of large-bowel diarrhea) is the predominant presenting sign, whereupon they may detect abdominal masses, prostatomegaly, rectal diverticula, and perineal hernias.

Fecal Culture

The difficulties interpreting fecal cultures have already been discussed. Culture of feces for salmonella and campylobacter is

particularly important in animals that develop large-bowel diarrhea during or immediately after kenneling with other dogs or cats. A positive culture for *Clostridium perfringens* is particularly likely if clostridial spores were noted on fecal smears. If the histopathologic picture is dominated by neutrophil infiltration and erosion or ulceration, bacterial colitis is a possibility and culture for enteric bacterial pathogens is warranted. If the histopathology shows pseudomembranous inflammation, culture for *Clostridium difficile* is indicated.

Endoscopy and Colon Biopsy

Rigid proctoscopy is preferred over flexible colonoscopy for the initial evaluation of uncomplicated large-bowel disease. Rigid proctoscopy entails less risks, time, and cost than colonoscopy, yet it is able to diagnose the majority of large-bowel diseases, because such diseases are commonly diffuse (e.g., colitis) and/or located within reach of a protoscope (e.g., adenocarcinoma). Flexible colonoscopy should be performed if a diagnosis is not apparent using rigid proctoscopy, if the clinician perceives an increased likelihood of upper colonic disease (e.g., palpable ileocolic thickening or heavy rectal bleeding without tenesmus), or if an accurate evaluation of the extent of the disease is needed. Diseases identifiable by colonoscopy but not proctoscopy include cecal inversion, occult *Trichuris* infection, and ileocolic neoplasia.

The colon may be biopsied with a suction biopsy instrument, speculum biopsy forceps, or pinch (endoscopic) biopsy forceps. If possible, full thickness colon biopsies should be avoided because the rate of healing is slower in the large bowel than in the small bowel, and the consequences of dehiscence are greater due to the higher bacterial numbers in the large bowel. As with small-bowel biopsy, biopsy of the colon rarely reveals the cause of the diarrhea, but does allow categorization of the disease process on which therapeutic and prognostic advice can be more soundly based.

Miscellaneous Diagnostic Tests

With reasonable frequency, colon biopsy shows little or no inflammation in spite of persistent signs of large-bowel disease. At present, this noninflammatory large-bowel dysfunction is an enigma. It is probably due to a group of diseases that are somewhat analogous to irritable bowel syndrome in humans and may have a psychogenic component. Possible pathomechanisms include exposure to secretagogues and deranged motility patterns. Increased fecal concentrations of unconjugated bile acids or hydroxylated fatty acids could be responsible for some of the cases. In the future, tests of bile acid absorption or colonorectal manometry may allow more specific diagnosis but at present, diagnosis is largely made by treatment trials. Therapies used have included removing identifiable stressors; increasing dietary fiber; use of bile acid chelators such as cholestyramine (not in cats); and administration of narcotic analgesics (diphenoxylate or loperamide), anticholinergics, or tranquilizers.

TENESMUS

Tenesmus refers to persistent or prolonged straining that is usually ineffectual and often painful. The most prevalent causes of tenesmus are listed in Table 5–24. The diagnostic approach to tenesmus is similar to that described for large-bowel diarrhea.

Clinical Examination

Clients often equate the clinical sign of straining with "constipation." In addition to history pertaining to the gastrointestinal tract, the clinician should obtain information concerning the normality, or otherwise, of urination. A description of the posture the patient adopts while straining may help localize the disorder. Female animals straining to urinate usually squat and hold their tail lower to the ground than those straining to defecate. Whether the tenesmus occurs before or after micturition or defecation can also aid differentiation. Obstructive disorders are more commonly associated with tenesmus before evacuation, whereas irritative disorders are often associated with persistent tenesmus after evacuation. In addition to physical examination of the large bowel, anus, and perineum, the clinician should carefully palpate the bladder and prostate and closely examine the vagina or penis for evidence of pain, discharges, masses, or calculi.

Diagnostic Procedures

The diagnostic procedures are similar to those described for the evaluation of large-bowel diarrhea. If the cause of the

Table 5–24

CAUSES OF TENESMUS
Large Bowel
Constipation (Table 26–4)
Colitis
Neoplasia
Miscellaneous large-bowel diseases (Table 5–22)
Rectal or anal foreign body
Perianal/perineal disorders
Perineal hernia
Perianal fistula
Anal sac abscess
Anal sac neoplasia
Genitourinary Tract
Cystitis or urethritis (especially FUS)
Cystic or urethral calculi
Prostatomegaly (neoplasia, hyperplasia, abscess)
Genitourinary neoplasia
Vaginal masses or foreign bodies
Dystocia
Caudal Abdominal Cavity Disorders
Abdominal cavity masses
Pelvic fractures
Pelvic osteosarcoma

tenesmus is localized to genitourinary disease, various additional diagnostic procedures such as urinary catheterization, urinary tract contrast radiography, urethroscopy, cultures of urine or prostatic fluid, and biopsy of the urinary tract, uterus, or prostate may be required.

MELENA AND HEMATOCHEZIA

Melena describes dark tarry stools resulting from digested blood. The blackening of the stool results from oxidation of hemoglobin to hematin or other hematochromes. The tarry appearance results from bacterial breakdown of hemoglobin. In dogs, 350 to 500 mg of hemoglobin per kg of body weight must enter the upper gastrointestinal tract before melena will develop.[23]

Melena usually results from bleeding into the pharynx, esophagus, stomach, or upper small intestine. However, it is not the site of origin, per se, that determines the color of blood in feces but instead the duration of passage through the gastrointestinal tract. For instance, it has been estimated that blood must be retained in the intestinal tract of humans for at least eight hours for it to turn black. Therefore, black stools can result from lower small-bowel or upper large-bowel bleeding if transit time of the blood is sufficiently slow (for example, bleeding proximal to a lower small-bowel neoplasm). In such cases, however, it is unusual for the stools to have a tarry appearance because there is usually insufficient blood lost from lower gastrointestinal tract lesions to result in tarry feces. It is also important to note that the transit time of blood in the gastrointestinal tract shortens as the volume of blood entering the tract increases. As a result of this phenomenon, very heavy upper gastrointestinal bleeds can result in large quantities of fresh blood in the feces instead of melena.

Hematochezia refers to the presence of streaks of red blood on the stool. Fresh blood adherent to the feces is strongly suggestive of lower large-bowel hemorrhage. The diagnostic evaluation of hematochezia is similar to that described earlier for the evaluation of large-bowel diarrhea, but, particularly in the absence of other signs of large-bowel disease, it should include coagulation tests. Important causes of gastrointestinal bleeding are listed in Table 5–25, and diagnostic procedures useful in the evaluation of patients with melena are listed in Table 5–26.

Confirmation of Melena

The first step in the diagnostic evaluation of melena is the objective confirmation of the problem. Subsequently, diagnostic evaluations are selected to first localize the site of bleeding and then define the cause.

The classic appearance of melena is of coal black, shiny, sticky, foul-smelling feces of tar-like consistency. On many occasions, however, feces will have some, but not all, of these classic features. For instance, there are a number of spurious reasons for black feces. Many normal animals consuming meat-based diets have black feces. Similarly, diets high in iron can cause black feces as can the use of some drugs such as salicylates, bismuth, and charcoal.

Therefore, it can become important to confirm the presence of digested blood by use of tests for fecal blood, such as the orthotolidine (Hematest) and guaiac (Hemoccult) tablet tests. These tests are qualitative, only moderately sensitive, and can generate false positive results. Recently, a highly sensitive, quantitative fluorometric assay of fecal hemoglobin has been described.

Clinical Examination

The patient's age helps determine the likelihood of gastrointestinal neoplasia. The history should include inquiry as to the usage of NSAIDS or prednisone, evidence of bleeding tendency, and the likelihood of trauma (avulsions, infarction). Clinical manifestations of gastrointestinal bleeding depend on the extent and rapidity of the hemorrhage and range from mild weakness to collapse. On occasion, life-threatening volumes of blood can accumulate within the gastrointestinal tract, with little or no visible signs of external blood loss. Clinical signs of gastrointestinal blood loss usually pertain primarily to anemia and hypovolemia, but on occasion they may help localize the site of hemorrhage. Thus, concomitant regurgitation suggests esophageal or pharyngeal disease, cough raises the likelihood of hemoptysis, and jaundice and ascites imply liver disease. Hepatic encephalopathy may occur following gastrointestinal hemorrhage in patients with liver disease. Hematemesis strongly suggests gastric or duodenal bleeding, but swallowed blood will also cause infrequent vomiting. The physical examination should include careful inspection of the nares and oropharynx for evidence of nasal or oropharyngeal sources of bleeding, and the skin of the abdomen and the mucous membranes for evidence of bleeding disorders. Fever occurs in 80% of humans with gastrointestinal hemorrhage of any cause.

Admission Laboratory Work

Along with the clinical examination, the complete blood count helps determine the severity and chronicity of the condition. Microcytic, hypochromic anemias are common following prolonged gastrointestinal blood loss. The rapidity with which the hematocrit declines after hemorrhage is variable, depending on such factors as hydration status and preexisting anemia. Significant decline can occur within one to two hours. The platelet count usually declines little as a result of

hemorrhage and in fact may rise as a result of increased platelet production. Leukocytosis and occasionally a leukemoid reaction can occur following hemorrhage. Reticulocytosis should be expected within two to four days.

The BUN to creatinine ratio rises after upper gastrointestinal hemorrhage due to the digestion and absorption of blood protein. Lower bowel hemorrhage has little effect on BUN, but will elevate blood ammonia. Slight hyperbilirubinemia is common in humans after gastrointestinal hemorrhage. The hyperbilirubinemia results from the breakdown of large quantities of heme. A fecal flotation for hookworm should not be neglected.

Tests Assisting Localization of Gastrointestinal Hemorrhage

In the absence of an endoscope, aspiration of esophageal or gastric content following the passage of a measured nasogastric tube may help localize the site of bleeding. The peroral string test has been successfully used for diagnostic purposes in the dog. One of the uses of this test in humans is the determination of the site of bleeding. To determine the level at which bleeding begins, the string is measured from the oral cavity to the proximal limit of the blood-stained string. Conversely, the level at which blood staining of the string is first detected is compared to the level at which bile staining of the string, or acidification of fluid absorbed into the string, is first detected.

In humans, endoscopy has an 80% to 90% accuracy rate for the detection of upper gastrointestinal lesions resulting in bleeding, if performed early in the diagnostic workup. Radiography is usually of less value than endoscopy in localizing the site of the bleeding. Selective celiac arteriography may be required to determine the site of intestinal bleeding due to vascular anomalies. Such anomalies are difficult to recognize at endoscopy or surgery and are an important cause of gastrointestinal hemorrhage in older humans. Tests using ^{99m}Technetium-labeled red blood cells may be used to locate the site of bleeding. Miscellaneous other diagnostic procedures of value are listed in Table 5–26.

BORBORYGMUS AND FLATULENCE

Borborygmus is a rumbling noise caused by the propulsion of gas through the gastrointestinal tract. Borborygmus and flatulence most commonly affect the dog. They usually result from dietary indiscretions, but on occasion in both species can herald more serious gastrointestinal disease.

The two most common sources of intestinal gas in dogs and cats are swallowed air and bacterial fermentation of nutrients such as carbohydrate and fiber. Additional sources are the chemical release of carbon dioxide from bicarbonates and diffusion of gas from the blood. The composition of intestinal gas is primarily nitrogen, oxygen, hydrogen, methane, and carbon dioxide, all of which have no odor. Odiferous potentially volatile substances such as ammonia, hydrogen sulfide, indole, skatole, mercaptans, volatile amines, and short chain fatty acids comprise less than 1% of intestinal gas. The transit time for gas is considerably shorter than that for liquids or solids. In humans, gas introduced into the stomach can be passed per rectum in as short a time as 15 minutes. Overdistension of the stomach or intestinal tract by gas can lead to considerable abdominal discomfort.

Excessive aerophagia can induce increased flatus and borborygmi. Diets high in legumes, such as soybean meal, also

Table 5–25

CAUSES OF MELENA AND GASTROINTESTINAL BLOOD LOSS

Swallowed Blood
  Hemoptysis
  Nasal adenocarcinoma
  Oropharyngeal neoplasia
Esophagus
  Laceration
  Ulceration
  Neoplasia
Stomach
  Widespread erosions
  Ulcers (drugs, stress, uremia, liver failure, mastocytosis, gastrinoma, hypoadrenocorticism)
  Severe gastritis
  Sharp foreign bodies
  Neoplasia (adenocarcinoma, leiomyosarcoma, lymphosarcoma, mastocytosis)
Upper Small Intestine
  Duodenal ulcers (drugs, stress, uremia, liver failure, mastocytosis, gastrinoma)
  Severe duodenitis
  Neoplasia (mast cell neoplasia, lymphosarcoma, adenocarcinoma)
  Foreign bodies
  Hookworms
Lower Small Intestinal and Proximal Colon
  Neoplasia
  Hookworms
Gastrointestinal Blood Vessels
  Laceration, varix, aneurysm, arteriovenous malformations, thrombosus, polyarteritis nodosa, SLE
Gastrointestinal Ischemia
  Shock
  Volvulus
  Intussusception
  Mesenteric avulsion
  Gastrointestinal infarction
Gastrointestinal Toxicosis
  "Magic" mushrooms
  Heavy metals
  Caustic agents
Liver (hemobilia)
  Hematoma that discharges into the biliary system
  Arteriobiliary fistula following penetrating trauma
  Hepatic cancer
  Liver failure
Pancreas
  Severe acute pancreatitis
Kidney
  Uremia
Hematologic disorders
  Thrombocytopenia
  Thrombocytopathy
  Clotting defects
  Von Willebrand's disease
  DIC
  Polycythemia
Drug administration
  Nonsteroidal anti-inflammatory drugs
  Glucocorticoids
  Iron preparation overdosage

Table 5–26

DIAGNOSTIC ENDEAVORS FOR THE EVALUATION OF APPARENT UPPER GASTROINTESTINAL BLEEDING

Clinical Examination	Usefulness
History	Trauma, drug usage
Physical examination	Nasal or oropharyngeal bleeding
Inspection of the stool	Melena vs. hematochezia
Admission Laboratory Work	
CBC	Severity and chronicity of blood loss; polycythemia
Reticulocyte count	Regenerative or nonregenerative anemia
Buffy coat	Mast cell neoplasia, lymphoma
Serum chemistry profile	Uremia, BUN to creatinine ratio, liver disease, multiple myeloma
Fecal flotation	Hookworms
Coagulation Tests	
Platelet count	Thrombocytopenia
Bleeding time	Thrombocytopenia, thrombocytopathy
OSPT, APTT	Clotting defects
Von Willebrand's test	Von Willebrand's disease
Fibrin degradation products	DIC
Procedures for Localization and Diagnosis of GI Bleeding	
Nasogastric intubation	Localize site of hemorrhage
Survey radiographs	GI masses, perforation
Ultrasound	GI mass lesions
Gastrogram	Gastric ulcers, masses
Scintigraphy	Localize site of bleeding
Arteriography	Aneurysm, thrombosis, arteriovenous malformation
Rhinoscopy/nasal radiographs	Nasal adenocarcinoma
Pharyngoscopy	Pharyngeal neoplasia
Bronchoscopy/chest rads	Hemoptysis
Upper GI endoscopy	Esophageal ulceration, esophageal neoplasia, gastric erosions, ulcers, neoplasia and severe gastritis, foreign bodies, varices, duodenal ulcers and neoplasms
Colonoscopy	Lower small intestinal and proximal colonic neoplasia
Exploratory surgery	Miscellaneous diagnosis and therapy

animals with lactase deficiency. Malassimilation can result in excessive intestinal gas.

The management of borborygmus and flatulence begins with a change to a highly digestible low-fiber diet of moderate protein and fat content. Suitable commercial products are available (for instance Prescription Diet i/d). Alternatively, the owner can prepare a homemade diet comprised of highly digestible protein and carbohydrate sources such as cottage cheese and rice appropriately balanced with vitamins and minerals. Reducing aerophagia by avoiding situations that provoke nervousness and by discouraging greedy eating, for instance by ensuring a dog does not have to compete for his food, may also be helpful. In the rare event that dietary manipulation is not successful, consider investigation of the patient as already described for the evaluation of small-bowel diarrhea. Alternatively, symptomatic pharmacologic management can be tried.

Pharmacologic management of excessive gaseousness relies on adsorbents, antifoaming agents, or digestive enzymes. Charcoal is the most commonly used adsorbent antiflatulent in people but is of questionable effectiveness and practicality. Simethicone (25 to 200 mg per dose, q 6 hours) is frequently used as a treatment for borborygmus, gaseous colic, and flatulence in human begins. It is an

are associated with gaseousness. Legumes contain large quantities of indigestible oligosaccharides. Unabsorbed oligosaccharides are fermented by clostridia and other bacteria to produce hydrogen, carbon dioxide, and methane. Spoiled diets and diets high in fat or poorly digestible protein are particularly likely to yield odiferous gases. The type and abundance of bacterial flora also affect the composition and quantity of flatus. Milk products may cause gaseousness in some antifoaming agent that reduces surface tension, allowing bubbles to coalesce so they may be more easily passed. It is not absorbed from the gastrointestinal tract and can be safely used in dogs and cats at or near the dose for human beings. Its effectiveness as an antiflatulent in dogs and cats is unknown. Antiflatulent enzyme supplements are claimed to assist the digestion of fermentable nutrients that are digested poorly by the gastrointestinal systems of monogastrics. Anecdotal reports suggest these enzyme supplements can reduce the severity of flatulence in cats and dogs.

ASCITES[24]

Ascites is an abnormal accumulation of fluid within the peritoneal cavity. The presence of ascites is usually detected by physical examination, radiography, or ultrasound. Ultrasound is the most sensitive technique, regularly detecting as little as 6.6 ml of fluid per kg body weight.[25] Paracentesis classifies the abdominal fluid, markedly reducing the list of diagnostic possibilities, and on occasion providing a diagnosis. The fluid may be transudative, exudative, hemorrhagic, bilious, chylous, pseudochylous, eosinophilic, or it may result from the accumulation of urine. Transudates are colorless fluids, with a specific gravity of less than 1.017, a WBC count of less than 3000/μl (mainly mononuclear), and a protein content of less than 3 g/dl (usually less than 1.5 g/dl). Capillary permeability and plasma protein concentration influence the level of protein in the fluid. Pure transudates are due to hypoalbuminemia. Modified transudates are a common cause of ascites. They share some features of transudates and exudates and usually have a clear or serosanguinous appearance. The most important cause of ascitic modified transudates is portal hypertension. Exudates have a cloudy appearance and variable color. They have a specific gravity of greater than 1.017, a protein content of greater than 3 g/dl, and a cell count of greater than 3000/μl (usually predominantly neutrophils). Exudates are usually due to inflammatory processes such as FIP, septic or chemical peritonitis, or necrosis (torsions, large tumors). Hemorrhagic abdominal effusions are characterized by a PCV, total protein, and white blood cell count similar to peripheral blood. Observation of erythrophagocytosis, hemosiderin-laden macrophages, or the absence of platelets indicates preexisting hemorrhage and rules out the possibility of misdiagnosed hemorrhagic effusion due to inadvertent puncture of the spleen, liver, or a blood vessel during paracentesis. Eosinophilic effusions are rarely reported in cats and dogs.[27] They can be classified as transudates or exudates. Many affected animals do not have a corresponding eosinophilia in the blood. Neoplasia and hypereosinophilic syndrome are the most common causes of eosinophilic ascites. Treatment is usually directed at the underlying cause. Rupture of the biliary tree is usually due to trauma or neoplasia. Bile is highly irritating and induces a chemical peritonitis. The ascitic fluid can be yellow-ocher in color and is usually exudative, containing many neutrophils. The diagnosis is confirmed by a highly positive bilirubin reaction on a urine dipstick immersed in ascitic fluid. Bilirubin crystals or bilirubin-laden macrophages may be observed in the ascitic fluid. Location of the leak requires scintigraphy or surgical exploration.

Chylous ascites is due to accumulation of lymph in the abdominal cavity. Pseudochylous ascites is due to the accumulation of fluid with a high content of phospholipid-protein material. Chylous fluid appears white when the lymph contains a high concentration of triglyceride-rich chylomicrons. Pseudochyle appears white because of the high phos-

Table 5–27

CAUSES OF ASCITES

Transudative Ascites
　Hypoalbuminemia (glomerulonephritis, liver failure, protein-losing enteropathy)
Modified Transudates
　Prehepatic portal hypertension: vascular occlusion from torsions, strangulations (hernias), neoplasia (abdominal carcinomatosis, mesothelioma, metastatic neoplasia, others)
　Hepatic portal hypertension: cirrhosis, hepatic thrombosis, neoplasia, hepatic AV fistula, hepatic venous abnormalities, toxoplasmosis, liver flukes
　Posthepatic portal hypertension: congestive heart failure, obstruction of the caudal vena cava ("kinked" caudal vena cava, acquired and congenital intraluminal obstructions, extraluminal obstructions, GDV)
Exudative Ascites
　Septic peritonitis (perforations of bowel, penetrating abdominal wounds, rupture of bowel, uterus, or abscess)
　Chemical peritonitis (pancreatitis, bile, urine)
　FIP
　Necrosis of neoplastic cells or organs
Hemorrhagic Ascites
　Trauma: ruptured liver or spleen, mesenteric avulsion
　Coagulopathies: warfarin toxicosis
　Vascular disorders: ruptured aneurysm
　Neoplasia: splenic hemangiosarcoma, ovarian neoplasia, hepatic neoplasia
Bile Ascites
　Rupture of biliary tract: trauma, necrotizing cholecystitis
Chylous Ascites
　Rupture of lymphatics: trauma, neoplasia
　Lymphatic hypertension: obstruction (congenital absence, neoplasia, cranial vena caval hypertension); increased lymph flow (hypoalbuminemia)
　Increased lymphatic permeability: perilymphatic inflammation (pancreatitis)
Pseudochylous Ascites
　Neoplasia
　Others?
Eosinophilic Ascites
　Neoplasia
　Hypereosinophilic syndrome
　Gastrointestinal perforation (rarely)

pholipid-protein content. Chylous fluid can also be clear and water-like when its lipids are solubilized in a micellar solution. Such solutions are free of protein, and the lipid content is demonstrated following staining with Sudan stain. Chylous ascites usually results from rupture or leakage of abdominal lymphatics due to trauma, lymphatic obstruction (congenital, neoplastic, adhesions), increased lymphatic flow, or increased lymphatic permeability. Pseudochylous effusions appear to be rare in the dog and cat. In humans, pseudochyle most commonly results from degenerating neoplastic, inflammatory, or mesothelial cells. Several tests can be used to differentiate chylous and pseudochylous effusions. Chyle forms a cream layer after standing, contains many lymphocytes, and has a cholesterol-to-triglyceride ratio less than 1. It will clear with ether and will not clear following centrifugation. Lipoprotein analysis should reveal chylomicrons.

The prevalent causes of ascites and the diagnostic procedures commonly employed for the evaluation of such patients are listed in Tables 5–27 and 5–28, respectively. Before embarking on a diagnostic workup, it behooves clinicians to note that patients with double compartment effusions (abdominal and pleural cavities) have a poor to grave prognosis.[26]

Table 5–28

DIAGNOSTIC PROCEDURES OF VALUE FOR DIAGNOSING ASCITES

PROCEDURE	USEFULNESS
GENERAL CBC	
Hematocrit	Hemorrhage
Differential	Sepsis, toxemia, hydration
Lymphocyte count	Lymphangiectasia
Serum chemistry profile	
BUN/creatinine	Uremia
Liver enzymes, BUN, albumin	Liver disease
Albumin	Hypoalbuminemia
Globulin	Protein-losing enteropathy, FIP
Urinalysis	Renal disease, proteinuria
Fluid analysis	
Cell count	Characterize effusion
Protein concentration	Characterize effusion
Cytology	Inflammation, neoplasia
Anaerobic/aerobic culture	Septic peritonitis
BUN, creatinine, potassium level	Urinary tract perforation
Bilirubin	Biliary tract perforation
Amylase	Pancreatitis, intestinal perforation
Triglyceride to cholesterol ratio	Chyle
Lipoprotein analysis	Chyle
TRANSUDATIVE ASCITES	
Urine protein/creatinine ratio	Proteinuria
Liver function test	Liver failure
Scintigraphy	Protein-losing enteropathy
Endoscopy	Protein-losing enteropathy
Thoracic radiography	Concomitant thoracic effusions
MODIFIED TRANSUDATE	
Thoracic radiography	Concomitant thoracic effusions, heart disease, diaphragmatic hernias
Abdominal ultrasonography	Masses, metastatic neoplasia, portal hypertension, liver disease, torsions
Cardiac ultrasonography	Heart disease
Portal pressures/CVP	Portal hypertension characterization
Portal venograms	Venous obstruction, shunts
Hepatic arteriograms	Hepatic AV fistula
Exploratory celiotomy	Neoplasia, torsions, strangulations
EXUDATIVE ASCITES	
Serum antibody/antigen tests	FIP
Serum amylase/lipase	Pancreatitis
Abdominal ultrasonography	Neoplasia, pancreatitis
Exploratory celiotomy	Necrotizing lesions, perforations
HEMORRHAGIC ASCITES	
PIVKA	Warfarin toxicosis
Clotting times	Warfarin toxicosis, clotting factor deficiencies
FDPs	DIC
Abdominal ultrasonography	Splenic neoplasia, other neoplasia, trauma
Exploratory celiotomy	Traumatic damage, neoplasia, vascular diseases
CHYLOUS ASCITES	
Lymphangiograms	Localize lymphatic obstruction, leakage
Exploratory celiotomy	Localize obstruction, leakage
BILE ASCITES	
Scintigraphy	Localize bile duct rupture
Exploratory celiotomy	Localize bile duct rupture

ABDOMINAL PAIN (ACUTE ABDOMEN)

Abdominal pain can be acute or chronic. The term *acute abdomen* is applied to painful abdominal disorders of acute onset.

Etiopathogenesis

The causes of abdominal pain are listed in Table 5–29. Abdominal pain may arise from the parietal peritoneum and abdominal wall (somatic pain), the abdominal viscera (visceral pain), or extra-abdominal tissues such as prolapsed discs (referred pain).

Visceral pain may originate in the visceral peritoneum, mesentery, gastrointestinal tract, liver, pancreas, urinary system, spleen, or reproductive organs. It can result from distension of a hollow viscus; swelling of an organ; traction on a mesentery; or inflammation, ischemia, or perforation of an abdominal structure. These perturbations cause pain by stimulation of nociceptors via stretch or exposure to mediators such as kinins, prostaglandins, and substance P.

In humans, visceral pain is reported to have a dull, gnawing, or cramping character and is usually poorly localized. In contrast, somatic pain is sharp, localized, and is aggravated by movement. These differing characteristics result from variations of the mode of transmission of the two different classes of pain. Visceral pain is transmitted by unmyelinated C nociceptive fibers. These fibers enter the sympathetic trunk and pass cranial or caudal in the trunk for variable distances before entering the rami communicans, to join the dorsal root of the spinal nerve and enter the spinal cord. There is thus extensive overlap of the spinal segments to which afferent fibers from one locale project. In contrast, transmission of somatic pain is by thinly myelinated A-delta fibers of spinal nerves. They project directly to their respective spinal cord segments with minimal overlap. The afferent pathway of nociception is complex and can be influenced by various inhibitory or facilitatory events at a number of different levels. The threshold for the sensation of painful stretch is lowered by the presence of kinins and prostaglandins at the nociceptors. Thus, mild distension or stretching, such as might occur with minor organ congestion or normal bowel contraction, may produce considerable pain in abdominal organs in which inflammation exists.

Diagnostic Approach

The diagnosis of abdominal pain begins with the clinical examination. The clinical findings dictate the urgency of the patient's condition and the order and extent of subsequent diagnostics. A rapid, accurate decision as to whether celiotomy is required for diagnosis or treatment can be critical to patient survival.

HISTORY. The animal with an acute abdomen is usually depressed, inappetant, and may have a hunched appearance. Other signs of abdominal disease, such as vomiting, diarrhea, and abdominal distension, are often present. Animals may adopt postures of relief such as the "praying" position. Occasionally they "dog-sit" or lie on cold surfaces for abnormally prolonged periods. Animals may cry out when the owner lifts them, may be unwilling to move, or conversely may behave in a distressed and agitated manner, sometimes verging on hysteria.

The history may suggest the cause of the abdominal pain.

Table 5–29

CAUSES OF ACUTE ABDOMEN

Abdominal Wall
  Strangulated hernias[s]: inguinal, scrotal, abdominal, umbilical, diaphragmatic, hiatal, mesenteric
  Trauma[s,m]
  Steatitis[m]
Peritoneum and Mesentry
  Abdominal abscess[s]
  Septic peritonitis[s]: perforated viscus, penetrating wounds (foxtails)
  Bile peritonitis[s]
  Urine peritonitis[s]
  Mesenteric traction[s,m]: large masses
  Mesenteric avulsion[s]
  Adhesion[s]
Gastrointestinal Tract
  Gastroenteritis[m]: viral, bacterial, toxic, hemorrhagic
  Gastric dilatation[m,s]
  Gastric dilatation-volvulus[s]
  Gastrointestinal gaseousness[m]
  Gastroduodenal ulceration[s,m]
  Anatomic gastrointestinal obstruction[s]: fb, stricture, intussusception
  Functional gastrointestinal obstruction[m]: ileus
  Gastrointestinal perforation or dehiscence[s]
  Intestinal volvulus[s]
  Mesenteric artery thrombosis[s]
  Colitis[m]
  Irritable bowel syndrome?[m]
  Cecal inversion[s]
  Neoplasia[s,m]
Liver
  Hepatitis[m]
  Hepatopathy[m]
  Neoplasia[s,m]
  Bile duct obstruction[s]: calculi, neoplasia, pancreatic abscess
  Biliary tree rupture[s]
  Liver abscess[s]
Pancreas
  Pancreatic abscess[m,s]
  Pancreatitis[m]
  Pancreatic neoplasia[s]
Urinary System
  Acute nephrosis[m]: ethylene glycol, aminoglycosides
  Acute nephritis and pyelonephritis[m]
  Renal calculi[s,m]
  Renal neoplasia[s,m]
  Urethral obstruction[s,m]: calculi, neoplasia, stricture
  Ureteral obstruction[s]: calculi, neoplasia, strictures
  Urinary tract rupture[s]
Spleen
  Torsion[s]
  Neoplasia[s]
  Trauma[s,m]
Reproductive Organs
  Uterine torsion or rupture[s]
  Pyometra[s,m]
  Ectopic pregnancy[s]
  Ovarian or prostatic cysts[s]
  Prostatic abscess[s]
  Prostatic cyst or neoplasia[s,m]
  Acute prostatitis[m]
  Testicular torsion[s]
Miscellaneous
  Abdominal hemorrhage[m,s]
  Hypoadrenocorticism[m]
  Mesenteric lymphadenopathy[m]
  Heavy metal poisoning[m]: lead, organophosphates
  Household agent toxicoses[m] (NSAIDs, corrosives, soaps and detergents, pine oil)
  Thoracic diseases: referred pain
  Vertebral or disc diseases

[s]Surgical therapy; [m]medical therapy.

Previous use of corticosteriods can lead to pancreatitis, colonic perforation, or gastric ulceration. Nonsteroidal medications can cause gastrointestinal ulceration. A history of tenesmus suggests the possibility of prostatic, urinary tract, or colonic diseases. Trauma and toxicities are more likely in pets allowed to wander. Pancreatitis is common in obese middle-aged dogs fed a high-fat diet. Unvaccinated young animals are more commonly afflicted with viral gastroenteritis. Gastrointestinal obstructions due to foreign bodies and intussusceptions are common in younger dogs and animals with access to bones, toys, string, and garbage. Large-breed dogs are prone to organ torsions. Urinary obstruction is a common cause of abdominal pain in male cats. Schnauzers may develop abdominal pain in association with their hyperlipidemia syndrome. Chondrodysplastic breeds may suffer apparent abdominal pain from disc prolapse.

Abdominal pain developing several days after trauma raises the possibility of perforation of bowel, rupture of biliary or urinary tract, or necrosis of pieces of liver or spleen. Spasmodic pain is commonly due to contractions of a hollow viscus. Pain associated with defecation suggests large-bowel, prostatic, or perianal disease. Postprandial pain can occur with gastrointestinal tract, pancreatic, and biliary disorders. Important examples include pancreatitis, biliary carcinoma, and the "magenblase syndrome." The latter refers to abdominal pain due to gaseous gastric distension resulting from excessive aerophagia.

PHYSICAL EXAMINATION. Rapid evaluation of the seriousness of the patient's condition is important. Hallmarks of severity include evidence of shock, hypothermia, tympany, hyperpnea, marked dehydration, weakness, and depression. In the presence of these signs urgent therapeutic intervention is essential.

Clinical signs of abdominal pain include a hunched stance and stilted gait. Areas of the physical examination that deserve emphasis include oral, rectal, orthopedic, neurologic, and abdominal examinations. The mouth is examined for linear foreign bodies and discolorations of the mucous membranes such as jaundice. Rectal examination detects pelvic abnormalities, such as prostatomegaly, and may reveal melena. Orthopedic and neurologic examinations detect diseases of the limbs and vertebral column that can cause a hunched appearance and gait abnormalities that mimic abdominal pain. The clinician should examine the skin for oil or abrasion, and the claws of cats for shredding consistent with road trauma. The patient is checked for undescended testicles (that can torse) or vaginal discharge suggestive of pyometra.

Abdominal palpation is performed in a careful and systematic manner. To begin, the clinician should run his or her fingertips through the hair of the entire abdomen. This facilitates detection of penetrating wounds (such as scabs from cat bites) and swellings (hernias, hematomas). The clinician must differentiate abdominal pain from intractability. More significance is attributed to pain responses elicited in stoic animals and to pain that is localized, repeatable, and evident after minimal manipulation. Determination is made whether the painful area is superficial (skin or abdominal wall), located in the cranial or caudal abdomen, or originates from a specific viscus. Superficial pain restricted to a well-defined area suggests somatic pain, perhaps of spinal cord, spinal nerve, or cauda equina origin. Cranial abdominal pain is common in pancreatitis. Generalized abdominal pain with board-like rigidity of the abdominal musculature suggests generalized peritonitis. Pain associated with acute tympany implies gas distension of stomach. Other palpable abnormalities, such as thickened bowel, abdominal masses, ascites, organomegaly, intussusception, and tympany, may reveal the cause of the acute abdomen or narrow the diagnostic possibilities. Abdominal auscultation may be a helpful adjunct. Failure to detect borborygmus after two to three minutes of auscultation suggests ileus.

Diagnostic Procedures

Diagnostic procedures of value for the evaluation of patients with abdominal pain are listed in Table 5–30. Diagnostics for urgent cases are usually limited to PCV, TP, urine specific gravity, reagent strip assessment of blood glucose and BUN, paracentesis, and abdominal radiographs or ultrasound. If available, serum electrolytes and blood gases are of value in tailoring fluid therapy. Diagnostics for more stable patients may be more extensive.

ADMISSION LABORATORY WORK. The CBC, serum chemistry profile, urinalysis, and blood gas analysis provide information that greatly helps with differential diagnosis and case management. The laboratory database may determine the organ(s) involved (liver, kidney, adrenal) and the type of disease process (inflammation, hemorrhage), and it may reinforce clinical assessment of severity (hypoglycemia, degenerative left shift, dehydration, acidosis, electrolyte imbalance). Lipase and amylase analysis aid detection of pancreatitis. Platelet number and tests of hemostasis may detect DIC. Fecal flotation may yield evidence of parasitism (hookworms, whipworms, *Nanophytes salmincola*). Toxicologic analyses may be indicated depending on the likelihood of exposure.

ABDOMINAL RADIOGRAPHS. Abdominal radiographs may reveal free gas in the abdomen, suggestive of intestinal or body wall perforation. The free gas often accumulates between the diaphragm and the liver. Generalized loss of abdominal detail in a well-fleshed animal indicates abdominal effusion. Organomegaly, masses, calculi, obstructive disorders, foreign bodies, organ torsions, pancreatitis, and skeletal abnormalities may be apparent.

ABDOMINAL ULTRASOUND. Abdominal ultrasound is a sensitive technique for the detection of abdominal masses, including intraorgan miliary masses (e.g., metastatic neoplasia), abdominal fluid, abscesses, cysts, mural thickenings, lymphadenopathy, biliary obstruction, biliary and urinary calculi, and pancreatic abscess. On occasion, portal hypertension or hydronephrosis may be apparent. Ultrasound-guided percutaneous biopsy or aspiration of organs, masses, cysts, or effusion may be appropriate.

PARACENTESIS. Paracentesis is indicated if abdominal fluid is detected during physical examination or diagnostic imaging. It provides fluid for culture, cytology, and chemical analysis, thus allowing the characterization of the effusion and markedly narrowing the diagnostic possibilities. Ultrasound guidance aids aspiration of localized collections of fluid.

FLUID ANALYSIS. Fluid analysis may include visual inspection, cytology, gram stain, aerobic, and anaerobic culture. Cell count, specific gravity, PCV, and concentration of total protein, potassium, creatinine, bilirubin, and amylase may also be determined. Fluid analysis may be suggestive of bowel perforation (mixed flora, vegetable matter, neutrophils), organ torsion or neoplasia (modified transudates, anaplastic cells), urine leakage (higher BUN, creatinine, or potassium in the abdominal fluid than in serum), bile peritonitis (bilirubin positive), trauma (blood), or pancreatitis (nonseptic exudate, high amylase). High amylase concentration in the abdominal fluid is not pathognomonic for pancreatitis; it can also occur following bowel perforation.

DIAGNOSTIC PERITONEAL LAVAGE. Diagnostic Peritoneal Lavage (DPL) is indicated if paracentesis fails to yield abdom-

Table 5–30

DIAGNOSTIC PROCEDURES FOR EVALUATING ABDOMINAL PAIN

PROCEDURE	USEFULNESS
CBC	Sepsis, toxemia, blood loss, hypoadrenocorticism
Serum chemistry profile	Uremia, liver disease, hyperlipidemia, electrolyte imbalance
Blood gas	Acid-base status
Urinalysis	Kidney, liver disease
Fecal flotation	Hookworms, Salmon poisoning, whipworms, liver flukes
Platelet count	DIC
OSPT, APTT, ACT	DIC
Fibrin degradation products	DIC
Lipase/amylase	Pancreatitis
Survey radiographs	Masses, perforation, organomegaly, calculi, foreign bodies, GDV, obstructions, gaseousness
Ultrasound	Masses, fluid, biliary and urinary calculi, kidney and liver disease, uterine and prostatic disease, GI obstructions, torsions
Paracentesis	Fluid analysis (see Ascites)
Diagnostic peritoneal lavage	Fluid analysis (see Ascites)
Excretory urography	Renal and ureteral diseases
Gastrogram	Gastric ulcers, masses
Upper GI contrast study	Obstruction, GI neoplasia
Scintigraphy	Biliary obstruction
Upper gastrointestinal endoscopy	Gastric ulcers, foreign bodies, neoplasia and severe gastritis, inflammatory bowel disease, duodenal ulcers and neoplasms
Colonoscopy	Colitis, colonic neoplasia, cecal inversion
Arteriography	Aneurysm, thrombosis
Exploratory celiotomy	Miscellaneous diagnosis and therapy

inal fluid because of its paucity, flocculent nature, or because of loculation. DPL is performed by lavaging the abdomen with a large volume of sterile isotonic fluid (20 ml/kg body weight). It is utilized to improve the yield and sensitivity of the abdominal tap, and is very useful for the early detection of conditions such as abdominal hemorrhage, bowel dehiscence or perforation, pancreatitis, and neoplasia. Because DPL is more time consuming, dilutes abdominal effusions, and causes more patient discomfort, it should be performed only if paracentesis is unsuccessful. DPL does not detect retroperitoneal injury. Diagnostic criteria for DPL have been established to account for the dilution effects of the infused fluid. For instance, significant intra-abdominal hemorrhage is probable if the microhematocrit of the lavage fluid is greater than 2%. Peritonitis is likely if the neutrophil count is greater than 1500/μl.

MISCELLANEOUS TESTS. Various diagnostic tests pertaining to specific organ systems may be indicated. Examples include excretory urography, liver function tests, gastrointestinal contrast procedures, fine needle aspiration, or biopsy of abdominal masses. Endoscopy facilitates detection of upper gastrointestinal lesions, such as ulceration or neoplasia, and lower bowel lesions such as colitis, neoplasia, and cecal inversion.

EXPLORATORY CELIOTOMY.[11] Abdominal surgery is required in some patients to establish the cause of the abdominal pain and in many patients for its treatment. The decision to operate may be based on a progressive and rapid worsening in a patient's condition or on the diagnosis of a disease amenable to surgical therapy. Conditions generally warranting surgery are listed in Table 5–29. In some situations, rapid surgical intervention is clearly indicated. In other situations, the clinician must balance the need for urgency with the benefit of adequate preoperative supportive care. Crystaloid fluid, blood, plasma, antibiotics, corticosteroids, or analgesic administration may be required in the preoperative period.

Treatment

Treatment of abdominal pain depend on the cause. Symptomatic management includes the use of analgesics. Concern regarding the effect of the narcotics on respiratory, pancreatic, and biliary function has limited their use for abdominal pain, although there is little firm evidence to suggest they complicate recovery provided they are used at appropriate doses. Suitable analgesics for cats and dogs with abdominal pain are butorphanol (0.2–0.4 mg/kg SQ q 8 hours), oxymorphone (0.05 mg/kg, SQ, q 8 hours), and buprenorphine (0.01 mg/kg, SQ, q 8 hours).

REFERENCES

1. Politzer JP, Devroede G, Vasseur C, et al. The genesis of bowel sounds: Influence of viscus and gastrointestinal content. Gastroenterology 71:282–285, 1976.
2. Martin DC, Beckloff GL, Arnold JD, et al. Bowel sound quantitation to evaluate drugs on gastrointestinal motor activity. J Clin Pharm 11:42–45, 1971.
3. Lang IM, Sarna, SK, Condon RE. Gastrointestinal motor correlates of vomiting in the dog: Quantification and characterization as an independent phenomenon. Gastroenterology 90:40–47, 1986.
4. Kantrowitz B, Biller D. Using radiography to evaluate vomiting in dogs and cats. Vet Med, August:806–813, 1992.
5. Penninck DG, Nyland TG, Kerr LY, et al. Ultrasonographic evaluation of gastrointestinal diseases in small animals. Vet Radiol 31:134–141, 1990.
6. Lamb CR. Abdominal ultrasonography in small animals: Intestinal tract and mesentery, kidneys, adrenal glands, uterus and prostate. J Small Anim Pract 31:295–304, 1990.
7. Feeney DA, Johnston GR, Walter PA. Abdominal ultrasonography—1989: General interpretation and masses. Sem Vet Med Surg 4:77–94, 1989.
8. Miyabayashi T, Morgan JP. Upper gastrointestinal examinations: A radiographic study of clinically normal Beagle puppies. J Small Anim Pract 32:83–88, 1991.
9. Wolvekamp WTC. Enteroclysis: A New Radiographic Technique for the Evaluation of the Small Intestine of the Dog. Iowa State University Press, Ames, 1989.
10. Boothe HW. Exploratory laparotomy in small animals. Comp Contin Ed Pract Vet 12:1057–1066, 1990.
11. Boothe HW, Slater MR, Hobson HP, et al. Exploratory celiotomy in 200 nontraumatized dogs and cats. Vet Surg 21:452–457, 1992.
12. Oettle GJ. Effect of moderate exercise on bowel habit. Gut 32:941–944, 1991.
13. Fine KD, Fordtran JS. The effect of diarrhea on fecal fat excretion. Gastroenterology 102:1936–1939, 1992.
14. Latimer KS. Cytologic evaluation of rectal mucosal scrapings. Proc 11th Am Col Vet Int Med Forum, May 1993, 39–41.
15. Williams DA, Reed DS, Perry P. Fecal proteolytic activity in clinically normal cats and in a cat with exocrine pancreatic insufficiency. J Am Vet Med Assoc 197:210–212, 1990.
16. Smith S. Ultrasound-guided biopsy. Sem Vet Med Surg 4:95–104, 1989.
17. Leveille R, Partington BP, Biller DS, et al. Complications after ultrasound-guided biopsy of abdominal structures in dogs and cats—246 cases (1984–1991). J Am Vet Med Assoc 203:413–415, 1993.
18. Eltringham WK, Roe AM, Galloway SW, et al. A laproscopic technique for full thickness intestinal biopsy and feeding jejunostomy. 34:122–124, 1993.
19. Harvey HJ. Complications of small intestinal biopsy in hypoalbuminemic dogs. Vet Surg 19:289–292, 1990.
20. Cook AK, Gilson SD, Fischer WD, et al. Effect of diet on results obtained by use of two commercial test kits for detection of occult blood in feces of dogs. Am J Vet Res 1749–1751, 1992.
21. Fossum TW. Protein-losing enteropathy. Sem Vet Med Surg 4:219–225, 1989.
22. Lifschitz CH, Shulman RJ. Intestinal permeability tests: Are they clinically useful? J Pediatr Gastroenterol Nutr 10:283–286, 1990.
23. Gilson SD, Parker BB, Twedt DC. Evaluation of two commercial test kits for detection of occult blood in feces of dogs. Am J Vet Res 51:1385–1387, 1990.
24. King LG, Gelens HCJ. Ascites. Comp Contin Ed Pract Vet 14:1063–1075, 1992.
25. Henley RK, Hager DA, Ackerman N. A comparison of two-dimensional ultrasonography and radiography for the detection of small amounts of free peritoneal fluid in the dog. Vet Radiol 30:121–124, 1989.
26. Steyn PF, Wittum TE. Radiographic, epidemiologic, and clinical aspects of simultaneous pleural and peritoneal effusions in dogs and cats—48 cases (1982–1991). J Am Vet Med Assoc 202:307–312, 1993.
27. Fossum TW, Wellman M, Relford RL, et al. Eosinophilic pleural or peritoneal effusions in dogs and cats: 14 cases (1986–1992). J Am Vet Med Assoc 202:1873–1876, 1993.

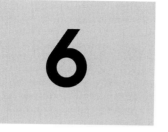

6

Procedures for the Evaluation of Pancreatic and Gastrointestinal Tract Diseases

DAVID A. WILLIAMS AND W. GRANT GUILFORD

INTRODUCTION

Numerous diagnostic procedures were referred to in Chapter 5. In this chapter the usefulness of these procedures is described in more detail, with particular reference to their indications, advantages, limitations, complications, contraindications, and methodology.

LABORATORY EVALUATION OF VOMITUS

Vomitus should be evaluated grossly for volume, content (food, mucus, bile, foreign ingested material), and odor (toxins, for example). Additional evaluations that may be useful include determination of pH and specific parasitologic, cytologic, virologic, and toxicologic procedures depending on circumstances. Consideration of the content and pH of suspect vomited material may help differentiate vomiting from regurgitation (Chapter 5).

Evidence for bile in vomitus makes pyloric obstruction unlikely. Small flecks of fresh blood may be present secondary to capillary trauma following repeated prolonged vomiting from any cause; if blood in vomitus has the appearance of "coffee grounds," however, this is usually an indication of significant upper gastrointestinal blood loss. (Chapter 5). Dogs and cats will occasionally vomit gastric or small intestinal parasites such as ascarids, *Physaloptera* spp., cestodes, and *Capillaria* spp.

Vomitus with an odor of feces can result from gastrointestinal obstruction, prolonged ileus, or coprophagia. "Vomited" food may smell of fermentation as a result of prolonged retention in the stomach or esophagus or of the ingestion of spoiled foods. Foul-smelling vomitus can also result from gastrointestinal necrosis.

Microscopic examination of vomitus will occasionally reveal the eggs of *Physaloptera* spp., the larvae or adult stages of *Ollulanus tricuspis,* spores of toxic fungi,[1] bacteria, and cellular remnants. Occasionally clusters of neoplastic cells will have sufficiently preserved morphology to be recognizable.

If poisoning is suspected, samples of vomitus can be submitted for toxicologic analysis. Toxins that may be detected include alpha-naphthyl thiourea (ANTU), phosphorus, zinc phosphide, arsenic, herbicides, and fungicides.

GASTRIC SECRETORY TESTING

Hydrochloric acid is an important component of gastric secretion. Gastric acid secretion may be normal, subnormal (hypochlorhydria), absent (achlorhydria), or increased (hyperchlorhydria). Changes in gastric acid secretion occur in association not only with gastric disease but also with other diseases such as gastrin-secreting pancreatic tumors, chronic renal disease, and intestinal resection.[2] The secretory activity of parietal cells cannot be assessed by examination of gastric biopsies. Several tests are available for assessment of gastric acid secretion, but the invasive nature, cost, limited indications, and low clinical yield of such tests have restricted their application in clinical veterinary medicine. These tests may prove useful in assessing the potential role of achlorhydria in small intestinal bacterial overgrowth and the potential role of gastric hypersecretion in patients with gastroduodenal ulcers and reflux esophagitis.[3]

Gastric Aspiration and pH Determination

The simplest gastric acid secretory test is the aspiration of gastric juice from a fasting patient by way of a naso- or orogastric tube, or endoscope, and the determination of the pH. In one study of healthy dogs, the pH of gastric fluid during the fasting state was found to range from 0.9 to 2.5.[4] Postprandial gastric pH was slightly higher (0.5–3.5) because of the buffering action of the food. In another study, the fasting gastric pH ranged from 0.8 to 8.0, with 70% of the dogs having a fasting gastric pH of less than 5.[3] If an acidic fasting gastric pH is detected, it proves the patient can secrete gastric acid. The observation of a low gastric pH, however, does not rule out hypochlorhydria or gastric hypersecretory states because the rate or total amount of gastric acid secretion is not measured, and pH in gastric fluid does not directly correlate to hydrogen ion "activity."[5]

In healthy dogs, basal gastric acid output is minimal during fasting. The bicarbonate in swallowed saliva and refluxed duodenal content may raise the pH of the gastric content toward neutrality. Thus, collection of gastric fluid with a near-neutral pH does not provide any evidence to support decreased gastric acid secretory capacity. Collection of a sample of gastric juice with near-neutral pH 15 to 30 minutes after pentagastrin or histamine stimulation, however, is diagnostic for achlorhydria. Within 15 minutes of pentagastrin administration (6 μg/kg), 100% of healthy dogs had a pH of less than 2.[3] Similarly, a near-neutral pH in the presence of raised serum gastrin levels suggests the raised gastrin is a result of achlorhydria and not gastrinoma.

It is important to recognize that the ability of the stomach to respond to exogenous secretagogues does not reflect actual acid secretion in a given patient in response to physiologic stimuli. Failure to secrete under such stimulation probably does reflect severely impaired gastric mucosa, but such a situation has not been reported in dogs or cats and must be extremely rare.[6]

Radiotelemetric Determination of Gastrointestinal pH

A radiotelemetric technique for the measurement of gastrointestinal pH has been used in the dog.[4] The technique allows continuous, accurate measurement of pH, but is disadvantaged by the restricted availability of the equipment and by potential misdiagnosis of achlorhydria resulting from the passage of the radiotelemetric capsule from the stomach into the duodenum.

Gastric Acid Output

Quantitative gastric acid secretory testing requires the placement of an indwelling tube in the pyloric antrum to allow the complete collection of gastric secretion during a defined time period. The technique may be performed by temporary pharyngostomy or by orogastric intubation using a specific anesthetic technique.[3]

BASAL GASTRIC ACID SECRETION. To assess basal acid output (BAO), gastric secretions are collected from the fasting stomach by continuous suction for two to four consecutive 15-minute collection periods. The samples are titrated with sodium hydroxide to pH 7 and the acidity expressed in mEq (mmol) of hydrogen ion produced per unit time. BAO is normally a fraction of 1 mEq of hydrogen ion per hour. The basal volume of gastric secretion is 0.37 to 2.95 mL/hour/kg$^{0.75}$. BAO analysis is of most use should the clinician wish to confirm a gastric hypersecretory state. The accuracy of this technique depends on appropriate tube placement, complete collection of gastric fluid, and minimal gastroduodenal reflux. Wide variations on repeated determinations from the same patient compromise the usefulness of this test. Increased BAO in humans is associated with stress, renal failure, duodenal ulcers, mastocytosis, increased intracranial pressure, and gastrinomas. In humans with gastrinomas, the BAO is usually 60% or more of the maximal acid secretory response to secretagogues. Similar findings have been reported with canine gastrinoma.[7]

MAXIMUM OR PEAK ACID OUTPUT. To determine peak acid output (PAO), gastric acid secretion is quantified during consecutive 15-minute periods following administration of secretagogues such as histamine, betazole, or pentagastrin. Subsequently either the two consecutive 15-minute collections giving the highest acid output are chosen and their acid output doubled to give PAO in mEq/hour, or alternatively, the acid outputs from the four consecutive samples are totaled to determine maximum acid output (MAO). Histamine stimu-

lates maximum secretion when a single dose of 0.320 mg/kg of histamine base is given subcutaneously. In human gastric acid secretory testing, the following subcutaneous doses for the different histamine formulations are used: 0.04 mg/kg histamine acid phosphate, 2.75 mg/kg histamine hydrochloride, and 0.014 mg/kg histamine base. The secretion rate peaks during the second hour after injection (Figure 6–1). The mean maximum rate of secretion by dogs weighing 4.5 to 28 kg is 14 to 40 mEq hydrogen ions/hour.[8] An almost linear positive correlation exists between parietal cell mass and maximal acid secretion.[8] H$_1$-receptor antagonists are given with histamine to minimize cardiovascular effects. The H$_1$-receptor antagonists do not interfere with gastric acid secretion.

Betazole (Histalog) is an analogue of histamine that can be used to stimulate acid secretion without need for an antihistamine. The dose of betazole for maximum acid secretion is 30 mg/kg body weight.[8] Much smaller doses (0.5 mg/kg SQ) are currently used during clinical testing in humans to minimize side effects.

Pentagastrin (Peptavlon) is a synthetic gastrin analogue that stimulates maximal acid output within 15 to 30 minutes in the dog when given at 6 μg/kg SQ or IV. Reference values for peak hydrogen ion output after pentagastrin stimulation are 1.5 to 3.61 mEq/hour/kg$^{0.75}$.[3] Pentagastrin is the preferred secretagogue for gastric acid secretory testing because of rapidity of action and minimal side effects.

The assessment of PAO or MAO can be used for the quantitative assessment of gastric hyposecretion or hypersecretion. Conditions associated with reduced gastric acid secretion in humans include gastritis, gastric carcinoma, and gastric polyps.

In a series of 111 dogs with signs of upper gastrointestinal disease, 18 were hypersecretory, 43 hyposecretory, and the remaining 50 patients had normal responses to stimulation with pentagastrin.[6] None of the dogs had achlorhydria. Pathologic changes observed in these three groups are summarized in Table 6–1. The underlying pathology tended to be more severe in the hyposecretory group. Given that the median age of the hyposecretory group of dogs was greater than that of the other groups, it was suggested this repre-

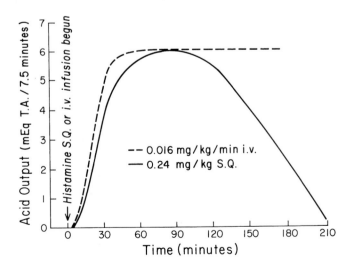

FIGURE 6-1. Gastric acid secretion following a single injection or continuous infusion of histamine (expressed as histamine base) in a large (30 kg) dog. Dogs weighing 5 to 10 kg have maximal secretory responses 35% to 85% as great when given the same doses. Total hourly secretion of titratable acid ranges from 15 mEq in 5 kg dogs to 40 mEq in 30 kg dogs.

sented a more chronic stage of a disease process.[6] Although of interest, these results do not support the value of gastric acid secretory testing in the routine investigation of dogs with signs of chronic upper gastrointestinal disease.

SERUM GASTRIN. Serum gastrin can be secreted by G cells in the pyloric antrum and duodenum or by neoplastic cells (gastrinomas), usually located in the pancreas. Radioimmunoassay kits for the measurement of human gastrin are probably valid for use in dogs and other species, but appropriate validation of individual kits with production of appropriate canine controls is desirable, as with any radioassay.[9] Blood for gastrin assay should be collected into a cold tube, the serum promptly separated from blood cells, and shipped frozen on dry ice. Normal fasting serum gastrin concentrations in the dog are less than approximately 100 pg/mL and in the cat 28 to 135 pg/ml.[3,7,9,10–13]

Serum gastrin concentration varies inversely with the concentration of hydrogen ions in the gastric lumen. In dogs and cats elevated serum gastrin has been reported in association with chronic, ulcerative, and atrophic gastritis, gastric dilatation-volvulus, pyloric stenosis, immunoproliferative small intestinal disease of Basenjis, renal failure, gastrinoma, antacids, gastric antisecretory drugs, and glucocorticoids.[14] Additional causes have been reported in humans (Table 6–2). Very high concentrations of gastrin (greater than 500 pg/ml) are generally considered diagnostic of gastrinoma in the dog, although in human patients serum gastrin concentrations greater than 500 pg/mL can also occur with gastric hyposecretory states such as atrophic gastritis.[14,15] Therefore, in a patient with a markedly elevated serum gastrin, it would seem prudent to ensure that gastric pH is low and perhaps perform an endoscopic examination and gastric biopsy to verify the presence of gastric mucosal hypertrophy or gastric/duodenal ulceration before surgical exploration for suspected gastrinoma. In those dogs with only moderately elevated gastrin levels in association with acidic gastric pH, various provocative tests of serum gastrin (serum gastrin response to a test meal, intravenous calcium infusion, or intravenous secretion infusion)[16] may be required to confirm gastrinoma (see APUDomas).

TESTS OF GASTROINTESTINAL NEUROMUSCULAR FUNCTION

At present, clinically applicable tests of gastrointestinal motor function in dogs and cats rely on the determination of gastric motility by way of fluoroscopy or on the evaluation of gastric emptying by way of contrast radiography or scintigraphy. These radiographic techniques are discussed in the section on gastrointestinal radiography.

In the experimental setting, gastrointestinal motor function of animals has been accurately examined by implanting bipolar electrodes in the gastric or intestinal wall for the measurement of myoelectrical activity and using strain gauges for the measurement of mechanical activity. These techniques can detect gastric dysrhythmias and electromechanical dissociation.[17] Cutaneous devices for recording the "electrogastrogram" are also becoming available.[18]

Gastrointestinal manometry is extensively used in human medicine for the diagnosis of esophageal and large-bowel motility disorders. The development of a peroral silicone pressure sensor device, which contains a series of pressure transducers encased in a 2.7 mm diameter flexible polyurethane sheath, now allows the accurate recording of gastric and small intestinal motility in clinical patients.[19]

The value of manometric techniques in veterinary clinical gastroenterology remains to be established. The techniques have been successfully used on an experimental basis in dogs for the evaluation of lower esophageal sphincter tone, gastric pressure, and anal sphincter tone.[20,21]

TESTS OF GASTRIC INFLAMMATION/FOOD SENSITIVITY

Serum pepsinogens (PGs) have been shown to be useful markers for gastritis in human patients.[22] In humans there are two immunologically distinct groups of pepsinogens, named PGI and PGII, the latter being produced only by pyloric glands in the gastric antrum; the ratio of changes in the concentrations of these zymogens reflects the distribution of the gastric inflammation.[22] In dogs, pepsinogen synthesis has been localized to gastric chief cells, but immunologically distinct PG groups have not been described.[23] Dog gastric lipase has also been localized in gastric mucosa, although in contrast to pepsinogen it originates from mucous pit cells.[23] Assays of pepsinogen or gastric lipase are both potentially useful markers for gastric disease; unfortunately it is likely that species-specific immunoassays will be required to detect serum concentrations of enzyme with sufficient accuracy and precision to be clinically useful.

The local response of the gastric mucosa to direct application of food antigens has recently been assessed using endo-

Table 6–1

GASTRIC ACID SECRETORY RESPONSES AND GASTROINTESTINAL ENDOSCOPIC AND HISTOLOGIC FINDINGS IN 111 DOGS WITH UPPER GASTROINTESTINAL DISEASE

GASTRIC ACID SECRETORY RESPONSE	REFLUX ESOPHAGITIS	GASTRITIS	GASTRIC ATROPHY	GASTRO-DUODENAL REFLUX	ENTERITIS
Hypersecretory n = 18	+ (n = 2)	++	–	–	++
Normal n = 50	–	++	–	–	++
Hyposecretory n = 43	+ (n = 2)	+++	++	+++	++

The number of + signs reflects severity and frequency of the findings in each group; a – sign indicates the abnormality was not observed. Data abstracted from Happé, 1982.[6] Unless otherwise indicated (n=) almost all dogs in each group exhibited(+) did not exhibit (–) a given abnormal finding.

Table 6–2

POSSIBLE CAUSES OF ELEVATED PLASMA
GASTRIN CONCENTRATION

Achlorhydria
Atrophic gastritis
Antral G cell hyperplasia
Antacids
Gastrinoma
Gastric antisecretory drugs
Gastric cancer
Gastric dilatation-volvulus
Gastric ulceration
Glucocorticoids
Hypercalcemia
Immunoproliferative small intestinal disease of Basenjis
Pyloric stenosis
Renal failure

scopic visualization.[24,25] Gastroscopic food sensitivity testing probably evaluates only immediate (type 1) hypersensitivities to foods, but this approach may nonetheless be useful in formulating therapeutic diets. It may be of particular value in investigation of dietary sensitivity in research centers.[26]

EXAMINATION OF FECES[27–30]

Feces from every patient with a gastrointestinal problem should be evaluated for physical appearance and for parasites. Biochemical analysis, occult blood tests, fecal cytology, fecal virology, and bacterial culture may be indicated in selected cases.

Gross Examination

PHYSICAL APPEARANCE.   Diarrhea is defined as an increase in the volume or frequency of bowel movements, or a change in consistency of the feces. The content of water and fiber determines fecal volume. Normal feces contain 60% to 70% water; an increase of 10% can produce a watery diarrhea. The bulk and weight of feces in normal dogs varies with the nature of the diet; dogs fed dry cereal–based food have bulkier, softer feces, which weigh approximately twice as much (20 g/kg body weight/day) as feces passed by dogs eating commercial meat-based canned food (10 g/kg body weight/day).[31,32] Normal feces are completely formed; the last part of the feces passed should be as well formed as the first. Normal feces have indentations, produced by colonic contractions, and contain scant or no mucus and no blood. The presence of fresh blood and mucus is suggestive of large-bowel disease, but this does not preclude the possibility of coexistent or underlying small-bowel disease (Chapter 5). Normal feces can contain recognizable foods that are known to be indigestible, such as whole grains of corn. Indigestible materials such as grass and hair are also commonly present. Small amounts of ingested hair are of no concern, but larger amounts may be a cause of gastrointestinal irritation, gastric impaction, or constipation. Undigested particles of digestible foods suggest hurried passage or maldigestion. Steatorrhea is not grossly recognizable until fecal fat content is extremely high, when fat may actually separate from the aqueous phase of the feces. In acute exudative inflammation, animals may pass fibrinous casts of their bowel. Tapeworm proglottides are often noted on the feces of dogs and cats by their owners.

COLOR.   The dark brown color of normal feces is imparted by bile pigments (stercobilin) that have been metabolized by intestinal bacteria. Complete absence of biliary secretions results in no fecal pigmentation, producing "acholic" or gray feces, a very rare finding that is usually associated with obstructive jaundice. Brown coloration of feces also depends on adequate intestinal bacterial activity. Patients with diarrhea may have reduced numbers of intestinal bacteria and rapid intestinal transit. The result is incomplete metabolism of bile pigments and altered fecal color to yellow, green, or light brown. Antibiotics that reduce the number of intestinal bacterial bacteria may also produce light-colored feces. The effect persists for only a few days, however, the longest time the microflora can be suppressed with antibiotics. Diet also influences fecal color. Diets containing predominantly milk proteins produce light-colored feces. Diets containing predominantly meat proteins produce dark-colored feces because of the metabolism of heme pigments contained in the meat. Upper gastrointestinal hemorrhage results in black, tarry feces, termed melena (Chapter 5). Excessive iron in feces causes a similar greenish black appearance. Some drugs pigment feces; charcoal, bismuth, and salicylates darken the feces, whereas antacids lighten them.

ODOR.   The odor of feces is produced by indoles and skatols—products of bacterial activity on tryptophan—and by mercaptans, hydrogen sulfide, methyl sulfides, and related by-products of the sulfur-containing amino acids. The odor is greatest in feces produced from diets containing a high amount of meat protein. The odor is diminished on easily digestible high-carbohydrate or milk-protein diets. Any diet or antibiotic modifying the bacterial microflora can affect fecal odor. Feces from patients with malabsorption can smell acrid or sour because of the presence of short-chain fatty acids produced by bacterial fermentation of unabsorbed carbohydrates and fatty acids.

Microscopic Examination (Table 6–3)

Feces are examined microscopically for evidence of malabsorption/maldigestion and of intestinal parasites and for evaluation of fecal cytology. Fecal examinations that may support suspected malabsorption are described later in this chapter in the section on tests for malabsorption.

FECAL AND RECTAL SCRAPE CYTOLOGY.   Cytologic examination of feces or scrapings of rectal mucosa can be helpful in

Table 6–3

MICROSCOPIC EXAMINATION OF DIRECT
SMEARS OF FECES

Parasites	Ascarids, Hookworms, Whipworms, Strongyloides, Giardia, Trichomonas, Coccidia, Entamoeba, Balantidium
Fat triglycerides	Sudan III stain
Fatty acids	Acetic acid + Sudan III stain
Starch granules	Lugol's solution stain
Protein, muscle fibers	Cytology stains
Inflammatory cells (white blood cells)	Cytology stains
Microorganisms	*Staphylococcus* spp. overgrowth *Clostridia* spp. overgrowth *Clostridium perfringens* spores *Histoplasma capsulatum* *Campylobacter*

the diagnosis of patients presenting with signs of large-bowel diarrhea. It is particularly useful in identifying patients infected with *Histoplasma* or invasive bacteria such as *Salmonella* sp. To perform fecal cytology, a fleck of mucus or a sample of feces from the surface of the stool is smeared thinly on a slide and stained with hematology stains. To perform rectal scrapes, a gloved finger or cotton-tipped applicator is is used manually to abrade the rectal mucosa. The material adherent to the scraping object is transferred to a microscope slide by rolling or smearing it across the slide.

Large numbers of fecal neutrophils are suggestive of acute colonic inflammation, such as may occur with invasive bacterial infections, and should prompt culture of the stool, especially if concomitant fecal blood is detected.[33] In humans, large numbers of leukocytes in the stool are most commonly associated with invasion of the mucosa by *Shigella*, *E. coli*, *Entamoeba histolytica*, *Salmonella*, and *Campylobacter*. *Shigella*, *Campylobacter*, and invasive *E. coli* cause the most severe purulent exudates in human patients but are rarely diagnosed in dogs and cats. The presence of eosinophils in a fecal smear supports eosinophilic colitis, and the presence of a mixed leukocyte population can appear with inflammatory bowel disease in human patients.[34] Such findings are uncommon in dogs and cats with intestinal disease. A study comparing the results of rectal scrape cytology with colonoscopic examination and colon biopsy in dogs with chronic large-bowel diarrhea found that rectal cytology did not permit differentiation of rectal neoplasia, noninflammatory colonic disease, and plasmacytic/lymphocytic colitis.[35] Rectal scrape cytology may be of benefit in the diagnosis of histoplasmosis, however, because *Histoplasma* organisms are sometimes identified in macrophages from rectal mucosal scrapes; organisms are rarely seen in simple fecal smears.

The presence of *Clostridium perfringens* spores (Figure 6–2) in a fecal smear is highly suggestive of diarrhea due to *Clostridium perfringens*– associated enterotoxicosis.[36] Fecal smears occasionally identify overgrowth of normal microorganisms in the rectum; in such cases a gram stain may provide some clues about the responsible bacteria, such as *Staphylococci* (gram-positive cocci) and *Clostridia* spp. (gram-positive bacilli). Unfortunately the significance of such overgrowth by a single organism is at present not clear.

Spirochetes are frequently seen in fecal smears of animals with diarrhea but are not believed to be pathogenic; they are part of the normal microflora of the colon. During diarrheic episodes, they are dislodged from the colonic crypts and can appear in large numbers in the feces. They

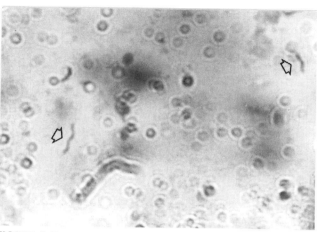

FIGURE 6-3. *Campylobacter* in fecal smear. From Green CE. Enteric bacterial infections. In CE Green (ed) Clinical Microbiology and Infectious Diseases of the Dog and Cat. WB Saunders, Philadelphia, 1984, Fig. 38–2, p. 626.

should not be confused with *Campylobacter*, which may also be seen in direct fecal smears. The latter have a characteristic "seagull-wing" appearance (Figure 6–3), and high numbers of the organism (at least 10^6 organisms per gram of feces) must be present in order to see one per high-power field. Identification is facilitated by staining with Wright's or Wright's-Giemsa stain. Mushroom toxicity has been diagnosed by detecting fungal spores in feces or vomitus.[1] *Candida* spp. may be visualized in its pseudomycelium and yeast forms, but it is a normal inhabitant of the gastrointestinal tract and is probably not of significance unless it is also present in other locations as part of a generalized opportunistic infection in an immunocompromised patient.[37]

Parasitology[38]

Microscopic evaluation of feces to identify intestinal parasites is indicated in all cases of diarrhea (Figure 6–4).

DIRECT SMEARS OF FECES. Examination of direct smears of feces readily identify the ova, oocysts, larvae, or trophozoites of some nematode and protozoal parasites. The direct smear is important in identifying *Strongyloides stercoralis* infection (because larvae rather than eggs are usually found in the stool) and trichomonas and entamoeba infections (because these protozoa have no form other than that of the trophozoite). Trophozoites are the active, feeding motile stage of protozoal parasites. The motility of trophozoites assists their identification in fecal smears and can aid in the diagnosis of protozoal disorders such as giardiasis.[39] Trophozoites are found only in fresh fecal samples; as feces cool from body temperature, the trophozoites encyst. Direct smears of feces for trophozoites are, therefore, best examined immediately after collection; trophozoites are most likely to be observed if aspirated duodenal juice is examined.[40] The fecal sample is placed on a warmed glass slide, diluted with a few drops of normal saline to improve visualization of motile structures, and examined at 40× magnification.[41] Addition of a drop of Lugol's iodine solution kills and immobilizes the parasites and stains various internal structures, thereby enhancing the morphology of the organ-

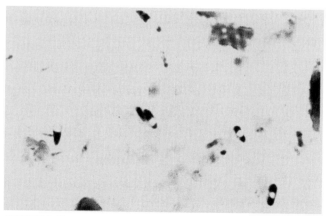

FIGURE 6-2. *Clostridium perfringens* spore.

isms. This also helps differentiate cysts from similar structures in feces, including plant cells, starch granules, and fungal spores, which do not contain internal structures. The primary limitations of fecal smear examinations are small sample size and the lack of concentration of parasites. A negative result does not rule out infection.

Examination of air-dried smears of fresh feces that have been stained with hematology stains will occasionally identify *Giardia* and *Entamoeba* trophozoites. Trichrome stains are very effective for the diagnosis of giardiasis using feces preserved in polyvinyl alcohol fixative.[42,43] Acid-fast stains may reveal *Cryptosporidia*.[44]

FECAL FLOTATIONS. Ova of nematode parasites and the cysts and oocysts of most protozoa are easier to find if they are concentrated by various flotation methods. The principal of the procedure is the dispersion of ova and fecal material in saturated sugar or salt solutions and their separation based on their differential density. Because most parasite ova have a lower density than these solutions, they will float to the surface of the solution, whereas the heavier fecal particulate matter will not float. The ova are collected on a coverslip in contact with the surface of the suspension. Separation of ova from fecal material can be hastened by centrifuging the suspension. Flotation solutions in use include sucrose and zinc sulfate solutions.[45] Sucrose solutions are not as dense as salt solutions, and fluke eggs and some nematode eggs will not float in them. Sheather's sugar centrifugation technique is useful for the identification of *Toxoplasma, Cryptosporidium,* and other coccidia, as well as hookworm, roundworm, tapeworm, whipworm, and *Capillaria,* although this solution will distort *Giardia* cysts.[44,45] Zinc sulfate flotation is a sensitive test for the diagnosis of giardiasis provided three fecal samples are examined.[39,41,43] Almost all fluke and nematode ova float in this solution, but the high density of this medium causes some ova to collapse. Tapeworm ova are not found in microscopic examinations unless the packets containing the ova are broken. Multiple fecal examinations are sometimes necessary to detect whipworm infection.

FECAL SEDIMENTATION. Fluke ova are best concentrated by sedimentation. Feces are dispersed in water, after which the mixture is strained and centrifuged. The supernatant is poured off, and a few drops of the sediment are examined microscopically for fluke ova. This technique, or variants thereof, is useful for the detection of *Nanophyteus salmincola,* the vector of *Neorickettsia helminthoica,* the agent of Salmon poisoning in dogs and of *Eurytrema, Platynosomum,* and *Amphimerus* fluke infections in cats. The eggs of *Nanophyteus salmincola* will also float in many standard flotation media, however. Modified fecal sedimentation techniques, including the formalin-ether sedimentation technique,[46] have been described. Care should be taken to differentiate *Diphyllobothrium latum* tapeworm ova from fluke eggs.

PRESERVATION OF FECES FOR PARASITOLOGIC EXAMINATION. If a delay between elimination and examination of the feces is anticipated, techniques can be used to preserve protozoal oocysts and helminth eggs.[45] Small amounts of uncooled formed stool may be mixed with equal volumes of 10% formalin or, alternatively, with three times the amount of polyvinyl alcohol. Vials containing polyvinyl alcohol fixative are commercially available (Fekal FK10, Trend Scientific). Polyvinyl alcohol fixation can preserve fecal specimens for months and does not interfere with subsequent staining, or with the formalin-ether sedimentation technique.[45,47]

IMMUNOASSAY FOR PARASITES. Giardiasis can be diagnosed by enzyme-linked immunosorbent assay (ELISA) of trophozoite antigens in feces, a method that is reported to be very sensitive and specific in human patients.[48] The fecal ELISA test avoids the problem of intermittent cyst formation and is probably more sensitive than performing a single zinc sulphate flotation examination. However, it is reported to be no better than a skilled observer performing zinc flotation three times.[41] The ELISA can be done using feces preserved by freezing or formalin fixation and mailed to a commercial laboratory.[41,49]

Fecal Culture

INDICATIONS. Routine bacteriologic cultures of feces from dogs and cats with diarrhea are not warranted in view of the rarity with which enteric pathogens are cultured, the difficulties involved with the interpretation of culture results, the self-limiting nature of many bacterial infections, and the inappropriateness of antibiotic therapy for many bacterial-mediated diarrheas. Furthermore, isolation and identification of enteric pathogens is a labor-intensive, expensive process that involves enrichment, plating, and identification steps performed sequentially over a three- to four-day period. On occasion, however, stool culture in animals with diarrhea may be helpful (Table 6–4). These include a history of exposure to bacterial pathogens, outbreaks of diarrhea among more than one pet in a household, concern about a public health hazard or nosocomial infection, and clinical, cytologic or biopsy evidence of bacteria-associated diarrhea. Clinical signs of infection with the currently known enteric bacterial pathogens are highly variable, but suspicion of infection should be aroused by dogs or cats that display an acute onset of a predominantly "large-bowel" diarrhea. Clinical or laboratory evidence of sepsis should further heighten suspicion. Positive culture for *Clostridium perfringens* is likely if spores are noted on cytologic examination of fecal smears[36,50]; however, a positive culture alone is meaningless because *C. perfringens* is a normal inhabitant of the gastroin-

Table 6–4

POTENTIAL INDICATIONS FOR BACTERIOLOGIC CULTURE OF FECES FROM CATS OR DOGS WITH DIARRHEA

Historical Findings
 Onset after exposure to spoiled or contaminated food products
 Onset after kenneling
 Onset after show attendance
 Onset after contact with an animal infected by a bacterial pathogen
 Outbreak of diarrhea among more than one pet of a household
Physical Exam Findings
 Acute onset of bloody diarrhea in association with evidence of sepsis (blood cultures also required)
Laboratory Work
 Evidence of sepsis (leukocytosis, leukopenia, hypoglycemia, etc.)
Fecal Smears
 Large number of fecal neutrophils especially if with fecal blood
 Bacterial overgrowth of the colon
 Clostridium perfringens spores
 Presence of "seagull-wing" bacteria (suspect *Helicobacter* spp.)
Colon Biopsy
 Evidence of suppurative or pseudomembranous inflammation
Public Health Hazard
 Young, elderly, or infirm humans in the household
Nosocomial Infection Hazard

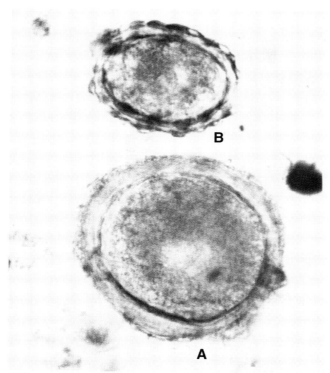

FIGURE 6-4. Parasites and parasitic ova found in the feces of small animals.

(A) Toxocara canis ovum × 800
(B) Ascaris lumbricoides ovum (spurious) × 800

(**FIGURE 6-4** *continued*)

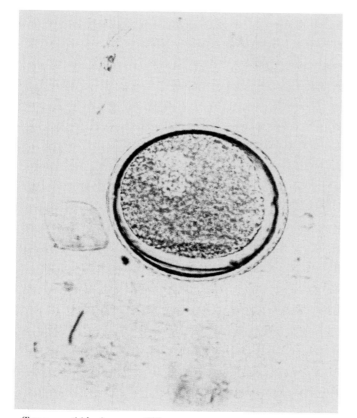

Toxocara cati (dog) ovum × 800

(**FIGURE 6-4** *continued*)

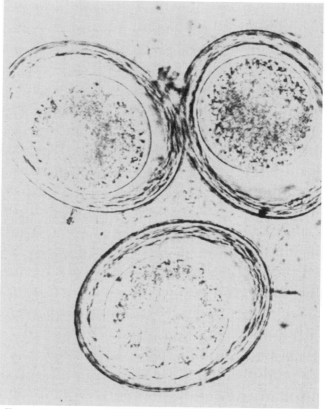

Toxascaris leonina (dog) × 800

Figure continued on following page

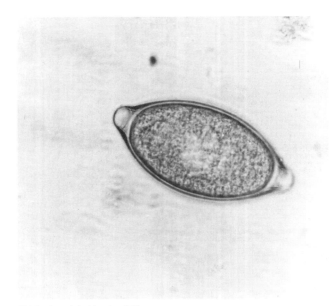

Trichuris vulpis (dog) × 800

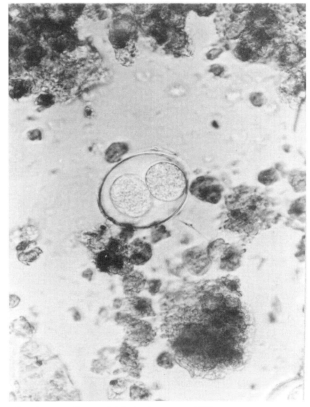

Cystoisospora (Isospora) felis (cat) oocyst × 800

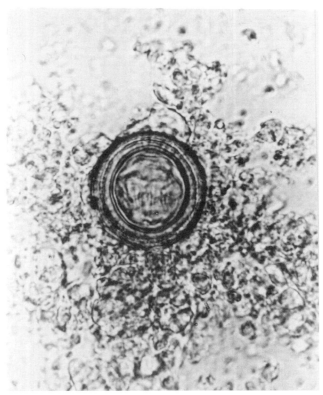

Taenia sp. (cat) ovum × 1300

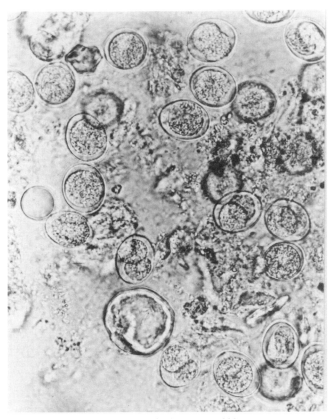

Cystoisospora (Isospora) ohioensis (dog) oocysts × 800

(**FIGURE 6-4** *continued*)

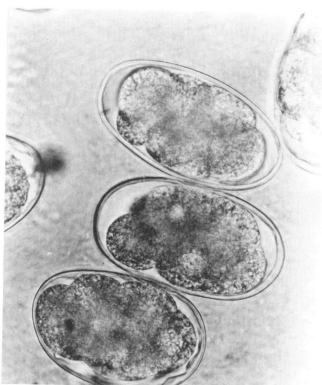

Ancylostoma caninum (dog) × 800

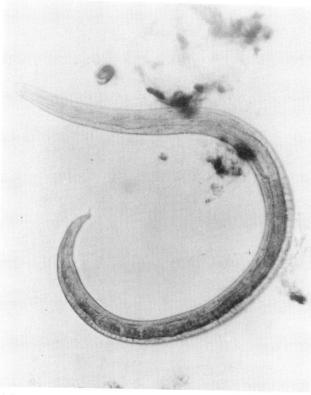

Aelurostrongylus abstrussus (cat) × 300

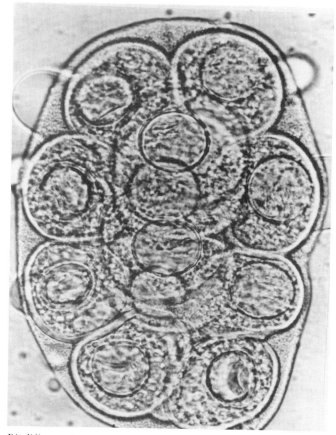

Dipylidium caninum (dog) egg packet × 300

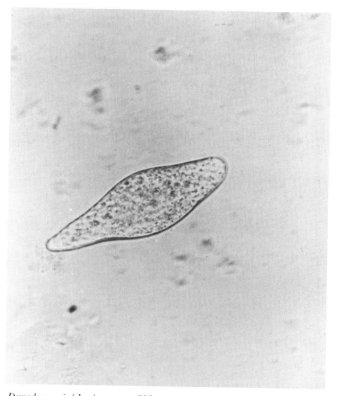

Demodex canis (dog) ovum × 800

(FIGURE 6-4 *continued)*

Figure continued on following page

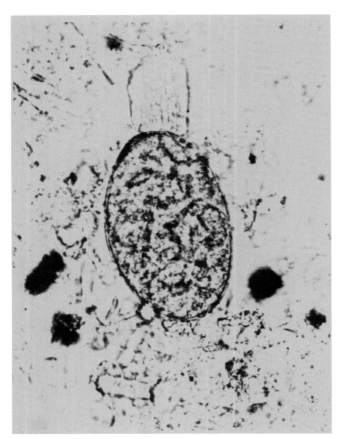

Nanophyetus salmincola (dog) ovum × 800

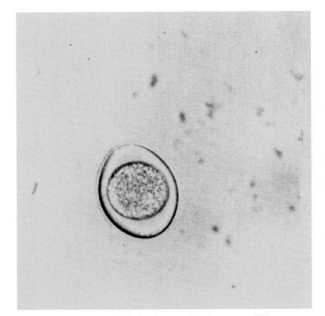

Cystoisosospora (Isospora) felis (cat) sporulated oocyst × 800

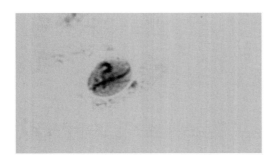

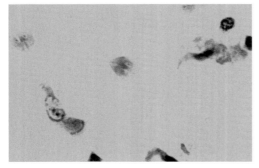

Giardia cyst and trophozoite

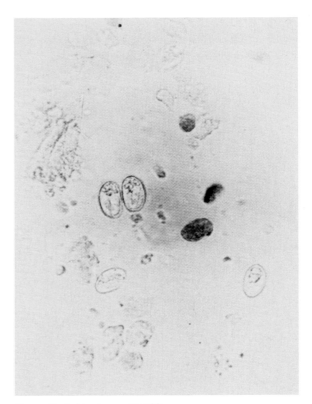

Sarcocystis sp. (dog) oocyst × 800

(**FIGURE 6-4** *continued*)

testinal tract. An assay for *C. perfringens* enterotoxin (Pet-RPLA Test, Oxoid Ltd., Hampshire, U.K.) can be used to confirm *C. perfringens* enterotoxin-associated diarrhea.[36,50–53] If a biopsy of the colon is dominated by neutrophil infiltration, erosion, and ulceration, bacterial colitis is a possibility. If the histopathology shows pseudomembranous inflammation, a culture for *Clostridium difficile* and an assay for its toxin may be rewarding.

Quantitative culture of fecal bacteria has no clinical application. Quantitative culture of duodenal fluid is of value, however, and is discussed in the section on endoscopy. Culture of feces for fungal organisms such as *Histoplasma capsulatum* is less reliable than serodiagnosis or identification of fungal elements by biopsy or fecal cytology.

In summary, in certain circumstances, culture of the feces for specific enteric pathogens is warranted, and on some occasions, antibiotic therapy of a patient based on culture of an enteric pathogen is appropriate. On most occasions, however, the feces are cultured to identify patients that may be carrying organisms such as *Salmonella* and therefore pose a public health risk.

TECHNIQUE. Appropriate sample submission protocol and culture techniques vary widely for the different enteric pathogens. The clinician must tell the laboratory which bacterial species to attempt to culture and must seek advice on the methods for collecting and submitting samples. Sterile cotton-tipped applicators that are supplied with transport media or enrichment broth are suitable for the submission of fecal samples for culture of aerobic enteric pathogens.[54–56] When these swabs are used, it is preferable to sample the surface of a fresh stool, including a portion of any mucus, exudate, or blood. Fecal samples for the culture of microaerophilic or anaerobic organisms should be very fresh. It is preferable to aspirate or remove the sample directly from the colon. Two to 10 g of solid feces or 3 to 10 mL of liquid feces should be submitted in sterile airtight vials to the laboratory without delay. If cotton-tipped swabs are used for the collection of these more fastidious bacteria, the swabs should be rubbed over the rectal mucosa and, once liberally coated with feces and exudate, placed immediately into transport media specifically suited for these organisms. Inadequate sample size is the most common error associated with fecal culture submission. Feces should be submitted for culture early in the course of diarrhea, because as time progresses the numbers of pathogens decline and their isolation becomes more difficult.[54–56]

INTERPRETATION. Because many normal flora can be opportunistic pathogens, and because many pathogens can be occasionally cultured from the feces of normal animals, the results of fecal cultures can be difficult to interpret. Furthermore, some pathogens such as certain *E. coli* can be diagnosed only by refined bacterial typing techniques. Interpretation of culture results is made easier if the laboratory provides a comparative estimate of the number of the bacterial pathogen in relation to other bacterial flora. It is often assumed a heavy and relatively pure growth of a known pathogen is significant, whereas light growths of pathogens among healthy mixed flora are of more doubtful significance, but definitive studies of these interpretations are lacking.

Fecal Virology

Because of the self-limiting nature of many gastrointestinal viral infections, or the presence of characteristic clinical or laboratory features (as in parvovirus infections), virologic studies of feces or vomitus are seldom utilized in small animal veterinary medicine. Identification of viral pathogens is indicated, however, when outbreaks of contagious diarrhea are being pursued in a kennel, cattery, or hospital situation, whereby identification of the viral agent may aid effective prophylactic procedures.

A number of procedures for the diagnosis of viral gastroenteritis from feces or vomitus have been utilized. These include virus isolation, immunofluorescence on cell culture, fecal hemagglutination, immunoassay (ELISA), electrophoretic methods, and electron microscopy.[54,57–60] Fecal hemagglutination, ELISA, and electron microscopy tests provide the most rapid diagnostic information and are preferred for clinical use. The sensitivity and specificity of most of these tests for the diagnosis of viral gastroenteritis in dogs and cats have not been adequately examined. Improved detection of viruses by electron microscopy after ultracentrifuge preparation of specimens has been reported in humans and some farm animals.[61,62] Using convalescent serum to aggregate the fecal virus particles before examination may also improve the sensitivity of electron microscopy.[63] These latter techniques hold promise for the rapid, accurate diagnosis of viral gastroenteritis in small animal patients. A fecal ELISA test is available for the detection of rotaviruses (Rotazyme, Abbott Laboratories, North Chicago, IL), and fecal hemagglutination tests and ELISA tests are widely utilized for the diagnosis of canine parvovirus.[60,64] Canine parvovirus ELISA tests are available in kit form (e.g., CITE Test, IDDEX, Inc., Portland, ME) and appear to be sensitive and specific, because in acute cases the amount of virus in feces is great. False negatives may occur in more chronic cases as a result of the decline in the number of viral particles excreted later in the course of the infection of clinical signs. It is likely that whatever technique is used for identification of any viral cause of diarrhea, diagnostic yield will be greater if samples collected early after the onset of clinical signs are submitted for analysis.

Biochemical Evaluation

FECAL WATER PERCENTAGE, pH, ELECTROLYTE CONCENTRATIONS, OSMOTIC GAP, AND OSMOLALITY. The percentage of water in feces provides an objective assessment of the severity of diarrhea. The percentage of stool weight present as water is determined by comparison of the wet weight of a stool sample with the weight of the same sample subjected to 48 hours of drying at 80° C in a vacuum oven.

Low fecal pH is suggestive of diarrhea due to carbohydrate malabsorption, although in clinical situations involving generalized malabsorption it is likely reductions in pH will be mitigated or masked by the buffering effects of unabsorbed fatty acids and amino acids.[65]

Fecal osmolality and electrolyte concentration are determined on an aliquot of stool water derived from the centrifugation of feces at approximately $10,000 \times g$ for 15 minutes. Fecal electrolyte concentration is used to diagnose congenital secretory diarrheas in human patients because in this situation fecal fluid is rich in monovalent electrolytes. Fecal electrolyte concentration in association with the fecal osmolality can be used to calculate the osmotic gap, which is expected to be large (>50 mOsm/kg) in osmotic diarrheas but small (<50 mOsm/kg) in secretory diarrheas. Fecal fluid osmolality, in human patients at least, is assumed to be the same as plasma osmolality for the purposes of this calculation; osmotic gap is therefore calculated by subtracting ([Na + K] × 2) from 290. Measured fecal fluid osmolality should not be used for this calculation because it can deviate from 290 mOsm/kg. Reductions below 290 mOsm/kg can reflect contamination of stool with water or dilute urine, whereas values above 290 mOsm/kg may arise due to contamination with concentrated urine or after ingestion of large amounts of bran. Most important, osmolality may also rise rapidly after passage of stool owing to bacterial metabolism of fecal carbohydrate during storage.[65,66]

Despite their relative ease of use and utility for the diagnosis of secretory and osmotic diarrheas in human patients, the value of fecal electrolyte and osmolality analysis in cats and dogs has yet to undergo objective evaluation. The osmolality, sodium concentration, and potassium concentration of feces from four normal cats were 622 to 927 mOsm/kg, 27 to 57 mEq/L, and 19 to 46 mEq/L, respectively.[67]

Fecal Blood. Feces may contain small amounts of blood insufficient to produce melena. A variety of chemical tests can identify such occult gastrointestinal bleeding. The qualitative tests for occult blood are sufficiently simple and inexpensive to be suitable for inclusion in the routine database. A positive occult blood test provides objective evidence for the presence of inflammatory, ulcerative, or neoplastic gastrointestinal disease that probably justifies further investigations to establish the underlying cause of the abnormality. Occult blood tests may also be used to differentiate true melena from other conditions that may cause artifactual coloration of feces.

Qualitative tests are based on the catalytic augmentation by hemoglobin and some of its breakdown products of the activity of the peroxidase enzyme catalyzing the conversion of hydrogen peroxide to water and oxygen.[68] Some chemicals can be oxidized during this reaction, forming colored products that are readily identified. Some tests contain orthotoluidine (Hematest, Ames Co.) or benzidine as the chemical oxidized to a colored product. Others use guaiac as the indicator chemical (Hemoccult, SmithKline Beecham Corp.). To avoid false positive results, diets should ideally not contain red meat for three days before testing. The sensitivities of both types of tests are probably adequate to detect most bleeding lesions.

False positive occult blood tests can occur if the patient is consuming oral iron preparations, aspirin, cimetidine, or significant quantities of vegetable heme proteins or red meat. Mutton-containing diets are particularly likely to cause false positive test results.[69] If there is any doubt as to the suitability of the diet for use during occult blood testing, a blended sample of the diet can be applied to the tablet to help determine if a false positive test is likely. Occult blood tests can remain positive for as long as a week after a single incidence of gastrointestinal hemorrhage.

A quantitative fluorometric assay of fecal hemoglobin has been used to detect fecal hemoglobin in dogs,[70] and immunoassays for human hemoglobin are available for use in human patients. These assays allow determination of the severity of gastrointestinal hemorrhage and have greater sensitivity and specificity than the peroxidase techniques. Unfortunately, intraluminal degradation of hemoglobin may lead to less than total detection of intestinal lesions causing gastrointestinal blood loss.[68]

Recent studies of human patients have indicated that assay of fecal alpha$_1$-protease inhibitor (alpha-1-antirypsin) presently provides the most sensitive and specific test for occult blood loss.[68] Unlike hemoglobin, this plasma protease inhibitor is resistant to intraluminal proteolytic degradation, so that when there is blood loss into the gut lumen it is eliminated immunologically intact in feces. The recent development of an immunoassay for the canine protein will allow evaluation of this approach in canine patients.[71]

TESTS FOR MALABSORPTION

Introduction

Clinical signs of weight loss, diarrhea, and failure of nutrient absorption are common to diseases in which digestion of food and/or subsequent absorption of nutrients are defective. These disorders are traditionally classified as either primary failure to digest the food (maldigestion) or primary failure to absorb the constituent nutrients (malabsorption). The principal cause of maldigestion is exocrine pancreatic insufficiency (EPI), whereas most cases of malabsorption are caused by small intestinal disease (SID).

This classification is somewhat misleading because failure of absorption is an inevitable consequence of defective digestion, and most diseases affecting the small intestine will inevitably impair the terminal processes of digestion that take place at the luminal surface of the intestinal mucosa. Nonetheless, this division does emphasize that the most useful application of tests of pancreatic and intestinal function is to distinguish patients with EPI from those with SID.

Established tests to evaluate dogs with suspected maldigestion or malabsorption include microscopic examination of feces for the presence of undigested food, several methods that indirectly assess fat absorption, assay of pancreatic enzyme activities in feces, bentiromide (N-benzoy-L-tyrosyl-p-aminobenzoic acid, BT-PABA), and xylose absorption tests. Many of these tests have found limited application due to unreliability (lack of sensitivity or specificity), practical constraints, or expense. Several new tests are now available for use in general practice, and other new approaches to diagnosis of small intestinal disease, although not widely available, have recently been described.

Many of these tests have drawbacks, one of the most common of which is limited sensitivity. This disadvantage, together with increased availability of gastrointestinal endoscopy, has led to an inappropriately reduced use of malabsorption tests for diagnosing SID. Endoscopy is not a replacement for malabsorption tests because the former detects morphologic disease only, whereas many of the latter procedures are tests of bowel function. It has been clearly demonstrated that many canine patients with SID have minimal or absent morphologic abnormalities while function as reflected by tests of absorptive capacity is abnormal.[72] Furthermore, even when morphologic changes are seen, the abnormalities are usually mild and nonspecific. Thus, ideal evaluation of suspected small-bowel disease requires both tests of specific functions and morphologic evaluation of intestinal biopsies.

Tests of Exocrine Pancreatic Function[73,74]

One of the major reasons for testing for diseases causing malabsorption is to distinguish patients with exocrine pancreatic insufficiency (EPI) from those with small intestinal disease. This is easily and reliably done by either assay of serum trypsin-like immunoreactivity (TLI) or assay of fecal proteolytic activity (FPA).

Serum Trypsin-like Immunoreactivity (TLI). Trypsinogen is synthesized exclusively by the pancreas, and measurement of the serum concentration of this zymogen by species-specific radioimmunoassay (Canine TLI Assay, Diagnostic Products Corp.) provides a good indirect index of pancreatic function in the dog.[73] This immunoassay detects both trypsinogen and trypsin, hence the use of the term *trypsin-like immunoreactivity* to describe the total concentration of these two immunoreactive species (Figure 6–5). Serum TLI concentration is both highly sensitive and specific for the diagnosis of canine EPI. Concentrations are dramatically reduced in dogs with EPI, whereas those in dogs with SID are not significantly different from normal (Figure 6–6).[73,75] Marked reductions in serum TLI (to less than 2 μg/L) may even precede signs of weight loss or diarrhea in dogs with pancreatic acinar atrophy, at a time when results of other tests (fecal proteolytic activity, bentiromide absorption) are still within the control ranges.[75–77]

A major advantage of this test is its simplicity. Analysis of a single serum sample obtained after food has been withheld for several hours is all that is required. Serum TLI is very stable, and samples can therefore be mailed without refrigeration to an appropriate laboratory. Administration of oral pancreatic extracts (usually of porcine origin) does not affect serum TLI concentration because trypsins from different species do not cross-react immunologically, and little, if any, intact enzyme is absorbed intact from the gut lumen. Withdrawal from enzyme supplementation prior to testing of dogs is therefore unnecessary. Although not documented, one can predict that serum TLI concentrations will be normal in those rare dogs with EPI due to tumors obstructing the pancreatic ducts or to congenital deficiencies of enzymes other than trypsinogen. Equivocal serum TLI concentrations in the range 2.5 to 5.2 μg/L sometimes reflect failure to withhold food prior to collecting blood. On retesting serum TLI concentrations in many such cases are either clearly consistent with EPI or normal.[76] Those few dogs with consistent "gray zone" serum TLI concentrations have variable responses to enzyme replacement therapy, may have subtotal acinar atrophy with degenerative ultrastructural changes, and in rare cases may even improve spontaneously.[76,78] Individual variation in extrapancreatic digestive capacity may explain the differing clinical courses in these patients.

Radioimmunoassays for trypsin are usually species specific, and assays for human TLI do not detect canine TLI. A specific radioimmunoassay for feline TLI has recently been developed.[79] Preliminary investigations using this assay have shown that there is no cross-reactivity between canine and feline TLI, that normal serum TLI values in cats are greater than those in dogs, and that serum TLI is subnormal in cats with EPI.[79]

FECAL PROTEOLYTIC ACTIVITY Fecal proteolytic activity has been used as an index of pancreatic enzyme activity for many years, but the reliability of the test varies widely depending on the assay method employed as well as on the precautions taken to minimize autodegradation of the rela-

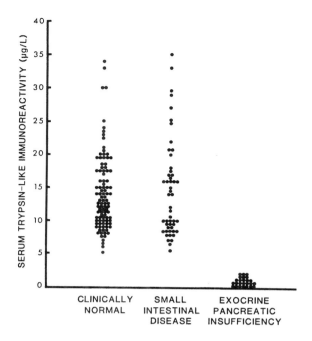

FIGURE 6-6. Serum trypsinlike immunoreactivity in 100 healthy dogs, 50 dogs with small intestinal disease and 25 dogs with exocrine pancreatic insufficiency. (Reproduced from Williams DA, Batt RM. Sensitivity and specificity of radioimmunoassay of serum trypsin-like immunoreactivity for the diagnosis of canine exocrine pancreatic insufficiency. J Am Vet Med Assoc 192:195, 1988.)

tively labile proteases in the fecal sample during the interval between collection and assay.[80] The widely used X-ray film digestion test is unreliable as performed in many laboratories. Gelatin digestion is difficult to evaluate with precision, and the test gives many false negative and false positive results, perhaps reflecting poor standardization of technique.[29,81–83] Proteolytic activity can be measured more precisely using dyed protein substrates such as azocasein, or by radial enzyme diffusion into agar gels containing casein substrate (Figure 6–7).[80,84–86] Fecal proteolytic activity as assessed by these methods is consistently low in most dogs and cats with EPI, but because both dogs and cats with normal pancreatic function occasionally pass feces with low proteolytic activity, either repeated determinations must be made (Figure 6–8), or, in dogs, the test can be performed on a single sample collected after feeding crude soybean meal for two days.[73,86,87] Some dogs with EPI have normal fecal proteolytic activity as assessed by this assay, but this is rare;[73,75] it is likely that a similar situation exists in cats.

Synthetic substrates degraded only by enzymes with trypsin or chymotrypsin-like specificities have been used to investigate the value of assay of true fecal trypsin or chymotrypsin activities in the identification of dogs with EPI.[29,88,89] Assay of chymotrypsin is reported to be preferable to that of trypsin because less chymotrypsin is degraded during intestinal passage. A spectrophotometric test kit for assay of fecal chymotrypsin is commercially available (Monotest Chymotrypsin, Boehringher Mannheim) and has been shown to be useful in dogs.[88] These assays require relatively expensive laboratory equipment and appear to offer no advantages over simple assays of general proteolytic activity based on azoproteins or radial enzyme diffusion.

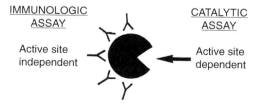

FIGURE 6-5. Assay of pancreatic enzymes and zymogens in serum. Catalytic assays detect degradation of specific substrates exposed to the active site of the molecule, and therefore measure activity. Immunoassays detect antigenic sites over the surface of the molecule and therefore measure enzyme or zymogen concentration. (From Ettinger SJ, Feldman EC. Textbook of Veterinary Internal Medicine, 4th ed. WB Saunders, Philadelphia, 1995, Fig. 107–9.)

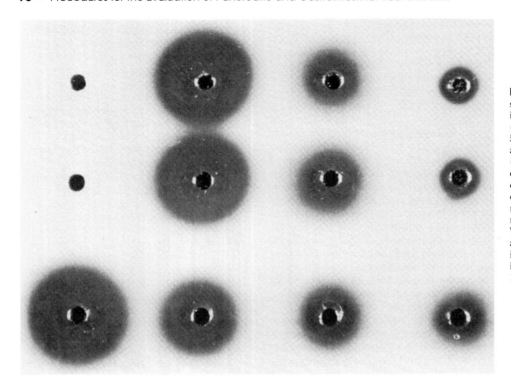

FIGURE 6-7. Radial enzyme diffusion plate showing proteolytic activity in cat feces. The lower 4 wells (left to right) are results of serial 50% dilutions of a sample with high activity. The upper 4 pair of wells (left to right) are results (duplicate determinations) using feces from a cat with EPI, and clinically normal cats with high, medium, and low normal fecal proteolytic activities, respectively. (Reproduced from Williams DA, et al. Fecal proteolytic activity in clinically normal cats and in a cat with exocrine pancreatic insufficiency. J Am Vet Med Assoc 197:210, 1990.)

Other Tests

Bentiromide (N-benzoyl-L-tyrosyl-p-aminobenzoic acid, or BT-PABA) Absorption Test. Chymotrypsin activity in the proximal small intestine may be assayed in vivo by the oral administration of the synthetic substrate bentiromide (Figure 6–9).[90] Free p-aminobenzoic acid (PABA) is released from this substrate by chymotrypsin, absorbed from the gut lumen, and subsequently excreted in the urine. Absorption may be assessed by measuring PABA either in plasma (Figure 6–10) or in urine.

The technique for the urinary bentiromide test in dogs is as follows. After an 18-hour fast the patient receives 0.25 mL (16.7 mg) of bentiromide/kg of body weight by stomach tube, followed by 25 to 100 mL water. This dose results in excretion of exogenous PABA that is 25 to 30 times as great as endogenous PABA and other aromatic amines in the urine.[90] Dogs are confined for 6 hours in a cage, after which urine is collected by catheterization of the bladder and analyzed for PABA. The test cannot be instituted in dogs that have been treated with chloramphenicol, diuretics, sulfonamides, and pancreatic extracts within 5 days of the test because these administrations will interfere with the validity of the results.[90] Dogs with evidence of renal insufficiency are also excluded because the excretion of PABA depends on intact renal function.

In clinically normal dogs, 6-hour PABA excretion of 63.1% ± 3.53 (mean ± SE) and 73.6 ± 13.7 (mean ± SD) have been reported.[81,90] PABA excretions of less than 46% are considered abnormal. Dogs with experimentally ligated pancreatic ducts excrete only 3.8% ± 0.6 (mean ± SE) of the administered dose.[90] This minimal PABA excretion represents the small concentration of measurable aromatic amines always found in the urine.

Dogs require pancreatic enzyme replacement therapy when their PABA excretion is less than approximately 16% (actual PABA, less the 3.8% background level of aromatic

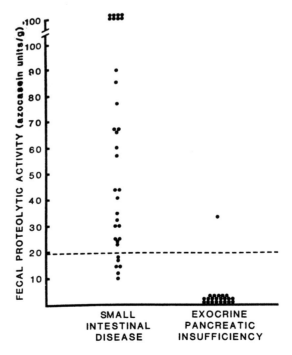

FIGURE 6-8. Fecal proteolytic activity determined by azocasein assay of 3-day collections from 34 dogs with small intestinal disease and 22 dogs with exocrine pancreatic insufficiency. The dashed line indicates the lower limit of the range of values in healthy dogs. (Reproduced from Williams DA, Batt RM. Sensitivity and specificity of radioimmunoassay of serum trypsin-like immunoreactivity for the diagnosis of canine exocrine pancreatic insufficiency. J Am Vet Med Assoc 192:195–201, 1988.)

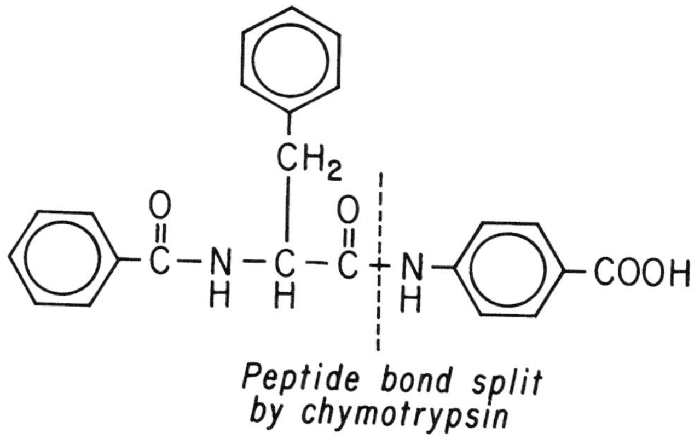

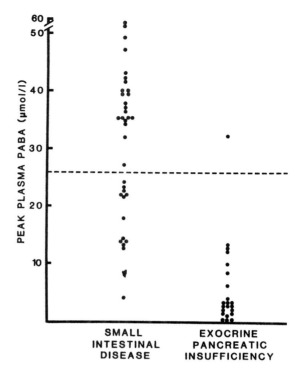

FIGURE 6-9. Chemical structure of N-benzoyl-L-tyrosyl-p-aminobenzoic acid (BT-PABA), used for pancreatic function test. The peptide bond at the dashed line is split by pancreatic chymotrypsin in the gut lumen, releasing free p-aminobenzoic acid (PABA, to the right of the dashed line), which is then absorbed into the blood and subsequently excreted in the urine.

amines).[81] Dogs with PABA excretions greater than 20% in 6 hours reportedly do not benefit from replacement therapy.[81] Dogs with PABA excretions of 20% to 46% have intestinal pancreatic enzyme activity that is significantly less than normal and are partially deficient, but their disease is subclinical. Urinary bentiromide test results may provide additional information as to whether enzyme replacement therapy is likely to be of benefit when results of plasma testing is equivocal.[81]

The plasma bentiromide absorption test is performed by oral administration of bentiromide at 16.5 mg per 10 mL of water per kg of body weight. Peak plasma PABA concentrations (mean ± SE) in normal dogs, dogs with small intestinal disease, and dogs with exocrine pancreatic insufficiency have been reported to be 31 ± 2.6, 25 ± 3.6, and 2.5 ± 0.8 μmol/L, respectively, in one study.[91] Another study yielded similar

FIGURE 6-11. Peak plasma p-aminobenzoic acid (PABA) concentration after combined bentiromide/xylose absorption testing of 35 dogs with small intestinal disease and 22 dogs with exocrine pancreatic insufficiency. The dashed line indicates the lower limit of the range of peak plasma PABA values in healthy dogs. (Reprinted from Williams DA, Batt R M. Sensitivity and specificity of radioimmunoassay of serum trypsin-like immunoreactivity for the diagnosis of exocrine pancreatic insufficiency. J Am Vet Med Assoc 192:195–201, 1988.)

plasma PABA concentrations but showed a 20% overlap between dogs with exocrine pancreatic insufficiency and those with small intestinal disease (Figure 6–11).[73,75,81,89–94]

In some dogs with SID, free PABA is not adequately absorbed or a "functional" pancreatic insufficiency may occur, possibly due to impaired release of pancreatic secretagogues from diseased intestinal mucosa.[73,91,92] Abnormal results may also occur as a result of delayed gastric emptying. For these reasons the BT-PABA test is usually combined with a simultaneous xylose absorption test. Normal xylose absorption indicates that gastric contents have passed into the small intestine.[91,92] Furthermore, SID severe enough to cause malabsorption of free PABA is likely to be associated with obvious xylose malabsorption. Markedly subnormal PABA absorption accompanied by normal xylose absorption is therefore clearly diagnostic for EPI. However, because xylose malabsorption is common in dogs with EPI, exocrine pancreatic function cannot be reliably assessed in those dogs with both abnormal xylose and PABA absorption on the basis of these tests alone.[91,92,95]

The explanation for the appreciable PABA absorption seen in some dogs with EPI is not known. Bacterial degradation could significantly increase BT-PABA hydrolysis in those individuals with bacterial overgrowth.[96] Alternatively, there may be compensatory synthesis of increased amounts of an intestinal peptidase with chymotrypsinlike substrate specificity.[97] One case has been described of a dog with clinical signs of malabsorption, pancreatic acinar atrophy observed at laparotomy, a normal serum PABA/bentiromide test result, normal

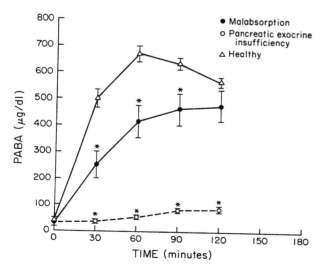

FIGURE 6-10. Plasma bentiromide test results in normal dogs, dogs with small intestinal disease (malabsorption), and dogs with exocrine pancreatic insufficiency. (Results are presented as mean ± SEM; *Significantly different (P < 0.05) from healthy dogs.) (Modified from Washabau RJ, et al. Use of pulmonary hydrogen gas excretion to detect carbohydrate malabsorption in dogs. J Am Vet Med Assoc 189:674–679, 1986.)

fecal proteolytic activity, but diagnostically low serum trypsin-like immunoreactivity.[75] The dog responded well to pancreatic enzyme replacement therapy.

An important limitation of the bentiromide test, however, is its impractical and time-consuming nature. The relatively high cost of the substrate, the requirement for either multiple blood sampling or collection of urine in a metabolism cage, and the technical expertise required for the PABA assay largely restricted its use to referral practices and institutions. The relatively high proportion of equivocal results also make this test less attractive than either assay of fecal proteolytic activity or serum TLI.

An advantage of the bentiromide absorption test over serum TLI assay is that it should detect EPI in those cases caused by obstruction to the flow of pancreatic juice. In these animals release of trypsinogen into the blood, and hence the concentration of serum TLI, may be normal.[98]

Combined bentiromide/xylose absorption test results in healthy cats vary considerably and differ from those seen in the dog, but a markedly abnormal result has been reported in a cat with EPI.[99–101] The diagnostic usefulness of the bentiromide/xylose test is probably limited in this species because of the wide variation seen in normal cats and practical constraints associated with the performance of the test itself.[100,101]

MICROSCOPIC EXAMINATION OF FECES. Evidence of undigested food (observation of fat droplets, starch grains, muscle fibers) is subjective and imprecise, and interpretation is complicated by the variation in fecal characteristics that occurs with different diets and with changes in intestinal transit time.[84,85,102,103] Fecal smears can be stained with Lugol's solution to identify undigested starch granules (that stain dark blue). These may be found in increased numbers with EPI, but there are no good studies to evaluate the reproducibility, sensitivity, or specificity of this test.

Although EPI is usually associated with steatorrhea, this is often not apparent on examination of Sudan III stained samples. It has been reported that the observation of "heavy" fecal fat, when present, is almost always associated with EPI, but this identifies less than 50% of affected dogs.[84] The majority of dogs with EPI have only "trace," "mild," or "moderate" fecal fat content. Quantitative assessment of fecal fat output is a more sensitive and specific indicator of steatorrhea, but neither the qualitative or quantitative tests reliably differentiate exocrine pancreatic insufficiency from other causes of fat malabsorption (Figure 6–12).[87] Microscopic evaluation of canine feces for the presence of "split" (i.e., digested) and "neutral" (i.e., undigested) fat, although theoretically attractive, does not appear to be useful in differentiating pancreatic from nonpancreatic steatorrhea.[102]

Plasma turbidity (lipemia) after oral administration of fat is often diminished or absent in dogs with fat malabsorption. Theoretically, EPI can be distinguished from other causes of fat malabsorption by repeating the test after addition of pancreatic extract to the fat meal. However, some dogs with EPI develop visually detectable lipemia after a fatty meal without addition of pancreatic extract, because even when pancreatic enzymes are absent, up to 80% of fat in a meal may be absorbed.[104–106] In addition, other poorly defined factors such as variations in gastrointestinal transit times, gastric lipase secretory capacity, and rates of lipid clearance from plasma make this test difficult to evaluate reliably. Finally, evidence indicates that absorption of free fatty acids after oral administration of hydrolyzed fat is decreased in canine EPI. Thus, development of lipemia may be impaired even when affected dogs are given fat with pancreatic enzymes.[102,107] Biochemical quantitation of serum triglyceride levels after oral fat adminis-

tration barely distinguishes dogs with EPI from healthy dogs, and the results of such testing in dogs with SID have not been reported.[108]

Miscellaneous Tests

STARCH TOLERANCE TEST. Oral administration of starch is followed by a small increase in blood glucose in normal dogs, but due to carbohydrate malabsorption the magnitude of this response is reduced in dogs with EPI.[84,95] However, evidence for amylase activity of intestinal origin in the dog[109,110] makes the sensitivity of this test questionable. Moreover, abnormal starch tolerance may also occur in dogs with small intestinal disease,[84] presumably because the degradation of starch and subsequent absorption of glucose involves brush border as well as pancreatic enzymes.

GLUCOSE TOLERANCE TEST. Oral and intravenous glucose tolerance is often abnormal in dogs with EPI but may occur as a result of malnutrition rather than EPI per se.[111–115] Because glucose intolerance is not seen in all cases[116] and may occur in some dogs with SID as well as with diseases remote from the gastrointestinal tract,[84] this test is of limited diagnostic value.

OTHER SERUM TESTS. Routine laboratory test results are generally not helpful in establishing the diagnosis of EPI. Serum alanine aminotransferase activities are mildly to moderately increased and may reflect hepatocyte damage secondary to increased uptake of hepatotoxic substances through an abnormally permeable small intestinal mucosa.[84,107,117] Other routine serum biochemical test results are unremarkable, except that total lipid, cholesterol, and polyunsaturated fatty acid concentrations are often

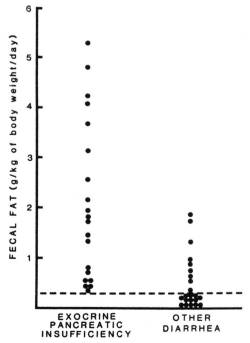

FIGURE 6-12. Fecal fat output in dogs with exocrine pancreatic insufficiency and dogs with chronic diarrhea due to other causes. The dashed line indicates the upper limit of normal in healthy dogs. (Modified from Burrows CF, et al. Determination of fecal fat and trypsin output in the evaluation of chronic canine diarrhea. J Am Vet Med Assoc 174:62, 1979.)

reduced.[84,89,107] Dogs with EPI display a remarkable ability to maintain normal serum protein concentrations even when severely malnourished. Mild lymphopenia and eosinophilia are occasionally seen in dogs with EPI, but complete blood count results are usually within normal limits, and major abnormalities should be perused as evidence of additional or alternative underlying disorders.[89,118]

Serum amylase, lipase and phospholipase, A_2 activities are generally normal or only slightly reduced in EPI, and these tests are not useful in identifying affected dogs.[89,107,119] Non-pancreatic sources of these enzymes are clearly present in dogs, and although their activities may increase in inflammatory disease of the pancreas, they do not decrease proportionately as the mass of functional exocrine pancreatic tissue declines.[120] For example, even though amylase secreted into the gut lumen in response to stimulation with cholecystokinin and secretin is reduced to less than 10% of the normal value in dogs with EPI, serum amylase activity is decreased only to approximately 66% of normal.[107,109] Quantitation of putative pancreas-specific isoamylase using either electrophoresis or selective inhibition has not yet proved to be reliable in the identification of dogs with EPI.[109,120,121]

Additional tests that reflect exocrine pancreatic function include serum vitamin assays (cobalamin, folate, vitamin A, vitamin E) and the radio-labeled triolein and cholesterol octanoate tests. These are used primarily as tests for SID, and they are discussed in further detail later.

In summary, assay of serum TLI or fecal proteolytic activity as described provide reliable tests for EPI in dogs. Serum TLI assay is a more specific test, however, because assay of fecal proteolytic activity gives a higher proportion of abnormal results in dogs with SID. The bentiromide test is impractical in most clinical situations and is neither as sensitive nor as specific as assay of serum TLI. Microscopic examination of feces for undigested food, assessment of fecal proteolytic activity by gelatin digestion, and plasma turbidity tests all give significant proportions of false negative and false positive results, and their use even as crude "screening" tests is not recommended. Assay of fecal proteolytic activity is the test of choice for use in cats, in the absence of an available feline TLI assay.

Tests of Fat Absorption

QUALITATIVE FECAL FAT TEST. Although it is reputed to be a simple and useful screening test for fat malabsorption in human patients,[122] results in canine studies are disappointing.[29,102] Only when steatorrhea is severe are results consistently positive, and numerous false positive results can be obtained.[29] This may reflect differences in digestive physiology between the two species, or perhaps failure to standardize the test procedure (diets, technician skill, and experience), as well as other differences between veterinary and human medical facilities.

For reproducible results it is probably best to perform this test after feeding a standardized diet containing a moderate fat content (approximately 8% as fed) for several days and to evaluate at least two fresh fecal samples. This will minimize variation due to diet.[85,103] The qualitative fecal fat test is performed in two parts. The "direct" test detects undigested fecal triglycerides; the "indirect" test detects "split" fats such as fatty acids.

To perform a direct fecal fat test a small piece of fresh feces is placed on a microscope slide, mixed well with a drop of Sudan III or IV, covered with a coverslip, and examined microscopically under 10× magnification. Undigested fat appears as large, refractile, red-orange droplets. Dogs with normal fat digestion will have few if any fat droplets (fewer than 3 droplets per low-powered field) in their feces. To perform the indirect fecal fat test, 1 to 2 drops of glacial acetic acid (36%) are placed on the edge of the coverslip of the slide previously examined for undigested fat and mixed with the sample of diluted feces. The slide is then heated to near boiling temperature, stopping when the first bubbles are seen to appear under the coverslip. The specimen is then examined while it is still warm. The acetic acid and heat convert fecal soaps into water-insoluble free fatty acids that aggregate into globules of sufficient size for visualization. Dogs with normal fat absorption will have fewer than 3 droplets of split fats per low power field.

Maldigestion is theoretically associated with a positive test for triglyceride and split fat; a positive test for split fats alone is suggestive of malabsorption. A comparison of the results of the direct and indirect tests therefore theoretically helps to differentiate between fat malabsorption and maldigestion, but in practice does not appear to be useful in differentiating pancreatic from nonpancreatic steatorrhea in either dogs[102] or cats.[123] In the past, use of this test has led to much over-diagnosis of EPI, and given the fact that steatorrhea is usually only mild, if present at all, in patients with SID, its use even as a simple screening test is highly questionable.

QUANTITATIVE FECAL FAT TEST. The quantitative fecal fat test is the most accurate test of fat malabsorption, but it must be remembered that steatorrhea is often not a feature of SID, and when present it is often mild.[84,89] Furthermore, although steatorrhea is sometimes very severe in patients with EPI, the method does not reliably differentiate between patients with EPI and those with SID (Figure 6–12).[29] Nonetheless, demonstration of steatorrhea in a patient with normal pancreatic function (as assessed earlier) is strong evidence for the presence of SID. Thus, this approach to diagnosis is very specific but not sensitive in such a population of patients.

To perform the test, a standard diet with a known amount of fat is fed for several days before collection of feces begins. All feces are collected for 72 hours, pooled, and stored refrigerated. The amount of fat in a representative sample is determined chemically, usually by the Van de Kamer method,[124] and the total fecal fat content is calculated. This test is very rarely used because it is time consuming, unpleasant to perform, expensive, and can be logistically frustrating in coprophagic animals. Normally, fecal fat output in dogs is no more than 5% to 10% of dietary fat ingested, with greater output when a cereal-base diet is fed.[31,84,91,125] In a study of dogs with chronic diarrhea fed a meat-base canned food, control dogs had fecal fat output of less than 0.3g/kg/day.[29]

Fecal fat output has been investigated in the cat.[126] Fat concentration in individual fecal samples was extremely variable, but dietary fat digestibility was 91.4 ± 5.0% and daily output was 0.35 ± 0.23 g/kg/day in normal cats.[126] An output of more than 3.5 g/day has been suggested as a cutoff value for definition of steatorrhea,[126] although greater output and surprisingly low fat digestibility in normal cats was reported in another study.[123] Despite extensive laboratory studies of fat balance and careful observation of the response to pancreatic enzyme replacement therapy in that study, it was not possible to clearly define if three cats with steatorrhea had EPI or SID, or both.

Quantitative fat measurement, although rarely useful in clinical practice, is one criterion for defining malabsorption and can be used as a criterion for diagnosis of SID in patients that do not have EPI. Another virtue of the test is that with appropriate control values it can be applied to many different species, including exotic species in which other tests may be impractical to perform. Newer assay methods, such as NMR spectrometry[127] or near infrared reflectance analysis,[128,129] that simplify sample preparation and analysis may make quantitative fecal fat analysis more practical in the future.

PLASMA TESTS OF LIPID ABSORPTION. The plasma turbidity test is a qualitative test that involves the administration of 3 or 6 ml/kg of corn oil to a fasted dog, followed by examination of plasma for lipemia 2 and 3 hours later. Clear plasma is said to identify animals with fat malassimilation. Unfortunately, postprandial lipemia is not consistently observed in normal dogs, and there is poor correlation of turbidity with the amount of lipid given.[130] This unpredictability probably reflects individual variation in the rate of gastric emptying, as well as of plasma lipid clearance. To improve the objectivity of the plasma turbidity test, a modification has been described in which serum triglyceride concentration is measured before and after the administration of vegetable oil.[108] However, this approach barely distinguishes dogs with EPI from healthy dogs, and because results may be abnormal in dogs without primary gastrointestinal disease,[108,131,132] it is unlikely that results of such testing in dogs with SID will be clinically useful.

Quantitative lipid absorption tests that have been described to identify dogs with lipid malabsorption and to identify those with primary maldigestion are the ^{131}I-triolein and the ^{131}I-oleic acid tests.[133] Although theoretically attractive, these tests are unfortunately poorly evaluated because of practical restraints related to the use of radioisotopes. The increased availability and use of stable isotopes in clinical medicine may facilitate further investigations using this type of approach.

Fat soluble vitamins A (retinol) and E (tocopherol) are only absorbed normally when fat absorption is normal. In human patients serum retinol concentration correlates well with results of quantitative fat absorption. Serum tocopherol concentration may be subnormal in dogs with EPI or enteropathy associated with small intestinal bacterial overgrowth.[134–137] A vitamin A response test protocol for use in dogs has been described, and failure of normal vitamin A absorption has been reported in canine patients with EPI.[138,139] Given the simplicity, economy, and availability of serum retinol and tocopherol assays, these approaches to diagnosis merit further evaluation.

In summary, assessment of lipid absorption by means of plasma lipid tests or fecal fat output tests have little practical clinical application outside of clinical research establishments, largely because of availability of more sensitive and specific techniques for diagnosis of EPI and the low prevalence of fat malabsorption in patients with SID.

BREATH TESTS FOR LIPID MALASSIMILATION. A variety of breath tests have been developed for the diagnosis of fat malabsorption in human patients. The most well established of these is the ^{14}C-triolein breath test.[140] ^{14}C-triolein is a triglyceride (glycerol trioleate), in which the 1 acyl moiety is labeled with ^{14}C. The adequacy of the digestion of the triglyceride and absorption and metabolism of the labeled oleic acid can be determined from the amount of $^{14}CO_2$ excreted in the breath. Subsequent administration of ^{14}C oleic acid to patients with abnormal ^{14}C-triolein tests helps determine the status of fatty acid absorption. The cholesteryl octanoate breath test is a similar procedure.[141] Given the increased use of breath tests in canine and feline patients, these methods or similar ones may find clinical application at least in research settings.

Tests of Carbohydrate Absorption

Carbohydrate absorption tests may be used to evaluate small intestinal mucosal disease, selective carbohydrate mal-

absorption due to brush border enzyme defects, and bacterial overgrowth.

FECAL REDUCING SUBSTANCES, pH, OSMOLALITY, AND STARCH. Qualitative tests for carbohydrates, designed for analysis of urine, have been used to identify carbohydrate malabsorption. Clinitest tablets (Ames) can be used to detect reducing substances such as glucose, galactose, fructose, maltose, and lactose (but not sucrose, lactulose, sorbitol, mannitol) in feces.[65] A fresh fecal sample is first liquified by the addition of two volumes of water. Fifteen drops of the fecal solution are placed in a test tube, to which a Clinitest tablet is added. A positive test is indicated by the development of green-orange color. A positive test, especially in the presence of a low fecal pH and a high fecal osmolality, is indicative of carbohydrate malassimilation.[65] The low pH and high osmolality are a result of the accumulation of unabsorbable, low molecular weight, acidic fermentation products of carbohydrate. The test must be performed on fresh feces because colonic bacteria rapidly metabolize carbohydrate, and for this reason the test probably has a low sensitivity. The value of this technique in the evaluation of dogs and cats with carbohydrate malabsorption is unknown.

XYLOSE ABSORPTION TEST. Xylose is a five-carbon monosaccharide that has been widely used to evaluate intestinal absorption. It is traditionally assumed xylose is an inert sugar not metabolized by mammalian cells, so that orally administered xylose absorbed across the intestine appears in peripheral blood and is in then excreted completely in urine. In theory, this frees interpretation of xylose absorption test results from extraintestinal variables that affect clearance of readily and variably metabolized sugars such as glucose. However, in dogs, only about 48% of xylose administered IV at a dose of 0.1 mg/kg is recovered in urine;[142] the balance is presumably metabolized in the liver and perhaps elsewhere.

The test is performed as follows. A 10% to 25% solution of D-xylose is given by stomach tube at a dose of 500 mg/kg body weight to fasted patients. Water is used to flush the tube and reduce the concentration of the solution. Blood samples for xylose assay are collected into heparin tubes before the sugar is given and subsequently at 1-hour intervals for 5 hours. In healthy dogs, the mean blood level of D-xylose at 60 minutes (mean ± SD) is 63 ± 12 mg/dl. All values above 45 to 50 mg/dl at 60 minutes are normal (Figure 6–13). Values between 45 and 50 mg/dl are in the gray zone. In another report, values greater than 45 mg/dl at 90 minutes were considered normal.[125]

Xylose is absorbed in the small intestine by at least four incompletely understood mechanisms (active transport, passive carrier-facilitated transfer, solvent drag through aqueous pores, and leakage through tight junctions), the balance of which varies between species.[84,92,101,139,143–149] The rate of xylose absorption is determined by the amount administered, the rate of gastric emptying, the extent of intraluminal bacterial metabolism of xylose, the surface area available for absorption in the small intestine, and the adequacy of intestinal circulation. Administration of a hypertonic solution may also delay gastric emptying and reduce absorption of D-xylose by means of its own contribution to osmotic pressure. These variables may all contribute to variation between control values derived in different centers. Other causes of delayed gastric emptying should be ruled out by history and radiographic procedures. If gastric emptying is normal, a reduction in the rate of xylose absorption may be a consequence of inadequate intestinal blood flow such as may occur with portal hypertension. Other factors affecting blood levels of xylose include sequestration of xylose in ascitic fluid and slowed clearance of xylose with renal insufficiency.[150] In

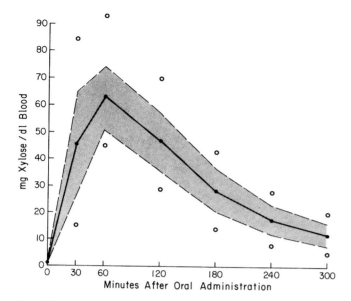

FIGURE 6-13. Xylose absorption test results in 32 normal dogs. Blood xylose concentrations from 0 to 5 hours after oral administration of 2 ml/kg of a 25% xylose solution. Mean (solid line) ± standard error (dashed line) shows peak at 60 minutes. The highest and lowest individual values are represented by open circles. A 1-hour blood xylose test can be done with any value less than 45 mg/dl being abnormal.

humans, concomitant administration of several drugs, such as NSAIDs and neomycin, may also reduce absorption.

Bacterial overgrowth may result in abnormally low blood xylose concentrations because of increased bacterial metabolism of xylose.[151] When low xylose absorption due to bacterial overgrowth is suspected, antibiotic therapy can be instituted and the xylose absorption test repeated in 48 hours. Figure 6–14 shows xylose absorption tests for a dog before and after antibiotic therapy. It must be emphasized that this is a very insensitive and low-yield test for canine small intestinal bacterial overgrowth, results being normal in most cases.[152-154]

In spite of these drawbacks, xylose absorption is considered a useful screening test in human patients, and abnormal xylose test results are usually associated with morphologically apparent intestinal disease. It appears to be a much less useful test in the dog, however, and probably in the cat too. This may reflect a relatively reduced dependence on active and facilitated transport mechanisms in dogs compared to human beings, perhaps in association with increased nonspecific absorption through tight junctions and aqueous pores. Absorption through these latter routes may even be increased in canine and feline patients with SID. Whatever the explanation, the xylose absorption test is generally regarded to have very low sensitivity for diagnosis of SID in dogs and cats. Plasma xylose concentrations are not consistently reduced in dogs with chronic SID and test results are also abnormal in many dogs with EPI (Figure 6–15).[73,95]

The xylose absorption test cannot be recommended for use in cats because of the high degree of individual variation in xylose absorption and the insensitivity of the test in documenting feline intestinal disease.[100,101] Endoscopic biopsy provides a more specific and sensitive technique for the detection of morphologically detectable mucosal disease in dogs and cats. Serum cobalamin and folate concentrations, despite their limitations, are more sensitive and specific than xylose absorption testing for detecting of functional abnormalities in patients with absent or minimal morphologic changes in intestinal biopsies.

DISACCHARIDE DIGESTION AND ABSORPTION TESTS. A test employing one or more disaccharides can be used to evaluate brush border enzyme functions indirectly in patients with carbohydrate malabsorption. The disaccharides lactose, sucrose, and maltose require digestion by brush border lactase, sucrase, and maltase before absorption of their constituent monosaccharides (glucose, galactose, and fructose).

After oral administration of 1 g of maltose, lactose, or sucrose/g body weight, blood glucose is measured at 30, 60, and 120 minutes. Normally, blood glucose increases by greater than 30 mg/dl at 30 minutes. With a deficiency of one or more of the disaccharidases, the increment is less than 10 mg/dl. A glucose-galactose absorption test is then conducted on the same patient by oral administration of the two monosaccharides followed by blood glucose determinations. When this test is normal and lactose tolerance is abnormal, there is a deficiency of lactase activity. The same controls are used to evaluate maltase and sucrase activity, employing the appropriate monosaccharides.

These tests are an indirect evaluation of brush border enzyme activity. They are rarely conducted in small animal patients and are difficult to interpret because of sparse control data,[84] and because blood glucose levels can be influenced by a number of potentially variable hormonal and metabolic factors that are not possible to control. The activity of brush border disaccharidases is best determined by direct assay of biopsies of the small intestine. Very sensitive assays are described that can be used to assay activities in very small pieces of tissue collected endoscopically.[155]

BREATH HYDROGEN TEST.[95,156-158] Results of a breath hydrogen test may be abnormal either when there is a carbohydrate malabsorption or when there is small intestine bacterial overgrowth; it is more sensitive than the xylose absorption test for detecting these abnormalities.[95,157,159] Mammalian cells do not metabolize carbohydrate to generate hydrogen, but many bacteria in the gut lumen do. Some of this hydrogen is absorbed into the bloodstream and subsequently excreted in breath. The normal minimal output of hydrogen in breath can increase either as a result of carbohydrate malabsorption, in

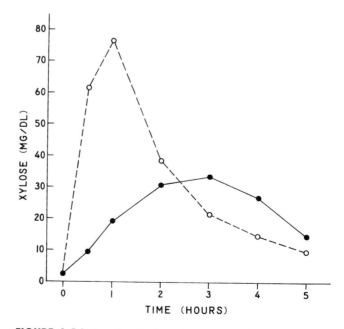

FIGURE 6-14. Results of xylose absorption testing in a dog with bacterial overgrowth of the small intestine. Initial xylose absorption test (solid line) was abnormal. After treatment with antibiotics a xylose absorption test was normal (dashed line).

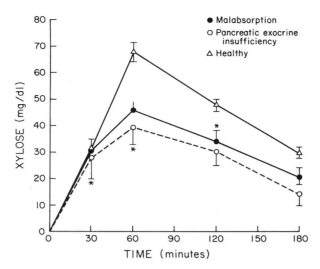

FIGURE 6-15. Xylose-absorption test results in normal dogs, a group of dogs with severe small intestinal disease, and dogs with exocrine pancreatic insufficiency. Results are presented as mean ± SEM. *Significantly different (P < 0.05) from healthy dogs. It should be emphasized that many dogs with chronic small intestinal disease have normal xylose absorption test results. (Modified from Washabau RJ, et al. Use of pulmonary hydrogen gas excretion to detect carbohydrate malabsorption in dogs. J Am Vet Med Assoc 189:674–679,1986.)

which case more substrate passes to the lower bowel and is fermented, or as a result of abnormal proliferation of bacteria in the upper small bowel, in which case dietary carbohydrate is metabolized by bacteria competing with the host for available nutrients. In animals with a normal bowel transit time, carbohydrate malassimilation, and no small intestinal bacterial overgrowth, the rise in breath hydrogen begins 4 to 6 hours after eating (Figure 6–16). If bacteria have overgrown the small bowel, increased breath hydrogen excretion is detected within 1 to 2 hours of eating (Figure 6–16). This early peak is more readily identified after oral administration of a readily fermentable sugar such as lactulose.[159]

The fraction of hydrogen in single samples of dog breath correlates with total hydrogen excretion, so data from single time points can be evaluated in clinical studies.[160] In one study healthy fasted dogs had a breath hydrogen concentration of 0.9 ± 0.1 ppm (mean ± SE), and a peak hydrogen concentration of 1.4 ± 0.2 ppm 8 hours after feeding.[156] In a group of dogs with carbohydrate malabsorption due to EPI, fasting expired hydrogen concentration (mean ± SE) was 3.3 ± 0.9 ppm, and increased to 28.8 ± 2 ppm 6.5 hours after feeding.[95] In the same study a group of dogs with chronic SID had fasting breath hydrogen concentrations of 5.3 ± 1.3 ppm, which increased to peak of 72.2 ± 18 ppm 7 hours after feeding.[95] Although there is variation between dogs on a given diet, the results from a given dog seem quite reproducible within narrow limits from day to day.[161]

Expired air is easily collected using an anesthetic induction mask, a non-rebreathing valve, and a 1 liter latex bag. Samples are collected hourly for up to 8 hours after feeding a carbohydrate-containing diet. A sample of expired air is withdrawn from the latex bag through a three-way sampling valve into a 35 cc syringe. Syringes are capped by a three-way valve and can be stored at room temperature for at least 12 hours without significant loss of hydrogen (hydrogen is lost at the rate of approximately 5% per day from new syringes). Hydrogen in the gas

samples is assayed using thermal conductivity gas chromatography or hydrogen-sensitive electrochemical cells.

The breath hydrogen test is potentially a very practical technique. Even though multiple samples are drawn, the sampling time is very brief and the sampling procedure very well tolerated by most dogs and cats. Hydrogen assay methodology is available at many human hospitals, and the sampling equipment is inexpensive, and easily acquired by any practice. The test has the potential to differentiate between dogs with bacterial overgrowth and those with carbohydrate malabsorption. Unfortunately, as yet insufficient data are available to assess the test's value in dogs and cats; preliminary results suggest the method represents a significant advance, certainly over xylose absorption testing and probably over assay of serum cobalamin and folate.

The test does have some limitations. Between 5% and 10% of human patients with carbohydrate malassimilation do not produce excessive hydrogen gas for a variety of reasons,[162,163] and it is possible the same will prove true in small animal medicine. The type of intestinal bacteria may influence the amount of hydrogen excreted, and variations in the diet markedly affect the breath hydrogen concentration because of differences in the digestibility of the carbohydrate and variable transit times. Other possible confounding factors include prior use of antibiotic therapy and enemas. A study

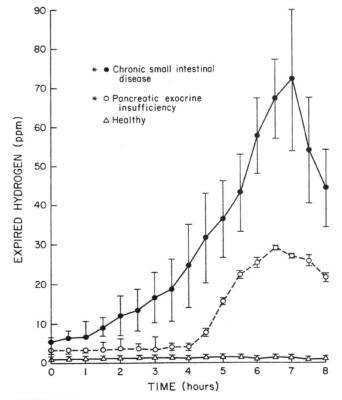

FIGURE 6-16. Breath hydrogen test results in healthy dogs, in dogs with pancreatic exocrine insufficiency (carbohydrate malassimilation and mild bacterial overgrowth), and in dogs with chronic small intestinal disease (carbohydrate malassimilation and marked bacterial overgrowth). Results are presented as mean ± SEM. * Significantly different (P < 0.05) from healthy dogs. (Reprinted from Washabau RJ, et al. Use of pulmonary hydrogen gas excretion to detect carbohydrate malabsorption in dogs. J Am Vet Med Assoc 189:674–679,1986.)

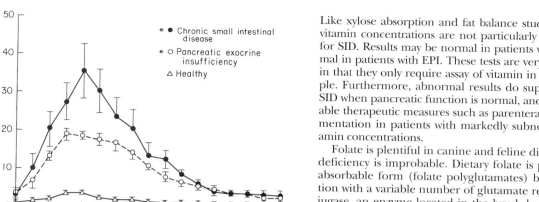

FIGURE 6–17. Breath hydrogen test results in healthy dogs, in dogs with pancreatic exocrine insufficiency, and in dogs with chronic small intestinal disease after oral administration of xylose. Results are presented as mean ± SEM; *Significantly different (P < 0.05) from healthy dogs. (Reprinted from Washabau RJ, et al. Use of pulmonary hydrogen gas excretion to detect carbohydrate malabsorption in dogs. J Am Vet Med Assoc 189:674–679, 1986.)

in humans found that breath hydrogen tests given after an oral glucose load in human patients had a sensitivity of 93% and a specificity of 78% for the diagnosis of bacterial overgrowth.[164] Breath hydrogen testing in dogs after oral sugar (xylose, lactulose, others) administration shows promise for having a high sensitivity and a high specificity for small intestinal bacterial overgrowth (Figure 6–17).

Tests for Protein Malassimilation

Tests for protein malassimilation are rarely performed because specific defects of protein malassimilation in the absence of fat or carbohydrate malassimilation have not been recognized, and in patients with pancreatic or intestinal disease, fat and carbohydrate malassimilation usually precedes protein malassimilation.

Fecal smears can be examined for undigested muscle fibers. These may appear in larger numbers in stools from dogs with EPI and dogs with rapid intestinal transit time. Cytologic stains may help identify muscle fibers, but the yield of this method is very low, particularly because many diets may have a minimal content of meat products.

The fecal excretion of nitrogen can be measured by the macro-Kjeldahl method. The nitrogen measured is the residue of both endogenous and dietary protein. Elevations can indicate poor digestibility of the diet, EPI, or protein-losing enteropathy (see scintigraphy).

It has been suggested that measuring breath hydrogen after the oral administration of glycoproteins may be useful for the detection of protein malabsorption, bacterial overgrowth, and protein-losing enteropathy.[165]

Miscellaneous Absorption Tests

SERUM COBALAMIN (VITAMIN B₁₂) AND FOLATE ASSAYS.[166–168] Serum concentrations of the water soluble vitamins folate and cobalamin are useful markers of intestinal absorptive function.

Like xylose absorption and fat balance studies, tests for serum vitamin concentrations are not particularly sensitive or specific for SID. Results may be normal in patients with SID and abnormal in patients with EPI. These tests are very practical, however, in that they only require assay of vitamin in a single serum sample. Furthermore, abnormal results do support a diagnosis of SID when pancreatic function is normal, and may indicate desirable therapeutic measures such as parenteral cobalamin supplementation in patients with markedly subnormal serum cobalamin concentrations.

Folate is plentiful in canine and feline diets, and nutritional deficiency is improbable. Dietary folate is present in a poorly absorbable form (folate polyglutamates) because of conjugation with a variable number of glutamate residues. Folate conjugase, an enzyme located in the brush border membrane of the jejunal mucosa, removes all but one glutamate residue before mucosal uptake.[133,169,170] Specific folate carriers located only in the proximal small intestine then transport folate monoglutamate into mucosal cells (Figure 6–18).

Malabsorption results in a subnormal serum folate concentration only when the defect is severe and has been present for a long enough time to deplete body stores. Subnormal serum concentrations, however, reflect the presence of disease affecting the proximal small intestine.[168] Disease restricted to the middle and/or distal segments of the small intestine does not impair folate absorption. Various drugs, including phenytoin and sulfasalazine, interfere with folate absorption in human beings, although little evidence suggests this is of significance in dogs.[171]

Serum folate concentrations can increase in dogs with small intestinal bacterial overgrowth (see later) as a result of folate synthesis by the abnormal microflora.[167,172–174] Overgrowth must be in the proximal small intestine for serum folate concentrations to increase; changes in the microflora

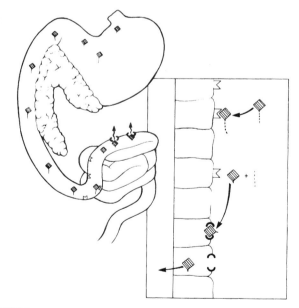

FIGURE 6–18. Normal absorption of dietary folate. Folate polyglutamates are converted to monoglutamate by the intestinal brush border enzyme folate conjugase. Folate monoglutamate is then absorbed by a carrier-mediated mechanism located only in the proximal segments of the small intestine. (Reprinted from Williams DA. Practical tests for pancreatic and small intestinal diseases. Managing Gastrointestinal Disorders, Veterinary Medical, 1989.)

distal to the site of absorption have no effect.[173,174] Dogs with exocrine pancreatic insufficiency often have elevated serum folate concentrations, which might reflect associated small intestinal bacterial overgrowth.[175] Alternatively, impaired pancreatic bicarbonate secretion may enhance folate absorption by decreasing the pH in the proximal small intestine.[176,177] Folate absorption is optimal at a mildly acid pH, and even minimal reductions in intraluminal pH promote uptake.[178]

Cobalamin is also plentiful in canine and feline diets. Dietary deficiency is highly improbable; indeed it is very difficult to induce cobalamin deficiency in most species.[179] However, severe malabsorption in human patients with gastrointestinal diseases leads to megaloblastic anemia and neurologic disease. Cobalamin malabsorption similarly occurs in some dogs with gastrointestinal disease, although there are no reports of clinical signs attributed to the vitamin deficiency.[168]

The mechanisms for cobalamin absorption in normal dogs and cats are similar to those in human beings (Figure 6–19). Gastric acid and pepsins release cobalamin from dietary protein. At the acid pH in the stomach, the free vitamin is bound by proteins called R proteins that are secreted in saliva and/or gastric juice. The R protein–bound cobalamin then passes into the duodenum where pancreatic proteolytic enzymes degrade the R protein and thereby release the cobalamin. At the neutral pH in the small intestine, the free cobalamin binds to intrinsic factor, a protein secreted largely in gastric juice in humans, but largely in pancreatic juice of dogs and cats.[180,181]

Cobalamin malabsorption only leads to a subnormal serum vitamin concentration when malabsorption is severe and has been present for a sufficiently long period of time to deplete body reserves. In human beings cobalamin malabsorption occurs in association with atrophic gastritis or gastric resection, chronic EPI, small intestinal bacterial overgrowth, and ileal disease or ileal resection.[169] Rare causes of malabsorption in human beings included failure to synthesize intrinsic factor, synthesis of nonfunctional intrinsic factor, and selective defects in ileal absorption.[169] In dogs and cats, both EPI and SID can cause subnormal serum cobalamin concentrations.[167,168] Pancreatic intrinsic factor probably maintains normal cobalamin absorption in dogs and cats with gastric disease.[180,181]

In patients with SID, cobalamin malabsorption can result from lesions affecting the intrinsic factor-cobalamin receptors in the distal small intestine. Disease restricted exclusively to the ileum is uncommon, and is more usually associated with generalized disease affecting additional segments of the intestine. Ileal resection will also lead to cobalamin malabsorption in dogs and cats, as it does in human beings.

Competition for cobalamin by abnormally high numbers of bacteria proximal to the ileum (small intestinal bacterial overgrowth) also predisposes to cobalamin malabsorption (see later).[169,182] An inherited selective malabsorption of cobalamin has recently been reported in Giant Schnauzers,[183–185] and a defect in cobalamin absorption is suspected in some Sharpei dogs.[186]

Several mechanisms may contribute to cobalamin malabsorption in EPI, including (1) failure of pancreatic enzymes to liberate cobalamin from binding by R protein, (2) failure to secrete pancreatic intrinsic factor, (3) abnormally acidic pH in the intestine secondary to reduced pancreatic bicarbonate secretion resulting in failure of intrinsic factor to bind cobalamin, and (4) competition for available cobalamin by intestinal microflora in dogs with coexisting small intestinal bacterial overgrowth. Whatever the mechanism, subnormal serum cobalamin concentrations are often subnormal in both dogs and cats with EPI. In some cases the deficiency is severe, and worsens even after otherwise effective therapy has corrected weight loss and diarrhea.[187]

It is very important to use a valid assay method for assay of serum cobalamin and folate in canine serum samples. A variety of bioassay or competitive-binding assay methods can be used.[166] Bioassays are more technically demanding, however, and generally less readily available. Many competitive-binding radioassay kits marketed for assay of vitamins in samples from human beings use alkaline denaturation to liberate cobalamin from endogenous binders in serum. There is marked species variation in these endogenous binding molecules and in their resistance to denaturation, and it has been shown that some kits marketed for use in human beings are not valid in other species.[188,189] Available evidence suggests that methods using boiling to denature endogenous binders and charcoal to separate bound from free vitamin (Dualcount Charcoal Boil B12/Folate, Diagnostic Products Corp.) are valid in the dog and cat.[189–191]

It is also important that control values for each species be derived in each laboratory using a suitable population of animals for each geographic location. These control populations should consist of healthy pet animals living in normal home environments because kenneled dogs often have different serum concentrations, perhaps because of coprophagy or differences in environmental flora. Control groups of animals should also be fed a variety of different foods in order to accommodate variation due to different vitamin contents and availabilities in different products.

Normal canine serum concentrations of cobalamin and folate using the charcoal boil competitive-binding assay mentioned earlier range from 225 to 860 ng/L and 6.7 to 17.4 µg/L, respectively.[74] Normal feline serum concentrations of cobalamin and folate determined by the same assay method range from 200 to 1680 ng/L and 13.4 to 38.0 µg/L, respectively (David A. Williams, GI Laboratory, Purdue University, W. Lafayette, IN 47907). Using *Euglena viridis* and protozoa bioassays, canine serum and whole blood cobalamin concentrations, respectively, have been reported to be 200 to 400 ng/L[168] and 135 to 950 ng/L.[192] Using *Lactobacillus casei* bioassay, canine serum and plasma folate concentrations, respectively, have been reported to be 4.8 to 13.0 µg/L[168] and 4.0 to 26.0 µg/L.[192]

There are no reports of clinical application of these assays to feline patients with intestinal or pancreatic disease. However, extremely low or undetectable serum cobalamin concentrations are common in cats with EPI that have been tested,[193] and many cats with inflammatory bowel disease have decreased serum cobalamin and/or folate.[191] Examination of intestinal biopsies from cats with subnormal serum cobalamin or folate usually reveals moderate to marked histologic abnormalities (that is, the tests appear to be specific, and more cats than dogs with abnormal values appear to have morphologic abnormalities in intestinal biopsies).[191] Elevations in serum folate appear to be much less common in cats than in dogs. These preliminary observations require further investigation.

TESTS OF BILE ACID MALABSORPTION.[194] Tests of bile acid malabsorption may be indicated when secretory diarrhea of the large bowel is suspected, such as in some cases of canine large-bowel diarrhea in which minimal or no inflammation is detected on biopsy. Various tests have been developed for detecting abnormal bile acid deconjugation and absorption in human beings. These include the ^{75}Se-selenohomocholyltaurine (SeHCAT) test (in which abdominal retention of the gamma-labeled conjugated bile acid is detected by counting radiation); the bile acid (^{14}C-cholyglycine) breath test (usually

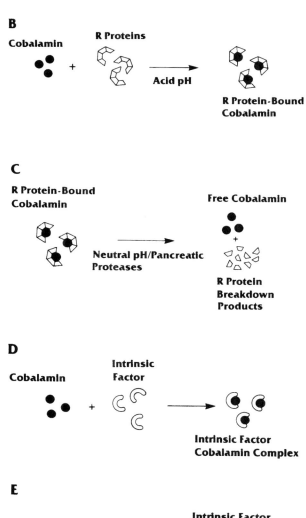

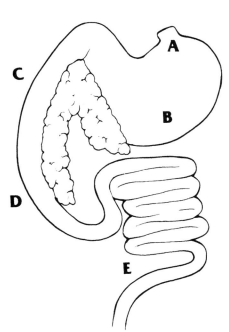

FIGURE 6-19. Normal absorption of dietary cobalamin. Cobalamin is liberated from dietary protein by acid and pepsins in the stomach, where it is bound by R proteins. Subsequent degradation of R protein by pancreatic proteases at neutral pH in the small intestine allows cobalamin to be bound by intrinsic factor. Cobalamin is absorbed only in the ileum where specific receptors for the intrinsic factor/cobalamin complex are located. (Reprinted from Williams DA. Practical tests for pancreatic and small intestinal diseases. Managing Gastrointestinal Disorders, Veterinary Medical Publishing Company, 1989.)

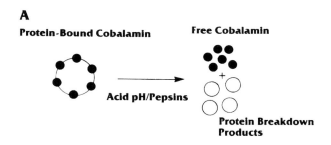

used as a test for abnormal deconjugation of bile acids in patients with small intestinal bacterial overgrowth); and a modification of the latter test in which the excretion of[14]C in stool after oral administration of the[14]C-labeled cholyglycine is determined.[65,194,195] In practice the most widely used technique to diagnose the possible role of bile acid malabsorption in diarrhea, even in human patients, remains a clinical trial with a bile acid binding resin such as cholestyramine (Questran; Mead Johnson). A good response to cholestyramine suggests, but does not prove, that bile acid malabsorption is a cause of the diarrhea. For these purposes, cholestyramine is administered at 200 to 300 mg/kg. If a response is to be seen, it usually occurs within days. Cholestyramine should be used very judiciously in cats because it may rapidly deplete them of taurine.

URINARY INDICAN AND NITROSONAPHTHOL TESTS. Urine indican levels have been used to identify intestinal disorders ranging from enterotoxemias to abnormal bacterial numbers and species colonizing the small intestine. Bacteria that possess tryptophanase activity metabolize tryptophan, ultimately producing indican that is eliminated in urine. Theoretically, the amount of indican produced is a function of the amount of tryptophan and the numbers of tryptophan-metabolizing bacteria in the small intestine.[196,197]

The nitrosonaphthol test detects compounds such as tyramine and 4-hydroxyphenylacetic acid generated as a result of bacterial degradation of tyrosine. Such degradation may occur with small intestine bacterial overgrowth, but also when there is increased delivery of substrate to the large bowel, such as with rapid transit time, gastrointestinal bleeding, and some liver diseases. A positive test result has been reported in 8 of 13 dogs with EPI, as well as in 8 of 12 dogs with small intestinal disease, and in each of 14 dogs with diarrhea of undetermined cause; only 2 of 21 dogs with large intestinal disease had positive test results. Eight of the dogs with diarrhea of undetermined cause were treated with antibiotics, with a favorable clinical result. The test may therefore be helpful in identifying patients with small intestinal disease that may benefit from antibiotic therapy.[198]

In practice, however, neither of these urinary tests have found widespread use, probably because they are not specific for the identification of patients with small intestine bacterial overgrowth. Abnormal test results are potentially obtained in any circumstances that result in delivery of excess tryptophan or tyrosine to the colonic microflora.[199–201]

Tests for Bacterial Overgrowth

Tests for small intestinal bacterial overgrowth (SIBO) are indicated as part of the evaluation of most patients with diarrhea. Approximately 50% of patients referred to a university gastroenterology referral service for investigation of suspected malabsorption were shown to have SIBO.[202] SIBO is particularly prevalent in German shepherd dogs. A test for EPI (serum TLI assay) should always accompany testing for SIBO because nearly all dogs with EPI do have SIBO, and EPI itself can affect some tests that may be used to obtain evidence for the presence of SIBO (such as serum cobalamin or folate assays).

Routine serum biochemical testing provides no specific information regarding SIBO, but some animals may manifest secondary hepatobiliary injury related to absorption of increased amounts of toxic bacterial products such as peptidoglycan-polysaccharide polymers.[203,204]

A diagnosis of bacterial overgrowth in the small intestine cannot be made by fecal culture because bacteria cultured from the feces, even in heavy growth, does not reflect microbial activity in the small bowel. A definitive diagnosis of bacterial overgrowth can, however, be made by quantitative anaerobic and aerobic culture of duodenal fluid aspirated by either peroral intubation (at endoscopy, suction capsule biopsy, or when a tube is passed specifically for this purpose), or by direct needle puncture during laparotomy.

An early abnormal peak of hydrogen output during breath hydrogen testing provides supportive evidence for bacterial overgrowth. Providing that exocrine pancreatic function is normal, observation of subnormal serum cobalamin concentration, elevated serum folate concentration, or a combination of these abnormalities is also supportive of this diagnosis.

CULTURE OF DUODENAL FLUID. Quantitative culture of fluid from the duodenum or jejunum is the gold standard for the diagnosis of bacterial overgrowth. Intestinal fluid may be collected by syringe and a needle at laparotomy, by an aspiration tube inserted into the duodenum through the operating channel of an endoscope, or through the lumen of a peroral suction capsule instrument (Quinton Instrument Company, Seattle, WA).[205] A 1 to 5 mL volume of duodenal fluid is withdrawn using gentle suction (this often takes 10 to 30 minutes to collect). The fluid is quantitatively cultured under both anaerobic and aerobic conditions, and the subsequent colonies grown should be speciated (Table 6–5). Bacterial colony counts greater than 10^5 colony-forming units (CFU) per mL in duodenal or jejunal fluid of fasted dogs are considered abnormal. The overgrowth may or may not include increased numbers of obligate anaerobic bacteria. In duodenal fluid from normal cats an unexpectedly high number of bacteria have been cultured, including large numbers of anaerobic bacteria.[206]

SERUM COBALAMIN (VITAMIN B_{12}) AND FOLATE ASSAYS. Increased numbers of many species of bacteria generate large quantities of folate, which is available for absorption via the specific carriers located in the upper small intestine. In con-

trast, most bacteria compete for available intraluminal cobalamin and thereby reduce its uptake in the distal small intestine (Figure 6–20). A high serum folate concentration, a low serum cobalamin concentration, or a combination of the two provides evidence suggestive of bacterial overgrowth.[74,168] Available evidence suggests that providing EPI has been eliminated by prior testing, these test results exhibit good specificity but relatively poor sensitivity for the diagnosis of small intestinal bacterial overgrowth in the dog. Thus, normal test results do not rule out the possibility of SIBO; but abnormal test results are supportive of this diagnosis. It is more common to see an increased serum folate than a reduced cobalamin; this combination of abnormalities, although relatively uncommon, is highly specific for SIBO. The sensitivity of these tests for subclinical SIBO appears to be relatively poor, especially for cobalamin,[207] perhaps reflecting the particular importance of obligate anaerobic bacteria in worsening the severity of clinical sequelae of bacterial overgrowth; obligate anaerobic bacteria are particularly effective at inhibiting absorption of cobalamin and at damaging small intestinal brush border membrane.[152,182,208–210]

Confounding factors in the interpretation of serum cobalamin and folate assays include (1) EPI, which may reduce the absorption of cobalamin and increase the absorption of folate by various mechanisms;[74] (2) severe mucosal disease, which can reduce the absorption of either of these vitamins and therefore inhibit folate absorption even in the face of enhanced bacterial synthesis; (3) low folate diets, which, although highly improbable, could theoretically reduce serum folate concentrations over a period of several weeks; and (4) therapeutic administration of vitamins, which can markedly elevate serum concentrations.[74,168]

THE ^{14}C-D-XYLOSE BREATH TEST. The ^{14}C-D-xylose breath test is a useful test for the diagnosis of bacterial overgrowth in humans.[195,211–214] The principle of the test is to give a sufficiently small amount of xylose, including a tracer dose of ^{14}C-D-xylose, to allow all the administered material to be absorbed in the small intestine, even in the face of small intestinal disease, so no sugar passes into the large bowel for degradation by colonic microflora. If there is bacterial overgrowth in the

Table 6–5

METHOD FOR QUANTITATIVE BACTERIOLOGIC CULTURE OF DUODENAL JUICE

1. Dilute 100 μL of juice in 10 mL of peptone broth, then culture 100 μL of this dilution (10^{-2} dilution) in duplicate on blood agar plates under both aerobic and anaerobic conditions.* Count and speciate colonies.
2. Dilute 100 μL of the 10^{-2} dilution further in 10 mL of peptone broth, then culture 100 μL of this dilution (10^{-4} dilution) in duplicate on blood agar plates under both aerobic and anaerobic conditions.* Count and speciate colonies.
3. If the same colony type is identified growing under both aerobic and anaerobic conditions, then only the greater of the two counts is included in calculation of the total because some species grow under both circumstances but often thrive better under one set of conditions; many facultative anaerobes are adapted to the oxygen-poor environment within the intestinal lumen and grow better under anaerobic conditions.
4. If there is no growth on the 10^{-2} dilution plates, then total counts are > 10^3 colony-forming units (CFU)/mL.
5. If colonies are too numerous to count on the 10^{-4} dilution plates, then total counts are > 10^8 CFU)/mL and there is massive small intestinal bacterial overgrowth.

*Use of additional selective media and conditions may increase the yield of organisms. These methodologic variations will lead to differences in control and patient data between laboratories.

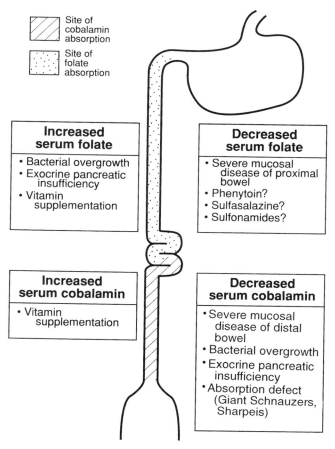

Site of cobalamin absorption

Site of folate absorption

Increased serum folate
• Bacterial overgrowth
• Exocrine pancreatic insufficiency
• Vitamin supplementation

Decreased serum folate
• Severe mucosal disease of proximal bowel
• Phenytoin?
• Sulfasalazine?
• Sulfonamides?

Increased serum cobalamin
• Vitamin supplementation

Decreased serum cobalamin
• Severe mucosal disease of distal bowel
• Bacterial overgrowth
• Exocrine pancreatic insufficiency
• Absorption defect (Giant Schnauzers, Sharpeis)

FIGURE 6–20. Schematic showing sites of cobalamin (vitamin B_{12}) and folate absorption in the small intestine; also tabulated are the problems that can alter serum cobalamin and folate concentrations.

upper small bowel, then some of the administered xylose will be degraded by bacteria with liberation of some of the labeled $^{14}CO_2$, which is subsequently absorbed into the blood and exhaled, where it can be trapped in the breath for subsequent counting in a beta scintillation counter. Control values have been reported in the dog.[215] The method requires further work to optimize the total dose of xylose administered and to evaluate the potential role of endogenous xylose metabolism. Nonetheless, the method can be adapted to take advantage of the increased availability of stable isotopes and may become more widely applicable in the future, even in practices without the capability to use radioisotopes.

SERUM UNCONJUGATED BILE ACIDS. Intraluminal bacteria deconjugate bile acids, and these bile acids are then passively absorbed across the entire small intestinal mucosa. Conjugated bile acids, in contrast, are absorbed by a specific carrier-mediated mechanism located only in the ileum.[194] It has been reported that the serum concentration of unconjugated bile acids is increased in patients with SIBO.[216–222] Unfortunately, assay of specific components of total bile acids is not widely available at this time, but technical advances may make the test more available in the future.

Tests of Gastrointestinal Permeability

Although the intestinal tract is traditionally thought of as a specialized absorptive surface, it also serves an important role as a barrier to keep unwanted substances from being absorbed to any great extent. This barrier function not only excludes large molecules, but also small molecules the size of mono- and disaccharides. Nonetheless, there is a low background absorption of such small molecules. Inert (essentially nonmetabolized) monosaccharides, such as rhamnose, and the hexitol mannitol (molecular weights approximately 150), for which no brush border transport mechanisms exist, apparently diffuse across the intestinal mucosa, probably through transcellular aqueous pores.[223] In contrast, ^{51}Chromium-labeled ethylenediaminetetraacetate(^{51}Cr-EDTA) and larger inert disaccharides such as cellobiose or lactulose (molecular weights approximately 300) cannot traverse these pores, but can cross the gut in small amounts by leaking through the tight junctions.[223–227] When these molecules enter the blood they undergo rapid glomerular filtration and are excreted in urine. Thus, absorption from the gut is reflected in urinary sugar output.

In many intestinal diseases it appears the tight junctions become more leaky, thereby increasing passive absorption through the intercellular route, while at the same time the surface area of the brush border membrane decreases, thereby decreasing absorption through the transcellular route. If absorption through the two routes is expressed as a ratio, this ratio tends to depart even further from normal than the change through either route evaluated alone, thereby increasing the sensitivity of the tests.[223] Expressing the ratio of passive absorption of two marker molecules has the additional advantage of correcting for errors potentially caused by bacterial degradation within the gut lumen, and variations in gastric emptying.[223,225] It would be difficult to account for these effects if changes in only a single marker molecule were evaluated.

At present, tests of gastrointestinal permeability have application primarily in research. Preliminary reports indicate this approach offers good sensitivity and specificity for diagnosis of small intestinal disease in the dog. It is likely that increased availability of newer analytical methods for sugars in human hospital laboratories will facilitate use of tests of intestinal permeability in veterinary patients in the future.

Tests for Protein-Losing Enteropathy

Excessive loss of plasma and other protein-containing tissues into the gastrointestinal tract is referred to as protein-losing enteropathy (PLE). It occurs in association with numerous disorders including idiopathic inflammatory enteropathies such as lymphocytic-plasmacytic, eosinophilic, or granulomatous gastroenteritis, gastrointestinal neoplasia, foreign bodies, intussusceptions, bacterial overgrowth in the small intestine, parasitic and fungal enteropathies, acute infectious (viral or bacterial) enteritis, nonspecific enteritis, intestinal lymphangiectasia, and immune-mediated diseases. The mechanism for protein loss may related to inflammation or erosion affecting the normal barrier function of the gut, or less commonly to acquired or congenital abnormalities in intestinal lymphatic drainage.[228–235]

The diagnosis of PLE is most commonly made by eliminating liver disease and protein-losing nephropathy as causes of hypoalbuminemia. If hypoglobulinemia accompanies hypoalbuminema, then PLE is nearly always the cause because hypoglobulinemia is rarely seen with protein-losing nephropathy. However, not all patients with PLE will have hypoglobulinema. For example, the PLE reported in Basenji dogs is characterized by hyperglobulinemia and hypoalbuminemia.[236] In dogs with histoplasmosis a significant increase in globulin production may occur as part of the inflammatory response; thus, serum levels of globulins may be normal or increased. Serum cobalamin and folate concentrations may provide additional evidence for gastrointestinal disease in equivocal cases. In many cases the diagnosis remains presumptive because patients are often poor candidates for anesthesia and intestinal biopsy because of malnutrition and hypoproteinemia, and/or the expense of plasma transfusion and exploratory surgery or endoscopy is prohibitive. Noninvasive tests that might reveal abnormal enteric loss in such patients include the ^{51}Cr-labeled albumin test and assay of fecal alpha$_1$-protease inhibitor.

[51]CR-LABELED ALBUMIN TEST. The gold standard for diagnosis of PLE is to quantitate loss of radioactive ^{51}Cr-labeled albumin into the gastrointestinal tract.[237,238] Although albumin lost into the gastrointestinal tract may be degraded by digestive enzymes and constituent amino acids reabsorbed, the chromium label is not reabsorbed and is excreted in feces. Thus, following administration of intravenous radioisotope to label albumin in vivo, quantitation of radioactivity in feces collected over several days provides an index of gastrointestinal protein loss. Obvious drawbacks such as the need for prolonged hospitalization in a metabolism cage in a facility approved for radioisotope use, the need to separate urine from feces, the necessity of handling large volumes of feces, safety concerns related to exposure to radioisotopes, and expense have all limited the application of this approach.

FECAL ALPHA-1-PROTEASE INHIBITOR. Assay of alpha$_1$-protease inhibitor alpha$_1$-PI) in a single sample of feces has been shown to be a reliable method to detect PLE in human patients.[239–243] This plasma protease inhibitor has a molecular weight similar to that of albumin, and is present in the vascular space, in the intercellular space, and in lymph. It is therefore lost into the gastrointestinal tract when there is leakage from these sites in disease states. Unlike albumin, however, alpha$_1$-PI is not degraded by enzymes when it is lost into the gut lumen by virtue of its broad-spectrum inhibition of digestive proteases; it is therefore passed in feces essentially intact, and can be detected using immunoassay methods.[244]

There are substantial species differences in the antigenic determinants of alpha$_1$-PI, and specific immunologic methods usually need to be developed for each species. A commercially available kit for human alpha$_1$-PI unfortunately does not detect canine alpha$_1$-PI. Preliminary investigation of a radial immunodiffusion assay for canine alpha$_1$-PI showed concentrations in feces to be increased in dogs with PLE[245] and prompted development of a more sensitive and accurate ELISA assay.[71] This assay is currently being used to study the fate of alpha$_1$-PI lost into the lumen of the canine gastrointestinal tract and shows promise as a new test for the diagnosis of PLE in dogs and for indirect quantitation of enteric protein loss.

Peroral String Test[246]

The peroral string test utilizes a 140 cm absorbent nylon yarn within a weighted gelatin capsule. The capsule is administered to the dog, and the free end of the yarn is tied to a piece of gauze tape that has been tied around the dog's mandible just cranial to the canine teeth. As the capsule passes by peristalsis into the duodenum, the yarn unwinds and soaks up gastrointestinal fluid, which is later analyzed once the yarn is retrieved from the dog's mouth.

The peroral string test (Entero-test, HDC Corp., Mountain View, CA) has been successfully used for the diagnosis of giardiasis in the dog.[246] In humans it has also been used for the diagnosis of *Strongyloides stercoralis,* enteropathogenic bacteria,

achlorhydria, and gastroesophageal reflux; for the acquisition of duodenal fluid for culture and cytology; and for the location of the site of gastrointestinal hemorrhage. To determine the level at which bleeding begins, the string is measured from the oral cavity to the proximal limit of the blood-stained string. Alternatively, the level at which blood staining of the string begins is compared to the level at which bile staining of the string, or acidification of fluid absorbed into the string, is first detected. The possibility of partial obstruction secondary to a linear foreign body exists should a dog swallow the string, but this has not been observed in humans following this eventuality.

GASTROINTESTINAL IMAGING TECHNIQUES

Introduction

Veterinary gastrointestinal radiography has been the subject of several reviews.[247–252,253–257] See these publications for a detailed description of correct radiographic technique and interpretation. This discussion focuses largely on the indications and limitations of gastrointestinal imaging techniques, with particular emphasis on newer techniques such as enteroclysis, ultrasound, and scintigraphy.

Imaging techniques are powerful tools for investigating gastrointestinal disease. Imaging techniques available to veterinary practitioners, either in their own practice or by referral to specialist hospitals, include radiography, fluoroscopy, ultrasonography, nuclear scintigraphy, computer-assisted tomography, and magnetic resonance imaging. Although some overlap occurs, each technique occupies a particular niche in the spectrum of application of diagnostic imaging modalities. Thus, gastrointestinal radiography is primarily suited to the detection of morphologic abnormalities that distort organ size or position; fluoroscopy is utilized to detect motility disorders; ultrasonography recognizes morphologic abnormalities resulting from altered tissue density as well as organ size and position; scintigraphy examines the integrity of gastrointestinal physiologic functions such as gastric emptying, biliary excretion, portal vein blood flow, and mucosal permeability; and computer-assisted tomography and magnetic resonance imaging provide detailed information regarding morphology.

Survey Radiographs

Survey pharyngeal, cervical, thoracic, and abdominal radiographs are often indicated for evaluating gastrointestinal problems. Their value in the investigation of patients with regurgitation, chronic vomiting, diarrhea, and abdominal pain is discussed in Chapter 5. Survey radiography assists the clinician in tentatively ruling out disorders such as gastrointestinal obstruction, adynamic ileus, intestinal perforation, or peritonitis. Furthermore, survey radiographs often provide valuable diagnostic clues, such as estimations of organ size and the presence or absence of masses or fluid. A retrospective study of patients with suspected gastric disease determined that survey abdominal radiographs had a 25% diagnostic yield, whereas positive contrast studies had a 40% yield.[258]

Contrast Radiographic Examination

INDICATIONS, CONTRAINDICATIONS, COMPLICATIONS. A major obstacle to effective gastrointestinal contrast radiogra-

Table 6–6

INDICATIONS FOR CONTRAST RADIOLOGY OF THE GASTROINTESTINAL TRACT

Liquid Barium Swallowing Study
  Dysphagia
  Regurgitation
  Suspected morphologic disorders of the pharynx and esophagus
  Suspected motility disorders of the pharynx and esophagus
Barium-Coated Food Swallowing Study
  Dysphagia
  Regurgitation
  Suspected morphologic disorders of the pharynx and esophagus
    (especially partial obstructions)
  Suspected motility disorders of the pharynx and esophagus
    (especially subtle motility abnormalities)
Positive Contrast Gastrogram
  Chronic vomiting
  Suspected gastric foreign bodies
  Suspected mural gastric lesions
  Suspected extramural masses impinging on the stomach
  Suspected overt gastric mucosal disease
  Suspected pyloric obstruction
  Assist location of stomach
Double-Contrast Gastrogram
  Chronic vomiting
  Suspected radiolucent gastric foreign bodies
  Enhance detail of gastric mucosa
Upper GI Contrast Study with Small-Bowel Follow-Through Evaluation
  Chronic vomiting
  Chronic bloating
  Chronic diarrhea (rarely of value)
  Suspected intestinal foreign body
  Suspected intestinal obstruction
  Suspected herniation
  Assist localization of abdominal masses
  Assess gastrointestinal transit time
Barium Meal
  Assess gastric emptying time
Barium-Impregnated Polyethylene Spheres
  Chronic vomiting
  Suspected pyloric obstruction
  Suspected intestinal obstruction
  Suspected gastrointestinal motility abnormality
  Assess gastric emptying time
  Assess orocolic transit time
Fluoroscopy
  Suspected gastrointestinal motility abnormality
Enteroclysis
  Chronic diarrhea
  Suspected intestinal partial obstruction
  Suspected intestinal motility abnormality
Air or Barium Enema
  Suspected large-bowel mass
  Suspected ileocecal abnormalities
  Assist localization of pelvic and abdominal masses
  Assist localization of gastrointestinal gas accumulations

phy is the mistaken belief that there is one contrast procedure which provides adequate evaluation for the entire upper gastrointestinal tract. For maximum diagnostic return, the veterinarian must select from as many as 10 different contrast techniques, each of which has different indications (Table 6–6).

Upper gastrointestinal contrast radiography and endoscopy are complementary procedures. Contrast procedures do not require anesthesia, and they provide a better estimation of luminal diameter (esophagus), mural masses, extramural compressive lesions, jejunal diseases, gastrointestinal motility, and gastric emptying. Endoscopy is more sensi-

tive for diagnosing mucosal diseases of the upper gastrointestinal tract and offers the important potential advantage of definitive diagnosis through biopsy, or specific therapy by way of removal of foreign bodies or dilation of strictures. In most cases of suspected esophageal disease, barium swallows are performed before endoscopy; in most cases of suspected gastroduodenal disease, endoscopic examination precedes the contrast procedure.[258] One prospective study in dogs showed gastroscopy to be superior to double-contrast gastrography for the diagnosis of gastric neoplasia, ulceration, and gastritis.[258]

Contraindications for contrast radiography include inadequate preparation (bowel cleansing) and rapid deterioration of a patient's condition. Complications include aspiration of contrast material and barium peritonitis from gastrointestinal rupture. Aspiration of contrast material is particularly common in patients with megaesophagus. Animals with megaesophagus should never be returned to their cages with an esophagus full of contrast material. The performance of a gastrogram delays upper gastrointestinal endoscopy by a minimum of 24 hours.

CONTRAST PROCEDURES FOR THE EVALUATION OF SWALLOWING. Contrast studies are done with barium as paste, liquid suspension, or mixed with food. The paste is a 70% (w/w) form containing a binding agent and can be administered with a syringe. It is used to outline the pharynx and cranial esophagus in animals with suspected pharyngoesophageal swallowing disorders. The suspension is used at a 30% (w/v) concentration for evaluating esophageal problems. Each of the three forms is given in small boluses and as frequently as necessary to satisfy that an accurate evaluation of pharyngoesophageal motility has been made and that obstruction is confirmed or ruled out.

If fluoroscopy is available, the passage of the barium contrast agents during swallowing can be observed. The study should include observation and recording of three to six complete swallows of liquid barium suspension followed by a similar number of barium-coated food boluses.

If esophageal perforation is suspected, a water-soluble iodinated contrast material should be used. Such materials are less irritating to the periesophageal tissues. If the swallow does not identify a perforation, the study should be repeated with a liquid barium suspension because esophageal perforations may be missed with water-soluble agents.

Swallowing studies are done without giving patients any chemical restraint. If sedation is necessary, low-dose acetylpromazine has a minimal adverse affect on swallowing, but such a low dose is not likely to ensure success in managing the patient.

CONTRAST PROCEDURES FOR THE ASSESSMENT OF GASTRIC MORPHOLOGY. Positive contrast gastrograms and double-contrast gastrograms are the most useful contrast procedures for the assessment of gastrointestinal morphology. Positive contrast gastrograms utilize a large volume of dilute barium suspension (10–20 ml/kg) with the intent of causing mild gastric distention. This technique is particularly useful for the detection of poorly distensible mural lesions. In combination with fluoroscopy, it allows evaluation of gastric motility. Positive contrast gastrograms allow the visualization of some mucosal detail, but double-contrast gastrograms are the preferred technique for the radiographic evaluation of the gastric mucosa.[255] Double-contrast gastrograms may be performed after most of the barium from the positive contrast gastrogram has left the stomach, or alternatively by instilling into the stomach 2 ml/kg of barium followed by sufficient air to ensure even gastric distention.

CONTRAST PROCEDURES FOR THE ASSESSMENT OF GASTRIC EMPTYING. Gastric emptying time may be assessed by contrast radiographic techniques. The gastric emptying of fluids and solids depends on markedly different physiologic mechanisms, and the emptying time of liquids has less clinical relevance. Normal gastric emptying times of liquids, using 10 ml/kg of 60% w/v barium suspension, have been reported to be 0.5 to 2 hours in dogs,[259] although another investigator, using a slightly different technique, has reported a range of 1 to 7 hours with a mean and standard error of 4 ± 0.2 hours.[258] Gastric emptying should begin within 45 minutes of administration of barium liquids.[258] Normal gastric emptying time of barium and food admixtures, using 7 ml/kg of 60% w/v barium sulfate suspension mixed with 8 g/kg of ground kibble has been reported to vary from 7 to 15 hours with a mean of 11 hours in mixed-breed dogs.[260] A similar study in beagles showed a barium-food mean gastric emptying time of 7 ± 0.74 hours.[261] The caloric density, nutrient composition, osmolality, and particle size of the test meal will affect emptying time and so must be standardized for consistent results. The emptying of 1 cm segments of radiopaque plastic tubing (0.2 cm diameter) that act as indigestible solids has been successfully used as a simple, accurate, and inexpensive means of detecting abnormal gastric emptying in humans.[262] The markers are given with a meal and the time determined for their complete emptying. A similar technique has been utilized in the dog.[263] A method employing barium-impregnated plastic spheres (BIPS, Ken Bowman Assocs, Diamond Bar, CA; Arnolds, Shrewsbury, U.K.) of 1.5 mm and 5 mm diameters has also been used to evaluate gastric emptying, intestinal transit, and the presence or absence of intestinal obstruction.[264] BIPS are discussed more fully in Chapters 15 and 25.

Fear, pain, metabolic derangements, and certain tranquilizers will delay gastrointestinal transit times. If tranquilization is required, use acetylpromazine (0.05–0.1 mg/kg SQ) for the dog. A tranquilization protocol that does not affect gastrointestinal motility yet provides safe and effective sedation has not been determined for the cat. Ketamine increases gastric motility and hastens transit time.[265]

More accurate techniques for the assessment of gastric emptying are available, but their use is restricted by their cumbersome nature or requirement for radionuclides. They include orogastric intubation methods and various scintigraphic techniques.

CONTRAST PROCEDURES FOR THE EVALUATION OF THE SMALL INTESTINE. The contrast procedure of choice for the examination of small intestinal morphology is enteroclysis (see later). Crude assessment of morphology may be acquired by use of liquid barium "follow-through" studies. In the absence of obstructive lesions, the rate of passage of contrast material through the gastrointestinal tract is a function of the frequency of peristaltic and segmental contractions of the stomach and intestine, the functional status of the pylorus, and the amount and viscosity of the contrast medium. As a result of these variables, gastrointestinal transit time is a poor measure of intestinal motility. Normal gastrointestinal transit and gastrointestinal emptying times using 10 ml/kg of 60% (w/v) liquid barium suspension in dogs have been reported to be 0.5 to 2 hours and 3 to 5 hours, respectively.[259] A transit time of greater than 4 hours is evidence of a transit defect in dogs. In the cat, transit is more rapid, ranging from 30 to 60 minutes.[265] As with gastric emptying, psychologic factors and drugs can delay transit. The fluoroscopic inspection of the barium-filled gastrointestinal tract during the barium "follow-through" study or enteroclysis provides the best assessment of intestinal motility.

CONTRAST PROCEDURES FOR EXAMINATION OF THE LARGE INTESTINE. In the absence of an endoscope, barium enemas can be useful for detecting morphologic abnormalities of the large bowel such as masses, strictures, diverticula, ileocecal inversion, and ileocecal intussusception. Insufflation of the colon with air (15–20 ml/kg) through a balloon-tipped catheter is a simple procedure to outline the large bowel and assist localization of colonic, pelvic or abdominal masses and abdominal gas accumulations; it may be utilized alone as a negative contrast procedure, or following barium administration as part of a double-contrast technique.

Fluoroscopy

Fluoroscopy, videofluorography, and cinefluorography are indicated for diagnosing gastric and intestinal motility disorders and differentiating swallowing disorders into oral, pharyngeal, cricopharyngeal, esophageal, and gastroesophageal phases. Only through fluoroscopy is it possible to assess the rate of gastrointestinal motility, the coordination of peristaltic movement, and the manner in which contrast medium is propelled through the gastrointestinal tract.[247,266] By evaluating esophageal motility, fluoroscopy helps determine the prognosis for patients with megaesophagus. Fluoroscopy can also be of value for various diagnostic and operative techniques, such as enteroclysis, balloon dilation of esophageal strictures, noninvasive suction biopsy of the small intestine, and fine needle aspiration of periesophageal thoracic masses.

Enteroclysis[266]

Enteroclysis entails the inflation of the small intestine with a dilute solution of barium through a tube placed directly into the duodenum under fluoroscopic guidance. The initial barium infusion is followed by an infusion of water. The result is a double-contrast study of the distended small bowel. Enteroclysis is indicated for the diagnosis of suspected small-bowel partial obstructions and for the further evaluation of patients with confirmed bacterial overgrowth. It also provides accurate information about mucosal morphology and small-bowel motility. A uniform progression of barium through the gastrointestinal tract (as can be assessed with enteroclysis) is a more important indicator of normal gastrointestinal motility than is the exact transit time.[252,266]

Food is withheld for 2 days and water for 2 hours prior to enteroclysis.[266] An enteroclysis solution containing 28% (w/v) barium sulfate is prepared by making a 3 to 5 (barium to water) dilution of the following suspension: barium sulphate 750 g, sodium citrate 15 g, sodium carboxy-methylcellulose 10 g, Tween-80 (polysorbate 80) 1 ml, silicon antifoam emulsion 1.5 ml, water (800 ml) to a final volume of 1000 ml. For smaller dogs, 21.5% w/v (2 to 5, barium to water) is preferred. Duodenal intubation is carried out under fluoroscopic guidance using a 135 cm long, 14 (French gauge) radiopaque polyvinyl catheter through which is inserted a lubricated flexible insertion guide wire. An infusion set, consisting of two disposable enema bags connected by a Y-shaped connector and fitted with clamps to allow individual delivery of either water or barium suspension, is fitted to the duodenal tube. The patient is sedated and placed in left lateral recumbency. A mouth gag is positioned and the tube maneuvered into the antrum and through the pylorus until the tip is positioned in the descending duodenum. The guide wire is removed, the tube taped in position, and the dog rotated to right lateral recumbency. The infusion bags are lifted to 60 cm above the tabletop and the barium suspension infused (giving an inward flow of 40 to 50 cc per minute and an infusion time of 5 to 15 minutes). Infusion of barium suspension is stopped when filling of the cecum and colon begins (usually amounts to 20–25 cc per kg). Radiographs of the complete contrast-filled small intestine are made using high kVp (90–125) and low mAs settings. The bags are then lowered to 20 to 30 cm above the table and the water infused (at a rate of 60–100 cc per minute). Radiographs (double contrast) are taken of the successively distended bowel loops using the technique just described. Occasionally, compression radiographs are taken of specific areas. The water infusion forces the contrast column into the large bowel, leaving a thin layer of barium coating the intestinal mucosa. Between 20 and 40 cc of water per kg with an infusion time of 5 to 10 minutes results in full distention of the intestinal loops as well as a transient ileus (removing artifactual "strictures" due to peristalsis). The infusion of water is continued until a sufficient degree of transradiancy and distention has been achieved throughout the small bowel. Termination of infusion of water results in partial collapse of the bowel. The rectum is then intubated and rectal fluid drained. In the hands of experienced personnel, the total fluoroscopy time is 10 minutes, and the total procedural time is 40 minutes. Measurements of wall thickness, lumen width, and villus border height are taken. The contrast column (before water) usually measures 12 to 13 mm in width in small dogs and 13 to 16 mm in large dogs. Villus border width (mucosal barium margination) does not exceed 1 mm. Intestinal wall thickness measures 1 to 1.25 mm exclusive of the height of the villus border. Following full distention, the diameter of the intestinal lumen ranges from 15 to 18 mm in small dogs to 18 to 24 mm in larger dogs.[266]

Contraindications for enteroclysis include compromised cardiovascular or renal function or evidence of gastrointestinal perforation. To avoid aspiration, the procedure must be abandoned if excessive gastroduodenal reflux of barium occurs. Complications recorded in a series of 270 enteroclysis procedures on dogs include failure of intubation (5.5%), excessive reflux (3.3%), bowel perforation (0.4%), and vomiting (1.0%).[266] The rate of infusion of the barium suspension is the most important technical aspect of the study and must be adjusted to achieve forward movement of an uninterrupted column of barium through the small bowel. Too rapid infusion of the barium can result in an ileus producing barium-filled, amotile bowel loops that result in a nondiagnostic study.

Disadvantages of enteroclysis are the requirements for fluoroscopy and technical expertise. Advantages of enteroclysis over the upper gastrointestinal study are the shorter examination time, greater accuracy for the detection of morphologic disorders of the intestine, and better ability to assess small intestinal motility (during the barium infusion phase of the study). Enteroclysis has been successfully used in dogs to diagnose enteritis, villus atrophy, duodenal ulcers, intussusception, foreign bodies, strictures, and gastrointestinal neoplasia.[266]

Ultrasonography

Ultrasonography uses the reflection of high-frequency sound waves from tissue interfaces to produce a visual image. Abdominal ultrasonography accurately depicts the size, shape, position, and spatial relationships of abdominal organs. Tissues of varying densities can be delineated, includ-

ing those within an organ. Detailed information on ultrasonographic equipment, technique, and interpretation may be found elsewhere.[267–272]

Abdominal ultrasound and radiographs are complementary examinations. In contrast to radiography, the ultrasound image is enhanced by ascitic fluid and compromised by gas within any distensible viscus. Ultrasound is more sensitive than radiography for the detection of abdominal masses including intraorgan miliary masses (e.g., metastatic neoplasia), abdominal fluid, abscesses, cysts, mural thickenings, lymphadenopathy, pancreatitis, biliary obstruction, and radiolucent biliary and urinary calculi. On occasion, portal hypertension or hydronephrosis may be apparent. Furthermore, ultrasound-guided percutaneous biopsy or aspiration of organs, masses, cysts, or effusion provide safe and effective methods to obtain diagnostic material.[273,274] Additional advantages of ultrasonography are its noninvasiveness, lack of ionizing radiation, and the ability to examine the entire abdominal cavity, not merely mucosal surfaces, as is the case with endoscopy. Disadvantages of ultrasonography include the inability to penetrate bone or air, the cost of the instrumentation, and the technical expertise required to perform examinations well.

Ultrasonography is indicated for the evaluation of nearly all potential gastrointestinal or abdominal problems. Ultrasonography is very useful for the detection and characterization of pancreatitis in the dog and cat.[275–279] The gastric limb of normal pancreas can often be visualized by ultrasonography and during acute pancreatitis it becomes swollen and is more easily visualized. In edematous or early hemorrhagic experimental pancreatitis, there is a generalized increase in size and echodensity in the pancreatic limbs, the changes often being more easily seen in the left limb due to duodenal gas interfering with inspection of the right limb. Ultrasonographic examination of the pancreas is facilitated by introduction of fluid into the abdominal cavity, as is visualization of the liver.[280]

The ultrasonographic appearance of the stomach and intestines of the dog has been described.[281] In skilled hands, ultrasonography can detect mural thickenings of the gastric body, pylorus, and intestinal tract. Intussusceptions have a characteristic appearance. Ultrasound also provides information on gastrointestinal motility and in humans has been used to assess gastric emptying time.[282]

Endoscopic ultrasonography is carried out by endoscopes mounted with an ultrasound transducer at their tip, or alternatively by the passage of newly developed ultrasound probes through the operating channel of the endoscope. These instruments provide cross-sectional images of the gastrointestinal tract. They are particularly valuable for detecting intramural lesions and evaluating local lymph nodes, as well as the right limb and head of the pancreas.[283]

Scintigraphy

Scintigraphy involves the administration of a radiopharmaceutical followed by scanning to determine the differential localization of the radionuclide within the tissues of the body. Nuclear imaging studies of the gastrointestinal tract are currently used in human medicine to investigate esophageal motility, gastroesophageal reflux, gastric emptying, and gastrointestinal transit time, and to detect gastrointestinal inflammation, bleeding, and protein loss. The most important applications of nuclear medicine in veterinary gastroenterology are the determination of gastric emptying time and the detection of hepatic vascular abnormalities, biliary obstruction, and gastrointestinal blood and protein loss.[284] Gastrointestinal nuclear scintigraphy has the ability to provide noninvasive, dynamic, quantitative information about organ function.[284] The most important limitations of scintigraphic techniques are their restricted availability and the necessity for several days of postprocedural hospitalization in a nuclear medicine facility until the patient has excreted sufficient radionuclide to be no longer a radiation hazard.

SCINTIGRAPHIC EVALUATION OF GASTRIC EMPTYING. Gastric isotope scanning studies are indicated to confirm gastric emptying disorders and are especially useful after endoscopy has failed to reveal a physical obstruction to gastric outflow in a patient whose clinical history suggests delayed gastric emptying. Gastric isotope scanning has become the preferred technique for assessing gastric emptying because of its noninvasive nature, fidelity to the physiologic process, and the ability to provide accurate quantitative or semiquantitative measurements of emptying of both liquids and solids.

Isotope scanning involves the ingestion by the patient of an intrinsically or extrinsically labeled liquid or solid meal. Gamma or scintillation counters determine the rate of emptying of the label; the counters are linked to computers to provide quantitative analysis of the scanning data. Isotopes that are most often used in humans include [113]mindium, [111]indium, ^{99m}Tc-labeled sulfur colloid attached to liver cubes, and ^{99m}Tc-labeled DTPA for liquid phase marking. In the dog, ^{99m}Tc disofennin has been mixed with baby food and kibble to provide a solid phase marker.[285] Other isotopes reportedly useful for the examination of emptying time in dogs include ^{14}C polyethylene glycol, [57]Co cyanocobalamin, and ^{99m}Tc-DPTA.[286–288] Liquids are more easily labeled than solids, but the emptying of liquids has less clinical significance. Some investigators prefer double isotope labeling to allow individual assessment of both liquid and solid emptying.

Scintigraphy requires considerable expertise to minimize technical problems, such as straying of the label from the ingesta to gastric mucus or mucosa, and to interpret the radionuclide data correctly. Various presentations of the data have been proposed, including the time it takes for 50% emptying (suitable for liquids only), the percentage of label emptied over a set time period, the area under the emptying curve, and certain mathematical analyses of the emptying curve.[285,287,289] Gastroesophageal reflux of the label invalidates the study.

SCINTIGRAPHIC EVALUATION OF GASTROINTESTINAL BLEEDING. Scintigraphy can aid in locating the site of gastrointestinal bleeding (see Chapter 5). In humans, various radionuclides have been utilized that vary in their sensitivities and half-lives in the bloodstream.[284] Agents with short half-lives are suitable for the detection of active but not recurrent bleeding. In dogs, the administration of [99m]Technetium-labeled red blood cells has been used successfully to locate the site of gastrointestinal bleeding.[290]

NONINVASIVE BIOPSY OF THE GASTROINTESTINAL TRACT [291–293]

A number of biopsy capsules and forceps have been designed to be passed through the mouth or the rectum to obtain samples of gastrointestinal tissues. Unless passed alongside an endoscope, noninvasive biopsy instruments do not allow directed biopsies. Therefore, noninvasive biopsy is indicated only for diagnosing gastrointestinal diseases with a diffuse rather than focal pattern. They are particularly useful if anesthesia is contraindicated, or if full thickness biopsy is considered undesirable because of debilitation. Multiple

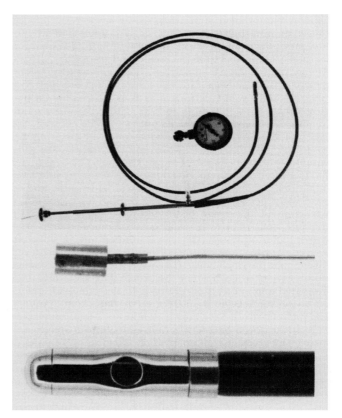

FIGURE 6–21. (above) Quinton biopsy instrument employing a Crosby capsule can be passed orally to obtain biopsies of the stomach and rectally to obtain biopsies of the colon (shorter cables are designed for colon biopsy). Close-up (below) shows the capsule with its port into which mucosal tissue is drawn in by vacuum and the knife with its wire that is drawn to cut a biopsy sample from the mucosa.

biopsies should be obtained from different sites to increase the chance of detecting patchy lesions. Noninvasive biopsy instruments sample only mucosa, unlike full thickness surgical biopsies, which also allow diagnosis of diseases located in the submucosa and muscularis. Suction biopsies are particularly desirable in the large bowel, where full thickness biopsies should be avoided if possible. As discussed in Chapter 5, biopsies of the gastrointestinal tract often do not yield a specific diagnosis. However, they do help rule out infectious (fungal) enteropathies, and often allow a categorization of the disease process on which therapeutic and prognostic advice can be more soundly based. Biopsies of the gastrointestinal tract are contraindicated in patients with bleeding tendencies.

Suction biopsy instruments (Quinton Instruments, Seattle, WA) (Figure 6–21) are the safest method for acquiring noninvasive biopsies. They may be used to obtain biopsies from the mucosa of the esophagus, stomach, small intestine, and large intestine. Noninvasive biopsy of the small intestine uses a single- or multiple-biopsy suction capsule (Quinton Instruments, Seattle, WA) that is passed under fluoroscopic guidance into the duodenum. These instruments are no longer commercially available, having to a large extent been superseded by advances in endoscopic technology.

Suction biopsy instruments possess a biopsy capsule at the end of a flexible insertion tube. The biopsy capsule contains a sliding cylindrical knife and a biopsy port. The knife is connected by wire to a handpiece. The biopsy technique requires good coordination between operators, one of whom applies suction to the instrument via a large syringe, sucking a piece of mucosa into the biopsy capsule (Figure 6–22). The second operator sections the aspirated tissue, applying traction to the biopsy knife by way of the handpiece. Cutting is best performed at suction pressures of 20 to 25 mm Hg. The biopsy capsule, containing the tissue sample, is removed from the lumen of the bowel, disassembled to retrieve the biopsy, and then reintroduced to obtain more samples. This device can be used to obtain tissue from the stomach and colon of the conscious animal with no need for sedation. Due to the relatively greater thickness of the canine intestinal mucosa, suction biopsy capsules with large ports are best suited for use in dogs. Reasons for unsuccessful biopsy include equipment failure, the immersion of the biopsy capsule in fecal debris, and failure to aspirate air from the viscus being biopsied. The latter may result from failure to apply the biopsy port of the capsule to a mucosal surface or inability of the tightly stretched mucosa to be suctioned into the capsule.

Speculum forceps biopsy instruments are a less desirable way to obtain noninvasive biopsies. They are occasionally used with rigid colonoscopes to biopsy the large bowel. They can be useful when the bowel is poorly cleansed and fecal debris prevents the successful operation of suction biopsy instruments. These biopsy instruments are potentially able to perforate the bowel, particularly in the hands of less skilled operators. It is important *never* to depress the bowel wall with the open jaws of the forceps and then take a biopsy. Rather, a three-stage biopsy technique should be used. This entails grasping the mucosa lightly with the biopsy jaws, gently pulling the mucosa toward the center of the bowel lumen, and then finally severing the tissue in the jaws of the forceps (Figure 6–23). In most cases this technique allows the serosal and muscular layers of the bowel to slip out from the grasp of the biopsy instrument's jaws, avoiding perforation.

Biopsy specimens should be handled gently, allowed to dry, and ideally placed on some support such as a piece of cardboard or tongue depressor to minimize contraction and preserve orientation. The mucosa should always be mounted upward, facing away from the surface of the support.

The most important complications of noninvasive biopsy are gastrointestinal perforation and hemorrhage. If perforation is suspected, it can usually be confirmed by the radiographic demonstration of free abdominal gas. If perforation has occurred, immediate abdominal lavage and surgical repair of the defect are indicated. Significant hemorrhage from a gastrointestinal biopsy site is not common, but when it does occur it can be easily overlooked because of the reservoir capacity of the bowel. It is therefore prudent to observe patients closely after biopsy for clinical evidence of hemorrhage. Most cases of biopsy-related gastrointestinal hemorrhage can be handled by administering fresh whole blood without the need for surgical intervention. In the case of large-bowel biopsy-induced hemorrhage, cessation of bleeding may be promoted by packing epinephrine-soaked sponges into the colon.

Cytologic and Histologic Examination of Gastric and Intestinal Biopsy Specimens

Mucosal biopsy specimens can be squashed between two microscope slides for cytologic examination, as well as processed for routine histologic examination. Microscopic examination may reveal inflammatory or neoplastic change,

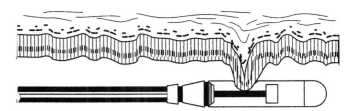

FIGURE 6–22. Drawing showing retrieval of mucosal biopsy with capsule biopsy instrument.

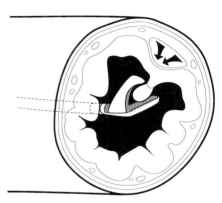

FIGURE 6–23. Biopsy of mucosa using forceps. Mucosa is pulled away from intestinal wall before mucosal tissue is severed.

as well as evidence of infection by organisms such as *Giardia, Histoplasma, Candida, Helicobacter,* or *Spirillum.*[294,295] In the absence of examination by a pathologist skilled in cytologic examination of mucosal biopsies, histologic examination is more likely to provide evidence of inflammatory change, and will also reveal information about mucosal architecture (villous atrophy, dilated lacteals, etc.).[125,296] It is important to remember, however, that in dogs at least, only about 50% of patients with chronic SID have histologic abnormalities;[72,125] in many cases the disease is functional and is revealed better by methods such as quantitative enzymology or tests of intestinal permeability.

Urease Activity in Gastric Biopsy Specimens

Helicobacteria pylori is now believed to be responsible for many cases of chronic gastritis, gastric ulceration, and even gastric carcinoma in humans.[297–301] Several methods are available to diagnose *H. pylori* infection, including histologic observation of the organism in gastric biopsies, culture of the organism, serologic testing, or demonstration of the marked urease activity of the organisms. The latter can be done using a ^{13}C or ^{14}C urea breath testing[302] or by direct demonstration of the urease activity in gastric biopsy. The latter is very easily done using rapid urease tests (CLO test, Tri-Med Specialties, Overland Park, KS) at the time of gastroscopy. A gastric biopsy specimen is placed in a medium that contains urea and an indicator that changes color when the pH rises; if the specimen contains urease activity (most likely due to *Helicobacter* in gastric biopsy specimens), the pH will rise and the substrate will change color over several hours. An association between gastric disease and *Helicobacter* infection appears increasingly probable in dogs and cats,[299,303-305] and several dogs with positive rapid urease test results have been observed, including one with a large and otherwise idiopathic gastric ulcer.[191] The urease activity assay is inexpensive and easily performed, and is likely to be the subject of studies in the future.

Evaluation of Brush Border Enzyme Activity

Unlike many other tissues of the body, serum concentrations of intestinal enzymes are not good markers of intestinal disease because damaged and dying mucosal cells are sloughed into the lumen of the bowel with minimal resorption of their contents in an intact form.[125,306] Brush border enzyme activity can, however, be assayed directly in biopsy samples. One indication for brush border enzyme analysis is the diagnosis of congenital disaccharidase deficiencies that can result in carbohydrate malabsorption and intolerance. Composition of the diet influences the levels of brush-border enzyme activity, and activities of these enzymes are decreased by acute enteritis or toxic insult that damages the mucosal surface.

Assay of brush border and other enterocyte marker enzymes has also been used as an objective method to assess biochemical pathology in dogs with acquired chronic small intestinal diseases.[167] This method clearly reveals abnormalities in the small intestine of dogs with signs of gastrointestinal disease but absent or minimal jejunal morphologic changes. For instance, in a series of German shepherd dogs with bacterial overgrowth, pronounced brush order enzyme defects were observed consistently, whereas only a few of the dogs had histologically recognizable lesions.[72,152] Similarly, wheat-sensitive enteropathy in the Irish setter is associated with only mild patchy villous atrophy and minimal inflammatory change, but distinct abnormalities in the specific activities of brush border marker enzymes can be recognized.[72] Finally, this method has been used to document small intestinal mucosal abnormalities in dogs with exocrine pancreatic insufficiency.[175,307]

PARACENTESIS AND DIAGNOSTIC PERITONEAL LAVAGE

Paracentesis

Paracentesis is indicated if abdominal fluid is detected during physical examination or diagnostic imaging. It provides fluid for culture, cytology, and chemical analysis. Ultrasound guidance aids aspiration of localized collections of fluid.

The preferred site for paracentesis is the caudal abdomen. In male dogs a suitable site is just to the right of the prepuce. In bitches and cats an analogous site can be used. The advantage of such a caudal placement is the avoidance of the omentum, which frequently blocks the lumen of needles placed more cranially. The disadvantage of this site is its proximity to the bladder, which should always be emptied before the procedure. If this site does not yield fluid, up to three other quadrants may be penetrated. Suitable needles for paracentesis are 1 to 2 inch, 14 to 20 gauge. The needle is best inserted slowly to assist judgment of depth and lessen the

likelihood of penetrating a viscus. Local anesthesia is usually not required.

Diagnostic Peritoneal Lavage

Diagnostic peritoneal lavage (DPL) is indicated if paracentesis fails to yield abdominal fluid. Using either an 18 gauge needle or a peritoneal lavage catheter and an intravenous administration set, 20 ml/kg of warm sodium chloride or lactated Ringer's solution is infused into the abdomen. If a needle was used it is removed and the animal's abdomen is gently manipulated while the patient's body position is altered as necessary to help distribute the infused fluid. After several minutes, either the abdominal tap is repeated or fluid is withdrawn via the catheter, and the abdominal fluid examined. Diagnostic criteria for DPL have been established to account for the dilution effects of the infused fluid. For instance, significant intra-abdominal hemorrhage is probable if the microhematocrit of the lavage fluid is greater than 2%. Peritonitis is likely if the neutrophil count is greater than $1500/\mu l$.

EXPLORATORY CELIOTOMY

Abdominal surgery is required in some patients to establish the cause of the gastrointestinal disease, and in many patients for its treatment. The rapidity with which a clinician must resort to exploratory celiotomy for diagnosis is largely a reflection of the diagnostic equipment and financial resources available. Celiotomy optimizes visual inspection and palpation of abdominal organs. Indications for celiotomy include rapid progressive decline in the condition of a patient with abdominal disease, suspected gastrointestinal perforation, and the need for multiple organ or full thickness biopsies. Celiotomy is required for the diagnosis of intestinal lesions out of reach of the endoscope, gastrinomas, and low-grade diseases of some organs such as chronic pancreatitis. Biopsies of the intestine should be taken even when it appears normal. Biopsy artifacts are reduced by placing the sample on a supporting surface before placement in formalin.[308]

It is important to note that in many dogs with chronic SID there are minimal histologic abnormalities.[72] Thus, examination of intestinal biopsies will not always provide definitive diagnostic information, even when disease is present. Many infectious, neoplastic, and severe inflammatory enteropathies will be eliminated with a high degree of confidence, however, allowing a more rational approach to nonspecific management.

Exploratory celiotomy is contraindicated if the diagnosis can be obtained by noninvasive means and/or if the patient is an unacceptable anesthetic risk. A major complication of full thickness biopsy of the gastrointestinal tract is wound dehiscence. The biopsy sites of debilitated animals are particularly likely to dehisce. In these patients, full thickness intestinal biopsy should be performed only after great circumspection, and preferably in association with parenteral nutrition support. Proper technique is essential for an effective surgical evaluation of the abdomen and its contents. Detailed description of the correct approach to the exploratory celiotomy is available.[309-311]

REFERENCES

1. Wilson RB, Holladay JA. Mushroom poisoning. Comp Cont Ed Prac Vet 9:791–793, 1987.
2. Goldschmiedt M, Feldman M. Gastric secretion in health and disease. In: Sleisenger MH, Fordtran JS (eds) Disease. Gastrointestinal Disease. Pathophysiology/Diagnosis/Management. WB Saunders, Philadelphia, 524–544, 1993.
3. Happé RP, de Bruijne JJ. Pentagastrin stimulated gastric secretion in the dog (orogastric aspiration technique). Res Vet Sci 33:232–239, 1982.
4. Youngberg CA, Wlodyga J, Schmaltz S, et al. Radiotelemetric determination of gastrointestinal pH in four healthy beagles. Am J Vet Res 46:1516–1521, 1985.
5. Walt RP. Twenty-four hour intragastric acidity analysis for the future. Gut 27:1–9, 1986.
6. Happé RP. Investigations into disorders of canine gastroduodenal function. Griffioen's, Nieuwegein, 1982.
7. Straus E, Johnson GF, Yalow RS. Canine Zollinger Ellison syndrome. Gastroenterology 72:380–381, 1977.
8. Marks IN, Komarov SA, Shay H. Maximal secretory response to histamine and its relation to parietal cell mass in the dog. Amer J Physiol 199:579–588, 1960.
9. Gabbert NH, Nachreiner RF, Holmes-Word P, et al. Serum immunoreactive gastrin concentrations in the dog. Basal and postprandial values measured by radioimmunoassay. Am J Vet Res 45:2351–2353, 1984.
10. Hall JA, Twedt DC, Curtis CR. Relationship of plasma gastrin immunoreactivity and gastroesophageal sphincter pressure in clinically normal dogs and in dogs with previous gastric dilatation-volvulus. Am J Vet Res 50:1228–1232, 1989.
11. Leib MS, Wingfield WE, Twedt DC, et al. Gastric distension and gastrin in the dog. Am J Vet Res 46:2011–2015, 1985.
12. Lee KY, Tai HH, Chey WY. Plasma secretin and gastrin responses to a meat meal and duodenal acidification in dogs. Am J Physiol 230:784–789, 1976.
13. Middleton DJ, Watson ADJ. Duodenal ulceration associated with gastrin-secreting pancreatic tumor in a cat. J Am Vet Med Assoc 183:461–462, 1983.
14. Breitschwerdt EB, Turk JR, Turnwald GH, et al. Hypergastrinemia in canine gastrointestinal disease. J Am Anim Hosp Assoc 22:585–591, 1986.
15. Brooks FP. Tests related to the stomach. WB Saunders, Philadelphia, 1985.
16. Wolfe MM. Diagnosis of gastrinoma: Much ado about nothing? Ann Intern Med 111:697–699, 1989.
17. Graves GM, Becht JL, Rawlings CA. Metoclopramide reversal of decreased gastrointestinal myoelectric and contractile activity in a model of canine postoperative ileus. Vet Surg 18:27–33, 1989.
18. Bellahsene BE, Schirmer B, McCallum R. Validation of cutaneous EGG recordings by comparing with recordings from intragastric surgically implanted electrodes. Gastroenterology 92:1313, 1987.
19. Mathias JR, Sninsky CA, Millar HK. Development of an improved multi-pressure sensor probe for recording muscle contraction in human intestine. Dig Dis Sci 30:119, 1985.
20. Strombeck DR, Turner WD, Harrold D. Eructation of gas through the gastroesophageal sphincter before and after gastric fundectomy in dogs. Am J Vet Res 49:87–89, 1988.
21. Strombeck DR, Harrold D. Anal sphincter pressure and the rectosphincteric reflex in the dog. Am J Vet Res 49:191–192, 1988.
22. Hunter FM, Correa P, Fontham E et al. Serum pepsinogens as markers of response to therapy for Helicobacter pylori gastritis. Dig Dis Sci 38:2081–2086, 1993.
23. Carrière F, Raphel V, Moreau H, et al. Dog gastric lipase: Stimulation of its secretion in vivo and cytolocalization in mucous pit cells. Gastroenterology 102:1535–1545, 1992.
24. Olsen JW, Guilford WG, Strombeck DR. Clinical use of gastroscopic food sensitivity testing in the dog. J Vet Int Med 5:132, 1991.
25. Elwood CM, Rutgers HC, Batt RM. Gastroscopic food sensitivity testing in 17 dogs. J Sm Anim Pract 35:199–203, 1994.
26. Hall EJ. Gatrointestinal aspects of food allergy: A review. J Sm Anim Pract 35:145–152, 1994.
27. Beeler MF, Kao YS. Laboratory Evaluation of Pancreatic Disorders. WB Saunders, Philadelphia, 1974.
28. Beeler MF, Kao YS. Examination of Feces. WB Saunders, Philadelphia, 1974.
29. Burrows CF, Merritt AM, Chiapella AM. Determination of fecal fat and trypsin output in the evaluation of chronic canine diarrhea. J Am Vet Med Assoc 174:62–66, 1979.
30. Drummey GD, Benson JA, Jones CM. Microscopic examination of the stool for steatorrhea. N Engl J Med 264:85 1961.
31. Merritt AM, Burrows CF, Cowgill L, et al. Fecal fat and trypsin in dogs fed a meat-base or cereal-base diet. J Am Vet Med Assoc 174:59–61, 1979.
32. Burrows CF, Merritt AM. Assessment of gastrointestinal function. In: Anderson NV (ed) Veterinary Gastroenterology. Lea & Febiger, Philadelphia, 16–42, 1992.
33. Siegel D, Cohen PT, Neighbor M, et al. Predictive value of stool examination in acute diarrhea. Arch Pathol Lab Med 111:715–718, 1987.
34. Pickering LK, DuPont HL, Olarte J, et al. Fecal leukocytes in enteric infections. Am J Clin Pathol 68:562–565, 1977.
35. Hay WH, Chickering WR, Roth L, et al. Rectal cytology as a diagnostic aid in the evaluation of large bowel diarrhea in dogs. ACVIM Proc 1046, 1988.
36. Twedt DC. Clostridium perfringens-associated enterotoxicosis in dogs. In: Kirk RW, Bonagura JD (eds) Current Veterinary Therapy. WB Saunders, Philadelphia, 602–604, 1992.
37. Greene CE, Chandler FW. Candidiasis. In: Greene CE (ed) Infectious Diseases of the Dog and Cat. WB Saunders, Philadelphia, 723–727, 1990.
38. Georgi JR. Parasitology for Veterinarians. WB Saunders, Philadelphia, 1974.
39. Zimmer JF, Burrington DB. Comparison of four techniques of fecal examination for detecting canine giardiasis. J Am Anim Hosp Assoc 22:161–167, 1986.
40. Pitts RP, Twedt DC, Mallie, KA. Comparison of duodenal aspiration with fecal floatation for diagnosis of giardiasis in dogs. J Am Vet Med Assoc 182:1210–1211, 1993.
41. Barr SC, Bowman DD. Giardiasis in dogs and cats. Comp Cont Ed Prac Vet 16:603–610, 1994.
42. Baker DG, Strombeck DR, Gershwin LJ. Laboratory diagnosis of Giardia duodenalis infection in dogs. J Am Vet Med Assoc 190:53–56, 1987.
43. Hahn NE, Glaser CA, Hird DW, et al. Prevalence of Giardia in the feces of pups. J Am Vet Med Assoc 192:1428–1429, 1988.
44. Current WL. Cryptosporidiosis. J Am Vet Med Assoc 187:1334–1338, 1985.
45. Lappin MR, Calpin JP, Prestwood AK. Laboratory diagnosis of protozoal infections. In: Green CE (ed) Infectious Diseases of the Dog and Cat. WB Saunders, Philadelphia, 751–757, 1990.
46. Bielsa LM, Greiner EC. Liver flukes (Platynosomum concinnum) in cats. J Am Anim Hosp Assoc 16:269–274, 1985.
47. Goldberg DM, Spooner RJ. Amylase, isoamylase and macroamylase. J Am Vet Med Assoc 13:56–75, 1975.
48. Knisley CV, Engelkirk PG, Pickering LK et al. Rapid detection of Giardia antigen in stool with the use of enzyme immunoassays. Am J Clin Pathol 91:704–708, 1989.
49. Barr SC, Bowman DD, Erb HN. Evaluation of two test procedures for diagnosis of giardiasis in dogs. Am J Vet Res 53:202–2031, 1992.
50. Twedt DC, Jones RL, Collins JK, et al. Clostridium perfringens enterotoxin associated with diarrhea in dogs. ACVIM Proc, 1046, 1989.
51. Carman RJ, Lewis JCM. Recurrent diarrhea in a dog associated with Clostridium perfringens type A. Vet Rec 112:342–343, 1984.
52. Kruth SA, Prescott JF, Welch MK, et al. Nosocomial diarrhea associated with enterotoxogenic Clostridium perfringens infection in dogs. J Am Vet Med Assoc 195:331–334, 1989.
53. Berry PR, Rodhouse JC, Hughes S, et al. Evaluation of ELISA, RPLA, and VERO cell assays for detecting Clostridium perfringens enterotoxin in faecal specimens. J Clin Pathol 41:458–461, 1988.
54. Greene CE. Gastrointestinal and intra-abdominal infections. In: Greene CE (ed) Infectious Diseases of the Dog and Cat. Saunders, Philadelphia, 125–145, 1990.
55. Jones RL. Laboratory diagnosis of bacterial infections. In: Greene CE (ed) Infectious Diseases of the Dog and Cat. WB Saunders, Philadelphia, 453–460, 1990.
56. Fox JG, Greene CE, Jones BR. Enteric and other bacterial infections. In: Greene CE (ed) Infectious Diseases of the Dog and Cat. WB Saunders, Philadelphia, 538–557, 1990.
57. Blacklow NR, Greenberg HB. Viral gastroenteritis. N Engl J Med 325:252–264, 1991.
58. Pollock RVH, Carmichael LE. Canine viral enteritis. In: Greene CE (ed) Infectious Diseases of the Dog and Cat. WB Saunders, Philadelphia, 268–287, 1990.
59. Muir P, Gruffydd-Jones TJ, Howard PE, et al. A clinical and microbiological study of cats with protruding nictitating membranes and diarrhoea: Isolation of a novel virus. Vet Rec 127:324–330, 1990.
60. Mildbrand MM, Teramoto YA, Collins JK, et al. Rapid detection of canine parvovirus in feces using monoclonal antibodies and enzyme-linked immunosorbent assay. Am J Vet Res 45:2281–2284, 1984.
61. Hammond GW, Hazelton PR, Chuang I, et al. Improved detection of viruses by electron microscopy after direct ultracentrifuge preparation of specimens. J Clin Microbiol 14:210–221, 1981.
62. Trampel DW, Kinden DA, Solorzano PL. Parvovirus-like enteropathy in Missouri turkeys. Avian Dis 27:49–54, 1984.
63. Ginsburg HS. Reoviruses and epidemic acute gastroenteritis virus. In: Davis BD, Dulbecco R, Eisen HN, et al. (eds) Microbiology. Harper Row, Hagerstown, 1206–1216, 1980.
64. Guy JS. Diagnosis of canine viral infections.. Vet Clin North Am: Small Anim Pract 16:1145–1156, 1986.
65. Fine KD, Krejs GJ, Fordtran JS. Diarrhea. In: Sleisenger MH, Fordtran JS (eds) Gastrointestinal Disease. WB Saunders, Philadelphia, 1043–1072, 1993.

66. Shiau YF, Feldman GM, Resnick RM, et al. Stool electrolyte and osmolality measurements in the evaluation of diarrheal disorders. Ann Intern Med 102:773–775, 1985.
67. Guilford WG. Unpublished observations.
68. Moran A, Lawson N, Morrow R, et al. Value of faecal alpha-1-antitrypsin, haemoglobin and a chemical occult blood test in the detection of gastrointestinal disease. Clin Chim Acta 217:153–161, 1993.
69. Cook AK, Gilson SD, Fischer WD, et al. Effect of diet on results obtained by use of two commercial test kits for detection of occult blood in feces of dogs. Am J Vet Res 53:1749–1751, 1992.
70. Boulay JP, Lipowitz AJ, Klausner JS, et al. Evaluation of a fluorometric method for the quantitative assay of fecal hemoglobin in the dog. Am J Vet Res 47:1293–1295, 1986.
71. Melgarejo T, Asem EK, Williams DA. Enzyme-linked immunoadsorbant assay for canine alpha$_1$-protease inhibitor (a$_1$-PI). J Vet Int Med 7:133, 1993.
72. Batt RM, Hall EJ. Veterinary gastroenterology: Chronic enteropathies in the dog. In: Pounder R (ed) Recent Advances in Gastroenterology. Churchill Livingstone, London, 131–152, 1988.
73. Williams DA, Batt RM. Sensitivity and specificity of radioimmunoassay of serum trypsinlike immunoreactivity for the diagnosis of canine exocrine pancreatic insufficiency. J Am Vet Med Assoc 192:195–201, 1988.
74. Williams DA. New tests of pancreatic and small intestinal function. In: Anonymous Veterinary Learning Systems (ed), Gastroenterology in Practice. Trenton, 62–69, 1993.
75. Williams DA, Batt RM. Exocrine pancreatic insufficiency diagnosed by radioimmunoassay of serum trypsin-like immunoreactivity in a dog with a normal BT-PABA test result. J Am Anim Hosp Assoc 22:671–674, 1986.
76. Westermarck E, Batt RM, Vaillant C, et al. Sequential study of pancreatic structure and function during development of pancreatic acinar atrophy in a German shepherd dog. Am J Vet Res 54:1088–1094, 1993.
77. Boari A, Williams DA, Famigli-Bergamini P. Observations on exocrine pancreatic insufficiency in a family of English setter dogs. J Sm Anim Pract 35:247–250, 1994.
78. Westermarck E, Rimaila-Pärnänen E. Two unusual cases of canine exocrine pancreatic insufficiency. J Sm Anim Pract 30:32–34, 1989.
79. Medinger TL, Burchfield T, Williams DA. Assay of trypsin-like immunoreactivity (TLI) in feline serum. J Vet Int Med 7:133, 1993.
80. Williams DA, Reed SD. Comparison of methods for assay of fecal proteolytic activity. Vet Clin Path 19:20–24, 1990.
81. Strombeck DR. New method for evaluation of chymotrypsin deficiency in dogs. J Am Vet Med Assoc 173:1319–1323, 1978.
82. Westermarck E. The diagnosis of pancreatic degenerative atrophy in dogs: A practical method. Acta Vet Scand 23:197–203, 1982.
83. Westermarck E, Sandholm M. Fecal hydrolase activity as determined by radial enzyme diffusion: A new method for detecting pancreatic dysfunction in the dog. Res Vet Sci 28:341–346, 1980.
84. Hill FWG. Malabsorption syndrome in the dog: A study of thirty-eight cases. J Sm Anim Pract 13:575–594, 1972.
85. Canfield PJ, Fairburn AJ, Church DB. Effect of various diets on fecal analysis in normal dogs. Res Vet Sci 34:24–27, 1983.
86. Williams DA, Reed SD, Perry LA. Fecal proteolytic activity in clinically normal cats and in a cat with exocrine pancreatic insufficiency. J Am Vet Med Assoc 197:210–212, 1990.
87. Williams DA. Exocrine pancreatic disease. In: (ed) Ettinger SJ Textbook of Veterinary Internal Medicine. WB Saunders, Philadelphia, 1528–1554, 1989.
88. Reusch C. Photometrische chymotrypsinbestimmung im kot des hundes. Tierarztl Prax 14:147–152, 1986.
89. Freudiger U Bigler B. The diagnosis of chronic exocrine pancreatic insufficiency by the PABA test. Kleintier-Praxis 22:73–79, 1977.
90. Imondi AR, Stradley RP, Wolgemuth R. Synthetic peptides in the diagnosis of exocrine pancreatic insufficiency in animals. Gut 13:726–731, 1972.
91. Batt RM, Mann LC. Specificity of the BT-PABA test for the diagnosis of exocrine pancreatic insufficiency in the dog. Vet Rec 108:303–307, 1981.
92. Rogers WA, Stradley RP, Sherding RG, et al. Simultaneous evaluation of pancreatic exocrine function and intestinal absorptive function in dogs with chronic diarrhea. J Am Vet Med Assoc 177:1128–1131, 1980.
93. Batt RM, Bush BM, Peters TJ. A new test for the diagnosis of exocrine pancreatic insufficiency in the dog. J Sm Anim Pract 20:185–192, 1979.
94. Strombeck DR, Harrold D. Evaluation of 60-minute blood p-aminobenzoic and concentration in pancreatic function testing of dogs. J Am Vet Med Assoc 180:419–421, 1982.
95. Washabau RJ Strombeck DR, Buffington CA, et al. Use of pulmonary hydrogen gas excretion to detect carbohydrate malabsorption in dogs. J Am Vet Med Assoc 189:674–679, 1986.
96. Gyr K, Felsenfeld O, Imondi AR. Chymotrypsin-like activity of some intestinal bacteria. Am J Dig Dis 23:413–416, 1978.
97. Sterchi EE, Green JR, Lentze MJ. Nonpancreatic hydrolysis of N-benzoyl-L-tyrosyl-P-aminobenzoic acid (PABA peptide) in the rat small intestine. J Pediatr Gastroenterol Nutr 2:539–547, 1983.
98. Bright JM. Pancreatic adenocarcinoma in a dog with maldigestion syndrome. J Am Vet Med Assoc 187:420–421, 1985.
99. Perry LA, Williams DA, Pidgeon G, et al. Exocrine pancreatic insufficiency with associated coagulopathy in a cat. J Am Anim Hosp Assoc 27:109–114, 1991.
100. Sherding RG, Stradley RP, Rogers WA, et al. Bentiromide:xylose test in healthy cats. Am J Vet Res 43:2272–2273, 1982.
101. Hawkins EC, Meric SM, Washabau RJ, et al. Digestion of bentiromide and absorption of xylose in healthy cats and absorption of xylose in cats with infiltrative intestinal disease. Am J Vet Res 47:567–569, 1986.
102. Zimmer JF, Todd SE. Further evaluation of bentiromide in the diagnosis of canine exocrine pancreatic insufficiency. Cornell Vet 75:426–440, 1985.
103. Canfield PJ, Fairburn AJ, Church DB. Fecal analysis for maldigestion in prancreatectomised dogs. Res Vet Sci 34:28–30, 1983.
104. Vermeulen C, Owens FM, Dragstedt LR. The effect of pancreatectomy on fat absorption from the intestines. Am J Physiol 138:792–796, 1943.
105. Pessoa VC, Kim KS, Ivy AC. Fat absorption in the absence of bile and pancreatic juice. Am J Physiol 174:209–218, 1953.
106. Douglas GJ, Reinauer AJ, Brooks WC, et al. The effect on digestion and absorption of excluding the pancreatic juice from the intestine. Gastroenterology 23:452–459, 1953.
107. Sateri H. Investigations on the exocrine pancreatic function in dogs suffering from chronic exocrine pancreatic insufficiency. Acta Vet Scand (suppl) 53:1–86, 1975.
108. Simpson JW, Doxey DL. Quantitative assessment of fat absorption and its diagnostic value in exocrine pancreatic insufficiency. Res Vet Sci 35:249–251, 1983.
109. Jacobs RM, Hall RL, Rogers WA. Isoamylases in clinically normal and diseased dogs. Vet Clin Path 11:26–32, 1982.
110. Stickle JE, Carlton WW, Boon GD. Isoamylases in clinically normal dogs. Am J Vet Res 41:506–509, 1980.
111. Hill FWG, Kidder DE. The oral glucose tolerance test in canine pancreatic malabsorption. Br Vet J 128:207–214, 1972.
112. Greve T, Anderson NV. The high-dose, intravenous glucose tolerance test (H-IVGTT) in dogs. Nord Vet Med 25:436–445, 1973.
113. Williams DA, Batt RM. Reversible intravenous glucose intolerance in canine exocrine pancreatic insufficiency. Proc 4th Ann Vet Med Forum ACVIM, Washington, DC, 14–19, 1986.
114. Smith SR, Edgar PJ, Pozefsky T, et al. Insulin secretion and glucose tolerance in adults with protein-calorie malnutrition. Metabolism 24:1073–1084, 1975.
115. Heard CRC. The effects of protein-energy malnutrition on blood glucose homeostasis. Wld Rev Nutr Diet 30:107–147, 1978.
116. Pfister K, Rossi GL, Freudiger U et al. Morphological studies in dogs with chronic pancreatic insufficiency. Virchows Arch [A] 386:91–105, 1980.
117. Walker WA, Isselbacher KJ. Uptake and transport of macromolecules by the intestine. Possible role in clinical disorders. Gastroenterology 67:531–550, 1974.
118. Van Kruiningen HJ. Pancreatic atrophy. In: Anonymous (ed) Comparative Gastroenterology. Chas. C. Thomas, Springfield, IL, 42–64, 1982.
119. Westermarck E, Lindberg LA, Sandholm M. Quantitation of serum phosphalipase A2 by enzyme diffusion in lecithin agar gels. A comparative study in man and animals. Acta Vet Scand 25:229–244, 1986.
120. Simpson KW, Simpson JW, Lake S, et al. Effect of pancreatectomy on plasma activities of amylase, isoamylase, lipase and trypsin-like immunoreactivity in dogs. Res Vet Sci 51:78–82, 1991.
121. Simpson JW, Doxey DL, Brown R. Serum isoamylase values in normal dogs and dogs with exocrine pancreatic insufficiency. Vet Res Commun 8:303–308, 1984.
122. Wright TL, Heyworth MF. Maldigestion and Malabsorption. WB Saunders, Philadelphia, 1989.
123. Nicholson A, Watson ADJ, Mercer JR. Fat malassimilation in three cats. Aust Vet J 66:110–113, 1989.
124. Van de Kamer JH, Huinink HTB, Weyers HA. Rapid method for the determination of fat in feces. J Biol Chem 177:347–355, 1949.
125. Hill FWG, Kelly DF. Naturally occurring intestinal malabsorption in the dog. Dig Dis 19(7): 649–665, 1974.
126. Lewis LD, Boulay JP, Chow FHC. Fat excretion and assimilation by the cat. Fel Pract 9:46–49, 1979.
127. Schneider MU, Demling L, Jones SA, et al. NMR spectrometry: A new method for total stool fat quantification in chronic pancreatitis. Dig Dis Sci 32:494–499, 1987.
128. Benini L, Caliari S, Bonfante F, et al. Fecal fat concentration in the screening of steatorrhea. Dig 53:94–100, 1992.
129. Caliari S, Benini L, Bonfante F, et al. Pancreatic extracts are necessary for the absorption of elemental and polymeric enteral diets in severe pancreatic insufficiency. Scand J Gastroenterol 28:749–752, 1993.
130. Brobst DF, Funk A. Simplified test of fat absorption in dogs. J Am Vet Med Assoc 161:1412–1417, 1972.
131. Van Den Broek AHM, Simpson JW. Fat absorption in dogs with demodicosis or zinc-responsive dermatosis. Res Vet Sci 52:117–119, 1992.
132. Simpson JW, Van Den Broek AHM. Fat absorption in dogs with diabetes mellitus or hypothyroidism. Res Vet Sci 50:346–348, 1991.
133. Kallfelz FA, Norrdin RW, Neal TM. Intestinal absorption of oleic acid I

and triolein I in the differential diagnosis of malabsorption syndrome and pancreatic dysfunction in the dog. J Am Vet Med Assoc 153:43–46, 1968.

134. Williams DA, Prymak C, Baughan J. Tocopherol (vitamin E) status in canine degenerative myelopathy. Proc 3rd Ann Vet Med Forum ACVIM, San Diego, May 1985, 154, 1985.

135. Williams DA. The pancreas: Exocrine pancreatic insufficiency. In: Anderson NV (ed) Veterinary Gastroenterology. Lea & Febiger, Philadelphia, 283–294, 1992.

136. Williams DA. Studies on the diagnosis and pathophysiology of canine exocrine pancreatic insufficiency. PhD thesis, University of Liverpool, England, 1985.

137. Williams DA. The pancreas: Exocrine pancreatic insufficiency. In Anderson NV (ed) Veterinary Gastroenterology. Lea & Febiger, Philadelphia, 570–594, 1992.

138. Coffin DL, Thordal-Christensen A. The clinical and some pathological aspects of pancreatic disease in dogs. Vet Med 48:193–198, 1953.

139. Hayden DW, VanKruiningen HJ. Control values for evaluating gastrointestinal function in the dog. J Am Anim Hosp Assoc 12:31–36, 1976.

140. Butler RN, Gehling NJ, Lawson MJ, et al. Clinical evaluation of the 14C triolein breath test: A critical analysis. Aust NZ J Med 14:111, 1984.

141. Cole SG, Rossi S, Stern A. Cholesteryl octanoate breath test. Gastroenterology 93:1372–1380, 1987.

142. Hall EJ. Unpublished observations.

143. Hill FWG, Kidder DE, Frew J. A xylose absorption test for the dog. Vet Rec 87:250–255, 1970.

144. Trinder P. Micro-determination of xylose in plasma. Analyst 100:12–15, 1975.

145. Levitt DG, Hakim AA, Lifson N. Evaluation of components of transport of sugars by dog jejunum in vivo. Am J Physiol 217(3):777–783, 1969.

146. Heyman M, Dumontier AM, Desjeux JF. Xylose transport pathways in rabbit ileum. Am J Physiol 238:326–331, 1980.

147. Cherbut C, Meirieu O, Ruckebusch Y. Effect of diet on intestinal xylose absorption in dogs. Dig Dis Sci 31(4):385–391, 1986.

148. Heyman M, Desjeux JF, Grasset E, et al. Relationship between transport of d-xylose and other monosaccharides in jejunal mucosa of children. Gastroenterology 80:758–762, 1981.

149. Merritt AM, Duelly P. Phloroglucinol microassay for plasma xylose in dogs and horses. Am J Vet Res 44(11):2184–2185, 1983.

150. Krawitt EL, Beeken WL. Limitations of the usefulness of the d-xylose absorption test. Am J Clin Pathol 63:261–263, 1975.

151. Simpson JW. Bacterial overgrowth causing malabsorption in a dog. Vet Rec 110:335–336, 1982.

152. Batt RM, McLean L, Comparison of the biochemical changes in the jejunal mucosa of dogs with aerobic and anaerobic bacterial overgrowth. Gastroenterology 93:986–993, 1987.

153. Batt RM, Needham JR, Carter MW. Bacterial overgrowth associated with a naturally occurring enteropathy in the German shepherd dog. Res Vet Sci 35:42–46, 1983.

154. Batt RM, Carter MW, Peters TJ. Biochemical changes in the jejunal mucosa of dogs with a naturally occurring enteropathy associated with bacterial overgrowth. Gut 25:816–823, 1984.

155. Peters TJ, Batt RM, Health JR, et al. The micro-assay of intestinal disaccharidases. Biochem Med 15:145–148, 1976.

156. Washabau RJ, Strombeck DR, Buffington CA, et al. Evaluation of intestinal carbohydrate malabsorption in the dog by pulmonary hydrogen gas excretion. Am J Vet Res 47:1402–1406, 1986.

157. Washabau RJ, Buffington CA, Strombeck DR. Evaluation and Management of Carbohydrate Malassimilation. WB Saunders, Philadelphia, 1986.

158. Rumessen JJ, Kokholm G, Gudmand-Hoyer E. Methodological aspects of breath hydrogen analysis. Scand J Clin Lab Invest 47:555–560, 1987.

159. Rutgers HC, Lamport A, Simpson KW, et al. Bacterial overgrowth in dogs with chronic intestinal disease. J Vet Int Med 7:133, 1993.

160. Ludlow CL, Bruyette DS, Davenport DJ, et al. Relationship between breath hydrogen fraction and calculated breath hydrogen excretion in healthy dogs. J Vet Int Med 8:152, 1994.

161. Ludlow CL, Bruyette DS, Davenport DJ, et al. Daily and individual variation of breath hydrogen excretion in healthy dogs. J Vet Int Med 8:150, 1994.

162. Vogelsang H, Ferenci P, Frotz S. Acidic colonic microclimate—possible reason for false negative hydrogen breath tests. Gut 29:21–26, 1988.

163. Thompson DG, Binfield P, DeBelder A, et al. Extraintestinal influences on exhaled breath hydrogen measurements during the investigation of gastrointestinal disease. Gut 26:1349–1352, 1985.

164. Kerlin P, Wong L. Breath hydrogen testing in bacterial overgrowth of the small intestine. Gastroenterology 95:982–988, 1988.

165. Perman J, Modler S. Glycoproteins as substrates for production of hydrogen and methane by colonic bacterial flora. Gastroenterology 83:388–393, 1982.

166. Williams DA. New tests of pancreatic and small intestinal function. Comp Cont Ed Prac Vet 9:1167–1174, 1987.

167. Batt RM. New approaches to malabsorption in dogs. Comp Cont Ed Prac Vet 8:783–795, 1986.

168. Batt RM, Morgan JO. Role of serum folate and vitamin B12 concentra-

tions in the differentiation of small intestinal abnormalities in the dog. Res Vet Sci 32:17–22, 1982.

169. Lindenbaum J. Malabsorption of vitamin B12 and folate. Curr Concepts Nutr 9:105–123, 1980.

170. Reisenauer AM, Chandler CJ, Halsted CH. Folate binding and hydrolysis by pig intestinal brush-order membranes. Am J Physiol 251:G481–G486, 1986.

171. Bunch SE, Easley JR, Cullen JM Hematologic values and plasma and tissue folate concentrations in dogs given phenytoin on a long-term basis. Am J Vet Res 51:1865–1868, 1990.

172. Davenport DJ, Sherding RG. Clinicopathologic parameters of an experimental model of small intestinal bacterial overgrowth. Proc 4th Ann Vet Med Forum ACVIM, Washington, DC, II, Sec. 14:7, 1986.

173. Bernstein LH, Gutstein S, Efron G, et al. Experimental production of elevated serum folate in dogs with intestinal blind loops: Relationship of serum levels to location of the blind loop. Gastroenterology 63:815–819, 1972.

174. Bernstein LH, Gutstein S, Efron G, et al. Experimental production of elevated serum folate in dogs with intestinal blind loops II. Nature of bacterially produced folate coenzymes in blind loop fluid. Am J Clin Nutr 28:925–929, 1975.

175. Williams DA, Batt RM, McLean L. Bacterial overgrowth in the duodenum of dogs with exocrine pancreatic insufficiency. J Am Vet Med Assoc 191:201–206, 1987.

176. Dutta SK, Russell RM, Iber FL. Impaired acid neutralization in the duodenum in pancreatic insufficiency. Dig Dis Sci 24:775–780, 1979.

177. Dutta SK, Russell RM, Iber FL. Influence of exocrine pancreatic insufficiency on the intraluminal pH of the proximal small intestine. Am J Dig Dis 24:529–534, 1979.

178. Russell RM, Dhar GJ, Dutta SK, et al. Influence of intraluminal pH on folate absorption: Studies in control subjects and in patients with pancreatic insufficiency. J Lab Clin Med 93:438–436, 1979.

179. Kark JA, Victor M, Hines JD, et al. Nutritional vitamin B12 deficiency in rhesus monkeys. Am J Clin Nutr 27:470–478, 1974.

180. Batt RM, Horadagoda NU, McLean L, et al. Identification and characterization of a pancreatic intrinsic factor in the dog. Am J Physiol 256:G517–G523, 1989.

181. Fyfe JC. Feline intrinsic factor (IF) is pancreatic in origin and mediates ileal cobalamin (CBL) absorption. J Vet Int Med 7:133, 1993.

182. Welkos SL, Toskes PP, Baer H, et al. Importance of aerobic bacterial in the cobalamin malabsorption of the experimental blind loop syndrome. Gastroenterology 80:313–320, 1981.

183. Fyfe JC, Jezyk PF, Giger U, et al. Inherited selective malabsorption of vitamin B12 in giant schnauzers. J Am Anim Hosp Assoc 50:533–539, 1989.

184. Fyfe JC, Ramanujam KS, Ramaswamy K, et al. Defective brush-border expression of intrinsic factor-cobalamin receptor in canine inherited intestinal cobalamin malabsorption. J Biol Chem 266(7):4489–4494, 1991.

185. Fyfe JC, Giger URS, Hall CA, et al. Inherited selective intestinal cobalamin malabsorption and cobalamin deficiency in dogs. Pediatr Res 39:24–31, 1991.

186. Williams DA. Markedly subnormal serum cobalamin in Shar-Pei dogs with signs of gastrointestinal disease. J Vet Int Med 5:133, 1991.

187. Williams DA. Exocrine pancreatic insufficiency. Walth Int Focus 2:9–14, 1993.

188. Schultz WJ. A comparison of commercial kit methods for assay of vitamin B12 in ruminant blood. Vet Clin Path 16:102–106, 1987.

189. Williams DA. Evaluation of radioassay methods for analysis of canine serum cobalamin and folate. J Vet Int Med 6:81, 1992.

190. Batt RM, McLean L, Rutgers HC, et al. Validation of a radioassay for the determination of serum folate and cobalamin concentrations in dogs. J Sm Anim Pract 32:221—224, 1991.

191. Williams DA. Unpublished observations.

192. Baker H, Schor SM, Murphy BD, et al. Blood vitamin and choline concentrations in healthy domestic cats, dogs, and horses. Am J Vet Res 47:1468–1471, 1986.

193. Williams DA: Feline exocrine pancreatic disease. Proc 12th Ann Vet Med Forum ACVIM, San Francisco, 617–619, 1994.

194. Hofmann AM. The enterohepatic circulation of bile acids in health and disease. In: Sleisenger, MH, Fordtran JS (eds) Gastrointestinal Disease. Pathophysiology/Diagnosis/Management. WB Saunders, Philadelphia, 127–150, 1993.

195. Suhr O, Danielsson A, Horstedt P, et al. Bacterial contamination of the small bowel evaluated by breath tests,75 Se-labelled homocholic-tauro acid, and scanning electron microscopy. Scand J Gastroenterol 25:841–852, 1990.

196. Aarbakke J, Schjonsby H. Value of urinary simple phenol and indican determinations in the diagnosis of the stagnant loop syndrome. Scand J Gastroenterol 11:409–414, 1976.

197. Toskes PP, Donaldson RM. Enteric bacterial flora and bacterial overgrowth syndrome. In: Sleisenger MH, Fordtran JS (eds) Gastrointestinal Disease. Pathophysiology/Diagnosis/Management. WB Saunders, Philadelphia, 1106–1118, 1993.

198. Burrows CF, Jezyk PF. Nitrosonaphthol test for screening of small intestinal diarrheal disease in the dog. J Am Vet Med Assoc 183:318–322, 1983.

199. Fordtran JS, Scroggie WB, Potter DE. Colonic absorption of tryptophan metabolites in man. J Lab Clin Med 64:125–132, 1964.

200. Van der Heiden C, Wadman SK, Ketting D, et al. Urinary and fecal excretion of metabolites of tyrosine and phenylalanine in a patient with cystic fibrosis and severely impaired amino acid absorption. Clin Chim Acta 31:133–141, 1971.

201. Van der Heiden C, Wauters EAK, Ketting D et al. Gas chromatographic analysis of urinary tyrosine and phenylalanine metabolites in patients with gastrointestinal disorders. Clin Chim Acta 34:289–296, 1971.

202. Batt RM, Rutgers HC. Unpublished observations.

203. Lichtman SN, Sartor RB, Keku J, et al. Hepatic inflammation in rats with experimental small intestinal bacterial overgrowth. Gastroenterology 98:414–423, 1990.

204. Lichtman SN, Sartor RB. Hepatobiliary injury associated with experimental small-bowel bacterial overgrowth in rats. Immunol Res 10:528–531, 1991.

205. Davenport DJ, Ludlow CL, Hunt J, et al. Effect of sampling method on quantitative duodenal cultures in dogs: Endoscopy vs. permucosal aspiration. J Vet Int Med 8:152, 1994.

206. Johnston K, Lamport A, Batt RM. An unexpected bacterial flora in the proximal small intestine of normal cats. Vet Rec 132:362–363, 1993.

207. Willard MD, Simpson RB, Fossum TW, et al. Characterization of naturally developing small intestinal bacterial overgrowth in 16 German shepherd dogs. J Am Vet Med Assoc 204:1201–1206, 1994.

208. Jonas A, Flanagan PR, Forstner GC. Pathogenesis of mucosal injury in the blind loop syndrome. Brush border enzyme activity and glycoprotein degradation. J Clin Invest 60:1321–1330, 1977.

209. Jonas A, Krishnan C, Forstner G. Pathogenesis of mucosal injury in the blind loop syndrome. Release of disaccharidases from brush border membranes by extracts of bacteria obtained from intestinal blind loops in rats. Gastroenterology 75:791–795, 1978.

210. Biemond I, Kreuning J, Jansen JBMJ, et al. Diagnostic value of serum pepsinogen C in patients with raised serum concentrations of pepsinogen A. Gut 34:1315–1318, 1993.

211. Toskes PP. Bacterial overgrowth of the gastrointestinal tract. Adv Intern Med 38:387–407, 1993.

212. King CE, Toskes PP. The use of breath tests in the study of malabsorption. Clin Gastrolenterol 12:591–610, 1983.

213. King CE, Toskes PP, Spivey JC, L et al. Detection of small intestine bacterial overgrowth by means of a 14C-D-xylose breath test. Gastroenterology 77:75–82, 1979.

214. King CE, Toskes PP. Comparison of the 1-gram [14C]xylose, 10-gram lactulose-H₂, and 80-gram glucose H₂ breath tests in patients with small intestine bacterial overgrowth. Gastroenterology 91:1447–1451, 1986.

215. Dill-Macky E, Williams DA. Breath 14CO₂ output following oral administration of 14C-D-xylose to healthy dogs. J Vet Int Med 3:132, 1989.

216. Einarsson K, Bergström M, Eklöf RN, et al. Comparison of the proportion of unconjugated to total serum cholic acid and the [¹⁴C]-xylose breath test in patients with suspected small intestinal bacterial overgrowth. Scand J Clin Lab Invest 52:425–430, 1992.

217. Bolt MJG, Stellaard F, Paumgartner G. Serum unconjugated bile acids in patients with small bowel bacterial overgrowth. Clin Chim Acta 181:87–102, 1989.

218. Muir P, Gruffydd-Jones TJ, Harbour DA. A preliminary assessment of postprandial unconjugated bile acids in serum of cats with chronic diarrhoea and vomiting. Vet Rec 130:119–121, 1992.

219. Salemans JMJI, Nagengast FM, Tangerman A, et al. Unconjugated serum bile acid levels in small intestinal bacterial overgrowth. Gastroenterology 100:A247, 1991.

220. Setchell KDR, Harrison DL, Gilbert JM, et al. Serum unconjugated bile acids: Qualitative and quantitative profiles in ileal resection and bacterial overgrowth. Clin Chim Acta 152:297–306, 1985.

221. Masclee A, Tangerman A, van Schaik A, et al. Unconjugated serum bile acid as a marker of small intestinal bacterial overgrowth. Eur J Clin Invest 19:384–389, 1989.

222. Salemans JMJI, Nagengast FM, Tangerman A, et al. Postprandial conjugated and unconjugated serum bile acid levels after proctocolectomy with ileal pouch-anal anastomosis. Scand J Gastroenterol 28:786–790, 1993.

223. Hall EJ, Batt RM. Differential sugar absorption for the assessment of canine intestinal permeability: The cellobiose/mannitol test in gluten-sensitive enteropathy of Irish setters. Res Vet Sci 51:83–87, 1991.

224. Hall EJ, Batt RM, Brown A. Assessment of canine intestinal permeability, using 51Cr-labeled ethylenediaminetetraacetate. Am J Vet Res 50:2069–2074, 1989.

225. Papasouliotis K, Gruffydd-Jones TJ, Sparkes AH, et al. Lactulose and mannitol as probe markers for in vivo assessment of passive intestinal permeability in healthy cats. Am J Vet Res 54:840–844, 1993.

226. Marks SL, Williams DA. Cumulative urinary recovery of orally administered 51Cr-EDTA in healthy dogs. ACVIM Proc, 1046: 1989.

227. Batt RM, Hall EJ, McLean L, et al. Small intestinal bacterial overgrowth

228. Tams TR, Twedt DC. Canine protein-losing gastroenteropathy syndrome. Comp Cont Ed Pract Vet 3:105–114, 1981.

229. Van Kruiningen HJ, Lees GE, Hayden DW, et al. Lipogranulomatous lymphangitis in canine intestinal lymphangiectasia. Vet Pathol 21:377–383, 1984.

230. Fossum TW, Sherding RG, Zack PM, et al. Intestinal lymphangiectasia associated with chylothorax in two dogs. J Am Vet Med Assoc 190 (1): 61–64, 1987.

231. Meschter CL, Rakich PM, Tyler DE. Intestinal lymphangiectasia with lipogranulomatous lymphangitis in a dog. J Am Vet Med Assoc 190 (4):427–430, 1987.

232. Fossum TW. Protein-losing enteropathy. Sem Vet Med Surg 4:219–225, 1989.

233. King CE, Toskes PP. Protein-losing enteropathy in the human and experimental rat blind loop syndrome. Gastroenterology 80:504–509, 1981.

234. Kobayashi K, Asakura H, Shinozawa T, et al. Protein-losing enteropathy in systemic lupus erythematosus. Observations by magnifying endoscopy. Dig Dis Sci 34:1924–1928, 1989.

235. Bai JC, Sambuelli A, Sugai E, et al. Gluten challenge in patients with celiac disease: Evaluation of a₁-antitrypsin clearance. Am J Gastroenterol 86:312–316, 1991.

236. Breitschwerdt EB, Halliwell WH, Foley CW, et al. A heredity diarrhetic syndrome in the basenji characterized by malabsorption, protein losing enteropathy and hypergammaglobulinemia. J Am Anim Hosp Assoc 16:551–560, 1980.

237. Waldmann TA. Protein-losing enteropathy. Gastroenterology 50:422–433, 1966.

238. Barton CL, Smith C, Troy G, et al. The diagnosis and clinicopathology features of canine protein-losing enteropathy. J Am Anim Hosp Assoc 14:85–91, 1978.

239. Crossley JR, Elliott RB. Simple method for diagnosing protein-losing enteropathies. Br Med J. 1:428–429, 1977.

240. Bernier JJ, Florent CH, Desmazures CH, et al. Diagnosis of protein-losing enteropathy by gastro-intestinal clearance of alpha₁-antitrypsin. Lancet 2:763–764, 1978.

241. Florent C, L'Hirondel C, Desmazures C, et al. Intestinal clearance of a₁-antitrypsin: A sensitive method for the detection of protein-losing enteropathy. Gastroenterology 81:777–780, 1981.

242. Karbach U, Ewe K, Bodenstein H. Alpha₁-antitrypsin, a reliable endogenous marker for intestinal protein loss and its application in patients with Crohn's disease. Gut 24:718–723, 1983.

243. Thomas DW, Sinatra FR, Merritt RJ. Random fecal alpha₁-antitrypsin concentration in children with gastrointestinal disease. Gastroenterology 80:776–782, 1981.

244. Brouwer J, Smekens F. Determination of a₁-antitrypsin in fecal extracts by enzyme immunoassay. Clin Chim Acta 189:173–180, 1990.

245. Williams DA. Evaluation of fecal alpha₁-protease inhibitor (a₁-PI) concentration as a test for canine protein-losing enteropathy (PLE). J Vet Int Med 5:133, 1991.

246. Hall EJ, Rutgers HC, Batt RM. Evaluation of the peroral string test in the diagnosis of canine giardiasis. J Sm Anim Pract 29:177–183, 1988.

247. Morgan JP, Silverman S. Techniques of Veterinary Radiography. Veterinary Radiology Associates, Davis, CA, 1982.

248. Aronson E, Carrig CB, Lattimer JC. Radiology of the gastrointestinal system. In: Jones BD, Liska WD (eds) Canine and Feline Gastroenterology. WB Saunders, Philadelphia, 380–486, 1986.

249. Burt JK. Contrast radiology of the gastrointestinal tract. Proc 8th Kal Kan Symp 8:57–63, 1984.

250. Thrall DE, Lewis RE. Gastrointestinal radiography. In: Anderson NV (ed) Veterinary Gastroenterology. Lea & Febiger, Philadelphia, 59–79, 1980.

251. Thrall DE. Textbook of Veterinary Diagnostic Radiology. WB Saunders, Philadelphia, 1986.

252. Brawner WR, Bartels FE. Contrast radiography of the digestive tract. Vet Clin North Am 13:599–626, 1983.

253. Allan GS. Radiology of the digestive system. Aust Vet Pract 17:25–34, 1987.

254. Kleine LJ. Interpreting radiographic signs of abdominal disease in dogs and cats—3. Vet Med 80:73–86, 1985.

255. Evans SM Double versus single contrast gastrography in the dog and cat. Vet Radiol 24:6–10, 1983.

256. Morgan JP. The upper gastrointestinal examination in the cat: Normal radiographic appearance using positive contrast media. Vet Radiol 22:159–169, 1981.

257. O'Brien TR. Radiographic Diagnosis of Abdominal Disorders in the Dog and Cat. WB Saunders, Philadelphia, 1978.

258. Jakovljevic S. Gastric radiology and gastroscopy in the dog. Vet Ann 28:172–182, 1988.

259. Miyabayashi T, Morgan JP, Atilola AO, et al. Small intestinal emptying times in normal Beagle dogs. Vet Radiol 27:164–168, 1986.

260. Burns J, Fox S. The use of barium meal to evaluate total gastric emptying time in the dog. Vet Radiol 27:169–172, 1986.

and enhanced intestinal permeability in healthy Beagles. Am J Vet Res 53:1935–1940, 1992.

261. Miyabayashi T, Morgan JP. Gastric emptying in the normal dog. Vet Radiol 25:187–191, 1984.

262. Feldman M, Smith HJ, Simon TR. Gastric emptying of solid radiopaque markers: Studies in healthy subjects and diabetic patients. Gastroenterology 87:895, 1984.

263. Hall JA, Willer RL, Seim III HB, et al. Gastric emptying of nondigestible radiopaque markers after circumcostal gastropexy in clinically normal dogs and dogs with gastric dilatation-volvulus. Am J Vet Res 53:1961–1965, 1992.

264. Allan FJ, Guilford WG. Radiopaque markers: Preliminary clinical observations. J Vet Int Med 8:151, 1994.

265. Hogan PM, Aronson E. Effect of sedation of transit time of feline gastrointestinal contrast studies. Vet Radiol 29:85–88, 1988.

266. Wolvekamp WTC. Enteroclysis: A new radiographic technique for evaluation of the small intestine of the dog. Iowa State University Press, Ames, 1989.

267. Nyland TG, Park RD, Lattimer JC. Gray-scale ultrasonography of the canine abdomen. Vet Radiol 22:220–227, 1981.

268. Nyland TG, Bernard WV. Application of abdominal ultrasound. Calif Vet 36:21–25, 1982.

269. Nyland TG, Park RD. Hepatic ultrasonography in the dog. Vet Radiol 24:77–84, 1983.

270. Rantanen NW, Ewing RL. Principles of ultrasound application in animals. Vet Radiol 22:196–203, 1981.

271. Lamb CR, Stowater JL, Pipers FS. The first twenty-one years of veterinary diagnostic ultrasound—a bibliography. Vet Radiol 29:37–45, 1988.

272. Wrigley RH, Konde LJ, Park RD, et al. Ultrasonic diagnosis of portacaval shunts in young dogs. J Am Vet Med Assoc 191 (4)421–424, 1987.

273. Hoppe FE, Hager DA, Poulos PW. A comparison of manual and automatic ultrasound-guided biopsy techniques. Vet Radiol 27:99–101, 1986.

274. Kerr LY. Ultrasound guided biopsy. Calif Vet 42:9–10, 1988.

275. Rutgers HC, Herring DS, Orton EC. Pancreatic pseudocyst associated with acute pancreatitis in a dog: Ultrasonographic diagnosis. J Am Anim Hosp Assoc 21:411–416, 1985.

276. Murtaugh RJ, Herring DS, Jacobs RM, et al. Pancreatic ultrasonography in dogs with experimentally induced acute pancreatitis. Vet Radiol 26:27–32, 1985.

277. Edwards DF, Bauer MS, Walker MA, et al. Pancreatic masses in seven dogs following acute pancreatitis. J Am Anim Hosp Assoc 26:189–198, 1990.

278. Simpson KW, Shiroma JT, Biller DS, et al. Ante mortem diagnosis of pancreatitis in four cats. J Sm Anim Pract 35:93–99, 1994.

279. Nyland TG, Mulvany MH, Strombeck DR. Ultrasonographic features of experimentally induced, acute pancreatitis in the dog. Vet Radiol 24:260–266, 1983.

280. Miles KG, Lattimer JC, Krause GF, et al. The use of intraperitoneal fluid as a simple technique for enhancing sonographic visualization of the canine pancreas. Vet Radiol 29:258–263, 1988.

281. Penninck DG, Nyland TG, Fisher PE, et al. Ultrasonography of the normal canine gastrointestinal tract. Vet Radiol 30:272–276, 1989.

282. Bateman DN, Whittingham TA. Gastric emptying measurement by real-time ultrasound. In: Weinbeck M (ed) Motility of the Digestive Tract. Raven Press, New York, 1982.

283. Rösch T, Classen M. Endoscopic ultrasonography: An added advantage in pancreatic diagnosis. Schweiz Med Wochenschr 123:1059–1068, 1993.

284. Koblik PD, Hornof WJ. Gastrointestinal nuclear medicine. Vet Radiol 26:138–142, 1985.

285. Hornof WJ, Koblik PD, Strombeck DR, et al. Scintigraphic evaluation of solid-phase gastric emptying in the dog. Vet Radiol 30(6):242–248, 1989.

286. Gue M, Fioramonti J, Bueno L. A simple double radio-labeled technique to evaluate gastric emptying of canned food meal in dogs. Gastroenterol Clin Biol 12:425–430, 1988.

287. Van den Brom WE, Happe RP. Gastric emptying of a radionuclide-labeled test meal in heathy dogs: A new mathematical analysis and reference values. Am J Vet Res 47:2170–2174, 1986.

288. Lawaetz O, Olesen HP, Andreasen R. Evaluation of gastric emptying by a simple isotope technique. Scand J Gastroenterol 16:737–748, 1981.

289. McCallum RW. Motor function of the stomach in health and disease. In: Sleisenger MH (ed) Gastrointestinal Disease. WB Saunders, Philadelphia, 675–713, 1989.

290. Metcalf MR. Scintigraphic gastrointestinal bleeding localization with[99m]Tc-labeled red blood cells: Clinical application in nine dogs. Vet Radiol 28:96–100, 1987.

291. Kasper JB, Chiapella AM. Gastrointestinal biopsy techniques. In: Anonymous (ed) Current Veterinary Therapy VII. WB Saunders, Philadelphia, 962–969, 1980.

292. Bradley RL. Digestive tract biopsy in dogs and cats. Mod Vet Pract 66:614–620, 1985.

293. Golden DL. Gastrointestinal endoscopic biopsy techniques. Semin Vet Med Surg 8:239–244, 1993.

294. Debongnie JC, Beyaert C, Legros G. Touch cytology, a useful diagnostic method for diagnosis of upper gastrointestinal tract infections. Dig Dis Sci 34:1025–1027, 1989.

295. Geyer C, Colbatzky F, Lechner J, et al. Occurrence of spiral-shaped bacteria in gastric biopsies of dogs and cats. Vet Rec 133:18–19, 1993.

296. Hart IR, Kidder DE. The quantitative assessment of normal canine small intestinal mucosa. Res Vet Sci 25:157–162, 1978.

297. Weinstein WM. Gastritis and gastropathies. In: Sleisenger MH, Fordtran JS (ed) Gastrointestinal Disease. Pathophysiology Diagnosis/Management. WB Saunders, Philadelphia, 545–571, 1993.

298. Soll AH. Gastric, duodenal, and stress ulcer. In: Sleisenger MH, Fordtran JS (eds) Gastrointestinal Disease. Pathophysiology/Diagnosis/Management. WB Saunders, Philadelphia, 580–679, 1993.

299. Lee A, Krakowka S, Fox JG, et al. Role of Helicobacter felis in chronic canine gastritis. Vet Pathol 29:487–494, 1992.

300. Lee A. Spiral organisms: What are they?. Scand J Gastroenterol [suppl] 26:9–22, 1991.

301. Dooley CP, Cohen H, Fitzgibbons PL, et al. Prevalence of Helicobacter pylori infection and histologic gastritis in asymptomatic persons. N Engl J Med 321:1562–1566, 1989.

302. Rauws EAJ, Royen EAV, Langenberg W, et al. ^{14}C-urea breath test in C. pylori gastritis. Gut 30:798–803, 1989.

303. Eaton KA, Dewhirst FE, Radin MJ, et al. Helicobacter acinonyx sp. nov., isolated from cheetahs with gastritis. Int J Syst Bacteriol 43:99–106, 1993.

304. Eaton KA, Radin MJ, Kramer L, et al. Epizootic gastritis associated with gastric spiral bacilli in cheetahs (Acinonyx jubatus). Vet Pathol 30:55–63, 1993.

305. Leblanc B, Fox JG, Le Net JL, et al. Hyperplastic gastritis with intraepithelial Campylobacter-like organisms in a beagle dog. Vet Pathol 30:391–394, 1993.

306. Goldberg DM. The enzymology of intestinal disease. Clin Biochem 20:63–72, 1987.

307. Batt RM, Bush BM, Peters TJ. Biochemical changes in the jejunal mucosa of dogs with naturally occurring exocrine pancreatic insufficiency. Gut 20:709–715, 1979.

308. Fenwick BW, Kruckenberg S. Comparison of methods used to collect canine intestinal tissues for histologic examination. Am J Vet Res 48:1276–1281, 1987.

309. Crowe DT. The steps to arresting abdominal hemorrhage. Vet Med 83:676–677, 1988.

310. Crowe DT. Dealing with visceral injuries of the cranial abdomen. Vet Med 83:682–699, 1988.

311. Crowe DT. What to do with disorders of the caudal abdomen. Vet Med 83:700–709, 1988.

7

Gastrointestinal Endoscopy

W. GRANT GUILFORD

INTRODUCTION

Endoscopy is the visual inspection of the viscera or cavities of the body with an optical instrument. The technique was first introduced into medicine over a century ago.[1] In the decade since the first reviews of veterinary endoscopy,[2-7] the popularity and applications of the procedure have increased considerably.[8-11]

INDICATIONS AND LIMITATIONS

General

Endoscopy is a minimally invasive, atraumatic technique that permits visual examination of gastrointestinal lesions and allows descriptive or photographic documentation of their severity and extent. Endoscopy provides biopsy, cytologic, and fluid samples for laboratory evaluation. It allows therapeutic interventions such as foreign body retrieval, bougienage, and gastrostomy tube placement. It has a low morbidity and mortality but should only be used after routine workup has failed to reveal a diagnosis. Endoscopy is most useful for the diagnosis of esophageal, gastric, upper small intestinal, and colonorectal disorders with a mucosal or luminal location. Endoscopy detects morphologic but not functional disease. It will not detect abnormal gastrointestinal motility, gastrointestinal hypersecretory disorders, and subcellular defects such as brush border enzyme deficiencies. Furthermore, mid–small intestinal disease and lesions of the submucosa or muscle layers are difficult to assess with an endoscope. The clinical problems commonly evaluated by upper and lower gastrointestinal endoscopy are listed in Tables 7–1 and 7–2, respectively. The most frequent gastrointestinal endoscopic procedure at the UCD VMTH is the gastroduodenoscopy.

Endoscopy Versus Contrast Radiography

Upper gastrointestinal contrast radiography and endoscopy are complementary procedures. Contrast procedures do not require anesthesia and provide a better estimation of luminal diameter (esophagus), gastrointestinal motil-ity, and gastric emptying rate. Contrast radiography is better able to detect mural masses, extramural compressive lesions, and jejunal diseases than endoscopy. In contrast, endoscopy is more sensitive for the diagnosis of mucosal diseases of the upper gastrointestinal tract and large bowel and offers the important advantage of definitive diagnosis through biopsy.[12,13]

Contraindications

With the exception of animals unfit for anesthesia, there are few absolute contraindications to performing gastrointestinal endoscopy. The procedure is not appropriate if bowel perforation is suspected because pressurization of the bowel with air during endoscopy may increase contamination of the surrounding tissues. Endoscopy is discouraged in inadequately prepared animals and in animals with bleeding diatheses.

Table 7–1

PRINCIPAL INDICATIONS FOR UPPER GASTROINTESTINAL ENDOSCOPY

Evaluation of dysphagia
Evaluation of regurgitation
Evaluation of chronic vomiting
Evaluation of hematemesis
Evaluation of melena
Evaluation of chronic diarrhea
Retrieval of esophageal foreign bodies
Bougienage of esophageal strictures
Retrieval of select gastric foreign bodies
Placement of percutaneous gastrostomy tubes

Table 7–2

PRINCIPAL INDICATIONS FOR LARGE-BOWEL ENDOSCOPY

Persistent hematochezia	Chronic diarrhea
Persistent tenesmus	Fecal incontinence
Persistent mucoid stools	Dyschezia

114

Table 7-3

MOST COMMON COMPLICATIONS OF
GASTROINTESTINAL ENDOSCOPY

Gastrointestinal perforation
Laceration of major blood vessels
Laceration of organs adjacent to the gastrointestinal tract
Decreased venous return due to gastric overdistension
Acute bradycardia
Gastric dilatation-volvulus
Mucosal hemorrhage
Transmission of enteropathogenic organisms
Bacteremias*

*Incidence uncertain in veterinary medicine.

Complications

The principal complications of gastrointestinal endoscopy are shown in Table 7-3. Perforation of the gastrointestinal wall with resultant mediastinitis, pleuritis, or peritonitis can result from forceful insertion of the endoscope without adequate vision of the lumen or, more commonly, from poor biopsy technique. Small perforations are difficult to detect by endoscopy. If a perforation is suspected, radiography should be performed immediately. Following perforation, large quantities of air rapidly enter the surrounding body cavity, and can be easily visualized on survey radiographs. Small amounts of free abdominal air without symptoms of perforation have, however, been reported in 1% of humans after colonoscopy.

Gastric dilatation-volvulus can occur following administration of oral lavage solutions or during recovery from endoscopic procedures, perhaps due to inadequate removal of insufflated air. In some animals, overdistention of the stomach with air during the procedure results in increased pyloroantral tone, significantly decreased tidal volume, compression of the caudal vena cava, and a rapid drop in venous return and blood pressure (Figure 7-1). Acute bradycardia, apparently due to vagovagal reflexes, can occur during endoscopy. This phenomenon most often occurs when the instrument enters the small intestine of small breeds. It is perhaps caused by overdistention of the intestinal tract or by excessive traction on the mesentery. Rupture of major blood vessels can occur during removal of foreign bodies and during bougienage. Rarely, considerable hemorrhage can follow biopsy procedures. Poorly disinfected scopes can transmit enteropathogenic organisms. Following routine endoscopy, oropharyngeal or colonic organisms can be transiently cultured from the blood of 3% to 8% of human patients. A similar bacteremia is likely to occur in dogs and cats undergoing endoscopy.

ENDOSCOPIC EQUIPMENT

Endoscopes

An appropriate selection of endoscopic equipment for a particular practice depends on the nature of the practice and requires an understanding of the range of equipment available and the purposes for which that equipment is best suited.

RIGID ENDOSCOPES. Modern rigid endoscopes consist of hollow plastic or metal insertion tubes with an accompanying

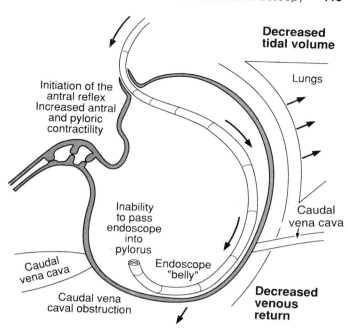

FIGURE 7-1. Schematic showing consequences of gastric overdistention.

light source, obturator, and insufflation bag (Figure 7-2). The plastic insertion tubes are disposable but can be reused. Most rigid endoscopes have a length of approximately 25 cm and an outside diameter of 2 cm. They are more durable, cheaper to purchase, and easier to use and clean than fiberoptic endoscopes. They are most commonly used for proctoscopy for which they are very effective. They allow visualization of the descending colon and rectum only. Rigid endoscopes can be used to examine the esophagus and are useful for removing esophageal foreign bodies.

FIBEROPTIC ENDOSCOPES. Flexible fiberoptic endoscopes consist of several sections: the insertion tube, hand piece, and so-called umbilical cord.

The insertion tube (Figure 7-3) is flexible and contains glass fiber bundles to transmit and receive light. Fiberoptic bundles are fragile and can be damaged by inappropriate handling. Broken fiberoptic light-receiving bundles leave black specks in the field of vision. Disruption of the spatial arrangement of light-receiving bundles (e.g., from a bite of the insertion tube) or leakage of water around the bundles (e.g., from perforation of the external cladding or the biopsy channel) lead to a blurred image. Breakage of light-transmitting fibers reduces the light intensity of transmitted light but otherwise does not affect image quality. The insertion tube also has a biopsy and suction channel, an air and water channel, and tip deflection cables. The air/water channel is for insufflation of the viscus under examination and cleaning of debris from the lens. Blockage of the air/water channel is a common problem and usually results from using nondistilled water in the wash bottle or impaction of mucosal debris in the channel tip. Mucosal debris can often be freed from the air/water channel by soaking the endoscope and then insufflating the channel with compressed air.

The hand piece has up/down and right/left deflection knobs for deflection of the distal tip of the insertion tube. Most endoscopes have brakes to lock the position of the deflection knobs. An air/water valve and suction valve are also located on the hand piece. Light pressure on the air/water valve results in insufflation. Depression of the

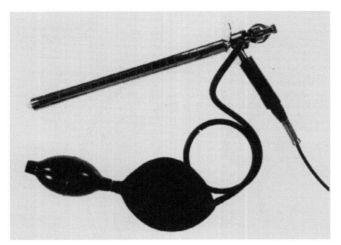

FIGURE 7-2. Welch Allyn sigmoidoscope.

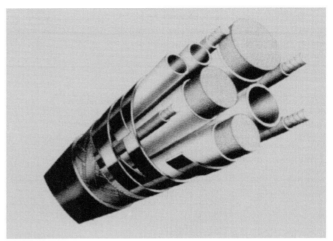

FIGURE 7-3. Cross section of endoscope insertion tube showing glass bundles, channels, and deflection cables.

air/water valve causes a jet of water to spray onto the endoscope lens for cleaning purposes. Depression of the suction knob results in suction of gas or fluid through the operating channel, provided a suitable suction pump has been attached to the endoscope. The umbilical cord of the endoscope conveys light from the light source to the endoscope via fiberoptic bundles.

Many types of fiberoptic endoscopes have been designed. Their suitability for different endoscopic procedures and for the diverse requirements of individual veterinary practices are discussed in the section on features of flexible endoscopes.

VIDEO ENDOSCOPES. The recently introduced video endoscope differs considerably from the fiberoptic endoscope. It has no fiberoptic bundles for receipt of light. Instead, a microelectronic chip (charge-coupled device), located on the distal tip of the instrument, receives the image, which is then transmitted by wires to a videoprocessor that reconstructs the image and relays it to a television monitor. This results in superior image resolution and a more robust scope. Video endoscopes allow better permanent documentation of examinations, create an atmosphere of team participation, facilitate coordination of biopsy and retrieval procedures, are less fatiguing, and greatly facilitate teaching. Video endoscopes are more expensive than a fiberoptic system, but their cost may be defrayed by greater longevity.

Features and Characteristics of Flexible Endoscopes

WORKING LENGTH. Pediatric gastroscopes, the most common type of endoscope used for upper gastrointestinal examinations in small animals, usually have a 100 to 110 cm working length. This working length is adequate for the majority of gastrointestinal examinations in small animal patients, with the exception of duodenoscopy of large-breed dogs, for which endoscopes of 125 cm or greater are ideal. Veterinarians frequently performing endoscopy on large-breed dogs will find the longer diameter endoscopes of the Schott and Storz companies a distinct advantage.

INSERTION TUBE DIAMETER. Gastrointestinal endoscopes range in diameter from approximately 7.5 to 16 mm. The smaller diameter scopes are easier to insert, but they have diminished clarity and brightness due to smaller and fewer

fiber bundles (other things being equal) and provide smaller biopsies. In general, for gastrointestinal endoscopy of dogs and cats the insertion tube diameter should be less than 10 mm. The smaller diameter endoscopes (< 8 mm) are very useful for feline duodenoscopy.

OPERATING CHANNEL. Endoscopes designed for therapeutics (e.g., polypectomy) often have two operating channels. One operating channel suffices for veterinary endoscopy. Most gastrointestinal endoscopes have 2 to 4 mm channels. Large-diameter operating channels facilitate significantly larger and better quality biopsy samples. The diameter of the operating channel and the length of the endoscope dictate the compatibility of through-the-scope accessories such as biopsy instruments.

TIP DEFLECTION. Most gastrointestinal endoscopes have four-way tip deflection. The maximum bending angle in each direction of deflection varies considerably with manufacturer and scope diameter. In general, gastrointestinal endoscopes should have at least 180° to 210° deflection in one direction and a minimum of 90° to 100° deflection in the other three directions. The greater the tip deflection, and the smaller the bending radius, the greater the maneuverability of the scope.

DIRECTION OF VIEW. Forward-viewing endoscopes are necessary for veterinary endoscopy. Side-viewing scopes, utilized for certain catheterization techniques in humans, have not found an application in veterinary patients.

ANGLE OF VIEW. Most scopes have a field of view of 90° to 120°. A wide angle of view facilitates orientation and panoramic examination, decreasing the likelihood of missing lesions due to tunnel vision.

OPTICS. The quality of an endoscope's optics is reflected in its depth of field, image resolution, image brightness, color rendition, evenness of illumination, image size, contrast range, and absence of artifacts such as flare. Acceptable depth of field for most purposes is 3 to 100 mm. Minimum visible distance greater than 3 to 5 mm compromises detailed examination of the mucosal surface and hinders pyloric intubation. Image brightness is of particular importance in a large viscus. Without adequate brightness the stomach, for instance, may appear dark, prohibiting a panoramic examination. A wide contrast range allows vision in both shadowed and exposed areas of the bowel.

HANDLING. Endoscopes must be comfortable to hold in one hand. Operating controls should be in effortless reach, and biopsy channels must accept instruments easily, even while the tip is deflected.

MISCELLANEOUS. Compatibility of an endoscope with any other endoscopy equipment owned by the practice is an advantage. The endoscope must be durable. Fully immersible endoscopes are easier to clean and may be more hardy.

Light and Vacuum Sources

Flexible endoscopes utilize halogen or xenon "cold" light sources of 150 to 300 watts. High light intensity is necessary for panoramic views of a large viscus and for photography. Light sources vary considerably in the sophistication with which they regulate illumination. The light source is also the source of pressure for air insufflation and water flushing. If there is no pressure in the air/water channel, check that the water bottle is connected to the light source and the cap of the water bottle is not leaking.

A vacuum source is necessary for the aspiration of gastrointestinal fluid and air. It is wise to avoid attempted aspiration of particulate matter such as food, gastric debris, or feces to prevent costly blockages of the operating channel. Many varieties of pumps are available.

Endoscopic Accessories

Biopsy forceps, retrieval equipment, and cleaning accoutrements are essential endoscopic accessories. Useful but not essential accessories include cytology brushes, polypectomy snares, balloon dilators or bougies, percutaneous endoscopic gastrostomy sets, camera equipment, videorecorders, procedure carts, endoscope storage cabinets, and endoscope washers.

BIOPSY EQUIPMENT. The biopsy equipment should include two or three pinch biopsy instruments. These instruments are flexible, through-the-endoscope forceps possessing at their distal end two opposing 2 to 3 mm oval or round cups with smooth or serrated edges. Opening and closing is controlled by a hand piece at the proximal end of the instrument. Spiked biopsy instruments can facilitate bowel biopsy but are not essential and compromise biopsy quality when the tip becomes burred. Pinch biopsy equipment provides targeted biopsies.

Suction biopsy capsules are the preferred instruments for nontargeted biopsy of the esophagus and descending colon. On occasion, hand-held speculum biopsy forceps with large-diameter biopsy cups may be necessary for biopsy of the colon. A variety of types and sizes are available. Speculum biopsy forceps are usually used with proctoscopes and are the least desirable way to biopsy the colon because of the risk of perforation.

RETRIEVAL EQUIPMENT. Retrieval equipment should include through-the-endoscope equipment such as a basket retrieval instrument and a three- or four-prong grasper and/or some form of jawed grasper, such as a rat tooth grasper. Polyp snares are also useful retrieval instruments. In addition, it is helpful to obtain some form of long semirigid grasping instrument (such as that available in many hardware stores) to be passed alongside a fiberscope or through a proctoscope for the removal of proximal esophageal foreign bodies.

CYTOLOGY BRUSHES. Shielded through-the-endoscope cytology brushes are available for attaining targeted brush cytology specimens. They can be helpful for the diagnosis of protozoal diseases.

BALLOON DILATORS AND BOUGIES. Suitable balloon dilators for gastrointestinal work have a 15 to 20 mm inflatable diameter with 6 to 8 cm lengths. Rigid bougies are tapered probes of variable diameter. On the rare occasions rigid bougies are needed in veterinary practice, they can often be borrowed from a local hospital.

CLEANING AND STORAGE EQUIPMENT. Cleaning equipment usually consists of cleaning brushes for passage through the operating channels of the scope and cleaning solutions such as glutaraldehyde. Gas sterilization is possible also. The manufacturer's recommendations should be followed closely and precautions with the use of glutaraldehyde should be rigidly adhered to. Endoscopes should be stored hanging up. Endoscopes stored in their cases do not drain well and can develop kinks in the insertion tubes because of prolonged storage in coils. Various hangers for endoscopes can be purchased. These are best mounted in a lockable cupboard.

ENDOSCOPIC TECHNIQUE

Patient Preparation

GASTROSCOPY. The patient should be fasted for 12 to 24 hours, or longer if there is evidence of delayed gastric emptying. Retained gastric material interferes with visualization, may plug the endoscope, and may result in aspiration during recovery.

COLONOSCOPY. Adequate preparation is essential for effective evaluation and biopsy of the mucosa. A period of fasting is essential. A 3 day fast is ideal (where possible, begun at home), 2 days will often suffice, and 1 day is rarely adequate. The most effective cleansing of the entire colon, with the least attendant artifacts, is attained by the use of intestinal lavage solutions (CoLyte, Endlaw Preps, NY; Golytely, Braintree Labs, MA).[14,15] These solutions contain polyethylene glycol, which acts as an osmotic agent, and replacement electrolytes. They are administered in volumes of 30 to 40 ml/kg by stomach tube two to three times over a period of 12 to 24 hours prior to the procedure. Two to 6 hours should separate stomach tubings, and the last administration should be greater than 12 hours prior to colonoscopy. Performing colonoscopy earlier than this does not allow adequate evacuation of the lavage solution from the colon. In addition, it is risky to perform anesthesia within 4 hours of administration of the lavage solution because the stomach often still contains a considerable amount of fluid. Pretreatment with acetylpromazine facilitates stomach tubing and reduces the likelihood of vomition. Metoclopramide administration prior to the stomach tubing may facilitate gastric emptying. Complications of intestinal lavage include vomition, aspiration of lavage solution, and gastric dilatation-volvulus. These complications are rare if the fluid volumes administered are less than 40 ml/kg. Use of lavage solutions is contraindicated in intractable animals and should be used with extreme caution in dogs with delayed gastric emptying, swallowing dysfunction, or a history of previous gastric dilatation-volvulus. Cheaper osmotic lavage solutions such as magnesium citrate, magnesium sulphate, and magnesium hydroxide should be avoided because of the risks of hypermagnesemia and volume contracture.

Enemas are less desirable for preparing the colon prior to colonoscopy.[14] They are less effective at cleansing (especially proximally), and they can produce artifactual mucosal erosions. In most animals, however, they are cheaper, easier, and less time consuming to administer (particularly to cats). It is important to avoid additives in the enemas. Soap, especially if in high concentrations, can induce colitis in humans. Hypertonic sodium phosphate enemas (Fleet) and rectal administration of bisacodyl laxatives both alter proctoscopic and histologic appearance of the mucosa. Furthermore, hypertonic sodium phosphate enemas have been associated with fatal hyperphosphatemia and hypernatremia in cats. Large cotton-tipped applicators (Scopettes, Birchwood, MN) can be used to swab out residual fecal material from the rectum.

RIGID PROCTOSCOPY. One to two days of fasting and two to three warm water enemas usually provide adequate preparation for protoscopy.

Anesthesia

Anesthesia is necessary for all endoscopic procedures, with the exception of proctoscopy with a rigid endoscope in which sedation can be used if anesthesia is unwarranted. Choice of anesthetic technique should be made with respect to the animal's general condition and presence or absence of intercurrent disease.

I have found anticholinergic premedication an advantage to reduce bowel motility and secretion but others believe atropine makes duodenal intubation more difficult.[16] Narcotic agents increase pyloric and cranial duodenal tone in humans, interfering with the easy passage of the scope.[17] My clinical impression is that a similar phenomenon occurs in dogs. If the clinical condition of the animal allows, I therefore avoid narcotics during gastrointestinal endoscopy.

Particular attention for signs of gastric overinflation are necessary. These include abdominal tympany, tachycardia, pale mucous membranes, and a precipitous drop in blood pressure. Significant cardiovascular and respiratory complications do not occur in all dogs with overdistended stomachs,[18] but failure to recognize and correct these complications in those animals in which they occur can lead to death of the patient. The anesthetist should also be alert for acute onset of bradycardia suggestive of vagovagal reflexes.

General Endoscope Technique

EQUIPMENT CHECK. Before introducing the scope, ensure that all functions are working, including tip deflection, lens wash, insufflation, and suction. Check that the image is focused and the lens clean. A reliable gag must always be placed in the mouth to protect the endoscope.

HOLDING THE ENDOSCOPE. The endoscope is held between thumb and first finger of the left hand with the umbilical cord in contact with the back of the hand and the control section nestled in the palm (Figure 7–4). In this manner, most endoscopists can comfortably manipulate the controls. The fingers of the left hand manage the insufflation and suction buttons and the thumb adjusts the up-down deflection knob. The right hand is used to advance and torque the scope and to make the occasional adjustment of the left-right deflection knob. An assistant is helpful to stabilize the instrument in a particular position in the bowel and necessary for efficient biopsy and retrieval procedures. Tyro endoscopists often rely on an assistant to advance the insertion tube of the endoscope while they use both hands to manipulate the controls. This habit is to be discouraged because it robs the endoscopist of the fine and coordinated motion necessary to intubate difficult pyloric canals.

MANEUVERING THE ENDOSCOPE. The tip of the endoscope is maneuvered by use of the up-down and left-right deflection knobs and by torquing the insertion tube. The up-down deflection direction of most endoscopes has greater bending capability than the left-right deflection direction. Torquing allows the up-down deflection direction of the endoscope to be maneuvered to the plane that is most beneficial for the negotiation of bends requiring maximal deflection of the endoscope tip. Torquing lessens the reliance of the endoscopist on the left-right deflection knob (the knob most difficult to reach). Torquing is often required to negotiate the pylorus and cranial duodenum.

Torque should be initiated by rotating the insertion tube not the hand piece (Figure 7–4). The hand piece should not be used to initiate torque because its larger diameter allows the generation of sufficient rotational force to damage the endoscope. Instead, the hand piece should passively follow the rotation of the insertion tube. If the hand piece and insertion tube are not rotated in the same direction and by the same degree, rotational stress is placed on the fiberoptics. Many endoscopists achieve the rotation of the hand piece and insertion tube as a unit by left or right movement of their upper body at the hips. Maximal torquing can result in impressive contortion. Greater resistance to torquing is experienced as more insertion tube is buried in the animal. It can be very difficult to elicit any meaningful rotational movement of the endoscope when the tip is in the distal duodenum.

THE SLIDE-BY TECHNIQUE. On most occasions, the endoscope should be advanced only if the bowel lumen is in clear view. One exception to this is the slide-by technique. This entails prior deflection of the endoscope tip in the perceived direction of a flexure, followed by *gentle* sliding of the endoscope over the mucosa of the greater curvature of the flexure. The lumen is temporarily lost to view, and a mucosal "redout" occurs. The impression of the mucosa sliding by the tip of the endoscope occurs and a tunnel view is not regained until the endoscope rounds the flexure. The slide-by technique is often necessary to round the cranial duodenal and left colic flexures. One disadvantage of this technique is that it will occasionally result in temporary obstruction of the insufflation/flush channel by shards of mucosa.

FREQUENT CAUSES OF DAMAGE TO ENDOSCOPES. Endoscopes are relatively fragile instruments and should be handled with care. They can be damaged by bites, collision with surfaces, inappropriate coiling, excessive insertion or torquing force, forceful passage of biopsy instruments, and repeated fluoroscopy. Bites can be prevented by conscientious placement of mouth guards. Collision with surfaces usually occurs when the weight of a loop of uninserted endoscope drags the tip of the endoscope out of the animal and whips the tip of the instrument against the floor or table leg. This abuse can be prevented if an assistant gently grips the insertion tube when the endoscopist removes his or her right hand from the instrument. In general, endoscopes should

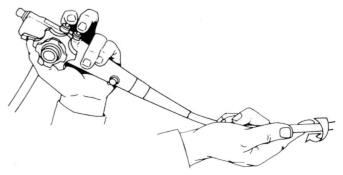

FIGURE 7–4. Scope handling. The endoscope should be held comfortably in the left hand. Torque should be applied from the insertion tube only.

not be coiled greater than 360° and should not be forced into tight bends. The latter often inadvertently occurs when a standing endoscopist leans forward over the table, intent on some endoscopic quest. This posture can kink severely the loop of uninserted insertion tube against the tabletop. The deflection cables of the endoscope can be stretched by over-rotation of the deflection knobs. The cables will also stretch if the deflection knobs are forcefully rotated against the deflection brakes.

PATIENT POSITIONING. For routine gastrointestinal endoscopy the patient is positioned in left lateral recumbency. In the case of upper gastrointestinal endoscopy this position facilitates examination of the pylorus. During large-bowel endoscopy this position assists examination of the ileocecal region and encourages drainage of fluid to the descending colon, where it can be aspirated.

Esophagoscopy

ENDOSCOPIC TECHNIQUE. Flexible endoscopes allow the most thorough examination of the esophagus, but rigid endoscopes can be used and have some advantages for the removal of sharp foreign bodies. To pass the endoscope into the esophagus the animal's neck is extended and the lubricated insertion tube is introduced into the mouth, dorsal to the endotracheal tube. With firm pressure the endoscope is then passed through the upper esophageal sphincter.

After entering the esophagus, the tip of the endoscope is drawn back until it just rests inside the upper esophageal sphincter and the esophagus is insufflated with air until sufficiently distended to visualize the lumen. As the esophagus dilates, the longitudinal mucosal folds of the proximal esophagus reduce in size and it is usually possible to see the lumen of the entire cervical esophagus. Once the esophagus is adequately distended, the endoscope is advanced. There is little resistance to movement of the endoscope in the esophagus and rapid aboral passage with a full luminal view can usually be managed by minor adjustments of the up-down deflection knob in combination with small torquing movements. At the junction of the cervical and thoracic esophagus there is a slight flexure. Once this is rounded, an uninterrupted view to the lower esophageal sphincter is usually attained.

Because of its durable epithelium, biopsy of the esophagus is more difficult than the biopsy of other parts of the gastrointestinal tract. A suction biopsy instrument is the safest and most effective method to biopsy the esophagus.

APPEARANCE OF THE NORMAL ESOPHAGUS. In the anesthetized animal the normal esophagus appears flaccid and may drape over the trachea and thoracic vasculature. Because of anesthesia-induced muscle paralysis, the esophageal lumen appears quite large and the endoscopist must be wary of diagnosing megaesophagus based on endoscopic appearance alone. The esophagus may contain small amounts of clear fluid. The presence of food is abnormal and the pooling of bile is unusual but not necessarily pathologic. The normal mucosa is pale and smooth. Submucosal vessels are usually not visible in the dog esophagus, but a network of superficial vessels is sometimes apparent in the esophagus of pups and cats. There may be a redundancy of tissue at the thoracic inlet that gives the impression of a diverticulum but can be largely obliterated by full extension of the neck. The distal few centimeters of the cat esophagus is characterized by a series of circumferential mucosal folds (the "herringbone" pattern) (Figure 7–5). These folds should not be confused with the radial fibrotic striations that occur in strictures. This

area of the cat esophagus may also occasionally undergo peristaltic contractions in spite of anesthesia.

The gastroesophageal junction usually has a slit-like appearance (Figure 7–6). Slight reddening at the gastroesophageal orifice may be observed in normal animals. This red coloration is due to the transition from esophageal to gastric mucosa. The lower esophageal sphincter is usually closed at the time of examination but occasionally may gape open. Little significance should be afforded to a patulous lower esophageal sphincter unless the surrounding esophageal mucosa shows evidence of esophagitis.

APPEARANCE OF THE ABNORMAL ESOPHAGUS. Dogs with megaesophagus usually have fluid and fermenting food retained in large esophageal folds. The folds are often so voluminous that it can be difficult to pass the endoscope to the lower esophageal sphincter. A similar problem arises with gastroesophageal intussusception because the endoscope continually passes into blind folds caused by the inversion of the stomach into the esophagus. Abnormalities suggestive of esophagitis include erythema, erosions, irregularity, and strictures. Esophageal strictures appear as circumferential narrowings of the esophageal lumen. If the lumen of the stricture is sufficiently wide, radial fibrotic striations are often visible in the stricture wall. Fibrous postinflammatory strictures usually have a smooth surface devoid of erosions. In contrast, stric-

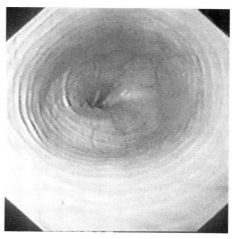

FIGURE 7–5. Normal lower esophagus of a cat. Note the radial mucosal striations.

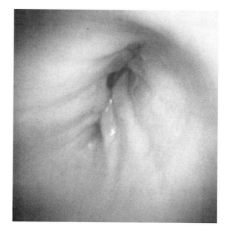

FIGURE 7–6. Normal lower esophageal sphincter of a dog.

tures due to neoplasia of the esophageal mucosa often have a friable appearance. Hiatal hernias sometimes appear as a ballooning of the distal esophageal wall into the esophageal lumen. The ballooning often occurs at the same rate as respiration. Leiomyomas often arise at the gastroesophageal junction. The growth of these masses sometimes everts gastric mucosa into the esophagus, providing an endoscopic clue to the presence of the tumor. Other esophageal tumors such as sarcomas and carcinomas are usually more obvious, appearing as friable and often ulcerating masses.

Gastroduodenoscopy

The large size of the stomach means the endoscopist must develop a systematic approach to gastroscopy; otherwise lesions will be missed. In order to facilitate pyloric intubation it is usual practice to pass the endoscope quickly to the pyloric antrum with minimal insufflation of the gastric body. On withdrawal of the endoscope from the duodenum, the antrum, body, lesser curvature, cardia, and fundus of the stomach are then carefully examined.

INITIAL PASSAGE OF THE ENDOSCOPE TO THE PYLORIC ANTRUM. Following examination of the esophagus, the endoscope is gently advanced through the gastroesophageal sphincter into the stomach. On entry into the stomach, the mucosa of the undistended stomach usually interferes with vision until the stomach is partially insufflated. The first part of the stomach wall that is visualized is the junction of the fundus and body. Slight deviation of the tip of the scope away from the mucosa will allow the endoscopist to obtain a panoramic view of the body of the stomach as it is inflating. It is important not to overinflate the stomach at this stage of the examination. Introduce sufficient air to just part the rugal folds. Overdistension of the stomach allows a "belly" to develop in the insertion tube that inhibits maneuverability of the endoscope and increases antral and pyloric contraction frequency by way of the antral reflex, both of which make passage of the endoscope into the duodenum more difficult.

Once the gastric body is partially inflated the orientation of the gastric rugal folds will become apparent. Most rugal folds run a convoluted course toward the pyloric antrum. The endoscope is advanced in the same direction as the rugal folds. This will direct the endoscope along the greater curvature of the stomach toward the incisura angularis, which appears as a crescent-shaped fold at the distal end of the gastric body (Figure 7–7). The incisura angularis is an important landmark. It is a narrow fold that divides the pyloric antrum from the lesser curvature of the gastric body.

EXAMINATION OF THE PYLORIC ANTRUM. Advancement of the endoscope into the pyloric antrum can sometimes present difficulties. In cats, the flexure between the body and antrum can be sufficiently acute so that vision will be temporarily lost as the endoscope slides into the antrum. In large dogs, particularly if their stomach is overdistended, as the endoscope is advanced there is a tendency for a loop of insertion tube to become "imbedded" in the distal greater curvature of the stomach. As forward pressure is applied to the endoscope at the mouth, the loop is forced further into the mucosa, resulting in little forward progress and a lack of control of the movement of the tip. At times, the loop becomes the leading edge of the endoscope, stretching the greater curvature and paradoxically drawing the tip away from the pylorus as the endoscopist applies forward pressure to the insertion tube. There can also be a tendency for the tip of the endoscope to flip over the incisura (toward the cardia) rather than under it (toward the pylorus).

These problems can usually be remedied by withdrawing the endoscope to the cardia, aspirating the majority of air from the stomach (leaving just sufficient air to provide limited vision), and then repeating the advance of the endoscope into the antrum. Another manipulation that can sometimes help is to use the deflection knobs to direct the tip of the endoscope flat against the mucosa. This may result in a temporary loss of view of the antrum but will open the loop of insertion tube slightly and often allows the insertion tube to slide more freely around the greater curvature and into the antrum. A third method to overcome this problem is for an assistant to apply firm pressure to the lower right body wall with the flat of the hands. The abdominal compression appears to flatten the flexure between the antrum and body, and sometimes assists passage of the endoscope into the antrum.

Once in the antrum, the tip of the endoscope is slowly advanced toward the pylorus. Vision may be temporarily obscured by rings of antral contraction. During this part of the examination, be sure the lesser curvature of the pyloric antrum is examined closely because lesions can be easily missed in this area, especially when using scopes with narrow angles of view.

PYLORIC INTUBATION. Adroit manipulation of the endoscope is often necessary to penetrate the pylorus. As the endoscope approaches the pylorus, the endoscopist should endeavor to maintain an en face view of the pyloric canal in the center of the field of vision. If the pylorus is in the center of the antrum, maintaining this view may simply require fine adjustments of one or both deflection knobs. If the pylorus is mounted off center (particularly to left of center), torquing of the endoscope (by rolling of the endoscopist's body to the left) is usually necessary. At times even this is insufficient and the patient must be temporarily repositioned to realign the pylorus.

As the tip of the endoscope contacts the pylorus, clear vision is usually temporarily lost, but the impression of a dark space (the pyloric canal) surrounded by pale red mucosa is often retained. As firm forward pressure is applied to the insertion tube the endoscopist should intermittently insufflate air and meticulously maintain the pyloric canal in the center of the field. The normal pylorus will usually dilate to accommodate the endoscope. As the pylorus begins to yield, downward and to the right deflection of the endoscope tip will assist entrance into the duodenum.

If the pylorus will not admit the endoscope, it may be relaxed with glucagon (0.05 mg/kg, not to exceed 1 mg, IV). Metoclopramide may assist pyloric intubation in some animals but in others it greatly enhances antral contractions creating a moving target. It was not found to aid pyloric intubation in a recent study in dogs[19] and in another study actually made pyloric intubation more difficult.[16] In the latter study,[16] glucagon was also not found to be effective for these purposes. This finding contrasts to my observations in endoscopy teaching laboratories. In my experience, glucagon is very effective in relaxing the pylorus, reducing antral contractions and allowing inexperienced endoscopists to gain entry to the duodenum. Glucagon is not expensive to purchase. In some animals, however, glucagon will induce a pronounced tachycardia, and it should be avoided in patients with cardiovascular problems.

It is important to note that many inexperienced endoscopists who have difficulty passing the endoscope into the duodenum are actually penetrating the pylorus successfully but are not rounding the cranial duodenal flexure (see later).

DETAILED EXAMINATION OF THE STOMACH. Once the endoscope has been passed into the duodenum (see later description) and appropriate diagnostic materials obtained, the endoscopist should withdraw the instrument to the stomach and examine the different areas of the stomach systematically to ensure no lesions are missed.

The detailed gastric examination is undertaken with sufficient insufflation to efface the majority of rugal folds. The endoscopist should be cognizant of the readiness with which the stomach inflates and the rugal folds disappear. If the stomach does not inflate, consider the possibility that air is exiting the stomach via the esophagus (firmly occlude by digital pressure if necessary), your equipment is not insufflating correctly, or the stomach is unable to distend due to extramural compression or an intramural lesion.

Particular care should be taken to observe the fundus, cardia, and lesser curvature, all areas of the stomach easily overlooked if the tip of the endoscope is single-mindedly passed to the pylorus along the greater curvature. These areas can be visualized by firm retroflexion of the endoscope away from the greater curvature as the tip nears the pyloric antrum. This maneuver (sometimes called the J maneuver) usually necessitates counterclockwise rotation of the up-down deflection knob to its fullest extent. If the expected view is not obtained, gentle advancement of the curved tip of the endoscope into the mucosa will usually guide the endoscope back on itself and achieve full retroflexion.

The J maneuver will provide a dramatic en face view of the incisura (Figure 7–8). Once the incisura is identified, to one side will be seen the pyloric antrum and to the other side will be seen the lesser curvature with the cardia identifiable in the distance (Figure 7–8). Small torquing motions of the retroflexed endoscope will allow the endoscopist to switch from a view of the antrum to a view of the cardia.

The cardia is easily identified by the presence of the insertion tube of the endoscope. Withdrawal of the retroflexed endoscope will bring the cardia into close proximity. If the antrum is in view when the retroflexed endoscope is withdrawn, the pylorus will come clearly into view. Pyloric intubation cannot be achieved by this maneuver, however.

If fluid is retained in the stomach it usually pools in the fundus and proximal greater curvature of the body. Pooled fluid assists identification of this area but inhibits visualization of the mucosa. Large volumes of retained fluid should be aspirated to facilitate mucosal examination and to prevent aspiration dur-

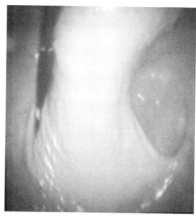

FIGURE 7–8. En face view of the incisura angularis with the cardia and pyloric antrum in view.

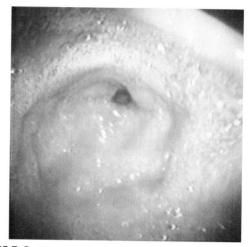

FIGURE 7–9. Normal pylorus of a dog.

ing recovery. Similarly, all air should be aspirated from the gastrointestinal lumen before the endoscope is withdrawn.

APPEARANCE OF THE NORMAL STOMACH. The normal stomach (Figure 7–7) may contain small amounts of clear or yellow-tinged fluid but after a 12 to 24 hour fast should be devoid of food. The mucosa is smooth. It has a bright pink to red color and is lighter in color in the pyloric region. Patches of erythema are sometimes seen. These are usually physiologic and are presumably due to variations in local blood flow. Submucosal vessels can be clearly observed in the fundus and cardia, but are usually not visible in the normal gastric body unless the stomach is overinflated. The lesser curvature is characterized by fewer and straighter mucosal folds than the greater curvature. There are usually no rugal folds in the pyloric antrum. The antrum is the only part of the stomach with contractions recognizable by endoscopy.

The pylorus of normal dogs has a wide variety of appearances (Figure 7–9). In general it should have clean margins, should not be obscured by excessive folds, and usually demonstrates rhythmical opening and closing. Occasionally gastroduodenal reflux of bile or foam will be noticed. This is a normal occurrence in many dogs and cats.

APPEARANCE OF THE ABNORMAL STOMACH. Chronic gastritis is the most frequent gastric abnormality detected by

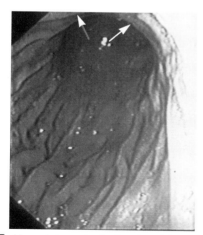

FIGURE 7–7. Normal stomach of a dog viewed from the cardia. The incisura angularis can be seen (arrows). In order to facilitate pyloric intubation it would be preferable to have insufflated the stomach considerably less than shown.

endoscopy. In mild gastritis, the mucosa may appear normal and the diagnosis is made histologically. More severe gastritis is characterized by mucosal thickening, granularity, friability, erosions, and subepithelial or frank hemorrhage.

Prominent rugal folds in the stomach body are usually due to ineffective insufflation, but hypertrophic gastropathy must be considered. In hypertrophic gastropathy, the rugae often appear thickened and have prominent light reflectivity suggestive of edema. In contrast to normal rugae, full insufflation of the stomach does not result in elimination of hypertrophic mucosal folds. Furthermore, the folds may be focal and may extend into the antrum, where it is unusual in normal animals to find many rugae. Mucosal erosions or ulcers may be apparent. In contrast, atrophic gastritis is characterized by a reduction in the number and size of rugal folds and by visible submucosal blood vessels in the gastric body.

Pyloric stenosis can be due to hypertrophy of the pyloric musculature. The hypertrophic pylorus usually has an enlarged, protuberant appearance with a small pyloric canal that is unable to accommodate the scope. Pyloric obstruction can also occur from focal hypertrophic gastritis affecting the pylorus or pyloric antrum. Failure to intubate the pylorus is usually due to technical problems and *not* an abnormal pylorus. The endoscopist should only suspect pyloric obstruction if the patient's history indicates delayed gastric emptying and if retained gastric ingesta or rugal hypertrophy are observed.

Gastric erosions are shallow areas of mucosal disruption. The bed of the erosion usually has a red or brown color from accumulated blood. Erosions are most often seen in association with inflammatory diseases of the stomach but may also result from stress or anti-inflammatory drugs. Foreign bodies will often excoriate the mucosa, producing erosions.

Gastric ulcers are mucosal disruptions that penetrate into the submucosa or deeper. They often have a raised, thickened margin. The bed of the ulcer is usually dark brown, due to accumulated blood, or dirty yellow or white due to accumulation of necrotic tissue. The first indication that an ulcer is present may be accumulation of digested (brown) blood in the gastric fundus. Most ulcers observed endoscopically by the author have been due to gastric adenocarcinoma, leiomyoma, or leiomyosarcoma. Ulcers resulting from gastric adenocarcinoma are usually associated with broad areas of induration. Ulcers due to leiomyomas are usually crater-like with raised margins. Drug-induced ulcers resulting from administration of NSAIDs or glucocorticoids are occasionally observed.

Gastric polyps are benign protuberances of the gastric mucosa. They are relatively uncommon. Gastric neoplasms can have a variety of appearances. They may ulcerate, as just described, or may appear as raised plaques or masses. Infiltrative neoplasms, such as lymphosarcoma, usually appear as diffusely thickened mucosa. The indurated mucosa often feels heavy and yields little as the endoscope or biopsy forceps contact it.

Parasites are occasionally encountered in the stomach. The most commonly recognized is Physaloptera, a short stout nematode. The parasite can be snared and removed after a short rodeo.

NEGOTIATING THE CRANIAL DUODENAL FLEXURE. As the endoscope enters the duodenum, vision is often obscured by the duodenal mucosa of the cranial duodenal flexure (Figure 7–10), but a change in mucosal coloration to a darker red or a yellow-tinged red (bile) may be noted. If the endoscope is freely moving, as indicated by the sliding of mucosa across the lens, forward pressure on the insertion tube is maintained for another 5 to 10 cm. Thereafter, methodical deflection of the tip of the endoscope and insufflation of air will usually achieve

a luminal view of the descending duodenum distal to the cranial duodenal flexure (Figure 7–11). Passage of the endoscope around the cranial duodenal flexure is often facilitated by a little clockwise torque. As the endoscopist becomes more experienced, more of the cranial duodenum will be clearly visualized as the endoscope rounds the cranial duodenal flexure.

EXAMINATION OF THE DUODENUM. After passing the pylorus and rounding the cranial duodenal flexure, the endoscopist should obtain a luminal view of the descending duodenum (Figure 7–11). Careful examination of the proximal duodenum may reveal the duodenal papillae (two in the dog, usually one in the cat) (Figure 7–12). Because the papillae are positioned immediately after the cranial duodenal flexure, they are often overlooked. If they are seen, they usually appear as small, white, relatively flat protuberances.

The endoscope should be slowly advanced down the descending duodenum until the majority of the working length is used. It is usually possible to reach the caudal duodenal flexure in all animals with the exception of large dogs. In cats, this flexure can be negotiated and the short ascending duodenum and the proximal jejunum examined. The mobility of the tip of the endoscope is reduced in the duodenum by the convolutions of the insertion tube in the stomach. As a result, the slide-by technique is usually required to negotiate flexures in the duodenum and jejunum. Torquing the instrument at this point is also difficult, particularly if there is excess belly in the insertion tube as it rounds the greater curvature.

Once the endoscope has reached its full working length and diagnostic samples have been obtained, it is withdrawn. It is during the retrograde passage of the endoscope that the best views of the gastrointestinal tract are obtained, but the endoscopist must always be cognizant that observed lesions may have been caused by the endoscope. Particular care must be taken to observe the cranial duodenal flexure, lesions of which may have been overlooked during pyloric intubation.

APPEARANCE OF THE NORMAL DUODENUM. The normal duodenal mucosa is redder than the stomach and may have a yellow tinge. Submucosal vessels are not apparent. The duodenal mucosa is more friable than that of the stomach. As a result, superficial linear mucosal erosions are frequently left in normal mucosa by the passage of the endoscope around flexures. The mucosa has a fine granular appearance due to the duodenal villi (Figure 7–11). Care must be taken in assessing duodenal granularity because this feature of the duodenum is markedly influenced by the degree of distension. Before judg-

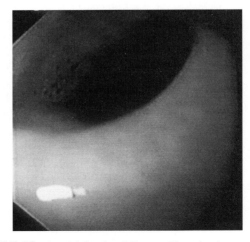

FIGURE 7–10. Cranial duodenal flexure. Note the downward and to the right orientation of the flexure.

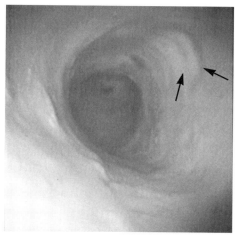

FIGURE 7-11. Normal descending duodenum of a dog. Note Peyer's patches (arrows).

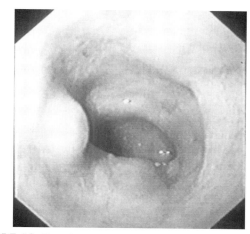

FIGURE 7-12. Prominent duodenal papilla.

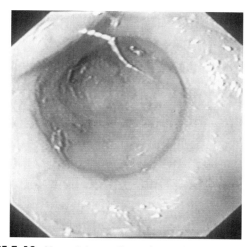

FIGURE 7-13. Normal descending colon and left colic flexure of a dog.

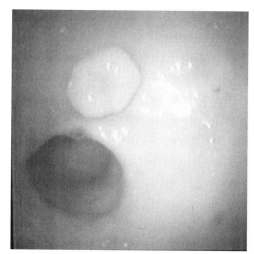

FIGURE 7-14. Normal ileocolic area of a dog. The cecum is seen at the bottom left of the picture. The ileocolic valve is the button-like protuberance immediately above the cecum.

ing granularity, the author prefers to distend the duodenum to its full extent and then to stop insufflating, allowing the duodenal diameter to settle slightly but not collapse.

Peyer's patches may be observed in the duodenum of dogs. They appear as large (several centimeters in length), pale, oval depressions in the mucosa (Figure 7–11). They are often multiple.

APPEARANCE OF THE ABNORMAL DUODENUM. Abnormal duodenal mucosa usually develops a pronounced granularity and friability. These abnormalities are most commonly associated with inflammatory bowel disease. The diseased duodenal mucosa usually bleeds freely when contacted by the endoscope. Passage of the endoscope around bends may leave deep excoriations. Infiltrative neoplasms, such as lymphosarcoma, usually result in marked duodenal thickening and irregularity. Adenocarcinoma may be infiltrative in behavior or result in annular obstructive lesions. Occasionally, circular patches of lipid-laden villi may be observed, characteristic of lymphangiectasia. Ascarid parasites are now and then encountered.

Endoscopy of the Large Bowel

RIGID PROCTOSCOPY. After digital examination of the anal area, the lubricated proctoscope is introduced through the anus with the obturator in place. The obturator is then removed, the glass viewing window is secured, and the colon is insufflated using the rubber insufflation bulb.

COLONOSCOPY. Before colonoscopy, a digital examination of the anus should be carried out to detect anal lesions that are otherwise easily missed. The tip of the endoscope is then introduced with a gloved hand into the rectum. The large bowel is insufflated, and once a luminal view is obtained the endoscope is steadily advanced toward the left colic flexure, which marks the junction between the descending and transverse colon (Figure 7–13). The flexure is usually rounded by the slide-by technique. Subsequently, the endoscope is further advanced toward the short, ascending colon. The flexure that unites the transverse and ascending colon, the right colic flexure, is sometimes not apparent, perhaps because cranial pressure of the endoscope forces the transverse colon cranially, a movement which tends to straighten the flexure. Once the ascending colon is entered it is generally possible to see the ileocolic valve and cecum (Figure 7–14). Skilled endoscopists can sometimes maneuver their scopes into the distal ileum. Careful examination of the ileocecal area is an integral part of the colonoscopic examination because it has a significant frequency of disease, including intussusception, cecal inversion, parasitism, and neoplasia.

APPEARANCE OF THE NORMAL COLON. The normal colonic mucosa is smooth and pink (Figure 7–13). Submucosal blood vessels should be clearly visible (Figure 7–15). There should be no evidence of erosions or ulcers, and the mucosa should not be obviously friable or bleed after gentle passage of the endoscope. There should be little mucus, no masses, and the colon should distend readily and evenly following insufflation.

APPEARANCE OF THE ABNORMAL COLON. One of the earliest signs of abnormal colonic mucosa is reduced visibility of submucosal vessels. This mucosal change is usually due to infiltration of the lamina propria with inflammatory cells. It may also be due to failure to insufflate the colon sufficiently. Submucosal vessels are also easily obscured by fecal material if the colon has been poorly prepared. Abnormal colonic mucosa is usually friable. Shallow erosions and/or scattered nodularity may be apparent. These abnormalities are most commonly associated with chronic colitis. Histiocytic colitis is characterized by deep well-demarcated erosions or ulcers. Infiltrative neoplasms such as lymphosarcoma usually result in marked mucosal thickening and irregularity. Adenocarcinoma usually appears as friable proliferative masses. Whipworms may be seen in the colon or cecum.

ANCILLARY ENDOSCOPIC TECHNIQUES

Brush and Touch Cytology

Brush cytology is a useful adjunct to endoscopic biopsy. It may improve diagnostic yield because superficial material that otherwise may be lost during processing is sampled. Thus, organisms such as protozoa that reside in the mucus of the gastrointestinal tract may occasionally be detected by brush cytology but not seen in biopsy specimens.[21] Furthermore, the brush ranges over a wider area than that examined by biopsy, and cytologic specimens may be rapidly evaluated.

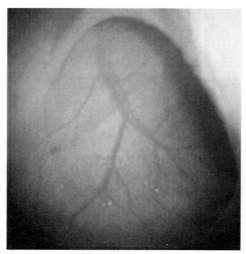

FIGURE 7-15. Submucosal vessels in the colon of a dog

Aspiration of Duodenal Fluid

Acquisition of duodenal fluid for culture and cytology is facilitated by use of aspiration kits (Har-Vet Inc., Spring Valley, WI), consisting of a stylet and sterilized plastic tubing. The plastic tubing is threaded down the endoscope and into the duodenum. The duodenal lumen is then collapsed and the tubing slowly drawn back to the endoscope tip as gentle suction is applied by way of a large-volume syringe. On most occasions, this technique will provide 0.25 to 1 mL of duodenal fluid. The fluid should be quickly transferred to a suitable anaerobic container for transfer to the microbiology lab.

Quantitative culture of duodenal fluid is an effective way to diagnose bacterial overgrowth of the small intestine. Colony counts of greater than 10^5 per mL are currently considered diagnostic of bacterial overgrowth.

Cytology of duodenal fluid is an accurate technique for the diagnosis of giardiasis. Occasionally cytology will reveal neoplastic cells. This is particularly true of lymphosarcoma.

Endoscopic Biopsy

Mucosal biopsy specimens should be acquired whenever a dog or cat is undergoing endoscopy for a chronic gastrointestinal complaint whether or not the mucosa looks normal. Interpretation of endoscopic biopsy specimens is somewhat subjective. As aptly put by Wilcox (1992), our ability to interpret endoscopic biopsy specimens has lagged far behind our ability to obtain them.[22] Where possible, the clinician is advised to work with one pathologist to improve consistency of histologic interpretations. If you are interested in the difficulties of biopsy interpretation, read the article by Wilcox (1992).[22]

DISCORDANCE BETWEEN BIOPSY RESULTS AND ENDOSCOPIC FINDINGS. In the author's experience and that of others,[23,24] the mucosa can appear endoscopically normal in spite of the presence of significant inflammatory or neoplastic disease. Conversely, mucosa that appears abnormal to the endoscopist may prove to be histologically normal in up to 29% of samples.[23] Endoscopically observed mucosal hemorrhage and erythema hold the least predictive value for histologic abnormality.[23] Excess mucosal friability and granularity are associated with histologic abnormality in approximately 80% of cases.[23] Possible reasons for discordance between endoscopy findings and biopsy are described in Table 7–4. The most obvious reason for discordance is inexperience of the endoscopist or pathologist. Unfortunately, however, there is also considerable variance in the pathologic significance afforded to histologic findings by different pathologists.[22]

ENDOSCOPIC VERSUS SURGICAL BIOPSY. Endoscopic biopsy of the gastrointestinal tract is less traumatic than surgical biopsy and does not carry the risk of wound dehiscence. Dehiscence is particularly likely in debilitated animals and is considered more frequent following surgery of the large bowel than small bowel.[25] However, surgical biopsy provides better quality mucosal samples for evaluating important morphologic features such as crypt depth and villus height by routine light microscopy. A microdissection technique can be used to obtain similar information from endoscopic biopsy specimens,[26] but this technique is not routinely performed in diagnostic laboratories. Surgical biopsy specimens are full thickness allowing detection of disease in the submucosa, neural plexi, and muscularis, all areas not sampled by endoscopic biopsy. Furthermore, during laparotomy, assessment and biopsy of the jejunum and other organs such as the pancreas and liver is possible.

Table 7–4

REASONS FOR DISCORDANCE OF BIOPSY AND
ENDOSCOPIC FINDINGS

Incorrect Endoscopic Assessment of Gastrointestinal Mucosa
Inexperience
Inadequate insufflation misread as mucosal thickening, mucosal
granularity, or obscured submucosal blood vessels
Scope-induced trauma misread as spontaneous disease
Incorrect Biopsy Evaluation by Pathologist
Inexperience
Unknown significance of mild inflammatory changes
Sample handling error
Nonrepresentative Biopsies
Poor biopsy technique
Biopsied incorrect aspect of a lesion (e.g., necrotic center)
Patchy mucosal lesions

ENDOSCOPIC PINCH BIOPSY. Endoscopic biopsy of the stomach and duodenum is performed with a pinch biopsy instrument. The tissue samples obtained are small (2–3 mm). Good biopsy technique and multiple samples are essential for diagnostic accuracy. The instrument must be sharp to avoid crush artifacts.

Where possible, the long axis of the biopsy instrument should be directed at a 90° angle to the mucosal surface to be sampled (Figure 7–16). This lessens the likelihood of obtaining only villus tips, a common result if the biopsy forceps are directed parallel with the mucosal surface. In the small bowel, attaining a perpendicular orientation with the biopsy forceps is easier if the tip of the endoscope is extended until it encounters a flexure, or if the bowel is partially collapsed by the aspiration of the majority of luminal air. If the pylorus cannot be negotiated, it is possible to obtain duodenal biopsies in a "blind" manner by passing the biopsy forceps through the pylorus while the endoscopic tip remains in the antrum.

Because histologic appearance varies between regions of the bowel, obtaining biopsies at consistent sites is likely to improve the ability of pathologists to differentiate normal from abnormal histology. For this reason, it is routine practice during upper gastrointestinal endoscopy to obtain biopsy specimens from any visible lesions and from the caudal duodenal flexure, pyloric antrum, incisura angularis, mid-greater curvature, and cardia.[23] At each site two or three biopsy samples are suggested and at least eight biopsies should be obtained from the duodenum. During lower gastrointestinal endoscopy, biopsy of visible lesions, cecum, ascending colon, orad transverse colon, orad descending colon, mid-descending colon, and aboral descending colon are advised.

It is often useful to obtain more than one pinch biopsy from the same site to increase the depth of the tissue sampled. This is particularly important when obtaining biopsies of masses because of the inflammatory reaction that commonly surrounds neoplasms. Biopsy of ulcerating lesions is best performed at their periphery to avoid the sampling of necrotic tissue. Furthermore, the crater of ulcers is often thin and easy to perforate.

SUCTION BIOPSY. Suction biopsy instruments are safe and effective for obtaining mucosal tissue from the esophagus. They are best suited for nontargeted biopsy of diffusely diseased tissue but, if the suction instrument is passed alongside the endoscope, targeted biopsies can occasionally be obtained. The biopsy technique is described in Chapter 6.

SPECULUM FORCEPS BIOPSY. Occasionally, hand-held biopsy instruments with large-diameter jaws are utilized for biopsy of the large bowel. In order to avoid perforation of the bowel, the open jaws of these instruments should never be pressed into the bowel wall during the biopsy. Instead, the three-stage biopsy technique should be used. This entails the following: Lightly grasp the mucosa with the jaws of the instrument, gently pull the mucosa toward the center of the bowel lumen, and then sever the tissue (see Chapter 6). In most cases this technique allows the serosal and muscular layers of the bowel to slip out from the grasp of the jaws, avoiding perforation.

HANDLING OF BIOPSY SPECIMENS. Endoscopic biopsy yields pieces of tissue that are small and easily damaged. They should be handled gently and should not be allowed to dry. I prefer to collect the samples on a saline-soaked piece of tissue paper or in the plastic cassette in which they will later be embedded for histology (Figure 7–17). After inspection for adequate number and size, they are then placed in formalin. Attempts to orient the samples on supports are unnecessary.[22]

Foreign Body Retrieval

RETRIEVAL EQUIPMENT. Retrieval equipment should include through-the-endoscope equipment such as a basket retrieval instrument, a snare, a three- or four-prong grasper, and/or a rat tooth grasper. In addition it is helpful to obtain some form of large, semirigid, or rigid grasping instrument for the removal of proximal esophageal foreign bodies. Suitable rigid retrieval instruments are available from most major surgical equipment manufacturers but are expensive. An economical alternative (designed for retrieval of objects lost in plumbing and engines) can often be found at local hardware shops.

INDICATIONS FOR ENDOSCOPIC FOREIGN BODY REMOVAL. Foreign bodies may be managed by conservative, endoscopic, or surgical means. Factors that influence this decision include the clinical appearance of the animal, the attentiveness with which the pet is observed by the owner, the type of foreign object, its anatomic location, and radiographic findings. Careful survey radiographic evaluation of the patient prior to endoscopy is recommended. Radiography assists localization of the foreign body and the detection of perforation. When sharp objects such as fishhooks are observed by radiography, the veterinarian should ascertain carefully if the foreign body remains in the

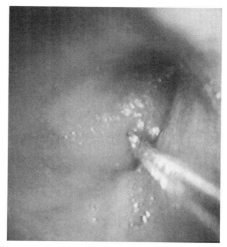

FIGURE 7–16. Good biopsy technique. The instrument is being orientated at 90° to the mucosa. The biopsy site is the caudal duodenal flexure.

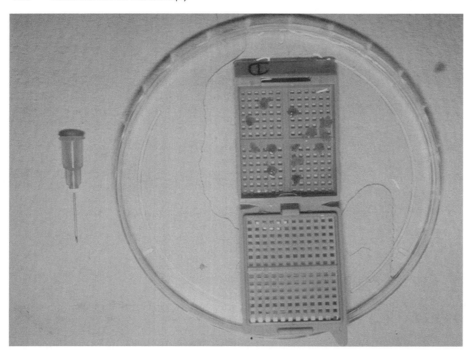

FIGURE 7-17. Endoscopic biopsy samples collected in a cassette prior to placing in formalin.

lumen of the gastrointestinal tract. Not uncommonly, sharp objects will penetrate the esophageal or gastrointestinal wall where they become inaccessible to the endoscope. If perforation of the gastrointestinal tract is detected, surgery, not endoscopy, is indicated.

All esophageal foreign bodies should be rapidly removed because they cause pain and dysphagia, and may result in esophageal stricture. Endoscopic removal is particularly desirable in view of the possible complications of esophageal surgery and thoracotomy. Timely endoscopic removal of all sharp objects from the stomach is recommended because of the risk of perforation of the stomach or, should the object leave the stomach, perforation of the intestine. To avoid gastrointestinal obstruction, the early endoscopic or surgical removal of gastric foreign bodies judged too large to pass through the gastrointestinal tract is suggested. Foreign bodies suspected of containing lead, zinc (such as pennies), or caustic materials (batteries) should be removed from the gastrointestinal tract immediately unless repeated radiographs reveal rapid progressive aboral transit. Obstructed, small intestinal foreign bodies usually cannot be reached by endoscopy and are best removed by surgery.

TECHNIQUE. Successful retrieval of foreign bodies requires considerable discretion, ingenuity, and technical prowess. Tightly wedged foreign bodies should never be forcibly removed. If a foreign object cannot be removed by firm traction, under direct endoscopic vision, then surgical removal is indicated. Forceful removal bears a great risk of laceration of the viscus or adjacent vessels or organs. Furthermore, tightly wedged foreign bodies usually have caused significant mucosal pressure necrosis that requires surgical inspection to determine its mural extent. Trial and error often determines the best retrieval instrument for a particular retrieval; however, certain generalizations may be made. For instance, basket retrieval instruments are only useful in a lumen of sufficient diameter to allow their expansion. Pronged graspers are of little value in the retrieval of foreign bodies with smooth surfaces. If the surface is smooth but indentable, strong jaw-tooth graspers are usually effective. Certain metals may be retrieved by magnetic extractors.

Endoscopic entrapment with suture material can be used to remove large foreign bodies, such as choke chains, from the stomach. To entrap a foreign body with suture material the following technique is used. With the endoscope removed from the animal, a biopsy or grasping instrument is passed through the biopsy channel until the instrument's jaws just appear. One end of a 2 meter length of sturdy suture material is grasped in the instrument's jaws and the endoscope passed to the foreign body. Using the grasping instrument, the suture material is passed through a hole in the foreign body and let go. The suture material is then regrasped on the other side of the foreign body and drawn out of the mouth by removal of the endoscope. The result is a loop of suture material that passes into the animal's mouth, through the foreign body and out the mouth again, enabling the object to be removed by gentle traction. Additional useful retrieval techniques include pulling esophageal foreign bodies into a preplaced rigid endoscope in the esophagus, thus aiding atraumatic removal of sharp objects; pushing obstinate esophageal foreign bodies into the stomach where they may be digested (for example, bones), better manipulated to an appropriate orientation for removal, or more easily removed surgically; placing a Foley catheter distal to the object and then using the inflated catheter to draw the foreign body out.

Bougienage and Balloon Catheter Dilation

Bougienage or balloon dilation of esophageal strictures is sometimes required. Endoscopy allows visual assessment and biopsy of strictures before dilation. This helps differentiate postinflammatory strictures, extraesophageal compressions, and strictures resulting from neoplasia, thus facilitating the selection of an appropriate therapy. Furthermore, endoscopy simplifies the placement of the bougie or balloon catheter directly into the orifice of the stricture, and allows assessment of the effect of the procedure on the mucosal tissue and luminal diameter. Dilation of strictures can be performed by balloon catheter or rigid dilators. Rigid bougies are less desirable than balloon dilators because they produce less radial force and more shearing forces;[27] however, they are still effective in many situations.

BALLOON CATHETER DILATION. As mentioned earlier, suitable balloon dilators for gastrointestinal work have a 15 to 20 mm inflatable diameter with a length of 6 to 8 cm. Smaller balloon diameters than 10 mm are of little value because they provide insufficient distension of esophageal strictures. Shorter lengths are inadequate for long strictures because they may not extend past the margins of the lesion and therefore are difficult to keep in position during inflation. Although designed to pass through the biopsy channel of the endoscope, some of the longer balloon catheter dilators are not sufficiently flexible at their tip to pass through gastroscopes and must be passed alongside the endoscope. Once the balloon has been centered in the stricture it is gradually inflated using a syringe. The progress of the dilation can be monitored by fluoroscopy (contrast media-filled balloon) or endoscopy. Manometers can be purchased to estimate pressures applied, but are not essential. Successful passage of a 10 mm diameter gastroscope through the previously strictured area is indicative of a successful procedure in small dogs and cats. Larger dogs require a slightly greater esophageal diameter to remain relatively symptom free.

BOUGIENAGE. Rigid bougies are used by increasing systematically the diameter of the bougie passed through the stricture. The stricture is dilated as widely as possible without the use of excessive force. The diameter of the largest bougie that is accommodated helps judge the success of the procedure. As an example, the comfortable passage of a 40 French diameter bougie through an esophageal stricture of a 20 kg dog would suggest adequate bougienage.

COMPLICATIONS OF DILATION OF STRICTURES. Complications of bougienage and balloon catheter dilation are not uncommon, particularly in inexperienced hands. Complications include perforation of friable esophageal tissues and the rupture of major periesophageal vessels entrapped by the inflammatory or neoplastic disease process that formed the stricture. Insufflation of the esophagus proximal to the stricture can lead to gastric overdistension from the passage of air through the stricture. If this occurs, gastric decompression can be achieved by trocarization of the stomach with a needle.

FOLLOW-UP THERAPY. Repeated dilation of esophageal strictures is required to maintain an adequate luminal diameter in most, but not all[28] patients. This repeat procedure is performed as soon as regurgitation recurs. In the first month of treatment, weekly dilation may be required but the frequency usually declines thereafter. Adjunctive medical therapy can be used to help prevent restricturing. If the cause of the stricture is reflux esophagitis, metoclopramide (0.2–0.4 mg/kg q 6–8 hours) and H_2 receptor agonists such as ranitidine (1–4 mg/kg q 12 hours) are useful. Corticosteroids are recommended by many to inhibit fibrosis but have been of little value in my experience.

Endoscopic Placement of Gastrostomy Tubes

INDICATIONS. Endoscopic placement of a gastrostomy tube is indicated for long-term (weeks to months) nutritional support of anorectic or dysphagic animals.[29,30] Gastrostomy tubes are not recommended in vomiting animals.

COMPLICATIONS. Complications of endoscopically placed gastrostomy tubes are rare, but include vomiting, delayed gastric emptying, aspiration pneumonia, pressure necrosis of the gastric wall, peritonitis, splenic perforation, and peristomal

infection.[29] Several of these complications may be reflective of the underlying disease rather than directly attributable to the gastrostomy tube. An increased risk of peritonitis due to failure of gastroabdominal adhesion following endoscopic placement of gastrostomy tubes has been noted in large debilitated dogs undergoing chemotherapy (RC Straw, personal communication, 1989). Gastrostomy tubes may be difficult to place endoscopically in fat animals.

TECHNIQUE. Endoscopic placement of gastrostomy tubes necessitates a brief anesthesia. Two techniques are in use: a percutaneous technique and a percutaneous-peroral technique. In both techniques, the animal is placed in right lateral recumbency so the stomach tube may be placed through the greater curvature of the stomach and the left body wall. The site of emergence for the catheter is just ventral to the 13th rib. The techniques are described here. The percutaneous-peroral technique has also been described elsewhere.[30–32]

The percutaneous-peroral technique is the most commonly used technique for the endoscopic placement of gastrostomy tubes in veterinary patients. A specially prepared Pezzar mushroom-tipped catheter (Bard, Benecia, CA) is used for this procedure. A suitably sized catheter for dogs is 18 to 24 F and for cats is 18 to 20 F. Economical gastrostomy kits containing already prepared catheters can be purchased from Mill Rose Labs (Mentor, OH 44060), or if desired the tubes can be prepared as shown in Figure 7–18.

Surgically prepare the left paracostal area centered just ventral to the distal end of the 13th rib. Introduce the endoscope into the stomach and carefully inflate this viscus until the abdomen is distended but not drum tight. Transilluminate with the endoscope to ensure the spleen is not between the stomach and body wall. Insert a 16 to 18 G, 1.5 to 2 inch nee-

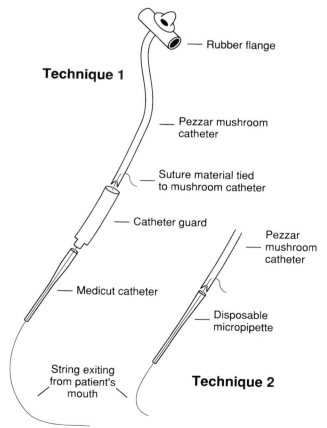

FIGURE 7–18. Percutaneous gastrostomy tube.

dle through the skin just ventral to the 13th rib and pass it through the body wall, gastric wall, and into the gastric lumen. Thread sturdy suture material of sufficient length to reach comfortably from mouth to last rib, through the catheter into the lumen of the stomach. Grasp the suture with an endoscopic retrieval instrument and withdraw the endoscope from the animal, thus drawing one end of the suture through the esophagus and out of the mouth. Be careful not to draw all of the suture into the stomach. At the mouth, the suture material is then passed through the lumen of the plastic pipette (tapered end first) and firmly tied to the end of the mushroom catheter. The suture material is then grasped at its point of exit from the abdominal wall and firm traction is applied to draw the entire catheter assemblage (pipette first) through the lumen of the mouth, esophagus, and stomach, and partially through the stomach and body wall. Further gentle traction on the catheter results in the distal (flanged) end of the catheter drawing the stomach wall against the body wall. It is anchored in this position by the second flange placed over the catheter at the skin surface. Bandage the catheter in place to prevent vandalism by the patient. After 6 to 7 days the catheter may be safely withdrawn. To remove the catheter, apply firm external traction and then cut the catheter as close to the distal tip as possible. The internal flange and mushroom tip usually pass uneventfully but can be removed endoscopically if so desired in small dogs and cats.

The second technique for placement of gastrostomy tubes by endoscopy is the percutaneous technique. This technique utilizes a wire guide and a trocar and peel-away sheath that are serially passed through the abdominal wall into the air-distended stomach (PEG set, Wilson-Cook, Winston-Salem, NC). After penetration of the stomach, the wire guide and trocar are removed and a lubricated Foley passed directly into the stomach through the peel-away sheath. Once the Foley is inflated, the sheath is peeled away and pressure is carefully applied to the inflated Foley catheter to draw the stomach against the body wall.

Both of these techniques have been successfully used by the author. The percutaneous technique has a slightly shorter operating time and avoids contamination of the abdomen with oropharyngeal secretions. The female end of the catheter need not be cut off, and the removal process does not leave any flanges in the gastrointestinal tract. An important disadvantage is that the Foley catheter provides a less secure initial bond of the stomach to the body wall in comparison to the percutaneous-peroral technique. The Foley balloon can rupture within three days resulting in a breakdown of the stoma and peritonitis.

For long-term use, the more cumbersome standard percutaneous endoscopic gastrostomy tubes can be replaced by low-profile button replacement tubes that sit flush with the skin surface. The use of one-step button tubes in dogs has also been described.[33]

Gastroscopic Food Sensitivity Testing

Gastroscopic food sensitivity testing is a diagnostic technique that specifically evaluates the acute response of the gastric mucosa to foods. Food extracts of 5000 to 15,000 PNU/mL are dripped onto the gastric mucosa by way of plastic tubing passed through the operating channel of an endoscope.[34] The mucosa is observed for 2 to 3 minutes for swelling. Mucosal swelling at the site of application suggests an immediate sensitivity to the food applied and indicates it should not be included in the diet of the animal under test. The technique is currently being evaluated in dogs and cats for the diagnosis of food allergy. It is discussed in Chapter 23.

LAPAROSCOPY

Indications and Limitations

Laparoscopy[35,36] is a valuable technique for inspecting the peritoneal cavity visually, but its use has declined somewhat with the advent of ultrasonography. The primary indication for laparoscopy is the biopsy of the liver and kidneys. Ultrasound-guided biopsy of these structures is less invasive and less time consuming. Laproscopic techniques for full thickness small intestinal biopsy and placement of enteral feeding tubes have been described in humans.[37] Application of these techniques to dogs and cats could prove very useful. Laparoscopy should not be considered a replacement for exploratory celiotomy because it provides restricted visualization of the abdominal organs and has limited therapeutic capability.

Contraindications and Complications

Laparoscopy is contraindicated in patients with obesity, diaphragmatic hernias, and coagulopathies. Complications are not common but include abdominal hemorrhage from laceration of an organ or vessel, subcutaneous emphysema, air embolism, hypercapnia if CO_2 is used as the distending gas, decreased cardiac output, infection at trocar sites, peritonitis (usually from penetration of bowel), pneumothorax, and biopsy-related morbidity.[38] Air embolism should be suspected if there is a sudden deterioration of the patient, if "mill wheel" murmurs are heard, or the penetration of the spleen or a major vessel with the Verres needle are noticed.

Equipment

Equipment required is a cold light source, a Verres needle, a trocar, a source of gas for distension of the abdomen (nitrous oxide, CO_2, or nitrogen in declining order of preference), a method of recording intra-abdominal pressure, an optical system (usually composed of a lens and a series of fiber bundles encased in a metal tube), biopsy instruments, and warm sterile saline (Figure 7–19).

Technique

Laparoscopy can be performed under general anesthesia or heavy sedation in association with local anesthesia. The patient is placed in left lateral recumbency to allow a right-lateral approach. This reduces the likelihood of damage to the spleen. The left-lateral approach should only be utilized if a left-sided lesion is suspected. The flank is surgically prepared and draped. A Verres needle is carefully inserted into the abdominal cavity. The mid-dorsal flank region is a suitable area for insertion. The clinician should ensure that the needle penetrates the peritoneum; otherwise, massive subcutaneous emphysema will ensue. Great care must be taken to avoid penetrating abdominal organs. If the spleen is pene-

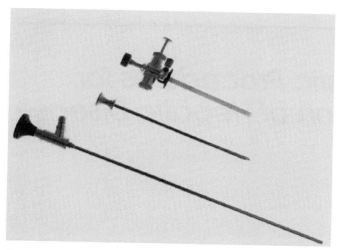

FIGURE 7-19. Laparoscopy equipment (Wolf) showing from top to bottom cannula passed through abdominal wall, trocar to aid in cannula passage, and laparoscope. Not shown is the light source and illuminating cable for the scope.

trated, fatal air embolism is likely. After the Verres needle is in place, the clinician should begin insufflation of the abdomen. Insufflation should be at a rate of less than 1 liter per minute and result in an intra-abdominal pressure of no greater than 20 mm Hg. Higher pressures decrease cardiac output.

Once the abdomen is tight to the touch, the skin is incised over the area of interest, the trocar is inserted into the laparoscope sleeve, and the trocar/sleeve is firmly driven through the body wall. Once the abdomen is penetrated, the trocar is removed, being careful not to lose insufflation, and the optical instrument is inserted. The entire assemblage is rotated cranially and caudally to view the entire extent of the visible abdomen. If the lens steams up, the optical system is withdrawn and warmed in warm sterile saline. Biopsy or aspiration instruments are inserted through separate trocars or, in the case of needle biopsy instruments, directly through the body wall.

REFERENCES

1. Hirschowitz BI. Development and application of endoscopy. Gastroenterology 104:337–342, 1993.
2. Johnson GF, Twedt DC. Endoscopy and laparoscopy in the diagnosis and management of neoplasia in small animals. Vet Clin N Am 7:77–92, 1977.
3. Johnson GF. Gastroscopy. In: Anderson NV (ed). Veterinary Gastroenterology. Lea & Febiger, Philadelphia, 84–88, 1980.
4. Johnson GF. Duodenoscopy. In: Anderson NV (ed). Veterinary Gastroenterology. Lea & Febiger, Philadelphia, 89–90, 1980.
5. Johnson JH. Endoscopes. In: Anderson NV (ed). Veterinary Gastroenterology. Lea & Febiger, Philadelphia, 77–79, 1980.
6. Happe RP, van der Gaag I. Endoscopic examination of esophagus, stomach, and duodenum in the dog. J Am Anim Hosp Assoc 19:197–206, 1983.
7. O'Brien JA. Esophagoscopy. In: Anderson NV (ed). Veterinary Gastroenterology. Lea & Febiger, Philadelphia, 81–83, 1980.
8. Tams TR. Small Animal Endoscopy. CV Mosby, St. Louis, 1990.
9. Jones BD (ed). Veterinary endoscopy. Vet Clin N Am 20:1199–1395, 1990.
10. Simpson KW. Gastrointestinal endoscopy in the dog. J Sm Anim Pract 34:180–188, 1993.
11. Twedt DC. Perspectives on gastrointestinal endoscopy. Vet Clin N Am 23:481–495, 1993.
12. Jakovljevic S. Gastric radiology and gastroscopy in the dog. Vet Ann 28:172–182, 1988.
13. Pariente EA, Kerlau M, Lanoe JL. Fibroscopie ou radiographie oeso-gastroduodenale de première intention? Une évaluation pragmatique. Nouv Press Med 10:3477–3480, 1981. Cited in: Schuman BM. Upper gastrointestinal endoscopy. In: Berk JE (ed) Gastroenterology. WB Saunders, Philadelphia, 564–580, 1985.
14. Richter KP, Cleveland MvB. Comparison of an orally administered gastrointestinal lavage solution with traditional enema administration as preparation for colonoscopy in dogs. J Am Vet Med Assoc 195:1727–1731, 1989.
15. Burrows CF. Evaluation of a colonic lavage solution to prepare the colon of the dog for colonoscopy. J Am Vet Med Assoc 195:1719–1721, 1989.
16. Matz ME, Leib MS, Monroe WE, et al. Evaluation of atropine, glucagon, and metoclopramide for facilitation of endoscopic intubation of the duodenum in dogs. Am J Vet Res 52:1948–1950, 1991.
17. Jaffe JH, Martin WR. Opioid analgesics and antagonists. In: Goodman GA, Goodman LS, Rall TW (eds) The Pharmacological Basis of Therapeutics. Macmillan, New York, 502, 1985.
18. Jergens AE, Riedesel DH, Ries PA, et al. Cardiopulmonary responses in dogs during endoscopic examination. J Vet Int Med 7:132, 1993.
19. Monroe WE, Leib MS, Matz ME, et al. Evaluation of metoclopramide hydrochloride as an aid for passage of a flexible endoscope into the duodenum of dogs. Am J Vet Res 53:149–152, 1992.
20. Church EM, Mehlhaff CJ, Patnaik AK. Colorectal adenocarcinoma in dogs: 78 cases (1973–1984). J Am Vet Med Assoc 191(6):727–730, 1987.
21. Debongnie JC, Beyaert C, Legros G. Touch cytology, a useful diagnostic method for diagnosis of upper gastrointestinal tract infections. Dig Dis Sci 34:1025–1027, 1989.
22. Wilcox B. Endoscopic biopsy interpretation in canine or feline enterocolitis. Sem Vet Med Surg 7:162–171, 1992.
23. Roth L., Leib MS, Davenport DJ, et al. Comparisons between endoscopic and histologic evaluation of the gastrointestinal tract in dogs and cats: 75 cases (1984–1987). J Am Vet Med Assoc 196:635–638, 1990.
24. Dennis JS, Kruger JM, Mullaney TP. Lymphocytic/plasmacytic gastroenteritis in cats: 14 cases (1985–1990). J Am Vet Med Assoc 200:1712–1718, 1992.
25. Martens MFWC, Hendriks TH. Postoperative changes in collagen synthesis in intestinal anastomoses of the rat: Differences between small and large bowel. Gut 32:1482–1487, 1991.
26. Goodlad RA, Levi S, Lee CY, et al. Morphometry and cell proliferation in endoscopic biopsies: Evaluation of a technique. Gastroenterology 101:1235–1241, 1991.
27. Burk RL, Zawie DA, Garvey MS. Balloon catheter dilation of intramural esophageal strictures in the dog and cat: A description of the procedure and a report of six cases. Sem Vet Med Surg 2:241, 1987.
28. Black AP. Balloon-catheter dilation of an oesophageal stricture in a cat. Australian Vet Pract 22:50–52, 1992.
29. Armstrong PJ, Hardie EM. Percutaneous endoscopic gastrostomy: A retrospective study of 54 clinical cases in dogs and cats. J Vet Intern Med 4:202–206, 1990.
30. Bright RM. Percutaneous endoscopic gastrostomy. Vet Clin N Am 23:531–545, 1993.
31. Mathews KA, Binnington AG. Percutaneous incisionless placement of a gastrostomy tube utilizing a gastroscope; preliminary observations. J Am Anim Hosp Assoc 22:601–610, 1986.
32. Sherding B, Johnson S. Interventional gastrointestinal endoscopy. Proc 11th ACVIM Forum, Washington, DC, 1993, 217–220.
33. Ferguson DR, Harig JM, Kozarek RA, et al. Placement of a feeding button ("One-Step Button") as the initial procedure. Am J Gastroenterol 88:501–504, 1993.
34. Guilford WG. Strombeck DR, Rogers G, et al. Development of gastroscopic food sensitivity testing in dogs. J Vet Intern Med 8:414–422, 1994.
35. Rothuizen J. Laparoscopy in small animal medicine. Vet Q 7:225–228, 1985.
36. Jones BD. Laparoscopy. In: Jones BD (ed) Veterinary Endoscopy. Vet Clin 20:1243–1263, 1990.
37. Eltringham WK, Roe AM, Galloway SW, et al. A laproscopic technique for full thickness intestinal biopsy and feeding jejunostomy. Gut 34:122–124, 1993.
38. Gilroy BA, Anson LW. Fatal air embolism during anesthesia for laparoscopy in a dog. J Am Vet Med Assoc 190:552–554, 1987.

8 Diagnostic Procedures for Evaluation of Hepatic Disease

SHARON A. CENTER

APPROACH TO THE PATIENT WITH LIVER DISEASE

The history and physical findings of a patient with hepato-biliary disease are often vague (Tables 8–1 and 8–2). This is particularly true when the underlying pathologic lesion does not induce cholestasis and is multifocal in distribution. As a result, liver disease is often discovered on the basis of routine hematologic, serum biochemical, and urine screening tests. A diagnostic algorithm appropriate for the clinical evaluation of a patient with hepatobiliary disease is provided in Figure 8–1. Diagnostic evaluation of an hepatic problem includes hematologic and biochemical tests and morphologic evaluation of the liver for definitive diagnoses. Biochemical tests

Table 8–1

HISTORICAL AND PHYSICAL SIGNS OF LIVER DISEASE

ACQUIRED			CONGENITAL
Early Signs	**Major Bile Duct Occlusion**	**Severe Hepatic Insufficiency**	**Portosystemic Vascular Anomaly**
Anorexia	Anorexia	Anorexia	Stunted body size
Vomiting	Vomiting	Vomiting	Abnormal behavior: lethargic
Diarrhea/constipation	Diarrhea/constipation	Diarrhea/constipation	Diarrhea/constipation
Weight loss	Weight loss	Weight loss	Weight loss
Pyrexia	Pyrexia	Pyrexia	Pyrexia
Normal bilirubinemia	Jaundice within 72 hours	Jaundice as disease advances	No jaundice
Polyruia/polydipsia	Polydipsia	Polyuria/polydipsia	Polyuria/polydipsia
Clear to yellow urine	Orange urine	Clear to orange urine	Clear urine, urobilinogen "+"
	Negative urobilinogen	Urobilinogen "+"	Copper-colored iris (cats)
	Bleeding tendencies	Bruising/bleeding tendencies	Normal coagulation
	Acholic (pale) feces	Brown to melanic feces	Brown feces
	Melanic feces if bleeding	Green feces	Melena: hookworms, coccidia
	Hepatomegaly	Hepatomegaly (cat)	Microhepatica
	firm, rounded borders	Normal to microhepatica (dog)	"Plump" kidneys
	Palpable gallbladder (cat)	Ptyalism (cats)	Cryptorchid (dogs)
	Gastroduodenal ulceration	Gastroduodenal ulceration	Rare gastrointestinal ulceration
	If chronic: > 6 weeks	If ↓ albumin and portal hypertension	Portal hypertension: ± ligation, AV fistula
	ascites	ascites	ascites rare unless hepatic AV fistula
		edema (rare in cat)	edema does not occur
		Hepatic encephalopathy	Hepatic encephalopathy
		stupor, lethargy, depression	amaurosis, stupor, depression,
		pacing, head pressing	head pressing
		rarely coma, seizures	pacing, aggression (esp. cats), ptyalism
			seizures with prolonged prodrome
		Hyperammonemia	Hyperammonemia
		usually coincides with HE signs	usually coincides with HE signs
		ammonium biurate crystalluria	ammonium biurate crystalluria
		cystic/renal calculi	cystic/renal calculi
		urinary tract obstruction	urinary tract obstruction
		pollakiuria, hematuria	pollakiuria, hematuria

From Center SA. Pathophysiology and laboratory diagnosis of hepatobiliary disorders. In: Ettinger SJ, Feldman EC (eds), Textbook of Veterinary Internal Medicine, 4th ed. Philadelphia, WB Saunders, 1995, 1267.

Table 8-2

CLINICAL MANIFESTATIONS OF HEPATIC ENCEPHALOPATHY IN COMPANION ANIMALS

COMMON SUBCLINICAL SIGNS	COMMON CLINICAL SIGNS	LESS COMMON SEVERE SIGNS
Anorexia	Personality changes	Amaurosis
Lethargy	irritability	(unexplained blindness)
Drowsiness	aggression	Disorientation
Ptyalism (cats especially)	dull responsivity	Somnolence → coma
Vomiting	inappropriate vocalizations	Seizures
Dietary related "illnesses"	Ataxia	protracted prodrome
Slow "learner"	Weakness	protracted postictus
difficult to house train	Aberrant responses to drugs	
	prolonged recovery	
	↑ sensitivity	
	tranquilizers	
	e.g., phenothiazines,	
	benzodiazepines	
	anesthetics	
	e.g., barbiturates	
	antihistamines	
	antibiotics	
	e.g., metronidazole	

---

include liver function tests and measurement of the activities of plasma enzymes originating in the liver. When the liver is screened for serious disease, the evaluation includes at least one function test in addition to the measurement of enzymes. The most common function test used in clinical practice is measurement of serum bile acids in the unfed and fed states. Other function studies include the sulfobromophthalein (BSP) retention test, clearance of indocyanine green (ICG), and measurement of blood ammonia concentration. These tests measure hepatocellular function and hepatic circulation, allowing the clinician to assess a completely different aspect of the liver from that gained by measuring the serum activities of hepatic enzymes.

The most important serum enzyme routinely measured that reflects the integrity of the compartmentalization function of hepatocytes is alanine aminotransferase (ALT). With hepatocyte damage, plasma ALT activity increases. However, a large number of other pathologic processes can cause increased release of ALT and other liver enzymes. Thus, increased liver enzyme activity is commonly seen in small animal practice and presents a major obstacle to accurate diagnoses. Enzyme activity can increase as a result of induction, reversible and irreversible changes in cellular membranes, and hepatocellular as well as biliary injury. Increased enzyme activity lacks specificity and provides no indication of functional capabilities. Interpretation of increased liver enzyme activity is particularly problematic in the dog because this species has a spectacular ability to undergo enzyme induction. Detection of increased liver enzymes in the dog warrants a search for other health problems and any history of exposure to inducing agents. In the cat, hyperthyroidism and diabetes mellitus must be ruled out before proceeding with further costly or invasive diagnostic tests. Medications and conditions associated with increased liver enzyme activity in the absence of serious hepatobiliary disease are common; these are discussed in Chapter 30 and later in this chapter.

In the course of a diagnostic evaluation, finding liver enzyme activity 1.5- to 2-fold normal, warrants reevaluation of a patient's physical condition for other organ system abnormalities and review of the medical history for administration of enzyme-inducing drugs. If nothing suspicious is discovered, symptomatic treatment is usually offered and reevalua-

tion is scheduled in 2 to 4 weeks. If liver enzymes remain abnormal on reevaluation or exceed 2.5- to 3-fold normal on initial testing, a liver function test is performed; fasting and postprandial serum bile acids are most commonly used. If hyperbilirubinemia is detected and hemolysis has already been discounted as a cause of jaundice, the evaluation of serum bile acids is unnecessary.

Documentation of abnormal liver function or hyperbilirubinemia attributed to hepatobiliary disease suggests the need for hepatic ultrasonographic evaluation and usually a liver aspirate and/or biopsy. If functional evaluations are normal, the animal is given symptomatic care until reevaluation of liver enzymes in 2 to 4 weeks. If abnormal enzyme activity persists and remains unexplained and/or abnormal serum bile acids are detected, ultrasonographic evaluation and biopsy are pursued at that time. Prior to liver aspirate or biopsy, the coagulation status of the patient must first be appraised. If a coagulation abnormality is detected (laboratory tests or mucosal bleeding time), parenteral vitamin K_1 should be given at least 12 hours before the procedure and the need and availability for a fresh whole blood transfusion be considered.

In the course of patient evaluation, it is important to remember that liver enzyme activity is a sensitive but rather nonspecific indicator of end-stage hepatic disease. Severe dysfunction associated with end stage cirrhosis and portosystemic vascular anomalies can exist in the absence of serum enzyme abnormalities. Furthermore, liver enzymes cannot be used as reliable prognostic indicators. However, sequential evaluations showing continued abnormal enzyme activity indicate continuing hepatobiliary disease, enzyme induction, or perturbed hepatocellular membrane permeability. Diminished enzyme activity may indicate improvement, resolution of an enzyme-inducing or releasing process, or a paucity of viable hepatocytes.

The nuances offered by each of the screening tests and the association of these findings with different disorders can be extremely helpful in formulating a list of diagnostic rule-outs. These details are discussed in the following sections.

Morphologic evaluation of the liver is required to identify specific pathologic processes and to determine patient management and prognosis. Gross morphologic evaluation is less

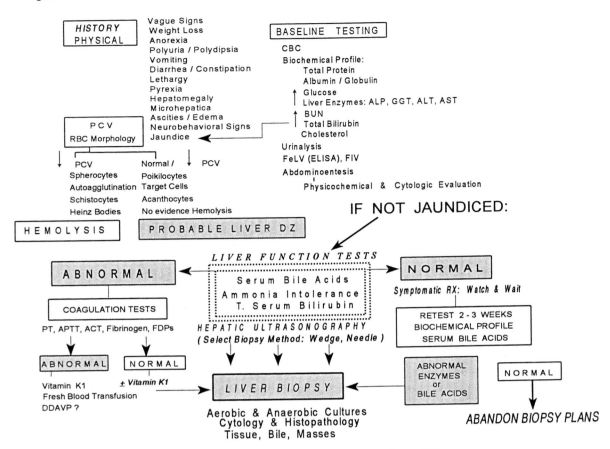

FIGURE 8-1. Diagnostic algorithm for diseases of the hepatobiliary system.

valuable than microscopic assessment. Microhepatica and hepatomegaly suggest hepatic disease (Table 8–3), but many patients with hepatobiliary disease have normal-sized livers. Once a patient is identified as having liver pathology, the only means of attaining a definitive diagnosis is through liver biopsy.

CLINICOPATHOLOGIC SCREENING TESTS USEFUL IN THE DIAGNOSIS OF HEPATOBILIARY DISEASE

Hematologic Evaluations

Hematologic changes may include the development of anemia, abnormal erythrocyte morphology, reduced platelet number or function, and the detection of jaundiced or lipemic plasma. When an inflammatory, septic, or necrotizing process is involved, systemic response may be indicated by development of a neutrophilic leukocytosis. Dogs with a glucocorticoid hepatopathy often will develop a stress leukogram.

A regenerative anemia is occasionally recognized due to blood loss associated with gastrointestinal ulceration and/or a coagulopathy. More commonly, anemia is nonregenerative (normocytic, normochromic). A nonregenerative anemia may develop due to inefficient utilization of marrow iron stores (anemia of chronic disease), decreased nutritional

intake of substances essential for erythropoiesis, reduced availability of micronutrients from the liver, inadequate erythropoietin, chronic blood loss associated with coagulopathy, or reduced erythrocyte surivival.[1-26]

Abnormal erythrocyte morphology has been recognized in humans, dogs, and cats with liver disease.[2-8] Morphologic changes may be induced by splenic dysfunction or the result of lipoprotein abnormalities. Abnormal splenic function has been attributed to lymphoreticular hyperplasia associated with altered systemic immune response and to changes in the splenic microcirculation due to portal hypertension. Microscopically observed changes in erythrocyte shape termed *poikilocytosis* is particularly common in the cat with liver disease. Target cells and spur cells (acanthocytes) have been observed in dogs with serious liver disorders. In humans, alterations in erythrocyte membrane fluidity and thus, deformability, are associated with changes in blood cholesterol, lipoproteins, phospholipids, lecithin, electrolytes, and vitamin E concentrations. A change in erythrocyte energy metabolism may also be associated with cell deformation. The susceptibility of feline erythrocytes to poikilocyte formation may be related to differing composition of phospholipids compared to other species and their increased susceptibility to oxidative injury.[27,28] Poikilocytes described in cats with liver disease include acanthocytes, elliptocytes (ovalocytes), keratocytes, schistocytes, and "blister cells."[7] Conformational changes typical of poikilocytosis in cats with liver disease are illustrated in Figure 8–2. Recognition of erythrocyte morphology changes requires prepara-

Table 8–3

DIFFERENTIAL DIAGNOSIS FOR ALTERATIONS IN HEPATIC SIZE

MICROHEPATICA	HEPATOMEGALY	

MICROHEPATICA

Decreased Hepatic Perfusion
  Hypotension
    severe dehydration
    shock
    hypoadrenocorticism
    endotoxemia
  Impaired portal vein perfusion
    congenital portal venous shunt
    portovascular dysplasia
    portal vein atresia
    portal venous thrombi
Hepatocellular Atrophy
  Congenital portosystemic anomaly
  Congenital portovascular atresia
Hepatocyte Destruction
  Cirrhosis (not biliary cirrhosis; dog)
  Severe necrosis (stromal collapse)

HEPATOMEGALY

Impaired Venous Outflow
  Cardiac disease
    congestive heart failure
    pericardial disease
    pericardial tamponade
    dirofilariasis
    atrial hemangiosarcoma
    cardiomyopathy
    arrhythmias
    cor triatrium (rare)
Venous Occlusion
  "Kinked" vena cava (congenital)
  Vena caval occlusion (trauma, stenosis)
  Hepatic vein thrombi
  Vena caval syndrome (Dirofilariasis)
  Budd-Chiari-like syndrome
  Venoocclusive-like disease
Reticuloendothelial Hyperplasia
  Immune-mediated disease
    anemia (immune, hemolytic)
    thrombocytopenia
    vasculitis (SLE, others)
  Infectious diseases
    bacterial
    protozoan
    mycotic
    rickettsial
    septicemia
  Nodular hyperplasia
    idiopathic (elderly dogs)
    hepatic regeneration
  Extramedullary hematopoiesis
    Bone marrow failure
    Severe chronic blood loss
  Erythrocytic parasitemia

Infiltrative Disorders
  Glycogen
    hyperadrenocorticism
    glycogen storage disease (rare)
  Lipid
    severe feline hepatic lipidosis
    diabetes mellitus
  Lipoprotein lipase deficiency (LPL) (cat)
  Neoplasia
    lymphosarcoma
    malignant histocytosis
    myeloproliferative disease
    hemangiosarcoma
    metastatic
    hepatocellular carcinoma (one large lobe)
    hepatoma (single, multiple)
  Amyloid (rare)
  Hemochromatosis (iron overload, rare)
  Storage diseases (lysosomal)
Inflammatory Disease
  Hepatitis (infectious, inflammatory)
  Acute necrosis/degeneration
  Cholangitis
  Cholangiohepatitis
  Cirrhosis (biliary, cat)
  Abscess
Extrahepatic Bile Duct Occlusion
  Pancreatitis (dog especially)
  Cholelithiasis
  inspissated bile syndrome (cat)
  Neoplasia (bile duct adenocarcinoma; cat)
Cystic Disorders
  Parenchymal cysts (isolated)
  Biliary cysts
  Polycystic biliary/parenchymal (cats especially)

From Center SA. Pathophysiology and laboratory diagnosis of hepatobiliary disorders. In: Ettinger SJ, Feldman EC (eds), Textbook of Veterinary Internal Medicine, 4th ed. Philadelphia, WB Saunders, 1995, 1265.

tion of a well-made blood smear because poorly prepared smears can result in artifactual conformational changes. The blood smear should be air dried as rapidly as possible and examined with a Wright's-Giemsa stain.

Erythrocyte microcytosis is associated with both acquired and congenital portosystemic shunting in the dog and cat.[13-16] An association with iron metabolism is suspected, although the pathogenetic mechanism has not been defined (see Chapter 35). The range of PCV and MCV documented in dogs and cats with congenital portosystemic vascular anomalies and dogs with cirrhosis associated with intrahepatic and extrahepatic shunting are shown in Figure 8–3.

Quantitative and qualitative platelet defects may be associated with hepatobiliary disorders, although they have not been well characterized in domestic species.[1,17-26] Thrombocytopenia may develop due to platelet sequestration, increased platelet destruction, or reduced marrow production of platelets. In humans, hypersplenism associated with portal hypertension can cause sequestration of from 60% to 90% of platelets at one time.[21,22] Thrombocytopathies, functional platelet abnormalities, have been characterized in humans with serious liver disease where it is proposed that an abnormal metabolic environment is primarily responsible.[21,22] It has also been suggested that the changes associated with liver disease augment expression of subclinical inherent platelet defects. Studies in the dog have shown reduced

platelet aggregation in animals with demonstrable bleeding tendencies and in dogs that had normal bleeding times.[18-20] Crude clinical evaluation of platelet function is possible by evaluating the buccal mucosal bleeding time and subjectively evaluating whole blood clot retraction.

SERUM BIOCHEMICAL EVALUATIONS

Serum Proteins

TOTAL PROTEIN. The liver is the primary site for synthesis of a majority of the plasma proteins and is the site of degradation or regulation for many others. The total serum protein concentration is influenced by liver disease in a number of diverse ways. For optimal diagnostic interpretation, the total serum protein concentration should be fractionated into albumin and total globulin moieties. This will permit identification of differential effects from either component.

ALBUMIN. Albumin is exclusively synthesized in hepatocytes; under normal circumstances this occurs at only 33% of its maximal capacity. There is a large reserve capacity for albumin synthesis, and liver injury must be severe and diffuse or extracorporeal losses must be prodigious for synthetic insufficiency to cause hypoalbuminemia. Albumin

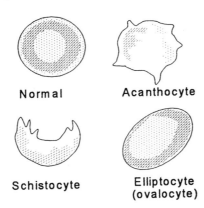

FIGURE 8–2. Common morphologic changes in erythrocytes in cats termed poikilocytosis.

homeostasis reflects the balance among the rates of synthesis, secretion, distribution, and degradation. The normal half-life of albumin in the dog is estimated at between 8 and 10 days. The many complexities associated with regulation of the serum albumin concentrations are comprehensively reviewed in Chapter 30.

Plasma albumin concentration has commonly been used as an indicator of liver function. Unfortunately, it is a nonspecific parameter because its concentration reflects so many other variables including (1) the rate of hepatic synthesis, (2) the rate of degradation, (3) the influence of pathologic extracorporeal excretion, and (4) the volume of distribution. Any chronically anorectic animal may have a minor decrease in serum albumin concentration as a result of reduced synthesis. Pathologic processes associated with considerable losses of albumin from the body include (1) proteinuria, (2) protein-losing enteropathy, and (3) exudative cutaneous lesions. In certain disease states, the volume of distribution of albumin expands as a result of third space fluid sequestration, which can lead to a lowered serum albumin concentration. In patients with cirrhosis associated with ascites, a low serum albumin concentration may be more reflective of an increased volume of distribution than of impaired hepatic synthesis.[30] In addition, sodium and water retention associated with cirrhosis may cause dilutional hypoalbuminemia, despite continued normal or increased rates of albumin synthesis.[31–35] In some of these patients, newly synthesized albumin may leak directly from hepatic lymph into ascites, thereby circumventing the vascular compartment. A diagnostic algorithm for the differential diagnosis of hypoproteinemia is provided in Chapter 30, Figure 30–7.

The actual serum concentrations of albumin and globulins of clinical patients with a variety of different hepatobiliary disorders are shown in Figure 8–4. Lowest albumin concentrations are seen in dogs with cirrhosis accompanied by ascites and dogs in fulminant hepatic failure, such as the Doberman pinscher with chronic active hepatitis. Loss into ascitic fluid (third space sequestration), reduced hepatic synthesis, and protein loss into the bowel are suspected causal mechanisms. Animals with congenital vascular anomalies and cats with lipidosis may have normal or only moderate decreases in their serum albumin concentration. The sequential changes in the plasma albumin and gamma globulin concentrations in dogs following experimental induction of severe hepatic injury (liver disease modeled with nitrosamine administration) is shown in Figure 8–5. As the albumin concentration progressively declines, the serum globulin concentration rises. This phenomenon is discussed in the next section. Overall, the sensitivity of albumin as a test for liver disease is poor (Figure 8–6).

An increased serum albumin concentration usually reflects the presence of dehydration. However, animals chronically treated with glucocorticoids can become mildly hyperalbuminemic probably as a result of glucocorticoid-induced protein synthesis. Some hypothyroid dogs also become hyperalbuminemic; the underlying mechanism is not understood.

GLOBULINS. The measured total serum globulin concentration represents a large number of different proteins. The majority of the nonimmunoglobulin serum globulins are synthesized and stored in the liver. This includes most of the gamma globu-

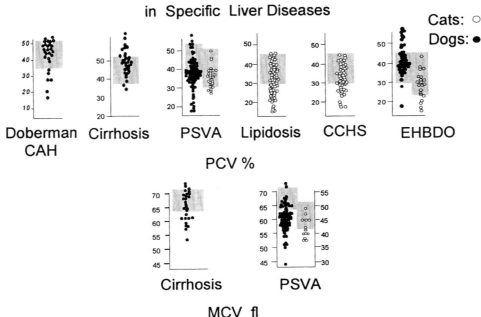

FIGURE 8–3. Scattergrams showing the PCV and MCV documented in dogs and cats with congenital portosystemic shunts and in dogs with hepatic cirrhosis. Data derived from the College of Veterinary Medicine, Cornell University. Normal range is shown by the shaded areas.

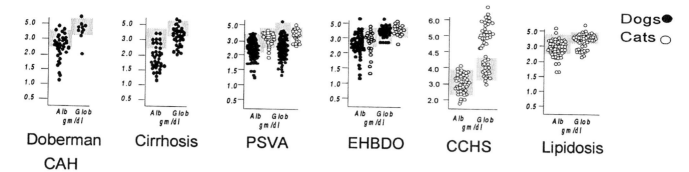

FIGURE 8–4. Scattergrams showing the serum albumin and globulin concentrations in dogs and cats with various acquired hepatobiliary disorders and with portosystemic vascular anomalies (PSVA). Doberman CAH denotes chronic active hepatitis in the Doberman pinscher, cirrhosis denotes dogs with cirrhosis and ascites, EHBDO denotes dogs and cats with extrahepatic bile duct obstruction, CCHS denotes cats with the cholangitis/cholangiohepatitis syndrome, and lipidosis denotes cats with severe hepatic lipidosis syndrome. Normal range is shown by the shaded areas. Data derived from the College of Veterinary Medicine, Cornell University.

lins and 50% of the beta globulins.[36] Many of these globulins function as "acute-phase proteins"; these are functionally diverse proteins normally present in only very small quantities.[37-43] The synthesis of acute-phase proteins is rapidly and markedly increased in response to tissue injury or inflammation. Although these proteins can contribute to an increased total serum globulin concentration, total globulins are not a good measure of liver synthetic function because of the large component comprised of immunoglobulins derived from other sources. The cellulose acetate electrophoretic separation of serum globulins has been studied in patients with liver disorders, but the results are not diagnostically useful because of the diverse overlap between protein moieties.

Hyperglobulinemia is common in animals with acquired hepatobiliary disorders. The magnitude of hyperglobulinemia may be great enough to mask hypoalbuminemia if only a total serum protein is determined. In addition to the acute-phase response, increased globulin concentrations also may develop as a result of an immunoreactive systemic response to reduced Kupffer cell function, disturbed B and T cell func-

tion, and development of autoantibodies (see Chapter 30).[44-46] The chronologic increase in the concentration of serum gamma globulins in the dog with experimentally induced liver disease created by ingestion of nitrosamines is shown in Figure 8–5. Generally, changes in globulin concentrations are mild and because this is a nonspecific response, they do not contribute much to the clinical diagnosis of hepatic disease.

ALPHA-FETOPROTEIN. Alpha-fetoprotein is the major plasma protein synthesized by the yolk sac and liver that is secreted into the blood during fetal life. This ability declines during the perinatal period so that little alpha-fetoprotein is detected in the blood of a healthy adult animal or human. However, development of rapidly growing hepatocellular, cholangiolar, or biliary epithelial tumors in humans or dogs, or marked parenchymal regeneration in the dog, can stimulate renewed production of this protein.[47-54] After a 70% hepatectomy in normal dogs, an increase in serum alpha-fetoprotein is detectable on postoperative day 4, reaching peak values between days 7 and 12. Values return to the normal range by 3 to 4 weeks.[50] Alpha-fetoprotein values are more consistently and chronically increased during hepatic regeneration than are conventional serum enzyme activities and the total bilirubin concentration. Determination of this

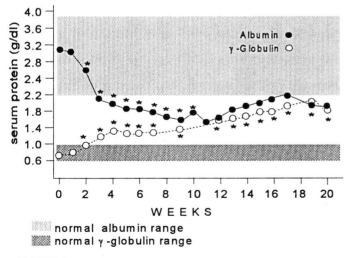

FIGURE 8–5. Changes in plasma albumin and globulin concentrations, before and after exposure of dogs to nitrosamines. Normal range is shown by the shaded areas.* Indicates significant changes from baseline values.

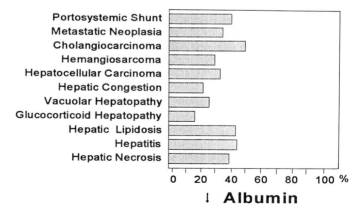

FIGURE 8–6. Sensitivity of serum albumin in detecting liver diseases in dogs.

protein has been proposed as a superior marker for hepatic regeneration in the dog but there has been little clinical work with alpha-fetoprotein as a routine diagnostic test.[50,51] In humans, increased serum alpha-fetoprotein concentrations also develop in patients with malignant disease of yolk-sac cell origin (gonadal carcinomas) and a variety of liver diseases including viral hepatitis, chronic active hepatitis, and cirrhosis.[47–49] Increased alpha-fetoprotein values were reported to function as a paraneoplastic marker in dogs with experimentally induced hepatic carcinomas,[52,53] and in dogs with naturally occurring cholangiocarcinoma, hepatocellular carcinoma, and hepatic lymphosarcoma.[54] Determination of alpha-fetoprotein is not routine. Analysis requires use of either radioimmunoassays or immunoenzymetric assays that have been validated for the dog.[54] Previous work has shown that there is partial but not complete cross reactivity with antibodies raised against human alpha-fetoprotein when applied to dog alpha-fetoprotein.[50]

Liver Enzymes

Increased serum activity of liver enzymes is common, and unfortunately is not necessarily associated with clinically significant liver disease. Enzymes customarily included in serum biochemical profiles include alanine aminotransferase (ALT, formerly SGPT), aspartate aminotransferase (AST, formerly SGOT), alkaline phosphatase (ALP), and gamma-glutamyltransferase (GGT). Major variables influencing the activity of liver enzymes in circulation include (1) their intracellular localization, (2) their rate of synthesis and baseline intracellular activity, (3) their size and tendency to leak from the cell if membrane permeability increases, (4) their serum half-life, and (5) the extent, rapidity, and severity of tissue damage. Increases in serum enzyme activity may be associated with (1) reversible or irreversible alterations in membrane permeability, (2) microsomal enzyme induction, or (3) structural injury resulting from hepatobiliary ischemia, necrosis, neoplasia, or cholestasis. Plasma activities of liver enzymes increase greatly with diffuse, rapidly developing, and severe cell damage. This increase in plasma enzyme activity is exaggerated when their molecular size is small, they are rapidly synthesized, and not bound to membranes or entrapped within organelles and can diffuse rapidly from the cell. The circulation of the liver promotes rapid egress of enzymes from the hepatobiliary structures because of the highly permeable nature of the sinusoidal endothelium. Increased activity of liver enzymes also reflects stimulated synthesis, an important adaptation for cell regeneration.[55,56] Induced liver enzyme synthesis is a normal response to growth, certain drugs, and biliary obstruction. The concentration of some enzymes increase because of delayed enzyme clearance; this is recognized for example with lipase, when renal function is compromised. It is not known whether delayed enzyme clearance influences liver enzyme activity.

Most enzymes are found in multiple tissues located in different parts of the body. As a result, disorders involving a diversity of tissues may contribute to increased plasma enzyme activity. Although the hepatocyte contains certain enzymes in abundant concentrations as compared to other tissues (most notably ALT, AST, and ALP), none of the enzymes routinely used for the detection of hepatobiliary disorders are unique for disease in this system.

As already implied, there are many different systemic conditions and medications that are associated with increased serum enzyme activity in the absence of serious hepatobiliary

Table 8–4

CONDITIONS ASSOCIATED WITH INCREASED SERUM ACTIVITY OF LIVER ENZYMES BUT NOT NECESSARILY WITH CLINICALLY IMPORTANT HEPATOBILIARY DISEASE

Bone Disorders
Growth (birth to 7 months)
Metabolic bone disease
Osseous neoplasia
Osteomyelitis

Endocrine Disorders
Diabetes mellitus
Hyperadrenocorticism
Hypoadrenocorticism
Hyperthyroidism (cats)
Hypothyroidism (dogs)

Gastrointestinal Disorders
Diarrhea
  acute or chronic
  small or large bowel
  viral enteritis
  infiltrative disease
Constipation: obstipation
Gastric dilatation/volvulus
Pancreatitis
Splenic torsion

Hypoxia
Cardiac failure
Pulmonary disease
Severe acute anemia
Severe chronic anemia
Drowning
Smoke inhalation

Hypotension
Cardiac disease
  cardiomyopathy
  arrhythmias
  end-stage mitral insufficiency
Pericardial disorders
Severe dehydration
Shock

Neoplasia
Enzyme induction
  paraneoplastic syndrome
  liver origin
  micrometastasis

Systemic Infections
Rickettsial diseases
Dirofilariasis
Viral (parvovirus, FIP, respiratory)
Pyelonephritis
Abscessation
Pyometra/prostatitis
Severe dental disease
Septicemia

Miscellaneous
Blunt abdominal trauma
Systemic tissue necrosis
Fever/hyperthermia
Hymenoptera stings
After general anesthesia
Severe muscle trauma
Malignant hyperthermia
Duchenne muscular dystrophy
Other myopathies

consequences. Important and representative examples are shown in Tables 8–4 and 8–5. Liver enzyme induction is common in the dog and is the major reason for confusion in determining the clinical significance of abnormal enzyme activity on biochemical screening profiles.

Different hepatobiliary disorders can cause proportionately different magnitudes of increased enzyme activity due to variations in enzyme localizations within the hepatic lobule. In certain disorders, these variations can be used to differentiate between broad diagnostic categories. Severe hepatic dysfunction associated with end-stage cirrhosis and congenital portosystemic vascular malformations can exist in the absence of serum enzyme abnormalities; Figure 8–7 demonstrates the fold increases realized in ALT, AST, and ALP in various hepatobiliary conditions in the dog and cat. Caution must be exercised in the interpretation of "quiet" liver enzyme activity. Enzymes should not be used as prognostic indicators unless they are sequentially monitored and histopathologic evaluation of a liver biopsy has been accomplished. Diminished enzyme activity may indicate (1) improvement in a pathologic condition, (2) resolution of an enzyme-inducing process, (3) discontinuation of an enzyme-inducing drug, or (4) a paucity of viable hepatocytes capable of releasing enzyme. Single measurements of enzyme activity should not be used as a basis for important clinical decisions.

Table 8–5

DRUGS CAUSING HEPATIC ENZYME INDUCTION AND INHIBITION

INDUCTION	INHIBITION	
Carbamazine	Amiodarone	Metronidazole
Clofibrate	Allopurinol	Parathion
Ethanol (acute)	*Chloramphenicol	Phenothiazines
Griseofulvin	*Cimetidine	Propylthiouracil
†Glucocorticoids	Ciprofloxacin	*Quinidine
Phenytoin	Cyclophosphamide	Ranitidine
*†Phenobarbital	Danazol	Sulfadiazine
Pentobarbital	Disulfiram	Sulfonamides
†Phenylbutazone	Griseofulvin	Tricyclic antidepressants
Piperonyl butoxide	Disulfiram	valproic acid
*Primidone	Ketoconazole (imidazole antifungals)	
Rifampin		
Spironolactone		
Tobacco smoke		

*Of particular importance in affecting metabolism of other drugs.
†Strong induction of liver enzyme activities notable in clinical patients.

ALT. Alanine aminotransferase (ALT) is a cytosolic enzyme regarded as liver specific in the dog and cat, although it is also present in the heart, kidneys, and muscle.[57,58] Concentration in the liver is 4 times that in the next most abundant site (cardiac muscle) and 10 times that in the kidney. In health, the concentration of ALT in the hepatocyte is 10,000 greater than that in plasma. In the dog, the serum half-life of ALT is reported as between 3 hours and 4 days.[59,60]

Because it is a cytosolic enzyme, immediate increase in serum ALT activity follows hepatocellular injury or altered cell membrane permeability. The magnitude of ALT increase generally correlates with the number of involved cells, although focal and diffuse disorders cannot be differentiated. Largest increases develop with hepatocellular necrosis and inflammation. Gradual and sequential decreases in ALT activity can be a sign of recovery. In acute liver disease, a 50% or more

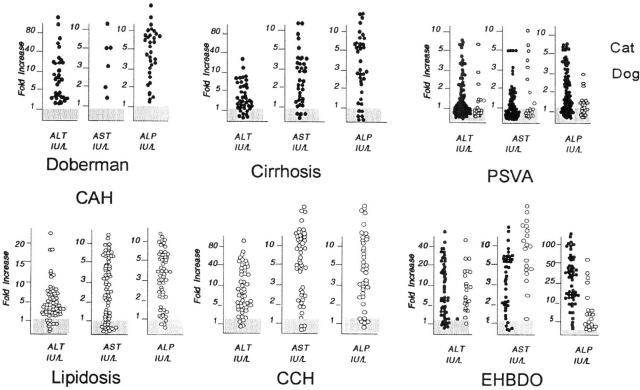

FIGURE 8–7. Scattergrams showing the serum activity of ALT, AST, and ALP in dogs and cats with various acquired hepatobiliary disorders and congenital portosystemic vascular anomalies (PSVA). Cirrhosis denotes dogs with cirrhosis and ascites, Doberman CAH denotes chronic active hepatitis in the Doberman pinscher, Lipidosis denotes cats with the severe hepatic lipidosis syndrome, CCHS denotes cats with the cholangitis/cholangiohepatitis syndrome, EHBDO denotes dogs and cats with extrahepatic bile duct obstruction. Data derived from the College of Veterinary Medicine, Cornell University.

decrease in serum ALT activity over several days is considered a good prognostic sign. As can be seen in Figure 8–7, some dogs and cats with severe disease have normal serum ALT activity. It is important ot remember that declining serum ALT activity may also represent a paucity of viable hepatocytes in chronic liver disease.[61]

After acute, severe, diffuse hepatocellular necrosis, serum ALT activity sharply increases within 24 to 48 hours up to 100-fold normal (or higher) to peak during the first 5 post-injury days.[61–67] If the injurious event resolves, ALT activity gradually declines to normal over 2 to 3 weeks. This is seen with CC1₄-induced liver injury but not with some other toxins that do not produce persisting necrosis. An example of the latter circumstance is the hepatic injury induced by acetaminophen where marked increases in plasma ALT and AST activities within 24 hours subsequently decrease within 72 hours to near normal values.[68] Hepatocellular necrosis induced by nitrosamines increases plasma ALT activity, but not significantly, until after one week of exposure (Figure 8–8). The increase persists for weeks until the necrosis resolves if administration of nitrosamines is discontinued.

Discordance between increased serum ALT activity and obvious histologic lesions is well recognized and is demonstrated in animals with portosystemic shunts. As shown in Figure 8–8, the experimental creation of a portosystemic shunt in the dog is followed by two- to fourfold sustained increases in the serum ALT activity for 40 weeks. However, histologic evaluation of liver tissue does not consistently show ongoing hepatic necrosis. Only small foci of cellular necrosis and residual lipogranulomas are observed in most cases.

Extrahepatic bile duct occlusion incurs a more gradual increase in ALT activity of lesser initial magnitude than that associated with necrosis. Within 3 days of major duct occlusion, ALT activity may increase 5- to 45-fold in cats and 20- to 70-fold in dogs.[62,63,67,69–72] Within 1 to 2 weeks, ALT may peak at increases 20- to 40-fold normal (sometimes higher in the dog), and up to 15- to 45-fold normal in the cat. Severe cholestasis induces hepatic necrosis and membrane alterations as a result of noxious effects of bilirubin and bile salts. After the initial 1 to 3 week increase, ALT activity

declines, but usually does not normalize. The peak serum ALT activity with spontaneous clinical disorders associated with biliary obstruction are of lesser magnitudes than those associated with experimentally induced obstruction. Initial values in experimental disease are markedly increased, but these tend to diminish faster and stabilize at lower, albeit abnormal levels.

In clinical cases, plasma ALT activity increases markedly and consistently with acute hepatic necrosis; the degree to which it increases roughly parallels the severity and extent of hepatocyte degeneration. The sensitivity of ALT for some disorders in the dog is shown in Figure 8–9. Unfortunately, the high sensitivity is not associated with high specificity in differentiating clinically significant changes in hepatic histology or function. Acute hepatic necrosis caused by infectious canine hepatitis increases plasma ALT activity to 30 times normal; activity peaks within four days.[73] Toxic hepatitis causes plasma ALT activity to increase, peak, and normalize sooner than infectious viral hepatitis. Chronic hepatitis, a persistent necroinflammatory disorder, is associated with varying severities of necrosis and fibrosis. The mean plasma ALT activity is often 10- to 12-fold normal, and the enzyme activity spontaneously fluctuates with the biologic behavior of the disease process. This fluctuation contrasts with the serum ALT activity associated with hepatic necrosis originating from a single acute injurious event or toxin exposure. In that circumstance, the serum ALT activity declines as injury resolves.

Microsomal enzyme induction in dogs generally causes smaller increases in ALT activity than necrosis or bile duct occlusion. Several anticonvulsant medications (phenobarbital, phenytoin, primidone) given in conventional therapeutic dosages may be associated with up to four-fold ALT increases. Following high-dose phenobarbital treatment (4.4 mg/kg TID) ALT has increased over 50-fold normal in certain individuals.[74] Whether large increases in ALT activity are consistently associated with morphologic evidence of liver injury is unknown. Administration of prednisone (4.4 mg/kg SID × 14 days) to dogs may result in ALT activity two- to fivefold normal within 1 week, and up to 10-fold normal within 2 weeks.[75,76] Dogs developing a glucocorticoid hepatopathy may have ALT activity increase up to 40-fold normal. After discontinuation of short-acting glucocorticoids, induced ALT activity may persist for several weeks.

In the dog, activities of serum ALT consistently increase with primary hepatic neoplasia (hepatocellular carcinoma, hepatocellular adenomas (hepatoma)), invasive secondary neoplasia, and nodular hyperplasia.[66,77–81] Values ranging from 3- to 35-fold normal have been observed in dogs with hepatocellular carcinoma. Such increases could be due to

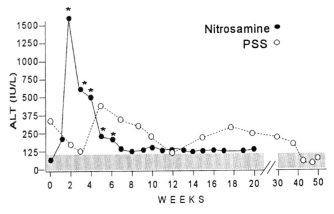

FIGURE 8–8 Changes in plasma ALT activity before and after exposure of dogs to nitrosamines and before and after surgical creation of portosystemic shunts (PSS). Normal range is shown by the shaded area. * Indicates significant change. Data derived from Strombeck DR, Harrold D, Rogers Q, et al. Plasma amino acids, glucagon, and insulin concentrations in dogs with nitrosamine-induced hepatic disease. Am J Vet Res 44:2028–2036, 1983. Schaeffer MC, Rogers QR, Buffington CA, et al. Long-term biochemical and physiologic effects of surgically placed portacaval shunts in dogs. Am J Vet Res 47:346–355, 1986.

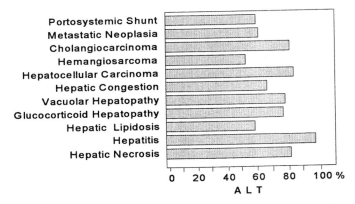

FIGURE 8–9. Comparison of the sensitivity of serum ALT activity in dogs with different hepatic disorders.

tumor-associated necrosis, compression and necrosis of adjacent normal hepatocytes, isoenzyme production, or abnormal membrane permeability in neoplastic cells (paraneoplastic enzyme liberation). Metastatic hepatic neoplasia in dogs and cats may be associated with normal or slight to moderate increases in serum ALT activity. In exceptional cases, values as high as 10-fold normal have developed.

In the dog, hepatic vacuolar hepatopathy, hepatic lipidosis, and chronic passive congestion cause slight increases in serum ALT activity. Mean increments five to six times normal are consistent with moderate hepatocellular degeneration, marked by ballooning degeneration or hydropic change on histopathologic evaluation. There are many systemic disease processes that secondarily affect the liver and invoke an increase in serum ALT activity usually associated with the degenerative or vacuolar hepatocellular change.

The serum activity of ALT in cats may be increased from 2- to 45-fold normal in hepatic necrosis, cholangitis, or cholangiohepatitis, 2- to 10-fold normal in hepatic lipidosis, and 2- to 5-fold normal in severe acute anemia, septicemia, and in feline leukemia virus–associated disorders (lymphosarcoma, myeloproliferative disease).

AST. Aspartate aminotransferase is present in substantial concentrations in a wide variety of tissues. In the dog and cat, highest tissue concentrations are present in the heart, liver, skeletal muscle, kidney, brain, and plasma.[58–60,64,82–85] The plasma half-time of AST is reported as 5 hours in the dog and 77 minutes in the cat.[59,83] Hepatic AST is located in the cytosol and associated with mitochondrial membranes. In humans, AST from hepatocellular mitochondria and cytosol are immunochemically distinct.[86] Although most of the circulating AST is of cytosolic origin, the majority of hepatocellular enzyme is the mitochondrial form. In humans, mitochondrial AST has a very short half-life in circulation; therefore, its presence in serum implies a severe ongoing hepatocellular insult.[86] It is unknown if similar AST isoenzyme identification would be useful in the dog or cat.

Increased serum AST activity can result from altered membrane permeability, necrosis, inflammation, and in the dog, microsomal enzyme induction. Liver disease–related AST activity parallels increased ALT activity. In some circumstances, AST activity becomes quiescent before ALT activity.[64] Increases in AST activity in the absence of abnormal ALT activity implicates an extrahepatic source of enzyme, most notably muscle injury.

Following acute diffuse severe hepatic necrosis, AST activity increases sharply during the first 3 days; 10- to 30-fold normal in dogs and up to 50-fold normal in cats.[64,67,87] If necrosis resolves, AST activity gradually declines over a period of 2 to 3 weeks. In dogs with 70% hepatectomy, the AST activity increased 3-fold during the first week, then declined to near normal activity during regeneration.[88] It is probable that increased serum AST activity was partially due to surgical injury to muscle tissue.

Complete extrahepatic bile duct occlusion is associated with a marked rapid increase in AST during the first week, up to 25-fold normal in the dog and to 20-fold normal in the cat. Enzyme activity may continue rising through 3 weeks or plateau and then gradually decline.[65–69] In experimentally induced obstructive jaundice, surgical trauma to muscle and viscera contribute to increased AST activity during the early postoperative period.

In some cats with liver disease, is seems that AST may be a more sensitive indicator of the hepatobiliary process than ALT. This observation has been made in individuals with hepatic necrosis, cholangiohepatitis, myeloproliferative disease, lymphosarcoma, and chronic bile duct obstruction.[69,87,89] A study of the diagnostic value of different liver enzymes in dogs with naturally developing hepatic disease indicated that increases in the AST activity was overall more sensitive than ALT.[90] This finding was corroborated by results of another study of the diagnostic utility of liver enzymes in dogs with histologically confirmed disease.[91] The contribution of AST activity from other tissues, particularly in animals with metastatic cancer, systemic inflammatory conditions, and in those with congestive heart failure, was suspected.

Dogs treated with glucocorticoids may have normal or only mild increases in the serum AST activity.[76] The induced enzyme activity resolves within several weeks after glucocorticoid withdrawal.

The serum activity of AST in dogs and cats with spontaneous clinical disorders is illustrated in Figure 8–7.

SORBITOL DEHYDROGENASE. Sorbitol dehydrogenase (SDH) is a cytosolic enzyme released during hepatic degeneration or necrosis. The concentration of SDH is greater in the liver than in all other tissues.[59] Although it may be a useful test for the recognition of hepatocellular injury, it seems to offer no advantage over determination of the serum ALT activity. There is also concern over its lability in vitro as compared to ALT; consequently, there has been little use of this enzyme in the small animal patient.

ARGINASE. Arginase is considered a liver-specific enzyme because it is present in higher concentrations in hepatocytes than in any other tissue. It is a major catalyst of the urea cycle with large quantities located in mitochondria; these can be released with hepatic necrosis.[92,93]

A simplified method for analysis of arginine has made this test applicable for clinical practice.[94] Simultaneous measurements of serum arginase and transaminase activity may provide prognostic information concerning the nature of an hepatic disorder. With acute necrosis, ALT and arginase are immediately released from hepatocytes, causing sharp increases in their respective activities.[95] If both plasma arginase and transaminase activities are continually increased, a progressive necrotizing lesion is likely.[92] In both dogs and cats, experimentally induced acute hepatic necrosis with CCl_4 results in a 500- to 1000-fold increase in arginase that persists for only 2 to 3 days. During recovery, leakage of transaminases but not arginase continues, ALT and AST activity remaining increased for 1 week or longer.[92,95,96]

Dogs treated with dexamethasone (3 mg/kg SID × 11 days) developed a transient increase (5- to 8-fold) in arginase activity by day 4. With chronicity of treatment, a steady increase in the serum arginase activity was observed. On termination of the study (day 12) the serum arginase activity was 10-fold normal.[97] It is possible that induction by glucocorticoids or the resulting catabolism caused the increase in arginase activity, as has been reported in other species.[93,97]

ALP. The alkaline phosphatases are a group of enzymes that catalyze the hydrolysis of a number of organic phosphate compounds to yield phosphate and an organic molecule. These enzymes operate best at an alkaline pH. Their exact role in physiologic processes remains ill defined. Increased serum ALP activity is the most common biochemical abnormality observed in chemistry profiles from ill dogs. In the dog, ALP has high sensitivity but low specificity as a test for liver disease.[98] In the cat, it has a lower sensitivity but is more specific.[99] Alkaline phosphatase is a membrane-bound enzyme present in many tissues.[82,85,100,101] The tissue containing the greatest amount of ALP is the intestinal mucosa, with lesser, yet substantial amounts also present in the renal cortex, placenta, liver, and bone. The ALP extracted from these tissues are distinctly different isoenzymes.[72,101–104] Three major isoenzymes are commonly identified in canine serum including a bone, liver, and a glucocorticoid-induced isoenzyme.[101] In the dog, the half-life of the placental, renal, and intestinal ALP is vey short, less than 6 minutes.[101,105] In the cat, the half-life of the intestinal isoenzyme is less than 2 minutes and because the structure of the placental and renal isoenzymes in the cat are similar, they are surmised to have a short half-life.[106–108] The isoenzymes with ultrashort half-lives are not routinely detected in sera of dogs or cats with increased ALP activity. The exception is the placental isoenzyme, which has been detected in late-term pregnant cats.[72] In the dog, liver and glucocorticoid isoenzymes are primarily responsible for serum ALP activity; the liver isoenzyme is primarily responsible in the cat. The half-life of the liver isoenzyme is about 6 hours in the cat; the half-lives of the liver and glucocorticoid isoenzymes in the dog approximate 70 hours.[101,104,105] The specific activity of ALP in liver extract from the normal dog has been reported as equal or twofold greater than that of the normal cat.[72,83] The comparatively smaller increases in ALP activity realized in cats than in dogs with hepatobiliary disorders is related to the different ALP half-life and liver content. Regardless of the small magnitudes of change, ALP remains an important and useful diagnostic test for feline hepatobiliary disease.[62,63,99] A magnitude of increased activity of two- to threefold normal is a strong indicator of clinically significant liver disease in the cat.

The use of ALP in the dog is complicated by the accumulation of different isoenzymes in the serum and the ease with which the hepatic and glucocorticoid enzymes are induced. Unfortunately, the clinical utility of ALP in the dog is not improved by using isoenzyme determination because of the liberal production of the glucocorticoid isoenzyme. The interpretation of ALP activity is less complicated in the cat than in the dog because there is no glucocorticoid isoenzyme and no substantial evidence of ALP induction by drugs.

The ALP bone isoenzyme increases as a result of osteoblast activity; it can thus be detected in serum of young growing animals and may be associated with bone tumors and secondary renal hyperparathyroidism. Increased ALP activity due to the bone isoenzyme usually doesn't exceed 4- to 6-fold normal in the dog.[101] Bone remodeling associated with neoplasia may not substantially affect serum ALP activity or may cause a two- to threefold increase. In the young cat, increased serum ALP activity attributable to bone isoenzyme may simulate enzyme activity realized with hepatobiliary disease.

The liver ALP isoenzyme is derived from membranes in the canalicular area.[109–111] This isoenzyme increases as a result of increased de novo hepatic synthesis, canalicular injury, and solubilization of membrane-bound protein by the detergent action of bile salts.[101,109–114] Increased enzyme synthesis may develop in response to primary or secondary hepatocellular disorders or drug exposure. It is proposed that the toxic effects of bile salts are involved in both the induction of increased synthesis as well as membrane solubilization and detachment of the enzyme or enzymes linked to subcellular components. Local accumulations of bile salts are believed to promote enzyme regurgitation into plasma by alteration of cell membrane permeability.[114]

Whereas ALT is immediately released from the cytosol in the circumstance of acute hepatocellular necrosis, membrane-bound ALP, which is present in lesser amounts within the cytosol, is not. Rather, it takes several days for induction of membrane-associated enzyme to gear up and spill into the circulation. Largest increases in serum ALP (liver and/or glucocorticoid isoenzymes as high as 100-fold normal or greater) are associated with diffuse or focal cholestatic disorders, primary hepatic neoplasms (hepatocellular carcinoma and bile duct carcinoma) and, in the dog, enzyme induction. Marked increases in the serum ALP activity were reported in dogs with mammary cancer; that report however did not clearly rule out osseous or hepatic metastasis.[115] Circumstantial evidence suggested a paraneoplastic effect because tumor resection was followed by long-term survival and reduction in serum ALP activity; this could have been the glucocorticoid isoenzyme. The serum activity of ALP may be normal or moderately increased in dogs with metastatic neoplasia involving the liver.

Following acute severe hepatic necrosis, ALP activity (dog or cat) increases 2- to 5-fold normal, stabilizes, and then gradually declines over 2 to 3 weeks.[60,62,63] After an acute insult, serum enzyme increases are less predictable in the cat than in the dog, and enzyme abnormalities appear to resolve faster. Plasma ALP activities increase in clinical patients with hepatic necrosis and chronic hepatitis, although not consistently; the increases that develop are usually three to six times the upper normal limits. Enzyme activity is believed to increase as a result of intrahepatic cholestasis caused by bile canalicular injury or collapse, membrane destruction, and hepatocellular swelling.

Extrahepatic bile duct obstruction in the dog results in serum ALP activity that increases within 8 hours. Values may reach 15-fold normal by 2 to 4 days and as much as 50- to 100-fold normal within 1 to 2 weeks. After this, ALP activity stabilizes and gradually declines, but not into the normal range.[66,70,71,116] In the cat, extrahepatic bile duct obstruction results in 2-fold increases within 2 days, as much as 4-fold increases within 1 week, and up to 9-fold increases within 2 to 3 weeks. After this, activity stabilizes and gradually declines, but never to the normal range.[69,72,117] Experimentally, cats with partial occlusion of the biliary tree (ligation of major hepatic ducts) develop serum ALP activity approximately half that observed in cats with complete common duct occlusion.[72] In contrast, even partial experimental occlusion of the biliary tree in the dog causes huge increases in the serum ALP activity. In both the dog and cat, however, similar magnitudes of serum ALP activities are realized in spontaneously developing intrahepatic cholestatic disorders as compared to disease or obstruction of the extrahepatic biliary tree (Figures 8–7, 8–10, and 8–11). Consequently, ALP activity cannot be used to differentiate between these cholestatic disorders.

Many different extrahepatic and hepatic conditions may promote increased production of the hepatic ALP isoenzyme, particularly in the dog. Hepatic parenchymal inflammation and systemic infection or inflammation may cause secondary intrahepatic cholestasis.[101,118–121] It is speculated that alterations in energy-dependent membrane pumps result in hepatocellular swelling and subsequent cholestasis by interference with microtubule assembly. Any involvement of biliary (canalicular) structure or function can stimulate ALP synthesis and disrupt local bile acid transport, causing subsequent appearance of enzyme in the systemic circulation. Obstruction of canalicular flow of bile is probably the major cause of the marked increases in ALP that develop in cats with the severe hepatic lipidosis syndrome (Figures 8–7 and 8–11). Increased hepatic and glucocorticoid isoenzyme synthesis occurs in response to many other systemic conditions in the dog and may cause ALP activity to increase up to fivefold normal or higher.

The glucocorticoid isoenzyme in the dog is produced in the liver in the area of the bile canaliculi.[110,111,113,122–124] It can be identified in serum by many different techniques; the most popular method today is by levamisole inhibition.[124] This isoenzyme develops in animals treated with glucocorticoids, in those with spontaneous or iatrogenic hyperadrenocorticism, dogs with hepatic or nonhepatic neoplasia, and most importantly, dogs with many different chronic ill-

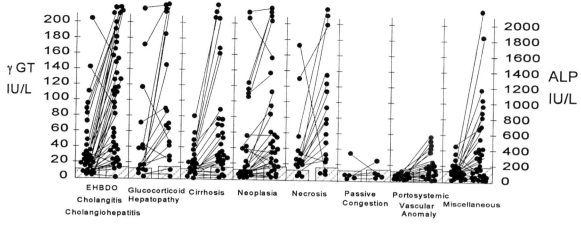

FIGURE 8-10. Serum activity of γ-glutamyl transpeptidase (γGT) and alkaline phosphatase (ALP) in cats with spontaneous clinical hepatobiliary disease confirmed by histomorphologic evaluation. The left column for each disease category shows actual γGT activity, the right column shows actual ALP activity. Straight lines connect data for a single patient. Hatched areas represent the normal reference range. Data derived from the College of Veterinary Medicine, Cornell University.[99]

nesses.[101,122,124] There is no reliable relationship between the magnitude of increased serum ALP activity due to the glucocorticoid isoenzyme and the presence of a steroid hepatopathy.[76] Serum ALP activity increases as early as 1 week following daily administration of prednisone (2 mg/kg SID),[125] as early as 2 days following daily administration of prednisone (4.4 mg/kg SID),[75] and as early as 3 days following daily administration of dexamethasone (2.2 mg/kg SID).[76] The initial increase in ALP activity is attributed to the liver isoenzyme.[110] Thereafter, the glucocorticoid isoenzyme continues to increase (Figure 8–12).[111] Different magnitudes of enzyme activity develop depending on the type of glucocorticoid administered, the dose, and the individual patient response.[75,101,126,127] Increases in serum ALP activity due to glucocorticoid isoenzyme usually exceed those associated with liver or bone isoenzymes. Following 14 consecutive daily doses of 4.4 mg/kg prednisone after which treatment was dis-

continued, dogs reached a maximum ALP activity of 64-fold normal by day 20 (Figure 8–13).[127] These values decreased gradually to 8-fold normal by day 56. This study is particularly relevant to clinical practice because commonly prescribed immunosuppressive dosages of prednisone were used. The production of the glucocorticoid ALP isoenzyme does not imply that a dog treated with cortisone has iatrogenic hyperadrenocorticism, a suppressed pituitary adrenal axis, or a clinically important glucocorticoid hepatopathy. The glucocorticoid isoenzyme increase in chronically ill dogs is likely the result of endogenous glucocorticoid release. In the author's experience, liver biopsy in many of these chronically ill dogs has shown a vacuolar-glucocorticoid hepatopathy in spite of normal low-dose dexamethasone suppression, ACTH response test, and in the absence of historical exposure to glucocorticoids. See Chapter 34 where vacuolar and glucocorticoid hepatopathies are comprehensively discussed.

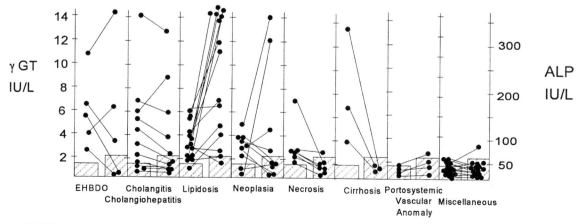

FIGURE 8-11. Serum activity of γ-glutamyl transpeptidase (γGT) and alkaline phosphatase (ALP) in dogs with spontaneous clinical hepatobiliary disease confirmed by histomorphologic evaluation. The left column for each disease category shows actual γGT activity, the right column shows actual ALP activity. Straight lines connect data for a single patient. Hatched areas represent the normal reference range. Data derived from the College of Veterinary Medicine, Cornell University.[99]

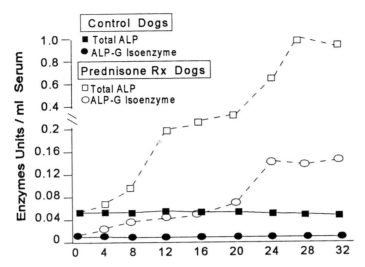

FIGURE 8-12. Serum activity of alkaline phosphatase following administration of prednisone (4 mg/kg/day for 32 days). Note the early increase in the liver isoenzyme and the later increase in the glucocorticoid isoenzyme. Data derived from Sanecki RK, Hoffmann WE, Gelberg HB, et al. Subcellular location of corticosteroid-induced alkaline phosphatase in canine hepatocytes. Vet Pathol 24:296–301, 1987.

The feline liver, by comparison, is relatively insensitive to glucocorticoids. Administration of prednisolone (5 mg BID PO) to normal cats for 30 days failed to elicit an increase in ALP activity in serum or liver tissue.[106] When cats received 2 mg/kg prednisolone SID for 16 days, changes in serum ALP activity did not occur or were minor. Morphologic hepatocellular alterations were rare and minor in some studies but were suggested to be consistent in one recent study.[128–131]

In the dog, the serum activity of the liver ALP isoenzyme may be increased by administration of the anticonvulsants: phenobarbital, primidone, and phenytoin.[74,132] Induced ALP activity usually increases 2- to 6-fold. During a 30 day study of drug administration to normal dogs, phenytoin (22 mg/kg TID) produced a uniform small increase in serum ALP activity. Phenobarbital (4.4 mg/kg TID) produced peak serum enzyme activity of 30-fold normal by 24 days and then declined. Primidone (17.6 mg/kg TID) produced a 5-fold increase in serum ALP activity by day 28. Healthy dogs receiving combination therapy (primidone and phenytoin) developed ALP increases that ranged from 2- to 12-fold normal, and some receiving high-dose phenobarbital had ALP activity 30- to 40-fold normal. In contrast to the dog, the administration of phenobarbital (0.25 grain BID) for 30 days in cats failed to elicit an increase in serum or liver tissue ALP activity.[106]

GGT. Gamma-glutamyltransferase, also known as gamma-glutamyl transpeptidase (GGT), is a glycoprotein believed to be important in amino acid membrane transport, foreign compound detoxification, and in glutathione metabolism.[134–137] Most body cells contain cytosolic and membrane-associated GGT. Highest tissue GGT concentrations in the dog and cat are in the kidney and pancreas[70,138] with lesser quantities in the liver, gallbladder, intestines, spleen, heart, lungs, skeletal muscle, and erythrocytes.[75] Serum GGT activity is largely derived from the liver.[138–142] There is considerable species variation in the localization of GGT within the liver. Hepatic microsomal localization has been shown for GGT in the dog where it is associated with the bile ducts and perilobular parenchyma.[138,143,144] Increased serum GGT activity is the result of increased de novo hepatic synthesis and regurgita-

tion or elution of enzyme from cell membranes.[145–147] The diagnostic performance of GGT in clinical cases has been examined.[70,98,99,149,150]

Studies of serum GGT activity in dogs and cats undergoing acute severe diffuse necrosis have shown either no change or a mild 1- to 3-fold increase that resolves over the ensuing 10 days. In the dog, extrahepatic bile duct obstruction causes serum GGT activity to increase 1- to 4-fold within 4 days and 10- to 50-fold within 1 to 2 weeks, after which time values may plateau or continue to increase as high as 100-fold.[65,70,148] In the cat, serum GGT activity may increase up to 2-fold within 3 days, 2- to 6-fold within 5 days, 3- to 12-fold within a week, and 4- to 16-fold within 2 weeks.[62,63]

Glucocorticoids and certain other microsomal enzyme inducing drugs may stimulate GGT production similar to their influence on hepatic ALP. Administration of dexamethasone (3 mg/kg SID) or prednisone (4.4 mg/kg SID IM) induced GGT activity within 1 week to 4- to 7-fold normal and up to 10-fold normal within 2 weeks.[75,97,127] The increased serum GGT activity in dogs given glucocorticoids is thought to be of hepatic origin. In comparison to glucocorticoid induction, dogs given anticonvulsants develop only a modest increase in serum GGT activity (up to 2- or 3-fold).[134]

Some cats with cirrhosis, major bile duct obstruction, or intrahepatic cholestasis have larger magnitudes of serum GGT increase as compared to ALP (Figure 8–11).[99] Cholestasis is thought to enhance the synthesis as well as the release of hepatic GGT. It is unknown whether glucocorticoids or other enzyme inducers clinically influence serum GGT activity in the cat. Experience of the author suggests this does not occur or is exceptional. It is noteworthy that some assays are relatively insensitive to the small increases in GGT that develop in cats with liver disease. Another problem is that a recommended normal range similar to that reported for the dog is used by many laboratories. In the author's opinion, this is erroneous. Feline GGT activity is normally very low. Small increases can easily be missed when a normal range has not been carefully validated.

In humans, a unique GGT isoenzyme is associated with hepatocellular carcinoma.[151] It is unknown if a similar phenomenon occurs in the dog or cat. However, eight- to 10-fold and higher increases in the serum GGT activity has been

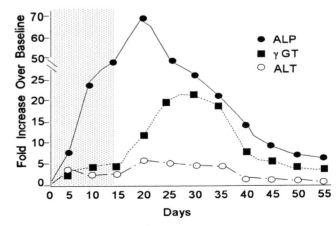

FIGURE 8-13. Enzyme induction over time due to glucocorticoid administration. Note the persistently increased enzyme activity following drug discontinuation that slowly resolves. Data derived from Badylak SF, Van Vleet JF. Sequential morphologic and clinicopathologic alterations in dogs with experimentally induced glucocorticoid hepatopathy. Am J Vet Res 42:1310–1318, 1981.

observed in some dogs with hepatocellular and biliary carcinomas.[70,90] Although GGT is useful as an indicator of hepatic metastasis in humans, it does not appear to be suitable for this purpose in either the dog or cat.[152]

Like ALP, GGT lacks specificity in differentiating between parenchymatous hepatic disease and occlusive biliary disease. It is not as sensitive in the dog as ALP but is more specific in the diagnosis of liver disease.[90,98] In the cat, GGT is more sensitive but less specific than ALP, and these two enzymes perform best when they are evaluated simultaneously.[99] The prediction of hepatic lipidosis in the cat is possible if the history, physical findings, and routine biochemical features are considered along with the GGT and ALP activities. In many cholestatic disorders in the cat, the magnitude of serum GGT exceeds that of ALP (Figure 8–11).[99] In severe feline hepatic lipidosis, usually a marked increase in ALP develops in the absence of substantial GGT activity. The mechanism for this difference is not known.

Neonatal animals of several species, including the dog, have been shown to have high serum activity of GGT.[153] This is related to colostrum ingestion and it is unclear if the increased serum enzyme activity is the result of absorption across the bowel wall of the very high GGT contained in colostrum or enzyme induction in the newborn stimulated by a substance contained in colostrum. Studies in newborn dogs deprived of colostrum but fed a milk replacer has documented this phenomenon in the dog (Figure 8–14).[153]

LACTATE DEHYDROGENASE (LDH). Lactate dehydrogenase has wide tissue distribution in all species. Highest tissue concentrations are present in skeletal muscle, heart, and kidney, with lesser amounts in the intestine, liver, lung, and pancreas. Each tissue has been shown to contain at least five different isoenzymes.[154] An LDH_5 isoenzyme predominates in the liver and is believed to be a major constituent of plasma LDH activity. Isoenzyme determination by electrophoresis and by spectrophotometry following pyruvate inactivation of the cardiac LDH isoenzyme can be accomplished.[154,155] Serum biochemical profile–reported LDH usually represents total LDH activity and thus has limited clinical application. High LDH activity is often seen in the presence of diffuse severe hepatic necrosis or inflammation and multicentric lymphosarcoma.

Miscellaneous Causes of Liver Enzyme Abnormalities

GLUCOCORTICOID EFFECTS One of the most common causes of increased liver enzyme activity in the dog is treatment with glucocorticoids. A glucocorticoid hepatopathy has been well characterized in dogs treated with glucocorticoids and in those with spontaneous or iatrogenic hyperadrenocorticism.[75,127,156–159] A comprehensive discussion of glucocorticoid hepatopathy in the dog is presented in Chapter 34. Enzymic changes induced with glucocorticoids depend on individual response, dose of drug, and on the particular drug used. Many variables influence the chronology of peak serum enzyme activities in relation to drug administration.[127] Continued enzyme induction after drug discontinuation probably depends on the persistence of high glucocorticoid concentrations in the circulation and/or their continued biologic effects.[160,161] Glucocorticoid enzyme induction has been shown to occur in dogs as a result of topical cutaneous, ocular, or otic medications containing glucocorticoids.[162–167] Most dogs seen in the clinical environment with enzyme induction

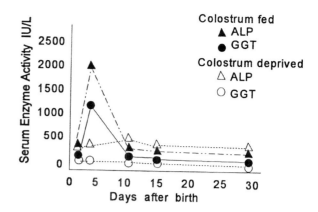

FIGURE 8–14. Serum activity of gamma-glutamyltransferase and alkaline phosphatase in neonatal dogs fed bitches colostrum or deprived natural colostrum and fed commercial puppy milk formula. Data derived from Aguilera-Tejero E, Mayer-Valor R, Gomez-Cardenas G. Spectrophotometric method for differentiation of cardiac and hepatic lactate dehydrogenase activities in dogs. Am J Vet Res 50:1128–1130, 1989.

as a result of glucocorticoid exposure do not develop hepatic dysfunction. There is no substantiated association between the degree of enzyme induction or the presence of a glucocorticoid hepatopathy.

ANTICONVULSANT MEDICATIONS The anticonvulsant drugs primidone, phenytoin, and phenobarbital, administered singly or in combination, cause variable increases in liver enzyme activity in the dog. Some dogs receiving chronic anticonvulsant therapy develop morphologic liver injury and functional impairment. The majority, however, only develop increased serum activities of ALP, ± ALT, AST, and GGT. Primidone and phenobarbital are more consistently associated with increased liver enzyme activity than phenytoin, perhaps owing to the ultrashort half-life of the latter drug in the dog. Combination anticonvulsant therapy with primidone and phenytoin or phenobarbital more consistently induces enzyme activity and to larger magnitudes than does single drug therapy.[134] Increased serum ALT and AST activity up to 2-fold baseline may develop with each drug used alone; combination therapy may induce transaminase activity 3- to 5-fold normal. Serum ALP activity is more remarkably and consistently affected. Changes in the serum ALP activity are discussed in the section dedicated to single enzyme activities. A significant linear association has been shown between primidone dose and the magnitude of serum ALT increase and between dose of primidone and of phenytoin and the magnitude of serum ALP activity.[134] This implies either a direct relationship between dose and enzyme induction or dose and liver injury. The GGT activity is infrequently altered in dogs receiving phenytoin but values twofold baseline may develop with primidone and combination treatment.[134] Delayed BSP plasma clearance was common in a group of clinical patients with seizure abnormalities treated long term with anticonvulsants.[133] Histologic examination of liver tissue could not be obtained for each patient and therefore the presence of morphologic disease was suspected but not confirmed. Based on cumulative clinical information regarding idiosyncratic drug toxicity in dogs on extended anticonvulsant therapy, the following recommendations are advised. Reevaluation including a thorough history, physical examination, and a complete biochemical assessment including liver enzymes, cholesterol, albumin, and total bilirubin is recommended at 6 month intervals. Serum bile acids (12 hour fasting and 2 hour postprandial) should be concurrently evaluated to appraise liver function. In dogs with reduced hepatic function, seizure medications should be changed to another alternative such as potassium bromide, which does not require hepatic biotransformation and is not known to be hepatotoxic. The author has seen epileptic dogs with apparent liver injury (abnormally increased serum bile acid values) associated with phenobarbital undergo functional recovery and resolution of serum enzyme activity and normalization of serum bile acid values when placed on potassium bromide as their exclusive anticonvulsant. Continued administration of traditional anticonvulsants in a patient that has acquired liver dysfunction, suspected to be related to the drug therapy, may result in eventual cirrhosis and intoxication evidenced by somnolence or coma due to impaired drug elimination. Trough concentrations of the anticonvulsant should be evaluated to rule out impending drug overdose. Severe hypocholesterolemia and hypoalbuminemia are poor prognostic signs in this subset of patients because these findings are associated with hepatic failure.

FELINE HYPERTHYROIDISM. Hyperthyroidism is usually associated with increased serum transaminases and ALP activity. This can distract the clinician from pursuing and treating the underlying endocrinopathy.[168] Careful palpation of the cervical area for a thyroid-associated mass and submission of a baseline T_4 specimen is essential in any aged cat showing increased liver enzyme activity. The origin of serum ALP in hyperthyroid cats was recently studied using agarose gel electrophoresis and was shown to be comprised of mainly the liver and bone isoenzymes.[169] An additional isoenzyme was identified for which a source remains unclarified. In hyperthyroid humans, the source of the enzyme has been identified as bone and liver.[170] Severe thyrotoxicosis is associated with changes in hepatic morphology due to cardiac failure, severe weight loss, or the direct toxic effects of thyroid hormone.[170–173] Similar considerations seem applicable to the cat. In most cases, only modest and nonspecific histologic lesions are found in liver tissue, including centrilobular fatty infiltration and mild focal necrosis.[172] Evidence of liver dysfunction is uncommon in humans and appears to be uncommon in the cat. Despite the increase in cardiac output that accompanies hyperthyroidism, the liver does not realize an increased blood flow.[173] At the same time, the splanchnic and hepatic oxygen consumption is increased owing to the raised metabolic rate. Any pre-existent hepatic disease may flourish under these circumstances. The liver enzyme abnormalities associated with hyperthyroidism in the cat resolve following restitution of a euthyroid status; within 6 weeks following I^{131} therapy, liver enzymes are within the normal range.

PASSIVE CONGESTION/CONGESTIVE HEART FAILURE. Acute and chronic passive congestion of the liver may result in mild to moderate increases in the serum ALP and transaminase activities.[174–176] Abnormal retention of BSP occurs owing to impaired hepatic circulation. These patients have normal serum bile acid concentrations unless they have chronic severe cardiac failure. In humans, reduced hepatic function develops in patients with severe congestive heart failure and is realized by prolonged coagulation times, hypoalbuminemia, and hyperbilirubinemia. Similar overt abnormalities are uncommon in the dog and cat with heart failure.

NEOPLASIA. Primary or secondary hepatic neoplasia are commonly associated with biochemical evidence of liver involvement. Increases in the transaminases, ALP, and GGT are variable. In a study of metastatic liver disease in the dog, AST was the most sensitive indicator of hepatic involvement, and ALT and ALP together detected liver disease in 70% of 95 dogs.[81] In another report of 15 dogs with metastatic hepatic

neoplasia, abnormalities included increased ALT in 46%, increased ALP in 50%, and hyperbilirubinemia in 46%.[80] Canine tumors associated with increased serum ALP activity include pancreatic adenocarcinoma, intestinal adenocarcinoma, leiomyosarcoma, giant cell tumor, adrenal cortical adenocarcinoma, mixed mammary tumor, hemangiosarcoma, lymphosarcoma, and oral carcinoma. Metastatic hepatic involvement seems likely in most instances, but the presence of unique isoenzymes cannot be discounted.[81,177] Laboratory findings reported in 8 dogs with primary hepatocellular carcinoma included increased ALT and ALP activity in all dogs.[80]

MISCELLANEOUS METABOLIC DISORDERS. Increased liver enzyme activity, particularly of ALP, is common in dogs with hypothyroidism, and dogs and cats with diabetes mellitus and pancreatitis.[177] Disorders associated with endotoxemia, septicemia, anoxia, hyperthermia, thromboembolism, changes in hepatic perfusion caused by hypotension, and microsomal enzyme induction in the dog may be associated with increased serum ALP, GGT, ALT, and AST activities. In most instances the magnitudes of increase do not exceed two- to threefold normal.

In addition to glucocorticoids and anticonvulsants, other drugs may cause transient increases in the serum activity of liver enzymes. A comprehensive list of drugs reported to be associated with hepatotoxicity is provided in Table 30–26. Increased transaminases and ALP may follow the administration of thiacetarsamide, ketoconazole, and danazol.[179,180] In each case, substantial hepatic necrosis has not been proven. It is difficult to induce extensive hepatic necrosis consistently in normal dogs given thiacetarsamide at therapeutic dosages.[178] Biochemical changes during ketoconazole therapy have been observed in dogs and have been extensively studied in humans.[179,180] A list of drugs associated with liver enzyme induction and suppression is provided in Table 8–5. Recently, idiosyncratic diazepam toxicity has been recognized in the cat. Affected animals undergo profound increases in liver enzymes, rapidly become jaundiced, and most cats have died.

Carbohydrate Metabolism

Fasting hypoglycemia is uncommon in liver disease because euglycemia can be managed with as little as 30% of the normal parenchymal mass and because the kidney is also capable of gluconeogenesis.[181,182] Causes of hepatogenic hypoglycemia are discussed in Chapter 30. Hepatogenic hypoglycemia should alert the clinician to consider acute fulminant hepatic failure, decompensated end-stage chronic liver disease, or severe portosystemic shunting.[181–183] In some dogs with portosystemic vascular anomalies, hypoglycemia has been recognized as the dominant clinical sign. Toy breeds appear to be at increased risk; these dogs may be presented as "fading puppies." Yorkshire terriers are more commonly presented with symptomatic hypoglycemia than other breeds of dogs with congenital portosystemic shunts. Hypoglycemia has also been reported as an uncommon complication of hepatic tumors in dogs.[77,80,183]

Some dogs with liver disease develop hyperglycemia rather than hypoglycemia. Hyperglucagonemia has been demonstrated in humans with hepatic insufficiency and has been suggested to occur in dogs with cirrhosis and concurrent glucose intolerance or diabetes mellitus.[184–187] Some dogs with hepatic insufficiency and an unusual vacuolar hepatopathy develop glucose intolerance and a dermatologic condition termed necrolytic migratory erythema. This syndrome is discussed in detail in Chapter 34.

Overall, blood glucose concentration is an insensitive indi-

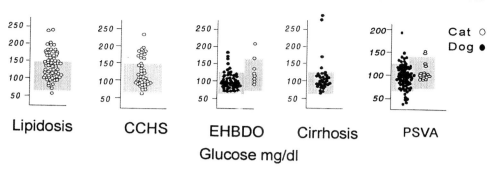

FIGURE 8–15. Scattergrams showing the serum glucose concentrations in dogs and cats with various acquired hepatobiliary disorders and congenital portosystemic vascular anomalies (PSVA). Lipidosis denotes cats with the severe hepatic lipidosis syndrome, CCHS denotes cats with the cholangitis/cholangiohepatitis syndrome, EHBDO denotes dogs and cats with extrahepatic bile duct obstruction. Cirrhosis denotes dogs with cirrhosis and ascites. Normal range is shown by shaded areas. Data derived from the College of Veterinary Medicine, Cornell University.

cator of hepatobiliary function because of the large hepatic reserve for maintaining euglycemia. In particular, cats are least likely to manifest hypoglycemia as a result of hepatic disease. The blood glucose concentration seen in a variety of hepatobiliary disorders in the dog and cat are shown in Figure 8–15. As is evident from this data, hypoglycemia is most common in dogs with cirrhosis and dogs with congenital portosystemic vascular anomalies. Fulminant hepatic failure, such as that seen in the Doberman pinscher with chronic active hepatitis, acute toxic and ischemic insults, infections, acquired portal systemic shunting, or extensive hepatic neoplasia are also each capable of causing symptomatic hypoglycemia. Because of the variety of metabolic interactions that can influence carbohydrate metabolism, finding hypo- or hyperglycemia is a nonspecific screening test. The differential diagnoses warranting consideration in a patient with fasting hypoglycemia are provided in Table 30–2.

Cholesterol and Lipid Metabolism

Lipid metabolism is complex and many facets depend, at least in part, on normal hepatic function. A thorough discussion of lipid metabolism is provided in Chapter 30.

Cholesterol, cholesterol esters, phospholipids, and triglycerides comprise the major plasma lipids. These water insoluble substances are transported in the circulation as lipoprotein complexes. Liver disease may disrupt the normal balance between the major lipid moieties and in the distributions within the lipoprotein classes. The use of lipid moieties as diagnostic indices for liver disease in veterinary medicine is poorly understood, with the exception of cholesterol and triglycerides. The poor sensitivity of the serum total cholesterol concentration as a test of hepatic disease is illustrated in Figures 8–16 and 8–17.

There is a great deal of discrepancy in the normal ranges for total cholesterol as reported on most biochemical screening profiles. The same procedure used in different laboratories has been applied against widely variant so-called normal ranges. One study reports that plasma cholesterol concentrations in healthy dogs range from 125 to 335 mg/dl;[193] another report uses an upper limit of normal as 250 mg/dl.[194] A similar problem complicates use of total cholesterol concentrations in cats. In one report the normal feline range for total cholesterol was 116 to 126 mg/dl, and 89 to 258 mg/dl by another investigator using the same method of cholesterol measurement.[194,195] Mild increases or decreases in the total cholesterol concentration are difficult to identify as a result of the normal range variation.

Total serum cholesterol (nonesterified and esterified cholesterol) is usually measured on routine screening profiles. In the normal dog, 60% to 80% of the circulating cholesterol is esterified.[188,189] Cholesterol esterification is catalyzed by acyl coenzyme A:cholesterol acyltransferase (ACAT) and lecithin-cholesterol acyltransferase (LCAT), which act on cholesterol incorporated in lipoproteins.[190,191]

Reduced LCAT has been shown in dogs with experimental liver injury as in humans with liver disease.[197–203] The decline in enzyme activity is attributed to synthetic failure. The net result is reduced plasma cholesterol esterification. The ratio of esterified to nonesterified cholesterol ranges from 0.64 to 0.88 (in control experimental dogs, mean ratio was 0.80).[189] In dogs with histologically confirmed liver disease, 90% had esterified to unesterified cholesterol ratios of less than 0.52. Dogs with acute hepatitis had the highest incidence of abnormal ratios. In descending order, this is followed by obstructive jaundice, hepatic cirrhosis, and hepatic neoplasia. In most circumstances, the abnormal cholesterol ester ratio was associated with hyperbilirubinemia. The degree of alteration in the ratio was not significantly associated with the estimated severity of the hepatic disease.

In humans, hypertriglyceridemia may develop in acute and chronic hepatitis and in cholestasis.[198,204] Obstructive jaundice may lead to hypercholesterolemia and hypertriglyceridemia; this has also been shown in the dog.[198,202,205,206] In a 1-week study of dogs with experimental bile duct obstruction,

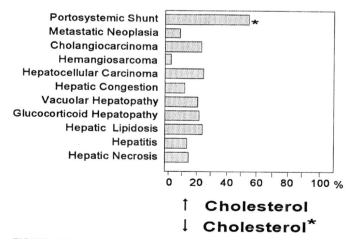

FIGURE 8–16. Comparison of the sensitivity of serum total cholesterol concentration in dogs with different hepatic disorders; the sensitivity for portosystemic shunts is for low-serum cholesterol and for all the other disorders is for high-serum cholesterol.

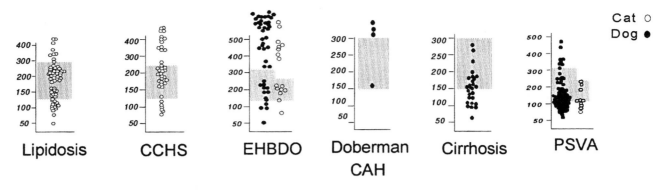

Total Cholesterol mg/dl

FIGURE 8–17. Scattergrams showing the serum total cholesterol concentrations in dogs and cats with various acquired hepatobiliary disorders and with portosystemic vascular anomalies (PSVA). Lipidosis denotes cats with the severe hepatic lipidosis syndrome, CCHS denotes cats with the cholangitis/cholangiohepatitis syndrome, EHBDO denotes dogs and cats with extrahepatic bile duct obstruction, Doberman CAH denotes chronic active hepatitis in the Doberman pinscher, Cirrhosis denotes dogs with cirrhosis and ascites. Normal range is shown by the shaded areas. Data derived from the College of Veterinary Medicine, Cornell University.

plasma cholesterol increased within 3 to 4 days and peaked by 5 to 6 days; mean values increased from a preobstruction value of 175 mg/dl to a peak value of 350 mg/dl.[67] In a longer term study, the serum cholesterol concentrations increased more gradually over a 14 day interval from 184 mg/dl to 322 mg/dl.[189] Hypercholesterolemia and hypertriglyceridemia developed as early as day 3 and remained through 17 days of observation. The concentration of plasma phospholipid doubled over 8 days after obstruction and then gradually returned to values 50% higher than normal. Studies of obstructive jaundice in the dog have shown either no change in cholesterol esterification or a transient (2 to 6 days postobstruction) decrease followed by a gradual rise to normal.[67,198] In one study, fractionation of total cholesterol into free and esterified moieties showed the free cholesterol concentration to increase four- or fivefold over normal. The percentage of total cholesterol represented in cholesterol esters decreased from approximately 80% in healthy dogs to 50% or less within 8 days of bile duct occlusion. The increase in unesterified cholesterol is attributed to increased reflux of cholesterol from the obstructed biliary system and to increased cholesterol synthesis; the latter mechanism is believed to be most important although the exact mechanism is not fully understood. Increased synthesis of cholesterol has been proposed to be related to the increased reflux of lecithin from the obstructed biliary system or to impaired feedback inhibition via chylomicron remnants.[206] Obstruction of the biliary system in the cat also produces an increase in the serum total cholesterol concentration, as can be seen in Figure 8–18. With complete bile duct obstruction, the plasma cholesterol concentration in the cat increases over three weeks, and then declines to the normal range by the seventh week of obstruction concurrent with development of cirrhosis and hepatic failure.[69]

Hypercholesterolemia may also be associated with metabolic derangements stemming from other primary disease processes such as hypothyroidism, diabetes mellitus, pancreatitis, hyperadrenocorticism, the nephrotic syndrome, familial hyperlipidemia, and renal insufficiency (in the cat). Disorders associated with abnormally increased or subnormal cholesterol concentrations are provided in Table 8–6.

An unusual lipoprotein may accumulate in patients with reduced LCAT activity and obstructive jaundice. This lipoprotein is an abnormal very low density lipoprotein (VLDL) (lipoprotein X) and is characterized by reduced cholestryl ester and triglyceride components.[196,202,204,207–209] This test has high sensitivity and specificity for severe cholestasis but is no better than serum bilirubin for that purpose. The most likely explanations for the occurrence of lipoprotein X include regurgitation of biliary lipids into plasma, substrate accumulation secondary to LCAT deficiency, or because lipoprotein X is a poor substrate for LCAT activity.[191] Lipoprotein X has been quantified in normal dogs following surgically created complete extrahepatic bile duct occlusion; it does not seem unique to particular species.[210]

Other studies of lipids in animals with hepatic disease are sparse. Experimentally induced hepatic necrosis in dogs (CCL$_4$) results in reduced serum triglyceride concentrations for 2 days.[192] Within 6 days of acute hepatic necrosis induced by CCl$_4$ in the dog[67] a transient decrease in cholesterol esters develops; the net result is an increase in the unesterified or free cholesterol to esterified cholesterol ratio. This resolves

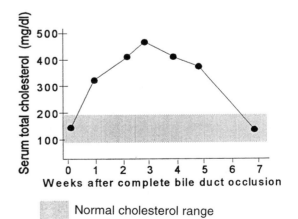

Normal cholesterol range

FIGURE 8–18. The sequential changes in the mean serum total cholesterol concentration in cats undergoing experimental extrahepatic bile duct occlusion. The shaded area represents the normal range. Data derived from Center SA, Baldwin BE, Tennant B, et al. Hematologic and biochemical abnormalities associated with induced extrahepatic bile duct obstruction in the cat. Am J Vet Res 44:1822–1829, 1983.

Table 8–6

DIFFERENTIAL DIAGNOSES FOR INCREASED AND DECREASED
SERUM CHOLESTEROL CONCENTRATION

↑ SERUM CHOLESTEROL	↓ SERUM CHOLESTEROL
Extrahepatic bile duct occlusion	GI malabsorption
Diabetes mellitus	protein-losing enteropathy
Pancreatitis	lymphangiectasia
Glucocorticoid excess	infiltrative bowel disease
endogenous and exogenous	GI maldigestion → fat malabsorption
Hypothyroidism	pancreatic exocrine insufficiency
Glomerular disease → nephrotic syndrome	Starvation/inanition
Renal insufficiency (cats)	Hypoadrenocorticism
Postprandial (mild increase)	Hepatic insufficiency
Idiopathic	cirrhosis
Schnauzers, Beagles, Shetland sheepdogs, others?	portosystemic vascular anomaly
	Drugs
	hypolipidemic agents (clofibrate)
	primidone

rapidly with tissue repair, and purportedly the regained capacity for hepatic LCAT synthesis.

Hypocholesterolemia is common in patients with hepatic insufficiency. Subnormal values of the total serum cholesterol concentration have been recognized in animals with congenital portosystemic vascular anomalies, acquired hepatic insufficiency, and dogs treated with anticonvulsant drugs in end-stage liver failure. Experimentally, after surgical creation of portacaval shunts, dogs develop a 40% to 45% decrease in the total cholesterol concentration.[211] The mechanism remains undetermined but is conjectured to involve decreased synthesis of cholesterol, triglyceride, or lipoproteins, or a shift in the localization of cholesterol away from the routinely measured pool.[187a,211–214] In dogs with surgically created shunts, the size of the shunting vessels, the extent of visceroportal shunting, and the longevity of patient survival seem to correlate with the severity of the hypocholesterolemia. It has been shown that this effect is reversible because patients with congenital portosystemic vascular anomalies normalize their serum total cholesterol concentrations after surgical correction of their vascular anomaly.

A moderate decline in serum cholesterol concentrations was shown in normal dogs treated with oral primidone. Normalization of cholesterol concentrations to pretreatment levels occurred within two weeks of drug discontinuation. Dogs with anticonvulsant-associated hepatic disease develop severe hypocholesterolemia as a sign of severely impaired hepatic function. Both esterified and nonesterified cholesterol fractions decline in hepatic failure. Sequential blood samples demonstrating persistent severe hypocholesterolemia in a patient with acquired hepatic insufficiency warrants a grave prognosis if other causes of low cholesterol can be discounted. The hypocholesterolemia noted in animals with portosystemic vascular anomalies or cirrhosis is associated with markedly increased concentrations of serum bile acids that verify the presence of hepatic insufficiency.

An idiopathic hyperlipidemic condition in Schnauzers has been reported[215] and a similar hyperlipidemic syndrome has been recognized in Shetland sheepdogs and Beagles. These canine syndromes are associated with profound hyperlipidemia, hypertriglyceridemia, and usually hypercholesterolemia. Affected dogs usually develop a severe vacuolated hepatopathy associated with marked increases in ALP activity and abnormal serum bile acid concentrations. The lipoprotein profiles in affected Schnauzers have been characterized.[216] These dogs usually have slow clearance of VLDLs.

Evaluation of Coagulation States

The liver plays a central role in the coagulation and fibrinolytic systems. A comprehensive discussion of the coagulation system as it relates to hepatobiliary disease is provided in Chapter 30; specific defects in coagulation factors reported in humans and dogs with different types of liver disease are provided in Table 30–14.

Tests evaluating the balance of the coagulation system (bleeding time, prothrombin time (PT), activated coagulation time (ACT), activated partial thromboplastin time (APPT), and thrombin time (TT)) can reflect the adequacy of hepatic function. Thrombocytopathia, or abnormal platelet function, can develop in patients with liver disease. Functional platelet defects are detected by evaluating a buccal mucosal bleeding time and assessing platelet aggregation. The latter assessments can be done crudely by evaluating the contraction of a whole blood clot in comparison to a normal animal or more accurately using an aggregometer.

Interpretation of coagulation tests is complicated by the diverse interactions among procoagulants, activators, inhibitors, and plasminogens and the growing understanding of the complexity and interdependence between the classical pathways.[218,219] During synthetic failure the onset of factor deficiency is determined by factor utilization, factor activation, and factor half-life. The factor half-lives vary from hours to days; the shortest lived factor is Factor VII of the extrinsic pathway (Table 30–11). Factor depletion to less than 30% of normal activity causes prolonged "bench" test clotting times and bleeding tendencies. Unfortunately, the sensitivity of these tests is low and they do not predict bleeding tendencies reliably.[218,219] Usually, factor depletion associated with liver disease is not as severe in its manifestations as many of the congenital factor deficiencies. Bleeding in patients with liver disease is primarily due to provocative local factors such as gastritis, ulcers, invasive procedures, or other medical problems rather than spontaneous hemorrhage associated with trivial trauma.[217] Only 15% of human patients with severe hepatic dysfunction evidence pathologic bleeding.[222] It is unknown what percentage of dogs or cats with liver disease demonstrate bleeding tendencies; however, it is prudent to anticipate a bleeding diathesis in any patient with hepatic insufficiency or major bile duct occlusion. Prolongation of the PT has been reported to be more common than prolongation of the other coagulation tests in humans with liver disease. Comparison of the PT and APTT in dogs with naturally occurring hepatic disease showed that abnormal clotting

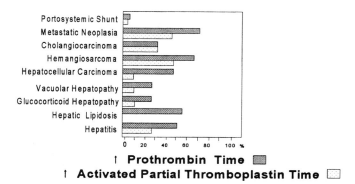

FIGURE 8-19. Comparison of the sensitivity of prolonged prothrombin time and activated partial thromboplastin time in dogs with different hepatic disorders.

times (prolongation or shortening) may develop, but that neither test consistently outperforms the other.[223] Prolonged coagulation times were more common than shortened times, but the predictive value of the tests was too low for use in screening or diagnostic capacities. The sensitivity of these tests was improved using dilutions of patient's citrated platelet-poor plasma. The sensitivity of the routinely evaluated PT and APTT for detection of specific hepatic disorders in the dog is shown in Figure 8–19. Actual test values for PT, APTT, and fibrinogen and fibrin degradation products in animals with various liver diseases are shown in Figure 8–20.

Specific factor deficiencies have been described in dogs with various types of liver disease; these are detailed in Chapter 30.[225-230] In a study of naturally occurring hepatic disease in dogs, changes in specific factors were more frequent than abnormalities in the PT or APTT or in serum liver enzyme activities. Single factor evaluation had discriminant value.[225] Unfortunately, assays for clotting factors are neither practical nor accomplished expediently in most clinical settings.

The prothrombin coagulant factors II, VII, IX, and X comprise a unique class of coagulation proteins that require activation by a vitamin K–dependent carboxylation reaction. This occurs primarily in the hepatocyte.[224,231-233] During factor activation, vitamin K is oxidized to its epoxide form, which then must be regenerated to the active moiety. This occurs in the hepatocyte; see the so-called vitamin K epoxidase cycle, shown in Figure 30–18. Vitamin K must be adequate in concentration and in its functional state if factors II, VII, IX, and X are to be normally activated. In the absence of vitamin K, these factors are present in plasma but lack coagulant activity.[233-237] The inactive proteins may be measured as evidence of insufficient vitamin K activation and are referred to as "proteins induced by vitamin K absence or antagonists" (PIVKA).[235-237] The presence of PIVKAs is estimated in citrated plasma using a functional assay (Thrombotest, Nycomed Pharma AS, Oslo, Norway). Vitamin K can be derived from performed dietary sources or be synthesized within the lower bowel by intestinal microbes. Liver conditions resulting in vitamin K deficiency include major bile duct obstruction, biliary fistula, and insufficient hepatic capacity to reactivate vitamin K. Prolongation of the PT is the

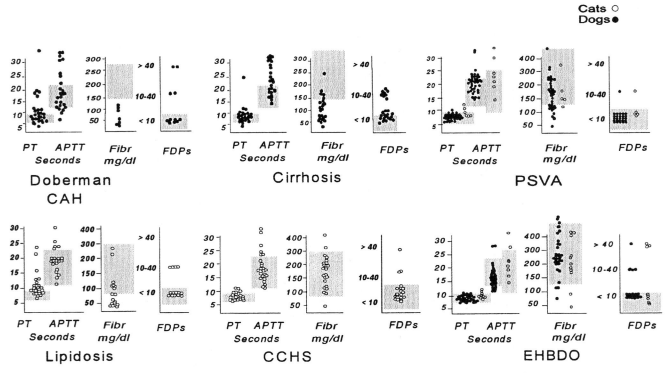

FIGURE 8-20. Scattergrams showing the prothrombin time (PT), activated partial thromboplastin time (APTT), fibrinogen (Fibr), and fibrin degradation products (FDPS) in dogs and cats with various acquired hepatobiliary disorders and with portosystemic vascular anomalies (PSVA). Doberman CAH denotes chronic active hepatitis in the Doberman pinscher, Cirrhosis denotes dogs with cirrhosis and ascites, Lipidosis denotes cats with the severe hepatic lipidosis syndrome, CCHS denotes cats with the cholangitis/cholangiohepatitis syndrome, EHBDO denotes dogs and cats with extrahepatic bile duct obstruction. Normal range is shown by the shaded areas. Data derived from the College of Veterinary Medicine, Cornell University.

first demonstrable abnormality of routine coagulation tests following vitamin K depletion. However, the APTT and ACT also often are prolonged in clinical patients with liver disease having coagulopathies responsive to Vitamin K. Determination of PIVKAs can demonstrate deficient factor activation before the PT and APTT become prolonged. The assessment of the PIVKA clotting time is used to determine the need for chronic vitamin K therapy in the patient with chronic hepatic insufficiency. If a PIVKA is shown to be responsive to vitamin K intervention, vitamin treatment is included as part of the chronic management strategy.

Although fibrinogen is exclusively synthesized in hepatocytes, its behavior as an acute-phase protein complicates its use as a measure of hepatic functional adequacy.[37,38,239] Increased fibrinogen synthesis may occur in response to acute or chronic inflammatory, infectious, or necrotizing hepatic or nonhepatic disorders. The liver has a huge capacity for fibrinogen synthesis and it is only with severe diffuse injury that synthetic failure is realized.

When liver disease is associated with disseminated intravascular coagulation (DIC), excessive formation of fibrin from fibrinogen occurs. Proteolysis of fibrin by plasmin releases fibrin monomers and other degradation products that are normally cleared by the reticuloendothelial system in the liver and spleen. If liver disease is severe enough to impair Kupffer cell function, fibrin breakdown products may accumulate. Fibrin degradation products (FDPs) are easily detected in plasma using immunologic techniques. In normal animals, bleeding into body cavities does not produce increased FDPs in the systemic circulation.[240] It is unknown if this is so in patients with hepatic failure or with inflammatory conditions complicated by hemorrhage into body cavities.

Low plasma antithrombin III (AT III) concentrations can develop in patients with hepatic disease, consumptive coagulopathy, or extracorporeal loss associated with a protein-losing enteropathy or nephropathy.[241,242–249] In the author's hospital, measurements of AT III in dogs with liver disease has shown that values decline as hepatic function worsens; values 50% of normal plasma activity are associated with a grave prognosis. Subnormal concentration of AT III in the patient with severe liver disease and evidence of DIC requires that heparin therapy be combined with transfusion of fresh blood or plasma.

In summary the hemostatic disorders that develop in the veterinary patient with hepatobiliary disease are complex. As in humans, the laboratory tests used to assess this system are insensitive and do not reliably reflect bleeding tendencies.[220,221,238] The mucosal bleeding time has been shown to correlate more closely than any bench test with the clinical behavior of impending coagulopathy.

Determination of Serum Bilirubin

The serum bilirubin concentration reflects a balance between the rate of heme pigment liberation, hepatocellular

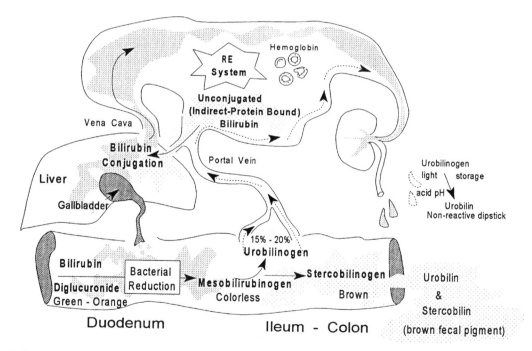

FIGURE 8–21. Diagram showing the metabolism of bilirubin pigments: derivation of hemoglobin pigment from senescent RBCs; dissociation of heme and globin in the reticuloendothelial cells of the bone marrow, spleen, or liver, formation of biliverdin, which is transformed into unconjugated bilirubin. Unconjugated bilirubin is circulated tightly bound to albumin. When delivered to the liver, active uptake, protein binding, transcellular transport, and eventual conjugation to glucuronide yield formation of conjugated bilirubin. Conjugated bilirubin is excreted through the patent biliary system into the gut at the time of gallbladder contraction. Conjugated bilirubin may be (1) deconjugated by bacterial glucuronidases, and subsequently absorbed, (2) digested into urobilinogen, which may be absorbed and undergo enterohepatic circulation (25%) or fecal elimination, or (3) digested into stercobilin, which imparts the normal fecal coloration. From Center SA. Pathophysiology and laboratory diagnosis of hepatobiliary disorders. In: Ettinger SJ, Feldman EC (eds), Textbook of Veterinary Internal Medicine, 4th ed. Philadelphia, WB Saunders, 1995, 1261–1312.

Table 8–7

DIFFERENTIAL DIAGNOSIS OF JAUNDICE

PREHEPATIC OR HEMOLYTIC JAUNDICE

Hemolytic Anemias
erythrocyte parasitemia:
  Babesia
  Haemobartonella
incompatible blood transfusion
neonatal isoerythrolysis
microangiopathic hemolytic anemia
  DIC
  vasculitis
  dirofilariasis
  vascular neoplasia (hemangiosarcoma)
congenital erythrocyte defects
  pyruvate kinase deficiency (Basenji)
  phosphofructose kinase deficiency
  hereditary stomatocytosis (Malamutes)
immune-mediated hemolytic anemia
  autoimmune hemolytic anemia
  SLE
  infectious disease associated
  idiopathic
  drug associated
infectious
  FeLV
  Ehrlichia
  dirofilariasis
  leptospirosis
  septicemia
heinz body anemias

onion toxicity	benzocaine (cats)
zinc toxicity	cetocaine (cats)
vitamin K_1	acetaminophen
propylene glycol	
methionine	
methylene blue	
phenazopyridine	

Increased Hemoprotein Liberation
body cavity hemorrhage
large hematoma formation and absorption
ineffective erythropoiesis
congenital porphyria (cats; rare!)

EXTRAHEPATIC JAUNDICE

Bile Duct Occlusion
cholecystitis
cholangitis
2° peribiliary disease
congenital malformations
  choledochal cysts
  multiple biliary cysts (cats)
intraluminal bile duct occlusion
  inspissated bile (cats)
  cholelithiasis
  trauma → blood clots
  neoplasia
1° and 2° biliary involvement
  pancreatic disease
  parasitic infection (flukes)

Ruptured Biliary Tract
(Bile Duct or Gallbladder)
trauma
cholelithiasis
cholangitis/cholecystitis
iatrogenic: hepatic biopsy

HEPATIC JAUNDICE

Miscellaneous Disorders

endotoxemia/sepsis	hemolytic disease → cholestasis
shock	anoxia → cholestasis
chronic passive congestion DIC	
hyperthyroidism (cat; rare!)	

Intrahepatic Cholestasis
infectious
  viral (FIP, Infectious Canine Hepatitis, Parvovirus)
  bacterial (leptospirosis, septicemia)
  mycotic
neoplasia
mechanical infiltrative—sinusoids, peribiliary
  paraneoplastic effects
drug associated

methyl testosterones	mebendazole
impeded androgens: Danazol	Thiacetarsemide
sulfa antibiotics	
anticonvulsants: phenytoin, primidone, phenobarbital	
acetaminophen	

specific hepatic disorders

cholangitis	cholangiohepatitis syndrome (cat)
cirrhosis	lobular dissecting hepatitis
chronic active hepatitis	breed-specific disorders
hepatic lipidosis (cats)	Bedlington terrier
idiopathic lipidosis	Doberman pinscher
2° to other disorders	West Highland white terriers
diabetes mellitus	Cocker spaniels
hepatic necrosis: many causes	severe steroid hepatopathy (dog only)

infiltrative disease
  (neoplasia, amyloid, infectious agents)

Impaired Hepatobiliary Bilirubin Processing: Congenital Defects

impaired uptake ± storage:	Gilbert's and Rotor's Dz (humans)
	Mutant South Down sheep
impaired conjugation:	Gunn rat. Gigler Najjar (humans)
	anorectic cats (?)
impaired excretion:	Mutant Corriedale sheep

From Center SA. Pathophysiology and laboratory diagnosis of hepatobiliary disorders. In: Ettinger SJ, Feldman EC (eds), Textbook of Veterinary Internal Medicine, 4th ed. Philadelphia, WB Saunders, 1995, 1285.

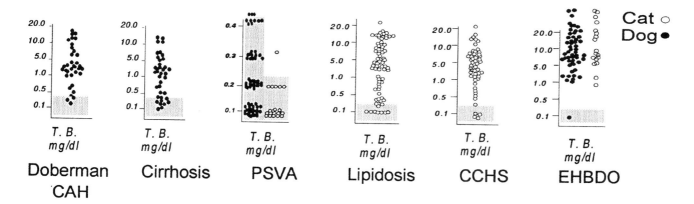

FIGURE 8-22. Scattergrams showing the total bilirubin concentrations in dogs and cats with various acquired hepatobiliary disorders and congenital portosystemic vascular anomalies (PSVA). Doberman CAH denotes chronic active hepatitis in the Doberman pinscher, Cirrhosis denotes dogs with cirrhosis and ascites, Lipidosis denotes cats with the severe hepatic lipidosis syndrome, CCHS denotes cats with the cholangitis/cholangiohepatitis syndrome, EHBDO denotes dogs and cats with extrahepatic bile duct obstruction. Normal range is shown by the shaded areas. Data derived from the College of Veterinary Medicine, Cornell University.

uptake, storage, conjugation, and biliary excretion. A general overview of bilirubin metabolism is given in Figure 8–21. Hyperbilirubinemia due to hemolytic processes is termed *prehepatic,* that due to hepatic parenchymal disease or insufficiency is termed *hepatic,* and that due to impaired bile excretion in the large biliary ducts is termed *posthepatic.* Diseases responsible for jaundice are shown in Table 8–7.

Unconjugated bilirubin is transformed into conjugated bilirubin by formation of glucuronide conjugates in the liver. Transport of bilirubin conjugates into canaliculi is energy dependent and the rate-limiting step of bilirubin excretion. When bilirubin has restricted entry into the biliary tract or when excessive liberation of heme pigments overwhelms the hepatobiliary processing/excretion of bilirubin, pigments regurgitate into the systemic circulation causing hyperbilirubinemia and jaundice. The plasma bilirubin concentrations increase only with moderate to severe parenchymal hepatic dis-

ease, and thus it is a relatively insensitive test for the detection of many liver diseases common in the dog. Comparatively, the cholestatic nature of feline liver disorders makes the total bilirubin a more sensitive test for liver disease in the cat than in the dog. The bilirubin values associated with selected clinical disorders in the dog and cat and the sensitivity of total bilirubin determinations are shown in Figures 8–22 and 8–23. The sensitivity of bilirubin for detecting significant parenchymal, cholestatic, or hepatic perfusion abnormalities is less than the sensitivity of fasting and postprandial bile acid concentrations in humans, the dog, and to a lesser extent the cat. Bile acid metabolism is disrupted by many of the same mechanisms that impair hepatic bilirubin processing, but the dynamics of the test permit detection of abnormalities at an earlier stage of injury.

Because conjugated bilirubin is less avidly protein bound than the unconjugated moiety, it can be excreted via glomeru-

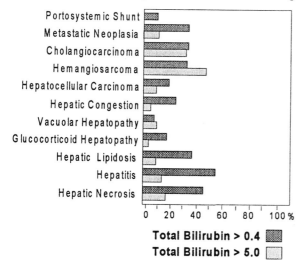

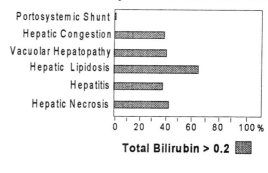

FIGURE 8-23. Comparison of the sensitivity of increased concentrations of total bilirubin in the diagnosis of hepatobiliary disorders in the dog and cat. For diseases in the dog, bilirubin values more than 0.4 mg/dl and more than than 5.0 mg/dl are shown. For diseases in the cat, bilirubin values more than 0.2 mg/dl are shown.

lar filtration. Dogs have a so-called low renal threshold for bilirubin elimination and thus routinely test positive for urine bilirubin; male dogs have a greater capacity than females to excrete bilirubin in urine.[250–252] Cats do not eliminate bilirubin in urine under normal circumstances; thus, finding urine bilirubin signals the presence of hyperbilirubinemia.[253] Excessive bilirubinuria generally indicates conjugated hyperbilirubinemia or reduced bilirubin-protein binding. Decreased protein binding can result from hypoalbuminemia or the competitive displacement of bilirubin from albumin by a variety of exogenous substances.[254] In the dog, urine bilirubin can be directly produced in the renal tubule cells from hemoglobin or biliverdin.[250,255–261]

After conjugation and transport into the biliary system, bilirubin is expelled into the intestines in bile. Conjugated bilirubin is not absorbed by enterocytes because of its poor lipid solubility. Rather, it is excreted in feces or metabolized by colonic bacteria to other products such as urobilinogens and stercobilinogens. A large amount of bilirubin in feces imparts a dark orange-brown to green stool color. The absence of bilirubin, such as occurs in extrahepatic bile duct occlusion, results in a pale tan or gray colored "acholic" stool. Acholic feces are seen in animals with complete obstruction of the biliary tract. However, if any gastroenteric bleeding develops, enough bilirubin pigment may enter the alimentary lumen to permit formation of stercobilins and conversion of acholic feces to a normal-appearing brown stool.

Urine Bilirubin and Urobilinogen

As discussed earlier, bilirubin is usually found in the urine of dogs. The renal threshold is so low that pigment appears in urine even when plasma bilirubin concentrations are normal. Detection of urine bilirubin is a semiquantitative assessment. The amount detected should be interpreted with consideration of the urine specific gravity. A large amount of bilirubin in concentrated urine is not unusual in the dog. The same amount in a dilute urine sample, however, may be due to prehepatic, hepatic, or posthepatic hyperbilirubinemia. Measurement of urine bilirubin concentrations in the context of anicteric plasma and a normal or near-normal PCV can help detect early liver disease.

Urine bilirubinuria is a more useful screening test in the cat as detection of urine bilirubin at any urine specific gravity in the cat is a strong indication of either an hepatobiliary or hemolytic disorder.[252,253] The sensitivity of urine bilirubin as a test for detection of hyperbilirubinemia and liver disease in cats has not been determined.

Nonhepatic or nonhemolytic processes can also increase urine bilirubin excretion. For example, small intestinal overgrowth can result in bacterial glucuronidases that deconjugate bilirubin-glucuronide in the gut. This leads to increased amounts of resorbed pigment, and potentially increased elimination of urine bilirubin. The use of the tablet method (Ictotest, R, Ames,) for the detection of bilirubinuria is more sensitive and reliable than the reagent strip method and is therefore the preferred procedure for clinical evaluation of feline urine.

Urobilinogen is a colorless product of enteric bacterial degradation of conjugated bilirubin. Approximately 20% undergoes enterohepatic circulation and biliary excretion.[262] A small fraction of absorbed urobilinogen is eliminated in urine where its detection provides evidence of alimentary formation and an intact enterohepatic circulation. The appearance of urobilinogen in urine is variable in each individual in that there is a diurnal cycle associated with food intake and gallbladder kinesis. The pH of the urine influences the urinary elimination of urobilinogen. In health, urobilinogen is both filtered through the glomerulus and secreted in the proximal renal tubule. Because it is a weak organic acid, is exists in an unionized and lipid soluble form in acidic urine. Thus, in acidic urine, passage through the distal tubules permits urobilinogen reabsorption. In alkaline urine, urobilinogen is largely ionized and little back diffusion occurs. Thus, little to no urobilinogen in acid urine is difficult to interpret, considering that small amounts may have been reabsorbed. It is also known that urobilinogen is unstable in acid urine and in light; as a result, prompt evaluation of a urine specimen is required for accurate estimation. As for urine bilirubin, the specific gravity of urine must be considered when the urobilinogen concentration is interpreted. Dilute urine may result in a urobilinogen concentration too low for detection with the conventionally used urine dipsticks.

Used as a test for the detection of liver disease, urobilinogen has its best application in the jaundiced patient where its absence implies a lack of bile duct patency. Unfortunately, the

Table 8–8

URINE UROBILINOGEN: TEST INTERPRETATION AND SHORTCOMINGS

True Positive
Reflects an intact enterohepatic circulation
  Bilirubin pigments reaching alimentary canal
  Bilirubin undergoing bacterial reduction to urobilinogen
  Intestinal absorption: 15% to 20% formed urobilinogen
  Verifies urobilinogen renal elimination routinely detected in healthy dogs and cats
  Hemolytic (Prehepatic) hyperbilirubinemia/jaundice
  Hepatobiliary (Hepatic) hyperbilirubinemia/jaundice
  Exaggerated positive test with constipation: ↑ deconjugation in gut leads to
    increased bilirubin for absorption

False Positive
Detected urobilinogen in complete bile duct occlusion
  GI hemorrhage
    endoparasitism
    gastroduodenal ulcer formation
    coagulopathy: factor deficiency, vitamin K deficiency

True Negative
Absence of bilirubin enterohepatic circulation
Complete extrahepatic bile duct occlusion
Rare in severe intrahepatic cholestasis

False Negative
Urobilinogen → ↑ urobilin (nonreactive with dipstick test)
  Urine exposure to light
  Prolonged urine storage
  Acid pH
Urine acidification: → ↓ renal tubule excretion
                      → ↑ renal tubule resorption
Dilute urine: insufficient concentration to detect
  ↓ Intestinal urobilinogen synthesis
  Deranged bacterial flora
    antibiotics
    bacterial overgrowth
    Intestinal malabsorption
    ↓ Intestinal transit time (diarrhea)

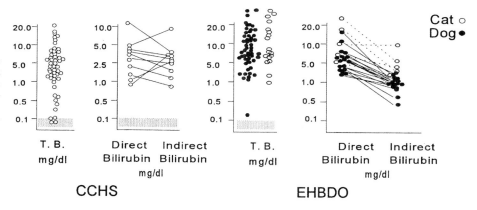

FIGURE 8-24. Scattergrams showing the concentrations of direct and indirect bilirubin in dogs and cats with cholestatic liver disease. Values for an individual animal are joined by an interconnecting line. Data derived from the College of Veterinary Medicine, Cornell University.

test has many shortcoming, in addition to the problems already discussed, which complicate its clinical application. These are summarized in Table 8–8. The alimentary urobilinogens that are not absorbed (approximately 80%) may undergo conversion to urobilins and stercobilins. These substances are responsible for the normal brown fecal pigmentation.

Van den Bergh Bilirubin Fractionation

The total serum bilirubin concentration can be fractionated into unconjugated and conjugated moieties using the van den Bergh reaction. Conjugated bilirubin reacts directly (direct bilirubin); unconjugated bilirubin does not (indirect bilirubin). Unconjugated bilirubinemia indicates increased heme pigment liberation and/or delayed hepatic bilirubin uptake, storage, or conjugation. Acute hemolytic disorders initially cause unconjugated bilirubinemia. However, if the liver is normal, a rapid rise in conjugated bilirubin soon follows. Several studies of dogs with either hemolytic or hepatobiliary jaundice have shown that van den Bergh bilirubin fractionation has no clinical value. Mean values and ranges for various disorders are provided in Table 30–17.[263–268] In Figure 8–24, the values of conjugated and unconjugated bilirubin determinations are shown for animals with major cholestatic disorders. Scrutiny of this diagram reveals that many of these animals have large unconjugated bilirubin concentrations, not unlike values associated with hemolytic (prehepatic) jaundice.

The reason the van den Bergh tests provides useless information is because of the formation of biliprotein complexes. These are covalently bound complexes that form when the serum bilirubin concentration increases. These remain in circulation until the involved protein is catabolized. The fraction of total bilirubin that the biliprotein comprises increases with chronicity of disease as the circulating biliprotein moieties continue to accumulate.[269–273] Measurement of total bilirubin or the fraction of direct-reacting bilirubin is meaningless unless the fraction of biliproteins is known. This phenomenon in conjunction with the apparent efficiency of bilirubin conjugation and the relatively late presentation of the veterinary patient in the course of a hemolytic disorder limits the clinical usefulness of bilirubin fractionation. A better estimate of the importance of hemolysis in the genesis of hyperbilirubinemia is accomplished by evaluating a patient's hematocrit, erythrocyte morphology, serum biochemical profile, and, when necessary, determination of serum bile acid concentrations.

Serum and Urine Bilirubin in the Differential Diagnoses of Jaundice

Although less sensitive than the liver enzymes in identifying hepatobiliary disorders, the concentration of total bilirubin is a more specific indicator of hepatic disease. Using bilirubin values adjunctively with the serum enzymes improves the diagnostic performance of each test. Jaundice becomes clinically detectable when bilirubin values exceed 1.5 to 2.0 mg/dl. Conjugated bilirubinemia is the principal cause of tissue jaundice in the dog and cat. The variety of conditions associated with jaundice in clinical practice are presented in Table 8–7. The diagnostic approach to the jaundiced patient is shown in Figure 8–25; a discussion of this algorithm follows.

Distinguishing whether hemolysis is the cause of jaundice is usually easy. Careful evaluation of the PCV, RBC morphology, and specific examination for parasites and staining erythrocytes for Heinz bodies and reticulocyte identification is routinely accomplished. If the patient is anemic, it should be determined on the basis of a reticulocyte count whether the anemia is regenerative or nonregenerative; the formula for correction of the reticulocyte count is provided in the algorithm. In clinical practice, the reticulocyte index is often used without regard for additional adjustments for cell maturation. A ratio more than 1.0 is usually regenerative. A well-prepared blood smear should be examined for spherocytes, poikilocytes, and schistocytes. Spherocytes suggest immune-mediated cell injury and should be followed up with evaluation of a direct Coombs test. Spherocytes can develop in association with other disorders besides immune-mediated hemolytic anemia; these include disorders causing shearing effects on red cell membranes (vasculitis, hemangiosarcoma), postadministration of a whole blood transfusion, and conditions associated with altered splenic function. Poikilocytes (acanthocytes) are seen in a number of conditions, including hemangiosarcoma, hyperlipidemia, and liver disease in both the dog and cat. Schistocytes indicate the presence of microangiopathy, which can be associated with vasculitis, vascular tumors (hemangiosarcoma), dirofilariasis, or DIC. Evaluation for RBC agglutination, indicative of immune-mediated hemolysis, may be done on EDTA-anticoagulated blood, one drop of blood mixed with several drops of physiologic saline. Examination of a coverslipped wet mount will reveal agglutination and permit differentiation from rouleau, which will disperse when pressure is applied to the surface of the coverslip. If a prehepatic cause of jaundice is denied by the evaluations just described, the clinician focuses attention on the hepatobiliary system and moves on

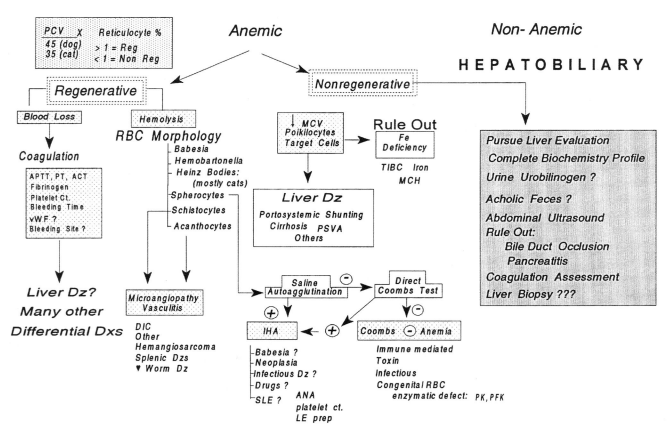

FIGURE 8–25. Algorithm showing the diagnostic approach to the small animal patient with hyperbilirubinemia or jaundice.

to the systematic evaluations according to the general algorithm provided in Figure 8–1.

When liver disease is responsible for jaundice, a severe diffuse cholestatic disorder or major bile duct obstruction should be suspected. When a primary cholestatic disorder is the underlying problem, jaundice usually develops earlier in the course of the disease than with parenchymal disease. Total bilirubin concentrations documented in dogs and cats with different forms of hepatobiliary disease are shown in Figure 8–22. As shown in this diagram, the total bilirubin concentration cannot differentiate between various disorders because there is wide overlapping in the bilirubin concentrations.

In extrahepatic bile duct obstruction, hyperbilirubinemia develops within several hours and jaundice may be detectable as early as 48 hours. Within 3 to 5 days of obstruction, serum bilirubin concentrations may increase 10- to 20-fold normal. With chronic bile duct obstruction exceeding 14 days, serum bilirubin levels may plateau at levels up to 50- to 70-fold normal and then gradually decrease, but not to normal concentrations.[65,67,69,71] In severe acute diffuse hepatic necrosis, bilirubin may increase twofold within 1 to 4 days but then declines if reparative processes and reserve capacity can reestablish normal liver function.

The clinical differentiation between intrahepatic and extrahepatic causes of jaundice is important because these conditions require profoundly different managements. Extrahepatic jaundice is a mechanical problem that often requires prompt surgical intervention. Intrahepatic cholestasis benefits from nonsurgical therapy; this condition may be worsened by

the stresses of general anesthesia and surgical exploration. Differentiating between extrahepatic and intrahepatic cholestasis cannot be accomplished on the basis of laboratory tests alone, but requires consideration of the information derived from the patient's history, physical examination, survey radiographs, and abdominal ultrasonography; see the diagnostic algorithm for evaluation of disorders of the biliary system in Chapter 37, Figure 37–2.

Cholangiography has not been useful as a routine test in dogs or cats. Ultrasonographic examination of the hepatobiliary structures is the most important noninvasive diagnostic evaluation that can be accomplished (see later). Liver function testing is superfluous if cholestasis is suspected on the basis of hyperbilirubinemia and other baseline laboratory tests. In differentiating intrahepatic from extrahepatic cholestasis, the complete clinical evaluation has better accuracy than any one test procedure. In two separate studies of methods used to differentiate intrahepatic from extrahepatic jaundice in humans, the collective clinical evaluations had better overall accuracy than did computed tomography, ultrasonography, or radioisotope scanning.[274,275]

Jaundice associated with pancreatitis is one of the most challenging cholestatic conditions to diagnose and manage. Affected animals may develop intrahepatic or extrahepatic jaundice or have components of each. Some patients develop occlusion of the common bile duct subsequent to focal peritonitis and ascending cholangitis. These may require surgical biliary diversion such as cholecystojejunostomy. Not all such patients require immediate surgical intervention. Sequential evaluation of the total bilirubin concentration is more useful

Table 8-9

DISORDERS ASSOCIATED WITH HYPERBILIRUBINEMIA IN THE CAT			
SERUM TOTAL BILIRUBIN CONCENTRATION			
1.0–3.0 mg/dl		**> 3.0 mg/dl**	
Disease	*Prevalence*	*Disease*	*Prevalence*
Renal disease	21%	Hepatic disease	68%
Infectious panleukopenia	13%	Lipidosis	(24%)
Gastrointestinal disease	12%	Hepatitis	(18%)
Hepatic disease	10%	Ill defined (toxic)	(16%)
Lymphosarcoma	10%	Biliary obstruction	(5%)
Trauma	10%	Hepatic neoplasia	(5%)
Feline infectious peritonitis	7%	Feline infectious peritonitis	14%
Pyometra	7%	Hemolytic anemia	7%
Other	7%	Lymphosarcoma	4%
		Others	7%

than measurements of liver enzymes, lipase, or amylase activities in deciding whether surgical therapy is indicated. Animals with serum bilirubin concentrations undergoing a continuous increase over a course of 7 to 10 days usually benefit from surgical intervention.

Cats ill from a variety of disorders may develop mild hyperbilirubinemia in the absence of overt hepatic disease or dysfunction. This phenomenon is not yet understood. It is possible the cat undergoes impaired hepatic biliary processing involving either the conjugation reactions or cytosolic pigment transport or storage when systemically ill or anorectic. The fact that many of these animals have normal serum bile acid concentrations suggests this is a problem with bilirubin processing. It appears that some of these cats develop liver disease as a consequence of their underlying primary disorder, and subsequently develop signs of liver dysfunction (increased total serum bile acids). Health problems associated with increased total bilirubin concentrations in cats lacking overt clinical evidence of hepatic disease are shown in Table 8–9. Unfortunately, evaluation of liver tissue, the gold standard for ruling in or out clinically significant hepatobiliary disease, has not been rigorously accomplished in this group of animals. Primary hepatic disease is more likely when the serum total bilirubin concentration is more than 3.0 mg/dl.

LIVER FUNCTION TESTS

The high sensitivity but relative lack of specificity of liver enzymes for detecting hepatobiliary disease makes it necessary to use other tests that provide information about liver function and circulation. When clinical signs remain unexplained after examination of routine tests, and liver disease is still highly suspected, to determine if clinically significant liver disease is present and/or to determine the propriety of liver biopsy, functions tests are done. Total serum bile acids, ammonia tolerance testing, and organic anion dye clearance are used in this regard.

It is important to remember that some liver diseases have increased liver enzyme activity as their single early test abnormality. Liver function may be normal. If continued liver enzyme activity is documented over several weeks and an underlying disease or condition remains undiscovered (in the dog, liver enzyme induction due to drug therapy, hyperadrenocorticism, or stress of disease is ruled out, and in the cat, hyperthyroidism is ruled out), a liver biopsy is still pursued.

Cholephilic Dyes: Sulfobromophthalein (BSP) and Indocyanine Green (ICG)

The organic anion water soluble cholephilic dyes sulfobromophthalein (BSP) and indocyanine green (ICG) have been used clinically to evaluate hepatic perfusion and hepatobiliary function. Their use has declined during the last decade owing to severe perivascular inflammation associated with extravasation of BSP during intravenous injection, so-called allergic anaphylactoid responses to BSP in human beings, the inconveniences associated with preparation and measurement of ICG, and most importantly, because of the numerous variables that influence plasma clearance calculations. Both dyes are high-extraction substances with clearance primarily determined by the rate of circulatory delivery to hepatocytes and hepatocyte dye excretion into the biliary tree. ICG may undergo capacity-limited elimination in the dog because experimental work has been unable to document the high-extraction ratio of 0.5 to 0.8 shown for humans.[276–282] The hepatic extraction ratio in healthy dogs is 0.09 to 0.24.[283,284] ICG entirely depends on hepatobiliary excretion, having a 97% recovery in bile. BSP has a bile recovery ranging between 50% and 80%.[276,277] Following intravenous injection, each dye is instantaneously bound to plasma proteins. The major binding proteins are albumin and an alpha-1-lipoprotein.[278]

Hepatobiliary excretion, shown in Figure 8–26, involves a complex series of processes, including (1) delivery to the hepatocyte, (2) uptake into the cell, (3) binding to cytosolic carrier proteins, (4) binding to cytosolic storage proteins, (5) biotransformation (BSP conjugation), (6) passage into the canalicular network, and (7) biliary excretion.[276–286] Abnormalities in any of these steps will alter the plasma dye disappearance. ICG is believed to be a better indicator of hepatic function than BSP. The avid protein binding of the former allows a more predictable volume of distribution and restricts its extrahepatic removal.[281,282] In addition, unlike BSP, ICG does not undergo an enterohepatic circulation.

Clinical use of BSP and ICG has been either as time-limited retention tests conducted after a single intravenous injection or as plasma clearance studies in which plasma samples are collected before and incrementally after a single intravenous dye injection. The most experience in clinical practice has been with the 30 minute percentage retention study using BSP in the dog and clearance of ICG in dogs and cats.

Despite the fact that plasma disappearance of these dyes is regarded as a sensitive indicator of abnormalities in hepatic perfusion or function, there are many shortcomings in such use;

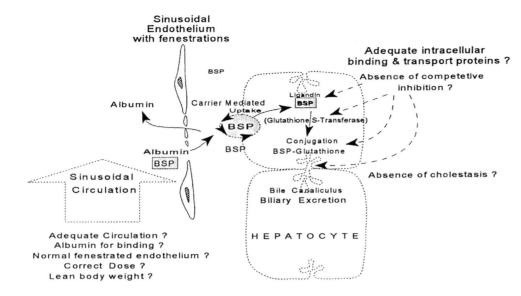

FIGURE 8-26. Diagram illustrating the variables influencing the hepatic uptake and metabolism of BSP and ICG.

these are detailed in Table 8–10, which corresponds to the following discussion.

Variables Influencing Clinical Utilization of BSP and ICG for Liver Function Testing

CIRCULATORY EFFECTS. Because they are high-extraction substances, the rate of circulation to the liver is an important determinant of their speed of plasma clearance. Reduced hepatic blood flow delivers less dye for hepatic uptake, causing prolonged dye retention. Any condition that impairs or slows hepatic blood flow has the potential to reduce the clearance of BSP or ICG. Extrahepatic portosystemic shunting, such as occurs with congenital portosystemic vascular anomalies, acquired portal hypertension, portal thromboem-

bolism, or portal vein occlusion, each predictably prolong plasma dye clearance. The presence of intrahepatic shunting, as occurs with cirrhosis when the sinusoids undergo capillarization and connective tissue becomes a barrier between the hepatocyte and its circulation, also causes a marked delay in plasma dye clearance. Any hepatic or posthepatic lesion interfering with flow from the hepatic veins into the vena cava and heart can also cause a marked decrease in dye clearance. Pericardial disease, pericardial tamponade, cardiac dysfunction, vena caval occlusion, or extensive pulmonary thromboembolism can each cause passive congestion in the liver that impairs hepatic perfusion and dye elimination. Severe hypotension associated, for example, with dehydration, shock, pancreatitis, Addison disease, or endotoxemia, can also diminish hepatic perfusion to the extent that plasma dye clearance is impaired.

Table 8–10

PROBLEMS ASSOCIATED WITH USE OF BSP AND ICG AS INDICATORS OF HEPATOBILIARY FUNCTION

PROBLEM	CAUSE	EFFECT
Miscalculated dose	Obesity Inaccurate weighing Ascites Edema	Dye overdosage ↑ percentage retention
↓ Protein binding	Hypoalbuminemia Competitive displacement	Extravascular dye dispersal Accelerated clearance
↓ Hepatic perfusion	Congestive heart failure Pericardial disease/tamponade Dirofilariasis Systemic hypotension Obstructed thoracic vena cava: tumor, stricture, kink	Delayed plasma clearance
Miscellaneous effects	Fever Hyperbilirubinemia Drugs interactions	Altered clearance Altered uptake, storage, excretion Competitive uptake/excretion Impaired binding to hepatic storage proteins Impaired BSP conjugation Altered hepatic perfusion

Table 8–11

HEPATIC FUNCTION TESTS: NORMAL VALUES FOR DOGS AND CATS

	DOSE	NORMAL VALUES
Sulfobromophthalein (BSP)	2.2 mg/kg IV	30 minute % retention ≤ 5.0% dog ≤ 2.0% cat
Indocyanine Green (ICG)	1.0 mg/kg IV 1.5 mg/kg IV	30 minute % retention ≤ 14.7 ± 5.0% dog ≤ 7.3 ± 2.9% cat
		Clearance mL/minutes/kg (0 to 15 minutes) 3.7 ± 0.7 dog 8.6 ± 4.1 cat
Ammonia Tolerance Test	100 mg/kg PO, (not to exceed 3 g)	30 minute < 50–100 µmol/L
	2.2 mL/kg 55 solution rectal catheter inserted 20 to 35 cm into colon	20, 40 minutes < 100 µmol/L
Total Serum Bile Acids	Endogenous test feed diet equivalent to: p/d* for dogs c/d* for cats	Fasting Postprandial < 5 µmol/L < 15.5 µmol/L dog ≤ 2 µmol/L < 10 µmol/L cat
		High sensitivity and specificity for histomorphologic lesions and portosystemic shunting with enzymatic analysis: values > 25 µm/L in dog values > 20 µm/L in cat

*Hills Pet Products, Topeka, KS.

PLASMA PROTEIN BINDING. ICG is more avidly bound to plasma proteins than BSP; approximately 90% of ICG is protein bound compared to 60% of BSP. Their extent of protein binding determines the degree of extravascular dispersal and renal excretion that can occur. Hypoproteinemia or any factor that serves to reduce protein binding of the organic anion dyes can influence their rate of plasma elimination. Substances competitive for protein binding, including certain drugs that are highly protein bound (e.g., aspirin) and hypoalbuminemia, permit extravascular dye dispersal and renal elimination. Although reduced protein binding does impair hepatic presentation and extraction of the dyes, the overbearing influence of extravascular dispersal facilitates plasma clearance. Severe hypoalbuminemia (≤ 1.5 g/dl) has been associated with normal BSP plasma retention percentages in animals with cirrhosis and with congenital portosystemic vascular anomalies.

HEPATIC UPTAKE, BSP CONJUGATION, AND HEPATIC STORAGE. The rate of plasma dye clearance is influenced by the rate of hepatic uptake. It is believed this is a carrier-mediated process facilitated by the presence of albumin or other binding protein(s). Certain cytoplasmic proteins, most notably a glutathione-S-transferase, serves as storage protein and facilitates the conjugation of BSP with glutathione. The cytosolic binding protein (also referred to as ligandin) also binds with other organic anions, including bilirubin. Approximately 75% of BSP is conjugated; the remainder is eliminated in unconjugated form. When the dose of BSP given exceeds the hepatocellular capacity for dye excretion in bile, the hepatocyte continues to uptake plasma dye and to store it in the cytosol (mainly in unconjugated form). When excessive quantities accumulate, small amounts may return to the plasma (regurgitation). When the hepatic uptake maximum is saturated, and cytosolic dye exceeds the rate of biliary elimination, the amount of dye regurgitating into plasma increases. Fortunately, the hepatocellular storage capacity for

ICG and BSP is great enough that it is never exceeded in normal animals given conventional diagnostic quantities.

EXCRETION INTO BILE. The most important rate limiting step in the hepatobiliary clearance of the organic anion dyes is their secretion into canaliculi. The nature of the transport mechanism for the organic anion dyes is not completely understood, although it is known that certain bile acids may facilitate the rate of elimination. The choleretic action of bile acids is thought to produce this effect. It is for this reason that dye retention studies are done during a fasting interval, to avoid bile acid facilitated dye elimination.

IMPORTANCE OF CORRECT DYE DOSAGE AND RAPID INTRAVENOUS BOLUS INJECTION. The dose of BSP and ICG recommended for function testing is provided in Table 8–11. It is important that lean body weight be used to calculate the correct diagnostic dose. Hepatic mass and intravascular volume is known to be proportional to lean body weight, and standard curves used for analysis of BSP are based on the dose calculated for this relationship.[285,286] In animals that are obese, or have edema or ascites, an inappropriately large dye dose may be given if this concept is not considered. Subsequently, the percentage retention will appear factitiously increased. This also occurs in healthy animals given an inappropriately large dye dose.

COMPETITIVE SUBSTANCES. As previously discussed, any substance or drug that competes for protein binding with BSP or ICG can alter the kinetics of plasma clearance. Certain drugs can also impair by competition the hepatic uptake and binding of the organic anion dyes to hepatic transport and storage proteins. The hepatocellular uptake of BSP and ICG is carrier mediated and is competitively inhibited by other organic anions, including bilirubin but not bile acids.[281,287] Some substances impair the conjugation of BSP, which slows its biliary elimination. Certain drugs that alter hepatic perfusion can impair or facilitate hepatic dye uptake. Bilirubin is the best recognized competitive substance that markedly slows the plasma clearance of the organic anion dyes. This occurs not only because of competition for hepatic uptake, but also due to competition for storage and biliary excretion. Neither retention nor plasma clearance studies using the organic anion dyes can differentiate the causes of jaundice in the dog and cat.

Clinical Applications

The many variables involved with the hepatic extraction, processing, and biliary excretion of the organic anion dyes has produced spurious test results in clinical patients. Neither BSP nor ICG are sensitive enough to use as screening tests for detection of mild to moderate liver disease. ICG can detect liver dysfunction following 60% but not 40% hepatectomy in the dog.[288]

Serum clearance of ICG has been shown to decrease in dogs with experimentally induced hepatic congestion and toxic hepatitis.[288-290] However, in some experimental models of liver injury, BSP appears to be a more sensitive indicator than ICG of induced hepatic damage.[67] For example, although CCl_4 and bile duct obstruction cause BSP retention times to increase to 6- to 10-fold within several days, they alter ICG retention to a lesser degree. Abnormalities in liver function following liver injury can be detected for longer periods with BSP than with ICG. In dogs with dimethylnitrosamine-induced progressive hepatic disease, BSP percentage retention and increased fasting and postprandial bile acid concentrations were abnormal hepatic function tests in dogs with mild histologic injury.[289] In dogs with moderate to severe injury, delayed ICG clearance, postprandial hyperammonemia, increased BSP percentage retention, and abnormal fasting and postprandial bile acids coexisted (Table 8–12).[289] Studies of the hepatic extraction of ICG in dogs with chronic dinitrosamine-induced liver injury have produced conflicting results.[289,290] One study suggests that chronic liver injury reduces ICG hepatic extraction; another suggests that injury impairs the rate of dye delivery to the hepatocyte. Following partial hepatectomy, hepatic regeneration correlates well with the return of normal ability to extract ICG, whereas abnormal BSP retention can persist. This is believed to reflect the disorganized sinusoidal configuration and altered microcirculation that may influence BSP uptake to a greater extent than ICG.

It is not possible to make judgments on the degree of hepatic damage or the nature of the damage when an abnormal BSP or ICG retention is found because both circulatory and hepatocellular variables contribute to dye elimination. In all forms of liver disease, BSP and ICG tests are poorly correlated with the degree of clinical signs of hepatic dysfunction. An animal with only 50% of its normal liver mass can be clinically normal and have profoundly increased BSP 30 minute percentage retention.

Similar to the finding with bile acids, BSP retention becomes abnormal prior to the overt onset of jaundice. This has been shown in dogs with experimentally induced complete bile duct obstruction. In dogs with a baseline normal BSP 30 minute retention of 2%, complete bile duct obstruction caused BSP retention to increase to 11% to 12% within two days.[67] It remained increased at 14% to 18% for another week, after which it decreased to 7%.

The increased sensitivity of BSP as compared to ICG for the detection of induced hepatic damage is likely related to its dependency on hepatic metabolism prior to elimination. The BSP retention time can be abnormal in the absence of any other biochemical or histomorphologic evidence of liver disease. The abnormal retention can result from a defect in one or more steps in liver metabolism of BSP. This type of defect has been reported in a dog.[291]

The sensitivity for detection and the quantitative estimation of functional liver mass with BSP and ICG are improved with large dye doses that saturate hepatic uptake and storage processes. Such doses are not advocated for use in clinical diagnostic testing. The information provided by measuring plasma dye concentration at a single point in time is of limited value because it represents the combined effects of hepatic blood flow, uptake, metabolism, and biliary excretion, and is subject to many inaccuracies. Monitoring plasma dye disappearance using several sequential measurements is a more sensitive and reliable method for detection of hepatobiliary dysfunction. In humans the initial fractional disappearance rate of BSP or ICG provides the best discrimination between normal controls and patients with liver disease; this is also suspected to be true in animals.[67,290,292,293] Clearance studies, however, are too cumbersome for routine clinical use because they require multiple venipunctures and carefully timed sample collection.

The plasma clearance of BSP and ICG is much faster in the cat than in the dog and it appears that ICG is the preferable dye for use in the cat.[294] Doses used for liver function testing and normal values for BSP and ICG percentage retention and clearance, respectively, are provided in Table 8–11.[294,295]

Ammonia and Urea as Function Tests

Determination of the blood ammonia concentration provides a measure of hepatic function. Urea is synthesized in the liver as the major metabolic end product of hepatic ammonia detoxification (see Chapter 30).

Because of the large functional reserve and tremendous regenerative capabilities of the liver, a reduced capacity to degrade ammonia does not develop until more than 70% of

Table 8–12

ALTERATION IN LIVER FUNCTION TESTS IN DOGS CHRONICALLY INTOXICATED WITH DINITROMETHYLAMINE[288] (MEAN ± SD)

| Function Test | DEGREE OF HISTOMORPHOLOGIC INJURY | | | Normal Value |
	Mild	Moderate	Severe	
BSP % (30 minutes)	18.2 ± 7.0	38.6 ± 16.6	25.2 ± 11.4	$< 5\%$
ICG mL/minutes/kg plasma clearance (60 minutes)	5.1 ± 3.6	0.8 ± 0.44	2.52 ± 2.0	5.6 ± 1.9
Postprandial NH_3 µg/dl	137.2 ± 201.2	329 ± 120	110 ± 126	$30 - 50$
Fasting bile acids µmol/L	56.7 ± 95.3	122 ± 92	50.4 ± 41.2	1 to 3
Postprandial bile acids µmol/L	148.9 ± 119.2	198 ± 105	197 ± 99	6 to 20

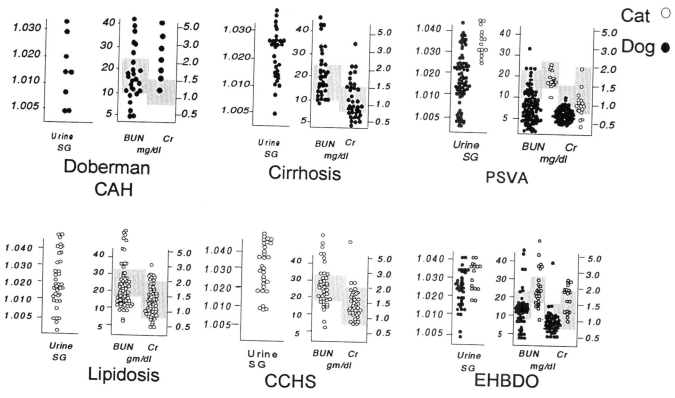

FIGURE 8-27. Scattergrams showing the serum BUN and creatinine concentrations in dogs and cats with various acquired hepatobiliary disorders and congenital portosystemic vascular anomalies (PSVA). Doberman CAH denotes chronic active hepatitis in the Doberman pinscher, Cirrhosis denotes dogs with cirrhosis and ascites, Lipidosis denotes cats with the severe hepatic lipidosis syndrome, CCHS denotes cats with the cholangitis/chlangiohepatitis syndrome, EHBDO denotes dogs and cats with extrahepatic bile duct obstruction. Normal range is shown by the shaded areas. Data derived from the College of Veterinary Medicine, Cornell University.

the normal hepatic synthetic capacity has been lost.[296] Insufficient ammonia detoxification can result from a reduction in hepatic mass, a decline in activity of hepatocellular enzymes, or portosystemic shunting of blood in which the delivery of ammonia to the liver is impaired. Experimentally, insufficient ammonia detoxification correlates better with derangements in portal circulation than with loss of functional hepatic mass.[295a,297–299] Ammonia intolerance is demonstrable in dogs with 60% hepatectomy but not with 40% hepatectomy.[288] In clinical patients, ammonia intolerance is most often encountered in those with congenital portosystemic shunts or acquired liver disease associated with intrahepatic or extrahepatic circulatory deviations.

A low blood urea nitrogen (BUN) concentration can reflect a reduced ability to synthesize urea. However, as a test of liver insufficiency, the BUN has low sensitivity and low specificity. There are too many extrahepatic variables that influence the BUN. The serum urea and creatinine concentrations in animals with various hepatic disorders are shown in Figure 8–27. An interesting phenomenon is the occurrence of both subnormal BUN and creatinine concentrations in dogs with portosystemic vascular anomalies. This phenomenon may be explained by experimental work in which portosystemic shunting has been associated with an increased GFR.

In exceptional cases, hyperammonemia develops as a result of unusual inborn metabolic aberrations.[301] Hyperammonemia has been reported in two dogs with suspected congenital absence of argininosuccinate synthetase, one of the urea cycle enzymes.[302] Hyperammonemia has been reported in cats fed an experimental high-protein diet devoid of arginine.[303,304] Because arginine is an essential amino acid for the cat, it is proposed that hyperammonemia developed from insufficient urea cycle activity. Obstructive uropathies complicated by infection with urease-producing bacteria have also been reported as a cause of hyperammonemia in humans[305,306] and in a dog.[307]

BLOOD AMMONIA DETERMINATIONS. Blood ammonia concentrations have been used as evidence of hepatic encephalopathy because they are one of the few cerebral toxins that can be quantified. Ammonia measurements have high specificity but low sensitivity for the detection of serious hepatic disease. Clinical laboratory determination of blood ammonia values requires laborious efforts at maintaining high quality control. Samples for ammonia determinations must immediately be stored on ice, centrifuged in a precooled environment, and assayed as soon as possible (within 1 hour is recommended). Insufficient separation of plasma from erythrocytes can invalidate ammonia measurements because red cells contain two- to threefold as much ammonia as plasma.[308–313] Ammonia may also generate in stored plasma, possibly due to hydrolysis of protein or other ammoniagenic substances.[311,313–318] A study of ammonia lability in feline blood showed that plasma samples may be stored frozen at −20° C for up to 48 hours before assay if promptly separated from erythrocytes.[317] A similar study with canine plasma indicated that storage for any length of time resulted in spurious high or low ammonia values.[318] Plasma samples for ammonia determinations cannot be sent through the mail for analysis. Use of dry chemistry systems for determining blood ammonia concentrations have also produced unreliable results in the author's experience. The concentration of ammonia in arterial blood seems to be more reliable than that in venous blood because venous samples may reflect regional circulatory changes and local tissue metabolism.[319,320] Occlusion of a vein for blood collection for too long an interval or vigorous muscular activity can result in increased venous ammonia concentrations.[299,320] Although arterial samples seem to be subject to fewer artifactual influences, such samples are technically difficult and injudicious to collect in patients with a potential for pathologic hemorrhage. As a result, venous samples are routinely used to measure blood ammonia concentrations in clinical patients.

The other major shortcoming of the measurement of blood ammonia concentrations is that hyperammonemia is not consistently demonstrable in patients with hepatic encephalopathy because other toxic substances are involved in the genesis of the syndrome. Ammonia tolerance is not adequately or uniformly assessed by measurement of fasting or postprandial plasma ammonia concentrations. Hyperammonemia is more consistently documented in patients with hepatic insufficiency or portosystemic shunting following a provocative test of hepatic ammonia detoxification.

AMMONIA TOLERANCE TESTING. Ammonia tolerance testing can be accomplished using solutions of ammonium chloride (NH_4Cl) administered orally, per rectum by catheter-administered enema, or by oral administration of a NH_4Cl powder in a gelatin capsule.[319,321,322] The gelatin capsule method yields results comparable to solutions administered orally or rectally and is technically simpler to perform. The standard oral tolerance test is conducted following oral administration of 100 mg/kg body weight of NH_4Cl in a dilute solution (concentration not to exceed 20 mg/mL and total dose of 3 g). Heparinized blood samples are obtained by collection into ammonia-free heparinized vacutainers before and 30 minutes after NH_4Cl administration. Use of concentrated solutions may induce vomiting, which will invalidate the test if a majority of the test solution is expelled. Occasionally, acute ammonia toxicity may be apparent by demonstration of hypersalivation and aberrant behavior. The oral test depends on normal gastric emptying and intestinal transit rates for optimal challenge of the patient's ability to extract ammonia from the portal circulation. The rectal tolerance test is conducted after a 12 hour fast and cleansing enema. Ammonium chloride is administered as a 5% solution at a dose of 2.2 mL/kg body weight by catheter at a depth of 20 to 35 cm in the rectum. Heparinized blood samples are collected before and at 20 and 40 minutes following NH_4Cl administration. Some animals expel the solution immediately. Those with preexistent diarrhea are poor subjects for the rectal tolerance test. Spurious hyperammonemia can result from solution administered too shallow in the colon as a result of absorption through hemorrhoidal veins.

The oral tolerance tests are more commonly used than the rectal test; it is believed that oral administration of ammonia produces a more consistent evaluation of ammonia detoxification as compared to rectal instillation. Rectal instillation may be used to diagnose portosystemic vascular anomalies, but the ammonia challenge via this route is not great enough to detect ammonia intolerance reliably in animals with acquired parenchymal dysfunction. Occasionally, ammonia intolerance in animals with portosystemic shunts involving splenic vasculature will miss detection using this method. Regardless of the type of test performed, a control sample from a fasted healthy animal should be concurrently evaluated to ensure proper procedures were used in managing blood samples and the ammonia assay was correctly performed. In normal animals, blood ammonia concentrations remain unchanged or increase up to twofold greater than baseline fasting values at 30 minutes after oral NH_4Cl administration. In animals with compromised hepatic function, fasting ammonia values may be normal or up to 10-fold normal. Following the administration of NH_4 blood ammonia concentrations usually range between 3- and 10-fold baseline values in patients with hepatic insufficiency or portosystemic shunting.

In conclusion, although evaluation of ammonia tolerance is useful in the diagnosis of hepatic insufficiency and hepatic encephalopathy, the technical difficulties associated with the test limit its application in most clinical situations. The comparable sensitivity in detecting hepatic insufficiency, the increased convenience, and the stability of bile acids during sample transport make the serum bile acid tolerance test more appropriate for routine clinical use. Each of these tests is more specific than BSP

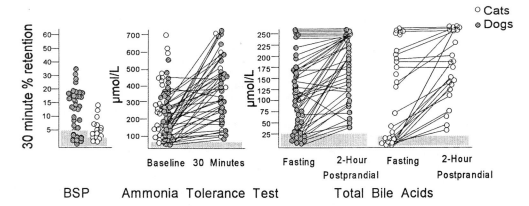

FIGURE 8-28. Scattergrams showing the BSP 30 minute percentage retention, blood ammonia concentrations before and after challenge with NH_4Cl, and fasting and postprandial serum bile acids in animals with congenital portosystemic vascular anomalies. Normal range is shown by the shaded areas. Data derived from the College of Veterinary Medicine, Cornell University.

or ICG for the detection of hepatic circulatory impairment because of the many variables that may influence organic anion pharmacokinetics (consult Table 8–10). Comparison of the performance of BSP, ammonia tolerance testing, and serum bile acids in the detection of portosystemic vascular anomalies is provided in Figure 8–28.

Uric Acid and Ammonium Urate Crystalluria/Calculi

Uric acid is a by-product of purine nucleotide catabolism.[323] Most dogs and cats transform uric acid to water soluble allantoin through the action of hepatic uricase. Some dogs, particularly Dalmatians, have an inborn error of uric acid metabolism whereby they cannot transform uric acid to allantoin. In animals with insufficient hepatic function, the serum concentration of uric acid may increase due to an acquired impairment in production of allantoin.[324,326] A tendency for hyperuricemia has been shown in dogs with experimentally produced portosystemic shunts.[300] Hyperuricemia also develops in patients with diffuse tissue destruction or inflammation causing increased catabolism of purine nucleotides.[327–331] Examples of such conditions include tissue infection and tumor lysis syndrome. Study of uric acid as a clinical test for liver disease in the dog showed it was a relatively insensitive measure of hepatic disease or function.[324,325] Its use has largely been abandoned because of limited clinical utility.

Ammonium urate crystalluria may develop in animals that have recurrent hyperammonemia. Ammonium biurate crystalluria and/or calculi, especially in young animals, dictates a thorough investigation for a congenital portosystemic shunt. Prior to the advent of ultrasonography, these radiolucent calculi were rarely detected unless clinical signs of urolithiasis were recognized. Routine use of abdominal ultrasonography has revealed the presence of renal and/or cystic calculi or sediment as a relatively common feature of a portosystemic vascular anomaly. Repeated examination of different urine specimens may be necessary to document ammonium biurate crystals in an individual patient. Recognition of ammonium urate crystalluria requires examination of urine sediment under 400× magnification with the microscope condenser lowered to improve sediment refraction. Crystals are usually golden brown, variably shaped, and commonly referred to as "thorn apple" in configuration. An example is shown in Figure 8–29. Clinical management of ammonium urate urolithiasis requires that liver function be appraised first. If hepatic insufficiency is detected, treatment should focus on liver disease. Interventional therapy with allopurinol has been suggested by some authors,[326] but there is no information on the safety or efficacy of its use in the veterinary patient with compromised liver function.

Serum Bile Acids

Measurement of total serum bile acids is a sensitive method of identifying hepatic disease associated with histologic lesions or impaired hepatic portal circulation. The physiology of bile acid metabolism is discussed comprehensively in Chapter 30.

Bile acids are exclusively synthesized in the liver. In humans, dogs, and cats, the major primary bile acids are cholic acid and chenodeoxycholic acid. Dehydroxylation of these moieties by intestinal microorganisms produces the more hydrophobic secondary bile acids; cholic acid is converted to deoxycholic

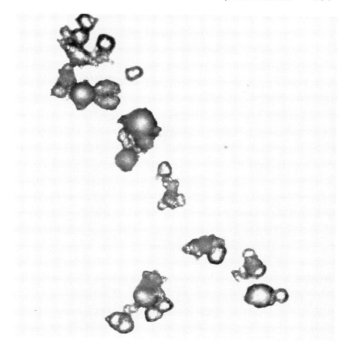

FIGURE 8-29. Photomicrograph showing the "thron apple" appearance of ammonium biurate crystalluria in urine from an animal with hyperammonemia due to hepatic insufficiency. (550× magnification)

acid and chenodeoxycholic acid to lithocholic acid. After synthesis, the primary bile acids are conjugated to an amino acid before excretion into bile; glycine and taurine are the major amino acid conjugates.[332] Approximately 95% of bile acids are absorbed in the ileum and return to the liver via the portal circulation. This enterohepatic circulation of bile acids is the basis for the provocative nature of the postprandial endogenous bile acid test.

Bile Acid Enterohepatic Circulation

After hepatic synthesis and conjugation, the primary bile acids undergo biliary excretion and are stored and concentrated in the gallbladder. Emptying of the gallbladder is usually, but not exclusively, initiated after meals following release of cholecystokinin. Cholecystokinesis can also occur sporadically such as during the night or a prolonged fast.[333–340] This variation causes some animals to have higher fasting than postprandial bile acid values. In health, the rate of intestinal absorption is the major factor determining serum bile acid concentrations in both fasting and postprandial intervals.[341,342] In a healthy animal, feeding induces only a very small postprandial increase in the total serum bile acid concentration as a result of the high efficiency of the enterohepatic circulation.[343] Bile salts returning to the liver in the portal circulation exceed the clearing capacity of the liver. It is this endogenous challenge that provides the clinical utility of the fasting and postprandial bile acid test. Animals with impaired hepatoportal perfusion, reduced hepatic mass, or cholestasis will develop high systemic bile acid concentrations. The dynamics of the enterohepatic circulation of bile acids are illustrated in Figure 8–30 and the many variables influencing the balance of this system are presented in Table 8–13.

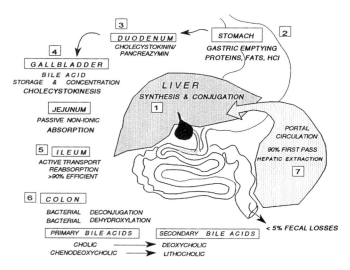

FIGURE 8–30. Bile acid enterohepatic circulation. Numbers correspond to variables discussed in Table 8–13 that influence the balance of this system. From Center SA. Serum bile acids in companion animal medicine. Vet Clin N Am (Sm Anim) 23:625–657, 1993.

Many factors influence the enterohepatic circulation of bile acids and can thereby influence individual and total serum bile acid concentrations. These include (1) the rate of bile acid synthesis, (2) meal synchronization and completeness of gallbladder emptying, (3) gastric emptying and intestinal transit rate, (4) the efficiency of ileal bile acid uptake, (5) the integrity of the portal circulation, (6) the function and patency of the biliary system, and (7) the enterohepatic cycling frequency. Variables that influence the use of an endogenous bile acid test and the ratio of trihydroxy to dihydroxy bile acids are summarized in Tables 8–13 and 8–14. The dynamics of the enterohepatic circulation influence the maximal bile acid concentration attained in the systemic circulation at a given point in time and thus influence the sensitivity of bile acid quantification as a test of hepatobiliary function. Individual variation in the components of the enterohepatic circulation may result in a submaximal challenge during the endogenous test. Rapid enterohepatic circulation, reduced intestinal absorption, incomplete gallbladder contraction, and an altered intestinal transit rate can each influence the optimal interval for postprandial sample collection. In order to best utilize serum bile acids as a clinical test, it is important to consider the variables that can alter their normal enterohepatic circulation and the optimal sampling interval for the provocative endogenous challenge. These are discussed in the section that follows.

Even though bile acid synthesis can become markedly reduced in the circumstance of serious liver disease, a number of variables collectively cause a marked increase in the serum bile acid concentrations. These include a more efficient enterohepatic cycling, reduced hepatic bile acid extraction, admixture of portal and systemic circulations due to portosystemic shunting, and regurgitation of bile acids due to cholestasis. Impaired hepatic synthesis of bile acids is always linked with an impaired ability to excrete bile acids into the canalicular system. As a result, there is no loss in test sensitivity when hepatic bile acid synthesis declines.

Chronic duodenal disease can be associated with mucosal injury severe enough to impair synthesis and release of cholecystokinin, the most important stimulus for gallbladder contraction. In such cases, normal meal-invoked cholecystokinesis does not occur and the enterohepatic circulation of bile

acids is altered. The optimal sampling interval for the bile acid test will vary from the normal dog.

Chronic diarrhea can alter small intestinal and colonic epithelium as a result of perturbed bile acid metabolism.[344] Some small-bowel disorders associated with bacterial overgrowth can alter enteric bile acid absorption. Increased bile acid deconjugation leads to rapid absorption of free bile acids in the proximal jejunum and subsequently, a reduced quantity of bile acids in the lower small bowel where they normally facilitate fat absorption. This results in steatorrhea and a perturbation of the appropriate diagnostic interval for postprandial sample collection. Loss or dysfunction of a critical volume of the terminal ileum as a result of inflammation or resection can cause bile acid malabsorption, which invalidates the use of the endogenous bile acid test. Severe diarrhea has also been observed to impair use of the endogenous bile acid test purportedly as a result of impaired absorption or enteric transit too rapid to permit bile acid absorption.

Impaired excretion of bile acids as a result of extrahepatic bile duct obstruction will prohibit their normal enterohepatic circulation. However, in this circumstance, the reflux of bile acids from hepatocytes into the ultrafiltrate in the perisinu-

Table 8–13

VARIABLES AFFECTING THE ENDOGENOUS SERUM BILE ACID TOLERANCE TEST

Dietary constituents: (2)*
  Inadequate fat or amino acid content for optimal cholecystokinin release, gallbladder contraction, and postprandial challenge of the enterohepatic circulation. Fiber binding of bile acids reduces their availability.

Inadequate meal consumption: (2)
  Food not consumed or insufficient ingested volume to optimally stimulate gastric emptying, gallbladder contraction, and ingesta/bile transport to the distal ileum at the 2 hour postprandial interval.

Delayed gastric emptying: (2)
  Results in a failure to stimulate gallbladder contraction and subsequently inadequate challenge of the enterohepatic circulation at the 2 hour postprandial interval.

Delayed intestinal transit: (2, 3, 5)
  Lack of optimal timing to evaluate optimally the postprandial challenge of the enterohepatic circulation.

Too rapid intestinal transit: (5, 6)
  Reduced intestinal absorption of bile acids and subsequently inadequate challenge of the enterohepatic circulation at the 2 hour postprandial interval.

Ileal disease or resection: (5)
  Reduced bile acid absorption resulting in an inadequate challenge of the enterohepatic circulation.

Small intestine malabsorption/maldigestion/steatorrhea: (5, 6)
  Altered bile acid absorption resulting in an inadequate challenge of the enterohepatic circulation.

Small intestinal bacterial overgrowth: (4, 5, 6)
  Bile acids metabolized reducing absorption of measured moieties.

Interdigestive gallbladder contraction: (3, 4)
  Normal physiologic variable; fasting bile acids more than postprandial values.

Delayed gallbladder contraction: (3, 4)
  Insufficient stimulation via cholecystokinin; absence of endogenous provocative challenge; fasting bile acids more than postprandial values.

Deviated or obstructed hepatoportal circulation: (7)
  Impaired presentation for bile acids for high extraction uptake by hepatocyte; spillover into the systemic circulation.

*Numbers correspond to those in Figure 8–30. From Center SA. Serum bile acids in companion animal medicine. Vet Clin N Am (Sm Anim) 23:625–657, 1993.

Table 8–14

INFLUENCE OF VARIABLES AFFECTING THE ENTEROHEPATIC CIRCULATION OF BILE ACIDS AND THEIR EFFECT ON THE ENDOGENOUS BILE ACID TEST

| | TOTAL SERUM BILE ACID CONCENTRATIONS | | |
	Fasting	Postprandial	Expected Qualitative Profile
Normal Subjects	Dog: < 5 μmol/L Cat: < 5 μmol/L	Dog: < 15 μmol/L Cat: < 10 μmol/L	Standard for comparison: trihydroxy > dihydroxy bile acids
Ileal dysfunction, ileal malabsorption	Subnormal	Subnormal, ↓ postprandial rise	↑ Unconjugated moieties
Fat malabsorption/maldigestion	Subnormal	Subnormal, ↓ postprandial rise	↑ Unconjugated moieties
Bacterial overgrowth	Variable	Variable	↑↑↑ Unconjugated moieties
Cholecystectomy, biliary diversion	Slightly ↑	Reduced rise, early postprandial rise	↑ Unconjugated moieties ↑ DCA vs. CA
Delayed gastric emptying	Slightly ↑; exceeds postprandial	Expected increase not realized	Normal
Rapid intestinal transit	Subnormal, variable	Subnormal	↓ Unconjugated
Delayed intestinal transit	May be increased; exceeds postprandial	Postprandial less than fasting value	↑ Unconjugated
Portosystemic shunting (congenital and acquired)	Normal after prolonged fast or ↑	Profound ↑↑↑; may see an acute change between fasting and postprandial values	↑ trihydroxy:dihydroxy ratio
Reduced hepatic mass	May be normal after prolonged fast or ↑	Profound ↑↑↑; may see an acute change between fasting and postprandial values	↓ trihydroxy:dihydroxy ratio ↑ sulfated moieties
Hepatic failure	Usually ↑	Profound ↑↑↑; may see an acute change between fasting and postprandial values	↓ trihydroxy:dihydroxy ratio ↑ sulfated moieties
Cholestasis	Profoundly ↑↑↑	Profoundly ↑↑↑; fasting and postprandial have similar values	May have ↓ unconjugated, ↑↑ sulfated, ↑↑ glucuronidated ↑ trihydroxy:dihydroxy ratio

soidal space of Disse carries them to the systemic circulation. Subsequently, the systemic concentration of bile acids becomes markedly increased.

Cholecystectomy and cholecystoduodenostomy or -jejunostomy do not invalidate use of the serum bile acid test. Both of these conditions increases the enterohepatic cycling of bile acids in the fasting state. The cholecystectomized patient has slightly high fasting serum bile acid concentration and slightly low, early, and a less acute postprandial serum bile acid increase. These patients develop increased quantities of secondary bile acids (dihydroxy bile acids) due to increased exposure to dehydroxylating intestinal anaerobes.

Although fecal losses of bile acids can increase when increased amounts of fiber are consumed, these losses do not deplete the bile acid pool and do not influence the clinical use of the serum bile acid test.

Shunting of portal blood to the systemic circulation has a profound effect on the serum bile acid concentration. As little as 5% of portal blood shunting around the liver can increase the fraction of bile acids escaping first-pass extraction by 100%.[345] Shunting of portal blood through the liver as a consequence of sinusoidal capillarization similarly limits the hepatic extraction of bile acids, causing markedly increased systemic concentrations. This has been repeatedly verified in dogs with congenital microscopic portovascular dysplasia; consult Chapter 35.

Variables known to impair the diagnostic utility of the organic anion indicator dyes (BSP and ICG) such as passive congestion, systemic hypotension, fever, hypoalbuminemia or hyperbilirubinemia, and administration of other organic anions (such as BSP or ICG), have not seemingly influenced the utility of serum bile acids to detect liver disease verified by

hepatic histology in the author's experience. If necessary, serum bile acid concentrations can be used to ascertain that jaundice is due to hepatobiliary disease rather than hemolysis. Serum bile acid values are normal when hemolysis is the single cause of hyperbilirubinemia. It is important to remember, however, that severe anemia can lead to hepatocellular injury and subsequently to reduced hepatic function.

Bile Acid Concentrations in Liver Disease

EXPERIMENTAL STUDIES. Experimental work has shown that serum bile acids are useful markers of impaired hepatic function or portal circulation. Results of an early study in dogs with CCl_4-induced hepatic injury showed that fasting bile acids increased from a normal value approximating 21 μmol/L to a maximum of 60 μmol/L.[346] These studies were done before sensitive and reliable methods were established for routine determination of bile acids that do not require organic extraction prior to analyses. These early studies probably were not as accurate as current methods permit. Later studies in dogs with liver injury induced by nitrosamines showed highly variable bile acid values that were often within the normal range; these studies did not use a provocative postprandial test.[293,347] A subsequent study of dinitrosamine-induced hepatic injury showed that total serum bile acids were as sensitive as BSP 30 minute percentage retention and superseded the sensitivity of ICG clearance and postprandial ammonia determinations (Table 8–12).[289] Dogs and cats with experimentally created complete bile duct obstruction develop profound increases in their serum bile acid concentrations,[69,348] and dogs with ligation of an hepatic duct develop modest increases in their fasting bile acid values.[97] Surgically created portosystemic shunts were shown to produce persistent but variable increases in the fasting serum bile acid concentrations in dogs lacking clinical signs.[300] Severe glucocorticoid hepatopathy induced by administration of large doses of dexamethasone in healthy dogs resulted in fasting bile acids 20-fold greater than normal.[97] This experimental work and a library of other studies investigating hepatic disease in animal models and in humans support the use of serum bile acids as a sensitive test of hepatic function and perfusion.

CLINICAL STUDIES. A large number of clinical patients have now been studied in which the histologic liver lesion has been characterized and used as the gold standard to verify the presence of significant hepatobiliary disease. These studies have clarified test reliability and predictive value. Interpretation of test "cutoff" values requires that the methodology used to quantify the bile acids be considered.

The diagnostic efficacy of fasting and 2 hour postprandial serum bile acid values in the dog and cat have established they are useful in the diagnosis of hepatobiliary disorders associated with histologic lesions or portosystemic shunting.[91,348–357] Overall, bile acid values have better specificity and predictive values than most routinely used tests confirming the presence of clinically significant liver disease. They improve the diagnostic performance of routine tests when used adjunctively.[91,341,352,353,356]

The total serum bile acid concentrations in dogs with histologically confirmed hepatobiliary diseases are shown in Figure 8–31. The following test performance statistics are *relevant only* for the direct enzymatic method for determining total serum bile acid values performed in a laboratory with optimal quality control aimed at elimination of test interference from lipemia (see later section on test methodology).[91,350,352,356] For all liver diseases associated with morphologic injury, specificity of fasting bile acids equals or exceeds 95% in the dog and cat at values more than 15 µmol/L. Specificity of postprandial bile acid values achieve 100% in the dog at more than 25 µmol/L and in the cat at more than 20 µmol/L. At these bile acid concentrations, the positive and negative predictive values are more than 92% in the dog and more than 97% in the cat in populations of animals in which liver disease was highly suspected on the basis of more routine information. In these studies, the overall test efficacy for fasting serum bile acids in the dog (n = 170) was 82% and in the cat (n = 108) was 66%, and for postprandial bile acids in the dog was 82% and in the cat was 81%.[91,356] In the dog a false positive test rate of only 2% was documented.[91]

The issue of whether fasting or postprandial serum bile acid values perform better remains controversial. The diagnostic efficacy of postprandial bile acid values in the dog are nearly identical to the fasting values in most disorders.[91] The diagnostic efficacy of postprandial values in the cat exceeds that of fasting values.[356] Postprandial values perform better in animals with portosystemic vascular anomalies, acquired shunts, or cirrhosis; these animals may have fasting bile acids within the normal range.[350,353,354,356] Use of both bile acid values provides the most reliable information in clinical patients because it reduces errors made due to gastrointestinal and gallbladder motility variables. The fact that early experimental work only involved fasting bile acid determinations compromised assessments of test efficacy.

Serum bile acid values cannot differentiate between liver disease because of the wide overlap in values among diseases (Figure 8–31). Particular patterns frequently (but not always) appear in the presence of shunting lesions, extrahepatic cholestasis, and intrahepatic cholestasis; these are shown in Figure 8–32. A normal liver rapidly clears bile acids so that only minor transient increases are realized in a postprandial serum sample. Deviation of the portal circulation, such as in portosystemic vascular anomalies or in some animals with cirrhosis, seriously impairs the enterohepatic bile acid cycle. Even though demonstrable extrahepatic portosystemic shunts may not exist, intrahepatic microcirculatory shunting occurs in cirrhosis due to sinusoidal changes and compres-

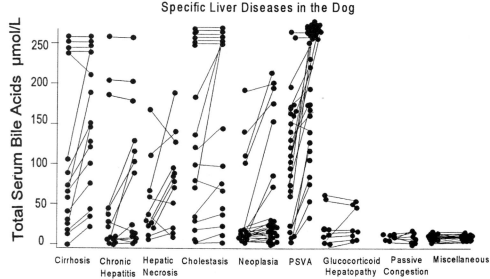

FIGURE 8–31. Scattergram showing the distribution of fasting and postprandial bile acid values in dogs with various hepatobiliary diseases. Data derived from the College of Veterinary Medicine, Cornell University.

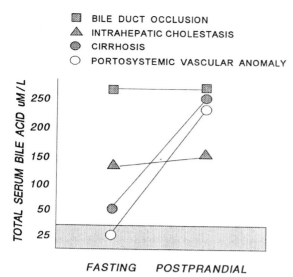

BILE DUCT OCCLUSION
INTRAHEPATIC CHOLESTASIS
CIRRHOSIS
PORTOSYSTEMIC VASCULAR ANOMALY

FIGURE 8–32. Diagram showing the "classic" patterns of fasting and postprandial bile acids in animals with various hepatobiliary disorders.

sion due to regenerative nodule formation. Diseases associated with cholestasis result in increased serum bile acid concentrations owing to reduced biliary bile acid excretion and regurgitation of bile acids into the systemic circulation. For these disorders, serum bile acids provide greater sensitivity in the early stages of disease than does determination of the total serum bilirubin concentration. This circumstance presents more commonly in the dog than in the cat.

The sensitivity of fasting and postprandial serum bile acids for particular canine and feline liver conditions is shown in Figure 8–33. Bile acids are not screening tests and should not be used alone to detect liver disease. Their best value is realized in combination with other more routine screening tests where they mutually improve test diagnostic utility. Combination of serum bile acid values with results of other liver tests may reveal useful diagnostic patterns. Abnormal bile acid concentrations in the absence of jaundice and increased liver enzyme activities indicate metabolically quiet liver disease associated with deranged hepatoportal perfusion or severely reduced hepatic mass. These findings typify occult cirrhosis, congenital portosystemic vascular anomalies, and microscopic portovascular dysplasia, especially when postprandial bile acid concentrations are greater than or equal to 250 μmol/L. A pattern typified by normal bile acid values in the presence of hyperbilirubinemia indicates prehepatic or

hemolytic jaundice. A pattern suggestive of glucocorticoid or vacuolar hepatopathy (in the dog only) includes marked increase in ALP activity, normal serum bilirubin, and normal to moderately increased bile acid values, coupled with the historical information or physical signs compatible with glucocorticoid excess. A pattern consistent with cholestasis includes marked enzyme abnormalities, especially increased ALP activity in the dog and increased ALP and GGT activities in the cat, moderate to marked hyperbilirubinemia, and marked increases in fasting and postprandial serum bile acid values. Animals with extrahepatic bile duct occlusion usually have bile acid values of more than 200 μmol/L and little if any difference exists between fasting and postprandial values. Animals with intrahepatic cholestasis often have increased fasting and postprandial bile acid values, but these are usually (but not always) lower than those associated with major bile duct occlusion. The pattern of intrahepatic cholestasis is extremely common in cats with liver disease including cholangitis, cholangiohepatitis, hepatic lipidosis, and neoplasia. A wide range of enzyme, bilirubin, and bile acid values are found in animals with primary and secondary hepatic neoplasia, depending on the extent and histologic distribution of the neoplastic process within the liver.

Bile acids cannot be used to estimate the severity or extent of liver injury. Quantification of bile acids only indicates the presence of "significant" hepatic injury. Relative changes in *abnormal* values *cannot* be used to quantify the improvement or worsening of a condition. A value is either abnormal or normal and has no linear relationship to extent of circulatory or tissue compromise due to the many variables involved.

Occasionally, clinically normal animals and animals with liver disease have fasting bile acid values that exceed the postprandial value. This is attributed to spontaneous gallbladder contraction during interdigestive intervals, delayed gastric emptying, slow intestinal transit, or differences from the norm in cholecystokinin release, alimentary response to cholecystokinin, or gastrointestinal tract flora. In consideration of these variables, it is noteworthy that differences in the optimal time of postprandial sample collection have been shown in humans with liver disease and in clinically normal dogs and cats.[358,359] Postprandial serum bile acid values may therefore be underestimated in some animals because sampling is not acquired at that individual's most optimal interval (when their enterohepatic challenge is maximized). Such individual variation can only be avoided by collecting blood samples frequently over a postprandial interval spanning 1 to 8 hours, which is unsuitable for clinical purposes.

A variety of uncommon factors may promote low serum bile acid values in the presence of hepatobiliary disease. Reduced flow of bile into the duodenum has been documented in some humans with early or transient obstruction

FIGURE 8–33. Comparison of the sensitivity of (fasting and postprandial) serum bile acid concentrations in dogs and cats with different hepatic disorders. A positive test was indicated by either value exceeding 25 μmol/L for dogs and 20 μmol/L for cats. Data derived from the College of Veterinary Medicine, Cornell University.

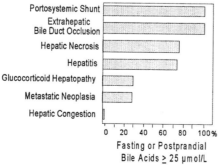

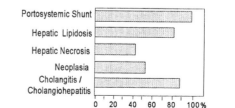

of the biliary tree. Intestinal malabsorption of bile acids will invalidate the test but this usually is obvious because the patient shows evidence of diarrhea and/or steatorrhea. In the author's experience, this is an uncommon complicating factor but has been seen in dogs with congenital vascular anomalies and severe hookworm or coccidia infestations. Failure of a patient to eat the test meal will result in an absence of enterohepatic bile acid cycling. This problem is avoided by visual confirmation that the test meal is consumed. Use of an inappropriate diet to invoke the enterohepatic bile acid cycle can also complicate test utilization.[357] Maintenance canine and feline diets for healthy animals usually contain sufficient protein and fat to trigger a normal enterohepatic cycle. Use of canned rations has been more reliable in the author's experience. It is also important to consider the quantity of food consumed. Too small an amount of food may fail to initiate proper cholecystokinin release, which initiates the test process. In the anorectic patient, blenderized food (liquified food fed with a dose syringe) is successful in standardizing food consumption. Minimal amounts of food for the endogenous bile acid test are 2 teaspoons for petite patients (≤ 10 lbs) and 2 tablespoons for larger patients. The clinician, however, should aim for a larger ingested volume if the animal is willing. In patients in which encephalopathic effects of protein are anticipated, a restricted protein food mixed with a small amount of corn oil can be used. The author has conducted many endogenous bile acid tolerance tests on dogs and cats with portosystemic vascular anomalies and with acquired hepatic insufficiency. Neuroencephalopathic complications from use of moderate amounts of canned maintenance rations are rare when they are not preceded by historical accounts of adverse food effects. In animals with congenital portosystemic vascular anomalies, a history of severe neuroencephalopathic signs contraindicates the feeding of normal maintenance rations.

Serum bile acid values are not indicated for use as screening tests. They should be used adjunctively with other routine tests when appropriate. Function tests are reserved for use when liver disease is suspected and the propriety of liver biopsy, colorectal scintigraphy, or mesenteric portography are being contemplated. In the author's experience, deciding to procure a liver biopsy on the basis of abnormal bile acid concentrations has led to earlier lesion characterization and few instances in which a histomorphologic lesion could not be characterized. One danger in the use of bile acids is when the laboratory evaluating the test does not eliminate lipemia from samples determined by the enzymatic method on automated analyzers. Spurious high and low values result and the test becomes virtually useless.

SERUM BILE ACID PROFILES. The percentage of individual bile acid moieties in serum and bile has been thoroughly studied in human beings with various types of liver injury.[359–368] Only limited information is available regarding bile acid profiles in serum and bile from dogs and cats with liver disease.[369–371] Serum bile acid profiles in normal dogs, dogs with portosystemic shunts, a dog with cholestatic neoplasia, normal cats, and cats with hepatic lipidosis and major bile duct occlusion have been characterized.[369–376] For further discussion of the alterations in serum bile acid profiles in patients with hepatic disease, see Chapter 30, the listed references, and Table 8–14.[369–376]

METHODS OF BILE ACID MEASUREMENT. Most laboratories use either the direct enzymatic method that quantifies total serum 3 alpha-hydroxylated bile acids or a radioimmunoassay (RIA) procedure that quantifies specific conjugated bile acid moieties.[377,378]

The enzymatic procedure has been clinically validated as a diagnostic test; bile acid values associated with histologic lesions have been statistically evaluated in populations of dogs and cats suspected of having hepatobiliary disease and having diagnoses-confirmed by liver biopsy.[91,349,350,352,355,356] This technique measures all 3 alpha-hydroxylated bile acids whether they are conjugated or not. It measures more bile acids than the RIA procedure(s). It provides a good estimate of serum bile acid concentrations because most of the common bile acids contain the 3 alpha-hydroxyl group. Test methodology requires that other dehydrogenases, such as lactic dehydrogenase (LDH), be inactivated before bile acids are measured and that hemolysis and lipemia be avoided. Hemolysis makes test end point indeterminable because hemoglobin overlaps with the absorbance spectra of the diformazen dye that forms in the reaction mixture and is related linearly to the quantity of bile acids in the sample being analyzed. Lipemia must be eliminated conscientiously from the test sample to avoid interference in the spectrophotometrically determined end point. This procedure requires vigilant quality control to avoid false positive and negative values. In some laboratories, the bile acid test has been adapted for automated analysis. These procedures may be invalid because of the interference with lipemia that does not receive the attention it requires. Comparison of test results among laboratories has shown marked variability in the quantities reported for a single sample due to these errors. It is the author's opinion that this test should be done by hand in order to obviate serious methodologic errors. Hemolysis can be avoided by collecting a blood specimen in heparin and harvesting plasma immediately. Blood should be placed in a vacutainer with the needle removed from the syringe to avoid hemolysis. Bile acids are stable in serum or plasma for prolonged periods and can be mailed to the laboratory routinely; this obvious advantage is why bile acids are used instead of ammonia determinations for estimating liver function. Separator tubes should not be used for mailing because even minor comingling of erythrocytes and serum during transport will result in hemolysis. The direct enzymatic method for bile acid analysis is linear up to bile acid concentrations of 250 μmol/L. The author does not advocate further dilution of samples for exact quantification because there is no evidence this information provides useful diagnostic information. This test is sensitive to values only as low as 2 μmol/L. Interassay variation is such that only whole number values rather than decimal values should be reported.

The most commonly used RIA procedure for the determination of serum bile acids in dogs and cats measures nonsulfated conjugated primary bile acids.[378] This kit has been validated for dog and cat sera. If an alternative RIA procedure is used, attention must be given to the specific bile acid moiety(ies) measured to ensure it (they) are bile acids prevalent in the dog and cat. The assay must be validated in these species before it can be applied to clinical patients. The most popular RIA procedure used is only linear up to 50 μmol/L and thus requires dilution and sample reevaluation if a high value is detected. Unfortunately, there are no comprehensive clinical studies detailing the useful cutoff values and clinical utility for both fasting and postprandial values using this procedure in animals with a variety of spontaneous hepatobiliary disorders. The diagnostic values published for the enzymatic procedure *cannot* be applied to results generated by RIA determination.

For a further discussion on assay methodologies see the previously published information.[357,376–378] Normal values for bile acids in dogs and cats determined by different authors with enzymatic and the RIA procedures are shown in Table 8–15.

Table 8–15

SERUM BILE ACID CONCENTRATIONS IN DOGS AND CATS WITHOUT HEPATOBILIARY DISEASE

	DOGS							CATS			
	Liver Biopsy*	Number	Mean	Median	SD	Sem	Range	Biopsy	Liver Number	Mean/Median	Range
Assay Method Enzymatic											
12 hour fasting	no	25	—	—	—	—	0–2.1[439]	yes	26	— / 2.5	0–16[104]
	yes	40	—	3.0	—	—	0–17.1[104]				
	no	15	2.46	—	1.31[447]	—		—			
	no	26	1.7	—	—	0.73	0–8.8[469]				
	no	13	—	1.0	—	—	0–14.8[466]				
2 hour postprandial	yes	40	—	6.0	—	—	0–21.9[104]	yes	26	— / 5.0	0–15[104]
	no	15	9.26	—	2.02[449]	—					
	no	26	6.8	—	1.9		0–30.6[469]				
	no	13	—	7.08	—	—	0–43.0[446]				
Radioimmunoassay											
12 hour fasting	yes	12	1.8	—	1.3	—	0–5.0[443]				
	yes	6	0.8	—	0.2[440]	—					
	no	22	4.2	—	—	0.7[470]	—				
	no	60	0.4	—	3.9	—	0.2–4.6[469]				
2 hour postprandial	no	37	3.7	—	3.9	—	0.5–25.5[469]				

*If a liver biopsy was not obtained, the health status was determined as healthy on the basis of routine physical, hematologic, biochemical, and urinalysis evaluations. Some studies were completed with clinical patients suspected of having liver disease; the controls were animals that did not have liver disease on the basis of liver biopsy. From Center SA. Serum bile acids in companion animal medicine. Vet Clin N Am (Sm Anim) 23:625–657, 1993.
SD = standard deviation; Sem = standard error of the mean

RADIOGRAPHIC, ULTRASONOGRAPHIC, AND NUCLEAR MEDICINE IMAGING OF THE HEPATOBILIARY SYSTEM

Radiography

The most important features of the liver that are visible using radiographs include alterations in size, position, shape, and variation in density.[379,380] Alteration of liver size is an important sign of liver disease (Table 8–3). Unfortunately, radiographic evaluation provides an imprecise estimate of liver dimensions. The position of adjacent viscera provides an approximation of liver size. The angle of the gas pocket in the stomach can be used as an anatomic landmark. In health, the gastric gas silhouette lies parallel to the intercostal spaces, following the arch of the ribs at about the tenth intercostal space. A small liver will shift the gastric gas pattern to a more upright location with cranial displacement reducing the distance between the stomach and diaphragm. A positional shift of the right kidney, pyloric antrum, proximal duodenum, and transverse colon to a more cranial location also may signify a reduced hepatic mass. Radiographic features of hepatomegaly include a rounding of the liver margins, extension of the liver lobes beyond the costal arch (particularly the left lateral lobe in the left lateral view), caudal-dorsal leftward displacement of the stomach, caudal displacement of the proximal duodenum and right kidney, and caudal medial displacement of the transverse colon.[381–389] The position of the tip of the liver and even the angle of the stomach gas shadow are influenced by the patient's thoracic conformation. Dogs with deep chests have a convex diaphragm with a steep slope; these animals have a liver tip within the costal arch and thus it tends to appear small. In dogs with a wide thorax, the liver tip may extend more caudally; these animals therefore tend to be evaluated with hepatomegaly. The position of the liver is influenced by the respiratory motion of the diaphragm. During inspiration the liver lobes move caudally; during expiration they move cranially, shifting the position of the liver in relation to the costal arch by 1 cm or more. Thoracic distention causing a caudal displacement of the diaphragm may create the appearance of hepatomegaly; diaphragmatic rupture or congenital peritoneopericardial diaphragmatic hernia may create the illusion of microhepatica. Positioning of the patient for radiography may also influence the perceived liver size. Right lateral recumbency promotes the caudal movement of the left hepatic mass and the impression of hepatomegaly.[379]

Several reports have suggested more reliable methods for estimating hepatic size.[386–389] These include the determination of the radiographic liver length measured as the length of the axis from the most cranial part of the diaphragm to the apex of the liver tip expressed as a ratio of vertebral length (T11). The length of the liver measured in this manner is not influenced by thoracic conformation. Analysis completed in one study has provided a regression formula that can be used to calculate the true liver volume in dogs. This requires determination of liver length and thoracic depth from a radiograph, and determination of thoracic width by measurement taken directly from the patient. Figure 8–34 provides a representation of data from dogs in which true liver weight was confirmed and was used to generate a regression formula for clinical use.

Radiographic assessment for surface irregularities is rewarding only in the caudoventral margins of the liver. This is enhanced by the presence of fat within the falciform ligament. Radiographs made with the patient in left lateral recumbency may result in a merging of the hepatic and splenic shadows, thus obscuring the ordinarily visible margins of the liver. Blunting or rounding of the liver margins suggests diffuse hepatomegaly. Irregular or bumpy liver margins indicate hepatic neoplasia, regenerative nodules, hepatic or biliary cysts, or other focal lesions. In some patients with major bile duct occlusion, the silhouette of the gallbladder may be identified. The radiographic appearance of a large biliary cyst is shown in Chapter 37, Figure 37–35.

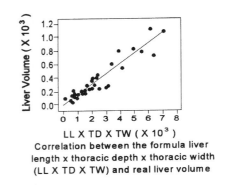

$$\text{True Liver Volume} = 11.62 + 0.154 \, (\text{LL} \times \text{TD} \times \text{TW})$$

LL = Liver length
TD = Thoracic depth
TW = Thoracic width
(external measurement)

Correlation between the formula liver length x thoracic depth x thoracic width (LL X TD X TW) and real liver volume

FIGURE 8–34. A method for estimating liver volume is shown. The liver length and thoracic depth are determined from a radiograph. The thoracic width is determined by measurement taken directly from the patient. The mathematical formula shown in the figure is applied. A representation of data from dogs in which true liver weight was confirmed and used to generate the regression formula is shown. Data derived from Lee R, Leowijuk C. Normal parameters in abdominal radiology of the dog and cat. J Sm Anim Pract 23:251–269, 1982.

The detection of gas in the common bile duct, gallbladder, or hepatic ducts may follow recent surgical intervention involving these structures (Figure 8–35). In these patients reflux of barium contrast material into the biliary system can also occur (Figure 8–36). Gas in these sites may also indicate infection with gas-producing organisms (anaerobes usually). Gas has been reported within the portal venous system following severe necrotizing or ulcerative gastroenteritis, paralytic ileus, gastric dilatation-volvulus, and portal thromboembolism. The presence of gas in the portal vasculature indicates discontinuity of the gastrointestinal microcirculatory bed, entry of alimentary gas, or infection with gas-producing organisms in a location where they have access to the portal circulation. Gas in hepatic vessels creates a linear branching pattern similar to an air bronchogram in the lung. Emphysematous cholecystitis, gas accumulation within the wall and lumen of the gallbladder, has been seen in dogs, some of which have had diabetes mellitus.[390–392] Rarely, pockets of gas within the hepatic parenchyma are recognized. These are usually associated with abscesses containing gas-forming organisms.

Occasionally, radiodense mineralized or calcified lesions are identified in the hepatobiliary tissues. Dystrophic mineralization may appear as multifocal intrahepatic densities and may be the sequela to necrosis or be associated with granulomas,

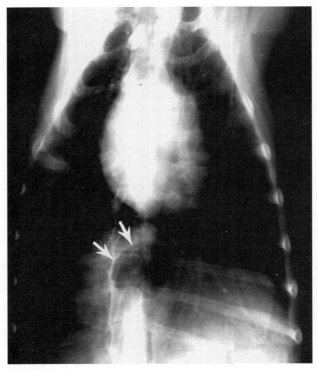

FIGURE 8–35. Dorsoventral radiograph showing a gallbladder filled with gas (arrows) in a dog with a cholecystojejunostomy. This dog was showing no clinical signs of retrograde cholecystitis.

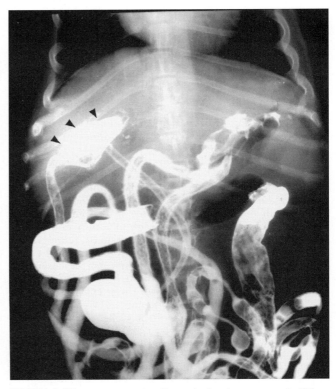

FIGURE 8–36. Dorsoventral radiograph showing retrograde filling of the gallbladder (arrows) with barium in a dog with a cholecystoduodenostomy. This dog was clinically ill, showing signs of abdominal discomfort, vomiting, and anorexia, possibly associated with ascending infection.

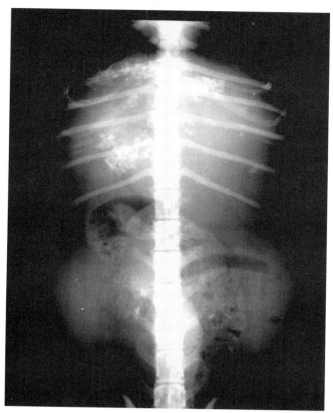

FIGURE 8–37. Dorsoventral abdominal radiograph of a dog showing multifocal hepatic dystrophic mineralization thought to be a sequela of an acute single incidence of hepatic necrosis/inflammation.

hematomas, neoplastic foci, or parasitic cysts (Figure 8–37). In addition, these also may represent choleliths within the gallbladder or major ducts or microcholeliths within the biliary ductules (Figure 8–38). The radiographic appearance of microlithiasis in a cat with cholangiohepatitis is shown in Chapter 37, Figure 37–3. Ultrasonographic evaluation assists in determining the nature and exact localization of mineralized lesions.

Pneumoperitoneography has been used to investigate the hepatic silhouette.[393] This technique is accomplished by injecting air, CO_2, or O_2 into the peritoneal space. The negative contrast is used to outline different areas of the liver by manipulation of patient position and exposure angles. This technique is no longer commonly used due to the increased availability and noninvasive nature of ultrasonographic imaging.

The use of positive contrast studies of the biliary tree has fallen out of favor in human medicine, with the exception of a few specific biliary tract disorders, because of the availability of ultrasonography and other improved imaging modalities. In veterinary medicine such studies were fraught with difficulties and were never frequently used; these are discussed in Chapter 37.

Arteriography and venography may be used to assess hepatic artery and portal vein vasculature. Arteriography requires selective catheterization of the celiac or anterior mesenteric artery. Selective catheterization of the celiac artery is used for hepatic artery injection when the presence of a congenital AV fistula requires documentation.[395,396] Today, confirmation of these malformations is accomplished by Doppler-assisted ultrasonography; Doppler easily demonstrates turbulent blood flow in the AV communication. Arteriography may be necessary to characterize the required extent of surgical resection.

Radiographic study of the portal circulation is usually accomplished by injection of contrast media into a mesenteric (jejunal) or splenic vein. These techniques are well described in the cited references and in Chapter 35.[397–399] Blind injections made into the splenic pulp are ill advised because of the potential for spleen infarction, hemorrhage, hematoma, or abscess formation. When radiographic methods are used to document the presence of a portosystemic vascular anomaly, both lateral and dorsoventral views should be obtained for correct vessel localization and identification. Portography can be used prior to surgery for shunt correction as an aid to vessel identification at the time of surgery if the surgeon is unsure about shunt location, and sometimes immediately after vessel ligation to verify correct occlusion. Because clinicopathologic features, ultrasonography, and colonic scintigraphy can be used to document the presence of a congenital shunt noninvasively, portography is reserved for the patient scheduled for surgical correction. In dogs, if the caudal extent of a congenital portosystemic shunt is cranial to vertebra T13, it probably is an intrahepatic anomaly.[398] Cats with portosystemic shunts commonly have left gastric vein anomalies.[401] These are easily located by an experienced surgeon and may be surgically attenuated without radiographic documentation.

Nuclear Imaging Procedures

Hepatic scintigraphy has been used in the dog to measure relative hepatic arterial and portal blood flow and to assess liver size.[400–410] One procedure involves hepatic radiocolloid uptake after intravenous injection (^{99m}Technetium sulfur colloid). Radiocolloid scanning uses the principle that particulate substances in the systemic circulation small enough to pass the capillary beds will be trapped by cells of the reticuloendothelial system (Kupffer cells). Although this procedure can derive quantitative information, it is not practical for routine use in clinical patients. Another scintigraphic procedure utilizes Technetium-labeled iminodiacetic acid analogues. These comprise a new class of organic anions that are taken

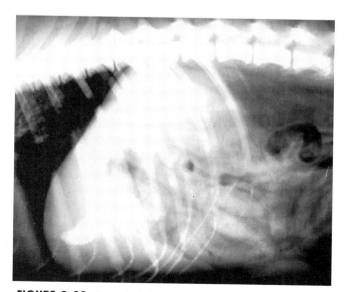

FIGURE 8–38. Lateral abdominal radiograph of a dog showing mineral density "sludge" in the gallbladder. This dog was clinically asymptomatic.

up and secreted by hepatocytes into bile by carrier-mediated mechanisms.[407] The amount of uptake and the rapidity of hepatic elimination depends on the structural configuration of the agent, the functional integrity of hepatocytes, and patency of the biliary system. Because gross anatomic changes may lag behind physiologic changes by weeks or months, there is enthusiasm among radiologists for imaging with these new agents.[407–410] Use in normal dogs and dogs with cholestatic disease has been reported.[402–406] The procedure has high sensitivity and specificity for differentiation of major bile duct occlusion from other forms of cholestasis.[408,410] The importance of these methods in veterinary clinical practice will increase during the next decade.

A more practical application of radio-labeled imaging is in use of ^{99m}Technetium pertechnetate (^{99m}TcO$_4$) for rectal portal scintigraphy in the diagnosis of portosystemic shunts.[399,400] A small amount of ^{99m}TcO$_4$-labeled solution is rapidly absorbed across the colon into the portal vein. In normal dogs the portal vein is visualized approximately 10 to 22 seconds following isotope deposition in the descending colon. In healthy dogs, the radioactivity reaches the liver before the heart. In animals with portosystemic shunts, some of the ^{99m}TcO$_4$ reaches the heart before or at the same time it reaches the liver. The severity of a shunt can be estimated by calculating a shunt fraction determined from the isotope's initial distribution. This represents the percentage of portal blood that bypasses the liver and can be calculated by computer analysis of scintigraphic images. Although shunt vessels can be seen crudely on the gamma camera image, the resolution possible with this method is inadequate to distinguish reliably between the various anatomic types. The only shortcoming of colonic scintigraphy is the underestimation of shunting phenomenon in splenic vein or splenic vein tributary shunts because colonic-derived venous blood does not normally pass through this vessel. This underestimation must be considered when applying this test to cats, given the high incidence of left gastric vein shunts in this species. Overall, this is an inexpensive, noninvasive test that has good clinical utility in confirmation of portosystemic shunting. It is available only at referral centers because it requires the availability of a gamma camera for data collection. This procedure is the only noninvasive method of differentiating animals with portal microvascular dysplasia from those with typical portosystemic problems; see Chapter 35 for a discussion of these hepatobiliary problems.

Ultrasonography of the Hepatobiliary System

The liver may appear normal on routine radiographic evaluation even when severely diseased. Comparatively, ultrasonography of the liver can add invaluable noninvasively obtained information to the patient's clinical data base.[411–422] However, grave errors in image interpretation can be made by the inexperienced operator. Use of this diagnostic modality is only possible if a person well experienced in ultrasonography and anatomy completes the examination. The recording of tapes by less experienced clinicians and referral of these images to an interpreting radiologist is fraught with inadequacies. Improper setting of the equipment and lack of a systematic approach to visceral inspection result in inaccurate assessments. Misdiagnosis of an obstructed biliary tree and assessment of increased hepatic echogenicity are two common and highly misleading mistakes.

Under optimal circumstances, ultrasonography is useful

Table 8–16

INDICATIONS FOR HEPATIC ULTRASONOGRAPHY

Investigation of:	Hepatomegaly
	Microhepatica
	Jaundice
	Abdominal effusion
	Mineral densities:
	gallbladder
	hepatic parenchyma

Confirmation of portosystemic vascular anomaly
Detection of portosystemic collateral shunting vessels
Confirmation of ascites
Survey for metastatic disease
Detection of portal thrombi (rare)

Unexplained:	Fever
	Abdominal pain
	Gastrointestinal signs
	↑ Liver enzymes
Evaluation of:	Treatment response
	Disease progression
Biopsy:	Method selection
	Biopsy guidance
	Postbiopsy observation for hemorrhage

for initial disease identification and subsequently as a method for monitoring disease progression. It can differentiate focal and diffuse liver disorders. Ultrasonographic findings provide meaningful information when considered in light of the clinical history, physical findings, laboratory test results, and realistic differential diagnoses. The clinician managing the case is in the best position to integrate the findings with collective case information in overall diagnostic and therapeutic application. For this reason, it is important that veterinary clinicians become familiar with the differential diagnoses associated with different ultrasonographic patterns (Table 8–17). It is important to remember that a normal ultrasound scan is common in a minimally affected liver and that abdominal effusion can enhance the hepatic image.

Specific indications for ultrasonography of the liver are given in Table 8–16. Ultrasonography can be used to assess liver size. Unfortunately, ultrasound criteria for the limits of normal liver size have not been established in small animals.[415] A small liver is usually difficult to image because of its position beneath the rib cage.

Ultrasonographic evaluation of the liver is the best method for detecting neoplastic metastasis and can be used for monitoring patient response to chemotherapy. Hepatic ultrasonography is indicated in the icteric patient when differentiation of extrahepatic biliary obstruction from intrahepatic disease is imperative. The technique is useful for detecting portosystemic shunts. Ultrasonographic examination of the liver and abdominal cavity is helpful in determining the origin of abdominal effusion. Dilated or engorged hepatic veins may distinguish passive congestion from intrahepatic portal hypertension. Ultrasound-guided biopsy collection is now a routine procedure in many clinical settings and has increased the safety and utility of percutaneous procedures for hepatic biopsy.

Optimal ultrasound examination requires a thorough and systematic examination of the abdominal cavity by a technically competent operator using appropriate equipment. A complete examination should routinely include inspection of the hepatic parenchyma, portal and hepatic veins, gallbladder, and intrahepatic biliary system. The margins of the liver should be smooth and sharp but these may be difficult to

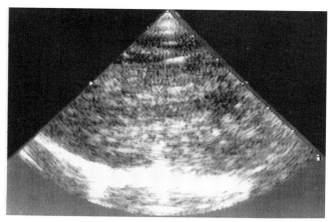

FIGURE 8-39. Ultrasonogram of the liver of a cat with chronic cholangitis/cholangiohepatitis. This sonogram shows a diffuse hyperechogenic appearance to the hepatic parenchyma. The liver occupies most of the central portion of the image. Courtesy Dr. A. Yeager, Section of Radiology, Department of Clinical Sciences, College of Veterinary Medicine, Cornell University.

evaluate. Margins are more easily visualized in the presence of ascites. The normal hepatic parenchyma has a homogenous medium level echogenicity compared relative to the renal cortex (right kidney is adjacent to the caudate lobe of the liver) and to the spleen. Usually, the liver parenchyma is the same (isoechoic) or slightly more echogenic (hyperechoic) than the renal cortex and less echogenic than the spleen.[411] A change in these echogenic relationships suggests architectural change in one or more of the compared organs. Estimation of the echogenicity of the liver in regard to the "standard comparison organs" (right renal cortex and spleen) is influenced by the operator experience, equipment settings, transducer, and the presence or absence of disease in the comparison organs. Unfortunately, subtle changes in hepatic parenchymal echogenicity resulting from diffuse disease can resemble those created by technical factors (Figure 8–39). Cats have kidneys that are more echogenic than dogs, which can complicate the assessment of relative hepatic echogenicity. Cats with hepatic lipidosis may have a substantial amount of fat in the renal epithelial cells that can further contribute to renal hyperechogenicity. In these patients hepatic echogenicity is usually compared to the adjacent faciform fat. The terms *anechoic, hypoechoic, hyperechoic,* and *mixed echogenicity* have been used to describe a lesion as it appears in relation to the "normal" surrounding tissue. Anechoic lesions lack internal echoes, hypoechoic abnormalities have reduced internal echoes, and hyperechoic lesions have increased internal echoes compared to normal liver parenchyma. Mixed patterns are described when combinations of anechoic, hypoechoic, and hyperechoic areas are detected within one lesion. During ultrasound imaging of the liver, a slight decrease in echogenicity from the ventral to dorsal part of the liver is accepted as normal (attenuation).[411,413]

In the normal liver, many anechoic/hypoechoic round structures can be visualized in the parenchyma that change to tubular structures when the transducer position is moved. These represent hepatic vessels, primarily the portal and hepatic veins. The hepatic arteries are difficult to visualize because of their small size, thicker walls, and small lumen. The caudal vena cava may be visualized adjacent to the diaphragm. The portal vein can be reliably seen in the porta hepatis ventral to the caudal vena cava, and then can be traced craniad into the hepatic parenchyma. Within the

parenchyma, portal veins appear "bright" owing to adjacent connective tissue. Although the presence of surrounding fat has been suggested as an additional contrasting material,[411] histologically and grossly there is little appreciable fat adjacent to these vessels. The portal vasculature appears throughout the hepatic parenchyma as linear (parallel) echogenicities.[411] Hepatic veins are recognized by their position adjacent to the diaphragm; these become larger as they approach the caudal vena cava. Within the hepatic parenchyma, the walls of the hepatic veins are not visualized like those of the portal veins. The normal intrahepatic biliary tree is usually not visible and so is not confused with vascular structures.

There are many diverse causes of diffuse liver disease that result in hyperechogenic, hypoechogenic, or mixed images (Table 8–17). The ultrasonographic findings characteristic of these hepatic diseases are discussed in later chapters.

Ultrasonography is particularly useful at detecting focal or multifocal lesions such as those due to metastatic neoplasia. Hepatic metastases are usually multiple, although solitary lesions also occur (Figure 8–40). Metastatic lesions are usually spherical because they grow equally in all planes from a single focus. Some neoplasias, for example, sarcomas, result in diffuse metastasis and thus create large ill-defined areas of increased or decreased echogenicity. A characteristic pattern of focal metastatic neoplasia is the target, or bull's-eye lesion, which consists of an echodense center surrounded by a sonolucent rim.[419,420] This pattern may be caused by a central region of necrosis and hemorrhage, surrounded by more homogenous, viable tumor tissue. Hepatic metastasis associated with extensive necrosis and/or hemorrhage may create a predominantly anechoic or hypoechoic pattern. This must be differentiated from hepatic abscesses or cysts (Figure 8–41).[419–423] It is important to remember that some types of diffuse infiltrative primary or secondary neoplasia are not reliably detected.

Clinicians must be cautious to differentiate nodular hyperplasia from metastatic neoplasia. Nodular hyperplasia may appear as a homogeneous or a diffuse mixed mass lesion with either increased or decreased echogenicity.[419,424] A rim or border to the lesion is usually ill defined; some nodules contain an anechoic central area that corresponds with necrosis. Nodular hyperplasia can present as a solitary finding or as multiple lesions. Unfortunately, the heterogeneity of lesion composition is consistent with a variety of ultrasonographic appearances.[424] It is suspected that the presence of nodular hyperplasia may not be detected in many animals because the echogenicity of the lesion is not distinct.[424] It becomes distinct when the lesions are large and contain areas of hemorrhage or fat-laden hepatocytes or macrophages.

Congenital portal vascular anomalies can be identified by experienced ultrasonographers in approximately 80% of the cases. Intrahepatic anomalies are more easily recognized than extrahepatic vascular anomalies. Operator technique and expertise determine the success of an ultrasonographic search for an anomalous extrahepatic shunting vessel. Systematic examination is required for success. Ultrasonography is helpful in making a diagnosis of acquired portosystemic shunts secondary to chronic liver disease. Portal veins near the porta hepatis become large and may appear slightly tortuous as a result of sinusoidal hypertension. When portal hypertension is associated with shunting through acquired portosystemic collaterals, tortuous vessels can often be visualized in the splenic or kidney regions. These can be difficult to image in some animals because of interference by alimentary gas.

Normal bile should be anechoic and produce posterior acoustic enhancement of the biliary structures.[411] Examination of the gallbladder commonly reveals the presence of

Table 8–17

CLASSIFICATION OF HEPATIC LESIONS IDENTIFIED BY ULTRASONOGRAPHY

FOCAL OR MULTIFOCAL

Hypoechoic
Metastatic neoplasia
Lymphosarcoma
Primary neoplasia (e.g., biliary carcinoma)
Hepatic nodular hyperplasia
Hepatitis
Telangiectasia
Regenerative nodules
Benign hepatic or biliary cyst(s)
Hematoma
Abscess
Hematoma

Hyperechoic
Primary neoplasia (hepatocellular carcinoma)
Metastatic neoplasia
Hepatic nodular hyperplasia
Peliosis hepatica
Glucocorticoid hepatopathy
Fatty infiltration
Foreign body
Gas-containing lesion
Dystrophic mineralization
Choleliths, micropholeliths

Complex
Primary neoplasia
Secondary neoplasia
Abscess
Hematoma
Focal necrosis

Double Rim Effect Gallbladder
Edema
Passive congestion
Hypoalbuminemia
Cholecystitis
Cholangiohepatitis
Ascites

DIFFUSE

Hypoechoic
Lymphosarcoma
Undifferentiated sarcoma
Hepatitis (suppurative)
Hepatic regeneration
Amyloidosis
Passive congestion
Histoplasmosis
Immune-mediated hemolytic anemia

Hyperechoic
Fibrosis (Cirrhosis?)
Lipidosis
Glucocorticoid hepatopathy
Lymphosarcoma

Extrahepatic Bile Duct Obstruction

Engorged gallbladder	24 hour
Dilated cystic duct	24 hour
↑ Common bile duct	48 hours
↑ Extrahepatic ducts	72 hours
↑ Intrahepatic ducts	5 to 7 days

Passive Congestion
Hepatomegaly
Dilated hepatic veins
Hepatic veins > portal veins
↑ Caudal vena cava (diaphragm level)

"sludged" or particulate biliary debris. At the present time this is considered not to correlate with disease in the dog or cat, but instead is considered a sign of fasting, anorexia, and temporary biliary stasis. However, if a patient is jaundiced or has present or historical laboratory indications of cholestatic disease, cholelithiasis, cholecystitis, and choledochitis should be considered. Compared to human beings, cholelithiasis is rare in the dog and cat. Ultrasonographic evaluation may localize and identify choleliths. This can be of particular value in the jaundiced patient and in animals with episodic gastrointestinal signs that might be attributable to cholelithiasis. Choleliths within the gallbladder are easily recognized using ultrasound (Figure 8–42). Changing the animal's position will demonstrate the gravitational effect on a cholelith. The size of a gallstone and its mineral content determine the degree of acoustic shadowing.[425] Choleliths within the common bile duct are difficult to recognize because of interference with bowel gas and because they are not surrounded by anechoic bile. Micropholeliths distributed throughout the hepatic parenchyma are sometimes detected in animals with chronic cholangiohepatitis. In these animals microlithiasis indicates a need for chronic choleresis and antibiotic therapy.

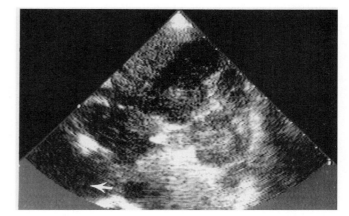

FIGURE 8–40. Ultrasonogram of the liver of a dog with multiple nodules having a mixed echogenic appearance. These lesions represented metastatic malignant carcinoma. Abdominal effusion is also present (arrow). Courtesy Dr. A. Yeager, Section of Radiology, Department of Clinical Sciences, College of Veterinary Medicine, Cornell University.

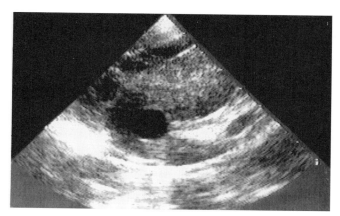

FIGURE 8–41. Ultrasonogram of the liver of a dog demonstrating a benign hepatic cystic lesion. The wall is thin, simple, and well demarcated, and the cyst is anechoic. A posterior acoustic enhancement is observed. Courtesy Dr. A. Yeager, Section of Radiology, Department of Clinical Sciences, College of Veterinary Medicine, Cornell University.

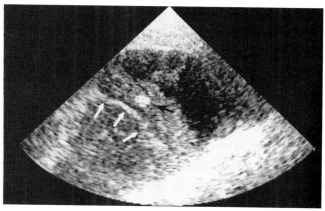

FIGURE 8–42. Ultrasonogram of the liver and gallbladder of a dog demonstrating a single echodense cholelith (black arrow) and sludged biliary debris. The wall of the gallbladder is delineated by white arrows. This animal had been showing intermittent signs of cholestatic liver disease. Courtesy Dr. A. Yeager, Section of Radiology, Department of Clinical Sciences, College of Veterinary Medicine, Cornell University.

The normal gallbladder varies in size with the fasting or fed condition of the patient. After a prolonged fast or in the anorectic patient, the gallbladder is usually distended and easily visualized. The gallbladder wall is usually barely visible. However, it becomes more echogenic and appears thicker when peritoneal fluid is present. The common bile duct may be seen adjacent to the portal vein in most normal animals and in the normal cat, appears more tortuous than in the dog. The remainder of the biliary tract is usually not visualized unless it is abnormal. Thickening of the gallbladder wall may occur due to edema, inflammation, or fibrosis. When the gallbladder wall becomes thickened, a double rim effect is produced by reflections from the inner and outer margins. Occasionally, sessile or polypoid lesions may be visualized within the gallbladder of dogs. Cystic hyperplasia of mucus-producing glands of the gallbladder may produce such lesions. Neoplastic lesions extending into the lumen of the gallbladder are rare in veterinary patients.

Ultrasonographic examination can be useful in differentiating biliary obstruction from hepatocellular jaundice.[426–428] The cause of obstruction may be discerned during examination in some cases (cholelith, mass, duct stricture). After extrahepatic bile duct occlusion, dilatation of the biliary tree occurs in a retrograde progression from the site of obstruction.[426] The gallbladder and cystic duct are rapidly engorged and this change is detectible within 24 hours. It must be remembered, however, that some patients with major bile duct occlusion have a nondistended gallbladder as a result of contraction associated with inflammation.[429] Enlargement of the common bile duct can usually be ascertained within 48 hours following obstruction (Figure 37–7). Dilatation of the extrahepatic ducts can be discerned in about 72 hours. Intrahepatic bile duct enlargement may be recognized after 5 to 7 days. The engorged intrahepatic ducts can usually be differentiated from portal veins by their irregular branching patterns and tortuosity. A detection of "too many tubes" is produced by increased numbers of engorged bile ducts adjacent to portal veins.[426] A partial bile duct occlusion produces similar but less severe ultrasonographic findings. Following resolution or surgical correction of major bile duct obstruction, the ultrasonographic feature of biliary tree dilation may persist indefinitely.

LIVER BIOPSY

Tissue examination is essential for definitive diagnosis of hepatobiliary disease. The only exception is the patient with a congenital portosystemic vascular anomaly where liver function testing, ultrasonographic evaluation, and colonic scintigraphy and/or portography confirm the disorder. In these patients, liver biopsy is still important because it is necessary to determine that acquired liver disease has not contributed to clinical signs. Liver biopsy is an invasive procedure that must be carefully considered before implementation. Of course, no biopsy is done if little additional useful information would be gained to assist in patient treatment. For example, a patient with highly suspected end-stage cirrhosis, in which the liver is small, liver function is profoundly deranged, the animal has tense ascites, ultrasonography discloses a multinodular hepatic appearance, and the risks of anesthesia and biopsy-related hemorrhage are great, probably would not benefit from this procedure. Liver biopsy should be pursued aggressively early in the development of progressive disease. The major indications for liver biopsy are listed in Table 8–18.

Major complications from liver biopsy experienced in veterinary and human patients ranges up to 3.5%. The frequency of complications and likelihood of retrieving a diagnostic specimen depends on the (1) procedure used, (2) nature of the patient's disease, and (3) experience of the clinician collecting the sample.[430–442] The decision on how to collect the biopsy specimen is individualized for the patient. Needle biopsy is preferred in most circumstances if the technology and expertise for accurate guidance and safety are available. In that circumstance, an invasive approach for biopsy collection, such as during a laparotomy, is reserved for animals suspected to have (1) resectable mass lesions, (2) disease or obstruction of the extrahepatic bile ducts requiring cholecystectomy or biliary diversion, (3) cholelithiasis requiring stone removal, (4) a need for multiple visceral biopsies or (5) portosystemic vascular anomaly with the intention of ligating the anomalous vessel. When needle biopsy of the liver is used, some clinicians prefer to feed a small quantity of corn oil (1 mL per kg body weight) 60 minutes before the procedure, in order stimulate gallbladder contraction and minimize the chance of its inadvertent perforation. This is usually

Table 8–18

CONSIDERATIONS WHEN PROCURING AN HEPATIC BIOPSY

INDICATIONS	CONTRAINDICATIONS OF NEEDLE BIOPSY
Hepatic failure of unknown cause	Focal cavitary lesion seen on ultrasound
Unexplained abdominal effusion/ascites	abscess: → abdominal contamination
Persistent abnormal liver enzyme activity	tumor: → hemorrhage, seeding
Persistent unexplained hyperbilirubinemia	(resectable lesion via laparotomy ?)
Unexplained hepatic insufficiency	Suspected extrahepatic bile duct obstruction
↑ serum bile acids ↓ glucose	laceration: → bile peritonitis
hyperammonemia ammonium biurates	(biliary diversion via laparotomy)
↓ cholesterol ↓ albumin	Small focal lesions
Confirm suspected hepatic lipidosis (cats)	< 1 cm diameter: → lesion missed
Unexplained, unequivocal ↓ or ↑ hepatic size	Lesions restricted to one liver lobe
Confirm or stage neoplasia	resectable lesion via laparotomy ?
Sequentially assess disease progression	Microhepatica
Sequentially assess response to treatment	requires unconventional needle approach
Evaluate for breed-related hepatopathy	Coagulopathy
	institute Vitamin K_1 ± transfusion
	Suspect severe end-stage cirrhosis: → no change in Rx
	laboratory data
	microhepatica
	severe tense unmanageable ascites

only necessary if a blind biopsy procedure is used, that is, a biopsy unassisted by ultrasound imaging.

Use of ultrasonographic guidance for tissue biopsy permits precise localization and sampling of focal lesions of at least 1 cm diameter. It also provides an accurate estimation of the safest depth for needle insertion and allows avoidance of large vascular and biliary structures.

FINE NEEDLE ASPIRATES

In some cases, a fine needle aspirate of liver tissue or biliary contents may provide a diagnosis. This is true for liver flukes if eggs are harvested, bacterial infection when bacteria are retrieved, idiopathic hepatic lipidosis, hepatic neoplasia when infiltrates are successfully harvested, and glucocorticoid hepatopathy. Examples of normal hepatic cytology and cytology showing macrovesicular and microvesicular hepatic lipidosis are shown in Figures 8–43, 8–44, and 8–45. The appearance of hepatocytes from a dog with a glucocorticoid hepatopathy are shown in Figure 34–16. However, in most

cases where a liver biopsy is warranted, tissue aspirates cannot be relied upon to provide a definitive diagnosis. For instance, in dogs with acute hepatitis or chronic active hepatitis and cats with cholangitis/cholangiohepatitis, tissue aspirates confirm the presence of hepatic inflammation in most cases, but cannot characterize the distribution of the lesion.

The method of fine needle aspirate can involve use of a 2.5–8 cm long 21 to 33 gauge needle attached to a 6 to 12 mL syringe. The needle is carefully thrust into the abdomen and then through the liver capsule into the parenchyma. Several vigorous aspirates are made. The needle may be backed out of the parenchyma and capsule and reinserted in a slightly different area. Care is taken not to tear the tissue by lateral motion of the needle. The needle is withdrawn from the tissues after negative pressure is relieved on the syringe. Contents of the needle are deposited on glass slides for cytologic evaluation and may also be collected for culture. An alternative method of fine needle sampling involves moving the needle rapidly back and forth 5 to 10 times within the target lesion without negative pressure. Enough tissue is harvested for one or two cytologic preps.[443]

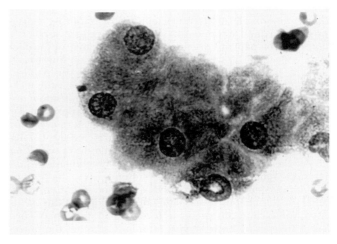

FIGURE 8-43. Photomicrograph showing the cytologic appearance of normal hepatocytes. (680×, modified Wright's-Giemsa stain)

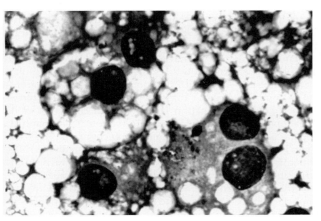

FIGURE 8-44. Photomicrograph showing the cytologic appearance of macrovesicular lipid vacuolation in the hepatocytes of a cat with the hepatic lipidosis syndrome. (900×, modified Wright's-Giemsa stain)

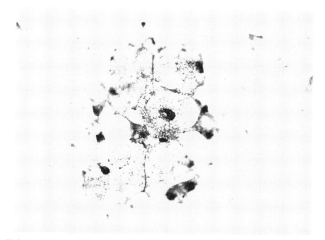

FIGURE 8-45. Photomicrograph showing the cytologic appearance of microvesicular lipid vacuolation in the hepatocytes of a cat with the hepatic lipidosis syndrome. (480×, modified Wright's-Giemsa stain)

Cholecystocentesis

In some animals, collection of bile will assist in ruling out a septic or parasitic process (flukes). Bile can be aspirated with ultrasonographic guidance using a spinal needle. The safest method for percutaneous bile aspiration is done using a parenchymal approach. The needle is inserted into hepatic parenchyma adjacent to the gallbladder and then penetrates the gallbladder. This offers local tissue pressure on the perforated surface of the gallbladder after needle withdrawal and entrapment of any small quantities of leaked bile.

Methods of Liver Biopsy

Methods of liver biopsy include (1) blind needle procedures, (2) ultrasonographic guided needle procedures, (3) laparascopic needle, pinch, or guillotine biopsy (biopsy secured with a pinch forceps or endoscopic biopsy forceps) techniques, or (4) laparotomy for wedge biopsy. A variety of methods for blind needle biopsy sample collection are described.

In general, needle biopsies pose a problem in sampling too few acinar units for accurate diagnosis of the severity of a lesion. An inadequate display of portal triads may hamper assessment of the extent of bridging fibrosis. This problem is particularly evident when evaluating a liver affected with macronodular cirrhosis. Connective tissue impedes adequate tissue extraction in a cirrhotic liver when a suction biopsy procedure is used (Menghini needle aspirate). Such needle biopsy specimens may appear shredded or fragmented when extracted from a fibrotic liver. If a patient has ascites, a lateral rather than a ventral midline approach should be used for needle procedures. This will minimize gravitational pooling of ascitic fluid into the subcutaneous tissues at the area of abdominal instrumentation. Following any biopsy procedure, the patient should be placed with the biopsy side down to attain visceral pressure on the biopsied area. It is hoped this will facilitate hemostasis.

ULTRASONOGRAPHIC-ASSISTED PROCEDURES. Ultrasonographic evaluation of the liver assists in deciding the best mode of tissue collection for the individual patient. Focal lesions as small as 1 cm may be sampled using a transducer-guided procedure. In deep-chested dogs, a small liver may be difficult to biopsy with an ultrasound-guided procedure. Alternatively, a transthoracic blind technique may be used, but a laparoscopic or laparotomy approach may be better with these patients.

The patient with a normal sized to large liver and many animals with microhepatica can be biopsied using an ultrasound-guided approach. With diffuse disease, an approach to the left liver lobes is used. The patient is fasted for 12 to 24 hours to minimize air and food within the stomach. After being placed under general anesthesia, the patient is positioned to optimize liver lobe accessibility; often the forequarters are slightly elevated. Use of a Vim Tru cut type needle in an automated biopsy gun (Figure 8-46A and B) allows the best control during biopsy acquisition. A 14 to 18 gauge needle is used. The sample is collected when respiratory movement is temporarily suspended by the anesthetist. These needles remove liver tissue by first isolating a core of tissue and removing it without relying on suction (Figure 8-46B). The depth of needle penetration into the liver and postbiopsy bleeding can be viewed on the ultrasound screen. The biopsy site should be inspected 15 minutes postbiopsy for signs of continued bleeding. Using the ultrasound equipment, pooling of fluid in the abdominal recesses indicates hemorrhage.

Collection of a needle biopsy should be avoided in the circumstance of large cavitary lesions or highly vascular masses suspected to be infectious or neoplastic. This avoids potential abdominal contamination and life-threatening hemorrhage. Instead, a fine needle aspirate using a spinal needle may be attempted if an owner will not permit open surgical tissue sampling. Of particular value with the ultrasonographic procedures is the ability to observe the biopsy site for hemorrhage. In humans, it is well established that life-threatening postbiopsy intrahepatic or subcapsular hematomas can develop during the first few hours following a procedure.[431–434] In humans, unexplained hypotension and tachycardia can follow needle biopsy procedures, unrelated to hemorrhagic complications.[432] Hematomas forming at the site of biopsy can be identified as hepatic ultrasonographic mass lesions for days to weeks following the procedure.

BLIND PERCUTANEOUS PROCEDURES. For blind needle tissue collection, the Menghini type of needle is preferred. This biopsy instrument, shown in Figure 8-47, consists of a needle, a needle guard, a blocking pin that inserts into the needle, and a blunt-ended stylet. This needle relies on suction to remove the biopsy from the liver rather than cutting as the Vim Tru cut needle does. The Menghini needle can be used for transabdominal and transthoracic approaches.

The transthoracic approach has been reported in dogs to be highly successful in tissue retrieval.[431] Complications are reportedly infrequent but have included perforation of the gallbladder or bile duct, collection of pulmonary and diaphragmatic tissues, and induction of pneumothorax or hemothorax.

Transthoracic liver biopsy is performed on the right side. The precise location is determined after evaluation of two radiographic views of the thorax and abdomen. The biopsy needle is passed through the 5th, 6th, or 7th intercostal space at a point slightly dorsal to the costochondral junction. After surgical preparation of the area, the biopsy site is infiltrated with an anesthetic if the animal is not under general anesthesia. It is preferable that the patient be under chemical restraint when needles are placed in the liver. A small incision is made to permit introduction of the biopsy needle through the skin. The Menghini needle is introduced into the subcutaneous intercostal structures at a right angle and with the stylet not completely within the needle hub. This allows the

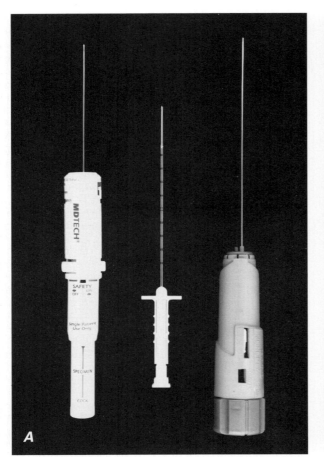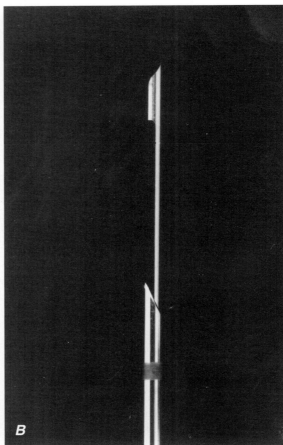

FIGURE 8-46. *(A)* Example of automated biopsy "guns" and Vim Tru cut biopsy needle (center) commonly used for ultrasonographically guided hepatic biopsy. The close-up photograph *(B)* shows the cutting apparatus of the Vim Tru cut type needle. Each of these automated needles shares this mechanism.

cutting edge of the biopsy needle to facilitate passing the needle into the pleural space, after which the stylet is pushed completely into the needle hub. The needle and stylet are then directed caudally and advanced to the level of the diaphragm. After making contact with the diaphragm the needle guard is adjusted and fixed at a point that is 1/2 inch (13 mm) from the skin. This limits the depth to which the needle will enter the liver when the biopsy is obtained. The stylet is removed, and a 12 mL syringe containing up to 5 mL sterile saline is attached. This procedure is done rapidly and with the tip of the needle against the diaphragm; both factors help minimize chances of a pneumothorax. The syringe is used to produce a negative pressure of about 3 mL, and at the end of expiration, the needle is rapidly thrust caudally into the liver up to the needle guard, and in a continuing motion, is removed rapidly from the body. The biopsy sample is drawn into the saline-filled syringe, from which it is transferred to a fixative solution of buffered formalin. The patient is placed on its right side for five minutes to cause the weight of the viscera to compress the biopsy site and facilitate hemostasis.

The transabdominal procedure is conducted on animals that are also in left lateral recumbency. The liver falls away from the uppermost part of the abdominal wall in this position, so a needle passed through this part at a right angle may not reach the liver. The approach is through the ventral abdominal wall at a site between the left lateral border of the xiphoid process and the left costal arch. This region is surgically prepared and infiltrated with a local anesthetic if the animal is not under general anesthesia. General anesthesia is preferred for the best patient control and to optimize safety of the procedure. A small skin incision is made to facilitate passage of the Menghini needle, with stylet and guard, through the abdominal wall. At this point, the stylet is removed and the blocking pin is inserted through the hub into the needle. A 12 mL syringe containing 5 mL sterile saline is attached, and a small amount of saline is flushed through the needle to wash away any blood or tissue collected inadvertently during needle placement. The needle is advanced in a craniodorsal direction until the surface of the liver is reached. The needle guard is adjusted to regulate the depth of penetration during the biopsy. A vacuum of 3 mL is produced with the syringe, and in one continuous motion the needle is rapidly thrust into the liver and removed from the body. The sample of liver tissue is transferred from the sterile saline to buffered formalin by simply flushing saline from the syringe through the needle.

An important difference between the two methods is that the blocking pin is used in the transabdominal approach and not in the transthoracic approach. The pin prevents the sample of tissue from being drawn into the syringe and minimizes the chances of it becoming fragmented. Another difference is the ability to flush the needle with the transabdominal approach and the omission of this step in the transthoracic approach. Flushing the needle reduces the chances of retrieving a sample of blood clot or nonhepatic tissue. The transtho-

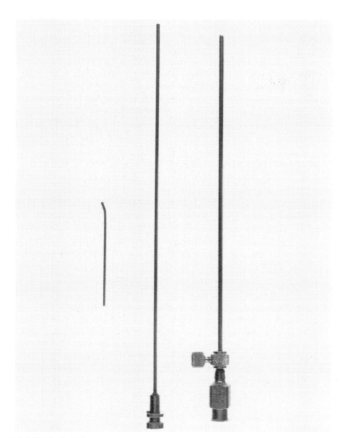

FIGURE 8–47. Menghini needle for blind percutaneous hepatic biopsy or for directed biopsy with a keyhole. Needle is shown with stylus that is removed after directing needle through abdominal wall and with pin that is placed in needle before biopsy is obtained.

racic approach also requires that the needle pass through the diaphragm without a stylet. The blind percutaneous procedures using the Menghini needle have been used in dogs by some clinicians routinely with relatively few procedure complications.[438–440]

KEYHOLE APPROACH. A keyhole approach in which the clinician can either see or feel the surface of the liver prior to biopsy collection is preferred by some clinicians. This involves a surgical incision just caudal to the xiphoid through which the index finger is inserted to facilitate the liver biopsy. This allows the operator to identify and avoid inadvertent laceration of gallbladder, major vessels, or other viscera. It also enables immobilization of a lobe of liver against the abdominal wall or other lobes so the biopsy needle will not simply push the lobe aside as it is thrust into the organ. This approach allows the clinician to identify by palpation abnormal surface contour of particular lobes and targeting of the biopsy needle to the most abnormal areas. Abnormalities in other abdominal organs can sometimes be identified. Either a Menghini or Vim Tru cut method or a cutting (pinch or guillotine) biopsy instrument can be used with this approach. The biopsy forceps used with an endoscope or hand-held guillotine-type biopsy instruments have been used. If a needle procedure is used, the needle is introduced through an incision separate from the keyhole opening used to immobilize or visualize the liver. If a cutting instrument is used, the liver must be visualized. An adaptation using an otoscope cone as a "mini-laparoscope" has also been described.[444]

LAPAROSCOPIC METHODS. A visual examination of the liver or a directed biopsy can be accomplished using laparoscopy. Isolated lesions can be sampled and the gross appearance of the liver can be evaluated. The liver is always biopsied during laparoscopy, regardless of its gross appearance, which is often misleading when compared to histology. The major disadvantages of laparoscopy are the expense of the equipment and the large amount of time required to become expert with the equipment so as to minimize the length of the procedure. The technique for laparoscopic collection of liver biopsy has been reviewed in detail.[29]

Complications and Contraindications to Liver Biopsy

The complications of liver biopsy are summarized in Table 8–19. The procedure is contraindicated if severe hemorrage is likely. Although the clinically significant incidence of coagulopathies is low in the dog or cat with liver disease, hemorrhage following liver biopsy is such a serious complication that clotting function is evaluated before every biopsy. Significant hepatic hemorrhage is possible (though seldom realized) following liver biopsy in dogs with even normal clotting tests. The bench coagulation tests are insensitive measures for detecting this complication. The buccal mucosal bleeding time seems better for predicting clinical bleeding in response to iatrogenic trauma. Patients showing bench test abnormalities, prolonged buccal mucosal bleeding times, or a propensity to bruise are given a blood transfusion concurrent with the biopsy procedure. Any jaundiced patient should in addition receive vitamin K_1 IM or SQ at least 12 to 24 hours preceding biopsy. Small dogs and cats receive 5 mg, dogs weighing between 10 and 40 lbs receive 10 mg, and large dogs, 15 to 20 mg. Two or three doses given at 12 hour intervals are appropriate. Many clinicians give a dose of vitamin K_1 to each patient scheduled for a liver biopsy irrespective of coagulation assessments. Serious postbiopsy bleeding is best detected by ultrasonography and/or abdominocentesis. In the circumstance of hemorrhagic shock, the PCV and total solids do not requilibrate fast enough to reflect loss of erythron mass. Vital signs will reveal tachycardia, blanching mucous membranes, and tachypnea. In dogs known to have von Willebrand factor deficiency, pretreatment immediately before the procedure with DDAVP (1-desamino-8-D-arginine vasopressin, Desmopressin acetate, USV Laboratories, Tarrytown, NY) at a dose of 1 to 5 µg/kg diluted in 10 to 20 mL of saline given IV slowly (over 10 minutes) or given SQ may help avert postbiopsy hemorrhagic complications.[445] This maximizes release of the active von Willebrand monomers from the endothelium to assist in coagulation. Only a short-term (hours) bene-

Table 8–19

COMPLICATIONS OF HEPATIC NEEDLE BIOPSY

Hemorrhage	Pneumothorax
Perforation of biliary structures	Hemothorax
gallbladder	Bile pleuritis/pleural effusion
common bile duct	Bacterial peritonitis
hepatic ducts	Septicemia
bile peritonitis	Development of hepatic AV fistula
scarring of major bile ducts	Anesthetic complications
Hemobilia	"Seeding" of malignancy
(bleeding into biliary tree)	
Abdominal viscera laceration	
Diaphragmatic puncture, laceration	

fit is realized. Repeated treatment within short intervals (hours) does not yield additional benefit. Use of DDAVP appears to benefit more than just von Willebrand disease in patients with liver disease and coagulopathies.[217] The mechanism(s) of these additional beneficial effects are not understood. If a blood transfusion is appropriate, only fresh blood should be administered. If possible, the donor should be pretreated with DDAVP. Using fresh blood optimizes platelet function, coagulation factor delivery, and avoids administration of high concentrations of ammonia as compared to previously stored blood. Optimally, the patient should be crossmatched to the donors; this requires anticipation of a potential transfusion at least a half day before the biopsy procedure is performed. Care must be given to the concern that cats with type B blood cannot be transfused with blood from the more prevalent type A donor cat.

A second major contraindication to needle biopsy is suspicion or evidence of an intrahepatic abscess. Needle penetration of abscesses may result in rupture and contamination of the peritoneal cavity. Release of endotoxins and microorganisms can lead to shock and bacteremia following the biopsy procedure. If cystic structures are identified on ultrasound evaluation and an abscess seems likely, exploratory laparotomy and liver lobe resection should be considered. Fortunately, cysts and abscesses are relatively uncommon problems.

A third major contraindication to needle liver aspirate or biopsy is the detection of a large vascular structure within the liver, suggesting the presence of either a highly vascular tumor or an arterioportal fistula. Because the latter condition is relatively rare, the former is usually first considered. Hemangiosarcoma can occur exclusively in the liver on early presentation. When biopsied, these tumors continue to ooze blood for hours, which may eventuate in hemorrhagic shock. A thoracic radiograph should be taken of any patient with a suspected liver mass or large well-vascularized hepatic lesion before collection of a liver biopsy is scheduled. If metastatic disease is obvious, acquisition of a liver biopsy is not pursued unless chemotherapy is considered an option. Biopsy in this circumstance would confirm the tumor type and permit selection of an appropriate chemotherapy protocol.

A fourth important contraindication to needle aspirate or biopsy of the liver is major bile duct occlusion. Laceration of the biliary tree during a biopsy procedure can lead to the devastating consequence of bile peritonitis.[436,437] Perforation of the biliary system in a patient with biliary tree obstruction can lead to fatal bile peritonitis. Vomiting and abdominal tenseness appear within a few hours of gallbladder perforation. In some cases, the rupture seals as a result of local inflammation and omental occlusion. If leakage continues, surgical exploration of the abdomen is critical. Ultrasonography can be used to detect the accumulation of leaked bile if it is loculated within the porta hepatis (Chapter 37). A more important contraindication to needle biopsy in the patient with suspected bile duct obstruction is that it delays definitive therapy that is possible during laparotomy. Evidence of bile duct obstruction is usually obvious to the experienced ultrasonographer. However, some patients will be misdiagnosed.

A final serious complication of hepatic biopsy is the devel-

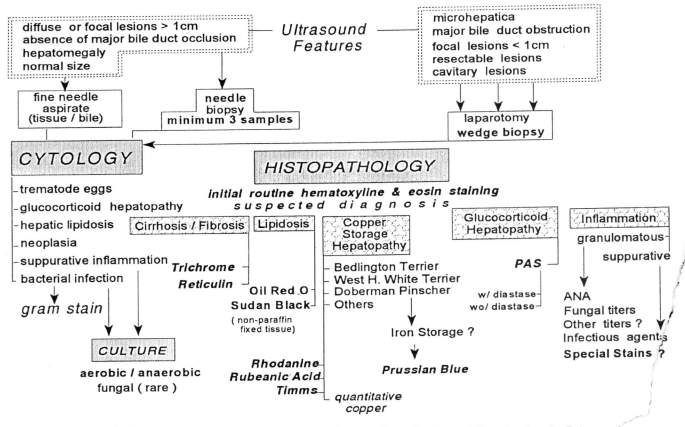

FIGURE 8–48. From Center SA. Pathophysiology and laboratory diagnosis of hepatobiliary disorders. In: Ettinger SJ, Feldman EC (eds), Textbook of Veterinary Internal Medicine, 4th ed. Philadelphia, WB Saunders, 1995, 1309.

opment of infection. The patient with hepatic disease severe enough to warrant biopsy usually has an increased susceptibility to infection. Although a surgical preparation is applied to the area of needle insertion, iatrogenic infection can develop. Transient bacteremia has been reported in humans undergoing percutaneous liver biopsy where hepatic abscessation or septic inflammation were not apparent and pre-biopsy blood cultures were sterile.[446] For this reason, a course of bactericidal antibiotics are given postbiopsy for a minimum of a week. Antimicrobials not reliant on hepatic metabolism and that attain good liver tissue and biliary concentrations are used; examples include metronidazole, enrofloxacin, or cefazolin.

OPTIMAL USE OF BIOPSY SPECIMEN. Once a biopsy is collected, optimal use of the sampled tissue requires some forethought. An algorithm for optimal biopsy utilization is provided in Figure 8–48. Considerations include (1) histopathologic evaluation, (2) cytologic evaluations, (3) cultures for aerobic, anaerobic, and fungal agents as guided by the considered differential diagnoses and cytologic information; (4) quantification of copper and/or iron tissue concentrations when metal storage–associated disorders are suspected, and (5) requests for special stains for collagen, reticulin, lipid, copper, iron, and infectious agents, as appropriate for the histologic lesions. An immediate preview of the cytologic features of sampled materials will permit better allocations of resources into cultures and may provide information important in immediate postbiopsy patient management. Bacteria are more easily identified on cytologic preparations than in histologic sections. Organisms are initially identified using routine stains (modified Wright's-

Giemsa, Diff Quik). A gram stain may be useful in prompting selection of initial antibiotic therapy before culture and sensitivity results are available. In some cases, despite recognition of bacterial organisms on cytology smears, culture results are negative. In such circumstances, the decision for long-term antimicrobial therapy will be made on the basis of the cytologic preparations.

If an ultrasonographic needle procedure is used, at least three and optimally seven separate specimens should be collected. The safety of collecting more than one biopsy can be assessed by watching for serious bleeding from the first biopsy site. A minimum of two biopsies are needed for histopathology.[546] If multiple specimens are collected, one-half of two specimens are used for cytology, one-half of two specimens are used for culture, and one biopsy is saved for metal (iron, copper, or zinc) quantification and/or special stains that require nonroutine tissue processing (such as fat or glycogen stains).

Laboratory Assessments in the Neonatal and Pediatric Patient

Clinicopathologic testing is sometimes necessary in neonatal and pediatric patients suspected of having hepatobiliary disease. There are certain features of the neonatal patient that are normal and could be misconstrued as indicating the presence of hepatobiliary disease. Most important are the reduced concentration of albumin seen during the first several weeks of life and the profound increases in the serum ALP and GGT activity that develop in the puppy that has

Table 8–20

NORMAL VALUES FOR ROUTINE BIOCHEMICAL INDICATORS OF HEPATOBILIARY DISORDERS IN PEDIATRIC DOGS AND CATS (MEDIAN AND (RANGE))

TEST	PUPPIES					KITTENS		
	1–3 days (n = 30)	2 weeks (n = 14)	4 weeks (n = 7)	8 weeks (n = 8)	Normal Adult Range	2 weeks (n = 24)	4 weeks (n = 8)	Normal Adult Range
BSP % 30 min retention	< 5	< 5	< 5	< 5	(0–5)	ND	ND	(0–3)
Bile Acids (μm/L)	< 15	< 15	< 15	< 15	(0–15)	ND	< 10	(0–10)
T. Bilirubin (mg/dl)	5 (0.2–1.0)	0.3 (0.1–0.5)	0 (0–0.1)	0.1 (0.1–0.2)	(0–0.4)	0.3 (0.1–1.0)	0.2 (0.1–0.2)	(0–0.2)
ALT (IU/L)	69 (17–337)	15 (10–21)	21 (20–22)	21 (9–24)	(12–94)	18 (11–24)	16 (14–26)	(29–91)
AST (IU/L)	108 (45–194)	20 (10–40)	18 (14–23)	22 (10–32)	(13–56)	18 (8–48)	17 (12–24)	(9–42)
ALP (IU/L)	3845 (618–8760)	236 (176–541)	144 (135–201)	158 (144–177)	(4–107)	123 (68–269)	111 (90–135)	(10–77)
GGT (IU/L)	1111 (163–3558)	24 (4–77)	3 (2–7)	1 (0–7)	(0–7)	1 (0–2)	2 (0–2)	(0–2)
T. Protein (g/dl)	4.1 (3.4–5.2)	3.9 (3.6–4.4)	4.1 (3.9–4.2)	4.6 (3.9–4.8)	(5.4–7.4)	4.4 (4.0–5.2)	4.8 (4.6–5.2)	(5.8–8.0)
Albumin (g/dl)	2.1 (1.5–2.8)	1.8 (1.7–2.0)	1.8 (1.0–2.0)	2.5 (2.1–2.7)	(2.1–2.3)	2.1 (2.0–2.4)	2.3 (2.2–2.4)	(2.5–3.0)
Cholesterol (mg/dl)	136 (112–204)	282 (223–344)	328 (266–352)	155 (111–258)	(103–299)	229 (164–443)	361 (222–434)	(150–270)
Glucose (mg/dl)	88 (52–127)	129 (111–146)	109 (86–115)	145 (134–272)	(65–110)	117 (76–126)	110 (99–112)	(63–144)

ALT = alanine aminotransferase, AST = aspartate aminotransferase, ALP = alkaline phosphatase, GGT = gamma-glutamyltranspeptidase, T. Protein = total protein, BSP = sulfobromophthalein. Center SA, Hornbuckle WE. College of Veterinary Medicine, 1987, Cornell University, Ithaca, NY, 14853 (reference 547).

ingested colostrum (Table 8–20).[448] During the first two days, low concentration of cholesterol has been shown in puppies. Hepatic function testing done in the young healthy puppy yields values within the adult normal range. Function testing with bile acids in normal young kittens also yields values within the adult normal range, although studies with BSP and ICG have not been completed.

REFERENCES

1. Steinberg SE, Hillman RS. The liver and hematopoiesis. In: Zakim D, Boyer TD (eds) Hepatology—a Textbook of Liver Disease. WB Saunders, Philadelphia, 537–545, 1982.
2. Douglass CC, McCall MS, Frenkel EP. The acanthocyte in cirrhosis with hemolytic anemia. Ann Intern Med 68:390–397, 1968.
3. Smith JA, Longergan ET, Sterling K. Spur-cell anemia: Hemolytic anemia with red cells resembling acanthocytes in alcoholic cirrhosis. N Engl J Med 271:396–398, 1964.
4. Grahn EP, Dietz AA, Stefani SS, et al. Burr cells hemolytic anemia and cirrhosis. Am J Med 45:78–87, 1968.
5. Silber R, Amorosi E, Lhowe J, et al. Spur-shaped erythrocytes in Laennec's cirrhosis. N Engl J Med 275:639–643, 1966.
6. Shull RM, Bunch SE, Maribei J, et al. Spur cell anemia in a dog. J Am Vet Med Assoc 173:978–982, 1978.
7. Christopher MM, Lee SE. Red cell morphologic alterations in cats with hepatic disease. Vet Clin Path 23:7–12, 1994.
8. Owen JS, Brown DJ, Harry DS, et al. Erythrocyte echinocytosis in liver disease. J Clin Invest 76:2275–2284, 1985.
9. Zieve L. Hemolytic anemia in liver disease. Medicine 45:497–505, 1966.
10. Cooper RA, Jandl JH. Destruction of erythrocytes. In Williams WJ, et al. (eds) Hematology, 3rd ed. McGraw-Hill, New York, 377–385, 1983.
11. Morse EE. Mechanisms of hemolysis in liver disease. Anim Clin Lab Sci 20:169–174, 1990.
12. Neerhout RC. Abnormalities of erythrocyte stromal lipids in hepatic disease. J Lab Clin Med 71:438–446, 1968.
13. Griffiths GL, Lumsden JH, Valli VO. Hematologic and biochemical changes in dogs with portosystemic shunts. J Am Anim Hosp Assoc 17:705–710, 1981.
14. Laflamme D, Mahaffey E, Allen S, et al. Microcytosis in dogs with portocaval shunt. Proc 8th ACVIM Forum, 1113, 1990, Washington, DC.
15. Bunch SE, Jordan HL, Sellon RK, et al. Iron status in 12 dogs with congenital portosystemic shunts. Proc 10th ACVIM Forum 809, 1992, San Diego.
16. Meyer DJ, Harvey JW. Hematologic changes associated with serum and hepatic iron alterations in dogs with congenital protosystemic vascular anomalies. J Vet Int Med 8:55–56, 1994.
17. Weiss HJ. Acquired qualitative platelet disorders. In Williams WJ, et al. (eds) Hematology, 3rd ed. McGraw-Hill, New York, 1356–1359, 1983.
18. Willis SE, Jackson ML, Meric SM et al. Evaluation of platelet aggregation in dogs with liver disease. (Abstract.) Proc 6 ACVIM Forum, 751, 1988.
19. Willis SE, Jackson ML, Meric SM, et al. Whole blood platelet aggregation in dogs with liver disease. Am J Vet Res 50:1893–1897, 1989.
20. Bowen DJ, Clemmons RM, Meyer DJ. Platelet functional changes secondary to hepatocholestasis and elevation of serum bile acids. Thromb Res 52:649–654, 1988.
21. Harker LA, Finch CA. Thrombokinetics in man. J Clin Invest 48:963–974, 1969.
22. Aster RH. Pooling of platelets in the spleen: Role in the pathogenesis of "hypersplenic" thrombocytopenia. J Clin Invest 45:645–657, 1966.
23. Thomas DP, Ream VJ, Stuart RK. Platelet aggregation in patients with Laennec's cirrhosis of the liver. N Engl J Med 276:1344–1348, 1967.
24. Thomas DP. Abnormalities of platelet aggregation in patients with alcoholic cirrhosis. Ann NY Acad Sci 201:243–250, 1972.
25. Mandel EE, Lazerson BA. Thrombasthesia in liver disease. N Engl J Med 265:56–61, 1961.
26. Stein SF, Harker LA. Kinetic and functional studies of platelets, fibrinogen, and plasminogen in patients with hepatic cirrhosis. J Lab Clin Med 99:217–230, 1982.
27. Nelson G. Lipid composition of erythrocytes in various mammalian species. Biochim Biphys Acta 144:221–232, 1967.
28. Weiss DJ. Susceptibility of canine, feline and human erthrocytes to oxidant mediated injury. Vet Clin Pathol 17:75–78, 1988.
29. Donohue TM, Jennett RB, Tuma DJ, et al. Synthesis and secretion of plasma proteins by the liver. In: Zakim D, Boyer TD (eds) Hepatology—a Textbook of Liver Disease. WB Saunders, Philadelphia, 124–136, 1990.
30. Hasch E, Jarnum S, Tygstrup N, et al. Albumin synthesis rate as a measure of liver function in patients with cirrhosis. Acta Med Scand 182:83–91, 1967.
31. Berson SA, Yalow RS. The distribution of I[131] labeled human serum albumin introduced into ascitic fluid: Analysis of the kinetics of a three compartment quaternary transfer system in man and speculation on possible sites of degradation. J Clin Invest 33:377–387, 1954.
32. Dykes PW. The rates of distribution and catabolism of albumin in normal subjects and in patients with cirrhosis of the liver. Clin Sci 34:161–183, 1968.
33. Sterling K. Serum albumin turnover in Laennec's cirrhosis as measured by I[131] tagged albumin. J Clin Invest 30:1238–1242, 1951.
34. Wilkinson P, Mendenhall CL. Serum albumin turnover in normal subjects and patients with cirrhosis measured by I[131]-labelled human albumin. Clin Sci 25:281–282, 1963.
35. Zimmon DS, Oratz M, Schreiberss, et al. Albumin to ascites: Demonstration of a direct pathway by passing the systemic circulation. J Clin Invest 48:2074–2078, 1969.
36. Kukral JC, Sporn J, Louch J, et al. Synthesis of alpha- and beta-globulins in normal and liverless dog. Am J Physiol 204:262–264, 1963.
37. Koj A. Metabolic studies of acute-phase proteins. In: Mariani G (ed) Pathophysiology of Plasma Protein Metabolism. Plenum Press, New York, London, 221–248, 1984.
38. Koj A. Liver response to inflammation and synthesis of acute phase plasma proteins. In: Gordon AH, Koj A (eds) The Acute Phase Response to Injury and Infection. Elsevier, New York, 139–246, 1985.
39. Harvey JW, West CL. Prednisone-induced increases in serum alpha-2- globulin and haptoglobin concentrations in dogs. Vet Pathol 24:90–92, 1987.
40. Harvey JW. Quantitative determinations of normal horse, cat and dog haptoglobins. Theriogenol 2–3;133–137, 1976.
41. Harvey JW. Comparison between serum haptoglobin and alpha-2-globulin concentrations in dogs. Vet Clin Path 15:4–5, 1986.
42. Ganrot K. Plasma protein response in experimental inflammation in the dog. Res Exp Med (Berl) 161:251–261, 1973.
43. Jain NC. Acute phase proteins. In: Kirk RW (ed) Current Veterinary Therapy X, WB Saunders, Philadelphia, 468:–471, 1989
44. Triger DR, Wright R. Immunological aspects of liver disease. In: Wright R, et al. (eds) Liver and Biliary Disease, 2nd ed. WB Saunders, Philadelphia, 215–232, 1985.
45. Canalese J, Gove CD, Gimson AES, et al. Reticuloendothelial system and hepatocyte function in fulminant hepatic failure. Gut 23:265–269, 1982.
46. Rimola A, Soto R, Bory F, et al. Reticuloendothelial system phagocytic activity in cirrhosis and its relation to bacterial infections and prognosis. Hepatology 4:53–58, 1984.
47. Ruoslahti E. Salaspuro M, Pihko H, et al. Serum α-alpha-feto-protein diagnostic significance in liver disease. Brit Med J 2:527–529, 1974.
48. Nayak SS, Kamath SS, Kundaje GN, et al. Diagnostic significance of estimation of serum apolipoprotein A along with alpha-fetoprotein in alcoholic cirrhosis and hepatocellular carcinoma patients. Clin Chim Acta 173:157–164, 1988.
49. Liaw Y-F, Chen T-J, Chu C-M, et al. Alpha-fetoprotein changes

in the course of chronic hepatitis: Relation to bridging hepatic necrosis and hepatocellular carcinoma. Liver 6:133–137, 1986.

50. Madsen AC, Rikkers LF, Moody RR, et al. Alpha-fetoprotein as a marker for hepatic regeneration in the dog. J Surg Res 28:71–76, 1980.
51. Madsen AC, Rikkers LF. Alpha-fetoprotein secretion by injured and regenerating hepatocytes in the dog. J Surg Res 37:402–408, 1984.
52. Hirao K, Matsumura K, Imagawa A, et al. Primary neoplasms in dog liver induced by diethylnitrosamine. Cancer Res 34:1870–1882, 1974.
53. Shinomiya Y, Hirao K, Matsumura K, et al. Alpha-fetoprotein during hepatocarcinogenesis in dogs treated with chemical carcinogens. In: Hirai H, Miyaji T (eds) GANN Monograph on Cancer Research: Alpha-fetoprotein and Hepatoma. University Park Press, Tokyo, 301–313, 1973.
54. Lowseth LA, Gillett NA, Chang I-Y, et al. Detection of serum α–fetoprotein in dogs with hepatic tumors. J Am Vet Med Assoc 199:735–741, 1991.
55. Pappas NJ Jr. Increased rat liver homogenate, mitochondrial, and cytosolic asparate aminotransferase activity in acute carbon tetrachloride poisoning. Clin Chim Acta 106:233–229, 1980.
56. Pappas NJ Jr. Source of increased serum asparate and alanine aminotransferase: Cyclohexinde effect on carbon tetrachloride hepatotoxicity. Clin Chim Acta 154:181–190, 1986.
57. Cornelius CE, Bishop J, Switzer J, et al. Serum and tissue transaminase activities in domestic animals. Cornell Vet 49:116–126, 1959.
58. Valentine BA, Blue JT, Shelley SM, et al. Increased serum alanine aminotransferase activity associated with muscle necrosis in the dog. J Vet Int Med 4:140–143, 1990.
59. Zinkl JG, Bush RM, Cornelius CE, et al. Comparative studies on plasma and tissue sorbitol, glutamic, lactic, and hydroxybutyric dehydrogenase and transaminase activities in the dog. Res Vet Sci 12:211–214, 1971.
60. Duncan JR, Prasse KW Liver. In: Veterinary Laboratory Medicine Clinical Pathology, 2nd ed. Ames, Iowa State University Press, 121–277, 1986.
61. Stolz A, Kaplowitz N. Biochemical tests for liver disease. In Zakim D, Boyer TD (eds) Hepatology–A Textbook of Liver Disease. WB Saunders, Philadelphia, 637–666, 1990.
62. Meyer D Serum gamma-glutamyltransferase as a liver test in cats with toxic and obstructive hepatic disease. J Am Anim Hosp Assoc 19:1023–1026, 1983.
63. Spano JS, August JR, Henderson RA, et al Serum gamma-glutamyl transpeptidase activity in healthy cats and cats with induced hepatic disease. Am J Vet Res 44:2049–2053, 1983.
64. Cornelius CE, Kaneko JJ. Serum transaminase activities in cats with hepatic necrosis. J Am Vet Med Assoc 137:62–66, 1960.
65. Noonan NE, Meyer DJ. Use of plasma arginase and gamma-glutamyl transpeptidase as specific indicators of hepatocellular or hepatobiliary disease in the dog. Am J Vet Res 40:942–947, 1979.
66. Hoe CM, Jabara AG. The use of serum enzymes as diagnostic aids in the dog. J Comp Path 77:245–254, 1967.
67. Van Vleet JF, JO Alberts Evaluation of liver function tests and liver biopsy in experimental carbon tetracholoride intoxication and extrahepatic bile duct obstruction in the dog. Am J Vet Res 29:2119–2131, 1968
68. Dixon MF, Fulker MJ, Walker BE, et al. Serum transaminase levels after experimental paracetamol-induced hepatic necrosis. Gut 16:800–807, 1975
69. Center SA, Baldwin BE, Tennant B, et al. Hematologic and biochemical abnormalities associated with induced extrahepatic bile duct obstruction in the cat. Am J Vet Res 44:1822–1829, 1983.
70. Shull RM, Hornbuckle W. Diagnostic use of serum gamma-glutamyltransferase in canine liver disease. Am J Vet Res 40:1321–1324, 1979.
71. Guelfi JF, Braun JP, Bernard P, et al. Value of so-called cholestasis markers in the dog. Res Vet Sci 33:309–312, 1982.
72. Everett RM, Duncan JR, Prasse KW. Alkaline phosphatase,

73. leucine aminopeptidase and alanine aminotransferase activities with obstructive and toxic hepatic disease in cats. Am J Vet Res 38:963–966, 1977.
73. Wigton DH, Kociba GJ, Hoover EA. Infectious canine hepatitis: Animal model for-viral-induced disseminated intravascular coagulation. Blood 47:287–296, 1976.
74. Sturtevant F, Hoffman WE, Dorner JL. The effect of three anticonvulsant drugs and ACTH on canine serum alkaline phosphatase. J Am Anim Hosp Assoc 13:754–757, 1977.
75. Badylak SF, Van Vleet JF. Tissue gamma-glutamyl transpeptidase activity and hepatic ultrastructural alterations in dogs with experimentally induced glucocorticoid hepatopathy. Am J Vet Res 43:649–655, 1982.
76. Dillon AR, Spano JS, Powers RD. Prednisolone induced hematologic, biochemical and histological changes in the dog. J Am Anim Hosp Assoc 16:831–837, 1980.
77. Magne ML, Withrow SJ. Hepatic neoplasia. Vet Clin N Am 15:243–256, 1985
78. Whiteley MB, Feeney DA, Whiteley LO, et al. Ultrasonographic appearance of primary and metastatic canine hepatic tumors: A review of 48 cases. J Ultrasound Med 8:621–630, 1989.
79. Trigo FJ, Thompson H, Breeze RG, et al. The pathology of liver tumors in the dog. J Comp Path 92:21–39, 1982.
80. Strombeck DR. Clinicopathologic features of primary and metastatic neoplastic disease of the liver in dogs. J Am Vet Med Assoc 173:267–269, 1978.
81. McConnell MF, Lumsden JH. Biochemical evaluation of metastatic liver disease in the dog. J Am Anim Hosp Assoc 19:173–178, 1983.
82. Boyd JW. The mechanisms relating to increases in plasma enzymes and isoenzymes in diseases of animals. Vet Clin Path 12:9–24, 1983.
83. Nilkumhang P, Thornton JR. Plasma and tissue enzyme activities in the cat. J Small Anim Pract 20:169–174, 1979.
84. Nagode LA, Frajola WJ, Loeb WF. Enzyme activities of canine tissues. J Am Vet Res 27:1385–1393, 1966.
85. Keller P. Enzyme activities in the dog: Tissue analyses, plasma values, and intracellular distribution. Am J Vet Res 42:575–582, 1981.
86. Morino Y, Kagamiyama H, Wada J. Immunochemical distinction between glutamic-oxalacetic transaminases from soluble and mitochondrial fractions of mammalian tissues. J Biol Chem 239:943–944, 1964.
87. Mia AS, Koger HD. Comparative studies on serum arginase and transaminases in hepatic necrosis in various species of domestic animals. Vet Clin Path 8:9–15, 1979.
88. Rikkers LF, Moody FG. Estimation of functional reserve of normal and regenerating dog livers. Surg 75:421–429, 1974.
89. Cornelius LM, DeNovo RC. Icterus in cats. In: Kirk RW (ed) Current Veterinary Therapy VIII. WB Saunders, Philadelphia, 822–829, 1983
90. Abdelkader SV, Hauge JG. Serum enzyme determination in the study of liver disease in dogs. Acta Vet Scand 27:59–70, 1986.
91. Center SA, ManWarren T, Slater MR, et al. Evaluation of twelve-hour preprandial and two-hour postprandial serum bile acids concentrations for diagnosis of hepatobiliary disease in dogs. J Am Vet Med Assoc 199:217–226, 1991.
92. Cornelius CE, Douglas GM, Gronwall RR, et al. Comparative studies on plasma arginase and transaminases in hepatic necrosis. Cornell Vet 53:181–191, 1963.
93. Cargill CF, Shields RP. Plasma arginase as a liver function test. J Com Path 81:447–454, 1971.
94. Mia AS, Koger HD. Direct colorimetric determination of serum arginase in various domestic animals. Am J Vet Res 173:1381–1383, 1978.
95. Cacciatore L, Antoniello S, Valentino B, et al. Arginase activity, arginine and ornithine of plasma in experimental liver damage. Enzyme 17:269–275, 1974.
96. Ugarte G, Pino ME, Peirano P. Serum arginase activity in subjects with hepatocellular damage. J Lab Clin Med 55:522–529, 1960.
97. DeNovo RC, Prasse KW. Comparison of serum biochemical and hepatic functional alterations in dogs treated with corti-

costeroids and hepatic duct ligation. Am J Vet Res 44:1703–1709, 1983.

98. Center SA, Slater MR, ManWarren T, et al. The diagnostic efficacy of serum alkaline phosphatase and γ-glutamyl transferase in the dog with histologically confirmed hepatobiliary disease: A study of 270 cases (1980–1990). J Am Vet Med Assoc 201:1258–1264, 1992.

99. Center SA, Baldwin BH, Dillingham S, et al. Diagnostic value of serum γ-glutamyl transferase and alkaline phosphatase in hepatobiliary disease in the cat. J Am Vet Med Assoc 188:507–510, 1986.

100. Fishman WH. Perspectives on alkaline phosphatase isoenzymes. Am J Med 56:617–649, 1974.

101. Hoffmann WE. Diagnostic value of canine serum alkaline phosphatase and alkaline phosphatase isoenzymes. J Am Anim Hosp Assoc 13:237–241, 1977.

102. Hoffmann WE, Dorner JL. Separation of isoenzymes of canine alkaline phosphatase by cellulose acetate electrophoresis. J Am Anim Hosp Assoc 11:283–285, 1975.

103. Saini PK, Peavy GM, Hauser DE, et al. Diagnostic evaluation of canine serum alkaline phosphatase by immunochemical means and interpretation of results. Am J Vet Res 39:1514–1518, 1978.

104. Hoffman WE, Dorner JL. Disappearance rate of intravenous injected canine alkaline phosphatase isoenzymes. Am J Vet Res 38:1553–1555, 1977.

105. Bengmark S, Olsson R. Elimination of alkaline phosphatases from serum in dog after intravenous injection of canine phosphatases from bone and intestine. Acta Chir Scand 140:1–6, 1974.

106. Hoffmann WE, Renegar WE, Dorner JL. Alkaline phosphatase and alkaline phosphatase isoenzymes in the cat. Vet Clin Path 6:21–24, 1977.

107. Hoffman WE, Dorner JL. Serum half-life of intravenously injected intestinal and hepatic alkaline phosphatase isoenzymes in the cat. Am J Vet Res 38:1637–1639, 1977.

108. Everett RM, Duncan JR, Prasse KW. Alkaline phosphatase in tissues and sera of cats. Am J Vet Res 38:1533–1538, 1977.

109. De Broe ME, Roels F, Nouwen EJ, et al. Liver plasma membrane: The source of high molecular weight alkaline phosphatase in human serum. Hepatology 5:118–128, 1985.

110. Sanecki RK, Hoffmann WE, Dorner JL, et al. Purification and comparison of corticosteroid-induced and intestinal isoenzymes of alkaline phosphatase in dogs. Am J Vet Res 51:1964–1968, 1990.

111. Sanecki RK, Hoffmann WE, Gelberg HB, et al. Subcellular location of corticosteroid-induced alkaline phosphatase in canine hepatocytes. Vet Pathol 24:296–301, 1987.

112. Seetharam S, Sussman NL, Komoda T, et al. The mechanism of elevated alkaline phosphatase activity after bile duct ligation in the rat. Hepatology 6:374–380, 1986.

113. Hadley SP, Hoffman WE, Kuhlenschmidt MS, et al. Effect of glucocorticoids on ALP, ALT and GGT in cultured dog hepatocytes. Enzyme 43:89–90, 1990.

114. Hatoff DE, Hardison WGM. Bile acid–dependent secretion of alkaline phosphatase in rat bile. Hepatology 2:433–439, 1982.

115. Hamilton JM, Wright J, Kight D. Alkaline phosphatase levels in canine mammary neoplasia. Vet Rec 93:121–123, 1973.

116. Aronsen KF, Hagerst F, Norden JG. Enzyme studies in dogs with extra-hepatic biliary obstruction. Scan J Gastroenterol 3:354–368, 1968.

117. McLain DL, Nagode LA, Wilson GP, et al. Alkaline phosphatase and its isoenzymes in normal cats and in cats with biliary obstruction. J Am Anim Hosp Assoc 14:94–99, 1978.

118. LaVia MF, Hill RB. Principles of Pathobiology. Oxford University Press, London, 27–30, 1971.

119. Oelberg DG, Lester R. Cellular mechanisms of cholestasis. Annu Rev Med 37:297–317, 1986.

120. Taboada J, Meyer DJ. Cholestasis associated with extrahepatic bacterial infection in five dogs. J Vet Int Med 3:216–221, 1989.

121. Righetti ABB, Kaplan MM. Disparate responses of serum and hepatic alkaline phosphatase and 5′nucleotidase to bile duct obstruction in the rat. Gastroenterology 62:1034–1039, 1972.

122. Hoffman WE, Dorner JL. A comparison of canine normal

123. Saini PK, Saini SK. Origin of serum alkaline phosphatase in the dog. Am J Vet Res 39:1510–1513, 1978.

124. Hoffman WE, Sanecki RK, Dorner JL. A technique for automated quantification of canine glucocorticoid-induced isoenzyme of alkaline phosphatase. Vet Clin Path 17:66–70, 1991.

125. Dorner JL, Hoffman WE, Long GB. Corticosteroid induction of an isoenzyme of alkaline phosphatase in the dog. Am J Vet Res 35:1457–1458, 1974.

126. Dillon AR, Sorjonen DC, Powers RD, et al. Effects of dexamethasone and surgical hypotension on hepatic morphologic features and enzymes of dogs. Am J Vet Res 44:1996–1999, 1983.

127. Badylak SF, Van Vleet JF. Sequential morphologic and clinicopathologic alterations in dogs with experimentally induced glucocorticoid hepatopathy. Am J Vet Res 42:1310–1318, 1981.

128. Scott DW, Kirk RW, Bentinck-Smith J. Some effects of short-term methylprednisolone therapy in normal cats. Cornell Vet 69:104–115, 1979.

129. Scott DW, Manning TO, Reimers TJ. Iatrogenic Cushing's syndrome in the cat. Feline Pract 12:30–36, 1982.

130. Middleton DJ, Watson AD, Howe CJ, et al. Suppression of cortisol responses to exogenous adrenocorticotrophic hormone and the occurrence of side effects attributable to glucocorticoid excess in cats during therapy with megestral acetate and prednisolone. Can J Vet Res 51:60–65, 1986.

131. Fulton R, Thrall MA, Weiser MG, et al. Steroid hepatopathy in cats. Proc Am Soc Vet Clin Pathol 23 [platform presentation], 1988.

132. Bunch SE, Castleman WL, Hornbuckle WE, et al. Hepatic cirrhosis associated with long-term anticonvulsant drug therapy in dogs. J Am Vet Assoc 181:357–362, 1982.

133. Bunch SE, Baldwin BE, Hornbuckle WE, et al. Compromised hepatic function in dogs treated with anticonvulsants. J Am Vet Med Assoc 184:444–448, 1984.

134. Bunch SE. Effects of anticonvulsant drugs phenytoin and primidone on the canine liver. Thesis, Cornell University, 81, 1983.

135. Albert Z, Orlowska J, Orlowski M, et al. Histochemical and biochemical investigations of gamma glutamyl transpeptidase in tissues of man and laboratory rodents. Acta Histochem 18:78–89, 1964.

136. Hanes CS, Hird FJ. Synthesis of peptides in enzymic reactions involving glutathione. Nature 166:288–292, 1950.

137. Hagenfeldt L, Larsson A, Anderson R. The gamma glutamyl cycle and amino acid transport. N Engl J Med 299:587–590, 1978.

138. Braun JP, Benard P, Burgat V, et al. Gamma glutamyl transferase in domestic animals. Vet Res Comm 6:77–90, 1983.

139. Shaw LM, London JW, Peterson LE. Isolation of gamma glutamyl transferase from human liver, and comparison with the enzyme from human kidney. Clin Chem 24:905–915, 1978.

140. Lum G, Gambino SR. Serum gamma glutamyl transpeptidase activity as an indicator of disease of liver, pancreas or bone. Clin Chem 18:358–362, 1972.

141. Naftalin L, Child VJ, Morley SA, et al. Observations on the site of origin of serum gamma-glutamyl transpeptidase. Clin Chim Acta 26:297–300, 1969.

142. Kokot F, Kuska J, Grzybek M. Gamma-glutamyl transpeptidase (GGTP) in the urine and intestinal contents. Arch Immunol Ther Exp 13:549–556, 1965.

143. Kokot F, Grzybek H, Kuska J. Experimental studies on gamma-glutamyl transpeptidase. IV. Histoenzymatic and biochemical changes in parenchymatous hepatitis in rabbits and in obstructive jaundice in dogs. Acta Med Pol 6:379–388, 1975.

144. Aronsen KF, Hagerstrand I, Norden JG. Enzyme histochemical studies of the liver remnant following partial hepatectomy in dogs. Acta Chir Scand 136:521–527, 1970.

145. Aronsen KF, Hagerstrand I, Norden JG. Enzyme studies in dogs with extra-hepatic biliary obstruction. Scand J Gastroenterol 3:355–368, 1968.

146. Moss DW. Clinical enzymology—a perspective. Enzyme 25:2–12, 1980.

147. Moss DW. Contribution of clinical enzymology to the study of hepatobiliary disease—the enzymologist's view. Clin Biochem 12:236–238, 1979.

148. Stein TA, Rurns GP, Wise L. Diagnostic value of liver function tests in bile duct obstruction. J Surg Res 46:226–229, 1989.

149. Colombo JP, Peheim E, Bachmann C, et al. Gamma-glutamyl transpeptidase in the rat liver after portacaval shunt. Pediatr Res 10:18–24, 1976.

150. Krebs C. Gamma-glutamyltransferase activity in the cat. Inaugural dissertation, Ludwig-Maximilans Universitat, Munchen, 122, 1979.

151. Sawabu N, Nakagen M, Ozaki K, et al. Novel gamma-GTP isoenzyme as diagnostic tool for hepatocellular carcinoma. Ann Acad Med 9:206–209, 1980.

152. Mircea P, Cucuianu M, Madarasan-Vulcan G, et al. Value of gamma-glutamyltransferase in the diagnosis of liver metastases. Rev Roum Med Med Int 19:339–345, 1981.

153. Center SA, Randolph JF, ManWarren T, et al. Effect of colostrum ingestion on gamma-glutamyltransferase and alkaline phosphatase activities in neonatal pups. Am J Vet Res 52:499–504, 1991.

154. Milne EM, Doxey DL. Lactate dehydrogenase and its isoenzymes in the tissues and sera of clinically normal dogs. Res Vet Sci 43:222–224, 1987.

155. Aguilera-Tejero E, Mayer-Valor R, Gomez-Cardenas G. Spectrophotometric method for differentiation of cardiac and hepatic lactate dehydrogenase activities in dogs. Am J Vet Res 50:1128–1130, 1989.

156. Fielder FG, Hoff EJ, Thomas GB. A study of the subacute toxicity of prednisolone, methylprednisolone, and triamcinalone in dogs. Toxicol Appl Pharmacol 1:305–314, 1959.

157. Thompson SW, Sparano BM, Diener RM. Vacuoles in the hepatocytes of cortisone-treated dogs. Am J Pathol 63:135–148, 1971.

158. Rogers WA, Reubner BH. A retrospective study of probable glucocorticoid-induced hepatopathy in dogs. J Am Vet Med Assoc 170:603–606, 1977.

159. Fittschen C, Bellamy JEC. Prednisone-induced morphologic and chemical changes in the liver of dogs. Vet Pathol 21:399–406, 1984.

160. Takeda Y, Ichihara A, Tanioka H, et al. The effect of corticosteroids on leakage of enzymes from dispersed rat liver cells. J Biol Chem 239:3590–3596, 1964.

161. Schulster D, et al. Molecular Endocrinology of the Steroid Hormones. Wiley, New York, 148–163, 273–292, 1976.

162. Roberts SM, Lavach JD, Macy DW, et al. Effect of ophthalmic prednisolone acetate on the canine adrenal gland and hepatic function. Am J Vet Res 45:1711–1714, 1984.

163. Glaze MB, Crawford MA, Nachreiner RF, et al. Ophthalmic corticosteroid therapy: Systemic effects in the dog. J Am Vet Med Assoc 192:73–75, 1988.

164. Meyer DJ, Moriello KA, Feder BM, et al. Effect of otic medications containing glucocorticoids on liver function test results in healthy dogs. J Am Vet Med Assoc 196:743–744, 1990.

165. Moriello KA, Fehrer-Sawyer SL, Meyer DJ, et al. Adrenocortical suppression associated with topical otic administration of glucocorticoids in dogs. J Am Vet Med Assoc 193:329–331, 1988.

166. Zenoble RD, Kemppainen RJ. Adrenocortical suppression by topically applied corticosteroids in healthy dogs. J Am Vet Med Assoc 191:685–688, 1987.

167. Moore GE, Mahaffey EA, Hoeing M. Hematologic and serum biochemical effects of long-term administration of anti-inflammatory doses of prednisone in dogs. Am J Vet Res 53:1033–1037, 1992.

168. Peterson ME, Kintzer PP, Cavanagh PG, et al. Feline hyperthyroidism: Pretreatment clinical and laboratory evaluation of 131 cases. J Am Vet Med Assoc 183:103–110, 1983.

169. Horney BS, Farmer AJ, Honor DJ, et al: Agarose gel electrophoresis of alkaline phosphatase isoenzymes in the serum of hyperthyroid cats. Vet Clin Path, 23:98–102, 1995.

170. Gavin LA, Cavalieri RR. Interrelationships between the thyroid gland and liver. In: Zakim D, Boyer TD (eds) Hepatology—A Textbook of Liver Disease. WB Saunders, Philadelphia, 508–515, 1982.

171. Beaver DC, Pemberton J. The pathologic anatomy of the liver in exophthalmic goitre. Ann Int Med 7:687–708, 1933.

172. Pipher J, Poulsen E. Liver biopsy in thyrotoxicosis. Acta Med Scand 127:439, 1947.

173. Meyers JD, Brannon ES, Holland BG. A correlative study of the cardiac output and the hepatic circulation in hyperthyroidism. J Clin Invest 29:1069–1077, 1950.

174. Hoe CM, O'Shea JD. The correlation of biochemistry and histopathology in liver disease in the dog. Vet Rec 77:1164–1171, 1965.

175. Cello JP, Grendell JH. The liver in systemic conditions. In: Zakim D, Boyer TD (eds) Hepatology—a Textbook of Liver Disease. WB Saunders, Philadelphia, 1411–1437, 1990.

176. Obrien PJ, O'Grady M, Lumsden JH, et al. Clinical pathologic profiles of dogs and turkeys with congestive heart failure, either noninduced or induced by rapid ventricular pacing, and turkeys with furazolidone toxicosis. Am J Vet Res 54:60–68, 1933.

177. Schall WD. Laboratory diagnosis of hepatic disease. Vet Clin N Am Sm Anim Pract 6:679–686, 1976.

178. Himes JA, Cornelius CE. Hepatic excretion and storage of sulfobromophthalein sodium in experimental hepatic necrosis in the dog. Cornell Vet 63:424–431, 1973.

179. Janssen PAJ, Symoens JE. Hepatic reaction during ketoconazole treatment. Am J Med Jan 24:80–85, 1983.

180. Heiberg JK, Svejgaard E. Toxic hepatitis during ketoconazole treatment. Br Med J 283:825, 1981.

181. Samols E, Holdsworth D. Disturbances in carbohydrate metabolism: Liver disease. In: Dickins F, et al. (eds) Carbohydrate Metabolism and Its Disorders, Vol. 2. Academic Press, New York, 289–336, 1968.

182. Owen OE, et al. Gluconeogenesis in normal, cirrhotic and diabetic humans. In Hanson RW, Mehlman MA (eds) Gluconeogenesis: Its Regulations in Mammalian Species. Wiley, New York, 533–558, 1976.

183. Strombeck DR, Krum S, Meyer D, et al. Hypoglycemia and hypoinsulinemia associated with hepatoma in a dog. J Am Vet Med Assoc 169:811–812, 1976.

184. Walton DK, Center SA, Scott DW, et al. Ulcerative dermatosis associated with diabetes mellitus in the dog: A report of four cases. J Am Anim Hosp Assoc 22:79–88, 1986.

185. Miller WH, Scott DW, Buerger RG, et al. Necrolytic migratory erythrema in dogs: A hepatocutaneous syndrome. J Am Anim Hosp Assoc 26:573–581, 1990.

186. Gross TL, O'Brien RD, Davis AP, et al. Glucagon-producing pancreatic endocrine tumors in two dogs with superficial necolytic dermatitis. J Am Vet Med Assoc 197:1619–1622, 1990.

187. Gross TL, Song MD, Havel PJ, et al. Superficial necrolytic dermatitis (necrolytic migratory erythema) in dogs. Vet Pathol 30:75–81, 1993.

187a. Francavilla A, Jones AF, Benichou J, et al. The effect of portacaval shunt upon hepatic cholesterol synthesis and cyclic AMP in dogs and baboons. J Surg Res 28:1–7, 1980.

188. Bloom F. The diagnosis and treatment of liver disease of the dog. N Am Vet 38:17–27, 1957.

189. Opitz M, Lettow E. Der cholesterinesterquotient im serujm leberkranker hunde. Berl Munch Tierarztl Wschr 89:28–32, 1976.

190. Erickson SK, et al. Rat liver acyl coenzyme A:cholesterol acyltransferase. Its regulation in vivo and some of its properties in vitro. J Lipid Res 21:930, 1980.

191. Cooper AD. Hepatic lipoprotein and cholesterol metabolism. In: Zakim D, Boyer TD (eds) Hepatology—Textbook of Liver Disease. WB Saunders, Philadelphia, 109–366, 1982.

192. Bass VD, Hoffman WE, Dorner JL. Normal canine lipid profiles and effects of experimentally induced pancreatitis and hepatic necrosis on lipids. Am J Vet Res 37:1355–1357, 1976.

193. Kaneko JJ. Normal values for blood chemistry used at VMTH in Davis, CA.

194. Kirk RW. Small animal practice. In: Kirk RW(ed) Current Veterinary Therapy XI. WB Saunders, Philadelphia, 1256, 1992.

195. Veterinary Medical Teaching Hospital, University of California at Davis, normal values.

196. Harry DS, Owen JS, McIntyre. Plasma lipoproteins and the liver. In: Wright R, Millward-Sadler GH, Alberti KGMM (eds) Liver and Biliary Disease, 2nd ed, WB Saunders, Philadelphia, 65–86, 1985.

197. Simon JB, Scheig R. Serum cholesterol esterification in liver disease: Importance of lecithin-cholesterol acyltransferase. N Engl J Med 283: 841–846, 1970.

198. Friedman M, Byers SO. Observations concerning the production and excretion of cholesterol in mammals. XVI. The relationship of the liver to the content and control of plasma cholesterol ester. J Clin Invest 34:1369–1374, 1955.

199. Fex G, Wallinder L. Liver and plasma cholesteryl ester metabolism after partial hepatectomy in the rat. Biochimica et Biophysica Acta 316:91–97, 1973.

200. Sugano M, Hori K, Wada M. Hepatotoxicity and plasma cholesterol esterification by rats. Arch Biochem 129:588–596, 1969.

201. Calandra S, Martin MJ, McIntyre N. Plasma lecithin: cholesterol acyltransferase activity in liver disease. Europ J Clin Invest 1:352–360, 1971.

202. Agorastos J, Fox C, Harry DS, et al. Lecithin-cholesterol acyltransferase and the lipoprotein abnormalities of obstructive jaundice. Clin Sci Mole Med 54:369–379, 1978.

203. Gjone E, Norum KR. Plasma lecithin-cholesterol acyltransferase and erythrocyte lipids in liver disease. Acta Med Scand 187:153–161, 1970.

204. Muller P, Fellin R. Hypertriglyceridaemia secondary to liver disease. Europ J Clin Invest 4:419–428, 1974.

205. Quarfordt SH, Oelschlaeger H, Krigbaum WR, et al. Effect of biliary obstruction on canine plasma and biliary lipids. Lipids 8:522–530, 1973.

206. McIntyre N, Harry DS, Pearson AJG. Progress report: The hypercholesterolemia of obstructive jaundice. Gut 16:379–391, 1975.

207. Milewski B, Palynyczko Z. Evaluation of the usefulness of serum lipoprotein-X (LP-X) detection test for the diagnosis of cholestasis in chronic liver diseases. Pol Arch Med Wewn 53:445–452, 1975.

208. Ritland S. Quantitative determination of the abnormal lipoprotein of cholestasis, LP-X, in liver disease. Scand J Gastroenterol 10:5–15, 1975.

209. Seidel D, Buff HU, Bleyl U. On the metabolism of lipoprotein-X (LP-X). Clin Chim Acta 66:195–207, 1976.

210. Bauer JE, Meyer DJ, Goring RL, et al. Cholestasis induced changes in canine serum lipids and lipoproteins. ACVIM Proc (abstract), 14–45, 1986.

211. Coyle JJ, Schwartz MZ, Marubbio AT, et al. The effect of portacaval shunt on plasma lipids and tissue cholesterol synthesis in the dog. Surgery 80:54–60, 1976.

212. Guzman IJ, Schneider PD, Coyle JJ. Combined hypolipidemia of portacaval transposition and ileal resection in the dog. Surg Gyn Obstet 150:475–480, 1980.

213. Coyle JJ, Guzman IJ, Varco RL. Cholesterol pool sizes and turnover following portacaval shunt in the dog. Surg Gyn Obstet 148:723–737, 1979.

214. Guzman IJ, Coyle JJ, Schneider PD, et al. The effect of selective visceral caval shunt on plasma lipids and cholesterol dynamics. Surgery 82:42–50, 1977.

215. Rogers WA, Donovan EF, Kociba GJ. Idiopathic hyperlipoproteinemia in dogs. J Am Vet Med Assoc 166:1087–1091, 1975.

216. Whitney MS, Boon GD, Rebar AH, et al. Ultracentrifugal and electrophoretic characteristics of the plasma lipoproteins of miniature schnauzer dogs with idiopathic hyperlipoproteinemia. J Vet Int Med 7:253–260, 1993.

217. Kelly DA, Summerfield JA. Hemostasis in liver disease. Sem Liver Dis 7:182–191, 1987.

218. Furie B, Furie BC. Molecular and cellular biology of blood coagulation. N Engl J Med 326:800–806, 1992.

219. Colman RW, Rubin RN. Blood coagulation. In Arias IM, Jakoby WB, Popper H, et al. (eds) The Liver: Biology and Pathobiology. Raven Press, New York, 1033–1042, 1988.

220. Ewe K. Bleeding after liver biopsy does not correlate with indices of peripheral coagulation. Dig Dis Sci 26:388–393, 1981.

221. Spector I, Corn M. Laboratory tests of hemostasis: The relation to hemorrhage in liver disease. Arch Intern Med 119:577–582, 1967.

222. Aledort LM. Blood clotting abnormalities in liver disease. In Popper H, Schaffner F (eds) Progress in Liver Diseases, Vol. 2. Grune & Stratton, New York, 350–362, 1976.

223. Badylak SF, Van Vleet JF. Alterations of prothrombin time and activated partial thromboplastin time in dogs with hepatic disease. Am J Vet Res 42:2053–2056, 1981.

224. Fiore L, Levine J, Deykin D. Alterations of hemostasis in patients with liver disease. In: Zakim D, Boyer TD (eds) Hepatology—a Textbook of Liver Disease. WB Saunders, Philadelphia, 546–571, 1990.

225. Badylak SF, Dodds WJ, Van Vleet JF. Plasma coagulation factor abnormalities in dogs with naturally occurring hepatic disease. Am J Vet Res 44:2336–2340, 1983.

226. Osbaldiston GW, Hoffman MW. Coagulation defects in experimental hepatic injury in the dog. Can J Comp Med 35:129–135, 1971.

227. Schenk WG, Fopeano J, Cosgriff JH, et al. The coagulation defect after hepatectomy. Surgery 42:822–826, 1957.

228. Furnival CM, Mackenzie RJ, MacDonald GA, et al. The mechanism of impaired coagulation after partial hepatectomy in the dog. Surg Gyn Obstet 143:81–86, 1976.

229. Green G, Poller L, Thompson JM, et al. Factor VII as a marker of hepatocellular synthetic function in liver disease. J Clin Pathol 29:971–975, 1976.

230. Dymock IW, Tucher JS, Woolf IL, et al. Coagulation studies as a prognostic index in acute liver failure. Br J Haematol 29:385–395, 1975.

231. Walllin R, Martin LF. Vitamin K dependent carboxylation and vitamin K metabolism in liver—the effects of warfarin. J Clin Invest 76:1879–1884, 1985.

232. Suttie JW. Recent advances in hepatic vitamin K metabolism and function. Hepatology 367–376, 1987.

233. Friedman PA. Vitamin K-dependent proteins. N Engl J Med 310:1458–1460, 1984.

234. Blanchard RA, Furie BC, Jorgensen M, et al. Acquired vitamin K-dependent carboxylation deficiency in liver disease. N Engl J Med 305;242–248, 1981.

235. Hemker HC, Muller AD. Kinetic aspects of the interaction of blood clotting enzymes: VI. Localization of the site of blood-coagulation inhibition by the protein induced by vitamin K absence (PIVKA). Throm Diath Haemorrh 20:78–87, 1968.

236. Gaudernack G, Prydz H. Studies on PIVKA-X. Thromb Diath Haemorrh 34:455–464, 1975.

237. Mount ME. Proteins induced by Vitamin K absence or antagonists (PIVKA). In: Kirk RW (ed) Current Veterinary Therapy IX. WB Saunders, Philadelphia, 513–515, 1986.

238. Koller F. Theory and experience behind use of coagulation tests in diagnosis and prognosis of liver disease. Scand J Gastroenterol (suppl 19) 8:51–61, 1973.

239. Ham TH, Curtis FC. Plasma fibrinogen response in man. Influence of the nutritional state, induced hyperpyrexia, infectious disease and liver damage. Medicine 14:413–445, 1938.

240. McCaw DL, Jergens AE, Turrentine MA, et al. Effect of internal hemorrhage on fibrin(ogen) degradation products in canine blood. Am J Vet Res 47:1620–1621, 1986.

241. Green RA. Clinical implications of antithrombin III deficiency in animal diseases. Comp Cont Ed 6:537–545, 1984.

242. Biggs R, Denson KW, Akwan N, et al. Antithrombin III, antifactor Xa and heparin. Brit J Haematol 19:283–305, 1970.

243. Rodzynek JJR, Preux C, Leautaud P, et al. Diagnostic value of antithrombin III and aminopyrine breath test in liver diseases. Arch Intern Med 146:677–680, 1986.

244. Feldman BF, Madewell BR, O'Neill S. Disseminated intravascular coagulation: Antithrombin, plasminogen, and coagulation abnormalities in 41 dogs. J Am Vet Med Assoc 179:151–154, 1981.

245. Raymond SL, Dodds WJ. Plasma antithrombin activity: A comparative study in normal and diseased animals. Proc Soc Exp Biol Med 161:464–467, 1979.

246. Mannucci L, Dioguardi N, Del Ninno E, et al. Value of Normotest and antithrombin III in the assessment of liver function. Scand J Gastroenterol 8 (suppl 19:103–107, 1973.

247. Duckert F. Behaviour of antithrombin III in liver disease. Scand J Gastroenterol 8 (suppl 19):109–112, 1973.

248. Boothe DM, Jenkins WL, Green RA, et al. Dimethylni-

trosamine-induced hepatotoxicosis in dogs as a model of progressive canine hepatic disease. Am J Vet Res 53:411–420, 1992.

249. Rodzynek JJ, Urbain D, Leautaud P, et al. Antithrombin III, plasminogen and alpha 2 antiplasmin in jaundice: Clinical usefulness and prognostic significance. Gut 25:1050–1056, 1984.

250. De Schepper J, Van Der Stock J. Influence of sex on the urinary bilirubin excretion at increased free plasma haemoglobin levels in whole dogs and in isolated normothermic perfused dog kidneys. Experientia 27:1264–1265, 1971.

251. Cameron JL, Stafford ES, Schraufer L, et al Bilirubin excretion in the dog. J Surg Res III:39–42, 1963.

252. Osborne CA, Stevens JB, Lees GE, et al. Clinical significance of bilirubinuria. Compend Contin Educ Pract Vet 2:897–903, 1980.

253. Lees GE, Hardy RM, Stevens JB, et al. Clinical implications of feline bilirubinuria. J Am Anim Hosp Assoc 20:765–771, 1984.

254. Yeary RA, Davis DR. Protein binding of bilirubin: Comparison of in vitro and in vivo measurements of bilirubin displacement by drugs. Tox Appl Pharm 28:269–283, 1974.

255. De Schepper J. Degradation of haemoglobin to bilirubin in the kidney of the dog. Tijdschr Diergeneesk 99:699–707, 1974.

256. De Schepper J, Van Der Stock J. Influence of sex on the urinary bilirubin excretion at increased free plasma haemoglobin levels in whole dogs and in isolated normothermic perfused dog kidneys. Experientia 27:1264–1265, 1971.

257. De Schepper J, Van der Stock J. Increased urinary bilirubin excretion after elevated free plasma haemoglobin levels. II. Variations in the calculated renal clearances of bilirubin in isolated normothermic perfused dog's kidneys. Arch Intern Physiol Biochim 80:339–348, 1969.

258. Van Der Stock J, De Schepper J. The urinary excretion of bilirubin after increased plasma hemoglobin concentration in dogs. Experientia 25:814–815, 1969.

259. De Schepper J, Van Der Stock J. Increased urinary bilirubin excretion after elevated free plasma haemoglobin levels. I. Variations in the calculated renal clearances of bilirubin in whole dogs. Arch Intern Physiol Biochim 80:279–291; 1972.

260. Royer M, Noir BA, Sfarcich D, et al. Extrahepatic bilirubin formation and conjugation in the dog. Digestion 10:423–434, 1974.

261. Fulop M, Braqeau P. The renal excretion of bilirubin in dogs with obstructive jaundice. J Clin Invest 43:1192–1202, 1964.

262. Gollan J, Schmid R. Bilirubin metabolism and hyperbilirubinemia disorders. In: Wright R, Millward-Sadler GH, ALberti KGMM (eds) Liver and Biliary Disease, 2nd ed. WB Saunders, Philadelphia, 301–359, 1985.

263. Eikmeier H. Diagnostische untersuchungen uber die lebererkrankungen des hundes. Zentbl Vet Med 7:22–58, 1960.

264. van den Ingh RSBAM, Rothuizen J, van den Brom WE. Extrahepatic cholestasis in the dog and the differentiation of extrahepatic and intrahepatic cholestasis. Vet Q 8:150–157, 1986.

265. Slappendel RJ. Hemolytic anemia in the dog. PhD thesis, University of Utrecht, 1978.

266. Rothuizen J. Hyperbilirubinemia in canine hepatobiliary disease. PhD thesis, University of Utrecht, 1985.

267. Rothuizen J, Van den Brom WE. Bilirubin metabolism in canine hepatobiliary and haemolytic disease. Vet Q 9:235–240, 1987.

268. Rothuizen J, van den Ingh T. Covalently protein-bound bilirubin conjugates in cholestatic disease in dogs. Am J Vet Res 49:702–704, 1988.

269. Van Hootegem P, Fevery J, Blanckaert N. Serum bilirubins in hepatobiliary disease: Comparison with other liver function tests and changes in the postobstructive period. Hepatology 5:112–117, 1985.

270. Gautam A, Seligson H, Gordon ER, et al. Irreversible binding of conjugated bilirubin to albumin in cholestatic rats. J Clin Invest 73:873–877, 1984.

271. Blanckaert N, D'Argenio G. Presence of bilirubin linked covalently to albumin in serum of patients with cholestasis. Gastroeterology 82:1222, 1982.

272. Wu TW, Sullivan SS. Biliprotein in adult icteric serum—demonstrated by an extension of the alkaline methanolysis procedure. Clin Chem 28:2398–2404, 1982.

273. Weiss JS, Gautam A, Lauff JJ, et al. The clinical importance of a protein-bound fraction of serum bilirubin in patients with hyperbilirubinemia. New Engl J Med 309:147–150, 1983.

274. Scharschmidt BF, Goldberg HI, Schmid R. Approach to the patient with cholestatic jaundice. N Engl J Med 308:1515–1519, 1983.

275. O'Connor KW, Snodgrass PJ, Swonder JE, et al. A blinded prospective study comparing four current noninvasive approaches in the differential diagnosis of medical versus surgical jaundice. Gastroenterology 84:1498–1504, 1983.

276. Cherrick GR, Stein SW, Leevy CM, et al. Indocyanine green: Observations on its physical properties, plasma decay and hepatic extraction. J Clin Invest 39:592–600, 1960.

277. Jablonski P, Owen JA. The clinical chemistry of bromosulfophthalein and other cholephilic dyes. In: Bodansky O, Stewart CP (eds) Advances in Clinical Chemistry. New York, Academic Press, 309–389, 1969.

278. Baker KJ. Binding of sulfobromophthalein (BSP) sodium and indocyanine green (ICG) by plasma α_1-lipoproteins. Proc Soc Exp Biol Med 957–963, 1966.

279. Paumgartner G, Probst P, Kraines R. Kinetics of indocyanine green removal from the blood (article 1). Ann NY Acad Sci 170:134–147, 1970.

280. Leevy CM, Bender J, Naylor J. Physiology of dye extraction by the liver: Comparative studies of sulfobromophthalein and indocyanine green (article 1). Ann NY Acad Sci 111:161–175, 1963.

281. Leevy CM, Smith F, Longieville J, et al. Indocyanine green clearance as a test for hepatic function. JAMA 200:236–240, 1967.

282. Paumgartner G. The handling of indocyanine green by the liver. Schwiz Med Wochenschr 107 (suppl 17):1–30, 1975.

283. Wheeler HO, Cranston WI, Meltzer JI. Hepatic uptake and biliary excretion of indocyanine green in the dog. Proc Soc Exp Biol Med 99:11–14, 1958.

284. Ketterer SG, Weigand BD, Rappaport E. Hepatic uptake and biliary excretion of indocyanine green and its use in estimation of hepatic blood flow in dogs. Am J Physiol 199:481–484, 1960.

285. Freston JW, Englert E. The influence of age and excessive body weight on the distribution and metabolism of bromsulphthalein. Clin Sci 33:301–312, 1967.

286. Ingelfinger FJ, Bradley SE, Medeloff AJ, et al. Studies with bromosulphthalein. I. Its disappearance from blood after a single intravenous injection. Gastroenterology 11:646–657, 1948.

287. Hunton DB, Bollman JL, Hoffman HN. The plasma removal of indocyanine green and sulfobromophthalein: Effect of dosage and blocking agents. J Clin Invest 40:1648–1655, 1948.

288. Prasse KW, Bjorling DE, Holmes RA, et al. Indocyanine green clearance and ammonia tolerance in partially hepatectomized and hepatic devascularized anesthetized dogs. Am J Vet Res 44:2320–2323, 1983.

289. Boothe DM, Brown SA, Jenkins WL, et al. Indocyanine green disposition in healthy dogs and dogs with mild, moderate, or severe dimethylnitrosamine-induced hepatic disease. Am J Vet Res 53:382–388, 1992.

290. Kawasaki S, Umekita N, Beppu T, et al. Hepatic transport of indocyanine green in dogs chronically intoxicated with dimethylnitrosamine. Toxicol Appl Pharmacol 309–317, 1984.

291. Strombeck DR, Qualls C. Hepatic sulfobromophthalein uptake and storage defect in a dog. J Am Vet Med Assoc 172:1423–1426, 1978.

292. Hacki W, Bircher J, Preisig R, et al. A new look at the plasma disappearance of sulfobromophthalein (BSP): Correlation with the BSP transport maximum and the hepatic plasma flow in man. J Lab Clin Med 88:1019–1031, 1976.

293. Strombeck DR, Harrold D, Rogers Q, et al. Plasma amino acids, glucagon, and insulin concentrations in dogs with nitrosamine-induced hepatic disease. Am J Vet Res 44:2028–2036, 1983.

294. Center SA, Bunch SE, Baldwin BH, et al. Comparison of sulfobromophthalein and indocyanine green clearances in the cat. Am J Vet Res 44:727–730, 1983.

295. Center SA, Bunch SE, Baldwin BH, et al. Comparison of sulfo-

bromophtalein and indocyanine green clearances in the dog. Am J Vet Res 44:722–726, 1983.

295a. Schimke RT. Studies on factors affecting the levels of urea cycle enzymes in rat liver. J Biol Chem 238:1012–1018, 1963.

296. Rudman D, DiFulco TJ, Galambos JT, et al. Maximal rates of excretion and synthesis of urea in normal and cirrhotic subjects. J Clin Invest 52:2241–2249, 1973.

297. Khatra BS, Smith RB III, Millikan WJ, et al. Activities of Krebs-Henseleit enzymes in normal and cirrhotic human liver. J Lab Clin Med 84:709–715, 1974.

298. Conn HO. Ammonia tolerance in assessing the potency of portacaval anastomoses. Arch Intern Med 131:221–226, 1973.

299. Stahl J. Studies of the blood ammonia in liver disease: Its diagnostic, prognostic, and therapeutic significance. Ann Int Med 58:1–24, 1963.

300. Schaeffer MC, Rogers QR, Buffington CA, et al. Long-term biochemical and physiologic effects of surgically placed portacaval shunts in dogs. Am J Vet Res 47:346–355, 1986.

301. Hsia YE. Inherited hyperammonemic syndromes. Gastroenterology 67:347–374, 1974.

302. Strombeck DR, Meyer DJ, Freedland RA. Hyperammonemia due to a urea cycle enzyme deficiency in two dogs. J Am Vet Med Assoc 166:1109–1112, 1975.

303. Morris JG. Nutritional and metabolic responses to arginine deficiency in carnivores. J Nutr 115:524–531,1985.

304. Rogers QR, Visek WJ. Metabolic role of urea cycle intermediates: Nutritional and clinical aspects. J Nutr 115:505–508, 1985.

305. Drayna CJ, Titcomb CP, Varma RR, et al. Hyperammonemic encephalopathy caused by infection in a neurogenic bladder. N Engl J Med 304:766–768, 1981.

306. Ullman MA, Hacker TA, Medani CR. Hyperammonemic encephalopathy and urinary obstruction. N Engl J Med 304:1546, 1981.

307. Hall JA, Allen TA, Fettman MJ. Hyperammonemia associated with urethral obstruction in a dog. J Am Vet Med Assoc 191:1116–1118, 1987.

308. Prytz B, Grossi CE, Rousselot LM. In vitro formation of ammonia in blood of dog and man. Clin Chem 16:277–278, 1970.

309. Reif AE. The ammonia content of blood and plasma. Anal Biochem 1:351–370, 1960.

310. Svensson G, Anfialt R. Rapid determination of ammonia in whole blood and plasma using flow injection analysis. Clin Chim Acta 119:7–14, 1982.

311. Seligson D, Hirahara K. The measurement of ammonia in whole blood, erythrocytes and plasma. J Lab Clin Med 49:962–970, 1957.

312. Davidovich A, Bartley EE, Bechtle RM, et al. Effects of storage temperature and mercuric chloride on preservation of blood samples for later determination of ammonia-N'. J Anim Sci 46:862–863, 1977.

313. Reinhold JG, Chung C. Formation of artifactual ammonia in blood by action of alkali: Its significance for the measurement of blood ammonia. Clin Chem 7:54–69, 1961.

314. Lathan JT, Bove Weirich FL. Chemical and hematologic changes in stored CPDA-1 blood. Transfusion 22:158–159, 1982.

315. Urainski CT, Goldfinger D, Pomerance JJ, et al. Ammonia accumulation in platelet concentrates during storage. Transfusion 21:113–117, 1981.

316. Barta E, Babusikova F. The concentration of ammonia in blood and plasma stored for transfusion. Resuscitation 10:135–139, 1982.

317. Ogilvie GK, Engelking LR, Anwer S. Effects of plasma sample storage on blood ammonia, bilirubin, and urea nitrogen concentrations: Cats and horses. Am J Vet Res 46:2619–2621, 1985.

318. Hitt ME, Jones BD. Effects of storage temperature and time on canine plasma ammonia concentrations. Am J Vet Res 47:363–364, 1986.

319. Rothuizen J, Van den Ingh, RSGAM. Rectal ammonia tolerance test in the evaluation of portal circulation in dogs with liver disease. Res Vet Sci 33:22, 1982.

320. Rothuizen J. Arterial and venous ammonia concentrations in the diagnosis of canine hepato-encephalopathy. Res Vet Sci 33:17–21, 1982.

321. Meyer DJ, Strombeck DR, Stone EA, et al. Ammonia tolerance test in clinically normal dogs and in dogs with portosystemic shunts. J Am Vet Med Assoc 173:377–379, 1978.

322. Davenport DJ, Sherding RG, Jacobs RM. Ammonia tolerance test: Comparison of three methods of ammonia administration. ACVIM Proc (abstract), 130, 1985.

323. Briggs OM, Harley EH. The fate of administered purines in the Dalmation coach hound. J Comp Path 96:267–276, 1986.

324. Hoe CM, Harvey DG. An investigation into liver function tests in dogs. II. Tests other than transaminase estimation. J Sm Anim Pract 2:109–127, 1961.

325. Morgan HC. A comparison of uric acid determinations and sulfobromsulfthalein retention tests as an index to canine liver dysfunction. Am J Vet Res 20:372–377, 1959.

326. Kruger JM, Osborne CA. Etiopathogenesis of uric acid and ammonium urate uroliths in non-Dalmation dogs. Vet Clin N Amer 16:87–126, 1986.

327. Wooliscroft JO, Colfer H, Fox IH. Hyperuricemia in acute illness: A poor prognostic sign. Am J Med 72:58–62, 1982.

328. Fox IH, Palella TD, Kelley WN. Hyperuricemia: A marker for cell energy crises. N Engl J Med 317:111–112, 1987.

329. Laing EJ, Carter RF. Acute tumor lysis syndrome following treatment of canine lymphoma. J Am Anim Hosp Assoc 24:691–696, 1988.

330. Page RL, Leifer CE, Matus RE. Uric acid and phosphorus excretion in dogs with lymphosarcoma. Am J Vet Res 47:910–912, 1986.

331. Page RL. Acute tumor lysis syndrome. Sem Vet Med Surg (Sm Anim) 1:58–60, 1986.

332. Haselwood GAD. The biological significance of chemical differences in bile salts. Biol Rev 39:537–574, 1964.

333. Nally CV, McMullin LJ, Clanachan AS, et al. Periodic gallbladder contraction maintains bile acid circulation during the fasting period: A canine study. Br J Surg 74:1134–1138, 1987.

334. Itoh Z, Takahashi I. Periodic contractions of the canine gallbladder during the interdigestive state. Am J Physiol 240:G183–189, 1981.

335. DiMagno EP, Hendricks JC, Go VLW, et al. Relationships among canine fasting pancreatic and biliary secretions, pancreatic duct pressure, and duodenal phase III motor activity-Boldyreff revisited. Dig Dis Sci 24:689–693, 1979.

336. Keane FB, DiMagno EP, Dozois RR, et al. Relationships among canine interdigestive exocrine pancreatic and biliary flow, duodenal motor activity, plasma pancreatic polypeptide, and motilin. Gastroenterology 78:310–316, 1980.

337. Traynor OJ, Dozois RR, DiMagno EP. Canine interdigestive and posprandial gallbladder motility and emptying. Am J Physiol 246:G426–432, 1984.

338. Scott RB, Strasberg SM, El-Sharkawy TY, et al. Regulation of the fasting enterohepatic circulation of bile acids by the migrating myoelectric complex in dogs. J Clin Invest 71:644–654, 1983.

339. Scott RB, Eidt PB, Shaffer EA. Regulation of fasting canine duodenal bile acid delivery by sphincter of Oddi and gallbladder. Am J Physiol 249:G622–633, 1985.

340. Mok HYL, von Bergmann K, Grundy SM. Kinetics of enterohepatic circulation during fasting: Biliary lipid secretion and gallbladder storage. Gastroenterology 78:1023–1033, 1980.

341. LaRusso NF, Korman MG, Hoffman NE, et al. Dynamics of the enterohepatic circulation of bile acids. N Engl J Med 291:689–692, 1974.

342. Barbara L, Roda A, Roda E, et al. Diurnal variations of serum primary bile acids in healthy subjects and hepatobiliary disease patients. Rendiconti di Gastroenterologia 8:194–198, 1976.

343. Vlahcevic ZR, Heuman DM, Hylemon PB. Physiology and pathophysiology of enterohepatic circulation of bile acids. In: Zakim D, Boyer T (eds) Hepatology—a Textbook of Liver Disease, 2nd ed. WB Saunders, Philadelphia, 341–377, 1989.

344. Gracey M, Papadimitriou J, Burke V, et al. Effects on small-intestinal function and structure induced by feeding a deconjugated bile salt. Gut 52:2353–2367, 1973.

345. Gilmore IT, Hofmann AF. Altered drug metabolism and elevated serum bile acids in liver disease: A unified pharmacokinetic explanation. Gastroenterology 78:177–178, 1980.

346. Anwer MS, Engelking IR, Gronwall R, et al. Plasma bile acid elevation following CCl_4 induced liver damage in dogs, sheep, calves and ponies. Res Vet Sci 20:127–130, 1976.

347. Hauge JG, Abdelkader SV. Serum bile acids as an indicator of liver diseases in dogs. Acta Vet Scand 25:495–503, 1984.

348. Rutgers HC, Stradley RP, Johnson SE. Serum bile acid analysis in dogs with experimentally induced cholestatic jaundice. Am J Vet Res 49:317–320, 1988.

349. Center SA, Baldwin BH, Erb HN, et al. Bile acid concentrations in the diagnosis of hepatobiliary disease in the dog. J Am Vet Med Assoc 187:935–940, 1985.

350. Center SA, Baldwin BH, deLahunta A, et al. Evaluation of serum bile acid concentrations for the diagnosis of portosystemic venous anomalies in the dog and cat. J Am Vet Med Assoc 186:1090–1094, 1985.

351. Johnson SE, Rogers WA, Bonagura JD, et al. Determination of serum bile acids in fasting dogs with hepatobiliary disease. Am J Vet Res 46:2048–2053, 1985.

352. Center SA, Baldwin BH, Erb H, et al. Bile acid concentrations in the diagnosis of hepatobiliary disease in the cat. J Am Vet Med Assoc 189:891–896, 1986.

353. Meyer DJ. Liver function tests in dogs with portosystemic shunts: Measurement of serum bile acid concentration. J Am Vet Med Assoc 188:168–169, 1986.

354. Jensen AL. Evaluation of fasting and postprandial total serum bile acid concentration in a dog with hepatobiliary disorders. J Vet Med A 38:247–254, 1991.

355. Aquilera-Tejero E, Mayer-Valor R, Gomez-Cardenas G. Plasma bile acids, lactate dehydrogenase and sulphobromophthalein retention test in canine carbon tetrachloride intoxication. J Sm Anim Pract 29:711–717, 1988.

356. Center SA, Joseph S, Erb HN. The diagnostic efficacy of fasting and 2-hour postprandial serum bile acids in cats (n = 108) with hepatobiliary disease. J Am Vet Med Assoc, in press.

357. Center SA, Leveille CR, Baldwin BH, et al. Direct spectrometric determination of serum bile acids in the dog and cat. Am J Vet Res 45:2043–2050, 1984.

358. Jensen AL. Variations in total bile acid concentrations in serum of dogs after a test meal. J Vet Med A 38:241–246, 1991.

359. Roda E, Aldini R, Mazzella G, et al. Enterohepatic circulation of bile acids after cholecystectomy. Gut 19:640–649, 1978.

360. Struthers JE, Mehta SJ, Kaye MD, et al. Relative concentrations of individual nonsulfated bile acids in the serum and bile of patients with cirrhosis. Dig Dis 22:861–865, 1977.

361. Patteson TE, Vlahcevic ZR, Schwartz CC, et al. Bile acid metabolism in cirrhosis. VI. Sites of blockage in the bile acid pathways to primary bile acids. Gastroenterology 79:620–628, 1980.

362. Poupon RY, Poupon RE, Lebree D, et al. Mechanisms for reduced hepatic clearance and elevated plasma levels of bile acids in cirrhosis. Gastroenterology 80:1438–1444, 1981.

363. Akashi Y, Mizazaki H, Yanagisawa J, et al. Bile acid metabolism in cirrhotic liver tissue-altered synthesis and impaired hepatic secretion. Clin Chim Acta 168:199–206, 1987.

364. Vlahcevic ZR, Juttijudata P, Bell CC, et al. Bile acid metabolism in patients with cirrhosis II. Cholic and chenodeoxycholic acid metabolism. Gastroenterology 62:1174–1181, 1972.

365. Yoshida T, McCormick WC, Sell L, et al. Bile acid metabolism IV. Characterization of the abnormality in deoxycholic acid metabolism. Gastroenterology 68:335–341, 1975.

366. Bremmelgaard A, Sjovall J. Bile acid profiles in urine of patients with liver diseases. Eur J Clin Invest 79:620–628, 1980.

367. Sjovall J. Bile acids in man under normal and pathological conditions. Clin Chim Acta 5:33–41, 1960.

368. Vlahcevic ZR, Goldman M, Schwartz CC, et al. Bile acid metabolism in cirrhosis. VII. Evidence for defective feedback control of bile acid synthesis. Hepatology 1:146–150, 1981.

369. Thompson MB, Chappell JD, Kunze DJ, et al. Bile acid profile in a dog with cholangiocarcinoma. Vet Pathol 26:75–78, 1989.

370. Thompson MB, Meyer DJ, Laflamme DP, et al. Serum bile acid concentrations and profiles in dogs with surgically created portocaval shunts. Vet Clin Path (abstract) 21:34, 1992.

371. Center SA, Thompson MB, Guida L, et al. 3α-hydroxylated bile acid profiles in clinically normal cats, cats with severe hepatic lipidosis, and cats with complete experimental extrahepatic bile duct occlusion. Am J Vet Res 54:681–688, 1993.

372. Taylor W. The bile acid composition of rabbit and cat gall-bladder bile. J Steroid Biochem 8:1077–1084, 1977.

373. Washizu T, Koizumi I, Kaneko JJ. Postprandial changes in serum bile acids concentration and fractionation of individual bile acids by high performance liquid chromatography in normal dogs. Jpn J Vet Sci 49:593–600, 1987.

374. Washizu T, Ikenage H, Washizu M, et al. Bile acid composition of dog and cat gall-bladder bile. Jpn J Vet Sci 52:423–425, 1990.

375. Washizu R, Tomoda I, Kaneko JJ. Serum bile acid composition of the dog, cow, horse and human. J Vet Med Sci 53:81–86, 1991.

376. Center SA. Serum bile acids in companion animal medicine. Vet Clin N Am (Sm Anim) 23:625–657, 1993.

377. Counsell LJ, Lumsden JH. Serum bile acids: Reference values in healthy dogs and comparison of two kit methods. Vet Clin Path 17:71–74, 1988.

378. Bunch SE, Center SA, Baldin BH, et al. Radioimmunoassay of conjugated bile acids in canine and feline sera. Am J Vet Res 45:2051–2054, 1984.

379. Kealy JK. The abdomen. In: Diagnostic Radiology of the Dog and Cat, 2nd ed. WB Saunders, Philadelphia, 26, 1987.

380. Obrien TR. Liver, spleen and pancreas. In: Obrien TR (ed) Radiographic Diagnosis of Abdominal Disorders in the Dog and Cat: Radiographic Interpretation, Clinical Signs, Pathophysiology. WB Saunders, Philadelphia, 396, 1978.

381. Gibbs C. Radiological features of liver diseases in dogs and cats. Vet Ann 21:239–249, 1981.

382. Suter PF. Radiographic diagnosis of liver diseases in dogs and cats. In: Kealy JK (ed) The Veterinary Clinics of North America (Small Animal Practice), Vol. 12. WB Saunders, Philadelphia, 153–173, 1982.

383. Wrigley RH. Radiographic and ultrasonographic diagnosis of liver disease in dogs and cats. In: Twedt DC (ed) The Veterinary Clinics of North America (Small Animal Practice), Vol. 15. WB Saunders, Philadelphia, 21–28, 1985.

384. Grandage J. The radiology of the dog's diaphragm. J Sm Anim Pract 15:1–17, 1974.

385. Lee R, Leowijuk C. Normal parameters in abdominal radiology of the dog and cat. J Sm Anim Pract 23:251–269, 1982.

386. Godshalk CP, Kneller SK, Badertscher RR, et al. Quantitative noninvasive assessment of liver size in clinically normal dogs. Am J Vet Res 51:1421–1426, 1990.

387. van Bree H, Sackx A. Evaluation of radiographic liver size in twenty-seven normal deep-chested dogs. J Sm Anim Pract 28:693–703, 1987.

388. Cockett PA. Radiographic anatomy of the canine liver: Simple measurements determined from the lateral radiograph. J Sm Anim Pract 27:577–589, 1986.

389. van Bree H, Jacobs V, Vanderkerckhove P. Radiographic assessment of liver volume in dogs. Am J Vet Res 50:1613–1616, 1989.

390. Lord PF, Wilkins RF. Emphysema of the gallbladder in a diabetic dog. J Am Vet Radiol Soc 13:49–52, 1972.

391. Burk RL, Johnson GF. Emphysematous cholecystitis in the non-diabetic dog: 3 case histories. Vet Radiol 21:242–245, 1980.

392. Meutzer RM: A comparative appraisal of emphysematous cholecystitis. Am J Surg 129:10–15, 1975.

393. Ticer JW. Abdomen. In: Radiographic Technique in Veterinary Practice, 2nd ed. WB Saunders, Philadelphia, 312, 1984.

394. Burgener FA, Fischer HW, Adams JT. Intravenous cholangiography in different degrees of common bile duct obstruction. An experimental study in the dog. Invest Radiol 97:383–386, 1975.

395. Suter PF. Portal vein anomalies in the dog: Their angiographic diagnosis. J Am Vet Radiol Soc 16:84–97, 1975.

396. Schmidt S, Suter PF. Angiography of the hepatic and portal venous system in the dog and cat: An investigative method. Vet Radiol 21:57–77, 1980.

397. Moon ML. Diagnostic imaging of portosystemic shunts. Sem Vet Med Surg (Sm Anim) 5:120–125, 1990.

398. Birchard SJ, Biller DS, Johnson SE. Differentiation of intrahepatic versus extrahepatic portosystemic shunts in dogs using positive-contrast portography. J Am Anim Hosp Assoc 25:13–17, 1989.

399. Daniel GB, Bright R, Ollis P, et al. Per rectal portal scintigraphy using[99m] technetium pertechnetate to diagnose portosystemic shunts in dogs and cat. J Vet Int Med 5:23–27, 1991.

400. Koblik PD, Komtebedde J, Yen C-K, et al. Use of transcolonic [99m]technetium-pertechnetate as a screening test for portosystemic shunts in dogs. J Am Vet Med Assoc 196:925–930, 1990.

401. Koblik PD, Hornof WJ, Breznock EM. Quantitative hepatic scintigraphy in the dog. Vet Radiol 24:226–231, 1983.

402. van den Brom WE, Rothuizen J. Quantitation of the hepatobiliary dynamics in clinically normal dogs by use of ^{99m}Tc-iminodiacetate excretory scintigraphy. Am J Vet Res 51:249–252, 1990.

403. Rothuizen J, van den Brom WE. Quantitive hepatobiliary scintigraphy as a measure of bile flow in dogs with cholestatic disease. Am J Vet Res 51:253–256, 1990.

404. Boothe HW, Hightower E, Boothe DM. Hepatobiliary scintigraphy in the diagnosis of extrahepatic biliary obstruction. Scientific Meeting ACVS (abstract), 59, 1990.

405. Boothe HW, Boothe DM, Komdov A, et al. Use of hepatobiliary scintigraphy in the diagnosis of extrahepatic biliary obstruction in dogs and cats: 25 cases (1982–1989). J Am Vet Med Assoc 20:134–141, 1992.

406. Kerr LY, Hornof WJ. Quantitative hepatobiliary scintigraphy using ^{99m}Tc-DISIDA in the dog. Vet Radiol 27:173–177, 1986.

407. Krishnamurthy S, Krishnamurthy GT. Technetium-99m-Iminodiacetic acid organic anions: Review of biokinetics and clinical application in hepatology. Hepatology 9:139–153, 1989.

408. Lieberman DA, Krishnamurthy GT. Intrahepatic versus extrahepatic cholestasis. Discrimination with biliary scintigraphy combined with ultrasound. Gastroenterology 90:734–743, 1986.

409. Shah KK, Shah KK, Fink-Bennett D, et al. Extrahepatic biliary obstruction versus intrahepatic disorder. Differentiation with hepatobiliary scintigraphy and ultrasonography. J Clin Gastroenterol 10:191–196, 1988.

410. Krishnamurthy GT, Lieverman DA, Brar HS. Detection, localization and quantitation of degree of common bile duct obstruction by scintigraphy. J Nucl Med 26:726–735, 1985.

411. Biller DS, Kantrowitz B, Miyabayashi T. Ultrasonography of diffuse liver disease. A review. J Vet Int Med 6:71–76, 1992.

412. Godshalk CP, Badertscher RR, Rippy MK, et al. Quantitative ultrasonic assessment of liver size in the dog. Vet Radiol 29:162–167, 1988.

413. Gosink BB, Lemon SK, Scheible W, et al. Accuracy of ultrasonography in diagnosis of hepatocellular disease. AJR 133:19–23, 1979.

414. Mittelstaedt CA. Abdominal Ultrasound. New York: Churchill Livingstone, 1–81, 1987.

415. Foster JK, Dewbury KC, Griffith AH, et al. The accuracy of ultrasound in the detection of fatty infiltration of the liver. Br J Radiol 53:440–442, 1980.

416. Scott WW, Donovan PJ, Sanders RC. The sonography of diffuse liver disease. Sem Ultrasound 11:219–225, 1981.

417. Yeager AE, Muhammed H. Accuracy of ultrasonography in the detection of severe hepatic lipidosis in cats. Am J Vet Res 53:597–599, 1992.

418. Kurtz AB, Rubin CS, Cooper HS, et al. Ultrasound findings in hepatitis. Radiology 136:717–723, 1980.

419. Nyland TG. Ultrasonic patterns of canine hepatic lymphoma. Vet Radiol 25:167–172, 1984.

420. Lamb CR, Hartzband LE, Tidwell AS, et al. Ultrasonographic findings in hepatic and splenic lymphosarcoma in dogs and cats. Vet Radiol 32:117–120, 1991.

421. Nyland TG, Park RD. Hepatic ultrasonography in the dog. Vet Radiol 24:74–84, 1983.

422. McArdle CR. Ultrasonic diagnosis of liver metastasis. J Clin Ultrasound 4:265–268, 1976.

423. Wooten WB, Green B, Goldstein HM. Ultrasonography of necrotic hepatic metastasis. Radiology 133:437–441, 1979.

424. Stowater JL, Lamb CR, Schelling SH. Ultrasonographic features of canine hepatic nodular hyperplasia. Vet Radiol 31:268–272, 1990.

425. Crow HC, Bartrum RJ, Foote SR. Expanded criteria for the ultrasonic diagnosis of gallstones. J Clin Ultrasound 4:289–292, 1976.

426. Nyland TG, Gillett NA. Sonographic evaluation of experimental bile duct ligation in the dog. Vet Radiol 23:252–260, 1982.

427. Malini S, Sabel J. Ultrasonography in obstructive jaundice. Radiology 123:429–433, 1977.

428. Zeman RK, Taylor KJW, Rosenfield T, et al. Acute experimental biliary obstruction in the dog: Sonographic findings and clinical implications. Am J Roentgenol 136:965–967, 1981.

429. Leopold GR. Ultrasonography of jaundice. In: Love L (ed) Abdominal Imaging. Radiol Clin N Am 27:127–136, 1979.

430. Zamcheck N, Klausenstock O. Liver biopsy. II. The risk of needle biopsy. N Engl J Med 26:1062–1069, 1953.

431. Piccinino F, Sagnelli E, Pasquale G, et al. Complications following percutaneous liver biopsy. A multicentre retrospective study on 68,276 biopsies. J Hepatology 2:165–173, 1986.

432. Minuk GY, Sutherland LR, Wiseman DA. Prospective study of the incidence of ultrasound-detected intrahepatic and subcapsular hematomas in patients randomized to 6 or 24 hours of bed rest after percutaneous liver biopsy. Gastroenterology 92:290–293, 1987.

433. Conn HO. Intrahepatic hematoma after liver biopsy. Gastroenterology 67:375–381, 1974.

434. Raines DR, Van Heertum RL, Johnson LF. Intrahepatic hematoma: A complication of percutaneous liver biopsy. Gastroenterology 67:284–289, 1974.

435. Pagliaro L, Rinaldi F, Craxi A, et al. Percutaneous blind biopsy versus laparoscopy with guided biopsy in diagnosis of cirrhosis: A prospective, randomized trial. Dig Dis Sci 28:39–43, 1983.

436. Conn HO. Liver biopsy in extrahepatic biliary obstruction and in other "contraindicated" disorders. Gastroenterology 68:817–821, 1975.

437. Morris JS, Gallo GA, Scheuer PJ, et al. Percutaneous liver biopsy in patients with large bile duct obstruction. Gastroenterology 68:750–754, 1975.

438. Jones BD, Hitt M, Hurst R. Hepatic biopsy. Vet Clin N Am 15:39–67, 1985.

439. Feldman EC, Ettinger SJ. Percutaneous transthoracic liver biopsy in the dog. J Am Vet Med Assoc 169:806–810, 1976.

440. Feldman EC, Ettinger SJ. Percutaneous transthoracic liver biopsy in the dog: A review of 75 cases. AAHA 13:17–22, 1977.

441. Edwards DF. Blind percutaneous liver biopsy: A safe diagnostic procedure. Calif Vet, 9–17, April 1977.

442. Hitt ME, Hanna P, Singh A. Percutaneous-transabdominal hepatic needle biopsies in 24 dogs. Am J Vet Res 53:785–787, 1992.

443. Menard M, Papageorges M. Technique for ultrasound-guided fine needle biopsies. Vet Rad Ultrasound 36:137–138, 1995.

444. Bunch SE, Polak DM, Hornbuckle WE. A modified laparoscopic approach for liver biopsy in dogs. J Am Vet Med Assoc 187:1032–1035, 1985.

445. Johnson GS, Krause KH, Turrentine MA, et al. DDAVP-induced increases in coagulation factor VIII and von Willebrand factor in the plasma of conscious dogs. J Vet Pharmacol Therap 9:370–375, 1986.

446. Le Frock JK, Ellis CA, Turchik JB, et al. Transient bacteremia associated with percutaneous liver biopsy. J Inf Dis 131:S104–S107, 1975.

447. Hess FA, Bnagi HR, Weiber ER, et al. Morphometry of dog liver: Comparison of wedge and needle biopsies. Europ J Clin Invest 3:451–458, 1973.

448. Center SA, Hornbuckle WE. The liver and hepatobiliary disorders. In: Hoskins JD (ed) Veterinary Pediatrics. WB Saunders, Philadelphia, 205–239, 1990.

9 Diseases of the Oral Cavity and Pharynx

W. GRANT GUILFORD

INTRODUCTION

Oropharyngeal diseases are common in dogs and cats. The oral cavity and pharynx can be damaged by a variety of processes including developmental disorders, infection, endocrine or metabolic disturbances, trauma, immune-mediated diseases, immunodeficiency, toxicoses, and neoplasia. In addition, several oropharyngeal diseases are of unknown cause. This chapter discusses diseases of the oropharynx, including salivary gland disorders. Dental diseases are not covered and readers interested in dentistry are referred to recent publications and specialist texts on this rapidly expanding field.[1-6] Oropharyngeal diseases, such as cricopharyngeal achalasia, that result in dysphagia are discussed in Chapter 11.

CLINICAL SIGNS

The clinical signs of oropharyngeal disease are listed in Table 9–1. They include inappetance, halitosis, ptyalism, oral hemorrhage, and oropharyngeal dysphagia. Animals with painful oropharyngeal lesions may be depressed, tilt their head to one side when eating, or refuse to eat or drink. They may show evidence of pain when swallowing (odynophagia), and are occasionally febrile (particularly when a penetrating foreign body has resulted in abscessation). They may paw at their mouth or face, and will occasionally develop paroxysms of rapid jaw chattering. Animals with dysphagia have difficulty drinking water and/or eating. They often gag or make multiple exaggerated attempts to swallow. Other clinical signs of pharyngeal dysfunction include immediate regurgitation during attempts to eat, nasal reflux, coughing, and sometimes dyspnea.

HISTORY AND PHYSICAL EXAMINATION

A thorough history and physical examination are the keys to diagnosis. Important historical findings include the rapidity of onset and duration of the signs, the likelihood of foreign body ingestion (especially bones and sticks) or access to products that might result in stomatitis (see later), and whether swallowing is normal. The physical examination should include careful scrutiny of the skin, pads, and mucocutaneous junctions for evidence of widespread inflammation supportive of autoimmune disease. In addition, skin and pad lesions can develop following exposure to caustic products or heavy metals such as thallium.

In many cases, careful examination of the oral cavity and pharynx will reveal the cause of the clinical signs. Anesthesia is frequently required for examination of the oropharynx in intractable animals and in those with painful lesions. However, if the veterinarian has a patient and gentle approach, it is possible to perform a satisfactory oropharyngeal examination successfully in many animals. Most animals resent having their jaws forced abruptly wide open, particularly if the animal's lips have been roughly forced against its teeth to encourage it to open its mouth. If this abrupt approach is taken, the veterinarian will usually, at best, get a fleeting glimpse of the oropharynx as the startled animal struggles from his or her grasp. As with any physical examination, inspection of the oral cavity should begin by reassuring the animal with a calm voice and gentle petting about the head. If the animal's behavior suggests the intention to bite, there is little point is proceeding further without anesthesia. It is my preference to begin the oral examination by flipping the gums up and examining the buccal mucous membranes, gingiva, and lateral surface of the teeth. The teeth should be carefully examined for evidence of fractures, caries, tartar, periodontal disease, and resorptive lesions. Next, the animal's head is tilted toward the lighting source in the room and its jaws are gently prised partly open to gain a view of the oral cavity, hard palate, tongue, and occlusal and medial surface of the teeth. To avoid creating unnecessary discomfort, the initial attempt to open the jaws is made without the assistance of pressing the animal's gums between its teeth. If the animal resists

Table 9–1

THE CLINICAL SIGNS OF OROPHARYNGEAL DISEASE

Abnormal chewing movements	Inability to open or close the jaws
Anorexia	Nasal discharge
Chattering jaw movements	Oral hemorrhage
Difficulty prehending food	Ptyalism or pseudoptyalism
Dysphagia or odynophagia	Pawing at the mouth or face
Halitosis	Retching or vomiting

this attempt, the gums can be used in this manner to encourage it to open its mouth. To facilitate complete examination of the tongue, the tongue base can be raised into view by dorsally directed digital pressure between the mandibular bones. Paresis of the tongue can usually be detected by observing its contractile activity, but occasionally checking muscular tone by attempting to draw the tip of the tongue from the mouth is useful. After inspecting the oral cavity, the last phase of the examination is observation of the pharynx, soft plate, and tonsils. The pharyngeal examination is left to last because it requires the jaws to be opened wide, and is the part of the examination most likely to provoke resentment from the patient. During the pharyngeal examination, the palate should be closely inspected for clefting and its length carefully evaluated (see later). In addition, it is helpful to palpate the soft palate (in an attempt to feel nasopharyngeal masses) and to check the gag reflex.

DIAGNOSIS

The cause of oropharyngeal disorders may be obvious from the history and clinical examination of the animal.[7] However, other investigations such as blood work, culture for infectious organisms, biopsy, radiographs, fluoroscopy, and possibly tests of immune function may also be required.

Complete blood counts and serum chemistry profiles are occasionally of value in the workup of animals with oropharyngeal diseases, particularly in the differential diagnosis of stomatitis (see later). Cultures of the oral cavity are difficult to interpret and are rarely performed. The oral cavity is home to large numbers of microorganisms in healthy animals.[8] The normal flora is dominated by anaerobic bacteria, such as *Bacteroides* and *Fusobacterium* spp., but large numbers of aerobic bacteria can also be cultured along with *Actinomyces,* mycoplasma, and ureaplasma organisms. In a cattery situation, culturing tonsillar swabs is occasionally of value for the definitive diagnosis of feline upper respiratory viruses or the identification of carriers.

Biopsy or fine needle aspiration are of great assistance in the diagnosis of ulcerative or proliferative oral lesions. They allow differentiation of neoplasms from inflammatory lesions, such as eosinophilic granuloma. In addition, biopsy is necessary to determine the type of neoplastic process present.

Survey radiographs may demonstrate fractured hyoid bones, temporomandibular ankylosis, foreign bodies such as bone fragments and needles, or distortion of the pharyngeal air space by masses. Retropharyngeal diseases may result in gas shadows, swelling, and loss of fascial lines in the retropharyngeal area.

Diagnosis of oropharyngeal disorders associated with dysphagia is described in Chapter 11. The investigation of dysphagia is begun by observing affected animals attempting to eat or drink. Fluoroscopy is necessary to differentiate the various types of functional pharyngeal disorders.

SYMPTOMATIC MANAGEMENT OF OROPHARYNGEAL DISEASES

Antimicrobial Therapy in Oropharyngeal Diseases

As already mentioned, the oral cavity carries a varied flora, but anaerobic organisms predominate. Antibiotic therapy is aimed at reducing the numbers of bacteria in the oral cavity, but should not be expected to sterilize the oral mucosa. Indis-

criminate use of antibiotics may predispose the animal to candidiasis.

A variety of antimicrobial agents have been used successfully in the treatment of oral disease. In particular, antimicrobials with a good anaerobic spectrum such as amoxicillin (10–20 mg/kg q 12 hours PO), metronidazole (10–20 mg/kg q 12 hours PO), and clindamycin (5–11 mg/kg q 12 hours PO) are effective. Spiramycin is a macrolide antibiotic that is excreted in high concentrations in the saliva. It has recently been claimed that a combination of metronidazole and spiramycin (Stomorgyl, Rhone Merieux) is more effective against oral infections in dogs and cats than either of these antibiotics used individually.[9,10] Mouthwashes with antiseptics, such as 0.1% to 0.2% chlorhexidine, have been found useful by some veterinarians as adjunct therapy in the treatment of oral infections. Poor compliance limits the value of these products, although swabbing the affected area with cotton-tipped applicators soaked in chlorhexidine is occasionally of value.

Feeding the Patient with Oral Disease

Many oral diseases are painful, prevent grooming, and impair appetite. Recovery of the patient is usually assisted if treatment of the underlying disorder is accompanied by appropriate nutritional support. At times animals with oral diseases can be coaxed to eat by measures such as warming the food and hand feeding. Alternatively, cats may be encouraged to eat with an intravenous injection of valium (1 mg) or oral administration of oxazepam (2.5 mg q 8–12 hours). Often, however, the provision of an adequate caloric intake requires the placement of a nasogastric, pharyngostomy, or gastrostomy tube (see Chapter 38). Specific indications for tube feeding include mandibular and facial fractures and severe stomatitis or glossitis.

Miscellaneous

Fluid therapy may be required in animals that are unwilling to eat or drink. Short courses of anti-inflammatory drugs are occasionally of value in the therapy of acute diseases of the oral cavity.

STOMATITIS

Introduction

Stomatitis is inflammation of the oral mucosa. On many occasions, stomatitis occurs concurrently with gingivitis (inflammation of the gums) or glossitis (inflammation of the tongue). Stomatitis is a frequent problem, particularly in cats, and can result from a variety of systemic and local causes (Table 9–2). The clinical signs of stomatitis are those of oral disease (see earlier and Table 9–1) and are similar no matter what the cause of the oral inflammation.

History, Physical Examination, and Diagnosis

Diagnosis of the cause of stomatitis is primarily made by history and the distribution and appearance of the lesions.

Acute onset of stomatitis in an otherwise healthy animal

supports ingestion of caustic or irritant chemicals, particularly if the oral lesions predominantly affect the tongue and pharynx and are relatively extensive (Figure 9–1). The likelihood of access to toxic chemicals, such as acids and alkalis, undiluted Zepharin,[11] heavy metals (including mercury[12] and thallium), paraquat, and phenols should be explored. Similarly, inquiry should be made as to whether the animal indulges in chewing irritant household plants because some, such as dieffenbachia, poinsettia, philodendron, and pine needles (Christmas trees), can result in stomatitis. Embedded fragments of plant material (e.g., cocklebur, burdock) or fiberglass have also been reported to cause stomatitis and gingival hyperplasia in dogs.[7,13–15] A history of a propensity to chew electric cords may suggest electrical injury as a cause of the stomatitis, particularly if the oral cavity lesion is acute in onset, linear in shape, and associated with pulmonary edema and cardiac arrhythmia. Electrical burns usually damage the hard palate, gingiva, and commissures of the lips and may result in extensive tissue sloghing.[16]

The dietary history will occasionally reveal the cause of the stomatitis (see Table 9–2). Oral trauma from chewing of bones will frequently result in scattered erosions of the oral

Table 9–2

CAUSES OF STOMATITIS

Dental Plaque/Calculus
Immune mediated
  Bullous pemphigoid
  Discoid lupus erythematosus
  Drug reactions
  Food sensitivity
  Idiopathic (lymphocytic-plasmacytic) stomatitis
  Pemphigus diseases
  Systemic lupus erythematosus
Immunodeficiency
  Neutrophil function defects
  Neutropenia
Microorganisms
  Bacteria (Bacteroides, spirochetes, tularemia, leptospirosis)
  Viruses (calici, herpes, distemper, canine adenovirus, papovavirus, FIV, FeLV)
  Protozoa (Trichomonas?)
  Fungal agents (Blastomycosis, candida; coccidioidomycosis, cryptococcus, histoplasma, sporotrichosis)
Metabolic diseases
  Diabetes mellitus
  Hypoparathyroidism
  Uremia
Neoplasia
Nutritional deficiencies
  Hypervitaminosis A
  Niacin
  Protein-calorie malnutrition
  Riboflavin
Physiochemical
  Caustic or irritant chemicals (acids, alkalis, phenols, petroleum products, benzalkonium chloride)
  Chemotherapeutic drugs
  Dilantin
  Foreign bodies (plant material, fiberglass, bone fragments, quills)
  Heavy metals (thallium, mercury)
  Insect bites
  Irritant plants (dieffenbachia, poinsettia, philodendron, pine needles)
  Electrical burns
  Persistent overgrooming
  Radiation therapy
  Trauma

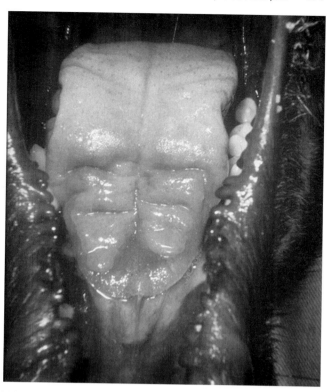

FIGURE 9–1. Ulcerative glossitis in a cat. The extensive glossitis resulted from the licking of a caustic substance from the cat's coat. (Courtesy of Dr. Elizabeth Lee, Massey University)

mucosa. Protein-calorie malnutrition predisposes patients to the development of stomatitis. Niacin and riboflavin deficiency can result in glossitis/stomatitis. Similarly, hypervitaminosis A will cause stomatitis in addition to the bony exostoses characteristic of the disorder. Recent vaccination raises the possibility of vaccine-induced oral inflammation. This is particularly likely if a modified live virus vaccine containing calicivirus or herpes virus is inadvertently deposited on the skin and then licked off by the cat.[16] A history of recent drug administration may also be relevant because drug reactions or chemotherapeutic agents can be a cause of stomatitis (Figure 9–2).

If the stomatitis is restricted to the gingival margin (gingivitis) and associated with dental plaque or calculus, the diagnosis is obvious and the stomatitis is likely to resolve following appropriate teeth cleaning procedures. Gingival inflammation is sometimes seen in the absence of dental disease, particularly in young cats. The cause of this intractable inflammation is often elusive, but serum tests for feline immunodeficiency virus should be performed because this virus can be responsible.

Chronic stomatitis restricted to the fauces and caudal gingiva of the mouth of cats is most likely due to chronic, idiopathic feline gingivitis-stomatitis-pharyngitis. In contrast, if the lesions predominantly involve the upper lip margin near one or both incisors, eosinophilic granuloma is the most likely diagnosis. Mucocutaneous oral lesions in cats or dogs are suggestive of the pemphigoid diseases, particularly if foot pads or mucocutaneous junctions in other parts of the body are also involved. Cats with scattered foci of ulcerative stomatitis predominantly affecting the tongue and hard palate are most likely affected by feline rhinotracheitis virus or calicivirus. The

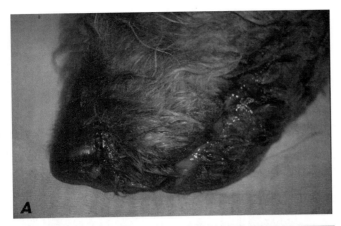

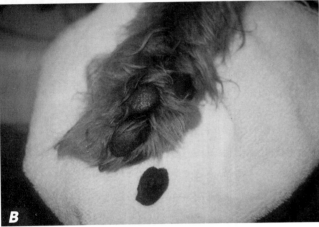

FIGURE 9-2. *(A and B)* Toxic epidermal necrolysis following administration of flucytosine for the treatment of CNS cryptococcosis in a dog. The oral mucosa, lips, and pads all sloughed within a few days of starting the treatment, resulting in euthanasia of the dog.

diagnosis is usually straightforward because cats affected by these viruses usually show additional signs such as sneezing and mucopurulent ocular and nasal discharge.

Occasionally, laboratory work is of value in the diagnosis of chronic stomatitis. Stomatitis secondary to uremia or diabetes mellitus should be ruled out by a serum chemistry profile and urinalysis. A complete blood count, antinuclear antibody test, and urinalysis can be useful if systemic lupus erythematosus is suspected. Leukopenia in a cat with stomatitis is suggestive of FIV or FeLV, a suspicion that can be confirmed by serum tests for these retroviral infections. Biopsy of intractable lesions is valuable to differentiate stomatitis from neoplastic processes of similar appearance (especially squamous cell carcinoma). In addition, biopsy will occasionally reveal the cause of the inflammation (e.g., fungal infections, embedded foreign material, Pemphigoid diseases), or will help classify idiopathic stomatitis as eosinophilic or lymphocytic-plasmacytic.

Acute Ulcerative Stomatitis

Acute ulcerative stomatitis is uncommon in the dog and cat.[13] It is sometimes referred to as Vincent's stomatitis or trench mouth. The disease is characterized by an acute onset of halitosis, salivation, severe gingivitis, and oral mucosal ulceration and necrosis. Periodontal disease with gingivitis, gingival recession, and generalized hyperemia may be prominent. The lesions are often covered by a grayish pseudomembrane of necrotic tissue.

The disease is thought to be initiated by mucosal invasion and damage by certain members of the normal oral flora, such as *Bacteroides melaninogenicus* or spirochetes.[17] Once mucosal ulceration has begun, other oral flora are likely to become involved. It is probable that a coexisting localized or systemic immunodeficiency is necessary to allow bacterial invasion of the mucosa. Ulcerative stomatitis can be recreated experimentally by applying dental debris from affected dogs to healthy dogs that have been immunosuppressed with corticosteroids.[17] Thus, any immunosuppressive disease is likely to predispose to acute ulcerative stomatitis.

Diagnosis is based on physical examination findings. Impression smears help rule out mycotic stomatitis and may reveal large numbers of spirochetes, an observation supportive of the diagnosis.[13] Treatment is symptomatic and consists of debridement of the necrotic area and administration of amoxicillin or metronidazole for 7 to 10 days. Mouthwashes with hydrogen peroxide (3% H_2O_2 diluted 1:1 with water) can also be useful.

Uremic Stomatitis

Stomatitis and oral ulceration occur in acute and chronic uremia. The lesions in acute uremia are more severe. Oral ulcers frequently develop over the "pressure points" (i.e., the labial mucosa overlying the carnasial and canine teeth). In addition, the distal tip of the tongue may undergo necrosis and slough due to the development of an arteritis (Figure 9-3). Treatment is directed at restoring and aiding renal function through fluid therapy and dietary modification.

Mycotic Stomatitis[13]

Mycotic stomatitis is rare and is usually caused by an overgrowth of *Candida albicans*. Candidiasis is often associated with long-term antibiotic treatment, immunodeficiency, or as a complication of other oral diseases. Other mucocutaneous junctions may be involved (e.g., vulva, nail beds). Physical examination reveals oral inflammation, ulceration, and, occasionally, creamy white plaque-like lesions on the tongue, oral mucosa, and mucocutaneous junction. Scraping the lesion reveals a raw bleeding mucosal surface, and yeast can be readily identified in stained smears, in biopsy samples, or by culture. Oral ketoconazole (10 mg/kg q 12–24 hours PO for 4 weeks) is a suitable treatment. Accessible lesions in the oral cavity can be treated topically with nystatin-containing ointments.

In addition to candida, mycotic stomatitis associated with cryptococcosis, sporotrichosis, blastomycosis, coccidioidomycosis, and histoplasmosis has been reported in cats and dogs.[16,18,19] Affected animals usually have fungal lesions in other parts of the body, such as skin, in addition to the oral lesions.

Nocardial Stomatitis

Nocardial stomatitis has been reported in dogs.[13] The disease results in severe halitosis, gingivitis, and oral ulceration. Lesions were most severe in the periodontal tissues, leading to loss of teeth. The lips, buccal mucosa, soft palate, and local

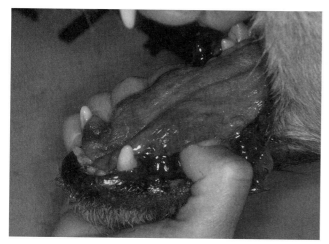

FIGURE 9–3. Stomatitis due to uremia in a 10-year-old dog. The tip and lateral margins of the tongue are undergoing necrosis and ulceration.

lymph nodes can also be involved. Diagnosis depends on culture of a heavy growth of *Nocardia* from the lesions and, preferably, histologic evidence of Nocardial infiltration into affected tissues. Treatment is based on prolonged courses (6 weeks) of sulfa antibiotics such as trimethoprim-sulfa.

Feline Respiratory Viruses

Herpes and calici viruses are common causes of acute ulcerative stomatitis in cats. As mentioned earlier, cats show sneezing, mucopurulent ocular and nasal discharge, depression, and painful ulcers on the tongue and hard palate. The ulcers are shallow and begin as small thin-walled vesicles. Occasionally, they can become quite extensive (Figure 9–4). Specific treatment is usually not required for the stomatitis but, instead, is directed at preventing secondary bacterial infection of the airway, resolving the conjunctivitis, and maintaining hydration and food intake. The carriage rate of calicivirus is high in cats with chronic stomatitis, but it seems unlikely that uncomplicated calicivirus infection causes chronic stomatitis (see later).[10,20–22]

Feline Leukemia and Immunodeficiency Viruses

Chronic gingivitis and stomatitis can occur in association with FeLV and especially FIV.[21–27] FIV is particularly common in uncastrated male cats or in other cats that fight frequently. Viral-induced suppression of the immune system is thought to be the cause of the stomatitis. Coinfection of FIV and calicivirus causes a particularly high prevalence of stomatitis and usually results in a more severe form of the disease.[22,29] It seems that FeLV is significantly less likely than FIV to precipitate stomatitis, even in the presence of chronic calicivirus infection.[22] Diagnosis is based on detection of FIV or FeLV antibody or antigen in circulation. Leukopenia or anemia may also be detected. Management of these diseases is palliative and includes antibiotics.

Chronic Feline Gingivitis-Stomatitis-Pharyngitis[10,16,28]

Chronic gingivitis-stomatitis-pharyngitis is a relatively common but intractable disease. It is most commonly seen in cats, but a similar disease occasionally affects dogs (Figures 9–5A, B, and C). The disease has a variety of different names in addition to chronic gingivitis-stomatitis-pharyngitis including chronic glossopharyngitis, lymphocytic-plasmacytic gingivitis-stomatitis, and plasma cell gingivitis-pharyngitis.

The cause(s) of the disease in these cats is unknown but an immune-mediated process is most likely, and in particular a hypersensitivity to oral bacterial antigens has been incriminated.[10] A large proportion of cats with chronic gingivitis-stomatitis-pharyngitis shed calicivirus but it seems unlikely that chronic calicivirus infection without the involvement of FIV results in a significant prevalence of stomatitis.[20–22,30] Most cats with chronic feline gingivitis-stomatitis-pharyngitis do not have a detectable FIV infection.

Cats of any age and breed can be affected, but young pedigree cats may be predisposed. Signs include anorexia, dysphagia, drooling, and halitosis. Intermittent exacerbations and relapses are common. Examination of the oral cavity shows proliferative and/or ulcerative stomatitis that can occur in a variety of localities including the gingiva, fauces, oropharynx, and tongue. The mucosa about the premolars and molars is usually more severely affected than that about the incisor and canine teeth. Laboratory abnormalities are nonspecific. Hyperglobulinemia is the most common, and electrophoresis may reveal a polyclonal elevation of gammaglobulin. Culture of the lesion fails to reveal any specific pathogen. Biopsy shows mucosal hyperplasia and heavy infiltration of plasma cells and lymphocytes in the mucosa and submucosa. Smaller numbers of neutrophils, eosinophils, and macrophages are also often present.

Chronic feline gingivitis-stomatitis-pharyngitis requires aggressive therapy. This can include teeth cleaning, debridement of necrotic tissue, and extraction of any adjacent teeth. Extraction of all the premolar and molar teeth may be necessary and often results in remission of lesions distant to the extracted teeth as well as those nearby. Administration of metronidazole (10–20 mg/kg q 12 hours PO) helps, at least on a temporary basis. A combination of metronidazole, aurothioglucose (Solganol-Schering: 1 mg/kg IM weekly until remission and then monthly for maintenance), and methylprednisolone acetate (20 mg SQ every 3 weeks for 3 months) has

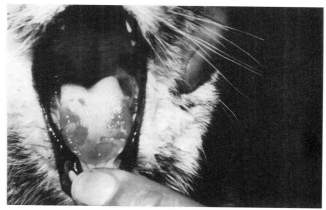

FIGURE 9–4. Extensive lingual ulceration in a young cat as a result of calicivirus infection. On most occasions, calicivirus will not produce stomatitis of the severity seen in this cat. (Courtesy of Dr. Elizabeth Lee, Massey University)

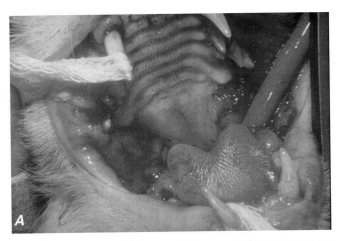

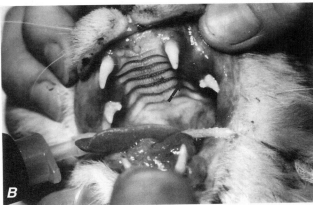

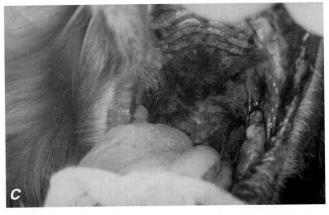

FIGURE 9–5. *(A)* Chronic feline gingivitis-stomatitis-pharyngitis. Marked ulceration of the gingiva and fauces is present. *(B)* Marked inflammation of the gingiva is present. *(C)* Chronic idiopathic stomatitis in a 7-year-old cocker spaniel. Lesions are similar to those of the cat in *(A)* and *(B)*. Deep ulceration is present in the fauces of the mouth.

every month during remission. The occasional urinalysis should be performed to check for proteinuria.

Other treatments reported to have beneficial results include dexamethasone (0.1–0.2 mg/kg PO q 24 hours until remission), megesterol acetate (1 mg/kg PO qod until remission and then once to twice per week thereafter), azathioprine (0.3 mg/kg PO qod), and chlorambucil (0.1–0.2 mg/kg PO q 24 hours until remission and then qod thereafter).[10] Great care is required with the use of megesterol acetate, azathioprine, and chlorambucil in cats because of the possibility of life-threatening side effects. The prognosis for chronic gingivitis-stomatitis-pharyngitis is guarded.

Immune-Mediated Disorders[10]

A variety of autoimmune and immune-mediated disorders cause stomatitis. These include contact dermatitis, pemphigus vulgaris, pemphigus foliaceous, bullous pemphigoid, systemic lupus erythematosus, discoid lupus erythematosis, and drug eruptions such as toxic epidermal necrolysis (Figure 9–2). Most of these conditions have similar oral manifestations and require biopsy for diagnosis. Control is achieved by removal of the inciting cause or by immunosuppressive therapy.

Feline Eosinophilic Granuloma Complex

Two components of feline eosinophilic granuloma complex affect the mouth. The most common is referred to as "indolent" or "rodent" ulcer and usually commences as a shallow erosion on the upper lip opposite the lower canine. Occasionally, indolent ulcers will affect the oral mucosa. The histologic appearance is that of chronic ulceration and, paradoxically, eosinophils are often not a prominent feature of the histopathology. Instead, the most frequent cell types are usually neutrophils, plasma cells, and other mononuclear cells.

Eosinophilic granuloma is the second component of the eosinophilic granuloma complex that is occasionally seen in the oral cavity. Lesions can occur on the lip, tongue, or hard and soft palate. They appear as circumscribed, raised, erythematous masses that can ulcerate. Squamous cell carcinoma is an important differential diagnosis. Differentiation is made by cytology of a scraping from the lesion or by obtaining a biopsy. In contrast to indolent ulcers, circulating eosinophilia is quite common in association with oral eosinophilic granulomas, and the histopathology of the lesion usually reveals granulomatous inflammation, often with a dominant eosinophilic infiltrate.

Treatment is either oral prednisone (1 mg/kg q 12 hours until remission, followed by decreasing dose over a 2–4 week period), intralesional triamcinolone (0.1–0.2 mg/kg), methylprednisolone acetate (20 mg SQ), or, less desirably, megesterol acetate (1 mg/kg PO qod until remission and then once or twice per week). In addition, rodent ulcer will often respond to antibiotics, such as trimethoprim-sulfa (30 mg/kg PO q 12 hours) or amoxicillin-clavulinic acid (32.5 mg PO q 12 hours). Intractable lesions may require surgical excision or radiation therapy.

Eosinophilic Granuloma of Siberian Huskies

Proliferative eosinophilic lesions of the tongue can occur in young Siberian huskies and are referred to as eosinophilic granulo-

given the author the best results in severe intractable cases. Other clinicians have also found these drugs useful, either in combination or used individually.[28] Care is needed with aurothioglucose. This gold salt is not licensed for use in cats and there is little information on efficacy and side effects in cats. No more than 20 consecutive weekly injections should be given. The first two injections should be test doses of 1 mg and then 2 mg. A CBC (including platelet count) should be checked for cytopenias every two weeks during induction and mas.[31] The cause is unknown but several affected dogs have been related. In an analogous manner to the feline disease, the lesions usually respond satisfactorily to 4 to 6 week courses of glucocorticoids. Recurrences can occur requiring further courses of glucocorticoids.

ORAL HEMORRHAGE

Any bleeding disorder can be associated with oral hemorrhage. Thrombocytopenia, von Willibrand disease, DIC, and anticoagulant rodenticide toxicity are the most common (Figure 9–6). When a bleeding disorder is the cause of the oral hemorrhage, petechia and bleeding are seldom restricted to the oral cavity. Diagnostic investigation may include assessment of platelet count, mucosal bleeding time, prothrombin time, activated partial thromboplastin time, and plasma level of factor VIII–related antigen and fibrin degradation products.

Bleeding restricted to the oral cavity is usually (but not always) due to a local disease process such as oral trauma, neoplasia, or severe ulcerative stomatitis. Occasionally, damage to the major palatine artery and overlying mucosa will result in recurrent bouts of severe oral bleeding.[32]

OROPHARYNGEAL FOREIGN BODIES

Foreign bodies not infrequently lodge in the oral cavity or pharynx. The most common types are bones, pieces of wood, string, grass blades, grass awns, fishhooks, and needles. The bones and pieces of wood usually become wedged transversely across the oral cavity between the dental arcades. If they remain chronically in this position they can lead to pressure necrosis of the palate. String and other linear foreign bodies often loop about the base of the tongue. Long blades of grass usually become lodged dorsal to the soft palate. How these grass blades reach such a position is a matter for speculation, but presumedly they are forced into the nasopharynx during retching or vomiting. Grass awns (foxtails) most frequently lodge in the nasal cavities, nasopharynx, gingival sulci, or tonsillar crypts. Occasionally, fragments of plant material will imbed in the oral mucosa and cause stomatitis (see earlier).[13]

Affected animals usually show signs of oral or pharyngeal discomfort. They may gag, expectorate, and retch or paw at their mouths and shake their heads. Ptyalism is common and at times profuse. Swallowing may appear painful. Linear foreign bodies may result in anorexia, vomiting, or abdominal pain.

Diagnosis of oral foreign bodies is usually made by physical examination under anesthesia. Careful examination of the base of the tongue is mandatory in order to detect linear foreign bodies, a potentially life-threatening problem (see Chapter 25). Detailed inspection of the tonsillar crypts may reveal the protruding tails of grass awns. Alternatively, the tonsillar crypts can be probed with a cotton-tipped applicator in an attempt to dislodge suspected foreign bodies. Nasopharyngeal foreign bodies are best visualized by use of a retroflexed endoscope. Another approach is to retract the soft palate with a spay hook and to inspect the nasopharynx with a dental mirror. Alternatively, vigorous flushing of the nasal cavity with saline with occasionally wash nasal or nasopharyngeal foreign bodies into the oropharynx. Prior to flushing the nasal cavity in this manner it is helpful to place swabs in the oropharynx to entrap any dislodged foreign bodies, and it is mandatory to ensure the endotracheal tube cuff is well inflated. Occasionally, radiography is helpful in localizing foreign bodies that have penetrated the pharynx.

The treatment of oropharyngeal foreign bodies centers on their expedient removal. A short course of antibiotics or anti-inflammatory drugs may be helpful to speed resolution of the clinical signs if the mucosal surface against which the foreign body was lodged is eroded or markedly inflamed.

OROPHARYNGEAL NEOPLASIA

The oropharynx is a common site of neoplasia in dogs and cats (see Chapter 27). In dogs, the most frequent oropharyngeal neoplasms are melanoma and squamous cell carcinoma, followed in prevalence by fibrosarcoma and epulides. Squamous cell carcinoma and fibrosarcoma are the most common feline oral neoplasms.[33] The most common sites of oropharyngeal neoplasia in dogs are the gingiva, palate, and tonsils.[34] Neoplasms of the feline oropharynx most commonly involve the tongue and gingiva.

Clinical Signs

The clinical signs of oral neoplasia include anorexia, drooling, dysphagia, and halitosis. Occasionally, the owner will notice bleeding from the mouth. Physical examination usually reveals a proliferative or ulcerative lesion in the oral cavity. In advanced cases, loosening of teeth in their sockets and facial deformation may be apparent.

Diagnosis

Diagnosis depends on biopsy of the oral mass. Regional lymph nodes should be palpated and those feeling abnormal should be aspirated with a fine needle to assist detection of metastasis. Oral radiography helps confirm the degree of bone lysis and the extent of the lesion.[35] The chest should be radiographed to check for pulmonary metastasis. In general, the prognosis is poorer for animals with large oral tumors or those with evidence of regional or distant metastasis.[34]

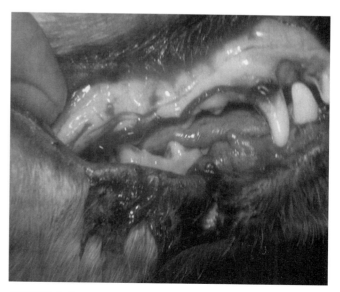

FIGURE 9–6. Gingival hemorrhage due to immune-mediated thrombocytopenia in a dog. (Courtesy of Dr. Elizabeth Lee, Massey University)

Squamous Cell Carcinoma

Squamous cell carcinoma can occur anywhere in the oropharynx including the gingiva, lips, palate, tongue, and tonsil. In dogs, the gingiva adjacent to the incisors and premolars in the lower jaw and the molars in the upper jaw are commonly affected. Squamous cell carcinoma is also the most common tongue tumor in dogs.[36] In cats, the tongue or sublingual area are commonly affected sites in addition to the gingiva. Squamous cell carcinoma of the oral mucosa can appear as a slowly progressive, localized, superficially ulcerative lesion or as a proliferative, expansile mass with or without ulceration. Occasionally, the tumor will appear concurrently in more than one place in the oral cavity. Invasion of nearby bone is common, but spread to local lymph nodes is slow to occur and distant metastasis is rare. In contrast, squamous cell carcinoma of the tongue and tonsil metastasize early.[36,37] Diagnosis is made by deep scrapings, fine needle aspiration, or biopsy of the affected area.

Treatment of squamous cell carcinoma involves wide surgical excision with or without adjuvant radiation therapy or chemotherapy (cisplatin). When the gingiva are involved, mandibulectomy or maxillectomy is advised because of the high likelihood of regional bone infiltration. When properly performed, these surgeries are cosmetically acceptable in spite of their radical nature. Squamous cell carcinoma affecting the tongue is also amenable to surgical therapy. Resection of 40% to 60% of the tongue of dogs is usually well tolerated, particularly if affected dogs are subsequently fed moist food and offered water in buckets sufficiently deep to allow immersion of their muzzle.[37] In cats, the usual location of the tumor in the base of the tongue makes surgical resection more difficult.

In dogs, the prognosis for gingival or palatine squamous cell carcinoma is good if complete surgical resection can be achieved but that for glossal or tonsillar squamous cell carcinoma is guarded to poor.[36,37] About 50% of dogs are alive one year postsurgery for squamous cell carcinoma of the tongue, the remainder succumbing to local recurrence and/or metastasis to regional nodes and lung.[37] Similarly, tonsil squamous cell carcinoma metastasizes early to the local lymph nodes (especially retropharyngeal) and the lungs and rapidly invades the surrounding pharyngeal tissue, making complete surgical excision difficult. In fact, many animals with tonsillar squamous cell carcinoma are first presented with the primary complaint of a subcutaneous pharyngeal swelling. In cats, both gingival and glossal squamous cell carcinoma have guarded prognoses following surgical treatment. However, adjuvant radiation therapy following hemimandibulectomy extends survival of cats with squamous cell carcinoma of the mandibular gingiva.[38]

Malignant Melanoma

Oral malignant melanomas most commonly originate on the gingival and buccal mucosa, and occasionally occur in the tongue.[36] They usually appear as proliferative, pigmented, friable masses (Figure 9–7), but amelanotic melanomas are also reasonably common. Local bone invasions and early metastasis are common.

Treatment is usually by aggressive surgical excision, but the prognosis is poor. Some evidence suggests that lingual melanoma may have a better prognosis than melanoma occurring elsewhere in the oral cavity.[36] Adjuvant radiation therapy may be valuable.[34]

Epulides

Epulides are an important group of oral neoplasms that occur along the gingival margin (Figure 9–8A). They are

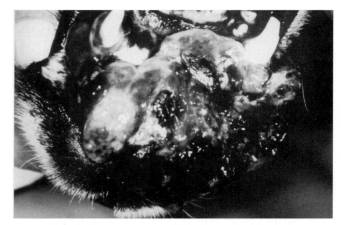

FIGURE 9–7. Malignant melanoma in a dog. (Courtesy of Dr. Hiliary Burbidge, Massey University)

most frequent in dogs but have also been reported in cats.[33] The prevalence of epulides is often underestimated.[34]

The histologic subclassification and terminology applied to these tumors is controversial. Most epulides can be classified as focal fibrous hyperplasia, peripheral ameloblastoma, peripheral odontogenic fibroma, or pyogenic granuloma.[39] Important differential diagnoses commonly mistaken for epulis include fibrosarcoma and squamous cell carcinoma (Figure 9–8B).[39] Previously used subclassifications of epulis including acanthomatous, ossifying, and fibrosing epulis have fallen into disfavor. Acanthomatous epulis is now thought by some to be a basal cell carcinoma derived from the gingival epithelium,[34] and by others to be a peripheral ameloblastoma.[39] Ossifying epulis and fibrosing epulis are derived from the periodontal ligament and are now referred to as peripheral odontogenic fibromas.[34,39]

From the clinical perspective, it is most important that the clinician and pathologist differentiate "acanthomatous epulis" from the other more benign epulides. Peripheral odontogenic fibromas do not invade bone whereas "acanthomatous epulis" is locally invasive into the surrounding bone. In keeping with their less aggressive behavior, peripheral odontogenic fibromas (and fibrous hyperplasia) have a more benign appearance (firm and smooth) than "acanthomatous epulides," which often ulcerate. Distant metastasis of epulides is rare and treatment is by surgical excision. Partial maxillectomy or mandibulectomy is required for the treatment of the acanthomatous form of the disease because wide surgical margins (approximately 1 cm) are necessary to prevent local recurrence.[34] Radiation therapy is also effective for the treatment of "acanthomatous epulis." The prognosis is favorable.

Fibrosarcoma

Fibrosarcoma of the oral cavity most commonly originates on the hard palate or maxilla (Figure 9–9). The mass is usually firm and in advanced cases may distort facial features. Occasionally, the tumor will be friable and ulcerated.[34] Local invasion of bone is common and metastasis to local lymph nodes and chest occurs readily. Treatment is by aggressive surgical excision (mandibulectomy or maxillectomy), preferably with adjuvant radiation therapy, but is usually only palliative. The median survival time following surgical resection is approximately 11 months.[40]

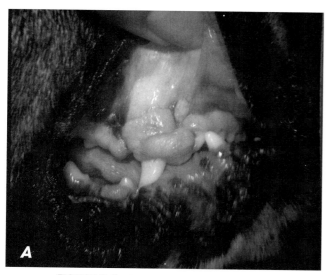 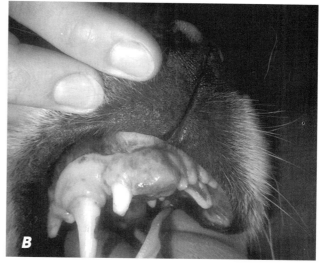

FIGURE 9–8. *(A)* Epulis in an elderly dog (Courtesy of Dr. Elizabeth Lee, Massey University). *(B)* Fibrosarcoma in an elderly dog. Note the similarity between epulis and fibrosarcoma in this case. (Courtesy of Dr. Elizabeth Lee, Massey University)

Oral Papillomatosis

Oral papillomatosis is occasionally seen in dogs.[41] The disease predominantly affects young dogs. It is characterized by the development of multiple benign cauliflower-like papillomas in the oral cavity (Figure 9–10). The lips, gingiva, tongue, and pharynx may be affected. The disease is induced by canine oral papillomavirus and is contagious with an incubation period of approximately 1 month. Scattered oral papillomas may be subclinical, but severe infections result in extensive lesions and dysphagia. The papillomas usually undergo spontaneous remission in 6 to 12 weeks followed by lifetime immunity. If sufficient papillomas are present to produce dysphagia, surgical removal of some of the papillomas is warranted. Cyclophosphamide (50 mg/m² PO for the first 4 days of each week for 6–8 weeks) or vincristine (0.8 mg/m² once per week for 6–8 weeks) can also be used successfully.[42]

Miscellaneous Oropharyngeal Neoplasms

Plasmacytomas occasionally affect the oral cavity of dogs.[43,44] They are usually solitary pink or red ulcerated nodules. Plasmacytomas are a distinct entity unrelated to multiple myeloma, and surgical excision is curative. Surgical excision of ectopic thyroid carcinoma involving the base of the tongue of dogs has recently been reported. No recurrence occurred.[45] Oral osteosarcoma has a more favorable prognosis than that of long bones, and has a median survival time following surgical resection of 13.6 months.[40] Miscellaneous other neoplasms of the oral cavity include lymphoma, mast cell tumors, myeloblastomas, hemangioma, hemangiosarcoma, and lingual rhabdomyoma.[46]

DISORDERS OF THE PALATE

Cleft Palate[47]

Cleft palate is a congenital disorder of cats and dogs that is due to incomplete fusion of the embryonic palatine processes. The result is a fissure in the midline of the palate that allows access of food and oral secretions into the

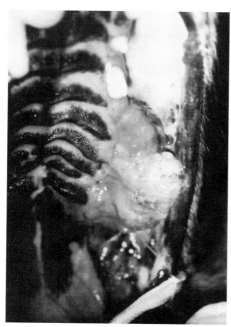

FIGURE 9–9. Fibrosarcoma in an elderly dog. (Courtesy of Dr. Elizabeth Lee, Massey University)

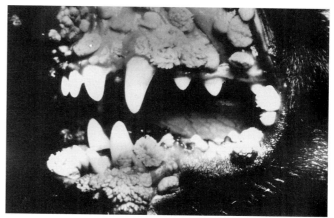

FIGURE 9–10. Oral papillomatosis in a dog. (Courtesy of Dr. Hiliary Burbidge, Massey University)

nasopharynx and nasal cavity. The hard palate is affected more frequently than the soft palate (Figure 9–11). The etiology of the disease is unknown. Cleft palate occurs sporadically in many breeds, suggesting the cause is an intrauterine insult such as a teratogen. In most breeds the heritability of the disorder does not appear to be high. However, breeding studies have shown evidence of an inherited pattern with incomplete penetrance in the Shih Tzu and possibly pointers and bulldogs.[47] In addition, there is evidence of a familial pattern in Siamese cats.[48]

Clinical signs are usually apparent from a young age. Affected pups and kittens may fail to thrive and will usually reflux milk from their noses during drinking. Coughing may also occur following drinking.

The diagnosis is made by physical examination. The most important differential diagnoses are congenitally short soft palate, pharyngeal motility abnormalities, and bronchoesophageal fistula.

The treatment is surgical repair of the palatine defect.

Elongated Soft Palate

Elongation of the soft palate predominantly results in airway rather than gastrointestinal disease, although affected animals may develop a degree of associated pharyngeal hyperplasia, gagging, and retching. The disease is most common in brachycephalic dogs. Diagnosis is made by physical examination. The caudal tip of the palate should just contact the rostroventral tip of the epiglottis. An elongated soft palate will extend dorsocaudally to the tip of the epiglottis and into the laryngopharynx and larynx. The treatment is surgical removal of the tip of the palate and repair of any concurrent abnormalities of the respiratory tract, such as everted laryngeal saccules and stenotic nares.

Congenitally Short Soft Palate

A short soft palate does not contact the epiglottis and thus fails to protect the nasopharynx from food and water during swallowing and drinking. The disease occurs in both cats and dogs, and the clinical signs are similar although less severe than cleft palate. In the author's experience, the predominant clinical sign is chronic nasal discharge, although the disorder can be subclinical. If the clinical signs warrant treatment, the palate can be elongated surgically.

PHARYNGEAL DISEASES

Pharyngitis

Primary pharyngitis is uncommon in the dog or cat, being more often associated with widespread oral, upper respiratory, or systemic disease. Causes of pharyngitis and pharyngeal edema include trauma, foreign bodies, insect stings, snake bites, allergic reactions, chemical or thermal injury, infections (especially the feline respiratory viruses), and immune-mediated disorders such as chronic gingivitis-stomatitis-pharyngitis. In addition, anecdotal evidence suggests that an antibiotic-responsive primary pharyngitis occurs in both dogs and cats.

Clinical signs of pharyngitis include inappetence, dysphagia, malaise, fever, and retching or vomiting. Diagnosis is usu-

ally by a combination of history and visual inspection of the oropharynx, which reveals inflamed pharyngeal mucosa.

Treatment is symptomatic and includes short courses of antibiotics (e.g., amoxicillin) and the maintenance of hydration and adequate food intake by the measures described earlier (see section on symptomatic management).

Tonsillitis

Primary tonsillitis is not very common. It occurs mainly in young dogs of the toy breeds and appears to be rare in cats. The etiology is unknown. Many different organisms have been cultured from the tonsillar area in affected animals, including Staphylococcal, Streptoccal, and *Proteus* spp., but no single organism has been consistently recovered. Affected dogs cough and gag, and often retch or expectorate small quantities of white foamy mucus that can be confused with vomitus by the client. Malaise, pyrexia, and inappetance may be present. The tonsils are usually hyperemic, mottled, and bulge from the crypts. Petechiation and white specks (focal abscesses) may be seen on the surface. It is important to note that the amount of tonsil protruding from the crypts varies greatly in normal dogs. Therefore observation of the tonsils protruding from their crypts is insufficient evidence in of itself to diagnose tonsillitis.

Tonsillitis is treated by a 7 to 10 day course of antibiotics (e.g., amoxicillin). Recurrence of primary tonsillitis is common even after treatment, but animals usually outgrow the disorder. Tonsillectomy is rarely required.

Secondary tonsillitis is more common than primary tonsillitis. It occurs in association with other conditions of the oral cavity, pharynx, and upper respiratory tract. In addition, an association between tonsillitis and diseases causing chronic vomiting, coughing, and regurgitation has been frequently

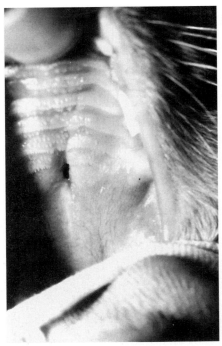

FIGURE 9–11. Cleft palate in a kitten. Note the small defect at the junction of the hard and soft palate. (Courtesy of Dr. Shane Guerin, Massey University)

reported. The clinical signs are the same as those of primary tonsillitis, but additional signs pertaining to the associated disease condition often predominate. Treatment is primarily directed at the underlying cause.

Tonsillar Neoplasia

Tonsillar neoplasms such as lymphosarcoma will occasionally result in massive bilateral enlargement of the tonsils, producing gagging, odynophagia, and dysphagia. Tonsillar squamous cell carcinoma is a highly malignant cause of unilateral tonsillar enlargement (see earlier). The tonsil quickly becomes fixed to the surrounding tissues. Diagnosis is made by physical examination. Fine needle aspiration or brush cytology is occasionally necessary to differentiate tonsillitis from tonsillar neoplasia. Treatment of tonsillar lymphosarcoma with standard lymphoma protocols (e.g., cyclophosphamide, vincristine, prednisone) is often rewarding, whereas treatment of tonsillar squamous cell carcinoma is usually unsuccessful.

Retropharyngeal Lymphadenopathy or Abscess

Retropharyngeal lymphadenopathy can result from pharyngitis, penetrating wounds of the pharynx, lymphosarcoma, and metastatic neoplasia from tumors situated anywhere in the head. Retropharyngeal abscess is usually due to penetration of the pharynx by a foreign body. Important clinical signs of these disorders include odynophagia and dysphagia. The disorders are discussed more fully in Chapter 11.

SALIVARY GLAND DISEASES

With the exception of sialoceles, salivary gland diseases are uncommon in dogs and cats. The most common salivary gland diseases are described here. The diagnostic approach to ptyalism and xerostomia is covered in Chapter 5.

Salivary Mucocele (Sialocele)[49,50]

Sialoceles are the most common salivary gland disease of dogs and cats. They result from leakage of saliva into the subcutaneous tissues of the neck, the pharyngeal wall, or the sublingual tissues (ranula). The sublingual glands or ducts are most frequently involved. The cause is not known, although trauma is considered most likely. The saliva accumulates in single or multiloculated cavities that form a fluctuant swelling. Cervical mucoceles usually develop just caudal and ventral to the mandible (Figures 9–12A and 9–12B). The swelling is usually slightly to one side of the neck but occasionally will be in the midline. Unlike cervical mucoceles, pharyngeal mucoceles often result in significant compromise of the patient's ability to eat or breathe (Figure 9–13). A ranula appears as an elongated swelling ventral and lateral to the tongue that eventually interferes with eating (Figure 9–14).

Diagnosis of sialoceles is confirmed by aspiration of a sample of the accumulated fluid. Typically, the fluid is mucoid with only low-grade inflammation unless the sialocele has

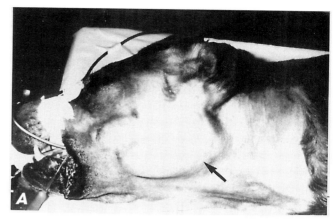

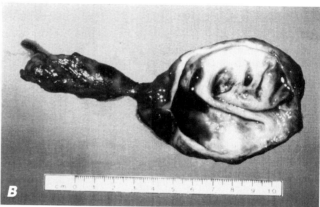

FIGURE 9–12. *(A)* Cervical sialocele in a dog. Note that the fluid-filled cyst is caudoventral to the mandible. (Courtesy of Dr. Steve Fox, Massey University). *(B)* Cervical sialocele from the dog in *(A)* after surgical removal. The cystlike structure has been opened to show the fibrous lining of the cavity. The sublingual salivary glands can be seen to the left. (Courtesy of Dr. Steve Fox, Massey University)

been subjected to repeated drainage attempts, whereupon inflammatory cells can become more numerous. Treatment of cervical mucoceles requires surgical drainage and removal of the mandibular and sublingual salivary glands on the same side as the lesion.[50] Occasionally, bilateral removal of these salivary glands is necessary to resolve the swelling. Ranula will often respond to marsupialization but occasionally the sublingual salivary tissue has to be removed.[50,51] Pharyngeal mucoceles are managed by marsupialization and resection of redundant pharyngeal tissue to reestablish a patent airway. Consideration should also be given to resection of the sublingual salivary tissue on the side of the pharyngeal swelling to help prevent recurrence.[50]

Sialodentitis

Inflammation of the salivary glands is rarely diagnosed. The cause is often not determined but, occasionally, blunt trauma, penetrating wounds, grass awns, or hematogenous spread of microorganisms, such as distemper, are responsible. The parotid and zygomatic glands appear to be the most commonly affected. Affected glands swell and are painful to the touch. Anorexia, fever, and pain on opening of the

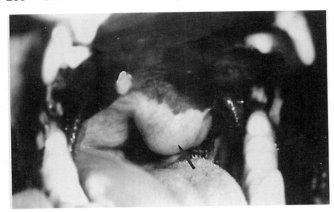

FIGURE 9-13. Pharyngeal sialocele in a dog. Note the pendulous swelling in the dorsal pharyngeal wall that is obstructing the pharynx. (Courtesy of Dr. Steve Fox, Massey University)

mouth are common. Periorbital inflammation and swelling can accompany zygomatic sialodentitis.[52] Diagnosis is by physical examination or fine needle aspiration. An important differential diagnosis is salivary adenocarcinoma. Antibiotic therapy is usually effective, although surgical drainage may be required if abscessation develops.

Salivary Gland Necrosis

Idiopathic salivary gland necrosis has been reported in a number of dogs, in particular those of terrier breeds such as the Jack Russell.[53-55] It is an uncommon disorder of unknown pathogenesis. Proposed causes have included ischemic necrosis secondary to vasculitis or avulsion of salivary vessels during fighting. Pressure necrosis due to swelling of the gland within its capsule or infarction secondary to a CNS abnormality have also been incriminated.[54,56] Affected animals develop persistent anorexia, ptyalism, gagging, vomiting, and/or regurgitation. Frequent swallowing, odynophagia, and depression are common. The mandibular salivary glands feel enlarged and firm but are usually nonpainful. Fine needle aspiration of the glands is unrewarding and diagnosis must be made by biopsy. Histology reveals large-scale infarction and necrosis of the salivary glands, which differentiates the condition from idiopathic hypersialism, a rare disorder that occurs in association with salivary gland enlargement but no necrosis.

Surgical resection of affected glands is sometimes palliative

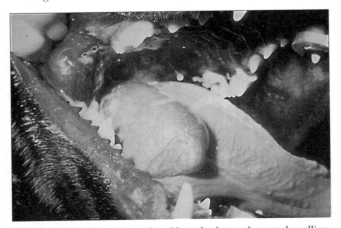

FIGURE 9-14. Ranula in a dog. Note the large elongated swelling ventrolateral to the tongue.

but often does not control the vomiting or regurgitation.[54,56] For unknown reasons, a good therapeutic response can occur to phenobarbital (3–4 mg/kg q 12 hours).[56] Spontaneous remission has also been reported.

Salivary Gland Neoplasia[57]

Salivary gland neoplasia is a relatively rare disorder. The parotid and mandibular glands of elderly dogs and cats are most frequently affected. Most salivary gland tumors are malignant, epithelial-derived neoplasms (e.g., carcinoma, adenocarcinoma). They result in extensive swelling and infiltration in the cervical, retropharyngeal, or retrobulbar areas. The swelling is usually not painful. If the zygomatic gland is involved, retrobulbar infiltration often results in exophthalmos. Occasionally, affected animals are presented for recurrent sialoceles, and the diagnosis is made when an attentive surgeon realizes remaining salivary tissue looks abnormal. The prognosis is poor because most salivary gland adenocarcinomas are advanced by the time of diagnosis and metastasize readily.

Miscellaneous Salivary Gland Diseases

Occasionally foreign bodies or sialoliths[58] will lodge in salivary ducts producing obstruction and glandular atrophy or, alternatively, rupture of the duct and a mucocele. Sjogren's syndrome, an autoimmune disease involving the salivary glands and lacrimal tissue, has been reported in dogs and is characterized by xerostomia and keratoconjunctivitis sicca.[59] Salivary gland fistula as a result of cutaneous wounds that damage the salivary glands can occur. Treatment requires removal of the affected gland.[51]

REFERENCES

1. Holmstrom SE. Canine dentistry: Periodontal disease. Comp Contin Ed Pract Vet 11:1485–1492, 1989.
2. Harvey CE, Orr HS (eds). Manual of Small Animal Dentistry. Brit Sm Anim Vet Assoc, Cheltenham, 1990.
3. Bojorab MJ, Tholen M. Small Animal Oral Medicine and Surgery. Lea & Febiger, Philadelphia, 1990.
4. Penman S. Dental conditions in the dog and cat. Vet Ann 30:223–232, 1990.
5. Lyon KF. An approach to feline dentistry. Comp Contin Ed Pract Vet 12:493–497, 1990.
6. Goldstein GS. Geriatric dentistry in dogs. Comp Contin Ed Pract Vet 12:951–960, 1990.
7. Anderson JG. Approach to diagnosis of canine oral lesions. Comp Contin Ed Pract Vet 13:1215–1226, 1991.
8. Love DN, Vekselstein R, Collings S. The obligate and facultatively anaerobic bacterial flora of the normal feline gingival margin. Vet Micro 22:267–275, 1990.
9. Guelfi JF, Legeay Y, Pages JP, et al. Comparative trial of Stomorgyl (N.D.), spiramycin and metronidazole in the treatment of oropharyngeal infections in dogs and cats. Rev Med Vet 141:985–990, 1990.
10. Diehl K, Rosychuk RAW. Feline gingivitis-stomatitis-pharyngitis. Vet Clin Am 23:139–153, 1993.
11. Bilbrey SA, Dulisch ML, Stallings B. Chemical burns caused by benzalkonium chloride in eight surgical cases. J Am Anim Hosp Assoc 25:31–34, 1989.
12. Greenwood JA, Studdert VP, Sullivan ND. Inorganic mercury poisoning in a dog. Aust Vet J 67:421–422, 1990.
13. McKeever PJ, Klausner JS. Plant awn, candidal, nocardial and necrotizing ulcerative stomatitis in the dog. J Am Anim Hosp Assoc 22:17–24, 1986.
14. Brown RM. Vegetative stomatitis. Mod Vet Pract, 856–858, Nov. 1985.
15. Greene RT, Harling DE, Dillman RC. Fiberglass-induced pyogranulomatous stomatitis in a dog. J Am Anim Hosp Assoc 23:401–404, 1987.

16. Wolf AM. Feline gingivitis, stomatitis, and pharyngitis. In: Kirk RW, Bonagura JD (eds) Current Veterinary Therapy XI. WB Saunders, Philadelphia, 568–572, 1992.

17. Mikx FHM, Maltha JC, van Campen GJ. Spirochetes in early lesions of necrotizing ulcerative gingivitis experimentally induced in Beagles. Oral Micro Immunol 5:86–89, 1990.

18. Dickson NJ. Disseminated feline cryptococcosis. Aust Vet J 19:98–101, 1989.

19. Fairley RA. Cryptococcus neoformans cases at Ruakura from 1985–1991. Surveillance, Ministry of Agriculture and Fisheries Bulletin, New Zealand 19:28, 1992.

20. Harbour DA, Howard PE, Gaskell RM. Isolation of feline calicivirus and feline herpesvirus from domestic cats 1980 to 1989. Vet Rec 128:77–80, 1991.

21. Knowles JO, Gaskell RM, Gaskell CJ, et al. Prevalence of feline calicivirus, feline leukaemia virus and antibodies to FIV in cats with chronic stomatitis. Vet Rec 124:336–338, 1989.

22. Tenorio AP, Franti CE, Madewell BR, et al. Chronic oral infections of cats and their relationship to persistent oral carriage of feline calici, immunodeficiency, or leukemia viruses. Vet Immunol Immunopathol 29:1–14, 1991.

23. Belford CJ, Miller RI, Mitchell G, et al. Evidence of feline immunodeficiency virus in Queensland cats: Preliminary observations. Aust Vet Pract 19:4–6, 1989.

24. Ishida T, Washizu T, Toriyabe K, et al. Feline immunodeficiency virus infection in cats of Japan. J Am Vet Med Assoc 194:221–225, 1989.

25. Friend SCE, Birch CJ, Lording PM, et al. Feline immunodeficiency virus: Prevalence, disease associations and isolation. Aust Vet J 67:237–243, 1990.

26. Shelton GH, Waltier RM, Connor SC, et al. Prevalence of feline immunodeficiency virus and feline leukemia virus infections in pet cats. J Am Anim Hosp Assoc 25:7–12, 1989.

27. Hosie MJ, Robertson C, Jarrett O. Prevalence of feline leukaemia virus and antibodies to feline immunodeficiency virus in cats in the United Kingdom. Vet Rec 125:293–297, 1989.

28. White SD, Rosychuk RAW, Janik TA, et al. Plasma cell stomatitis-pharyngitis in cats: 40 cases (1973–1991). J Am Vet Med Assoc 200:1377–1380, 1992.

29. Waters L, Hopper CD, Gruffydd-Jones TJ, et al. Chronic gingivitis in a colony of cats infected with feline immunodeficiency virus and feline calicivirus. Vet Rec 132:340–342, 1993.

30. Knowles JO, McArdle F, Dawson S, et al. Studies on the role of feline calicivirus in chronic stomatitis in cats. Vet Micro 27:205–219, 1991.

31. Madewell BR, Stannard AA, Pulley LT, et al. Oral eosinophilic granuloma in Siberian Husky dogs. J Am Vet Med Assoc 177:701–703, 1980.

32. Wildgoose WH. Palatine arterial haemorrhage in a cat. Vet Rec 126:273, 1990.

33. Stebbins KE, Morse CC, Goldschmidt MH. Feline oral neoplasia: A ten-year survey. Vet Path 26:121–128, 1989.

34. White RAS. The alimentary system. In: White RAS (ed) Manual of Small Animal Oncology. British Small Animal Veterinary Association, Cheltenham, 237–263, 1991.

35. Frew DG, Dobson JM. Radiological assessment of 50 cases of incisive or maxillary neoplasia in the dog. J Sm Anim Pract 33:11–18, 1992.

36. Beck ER, Withrow SJ, McChesney AE, et al. Canine tongue tumors: A retrospective review of 57 cases. J Am Anim Hosp Assoc 22:525–532, 1986.

37. Carpenter LG, Withrow SJ, Powers BE, et al. Squamous cell carcinoma of the tongue in 10 dogs. J Am Anim Hosp Assoc 29:17–24, 1993.

38. Hutson CA, Willauer CC, Walder EJ, et al. Treatment of mandibular squamous cell carcinoma in cats by use of mandibulectomy and radiotherapy: Seven cases (1987–1989). J Am Vet Med Assoc 201:777–781, 1992.

39. Verstraete FJM, Ligthelm AJ, Weber A. The histological nature of epulides in dogs. J Comp Path 106:169–182, 1992.

40. Kosovsky JK, Matthiesen DT, Marretta SM, et al. Results of partial mandibulectomy for the treatment of oral tumors in 142 dogs. Vet Surg 20:397–401, 1991.

41. Sundberg JP, Reszka AA, Williams ES, et al. An oral papillomavirus that infected one coyote and three dogs. Vet Path 28:87–88, 1991.

42. Calvert CA. Canine viral and transmissible neoplasms. In: Green CE (ed) Clinical Microbiology and Infectious Diseases of the Dog and Cat. WB Saunders, Philadelphia, 461–478, 1984.

43. Rakich PM, Latimer KS, Weiss R, et al. Mucocutaneous plasmacytomas in dogs: 75 cases (1980–1987). J Am Vet Med Assoc 194:803–810, 1989.

44. Clark GN, Berg J, Engler SJ, et al. Extramedullary plasmacytomas in dogs: Results of surgical excision in 131 cases. J Am Anim Hosp Assoc 28:105–111, 1992.

45. Lantz GC, Salisbury SK. Surgical excision of ectopic thyroid carcinoma involving the base of the tongue in dogs: Three cases (1980–1987). J Am Vet Med Assoc 195:1606–1608, 1989.

46. Sebernik N, Appleby EC. Breed prevalence and sites of hemangioma and hemangiosarcoma in dogs. Vet Rec 129:408–409, 1991.

47. Harvey CE. Palate defects in dogs and cats. Comp Contin Ed Pract Vet 9:404–420, 1987.

48. Noden DM. Normal development and congenital birth defects in the cat. In: Kirk RW, Bonagura JD (eds) Current Veterinary Therapy XI. WB Saunders, Philadelphia, 1248–1257, 1992.

49. Bellenger CR, Simpson DJ. Canine sialocoeles—60 clinical cases. J Sm Anim Pract 33:376–380, 1992.

50. Brown NO. Salivary gland diseases. Prob Vet Med 2:281–294, 1989.

51. Knecht CD. Diseases of the salivary glands in the dog. In: Burrows CF (ed) Gastroenterology in Practice. The Compendium Collection. Vet Learning Systems, Trenton, NJ, 234–238, 1993.

52. Simison WG. Sialdentitis associated with periorbital disease in a dog. J Am Vet Med Assoc 202:1983–1985, 1993.

53. Kelly DF, Lucke VM, Denny HR, et al. Histology of salivary gland infarction in the dog. Vet Path 16:438–443, 1979.

54. Cooke MM, Guilford WG. Necrotizing sialoadenitis in a wire-haired fox terrier. NZ Vet J 40:69–72, 1992.

55. Mawby DI, Bauer MS, Lloyd-Bauer PM, et al. Vasculitis and necrosis of the mandibular salivary glands and chronic vomiting in a dog. Can Vet J 32:562–564, 1991.

56. Chapman BL, Malik R. Phenobarbitone-responsive hypersialism in two dogs. J Small Anim Pract 33:549–552, 1992.

57. Carberry CA, Flanders JA, Harvey HJ, et al. Salivary gland tumors in dogs and cats: A literature and case review. J Am Anim Hosp Assoc 24:561–567, 1988.

58. Mulkey C, Knecht CD. Parotid salivary cyst and calculus in a dog. J Am Vet Med Assoc 159:1174, 1971.

59. Quimby FW, Schwartz RS, Poskitt T, et al. A disorder of dogs resembling Sjogren's syndrome. Clin Immunol Immunopathol 12:471–476, 1979.

10

Pharynx and Esophagus: Normal Structure and Function

DONALD R. STROMBECK AND W. GRANT GUILFORD

INTRODUCTION

The act of swallowing is initiated voluntarily by muscles of the tongue and head that propel a bolus of food from the oral cavity to the oropharynx. Movement of the bolus from the pharynx to the stomach and through the remainder of the alimentary canal is almost entirely reflex. An appreciation of the physiology of swallowing is necessary to understand the causes and treatment of dysphagia.

ANATOMY OF THE PHARYNX[1,2]

The pharynx is a funnel-shaped connection between the oral cavity and the esophagus, and between the nasal cavity and the larynx. Figure 10–1 shows a cross section of the pharynx and its related structures. The boundaries of the pharynx are defined ventrally by the root of the tongue, dorsally by the floor of the cranium and cervical flexor muscles, and laterally by pharyngeal constrictor muscles. The soft palate divides the rostral part of the pharynx into a dorsal cavity (the nasopharynx) and a ventral cavity (oropharynx). The common cavity caudal to the end of the soft palate is called the laryngopharynx. The pharynx has four apertures that open and close in an integrated fashion during swallowing and respiration. An opening connects the oropharynx with the oral cavity (aditus pharyngis), the nasal passages with the nasopharynx, the laryngopharynx with the larynx (aditus laryngis), and the laryngopharynx with the esophagus.

The muscles that form the lateral walls of the pharynx are primarily constrictors. These include the pterygopharyngeus and palatopharyngeus muscles, which constrict the rostral pharynx, and the thyropharyngeus and cricopharyngeus muscles, which constrict the middle and caudal pharynx, respectively. The cricopharyngeus muscle and the caudal part of the thyropharyngeus muscle form the pharyngoesophageal sphincter. The pharynx is dilated by one muscle, the stylopharyngeus, which also acts to draw the pharynx forward. The pharyngeal muscles are striated and contract reflexly, following pharyngeal stimulation. They are innervated by branches of the glossopharyngeal and vagus nerves.

Three sets of muscles control the function of the soft palate. The tensor veli palatini stretches the palate between the pterygoid

bones. The levator veli palatini raises the caudal part of the soft palate, and the palatinus shortens the palate and curls the caudal border ventrally. These muscles are innervated by branches of the trigeminal nerves.

ANATOMY OF THE ESOPHAGUS[1,2]

The esophagus is divided into cervical, thoracic, and abdominal portions. The anatomic relationship of the esophagus with other structures is shown in Figures 10–2 and 10–3. The cervical esophagus lies ventral and to the left of the ventral spinal muscles, and dorsal and to the left of the trachea. The thoracic esophagus includes that portion of the esophagus from the thoracic inlet to the diaphragm. The thoracic esophagus initially lies to the left of the trachea but comes to lie dorsal to the trachea at its bifurcation. At this point it crosses to the right of the aortic arch and passes caudally in

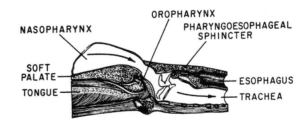

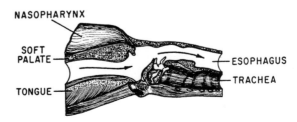

FIGURE 10-1. Drawing of sagittal section of pharynx, larynx, trachea, and esophagus. Upper drawing shows relative positions of structures during respiration. Lower drawing shows relative positions during swallowing.

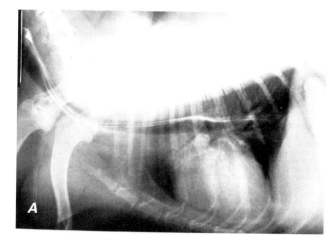

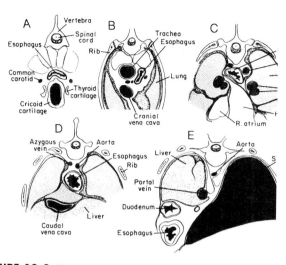

FIGURE 10–3. Topographic anatomy of the canine showing the relationship of the esophagus to adjacent structures at different transverse planes through the cervical, thoracic, and abdominal regions. The level of each plane corresponds to those bearing the same designations in the radiographs in Figure 10–2. (Level A not shown.)

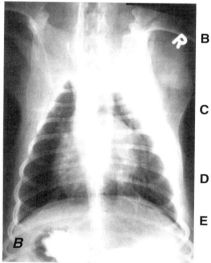

FIGURE 10–2. (A) Lateral and dorsoventral (B) radiographs of a dog after having swallowed a bolus of liquid positive-contrast medium. Transverse planes designated B, C, D, and E correspond to those with the same identification in the drawings of transverse sections shown in Figure 10–3.

the median plane. There is a short segment of abdominal esophagus between the diaphragm and the stomach. The wall of the esophagus is thickest in the cervical and abdominal portions. The esophagus is least distensible at the points where it enters and leaves the thoracic cavity.

The esophagus consists of four layers: the adventitia, muscularis, submucosa, and mucosa. The thin fibrous adventitia covers the esophageal muscle. The muscularis of the canine esophagus is composed of two oblique layers of striated muscle throughout its entire length. The only smooth muscle in the esophagus of the dog is the muscularis mucosae, which contributes little if anything to peristalsis. The tunica muscularis of the cranial feline esophagus consists of striated muscle, but the caudal thoracic and abdominal sections contain increasing quantities of smooth muscle until the final 2 to 3 cm of the esophagus are entirely smooth. The striated muscle of the feline esophagus consists of two layers that are oblique in the proximal portion and become spiral in the distal portion. In the caudal feline esophagus, the muscle forms a distinct inner, circular layer and an outer, longitudinal layer.

The submucosal layer of the esophagus contains mucus glands and loosely binds the mucosal and muscular layers together. This allows the relatively inelastic mucosal coat to be thrown into prominent longitudinal folds in the dog, and transverse folds in the caudal thoracic esophagus of the cat (the serrated or herringbone pattern; see Figure 7–7). The mucosal layer has a stratified squamous epithelium that contains openings for the ducts of the esophageal mucus glands.[3] In the caudal half of the esophagus the mucosa is bounded by the muscularis mucosae.

Blood to the cervical esophagus is supplied by the thyroid arteries. The cranial part of the thoracic esophagus receives blood from the bronchoesophageal artery. The remainder of the esophagus is supplied by branches from the aorta, intercostals, and gastric artery. Venous drainage of the esophagus occurs via satellite vessels of the arteries that supply it.

The vagus nerve and its associated branches innervate the esophagus. The vagus contains somatic motor nerves to the esophageal striated muscle, autonomic nerves to the esophageal smooth muscle, and general visceral afferent nerves from esophageal sensory receptors. Sympathetic nerves, accompanying the vascular supply, also innervate the esophagus. The sensory innervation of the cat esophagus has recently received detailed study.[4] Afferents from the striated muscle, smooth muscle, and lower esophageal sphincter distribute to spinal segments C1-T8, C5-L2, and T1-L3, respectively. Each level of the esophagus has a distinct but overlapping sensory projection to the spinal cord.

ANATOMY OF ESOPHAGEAL SPHINCTERS

Pharyngoesophageal Sphincter

The aperture between the oropharynx and the esophagus remains closed except when a bolus of ingesta passes through. The cricopharyngeus muscles and the caudal part of the thyropharyngeus muscles maintain this closure. These muscles lie dorsal to the esophagus. Their origins are the lateral surface of the cricoid cartilage and the oblique line of the thyroid lamina. The two muscles insert on the median dorsal raphe. The pharyngoesophageal sphincter (PES) is formed dorsally and laterally by the two muscles and ventrally by the cricoid cartilage. The motor fibers to the cricopharyngeus and thyropharyngeus muscles are in the glossopharyngeal nerve and the pharyngeal branches of the vagus nerve.[5–7]

Gastroesophageal Junction and Sphincter

GES sphincter tone, in conjunction with the anatomy of the gastroesophageal junction, prevents regurgitation of gastric contents into the esophagus. The GES is a physiologic rather than an anatomic sphincter because it does not consist of a specialized large mass of muscle. In dogs, the GES consists of an outer layer of longitudinal striated muscle fibers and an inner layer of circular smooth muscle that merges with the inner striated muscle layer of the adjacent esophagus. The longitudinal muscle layer merges with the smooth muscle of the stomach about 2 mm caudal to the junction of gastric mucosa with esophageal stratified squamous epithelium. Manometric studies of the dog GES have detected a high-pressure zone of about 3 cm in length (range 1–5 cm).[8] In cats the GES consists of only smooth muscle.[9]

The anatomic features of the gastroesophageal junction contribute to the prevention of reflux (see later). These features include 1) interdigitating rugal folds that converge near the gastroesophageal junction and continue into the terminal esophagus, (2) the right diaphragmatic crus, which serves as a muscular sling, (3) the oblique implantation of the distal esophagus into the stomach, (4) the muscular sling provided by the smooth muscle bundles of the lesser gastric curvature around the left side of the gastroesophageal junction, and (5) the compression exerted on the short intraabdominal esophageal segment by positive intra-abdominal pressure (Figure 10–4).[10]

Vagal fibers innervate the gastroesophageal junction and sphincter. Somatic efferents pass to the striated fibers from the nucleus ambiguus in the brain stem. Parasympathetic fibers derived from the dorsal motor nucleus of the vagus innervate the smooth muscle fibers. In addition, sympathetic fibers may play a role in regulating sphincter function.[11] Lastly, the smooth muscle of the GES has an intrinsic nervous system that consists of the nerve plexuses of Auerbach and Meissner.

PHYSIOLOGY OF SWALLOWING

Swallowing consists of a series of sequential well-coordinated events that transport food and liquids from the mouth to the stomach. This process has been divided into three major phases: oropharyngeal, esophageal, and gastroesophageal. The oropharyngeal phase is further subdivided into oral, pharyngeal, and cricopharyngeal stages, with each stage related to the action of a particular group of structures. Following the prehension of food, the voluntary oral stage is initiated in which a bolus is formed in the oropharynx and is passed in an aboral direction to the base of the tongue. Pharyngeal contact by the bolus next stimulates a series of rapid pharyngeal peristaltic contractions that propel the bolus from the base of the tongue to the laryngopharynx. This is the second, or pharyngeal, stage of the oropharyngeal phase.

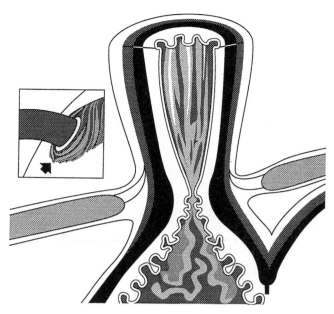

FIGURE 10–4. Competence of the GES junction to prevent reflux is maintained by rugal folds, muscular sling fibers, (see insert) oblique angle of distal esophagus and stomach, and compression of intra-abdominal esophagus by stomach.

Pharyngeal Phase of Swallowing[12,13]

Because the pharyngeal phase of swallowing must move the bolus from the pharynx only into the esophagus, the other three major pharyngeal openings through which the bolus might pass must be closed. The pathway between the oral cavity and oropharynx is closed by muscles of the mouth and tongue. The orifice between the oropharynx and the nasopharynx is reflexly closed by elevating the soft palate and approximating the palatopharyngeal folds. That is accomplished by simultaneous contraction of the levator palati and palatopharyngeal muscles. The opening to the trachea is protected by closure of the glottis and tipping of the epiglottis in such a manner as to divert food away from the glottis. To accomplish this, the larynx is drawn in a cranial direction by the thyroglossal and mylohyoid muscles. The epiglottis is then pushed back over the laryngeal orifice by the tongue.

The movement of a bolus through the pharynx is accomplished by an orderly sequential contraction of the pharyngeal muscles, beginning in the rostral part of the pharynx and proceeding aborally. The reflex motor events that begin in the pharynx are initiated by the stimulation of numerous sensory receptors located in specific areas of the palate, pharynx, and epiglottis. The receptors' nerve fibers are found in the maxillary branch of the trigeminal nerve, in the glossopharyngeal nerve, and in the superior laryngeal nerve. The afferent pathways carrying the information from these receptors to the brain stem are shown in the reflex arc diagrammed in Figure 10–5. Sequential firing in the nuclei of the cranial motor nerves evokes contraction of the buccal, tongue, pharyngeal, and esophageal muscles. The neural reflex produces the initial response in the rostral constrictors of the pharynx. The bolus is propelled aborally by the sequential contraction of constrictors of the remainder of the pharynx. Respiration is suspended during the pharyngeal phase of swallowing because the two events cannot occur simultaneously.

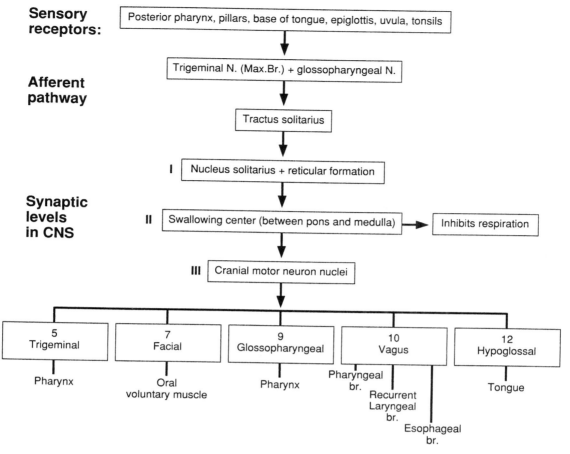

Sensory receptors: Posterior pharynx, pillars, base of tongue, epiglottis, uvula, tonsils

Afferent pathway Trigeminal N. (Max.Br.) + glossopharyngeal N.

Tractus solitarius

Synaptic levels in CNS

I Nucleus solitarius + reticular formation

II Swallowing center (between pons and medulla) → Inhibits respiration

III Cranial motor neuron nuclei

| 5 Trigeminal | 7 Facial | 9 Glossopharyngeal | 10 Vagus | 12 Hypoglossal |
| Pharynx | Oral voluntary muscle | Pharynx | Pharyngeal br. / Recurrent Laryngeal br. / Esophageal br. | Tongue |

FIGURE 10–5. Scheme of swallowing reflex showing afferent pathways, central synapses, and pathways of motor fibers.

The sequential motor events in the pharynx are controlled by a central generator.[12] The entire sequence of pharyngeal swallowing is completed without peripheral feedback. In contrast, esophageal motor events are completed only with peripheral feedback. Two functionally distinct central pattern generators are present for the pharyngeal and esophageal phases of swallowing. The presence of two central generators explains why many swallowing problems cause either pharyngeal or esophageal abnormalities, but not both. The central pattern generator is triggered by patterned sensory inputs over specific branches of the glossopharyngeal and vagal nerves. The particular sensory pattern determines which motor response is evoked in the pharynx. Different patterns of stimulation by the same sensory modality (touch) on the same pharyngolaryngeal region can evoke motor responses as disparate as gagging, laryngeal adduction, or swallowing.[12]

Solid boluses are more effective than liquids in stimulating pharyngeal receptors to initiating swallowing. In healthy animals, fluoroscopy reveals that multiple swallowing attempts may be necessary to stimulate deglutition of water or saline. Oil does not stimulate swallowing. Thus, mineral oil given orally is often aspirated into the trachea without stimulating deglutition.

The smooth muscle in the muscularis mucosa may participate in sensory function. The neural structures found in the intrinsic nervous system of the esophageal mucosa resemble sensory receptors in other tissues.[14] Motility in the muscularis mucosa may assist the sensory receptors in monitoring pro-gression of a bolus and reinforcing the peristaltic wave carrying it to the stomach.

Pharyngoesophageal Sphincter Function

During a normal swallow, as contraction of the pharyngeal and palatine muscles closes the three openings from the pharynx into the mouth, nasopharynx, and larynx, the cricopharyngeus and thyropharyngeus muscles relax to open the orifice into the esophagus. These muscles remain contracted at all other times, maintaining closure of the pharyngoesophageal sphincter. When this sphincter is functioning normally, the thyropharyngeus and cricopharyngeus muscles relax in anticipation of the bolus of food, and remain relaxed long enough to allow the entire bolus to enter the esophagus. The sphincter closes promptly after passage of the bolus. The interval the sphincter remains relaxed is determined by a central neural mechanism that senses the volume of the bolus propelled from the pharynx. During closure the sphincter shows phasic rather than tonic activity.[15] This generates a pressure in the sphincter higher than that on either side of the pharynx or esophagus. The high-pressure zone helps protect against esophagopharyngeal reflux and aspiration of intraesophageal contents. The pressure is highest during inspiration and predeglutition.[16]

Conditions in the esophagus affect pressure within the pharyngoesophageal sphincter.[17,18] The pressure increases when the cervical esophagus is distended by liquid or its mucosal surface is bathed by acid solution. The increase in PES pressure following gastric reflux protects against regurgitation and tracheobronchial aspiration of fluid. In contrast to fluid, air in the esophagus causes PES pressure to fall, permitting eructation of gas.[19]

Esophageal Phase of Swallowing[12,13,20]

The peristaltic wave generated in the pharynx is propagated through the esophagus and carries the bolus aborally to the GES (primary peristalsis). If the primary peristaltic wave fades before the bolus of food reaches the stomach, a secondary peristaltic wave is rapidly generated by local esophageal distension to complete the passage of the bolus to the stomach. In contrast to primary peristalsis, secondary peristalsis begins in the esophagus cranial to the bolus. It is otherwise indistinguishable from primary peristalsis by manometric evaluations.[31]

The esophagus is a flaccid tube at rest, offering little resistance to the passage of most substances. Hence, even a relatively weak peristaltic wave can readily and rapidly propel a bolus of liquid throughout the length of the esophagus. A bolus of food encounters more resistance to passage, and therefore needs a more sustained wave of peristalsis. Esophageal speed of peristalsis in the dog is 80 to 100 cm/second during water-induced swallows.[21] In the cat the transit rate of a bolus of food is slower than in the dog because smooth muscle contracts more slowly than striated muscle. The speed of esophageal contractions is 1 to 2 cm/second in sedated cats during liquid-stimulated swallows.[22] The rate in both species is slower in the caudal esophagus.

Control of the Esophageal Phase of Swallowing

The esophageal phase of swallowing is composed of a precisely coordinated series of sequential contractions mediated by a long and vulnerable reflex arc that consists of sensory receptors in the esophagus, visceral afferent fibers in the vagus and glossopharyngeal nerves, the nucleus solitarius in the brain stem, upper motor neurons in the swallowing center (located in the medial part of the lateral reticular formation[23]), efferent vagal parasympathetic neurons from the dorsal vagal motor nucleus, efferent vagal somatic neurons from the nucleus ambiguus, and the muscle of the esophagus. There are connections between the swallowing and respiratory centers because respiration must be inhibited during deglutition. The control of all phases of swallowing is shown in Figure 10–5, and reflex control of the esophageal phase is shown in Figure 10–6. Recent evidence has suggested that nitric oxide is important in the organization of esophageal peristalsis. Specifically, studies in opossums have shown that inhibitors of nitric oxide production eliminate the latency gradient along the esophageal body necessary for peristaltic contraction.[24]

Unlike most other parts of the gastrointestinal tract, coordinated motor function of the esophagus in dogs and cats depends on extrinsic nervous innervation. If the vagi are sectioned in the cervical region, the distal part of the esophagus dilates, retains food, and has feeble simultaneous repetitive contractions during swallowing.[25] Cutting the vagi in the hilar region or cutting some of the multiple vagal esophageal branches results in similar dysfunction distal to the level of section. Thus, interruption of the efferent fibers paralyzes the esophagus. Denervation also produces the histologic changes of striated muscle atrophy that occur whenever this type of tissue loses its nerve supply.[26] Paralysis of the esophagus occurs also when the nucleus ambiguus is bilaterally destroyed in the dog, although not when the dorsal motor nucleus of the vagus is destroyed.[27] In contrast, cats that have the dorsal motor nucleus destroyed lose coordinated motor activity in the esophagus.[27] This difference is due to the differing proportions of striated and smooth muscle in the dog and cat esophagus.

The swallowing reflex in dogs must have sensory reinforcement from an esophageal bolus; otherwise the peristaltic wave initiated at the pharynx will not progress to the stomach. Thus, if a fistula is created in the lower cervical area of the esophagus to divert a swallowed bolus to the outside, peristalsis will be observed in the esophagus down to the fistula, but none will be evident in the distal part.[28] Interference with sensory reinforcement of the swallowing reflex might underlay the observation that esophagitis in dogs and cats results in severely disordered motor activity.[29,30] The size of the bolus also influences the vigor of the peristaltic wave. Large boluses of food usually pass uninterruptedly down a normal esophagus, whereas peristaltic waves will sometimes be incomplete when a dog or cat swallows a liquid.

Function of the Gastroesophageal Sphincter and Junction[12,21,32,33]

The gastroesophageal sphincter (GES) is important in ensuring unidirectional flow between the esophagus and stomach (Figure 10–7). The GES maintains a high-pressure zone between the esophagus and stomach. The GES relaxes and opens during swallowing. Fibers in the vagus reflexly mediate relaxation, which can be detected up to 5 seconds before a bolus reaches the sphincter. The relaxed sphincter opens when the bolus arrives. After the bolus passes, the sphincter contracts and prevents reflux of gastric contents into the esophagus. The sphincter is not the only mechanism that prevents gastroesophageal reflux. For example, if the sphincter is replaced experimentally by a narrow stomach

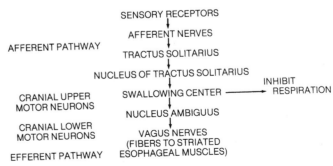

FIGURE 10–6. Neural pathway for the esophageal phase of swallowing in the dog. Sensory receptors are primarily in the pharynx. Motor fibers to esophageal muscles are somatic nerves in the vagus. Cats differ in that the caudal esophagus is made up of smooth fibers supplied by parasympathetic fibers in the vagus which have their origin in the dorsal motor nuclei of the vagus.

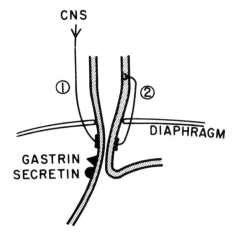

FIGURE 10-7. Diagram of gastroesophageal sphincter. Pressure in the sphincter is higher than in the esophagus at both the cranial and caudal ends. Pressure is maintained by vagal activity. During deglutition, vagal activity causes an immediate drop in pressure, via (1). When the bolus arrives at the end of the esophagus, a neural reflex causes the sphincter to open (2). The sphincter also responds to gut hormones via receptors for gastrin and secretin families.

tube, a high-pressure zone persists between the esophagus and stomach, preventing gastroesophageal reflux.[34]

The short segment of esophagus within the abdominal cavity is important in preventing gastroesophageal reflux. This segment acts as a flutter valve. When abdominal pressure increases, there is a potential for reflux caused by increasing pressure within the stomach. However, the increase in abdominal pressure is transmitted equally to the intra-abdominal segment of the esophagus, causing the segment to close, and preventing reflux. The pressure is normally greater in the lumen of the gastroesophageal sphincter than in the esophagus or stomach. When equal increments of pressure are added to both the sphincter (which is primarily in the abdominal cavity) and the stomach, the final pressure is still greater in the sphincter than in the stomach, and reflux does not occur. Increases in intra-abdominal pressure in cats result in comparable increases in both intragastric and GES pressures, so GES pressure continues to exceed intragastric pressure.[35] If the intra-abdominal segment of esophagus, including the sphincter, moves into the thorax as a result of a hiatal hernia, the flutter valve function is lost, and an increase in intra-abdominal pressure results in gastroesophageal reflux.

The angle at which the esophagus enters the stomach affects the ease with which gastric contents can reflux into the esophagus. The esophagus enters the empty stomach at an almost perpendicular angle. When the stomach is distended, however, the angle becomes very acute. Gastric distention results in compression of the esophagus by the fundus. This creates a valve whereby intragastric pressure maintains closure of the gastroesophageal junction (Figure 10–8). The oblique gastric muscle fibers at the junction contribute to the valve's competence (Figure 10–4). Contraction of these fibers accentuates the acuteness of the angle. However, removal of these "sling" fibers does not result in gastroesophageal reflux.

The diaphragm contributes to the competence of the gastroesophageal valve by helping maintain the oblique entry of the esophagus into the stomach and by contracting the crura of the diaphragm. Cutting the crural fibers results in the development of reflux esophagitis in dogs.

Mucosal folds in the cardia and the phrenoesophageal membrane are also thought to contribute to maintaining closure of the gastroesophageal valve (Figure 10–4). Many of the anatomic features of the gastroesophageal junction are important for normal function of the gastroesophageal sphincter, although the sphincter itself is controlled by the nervous system and, possibly, by peptide hormones.

Neurologic Regulation of Gastroesophageal Sphincter Function[21,32,36,37]

As described earlier, the dog's gastroesophageal sphincter consists of an outer layer of striated muscle and an inner layer of smooth muscle. The cat's gastroesophageal sphincter is composed entirely of smooth muscle. Striated muscle fibers are responsible for rapid closure of the sphincter; smooth muscle fibers maintain tonic closure. The sphincter opens and closes in response to neural activity associated with swallowing but can also function independently of swallowing.

Normal GES pressure in dogs is maintained at approximately 50 mm Hg by at least two excitatory neural influences. One is a vagal cholinergic mechanism that is blocked by vagotomy or by cooling of the vagus nerves, in which case GES pressure falls to approximately 28 mm Hg. Vagotomy does not completely paralyze the smooth muscle of the GES because it contains intrinsic nervous elements that impart some function, as well as autonomous smooth muscle tone. The second excitatory neural influence on GES function is a nonvagal mechanism mediated by both alpha-adrenergic and cholinergic (blocked by atropine) receptors. Both of the neural mechanisms contain a nicotinic ganglionic pathway. Atropine reduces GES pressure to approximately 13 mm Hg. This reduction is greater than that caused by vagotomy alone, and supports the belief there is a nonvagal as well as a vagal cholinergic control of GES pressure. Vagotomy also impairs relaxation and contraction of the GES associated with swallowing. As mentioned earlier, the GES normally relaxes at the onset of swallowing, a reflex mediated by vagal nerve fibers. Blockers of cholinergic or adrenergic activity have no effect on this vagally mediated sphincter relaxation, an observation that suggests a different neurotransmitter is involved. Vasoactive intestinal polypeptide (VIP) is a likely mediator of GES relaxation.[52,53] Sphincter muscle and its neural plexuses are

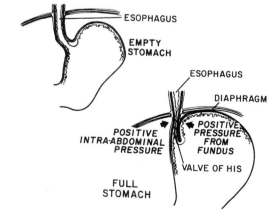

FIGURE 10-8. Schematic to show how filling of the stomach closes the gastroesophageal junction to form the valve of His.

associated with VIP-immunoreactive cells. Recent evidence has also implicated derivatives of nitric oxide.[24]

Other factors also regulate GES function, but these factors are much less effective than the control exerted by the extrinsic nervous system. The intrinsic properties of circular muscle from the sphincter have been studied in muscle-strip preparations. When graded tension is applied to these strips, resistance to stretch increases. The strips show a decrease in tension when they are stimulated electrically. Because the response is blocked by tetrodotoxin, it is thought to be mediated by the intrinsic nervous system of the GES. The intrinsic neural mechanisms in the smooth muscle can produce GES inhibition and contraction, and the myogenic mechanisms contribute to resting tone and may participate in GES relaxation and contraction. Although many peptide hormones and biogenic amines affect GES pressure, the extrinsic and intrinsic neural mechanisms are primarily responsible for basal GES tone.

Moderately increased intragastric pressure, whether produced by food, water, or abdominal compression, causes GES pressure to increase and remain above intragastric pressure.[38] This reflex protects against gastroesophageal reflux when intra-abdominal and intragastric pressure is raised, and may be partly vagally medicated. Another part of the response is produced by the flutter valve action of the GES, discussed earlier. In contrast, marked increases in intragastric pressure result in GES relaxation. Stimulation of intramural gastric nerves causes the GES relaxation, presumably permitting venting of gastric contents to prevent stomach rupture.[39]

The GES is still able to open and close (although not in a coordinated fashion with esophageal peristalsis) when all connections with the central nervous system are removed. The function is lost, however, when a circular cuff of muscle is removed from the esophagus just cranial to the sphincter, indicating the caudal esophagus exerts some control over GES function. Similarly, this esophageal-dependent control of sphincter function is lost when the caudal part of the esophagus is diseased. Esophagitis produced in experimental animals causes GES pressure to fall.[51] The inflammation disrupts the reception of sensory information that maintains GES closure.[40] Distention of the caudal esophagus stimulates GES relaxation by a reflex mediated through the vagus.[41]

Feeding and GES Function

The GES pressure of approximately 50 mm Hg varies little from day to day in an unfed individual. Feeding increases the pressure by increments up to 20 mm Hg. This postprandial response seems appropriate for preventing gastroesophageal reflux during times of maximum secretion of pepsin and hydrochloric acid, both of which can cause esophagitis. Part of the increased postprandial GES pressure is presumably mediated neurologically by the gastric pressure–dependent mechanisms just described. However, GES pressure is also influenced by hormones released in the postprandial and fasting states.

The GES has receptors for gastrin, histamine, and acetylcholine.[42] Whereas the cholinergic mechanisms are primarily responsible for maintaining GES pressure in the unfed state, an interaction of events at gastrin, histamine, and cholinergic receptors is largely responsible for the increase in GES pressure after feeding.[43] Histamine mediates its effect at H_1-receptors rather than H_2-receptors because diphenhydramine but not cimetidine prevents the postprandial increment in GES pressure. In addition to gastrin, other peptide hormones released during feeding have been shown to increase GES

pressure (Table 10–1). They include pancreatic polypeptide, motilin, and substance P.[44–46] Motilin is released during the unfed state and stimulates the interdigestive or migrating myoelectric complex that begins in the GES and increases GES pressure for short periods once every 1.5 to 2 hours.

A number of peptide hormones that reduce GES pressure are also released during the fed state. Despite the release of these inhibitory peptides the increment of approximately 20 mm Hg is maintained. Under normal conditions they are probably unimportant for regulating GES pressure. In many cases the inhibitory effects of these hormones reflect a GES response to infusion of pharmacologic amounts of hormone. Secretin is a competitive inhibitor of the action of gastrin on the gastroesophageal sphincter. Secretin also inhibits the release of gastrin. Some experiments have shown that alkalinization of the stomach can increase sphincter pressure by reciprocal changes in secretion of the two hormones gastrin and secretin. Glucagon has an inhibitory effect similar to that of secretin. Cholecystokinin has variable effects on sphincter tone.[24] Thus, gastroesophageal pressure is regulated by a number of gastrointestinal tract hormones that compete for receptor sites. That finding is consistent with the hypothesis that any organ which can be shown to respond to one gastrointestinal hormone will respond to all of them.[47]

The GES pressure after feeding is influenced by the type of food consumed. Protein meals increase GES pressure, presumably because protein is a potent stimulus for gastrin release. High-fat diets decrease GES pressure due to the lipid's effect of stimulating cholecystokinin's (and possibly other hormone's) release. Fat inhibits the gastrin-mediated increase in GES pressure. Other foods occasionally fed small animals can decrease GES pressure (Table 10–2). Food selection is important to successful management of animals with reduced GES pressure and reflux esophagitis.

Eructation and GES Function

Eructation of gas stimulates GES relaxation and opening via a vagal pathway that is not blocked by anticholinergic drugs.[54,55] The mechanism is probably the same as that described earlier for GES opening during swallowing, namely a nonadrenergic, noncholinergic efferent neural pathway to release VIP. Relaxation of the cranial diaphragm, an event also seen with swallowing, accompanies the GES changes.[56,57] The sensory receptors for initiating eructation are not located in the gastric fundus or in the gastric antrum.[58,59] Distention of the cardia by gas and not fluid is necessary for eructation; preventing such distention inhibits eructation.[60,61] As would be expected, changes in body position to maximize the opportunity for gas to accumulate in the cardia results in

Table 10–1

HORMONES AND CHEMICALS WITH EFFECTS ON GES PRESSURE

EXCITATORY	INHIBITORY
Gastrin	Cholecystokinin
Substance P	Secretin
Motilin	VIP
Histamine	Somatostatin
Met-enkephalin	Glucagon
Bombesin	Prostaglandins
Serotonin	Histamine
Cholinergics	Anticholinergics
Alpha-adrenergics	Beta-adrenergics
	Estrogens, progesterone

Table 10-2

FOODS AFFECTING GES PRESSURE

INCREASE	DECREASE
Proteins	Fats
	Chocolate
	Citrus juices
	Tomato juice
	Spices (?)

more frequent eructation.[62] During eructation the reflex changes also include relaxation and opening of the pharyngoesophageal sphincter.[63]

The GES relaxes transiently to permit eructation of gas at a frequency that is greater following a meal. Relaxations to vent gas from the stomach allow liquid contents to reflux into the esophagus. In normal dogs, over a 3 hour period there can be as many as 40 episodes of gastroesophageal reflux of acid.[64] The majority (77%) of refluxes are not associated with GES relaxation stimulated by swallowing. The acid reflux episodes are correlated with gas eructation. In another study in dogs, when the gastric gas cap was dorsal to the esophagus at the onset of eructation, some ingesta invariably accompanied gas into the esophagus.[56] Ninety percent of the eructations were followed by a relatively slow (17 cm/second) peristaltic wave that returned the refluxed material to the stomach. Similar patterns, but less frequent, of reflux are recorded in unfed dogs. The total time the esophagus is acidified is up to 3%; the time is determined by how rapidly and efficiently esophageal peristalsis clears the acid from the esophagus. The time of esophageal acidification is greater in the third hour than the first two hours after feeding. Thus, to a certain extent gastroesophageal reflux is a normal event.

Influence of Drugs on GES Function

Drugs have an important effect on the gastroesophageal sphincter. Pre- and postoperative drugs including acepromazine, atropine, xylazine, and diazepam lower GES pressure in dogs.[48,49] Metoclopramide, meperidine, cisapride, and bethanechol increase GES pressure in dogs.[43,49] The circular muscle of the sphincter is normally more sensitive to acetylcholine and norepinephrine than is other smooth muscle.[50] Catecholamines (epinephrine or norepinephrine) sometimes increase GES pressure and induce phasic contractions in the dog, but sometimes GES pressure is reduced.[43] Blocking these effects with either alpha-adrenergic or beta-adrenergic antagonists shows that stimulation or alpha-adrenergic receptors increases GES pressure and stimulation of beta-adrenergic receptors reduces GES pressure. Adrenergic neurons may contribute to the maintenance of GES pressure in cats.[11] Other chemicals such as serotonin increase GES pressure in dogs, and some such as domperidone cause strong and markedly phasic contractions.[43]

Age-Related Changes in Swallowing

Maturation of swallowing function does not occur for several months following birth.[12] Studies show the sensory systems for swallowing are well developed in the fetus, but the maturation of the control of swallowing continues after birth.

For example, stimulation of the superior laryngeal nerve in kittens up to a week old does not evoke the pharyngeal phase of swallowing consistently. Stimulation of the same nerve in puppies does not elicit a complete glottis closure; in fact, closure of the glottis is incomplete during swallowing in puppies up to 6 weeks old. Other studies show GES pressure to increase gradually in kittens so that by 6 weeks the pressure is one-half that of adults.[65] Similar maturation delays are found in pups.[19] It is evident that age-determined delays in maturation of swallowing must be considered when evaluating young pups and kittens for apparent swallowing abnormalities.

REFERENCES

1. Miller ME, Christensen GC, Evans HE. Anatomy of the Dog. WB Saunders, Philadelphia, 1964.
2. Nickel R, Schummer A, Seiferle E, et al. The Viscera of Domestic Mammals. Springer Verlag, New York, 1973.
3. Henk WG, Hoskins JD, Abdelbaki YZ. Comparative morphology of esophageal mucosa and submucosa in dogs from 1 to 337 days of age. Am J Vet Res 47:2658–2665, 1986.
4. Collman PI, Tremblay L, Diamant NE. The distribution of spinal and vagal sensory neurons that innervate the esophagus of the cat. Gastroenterology 103:817–822, 1992.
5. Lund WS. A study of the cricopharyngeal sphincter in man and in the dog. Ann R Coll Surg Eng 37:225–246, 1965.
6. Venker-van Haagen AJ, Hartman W, Wolvekamp WThC. Contributions of the glossopharyngeal nerve and the pharyngeal branch of the vagus nerve to the swallowing process in dogs. Am J Vet Res 47:1300–1307, 1986.
7. Suter PF. Watrous BJ. Oropharyngeal dysphagias in the dog I. Vet Radiol 21:24–39, 1980.
8. Evander A, Little AG, Riddle RH, et al. Composition of the refluxed material determines the degree of reflux esophagitis in the dog. Gastroenterology 93:280–286, 1987.
9. Clerc N. Histological characteristics of the lower esophageal sphincter in the cat. Acta Anat 117:201–208, 1983.
10. Watrous BJ, Suter PF. Normal swallowing in the dog: A cineradiographic study. Vet Radiol 20:99–109, 1979.
11. Behar J, Kersein M, Biancani P. Neural control of the lower esophageal sphincter in the cat: Studies on the excitatory pathways to the lower esophageal sphincter. Gastroenterology 82:680–688, 1982.
12. Miller AJ. Deglutition. Physiol Rev 62:129–184, 1982.
13. Doty RW. Neural organization of deglutition. In: Code CF (ed) Handbook of Physiology, Sec. 6; Alimentary Canal, Vol. 4. American Physiological Society, Washington, DC, 1861–1902, 1968.
14. Christensen J. Origin of sensation in the esophagus. Am J Physiol 246:G221–G225, 1984.
15. Levitt MN, Dedo HH, Ogura JH. The cricopharyngeus muscle, an electromyographic study in the dog. Laryngoscope 75:122–136, 1965.
16. Palmer ED. Disorders of the cricopharyngeus muscle: A review. Gastroenterology 71:510–519, 1976.
17. Freiman JM, Diamant NE. Upper esophageal sphincter (UES) response to esophageal distension and acid, and its alteration with nerve blockade. Gastroenterology 70:970, 1976.
18. Frieman JM, El-Sharkawy TY, Diamant NE. Effect of bilateral vagosympathetic nerve blockade on response of the dog upper esophageal sphincter (UES) to intraesophageal distention and acid. Gastroenterology 81:78–84, 1981.
19. Strombeck DR. Unpublished observations.
20. Code CF, Schlegel JF. Motor action of the esophagus and its sphincters. In: Code CF (ed) Handbook of Physiology, Sec. 6, Alimentary Canal, Vol. 4. American Physiological Society, Washington, DC, 1821–1839, 1968.
21. Gaynor F, Hoffner RE, Nichols MF, et al. Physiologic features of the canine esophagus: Effects of tranquilization on esophageal motility. Am J Vet Res 41:727–732, 1980.
22. Correnti FS, Little AG, Calleja IJ, et al. Manometric evaluation of the feline esophagus. J Surg Res 41:312–318, 1986.
23. Nakayama S, Neya T, Watanabe K, et al. Effects of electrical stimulation and local destruction of the medulla oblongata on swallowing movements in dogs. Rendic Gastroenterol 6:6–11, 1974.
24. Tobin RW, Pope CE. Esophageal motility. Curr Op G 9:622–628, 1993.
25. Carveth SW, Schlegel JF, Code CF, et al. Esophageal motility after vagotomy, phrenicotomy, myotomy, and myomectomy in dogs. Surg Gynecol Obstet 114:31–42, 1962.
26. Lynch VP, Schlegel JF, Ellis FH. Autotransplantation of the canine esophagus. Surg Gynecol Obstet 138:396–400, 1974.
27. Higgs B, Kerr FWF, Ellis FH. The experimental production of esophageal

achalasia by electrolytic lesions in the medulla. J Thor Cardio Surg 50:613–625, 1965.

28. Janssens J, Valembois P, Vantrappen G, et al. Is the primary peristaltic contractions of the canine esophagus bolus dependent? Gastroenterology 65:750–756, 1973.

29. Henderson RD, Mugashe F, Jeejeebhoy KN, et al. The role of bile and acid in the production of esophagitis and the motor defect of esophagitis. Ann Thorac Surg 14:465–473, 1972.

30. Liebermann-Meffert D, Klaus D, Vosmeer S, et al. Effect of intraesophageal bile and acid (HCL) perfusion on the action of the lower esophageal sphincter. Scand J Gastroenterol 19(suppl 92):237–241, 1984.

31. Janssens J, Valembois P, Hellemans J, et al. Studies on the necessity of a bolus for the progression of secondary peristalsis in the canine esophagus. Gastroenterology 67:245–251, 1974.

32. Arimori M, Code CF, Schlegel JF, et al. Electrical activity of the canine esophagus and gastroesophageal sphincter. Amer J Dig Dis 15:191–208, 1970.

33. Botha GSM. The Gastro—Oesophageal Junction: Clinical Applications to Oesophageal and Gastric Surgery. Little, Brown, Boston, 1962.

34. Moossa AR, Hall AW, Wood RAB, et al. Effect of pentagastrin (PG) infusions on gastroesophageal manometry and reflux status, before and after esophagogastrectomy. Abstract 80, Meeting Society for Surgery of the Alimentary Tract, Miami, 1976.

35. Boyle JT, Altschuler SM, Nixon TE, et al. Responses of feline gastroesophageal junction to changes in abdominal pressure. Am J Physiol 253:G315–G322, 1987.

36. Goyal RK, Rattan S. Neurohumoral, hormonal, and drug receptors for the lower esophageal sphincter. Gastroenterology 74:598–619, 1978.

37. Pope CE. Pathophysiology and diagnosis of reflux esophagitis. Gastroenterology 70:445–454, 1976.

38. Boyle JT, Altschuler Nixon TE, et al. Responses of feline gastroesophageal junction to changes in abdominal pressure. Am J Physiol 253:G315–G322, 1987.

39. Schulze-Delrieu K. Intrinsic reflexes between the esophagus and stomach. Gastroenterology 91:1568–1569, 1986.

40. Biancani P, Barwick K, Selling J, et al. Effects of acute experimental esophagitis on mechanical properties of the lower esophageal sphincter. Gastroenterology 87:8–16, 1984.

41. Price LM, El-Sharkawy TY, Mui HY, et al. Effect of bilateral cervical vagotomy on balloon-induced lower esophageal sphincter relaxation in the dog. Gastroenterology 77:324–329, 1979.

42. Zwick R, Bowes KL, Daniel EE, et al. Mechanism of action of pentagastrin on the lower esophageal sphincter. J Clin Invest 57:1644–1651, 1976.

43. Strombeck DR, Harrold D. Effect of gastrin, histamine, serotonin, and adrenergic amines on gastroesophageal sphincter pressure in the dog. Am J Vet Res 46:1684–1690, 1985.

44. Coltharp W, Maher JW, Maher MS, et al. The effect of truncal vagotomy on the response of the canine lower esophageal sphincter to varying doses of pancreatic polypeptide. Surgery 103:620–623, 1988.

45. Meissner AJ, Bowes KL, Zwick R, et al. Effect of motilin on the lower oesophageal sphincter. Gut 17:925–932, 1976.

46. Reynolds JC, Ouyang A, Cohen S. A lower esophageal sphincter reflex involving substance P. Am J Physiol 246:G346–G354, 1984.

47. Grossman ME. Gastrin and its activities. Nature (London) 228:1147–1150, 1970.

48. Strombeck DR, Harrold D. Effects of atropine, acepromazine, meperidine, and xylazine on gastroesophageal sphincter pressure in the dog. Am J Vet Res 46:963–965, 1985.

49. Hall JA, Magne ML, Twedt DC. Effect of acepromazine, diazepam, fentamyl-droperidol, and oxymorphone on gastroesophageal sphincter pressure in healthy dogs. Am J Vet Res 48:556–557, 1987.

50. Misiewicz JJ. Symposium on gastroesophageal reflux and its complications. Sec. 4, Pharmacology and therapeutics. Gut 14:243–246, 1973.

51. Eastwood GL, Castell DO, Higgs RH. Experimental esophagitis in cats impairs lower esophageal sphincter pressure. Gastroenterology 69:146–153, 1975.

52. Behar J, Field S, Marin C. Effect of glucagon, secretin, and vasoactive intestinal polypeptide on the feline lower esophageal sphincter: Mechanisms of action. Gastroenterology 77:1001–1007, 1979.

53. Biancani P, Walsh JH, Behar J. Vasoactive intestinal polypeptide. A neurotransmitter for lower esophageal sphincter relaxation. J Clin Invest 73:963–967, 1984.

54. Martin CJ, Patrikios J, Dent J. Abolition of gas reflux and transient lower esophageal sphincter relaxation by vagal blockade in the dog. Gastroenterology 91:890–896, 1986.

55. Strombeck DR, Harrold D, Ferrier W. Eructation of gas through the gastroesophageal sphincter before and after truncal vagotomy in dogs. Am J Vet Res 48:207–210, 1987.

56. Heywood LH, Wood AKW. A radiographic and electromyographic study of eructation in the dog. Gastroenterology Abstracts 192, 1988.

57. Altschuler SM, Boyle JT, Nixon TE, et al. Simultaneous reflex inhibition of lower esophageal sphincter and crural diaphragm in cats. Am J Physiol 249:G586–G591, 1985.

58. Strombeck DR, Turner WD, Harrold D. Eructation of gas through the gastroesophageal sphincter before and after gastric fundectomy in dogs. Am J Vet Res 49:87–89, 1988.

59. Franzi SJ, Martin CJ, Dent J, et al. Localization of the gastric trigger zone that induces transient lower esophageal sphincter relaxation in the dog. Gastroenterology 95:865, 1988.

60. Menguy R. A modified fundoplication which preserves the ability to belch. Surgery 84:301–307, 1978.

61. Strombeck DR, Griffin DW, Harrold D. Eructation of gas through the gastroesophageal sphincter before and after limiting distension of the gastric cardia or infusion of a β-adrenergic amine in dogs. Am J Vet Res 50:751–753, 1989.

62. Little AF, Martin CJ, Dent J, et al. Postural suppression of transient lower esophageal relaxations and gastroesophageal reflux in the dog. Gastroenterology reflux in the dog. Gastroenterology 90:1522, 1986.

63. Kahrilas PJ, Dodds WJ, Dent J, et al. Upper esophageal sphincter function during belching. Gastroenterology 91:133–140, 1986.

64. Patrikos J, Martin CJ, Dent J. Relationship of transient lower esophageal sphincter relaxation to postprandial gastroesophageal reflux and belching in dogs. Gastroenterology 90:545–551, 1986.

65. Hillemeier C, Gryboski J, McCallum R, et al. Developmental characteristics of the lower esophageal sphincter in the kitten. Gastroenterology 89:760–766, 1985.

11 Diseases of Swallowing

W. GRANT GUILFORD AND DONALD R. STROMBECK

CLINICAL SIGNS OF SWALLOWING DISORDERS

Swallowing disorders usually result in regurgitation and difficulty in swallowing food and/or water (dysphagia). Repeated or exaggerated swallowing movements accompanied by extension, flexion, or twisting of the head and neck may be observed. The physical condition of animals with dysphagia varies from normal to emaciated, depending on the severity of the disease process. Other clinical signs of swallowing dysfunction include painful swallowing (odynophagia), drooling (ptyalism and pseudoptyalism), halitosis, nasal discharge, cough, and dyspnea. Halitosis is usually due to retention of food in the esophagus but occasionally results from the presence of a necrotizing lesion in the esophagus or pharynx. The nasal discharge can be due to regurgitation of ingesta into the nasopharynx or to inhalation pneumonia, a frequent complication of dysphagia. Pneumonia typically causes a soft moist cough. Paroxysms of harsh coughing associated with eating or drinking should raise the possibility of a bronchoesophageal fistula. Dyspnea associated with regurgitation usually results from inhalation pneumonia, reduced pulmonary compliance due to dilation of the thoracic esophagus, and perhaps from acute bronchospasm secondary to inhalation of small quantities of food or gastric secretions. Polyphagia or anorexia and weight loss may accompany dysphagia. Anorexia is common with esophagitis, esophageal foreign bodies, and esophageal neoplasia, whereas a voracious appetite is customary in young dogs with idiopathic megaesophagus. In contrast to vomiting, regurgitated food is frequently *immediately* reconsumed. Rarely, dysphagia can be associated with cervical cellulitis or a draining fistulous tract secondary to esophageal perforation.

The clinical signs present in a particular animal are determined by chronicity and degree of pharyngeal, esophageal, or respiratory involvement. Signs vary widely in severity in different patients, and at times the diagnosis is elusive because respiratory signs predominate or the clinician mistakenly identifies regurgitation as vomiting. The differentiation of regurgitation and vomiting is discussed in detail in Chapter 5. It is as well to reiterate, however, that regurgitation is characterized by the passive reflux of undigested food. Abdominal heaving is not required, and the regurgitated food is usually bile free and may be passed in a tubular shape. Not uncommonly, animals with dysphagia regurgitate foam and saliva instead of food. The regurgitation of these fluids is often associated with the loud, harsh sounds of expectoration as the animal attempts to clear regurgitated material from the laryngopharynx. It is important to note that regurgitation and vomiting cannot be differentiated by the time of occurrence after eating. Similarly, refluxed material with an alkaline pH may have been vomited or regurgitated (see Chapter 5).

DIAGNOSIS OF SWALLOWING DISORDERS

The differentiation of swallowing disorders begins with subtle differences in history and physical examination. Definitive diagnosis depends on various diagnostic procedures including radiographic techniques (e.g., contrast studies and fluoroscopy), endoscopy, biopsy, and occasionally manometry, electromyography, and exploratory surgery.

History

The age of onset of the dysphagia and the patient's breed should be determined. Congenital problems are usually due to idiopathic megaesophagus or vascular ring anomalies, but occasionally foreign bodies or cricopharyngeal achalasia will be diagnosed. If the animal shows signs of dysphagia in adulthood, the likelihood of a recent anesthesia or exposure to caustic chemicals, foreign bodies, or toxic agents should be evaluated. Reports of concurrent muscle weakness or neurologic disorders should alert the clinician to an extraesophageal disease process that may underlie the esophageal disease. Acute onset of signs in either a young or older animal is consistent with the presence of a foreign body. Chronic or slowly worsening regurgitation is more suggestive of gastroesophageal reflux or a developing esophageal stricture. Knowledge of the patient's breed can be helpful because breed predispositions to megaesophagus have been recognized (see later).

Information regarding the animal's ability to retain liquids, soft food, or solid food should be sought. Animals with physical obstructions of the esophagus can often tolerate liquids but not solids whereas animals with motility abnormalities of the esophagus will usually have difficulty swallowing liquids in addition to some types of solid foods. Recording the type of food causing the most clinical evidence of dysphagia is also important should a barium swallow be deemed necessary for diagnosis. Barium swallows should be performed not only with barium suspension but also with barium-coated food. The food used in the swallowing study should be the food the patient has the most difficulty swallowing. If this simple precaution is not taken, many cases of swallowing dysfunction will not be detected by barium swallows.

It is essential to obtain an accurate description of the dysphagia.[1] If the client is unable to provide an adequate description, the veterinarian should observe the animal ingesting whatever food (or liquid) the animal has difficulty swallowing. Close observation will usually separate prehension difficulties from swallowing dysfunction. Animals with pharyngeal problems (including cricopharyngeal achalasia) usually regurgitate immediately whereas those with esophageal disease often have more delayed regurgitation. Evidence of pain during swallowing is consistent with esophagitis, neoplasia, or foreign bodies but is uncommon with motility abnormalities.

Physical Examination

Physical examination of patients with swallowing problems must include careful examination of the pharynx (using sedation or anesthesia if necessary). The pharynx and neck should be carefully palpated for masses, asymmetry, or pain. On occasion, a dilated cervical esophagus can be revealed by compressing the animal's chest while briefly occluding its nostrils. This forces air from the thoracic esophagus into the neck and can cause a ballooning of the cervical esophagus in affected animals. The chest should be auscultated carefully for evidence of inhalation pneumonia.

Radiology

Radiographic examination of the pharynx and esophagus is an essential procedure for both diagnosis and differential diagnosis of swallowing disorders. Cervical and thoracic survey films and static or dynamic contrast studies are used.[2]

Survey radiographs in lateral and ventrodorsal projections are taken of the pharyngeal to cranial abdominal regions to examine the pharynx and entire esophagus. A right ventrodorsal oblique projection that reduces superimposition of the esophagus on the thoracic vertebrae may also be of value. A high mAs-low kVp technique should be used to evaluate the cervical esophagus, whereas a high kVp-low mAs technique should be used to evaluate the thoracic soft tissue structures.

Contrast studies are usually performed with a liquid barium suspension and barium mixed with food. The suspension (approximately 30% w/v concentration) is useful for evaluating animals with a history of regurgitating liquids. It is carefully administered by syringe in small boluses as frequently as necessary to evaluate pharyngoesophageal function accurately. If a perforation of the esophagus is suspected, a water-soluble iodinated contrast material (e.g., Gastrografin, Schering) should be used. Such materials are less irritating to the periesophageal tissues but can cause acute pulmonary edema if they gain access to the lungs. If the water-soluble contrast agent does not identify a perforation, the study should be repeated with a large volume of liquid barium suspension because water-soluble agents occasionally fail to reveal

esophageal perforations.[3] Barium powder mixed with food is used in evaluating animals with a history of regurgitating food. As already discussed, the food used in the study should be determined by the history. A palatable food and a fasted patient help ensure a successful study.

If fluoroscopy is available, the passage of the barium contrast agents during swallowing can be observed. The study should include recording of three to six complete swallows of liquid barium suspension followed by a similar number of barium-coated food boluses.

Swallowing studies are best done without tranquilization. If sedation is necessary, low-dose acetylpromazine can be tried, and will have minimal influence on swallowing function. Unfortunately, more effective sedation protocols usually affect swallowing.

Radiographic Interpretation[2,4,5]

The pharynx of normal animals is evident on radiographs because it is air filled. The size of the air-filled space can be decreased by local inflammation or neoplasia, laryngeal edema, and elongation of the soft palate. Pharyngeal size may appear increased with dysfunction of the pharynx or pharyngoesophageal sphincter, chronic respiratory (inspiratory) disease, and chronic, severe megaesophagus. Pharyngeal disease can also alter contrast in the pharyngeal region and may displace the larynx.

The normal esophagus is not visible on survey radiographs. An exception occurs following aerophagia due to excitement, nausea, dyspnea, or anesthesia.[6] The presence of luminal air results in a radiolucency that allows visualization of part or all of the course of the esophagus and reveals some details of mucosal topography. Luminal air may also collect as a result of esophageal diseases, such as strictures or motility disturbances (megaesophagus). Several radiographic features aid differentiation between benign and pathologic accumulations of gas. Gas accumulations following aerophagia due to excitement or struggling are usually transient, and gas is often present in both the stomach and esophagus. Esophageal gas accumulation during anesthesia is usually generalized and uniform, and outlines an esophagus of normal diameter and smooth mucosal borders. In contrast, air accumulation in the diseased esophagus is usually persistent and may be irregular in shape due to esophageal masses or retained liquid or food.

Contrast media is not retained in the normal pharynx. Radiographs taken immediately after the administration of a barium suspension show at most a few streaks of contrast remaining in the pharynx. In normal animals, fluoroscopy demonstrates the formation of a bolus in the pharynx, pharyngeal constriction, and propulsion of the bolus through the pharyngoesophageal sphincter into the esophagus. Contrast materials are rapidly cleared from the normal esophagus by a series of brisk, aborally progressive peristaltic waves. Any persistent pooling of contrast material in the esophagus should be regarded as abnormal. Pooling of contrast material in the esophagus at the level of the heart base suggests esophageal obstruction due to a vascular ring abnormality. The degree of dilatation revealed by the contrast medium and the amount of motility noted on fluoroscopy provide important prognostic information. Once severe esophageal dilatation is present, function is unlikely to be regained. Absence of motility is associated with a poor but not hopeless prognosis. It is important to realize that a hypomotile esophagus has sometimes been demonstrated in excited, dyspneic, or nauseated dogs and in young dogs with no signs of regurgitation. It is also a feature of esophagitis.

Detection of an irregular esophageal mucosal border suggests an intramural lesion. In cats, however, the mucosa of the caudal third of the esophagus has a characteristic irregular radial ("herringbone") pattern that should not be misinterpreted as esophagitis. Other radiographic features suggestive of particular esophageal diseases are detailed along with the description of the disease.

Endoscopy, Esophageal Manometry, and Electromyography

Endoscopy (esophagoscopy) with either rigid or flexible fiberoptic instruments is an increasingly important tool in evaluating esophageal diseases. The technique is described in Chapter 7.

Esophageal manometry is a useful technique to evaluate esophageal pressure and motor function. It is currently being utilized extensively in human medicine and on research animals but has not been widely applied in clinical veterinary medicine at this time.

Electromyography is occasionally helpful in localizing the dysphagia and diagnosing the cause.

OROPHARYNGEAL AND PHARYNGOESOPHAGEAL SWALLOWING DISEASES[4,7–9]

Clinical Synopsis

Diagnostic Features

- Swallowing difficulty
- Immediate regurgitation
- Gagging and/or coughing
- Rabies status should be evaluated
- Pharyngeal exam and barium swallow with fluoroscopy confirm diagnosis
- Multitude of possible primary causes

Treatment

- Address primary cause if diagnosed
- Experiment with diet consistency
- Cricopharyngeal myotomy only if cricopharyngeal achalasia diagnosed definitively

Classification

Pharyngeal dysfunction may result from functional or structural disorders. Functional disorders are due to neuromuscular diseases (Table 11–1) and are often classified as oral, pharyngeal, cricopharyngeal (upper esophageal sphincter), and pharyngoesophageal dysphagia. This classification has limited value because many functional swallowing problems concurrently involve the pharynx, upper esophageal sphincter (UES), and cranial esophagus. This is not surprising because the swallowing center collectively integrates coordinated motility in the pharynx, UES, and cranial esophagus via a single generator.[10] Lesions must be very selective to dam-

Table 11–1

CAUSES OF OROPHARYNGEAL DYSPHAGIA*

DISORDER	CAUSES
Pharyngeal edema	Pharyngitis, trauma, insect stings, snake bites, allergy, chemical or heat injury
Trauma and foreign bodies	Bite wounds, gunshot wounds, hematoma fracture and dislocation of hyoid bones
Intraluminal masses	Elongated, inflamed soft palate; tonsillitis; cysts; sialoceles; neoplasms of epiglottis, tonsils, pharyngeal wall, or soft palate
Extraluminal masses	Retropharyngeal lymphadenopathy, retropharyngeal or pharyngeal wall abscesses, salivary gland enlargement, neoplasms, thyroid tumors, lymphosarcoma
Functional disorders	Neuropathies of cranial nerves V, VII, IX, X; hydrocephalus, brain stem lesions, rabies, cricopharyngeal achalasia, myasthenia gravis, botulism, CNS lesions, idiopathic multiple neuromuscular dysfunctions
Miscellaneous disorders	Glossal neoplasia, congenitally short or cleft palate, muscular dystrophy in Bouviers

*See also Table 5–11.

age only one part of the pharyngeal and upper esophageal phase of swallowing.

Structural abnormalities of the pharynx have a variety of causes including foreign bodies, neoplasia, retropharyngeal lymphadenopathy, tonsilitis, and pharyngeal swelling due to inflammation, edema, or trauma (Table 11–1).[11]

Clinical Signs and Diagnosis

Clinical signs of pharyngeal dysfunction include ptyalism, pseudoptyalism, retching, gagging, multiple exaggerated attempts to swallow, immediate regurgitation during attempts to eat, nasal reflux, coughing, and sometimes dyspnea. Animals with painful oropharyngeal lesions may be depressed and refuse to eat or drink. They often show odynophagia, and may be febrile (particularly when a penetrating foreign body is the cause). In contrast, animals with functional abnormalities of the pharynx are usually bright and alert, show no evidence of pain, and maintain a good appetite.

Diagnosis is made by the methods described earlier. Physical examination of the oropharyngeal and cranial cervical region occasionally reveal lesions but on most occasions no obvious problems will be identified. Survey radiographs may demonstrate fractured hyoid bones, foreign bodies such as bone fragments and needles, or distortion of the pharyngeal air space by masses. Retropharyngeal diseases may result in gas shadows, swelling, and loss of fascial lines in the retropharyngeal area. Fluoroscopy is necessary to differentiate the various types of functional pharyngeal disorders.

Oral Dysphagia

Oral dysphagia is an infrequent problem. The usual cause is loss of motility of the tongue. Affected animals may chew food abnormally and have difficulty drinking water and eating. Frequently they must bury their muzzle in water and food to force enough into the pharynx for swallowing. Tongue atrophy, due to hypoglossal nerve damage, may be evident. Paresis of the tongue interferes with the ability to propel water and food into the pharynx. A similar clinical picture is seen with some cases of idiopathic trigeminal neuropathy. In some dogs with trigeminal paralysis the jaw drop is sufficient to interfere with oral function but insufficient to be noticed by cursory clinical examination.

Diagnosis of oral dysphagia is usually made by observing affected animals attempting to eat or drink. Pharyngeal and UES dysfunction can be ruled out by manually placing food in the pharynx and observing whether it is swallowed. If necessary the same kind of evaluation can be made fluoroscopically. Once the site of the dysphagia has been confirmed, a search for underlying causes of damage to the tongue (such as neoplasia) or hypoglossal nerve (such as hydrocephalus or brain stem lesions) should be considered (Table 11–1). Unfortunately, on most occasions the cause of hypoglossal nerve dysfunction is not identified, and treatment remains symptomatic.

Symptomatic relief of oral dysphagia can usually be obtained by offering water in deep buckets and food as "meatballs." The buckets of water allow the affected animal to immerse its muzzle when drinking. Most animals soon learn to throw meatballs to the back of the pharynx by rapidly lifting their muzzle after prehension. If necessary, nutritional homeostasis can be maintained with a gastrostomy tube.

The prognosis for return to normal function is poor (with the exception of oral dysphagia due to idiopathic trigeminal nerve paralysis). Some animals can lead relatively normal lives, however, provided their nutrients are provided in the manner just described.

Pharyngeal Dysphagia

Pharyngeal dysphagia results from a loss of normal pharyngeal motility and/or a failure to propel pharyngeal contents through the UES. Inadequate closure of the glottis and nasopharyngeal and oropharyngeal orifices often accompanies the dysphagia. The clinical signs are those of pharyngeal dysphagia (described earlier) and include immediate regurgitation, repeated attempts to swallow, gagging, coughing, and nasal reflux. Some animals retain food in the pharynx for many hours after eating. Aspiration pneumonia is common (Figure 11–1). Anorexia and odynophagia are usually absent when the disorder is due to a motility abnormality. Occasionally, atrophy of the temporal and masseter muscles accompany the pharyngeal muscular dysfunction.

Many causes of pharyngeal dysphagia have been described (Table 11–1). Occasionally the cause is due to an anatomic obstruction by a mass or a foreign body. Rabies should always be considered a possible diagnosis. Bouviers have a high prevalence of dysphagia due to pharyngeal and/or esophageal muscle degeneration.[12] On most occasions, however, pharyngeal dysfunction is functional and attributed to an idiopathic neuromuscular dysfunction. The most likely site of the defect is the central nervous system (involving nuclei of the glossopharyngeal and vagus nerves) or the sensory input for the pharyngeal phase of swallowing. Sensory input primarily comes from areas of the caudal pharynx via the glossopharyngeal nerve.

Diagnosis of pharyngeal dysphagia is made by fluoroscopy. Fluoroscopy reveals slow and incomplete constriction of the pharyngeal cavity and failure of the UES to open with each

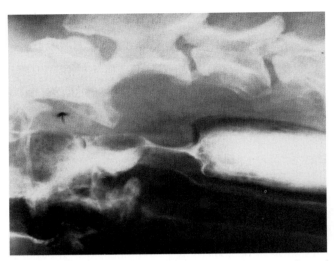

FIGURE 11–1. Lateral spot film made of pharyngoesophageal sphincter during a positive-contrast study made under fluoroscopic control. During each inspiration the contrast medium was aspirated into the larynx. Cough reflex was not evident; aspiration pneumonia was a problem.

swallow so that air and contrast persist throughout all swallowing attempts. Incomplete rostral and dorsal movement of the glottis and laryngeal aspiration of contrast medium are often seen. The laryngeal aspiration of fluid is not associated with the normally expected gagging and coughing.

Unless an underlying cause for the dysphagia can be identified, the prognosis is poor. Symptomatic relief can occasionally be achieved by varying the consistency of the food. A gastrostomy tube can be placed if necessary. Antibiotics are often required for concurrent inhalation pneumonia. Cricopharyngeal myotomy is contraindicated. Myotomy of the cricopharyngeus muscle in dogs with no obvious cricopharyngeal dysfunction invariably results in worsening of the condition and places the dog at greater risk for aspiration pneumonia.

Cricopharyngeal Dysphagia (Achalasia)

Cricopharyngeal dysphagia is characterized by a failure of the UES to relax (achalasia) or a lack of coordination between UES relaxation and pharyngeal contraction. Cocker spaniels and poodles may be predisposed. Affected dogs are bright and alert but show the clinical signs of pharyngeal dysfunction just described. Odynophagia is usually absent. The clinical signs most often appear at the time of, or shortly after, weaning. This has lead to the belief that the dysphagia is a congenital neuromuscular defect perhaps resulting from failure of part of the swallowing reflex to develop completely. Because most young dogs with cricopharyngeal dysphagia show concurrent pharyngeal dysphagia and motility deficits of the cranial part of the esophagus, a likely site for the swallowing dysfunction is the central nervous system. Alternatively, a lack of sensory input from the pharynx may be responsible.

Other suggested causes for cricopharyngeal dysphagia have included cricopharyngeal hypertrophy or myositis, leading to atrophy and fibrosis of the cricopharyngeus muscle. In young dogs, biopsy of the cricopharyngeus muscle usually does not show any of these pathologic changes, but these processes may

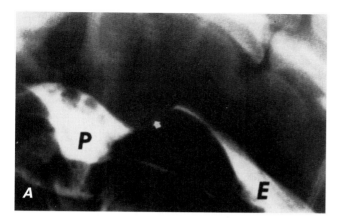

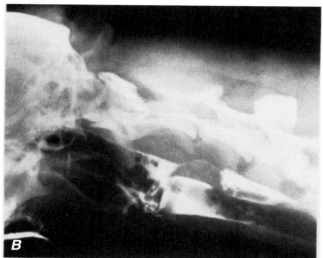

FIGURE 11-2. Dog with cricopharyngeal dysphagia. Lateral radiographs made when dog was swallowing a liquid positive-contrast medium. Radiograph *A* shows retention of contrast medium in the pharynx (P). Radiograph *B* shows same animal with aspiration of positive-contrast medium into upper airway. This illustrates that the normal integration of respiratory and swallowing was abnormal. Myotomy of the cricopharyngeus muscle resulted in a remission of all clinical signs, but follow-up cinefluoroscopic studies revealed a persistent motility problem in the pharynx and cranial part of the cervical esophagus. E = Esophagus.

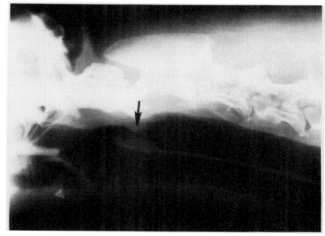

FIGURE 11-3. Lateral cervical radiograph shows dilated esophagus with open pharyngoesophageal sphincter (arrow).

trast in the cranial end of the cervical esophagus. Following repeated swallowing attempts, only small amounts of ingesta pass through the UES. In many cases swallowing liquids is almost as difficult as swallowing solid food.

Cricopharyngeal dysphagia is managed by myotomy of the cricopharyngeus muscle. The response to surgery is rapid and complete in at least 70% of affected dogs. Older dogs and those with a loss of coordination between pharyngeal and UES function are less likely to respond well to surgery.

Dysphagia with Multiple Functional Abnormalities

Most dogs with functional pharyngeal dysphagia have a complicated, mixed dysfunction with aspects of oral, pharyngeal, and cricopharyngeal dysphagias. The clinical signs and radiographic and fluoroscopic findings are a mix of those observed in the specific dysphagias described earlier. As the condition increases in severity, chalasia (failure of the UES to close) can occasionally be identified on survey radiographs of the cranial cervical region (Figure 11–3).

Management of dysphagia due to multiple pharyngeal dysfunctions is difficult, and the prognosis is generally poor. The consistency of the food should be altered to determine what is best tolerated. As noted earlier, nutritional homeostasis can be maintained with a gastrostomy tube if necessary. Unless cricopharyngeal achalasia is the principal component of the mixed dysfunction, cricopharyngeal myotomy is contraindicated.

Pharyngitis and Tonsillitis

Pharyngitis and pharyngeal edema from a variety of causes can interfere with swallowing. Causes of pharyngitis and pharyngeal edema include trauma, stings, snake bites, allergic reactions, chemical or heat injury, infections, and idiopathic disorders such as feline glossopharyngitis. Diagnosis is usually made by a combination of history and physical examination. Management is described in Chapter 9.

Tonsillitis and tonsillar neoplasia can produce dysphagia. Diagnosis is made by physical examination. Fine needle aspiration or brush cytology is occasionally necessary to differentiate tonsillitis from tonsillar neoplasia (see Chapter 9).

be responsible for the occasional reported case of adult-onset cricopharyngeal dysphagia. Other potential causes of adult-onset cricopharyngeal dysphagia include trauma, acquired neuromuscular disorders, and neoplasia. Rarely, cricopharyngeal dysphagia can also be a manifestation of generalized neuromuscular diseases such as polyneuropathies, polymyositis, muscular dystrophy, and myasthenia gravis.

Clinical signs do not differentiate pharyngeal dysphagia and cricopharyngeal dysphagia. Physical examination of the pharynx in dogs with cricopharyngeal achalasia is unremarkable. No unusual resistance or pressure is encountered at the UES on digital examination. Diagnosis of cricopharyngeal dysphagia is made by fluoroscopy. Intermittent or persistent failure of the UES to relax and dilate despite adequate bolus formation and adequate pharyngeal contractions is observed (Figure 11–2). Contrast is retained in the pharynx and in many cases spills into the oropharynx, nasopharynx, or larynx and trachea. Affected dogs often show retention of con-

Pharyngeal Foreign Bodies

Pharyngeal foreign bodies result in acute onset of dysphagia. Affected animals usually show pharyngeal discomfort. They may gag and retch or paw at their mouths. Ptyalism is common and at times profuse. Swallowing appears painful. Diagnosis is usually made by physical examination under anesthesia. Pharyngeal foreign bodies are described in more detail in Chapter 9.

Retropharyngeal Abscess

Penetration of the pharynx by foreign bodies or bites can lead to retropharyngeal abscesses. Clinical signs are malaise, anorexia, dysphagia, and odynophagia. Affected animals are sometimes unwilling to turn their neck. Physical examination may reveal fever and neck pain, but the abscess cannot usually be palpated. Occasionally a bite wound may be found. Diagnosis depends heavily on history. Inquiry should be made as to whether the animal is fed bones or chases sticks. Radiography may reveal evidence of a retropharyngeal mass effect. Ultrasound examination with fine needle aspiration may confirm the presence of an abscess. Shards of wood in the pharynx are usually not detected by radiographs, and exploratory surgery is necessary to confirm the diagnosis. Treatment is by surgical drainage and administration of broad-spectrum antibiotics.

Retropharyngeal Lymphadenopathy

The medial retropharyngeal lymph nodes are large glands (2–4 cm in length) situated on the dorsolateral surface of the pharynx. They drain the oral cavity, tonsils, pharynx, nasal cavity, larynx, esophagus, parotid, and mandibular lymph nodes, and the muscles of the head, hyoid apparatus, tongue, and cranial neck.

Retropharyngeal lymphadenopathy produces similar clinical signs to retropharyngeal abscess. Causes include pharyngitis, penetrating wounds of the pharynx, lymphosarcoma, and metastatic neoplasia from tumors situated anywhere in the head. Diagnosis is usually made by radiography, ultrasound, fine needle aspiration, and/or exploratory surgery.

MEGAESOPHAGUS[4,13–16]

Clinical Synopsis

Diagnostic Features

- Regurgitation
- Dilated esophagus observed by survey or contrast radiography
- Concurrent bronchopneumonia is common
- Multitude of possible primary causes

Treatment

- Address primary cause if diagnosed
- Treat secondary pneumonia if present
- Feed high-calorie diet from raised receptacle
- Experiment with diet consistency

Megaesophagus is a descriptive term for esophageal dilatation, a manifestation of a number of distinct diseases of varied causes. Congenital idiopathic megaesophagus refers to a dilatation of unknown cause that manifests at or shortly after weaning. Adult-onset idiopathic megaesophagus is a dilation with onset after maturity. Secondary or acquired megaesophagus describes all other forms of esophageal dilation where a cause can be identified.

Epidemiology

Esophageal dilation is the most important cause of regurgitation in the dog and cat. It is seen with reasonable frequency in referral institutions. Seventy-nine and 125 dogs with generalized megaesophagus were presented to the University of Pennsylvania Veterinary Hospital and the University of California at Davis Veterinary Teaching Hospital, respectively, over 8 year periods.[14,17] Over a period of 8 years, 53 cases of canine megaesophagus were presented to the University of Missouri Veterinary Teaching Hospital, representing approximately 1 case per 1000 of total visitations. The prevalence of esophageal dilatation in cats is lower than in dogs, but several reports have been published.[18–20,31] At the University of California VMTH, megaesophagus in cats is seen at a rate of less than 1 case per 1000 cats seen.

Congenital idiopathic megaesophagus is generally accepted as the most common form of megaesophagus in dogs (Table 11–2). In one recent survey of 50 cases, however, only 36% were congenital.[13] In a similar number of dogs with megaesophagus seen at the University of Missouri Veterinary Teaching Hospital, only one-third were less than one year of age at presentation. These numbers are likely to be biased because mature dogs with acquired megaesophagus are more likely to be referred to teaching hospitals than young pups with congenital idiopathic megaesophagus.

Idiopathic megaesophagus is known to be inherited in the wirehaired fox terrier[21,22] and miniature schnauzer.[23] The inheritance mode in wirehaired fox terriers is simple autosomal recessive,[21] whereas that in miniature schnauzers is compatible with a simple autosomal dominant or a 60% penetrance autosomal recessive pattern.[23] A breed predisposition

Table 11–2

AGE DISTRIBUTION OF DOGS WITH MEGAESOPHAGUS AT UNIVERSITIES OF PENNSYLVANIA AND CALIFORNIA REPORTED AS PERCENTAGE OF TOTAL CASES RECORDED

	10 WK	1 YR	2 YR	7 YR	15 YR
Pennsylvania	67%	13%	20%		
California	55%		10%	25%	10%

BREED PREVALENCE OF MEGAESOPHAGUS IN DOGS AT UNIVERSITIES OF PENNSYLVANIA AND CALIFORNIA REPORTED AS A MULTIPLE OF NORMAL PREVALENCE

	IRISH SETTER	GREAT DANE	GERMAN SHEPHERD
Pennsylvania	2	8	2
California	2	10	2

exists for the German shepherd, Great Dane, Irish setter, and Chinese sharpei (Table 11–2).[14,17,24,25] The high incidence of idiopathic megaesophagus in these breeds suggests a hereditary basis, as does the report of megaesophagus in litters of German shepherds,[26] Great Danes,[27] and sharpeis.[24] Numerous other breeds of dogs, both large and small, have been affected by the disease,[14,17,21,28] including a litter of Newfoundlands[29] and a litter of greyhounds.[30] Breeding of dogs affected by idiopathic congenital megaesophagus (or other close relatives) should be discouraged. No breed dispositions have been recognized for adult-onset idiopathic or acquired megaesophagus. There is some evidence, however, that idiopathic esophageal dilatation may also be inherited in the cat[31] and that Siamese-related breeds are predisposed.[32]

Etiopathogenesis of Congenital Idiopathic Megaesophagus

The etiopathogenesis of congenital idiopathic megaesophagus (CIM) remains unknown. Two suggested reasons for the development of the esophageal dilatation are paralysis of the muscle of the esophageal body, or abnormal opening of the gastroesophageal sphincter (GES) due to sphincter hypertonicity (achalasia).

The term *achalasia* was once widely used in dogs for what is now collectively called megaesophagus. Little evidence has been forthcoming, however, to suggest that failure of the GES to open is an important cause of CIM in dogs or cats (Figure 11–4).[14,33-38] Nevertheless, abnormal gastroesophageal sphincter function may complicate megaesophagus via damage to the esophageal segment immediately cranial to the GES.[33] Distention of this segment in the normal esophagus evokes GES relaxation whereas distention of a dilated segment results in no GES response. Although not the primary cause of megaesophagus, dogs with the fluoroscopic features of achalasia have occasionally been seen at the University of California at Davis VMTH. In these dogs, fluoroscopy showed a moderately dilated caudal thoracic esophagus with adequate, but not normal, peristaltic motility. When food reached the GES, the sphincter did not open, and the bolus moved back and forth a number of times before the GES finally relaxed to allow passage of all or part of the bolus. These observations suggested a lack of coordination between esophageal and GES function and may have been due to a sensory deficit in the caudal esophagus.

It is now considered that the pathogenesis of CIM most often involves loss of peristaltic function in the esophageal body. A defect in any part of the neural reflex that controls the pharyngeal and esophageal phases of swallowing can result in esophageal motor dysfunction. This reflex pathway includes sensory receptors in the pharynx and esophagus, afferent nerve fibers in the glossopharyngeal and vagus nerves, the tractus solitarius that leads to the nucleus solitarius, the swallowing center, which is located in the medial part of the lateral reticular formation,[39] lower motor neurons in the nucleus ambiguus, efferent somatic and parasympathetic nerve fibers in the vagus, the myoneural junction, esophageal striated muscle, and to a much lesser extent esophageal smooth muscle. Thus, it is not surprising that megaesophagus can be produced experimentally in dogs by cutting the vagus nerves or by bilateral destruction of the nucleus ambiguus.[40] In the spontaneously occurring idiopathic disease, however, there is no evidence of denervation myopathy or sufficient denervation potentials to suggest the presence of an axonopathy of the efferent limb of the swallowing response.[24,36,41] Furthermore, stimulation of the vagus nerves in dogs with idio-

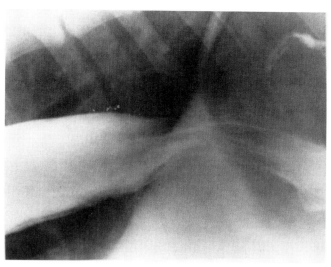

FIGURE 11-4. Megaesophagus in an 8-year-old German shepherd. Lateral spot film made of gastroesophageal junction during a positive-contrast study made under fluoroscopic control. Figure illustrates normal function of the gastroesophageal sphincter that has been documented in dogs with megaesophagus.

pathic megaesophagus results in contraction of the esophagus, indicating that at least some of the motor units are intact.[24] Central nervous system lesions also seem unlikely to be an important cause of the lack of peristalsis in dogs with CIM. Serial sections of the brain stem from one dog with megaesophagus were reported to have fewer cell bodies in the nucleus ambiguus,[42] but other studies have failed to support this observation.[43]

Current evidence favors the afferent limb of the reflex as the site of the lesion in CIM.[44,45] An experimental model of afferent nerve injury in dogs (acrylamide toxicity) produces a syndrome indistinguishable from CIM.[45] Afferent lesions can account for esophageal asperistalis because sensory reinforcement from an intraluminal bolus is necessary for normal esophageal peristaltic activity in dogs.[45,46] The initial abnormality observed as deafferentation develops is a failure of secondary peristalsis, and then a progressive decrease in the proportion of swallows that initiate esophageal peristalsis and a gradual increase in esophageal diameter.[45] Studies on other visceral reflexes in dogs with congenital idiopathic megaesophagus provide additional support for a sensory defect.[44] Distending the normal cranial esophagus or bathing it with acid causes upper esophageal sphincter pressure to increase. This protective reflex is absent in dogs with idiopathic megaesophagus. Furthermore, evidence shows that some of the respiratory reflexes mediated by afferent fibers in the vagus are abnormal in some dogs with megaesophagus.[36] These observations provide an explanation for the high frequency of aspiration pneumonia in dogs with megaesophagus.

The cause of the putative neurologic lesion in CIM is completely unknown. Karyotyping has not revealed any chromosomal abnormality in pups with the problem, but an inherited defect remains probable in some breeds.[47] A delay in the maturation of the esophageal innervation has been suggested. This would explain why young dogs may improve with careful feeding management.[48]

Recently, it has been observed that the viscoelastic properties of the esophageal wall in dogs with megaesophagus is altered.[49] Specifically, esophageal compliance is increased in megaesophagus, and it is possible that esophageal afferent function might be further compromised by this change.[49] The increased compliance is likely to depress the level of activity of the esophageal stretch receptors following distension of the esophagus by an intraluminal bolus.[49]

Megaesophagus of unknown cause has also been reported in the cat.[31,50,51] The problem may be inherited,[31] and little is known about the site of the lesion(s) or of the pathogenesis.

Etiopathogenesis of Secondary Megaesophagus

Numerous disease conditions have been associated with, or proposed as a cause for, esophageal dilatation (Table 11–3). Any disruption of esophageal muscle or of the central, afferent, or efferent pathways that control esophageal motility could result theoretically in megaesophagus by interfering with the act of swallowing. Many such disruptions, either disease or experimentally induced, have already been shown to cause megaesophagus. For instance, myositis and myopathy associated with a variety of diseases, including SLE,[13,52] trypanosomiasis,[53] glycogen-storage disease,[54] polymyositis,[13,55] advanced dermatomyositis,[56] cachexia,[32] dystrophin deficiency,[57] and a familial polymyopathy in English springer spaniels,[58] have produced sufficient esophageal muscle damage to cause megaesophagus.

Neuromuscular junction disease in botulism,[59,60] tetanus,[61] congenital or acquired myasthenia gravis,[13,62–65] and chronic anticholinesterase administration[66] have been shown to produce esophageal dilatation. Of these neuromuscular disorders, an acquired myasthenia gravis demonstrating selectivity for esophageal, pharyngeal, and facial muscles is a particularly common cause of megaesophagus.[65] In one study this selective myasthenia gravis was diagnosed in approximately one-third of dogs presenting with megaesophagus with German shepherds and golden retrievers predisposed.[65] Because of the selective muscular involvement, affected dogs do not show the generalized muscle weakness of classic myasthenia gravis. It is also important to note that up to half of the dogs with this disorder undergo clinical improvement.

Various types of peripheral neuropathies, including polyradiculoneuritis,[13] ganglioradiculitis,[67] dysautonomia,[68,69] demyelinating neuropathies (such as thallium toxicosis),[70] and axonopathies such as canine giant axonal neuropathy,[71] spinal muscular atrophy,[72] and polyneuritis[32] have produced megaesophagus. Megaesophagus has also been associated with lead toxicity.[20,73] The probable cause was a vagal polyneuropathy. Bilateral vagal damage due to trauma, neoplasia, or surgery may cause esophageal dilatation. Megaesophagus has been observed caudal to areas of mediastinitis subsequent to esophageal perforation from foreign bodies.[74] The dilatation was transient; the presumed cause was interference of vagal function by mediastinal cellulitis.[74] A similar finding was reported subsequent to a bronchoesophageal fistula in a dog.[75]

Central nervous system lesions have been established as causes of megaesophagus in dogs and cats. In dogs, both congenital[42] and experimental[40] lesions of the nucleus ambiguus were responsible. In cats, the lesions (experimental) were in the dorsal motor nucleus of the vagus[40,76] and the ventromedial nucleus of the hypothalamus.[77] The difference between the sites of the CNS lesions that cause megaesophagus in dogs and cats is a reflection of the difference in the proportion of the esophageal striated and smooth muscle between the species and therefore the respective importance of the somatic and autonomic nervous system in esophageal inner-

Table 11–3

DISEASES ASSOCIATED WITH AND CAUSES OF MEGAESOPHAGUS

Neuromuscular
  Idiopathic megaesophagus (hereditary?)
  Myasthenia gravis (generalized and selective)
  SLE
  Polymyositis and polymyopathy (immune mediated; familial in Springer spaniels)
  Dystrophin deficiency
  Glycogen storage disease Type II
  Dermatomyositis
  Giant cell axonal neuropathy
  Polyradiculoneuritis
  Immune-mediated polyneuritis
  Ganglioradiculitis
  Dysautonomia
  Spinal muscle atrophy
  Bilateral vagal damage (surgical, traumatic, neoplastic)
  Familial reflex myoclonus
  Cervical vertebral instability with leukomalacia
  Brain stem trauma, neoplasia, or vascular accident
  Botulism
  Distemper
  Tetanus
Esophageal Obstructive Diseases
  Neoplasia
  Vascular ring abnormalities
  Extraesophageal compression
  Strictures, granulomas, foreign bodies
Toxic
  Lead
  Thallium
  Anticholinesterase
  Acrylamide
Miscellaneous
  Mediastinitis
  Bronchoesophageal fistula
  Cachexia
  Pyloric stenosis
  Gastric heterotopia
  Addison disease
  Hypothyroidism?
  Pituitary dwarfism
  Trypanosoma cruzi infection
  Thymoma

vation. Other CNS diseases that have been associated with megaesophagus include cervical vertebral instability with leukomalacia or stroke, and choroid plexus carcinoma with hydrocephalus.[13] Distemper has been cited as a cause of megaesophagus in two dogs.[13,21] The pathogenesis probably relates to distemper-induced CNS lesions of the medulla or cranial nerve pathways. Familial reflex myoclonus of Labrador retrievers has been associated with megaesophagus.[78] No pathogenesis was determined.

Hypothyroidism is often cited as a possible cause of megaesophagus. However, very few dogs with hypothyroidism appear to develop megaesophagus. Misdiagnosis of hypothyroidism is likely in megaesophagus because euthyroid dogs with idiopathic megaesophagus can have particularly low serum-free thyroxine and total thyroxine levels.[79] Notwithstanding this comment, one hypothyroid dog with megaesophagus regained normal esophageal function following thyroid medication.[80] Addison disease can be associated with transient megaesophagus.[81–84] Esophageal asthenia presumably occurs for the same reasons as the skeletal muscle weakness characteristic of hypoadrenocorticism. Some authors believe any shock-like condition can result in megaesopha-gus.[85] Some canine pituitary dwarfs have a concurrent megae-sophagus.[81]

Most obstructive esophageal diseases (neoplasia, granulo-mas, vascular rings, strictures, periesophageal masses, and for-eign bodies) can lead to megaesophagus if they are of suffi-ciently chronic duration.[86] The pathogenesis probably relates to the physical dilatation of the esophagus by accumulating ingesta cranial to the obstruction. Neoplastic invasion of the esophagus can, however, cause motility disturbances,[87] which may contribute to the pathogenesis of the dilatation.

Thymomas are occasionally associated with myasthenia gravis and polymyositis in dogs and cats[88,89] and therefore have the potential to cause megaesophagus. Difficulty swallowing and retention of barium in the esophagus (caudal and cranial to the thymoma) were reported in two cats and several dogs with myasthenia gravis.

A series of cats has been reported with esophageal dysfunc-tion associated with abnormal gastric retention of food.[18] The clinical signs of persistent vomiting were corrected with a pyloromyotomy, and normal esophageal function returned. A cause for this reversible megaesophagus was not identified. It is possible that the chronic vomiting induced an esophagitis, which in turn caused the megaesophagus. Esophagitis has been shown to cause a loss of gastroesophageal sphincter competence[90] and deranged esophageal motility.[91] Megae-sophagus associated with gastric heterotopia (gastric mucosa lining the esophagus) has also been reported in the cat.[92]

Clinical Signs of Megaesophagus

Clinical signs of megaesophagus include regurgitation, enlargement of the esophagus in the cervical region, halito-sis, salivation, poor body condition, and respiratory diffi-culty.[13,14,17,28]

Not all dogs with megaesophagus regurgitate,[21,28] although this is by far the most consistent clinical sign. The frequency of regurgitation varies greatly from once every two to three days to greater than 10 times per day.[28] Regurgitation may be seen immediately after feeding or may occur up to 18 or more hours later. Regurgitation is delayed if the animal is inactive or if the esophageal dilation is marked.[32] Occasion-ally, however, regurgitation can occur during sleep.[86] Dogs with megaesophagus regurgitate both solids and fluids, in contrast to dogs with partial esophageal obstructions (caused by foreign bodies, strictures), in which fluids are often better tolerated. If retained for prolonged periods, the regurgitated ingesta may ferment. Retained fermenting ingesta may cause halitosis and produce gurgling sounds detectable by the owner.[21]

Profuse salivation may occur, presumably resulting from dysphagia. Such salivation may create the impression of nau-sea, more suggestive of nonesophageal disease. The poor body condition seen in some dogs is not a consistent finding. Up to half of the dogs in one study were presented in good body condition.[14]

Accumulation of food in the thoracic esophagus may pro-duce respiratory distress, especially in association with aspira-tion pneumonia. Signs of aspiration pneumonia, including mucopurulent nasal discharge, soft cough, respiratory crack-les, dyspnea, and pyrexia, may be seen. Dogs with megae-sophagus may die acutely due to intussusception of the stom-ach into the esophagus.

Other clinical signs exhibited by animals with mega-esophagus may reflect the underlying cause rather than the megaesophagus per se. For instance, muscle pain and weakness

may occur in dogs with megaesophagus associated with polymyositis.[55] Vomiting was the predominant sign in cats in which megaesophagus was secondary to pyloric dysfunction.[18] Weakness exacerbated by exercise occurs in both cats[63] and dogs[85] with megaesophagus associated with advanced myasthe-nia gravis and in dogs with megaesophagus due to polymyopa-thy.[93] Profound depression was the predominant clinical sign in a dog with megaesophagus associated with lead poisoning.[73] Ataxia and weakness were important signs in a group of dogs with megaesophagus and neuropathy.[71] Dilated pupils and dry mucous membranes accompany the megaesophagus in cats and dogs with dysautonomia.[68,69]

Diagnosis of Megaesophagus

The biggest barrier to the diagnosis of megaesophagus is fail-ure to distinguish regurgitation from vomiting during history taking. Once regurgitation (and/or dysphagia) are determined to be the primary complaint, megaesophagus is usually differ-entiated from the other causes of regurgitation by radiography. After megaesophagus has been identified, consideration should be given to further diagnostic workup to determine the cause of the megaesophagus because treatment and prognosis depend to some extent on accurate diagnosis of the cause. The history may give a clue to the cause of the regurgitation. Vascular ring abnormalities and cricopharyngeal dysphagia are more likely in younger dogs than in older dogs. A history of tolerance of fluids but not solids is more indicative of obstructive esophageal dis-ease than megaesophagus. Regurgitation immediately after eat-ing is suggestive of pharyngeal or cranial cervical esophageal disease. The important differential diagnoses of regurgitation are shown in Table 5–13.

RADIOGRAPHIC EVALUATION.[2,4] The diagnosis of megae-sophagus rests on radiographic procedures. Most cases can be identified by survey radiography because of the presence of air, fluid, or food in the dilated esophagus. Examples of these findings are shown in Figures 11–5 and 11–6. As discussed in the radiography section, the presence of air in the esophagus must be interpreted carefully because it can result from causes other than megaesophagus. In questionable cases, positive-contrast medium can be used to confirm a diagnosis of megaesophagus. Contrast procedures are particularly helpful for the diagnosis of obstructive esophageal diseases. It is advis-able to drain the majority of barium liquid from the esopha-gus after the procedure to minimize the likelihood of inhala-tion of the barium solution. Fluoroscopy is essential for the diagnosis of functional esophageal diseases not associated with esophageal dilatation and has some prognostic value in megaesophagus via assessment of the severity of peristaltic dys-function. It is worthy of note that the extent of esophageal involvement is often poorly correlated with the degree of clini-cal signs. Some animals with an esophagus dilated throughout its length show few clinical signs, whereas others with a short dilated segment regurgitate frequently.

ESOPHAGOSCOPY. Esophagoscopy can be used to diagnose megaesophagus but is less reliable than radiography and fluo-roscopy. Because of anesthesia-induced muscle paralysis, the esophageal lumen appears quite large in normal animals and the endoscopist must be wary of diagnosing megaesophagus based on endoscopic assessment of esophageal diameter alone. In addition to a voluminous esophagus, animals with megae-sophagus usually have fluid and fermenting food retained in large esophageal folds. In our opinion, the primary role of esophagoscopy in the diagnosis of megaesophagus is to rule out underlying causes such as esophagitis, neoplasia, and radi-olucent foreign bodies.

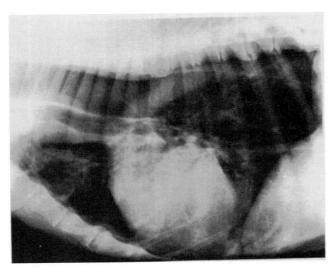

FIGURE 11-5. Megaesophagus, 4-year-old Great Dane. Lateral thoracic radiograph shows dilated air-filled esophagus.

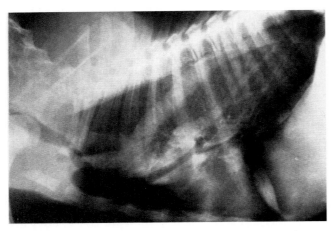

FIGURE 11-6. Lateral radiograph of pup with megaesophagus. Retention of fluid and food in the dilated esophagus increases the density of the structure and enhances its radiographic appearance.

ACETYLCHOLINE RECEPTOR ANTIBODY TEST. Myasthenia gravis (both generalized and selective) can be detected by the acetylcholine receptor antibody test. Esophageal dysfunction due to myasthenia gravis can precede the weakness characteristic of the generalized disease, and esophageal weakness is often the only manifestation of the selective form of the disease. For this reason, and because of the high prevalence of selective acquired myasthenia gravis in adult dogs with megaesophagus, the acetylcholine receptor antibody test should be performed routinely in this group of patients to rule out myasthenia gravis before a diagnosis of idiopathic megaesophagus is made.

MISCELLANEOUS DIAGNOSTIC PROCEDURES. Due to the varied nature of the possible causes of megaesophagus, the diagnostic approach to identify specific causes of secondary megaesophagus must be very broad based. Useful tests are detailed in Table 5-12. Not all of these tests are necessary in the workup of every animal. For instance, in most cases of congenital megaesophagus little additional diagnostic effort is justified after vascular ring anomalies and esophageal foreign bodies have been ruled out. In adult-onset megaesophagus, however, intensive diagnostic effort is more likely to be rewarded with the discovery of a potentially treatable underlying cause.

Botulism may be confirmed by mouse bioassay techniques. SLE may be detected by the presence of supportive systemic signs and positive ANA tests. Neuropathies may be diagnosed by the presence of other peripheral nerve involvement and if necessary by nerve and muscle biopsies. Myositis and myopathy may be proven by EMG findings, serum chemistry results, and muscle biopsy. Lead, thallium, and anticholinesterase toxicities may be diagnosed by history, clinical signs, and toxicologic assays. Dysautonomia is usually obvious on physical examination but can be confirmed by various ocular response tests. Obstructive esophageal diseases and miscellaneous causes such as mediastinitis may be diagnosed by esophagoscopy and radiographic procedures. In summary, idiopathic megaesophagus is a diagnosis of exclusion that, particularly in adult animals, can be reached only after an extensive workup.

PATHOLOGIC EVALUATION. Muscle from the dilated esophagus is usually histologically normal. Chronic dilatation can, however, cause secondary inflammatory changes. The esophageal mucosa will usually show evidence of esophagitis when food and liquids have been retained for more than a short time. Pathologic changes have not been demonstrated in either the vagus nerves or serial sections of the brain stem treated with both conventional and special stains.[47]

Treatment of Megaesophagus

If possible, treatment of megaesophagus is directed at the primary cause. For instance, esophageal obstruction may be relieved by esophagoscopy, bougienage, or surgery. SLE and immune-mediated polymyositis and polyneuritis may respond to immune suppression. Generalized myasthenia gravis may be treated with prednisone or azathioprine and long-acting anticholinesterase agents such as neostigmine and pyridostigmine (1–3 mg/kg q 8–12 hours). Care is necessary when using prednisone and anticholinesterases concurrently, as exacerbation of weakness can result during the initial phases of this combination therapy. Furthermore, prednisone may exacerbate subclinical inhalation pneumonia. Myasthenia gravis selectively involving the esophagus may recover spontaneously with symptomatic therapy (see later), but pyridostigmine is occasionally of value. Removal of a thymoma may result in resolution of myasthenia gravis and clinical improvement in esophageal function. Toxic causes of megaesophagus may be treated by removal of the offending agent and/or use of specific antidotes.[20] Megaesophagus secondary to pyloric stenosis may respond to pyloromyotomy.[18] Megaesophagus resulting from mediastinitis will improve with appropriate antibiotic therapy.

Symptomatic therapy is indicated in idiopathic megaesophagus and as an adjunct to the treatment of secondary megaesophagus regardless of cause. Symptomatic treatment reduces the frequency and/or severity of the common complications of megaesophagus such as aspiration pneumonia, overdilatation of esophageal muscle by large amounts of retained ingesta, and esophagitis secondary to fermenting retained ingesta.

The symptomatic management of megaesophagus centers on the feeding and watering of affected animals from an elevated container to enlist the aid of gravity in moving food through the paralyzed section of esophagus. High-caloric-density liquid gruels are usually fed because liquid meets less resistance in the esophagus than solids. It is important to note, however, that a number of animals will show fewer clinical signs when solid, rather than liquid, food is fed (perhaps because of greater stimulation of afferent pathways by the solid food bolus). Cachectic and anorectic patients, and those with a secondary esophagitis, will benefit from the placement of a gastrostomy tube for nutritional support. The gastrostomy tube provides rest for the esophagus and a rapid return to positive nitrogen balance. The authors have seen several dogs with megaesophagus whose condition resolved after several weeks of feeding via a gastrostomy tube. Animals with a concurrent inhalation pneumonia should receive antibiotics. Transtracheal wash results help guide the choice of antibiotic.

Many drugs have been used unsuccessfully in an attempt to augment esophageal peristalsis in dogs with idiopathic megaesophagus. These unsuccessful drugs include cholinergics such as urecholine and bethanecol, and dopamine antagonists such as metoclopramide. Because of the increased smooth muscle content of cat esophagus in comparison to dog esophagus, it is possible these drugs will be more beneficial in the treatment of feline megaesophagus. The role of cisapride in the treatment of canine and feline megaesophagus also needs to be addressed.

Reduction of gastroesophageal sphincter (GES) pressure could theoretically benefit animals with megaesophagus associated with unusually high resting pressure or those with failure of GES relaxation during swallowing. Furthermore, reducing normal GES pressure may aid the passage of food when esophageal motility is weak and ineffective. Anticholinergics reduce GES pressure to less than a third of normal. One older study reports antispasmodics improved several pups with congenital idiopathic megaesophagus.[27] Unfortunately, however, anticholinergics have met with little success in our hands. Furthermore, this class of drug can be detrimental in the presence of inhalation pneumonia, and by reducing GES tone may predispose animals with megaesophagus to reflux esophagitis. Lastly, anticholinergics may reduce motility in the smooth muscle part of the feline esophagus. Similarly, calcium channel antagonists, such as nifedipine, are unlikely to be beneficial in the treatment of megaesophagus because they have no significant effect on gastroesophageal sphincter tone in the dog.[94]

The surgical treatment of idiopathic megaesophagus is a controversial subject. Some authors think it is a worthwhile procedure,[95–97] whereas others, on the basis of pathophysiologic arguments and clinical experience, believe it is of no value.[14,17,35] Surgical treatments for megaesophagus incorrectly assume that achalasia causes the megaesophagus. As a consequence, a myotomy has been recommended. At Pennsylvania, 40% of dogs with megaesophagus underwent surgery, and because the results were poorer than in untreated dogs, surgery is no longer recommended. From 1967 to 1975, 18% of the cases of canine megaesophagus at the VMTH in Davis were treated surgically, with poor results. There is no rationale for a myotomy unless radiographic studies reveal loss of coordinated GES function or a stricture at the gastroesophageal junction. Surgery would also be indicated if manometric studies show GES pressure to be high and pressure reduction is not demonstrated during swallowing. In the unlikely event that an anticholinergic trial produces symptomatic improvement in megaesophagus, surgery may also be indicated to create a permanent reduction in GES tone without the need for chronic anticholinergic medication. Complications of GES myotomies have included gastroesophageal reflux and herniation of the stomach into the esophagus. If surgery is undertaken, the modified short Heller's esophagomyotomy appears to be the procedure of choice because it reduces GES pressure but still maintains enough GES competency to prevent esophageal reflex.[98] After surgery animals must still be fed from an elevated bowl.[99]

Prognosis of Megaesophagus

The prognosis depends on the cause of the megaesophagus and the age of onset of the clinical signs. Dogs with CIM should receive a guarded prognosis. There is a tendency for the esophageal function of young animals to improve as they mature.[48] Recovery rates in young dogs of 20% to 46% have been reported. Recovery is more likely if the condition is recognized early and appropriate dietary management is instituted because chronic dilatation from accumulated ingesta results in irreversible damage to the esophagus. Miniature schnauzer pups with hereditary esophageal dysfunction usually recover clinically and radiographically if they survive the first few weeks of life.[23]

Adult-onset idiopathic megaesophagus has a poor prognosis but on rare occasions can be transient.[100] The prognosis for secondary megaesophagus depends on the cause. Dogs with megaesophagus due to primary diseases such as myasthenia gravis, polyradiculoneuritis, polymyositis, and SLE can recover swallowing function following appropriate therapy.[13] Myasthenia gravis selectively involving the esophagus has a favorable prognosis; up to one-half of affected dogs recover with supportive therapy. Megaesophagus secondary to Addison disease, botulism, bronchoesophageal fistula, and mediastinitis has a favorable prognosis if treated early. The prognosis of megaesophagus associated with obstructive esophageal diseases, such as vascular anomalies, is guarded to poor unless the correction of the obstruction precedes significant esophageal dilatation. Relief of the obstruction usually results in some clinical improvement, but the dilated esophagus rarely regains normal function.[101] The prognosis of megaesophagus in cats with dysautonomia is poor. Although up to 30% of cats with dysautonomia return to clinical normality, the presence of significant megaesophagus in an affected cat markedly worsens its chances of recovery.[68] Similarly, the prognosis of cats with megaesophagus associated with pyloric dysfunction is poorer than those with pyloric dysfunction alone.[18] Some cats with pyloric dysfunction–associated megaesophagus do, however, show improved clinical signs and reduced esophageal diameter after pyloromyotomy.[18]

The prognosis of megaesophagus from any cause is adversely affected by evidence of concurrent inhalation pneumonia and debilitation, and by the absence of any esophageal motility. In summary, the prognosis of megaesophagus with few exceptions is guarded to poor.

ESOPHAGEAL MOTILITY ABNORMALITIES

Clinical Synopsis

Diagnostic Features

- Regurgitation
- Esophagus of normal diameter on contrast radiography
- Fluoroscopy reveals dysperistalsis
- Multitude of possible primary causes

Treatment

- Address primary cause if diagnosed
- Feed high-calorie diet from raised receptable
- Experiment with diet consistency

Abnormal esophageal peristalsis can occur without the development of megaesophagus. The prevalence of esophageal motility abnormalities is unknown, but in dogs seen at the Massey University Veterinary Clinic the condition is diagnosed with equal frequency to megaesophagus. There is a high prevalence of subclinical esophageal motility abnormalities in the sharpei breed.[25] As mentioned earlier, Bouviers can develop abnormal esophageal motility secondary to a muscular dystrophy.[12]

The clinical signs of esophageal dysperistalsis are similar in nature to megaesophagus but are usually less severe. Appetite is usually unaffected, but anorexia is occasionally observed. The reluctance to eat may be due in part to painful spasms induced in the esophagus when a bolus is swallowed. Signs of esophageal colic can be correlated with fluoroscopic demonstration of spastic contractions of the esophagus around a bolus of food. Occasionally the principal clinical signs of affected animals are related to the respiratory system and include signs such as cough and episodic dyspnea perhaps from inhalation of gastroesophageal content.

The causes of esophageal motility abnormalities are thought to be similar to those of megaesophagus. Indeed, it is likely that many cases of megaesophagus are preceded by a period in which esophageal motility is deranged but esophageal dilatation has not yet developed. Most esophageal motility problems diagnosed at Massey University have been idiopathic, but we have also recognized dysperistalsis secondary to esophagitis and mediastinitis. Esophagitis is a particularly well-described cause of esophageal motility abnormalities in cats and dogs.[90,91] The dysmotility resulting from the inflammatory process may cause generalized esophageal dysfunction or may involve only short segments of the esophagus. The latter most commonly occurs following impaction of a foreign body in the affected esophageal segment. The pathogenesis of the motility disorders resulting from esophagitis is not known but may relate to loss of sensory reinforcement of the swallow due to damaged esophageal sensory receptors in the inflamed esophagus. Damage to the striated muscle and intrinsic nervous system of the esophagus via ischemia and subsequent inflammation is the most likely cause of the segmental motility disorders seen following esophageal obstruction by a foreign body.

The diagnosis of esophageal dysperistalsis can only be made via fluoroscopy (Figure 11–7). Studies must be performed with both food and liquid. The most common motility disorder is a diffuse loss of the normal esophageal peristaltic activity (dysperistalsis). This activity is replaced by random and uncoordinated contrac-

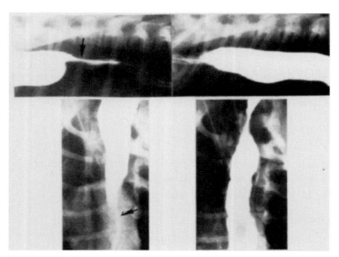

FIGURE 11–7. Esophageal motility disorders in an 18-month-old Toy poodle. Lateral and ventrodorsal radiographs were made under fluoroscopic control at different intervals after oral administration of positive-contrast medium. Comparison of the views illustrates that segments of the esophagus appearing to have megaesophagus are able to generate peristalsis, and the esophagus appears to be of a normal size after the bolus moves caudally. In addition, segments that do not appear to have megaesophagus (arrows) are abnormally dilated when the bolus of contrast medium moves into the segment. This type of lesion can be segmental or diffuse. There is often poor correlation between severity of lesions and degree of clinical signs.

tions that result in variable degrees of retention of food or liquid in the esophagus and frequently reverse peristalsis. Occasionally, spasms of the esophagus around a bolus of food are seen (esophageal colic). At times the motility defect will involve only a few centimeters of the esophagus. These defects may be so subtle that they are difficult to identify by radiographic procedures. Once the cause of the regurgitation is determined to be an esophageal motility disorder, affected animals should receive the same diagnostic workup recommended for those with megaesophagus. Endoscopy and/or endoscopic biopsy may reveal esophagitis but are otherwise normal.

Esophageal motility abnormalities are treated in the same manner as megaesophagus. Attention is given to both the primary cause (if identified) and to symptomatic nutritional management. In addition, we have seen several encouraging clinical responses to cisapride (0.25 mg/kg q 8–12 hours), although these observations must be tempered by caution because cisapride is not thought to have significant effect on the striated esophageal muscle found throughout the canine esophagus.

The prognosis is guarded. The clinical signs of many animals can be controlled by appropriate dietary choices, and some patients undergo spontaneous recovery of esophageal function up to six weeks after onset of the problem.

ESOPHAGITIS

Clinical Synopsis

Diagnostic Features

- Inappetence and subtle signs of swallowing discomfort
- Restlessness and repeated swallowing
- Intermittent regurgitation
- May be history of ingestion of irritant drugs or caustic agents
- Radiography or fluoroscopy may reveal gastroesophageal reflux and/or hiatal hernia
- Endoscopy may show hyperemia, erosions, fibrosis, or strictures
- Suction biopsy of esophagus may be diagnostic even if endoscopy normal

Treatment

- Neutralize any caustic agents
- Sucralfate slurries (0.25–1 g per animal q 8 hours)
- Ranitidine (2–3.5 mg/kg q 12 hours) or omeprazole (0.5–2 mg/kg q 24 hours in dogs)
- Metoclopramide (0.2–0.4 mg/kg q 6–8 hours) or cisapride (0.25 mg/kg q 6–8 hours)

The prevalence of acute esophagitis is thought to be low. It is likely, however, that the prevalence of esophagitis is underestimated because of the subtle clinical signs, limited use of endoscopy by the practicing veterinarian, and subtle radiographic findings associated with the disorder.

Etiopathogenesis

Inflammation of the esophagus may result from a variety of acute or chronic insults, the most frequent of which is gastroesophageal reflux. Other causes of esophagitis include thermal burns, acute and persistent vomiting, foreign body obstruction, infectious agents, and the ingestion of chemical irritants. The esophagus appears to be more susceptible to alkaline corrosives, such as sodium hydroxide, than acidic corrosives. It can also be damaged by quaternary ammonium cleaning agents and button batteries.[102] The latter produce damage by a combination of pressure necrosis, direct corrosive action, and low-voltage burn.[103] Infectious causes for esophageal inflammation are uncommon. Primary infectious esophagitis has been reported in immunocompromised patients and as a sequela to systemic phycomycosis in the dog.[104] Acute esophagitis with ulcerations has been observed in some cats with caliciviral upper respiratory infection.[105]

GASTROESOPHAGEAL REFLUX. Gastroesophageal reflux is a normal event in dogs and probably cats. Gastroesophageal reflux and regurgitation is particularly common in young animals. The GES is incompetent at birth, and in cats and dogs GES pressure at six weeks is only one-half of that in adults.[47,106] Mild gastrocesophageal reflux occurs during swallowing and belching. However, in healthy adult dogs, reflux occurs primarily during transient periods of marked GES relaxation that appear approximately once an hour in both unfed and fed animals.[107] The transient refluxes occur following complete GES relaxation rather than just low resting GES pressure.[108,109] Reflux will occur only if GES pressure falls to that in the stomach (i.e., if barrier pressure becomes zero or below). It is for this reason that individuals with lower than normal basal GES pressure do not necessarily have an increased frequency of reflux. Similarly, drugs that reduce (but do not eliminate) resting GES pressure do not necessarily increase the frequency of gastroesophageal reflux.

The frequency of transient GES relaxation in dogs is determined by noncholinergic vagal activity and by intragastric pressure.[110-111] Raised intragastric pressure following fundic contractions appears to be a stimulus for the transient GES relaxation.[112-114] The competence of the sphincter is suppressed by movement of the intra-abdominal segment of esophagus and cardia into the thoracic cavity, followed by contraction of the diaphragm and abdominal muscles. In the dog, contraction of the striated longitudinal muscles of the esophagus accomplishes cranial translocation of the gastroesophageal sphincter (it is noteworthy that tetanus has been associated with hiatal hernia,[61,115] perhaps through this mechanism). Because this physiologic sliding hernia depends on contraction of the longitudinal esophageal muscles, it follows that their denervation would eliminate the event. Indeed, in experimental studies, selective vagotomy of the muscles of the caudal esophagus has been shown to abolish transient GES relaxation.[116] Transient GES relaxation provides a physiologic mechanism to overcome the competence of the gastroesophageal sphincter. This mechanism is necessary during vomition and eructation, but an increase in frequency or persistence of this physiologic response will result in reflux esophagitis.

A major determinant of whether esophagitis develops is the length of time until normal esophageal pH is restored. Esophagitis will follow gastroesophageal reflux only if the refluxed contents are not cleared rapidly from the esophagus.[109] During gastroesophageal reflux in healthy animals, the pH of the esophagus becomes acidic for approximately 5 to 30 seconds (some studies have reported longer acidification times). After reflux, primary and secondary esophageal peristalsis removes acidic fluid and brings swallowed saliva to the acidified regions of the esophagus. The bicarbonate-rich saliva neutralizes and dilutes the acid. Primary esophageal peristalsis is stimulated by the swallowing of saliva, and secondary peristalsis is stimulated by distension of the esophagus. It is not known whether acid pH per se stimulates secondary peristalsis, but it is believed to stimulate nonpropagating esophageal contractions that do not clear the esophagus. Primary abnormalities in esophageal motility (and acid clearance) have been observed in some people with reflux gastritis.[117]

Effective barriers against the intercellular diffusion of acid and the regulation of intracellular pH by Na^+-H^+ exchange mechanisms assist esophageal mucosal defense against reflux.[117] Rapid clearance by esophageal blood flow of hydrogen ions that have diffused across the esophageal mucosa provides another defense mechanism.

FACTORS PREDISPOSING TO REFLUX ESOPHAGITIS. Swallowing and secretion of saliva are markedly reduced during sleep and anesthesia, resulting in an increased risk for the development of esophagitis during these periods. Paradoxically, the frequency of transient GES relaxations increases at night in humans, further increasing the likelihood of esophagitis during sleep.[118] Furthermore, many preanesthetic agents including anticholinergics, acetylpromazine, narcotic analgesics, diazepam, and most commonly used induction agents reduce GES pressure[119-124] predisposing to (but not necessarily causing) gastroesophageal reflux.[123,125] Thoracotomy procedures, however, do result in esophageal acidification, presumably because of gastroesophageal reflux.[125]

Any changes in the anatomic factors that contribute to the high-pressure zone in the GES can increase reflux frequency. These factors are discussed in Chapter 10 and include the abdominal esophagus and the diaphragmatic crus. It is little wonder, therefore, that hiatal hernias disrupt this relationship, increasing the risk for reflux. The greater the amount of stomach herniated through the esophageal hiatus, the more severe the esophagitis.[126]

Increased frequency of gastric contractions and increased gastric volume can increase reflux frequency. Reflux can be demonstrated in many cases of gastric outflow obstruction. Conversely, reflux esophagitis can result in slower gastric emptying.[127] Therefore it can be difficult for clinicians to determine whether the esophagitis or the delayed gastric emptying developed first.

Esophagitis compromises GES function and acid clearance from the esophagus leading to a vicious circle that perpetuates the esophagitis. Esophagitis causes a loss of GES smooth muscle tone, and with it the antireflux barrier.[128] As reflux frequency increases so does the duration of transient GES pressure reductions. In cats, bile and acid perfusion of the esophagus reduces GES pressure and swallowing pressure. Esophageal contractions become weak and uncoordinated, and no peristaltic waves are evident. Abnormal motility persists for more than two days following the insult, although GES pressure can return earlier.[129]

PATHOGENESIS OF REFLUX ESOPHAGITIS. The acid, pepsin, trypsin, bile acids, and lysolecithin in refluxed gastric fluid can be injurious to the esophageal mucosa. Acid is the most important factor leading to esophageal damage,[117] but a combination of these constituents is necessary for marked damage. Acid reflux stimulates proliferation of the basal epithelium of the canine esophagus but no erosions or inflammation.[130] Reflux of acid combined with pepsin or bile acids causes severe ulcerative changes within 20 to 60 minutes.[131,132] Perfusion of the esophagus with bile acids increases the mucosal permeability to acid but causes only minor if any morphologic changes. Bile acids must be in an acidic solution to produce damage, and there is some question as to whether any of the small amounts of bile commonly resident in the stomach of dogs appear in the refluxed fluid.[133] Trypsin at pH 7.5 damages the esophageal mucosa more severely than bile acids or pepsin do.[134,135] Whether such alkaline conditions ever prevail during gastroesophageal reflux is unknown. Recent studies in dogs show that the most severe esophagitis is caused by reflux of gastric juice during maximal gastric stimulation in the absence of duodenogastric reflux.[136] In the presence of duodenogastric reflux (for example, as occurs prior to vomiting), less severe esophageal changes occur. It appears the mixture of gastric and duodenal content neutralizes acid and creates a medium of intermediate pH unsuitable to the activity of either pepsin or trypsin.[136]

PATHOGENESIS OF DRUG OR CHEMICAL-INDUCED ESOPHAGITIS. Out of a small number of drugs evaluated in cats, a high percentage caused esophagitis (Table 11–4).[137] Drugs in tablet form pass through the esophagus more easily than capsules. In humans, 65% of capsules taken without water lodge and dissolve in the esophagus; taken with water 9% lodge in the esophagus. Oral medications given to dogs and cats are more likely to remain in the esophagus because liquids are usually not taken with the medicine. Many of the drugs causing esophageal injury in humans are also used in small animals.[138] It is noteworthy that a high frequency of nonsteroidal anti-inflammatory use has been observed in humans with reflux esophagitis.[117]

Esophageal damage from drugs and chemicals is caused by changes in mucosal pH, hyperosmolarity, and, at times, by unknown means. Clinicians should consider lubricating capsules routinely with palatable oils or syringing water into an animal's oral cavity following administration of capsules to minimize the risk of esophageal retention of injurious drugs. This is particularly important when esophageal motility may be abnormal because of esophageal disease, persistent vomiting, or in very young or old animals.

Clinical Signs

The damage in mild esophagitis is usually limited to the mucosa and is most often self-limiting once the inciting process is removed. Clinical signs of esophageal discomfort are mild or nonexistent, and the esophageal mucosa heals quickly without significant fibrosis. Severe esophagitis due to such causes as caustic burns results in painful swallowing, hypersalivation, depression, and, at times, polydipsia. Involvement of the muscular layers is uncommon but can lead to serious complications such as persistent ulceration, stricture formation, and esophageal perforation. Physical examination is usually nondiagnostic.

The clinical signs associated with reflux esophagitis are usually subtle. Discomfort during swallowing may be apparent. This may lead to reluctance to eat and at worse anorexia. Clinically apparent episodes of reflux are particularly common on an empty stomach, perhaps because food buffers acid in the stomach. During the periods of reflux the animal may be restless and appear uncomfortable. Repeated swallowing attempts may be made and regurgitation occasionally occurs. Severely affected animals show weight loss, excessive salivation, and regurgitation of viscid saliva-like fluid that may contain blood.

Diagnosis

Laboratory work and survey radiographs are usually unremarkable. Severe cases may show radiographic evidence of GES chalasia, hiatal hernia, or stricture formation. Contrast radiog-

Table 11–4

DRUGS CAUSING ESOPHAGITIS
Alprenolol (beta blocker)
Ascorbic acid
Ferrosuccinate
Ferrosulfate
Doxycycline
Nonsteroidal anti-inflammatories (NSAIDs)
Potassium chloride
Tetracycline

raphy using fluoroscopy may reveal gastroesophageal reflux and varying degrees of esophageal dysperistalsis secondary to esophagitis. Unfortunately, the reflux is often episodic and may not be apparent during the fluoroscopy. Endoscopy will identify animals with severe esophagitis, but the esophagus of mildly affected animals will look grossly normal. Severely affected areas of the esophagus are often hyperemic and may have mucosal erosions. If the esophagitis is chronic, radial fibrotic striations progressing to overt stricturing may be apparent (Figure 11–8). In animals with reflux esophagitis, not surprisingly, the majority of the damage is visible just cranial to the GES (Figure 11–8).

Biopsy of the esophageal mucosa is the most reliable diagnostic procedure for identifying esophagitis. Biopsy samples are best obtained with a suction capsule biopsy instrument. Pinch biopsies obtained via endoscopy are usually inadequate for diagnostic purposes because the esophageal mucosa is often too tough to be cut by endoscopic biopsy forceps. Biopsy samples are especially useful in identifying patients with esophagitis that have a grossly normal mucosa. In acute cases of esophagitis, epithelial necrosis and neutrophil infiltration may be observed. In chronic cases, thickening of the basal epithelial layer and elongation of the papilla toward the luminal surface are more typical (Figures 11–9 and 11–10).[136,139] In the author's experience these morphologic abnormalities are frequently missed by inexperienced pathologists. It is worthy of note that chronic inflammatory changes can include intraepithelial infiltration by eosinophils.[140] Furthermore, biopsy of the esophagus is useful for ruling out heterotopic gastric mucosa that can cause esophagitis and stricture.[141]

In humans, manometry of the GES and continuous monitoring of esophageal pH have been used successfully for diagnosis

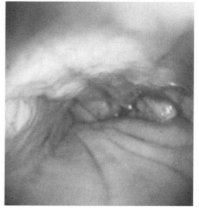

FIGURE 11–8. Endoscopic picture of chronic reflux esophagitis in a dog. Note the radial bands of fibrous tissue and the granular appearance to the mucosa.

of gastroesophageal reflux and reflux esophagitis. Continuous esophageal pH measurements are particularly useful, with the diagnosis of reflux esophagitis being based on the number and duration of the episodes of reflux. These techniques have not, as yet, enjoyed successful application to animals.

Treatment

In acute esophagitis, the esophagus is rested by fasting the animal for 1 to 2 days. Thereafter a low-fat diet is fed because high dietary fat content reduces GES pressure and may exacerbate reflux. A high dietary protein content may also be useful because such a diet increases GES pressure. Unfortunately, high-protein diets are also a potent stimulus for gastric acid secretion, potentially offsetting their beneficial effects on GES tone. Chocolate treats should be avoided because chocolate reduces GES pressure.

If the esophagitis is due to the ingestion of caustic agents, emesis should not be induced. Unabsorbed acids may be neutralized with magnesium oxide solution (1:25 dilution with warm water) or milk of magnesia. A weak acid such as vinegar (1:4 diluted with water) or lemon juice administered orally is recommended following the ingestion of caustic alkalis.

Medical management of reflux esophagitis includes the use of inhibitors of gastric acid secretion. Cimetidine (5 mg/kg q 8 hours) and ranitidine are useful for the treatment of mild to moderate esophagitis, but evidence from clinical trials in humans suggest that in intractable esophagitis a better choice might be omeprazole.[117,142] Esophageal erosions can be treated with colloidal bismuth suspensions or sucralfate.[143–145] The sucralfate acts as a protectant by binding to denuded mucosa.

Drugs that increase GES pressure in dogs (and probably cats), such as metoclopramide[146] and cisapride, are a useful adjunct to gastric acid inhibitors in the treatment of reflux esophagitis. The value of metoclopramide is limited in chronic

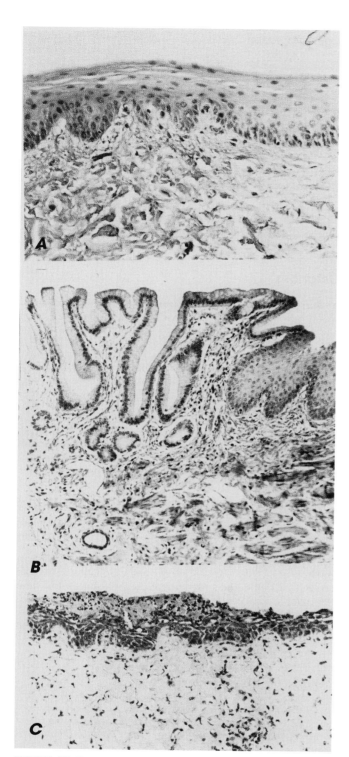

FIGURE 11-9. *(A)* Biopsy of normal esophageal mucosa obtained with capsule. *(B)* Photomicrograph of junction of gastric and esophageal mucosa at the gastroesophageal junction from a normal dog. *(C)* Biopsy of esophagus at the gastroesophageal sphincter obtained with capsule. Shows an esophagitis characterized by infiltration by neutrophils and necrosis of surface of epithelium. Typical changes caused by reflux of gastric contents into the esophagus.

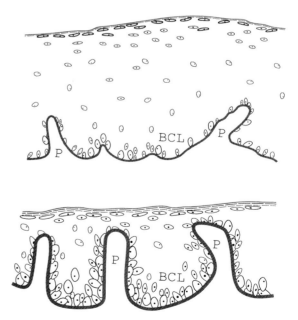

FIGURE 11-10. Drawing showing biopsy appearance of normal canine esophagus (above) and of dog with reflux esophagitis. Changes are seen for thickness of basal lamina (BCL) and for depth of papilla (P).

cases by its short duration of activity in dogs (only 1.5–2.0 hours when given orally). Cisapride may prove to be more effective than metoclopramide.[147] Cisapride reduces the frequency of recurrence of reflux esophagitis in humans[148] and may have a role in the treatment of esophagitis in the dog and cat. The therapeutic dose of cisapride in dogs and cats has not been established, but we have used the drug successfully for esophagitis at a dose of 0.25 mg/kg q 8 hours in dogs. Anticholinergic drugs are contraindicated. In addition to reducing GES pressure in both fed and unfed dogs and cats, they reduce motility in the caudal feline esophagus and impair the animal's ability to clear refluxed fluid back into the stomach.

A variety of surgical procedures have been used in humans to treat intractable reflux esophagitis. In dogs and cats, the procedure of choice to create a lower esophageal high pressure zone is Nissen fundoplication. Surgical correction of hiatal hernias may also be required (see later).

ESOPHAGEAL FOREIGN BODIES AND ESOPHAGEAL PERFORATION

Clinical Synopsis

Diagnostic Features

- Anorexia, drooling, odynophagia, and regurgitation
- Fever and/or evidence of sepsis suggests esophageal perforation
- Cough suggests concurrent airway-esophageal fistula or pneumonia
- Diagnosis by survey or contrast radiography

Treatment

- Endoscopic removal preferred
- Surgical removal necessary if endoscopy unsuccessful
- Surgical exploration, repair, and drainage are indicated if a large esophageal defect, nonlocalized mediastinitis, or evidence of sepsis are detected
- Broad-spectrum antibiotics are required

Esophageal foreign bodies are a common cause of dysphagia and regurgitation.[149–152]. The condition is more common in dogs than in cats,[150] presumably because of the more discriminatory eating habits of cats. Small breeds of dogs may be predisposed.[3] The foreign bodies encountered most frequently are bones and fishhooks, although other objects, such as furballs, chew toys, large chunks of food, needles, fabrics, and stones, are occasionally found (Figure 11–11).[152,153] Foreign bodies usually lodge in the esophagus at the thoracic inlet, the base of the heart, or the diaphragmatic hiatus. These are the points of least distensibility. Persistent lodgment of a foreign body can lead to pressure necrosis of the esophageal wall (Figure 11–12) and subsequent stricture. Full thickness necrosis leads to perforation, mediastinitis, pleuritis, and at times pneumonia.

Clinical Findings

Observations by the owner often provide important diagnostic information. A history of indiscriminate eating behavior or ingestion of bones raises the likelihood of an esophageal foreign body. Anorexia, odynophagia, and hypersalivation are the most common signs, but dysphagia, retching, gagging, and regurgitation of saliva are also frequently seen. With most esophageal foreign bodies, the anorexia is likely the result of pain. The pain arises from distention of the esophagus and esophageal spasm about the foreign body. It is exacerbated by swallowing and, at times, by pressure on the sternum as can occur when lifting the animal. A history of cough developing a few days after the initial clinical signs is strongly suggestive of the development of a secondary inhalation pneumonia or a bronchoesophageal fistula. Prolonged duration of signs increases the likelihood of esophageal perforation.

Physical examination of animals with esophageal obstruction is usually nondiagnostic. Affected animals may drool, adopt a hunched posture, or show reluctance to swallow. Body temperature may be elevated if mediastinitis has occurred. The examination should include careful attention to the base of the tongue and pharynx for linear foreign objects that may extend into the esophagus.

Diagnosis

The diagnosis of esophageal foreign bodies depends heavily on history and can usually be confirmed with survey chest radiographs. A few animals require contrast procedures and/or endoscopy for diagnosis.

The radiographic examination should include the entire esophagus. Radioopaque foreign bodies are readily visualized, but when sharp objects (e.g., fishhooks) are observed by radiography, the veterinarian should carefully ascertain if the foreign body remains in the lumen of the gastrointestinal tract. Not uncommonly, sharp objects will penetrate the esophageal or gastrointestinal wall where they become inaccessible to endoscopic removal. Radiolucent foreign bodies will occasionally cause accumulation of gas and fluid cranial to the obstruction that can be recognized on survey films. If necessary, positive contrast procedures can be used to outline radiolucent foreign bodies and detect perforations.

Perforation of the esophagus should be suspected when accumulation of gas or fluid in the cervical area, pleural cavity, or mediastinum is observed but this is not seen consistently.[3] A left-shifted leukogram (and fever) often accompanies perforation but will also occur with inhalation pneumonia, a frequent complication of esophageal disease of any type. Esophograms may reveal the perforation but false negatives occur in up to 15% of studies (especially if a foreign body is still present in the perforation at the time of radiography).[3] The interpretation of positive-contrast studies of the esophagus was described earlier.

Treatment

All esophageal foreign bodies should be rapidly removed because they cause pain and dysphagia, and may result in esophageal perforation or stricture. The degree of mucosal damage is usually proportional to the duration of the foreign body entrapment. Endoscopic removal is particularly desirable in view of the possible complications of esophageal surgery and thoracotomy. However, if perforation of the esophagus is suspected, surgery, not endoscopy is preferred (see later). Both endoscopy and surgery result in successful removal of esophageal foreign bodies in approximately 85% of affected dogs and cats.[149,150,154] Glucocorticoid therapy to minimize the likelihood of stricturing following retrieval of esophageal foreign bodies has been recommended, but in the opinion of the authors and others[152] is rarely necessary.

Successful endoscopic retrieval of foreign bodies requires considerable skill and discretion. The technique is described

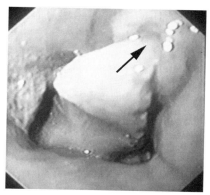

FIGURE 11–11. Endoscopic picture of a bone lodged in the esophagus of a dog. The bone had been swallowed four days previously. Note the point of mucosal perforation (arrow).

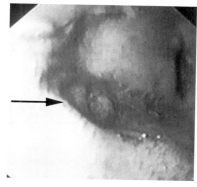

FIGURE 11–12. Endoscopic picture of the gastroesophageal sphincter region of a dog's esophagus. Note the mucosal erosions caused by a bone that had been lodged at this site for several days. The arrow indicates an area of necrosis from which a bronchoesophageal fistula developed.

in Chapter 7. Assessment of esophageal damage should follow endoscopic removal of the foreign body. The esophageal mucosa should be visualized throughout its entire length. Hyperemia and mild ulceration are common endoscopic findings. Careful attention can be necessary to detect small esophageal perforations. Survey thoracic radiographs should be performed following endoscopic removal of tightly wedged foreign bodies to assist detection of pneumothorax or pneumomediastinum secondary to esophageal perforation.

Minor tears, lacerations (less than 1 cm in length), or ulcerations of the esophagus can be handled conservatively with broad-spectrum antibiotic cover (for mediastinitis) and esophageal rest via placement of pharyngostomy or gastrostomy tubes for nutritional support. Large defects in the esophageal wall, defects of any size with concurrent signs of sepsis, nonlocalized mediastinitis, or other thoracic cavity involvement require surgical exploration and repair. Surgical management should include placement of thoracic drains.[132]

Prognosis

The prognosis is guarded to good. However, at least one-third of animals with esophageal foreign bodies develop complications. Esophageal perforation from lacerations and esophageal necrosis can lead to mediastinitis, which should carry a guarded prognosis.[3,132] Trauma from foreign bodies with sharp edges can cause laceration of major blood vessels adjacent to the esophagus, resulting in severe hemorrhage. Septicemia can occur following esophageal perforation. Esophageal strictures or diverticula and local deficits in motility can occur a week or more after foreign body removal. Unusual chronic complications of esophageal foreign body impaction include bronchoesophageal fistula, pericarditis, and persistent esophageal ulcers.

ESOPHAGEAL STRICTURE

Clinical Synopsis

Diagnostic Features

- Regurgitation (particularly regurgitation beginning 1 to 3 weeks after a general anesthesia)
- Liquids are tolerated better than solid food

- Narrowing of esophageal lumen demonstrated by contrast radiography
- Fibrous or neoplastic stricture differentiated by endoscopic biopsy

Treatment

- Balloon bougienage

Narrowing of the esophageal lumen due to proliferation of fibrous or neoplastic tissue within the esophageal wall is referred to as esophageal stricture.

Etiopathogenesis

Inflammation or disruption of the epithelium without damage to the deeper structures usually does not stimulate the formation of fibrous tissue. Erosions that extend through the lamina propria into the muscle layers, however, usually result in scar tissue. In severely damaged tissue, fibroblasts appear within 24 hours of the insult, and collagen fibers are formed within one week. Even though fibrotic changes begin early, clinical signs may not appear until after fibrous tissue matures and reduces the diameter of the esophageal lumen.

Esophageal strictures are usually secondary to reflux esophagitis, chemical burns, or circumferential trauma from an esophageal foreign body. It is noteworthy that use of undiluted benzalkonium chloride (Zepharin) on cats has been reported to cause severe skin burns, oral ulceration, esophagitis, and stricture.[155] Occasionally neoplasia will cause esophageal stricture.

Most esophageal strictures caused by reflux esophagitis are due to reflux occurring during general anesthesia. Proposed predisposing factors for gastroesophageal reflux during anesthesia include head-down body position and use of preanesthetic or induction agents that decrease pressure in the gastroesophageal sphincter.[156] As mentioned earlier, however, lower GES pressures need not result in an increased frequency of reflux.[125]

Clinical Signs

The clinical signs associated with esophageal stricture are similar to those seen with all other esophageal problems and include dysphagia, regurgitation, and pseudoptyalism. Liquids are tolerated better than solid food. Regurgitation usually appears abruptly and is then seen consistently. Not uncommonly, the regurgitation begins one to three weeks after a minor surgical procedure. In contrast to esophageal foreign bodies, anorexia and esophageal colic are usually not seen unless the cause of the stricture is esophageal neoplasia or there is an associated esophagitis. It has been shown in humans that the severity of dysphagia is not only correlated to the diameter of the esophageal stricture but also to the severity of any associated esophagitis.[157] Physical examination of affected animals is usually unremarkable.

Diagnosis

Contrast radiography will reveal esophageal stenosis with a dilated proximal esophagus. Occasionally, fluoroscopy or endoscopy is necessary to detect less pronounced esophageal stenosis. Differential diagnoses for esophageal stenosis include esophageal strictures, periesophageal masses, vascular anomalies, or adhesions that constrict the lumen of the esophagus from outside its wall. Endoscopy will confirm the presence of a stricture, and help differentiate fibrous (postinflammatory strictures) from neoplastic strictures (Figure 11–13). Neoplastic strictures are often eccentric whereas many fibrous strictures are concentric. If they involve the mucosa, neoplastic strictures tend to be erosive and more friable than fibrous strictures. Neoplastic and fibrous strictures can usually be differentiated by endoscopic biopsy unless the stricture is caused by an esophageal neoplasm that does not involve the mucosa (e.g., a leiomyoma), whereupon surgical exploration may be required to make the diagnosis.

Management

Fibrous esophageal strictures are best treated by balloon catheter dilatation (Figure 11–13).[158–160] Rigid bougies are less desirable than balloon dilators because they produce less radial force and more shearing forces; however, they are still effective in many situations. The techniques of balloon dilation and bougienage are described in Chapter 7. Endotracheal tubes can be used as dilators for cervical strictures in small dogs and cats.[161] Esophageal strictures may require repeated dilation, particularly if rigid bougies are used instead of a balloon dilator. The repeat dilation procedure is performed when and if the animal becomes clinical rather than to any other set schedule. Some strictures may require as many as four dilation procedures at 5 to 7 day intervals.[162] Some authors recommended the use of postdilation antibiotics and corticosteroids to help prevent bacterial invasion of the damaged esophageal mucosa and the reformation of fibrous tissue.[162,163] Experimental work has suggested that large doses of corticosteroids administered with antibiotics for 2 to 3 weeks beginning at the time of esophageal injury prevent stenosis of the esophagus.[164] However, good results following balloon catheter dilation of mature strictures can be obtained without the use of corticosteroids. Placement of a large-diameter pharyngostomy tube for 1 to 2 weeks after dilation of the stricture has also been recommended. The tube acts as a splint and prevents reformation of the stricture. Because large-bore pharyngostomy tubes are not well tolerated by most patients, we prefer not to use them, instead opting for repeated balloon dilation should this be necessary.

Following successful stricture dilation, most animals can tolerate soft foods. Feeding of gruels is usually unnecessary. Temporary nutritional support via a gastrostomy tube may be advantageous particularly if the stricture is associated with a severe esophagitis.

Several surgical techniques for the treatment of esophageal strictures have been described.[132,165] Surgical resection of the stenotic area is seldom successful and in our experience surgical management is much less successful than balloon dilation. Treatment of strictures due to esophageal neoplasia is described later in the discussion of neoplasms of the esophagus.

Prognosis

The prognosis for esophageal strictures is guarded, but balloon catheter dilation of fibrous esophageal strictures can be expected to produce good results on most occasions. Complications of bougienage are described in Chapter 7.

VASCULAR RING ANOMALIES[4,166–169]

Clinical Synopsis

Diagnostic Features

- Regurgitation (particularly regurgitation beginning just after weaning)
- Liquids are tolerated better than solid food
- Narrowing of esophageal lumen at heart base demonstrated by contrast radiography

Treatment

- Surgical transection of the vascular ring

Etiopathogenesis

Vascular rings caused by congenital anomalies of the aortic arches may constrict the esophagus and result in signs of obstruction. The aortic arch normally develops from the left fourth aortic arch and left dorsal aortic root in the embryo. The left sixth arch forms the ductus arteriosus, and the right fourth arch forms part of the right subclavian artery. In normal development, the aortic arch, ductus arteriosus, and pulmonary artery are positioned to the left of the esophagus, where they offer no resistance to swallowing. When the embryonic aortic arches develop abnormally, vascular rings can constrict the esophagus. Anomalies of the major vessels are common in canine anatomy specimens, with a prevalence of 20%. Few of these are vascular ring anomalies, and only a small fraction of the anomalies cause clinical signs of esophageal obstruction.

The most common vascular ring anomaly is caused by development of the aorta from the right fourth aortic arch instead of the left fourth aortic arch (PRAA). In this situation the esophagus becomes trapped between the heart ventrally, the aorta on the right, the pulmonary artery on the left, and the ductus arteriosus (ligamentum arteriosus) that connects these two vessels and crosses the dorsal border of the esophagus (Figure 11–14).

A variation of this anomaly occurs with retention of both arches, in which case the right arch forms a functional aortic arch and the left arch forms a remnant. Another clinically significant anomaly results if the left subclavian artery originates from the right aortic arch. The final position of the vessel is such that it has to pass to the left and over the esophagus to follow its normal pathway, resulting in a constriction of the

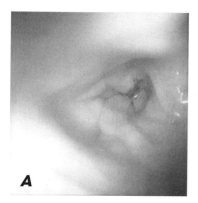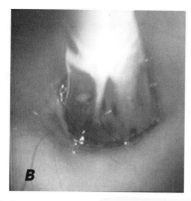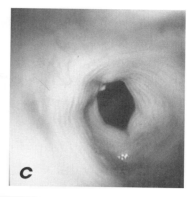

FIGURE 11-13. Endoscopic pictures of balloon dilation of an esophageal stricture in a cat. The cat developed the stricture following a general anesthesia. *(A)* The fibrous stricture before dilation, *(B)* The balloon positioned in the stricture and being inflated, *(C)* The dilated stricture—note the radial fibrous rings of the stricture and the normal esophageal diameter beyond the stricture.

esophagus. Esophageal abnormalities associated with a variety of other vascular anomalies have also been described.[170,171]

It is probable that vascular ring anomalies have an inherited basis. German shepherds and Irish setters have three times and ten times, respectively, the predicted risk of the normal population. Boston terriers are also at a higher than expected risk. Vascular rings are considerably less common in the cat, but persistent right aortic arch and constriction by ligamentum arteriosum have been described.

Clinical Signs

The most common clinical sign in affected animals is an acute onset of regurgitation at the time of weaning to solid foods. In 90% of all dogs with PRAA, the condition is identified before the age of six months.[169] Regurgitation usually occurs shortly after eating in the early stages of the disease, but as esophageal dilation progresses the regurgitation may become delayed. Affected puppies are malnourished, weak, and stunted. The food-filled esophagus may occasionally be palpated at the thoracic inlet. Coughing with respiratory distress is common and is indicative of a secondary aspiration pneumonia.

Diagnosis

The most important differential diagnosis is idiopathic megaesophagus. Unlike idiopathic megaesophagus, contrast radiography will usually reveal that the esophagus distal to the heart base is of normal diameter (Figure 11–15) whereas that cranial to the heart base is dilated to various degrees. Endoscopic evaluation of the esophagus will reveal an area of stenosis at the heart base without evidence of esophageal stricture. Examination of the esophagus by fluoroscopy reveals a loss of motility in the cranial portion of the esophagus, proportional to the degree of dilation. Esophageal motility caudal to the stricture can be normal or abnormal.

Treatment

Treatment consists of transection of the constricting bands forming the vascular ring. The prognosis for a complete

recovery is poor. Up to 50% of affected dogs continue to show occasional clinical signs after the surgery and as many as 40% do not survive long after surgery or are euthanized. Complications are common because of the initial malnourished and debilitated condition of the animal and the high incidence of concurrent aspiration pneumonia.[101] Permanent esophageal dilatation cranial to the constriction, as a result of irreversible degenerative changes in the esophagus, is common (Figure 11–15). Occasionally, esophageal dilatation develops caudal to the vascular ring, most probably due to interference with vagal function. Dogs with permanent esophageal disease following surgery should be managed as described for patients with megaesophagus.

MISCELLANEOUS CAUSES OF ESOPHAGEAL OBSTRUCTION

Periesophageal structures can enlarge and cause clinical signs of esophageal dysfunction. Esophageal compression can result from mediastinal masses such as enlarged bronchial or mediastinal lymph nodes (Figure 11–16). Tumors of the thoracic cavity, such as lymphosarcomas, thymomas, and heart-

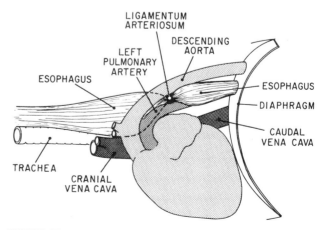

FIGURE 11-14. Drawing of thoracic structures in a pup with persistent right aortic arch that is constricting the esophagus and causing regurgitation.

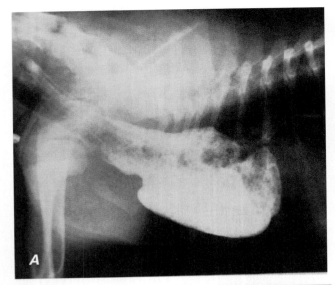

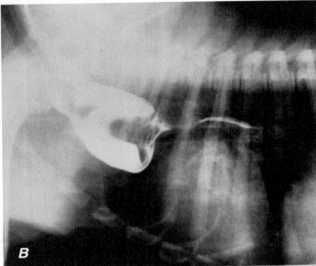

FIGURE 11-15. Persistent right aortic arch in 4-month-old Dalmatian. Lateral radiograph *(A)* was made following administration of contrast medium and shows dilated esophagus. The dilatation was caused by a stricture around the esophagus at the base of the heart. The stricture was surgically corrected and the dilatation was reexamined six weeks later. The later radiograph *(B)* illustrates that the dilatation in the esophagus persists. The clinical signs of regurgitation persist in many dogs following surgical correction of vascular anomalies that constrict the esophagus.

base tumors, are frequently associated with signs of esophageal obstruction. Neoplasms in the retropharyngeal and cervical area can compress the esophagus and produce clinical signs of obstruction.

Survey radiographs usually demonstrate a periesophageal mass. Contrast radiography confirms esophageal stenosis associated with the periesophageal mass. Esophagoscopy will reveal either luminal stenosis with no mucosal involvement or stricture formation if the mass has invaded the esophageal lumen. Treatment is directed toward the cause of the compressive lesion.

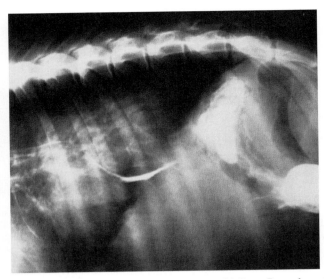

FIGURE 11-16. Mediastinal mass in 4-year-old Great Dane, lateral view. Clinical signs included dysphagia and regurgitation. The radiograph, made with the dog swallowing a positive-contrast medium, shows a ventral deviation of the esophagus that causes partial occlusion of the lumen. The mediastinal mass was caused by a migrating plant awn.

ESOPHAGEAL DIVERTICULA

Clinical Synopsis

Diagnostic Features

- Small diverticula may be subclinical
- Clinical signs of large diverticula include postprandial dyspnea, regurgitation, anorexia, fever, and/or weight loss
- Survey radiographs may reveal an air- or food-filled mass associated with the esophagus
- Barium swallow demonstrates a diverticulum

Treatment

- Surgical excision and reconstruction of the esophageal wall

Esophageal diverticula are pouch-like dilatations of the esophageal wall. They may be acquired or congenital and are rarely diagnosed in dogs and cats.[172] Esophageal diverticula are usually located at the thoracic inlet or in the thoracic esophagus just cranial to the diaphragm (epiphrenic location). Congenital diverticula are thought to develop due to congenital weakness of the esophageal wall, abnormal separation of tracheal and esophageal embryonic buds, or eccentric vacuole formation in the esophagus.[4] Acquired forms are subdivided into pulsion and traction diverticula, on the basis of their etiopathogenesis. Pulsion diverticula result from increased intraluminal pressure whereas traction diverticula are usually caused by contraction of periesophageal fibrous tissue.

Pulsion Diverticula

Increased esophageal intraluminal pressure, along with food accumulation and deep esophageal inflammation, is thought to lead to mucosal herniation and formation of pulsion diverticula. Proposed causes of pulsion diverticula include esophageal stenosis or a segmental abnormality of esophageal peristalsis.[150] Predisposing diseases include esophagitis, esophageal stricture, foreign bodies, vascular ring anomalies, megaesophagus, and hiatal hernia. Histologically, the wall of a pulsion diverticulum generally consists of only esophageal epithelium and connective tissue. Pulsion diverticula are found most often in the epiphrenic region.[172,173]

Traction Diverticula

In humans, traction diverticula usually result from inflammatory processes involving the trachea, bronchi, or hilar lymph nodes. In the authors' experience, the most common cause of traction diverticula in dogs is periesophageal inflammation resulting from perforation by foreign bodies. The inflammation leads to the production of fibrous tissue that later contracts, everting the esophageal wall into a pouch. Traction diverticula can occur anywhere along the esophagus. In contrast to a pulsion diverticulum, the traction diverticulum histologically consists of all four esophageal layers (adventitia, muscle, submucosa, and mucosa).

Diagnosis

Esophageal diverticula must be differentiated from the esophageal redundancy that is sometimes seen at the thoracic inlet of healthy young dogs, Chinese sharpeis, and dogs of brachycephalic breeds. Small amounts of contrast material or gas may accumulate in the redundancy, but repeat radiography with the neck extended removes the majority of the esophageal "slack" and results in a significant reduction in the size of the false diverticulum.

Small diverticula may be of little clinical significance. However, once a diverticulum is formed, it has the potential to accumulate ingesta. Esophageal impaction leads to chronic inflammation of the diverticulum which, in turn, can cause mucosal ulceration and ultimately rupture of the diverticulum with resultant mediastinitis.

Diverticula that cause clinical signs are usually large and multilobulated and may be inflamed or filled with food, bone, or foreign bodies.[4] Typical signs are distress or gasping shortly after eating, postprandial regurgitation, intermittent anorexia, fever, weight loss, and thoracic or abdominal pain. Diverticula can be identified on survey radiographs as either air- or food-filled masses in the area of the esophagus. Contrast procedures will demonstrate pooling of contrast in the diverticulum. Esophagoscopy confirms the diagnosis and identifies associated complications such as ulceration and scarring.

Management

Small diverticula, without other esophageal lesions, may be treated conservatively by using a soft bland diet, feeding the animal in an upright position, and providing ample liquids to minimize food accumulation in the pouch. Large diverticula require surgical excision and reconstruction of the esophageal wall, which warrants a less favorable prognosis. Any underlying cause must be treated appropriately.

ESOPHAGEAL NEOPLASIA

Clinical Synopsis

Diagnostic Features

- Slowly progressive regurgitation and weight loss
- Survey radiographs may reveal a dilated esophageal segment
- Barium swallow demonstrates esophageal stenosis
- Diagnosis confirmed by endoscopic, surgical, or percutaneous needle biopsy

Treatment

- Surgical excision of benign lesions
- Palliation of malignant lesions with bougienage and/or radiation therapy
- Treatment of *Spirocerca lupi* if present (see text)

Neoplasia of the esophagus, whether primary or metastatic, is uncommon in dogs and cats. Metastatic esophageal cancers are diagnosed more frequently than primary tumors but are still uncommon.[85] Metastatic tumors affecting the esophagus include thyroid carcinoma, bronchial carcinoma, gastric carcinoma, squamous cell carcinoma (especially tonsillar), and mammary adenocarcinoma.[174] In cats and dogs the most frequent primary esophageal cancers are squamous cell carcinomas and fibrosarcomas.[175,176] The esophageal sarcomas in dogs are usually associated with the parasite *Spirocerca lupi*.[176] Other reported primary tumors include leiomyosarcoma, osteosarcoma, and undifferentiated carcinomas.[174,178] Benign tumors are uncommon in the esophagus with the exception of leiomyomas, which have a high prevalence in older dogs and are usually found at the gastroesophageal junction.[174,177] With the exception of spirocercosis, the cause of esophageal cancer is usually not established. In humans, contamination of diets with nitrosamines has been implicated, however.

In the United States, *Spirocerca lupi* frequently result in esophageal fibrosarcomas, some of which undergo metaplastic transformation into osteogenic sarcomas.[176] The malignant lesions are found in the thoracic esophagus, the site typically occupied by this parasite. Interestingly, the association between *S. lupi* and esophageal neoplasia is not seen in all countries.

Adult *S. lupi* live in the wall of the esophagus. The parasite lays eggs that pass into the lumen of the esophagus and are subsequently eliminated from the body in feces. Eggs ingested by coprophagic beetles hatch, after which the larvae encyst in the beetle. This stage is infective for dogs. Alternately, the larvae can be ingested by rodents and birds that act as transport hosts in which they reencyst. Dogs are the definitive host. After ingestion of the beetle or transport host, the encysted larva is freed, invades the wall of the stomach, and migrates to the aorta by following the adventitia of arteries. The larvae concentrate in the thoracic aorta and migrate through small vessels to the esophagus, where they mature. Larvae that migrate mistakenly to other tissues become encysted. Larval migration and worm nodules in the esophagus can cause spondylitis in the adjacent bodies of vertebrae and aortic aneurysms as well as granulomatous lesions and neoplasia in the esophagus (Figure 11–17). Hypertrophic osteopathy has been reported in dogs with esophageal fibrosarcoma with and without pulmonary metastasis.[179]

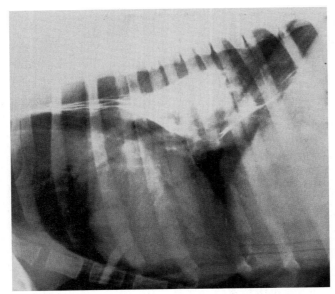

FIGURE 11-17. Lateral radiograph of dog with esophageal granuloma due to *Spirocerca lupi*. Spondylitic lesions are also evident. (Courtesy of Dr. J.E. Bartels, School of Veterinary Medicine, Auburn University)

Clinical Signs

Esophageal tumors usually occur in dogs and cats over six years of age. The clinical signs of esophageal neoplasia are those of a slowly progressive esophageal stenosis. Regurgitation, dysphagia, drooling, odynophagia, and weight loss are frequently seen. The clinical signs of dogs with spirocercosis can be quite variable including respiratory distress and hemothorax from rupture of the thoracic aneurysm.[180]

Diagnosis

Radiographic procedures may reveal evidence of esophageal stenosis in affected animals. The earliest and most consistent radiographic sign is retention of intraluminal gas cranial to the tumor. Other abnormalities observed on survey films can include displacement of periesophageal structures and soft tissue or mineral densities in the mediastinum. Positive-contrast radiography may delineate a stenotic area but endoscopy is necessary to allow visualization of the mass and permit biopsy.

Occasionally cancers of the esophagus will result in generalized esophageal dysmotility detectable by fluoroscopy. Diagnosis of *S. lupi* is based on observation of embryonated eggs in fecal flotations, thoracic radiography, and esophagoscopy.[180]

Treatment

Surgical resection of benign tumors can be curative. Malignant tumors, however, carry a poor prognosis. Surgical intervention is often not practical because of a high rate of postoperative stricture. Radiation therapy may be palliative but radiation-induced esophagitis is a potential sequela. Bougienage of neoplastic strictures may produce palliation but great care is required to avoid esophageal perforation.

Treatment of *S. lupi* infections has included the use of disophenol, diethylcarbamazine, and dithiazine iodide,[176,180]

and the surgical removal of the esophageal granulomas.[180] Fenbendazole and related compounds may be a useful adjunct, because they are effective against spirocerca larvae in extraintestinal tissue.

AIRWAY-ESOPHAGEAL FISTULA

Clinical Synopsis

Diagnostic Features

- Regurgitation
- Paroxysmal cough particularly after eating or drinking
- Survey radiographs may reveal bronchopneumonia in a single lobe
- Contrast study or esophagoscopy sometimes reveals fistula
- Fistula between airway and esophagus confirmed by thoracotomy

Treatment

- Lobectomy and repair of esophageal deficit

Fistula between the esophagus and airways have occasionally been reported in dogs. Bronchoesophageal fistula are the most commonly reported type of fistula, but tracheoesophageal and pulmonary-esophageal fistula can also occur.[181,182] Esophageal fistula usually develop secondary to foreign body perforation. The right caudal bronchus is frequently involved. A congenital form of esophageal fistula, probably due to incomplete separation of the esophagus and airways during embryonic development, has also been reported, and Cairn terriers may be predisposed.[4,183]

Clinical signs of esophageal fistula include coughing, regurgitation, and dysphagia. Coughing associated with drinking or eating is frequently observed but may not be present in all cases.[182] Anorexia, lethargy, weight loss, and pyrexia are also observed and are attributable to mediastinitis or bronchopneumonia. Crackles may be auscultated over affected lung regions on physical examination.

Survey thoracic radiographs may demonstrate radiopaque foreign bodies in the esophagus or bronchus, pulmonary consolidation, and pleural fluid accumulation (Figure 11-18). Localized lung pathology adjacent to an esophageal foreign body should always alert the clinician to the possibility of a fistula.[3] Contrast esophagrams will often confirm the presence of the respiratory tract communication (Figure 11-19), but false negative studies can occur.[182] Be wary of excessive contamination of the pulmonary system with hyperosmolar contrast radiography solutions because pulmonary edema may result. Esophagoscopy and bronchoscopy should be attempted but may prove futile in identifying the origin of the fistulous tract.

Surgical correction of the fistulous tract should be attempted. Lobectomy is often required because of foreign bodies in the airway, consolidated pulmonary tissue, or bronchopneumonia. If the animal survives the immediate postsurgical period the prognosis is good.

HIATAL HERNIA

Clinical Synopsis

Diagnostic Features

- Sharpeis are predisposed
- Congenital or acquired forms are observed

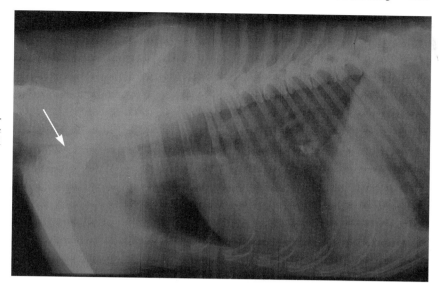

FIGURE 11–18. Radiograph demonstrating calcified material in the right caudal lung lobe (arrow). Surgery revealed a bronchoesophageal fistula and a piece of bone wedged in the airway.

- Signs include regurgitation, vomiting, dyspnea, and hypersalivation
- Survey or contrast radiography usually reveals herniation at esophageal hiatus, but fluoroscopy may be required

Treatment

- Congenital form requires restorative surgery
- Acquired form often can be managed with H$_2$ blockers (e.g., cimetidine 5 mg/kg q 8 hours), sucralfate (0.25–1 g per animal q 8 hours), and/or metoclopramide (0.2–0.4 mg/kg q 6–8 hours)   *Cisapride*

The diaphragmatic perforation through which the esophagus passes is called the esophageal hiatus. The esophagus is attached to the hiatus by a phrenicoesophageal ligament (Figure 11–20), which normally allows only minor cranial movement of the abdominal esophageal segment. Congenital or acquired lesions of the hiatus can lead to an axial (sliding) hiatal hernia, paraesophageal hiatal hernia, or a combination of axial and paraesophageal hiatal hernias (Figure 11–20).[184–188]

Hiatal (sliding) hernias result from a stretching of the phrenicoesophageal ligament allowing herniation of the abdominal esophagus, gastroesophageal junction, gastric cardia, and, at times, other parts of the stomach or other abdominal organs into the thoracic cavity via the hiatus (Figure 11–20). At times, the herniated organs may move back and forth from the thoracic to abdominal cavity creating diagnostic difficulty. Gastroesophageal reflux often accompanies hiatal hernia in dogs and cats, and frequently results in an accompanying esophagitis. The cause of the esophagitis may be increased frequency of reflux and/or slower clearance of refluxed material.[117] Both congenital and acquired forms of hiatal hernia are recognized. The congenital form of the disease is most common[187] and is best described in young Sharpei dogs.[25,184,185,188,189] Hiatal hernias can be acquired as a result of trauma and have also been reported in association with tetanus.[61,115]

Paraesophageal hiatal hernias are rare and involve displacement of a portion of the stomach (usually the fundus) through the hiatus without cranial displacement of the gastroesophageal junction (Figure 11–20).[184,186] Paraesophageal hernias do not usually lower GES pressure and may be sub-

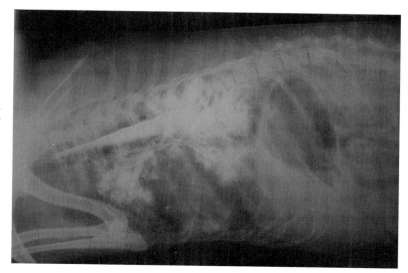

FIGURE 11–19. Radiographic demonstration of a bronchoesophageal fistula. The contrast material (Gastrograffin) was given per os and can be clearly seen entering the airway. Life-threatening pulmonary edema was precipitated in this patient.

clinical unless a large part of the stomach (or other abdominal organs) herniate and are strangulated.

Clinical Signs and Diagnosis

The clinical signs associated with hiatal (sliding) hernias in dogs and cats primarily result from reflux esophagitis (see earlier), and can include occasional or persistent regurgitation, vomiting, dyspnea, and hypersalivation. Abdominal pain may be evident on palpation. Occasionally, affected animals are asymptomatic.[187] The clinical signs are usually more severe with the congenital form of the disease. In congenital hiatal hernia, survey radiographs usually reveal a caudodorsal intrathoracic soft tissue opacity suggestive of a hiatal hernia (Figure 11–21). Many dogs with congenital hiatal hernias also have secondary esophageal dilation and alveolar infiltrates. Occasionally, the hiatal hernia is associated with a shortened esophagus.[184,187] Chronic gastroesophageal reflux can lead to a shortened esophagus by causing esophageal scarring, resulting in the GES and gastric cardia becoming irreducibly fixed in the thorax.[184]

In the acquired disease, one or more barium esophograms or fluoroscopy are often required to confirm the diagnosis. It is noteworthy that radiographs of dogs and cats taken during vomition may lead to an incorrect diagnosis of hiatal hernia because it is common for the stomach to invaginate into the esophagus during vomiting.

Treatment

Medical management of congenital hiatal hernia is usually ineffective and restorative surgery is frequently required.

Postoperative complications and mortality can be high. The surgical technique must be chosen carefully to obtain relief of clinical signs but avoid complications such as gastric tympany due to inability to eructate.[184,190] Successful techniques have included diaphragmatic crural apposition, esophagopexy, modified Nissen fundoplication, and left fundic tube gastropexy.[184,185,189,190] The necessity for antireflux procedures such as fundoplication in addition to surgical restoration of normal anatomy has not been established in dogs.[190]

In contrast to animals with congenital hiatal hernia, those with acquired lesions often respond well to medical management.[185] Affected dogs and cats should be fed frequently in small quantities (to minimize gastric pressure and the likelihood of reflux). As for reflux esophagitis, low-fat diets are probably advantageous. Useful medical management includes sucralfate, H_2 blockers, and motility modifiers such as metoclopramide.[185] Animals with large acquired hiatal hernias or those that do not respond to medical management should be considered surgical candidates.

Gastroesophageal Intussusception

Gastroesophageal intussusception describes the invagination of all or parts of the stomach into the thoracic esophagus. In severe cases, the spleen and pancreas may be herniated as well. In contrast to axial hiatal hernias, the gastroesophageal junction does not displace into the thorax. Idiopathic megaesophagus or incompetency of the GES may predispose dogs to this disorder.[86,191]

Although uncommon, gastroesophageal intussusception is most often seen in large breed dogs less than three months of

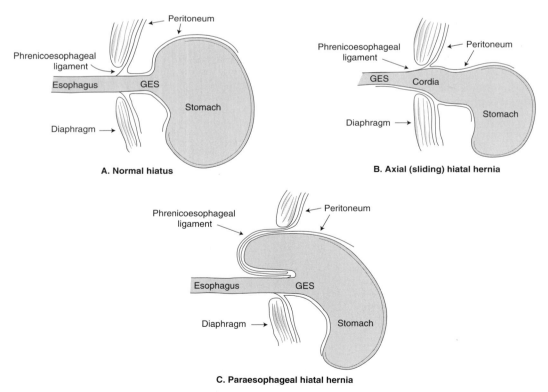

FIGURE 11–20. Classification of hiatal hernias. *(A)* Normal hiatus, *(B)* Axial (sliding) hiatal hernia, *(C)* Paraesophageal hiatal hernia. (Modified from Williams JM (1990)[188])

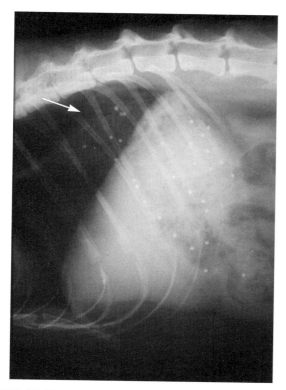

FIGURE 11–21. Radiograph of a hiatal hernia (arrow) in a domestic shorthaired cat. The hernia contains a small number of barium-impregnated plastic spheres (BIPS, Ken Bowman Assocs, Diamond Bar, CA). The cat's primary clinical sign was vomiting and the BIPS were being used for a gastric-emptying study when the hernia was discovered.

age.[192,193] German shepherds, in particular, are predisposed. The clinical signs are of esophageal obstruction and mortality is very high. Acute regurgitation, dyspnea, and hematemesis may be seen. Affected dogs may die acutely, presumably because of poor venous return, shock, and/or gaseous distension of the herniated stomach within the chest. Diagnosis is usually made by radiography. One of the author's (WGG) has diagnosed the condition via endoscopy. The endoscopy revealed a dilated esophagus packed full of redundant mucosal folds among which it was difficult to find the GES. Following continued insufflation of the esophagus (with the cranial esophagus held closed by digital pressure), the folds of mucosa began to move caudally until they finally popped through the GES leaving a residual megaesophagus. Successful surgical treatment has also been reported using a belt loop gastropexy.[194]

REFERENCES

1. Peeters ME, Venker-van Haagen AJ, Wolvekamp WThC. Evaluation of a standardized questionnaire for the detection of dysphagia in 69 dogs. Vet Rec 132:211–213, 1993.
2. Stickle RL, Love NE. Radiographic diagnosis of esophageal diseases in dogs and cats. Sem Vet Med Surg 4:179–187, 1989.
3. Parker NR, Walter PA, Gay J. Diagnosis and surgical management of esophageal perforation. J Am Anim Hosp Assoc 25:587–595, 1989.
4. Suter PF. Thoracic Radiography. PF Suter, Wettswil, Switzerland, 295–349, 1984.
5. Watrous BJ. Clinical presentation and diagnosis of dysphagia. Vet Clin N Am 13:437–459, 1983.
6. Harvey CE, O'Brien JA. Esophageal disease and disorders. Proc Am Anim Hosp Assoc 155–161, 1975.
7. Watrous BJ, Suter PF. Normal swallowing in the dog: A cineradiographic study. Vet Radiol 20:99–109, 1979.
8. Suter PF, Watrous BJ. Oropharyngeal dysphagias in the dog: A cinefluo-rographic analysis of experimentally induced and spontaneously occurring swallowing disorders. I. Oral and pharyngeal stage dysphagias. Vet Radiol 24:11–24, 1983.
9. Watrous BJ, Suter PF. Oropharyngeal dysphagias in the dog: A cinefluo-rographic analysis of experimentally induced and spontaneously occurring swallowing disorders. II. Cricopharyngeal stage and mixed oropharyngeal dysphagias. Vet Radiol 24:11–24, 1983.
10. Miller AJ. Deglutition. Physiol Rev 62:129–184, 1982.
11. White RAS, Lane JG. Pharyngeal stick penetration injuries in the dog. J Sm Anim Pract 29:13–35, 1988.
12. Peeters ME, van Haagen AJV, Goedegeburre SA, et al. Dysphagia in Bouviers associated with muscular dystrophy; evaluation of 24 cases. Vet Q 13:65–73, 1991.
13. Boudrieu RJ, Rogers WA. Megaesophagus in the dog: A review of 50 cases. J Am Anim Hosp Assoc 21:33–40, 1985.
14. Harvey CE, O'Brien JA, et al. Megaesophagus in the dog: A clinical survey of 79 cases. J Am Vet Med Assoc 165:443–446, 1974.
15. Strombeck DR. Pathophysiology of esophageal motility disorders in the dog and cat. Vet Clin N Am 8:229–244, 1984.
16. Leib MS. Megaesophagus in the dog. In: Kirk RW (ed) Current Veterinary Therapy IX. WB Saunders, Philadelphia, 848–851, 1986.
17. Strombeck DR. Diseases of swallowing. In: Strombeck DR, Guilford WG (eds), Small Animal Gastroenterology. Stonegate 2, Davis, CA, 50–67, 1979.
18. Pearson H, Gaskell CJ, et al. Pyloric and oesophageal dysfunction in the cat. J Sm Anim Pract 15:487–501, 1974.
19. Hoenig M, Mahaffey MB, Parnell PG, et al. Megaesophagus in two cats. J Am Vet Med Assoc 196:763–765, 1990.
20. Maddison JE, Allan GS. Megaesophagus attributable to lead toxicosis in a cat. J Am Vet Med Assoc 197:1357–1358, 1990.
21. Osborne CA, Clifford DH, Jessen C. Hereditary esophageal achalasia in dogs. J Am Vet Med Assoc 151:572–581, 1967.
22. Strating A, Clifford DH. Canine achalasia with special reference to hereditary. Southwest Vet 19:135–137, 1966.
23. Cox VS, Wallace LJ, et al. Hereditary esophageal dysfunction in the Miniature Schnauzer dog. Am J Vet Res 41:326–330, 1980.
24. Knowles KE, O'Brien DP, Amann JF. Congenital idiopathic megaesophagus in a litter of Chinese Shar Peis: Clinical, electrodiagnostic, and pathological studies. J Am Anim Hosp Assoc 26:313–318, 1990.
25. Stickle R, Sparschu G, Love N, et al. Radiographic evaluation of esophageal function in Chinese Shar Pei pups. J Am Vet Med Assoc 201:81–84, 1992.
26. Breshears DE. Esophageal dilation in six-week-old male German Shepherd pups. VM/SAC 60:1034–1036, 1965.
27. Palmer CS. Achalasia or cardiospasms in Great Dane puppies. VM/SAC 63:574–578, 1968.
28. Leib MS. Megaesophagus in the dog. Comp Cont Ed Pract Vet 5:825–833, 1983.
29. Schwartz A, Ravin CE, et al. Congenital neuromuscular esophageal disease in a litter of Newfoundland puppies. J Am Vet Radiol Soc 17:101–103, 1976.
30. Spy GM. Megaesophagus in a litter of Greyhounds. Vet Rec 75:853–854, 1963.
31. Clifford DH, Soifer FK, et al. Congenital achalasia of the esophagus in four cats of common ancestry. J Am Vet Med Assoc 158:1554–1560, 1971.
32. Watrous BJ. Esophageal disease. In: Ettinger SJ (ed) Textbook of Veterinary Internal Medicine. WB Saunders Philadelphia, 1191–1233, 1983.
33. Diamant N, Szczepanski M, Mui H. Manometric characteristics of idiopathic megaesophagus in the dog: An unsuitable animal model for achalasia in man. Gastroenterology 65:216–223, 1973.
34. Gray GW. Acute experiments on neuroeffector function in canine esophageal achalasia. Am J Vet Res 35:1075–1081, 1974.
35. Sokolvsky V. Achalasia and paralysis of the canine esophagus. J Am Vet Med Assoc 260:943–955, 1972.
36. Strombeck DR, Troya L. Evaluation of lower motor neuron function in two dogs with megaesophagus. J Am Vet Med Assoc 169:411–414, 1976.
37. Clifford DH, Gyorkey F. Myenteric ganglial cells in dogs with and without achalasia of the esophagus. J Am Vet Med Assoc 150:205–211, 1967.
38. Clifford DH. Myenteric ganglial cells of the esophagus in cats with achalasia of the esophagus. Am J Vet Res 34:1333–1335, 1973.
39. Nakayama S, Neya T, et al. Effects of electrical stimulation and local destruction of the medulla oblongata on swallowing movements in dogs. Rendic Gastroenterol 6:6–11, 1974.
40. Higgs B, Kerr FWF, Ellis FH. The experimental production of esophageal achalasia by electrolytic lesions in the medulla. J Thor Cardio Surg 50:613–625, 1965.
41. Rogers WA, Fenner WR, Sherding RG. Electromyographic and esophagomanometric findings in clinically normal dogs and in dogs with idiopathic megaesophagus. J Am Vet Med Assoc 174:181–183, 1979.
42. Clifford DH, Pirsch JG, Mauldin ML. Comparison of motor nuclei of the vagus nerve in dogs with and without esophageal achalasia. Proc Soc Exp Biol Med 142:878–882, 1973.

43. Leipold H. Unpublished observations cited by Guffy MM. Esophageal disorders. In: Ettinger SJ (ed) Veterinary Internal Medicine. WB Saunders, Philadelphia, 1975.

44. Tan BJK, Diamant NE. Assessment of the neural defect in a dog with idiopathic megaesophagus. Dig Dis Sci 32:76–85, 1987.

45. Satchell PM. The neuropathic oesophagus. A radiographic and manometric study on the evolution of megaesophagus in dogs with developing axonal neuropathy. Res Vet Sci 48:249–255, 1990.

46. Janssens J, Valembois P, Hellemans J, et al. Studies on the necessity of a bolus for the progression of secondary peristalsis in the canine esophagus. Gastroenterology 67:245–251, 1974.

47. Strombeck DR. Unpublished observations, 1990.

48. Diamant N, Szczepanski M, Mui H. Idiopathic megaesophagus in the dog: Reasons for spontaneous improvement and a possible method of medical therapy. Can Vet J 15:66–71, 1974.

49. Holland CT, Satchell PM, Farrow BRH. Oesophageal compliance in naturally occurring canine megaesophagus. Aust Vet J 70:414–420, 1993.

50. Forbes DC, Leishman DE. Megaesophagus in a cat. Can Vet J 26:354–356, 1985.

51. Crawley AJ, Gendreau CL. Esophageal achalasia in a cat. Can Vet J 10:195–197, 1969.

52. Krum SH, Cardinet GH, et al. Polymyositis and polyarthritis associated with systemic lupus erythematosis in a dog. J Am Vet Med Assoc 170:61–64, 1977.

53. Marsden PD, Hagstrom JWC. Experimental *Trypanosoma cruzi* infection in beagle puppies. Trans Royal Soc Trop Med Hyg 62:816, 1968.

54. Walvort HC, VanNess JJ, et al. Canine glycogen storage disease type II: A clinical study of four affected Lapland dogs. J Am Anim Hosp Assoc 20:279–286, 1984.

55. Kornegay JN, Gorgacz EJ, et al. Polymyositis in dogs. J Am Vet Med Assoc 176:431–438, 1980.

56. Haupt KH, Prieur DJ, et al. Familial canine dermatomyositis: Clinical, electrodiagnostic, and genetic studies. Am J Vet Res 46:1861–1869, 1985.

57. Gaschen FP, Hoffman EP, et al. Dystrophin deficiency causes lethal muscle hypertrophy in cats. J Neurol Sci 110:149–159, 1992.

58. Holland CT, Canfield PJ, et al. Dyserythropoiesis, polymyopathy, and cardiac disease in three related English Springer spaniels. J Vet Int Med 5:151–159, 1991.

59. Darke PGG, Roberts TA, et al. Suspected botulism in foxhounds. Vet Rec 99:98–100, 1976.

60. Van Nes JJ. Electrophysiological evidence of peripheral nerve dysfunction in six dogs with botulism type C. Res Vet Sci 40:372–376, 1986.

61. Dieringer TM, Wolf AM. Esophageal hiatal hernia and megaesophagus complicating tetanus in two dogs. J Am Vet Med Assoc 199:87–89, 1991.

62. Knauer CM, Carbone JV, et al. Alimentary tract and liver. In: Krupp MA, Chatton MJ, Werdegar D (eds) Current Medical Diagnosis and Treatment. Lange, Los Altos, 352–432, 1985.

63. Mason KV. A case of myasthenia gravis in a cat. J Sm Anim Pract 17:467–472, 1976.

64. Miller LM, Lennon VA, et al. Congenital myasthenia gravis in 13 smooth Fox terriers. J Am Vet Med Assoc 182:694–702, 1983.

65. Shelton GD, Willard MD, Cardinet GH, et al. Acquired myasthenia gravis, selective involvement of esophageal, pharyngeal and facial muscles. J Vet Int Med 4:281–284, 1990.

66. Harris LD, Ashworth WD, Ingelfinger FJ. Esophageal aperistalsis and achalasia produced in dogs by prolonged cholinesterase inhibition. J Clin Invest 39:1744–1751, 1960.

67. Cummings JF, deLahunta A, Mitchell WJ. Ganglioradiculitis in the dog. Acta Neuropathol 60:29–31, 1983.

68. Sharp, NJH, Nash AS. Feline dysautonomia. In: Kirk RW (ed) Current Vet Therapy IX. WB Saunders, Philadelphia, 802–804, 1986.

69. Schrauwen E, van Ham L, Maenhout T, et al. Canine dysautonomia: A case report. Vet Rec 128:524–525, 1991.

70. Zook BC, Gilmore CE. Thallium poisoning in dogs. J Am Vet Med Assoc 151:206–217, 1967.

71. Duncan ID, Griffiths IR. Canine giant axonal neuropathy; some aspects of its clinical, pathological and comparative features. J Sm Anim Pract 22:491–501, 1981.

72. Shell LG, Jortner BS, Leib MS. Spinal muscular atrophy in two Rottweiler littermates. J Am Vet Med Assoc 190:878–880, 1987.

73. Zook BC. The pathologic anatomy of lead poisoning in dogs. Vet Pathol 9:310–327, 1972.

74. O'Brien JA, Harvey CE, Brodey RS. The esophagus. In: Anderson NV (ed) Veterinary Gastroenterology. Lea & Febiger, Philadelphia, 372, 1980.

75. Van Ee RT, Dodd VM, et al. Bronchoesophageal fistula and transient megaesophagus in a dog. J Am Vet Med Assoc 188:874–875, 1986.

76. Cassella RR, Brown AL, et al. Achalasia of the esophagus: Pathologic and etiologic considerations. Am Surg 160:474–487, 1964.

77. Hara T. Experimental study on the pathogenesis of achalasia. Jpn J Smooth Mus Res 5:33–36, 1969.

78. Fox JG, Averill DR, et al. Familial reflex myoclonus in Labrador retrievers. Am J Vet Res 45:2367–2370, 1984.

79. Nelson RW, Ihle SL, et al. Serum free thyroxine concentration in healthy dogs, dogs with hypothyroidism, and euthyroid dogs with concurrent illness. J Am Vet Med Assoc 198:1401–1407, 1991.

80. Pidgeon G. Unpublished observations, 1987.

81. Chastain CB, Ganjam VK. Clinical Endocrinology of Companion Animals. Lea & Febiger, Philadelphia, 1986.

82. Feldman EC, Tyrrell JB. Hypoadrenocorticism. Vet Clin N Am 7:555–581, 1977.

83. Schaer M, Riley WJ, et al. Autoimmunity and Addison's disease in the dog. J Am Anim Hosp Assoc 22:789–794, 1986.

84. Bartges JW, Nielson DL. Reversible megaesophagus associated with atypical primary hypoadrenocorticism in a dog. J Am Vet Med Assoc 201:889–891, 1992.

85. Roudebush P, Jones BD, Vaughan RW. Medical aspects of esophageal disease. In: Jones BD (ed) Canine and Feline Gastroenterology. WB Saunders, Philadelphia, 54–80, 1986.

86. Hoffer RE. Surgical esophageal disease. In: Bojorab MJ (ed) Pathophysiology in Small Animal Surgery. Lea & Febiger, Philadelphia, 90–100, 1981.

87. Ridgeway RL, Suter PF. Clinical and radiographic signs in primary and metastatic esophageal neoplasms of the dog. J Am Vet Med Assoc 174:700–704, 1979.

88. Carpenter JL, Holzworth J. Thymoma in 11 cats. J Am Vet Med Assoc 181:248–251, 1982.

89. Darke PGG, McCullagh KG, Geldart PH. Myasthenia gravis, thymoma and myositis in a dog. Vet Rec 97:392–394, 1975.

90. Eastwood GL, Castell DO, Higgs RH. Experimental esophagitis in cats impairs lower esophageal sphincter pressure. Gastroenterology 69:146–153, 1975.

91. Henderson RD, Mugashe F, et al. The role of bile and acid in the production of esophagitis and the motor defect of esophagitis. Ann Thorac Surg 14:465–473, 1972.

92. Bishop LM, Kelly DF, et al. Megaloesophagus and associated gastric heterotopia in the cat. Vet Pathol 16:444–449, 1979.

93. Guilford WG. Unpublished observations, 1986.

94. Washabau RJ. Effects of calcium channel antagonism (nifedipine or verapamil) and guanylate cyclase activation (sodium nitroprusside) on canine lower esophageal sphincter function. Abstract, Proc 11th Am Cl Vet Int Med, Washington, DC, 943, 1993.

95. Hofmeyer CFB. An evaluation of cardioplasty for achalasia of the esophagus in the dog. J Sm Anim Pract 7:281–287, 1966.

96. Hoffer RE. Primary esophageal neuromuscular diseases. In: Jones BD (ed) Canine and Feline Gastroenterology. WB Saunders, Philadelphia, 89–100, 1986.

97. Hoffer RE, MacCoy DM, et al. Management of acquired achalasia in dogs. J Am Vet Med Assoc 175:814–817, 1979.

98. Hoffer RE, MacCoy DM, et al. Physiologic features of the canine esophagus: Effect of modified Heller's esophagomyotomy. Am J Vet Res 41:723–726, 1980.

99. Hofmeyr CFB. An evaluation of cardioplasty for achalasia of the oesophagus in the dog. J Sm Anim Pract 7:281–301, 1966.

100. Hendricks JC, Maggio-Price L, Dougherty JF. Transient esophageal dysfunction mimicking megaesophagus in three dogs. J Am Vet Med Assoc 185:90–92, 1984.

101. Shires PK, Lui W. Persistent right aortic arch in dogs: A long-term follow-up after surgical correction. J Am Anim Hosp Assoc 17:773–776, 1981.

102. Hovda LR. Toxicities from common household agents. Proc 11th Am Col Vet Int Med Forum, Washington, DC, 282–285, 1993.

103. Studley JGN, Linehan IP, et al. Swallowed button batteries: Is there a consensus on management? Gut 31:867–870, 1990.

104. Alder PL. Phycomycosis in fifteen dogs and two cats. J Am Vet Med Assoc 174:1217–1223, 1979.

105. O'Brien TR. Radiographic Diagnosis of Abdominal Disorders in the Dog and Cat: Radiographic Interpretation—Clinical Signs—Pathophysiology. WB Saunders, Philadelphia, 1978.

106. Hillemeier C, Gryboski J, et al. Developmental characteristics of the lower esophageal sphincter in the kitten. Gastroenterology 89:760–766, 1985.

107. Patrikios J, Martin CJ, Dent J. Relationship of transient lower esophageal sphincter relaxation to postprandial gastroesophageal reflux and belching in dogs. Gastroenterology 90:545–551, 1986.

108. Dodds WJ, Dent J, et al. Mechanisms of gastroesophageal reflux in patients with reflux esophagitis. New Engl J Med 307:1547–1552, 1982.

109. Dodds WJ, Hogan WJ, et al. Pathogenesis of reflux esophagitis. Gastroenterology 81:376–394, 1981.

110. Strombeck DR, Harrold D, Ferrier W. Eructation of gas through the gastroesophageal sphincter before and after truncal vagotomy in dogs. Am J Vet Res 48:207–210, 1987.

111. Martin CJ, Patrikios J, Dent J. Abolition of gas reflux and transient lower esophageal sphincter relaxation by vagal blockade in the dog. Gastroenterology 91:894–896, 1986.

112. Sarna SK, Gleysteen JJ, Ryan RP. Fundic motor activity and its role in gastroesophageal reflux. Gastroenterology 91:1615, 1986.

113. Boyle JT, Altschuler SM, et al. Responses of feline gastroesophageal junc-

tion to changes in abdominal pressure. Am J Physiol 253:G315–G322, 1987.

114. Holloway RA, Hongo M, et al. Gastric distention: A mechanism for postprandial gastroesophageal reflux. Gastroenterology 89:779–784, 1985.
115. van Ham L, van Bree H. Conservative treatments of tetanus associated with hiatus hernia and gastro-oesophageal reflux. J Sm Anim Pract 33:289–294, 1992.
116. Edwards MH. Selective vagotomy of the canine oesophagus—a model for the treatment of hiatal hernia. Thorax 31:185–189, 1976.
117. Hetzel DJ, Heddle R. Gastroesophageal reflux disease, pH monitoring, and treatment. Curr Opin G 9:629–640, 1993.
118. Gill RC, Kellow JR, Windgate DL. Gastroesophageal reflux and the migrating motor complex. Gut 28:929–934, 1987.
119. Hall AW, Moosa AR, et al. The effects of premedication drugs on the lower oesophageal high pressure zone and reflux status of Rhesus monkeys and man. Gut 16:347–352, 1975.
120. Misiewicz JJ. Symposium on gastroesophageal reflux and its complications. Sec. 4, Pharmacology and therapeutics. Gut 14:243–246, 1973.
121. Pope CE. Pathophysiology and diagnosis of reflux esophagitis. Gastroenterology 70:445–464, 1973.
122. Strombeck DR, Harrold D. Effects of atropine, acepromazine, meperidine, and xylazine on gastroesophageal sphincter pressure in the dog. Am J Vet Res 46:963–965, 1985.
123. Hashim MA, Waterman AE. Effects of thiopentone, propofol, alphaxalone-alphadolone, ketamine and xylazine-ketamine on lower oesophageal sphincter pressure and barrier pressure in cats. Vet Rec 129:137–139, 1991.
124. Waterman AE, Hashim MA. Effects of thiopentone and propofol on lower oesophageal sphincter and barrier pressure in the dog. J Sm Anim Pract 33:530–533, 1992.
125. Roush JK, Keene BW, Eicker SW, et al. Effects of atropine and glycopyrrolate on esophageal, gastric, and tracheal pH in anesthetized dogs. Vet Surg 19:88–92, 1990.
126. Baue AE, Hoffer RE. The effects of experimental hiatal hernia and histamine stimulation on the intrinsic esophageal sphincter. Surg Gynecol Obstet 125:791–799, 1967.
127. Carvalho P, Richter H, et al. Gastroesophageal reflux (GER) slows gastric emptying in dogs. Gastroenterology 94:A61, 1989.
128. Biancani P, Barwick K, et al. Effects of acute experimental esophagitis on mechanical properties of the lower esophageal sphincter. Gastroenterology 87:8–16, 1984.
129. Liebermann-Meffert D, Klaus D, et al. Effect of intraesophageal bile and acid (HCl) perfusion on the action of the lower esophageal sphincter. Scand J Gastroenterlgy 19(suppl 92):237–241, 1984.
130. DeBacker A, Haentjens P, Willems G. Hydrochloric acid: A trigger of cell proliferation in the esophagus of dogs. Dig Dis Sci 30:884–890, 1985.
131. Salo JA, Lehto VP, Kivilaakso E. Morphological alterations in experimental esophagitis. Dig Dis Sci 28:440–448, 1983.
132. Flanders JA. Problems and complications associated with esophageal surgery. Prob Vet Med 1:183–194, 1989.
133. Mittal RK, Reuben A, et al. Do bile acids reflux into the esophagus? Gastroenterology 92:371–375, 1987.
134. Lillemoe KD, Johnson LF, Harmon JW. Alkaline esophagitis: A comparison of the ability of components of gastroduodenal contents to injure the rabbit esophagus. Gastroenterology 85:621–628, 1983.
135. Salo JA, Kivilaakso E. Contribution of trypsin and cholate to the pathogenesis of experimental alkaline reflux esophagitis. Scand J Gastroenterol 19:875–881, 1984.
136. Evander A, Little AG, et al. Composition of the refluxed material determines the degree of reflux esophagitis in the dog. Gastroenterology 93:280–286, 1987.
137. Carlborg B, Densert O. Esophageal lesions caused by orally administered drugs. Eur Surg Res 12:270–282, 1980.
138. Bonavina L, DeMeester TR, et al. Drug-induced esophageal strictures. Ann Surg 206:173–183, 1987.
139. Cassidy T, Geisinger KR, et al. Continuous versus intermittent acid exposure in production of esophagitis in feline model. Dig Dis Sci 37:1206–1211, 1992.
140. Winter HS, Madara JL, et al. Intraepithelial eosinophils: A new diagnostic criterion for reflux esophagitis. Gastroenterology 83:818–823, 1982.
141. Steadman C, Kerlin P, et al. High esophageal stricture: A complication of "inlet patch" mucosa. Gastroenterology 94:521–524, 1988.
142. Bate CM, Keeling PWN, et al. Comparison of omeprazole and cimetidine in reflux oesophagitis: Symptomatic, endoscopic, and histologic evaluations. Gut 31:968–972, 1990.
143. Borkent MV, Beker JA. Treatment of ulcerative reflux oesophagitis with colloidal bismuth subcitrate in combination with cimetidine. Gut 29:385–389, 1988.
144. Katz PO, Geisinger KR, et al. Acid-induced esophagitis in cats is prevented by sucralfate but not synthetic prostaglandin E. Dig Dis Sci 33:217–224, 1988.
145. Elsborg L, Jorgensen F. Sucralfate versus cimetidine in reflux oesophagitis. A double-blind clinical study. Scan J Gastroenterol 26:146–150, 1991.
146. Strombeck DR, Harrold D. Effect of gastrin, histamine, serotonin, and

147. Strombeck DR, Turner WD, Harrold D. Eructation of gas through the gastroesophageal sphincter before and after gastric fundectomy in dogs. Am J Vet Res 49:87–89, 1988.
148. Blum AL, Adami B, et al. Effect of cisapride on relapse of esophagitis. Dig Dis Sci 38:551–560, 1993.
149. Pearson H. Symposium on conditions of the canine esophagus. I. Foreign bodies in the oesophagus. J Sm Anim Pract 7:107–116, 1966.
150. Ryan WW, Greene RW. The conservative management of esophageal foreign bodies and their complications. A review of 66 cases in dogs and cats. J Am Anim Hosp Assoc 11:243–249, 1975.
151. Zimmer JF. Canine esophageal foreign bodies: Endoscopic, surgical, and medical management. J Am Anim Hosp Assoc 20:669–677, 1984.
152. Spielman BL, Shaker EH, Garvey MS. Esophageal foreign body in dogs: A retrospective study of 23 cases. J Am Anim Hosp Assoc 28:570–574, 1992.
153. Squires RA. Oesophageal obstruction by a hairball in a cat. J Sm Anim Pract 30:311–314, 1989.
154. Knight GC. Transthoracic oesophagotomy in dogs: A survey of 75 operations. Vet Rec 75:264–266, 1963.
155. Bilbrey SA, Dulisch ML, Stallings B. Chemical burns caused by benzalkonium chloride in eight surgical cases. J Am Anim Hosp Assoc 25:31–34, 1989.
156. Pearson H, Darke PGG, et al. Reflux esophagitis and stricture formation after anesthesia: A review of seven cases in dogs and cats. J Sm Anim Pract 19:507–519, 1978.
157. Dakkak M, Hoare RC, et al. Oesophagitis is as important as oesophageal stricture diameter in determining dysphagia. Gut 34:152–155, 1993.
158. Sooy TE, Adams WM, et al. Balloon catheter dilatation of alimentary tract strictures in the dog and cat. Vet Radiol 28:131–137, 1987.
159. Hardie EM, Greene RT, et al. Balloon dilatation for treatment of esophageal stricture: A case report. J Am Anim Hosp Assoc 23:547–550, 1987.
160. Burk RL, Zawie DA, Garvey MS. Balloon catheter dilation of intramural esophageal strictures in the dog and cat: A description of the procedure and a report of six cases. Sem Vet Med Surg 2:241–247, 1987.
161. Harvey CE. Conservative treatment of acquired esophageal stricture. In: Slatter DH (ed) Textbook of Small Animal Surgery. WB Saunders, Philadelphia, 661–662, 1985.
162. Sherding B, Johnson S. Interventional gastrointestinal endoscopy. Proc 11th Am Col Vet Int Med Forum, Washington, DC, 217–220, 1993.
163. Strombeck DR. Diseases of swallowing. In: Strombeck DR, Guilford WG (eds) Small Animal Gastroenterology. Stonegate, Davis, CA, 140–166, 1990.
164. Pope CE. Involvement of the esophagus by infections, systemic illnesses, and physical agents In: Sleisenger MH, Fordtran JS (eds) Gastrointestinal Disease. WB Saunders, Philadelphia, 1973.
165. Johnson KA, Maddison JE, Allan GS. Correction of cervical esophageal stricture in a dog by creation of a traction diverticulum. J Am Vet Med Assoc 201:1045–1048, 1992.
166. VanGundy T. Vascular ring anomalies. Comp Contin Educ Pract Vet 11:36–48, 1989.
167. Leipold HW. Nature and causes of congenital defects of dogs. Vet Clin N Am 8:47–77, 1977.
168. Patterson DF. Epidemiologic and genetic studies of congenital heart disease in the dog. Circ Res 23:171–202, 1968.
169. Patterson DF. Canine congenital heart disease: Epidemiology and etiological hypothesis. J Sm Anim Pract 12:263–287, 1971.
170. Griffiths D. Three cases of aberrant right subclavian artery in the dog. Acta Vet Scand 30:355–357, 1989.
171. Hurley K, Miller MW, et al. Left aortic arch and right ligamentum arteriosum causing esophageal obstruction in a dog. J Am Vet Med Assoc 203:410–412, 1993.
172. Pearson H, Gibbs C, Kelly DF. Oesophageal diverticulum formation in the dog. J Sm Anim Pract 19:341–355, 1978.
173. Lantz GC, Bojrab MJ, Jones BD. Epiphrenic esophageal diverticulectomy. J Am Anim Hosp Assoc 12:629–635, 1976.
174. Ridgway RL, Suter PF. Clinical and radiographic signs in primary and metastatic esophageal neoplasms of the dog. J Am Vet Med Assoc 174:700–704, 1979.
175. Vernon FF, Roudebush P. Primary esophageal carcinoma in a cat. J Am Anim Hosp Assoc 16:547–550, 1980.
176. Fox SM, Burns J, Hawkins J. Spirocercosis in dogs. Comp Contin Educ Pract Vet 10:807–822, 1988.
177. Culbertson R, Branam JE, Rosenblatt LS. Esophageal gastric leiomyoma in the laboratory beagle. J Am Vet Med Assoc 183:1168–1171, 1983.
178. McCaw D, Pratt M, Walshaw R. Squamous cell carcinoma of the esophagus in a dog. J Am Anim Hosp Assoc 16:561–563, 1980.
179. Baily WS. Parasites and cancer—sarcoma in dogs associated with *Spirocerca lupi.* Ann NY Acad Sci 180:890–923, 1963.
180. Harmelin A, Perl S, et al. Spirocerca lupi—review and occurrence in Israel. Israel J Vet Med 46:69–73, 1991.
181. Caywood DD, Feeney DA. Acquired esophagobronchial fistula in a dog. J Am Anim Hosp Assoc 18:590–594, 1982.

182. Park RD. Bronchoesophageal fistula in the dog: Literature survey, case presentations, and radiographic manifestations. Comp Cont Ed Pract Vet 6:669–677, 1984.

183. Basher AWP, Hogan PM, et al. Surgical treatment of a congenital bronchoesophageal fistula in a dog. J Am Vet Med Assoc 199:479–482, 1991.

184. Ellison GW, Lewis DD, et al. Esophageal hiatal hernia in small animals: Literature review and a modified surgical technique. J Am Anim Hosp Assoc 23:391–399, 1987.

185. Washabau RJ. Diagnosis and management of hiatal hernia. Proc 11th Am Col Vet Int Med Forum, Washington, DC, 429–431, 1993.

186. Miles KG, Pope ER, Jergens AE. Paraesophageal hiatal hernia and pyloric obstruction in a dog. J Am Vet Med Assoc 193:1437–1439, 1988.

187. Bright RM, Sackman JE, et al. Hiatal hernia in the dog and cat: A retrospective study of 16 cases. J Sm Anim Pract 31:244–250, 1990.

188. Williams JM. Hiatal hernia in a shar-pei. J Sm Anim Pract 31:251–254, 1990.

189. Callan MB, Washabau RJ, et al. Congenital esophageal hiatal hernia in the Chinese shar-pei dog. J Vet Int Med 7:210–215, 1993.

190. Prymak C, Saunders HM, Washabau RJ. Hiatal hernia repair by restoration and stabilization of normal anatomy. Vet Surg 18:386–391, 1989.

191. Pollock S, Rhodes WH. Gastroesophageal intussusception in an Afghan hound: A case report. J Am Vet Radiol Soc 11:5–14, 1970.

192. Rowland MG, Robinson M. Gastroesophageal intussusception in an adult dog. J Sm Anim Pract 19:121–125, 1978.

193. Leib MS, Blass CE. Gastroesophageal intussusception in the dog: A review of the literature and a case report. J Am Vet Med Assoc 20:783–790, 1984.

194. Clark GN, Spodnick GJ, et al. Belt loop gastropexy in the management of gastroesophageal intussusception in a pup. J Am Vet Med Assoc 201:739–742, 1992.

12 | Gastric Structure and Function

W. GRANT GUILFORD AND DONALD R. STROMBECK

INTRODUCTION

The stomach serves as a reservoir that temporarily stores food and controls the rate at which ingesta enters the small intestine. It assists the digestion of food by secreting acid and enzymes, and by mixing and grinding food.

ANATOMY

Surface Anatomy[1-3]

The stomach is divided into five regions: cardia, fundus, body, antrum, and pylorus (Figure 12–1). The cardia is the point of entrance of the intra-abdominal segment of esophagus into the stomach. The fundus is a large blind outpocketing that is cranial, dorsal, and to the left of the cardia. The body is the large middle portion of the stomach between the fundus and antrum. The antrum is the distal third of the stomach, with the pylorus as its most terminal part. The boundaries between these regions are arbitrary. More properly, the stomach is better described as consisting of a proximal and a distal part. The proximal segment stores food temporarily and secretes the digestive juices. The distal part of the stomach regulates the release of hydrochloric acid, grinds food particles, and empties the stomach. The distal segment also includes the pylorus, an anatomical sphincter situated between the stomach and duodenum. The pylorus and antrum not only regulate the entry of solid food into the small bowel but also prevent the reflux of duodenal contents.

Topographic Anatomy

The stomach lies predominantly to the left of the median plane (Figures 12–2 and 12–3). The greater curvature of the stomach, the convex surface that stretches from cardia to pylorus, faces caudally, ventrally, and to the left. The lesser curvature, the short, predominantly concave surface between the cardia and pylorus, faces cranially, dorsally, and to the right. At approximately its midpoint, the concave surface of the lesser curvature forms the incisura angularis, a tissue protuberance that separates the antrum and cardia. The incisura is more pronounced in the empty stomach.

Movement of the stomach is restricted because the gastroe-sophageal junction is fixed where it passes through the diaphragm, and displacement of the pylorus is limited by the hepatogastric ligament of the lesser omentum. Additionally, displacement of the pylorus is further constrained by the hepatoduodenal ligament of the lesser omentum, and the mesoduodenum and bile duct that limit movement of the duodenum.

The empty stomach is located within the costal margin and cannot be palpated during the physical examination. The proximal half of the stomach expands rapidly during the ingestion of food. The fundus is filled first, accompanied by gastric distention in the caudodorsal direction. With subsequent filling, expansion of the stomach is caudoventral. In spite of this dilation, the full stomach usually remains difficult to palpate but, if the examiner hooks his or her fingers under

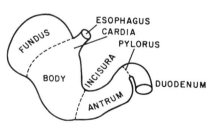

EMPTY STOMACH

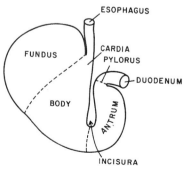

FULL STOMACH

FIGURE 12–1. Diagram of cross section of stomach showing anatomic and functional regions. Above: Empty stomach. Below: Full stomach, showing that increase in size is due to changes in the proximal part of the stomach.

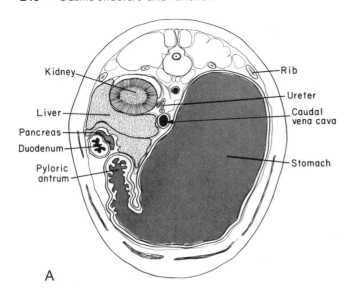

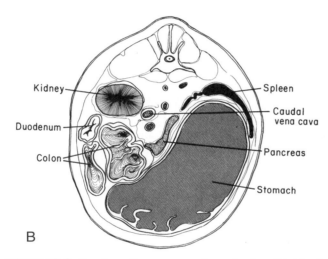

FIGURE 12–2. Drawings of transverse sections of a dog. *(A)* at level of vertebrae T13 to L1. *(B)* at level of vertebrae L1 to L2.

the costal arch, a doughy feeling gastric border can be delineated in some animals (particularly cats).

The parietal surface of the stomach is related to the liver and to the left and ventral abdominal wall (Figure 12–2). The visceral surface of the stomach is smaller than the parietal surface, and lies immediately ventral and to the left of the intestine, pancreas, and left kidney. The fundus lies under the vertebral ends of the eleventh and twelfth ribs. The pylorus lies at a point opposite the ventral part of the ninth rib and to the right of the median plane. It is related to the pancreas and to the portal fissure of the liver.

Gross Anatomy

The wall of the stomach consists of serosal, muscular, submucosal, and mucosal layers. In the empty stomach, the mucosa and submucosa are thrown up into folds called gastric plicae or rugae. This folding is facilitated by contraction

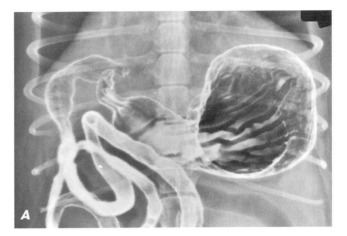

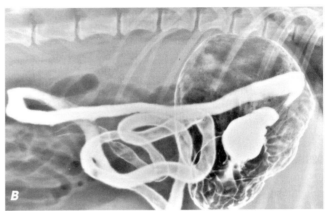

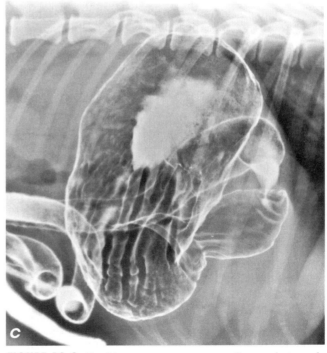

FIGURE 12–3. Double contrast gastrogram of normal stomach, pylorus, and duodenum. *(A)* Dorsoventral view. *(B)* Lateral view with right side down. *(C)* Lateral view with left side down. (Reproduced by permission of W. Th. C. Wolvekamp)

of the muscularis mucosa, a thin layer of smooth muscle dividing the submucosa and mucosa. In general, the folds run parallel with the greater curvature, extending between the cardia and the start of the antrum. Rugae are most obvious in the body of the stomach. In contrast, the antrum of healthy animals is largely free of rugal folds. The rugae become thinner as the stomach fills, stretching the mucosa and submucosa over a larger surface area.

The muscular layer of the stomach can be subdivided into an outer layer of longitudinally arranged muscle fibers and an inner layer of circularly arranged muscle fibers. In the body and fundus of the stomach, a third, obliquely oriented, muscle fiber layer is found adjacent to the submucosa. The outer longitudinal layer is continuous with muscle fibers in the esophagus and found primarily along the greater and lesser curvatures of the gastric body and throughout the antrum. The circular layer of muscle fibers is found throughout the stomach except the fundus. This layer is the most complete and well developed of all the muscle layers in the stomach. It extends into the gastroesophageal junction and forms part of the gastroesophageal sphincter. The circular muscle layer is particularly well developed in the antrum, facilitating the grinding function of this area of the stomach.[4] It is thickest in the lesser curvature and becomes thinner as it fans out over the larger surface area of the greater curvature. Fibers from the circular layer merge with the muscle fibers of the pyloric sphincter. The pylorus is considered a distinct anatomic sphincter because there are a greater number of muscle fibers encircling the pylorus than the antrum or duodenum. However, the entire mass of muscle in the antrum and pylorus behaves as a single functional unit.[4] A connective tissue septum separates the circular fibers of the pylorus from those of the duodenum.

CIRCULATION. Blood is supplied to the stomach by branches of the celiac trunk, the first visceral branch of the abdominal aorta. These branches are the hepatic and splenic arteries, giving rise to the right and left gastroepiploics, which run along the greater curvature and anastomose with one another. The lesser curvature contains the anastomosing branches of the right and left gastric arteries. The former is a branch of the hepatic trunk, and the latter is a branch of the celiac trunk. Venous drainage from the stomach occurs via the gastrosplenic vein on the left and the gastroduodenal vein on the right. Venous blood flows through the portal circulation to the liver. The microvascular arrangement of the gastric mucosa of the dog and cat has been described.[5,6] Lymphatic drainage is through the hepatic lymph nodes after passing through the gastric and splenic lymph nodes.

INNERVATION. The stomach is innervated by the vagal and splanchnic nerves. The vagal trunks lie dorsal and ventral to the esophagus as they pass through the diaphragm. The ventral vagus sends branches to the pylorus and to the liver in addition to the lesser curvature of the stomach. The dorsal vagus sends fibers to the lesser curvature and the ventral wall of the stomach. The splanchnic nerves follow the gastric branches of the celiac artery to innervate the stomach.

The predominant nerve fibers in the vagi are afferent fibers that are components of visceral reflex pathways. The vagal nerves also carry parasympathetic fibers involved in contractile and secretory activity in the stomach. The splanchnic nerves contain predominantly sympathetic efferent fibers that play an important role in the control of gastric blood flow and modulate gastric motility and bicarbonate secretion.[7] In addition, the splanchnic nerves contain smaller numbers of afferent fibers involved in the transmission of visceral pain.

MICROSCOPIC STRUCTURE[8]

The inner surface of the stomach is lined with a single layer of columnar mucus-secreting cells, as shown in Figure 12–4. Remarkably, this one cell layer is capable of maintaining a barrier that keeps hydrochloric acid and digestive enzymes contained within the lumen and prevents the loss of abnormal amounts of plasma constituents into the stomach (other important components of the gastric mucosal barrier are discussed later). The epithelium of the mucosa is invaginated to form pits that are also lined with mucus-secreting cells. At a short distance from the gastric surface, the epithelial lining of the pits changes, and specialized cells begin to appear. This transition marks the beginning of the gastric glands, which secrete a variety of substances into the lumen of the stomach and the blood.

Gastric Glands of the Proximal Stomach

Gastric glands vary in structure with the region of the stomach. In general, there is no sharp line of demarcation where cells of one type abruptly cease. The predominant glands in the cardiac region are mucous glands. They are branched tubular glands that have three to seven branches opening into each gastric pit. Although they have been termed cardiac glands, they are not limited to the cardiac region of the stomach, but are also found in the antrum.

The gastric glands in the proximal part of the stomach (fundus and body) are represented in Figure 12–4. These glands are branched and tubular. Several may open into the same pit. They are differentiated into three regions: an isthmus, neck, and base. The isthmus is the region of the gland closest to the lumen of the stomach. From the isthmus, the lumen of the gland narrows to form the neck, and then widens again at the base of the gland. The cell types in the gastric glands of the proximal stomach are oxyntic (parietal), chief, mucous neck, and endocrine.

Gastric Glands of the Distal Stomach

The gastric glands of the antrum are different from those in the fundus and body. These simple branched tubular glands are formed by mucous neck cells. No chief cells and only a few oxyntic cells are found. The glands contain endocrine cells that stain for biogenic amines and peptide hormones. Gastrin, the endocrine mediator of hydrochloric acid secretion, is synthesized and secreted by an endocrine cell (G cell) in the gastric glands of the antrum.

Cell Types of Gastric Glands

OXYNTIC CELLS. Oxyntic cells are most abundant in the isthmus and neck of the glands of the proximal stomach. They are responsible for the secretion of hydrochloric acid. Their structure is shown in Figure 12–5. They are large cells, oval or pyramid shaped, that stain deeply with eosin. Intracellular canaliculi, produced by invaginations of the luminal cell surface, can be seen with light microscopy. Some of these channels extend almost to the base of the cell. Electron microscopy reveals microvilli lining both the luminal border of the oxyntic cell and the network of canals traversing the

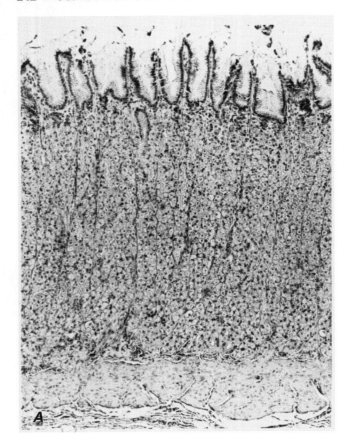

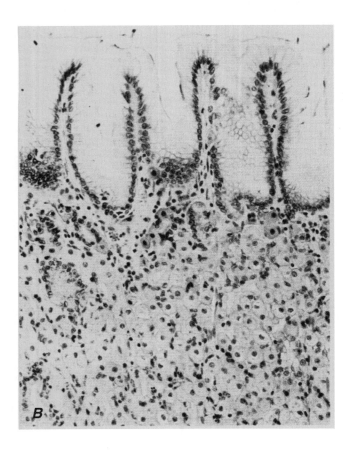

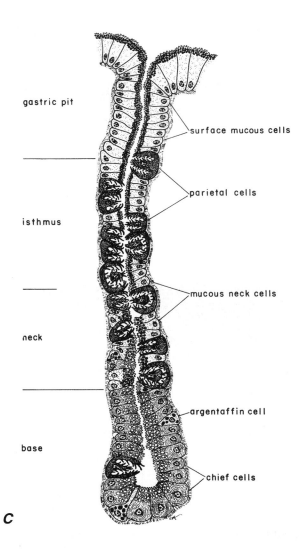

gastric pit

surface mucous cells

isthmus

parietal cells

mucous neck cells

neck

base

argentaffin cell

chief cells

C

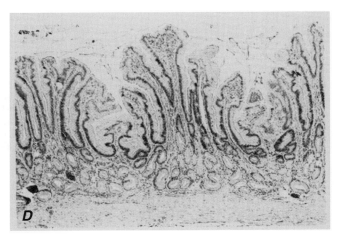

FIGURE 12–4. (*A* and *B*) Glands from body of normal canine stomach. Compare with (*C*) for anatomic details. (*C*) Diagram of gastric gland (from Ito S, Winchester RJ. J Cell Biol 16:541, 1963; by copyright permission of The Rockefeller University Press). (*D*) Mucosa from normal gastric cardia.

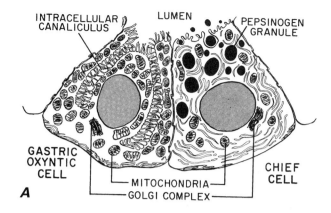

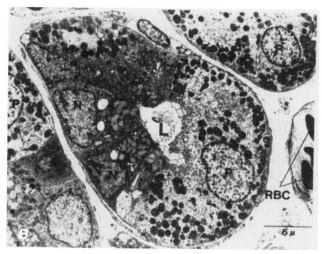

FIGURE 12-5. *(A)* Schematic drawing of gastric oxyntic and chief cells, which respectively secrete hydrochloric acid and pepsinogen. *(B)* EM of normal stomach. L = lumen of gastric gland, P = nucleus of parietal or oxyntic cell, N = nucleus of chief cell. ×2620.

cells. The microvilli greatly magnify the surface area of the cell, which is important in maximizing secretory capacity. During active secretion of hydrochloric acid, the canaliculi swell as the flow of hydrochloric acid to the cell surface increases.

The remainder of the intracellular structures of the oxyntic cell are indicative of its primary function as an ion transporter. The cell contains many mitochondria, which are necessary to provide the energy for ion transport against a large concentration gradient. The Golgi complex is poorly developed because oxyntic cells, unlike chief cells, are not involved with the synthesis, packaging, and secretion of macromolecules. Smooth endoplasmic reticulum is present in an amount inversely proportional to the quantity of canaliculi. The smooth endoplasmic reticulum may contribute to the secretion of ions in an analogous way to the canaliculi.

CHIEF CELLS. The chief cell is the predominant cell type in the deepest part of the glands of the proximal stomach (Figure 12–4). It is the source of pepsinogen. The basal part of the cell appears basophilic because of the abundant RNA in the rough endoplasmic reticulum. The apical part of the cell appears vacuolated as a result of the storage of zymogen granules that do not stain. The chief cell is designed for the synthesis, packaging, and transport of macromolecules. Thus, it is richly supplied with rough endoplasmic reticulum for protein synthesis and Golgi complexes for packaging of pepsinogen prior to storage and transport. The chief cell has

fewer mitochondria than oxyntic cells. The luminal surface of the chief cell contains microvilli to facilitate secretion.

MUCOUS NECK CELLS. Mucus-secreting cells are found in the gastric glands that contain oxyntic and chief cells. Because they are morphologically dissimilar and stain differently from surface mucous cells, they are considered a distinct epithelial cell type. In contrast to the columnar epithelial shape of the surface mucous cells, these mucous neck cells in the gastric glands of the body are smaller and are deformed by adjacent oxyntic cells. The width of the cell is constricted at either the apical or basal end. The presence of mucus granules can make it difficult for conventional stains to differentiate these cells from chief cells. The mucous neck cells are similar to surface mucous cells in intracellular structure. However, the mucus granules of the neck cells differ in size and density from those of the surface cells. The difference is reflected by different staining properties for the two types of mucus, indicating differences in structure and possible differences in function.

ENDOCRINE CELLS. Endocrine cells are found in the basal region of the gastric glands. They have a broad base, and the apex of the cell does not border on the lumen of the gland. This position is consistent with the view that they secrete their granules into the extracellular space and subsequently into the circulation instead of into the gland's lumen. Because many of the endocrine cells in the gastric glands of the fundus and body stain with silver, they have been called argentaffin cells. Their ability to stain with chromium salts results in their other designation, enterochromaffin cells. These cells contain biogenic amines, with serotonin the most abundant. Most of the serotonin in the body is found in the gastrointestinal tract. The physiologic role of these rich stores is unknown, but serotonin appears to have a role in the initiation and maintenance of peristalsis and in vasodilation following tactile stimulation of the mucosa.[9] As mentioned earlier endocrine cells in the distal stomach secrete the peptide hormone gastrin.

Pyloric Microstructure

The ultrastructure and immunocytochemistry of the canine pylorus has been described.[10] The pylorus is richly innervated and many pyloric neurons contain VIP.

Development of the Stomach

The epithelium of the stomach is derived from entoderm whereas the connective tissue and muscular tissues are derived from visceral mesoderm. Primitive gastric pits develop early in gestation and are followed by the appearance of parietal and chief cells, the cellular origin of which is unsure.[11] In humans, the capability to secrete enzymes develops before that of acid secretion, but both are detectable before birth.[11] In contrast, gastric motility does not develop until as late as 4 months in human infants.[11] Gastrin and possibly other hormones have a trophic effect on the developing sphincter muscles.[12]

MOTILITY[14,15]

Motility of the Different Gastric Regions

PROXIMAL STOMACH. Each area of the stomach has a different motor function (Figure 12–6). The fundus contributes

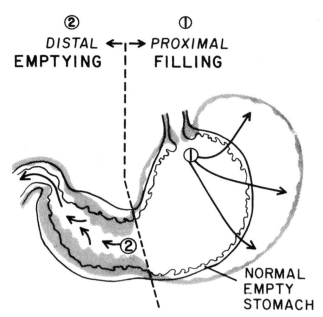

FIGURE 12-6. Schematic of stomach showing motor functions of each region. The proximal part is designed to adapt to entrance of food, and the distal part is concerned with vigorous motor activity to empty stomach.

to the reservoir function of the stomach by dilating in response to the entry of food. By a process referred to as "receptive relaxation," swallowing induces a decrease in fundic motor activity and pressure. If pressure begins to increase in the fundus, a second reflex (referred to as "gastric accommodation") is initiated and results in further relaxation of the fundus. As a consequence of these reflexes, the fundus can dilate to accommodate the entrance of food into the stomach. These reflexes are vagally mediated, and the neurotransmitters VIP and nitric oxide appear to play an important role.

Motility of the fundus has an important role in determining the gastric emptying rate of fluids.[13] In normal dogs, modest increases in gastric volume do not raise intragastric pressure above 10 cm of water. However, if the fundus is surgically removed, intragastric pressure increases above this level following comparable changes in gastric volume.[14] One effect of increased intragastric pressure is an increase in the rate of gastric emptying of liquids.

The body of the stomach also dilates to accommodate changes in the volume of its contents, facilitating gastric reservoir function. During digestion, however, phasic motility increases in the body of the stomach in order to mix contents and move them toward the antrum.

DISTAL STOMACH. Motility in the distal stomach of dogs has been examined by a number of cineradiographic studies.[15] The motility patterns of the antrum serve its role as a grinding mill that actively churns gastric contents and propels them aborally. Motor activity is more frequent and more vigorous in the antrum than in other parts of the stomach. The pylorus is an integral part of the antral grinding mill, helping to delay gastric emptying of particulate food and to prevent excessive duodenogastric reflux.[4,15] Peristaltic waves travel from the body of the stomach and spread over the antrum. The final 3 to 4 cm of the antrum contract vigorously and simultaneously. As the antrum and pylorus begin to con-

tract, the pylorus, having a narrower lumen, closes before the antrum has completed its contraction. It remains partially closed throughout the continuation of antral contraction, allowing small amounts of finely ground liquid chyme to pass into the duodenum but resulting in retrograde propulsion into the proximal antrum of the majority of liquid and nonliquid antral contents. It is this forceful retrograde propulsion that grinds food into appropriate-sized particles to enter the small intestine. Through this mechanism, the pylorus *and* antrum have a major influence on the gastric emptying rate of solid food and, to a lesser extent, liquids.[16]

Closure of the pylorus during antral grinding is facilitated by sliding of the loose pyloric antral mucosa into the pyloric canal to form a plug. The size of the mucosal plug can have an important effect on gastric emptying. Hyperplasia of the gastric mucosa due to chronic gastritis or other gastric disorders can markedly compromise pyloric outflow.

It is important to emphasize that the pylorus does not control gastric emptying rate by acting as a tonically contracted sphincter that opens occasionally to allow chyme to pass. Instead, the pylorus and antrum function as a single muscle unit during the grinding of food. Notwithstanding these comments, the pylorus is capable of acting independently of the antrum under certain circumstances. Contraction of the longitudinal muscle layer of the pylorus can cause the pyloric canal to open. The stimuli for this contraction are unknown. Furthermore, the circular muscle of the pylorus can contract independently of activity in the antrum. The canine pylorus shows independent phasic contractions at rates of 1 to 15 per minute that maintain a zone of pressure about 11 mm Hg higher than the stomach and duodenum.[17] The regulation of this motility is different from the regulation of antral motility.[18]

Regulation of Motility[15,19–22]

The smooth muscle of the stomach can contract without extrinsic or intrinsic innervation. However, the loss of regulation by these nervous systems results in random uncoordinated activity. In the normal animal, gastric motor function depends on a highly coordinated series of events that are neurally and hormonally regulated. Understanding this regulation requires knowledge of the physiology of gastric smooth muscle and of its intrinsic and extrinsic innervations.

ELECTRICAL ACTIVITY OF GASTRIC MUSCLE.[23] An electrically active area of gastric muscle, called the pacemaker, provides the first level of regulation of stomach motor function. The pacemaker is located on the greater curvature at the junction of the fundus and body of the stomach.[24,25] It generates electrical potentials that spread via the longitudinal smooth muscle of the stomach to end at the pylorus. These spreading potentials are referred to as the "electrical activity," "pacesetter potentials," "basic electrical rhythm," or "slow electric waves." They occur at a rate of approximately five per minute in the dog. The basic electrical rhythm is of myogenic origin, as demonstrated by its persistence after anatomic or pharmacologic denervation. The basis of its generation is unknown, but it has been likened to the cardiac pacemaker in the sinoatrial node. The potential is propagated by contacts between smooth muscle cells arranged in a syncytium, and by the nervous system that is distributed throughout the gastric muscles

"Fast-wave" or "electrical response activity" appears as spikes (action potentials) superimposed on the basic electrical rhythm (Figure 1–1). When fast-wave activity coincides with slow-wave peaks the depolarization threshold of the gastric muscle is reached, and contraction occurs. Thus, slow-wave frequency determines the duration and rate of muscle contraction. Not surprisingly, the frequency of contractions of gastric muscle is about five per minute in dogs.

The presence and the location of the pacesetter is important for normal emptying. Without the pacesetter, coordinated gastric motility is not possible. When another pacesetter is placed experimentally in the pylorus of a normal dog so the electrical activity spreads in an aboral direction, gastric emptying is slowed.[26]

Slow-wave activity generated by the pacemaker does not control the fundus. No pacesetter or action potentials are recorded from the fundus. Motility in the fundus is evident as tonic rather than phasic contractions. The tonic contractions initiate and sustain increased intragastric pressure for promoting emptying of liquids.

MODIFICATION OF GASTRIC ELECTRICAL ACTIVITY.[27-29] A number of factors that affect gastric function do so by influencing the basic electrical activity. Truncal vagotomy causes the slow wave to become disorganized and develop an abnormal shape. Electrical stimulation can increase slow-wave activity, although not above 7 cycles per minute. The frequency of the basic electrical rhythm is increased by gastrin and decreased by secretin. In addition, fast-wave activity is augmented by gastrin and cholecystokinin (CCK) and decreased by secretin. A rise in temperature increases the frequency of slow waves. The frequency of fast waves increases after feeding, whereas gastric electrical activity can be absent for as long as 6 hours after surgery. In general, naturally occurring pathologic problems delay gastric emptying more often than speeding it.

CONTROL OF MOTILITY BY EXTRINSIC NERVES AND HORMONES. The autonomic nervous system and gastrointestinal hormones play an important part in the extrinsic control of gastric motor activity (Figure 12–7). Stimulation of vagal cholinergic fibers results in gastric contraction over most of the stomach. It follows that anticholinergic drugs inhibit gastric motility, and cholinergic agents stimulate it. However, some vagal fibers inhibit motility. For instance, vagal activity is responsible for receptive relaxation of the fundus. Noncholinergic nonadrenergic vagal nerve fibers, whose neurotransmitters are most likely vasoactive intestinal polypeptide (VIP) and nitric oxide (NO), appear to mediate the relaxation.[30] It is thought that cotransmission of VIP and NO occurs with the former mainly being released by long-lasting stimulation and the latter being released by both long and short bursts of stimulation.[30] The sympathetic innervation of the stomach does not have a major role in normal gastric motor function. However, sympathetic stimulation inhibits gastric motor activity following surgery and during stressful situations. Furthermore, sympathetic fibers may partially mediate inhibition of antral motility under normal circumstances.

Gastrin inhibits motility in the fundus and stimulates it elsewhere in the stomach. This has the effect of decreasing intragastric pressure and allowing the stomach to store ingesta temporarily. Cholecystokinin has a similar, although weaker, effect. Secretin, glucagon, gastrointestinal inhibitory polypeptide, somatostatin, and VIP inhibit motility in all parts of the stomach. These hormones, along with neurogenic mechanisms, are involved in the regulation of the gastric emptying of food (see later) by their effects on gastric motility.

Acid that enters a breach in the gastric mucosa can stimulate gastric motility. The acid acts either on the neurons in the intrinsic plexuses or directly on gastric muscle. This phenomenon contributes to the gastric muscle spasms that are associated with gastritis or gastric ulcerations.

REFLEXES FOR GASTRIC PROTECTION. Marked distention of the stomach stimulates spontaneous gastroesophageal sphincter (GES) relaxation, relaxation of the body of the stomach,

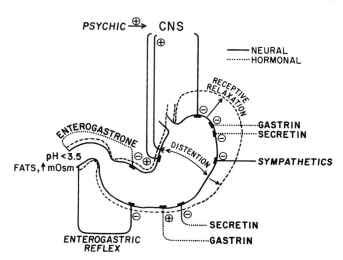

FIGURE 12–7. Neural and endocrine control of gastric motility. Both neural activity and endocrines cause relaxation (–) of proximal part of stomach. Distention of body of stomach stimulates (+) motility in antrum. The effect of reflexes and hormones from the duodenum is to inhibit gastric motility and emptying.

and contraction of the pylorus (take note, endoscopists). These reflexes prevent the dumping of contents into the duodenum and allow the stomach to accommodate a larger volume. The reflexes also permit venting of contents into the esophagus, which protects against gastric rupture. The relaxation of the GES and stomach following gastric overdistension is mediated by intramural gastric nerves, and the pyloric contraction may be due to cholinergic fibers, some possibly carried in the vagus.[31-33]

Regulation of Gastric Emptying[13,34]

In recent years it has become apparent that the two-compartment model of gastric emptying, in which the fundus controls the emptying of liquids and the antropylorus controls the emptying of solids, is an oversimplification. The emptying of gastric contents is a function of the driving force to generate intraluminal pressure and the resistance to movement of chyme. The primary determinants of intragastric pressure are motility of the body and antrum and the degree of relaxation of the fundus. The resistance to movement of chyme is determined by muscular activity of the antrum and pylorus and the viscosity of the ingesta.

ROLE OF THE FUNDUS. As already discussed, the muscular tone in the fundus is a primary determinant of intragastric pressure. This in turn influences the gastric emptying rate of liquids because the pressure gradient between stomach and duodenum has an important influence on the rate at which liquids will leave the stomach.[13] The fundus does not exert exclusive control of the emptying of fluids; duodenal motor activity (and duodenal pressure) are also important. Furthermore, it is now known that liquids can still leave the stomach when the pressure gradient between stomach and duodenum is abolished[35] suggesting there are other mechanisms in addition to fundic tone controlling the emptying rate of liquids. It is likely that the ratio of antral contractility to duodenal contractility is one such mechanism.

ROLE OF THE PYLORUS. The role of the pylorus in regulating the emptying of the stomach has been controversial.[36,37]

The pylorus does not regulate the emptying of liquids from the stomach, because permanent placement of a noncollapsible open tube through the sphincter does not increase the rate at which liquids leave the stomach of dogs and cats.[16] Furthermore, in the presence of a functionally normal antrum, the sieving function of the pylorus is not necessary to control the emptying rate of solids. Isolated pyloric pressure waves have been observed but do not necessarily inhibit gastric emptying. In fact, they may promote the gastric emptying of solids, forming part of an antropyloroduodenal pump.[38]

In the normal animal, the pylorus and antrum usually function as a unit and together have an important function in regulating the emptying of solid food. As discussed earlier, gastric digestion and grinding in the antropyloral mill must reduce solid food to a liquid suspension before it can pass through the small pyloric opening. In dogs, the suspended particles of food are usually less than 2 mm in size before they leave the stomach.[39–41]

Although the pylorus does not close completely during digestion, the pyloric canal can be narrowed, contributing to the control of gastric emptying rate. Pyloric tone is maintained by its intrinsic mechanical properties.[42] However, chyme entering the duodenum stimulates tonic and phasic contractions of the pylorus and reduces pyloric diameter, particularly if the chyme is rich in hydrochloric acid, triglycerides, or fatty acids.[43,44] These events may be mediated by cholinergic nerves passing from the duodenum to the pylorus.[17,45] This possibility is supported by the observation that atropine reduces phasic activity in the sphincter. Peptide hormones such as secretin and CCK induce pyloric contraction but are without any physiologic relevance.[46] Furthermore, histamine stimulates contraction via myogenic H_1 receptors.[47]

In contrast, stimulation of the antrum completely abolishes phasic activity and reduces tonic activity in the pylorus.[17] Pyloric relaxation induced by antral stimulation may be coordinated with antral peristaltic activity to facilitate gastric emptying. Furthermore, during gastric housekeeping contractions (see later) the pylorus of fasted dogs usually gapes open, allowing the evacuation of large indigestible particles. Relaxation of the pylorus is mediated by antral nerves with both nonadrenergic, noncholinergic, and phentolamine-sensitive pathways. VIP-mediated relaxation is likely to be important and NO-mediated relaxation also plays a role.[10,48]

ROLE OF THE ANTRUM. The primary determinant of the gastric emptying rate of solids is antral motility.[15] The factors regulating antral motility are the same as those regulating phasic and tonic contractions in the pylorus. Feeding initially stimulates antral motility. However, once acid and nutrients enter the duodenum, antral motility is reduced. Lipids in the duodenum have the most potent suppressive effect on antral motility; protein has a modest effect, and carbohydrates have no effect.[49] In addition, hyperosmolar chyme in the duodenum also inhibits antral motility. Furthermore, carbohydrate and fat in the distal small intestine also reduce gastric tone (see later).

COORDINATION OF ANTRAL, PYLORIC, AND DUODENAL MOTILITY. Antral, pyloric, and duodenal motility must be coordinated for chyme to leave the stomach. The coordination of antropyloroduodenal motility is a major determinant of the emptying rate of both solids and liquids.[50,51] Sophisticated coordination is necessary because the gastric pacesetter drives motility in the stomach at a frequency of 5 per minute, whereas a separate pacesetter drives motility in the duodenum at a frequency of 18 per minute. In the digestive state the frequency of isolated pyloric pressure waves is threefold that of the interdigestive period, but the contractions of the pylorus and duodenal bulb are inhibited when peristaltic waves travel across the antrum.[51] The coordination of low-frequency antral contractions (about one wave per minute) with duodenal and pyloric relaxation results in carefully controlled, intermittent gastric emptying. In the interdigestive state, antral waves occur about twice per minute, isolated pyloric pressure waves are less frequent than in the digestive period, and antral waves remain closely correlated with inhibition of pyloric and duodenal contractions.[51,53] This pattern facilitates the efficient clearing of indigestible solids from the stomach. In the unfed state, coordination of gastric and duodenal motility is optimal during phase 3 of the migrating motor complex. Duodenal contraction before pyloric contraction results in reflux of chyme into the antrum. The mechanisms for antral-duodenal coordination do not appear to involve intrinsic myoneural or luminal factors.[54,55]

REFLEXES CONTROLLING GASTRIC EMPTYING. The reflex mechanisms to reduce motility and delay emptying are more highly developed than those to facilitate motility. The stimulators and inhibitors of gastric motility are both neural and endocrine.

The reflexes involved in stimulating gastric motility have receptors both within and outside the stomach. The primary factors that initiate and maintain motility after a meal are vagal activity and distention of the stomach. A cephalogastric reflex is present by which the sight, smell, and taste of food increase gastric antral motility and inhibit gastric fundic motility via vagal fibers. A gastro-gastric reflex, employing both the afferent pathways in the vagus, is present to stimulate motility of the gastric body and antrum. The stimulus for this reflex is distension of the gastric body. Distension of the gastric antrum with small volumes of fluid increases antral contractions whereas distension of the antrum with volumes larger than 12.5 ml (in dogs) results in inhibition of contractions in the gastric body.[56] Vagotomy abolishes both of these reflexes. Some recovery of gastric function is observed with time, and the motor function that remains results from the inherent property of the muscle to respond to stretching.

As mentioned earlier, nutrients and acid in the upper small intestine inhibit antral motility and slow gastric emptying.[57–59] These so-called enterogastric reflexes have receptors that respond to mechanical (distention), physical (hypertonicity), and chemical (pH less than 3.5) stimuli. The antral relaxation induced by intestinal nutrients is mediated in part by a nonadrenergic noncholinergic neural pathway in the vagus,[60,61] but hormones such as secretin and CCK may play a role. Other possible inhibitors include gastrin, gastric inhibitory polypeptide, glucagon, VIP, and somatostatin, although the importance of the latter in dogs has been recently challenged.[62] Acid in the duodenum releases secretin, which inhibits motility in all parts of the stomach. Similarly, fats and proteins in the duodenum stimulate CCK release, which inhibits motility in the fundus and antrum and slows gastric emptying in dogs. Gastrin delays gastric emptying by reducing motility in the fundus. In addition, in cats, gastrin and CCK are associated with a decrease in the frequency of high-amplitude pressure peaks and an increase in frequency of low-amplitude (mixing contractions) in the antrum.[63] Furthermore, gastrin and CCK increase the frequency of spike bursts in the duodenum, potentially slowing gastric emptying. It is noteworthy that the collective inhibitory effects of the hormones just listed were once attributed to a single hormone, called "enterogastrone."

Nutrients in the lower small bowel as well as the duodenum reduce gastric emptying rate (the "ileal brake"). The ileal brake presumably functions to minimize the rate of entry of malabsorbed nutrients into the large bowel where they can induce diarrhea. Furthermore, nutrients in the colon or balloon distension of the colon inhibit gastric emptying.[64,65] There is some data to suggest that glucose sensors in the distal small bowel more potently inhibit stomach emptying of solid foods than glucose sensors in the proximal small bowel.[66] Perfusion of the ileum with the hydrolytic products of starch inhibits gastric emptying whereas perfusion with unhydrolyzed starch is without effect.[66] Fatty acids and triglycerides in the ileum also inhibit gastric emptying.[67] The mechanisms underlying the ileal brake are under investigation. In humans, perfusion of the ileum with triglyceride reduces propagated antropyloroduodenal pressure waves and increases isolated pyloric pressure waves.[68]

SUMMARY OF DIETARY INFLUENCES ON GASTRIC EMPTYING. Although the presence of protein, carbohydrate, and fat in the small intestine can all affect gastric emptying rate, fat has the most potent effect. As discussed, fats reduce emptying by inhibiting antral and fundic motility and by stimulating tonic and phasic pyloric contractions. Collectively, the influences of these macronutrients on gastric emptying result in isocaloric gastric emptying rates. That is, isocaloric meals of fat, carbohydrate, or protein all take the same time to empty.[15,69]

It is worth noting the linear relationship between the volume of solution emptied from the stomach per unit time and the total volume ingested.[70] However, the resistance to flow of ingesta can be increased by the addition of viscous fibers, such as pectin, to the diet. Furthermore, diets of high viscosity induce weaker antral contractions than low-viscosity diets.[71] As a result, meals of high viscosity have a slower gastric emptying rate than low-viscosity meals.[71,72]

GASTRIC EMPTYING OF NONDIGESTIBLE SOLIDS. The gastric emptying of nondigestible solids in dogs, and probably cats, is determined by particle size (and shape), pyloric diameter, and hydrodynamics.[50] The majority of digestible solids are emptied from the stomach only after they have been triturated to particle sizes of less than 1 mm diameter.[50] Large indigestible particles (more than 7 mm) do not leave the stomach until the interdigestive period and the onset of the migrating motility complex.[50] Therefore, the major determinant of the gastric emptying rate of large particles is the duration of the fed state, which in turn is dictated by meal size.[50] Intermediate diameter nondigestible solids (around 1–5 mm) empty from the stomach during the digestive period. Intermediate-sized particles of high buoyancy tend to empty faster than particles of similar size but low buoyancy.[50] Buoyancy is in turn determined by the density of the particles and the density (or viscosity) of the fluid in which they are suspended.

Gastric Interdigestive Motility (Housekeeeping Contractions)

Gastric motility in unfed dogs is driven by the interdigestive motor complex (IDMC). Slowly moving peristaltic waves of the IDMC pass over the antrum and pylorus and into the duodenum at regular intervals. During these strong antral contractions the pylorus undergoes maximum relaxation, allowing the evacuation of residual large-diameter particles of indigestible material from the stomach.[43,73] These large-particulate materials are prevented from leaving the stomach during the digestive period by the small diameter of the pyloric canal. Because the IDMC clear the stomach of indigestible material of this nature and reduce the number of gastric bacteria, they are aptly referred to as the housekeeping contractions. IDMC have yet to be clearly demonstrated in cats, but a similar motility pattern is likely to occur.

Duodenogastric Reflux

Reflux of duodenal contents through the pylorus and into the stomach is believed by some to be normal and by others to lead to gastritis.[73,74] Although duodenogastric reflux has been associated with clinical signs and gastritis in dogs, the relationship between the two is not clear.[76] Normal unfed dogs reflux 0.15 mL of duodenal contents per minute; in the fed state the reflux increases to about 1.0 mL per minute.[77,78] Segmental contractions of the duodenum produce reflux when the pylorus is open.[79] The pylorus is an important determinant of antroduodenal resistance, but it does not appear to play an indispensable role in the control of duodenogastric reflux.[80] Placing a tube in the pylorus to keep the sphincter open does not change the rate of duodenogastric reflux in unfed or fed dogs.[77] Antral motility may be the most important factor determining the frequency of duodenogastric reflux. Duodenogastric reflux increases when antral motility reduces.[81] Antral motility prevents reflux by generating a higher pressure in the antrum than in the duodenum. Antral motility is also important for clearing reflux contents from the antrum. It is worthy of note that drugs such as aspirin and indomethacin disrupt normal antral and pyloric motility, resulting in an increase in duodenogastric reflux.[82,83]

GASTRIC SECRETION

Gastric secretions play an important role in the initiation of protein digestion, in the intestinal absorption of calcium, iron, trace materials, and vitamin B_{12}, in the sterilization of food, and in the maintenance of the normal bacterial flora in the gastrointestinal tract. Gastric secretion is closely controlled by overlapping neural, endocrine, and paracrine mechanisms.[84] The secretions are a composite of macromolecular and electrolyte components.

Macromolecular Component of Gastric Secretion[85–87]

PEPSIN. The chief cells of the stomach secrete pepsinogen, which is an inactive precursor of the proteolytic enzyme pepsin. Hydrochloric acid converts the enzyme to its active form. This is accomplished by cleavage of small basic peptides from the pepsinogen molecule. Once formed, pepsin can catalyze its own formation from pepsinogen. A number of electrophoretically and immunologically distinct pepsinogens can be identified in canine gastric secretions. Small amounts of gastric chief cell–derived pepsinogen are found in the blood and urine of dogs. The significance of circulating pepsinogen is unknown.

Pepsin degrades proteins by splitting peptides at the bond between an amino group of one amino acid and the carboxyl group of an aromatic amino acid. The products formed are primarily polypeptides. Pepsin has a pH optimum of 2.0. When chyme enters the duodenum, the proteolytic activity of pepsin ceases because the enzyme is irreversibly inactivated at neutral pH. Pepsin is most active on collagen, and therefore it is relatively more important in the initiation of the digestion of meat rather than vegetable protein. In contrast to the proteolytic pancreatic enzymes, pepsinogen is not essential for the digestion and absorption of a meal. Perhaps the most important function of pepsin is the liberation of peptides that are more potent stimulants of gastrin and CCK release than intact proteins. Thus, pepsin activity contributes to the regulation of the overall process of digestion.

PEPSINOGEN SECRETION. Secretion of pepsinogen is controlled by an interplay of neural, hormonal, and paracrine factors.[88] Stimulatory agents include vagal cholinergic neurotransmitters, cholinergic agonists, histamine, CCK, secretin, gastrin, and VIP. After interacting with receptors on the chief cells, these agents result in inositol triphosphate-mediated intracellular calcium release, which in turn activates calcium-calmodulin-dependent protein kinases, and eventually results in the release of pepsinogen.[88] Furthermore, when the gastric mucosal barrier to hydrochloric acid is damaged, the secretion of pepsinogen is increased. [89] This may be important in the development of gastric ulceration.

The observation that histamine stimulates pepsinogen secretion suggests chief cells may have histamine receptors (H_2). Alternatively, histamine may stimulate pepsinogen secretion indirectly by initiating an acid-induced local cholinergic reflex in the gastric mucosa. Gastrin stimulates pepsinogen secretion indirectly by stimulating the release of both histamine and hydrochloric acid. Pepsinogen secretion is inhibited by somatostatin, peptide YY, and neuropeptide Y.[88]

OTHER GASTRIC ENZYMES. Other enzymes found in gastric secretions exhibit lipase,[90] gelatinase, lysozyme, urease, neuraminidase, and carbonic anhydrase activity. As yet, none of these are known to be important in normal gastric activities.

INTRINSIC FACTOR. The stomach secretes a mucoprotein called intrinsic factor that must bind to vitamin B_{12} before the latter can be absorbed in the distal small intestine. Intrinsic factor has been identified in the cytoplasm of the oxyntic cell of cats, and is secreted by the stomach and pancreas of dogs.[91] Humans with atrophic gastritis frequently have a deficiency of intrinsic factor, leading to vitamin B_{12} deficiency and pernicious anemia, neither of which is recognized as a problem in cats or dogs.

MUCUS. Gastric mucus is produced by the crypt and surface epithelial cells. Mucus is composed of glycoproteins and small amounts of mucopolysaccharides. It is an important component of gastric juice, and forms a continuous protective covering over the epithelium, stabilizing the microenvironment of the mucosal surface. The protective function of mucus depends on properties such as gelation, adhesiveness, ability to form a film, and viscosity. These properties are determined by the chemical composition of its components and by the three-dimensional structure of mucus.[92] The latter is disrupted by the acidity and high ionic concentrations of gastric secretions. Fortunately, a neutral pH is present at the mucosal surface of the stomach. As a result, mucus maintains its gel structure and can fulfill its protective role. However, mucus must be constantly synthesized and secreted to maintain the protective coating. Further from the mucosal surface, the acidity and the high ionic concentrations of gastric secretions (but not the pepsin content) degrade mucus. Furthermore, mucus components are highly soluble because of their carbohydrate concentration. Thus, they can be readily detached and lost from the gel on the mucosal surface.

Mucus protects the gastric mucosa by trapping a layer of alkaline fluid against the epithelial surface. In addition, sulfated forms of mucus protect epithelial cell membranes against the activity of pepsin. The sulfated polysaccharides in the mucus gel bind to protein constituents of the cell membrane and protect them against proteolytic degradation. Sulfated glycoproteins and mucopolysaccharides are present only in small quantities in mucus, yet they are likely to have an important protective function via this inhibitory action. Amylopectin sulfate is a synthetic sulfated polysaccharide that binds to the gastric mucosal surface and to mucus at low pH. This sulfated sugar has been shown to accelerate the healing of gastric ulcers and to prevent the recurrence of duodenal ulcers in experimental animals.[93,94]

The mucosal mucus layer acts as a fine meshwork that retards the passage of macromolecules but permits the movements of electrolytes and small molecules. The mucus polysaccharides have a number of charged groups that provide them with the properties of an ion exchanger. The ion-exchange capacity controls the composition of the fluid in immediate contact with the mucosa. This selective permeability is extended to provide a barrier against microorganisms. Gastric mucin protects against infectious agents by aggregating microorganisms, interacting with bacterial enzymes to inhibit their activity, binding enterotoxins, and interacting with secretory immunoglobulins to protect the mucosa.[87,95]

Cholinergic nerve activity stimulates gastric mucin secretion. Similarly, topical application of acetylcholine to canine gastric mucosa results in an increase in the mucous gel on the epithelial surface. Peptide hormones do not affect mucin secretion in the stomach. Some prostaglandins stimulate release of mucin as part of their cytoprotective properties. Inflammation, toxins, and chemicals stimulate mucin release in pathologic situations.

Electrolyte Component of Gastric Secretions[96]

The primary electrolytes secreted by the gastric mucosa during stimulation are hydrogen and chloride. In addition, the gastric mucosa secretes significant quantities of sodium and potassium, the concentrations of which vary with the rate of acid secretion. Smaller amounts of bicarbonate, phosphate, calcium, and magnesium are also secreted in gastric juice.

HYDROGEN-ION SECRETION.[97-100] The oxyntic cell secretes hydrochloric acid by a mechanism depicted in Figure 12–8. Hydrogen ions are transported by oxyntic cells from a concentration of 5×10^{-5} mEq/L in plasma to a concentration of 160 mEq/L in gastric secretions. Transport against such a large concentration gradient requires considerable energy. For instance, the secretion of 1 L of hydrochloric acid at a concentration of 160 mEq/L requires 1500 calories of energy. Hydrogen ion is secreted via a potassium ion exchange process using energy derived from hydrolysis of ATP by a membrane-bound ATPase. The primary substrate for this energy is glucose, which is oxidized through the hexose monophosphate shunt pathway. Oxygen is necessary to sustain optimum secretion, although anaerobic metabolism of glucose will support some secretion.

Secreted hydrogen ions are derived from carbonic acid following the hydration of carbon dioxide to form carbonic acid, a conversion catalyzed by the enzyme carbonic anhydrase. A small amount of carbonic acid can be formed without aid of the enzyme, although not enough to sustain normal rates of acid secretion. Thus, large amounts of carbonic anhydrase are present in the oxyntic cell, and treatment with a carbonic anhydrase inhibitor reduces secretion of hydrogen ions. Bicarbonate is produced following the ionization of carbonic acid. Its intracellular level increases with transport of hydrogen ions from the oxyntic cell. Some of the excess bicarbonate diffuses to the extracellular fluid and into the plasma. The movement of a large amount of bicarbonate into the plasma during gastric secretion is called the alkaline tide because it causes the pH of plasma to increase.

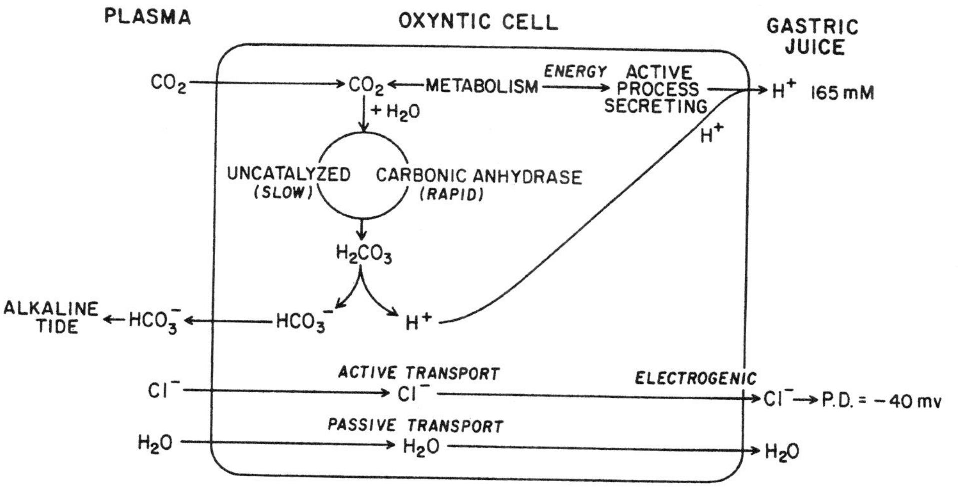

FIGURE 12-8. Schematic diagram showing the gastric oxyntic (parietal) cell's mechanisms to secrete hydrogen and chloride ions. Active transport of chloride ions creates electrical potential difference of 40 mv, with the luminal border negative.

CHLORIDE SECRETION. Chloride is transported across the apical surface of the oxyntic cell via an energy-dependent mechanism. The net movement of chloride to the lumen of the gland exceeds that of hydrogen ions, causing the mucosal surface to be electrically negative with respect to the serosal side of the cell. The potential difference that is generated is greater in the body of the stomach (−64 mv) than the antrum (−48 mv) and the duodenum (−11 mv). The chloride concentration is about 110 mEq/L in plasma and 165 mEq/L in gastric secretions. As a result of this comparatively low concentration gradient, it takes less energy to secrete chloride than hydrogen ions. A variety of agents can increase the permeability of the mucosal barrier. If the barrier to chloride decreases, the back-diffusion of chloride into the mucosa causes the gradient to disappear and the potential difference to fall to zero.

POTASSIUM SECRETION. The concentration of potassium in gastric secretions is 10 to 20 mEq/L, which is greater than that in plasma (4.0 to 5.0 mEq/L). The concentration of potassium in gastric juice increases with increased rates of gastric secretion, but after a prolonged period of secretion the levels fall, presumably because intracellular oxyntic cell potassium is depleted. Most potassium in gastric secretions is derived from cellular rather than plasma potassium. Some gastric juice potassium is derived from desquamated cells. A special secretory mechanism is not necessary for potassium secretion. The hydrated forms of potassium ions are relatively small, and the large potential difference across the mucosa is sufficient to cause passive movement of a large amount of positively charged potassium into the gastric secretions. Normal plasma potassium levels are necessary for hydrochloric acid secretion to occur at standard rates, but this appears to be related to the maintenance (by potassium) of the normal structure and function of the oxyntic cells.

SODIUM SECRETION. The sodium concentration of gastric juice varies inversely with that of hydrogen ion. Some sodium is added by the secretion of alkaline fluid from mucous surface cells. Sodium is also added by diffusion down an electrochemical gradient from the interstitial fluid. Sodium is the most abundant cation diffusing from interstitial fluid. During active secretion, oxyntic cells produce a 165 mM hydrochloric acid solution. With time, however, interstitial fluid and gastric secretion equilibrate so that their compositions become more similar. The degree to which oxyntic cell secretions become like plasma is determined by how long secretions remain in

the ducts (Figure 12–9). At high rates of secretion the hydrochloric acid content is modified very little, and the final secretion may contain 120 to 150 mM hydrogen ion per liter (Figure 12–10). When the rate of secretion is very low, however, the composition of the final gastric fluid has had much more opportunity to be modified, and the hydrochloric acid concentration is very low.

BICARBONATE SECRETION.[101] The surface mucosal cells secrete bicarbonate derived from that produced in oxyntic cells during secretion of hydrogen ions. Bicarbonate diffuses into capillaries below the basement membranes of oxyntic cells. The same capillaries extend into the area under mucosal surface cells, where the high blood bicarbonate diffuses out along a concentration gradient and into the surface mucosal cells. From here, the bicarbonate is secreted into the mucus layer on the surface. The mucosal capillaries have large pores that facilitate the diffusion of bicarbonate.

The amount of bicarbonate available for secretion is determined by the acid secretory activity of oxyntic cells, the blood bicarbonate concentration, and capillary blood flow in the tissue. Reduction in acid secretion can reduce bicarbonated secretion to the point that protection against acid in the stomach is inadequate. Acid placed in the stomach during histamine stimulation of acid secretion results in no gastric damage. Acid placed in the stomach during inhibition of acid secretion by cimetidine results in mucosal ulceration, perhaps because of the secretion of insufficient mucosal bicarbonate to maintain bicarbonate concentration in the surface mucus layer.

Prostaglandins stimulate bicarbonate secretion by gastric mucosal cells. Prostaglandins are more effective stimulants when applied to the mucosal surface than when injected intravenously. Cholinergic agents also stimulate secretion of bicarbonate, whereas anticholinergics block both the prostaglandin and cholinergic-stimulated secretion. Drugs inhibiting prostaglandin synthesis, such as salicylates and ibuprofen, inhibit bicarbonate secretion in some species of animals. Peptide hormones such as pancreatic polypeptide, CCK, gastrin, and neurotensin stimulate bicarbonate secretion. Secretion is stimulated also by calcium and is inhibited by the carbonic anhydrase inhibitor acetazolamide.

Acid bathing the mucosa stimulates gastric bicarbonate secretion. Some, but not all, studies suggest this response is mediated by prostaglandins. Cholinergic pathways in the vagus nerve can also stimulate gastric bicarbonate secretion, particularly during the cephalic phase of secretion.

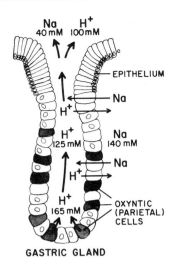

FIGURE 12–9. Diagram of gastric gland, showing hydrochloric acid secretion equilibrated with extracellular fluid as primary secretion moves out into lumen of stomach. Degree of equilibration is determined by rate of secretion and permeability of cells lining gastric gland.

Regulation of Acid Secretion

Gastric acid secretion is closely regulated by neurotransmitters, peptide hormones, and paracrines. These mechanisms are closely integrated and it appears their effects are largely mediated by the release of histamine, possibly from enterochromaffin-like cells.[11]

ACTIVATION OF OXYNTIC CELL SECRETION.[94–100] Gastric acid secretion is stimulated by three main mediators: gas-

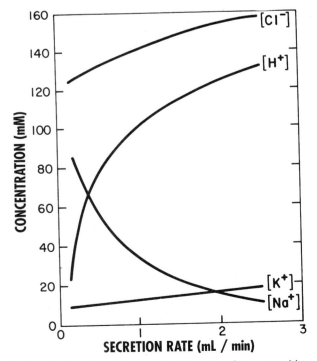

FIGURE 12–10. Graph showing that the electrolyte composition of gastric juice is a function of rate of secretion. As the rate increases, the juice comes to contain very little sodium. The concentration of potassium, however, is always greater than in the extracellular fluid.

trin, histamine, and acetylcholin Stimulation of receptors for all of these mediators is necessary for optimum acid secretion. For example, gastrin cannot stimulate oxyntic cells to secrete unless histamine and acetylcholine are bound to their oxyntic cell receptors at the same time. Selectively blocking any one of the three receptor sites markedly reduces the secretory response when any of the other two receptors is stimulated.

Histamine in the gastric mucosa is located in enterochromaffin-like cells and mast cells, the proportion of which varies with species.[84] The histamine receptor on the oxyntic cell is of the H_2 histamine receptor subclass. Analogues of histamine, such as cimetidine and ranitidine, bind to the oxyntic cell's H_2 receptor sites, but do not stimulate secretion of acid. Instead, they reduce gastric acid secretion because these drugs prevent histamine binding to the oxyntic cell. Through this mechanism, H_2 blockers are able to inhibit the secretory response to gastrin, food, cholinergics, and insulin.

The acetylcholine receptor on the parietal cell is of the M_3 (muscarinic) subtype and can interact with any cholinergic agent to cause secretion. Blocking this receptor with atropine inhibits hydrochloric acid secretion induced by cholinergic agents. Furthermore, atropine also inhibits the secretory response to both gastrin and histamine. It is possible that the secretory effects of acetylcholine are also mediated in part by the stimulation of histamine release from enterochromaffin cells.

The gastrin receptors involved in gastric acid secretion were previously thought to reside on the parietal cell. It now seems likely, however, that the gastrin receptor is located on nearby endocrine cells (probably enterochromaffin-like cells) and that gastrin stimulates gastric acid secretion by release of histamine from these cells (Figure 12–11).[11,84] Gastrin activity can be blocked by proglumide, a selective antagonist of receptor binding by the gastrin-CCK family of peptide hormones. Cholecystokinin can bind to gastrin receptors but acts as a competitive inhibitor of secretion by preventing interaction of gastrin with its receptor.

The interaction of histamine, gastrin, and acetylcholine, and their receptors, stimulates acid secretion via increasing the intracellular concentration of cyclic AMP (histamine) and calcium (gastrin and cholinergic agonists) (Figure 12–11).[84] An ATPase on the mucosal border mediates acid secretion. Drugs such as omeprazole block transport by this ATPase.[102]

The oxyntic cell also has receptors for secretin, which acts as an inhibitor of acid secretion. Secretin and CCK appear to mediate the inhibition of gastric acid secretion that occurs in response to intraintestinal lipid.[84] Prostaglandins inhibit gastric acid secretion by both central (CNS) and local (direct inhibition) mechanisms.[103,104] Dopamine inhibits basal acid secretion whereas metoclopramide and other dopaminergic antagonists increase gastric acid secretion.[105]

NEURAL AND HUMORAL CONTROL OF GASTRIC SECRETION. Control of gastric secretion involves a complex interaction of many neural and humoral factors that dictate secretion at controlled rates at the proper time. Events occurring in parts of the gastrointestinal tract other than the stomach and in other systems of the body have an important role in regulating normal gastric secretion. The control is highly organized, so that secretion during interdigestive periods is minimal and the rate of secretion during a digestive period is programmed to the quantity and type of nutrients fed. In the resting state there is a continuous low level of vagal stimulation of the stomach, and gastrin is always present in the plasma. The background level of each is sufficient to stimulate the secretion of a small amount of gastric juice that, in dogs, is less

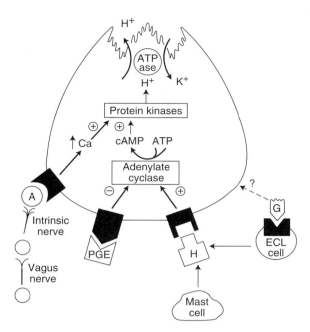

FIGURE 12-11. Current concept of oxyntic cell activation showing mechanisms for stimulating and inhibiting hydrogen ion secretion. A = acetylcholine, PGE = prostaglandins of the E series, H = histamine interacting on H_2 receptor, G = gastrin, and ECL = enterochromaffin-like cells. The gastrin receptors are now thought to reside on nearby enterochromaffin-like cells.

than 1% of the maximum capacity for acid secretion. The rate of secretion oscillates in the resting state, as would be expected when excitatory and inhibitory influences are balanced. There is a small increase in secretion as the interdigestive myoelectric complexes pass through the stomach. The process of feeding stimulates secretion to rise over basal levels, and the increased rate is maintained until the stomach is empty. Mechanisms controlling acid secretion have their effect at three separate sequential times during the digestive process. The overall regulation of gastric secretion is illustrated in Figure 12–12.

Cephalic Phase.[106–108] The anticipation, sight, taste, smell, and chewing of food stimulate the initial phase of gastric secretion. This is a reflex response mediated by higher cortical areas of the brain. The parasympathetic fibers to the stomach are in the vagus nerve. The fibers terminate on gastrin-secretion G cells, oxyntic cells, and chief cells stimulating the secretion of gastrin, hydrochloric acid, and pepsin. The vagally stimulated release of gastrin is somewhat resistant to inhibition with atropine. This neural mechanism is the major stimulus for the secretion of pepsin, but has a relatively minor influence on the release of gastrin and hydrochloric acid.

Hypoglycemia, acting through CNS receptors, results in vagally mediated gastric secretion of acid. In contrast, hyperglycemia suppresses serum gastrin levels and gastric acid production.[109] Other CNS stimulants of gastric secretion include thyrotropin-releasing hormone and neuropeptide Y.[84] Futhermore, elevated intracranial pressure stimulates gastric acid secretion. This may partly explain the high incidence of upper gastrointestinal erosions and ulcers in humans with head trauma.[84] CNS inhibitors of gastric acid secretion include GABA, tachykinins, and prostaglandin E_2.

Gastric Phase. The most important determinants of gastric secretion are events that occur in the stomach. The most potent stimulus of gastric acid secretion during the gastric phase is the release of gastrin. The main stimulus for gastrin release is mechanical distention of the antrum. The mechanism involved has been called the pyloropyloric reflex. Distension of the body of the stomach also causes gastrin release (the oxynto-pyloric reflex). Also present is an oxynto-oxyntic reflex, by which distension of the body of the stomach causes direct stimulation of the oxyntic cell. These reflexes have both long (vagovagal reflex) and short intramural neural pathways.

L-amino acids can directly stimulate oxyntic cells to secrete.[110] This local secretory response is gastrin independent but is sensitive to distension of the mucosa (which increases it) and to low pH (which reduces it). Amino acids given intravenously also stimulate gastric acid secretion by a cholinergic and gastrin-independent mechanism that is sensitive to gastric distension and pH.[111] Chemicals can also stimulate acid secretion via gastrin-mediated mechanisms. Amino acids of the sarcosine series, primarily glycine, serine, and alanine; proteins, especially liver, meat, and meat extracts; acetic and propionic acids; and bile acids can all stimulate acid secretion by this means. The type of protein fed influences the amount of acid secreted. Thus, acid secretion is 30% to 40% less when soy protein rather than meat protein is consumed. The release of gastrin by these chemicals involves neural pathways and can be blocked with local anesthetic placed on the antral mucosa.

Gastrin release is inhibited when the pH of the contents of the antrum is 3.0 or lower. At low pHs even the most potent stimulators of gastrin release are ineffective. This control mechanism is important in regulating hydrochloric acid secretion. Cholinergic and noncholinergic neural pathways may mediate the inhibitory effect. Stimulation of the fundic mucosa appears to inhibit gastric release.[113] Hormones released during the intestinal phase of digestion and absorption may also produce some of the inhibition. Hormones that inhibit acid secretion include somatostatin, secretin, gastric inhibitory peptide, enteroglucagon, and peptide YY.

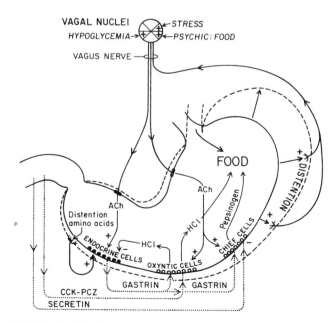

FIGURE 12-12. Diagram showing neural and endocrine control of gastric secretion of acid and pepsinogen. Illustrates cephalic, gastric, and intestinal phases. See text for description.

Intestinal Phase.[106] Events in the intestine can stimulate or inhibit gastric secretion. Food in the small intestine stimulates hydrochloric acid secretion in the vagally innervated or denervated stomach. Stimulation is due to distension of the intestine and the presence of the digestive products of proteins. The response appears to be mediated by a humoral agent called entero-oxyntin. It is biologically distinct from gastrin and not dependent on vagal innervation for its release from the mucosa.

Three small intestinal factors that inhibit acid secretion have been identified: acid, fat, and hyperosmolar solutions.[106] The bulbofundic reflex is stimulated by acid in the duodenum. Humoral agents belonging to the secretin family are released by the intestinal mucosa and inhibit gastric secretion. These hormones include gastrointestinal inhibitory polypeptide, vasoactive intestinal peptide, and glucagon. They all inhibit both hydrochloric acid and pepsinogen secretion, with the exception of secretin, which stimulates pepsinogen secretion. The mechanism of secretin release is well known, with receptors that respond primarily to acid in the duodenum.

Fat in the intestine causes inhibition of gastric secretion by a humoral means, and the phenomenon has been attributed to "enterogastrone." Fats, amino acids, and oral glucose (to a lesser degree) stimulate the release of gastrointestinal inhibitory polypeptide and probably vasoactive intestinal peptide. It is likely that the enterogastrone effect is mediated by a combination of these hormones in concert with neurotensin and peptide YY. Gastrointestinal inhibitory polypeptide and vasoactive intestinal peptide inhibit the secretion of pepsin and also the secretion of acid stimulated by pentagastrin, histamine, and insulin. Neurotensin, a potent inhibitor of pentagastrin-stimulated acid secretion, is released by fat in the small intestine. It may be the most important mediator of the enterogastrone response. Fat in the intestine also inhibits gastrin release.[114]

A number of other peptide hormones have some control over regulation of gastric secretion, although it is not known whether they are physiologically important. For example, bulbogastrone, a humoral factor distinct from secretin and CCK, is released by acid in the first part of the duodenum. Urogastrone, a substance found in the urine, is produced at an unknown site and inhibits the secretion of gastric juices. It is noteworthy that extensive resection of the small intestine results in hypersecretion of gastric acid. It is postulated that either an inhibitor of gastrin release has been removed or that an important function of the small intestine is to remove and degrade gastrin.[115]

Events in the colon can influence gastric secretion. Infusion of the canine colon with liver extract, sodium oleate, or hydrochloric acid inhibits gastric acid secretion.[116]

Relationship of Gastric Blood Flow and Secretion[117]

When gastric secretion of fluid and electrolytes is stimulated, mucosal blood flow must increase in order to provide the constituents of the secretion and the energy to produce it. Thus, not surprisingly, gastric blood flow increases in response to gastric distension and to the presence of food in the stomach. The potent vasodilator, nitric oxide, appears to be an important mediator of this phenomenon.[118] The increase in gastric blood flow stimulated by food is most marked immediately after ingestion and rapidly tails off toward preprandial values.[117] Most of the blood flow is directed to the mucosa, increasing in parallel with increases in secretion. The control of gastric blood flow is described in the chapter on integration of function.

GASTRIC MUCOSAL BARRIER[101,119–121]

The gastric mucosa is a barrier that separates and compartmentalizes the gastric juices and the interstitial fluid. The barrier has three physiologic components: (1) It is a barrier to the movement of cellular elements of the blood, such as erythrocytes; (2) it acts to minimize losses of important macromolecules, such as plasma proteins, from blood into gastric secretions; and (3) it is is a highly specialized semipermeable membrane that controls the rate of movement of water and ions. Of particular importance is the low permeability of the gastric mucosa to hydrogen and sodium ions.

The mucosal barrier consists of a layer of mucus, the cell membranes of the gastric epithelial cells, and the subepithelial vasculature. The integrity of the mucosal barrier is often evaluated by its electrical potential difference and resistance between the luminal and basal sides of the cells. Both potential difference and the resistance fall with injury, but they also decrease during acid secretion. Thus, evaluation of these parameters are of questionable value in assessing mucosal damage.

GASTRIC MUCUS-BICARBONATE LAYER. The mucus that is secreted onto the surface of the mucosal cells contributes to the gastric mucosal barrier. It protects the cell membrane by forming a barrier between the cell wall and proteolytic enzymes. Mucus is not, in and of itself, a barrier to the movement of hydrogen ions, but the alkaline secretions contained by the mucus do play a barrier role against hydrogen ions. The gastric mucus layer contains a bicarbonate-rich fluid that is derived from oxyntic cells and plasma bicarbonate. Hydrogen ions are neutralized as they back-diffuse through the mucus and unstirred water layers. Hydrogen ions reacting with bicarbonate form carbonic acid, which is converted to carbon dioxide and water for disposal. The latter step is catalyzed by carbonic anhydrase in the gastric epithelial cells.

In addition to holding bicarbonate-rich fluids, the layer of mucus protects the gastric surface by virtue of its physical properties. Mucus adheres tenaciously to underlying epithelial cells. Mucus also has a high viscosity, lubricating the mucosa and preventing the shear and stress of gastric digestion from disrupting the integrity of the continuous mucus coat and the epithelial surface. Furthermore, the hydrophobicity of the gastric surface appears to play an important role in the protection of the mucosa. Surface hydrophobicity is closely related to the secretion of surface-active phospholipids secreted into the mucus by the surface mucous cells of the gastric mucosa.[122]

The mucus layer increases in thickness following a variety of stimuli. The increase appears to be a defensive response to injurious agents. The mucus layer provides the right microenvironment for epithelial repair (see later). Removal of the mucus cap delays healing.

The rate of gastric mucus secretion is reduced and its composition is changed by corticosteroids, ACTH, aspirin, phenylbutazone, and indomethacin. These drugs are often associated with the development of gastric erosions and ulcers, and it has been suggested their deleterious effects are due, at least in part, to their effect on mucus.[123]

GASTRIC EPITHELIAL CELLS. Following breakdown of the mucus and epithelial membrane barriers, intracellular epithelial bicarbonate protects against back-diffusing acid in the epithelial cells. Also of importance is the correct functioning of electrolyte pumps, such as the Na^+/H^+ and Cl^-

/HCO⁻₃ exchangers on the basolateral epithelial membrane, which can regulate intracellular pH. It is noteworthy that although the junctions between epithelial cells appear on electron micrographs as an impermeable union that completely surrounds and cements one cell to another (thus the term *tight junctions*), these junctions are in fact quite permeable to water and ions.

MUCOSAL BLOOD FLOW. The mucosal barrier depends on the maintenance of normal mucosal blood flow. Exposure of gastric epithelium to acid or irritants results in reactive hyperemia.[118] The increased blood flow supplies plasma bicarbonate and removes injurious products such as back-diffused acid and inflammatory mediators. Mediators involved in reactive hyperemia appear to be calcitonin gene-related peptide and nitric oxide.[118]

Hemorrhagic shock reduces mucosal blood flow, and when combined with bile acids bathing the mucosal surface, causes gastric ulceration. Drugs such as isoproterenol, given to increase mucosal blood flow, prevent ulceration.

Reduction of plasma bicarbonate concentrations compromises maintenance of the bicarbonate barrier. Luminal pH of gastric contents is less than 2.0 in normal fed animals. When systemic acidosis reduces blood pH to 7.0 or less, gastric ulcers develop even if the luminal pH is 3.5. It is thought that not enough bicarbonate is provided by the circulation during severe acidosis to neutralize back-diffusing hydrogen ions. Thus, a combination of acidosis and reduced mucosal blood flow will invariably cause gastric ulceration. The protective effects of prostaglandins on the gastric mucosa (and the detrimental effects of NSAIDs) have been attributed, in part, to effects on gastric mucosal blood flow. In addition, prostaglandins stimulate mucus and bicarbonate secretion.

ADAPTIVE CYTOPROTECTION. Adaptive cytoprotection refers to the ability of the gastroduodenal mucosa to adapt to exposure to an irritant. The mechanisms underlying this mucosal adaption are poorly understood, but stimulation of local production of prostaglandins appears to be involved.[118] It is probable that the prostaglandins are protective by stimulation of mucosal blood flow and mucus secretion, but many other possible beneficial effects have been cited.[119]

EPITHELIAL RENEWAL. The epithelial cells of the gastric mucosa are rapidly renewed. The surface mucous cells are replaced by migration of cells from the wall of the pits to the surface, a process that is completed in three days. The mucous neck cells do not migrate, and they are renewed in one week. Oxyntic and chief cells turn over more slowly. The development and maintenance of gastric mucosa depend on the trophic effects of hormones and is encouraged by a variety of growth factors, including epidermal growth factor, transforming growth factor alpha, fibroblast growth factors, and insulin-like growth factors.[19,118,124-126]

Minor injury and loss of surface mucosal cells are repaired rapidly by the process of epithelial restitution (reconstitution). Epithelial cells adjacent to or just beneath lost cells migrate over the basement membrane to cover the defect.[119] It takes as little as 30 minutes for restitution to occur. Luminal pH of 3.0 or less inhibits restitution unless a high concentration of bicarbonate is available on the basal side of the cell. Fortunately, damaged mucosa releases increased quantities of bicarbonate into the gastric lumen.[127] Restitution requires the presence of calcium that may be necessary for microfilament function during migration or attachment of cells filling the breach. It is likely that polyamines, transglutaminases, transforming growth factor alpha, and epithelial growth factor and/or its receptor are involved in restitution.[118] The process does not appear to be mediated by prostaglandins.

Deeper injury requires a full inflammatory response and cellular proliferation before the mucosal defect is covered. After the mucosal defect is covered by the proliferation and migration of the surface mucous cells from the edges of the defect, invagination of the new epithelium occurs to form gastric pits and glands. The surface mucous cells lining the glands are transformed into mucous neck cells that are then thought to differentiate to oxyntic and chief cells. Healing of gastric ulcers and erosions is discussed in more detail in Chapters 14 and 15.

REFERENCES

1. Code CF, Carlson HC. Motor activity of the stomach. In: Code CF (ed) Handbook of physiology, Sec. 6, Alimentary Canal, Vol 4. American Physiological Society, Washington, DC, 1903–1916, 1968.
2. Miller, ME, Christensen GC, Evans HE Anatomy of the Dog. WB Saunders, Philadelphia, 1964.
3. Sisson S, Grossman JD. Anatomy of Domestic Animals, 4th ed. WB Saunders, Philadelphia, 1953.
4. Edwards DAW, Rowlands EN. Physiology of the gastroduodenal junction. In: Code CF (ed) Handbook of Physiology, Sec. 6; Alimentary Canal, Vol. 4. American Physiological Society, Washington, DC, 1985–2000, 1968.
5. Marais J, Anderson BG, Anderson WD. Comparative mucosal microvasculature of the mammalian stomach. Acta Anat 134:31–34, 1989.
6. Prokopiw I, Hynna-Liepert TT, Dinda PK, et al. The microvasculature anatomy of the canine stomach. Gastroenterology 100:638–647, 1991.
7. Frandriks L, Jonson C. Influences of the sympatho-adrenal system on gastric motility and acid secretion and on gastroduodenal bicarbonate secretion in the cat. Acta Physiol Scand 135:285–292, 1989.
8. Ito S. Functional gastric morphology. In: Johnson LR (ed) Physiology of the Gastrointestinal Tract. Raven Press, New York, 817–851, 1987.
9. Guilford WG. The enteric nervous system: Function, dysfunction and pharmacological manipulation. Sem Vet Med Surg 5:46–56, 1990.
10. Daniel EE, Berezin I, Allescher HD, et al. Morphology of the canine pyloric sphincter in relation to function. Can J Physiol Pharmacol 67:1560–1573, 1989.
11. Marks IN, Louw JA, Young GO. Acid secretion, 1932–92: Advances, adaptations, and paradoxes. Scand J Gastroenterol 27(suppl 193):7–13,1992.
12. Dodge JA, Karim AA. Induction of pyloric hypertrophy by pentagastrin. Gut 17:280–284, 1976.
13. Kelly K. Gastric emptying of liquids and solids: Rates of proximal distal stomach. Am J Physiol 239:G71–G76, 1980.
14. Wilbur BG, Kelly KA. The effect of gastric fundectomy on canine gastric pacesetter potential, transmural pressure, and emptying. Gastroenterology 62:863, 1972.
15. Meyer JH. Motility of the stomach and gastroduodenal junction. In: Johnson LR (ed) Physiology of the Gastrointestinal Tract. Raven Press, New York, 613–629, 1987.
16. Stemper TJ, Cooke AR. Effect of a fixed pyloric opening on gastric emptying in the cat and dog. Am J Physiol 230:813–817, 1976.
17. Allescher HD, Daniel, EE, Dent J, et al. Extrinsic and intrinsic neural control of pyloric sphincter pressure in the dog. J Physiol 401:17–38, 1988.
18. Golenhofen K, Ludtke FE, Milenov K, et al. Excitatory and inhibitory effects on canine pyloric muscle. In: Christensen J (ed) Gastrointestinal Motility. Raven Press, New York, 203–210, 1980.
19. Willems G, Vansteenkiste Y, Limbosch JM. Stimulating effect of gastrin on cell proliferation kinetics in canine fundic mucosa. Gastroenterology 62:583–589, 1972.
20. Daniel EE, Irwin J. Electrical activity of gastric musculature. In: Code CF (ed) Handbook of Physiology, Sec. 6, Alimentary Canal, Vol. 4. American Physiological Society, Washington DC, 1969–1984, 1967.
21. Duthi HL. Electric activity of gastrointestinal smooth muscle. Gut 15:669–681, 1974.
22. Thomas JE, Baldwin MV. Pathways and mechanisms of regulation of gastric motility. In: Code CF (ed) Handbook of Physiology, Sec. 6, Alimentary Canal, Vol. 4. American Physiological Society. Washington, DC,1937–1968, 1968.
23. Publicover NG, Sanders KM. Myogenic regulation in gastric smooth muscle. Am J Physiol 248:G512–G520, 1985.
24. Weber J, Kohatsu S. Pacemaker localization and electrical conduction patterns in the canine stomach. Gastroenterology 59:717–726, 1970.
25. Kelly KA, Code CF. Canine gastric pacemaker. Am J Physiol 220:112–118, 1971.
26. Sarna SK, Bowes KL, Daniel EE. Gastric pacemakers. Gastroenterology 70:226–231, 1976.
27. Kim CH, Azpiroz F, Malagelada JR. Characteristics of spontaneous and

drug-induced gastric dysrhythmias in a chronic canine model. Gastroenterology 90:421–427, 1986.

28. Gullikson GW, Okuda, H, Shimizu M, et al. Electrical arrhythmias in gastric antrum of the dog. Am J Physiol 239:G59–G68, 1980.

29. Kim CH, Zinsmeister AR, Malagelada JR. Mechanisms of canine gastric dysrhythmia. Gastroenterology 92:993–999, 1987.

30. Barbier AJ, Lefebvre RA. Involvement of the L-arginine: Nitric oxide pathway in nonadrenergic noncholinergic relaxation of the cat gastric fundus. J Pharmacol Exp Ther 266:172–178, 1993.

31. Schulze-Delrieu K. Intrinsic reflexes between the esophagus and stomach. Gastroenterology 91:1568–1569, 1986.

32. DePonti F, Azpiroz F, Malagelada JR. Reflex gastric relaxation in response to distention of the duodenum. Am J Physiol 252:G595–G601, 1987.

33. Glise H, Abrahamsson H. Reflex vagal inhibition of gastric motility by intestinal nociceptive stimulation in the cat. Scand J Gastroenterol 15:769–774, 1980.

34. Hinder RA, San-garde BA. Individual and combined roles of the pylorus and the antrum in the canine gastric emptying of a liquid and digestible solid. Gastroenterology 84:281–286, 1983.

35. Miller J, Kauffman G, Elashoff J, et al. Search for resistances controlling gastric emptying of liquid meals. Am J Physiol 241:G403–425, 1981

36. Winans CS. The fickle pylorus. Gastroenterology 70:622–623, 1976

37. Weisbrodt NW. The pylorus: Keeper of the gate? Gastroenterology 82:995–996, 1982.

38. Haba T, Sarna SK. Regulation of gastroduodenal emptying of solids by gastropyloroduodenal contractions. Am J Physiol 264:G261–G271, 1993.

39. Meyer JH, Thomson JB, Cohen MB, et al. Sieving of solid food by the canine stomach and sieving after gastric surgery. Gastroenterology 76:804–813, 1979.

40. Ohashi H, Meyer JH. Effect of peptic digestion on emptying of cooked liver in dogs. Gastroenterology 79:305–310, 1980.

41. Meyer JH, Dressman J, Fink A, et al. Effect of size and density on canine gastric emptying of nondigestible solids. Gastroenterology 89:805–813, 1985.

42. Biancani P, Zabinski MP, Kerstein MD, et al. Mechanical characteristics of the cat pylorus. Gastroenterology 78:301–309, 1980.

43. Ehrlein HJ. Motility of the pyloric sphincter studied by the inductograph method in conscious dogs. Am J Physiol 254:G650–G657, 1988.

44. Kumar D, Ritman EL, Malagelada JR. Three-dimensional imaging of the stomach: Role of pylorus in the emptying of liquids. Am J Physiol 253:G79–G85, 1987.

45. Mir SS, Telford GL, Mason GR, et al. Noncholinergic nonadrenergic inhibitory intervention of the canine pylorus. Gastroenterology 76:1443–1448, 1979.

46. Phaosawasdi K, Fisher RS. Hormonal effects on the pylorus. Am J Physiol 243:G330–G335, 1982.

47. Biancani P, Cilalzi LK, McCallum RW. Mechanism of histamine-induced excitation of the cat pylorus. J Clin Invest 68:582–588, 1981.

48. Bayguinov O, Sanders KM. Role of nitric oxide as an inhibitory neurotransmitter in the canine pyloric sphincter. Am J Physiol 264:G975–983, 1993.

49. Azpiroz F, Malagelada JR. Intestinal control of gastric tone. Am J Physiol 249:G501–G509, 1985.

50. Sirois PJ, Amidon GL, Meyer JH, et al. Gastric emptying of nondigestible solids in dogs: A hydrodynamic correlation. Am J Physiol 258:G65–G72, 1990.

51. Heddle R, Miedema BW, Kelly KA. Integration of canine proximal gastric, antral, pyloric, and proximal duodenal motility during fasting and after a liquid meal. Dig Dis Sci 38:856–869, 1993.

52. Ehrlein HJ, Hiesinger E. Computer analysis of mechanical activity of gastroduodenal junction in unanesthetized dogs. J Exp Physiol 67:17–29, 1982.

53. Malbert CH, Ruckebusch Y. Duodenal bulb control of the flow rate of digesta in the fasted and fed dog. J Physiol 409:371–384, 1989

54. Tanaka M, Hakim NS, Van Lier Ribbink J, et al. Coordination of motility across the pylorus: Role of myoneural and enteric continuity. Gastroenterology 95:891, 1988.

55. Ribbink JA-van-L, Sarr MG, Tanaka M. Neural isolation of the entire canine stomach in vivo: Effects on motility. Am J Physiol 257:G30–40, 1989

56. Grundy D, Hutson D, Rudge LJ, et al. Pre-pyloric mechanisms regulating gastric motor function in the conscious dog. J Exp Physiol 74:857–865, 1989.

57. Allescher HD, Daniel EE, Dent J, et al. Neural reflex of the canine pylorus to intraduodenal acid infusion. Gastroenterology 96:18–28, 1989.

58. Lin HC, Doty JE, Reedy TJ, et al. Inhibition of gastric emptying by glucose depends on length of intestine exposed to nutrient. Am J Physiol 256:G404–G411, 1989.

59. Hunt JN, Knox MT. The slowing of gastric emptying by nine acids. J Physiol 201:161–179, 1969.

60. DePonti F, Azpiroz F, Malagelada JR. Reflex gastric relaxation in response to distention of the duodenum. Am J Physiol 252:G595–G601, 1987.

61. Azpiroz F, Malagelada JR. Vagally mediated gastric relaxation induced by intestinal nutrients in the dog. Am J Physiol 251:G726–G735, 1986.

62. Lloyd KCK, Maxwell V, Ohning G, et al. Intestinal fat does not inhibit gastric function through a hormonal somatostatin mechanism in dogs. Gastroenterology 103:1221–1228, 1992.

63. Roche M, Descroix-Vagne M, Benouali S, et al. Effect of some gastrointestinal hormones on motor and electrical activity of the digestive tract in the conscious cat. Br J Nutr 69:371–384, 1993.

64. Nightingale JMD, Kamm MA, van der Sijp JR, et al. Disturbed gastric emptying in the short bowel syndrome. Evidence for a 'colonic brake.' Gut 34:1171–1176, 1993.

65. Youmans WB, Meek WJ. Reflex and humoral inhibition in unanesthetized dogs during rectal stimulation. Am J Physiol 120:750–757, 1937.

66. Lin HC, Kim BH, Elashoff JD, et al. Gastric emptying of solid food is most potently inhibited by carbohydrate in the canine distal ileum. Gastroenterology 102:793–801, 1992.

67. Brown NJ, Read NW, Richardson A, et al. Characteristics of lipid substances activating the ileal brake in the rat. Gut 31:1126–1129, 1990.

68. Fone DR, Horowitz M, Read NW, et al. The effect of terminal ileal triglyceride infusion on gastroduodenal motility and the intragastric distribution of a solid meal. Gastroenterology 98:568–575, 1990.

69. McHugh PR, Moran TH. Calories and gastric emptying: A regulatory capacity with implications for feeding. Am J Physiol 236:R254–R260, 1979.

70. Strunz UT, Grossman MI. Effect of intragastric pressure on gastric emptying and secretion. Am J Physiol 234:E552–E555, 1980.

71. Prove J, Ehrlein HJ. Motor function of gastric antrum and pylorus for evacuation of low and high viscosity meals in dogs. Gut 23:150–156, 1982.

72. Sandhu KS, El Samahi MM, Mena I, et al. Effect of pectin on gastric emptying and gastroduodenal motility in normal subjects. Gastroenterology 92:486–492, 1987.

73. Defilippi CC, Gomez E. Continuous recording of pyloric sphincter pressure in dogs. Dig Dis Sci 30: 669–674, 1985.

74. Heading RC. Duodenogastric reflux. Gut 24:507–509, 1983.

75. Ritchie WP. Alkaline reflux gastritis: A critical reappraisal. Gut 25:975–987, 1984.

76. Happe RP, van Den Brom WE. Duodenogastric reflux in the dog, a clinicopathological study. Res Vet Sci 33:280–286, 1982.

77. Muller-Lissner SA, Schattenmann G, Siewert JR, et al. Effect of a transpyloric tube on gastric emptying and duodenogastric reflux in the dog. Digestion 28:176–180, 1993.

78. Muller-Lissner SA, Blum AL. To-and-fro movements across the canine pylorus. Scand J Gastroenterol 19(suppl 92):1–3, 1984.

79. Code CF, Steinbach JH, Schlegel JF, et al. Pyloric and duodenal motor contributions to duodenogastric reflux. Scand J Gastroenterol 19(suppl 92):13–16, 1984.

80. Mearin F, Azpiroz F, Malagelada JR, et al. Antroduodenal resistance to flow in the control of duodenogastric bile reflux during fasting. Gastroenterology 93:1026–1033, 1987.

81. Defilippi C, Mamani N, Gomez E. Relationship between antropyloric and intestinal motility and duodenogastric reflux in fasting dogs. Dig Dis Sci 32:171–176, 1987.

82. Pantoja JL, Defilippi C, Valenzuela JE, et al.: Nonsteroidal anti-inflammatory drugs: Effect on pyloric sphincter and duodenogastric reflux. Dig Dis Sci 24:217–220, 1979.

83. Dooley CP, Mello WD, Valenzuela JE. Effects of aspirin and prostaglandin E_2 on interdigestive motility complex and duodenogastric reflux in man. Dig Dis Sci 30:513–521, 1985.

84. Schubert ML. Control of gastric acid secretion. Curr Opin G 8:895–906, 1992.

85. Hersey SJ. Pepsinogen secretion. In: Johnson LR (ed) Physiology of the Gastrointestinal Tract. Raven Press, New York, 947–957, 1987.

86. Donaldson RM. Intrinsic factor and the transport of cobalamin. In: Johnson LR (ed) Physiology of the Gastrointestinal Tract. Raven Press, New York, 959–973, 1987.

87. Neutra MR, Forstner JF. Gastrointestinal mucus: Synthesis, secretion, and function. In: Johnson LR (ed) Physiology of the Gastrointestinal Tract. Raven Press, New York, 975–1009, 1987.

88. Raufman JP. Regulation of pepsinogen secretion. Curr Opin G 8:907–910, 1992.

89. Johnson LR. Pepsin output from the damaged canine heidenhain pouch. Am J Dig Dis 16:403–407, 1971.

90. Carriere F, Raphel V, Moreau H, et al. Dog gastric lipase: Stimulation of its secretion in vivo and cytolocalization in mucous pit cells. Gastroenterology 102:1535–1545, 1992.

91. Batt RM, Horadagoda NU. Role of gastric and pancreatic intrinsic factors in the physiologic absorption of cobalamin in the dog. Gastroenterology 94:A1339, 1986.

92. Schrager J. The chemical composition and function of gastrointestinal mucus. Gut 11:450–456, 1970.

93. Kim YS, Bella A, Whitehead JS, et al. Studies on the binding of amylopectin sulfate with gastrin mucin. Gastroenterology 69:138–145, 1975.

94. Zimmon DS, Mazzola V. Amylopectin sulphate (SN–263) coats the gastric mucosal surface. Gut 14:847–849, 1973.

95. Strombeck DR, Harrold D. Binding of cholera toxin to mucins and inhibition by gastric mucin. Infect Immun 10:1266–1272, 1974.

96. Hunt JN, Wan B. Electrolytes of mammalian gastric juice. In: Code CF (ed) Handbook of Physiology, Sect. 6, Alimentary Canal, Vol. 2. American Physiological Society, Washington, DC, 781–804, 1967.

97. Forte JG, Wolosin JM. HCL secretion by the gastric oxyntic cell. In: Johnson LR (ed) Physiology of the Gastrointestinal Tract. Raven Press, New York, 853–863, 1987.

98. Sachs G. The gastric proton pump: The H^+, K^+-ATPase. In: Johnson LR (ed) Physiology of the Gastrointestinal Tract. Raven Press, New York, 865–881, 1987.

99. Soll AH, Berglindh T. Physiology of isolated gastric glands and parietal cells: Receptors and effectors regulating function. In: Johnson LR (ed) Physiology of the Digestive Tract. Raven Press, New York, 883–909, 1987.

100. Wolfe MM, and Soll AH. The physiology of gastric acid secretion. N Eng J Med 26:1707–1715, 1988.

101. Flemstrom G. Gastric and duodenal mucosal bicarbonate secretion. In: Johnson LR (ed) Physiology of the Gastrointestinal Tract. Raven Press, New York, 1011–1029, 1987.

102. Konturek SJ, Cieszkowski M, Kwiecien N, et al. Effects of omeprazole, a substituted benzimidazole, on gastrointestinal secretions, serum gastrin, and gastric mucosal blood flow in dogs. Gastroenterology 86:71–77, 1984.

103. Nezamis JE, Robert A, Stowe DF. Inhibition by prostaglandin E of gastrin secretion in the dog. J Physiol (London) 218:369–383, 1971.

104. Robert A. Prostaglandins and the digestive system. In: Les Prostaglandins, INSERM Symposium, Paris, 297–315, 1973.

105. Glavin GB, Szabo S. Dopamine in gastrointestinal disease. Dig Dis Sci 35:1153–1161, 1990.

106. Debas HT. Peripheral regulation of gastric acid secretion. In: Johnson LR (ed) Gastrointestinal Tract. Raven Press, New York, 931–945, 1987.

107. Tache Y. Central nervous regulation of gastric acid secretion. In: Johnson LR (ed) Physiology of the Gastrointestinal Tract. Raven Press, New York, 911–930, 1987.

108. Powers MA, Schiffman SS, Lawson DC, et al. The effect of taste on gastric and pancreatic responses in dogs. Physiol Behav 47:1295–1297, 1990.

109. MacGregor IL, Deveney C, Way LW, et al. The effect of acute hyperglycemia on meal-stimulated gastric, biliary, and pancreatic secretion and serum gastrin. Gastroenterology 70:197–202, 1976.

110. Konturek SJ, Tasler J, Obtulowiez W, et al. Comparison of amino acids bathing the oxyntic gland area in the stimulation of gastric secretion. Gastroenterology 70:66–69, 1975.

111. Konturek SJ, Tasler J, Cieszkowski M, et al. Comparison of intravenous amino acids in the stimulation of gastric secretion. Gastroenterology 75:817–824, 1978.

112. McArthur KE, Walsh JH, Richardson CT. Soy protein meals stimulate less gastric acid secretion and gastrin release than beef meals. Gastroenterology 95:920–926, 1988.

113. Soon-shiong P, Debas HT. Fundic inhibition of acid secretion and gastrin release in the dog. Gastroenterology 79:867–872, 1980.

114. Rayford PL, Konturek SJ, Thompson JC. Effect of duodenal fat on plasma levels of gastrin and secretin and on gastric acid responses to gastric and intestinal meals in dogs. Gastroenterology 75:773–777, 1978.

115. Wickbom G, Landor JH, Bushkin FL, et al. Changes in canine gastric acid output and serum gastrin levels following massive intestinal resection. Gastroenterology 69:448–452, 1975.

116. Seal AM, Debas HT. Colonic inhibition of gastric acid secretion in the dog. Gastroenterology 79:823–826, 1980.

117. Kato M, Naruse S, Takagi T, et al. Postprandial gastric blood flow in conscious dogs. Am J Physiol 257: G111–G117, 1989.

118. Wallace JL, Bell CJ. Gastroduodenal mucosal defense. Curr Opin G 8:911–917, 1992.

119. Silen W. Gastric mucosal defense and repair. In: Johnson LR (ed) Physiology of the Gastrointestinal Tract. Raven Press, New York, 1055–1069, 1987.

120. Davenport HW. Physiological structure of the gastric mucosa. In: Code CF (ed) Handbook of Physiology, Sec. 6; Alimentary Canal, Vol. 2. American Physiological Society, Washington, DC, 759–779, 1967.

121. Moody FG, Cheung LY, Simons MA, et al. Stress and the acute gastric mucosal lesion. Am J Dig Dis 21:148–154, 1976.

122. Lichtenberger LM. Mechanisms of gastric mucosal protection. Proc 11th ACVIM Forum, 74–79, 1993.

123. Menguy R. Gastric mucus and the gastric mucous barrier. Am J Surg 117:806–812, 1969.

124. Lemoine NR, Leung HY, Gullick WJ. Growth factors in the gastrointestinal tract. Gut 33:1297–1300, 1992.

125. Zumkeller W. Relationship between insulin-like growth factor-I and -II and IGF-binding proteins in milk and the gastrointestinal tract: Growth and development of the gut. J Pediatr Gastroenterol Nutr 15:357–369, 1992.

126. Sottili M, Sternini C, Brecha NC, et al. Transforming growth factor alpha receptor binding sites in the canine gastrointestinal tract. Gastroenterology 103:1427–1436, 1992.

127. Guttu K, Rosok B, Svanes K, et al. Release of bicarbonate from damaged and restituted gastric mucosa in the cat. Gastroenterology 105:74–83, 1993.

13

Vomiting: Pathophysiology and Pharmacologic Control

DONALD R. STROMBECK AND W. GRANT GUILFORD

INTRODUCTION

Vomiting is the most common cause of reflux of fluid and food from the gastrointestinal tract. It is differentiated from regurgitation, gagging, and expectoration as described in Chapter 5.

MECHANICAL EVENTS DURING VOMITING[1-5]

Vomiting is a reflex act that includes prodromal signs of nausea. These include depression, anxiety, shivering, hiding or seeking attention, yawning, and lip licking. Animals usually stand with their heads lowered and begin to hypersalivate. Salivation stimulates swallowing, and the repeated swallowing movements stimulate relaxation of the gastroesophageal sphincter in preparation for ejection of gastric contents, In addition, salivary bicarbonate may assist neutralization of gastric acid prior to vomiting.

At about this time, a number of motor events occur in the small intestine. Initially there is a short period of relaxation of intestinal motor activity. This is followed by a high-amplitude, monophasic, retrograde peristaltic contraction with a mean pressure (in dogs) of 230 cm of H_2O, a mean duration of 7.5 seconds and a mean velocity of 4.5 cm/second.[5] This reverse peristaltic wave is referred to as a "retrograde giant contraction" (RGC).[5] Immediately following the RGC, intestinal motor activity is again inhibited. The function of the RGC is unknown, but the reverse peristalsis moves intestinal contents into the stomach and may assist neutralization of gastric content prior to vomiting. These reflex events in the small intestine occur in spontaneous vomiting and in vomiting induced by emetic agents, such as apomorphine, that act on the chemoreceptor trigger zone, and hypertonic saline and copper sulfate, which stimulate mucosal receptors.

Retching begins with the onset of the RGC. Retching consisting of forceful contractions of the abdominal muscles and diaphragm with the glottis closed, resulting in rapid increases of pressure in the gastrointestinal tract.[5] The reflex changes in the small intestine are followed by disordered gastric antral contractions and then by retrograde antral contractions. At the same time, motility is inhibited in the body of the stomach, causing it to relax. In addition, there is reflexive relaxation of the gastroesophageal sphincter, pharyngoesophageal sphincter, and the esophageal body.[3,6] To facilitate gastroesophageal sphincter relaxation the intra-abdominal segment of the esophagus containing the gastroesophageal sphincter moves into the thoracic cavity via a vagally mediated contraction of the longitudinal muscles of the esophagus. This movement inhibits the gastroesophageal sphincter's ability to prevent gastroesophageal reflux. In contrast, motility is inhibited in the circular muscles of the esophagus and the cricopharyngeal muscle fibers forming the pharyngoesophageal sphincter.

The driving force for expulsion of gastric contents is contraction of the abdominal muscles and diaphragm. The force of this contraction generates enough inertia to propel the contents out from the flaccid stomach and through the esophagus and oral cavity. The small intestine and stomach do not develop pressure capable of ejecting their contents from the alimentary tract. As vomitus passes through the pharyngeal cavity, the glottis and nasopharyngeal orifice are closed, preventing pulmonary aspiration and nasal regurgitation.

NEURAL REFLEX OF VOMITING[1-4]

The Vomiting Center and Integration of the Reflex

Vomiting is a reflex act involving neural pathways that synapse in the medulla at the site of the vomiting center. This center contains a group of neurons associated anatomically with neural centers for the control of respiration, salivation, and swallowing. The act of vomiting is integrated with these other functions. For example, hypersalivation is a purposeful response preceding vomiting, and respiration must be inhibited during vomiting to prevent aspiration pneumonia. Stimulation of neurons in the vomiting center produces vomiting, and destruction of the nuclei prevents vomiting. The vomiting reflex is schematically represented in Figure 13–1.

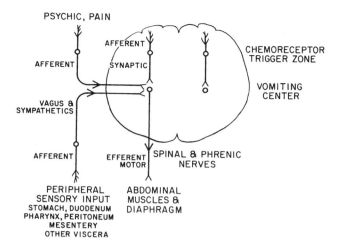

FIGURE 13-1. Diagrammatic cross section of brain stem at level of the vomiting center. Afferent input is via three main pathways. The act of vomiting requires a normal efferent pathway in the spinal and phrenic nerves to the abdominal muscles and diaphragm.

Receptors and Afferent Pathways

The vomiting center receives afferent input from peripheral receptors in the viscera, from the chemoreceptor trigger zone in the floor of the fourth ventricle, from the vestibular apparatus, and from the higher centers such as the cortex. As a result of this extensive innervation, a diverse number of different problems can cause vomiting (Table 5–14).

The peripheral receptors of the vomiting reflex are located in organs throughout the body. Particularly important receptors reside in the abdominal viscera, and especially in the duodenuem, a structure that has been called the organ of nausea. Osmoreceptors in the duodenum are stimulated by overly rapid gastric emptying and can cause vomiting. This is a protective response to prevent gastric dumping that could damage the intestinal mucosa. Acute distention or irritation of small intestinal mucosa can also stimulate the vomiting reflex. Causes include acute erosions, chronic ulceration, inflammation, chemical irritation, and distention secondary to gas accumulation or obstruction. Distention of the small intestine (particularly the cranial small intestine) induces vomiting more readily than distention of the stomach. Inflammation in other abdominal organs, such as the pancreas, can also cause vomiting.

The afferent fibers for abdominal vomiting receptors are found in the vagal and sympathetic nerves. Most of the afferent fibers from the stomach and duodenum are in the vagi, and those from the remainder of the intestine are in the sympathetics. The neurotransmitters involved in the visceral afferent nervous system appear to be noncholinergic. As a result, anticholinergics do not block visceral afferent transmission.

The chemoreceptor trigger zone (CTZ) is located on the floor of the fourth ventricle, astride the opening of the spinal canal (Figure 13–1). The CTZ mediates vomiting associated with many drugs (Table 13–1), such as apomorphine and cardiac glycosides, and with toxemias and metabolic diseases, such as uremia. The vestibular apparatus is responsible for vomiting associated with motion sickness or vestibular disease.

Higher centers in the central nervous system can also be involved in the initiation of vomiting. These centers mediate the vomiting that occasionally occurs in response to acute stressful events. It is noteworthy, however, that chronic stress has not been established as a cause of persistent intermittent vomiting in animals. Additionally, bitches that rear their pups under strictly defined conditions show vomiting that is considered physiologic. The vomiting is described as epimeletic and is defined as caregiving behavior with the biologic function of feeding the pups.[7] This behavior occurs regularly in wild animals, and there is some evidence it can be acquired by male dogs that are quartered near pups and their nest pen.

Efferent Pathways

The motor events of vomiting are mediated by the autonomic nervous system (innervating smooth muscle) and the somatic nervous system (innervating somatic muscles). Vagotomy abolishes all of the gastrointestinal reflexes of vomiting but none of the prodromal or somatomotor responses. Thus, vomiting is still possible when autonomic control is removed, because the primary role of the autonomic nervous system during vomiting is to inhibit motility in the gastric body, esophagus, and esophageal sphincters rather than to provide the contractile force of the vomiting act. Similarly, anticholinergics inhibit the RGC but do not interfere with any other responses in the vomiting reflex. Consequently, anticholinergics have little value as antiemetics. In contrast, denervation of the abdominal and diaphragmatic muscles renders an animal incapable of vomiting.

PHARMACOLOGIC MANAGEMENT OF VOMITING[1-8]

Antiemetics are indicated for the control of intractable vomiting causing distress to the patient or its owner. Antiemetics are not necessary when the vomiting is intermittent, and correction of fluid and electrolyte balance can easily be accomplished. It is important to remember that antiemetics are symptomic treatments. Very often, more long-lasting success is achieved if the therapy can be directed at the underlying cause of the vomiting rather than the vomiting itself.

Antiemetic agents vary in their site or sites of action. This in turn influences their effectiveness as antiemetics in different clinical situations. The most generally effective antiemetics are drugs, such as phenothiazine derivatives, which inhibit neural transmission through the vomiting center (Table 13–2).[9] The phenothiazine antiemetics also inhibit neural activity of the CTZ and have weak anticholinergic activity. Because of their inhibitory effects on all the CNS centers involved in vomiting, the phenothiazines are effective antiemetics for most causes of vomiting. The antiemetic effects of phenothiazines occur at drug levels much less than necessary to produce tranquilization. They must be used with caution in dehydrated patients because they are alpha adrenergic receptor blockers, and can therefore aggravate hypotension. In general, the antiemetic properties (and side effects) of phenothiazines are dose related. If control of vomiting is not achieved at low doses, the dose can be judiciously increased until a beneficial effect is observed or significant side effects are encountered.

Table 13-1

DRUGS CAUSING VOMITING IN CATS AND DOGS

Cats

Amoxicillin	n-Butyl chloride
Aspirin	Phenylbutazone
Bethanechol	Piperazine
Cephalexin	Praziquantel
Chloramphenicol	Sulfisoxazole
Dichlorophene	Tetracycline
Erythromycin	Toluene
Glycobiarsol	Trimethroprim/sulfadiazine
Lincomycin	

Dogs

Aminophylline	Mebendazole
Amoxicillin	Meclofenamic acid
Ampicillin	Corticosteroids
Arecoline	Neostigmine/physostigmine
Aspirin	(ophthalmic)
Bunamidine	Nitrofurantoin
Butorphanol	Phenylbutazone
Calcium edetate	Phenytoin
Chloramphenicol	Praziquantel
Dichlorophene	Primidone
Dichlorovos	Pyrantel pamoate
Diethylcarbamazine	Pyridostigmine
Digoxin	Ronnel
Dinoprost tromethamine	Styrylpyridinium
Dithiazine iodide	Sulfamerazine/sulfapyridine
Glycobiarsol	Tetrachlorethylene
Hetacillin	Tetracycline
Ibuprofen	Thiacetarsamide
Levamisole	Toluene
Lincomycin	Triamcinolone
	Trimethoprim/sulfadiazine
	Uredofos

In contrast to phenothiazines, antihistamines, such as diphenhydramine, primarily inhibit vomiting by blocking H_1 receptors in the vestibular apparatus and, to a lesser extent, the CTZ (Table 13-2). As a result, their primary effectiveness is in the treatment of vomiting from motion sickness.

Dopaminergic antagonists such as metoclopramide and domperidone primarily act at the CTZ and inhibit vomiting due to blood-borne emetic agents such as bacterial or uremic toxins. These drugs also inhibit the gastrointestinal myoelectrical changes associated with vomiting and promote gastric emptying.[10] Vomiting due to functional diseases causing delayed gastric emptying may respond to dopamine antagonists or to other prokinetic drugs such as low-dose erythromycin (1–5 mg/kg PO q 8 hours). Trimethobenzamide (Tigan, Smith Kline Beecham) is a potent inhibitor of the CTZ. It has met with mixed success in small animals.[8]

Opiate receptors are found in the vomiting center, and drugs binding to these receptors can inhibit vomiting. Morphine stimulates vomiting in dogs, but after one or two vomits further vomiting is inhibited. Narcotics such as fentanyl penetrate the brain rapidly and, after binding to opiate receptors in the vomiting center, inhibit vomiting. Butyrophenones, such as droperidol and haloperidol, and diphenylbutylpiperidines, such as primozide and penfluridol, are effective in blocking vomiting induced by drugs such as narcotics. At higher doses the butyrophenones also block vomiting at the vomiting center. Pimozide is long acting, and is able to prevent drug-induced vomiting in dogs for up to six days.

The anticholinergic drugs used commonly by veterinarians are rarely effective as antiemetics. If vomiting is initiated by contraction or spasm of smooth muscle in the gastrointestinal tract, anticholinergics will occasionally be able to relieve the spasm and reduce the stimulus to vomit. Anticholinergic drugs do not prevent the vomiting caused by stimulation of peripheral receptors through other means, such as inflammation. Furthermore, because this class of drug reduces gastrointestinal motility, they may actually be contraindicated in vomiting because they may exacerbate the hypomotility of the gastric body.

Continued vomiting despite antiemetic therapy is a danger sign that serious diseases, such as intestinal obstruction, have been overlooked.

CAUSES OF VOMITING[1-4]

Causes of vomiting are listed in Table 5–14. The most frequent are abdominal problems that stimulate receptors in the gastrointestinal tract, liver, pancreas, urinary tract, internal genitalia, and mesentery. Inflammation of any of those organs can stimulate the vomiting reflex. Inflammation that stimulates receptors in the pharynx can also induce vomiting.

Interference with normal gastric emptying and obstruction of the intestinal tract results in vomiting. This reflex is in part stimulated by distention of the bowel and irritation of its mucosa. The reflex is also stimulated by toxins absorbed from the gut that act on the CTZ. Phenothiazine antiemetics reduce but do not eliminate vomiting caused by obstruction of the pylorus and small intestine, whereas anticholinergics have no effect.

Many systemic diseases can cause vomiting, including infectious diseases such as parvovirus infection, canine and feline distemper, infectious canine hepatitis, leptospirosis, salmon poisoning, and a host of others. Vomiting in these

Table 13-2

ANTIEMETIC DRUGS AND DOSES

DRUG (SITE OF ACTION)	DOSAGE FOR DOGS (D) AND CATS (C)
Triethylperazine (VC) (Torecan)	0.25 mg/kg IM q 8 hours (D) 0.5 mg/kg rectal q 8 hours (D) 0.125 mg/kg IM q 8 hours (C)
Chlorpromazine (VC) (Thorazine)	0.5–4 mg/kg SC q 8 hours (D,C) 1.0 mg/kg rectal q 8 hours (D)
Prochlorperazine (VC) (Compazine)	0.1–0.5 mg/kg SC q 8 hours (D,C)
Diphenhydramine (CTZ) (Benadryl)	2.0–4.0 mg/kg PO, IM q 8 hours (D,C)
Dimenhydrinate (CTZ) (Dramamine)	8 mg/kg PO, IM q 8 hours (D,C)
Trimethobenzamine (CTZ) (Tigan)	3 mg/kg IM q 8–12 hours (D)
Metoclopramide (CTZ) (Reglan)	0.2–0.5 mg/kg PO, SC q 6 hours (D,C) 1–2 mg/kg daily slow IV (D,C) 1.3 µg/kg/minutes (D,C)
Haloperidol (CTZ) (Haldol)	0.02–0.1 mg/kg IM (D)
Fentanyl (CTZ) (Sublimaze)	0.01 mg/kg SC (D)
Dexamethasone (?) (Azium)	0.1 mg/kg SC, IV (D)

cases is stimulated through both peripheral and central receptors.

Cardiomyopathy and congestive heart failure can produce vomiting. The reasons for this are uncertain but may relate to impaired gastrointestinal and hepatic function due to circulatory disturbances, and perhaps to poor central nervous perfusion. Vomiting is often aggravated if the heart disease is managed with cardiac glycosides, which can stimulate vomiting through both central and peripheral receptors.

Fluid and electrolyte imbalances are frequently a factor in the persistence of vomiting. Acidosis as seen in renal disease and diabetes is associated with vomiting. Depletion of body potassium contributes to a loss of normal gastrointestinal motility, helping to perpetuate vomiting. Hyponatremia and hypercalcemia can also cause vomiting.

Endocrine imbalances cause vomiting indirectly by metabolic changes and directly by altered hormone levels. Adrenocortical insufficiency results in both hyponatremia and hyperkalemia; the altered ratio of these ions and a concomitant gastritis cause vomiting that is probably mediated through central and peripheral receptors. Diabetes mellitus is frequently associated with vomiting, perhaps due to ketoacidosis and/or electrolyte imbalances. In addition to endogenous metabolites that act as toxins, many drugs (see later and Table 13–1), chemicals, and bacterial toxins (such as staphylococcal enterotoxin) stimulate the CTZ to cause vomiting.

Diseases of the CNS can stimulate vomiting. Examples include increased intracranial pressure associated with tumors, infections, inflammation, hemorrhage, edema, and hydrocephalus. Expansile tumors or inflammatory diseases in the brain stem can cause vomiting without increasing CSF pressure. Vestibular disturbances stimulate vomiting. The stimuli originates in the utricular maculae of the labyrinth and is transmitted by the auditory nerve of the vestibular nuclei to the uvula and nodulus of the cerebellum, and thence to the VC.

Psychogenic causes of vomiting may be important in some animals. Vomiting induced by pain can be due to a thalamic reflex. Such reflexes can be facilitated by psychogenic factors originating from a higher CNS center. Trauma and shock frequently cause vomiting by stimulation through multiple afferent pathways.

Vomiting Due to Chemotherapeutics

Nausea and vomiting are frequent complications of cancer chemotherapy. They are particularly common with cisplatin, doxorubicin, and methotrexate. Individual susceptibility to these side effects varies widely and is influenced by dosage, route, and rate of administration.[11] Vomiting may occur within a few hours of treatment or may be delayed for 24 hours or more. It may persist for several days. Vomiting results from either stimulation of the CTZ or direct toxicity to the gastrointestinal tract. Direct toxicity is primarily due to an inhibition of rapidly dividing cells in the oral, gastric, and intestinal mucosa, but vincristine can induce ileus and a number of drugs can cause pancreatitis.[11] In addition to vomiting, adverse effects of chemotherapeutic drugs include stomatitis and diarrhea. The diarrhea usually occurs 1 to 10 days after drug administration.[11] It may be suggestive of malabsorption (small-bowel-type diarrhea) or colitis (muco-hemorrhagic).

Antiemetics affecting the CTZ are considered the most effective treatment for chemotherapy-induced vomiting.[11] Metoclopramide is more effective than phenothiazine antiemetics in the inhibition of vomiting from cisplatin therapy in dogs,[12] but metoclopramide should not be expected to prevent cisplatin-induced vomiting entirely. Butorphanol (0.4 mg/kg IM) has been useful in the prevention of cisplatin-induced vomiting in dogs when given at the beginning and end of the infusion period.[13] Phenothiazine antiemetics have not proven to be very effective antiemetics in humans receiving chemotherapy for cancer.[14] However, in the present author's experience they can be useful as adjunctive agents, particularly at high doses (e.g., chlorpromazine at 1.0 mg/kg SQ). Corticosteroids may have antiemetic activity with some chemotherapeutics, although their effectiveness has been questioned.

Preprandial Vomiting Syndrome, Early Morning Vomiting, Bilious Vomiting, Reflux Gastritis

Occasionally, otherwise healthy dogs will present with a history of intermittent vomiting on an empty stomach. The vomiting usually doesn't occur every day but, when it does occur, the dog usually vomits in the early morning (i.e., when the stomach is most likely to be empty). The dogs vomit bile, and as soon as the owner feeds them the vomiting stops and does not recur until the stomach is again empty. Physical examination is unremarkable, and diagnostic tests, including gastric and small intestinal biopsy, are most often normal. Endoscopy may reveal considerable amounts of bile in the stomach, but there are usually no other gross abnormalities. The observation of increased quantities of bile in the stomach has led some authorities to call this syndrome reflux gastritis. Unfortunately, whether the accumulation of bile is a cause or effect of the disease is not known. In our opinion, the latter is more likely. That is, bile has entered the stomach as a result of the duodenal retrograde giant contractions that occur immediately prior to vomiting (see earlier).

The cause of the preprandial vomiting syndrome is unknown. It is of interest to note, however, that the threshold of the VC is lowest during phase 2 of the migrating motor complex, an intestinal motility pattern that occurs during fasting.[5] As a result, emetic stimuli of any cause are more likely to result in vomiting if the stomach is empty. This observation suggests that preprandial vomiting may be an early manifestation of a number of different disorders.

Preprandial vomiting syndrome is treated by ensuring that affected dogs have food in their stomach during the period when most of the vomiting episodes are occurring. This can usually be achieved by feeding a meal last thing at night or by rising early to provide a snack for the dog. A search for any underlying causes is warranted if the vomiting becomes difficult to control by dietary management.

References

1. Code DF, Schlegel JF. Motor action of the esophagus and its sphincters. In: Code CF (ed) Handbook of Physiology, Sec. 6, Alimentary Canal, Vol. 4, 1821–1839, American Physiological Society, Washington, DC, 1968.
2. Daniel EE. Pharmacology of the gastrointestinal tract. In: Code CF (ed) Handbook of Physiology, Sec. 6, Alimentary Canal, Vol. 4, 2267–2324, American Physiological Society, Washington, DC, 1968.
3. Lang IM, Sarna SK, Condon RE. Gastrointestinal motor correlates of vomiting in the dog: Quantification and characterization as an independent phenomenon. Gastroenterology 90:40–47, 1986.
4. Thompson DG, Malagelada JR. Vomiting and the small intestine. Dig Dis Sci 27:1121–1125, 1982.

5. Defilippi C, Gomez E, Cumsille F. Relationship between small intestinal fasting motility and vomiting in dogs. Dig Dis Sci 35:406–410, 1990.
6. Lang IM, Marvig J, Srana SK, et al. Gastrointestinal myoelectric correlates of vomiting in the dog. Am J Physiol 251:G83–G838, 1986.
7. Korda P. Epimeletic (caregiving) vomiting in dogs: A study of the determining factors. Acta Neurobiol Exp 34:277–300, 1974.
8. Richter KP. Treating acute vomiting in dogs and cats. Vet Med, 814–818, August 1992.
9. DeNovo RC. Therapeutics of gastrointestinal diseases. In: Kirk RW (ed) Current Veterinary Therapy IX: Small Animal Practice. WB Saunders, Philadelphia, 862–872, 1986.
10. Lee KY, Park HJ, Chey WY. Studies on mechanism of retching and vomiting in dogs. Dig Dis Sci 30:22–28, 1985.
11. Gorman NT. Chemotherapy. In: White RAS (ed) Manual of Small Animal Oncology, British Small Animal Veterinary Association, Cheltenham, 127–159, 1991.
12. Gylys JA, Dorna KM, Buyniski JP. Antagonism of cisplatin induced emesis in the dog. Res Comm Chem Pathol Pharmacol 23:61–68, 1979.
13. Madewell BR, Simonson ER. Special considerations in drug presentation and administration. In: Kirk RW, Bonagura JD (eds) Current Veterinary Therapy X. WB Saunders, Philadelphia, 475–482, 1989.
14. Laszlo J. Emesis as a critical problem in chemotherapy. N Eng J Med 305:948–949, 1981.

14 Acute Gastritis

W. GRANT GUILFORD AND DONALD R. STROMBECK

Clinical Synopsis

Diagnostic Features

- Transient vomiting of acute onset exacerbated by eating or drinking
- Physical examination nondiagnostic
- Laboratory database may reveal systemic cause
- Gastric biopsy shows predominantly epithelial erosion, ulceration, and necrosis
- Recovery from primary acute gastritis is usually spontaneous and rapid

Standard Treatment

- NPO or no food for 24 to 48 hours
- Parenteral fluid therapy as required
- Gastroprotective drugs: sucralfate (cats: 125–250 mg q 8–12 hours; dogs: 250–1000 mg q 6–12 hours) or bismuth products (see text for doses)
- Cimetidine (5 mg/kg PO SC or IV q 6–8 hours) or ranitidine (1–4 mg/kg PO SC or IV q 8–12 hours) for 7 days if signs of hematemesis or melena
- Chlorpromazine (0.5–4.0 mg/kg SC q 8 hours) for 1 to 3 days if vomiting persistent or severe
- Subsequently feed easily digestible, "hypoallergenic" diet for 3 to 7 days

INTRODUCTION

Acute gastritis is a common problem in dogs and cats and is usually manifested by an acute onset of anorexia, and vomiting. The disease can result from a wide variety of causes (Table 14–1) including infectious organisms, toxins, allergens, and metabolic diseases. Acute gastritis can be differentiated into primary and secondary gastritis. It is often difficult to determine whether acute gastritis is due to agents acting directly on the gastric mucosa (primary gastritis) or is secondary to disease in another body system (secondary gastritis). Furthermore, acute gastritis must be differentiated from other problems that produce acute vomiting such as pancreatitis, hepatitis, intestinal obstruction, and toxicities (see Chapter 5).

PATHOGENESIS OF MUCOSAL DISRUPTION: GENERAL FEATURES

The structure and function of the gastric mucosal barrier has been described in Chapter 12. When the integrity of the barrier is compromised, the rate of back diffusion of gastric acid increases. A cascade of pathologic changes follows, damaging mucosal cells and disrupting subepithelial structures and functions (Figures 14–1 and 14–2). An early event following a serious noxious insult is sloughing of the surface epithelial cells which are rapidly replaced by restitution. Back-diffusing hydrochloric acid stimulates neural plexuses in the intrinsic nervous system. This stimulates motility in gastric smooth muscles predisposing to spasm. The oxyntic and chief cells respond to stimulation of the plexuses with increased secretion of acid and pepsinogen, respectively. In addition, back-diffusing acid, pepsin, and perhaps lipases directly stimulate mast cells, endothelial cells and neutrophils to release histamine, leukotrienes, platelet activating factor, proteolytic enzymes, oxidants and a variety of other mediators. Histamine, in turn, is a potent stimulator of acid secretion by the oxyntic cell, setting in motion a vicious circle of increased acid secretion, stimulating further acid and pepsinogen secretion.[1] Futhermore, histamine and the other mediators released promote vasodilation, venoconstriction, increased capillary permeability, edema, translocation of white blood cells and erythrocytes, capillary plugging, and eventually ischemia and necrosis of cells deeper in the mucosa.[2] In addition, extravasation of plasma fluid occurs through the damaged

Table 14–1

ETIOLOGY OF ACUTE GASTRITIS

PRIMARY GASTRITIS	SECONDARY GASTRITIS
Dietary indiscretion	Infectious diseases and sepsis
Food sensitivity	Stress and trauma
Drugs	Brain lesions
Toxic chemicals	Renal failure
Toxic plants	Liver failure
Bacterial toxins	Circulatory compromise
Fungal toxins	Disseminated intravascular coagulation
Bacteria	Hypoadrenocorticism
Viruses	

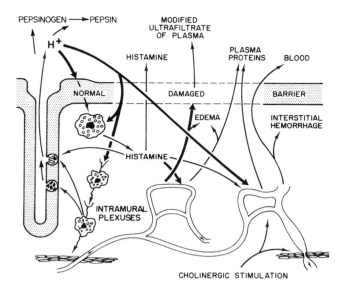

FIGURE 14-1. Early model of the pathophysiologic consequences of the back diffusion of acid through the broken mucosal barrier. (From Davenport HD. Fluid produced by gastric mucosa damage by acetic and salicylic acids. Gastroenterology 50:487–499, 1966.)

mucosal barrier and into the lumen of the stomach. This fluid modifies the primary gastric secretions, reducing its acidity and providing access of antiproteases and immunoglobulins to the mucosal surface. When the gastric mucosal barrier is damaged, protein-losing gastropathy initially occurs through the intercellular spaces (via the so-called tight junctions) and, if damage is more severe, through areas of mucosa denuded of epithelium.

ETIOLOGY AND PATHOGENESIS OF PRIMARY GASTRITIS

Infectious Agents

The contents of the fasting stomach are essentially sterile because of the acidic environment.[3] Gastric bacterial numbers rise transiently after a meal to approximately 10^5 per gram of stomach contents. The microorganisms found in the stomach after eating are derived from food and the oral cavity. They include *Streptococci, Enterobacter, Bacteroides, Bifidobacteria* spirochetes, vibrios, actinomyces, corynebacteria, and yeasts. This transient postprandial contamination of the stomach with increased numbers of normal flora does not cause acute gastritis; nor does more persistent gastric bacterial overgrowth resulting from gastric hypoacidity due to vagotomy[4,5] or H_2 antagonists.

Although the normal flora are not primary causes of acute gastritis, they are potential invaders when erosions or ulcers break the mucosal barrier. The pH of gastric contents approaches neutrality during gastritis because much of the acid secreted is lost due to excessive back diffusion. In addition, the influx of interstitial fluid buffers the acid and raises the pH. Consequently, gastric bacterial numbers will increase and in the presence of a damaged mucosal barrier will enhance the potential for invasion and perpetuation of the gastritis. Inflammatory gastric lesions containing microorganisms are occasionally reported in animals.[6,7]

Pathogenic bacteria given orally to normal animals rarely cause gastritis because they are usually unable to colonize the gastrointestinal tract. An important exception to this are certain spiral-shaped bacteria. Spiral bacteria have been recognized in the gastric mucosa of dogs and cats for many years and are generally believed to be normal inhabitants.[8] Some

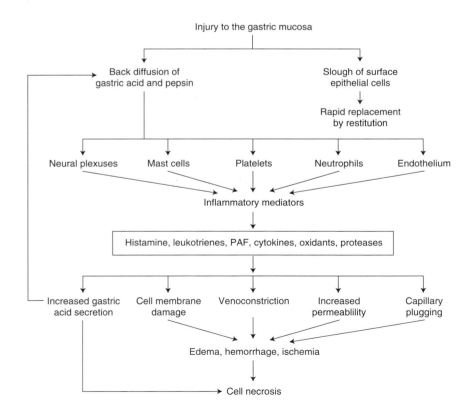

FIGURE 14-2. Expanded version of the Davenport model for gastric mucosal injury. The newer paradigm incorporates many more cell types and their mediators than the early model, but the central events remain similar. (Modified from Jacobson ED, Gastroenterology 102:1792, 1992.)

species of spiral bacteria, however, appear to have a pathogenic potential. Gastritis associated with these organisms is discussed in more detail in Chapter 15.

Pathogenic viruses are a common cause of acute gastritis in dogs and cats. Incriminated viruses include parvovirus, coronavirus, distemper virus, rotavirus, and a variety of other enteric viruses.

Bacterial and Fungal Toxins

Food poisoning resulting from contamination of food with bacterial or fungal toxins can cause acute gastritis.[3,9] Enterotoxins produced by staphylococci, *Clostridium perfringens, E. coli,* and *Klebsiella*[3] have been incriminated. Food poisoning is most frequent in animals that scavenge ("garbage can" gastroenteritis) or are offered food that has been improperly stored, prepared, or preserved (see Chapter 23).

Physical Damage

Physical stresses are occasional causes of gastritis. Hypertonic solutions can disrupt the gastric mucosal barrier and produce gastritis. Conventional diets have an osmolarity of 500 to 600 mOsm, twice that of the body fluids, but do not cause excessive osmotic stress to normal gastric mucosa. Monomeric enteral diets have a very high osmolality and can cause vomiting and gastritis if given in large amounts.

Gastric foreign bodies cause gastritis via direct irritation of the mucosa. They can also distend the antrum, which stimulates gastrin release and gastric acid secretion, eventually resulting in mucosal ulceration. In addition, gastric foreign bodies may obstruct the gastric outlet, resulting in retention of gastric contents and gastritis through a similar mechanism. This situation is similar to the hyperacidity-induced gastritis associated with gastric-outlet obstruction from tumors, pyloric stenosis, and gastric atony.

A temperature above 125° F for only seconds injures the gastric mucosa of dogs.[10] Irradiation can cause gastritis and is most likely to occur following radiation therapy for control of neoplasia. Gastric ulcers and/or perforation are likely once treatment doses approach 4500 CGy.[11]

Chemicals

Gastritis can develop from the inadvertent ingestion of a variety of toxic chemicals (Tables 14–2, 14–3, 18–9). Chemicals causing gastritis include plant toxins, floor finishes, cleaning agents, fertilizers, and heavy metals. Ingested drugs and other chemicals can cause gastritis by disrupting cell structure and interfering with cell function. Some chemicals can solubilize cell lipids or denature cell proteins. Many plants contain chemicals that cause gastrointestinal disorders (Tables 14–2 and 18–9). Similarly, many household chemicals can cause gastrointestinal signs if swallowed (Table 14–3 and 18–9). Often toxic agents have effects on additional systems, such as the cardiovascular and nervous systems, which can assist diagnosis (Table 18–9).

Drugs[12]

Many commonly used drugs can cause vomiting in cats and dogs (Table 13–1). Some drugs stimulate vomiting via effects

Table 14-2

PLANTS WITH GASTROINTESTINAL EFFECTS

Amaryllis	Euonymous
Daffodil	Holly
Hyacinth	Honeysuckle
Mushrooms	Mistletoe
Wisteria	Privet
English ivy	Spurges
Buckeye, horse chestnut	Yellow allamdanda
Mock orange	Yew
Rain tree (monkey pod)	Black locust
Daphne	Castor bean
Iris, flag	Sandbox tree, monkey pistol
Four o'clock	Ground cherry
Lords and ladies	Jasmine
Azalea, rhododendron	Nightshades: bittersweet, eggplant,
Bird of paradise	Jerusalem cherry, potato
Common box	
Poinsettia	

on the vomiting center, whereas others cause vomiting by damaging the gastric mucosa. The pathogenesis of drug-induced lesions is complex and often involves multiple mechanisms for each drug. In general, drugs damage the mucosa by altering gastric mucosal protective mechanisms. Protective mechanisms that can be compromised by drugs include mucus secretion, mucus-gel formation, and bicarbonate secretion. Drugs can alter the permeability of cell membranes, hydrogen ion back diffusion, the production of bicarbonate within the cell, and the ability of mucosal cells to generate energy and transport cations. Other protective mechanisms that can be altered by drugs include mucosal blood flow and the capacity to renew the superficial epithelium. The most well-studied drug-induced injury results from administration of nonsteroidal anti-inflammatory drugs (see later).

Heavy doses of glucocorticoids can cause gastric mucosal damage in dogs.[13,14] Glucocorticoids inhibit mucus secretion and alter mucus viscosity.[15] They also inhibit phospholipase

Table 14-3

HOUSEHOLD CHEMICALS WITH GASTROINTESTINAL EFFECTS

PRODUCT	CHEMICAL COMPOSITION
Deicer (automotive)	Ethylene glycol and isopropanol
Denture cleaners	Sodium perborate
Deodorants	Aluminum chloride, aluminum chlorhydrate
Detergents (anionic)	Sulfonated or phosphorylated forms
Detergents (cationic)	Quaternary ammonium with alkyl or aryl substituent groups
Fireworks	Oxidizing agents (nitrates, chlorates); metals (mercury, antimony, copper, strontium, barium, phosphorus)
Fire extinguisher (liquid)	Chlorobromomethane, methyl bromide
Fireplace colors	Heavy metal salts: copper rubidium, cesium, lead, arsenic, selenium barium, antimony, zinc
Fluxes (solder)	Acids (hydrochloric, glutamic, salicylic, boric)
Laundry bleach	Sodium hypochlorite
Matches	Potassium chloride
Pine oil disinfectants	Pine oil, 5% to 10%; phenols, 2% to 6%
Radiator cleaners	Oxalic acid (100% to 400%)
Rubbing alcohol	Ethyl alcohol
Thawing salt	Calcium chloride

activity, thereby reducing the synthesis of cytoprotective prostaglandins. Lastly, glucocorticoids decrease epithelial cell turnover. In one study, administration of moderately high doses of dexamethasone (0.6 mg/kg q 24 hours for 14 days) was associated with hyperemia and edema of all layers of the stomach wall, proliferation of the surface and gastric pit epithelium, cystic transformation of the mucosal glands, and lymphocytic infiltrations in the lamina propria.[16] Concurrent administration of glucocorticoids and nonsteroidal antiinflammatory drugs is particularly damaging.[17]

Antibiotics can damage the gastric mucosa by inhibiting protein synthesis (neomycin, tetracyclines) and through allergic mechanisms. Some topical medications contain chemicals that cause gastritis when licked and swallowed by the patient.

Nonsteroidal Anti-Inflammatory Drugs (NSAIDs)

Nonsteroidal anti-inflammatory drugs have a number of adverse consequences on the gastrointestinal tract including mucosal erosion, ulceration, perforation, and hemorrhage. Minor lesions are subclinical but anorexia, vomiting, diarrhea, pallor, abdominal pain, hematemesis, hematochezia, and melena may be seen. Dogs and cats are particularly sensitive to NSAIDs. In dogs, this sensitivity may be due to higher gastrointestinal absorption rates, a longer drug half-life, and more extensive enterohepatic cycling than many other species.[18,19] In cats, sensitivity to aspirin is due to poor glucuronyl transferase activity. It is worthy of note that breed differences may occur in NSAID half-lives.

In dogs, NSAIDs-induced lesions tend to be most frequent in the gastric antrum and pylorus but can occur elsewhere in the stomach, and in the duodenum, jejunum, and colon.[17,20] In general, they are more severe proximally in the intestine and decrease distally.[17] Many of the NSAIDs-induced gastric perforations have occurred in the pyloric antrum. The reason for the apparent susceptibility of the antrum to ulceration is unclear but may be partly explained by the observation that the antral microvasculature of dogs has a paucity of horizontal interconnections between superficial capillaries in comparison to the gastric body.[21] Thus, in contrast to the gastric body, stasis or thrombosis of superficial capillaries of the antrum is likely to render a large portion of the antral mucosa ischemic because of lack of anastomoses.[21]

Grossly, the gastrointestinal lesions induced by NSAIDs consist predominantly of shallow, circular, or linear erosions, hemorrhages, and, particularly in the duodenum and jejunum, mucosal reddening (Figure 14–3). Occasionally, deep ulcers penetrating into the muscularis layers or through the full thickness of the stomach or intestine are observed. These ulcers are usually associated with large amounts of digested blood in the stomach. Histologically, a generalized increase in mixed inflammatory cell types is seen in the superficial mucosa of the stomach and small intestine.[17] The erosions are characterized by minimal inflammatory response with little connective tissue proliferation or epithelial regeneration at their margins.[17] The histologic appearance of the ulcers is similar, but microthrombi, more extensive necrosis, acute hemorrhage of the eroded edges, and deeper penetration (through the muscularis mucosa) become apparent.[17,22] Small intestinal villi become blunted and some develop necrosis of the tips.[17] The pathogenesis of NSAIDs-induced lesions is multifactorial and includes direct toxicity to the gastric epithelium, increased back diffusion of acid, decreased synthesis of prostaglandins, bicarbonate, and mucus, reduced

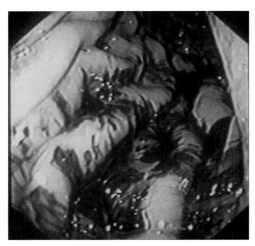

FIGURE 14–3. Endoscopic appearance of NSAIDs gastritis induced by aspirin. Note the extensive hemorrhage arising from mucosal lesions.

mucosal blood flow, and microvascular injury. Most studies on the pathogenesis of NSAIDs-induced injury have been performed on aspirin.

At the acidic pH of gastric contents, aspirin is unionized and rapidly enters the gastric epithelial cells. Intracellularly, where cytosolic pH is close to neutral, aspirin ionizes and is trapped inside the cell where it rapidly accumulates. High concentrations of this acidic molecule alter mucosal ion transport and eventually damage cell structure, disrupting the mucosal barrier (Figure 14–4). Aspirin impairs gastric mucus and bicarbonate secretion and delays cell renewal, all of which further compromise the gastric mucosal barrier.[23] Exfoliation of superficial epithelial cells follows. Disruption of the gastric barrier by aspirin causes increased back diffusion of hydrogen ions with the attendant adverse consequences described earlier (Figures 14–1 and 14–2).

Vascular damage becomes apparent early in the course of NSAIDs gastropathy and may in part be mediated by NSAID-induced increase in neutrophil adherence to the vascular endothelium.[24,25] Mucosal blood flow is decreased, further jeopardizing mucosal protection.[26,27] Stress potentiates the ulcerogenic effects of aspirin presumedly by further reducing gastric mucosal blood flow. Eventually gastric bleeding develops as a result of vascular damage, vascular stasis, and inhibition of platelet function.

Aspirin produces some of its damaging effects by blocking cyclooxygenase and inhibiting prostaglandin synthesis. As discussed in Chapter 12, prostaglandins have many protective influences including inhibition of gastric acid secretion, enhancement of mucosal blood flow, stimulation of bicarbonate and mucus secretion by the gastroduodenal mucosa, and maintenance of gastric mucosal hydrophobicity.[28] In addition, prostaglandins are involved in regulating gastric epithelial turnover and repair. Therefore, not surprisingly, administration of synthetic prostaglandin analogues reduces aspirin-induced injury to the gastric mucosa (see later).[29,30] The blockage of cyclooxygenase not only deprives the mucosa of cytoprotective prostaglandins but may divert arachidonic acid metabolism toward synthesis of leukotrienes that have been implicated in the production of NSAIDs gastropathy.[27]

Most other NSAIDs cause adverse effects to the gastric mucosa by mechanisms similar to aspirin. Phenylbutazone and indomethacin frequently cause gastric lesions.[31,32] The severity of the lesions induced by indomethacin can be

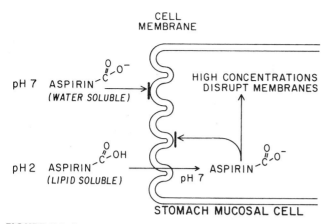

FIGURE 14-4. Schematic showing the effects of aspirin on the stomach. At a low pH, aspirin is almost all unionized and lipid soluble and can therefore enter the mucosal cell with ease. Once inside, it is ionized by the higher intracellular pH and does not readily leave the cell, eventually raising the intracellular aspirin concentration to the point where it damages the cell.

reduced (but not eliminated) by copper chelation of the indomethacin.[33] Similarly, flunixin meglumine, ketoprofen, ibuprofen, naproxen, indoprofen, cinchophen, and piroxicam can produce gastric lesions in dogs and cats (Table 14-4). At times, the lesions produced by flunixin meglumine, indomethacin, phenylbutazone, ibuprofen, naproxen, piroxicam, and aspirin, when administered at or near commonly used therapeutic dosages, can be severe and result in perforation of the gastric wall or severe melena.[22,32,34-38] For instance, ibuprofen is likely to induce gastrointestinal irritation and hemorrhage at a dose of 8 mg/kg/day that is not much greater than the usual therapeutic dose of the drug (5 mg/kg/day).[19] Gastric perforation in a dog has been associated with the use of ibuprofen at a dose of 14 mg/kg PO q 6 hours for 2 days.[22] The ulcerogenic properties of flunixin and other nonsteroidals such as cinchophen are exacerbated by concurrent administration with glucocorticoids.[17,18] Therefore, as a general rule, glucocorticoids and NSAIDs should not be administered together.

The adverse effects of NSAIDs can be minimized by giving the drugs with a meal, presumedly because of the buffering effects of the food and the increased mucosal blood flow that accompanies eating. Similarly, the use of buffered aspirin affords some protection against NSAIDs gastropathy but the small quantity of buffer in such tablets is unlikely to be as pro-

tective as a meal. Parenteral or rectal administration of NSAIDs minimizes the direct irritative effects on the gastric mucosa of many NSAIDs but does not prevent NSAIDs-induced mucosal injury.[17,39] Misoprostol, a synthetic prostaglandin analogue (PGE_2), reduces NSAIDs-induced injury to the gastric mucosa of dogs (see later).[29,30,41] The dose of misoprostol used is 1 to 3 μg/kg PO q 6 to 8 hours. Misoprostol is superior to H_2 blockers for the prevention of NSAIDs-induced mucosal damage but can produce transient diarrhea. In contrast, other commonly used gastroprotective drugs such as H_2 blockers, omeprazole, and sucralfate have little protective effects against NSAIDs-induced injury in dogs.[40-42] However, clinical experience in humans and dogs suggests these agents will accelerate healing of NSAIDs-induced ulcers once the NSAID therapy has been discontinued.[43,44]

Allergens

Allergens ingested following a previous sensitization can cause acute gastritis. Food allergy is most often attributed to immediate hypersensitivities but delayed hypersensitivities are also likely (see Chapter 23). Clinical signs usually appear rapidly and can include vomiting, urticaria, respiratory distress, and cardiovascular signs. In most cases only vomiting is observed, with no systemic signs apparent. Diagnosis is made by elimination challenge trials and can be assisted by gastroscopic food sensitivity testing.

ETIOLOGY AND PATHOGENESIS OF SECONDARY GASTRITIS[45,46]

A wide variety of systemic disorders or dysfunctions of other parts of the gastrointestinal tract can lead to secondary gastritis. The acute gastric mucosal lesions resulting from these disorders are usually due to increased secretion of hydrochloric acid, reduced mucosal blood flow, gastroduodenal reflux, and/or alteration of the mucus-bicarbonate mucosal barrier (Figure 14-5).

Gastric Hyperacidity Disorders

The development of acute gastric lesions depends to a large extent on the presence of gastric acid, regardless of the primary cause of the gastric damage.[47] Hypersecretion of

Table 14-4

DRUG	EROSIONS	PERFORATION	SEVERE HEMORRHAGE
Aspirin	Yes	Yes	Yes
Cinchophen	Yes	?	Yes
Copper indomethacin	Yes	?	?
Flunixin meglumine	Yes	Yes	Yes
Ibuprofen	Yes	Yes	Yes
Indomethacin	Yes	Yes	Yes
Indoprofen	Yes	?	?
Ketoprofen	Yes	?	?
Meclofenamic acid	Yes	?	Yes
Naproxen	Yes	Yes	Yes
Piroxicam	Yes	?	Yes
Phenylbutazone	Yes	?	Yes

NSAIDS KNOWN TO CAUSE GASTRODUODENAL INJURY IN DOGS

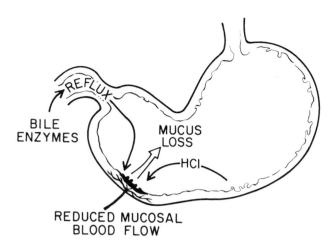

Table 14–5

CAUSES OF GASTRIC HYPERACIDITY
Gastrinomas
Mastocytoma
Head injury
Renal failure
Liver failure

FIGURE 14–5. Pathogenesis of acute mucosal lesions involves the interaction of (1) reflux of duodenal contents, (2) loss of normal mucus barrier, (3) secretion of hydrochloric acid, and (4) reduction in mucosal blood flow.

acid, without prior gastric injury, can also cause acute gastric lesions.[48] Gastric hyperacidity can result from a large number of different causes (Table 14–5). Secretion of excessive gastrin or histamine often underlies the increased acid secretion. Excessive gastrin is released from gastrinomas and other APUD tumors (see Chapter 27) and results in gastric mucosal ulceration.[48–50] Mastocytomas of all grades and sizes release large amounts of histamine and often result in gastric erosions or ulcers.[51–53]

In humans, head injuries are associated with increased gastric acid secretion and gastric ulceration. Gastric ulceration can also be seen in animals with head injury. The acid hypersecretion associated with head injury probably results from stimulation of oxyntic and G cells via vagal pathways originating in the CNS. The hypersecretion can be reduced by anticholinergic drugs.[54] Gastric hypersecretion is also of proposed importance in the pathogenesis of the gastric lesions associated with kidney and liver disease (see later).

Disorders Reducing Gastric Mucosal Blood Flow

Any disorder reducing mucosal blood flow predisposes to gastric ulceration by compromising the mucosal barrier (see Chapter 12). The decrease in mucosal flow most commonly results from stress, shock, portal hypertension, and/or disseminated intravascular coagulation. Mucosal blood flow is reduced in these conditions by hypovolemia, sympathetically mediated vasoconstriction, circulating catecholamines, and release of a variety of vasoactive agents.[55] Histamine release, stimulated by catecholamines and stress-induced vagal activity, contributes to the gastric lesions by causing vasodilation and vascular stasis in addition to stimulating acid secretion.[56] Serotonin (a vasoactive amine found in gastric mucosa), vasopressin (a vasoactive peptide released during shock), thromboxane (a potent vasoconstrictor and platelet aggregator), and leukotrienes (chemoattractant for neutrophils) may also play a role in reducing mucosal blood flow in some conditions. Ultimately, mucosal blood flow depends on the balance

between these mediators that reduce blood flow and those with vasodilatory and/or antiaggregatory properties such as vasodilator neuropeptides (e.g., VIP and calcitonin gene-related peptide), prostacyclin, and nitric oxide.[25,57] Once blood returns to the ischemic mucosa, reperfusion injury, mediated by oxygen-derived free radicals, may contribute to the mucosal damage (see Chapter 16).[58,59]

Disorders Causing Gastroduodenal Reflux

It has been suggested that dogs, and to a lesser extent, cats, can develop gastritis as a result of chronic gastroduodenal reflux (reflux gastritis). Certainly dogs and cats with gastritis frequently have bile-stained vomitus, signifying gastroduodenal reflux. Furthermore, there is no doubt that a syndrome exists in which dogs chronically vomit bile on an empty stomach (see Chapter 13). Unfortunately, however, there is little evidence to establish whether bile reflux is a cause or a consequence of the vomiting in this syndrome and, in general, the clinical significance of gastroduodenal reflux in dogs and cats is unknown.

As described in Chapter 12, some gastroduodenal reflux is normal in dogs and probably cats. In addition, gastroduodenal reflux is an inherent component of the vomiting reflex, no matter what the initiating cause of the vomiting (see Chapter 13). Furthermore, at least in some studies, dogs surgically altered to have chronic duodenogastric reflux do not necessarily develop any significant lesions in the antral mucosa although they do develop severe hyperemia and foveolar hyperplasia in the fundus.[60–62] Moreover, some studies have suggested that bile can act as a mucosal protective, perhaps because of its rich bicarbonate content.[63] In an alkaline environment, bile and gastric and pancreatic enzymes do not damage the gastric mucosa. The pKa of bile acids is around 4, so that the ionized form prevails at a higher gastric pH. At a pH lower than 4, bile acids are largely unionized, and, being lipid soluble, they can enter cells with ease to cause damage.

These observations cast doubt on the authenticity of the diagnosis of so-called reflux gastritis. However, many studies have shown that bile and to a lesser extent other components of duodenal juice, such as lysolecithin and pancreatic enzymes, can have damaging effects on gastric mucosa.[64–69] Bile acids are detergents that can solubilize lipid cell membranes and inhibit ion transport systems. In contrast to the observations mentioned in the preceding paragraph, other experiments have shown deleterious effects of gastroduodenal reflux in dogs. For instance, diversion of bile into the canine stomach causes histologic changes that include mucus depletion and epithelial cell degeneration within 3 months and mucosal atrophy at 6 months.[70] Furthermore, duodenogastric reflux in dogs following cholecystectomy is associated with a gastritis.[69] In addition, lysolecithin, a potent membrane-toxic phospholipid formed by the action of pancreatic phospholipase on lecithin in bile, causes increased gastric mucosal permeability for hydrogen and sodium ions in dogs.[71] Thus, it would seem that reflux gastritis may indeed be a clinical entity in dogs and perhaps cats.

Any disorders of the duodenum, antrum, and pylorus that interfere with the mechanisms minimizing gastroduodenal reflux could theoretically predispose an animal to reflux gastritis (the prevention of gastroduodenal reflux is described in Chapter 12). In humans, the problem is most commonly recognized following pyloroplasty procedures and results in nausea, frequent bilious vomiting, and midepigastric abdominal pain.[72] In dogs and cats, the clinical signs of reflux gastritis are likely to be similar. The disorder is most likely to cause clinical signs in fasting animals. Reflux of duodenal fluid is more frequent in fed than unfed animals, but reflux is likely to be more damaging in unfed animals because no food is present to dilute or buffer the refluxed material. Furthermore, the refluxed material is likely to be retained for longer periods in the fasting state because antral contractions occur only infrequently in the interdigestive period. In addition, as described in Chapter 12, the vomiting reflex has a lower threshold in the fasting state. The use of some drugs may predispose to reflux gastritis. For instance, drugs reducing antral motility (such as anticholinergics) can increase the amount of refluxed fluid and the time it remains in the stomach. Other drugs such as aspirin can disrupt the interdigestive migrating motor complex so the stomach is not cleared of refluxed fluid.[73]

Disorders Compromising the Mucus-Bicarbonate Mucosal Layer[74]

Compromise of the mucus-bicarbonate layer by systemic events can predispose to secondary gastritis. The structure and function of this protective layer is described in Chapter 12. Acidosis creates a high risk for gastric ulceration by reducing the delivery of plasma bicarbonate to the gastric mucosa. Acidosis is likely to contribute to the gastric lesions observed in dogs with shock or renal failure. Reduction in mucosal blood flow compromises the high pH microenvironment of the mucus-bicarbonate layer as does the administration of NSAIDs.[75]

Stress Erosions and Ulcers

Gastric mucosal erosions develop in animals following a variety of stressful disorders including trauma, shock, sepsis, psychologic stress, and head injury. They are often termed "stress erosions" or "stress ulcers." Stress erosions are usually not clinically apparent until they extend through the muscularis mucosa to produce gastric ulcers.

The pathophysiology of stress erosions remains controversial more than 60 years after their original description.[76] The major factors implicated are a decrease in mucosal blood flow, a reduction in mucus and prostaglandin secretion, and an increase in gastric acid secretion.[76] In addition, stress ulceration in rats is accompanied by a reduction in the mucosal synthesis of DNA, implying reduced mucosal turnover and repair.[76] Eventually, the role of mucosal protectants, such as epidermal growth factor, sulfhydrals and polyamines, and CNS neurotransmitters such as thyrotropin-releasing hormone (a neuropeptide that exacerbates stress ulcers) may also be defined.[25,76,77] Of these factors, stress-induced decrease in mucosal blood flow seems to play the central role.[54]

As already discussed, stress-induced reductions in mucosal blood flow are mediated by increased sympathetic activity and circulating catecholamines. These vasoconstrictors do not reduce blood flow uniformly throughout the different layers of the mucosa but instead produce focal areas of ischemia.[78] The focal nature of the ischemia may be due to focal spasms of the muscularis mucosae inducing compression of the submucosal blood vessels as they pass through the muscularis mucosae to supply the mucosa.[79] The decreased mucosal blood flow results in focal areas of gastric damage as a result of failure to remove back-diffusing acid, decreased delivery of bicarbonate, and breaks in the mucus-bicarbonate layer overlying the ischemic foci. The latter result from both the reduced delivery of bicarbonate and the decreased production of mucus by the stomach.[56] The mucosa may be further damaged when blood returns to the ischemic tissues by the generation of oxyradicals (ischemia-reperfusion injury). In stress-induced ulceration, reperfusion injury would be of most importance in animals undergoing chronic intermittent periods of stress. These animals would be likely to undergo frequent ischemia-reperfusion incidents.

It is probable that the pathogenesis of stress ulcers in most clinical cases involves not only decreased mucosal blood flow but also a combination of other factors. For instance, stress induced by hypothermia or restraint reduces mucosal blood flow but in addition stimulates gastric acid secretion and strong gastric contractions, both of which may contribute to the pathogenesis of the lesions.[56,80] Similarly, the cause of stress erosions associated with sepsis also appears to be multifactorial, and is likely to include reduced mucosal circulation, increased acid and pepsin secretion, and reduced effectiveness of the mucous barrier.[81,82] Furthermore, infected emboli may play a role, and sepsis may initiate DIC and mucosal thrombosis. The ulceration induced by sepsis is at times pronounced and is complicated by the bleeding tendencies of DIC sometimes culminating in severe gastrointestinal hemorrhage.

Inhibitors of gastric acid secretion reduce the severity of stress erosions as does tube feeding. Glucose, lipids, and proteins all can individually prevent the development of stress erosions.[80] The mechanisms by which feeding prevents gastric erosions are probably multifactorial and are likely to include increased mucosal blood flow, increased mucus secretion, decreased gastric acidity (buffering), and perhaps decreased strength of gastric contractions.[80] Whatever the mechanism, these observations provide more support for early use of enteral nutrition in stressed and anorexic hospitalized patients.

Renal Disease

Gastric erosions and ulcers are common in patients with chronic renal disease (Figure 14–6). The pathogenesis of these lesions is multifactorial, involving some or all of decreased mucosal blood flow and mucus-gel thickness, gastric hypersecretion, gastroduodenal reflux, and acidosis.[83,84] Decreased mucosal blood flow caused by diffuse vascular injury appears to be the most important factor.[83,84] Gastric mucosal acidosis from increased back diffusion of acid has been detected in humans and laboratory animals with renal disease and has been attributed to compromise of the mucus-gel layer, impaired epithelial tight junctions, and decreased mucosal blood flow.[84] Controversy surrounds the importance of gastric acid hypersecretion in the pathogenesis of uremic gastritis.[83] Chronic renal disease or bilateral nephrectomy result in hypergastrinemia.[85] The hypergastrinemia has been attributed to the kidney's important role in the degradation of gastrin, and it has been suggested that the hypergastrine-

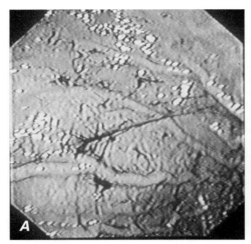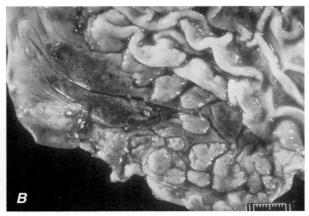

FIGURE 14-6. *(A)* Endoscopic appearance of early uremic gastritis in a dog. Scattered gastric hemorrhage can be seen in the gastric body. In addition, increased light reflectivity is present and suggests mucosal edema. *(B)* Necropsy specimen of chronic uremic gastritis. Note the areas of calcification, congestion, and hemorrhage. (Courtesy of Dr. Keith Thompson)

mia is the stimulus for gastric acid hypersecretion. However, studies in humans have suggested that gastric hyposecretion, rather than hypersecretion, is the norm for patients with chronic renal disease.[84] Low gastric acid secretion is, in turn, a potent stimulus for gastrin secretion.

High gastric ammonia levels have been suggested to contribute to the gastric damage induced by uremia.[86] The ammonia is produced from urea that has diffused from the interstitial fluid into the stomach. Ureases in bacteria and gastric mucosal cells convert the urea to ammonia. Recently, this hypothesis was examined in a small number of dogs infused intravenously with urea in sufficient quantities to produce very high plasma urea levels (3000 mg/dl).[87] After urea infusion, gastric urea content increased to 50% of the plasma level but the rise in gastric ammonia was relatively small (from 6.0 mg/dl to 17 mg/dl).[87] This study suggests that gastric ammonia is unlikely to reach toxic levels at the plasma urea concentrations more commonly found in animals with renal disease.

Inspection of the stomach of affected animals shows edema and thickening of the rugal folds often with focal areas of erosion or ulceration (Figure 14–6). As the condition progresses, severe mucosal congestion develops, resulting in a dark red color. Accumulations of digested blood are usually present. A prominent histopathologic feature of uremic gastritis is the presence of calcium phosphate deposits in the mucosa and submucosa. These mineral deposits are particularly common on the basement membrane of gastric glands and blood vessels (Figure 14–7). They are thought to occur as a result of the high serum phosphorus concentration and rapid mobilization of calcium that occur during renal disease. Precipitation occurs preferentially in the stomach because of the alkaline tissue environment produced by bicarbonate diffusing into the interstitial fluid during the secretion of hydrochloric acid. When calcium phosphate is in solution at a supersaturated level, the increase in pH causes precipitation. Additional histologic features of uremic gastritis are edema of the lamina propria, congestion, and hemorrhage. Eventually the gastric glands of uremic animals atrophy.[88]

Hepatic Disease

Acute and chronic hepatic disease can cause lesions in the gastric mucosa.[51,89] The pathogenesis of the gastric damage is controversial. In acute hepatitis the gastric lesions appear to be due primarily to reduced blood flow, usually as a result of thrombosis caused by DIC.[90] The liver is rich in thromboplastin, which is released during acute hepatitis. Thromboplastin initiates the clotting cascade, causing widespread thrombosis and resultant gastric erosion and ulceration. Furthermore, failure of the damaged liver to remove activated clotting factors from circulation further exacerbates the clotting tendency (see Chapter 30).

The pathogenesis of the gastric lesions in chronic liver disease is multifactorial involving gastric hypersecretion, decreased mucosal blood flow, and gastric vascular ectasia (see Chapter 30).[91] Dogs with hepatic cirrhosis secrete more gastric hydrochloric acid after portal circulation is partially shunted around the liver.[92] The cause of the increased gastric acid secretion is unknown. In some, but not all, studies of liver failure, blood levels of histamine and gastrin increase and may be responsible for the increased acid secretion (see Chapter 30). Decreased mucosal blood flow occurs in chronic liver disease as a result of portal hypertension, microvascular shunting, and thrombosis and dysplasia of gastric vessels (see Chapter 30).

Hypoadrenocorticism

Dogs with hypoadrenocorticism develop gastritis, gastric erosions and ulcers, and at times significant gastric hemorrhage.[93] The reasons for these gastric lesions are not clear but it appears that glucocorticoids are necessary for gastric cytoprotection. For instance, without glucocorticoid secretion, prostaglandins do not protect against aspirin damage to the mucosa.[94]

CLINICAL FINDINGS

Vomiting is a consistent sign of acute gastritis. It usually follows soon after drinking or eating and occurs less frequently if the patient is given nothing to eat or drink. The vomitus usually contains mucus, and it is often bile stained. Small amounts of fresh blood are occasionally seen. More severe gastric bleeding is manifested by large volumes of digested blood in the vomitus

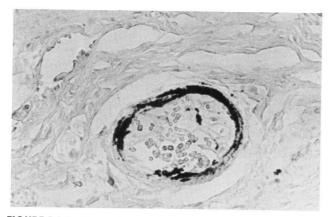

FIGURE 14-7. Photomicrograph of a blood vessel in the gastric submucosa from a dog with uremic gastritis. A calcium stain outlines mineral deposits in the vessel wall.

("coffee grounds") and by melena. Variable degrees of anorexia and depression occur. Abdominal pain is occasionally manifested by the assumption of a hunched stance or a praying position. It is important to note, however, that cranial abdominal pain is not pathognomonic for acute gastritis. Shivering is occasionally observed in dogs with gastritis and has also been attributed to abdominal pain. Abdominal sounds frequently increase, especially before the onset of vomiting. Vomiting animals often crave water, although little of the ingested water is retained. Fever is infrequent with primary acute gastritis.

Physical examination of the patient with acute gastritis often reveals signs of mild dehydration but is usually otherwise unremarkable. The empty stomach is situated too far cranially to be palpated, but mild cranial abdominal pain is occasionally detected. Not infrequently, the abdominal examination provokes vomiting.

LABORATORY FINDINGS

Laboratory tests in animals with primary gastritis are usually unremarkable with the exception of mild hemoconcentration and electrolyte imbalances. A complete blood count and serum chemistry panel is warranted if the clinician is suspicious of serious gastrointestinal bleeding or secondary gastritis due to liver or kidney disease, or wishes to check for other causes of vomiting such as acute pancreatitis.

RADIOGRAPHIC FINDINGS

Survey abdominal radiographs are usually unremarkable in animals with gastritis. In addition, gastric ulceration is difficult to identify even with contrast studies. In animals with acute onset of vomiting, radiographic procedures are used most often to rule out foreign bodies or small intestinal obstruction as the cause of the vomiting (see later).

BIOPSY AND PATHOLOGY FINDINGS

Biopsy samples are seldom taken from the gastric mucosa of animals with acute gastritis. As mentioned earlier, acute gastritis is characterized histologically by necrosis and hemorrhage (Figure 14–8).

DIAGNOSIS

A tentative diagnosis of acute gastritis is usually made on the basis of clinical findings. Definitive diagnosis of acute gastritis is rarely made and the specific cause of the gastric inflammation is seldom identified. Because acute gastritis is a common problem, symptomatic treatment of vomiting animals for presumptive acute gastritis is frequently undertaken. This approach is entirely acceptable, provided there are no warning signs of serious gastrointestinal diseases such as small intestinal obstruction (see Chapter 5 for warning signs).

If a gastrointestinal foreign body or obstruction is strongly suspected, survey abdominal radiographs should be taken immediately. Radiopaque foreign bodies are readily identifiable on survey radiographs, but radiolucent foreign bodies will be recognized only with contrast radiographic procedures (Figure 14–9). Small intestinal obstructions can be recognized by survey film abnormalities or by contrast studies with barium-impregnated polyethylene spheres (BIPS—Ken Bowman Associates, Diamond Bar, CA) or barium sulfate liquid.

If foreign bodies or obstructions are not highly likely, survey radiographs may be delayed until the response to symptomatic management is assessed. Rapid remission of signs is consistent with the diagnosis of acute gastritis. If signs do not begin to resolve after 24 to 48 hours of symptomatic management, further diagnostic work, including a complete blood count, serum chemistry profile, and radiography, should be performed to investigate the possibility of pancreatitis, liver disease, uremia, or gastrointestinal obstruction.

The convenience of administration and minimal cost of

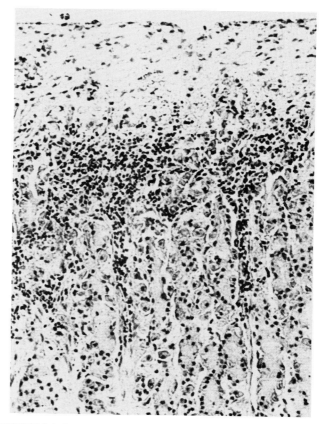

FIGURE 14-8. Photomicrograph of gastric mucosa from dog with signs of gastritis. Cells in luminal one-third are necrotic. Hemorrhage is evident in middle section, especially at border between necrotic cells and viable cells.

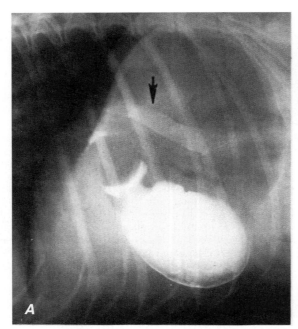 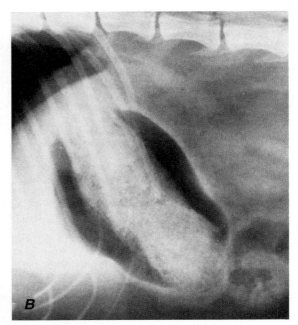

FIGURE 14-9. *(A)* Lateral radiograph of abdomen of Sheltie with clinical signs of intestinal obstruction. Positive contrast medium was given and appears in the caudal or distal part of the stomach. The pyloric antrum contains a filling defect that has a smooth circular outline, the shape of a ball. A minimal amount of the contrast is seen in the first part of the duodenum (arrow), which suggests the gastric outlet obstruction is not complete. The dog was induced to vomit a rubber ball. *(B)* Lateral radiograph of abdomen of 7-year-old cat. Stomach is in its normal position and contains an intraluminal mass. Radiographic density is that of fluid rather than bone or metal. Gastric wall is of normal thickness so there is probably no mural involvement. Most likely diagnosis is gastric foreign body, probably a hairball. This case shows the advantage of using air as a contrasting agent.

BIPS (Figure 14–10A) has led one of the authors (WGG) to routinely use this contrast agent during the first 24 hours of symptomatic management of acutely vomiting animals in which a gastrointestinal obstruction is possible. If the animal has responded to symptomatic management by the next morning, no radiographs are taken. However, if the animal has not made the expected response to treatment, a survey radiograph is taken (Figure 14–10B). The survey radiograph provides the usual anatomic information but, in addition, the BIPS yield functional information about gastrointestinal transit rates (and the need for prokinetic drugs) and assist in the detection of gastrointestinal obstructions (see Chapter 25).

MANAGEMENT OF ACUTE GASTRIC LESIONS

The theoretical goals in treating acute gastric lesions are to replace fluid and electrolyte losses; rest the stomach; minimize vomiting and abdominal pain; relieve gastric smooth muscle spasm; protect the mucosa from hydrochloric acid, pepsin, and bile acids; minimize duodenogastric reflux; control hemorrhage; limit the inflammatory process; treat the primary cause where identifiable; and encourage healing.

FLUID THERAPY. The fluid, electrolyte, and acid-base derangements that accompany vomiting range from mild to moderate in severity. Correction of these abnormalities is of prime importance in the therapy of acute gastritis. The fluid therapy of vomiting is discussed in detail in Chapter 39. In general, a balanced electrolyte solution such as lactated Ringer's solution is used. A minimum of 10 to 20 mEq/L of potassium chloride is added to the fluids unless there is clinical or laboratory evidence of diseases that can cause hyperkalemia (such as renal failure or hypoadrenocorticism). The additional potassium is required to replace the high losses of potassium in the vomitus.

If the acute gastritis is mild and the vomiting infrequent, oral rehydration solutions (ORS) may be valuable. The primary advantage of ORS is their minimal cost in comparison to parenteral fluid therapy. Food-based oral rehydration therapy is particularly attractive because of the low osmolality of the food-based ORS solutions in comparison to ORS based on dextrose (see Chapter 39). The ORS should be provided as frequent small boluses to quench the patient's thirst but avoid significant gastric distension that might stimulate vomiting.

DIETARY MANAGEMENT. Animals with acute gastritis should receive nothing per os for 12 to 36 hours. Feeding stimulates secretion of hydrochloric acid, increasing the amount of acid available for back diffusion and accelerating mucosal damage. Furthermore, even minor distention of an acutely inflamed stomach (with food or water) usually initiates the vomiting reflex.

At the conclusion of the fast, food should be offered in small quantities at frequent intervals. Careful selection of foods minimizes the probability of relapse. The ideal food for animals in the recovery stage of gastritis is nonabrasive, minimizes gastric acid stimulation, is hypoallergenic, empties rapidly from the stomach, and is not markedly hypertonic.

Carbohydrates stimulate the secretion of gastric juices less than do other nutrients. Isotonicity is easier to maintain in the stomach when carbohydrate is fed as starch rather than mono- or disaccharides. Therefore, an easily digested starch (such as rice) should be used, rather than a sugar solution. If glucose-based oral rehydration solutions are used in the early phases of treatment they should not contain greater than 10% dextrose.

Ideally, the protein content of the therapeutic diet should be kept as low as possible during the first few days of feeding because protein comprises the majority of dietary antigenic-

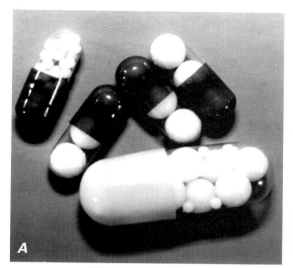

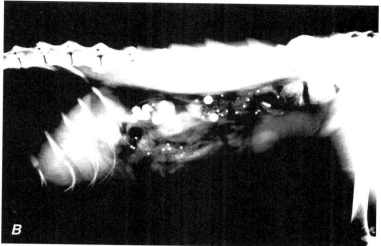

FIGURE 14–10. *(A)* Barium-impregnated polyethylene spheres (BIPS) are radiopaque markers of two sizes (1.5 and 5.0 mm diameter) used to quantitate the gastric emptying and orocolic transit time of food and to detect gastrointestinal obstructions. They are administered by capsule and their progress through the bowel is monitored by one or more abdominal radiographs. *(B)* Lateral abdominal radiograph of the abdomen of a cat presented for vomiting. BIPS were administered the previous evening because of concern the cat may have had an obstruction, although nothing definitive could be palpated. This radiograph was taken the next morning and all BIPS were now in the colon, indicating the cat did not have an obstruction.

ity, and amino acids are the most potent stimulators of gastric acid secretion. Unfortunately, very low-protein diets adversely affect palatability. The type of protein fed is also worth considering. It may be advantageous to change to a novel dietary protein source to reduce the likelihood of acquired food sensitivity to a dietary staple (see Chapter 24). The therapeutic diet should be low in fat to hasten gastric emptying. For the same reason, easily triturated diets are of value. Suitable diets fulfilling the criteria just outlined include cottage cheese or diced chicken and rice (see Chapter 38).

INHIBITION OF GASTRIC ACID SECRETION. For most patients with acute gastritis, a period of fasting provides sufficient inhibition of gastric acid secretion, and antacids or drugs such as H_2 blockers are unnecessary. However, in animals with sufficient gastric erosion or ulceration to cause melena or the vomiting of digested blood, inhibitors of gastric acid secretion are indicated. Commonly used acid inhibitors include cimetidine (5 mg/kg PO, SC or IV q 6–8 hours) or ranitidine (1–4 mg/kg PO, SC or IV q 8–12 hours) for 3 to 7 days. These drugs and other inhibitors of acid secretion are discussed in detail in Chapter 15.

ANTIEMETICS. Most animals with acute gastritis do not need antiemetics because their vomiting becomes infrequent when food and water are withheld. However, antiemetics are needed in patients with persistent vomiting because unrelenting vomiting quickly becomes distressing to them and their owners. In addition, antiemetics may be needed to minimize the need for fluid therapy in intractable patients or in those patients whose owners have limited budgets. The pathophysiologic background to the use of antiemetics is discussed in Chapter 13. A number of antiemetics are available for use.[95,96] These drugs must be administered with the understanding that they offer symptomatic control and do not treat the primary cause of the vomiting.

The phenothiazine derivatives, such as chlorpromazine and prochlorperazine, are the most effective antiemetics for managing animals with gastrointestinal problems (Table 14–6). These antiemetics inhibit activity at both the chemoreceptor trigger zone and, at higher doses, the emetic center. This results in antiemetic properties in a broad spectrum of diseases. Vomiting is inhibited in a dose-related manner by

phenothiazines. If the initial dose used fails to control the vomiting, the dose can be increased in a stepwise fashion until control is obtained. Caution is needed, however, because phenothiazines are alpha-adrenergic antagonists and therefore have hypotensive effects, particularly at high doses or in the presence of hypovolemia.

Metoclopramide acts as a dopamine antagonist at the CTZ and peripheral receptors. As a result, the drug has antiemetic properties and stimulates gastrointestinal motility. This prokinetic effect may contribute to the antiemetic effects of the drug. Because metoclopramide does not directly affect the vomiting center it does not have as broad a spectrum of activity as phenothiazines in the control of vomiting. In addition, metoclopramide has a relatively short half-life (approximately 1.5 hours), and so it must be administered frequently or as an infusion. Moreover, experimental evidence indicates that dopamine antagonists, such as metoclopramide, predispose the gastric and duodenal mucosa to ulceration, perhaps by reducing mucosal blood flow or by increasing basal gastric secretion.[97] For these reasons, metoclopramide is not the ideal or most effective antiemetic for dogs and cats. The dose of metoclopramide is 0.2 to 0.4 mg/kg PO, IM, or SC. When used as a continuous infusion the dose is 1 to 2 mg/kg/24 hours IV. Adverse reactions to metoclopramide include transient (2–3 days) sedation, vertigo, nervousness, and twisting movements of the head and neck or limbs.[98] In the event of overdosage, diphenhydramine will reduce the extrapyramidal signs. Metoclopramide is contraindicated in epileptic patients and should be used with care in patients with renal disease and those receiving cimetidine, digoxin, narcotics, tetracyclines, and tranquilizers.

A number of other dopamine antagonists act on the CTZ to inhibit vomiting. Domperidone (Motilium, Janssen) is an effective antiemetic in dogs.[99] It is a similar drug to metoclopramide but has the advantage of fewer CNS side effects. Butyrophenones such as droperidol and haloperidol and diphenylbutylpiperidines such as pimozide and penfluridol are effective in blocking vomiting induced by chemicals such as narcotics. At higher doses the butyrophenones also block vomiting at the vomiting center. Butyrophenones are generally considered potent antiemetics with similar efficacy to the phenothiazines.

Pimozide is a long-acting antiemetic and is able to prevent drug-induced vomiting in dogs for up to 6 days.

The antihistamines diphenhydramine and dimenhydrinate inhibit some forms of vomiting mediated through the CTZ by an action at H_1 receptors. These drugs are also used to prevent motion sickness via their effects on the vestibular apparatus and central muscarinic activity. Contrary to popular belief, the H_2 receptor antagonists do not possess antiemetic properties per se.

Although acetylcholine is the primary neurotransmitter in the emetic center, most anticholinergic drugs do not have demonstrable antiemetic properties because they do not cross the blood-brain barrier. Isopropamide (Darbazine, Norden) and aminopentamide (Centrine, Bristol) are two anticholinergics that can penetrate into the CNS and act as antiemetics. Unfortunately, their antiemetic properties are modest, and because this class of drug reduces gastrointestinal motility (which is already compromised in vomiting animals) they are a poor choice of antiemetic.

Other drugs used as antiemetics include dexamethasone, which has an unpredictable effect by an unknown mechanism. Bismuth subsalicylate may occasionally be effective as an antiemetic, but the mechanism is unknown. Trimethobenzamide (Tigan, Beecham) is believed to act at the CTZ and is generally considered less effective than the centrally acting antiemetics.

Failure to respond to antiemetic therapy should prompt reevaluation of the diagnosis and the dose and type of emetic used. In the case of phenothiazine antiemetics, a dose increase may provide more effective control. If metoclopramide is failing to control the vomiting, a change of antiemetic to a more broad-spectrum drug such as chlorpromazine or an increase in the frequency of administration may be advantageous. Some animals that do not respond to antiemetic therapy have more serious gastrointestinal diseases than gastritis, such as small intestinal obstruction.

ANTIBIOTICS. In animals with gastritis, proliferation of microorganisms in the stomach is possible as a result of failure to maintain the low pH necessary to prevent bacterial growth. Moreover, the use of antacids or inhibitors of acid secretion further increases gastric pH, encouraging more prolific bacterial growth.[100] In spite of these observations, most animals with uncomplicated acute gastritis do not require antibiotic therapy. However, in animals with severe mucosal disruption, antibiotics may be indicated to prevent mucosal invasion by bacteria, which are thriving where they normally would not survive. Therefore, antibiotic therapy is justified when there is clinical evidence of extensive mucosal disruption, such as hematemesis. Penicillin derivatives are a good choice because the most likely source of bacteria contaminating the stomach is the oral cavity, a site that has high numbers of anaerobic flora. Antibiotic therapy is of paramount importance when mucosal lesions perforate the gastric wall and bacteria contaminate the abdominal cavity. In this situation, antibiotics with a broad spectrum of effectiveness against anaerobes (e.g., metronidazole) and gram negative bacteria (e.g., gentamicin) are necessary to prevent abdominal abscessation and sepsis.

LOCALLY ACTING PROTECTANTS. Little evidence indicates that nonspecific gastric protectants, such as kaolin and pectin, hasten the recovery of acute mucosal lesions. Any beneficial effect they might have is not due to a mucosal "coating" action (as was once hypothesized) but is instead ascribed to the absorption of injurious products such as microbial toxins.

Sucralfate. Sucralfate (Carafate) is the aluminum salt of a sulfated derivative of sucrose. The drug is indicated for topical treatment of gastric and duodenal lesions.[101,102] Uncontrolled trials in dogs and cats with vomiting have suggested a beneficial effect.[103] In an acidic environment, the molecule dissociates into aluminum and sucrose sulfate. The negatively charged sulfate groups bind to the positively charged exposed proteins of disrupted epithelial surfaces, providing a protective barrier against the action of acid and pepsin. In addition, sucralfate inhibits pepsin activity and binds bile acids. Although it contains aluminum, sucralfate is not an antacid per se. However, the drug stimulates bicarbonate and mucus secretion by surface mucosal cells and also appears to reduce parietal cell responsiveness to secretagogues.[104] Sucralfate also increases the viscosity of gastric mucus and improves its ability to impede hydrogen ion diffusion.[105] In addition, sucralfate stimulates the release of prostaglandins. Among other functions, the latter facilitate mucosal blood flow and mucosal repair. Furthermore, sucralfate is thought to enhance binding of epithelial growth factor to eroded mucosa and to improve gastric mucosal hydrophobicity.[102,104]

Sucralfate is not absorbed from the gastrointestinal tract and has no toxic side effects. Esophageal impaction, slight delays in gastric emptying, and constipation have been reported in humans taking the drug. The dose of sucralfate in cats is usually 0.12 g to 0.25 g (125–250 mg) every 8 to 12 hours. The dose in dogs is usually 0.25 g to 1 g every 6 to 12 hours. Great care is required when using sucralfate with other drugs because of a high frequency of drug interactions. The binding properties of sucralfate reduce the absorption of many drugs including tetracyclines, fluoroquinilones, and cimetidine. Furthermore, the effectiveness of sucralfate is inhibited (but not eliminated) in an alkaline environment.[106] Thus, it is common practice to give sucralfate 1 to 2 hours prior to the use of antacids or drugs that inhibit gastric acid secretion, such as cimetidine.

Bismuth. Colloidal bismuth subcitrate (De-Nol), and bismuth subsalicylate (Pepto-Bismol) are valuable for the treatment of acute gastritis. Both drugs have been shown experimentally to reduce stress ulceration in rats but, with the exception of the United States, in humans colloidal bismuth subcitrate has become the bismuth compound of choice for upper gastrointestinal lesions whereas bismuth subsalicylate is predominantly used for acute diarrheal diseases.[107] Their beneficial effects in gastrointestinal disease have been attributed to their cytoprotective and demulcent properties.[107] Colloidal bismuth subcitrate appears to have a selective coating affinity for ulcers although this finding has been disputed.[107] The drug can form a complex with gastric glycoproteins that strengthens the mucosal barrier by retarding hydrogen ion diffusion.[107] It also diminishes the output of pepsin. In addition, bismuth compounds have antibacterial activity against helicobacter-like organisms (and possibly other bacteria).[107]

Bismuth products have a high degree of safety when used for short courses at standard doses. For acute gastritis in dogs and cats, a suitable dose of colloidal bismuth subcitrate is 1 to 3 mg/kg three to four times per day. Careful dosing is required with barium subsalicylate because the salicylate moiety is released by gastric acid and absorbed in the stomach and duodenum. In humans, the pharmacokinetics of salicylate in bismuth subsalicylate is identical to an equivalent dose of aspirin (Pepto-Bismol contains approximately 9 mg of salicylate per mL).[107] A suitable dose of Pepto-Bismol for cats is 0.5 mL/kg q 12 hours and for dogs is 1 mL/kg q 8 hours for 3 to 5 days. In addition to the salicylate, a small amount of the administered bismuth is absorbed from the intestine and sequestered in multiple sites about the body before being slowly excreted in the urine.[107] As a result, bismuth toxicity is possible, particularly in patients with reduced renal function

Table 14–6

ANTIEMETIC DRUGS AND DOSES

DRUG (SITE OF ACTION)	DOSAGE FOR DOGS (D) AND CATS (C)
Chlorpromazine (VC, CTZ) (D,C) (Thorazine)	0.5–4.0 mg/kg q 6–8 hours, SC, IM, IV 3–4 mg/kg q 6–24 hours PO (D,C) 1.0 mg/kg q 8 hours, rectal (D)
Prochlorperazine (VC, CTZ) (Compazine)	0.1–0.5 mg/kg q 6–8 hours, SC, IM, IV, PO (D,C)
Diphenhydramine (CTZ) (Benadryl)	2.0–4.0 mg/kg q 8 hours PO, IM (D,C) 1–2 mg/kg q 8–12 hours IV
Dimenhydrinate (CTZ) (Dramamine)	3–8 mg/kg q 8 hours PO, IM (D,C)
Trimethobenzamine (CTZ) (Tigan)	3 mg/kg q 8 hours PO, IM (D)
Metoclopramide (CTZ) (Reglan; Maxalon)	0.2–0.5 mg/kg q 6–8 hours PO, SC (D,C) 1–2 mg/kg daily slow IV (D,C) 1.3 µg/kg/minutes (D,C)
Haloperidol (CTZ) (Haldol)	0.02–0.1 mg/kg IM (D)
Droperidol (CTZ)	0.5–1.0 mg/kg q 8 hours IM, IV (D)
Dexamethasone (?) (Azium)	0.1 mg/kg SC, IV (D)

that are receiving long courses. Because of this possibility, human physicians have advised that treatment periods with bismuth-containing products should last no longer than 6 to 8 weeks followed by 8 week bismuth-free intervals.[107] In the absence of comparable data in dogs and cats, similar recommendations would seem advisable.

It is worthy of note that ingestion of bismuth products causes the feces to blacken, a change that can lead to a misdiagnosis of melena. The cause for the blackening is the formation of bismuth sulfide in the colon.[107]

REFERENCES

1. Johnson LR. Pepsin output from the damaged canine heidenhain pouch. Am J Dig Dis 16:403–407, 1971.
2. Jacobson ED. Circulatory mechanisms of gastric mucosal damage and protection. Gastroenterology 102:1788–1800, 1992.
3. Drasar BS, Hill MJ. Human Intestinal Flora. Academic Press, London, 1974.
4. Broido PW, Gorbach SL, Condon RE, et al. Upper intestinal microflora control. Arch Surg 106:90–93, 1973.
5. Smith HW. Survival of orally administered E. coli K₁₂ in alimentary tract of man. Nature 255:500–502, 1975.
6. Osborne AD, Wilson MR. Mycotic gastritis in a dog. Vet Rec 85:487–488, 1969.
7. Howard EB. Acute mycotic gastritis in a dog. VM/SAC 61:549–552, 1966.
8. Henry GA, Long PH, Burns JL, et al. Gastric spirillosis in Beagles. Am J Vet Res 48:831–836, 1987.
9. Food-borne diseases. Outbreaks due to microbial toxins in wheat and fish. Weekly Epidemiological Record 64:145–146, 1989.
10. Davis RE, Ivy AC. Thermal irritation in gastric disease. Cancer 2:138–143, 1949.
11. Maudlin N. Basic principles of radiotherapy. Proc 11th ACVIM Forum, Washington DC, 854–856, 1993.
12. Cheli R, Perasso A, Giacosa A. Gastritis. Springer-Verlag, New York, 36–44, 1987.
13. Crawford LM, Wilson RC. Melena associated with dexamethasone therapy in the dog. J Sm Anim Pract 23:91–97, 1982.
14. Sorjonen DC, Dillon AR, Powers RD, et al. Effects of dexamethasone and surgical hypotension on the stomach of dogs: Clinical, endoscopic, and pathologic evaluations. Am J Vet Res 44:1233–1237, 1983.
15. Menguy R, Masters YF. Effect of cortisone on mucoprotein secretion by the gastric antrum of dogs: Pathogenesis of steroid ulcer. Surgery 54:19–27, 1963.
16. Pavicevic D, Knezevic M. Character of the gastrointestinal lesions in dogs after experimental treatment with dexamethasone. Veterinarski-Glasnik 45:11–12, 831–836, 1991.
17. Dow SW, Rosychuk AW, McChesney AE, et al. Effects of flunixin and flunixin plus prednisone on the gastrointestinal tract of dogs. Am J Vet Res 51:1131–1138, 1990.
18. McKellar QA, May SA, Lees P. Pharmacology and therapeutics of non steroidal anti-inflammatory drugs in the dog and cat: 2 individual agents. J Sm Anim Pract 32:225–235, 1991.
19. Jones RD, Baynes RE, Nimitz CT. Nonsteroidal anti-inflammatory drug toxicosis in dogs and cats: 240 cases (1989–1990). J Am Vet Med Assoc 201:475–477, 1992.
20. Stewart THM, Hetenyi C, et al. Ulcerative enterocolitis in dogs induced by drugs. J Pathol 131:363–378, 1980.
21. Prokopiw I, Hynna-Liepert TT, Dinda PK, et al. The microvascular anatomy of the canine stomach. Gastroenterology 100:638–647, 1991.
22. Godshalk CP, Roush JK, Fingland RB, et al. Gastric perforation associated with administration of ibuprofen in a dog. J Am Vet Med Assoc 201:1734–1736, 1992.
23. Menguy R. Gastric mucus and the gastric mucous barrier. Am J Surg 117:806–812, 1969.
24. Wallace JL. Non-steroidal anti-inflammatory drug gastropathy and cytoprotection: Pathogenesis and mechanisms re-examined. Scand J Gastroenterol suppl 192:3–8, 1992.
25. Wallace JL, Bell CJ. Gastroduodenal mucosal defense. Curr Opin G 9:902–908, 1993.
26. Cheung LY, Moody FG, Reese RS. Effect of aspirin, bile salt, and ethanol on canine gastric mucosal blood flow. Surgery 77:786–792, 1975.
27. Borda IT. The spectrum of adverse gastrointestinal effects associated with nonsteroidal anti-inflammatory drugs. In: Borda IT, Koff RS. (eds) NSAIDs: A Profile of Adverse Effects. Mosby Year Book, St Louis, 25–80, 1992.
28. Lichtenberger LM, Richards JE, Hills BA. Effect of 16, 16-dimethyl prostaglandin E₂ on the surface hydrophobicity of aspirin-treated canine gastric mucosa. Gastroenterology 88:308–314, 1985.
29. Murtaugh RJ, Matz ME, Labato MA, et al. Use of synthetic prostaglandin-E₁ (Misoprostol) for prevention of aspirin-induced gastroduodenal ulceration of arthritic dogs. J Am Vet Med Assoc 202:251–256, 1993.
30. Johnston SA, Leib MS, Forrester SD. Misoprostol prevents endoscopically detectable gastric and duodenal mucosal injury in dogs receiving aspirin. Proc 11th ACVIM Forum, Washington DC, 945, 1993.
31. Urquhart J. Two cheers for NSAIDs. Gut 27:1287–1291, 1986.
32. Gilmour MA, Walshaw R. Naproxen-induced toxicosis in a dog. J Am Vet Med Assoc 191:1431–1432, 1987.
33. Forsyth SF, Guilford WG. Unpublished observations, 1994.
34. Daehler MH. Transmural pyloric perforation associated with naproxen administration in a dog. J Am Vet Med Assoc 189:694–695, 1986.
35. Storset A. Adverse effects of phenylbutazone on dogs. Norsk-Veterinaertidsskrift 102:42–43, 1990.
36. Gfeller RW, Sandors AD. Naproxen-associated duodenal ulcer complicated by perforation and bacteria- and barium sulfate-induced peritonitis in a dog. J Am Vet Med Assoc 198:644–646, 1991.
37. Spellman PG. Gastrointestinal reaction to piroxicam. Vet Rec 130:211, 1992.
38. Vonderhaar MA, Salisbury SK. Gastroduodenal ulceration associated with flunixin meglumine administration in three dogs. J Am Vet Med Assoc 203:92–95, 1993.
39. Ligumsky M, Sestieri M, Karmeli F, et al. Rectal administration of nonsteroidal antiinflammatory drugs. Gastroenterology 98:1245–1249, 1990.
40. Jenkins CC, DeNovo RC, Patton CS, et al. Comparison of effects of cime-

tidine and omeprazole on mechanically created gastric ulceration and on aspirin-induced gastritis in dogs. Am J Vet Res 52:658–661, 1991.

41. Paola JP, Sherding RG, Johnson SE, et al. Endoscopic comparison of protective effects of omeprazol versus cimetidine versus misoprostol versus sucralfate on gastric mucosal injury induced by flunixin plus prednisone in dogs [abstract]. Proc 12th ACVIM Forum, San Francisco, 981, 1994.

42. Boulay JP, Lipowitz AJ, Klausner JS. Effect of cimetidine on aspirin-induced gastric hemorrhage in dogs. Am J Vet Res 47:1744–1746, 1986.

43. Lancaster-Smith MJ, Jaderberg ME, Jackson DA. Ranitidine in the treatment of non-steroidal anti-inflammatory drug associated gastric and duodenal ulcers. Gut 32:252–255, 1991.

44. Wallace MS, Zawie DA, Garvey MS. Gastric ulceration in the dog secondary to the use of nonsteroidal antiinflammatory drugs. J Am Anim Hosp Assoc 26:467–472, 1990.

45. Silen W. What is cytoprotection of the gastric mucosa? Gastroenterology 94:232–235, 1988.

46. Fromm D. Mechanisms involved in gastric mucosal resistance to injury. Ann Rev Med 38:119–128, 1987.

47. Zinner MJ, Turtinen L, Gurll NJ. The role of acid and ischemia in production of stress ulcers during canine hemorrhagic shock. Surgery 77:807–816, 1975.

48. McGuigan JE. The endocrine ulcer concept. Am J Dig Dis 21:144–147, 1976.

49. Shaw DH. Gastrinoma (Zollinger-Ellison syndrome) in the dog and cat. Can Vet J 29:448–451, 1988.

50. Straus E, Johnson GF, Yalow RS. Canine Zollinger-Ellison syndrome. Gastroenterology 72:380–381, 1977.

51. Murray M, Robinson PB, McKeating FJ, et al. Peptic ulceration in the dog: A clinico-pathological study. Vet Rec 91:441–447, 1972.

52. Ritchie WP, Breen JJ, Grigg DI. Prevention of stress ulcer by reducing gastric tissue histamine. Surgery 62:596–600, 1967.

53. Fox LE, Rosenthal RC, Twedt DC, et al. Plasma histamine and gastrin concentrations in 17 dogs with mast cell tumors. J Vet Int Med 4:242–246, 1990.

54. Moody FG, Cheung LY, Simons MA, et al. C. Stress and the acute gastric mucosal lesion. Am J Dig Dis 21:148–154, 1976.

55. Nicoloff DM, Peter ET, Leonard AS, et al. Catecholamines in ulcer provocations: Their possible role in stress ulcer formation. J Am Med Assoc 191:383–385, 1965.

56. Cho CH, Koo MWL, Garg GP, et al. Stress-induced gastric ulceration: Its aetiology and clinical implications. Scan J Gastroenterol 27:257–262, 1992.

57. Stark ME, Szurszewski JH. Role of nitric oxide in gastrointestinal and hepatic function and disease. Gastroenterology 103:1928–1949, 1992.

58. Perry MA, Wadhwa S, Parks DA, et al. Role of oxygen radicals in ischemia-induced lesions in the cat stomach. Gastroenterology 90:362–367, 1986.

59. Itoh M, Guth PH. Role of oxygen-derived free radicals in hemorrhagic shock-induced gastric lesions in the rat. Gastroenterology 88:1162–1167, 1985.

60. Fontolliet C, Mosimann F, Diserens H, et al. modifications of the gastric mucosal barrier induced by experimental duodenogastric reflux: an electron microscopic study. Scand J Gastroenterol 19 (suppl 92):75–77, 1984.

61. Diserens H, Krstic R, Burri B, et al. The gastric mucosa in experimental duodenogastric reflux. Scand J Gastroenterol 19 (suppl 92):133–135, 1984.

62. Burri B, Mosimann F, Diserens H, et al. A long-term study of different types of experimental alkaline reflux and the effects of its suppression in dogs. Scand J Gastroenterol 19(suppl 92):81–86, 1984.

63. Rhodes J, Davies HA, Wheeler MH, et al. Bile diversion from the duodenum: Its effect on gastric pancreatic function. Scand J Gastroenterol 19 (suppl 92):221–223, 1984.

64. Lawson HH. Effect of duodenal contents on the gastric mucosa under experimental conditions. Lancet 1:469–472, 1964.

65. DenBesten L, Hamza KN. Effect of biles salts on ionic permeability of canine gastric mucosa during experimental shock. Gastroenterology 62:417–434, 1972.

66. Djahanguiri B, Abtahi FS, Hemmati M. Prevention of aspirin-induced gastric ulceration by bile duct or pylorus ligation in the rat. Gastroenterology 65:630–633, 1973.

67. Black RB, Rhodes J, Hole D. Measurement of bile damage to the gastric mucosa. Am J Dig Dis 12:411–415, 1973.

68. Duane WC, Wiegand DM. Mechanisms by which bile salt disrupts the gastric mucosal barrier in the dog. J Clin Invest 66:1044–1049, 1980.

69. Brough WA, Taylor TV, Torrance HB. The effect of cholecystectomy on duodenogastric reflux in dogs and humans. Scand J Gastroenterol 19(suppl 92):242–244, 1984.

70. Thomas WEG. Gastric morphological and functional changes produced by bile in the canine stomach. Eur Surg Res 13: 125–133, 1981.

71. Duane WC, McHale AP, Sievert CE. Lysolecithin-lipid interactions in disruption of the canine gastric mucosal barrier. Am J Physiol 250:G275–G279, 1986.

72. Markowitz JF. Duodenogastric reflux: The state of the art. J Pediatr Gastroenterol Nutr 10:287–289, 1990.

73. Dooley CP, Mello WD, Valenzuela JE. Effects of aspirin and prostaglandin E_2 on interdigestive motility complex and duodenogastric reflux in man. Dig Dis Sci 30:513–521, 1985.

74. Rees WDW. Mucus-bicarbonate barrier—shield or sieve. Gut 28:1553–1556, 1987.

75. Wallace JL, Mcknight GW. The mucoid cap over superficial gastric damage in the rat. Gastroenterology 99:295–304, 1990.

76. Konturek PK, Brzozowski T, Konturek SJ, et al. Role of epidermal growth factor, prostaglandin, and sulfhydrals in stress-induced gastric lesions. Gastroenterology 99:1607–1615, 1990.

77. Hernandez DE. Neurobiology of brain—gut interactions. Implications for ulcer disease. Dig Dis Sci 34:1809–1816, 1989.

78. Lucas CE, Sufawa C, Friend W, et al. Therapeutic implications of disturbed gastric physiology in patients with stress ulcerations. Am J Surg 123:25–34, 1972.

79. Piasecki CK, Thrasivoulou C. Spasm of gastric muscularis mucosae might play a key role in causing focal mucosal ischemia and ulceration. Dig Dis Sci 38:1183–1189, 1993.

80. Kleiman-Wexler RL, Ephgrave KS, Broadhurst KA. Effects of intragastric and intravenous glucose on restraint model of stress ulceration. Dig Dis Sci 37:1860–1865, 1992.

81. Douglass HO, Falk GA, LeVeen HH. Infection: A cause of acute peptic ulceration in hypersecreting animals. Surgery 68:827–830, 1970.

82. Odonkor P, Monat C, Himal HS. Prevention of sepsis-induced gastric lesions in dogs by cimetidine via inhibition of gastric secretion and by prostaglandin via cytoprotection. Gastroenterology 80:375–379, 1981.

83. Quintero E, Kaunitz J, Nishizaki Y, et al. Uremia increases gastric mucosal permeability and acid back-diffusion injury in the rat. Gastroenterology 103:1762–1768, 1992.

84. Diebel L, Kozol R, Wilson RF, et al. Gastric intramucosal acidosis in patients with chronic kidney failure. Surgery 113:520–526, 1993.

85. Falcao HA, Wesdorp RIC, Fischer JE. Gastrin levels and gastric acid secretion in anephric patients and in patients with chronic and acute renal failure. J Surg Res 18:107–111, 1975.

86. Merrill JP, Hampers CL. Uremia. Eng J Med 282:953–961, 1970.

87. Meyer H, Schunemann C, Grubler B. Intestinal urea metabolism in experimental uraemia. Adv Anim Physiol Anim Nutr 19:78–85, 1989.

88. Cheville NF. Uremic gastropathy in the dog. Vet Pathol 16:292–309, 1979.

89. Kirk AP, Dooley JS, Hunt RH. Peptic ulceration in patients with chronic liver disease. Dig Dis Sci 25:756–760, 1980.

90. Roberts HR, Cederbaum AI. The liver and blood coagulation physiology and pathology. Gastroenterology 63:297–320, 1972.

91. Quintero E, Pique JM, Bombi JA, et al. Gastric mucosal vascular ectasias causing bleeding in cirrhosis. Gastroenterology 93:1054–1061, 1987.

92. Hein MF, Silen W, Skillman JJ, et al. The effect of portacaval shunting on gastric secretion in cirrhotic dogs. Gastroenterology 44:637–641, 1963.

93. Medinger TL, Williams DA, Bruyette DS. Severe gastrointestinal tract hemorrhage in three dogs with hypoadrenocorticism. J Am Vet Med Assoc 202:1869–1872, 1993.

94. Szabo S, Gallagher GT, Horner HC, et al. Role of the adrenal cortex in gastric mucosal protection by prostaglandins, sulfhydryls, and cimetidine in the rat. Gastroenterology 85:1384–1390, 1983.

95. Willard MD. Some newer approaches to the treatment of vomiting. J Am Vet Med Assoc 184:590–592, 1984.

96. Forrester SD, Merton Boothe D, Willard MD. Clinical pharmacology of antiemetic and antiulcer drugs. Sem Vet Med Surg 4:194–201, 1989.

97. Glavin GB, Szabo S. Dopamine in gastrointestinal disease. Dig Dis Sci 35:1153–1161, 1990.

98. Neer MT. Drug-induced neurologic disorders. Proc 11th ACVIM Forum, Washington DC, 861–869, 1993.

99. Lee KY, Park HJ, Chey WY. Studies on mechanism of retching and vomiting in dogs. Dig Dis Sci 30:22–28, 1985.

100. Howden CW, Hunt RH. Relationship between gastric secretion and infection. Gut 28:96–107, 1987.

101. Colin-Jones DG. There is more to healing ulcers than suppressing acid. Gut 27:475–480, 1986.

102. Tarnawski A, Erickson RA. Sucralfate—24 years later: Current concepts of its protective and therapeutic actions. Eur J Gastroenterol Hepatol 3:795–810, 1991.

103. Steiner K, Sailer H. Sucralfate: A cytoprotective agent for treating vomiting and diarrhoea in dogs and cats. Kleintierpraxis 32:35–38, 1987.

104. Rees WDW. Prevention of peptic ulcer relapse by sucralfate: Mechanisms of action. Scand J Gastroenterol 27 (suppl 191): 4–6, 1992.

105. Slomiany BL, Laszewicz W, Slomiany A. Effect of sucralfate on the viscosity of gastric mucus and the permeability to hydrogen ion. Digestion 33:146–151, 1986.

106. Konturek SJ, Brzozowski T, Mach T, et al. Importance of an acid milieu in the sucralfate-induced gastroprotection against ethanol damage. Scand J Gastroenterol 24:807–812, 1989.

107. Gorbach SL. Bismuth therapy in gastrointestinal diseases. Gastroenterology 99:863–875, 1990.

15 Chronic Gastric Diseases

W. GRANT GUILFORD AND DONALD R. STROMBECK

CHRONIC GASTRITIS: INTRODUCTION

Chronic gastritis is an important cause of vomiting in dogs and cats. The prevalence of the disease in the general pet population is unknown, but in a study of clinically normal young beagles, 9% of the dogs were found to have microscopic evidence of chronic gastric inflammation.[1] It is likely that the prevalence of chronic gastritis in pets is equal to or higher than this value. The prevalence of the disease is probably greater than at first thought because dogs with chronic gastritis often vomit only infrequently in spite of quite severe gastric inflammation. Furthermore, in many cases, biopsy is required to make the diagnosis because dogs with chronic gastritis frequently do not have gross lesions in the stomach.[1] As a result, necropsy surveys that do not include histologic examination of the stomach will underestimate the prevalence of the disease.

Classification

An etiologic classification of gastritis can be made if the primary cause is identified. Etiologic diagnoses include gastritis due to food allergy, fungal infections, nonsteroidal anti-inflammatory drugs (NSAIDs), uremia, and *Helicobacter felis* (Table 15–1). However, in most cases of chronic gastritis, the cause is never determined. In the absence of a recognizable primary cause, chronic gastritis is usually subclassified according to the histologic appearance or, less commonly, according to breed associations (Table 15–1). Factors considered by pathologists when classifying idiopathic gastritis include the type of cellular infiltrate, the area of the mucosa affected (i.e., superficial and/or deep; focal or generalized), the severity of the inflammation, the mucosal thickness, and, to a limited extent, topography (e.g., antrum, body, etc.). On this basis, idiopathic chronic gastritis is frequently subdivided into the following categories: nonspecific (lymphocytic-plasmacytic) gastritis, eosinophilic gastritis, and granulomatous gastritis. Nonspecific gastritis can be further subdivided into atrophic gastritis, hypertrophic gastritis, simple superficial gastritis, and simple diffuse gastritis (Table 15–1). Note that the classification used for idiopathic gastritis is an arbitrary system imposed on inflammatory gastric diseases that have overlapping clinicopathologic features. Furthermore, in both human and veterinary medicine, there

is disagreement about the basis on which subclassification of gastritis should be made and the value to the clinician of current classification systems based solely on histologic findings rather than a combination of clinical, endoscopic, and histologic findings.[2-4] The latter holistic approach is more likely to provide a classification system that assists clinicians to advise appropriate therapy and prognosis.[2]

Table 15–1

VARIOUS CLASSIFICATIONS OF CHRONIC GASTRITIS IN DOGS AND CATS*+

Etiologic Classification
Allergic gastritis
Drug-associated gastritis (NSAIDs)
Foreign body–induced gastritis
Mycotic gastritis
Parasitic gastritis
Reflux gastritis
Spiral bacteria–associated gastritis
    Gastrospirillum hominis
    Helicobacter felis
Toxic gastritis
Uremic gastritis

Breed-Associated Gastritis
Basenji
Drentse patrijshond
Norwegian Lundehund

Histologic Classification (Idiopathic Chronic Gastritis)
Eosinophilic gastritis: dominant infiltrate is eosinophil
Granulomatous/histiocytic gastritis: dominant infiltrate is macrophage
Nonspecific gastritis: dominant infiltrate is round cells
    simple superficial gastritis: round cell infiltrate in the superficial mucosa with a normal mucosal thickness
    simple diffuse gastritis: round cell infiltrate throughout the mucosa with normal mucosal thickness
    atrophic gastritis: decreased mucosal thickness with or without a round cell infiltrate
    hypertrophic gastritis: increased mucosal thickness with or without a round cell infiltrate

*Many of these classifications have overlapping clinicopathologic features.
+These classifications may be further qualified by whether they are erosive or nonerosive and focal or generalized.

CHRONIC NONSPECIFIC GASTRITIS

Clinical Synopsis

Diagnostic Features

- Persistent intermittent vomiting exacerbated by eating or drinking
- Physical examination usually unremarkable
- Laboratory database required to rule out a systemic cause
- Gastric biopsy samples show variable infiltration with inflammatory cells (especially lymphocytes) and occasional changes in mucosal thickness
- Spontaneous recovery is unusual

Standard Treatment

- NPO or no food for 24 to 48 hours
- Easily digestible, hypoallergenic diet for 2 to 4 weeks
- Gastroprotective drugs: sucralfate (cats: 125–250 mg q 8–12 hours; dogs: 250–1000 mg q 6–12 hours) or colloidal bismuth subcitrate (1–3 mg/kg q 6-8 hours) for up to 8 weeks
- Cimetidine (5–10 mg/kg PO, SC, IV q 8 hours) or ranitidine (1–4 mg/kg PO, SC, IV q 8–12 hours) for 1 to 2 weeks if signs of hematemesis or melena observed
- Prednisone (1–2 mg/kg PO q 12 hours for 1–2 weeks followed by decreasing doses over an additional 2–3 months) if lymphocytic and/or plasmacytic infiltrates are heavy and remission not obtained by controlled diet
- Additional drugs sometimes required include antibiotics, prokinetics, and antiemetics (see text).

Chronic "nonspecific" gastritis is characterized by inflammatory infiltration of the gastric mucosa with lymphocytes, plasma cells, and lesser numbers of other inflammatory cells ("round" cells). As mentioned earlier, chronic nonspecific gastritis is usually further subdivided according to the area of the mucosa affected (superficial or diffuse gastritis) and whether the mucosa is of normal thickness (simple gastritis), increased thickness (hypertrophic gastritis), or decreased thickness (atrophic gastritis).[4] In the authors' experience, superficial and diffuse chronic gastritis without marked alteration in mucosal thickness are the most common forms of chronic gastritis, far exceeding the number of cases of atrophic or hyperplastic gastritis.

Etiopathogenesis

The etiology and pathogenesis of chronic nonspecific gastritis in dogs and cats is unknown. However, experimental studies in animals and clinical observations in humans with gastritis strongly suggest that immune-mediated and/or autoimmune processes are involved. Chronic gastritis can be produced experimentally by using a mucosal irritant to initiate an immune-mediated pathologic process. Chronic gastritis can also be induced in dogs by intravenous injection of human gastric juices[5] or by intradermal or subcutaneous injections of autologous or homologous gastric juice (see later).[6-8] Furthermore, autoimmune gastritis can be produced in experimental animals by perinatal thymectomy.[10] Perinatal thymectomy inhibits the development of self-tolerance, probably due to a loss of suppressor T lymphocytes. The inflammatory response in the stomach initiated by thymectomy includes both T and B lymphocytes and eventually leads to either mucosal atrophy or hypertrophy. At times, immune-mediated reactions (in particular the Arthus reaction) can result in gastric ulceration.[11]

In humans, a relationship is seen between chronic gastritis and a number of autoimmune diseases.[9] Laboratory evaluations in affected people demonstrate autoantibodies and cell-mediated immune responses to antigens in the gastric mucosa analogous to findings in animal models.

EXPERIMENTAL CANINE MODEL. An experimental model of chronic gastritis in dogs given intradermal injections of homologous gastric juice in Freund's complete adjuvant has received detailed description.[8] The initial morphologic change, appearing within 2 weeks, is an infiltration of the superficial part of the lamina propria by chronic inflammatory cells, producing a superficial gastritis. Over the next 2 to 4 weeks, inflammatory cells infiltrate the deeper mucosa to a marked degree (Figure 15–1). Fibrosis, with degeneration of oxyntic and chief cells, appears 5 to 10 weeks after immunization. Paralleling the morphologic changes is a reduced ability to secrete hydrochloric acid. The pathologic changes are associated with the appearance of delayed or cell-mediated hypersensitivity. Within 2 weeks of immunization, the dogs show positive skin tests and evidence of cell-mediated immune reactions to gastric juice. Circulating autoantibodies do not appear until 3 to 6 weeks after immunization. This study suggests that both cell-mediated immunity and, to a lesser extent, humoral immunity may play a role in the pathogenesis of the gastritis in this model. Cell-mediated immune reactions against a number of different antigens in the gastric juice, including those in oxyntic cells, can be demonstrated. All the pathologic changes are reversible on removel of the stimulus, and gastric morphology returns to normal. Chronic gastritis can also be produced by injections of gastric juice without Freund's adjuvant, although it takes longer to develop.

SUMMARY OF ETIOPATHOGENESIS The preceding observations suggest that spontaneously occurring chronic nonspecific gastritis (with or without ulceration) may often have an immune-mediated pathogenesis. Defects in the gastric mucosal barrier from any cause allow gastric contents to be absorbed into the mucosa and could potentially stimulate similar immune responses to those observed in experimental models. Alternatively, a breakdown in tolerance to self-tissues could result in a true autoimmune (rather than immune-mediated) gastritis.

Pathophysiology

As discussed in Chapter 14, gastric inflammation compromises all the major functions of the stomach. Gastric motility is deranged and the reservoir function of the stomach impaired, resulting in vomiting, delayed gastric emptying or, alternatively, dumping of gastric contents into the duodenum. Widespread inflammation of the mucosa interferes with gastric secretory functions and, in some chronic cases, can result in mucosal proliferation that can interfere with gastric emptying. Plasma proteins are lost through the inflamed mucosa into the gastric lumen. The loss of proteins is particularly marked in the face of gastric erosion or ulceration. In addition, experiments in dogs have demonstrated that protein loss is marked following gastric hypersensitivity reactions.[12] In the latter situation, the leakage is through the so-called tight junctions between epithelial cells and can be minimized by administration of corticosteroids and, in particular, azathioprine.[12]

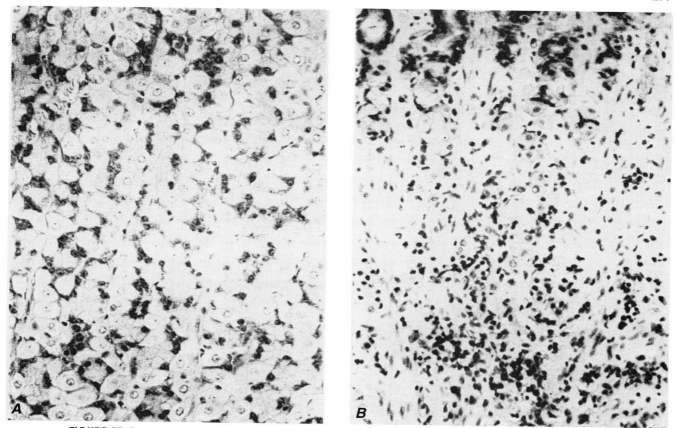

FIGURE 15-1. *(A)* Photomicrograph of gastric fundic mucosal biopsy from a normal untreated dog. *(B)* Photomicrograph of gastric fundic mucosal biopsy taken 3 weeks after immunization with autologous gastric juice. Reveals chronic inflammatory infiltrate and atrophy of gastric glands (KJB Krohn, Clin Exp Immunol 14:237–245, 1973; by permission of Blackwell Scientific Publications).

Subclassifications of Chronic Nonspecific Gastritis

CHRONIC SUPERFICIAL GASTRITIS.[9] The gross lesions of superficial gastritis include mucosal reddening, excessive mucus, edema, and sometimes aphthae-like small erosions. At times, however, no gross lesions will be recognizable. Histology shows epithelial cells of variable height and occasional microerosions. Mucous neck cells often have degenerative changes but deeper glandular cells are normal. The superficial interstitial tissue (between the gastric pits) is infiltrated by inflammatory cells. Plasma cells and lymphocytes are the dominant inflammatory cell type. With time, the surface epithelia can be destroyed and replaced by fibrous tissue, leaving the inner part of the mucosa relatively normal. Both gross and histologic lesions are often patchy, indicating that multiple biopsy specimens are needed for reliable diagnosis.

As described earlier, experimental immune-mediated gastritis in dogs intially involves the superficial mucosa and then progress to involve the entire mucosa. This suggests that superficial gastritis may be an early phase of diffuse chronic gastritis. Although this may occur in some cases, a follow-up study of gastritis in dogs has shown that on many occasions superficial gastritis resolves without progression to diffuse gastritis, implying that the superficial inflammation is usually a transient reaction to a noxious agent in the stomach.[4]

CHRONIC SIMPLE DIFFUSE GASTRITIS.[9] The gross lesions of chronic simple diffuse gastritis are similar to those of superficial gastritis. The histologic changes are also similar but are more extensive involving the full thickness of the mucosa, with lymphocytes and plasma cells again the dominant inflammatory cell type (Figure 15–2). In contrast to superficial gastritis, the lesions tend to be less patchy and more per-

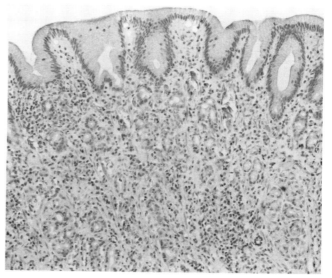

FIGURE 15-2. Mild chronic gastritis. There is mild infiltration with mononuclear cells and a slight decrease in oxyntic and chief cell numbers.

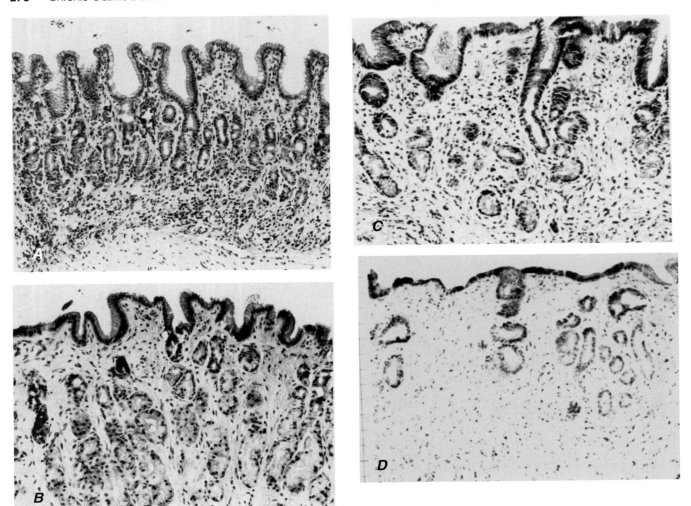

FIGURE 15-3. *(A)* Moderate atrophic gastritis. Tissue from body of stomach shows deepening of gastric pits with elongation of ridges to produce papillary effect, reduced numbers of oxyntic and chief cells, chronic inflammation throughout but especially in basal area where glandular cells have disappeared. Overall mucosal thickness is reduced. *(B)* Mild gastric atrophy. Glandular epithelium is slightly reduced with no replacement of oxyntic and chief cells by goblet cells. Little evidence of inflammation. *(C)* Moderate gastric atrophy. Gastric pits are deepened. Oxyntic and chief cells are replaced almost entirely by globlet cells. Few glandular cells of any type remain. *(D)* Severe gastric atrophy. Reduced numbers of gastric glands. Deepening of one gastric pit. Evidence for intestinal metaplasia in epithelia of both surface and glands. The appearance of cells resembling intestinal epithelium with absorptive properties is associated with increased cell turnover. The accelerated rate of proliferation by mucous neck cells affects their differentiation to oxyntic and chief cells so that intestinal epithelial type cells are produced. Corticosteroid therapy may reverse this pathology. Little evidence for inflammation. *(E)* Severe atrophic gastritis. There is diffuse infiltration by inflammatory cells that extends to submucosa. Intestinal glands have almost disappeared. Intestinal metaplasia evident by intestinal-like epithelium replacing both surface and glandular epithelium. *(F)* Severe atrophic gastritis. Changes similar to and more severe than Figure 15–3E except for inflammation, which is minimal.

sistent.[4] Unlike atrophic or hypertrophic gastritis the mucosal thickness remains normal.[4]

ATROPHIC GASTRITIS.[9] The gastric mucosa of dogs with atrophic gastritis appears discolored and thin. Submucosal blood vessels can be seen through the thinning mucosa. Histology shows changes similar to those in superficial gastritis but more extensive and more severe (Figures 15–3A–F). The gastric mucosal parenchyma is reduced, and inflammatory cells can usually be observed in the mucosal remnants. The mucosal epithelium is generally flat, consisting of elongated cells that have oval-shaped nuclei. Metaplastic cells are frequent and many goblet or enterocyte-like cells appear. The gastric pits are shortened and tortuous, and special staining of surface mucosal cells shows abnormal mucus. Cells staining with PAS decrease in number, and acid mucopolysaccha-

rides appear. Increased numbers of lymphocytes and plasma cells occasionally extend through the muscularis mucosae into the submucosa. The reduction in parenchymal thickness results from loss of glands and their cells. Residual glands are ectatic and their cells are deformed, showing vacuolar degeneration and sometimes substitution by metaplastic cells more reminiscent of the type of epithelium seen in the small intestine. Surprisingly, clinical[4] and experimental studies in dogs have shown that on removal of the cause, most of these histologic changes (including fibrosis) can return to normal.

End-stage gastric mucosal atrophy results in reduced secretion of gastric juices and a loss of nutritional homeostasis. The nutritional compromise does not result from poor digestion, per se, because hydrochloric acid and pepsinogen are not essential for the digestion of macronutrients. Acid secre-

(**FIGURE 15-3** *continued*)

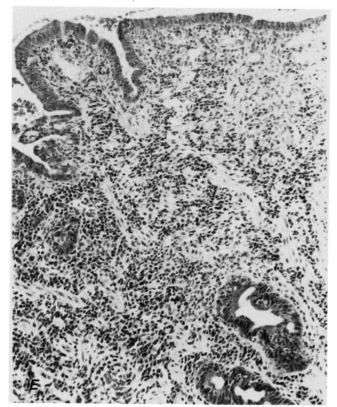

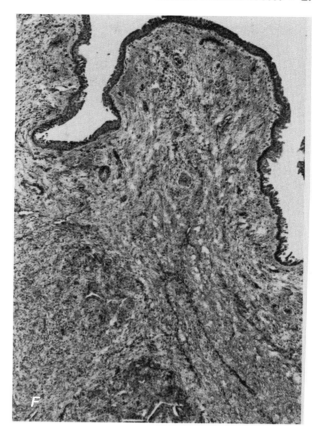

tion is necessary, however, for the suppression of bacterial growth in the small intestine. Thus, achlorhydria results in small intestinal bacterial overgrowth, which in turn leads to malabsorption and a loss of nutritional homeostasis. Unlike in humans, atrophic gastritis does not produce vitamin B_{12} deficiency in dogs. It is possible, however, that calcium and iron deficiency may occur because normal gastric acid secretion is required for absorption of calcium and iron.

HYPERTROPHIC GASTRITIS. Hypertrophic gastritis is characterized grossly by diffuse or focal mucosal proliferation (Figure 15–4). In the focal form of the disease the lesion can appear as one or many polyoid-like masses or as a discrete area of rugal enlargement (Figure 15–5). In some cases the hypertrophy is associated with gastric ulceration. The most common form of the disease is focal proliferation of the antral mucosa as a component of the antral pyloric hypertrophy syndrome (see later). Widespread mucosal enlargement of the gastric body is less frequent, and is most commonly reported in basenjis (see Chapter 24).

Histologically, hypertrophy and hyperplasia of the mucosa are apparent (Figures 15–6A–C). The glandular epithelium is hyperplastic and at times metaplastic. Proliferation of epithelial cells increases the surface area of the mucosa and throws it up into folds. Increased numbers of mucous cells contribute to the mucosal thickening, and retention of material in mucous cysts is sometimes found. These mucosal changes are usually the dominant microscopic finding. However, the mucosal hyperplasia is often accompanied by variable amounts of fibrous tissue and inflammatory cells such as lymphocytes, plasma cells, and lesser numbers of eosinophils and neutrophils.

Hypertrophic gastritis is most common in basenjis and other small-breed dogs such as the Lhasa apso, Shih tzu, Maltese, and miniature poodle.[13-15] The disease has recently been recorded in association with stomatocytosis in two families of the Drentse patrijshond breed.[16] Hypertrophic gastritis usually affects older dogs and males are predisposed.

The cause of the mucosal hypertrophy is unknown but, as demonstrated by the breed associations and the canine model discussed earlier, hereditary and immune-mediated factors may be involved. In addition, exposure of the gastric mucosa to chronic irritation can cause mucosal hypertrophy and hyperplasia.[17] Differential diagnoses include focal mucosal hypertrophy caused by chronic administration of salicylates. Mucosal hypertrophy and hyperplasia can also be seen in dogs and/or cats as a result of gastrinomas, mast cell neoplasia, *Ollulanus tricupis,* campylobacter-like organisms, idiopathic antral mucosal G cell hyperplasia, chronic omepra-

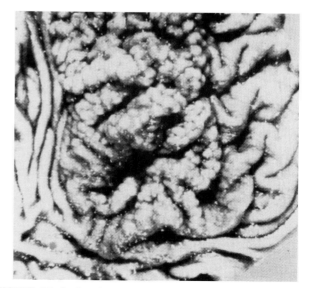

FIGURE 15-4. Gastric mucosal hypertrophy. Numerous folds produced by hypertrophy can cause gastric-outlet obstruction.

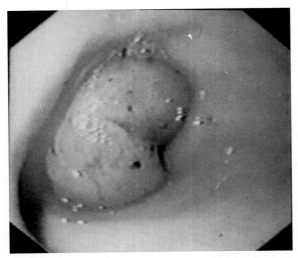

FIGURE 15–5. Endoscopic appearance of focal mucosal hyperplasia at the pylorus of an elderly Shih tzu with clinical signs of delayed gastric emptying. The diagnosis was antral pyloric hypertrophy syndrome, and response to pyloroplasty was good.

zole use, or gastric retention resulting from gastric-outlet obstruction.[18,19,21] Gastric retention stimulates release of gastrin, a hormone that is trophic for mucosa in the body of the stomach. Lastly, contraction of the muscularis musosae and/or gastric muscle can cause folding of the gastric mucosa, giving the appearance of mucosal hypertrophy.

Hypertrophic gastritis in dogs has been compared to Ménétrier's disease in humans.[22,23] Similarities include the gross and morphologic features, the presence of protein-losing gastropathy, and infiltration of mucosa and submucosa with lymphocytes and plasma cells. The pathogenesis of the problem in humans may involve an immune-mediated mechanism because the gastric mucosa contains an increased number of IgM-bearing cells.[24] Gastrin levels are normal in humans with Ménétrier's disease.[25]

Clinical Findings

The clinical signs in animals with chronic nonspecific gastritis include vomiting, weight loss (usually mild), anorexia, and depression. As mentioned previously, vomiting is the most consistent clinical sign but is not always seen. The vomiting is often intermittent and may consist of food or bile-stained mucoid liquid. Not uncommonly it is initiated by feeding, but in dogs with hypertrophic gastritis the vomiting may be delayed for hours after eating (due to delayed gastric emptying from gastric outlet obstruction). Hematemesis and melena are unusual unless the gastritis is associated with significant mucosal erosion or ulceration. Diarrhea is uncommon in uncomplicated chronic nonspecific gastritis but is frequently seen in animals whose gastritis is associated with concomitant lymphocytic-plasmacytic infiltration of the intestines (inflammatory bowel disease; see Chapter 24). Furthermore, advanced atrophic gastritis and hypertrophic gastritis will occasionally cause diarrhea as a result of small intestinal bacterial overgrowth or inactivation of pancreatic enzymes, respectively. The clinical signs of chronic gastritis are usually subtle early in the disease, and many patients are not presented for treatment until the problem is in an advanced stage.

Physical findings are most often unremarkable. Clinical evidence of weight loss and anemia may be found. Skin and hair coat are often poor.

Diagnosis

LABORATORY FINDINGS. The laboratory findings in animals with chronic gastritis are usually nonspecific. Anemia, leukocytosis, a stress leukogram, and hypoproteinemia are occasionally seen. The anemia has a variety of causes. Regenerative anemia along with melena can occur following gastric bleeding. Normocytic, normochromic, nonregenerative anemia is common and presumedly due to the "anemia of chronic disease." Occasionally, microcytic hypochromic anemia is present in animals with chronic gastritis and is probably due to iron deficiency from poor iron absorption or repeated blood loss. The hypoproteinemia is usually due to loss of both albumin and globulins into the gastric lumen. Measurement of electrolytes and blood gases is most commonly unremarkable, but hypokalemia, hypochloremia, and alkalosis can be seen in animals with antral pyloric hypertrophy syndrome.[15]

DIAGNOSTIC IMAGING. Survey radiographs are usually unremarkable. Contrast radiographic studies are occasionally abnormal if the chronic gastritis has produced gastric retention and/or gastric mucosal hypertrophy. In advanced gastritis, evaluation of gastric motility by fluoroscopy may show loss of normal motility. Ultrasonography is useful in demonstrating focal or diffuse thickening of the gastric wall or pylorus.

ENDOSCOPY FINDINGS. Endoscopy is the method of choice for diagnosis of chronic nonspecific gastritis. The mucosa may be grossly normal but in many cases abnormalities will be been (Table 15–2). Mucosal granularity and friability are the most frequent lesions observed endoscopically (Figure 15–7). Occasionally, heavy accumulations of mucus, patchy mucosal hyperemia, or scattered erosions are present. As mentioned earlier, mucosal hypertrophy suggests hypertrophic gastritis whereas the observation of submucosal vessels indicates atrophic gastritis (provided the stomach is not overinflated during endoscopic examination). Erosions and ulcers are identified more reliably with endoscopy than with radiographic studies.

Endoscopy is particularly advantageous for the retrieval of biopsy samples from focal areas of abnormal mucosa. Even when the gross appearance of the mucosa is normal, biopsy specimens should be taken because the mucosa of animals with superficial gastritis as well as chronic diffuse gastritis can appear grossly normal.

The endoscope should be passed through the pylorus, and the duodenum examined and biopsied. Not uncommonly lymphoplasmacytic infiltrates in the stomach are accompanied by similar infiltrates in the small bowel. Such cases are described in Chapter 24.

SERUM GASTRIN LEVEL. If the endoscopic appearance is of generalized rugal hypertrophy with ulceration, the clinician should consider obtaining a serum gastrin level. Although results must be interpreted carefully (see Chapter 6), high serum gastrin levels in a nonazotemic patient suggest the hypertrophic gastritis is secondary to hypergastrinemia and should prompt exploration of the pancreas for a gastrinoma.

BIOPSY AND PATHOLOGY FINDINGS. Histologic evaluation of gastric tissue is necessary to detect mild chronic gastritis, to differentiate more severe cases of gastritis from other gastric diseases such as neoplasia, and to determine the specific type and severity of gastritis present (both of which influence prognosis). Multiple biopsy samples are necessary because chronic nonspecific gastritis (in particular superficial gastri-

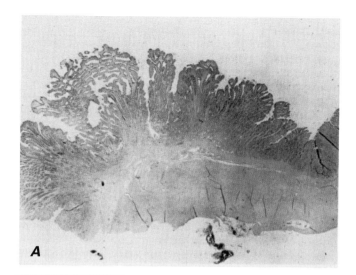

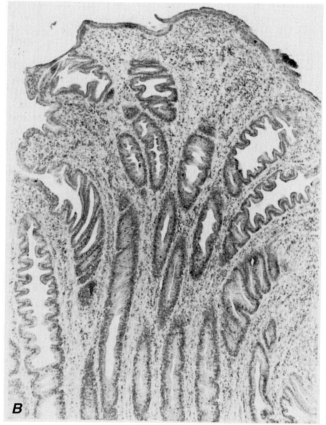

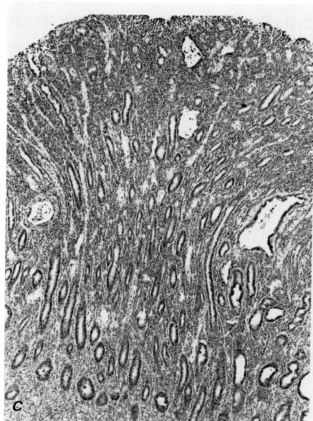

FIGURE 15-6. *(A)* Gastric mucosal hypertrophy. Cross section of stomach wall shows thickening that grossly resembled neoplastic process at surgery. *(B)* Gastric mucosal hypertrophy. Microscopic view of gross specimen in Figure 15–4. Greatly thickened antral mucosa produced by marked hyperplasia of epithelial cells that typify intestinal metaplasia throughout section. Increased lamina propria contain fibrous connective tissue and moderate numbers of inflammatory cells. Lesions caused signs of gastric-outlet obstruction that were corrected successfully by surgical excision. *(C)* Gastric mucosal hypertrophy. Changes in epithelium similar to Figure 15–6B except for marked infiltration by inflammatory cells.

subclassifications. Representative examples of the histologic findings are provided in Figures 15–2, 15–3, and 15–6. It is worth reiterating that mild chronic nonspecific gastritis may show superficial or deep inflammation and perhaps edema as the only changes. In more severe nonspecific gastritis, epithelial erosions develop and bands of inflammatory cells dissect and destroy the glandular mucosa, resulting in replacement by fibrous tissue and eventually atrophic gastritis or, alternatively, mucosal proliferation and hypertrophic gastritis.

Management

FLUID THERAPY. Treatment of chronic nonspecific gastritis is largely symptomatic. In comparison to acute gastritis, fluid, electrolyte, and acid-base derangements are less common with chronic gastritis, and fluid therapy is of less importance. However, occasional animals undergoing an acute flare-up of their disease, or those that develop marked gastric-outlet obstruction from hypertrophic gastritis, do need parenteral fluid therapy with lactated Ringer's or normal saline, respectively (see Chapter 39). Oral rehydration solutions may

tis) often has a patchy distribution. Endoscopy is the method of choice for obtaining gastric biopsy samples. Full thickness (surgical) biopsy of the stomach wall is seldom required because chronic gastritis invariably involves the mucosa. Full thickness biopsy of the stomach wall is indicated, however, if thickening of the gastric wall has been demonstrated by radiography or ultrasound, or it is considered necessary to perform a celiotomy because of some other particular aspect of the case (e.g., inspection of the pancreas to rule out pancreatitis).

The pathologic findings characteristic of the different forms of chronic nonspecific gastritis have already been described in the sections devoted to the different gastritis

Table 15–2

GASTRIC LESIONS SEEN DURING ENDOSCOPY

LESION	CAUSE
Hyperemia	Physiologic increased blood flow; inflammation; low-intensity illumination
Paleness	Anemia; mucosal atrophy; excess illumination
Hyperreflectivity	Edema, excess illumination
Submucosal vessels (body and antrum)	Atrophic gastritis; overinflation
Friability	Inflammation
Lack of mucosal pliancy	Infiltration
Petechia/ecchymosis	Intramucosal hemorrhage
Bleeding	Mucosal or mucosal-submucosal disruption; coagulopathy
Erosions	Mucosal disruptions
Ulcers	Mucosal-submucosal disruption
Rugal hypertrophy	Failure to insufflate; hypertrophic gastritis; hypergastrinemia
Polyps	Epithelial hyperplasia; submucosal masses
Pyloric stenosis	Neoplasia; hypertrophy
Altered luminal shape	Neoplasia; extrinsic compression; scarring from healed ulcer

also be helpful during acute flare-ups. They should be provided as frequent small boluses to quench the patient's thirst but avoid significant gastric distension that might stimulate vomiting.

NUTRITIONAL MANAGEMENT. The initial step in the management of chronic nonspecific gastritis is the feeding of a controlled diet. The same dietary recommendations made for acute gastritis are suitable for use in animals with chronic gastritis (see Chapter 14). Small meals fed frequently lessen the likelihood of vomiting. The food offered should preferably be nonabrasive, minimize gastric acid secretion, and empty rapidly from the stomach. To encourage rapid gastric emptying, the food should be easily triturated and low in fat. A selected (novel) protein diet should be used in case a

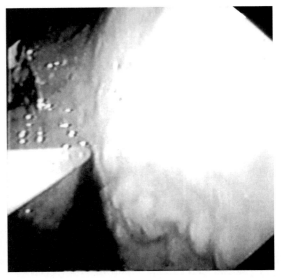

FIGURE 15–7. Endoscopic picture of chronic gastritis in a 5-year-old Russian blue with moderately severe chronic gastritis. An oblique view of the mucosa has been taken to highlight the mucosal granularity. An aspiration catheter is observed in the left of the picture.

dietary sensitivity initiated or is perpetuating the disease (see Chapter 24). Suitable diets fulfilling these criteria include various commercial selected protein diets or homemade diets such as cottage cheese, tofu or diced chicken, and rice (see Chapter 38).

LOCALLY ACTING PROTECTANTS. Sucralfate (Carafate) is indicated for the topical treatment of chronic nonspecific gastritis. The drug is well tolerated and has a number of potentially beneficial effects (see Chapter 14). The dose of sucralfate in cats is usually 0.12 g to 0.25 g (125–250 mg) every 8 to 12 hours. The dose in dogs is usually 0.25 g to 1 g given every 6 to 12 hours. Colloidal bismuth subcitrate (De-Nol, Parke Davis) is also probably of value for the treatment of chronic gastritis. As discussed in the previous chapter, it has mucosal cytoprotective properties and in addition has antibacterial activity against helicobacter-like organisms (and possibly other bacteria). A suggested dose of colloidal bismuth subcitrate is 1 to 3 mg/kg PO q 6 to 8 hours. Because a small amount of the administered bismuth is absorbed from the intestine and sequestered in the body before being slowly excreted, it would seem advisable to restrict therapy with bismuth-containing products to courses shorter than 6 to 8 weeks followed by 8 week bismuth-free intervals (see Chapter 14). Blackening of the stool will occur in patients receiving bismuth and should not be confused with melena.

ACID INHIBITION. Inhibition of gastric acid secretion is rarely necessary for the treatment of chronic nonspecific gastritis unless there is clinical, endoscopic, or histologic evidence of concomitant gastric erosions or ulceration (see later). Gastric acid inhibitors may even be contraindicated because achlorhydria or hypochlorhydria can accompany chronic gastritis, in particular the atrophic form of the disease. Drugs that further reduce gastric acid secretion may compound the bacterial overgrowth that complicates atrophic gastritis. The increased gastric bacterial numbers coincident with suppression of acid secretion may provide additional antigenic stimulation to an already inflamed mucosa. The potential for exacerbating the chronic inflammation is further increased by the propensity of H_2 blockers to inhibit T suppressor activity.[26] Of the different types of chronic gastritis, hypertrophic gastritis is the form of the disease in which inhibitors of acid secretion are most often useful.

ANTIEMETICS. Most animals with chronic nonspecific gastritis do not need antiemetics because their vomiting is infrequent and is further reduced by good nutritional management. Antiemetics are occasionally required during acute exacerbations of the disease (see Chapters 13 and 14). They are ineffective if the vomiting is due to gastric-outlet obstruction.

PROKINETICS. Prokinetic drugs, such as metoclopramide (0.4 mg/kg PO q 6–8 hours), cisapride (0.25–0.5 mg/kg PO q 8 hours), or erythromycin (1–5 mg/kg PO q 8 hours), may be of value in animals with chronic gastritis that have delayed gastric emptying due to secondary gastric motility abnormalities (see later). Caution is required in their use, however, because they are unlikely to be successful and may even be deterimental if the delayed gastric emptying has resulted from gastric-outlet obstruction secondary to mucosal hyperplasia.

ANTIBIOTICS. Routine antibiotic use in chronic nonspecific gastritis is not necessary. However, antibiotics may be indicated to prevent mucosal invasion by bacteria in animals with extensive mucosal erosions, particularly if they are also receiving acid inhibitors. Furthermore, if helicobacter-associated gastritis is suspected (see later) antibiotics may also be indicated. Penicillin derivatives are a good choice because anaerobic bacteria are likely to contaminate the stomach from the oral cavity, and because *Helicobacter* spp. are sensitive to high doses of pencillins.

IMMUNOSUPPRESSIVE DRUGS. Corticosteroids are indicated for the treatment of chronic nonspecific gastritis that does not respond to controlled diets or mucosal protectants. Their use is based on the premise that the gastric inflammation is immune mediated, but they are also reputed to have a trophic effect on parietal cell mass. They are particularly useful if the lymphocytic and plasmacytic infiltrates are heavy. Prednisone is initially used at immunosuppressive levels (1–2 mg/kg PO 12 hours) for 1 to 2 weeks before the dose is gradually reduced over a period of 2 to 3 months until the animal can be safely weaned off the drug. Animals with chronic, simple, nonspecific gastritis usually respond rapidly to corticosteroids. In contrast, patients with atrophic or hyperplastic gastritis do not respond as readily to corticosteroids. In severe cases of chronic gastritis, azathioprine may be a valuable adjunct to the corticosteroids. More information about the use of corticosteroids and azathioprine including precautions and likely side effects can be found in Chapter 24 (inflammatory bowel disease).

The use of glucocorticoids in animals with gastric erosions or ulcers is debatable. In the authors' experience, glucocorticoids in this situation have not exacerbated the ulceration and, with or without H$_2$ blockers and protectants such as sucralfate, have seemingly led to recovery of the mucosa. Glucocorticoids usually do not produce clinically significant gastroduodenal ulcerations unless administered in the face of another factor that predisposes to mucosal damage (e.g., NSAIDs, neurologic disease, shock).[27] Great circumspection is required, however, before corticosteroids or other immunosuppressive drugs are used when deep gastric ulcers are present. Perforation of an ulcer while a patient is receiving immunosuppressant drugs usually results in death because the patient's immune system is compromised and the early signs of perforation (such as abdominal pain) are hidden, resulting in too late a diagnosis for effective therapy.

SURGERY. Surgical resection of focal areas of mucosal hyperplasia usually meets with success. Pyloroplasty procedures are often required when mucosal hypertrophy is resulting in pyloric outflow obstruction (see later).

EOSINOPHILIC GASTRITIS

The clinical signs and diagnosis of eosinophilic gastritis are similar to those of chronic nonspecific gastritis. Many, but not all, animals with the disease have a peripheral eosinophilia. The detection of eosinophilia in a vomiting animal is strongly indicative of eosinophilic gastritis or eosinophilic gastroenteritis but hypoadrenocorticism and mastocytosis are important differential diagnoses. In addition, gastrointestinal parasitism and incidental causes of eosinophilia, such as flea allergic dermatitis, must be ruled out.

The hallmark of eosinophilic gastritis is infiltration of the gastric mucosa with an inflammatory infiltrate dominated by eosinophils (Figures 15–8A and B). In dogs, the eosinophilic infiltrates are often found in other parts of the gastrointestinal tract, a condition referred to as eosinophilic gastroenteritis (see Chapter 24). In cats, eosinophilic gastritis is often just one component of an even more generalized eosinophilic disease referred to as the hypereosinophilic syndrome (see Chapter 24).

Occasionally, the eosinophilic infiltration is granulomatous in nature and can be associated with necrosis, edema, and fibrosis (see Chapter 24).[28] The granulomatous lesions can occur as one or several foci or, alternatively, may be spread diffusely throughout the stomach. They usually involve the mucosa but can extend throughout all layers of the stomach. At times, the mucosa is spared and only the submucosa and muscle layers are affected. The wall of the stomach can become greatly thickened, resembling a gastrc neoplasm (Figure 15–9A).

The etiopathogenesis of eosinophilic gastritis is unknown but hypersensitivity to dietary antigens is a likely cause of some cases. Dietary elimination trials are not successful in a considerable number of affected animals, however, suggesting the disease may also result from an immune response to other antigens such as migrating parasites (see Table 24–4). A recent report described a high prevalence of superficial eosinophilic gastritis in beagles fed a particular commercial diet.[29] Macrophages containing foreign material were a prominent histologic finding in these dogs, intimating that some cases of eosinophilic infiltration may be initiated by for-

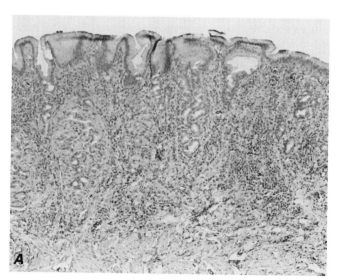
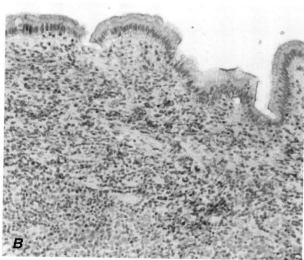

FIGURE 15–8. *(A)* Moderate chronic gastritis, typical of eosinophilic gastritis. Widespread infiltration of all regions of mucosa by mononuclear cells and eosinophils. *(B)* Chronic eosinophilic granulomatous gastritis. Biopsy shows marked infiltration by eosinophils and mononuclear cells.

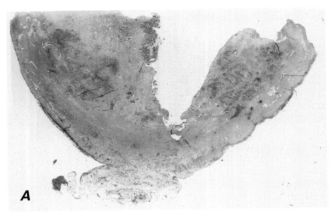

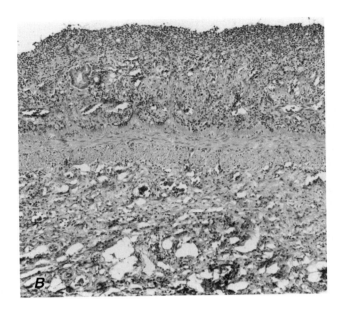

FIGURE 15-9. *(A)* Chronic granulomatous gastritis showing greatly thickened wall of stomach. The extent of the increased thickness is appreciated by the thickness of the mucosa that covers a small part of the luminal surface on the left center of section. *(B)* Severe chronic histiocytic gastritis (cat). Total disruption of normal mucosal architecture by diffuse infiltration of large foamy histiocytes. Neutrophils predominate near luminal surface. Cells were not found in submucosa where edema is marked. Similar lesions were found in the pancreas. Remainder of findings were unremarkable. Cause was undetermined.

eign body reactions. Further discussion of the etiopathogenesis of eosinophilic gastritis may be found in Chapter 24.

The treatment of eosinophilic gastritis is similar to that of chronic nonspecific gastritis. Some dogs and cats with the disease can be managed successfully with a selected protein hypoallergenic diet such as cottage cheese or chicken and rice. Many affected animals require corticosteroids, however. In dogs, the dose used is similar to that recommended for chronic nonspecific gastritis and eosinophilic gastroenteritis (initially 1–2 mg/kg PO q 12 hours). In cats, higher doses of corticosteroids are often required (initially 2–3 mg/kg PO q 12 hours), presumably because of the presence of concomitant hypereosinophilic syndrome. In dogs or cats with intractable eosinophilic gastritis, azathioprine is sometimes required (see Chapter 24). Surgical resection in association with controlled diets is usually successful in dogs with eosinophilic granulomatous masses.[28]

The prognosis for animals with eosinophilic gastritis is good. Most respond to dietary manipulation and corticosteroid therapy, but control rather than cure is often the ultimate result. Most animals must remain on controlled diets and many require low-dose maintenance glucocorticoid or azathioprine therapy. Even in dogs with surgically resected eosinophilic granulomas, the lesions can recur several years later if the dogs are returned to conventional dog foods.

GRANULOMATOUS/HISTIOCYTIC GASTRITIS

Chronic granulomatous gastritis is characterized clinically by the signs of chronic gastritis and histologically by granulomatous infiltration. The inflammation can form a localized granulomatous mass, often with an eosinophilic component as described earlier (Figure 15–9A). Alternatively, the inflammation can be more diffused throughout the stomach (Figure 15–9B). In addition, histiocytic gastritis has been associated with amyloidosis in a dog.[30]

Granulomatous inflammation has a number of known causes (see Table 24–5). Important considerations in the stomach include neoplasia, parasites (such as Gnathostoma nematodes), fungal diseases (including phycomycosis, histoplasmosis, and cryptococcosus), FIP, and foreign material.[31]

Treatment should be directed at any recognizable underlying cause. If no cause is apparent the gastritis should be treated in an analogous fashion to chronic nonspecific gastritis.

GASTRITIS ASSOCIATED WITH SPIRAL-SHAPED BACTERIA

Spiral-shaped organisms were identified in the stomach of dogs and cats over a century ago and since that time have at one time or another been suspected as a cause of chronic gastric disease.[32,33] In recent times, the discovery of the important role of the spiral-shaped organism *Helicobacter pylori* in human antral gastritis and peptic ulcer disease has again stimulated interest in spiral organisms as a cause of chronic gastritis in cats and dogs, and as a potential zoonosis

Spiral-shaped bacteria are common inhabitants of the gastric mucosa of dogs and cats.[32,34–37] The bacteria have been most commonly detected in the fundic mucosa, but they can colonize all parts of the stomach and, to a lesser extent, the duodenum and lower gastrointestinal tract.[32,37–39] They reside in the surface mucus, glandular lumina, and intracellular canaliculi of parietal cells.[37] The nomenclature pertaining to these organisms is receiving clarification. Initially they were referred to as *Spirillia* spp., of which a variety of morphologic forms were recognized.[32] Subsequently, they were given the name *Gastrospirillum hominis* (and lately *Helicobacter heilmannii*).[37] Recently it has been determined that in addition to *G. hominis,* a spiral-shaped bacteria closely related to *H. pylori* occurs in the stomachs of dogs and cats.[36,38] Because the organism was first identified in cats it is now called *Helicobacter felis.*[38] Both *G. hominis* and *H. felis* are tightly spiraled organisms but *H. felis* has characteristic entwined periplasmic fibrils.[35,36,38] The bacteria can be transmitted readily between animals housed in close proximity.[38] The route of transmission is unknown but a direct oral-oral or anal-oral route is likely.[37,38] Culture of facilities in which infected animals were housed and the animal's food and water were negative in one study.[38]

Although the clinical significance of gastric spiral-shaped bacteria in cats and dogs is unknown, it is clear the organisms are not completely saprophytic because in most but not all infected animals these bacteria have been associated with mild histologic changes in the stomach. These abnormalities have included dilation of the glandular lumens and intracellular canaliculi harboring the organisms.[37] Degenerative changes, such as vacuolization of the cytoplasm of the surface epithelium and necrosis of isolated glands, are observed in some cases.[37,39] In most infected animals, spiral-shaped bacteria are associated with low-grade inflammatory changes such as increased intraepithelial neutrophils and lymphocytes, mild mucosal edema and infiltration of the lamina propria with small numbers of lymphocytes, and lesser numbers of plasma cells and eosinophils.[37,38] Lymphoid nodules are prominent but mucosal erosions are infrequent.[37,38]

The pathogenesis of Helicobacter gastritis in humans is slowly being elucidated. The organism appears to be mucolytic and may secrete a cytotoxin. It also generates high quantities of ammonia from urea (a property used to assist diagnosis of *H. pylori*; see later) and possesses a phospholipase that is capable of markedly reducing the hydrophobicity of the gastric mucosa.[40] The organism can survive in the stomach because it interferes with acid secretion.

Although there is little doubt the spiral-shaped organisms of the dog and cat stomach can cause mild histologic abnormalities, there is to date only scant evidence that this mild gastritis can cause clinical signs. Spiral-shaped bacteria have been identified in 41% to 100% of all clinically healthy cats and dogs examined.[32,34,37] In a recent study, spiral-shaped bacteria were demonstrated histologically in the stomachs of similar numbers of healthy cats (41.4%) and cats with recurrent vomiting (56.6%).[37] In the latter study, most of the clinically healthy cats that harbored the spiral bacteria had a subclinical gastritis recognizable by gastric biopsy.[37] However, a recent report has described bloody diarrhea in a group of Persian cats with lymphocytic-plasmacytic gastroenterocolitis associated with a spiral-shaped organism.[39] The organism was observed in the gastrointestinal lumen and intracellularly in the gastric and colonic epithelium. The organism could not be cultured and its significance is unknown, but it is noteworthy that cells containing the organism were frequently undergoing degeneration, suggesting the organism was not a commensal. Experimental infection of dogs with *H. felis* produces a mild gastritis but no clinical signs develop.[38] Therefore, with the exception of the report of Feinstein (1992), most evidence suggests the usual consequence of exposure to spiral-shaped bacteria is a subclinical gastritis. Whether chronic exposure to the organisms predisposes infected animals to peptic ulceration or gastric neoplasia (as the bacteria do in humans) remains to be established. Furthermore, it is possible that spiral-shaped organisms predispose their hosts to food allergy, more severe gastritis, or even inflammatory bowel disease either in their own right or in association with other agents that injure the gastrointestinal mucosa. An example of such an injurious interaction is the observation that *Helicobacter* predispose humans to NSAIDs-induced gastropathy.[41]

Diagnosis of gastritis associated with spiral-shaped bacteria is usually made by light or electron microscopy. Warthin-Starry–stained sections facilitate identification.[38] Gastric mucosal scrapings can be examined by dark-field microscopy for motile helical organisms.[32] *H. felis* can also be cultured from infected tissues.[35,38] Screening of biopsy samples for ure-

ase activity (see Chapter 6) is a rapid way of identifying animals colonized with *H. felis* or *G. hominis*.[38]

The treatment of *H. pylori*–associated ulcers in people now centers around two major protocols. "Triple therapy" refers to amoxicillin or tetracycline (7 mg/kg PO q 6 hours of either drug) along with bismuth and metronidazole (approximately 4 mg/kg PO q 6 hours) used for approximately 16 days.[42] Doxycycline cannot be substituted for tetracycline in the triple therapy approach. A newer protocol, also showing a low relapse rate, consists of amoxicillin (approximately 7 mg/kg PO q 6 hours) and omeprazole (approximately 0.5–1.0 mg/kg PO q 24 hours) for 1–2 weeks.[42] The antimicrobial effect of amoxicillin is thought to be enhanced by the profound acid suppression of omeprazole.[45] Similarly, preliminary studies in cats have shown that *H. felis* can be transiently eliminated with 4 weeks of bismuth or 10 days of metronidazole therapy and that 10 days of ampicillin treatment will reduce numbers.[35]

It seems likely that the spiral-shaped bacteria of dogs' and cats' stomachs have zoonotic potential. Spiral bacteria with the characteristics of *H. felis* and *G. hominis* have been detected in humans with chronic gastritis.[35,43] In addition, *H. pylori* can colonize the stomach of dogs and cats and is associated with a low-grade gastritis.[44]

GASTRITIS DUE TO MISCELLANEOUS MICROORGANISMS

Chlamydia have been identified in both clinically normal cats and cats with signs of gastric disease.[45] The importance of the organism as a gastric pathogen is unknown.

Zygomycosis (phycomycosis) has been reported as a cause of chronic gastritis in dogs.[46,47] It is unknown whether fungi can initiate gastritis or whether they are opportunists that multiply when the normal defense mechanisms are compromised by mucosal injury. The signs are those of chronic gastritis, but not infrequently an abdominal mass is palpable. Diagnosis is made by biopsy or fungal culture of the affected tissues. Surgical excision of localized infections is the only reported successful treatment.

PARASITIC GASTRITIS

OLLULANUS TRICUSPIS. Ollulanus is a gastric nematode of cats that has a worldwide distribution. The prevalence of the parasite has been reported to range between 4% and 40% of cats in different geographical areas.[51] Dogs have also been reported to be infected with *Ollulanus tricuspis* but the prevalence is very low. Infections with the parasite can be inapparent but in other cases are associated with anorexia, vomiting, and chronic hypertrophic, fibrosing gastritis.[19,48–52]

Infection with the parasite is infrequently identified because routine parasitologic, endoscopic, and necropsy examinations usually fail to detect it. The parasite's very small size and unusual life cycle precludes easy identification. Neither adult nor larval parasites are usually passed in feces. The organisms are vomited, and transmission is due to uninfected cats eating the vomitus. Microscopic examination of vomitus is the only reliable method of antemortem diagnosis.[51] If need be, cats suspected of being infected with the parasite can be given emetic agents (e.g., xylazine 0.2 mg/kg IV, SC; or sodium carbonate crystals 40 mg/kg PO) to provide vomitus for examination.[52] Infected animals can also be identified by surgical biopsy and histology of the gastric mucosa, but up to 50% of infected cats do not show the organism even after three histologic sections have been examined. In another study. punch sampling (ten 4 mm samples) of the mucosa of infected cats was positive in only 29% of animals.[51] The gastric mucosa is usually normal on gross inspection but occasionally hypertrophic rugae covered in 2 to 3 mm nodules are observed.[51,52]

Little information is available on treatment of *O. tricuspis* although experimentally infected kittens had their infection eliminated following fenbendazole 10 mg/kg PO q 24 hours for 2 days.[50] Oxfendazole (10 mg/kg PO q 12 hours for 5 days) appears successful at eliminating the parasite from naturally infected cats whereas less frequent administration (10 mg/kg PO; two doses given 14 days apart) reduced but did not eliminate infection.[52]

PHYSALOPTERA SPECIES. *Physaloptera* are small stout nematodes that have a wide distribution in the world. A number of different *Physaloptera* species are known to cause chronic vomiting in dogs and cats.[53–55] In most, but not all reports, the prevalence of *Physaloptera* in dogs and cats is considered to be low. The frequency of inapparent (subclinical) infections is under debate but the consensus is that the parasite is an infrequent cause of chronic vomiting in cats and dogs. Diagnosis is usually made by fecal flotation, but it appears *Physaloptera* eggs may be difficult to isolate consistently by routine fecal flotation methods.[54] Endoscopy will usually reveal the 1 to 4 cm long, white parasites in the fundus and pyloric antrum. Bleeding erosions where the parasite was previously embedded may also be apparent. A single dose of pyrantel pamoate (5 mg/kg PO) eliminates *Physaloptera* from dogs whereas two doses of pyrantel pamoate (5 mg/kg) given 3 weeks apart appears to be effective in cats.[54–56] Prevention is difficult but requires blocking access to the intermediate and transport hosts such as cockroaches, crickets, beetles, and mice.

GNATHOSTOMA SPECIES. Infection with *Gnathostoma* nematodes has been described in cats worldwide.[57] The organism produces a granulomatous mass in the stomach wall that may or may not cause clinical signs. Occasionally death from gastric perforation occurs. Fecal examinations can reveal parasitic ova. Successful treatment of experimentally infected cats with several injections of disophenol has been reported.[57] Surgical resection of the gastric mass containing the parasite is also effective.

SPIROCERCA LUPI. *S. lupi* will occasionally infect the stomach of dogs and cats.[58] The resultant gastric nodule can be associated with vomiting. Treatment is surgical removal of the nodule.

AONCHOTHECA PUTORII. *A. putorii* is a parasitic nematode of the stomach and small intestine of many wild mammals including hedgehogs and mustelids. It has been observed in cats in North America and Europe. Infections with *A. putorii* can be inconsequential or can lead to chronic nodular hyperplastic gastritis with gastric perforation.[59] Diagnosis is made by finding bioperculated elongated eggs (similar to those of *Capillaria aerophilia*) in the feces.[59] Treatment is resection of the affected area of the stomach.

REFLUX GASTRITIS

As described in Chapters 13 and 14, reflux of duodenal contents into the stomach has been suggested as a cause of gastric damage and vomiting.[60–62] As previously mentioned, duodenogastric reflux is a normal event in dogs and probably also in cats. Furthermore, increased duodenogastric reflux may be a consequence of gastric disease rather than a pri-

mary cause. However, there remains a possibility that the clinical entity of reflux gastritis does exist and is a reasonably common cause of chronic vomiting on an empty stomach in otherwise healthy dogs. Vomiting of this nature can usually be prevented by feeding the animal more frequently.

CHRONIC GASTRITIS ASSOCIATED WITH HEPATIC AND RENAL DISEASE

Over 50% of humans with chronic renal insufficiency have superficial gastritis and a smaller number develop preatrophic or atrophic gastritis.[9] In a similar manner, chronic gastritis, erosions, and ulceration develop in animals with hepatic or renal insufficiency. See Chapter 14 for additional discussion of the gastric damage associated with these disorders.

CHRONIC GASTRITIS ASSOCIATED WITH ENDOCRINE DISEASES

Endocrine diseases are sometimes associated with chronic gastritis. Chronic gastritis with achlorhydria has been observed in humans with hypothyroidism and it has been suggested these two diseases are manifestations of a related autoimmune disease.[63] Surprisingly, similar gastric changes are found in humans with hyperthyroidism.[9] A form of chronic gastritis with achlorhydria and evidence of mucosal metaplasia has been observed in humans with diabetes mellitus. Chronic gastritis also occurs in humans and dogs with hypoadrenocorticism (see Chapter 27).

DRUG-INDUCED GASTRITIS

Prolonged administration of some drugs can cause chronic gastritis. Corticosteroids and NSAIDs are the most commonly implicated drugs. Drug-induced gastritis is discussed more fully in Chapter 14.

ALLERGIC GASTRITIS

As described in Chapter 23, food allergy is considered a likely cause of acute and perhaps chronic gastritis. Food allergic gastritis can be diagnosed only by properly conducted elimination challenge trials (see Chapter 23).

GASTRIC ULCERATION

Clinical Synopsis

Diagnostic Features

- Intermittent vomiting, hematemesis, and melena are common
- Abdominal pain is sometimes apparent
- Physical examination may suggest anemia
- Laboratory database may reveal systemic cause
- Diagnosis is confirmed by endoscopy or contrast study
- Biopsy is essential to differentiate peptic and neoplastic ulcers

Standard Treatment

- Treat primary cause if identified
- High carbohydrate, non-abrasive diet for 8 weeks
- Ranitidine (1–4 mg/kg PO, SC. IV, q 12 hours) or omeprazole (0.7–2 mg/kg PO 24 hours) for 4 to 8 weeks
- Blood transfusions as required
- Adjunctive therapy required in some patients includes antiemetics, prokinetics, sucralfate, antibiotics, and/or colloidal bismuth subcitrate

The structure and function of the gastric mucosal barrier and the etiopathogenesis of gastric erosions is described in Chapter 14. The following discussion focuses on gastric ulcers. Gastric ulcers are chronic mucosal defects that, in contrast to gastric erosions, breach the muscularis mucosa exposing the submucosa or deeper layers of the stomach. The nonacid-producing parts of the stomach (fundus and particularly the antrum) are most commonly affected by ulcers.

Ulcer Etiopathogenesis and Healing[64]

The causes and pathogenesis of gastric ulceration (Table 15–3) are similar to those of gastric erosion (see Chapter 14) but for poorly understood reasons the reparative mechanisms of the mucosa are overwhelmed, and deep, indolent lesions develop. Superficial gastric mucosal injury heals rapidly, usually within several hours of the injury. A layer of mucus, fibrin, and cellular debris forms above the lesion trapping plasma and bicarbonate against the mucosa and increasing the pH at the damaged mucosa to 4 to 6. In this protected microenvironment, surface mucous cells from the edge of the lesion slide over the epithelial defect. This is followed by cellular proliferation to restore subepithelial structure. The rapidity of restitution is thought to be important in preventing deeper mucosal injury from gastric acid and other injurious agents. Restitution in the stomach and duodenum is facilitated by reduced gastric acid secretion but is inhibited by NSAIDs.

Gastric ulcers heal more slowly than gastric erosions, usually requiring several weeks to resolve. Necrotic mucosa sloughs and granulation tissue fills the ulcer bed. Mucus and bicarbonate are actively secreted from the mucosa surrounding the ulcer, protecting the ulcer bed from further injury. The granulation tissue organizes, developing a predominance of fibroblasts and endothelial cells, and epithelium slides across the surface of the maturing connective tissue. The cells for the re-epithelialization are derived from gastric glands at the ulcer margin that dilate and become lined with poorly differentiated, rapidly proliferating cells. Eventually glandular structures are restored. Reduced gastric acidity favors ulcer healing directly by decreasing tissue damage from acid and indirectly by decreasing damage from pepsin, which is less active at higher pH.

Gastric re-epithelialization appears to proceed under the influence of epidermal growth factor (EGF). EGF encourages rapid epithelial turnover and also inhibits gastric acid secretion.[65] The source of EGF is likely to be a specific ulceration association cell lineage (UACL). It has been recently proposed that after ulceration (gastric and intestinal) UACL, secreting EGF and transforming growth factor alpha, grow out from adjacent glands and ramify to form a new gland.[66] Groups of cells adjacent to the UACL are then stimulated to produce trefoil peptides (a GI specific group of proteins), to

Table 15–3

CAUSES OF GASTRODUODENAL ULCERATION IN DOGS AND CATS

Primary Gastroduodenal Diseases
  Chemical toxins
  Chronic gastritis
  Gastric dilatation-volvulus
  Helicobacter spp.?
  Inflammatory bowel disease
  Neoplasia*
  Pyloric outlet obstruction
Gastric Hyperacidity Disorders
  Gastrinomas
  Mast cell tumors
  Other APUD tumors
Drugs*
  NSAIDs
  Corticosteroids
Miscellaneous Disorders
  Acute pancreatitis
  Cyclic hematopoiesis
  DIC*
  Hypoadrenocorticism
  Kidney failure*
  Liver failure*
  Neurologic diseases
  Shock*
  Stress
  Trauma

*Most common causes of gastric ulceration in dogs and cats.

divide, and to repopulate the ulcerated mucosa.[66] Administration of exogenous EGF hastens ulcer healing in dogs.[64] Similarly, transforming growth factor alpha is capable of accelerating healing in rat models of gastric mucosal injury.[42] Stimulation of angiogenesis in the granulation tissue of the ulcer bed with fibroblast growth factor also accelerates ulcer healing.[64,66]

EGF acts, at least in part, by stimulating polyamine formation in the gastric mucosa.[67] Polyamines, such as putrescine, spermidine, and spermine are essential for cell growth. The concentration of polyamines in tissues is regulated by ornithine decarboxylase, an enzyme whose activity has been shown to increase markedly in the submucosa of the ulcer base of dogs.[68] Inhibition of polyamine synthesis delays ulcer healing in dogs.[68]

Ulcer pain results from exposure of sensitive nerve endings to acid and from changes in gastric motility.[69] In humans, relief of symptoms does not mean the ulcer crater has healed.[69] Bleeding is initially caused by the erosion of superficial capillaries and venules, and eventually by arterial erosion.[69] Once arterial erosion has occurred the bleeding becomes severe and is not controllable by inhibition of acid secretion.[69]

Clinical Findings

No age, sex, or breed predilections have been identified for gastric ulceration. NSAIDs administration is frequently identified in the history. The clinical signs of gastric ulcers are highly variable. At times animals show little if any evidence of ill health. Vomiting is the clinical sign most commonly observed.[27,69] The vomitus may contain fresh or digested blood ("coffee grounds"). Occasionally anorexia and cranial abdominal pain are exhibited. In some patients the abdominal pain is less apparent after feeding, presumedly because of the buffering action of food. Delayed gastric emptying has been observed in humans and dogs with gastric ulcers.[70] Melena and clinical evidence of anemia may be apparent. Clinical signs of liver or kidney failure, two common causes of gastric ulceration, may be present. If the ulcer perforates, the clinical examination is indicative of peritonitis and septic shock.

Diagnosis

The diagnosis of gastric ulceration is usually made once evidence of upper gastrointestinal hemorrhage (hematemesis or melena) has been detected. The causes of melena are listed in Table 5–25 and the diagnostic evaluation of melena is described in Chapter 5. Some additional points of particular relevance to gastric ulceration are made here.

LABORATORY FINDINGS. The laboratory findings associated with gastric ulcers may indicate the underlying cause of the mucosal damage (e.g., azotemia or evidence of liver damage) or may simply reflect hemorrhage (low PCV and TP, positive fecal occult blood). The anemia resulting from gastric ulceration can be regenerative, but normocytic, normochromic, nonregenerative anemia and microcytic, hypochromic, nonregenerative anemia are also common.[27] The latter type of anemia is probably a result of iron-deficiency anemia as a result of chronic bleeding.[27] Neutrophilia with or without a left shift is also often observed in dogs with gastroduodenal ulceration.[27] The BUN to creatinine ratio is often raised following the loss of large volumes of blood into the upper gastrointestinal tract (see Chapter 5).

DIAGNOSTIC IMAGING. After ruling out systemic diseases (such as renal failure), endoscopy is the investigational procedure of choice when gastric ulceration is suspected. In the absence of an endoscope, contrast radiography (specifically a liquid or double-contrast gastrogram) can be valuable, but even in experienced hands these radiographic procedures are less sensitive than endoscopy. Furthermore, if contrast radiography does identify an ulcer, the owner's expenses do not finish there because follow-up endoscopic or surgical inspection and biopsy is then required to confirm the radiographic diagnosis and differentiate peptic (benign) from neoplastic ulcers.

The methodology of gastrointestinal contrast procedures is described in Chapter 6. If the radiographic position allows the ulcer to be visualized in profile, contrast material will be seen filling a crater in the gastric wall. If the crater is observed en face, persistent pooling of contrast may be observed in one area of the stomach.

ENDOSCOPIC APPEARANCE. Any solitary gastric ulcer recognized endoscopically should be viewed with a great deal of suspicion of neoplasia. In contrast to humans, in whom peptic ulceration is common, gastric neoplasia[4] is the most common cause of large localized gastric ulceration in dogs with otherwise normal stomachs. Other common causes of gastric ulceration such as NSAIDs therapy and kidney and liver failure usually cause more generalized gastric mucosal disease. Gastric adenocarcinomas most commonly appear on the lesser curvature of the stomach whereas peptic ulcers (i.e., those due to gastric hyperacidity) usually occur in the antrum or duodenum. Ulcerating gastric adenocarcinomas most often have an infiltrative appearance characterized by diffuse mucosal thickening around the ulcer bed (Figure 15–10). In contrast, peptic ulcers tend to be more localized with raised margins and a deep ulcer bed. NSAIDs-, glucocorticoid-, and stress-induced mucosal damage are usually associated with multiple superficial erosions but occasionally deep ulcers will

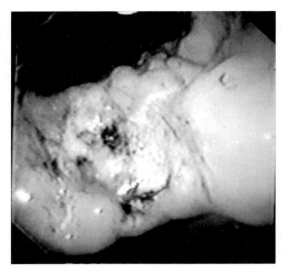

FIGURE 15–10. Ulcerating gastric adenocarcinoma in a Belgian shepherd. The cancer has infiltrated the lesser curvature (incisura angularis) of the stomach. This is the site of predelection for gastric adenocarcinomas.

appear, particularly at the antrum/body junction or in the antrum or pylorus.[27]

ENDOSCOPIC BIOPSY. As discussed in Chapter 7, endoscopists must be careful not to biopsy the center of the ulcer because the ulcer bed is often very friable and can be easily perforated by the biopsy instrument. Instead, the biopsy specimens should be obtained from the periphery of the lesion. To increase the depth of the biopsy, and therefore facilitate detection of any neoplastic tissue, double bites at the same biopsy site are recommended. Superficial biopsy specimens often give misleading results because they may only sample the inflammatory reaction that surrounds most tumors.

SERUM GASTRIN LEVEL. As discussed in the section on hypertrophic gastritis, if the endoscopic appearance is of generalized rugal hypertrophy with ulceration, the clinician should consider obtaining a serum gastrin level to assist the diagnosis of gastrinoma.

SUSPECTED GASTRIC PERFORATION. If clinical signs of peritonitis are observed during the physical examination of an animal with a suspected ulcer, the diagnostic procedures of choice are survey radiography and abdominal paracentesis in an attempt to confirm gastrointestinal perforation and septic peritonitis. Contrast radiography with iodinated contrast agents can be attempted to confirm a suspected perforation but are rarely performed because of time limitations. Instead, when there is a high index of suspicion of gastric perforation, the animal is usually prepared rapidly for abdominal exploration. Similarly, endoscopy is contraindicated in this situation because the pressurization of the gastrointestinal tract with air during the examination increases the contamination of the abdominal cavity with gastrointestinal contents. Perforated ulcers are usually readily confirmed by celiotomy. Occasionally, omental sealing of the ulcer is observed.[27]

Treatment of Gastric Ulcers

Management of gastric ulcers currently centers around treatment of the primary cause (if identified), inhibition of acid secretion, and, if necessary, control of gastric hemorrhage. In the future, the importance of antibiotics effective against gastric spiral-shaped organisms will be defined and the administration of mucosal growth factors may become more commonplace.

DIETARY MANAGEMENT. The dietary management of gastric ulcers is similar to that of acute gastritis discussed in Chapter 14. Suitable diets include cottage cheese and rice or chicken and rice.

INHIBITION OF GASTRIC ACID SECRETION.[71,72] For many years the axiom "no acid, no ulcer" has pervaded the medical literature. Recent experience, however, has revealed this axiom is only partly true. Mucosal lesions can develop in the absence of gastric acid.[73] Nevertheless, it is clear that acid exacerbates and perpetuates gastric mucosal lesions and that inhibitors of gastric acid secretion encourage their resolution. Drugs commonly used to achieve this aim are listed in Table 15–4. They are often classified into three groups: receptor antagonists that block the interaction of secretagogues with their receptors (e.g., anticholinergics, H_2-receptor antagonists); drugs that act on cellular metabolism to inhibit hydrogen ion secretion (e.g., prostaglandins); and "proton pump" inhibitors such as omeprazole that inhibit the H^+/K^+ATPase in the apical oxyntic cell membrane.

Anticholinergics.[74] Two types of muscarinic cholinergic receptors (M_1 and M_2) have been described. Atropine and most other anticholinergics act on both types of receptors, resulting in inhibition of acid secretion and and gastric motility. The latter is undesirable because, in an analogous manner to vagotomy,[75] it results in gastric retention that is a stimulus for vomiting (particularly in the inflamed stomach). Furthermore, antral distention encourages gastric acid secretion, partially counteracting the inhibitory effects of anticholinergics on the neural mechanisms that stimulate gastric acid secretion. As a result, anticholinergics such as atropine reduce the acid output stimulated by food by only 30%. Moreover, anticholinergics have a relatively minor influence on basal acid secretion in healthy individuals, and their ability to reduce the elevated basal level of acid secretion in animals with gastritis has been questioned.

To partly overcome, these problems, a selective M_1 receptor antagonist called pirenzepine was developed. Pirenzepine inhibits gastric acid secretion without the undesirable effects on gastric motility mediated by drugs acting on M_2 receptors. Pirenzepine is more potent than other anticholinergics and reduces stimulated acid secretion by 50% to 60%. The drug has not found wide usage in veterinary practice.

Prostaglandins. Prostaglandin E analogues inhibit gastric acid secretion in dogs.[76] The drugs inhibit adenylate cyclase, reducing cyclic AMP production and thereby reducing the protein kinase activity essential to hydrogen ion generation. They also have a variety of other benefical effects (such as improved blood flow and trophic effects) that have proven

Table 15–4

DRUGS INHIBITING GASTRIC ACID SECRETION

DRUG	DOSAGE FOR DOGS (D) AND CATS (C)
Cimetidine (Tagamet)	5–10 mg/kg PO, SC q 6–8 hours (D,C)
Ranitidine (Zantac)	10 mg/kg slow IV infusion over 30 minutes 1–4 mg/kg PO, SC, IV q 8–12 hours (D,C)
Famotidine (Pepcid)	0.3–0.6 mg/kg PO q 8–12 hours (D)*
Misoprostol (Cytotec)	1–3 µg/kg q 8–12 hours PO (D)
Omeprazole (Losec, Prilosec)	0.7–2 mg/kg PO q 24 hours (D)*

*Dose established in experimental dogs.

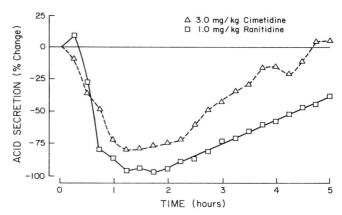

FIGURE 15–11. Graph of acid secretion in dogs during stimulation by histamine and inhibition by cimetidine or ranitidine.

valuable in managing mucosal lesions.[77] Misoprostol (Cytotec, Searle) is an analogue of prostaglandin E_1 that is available for human use in scored tablets of 100 µg. It is the drug of choice for NSAIDs-induced ulceration (see Chapter 14) and may have a role in the treatment of stress erosion or ulcers.[72,78] The usual dose is 1 to 3 µg/kg q 6 to 8 hours. Side effects of misoprostol include diarrhea, abdominal discomfort, and abortion.

H_2-Receptor Antagonists. Many analogues of histamine have been synthesized and evaluated as inhibitors of gastric acid secretion.[71] They inhibit acid secretion by binding to H_2-histamine-receptor sites on the oxyntic cell and preventing interaction of the receptor with histamine.

Cimetidine (Tagamet, Smith Kline Beecham) was the first H_2-receptor antagonist used in dogs, shortly followed by ranitidine, and more recently a host of others. Cimetidine inhibits histamine-stimulated gastric acid secretion in dogs at doses of 3.0 mg/kg or above.[79] Inhibition peaks at 75% within 1.5 hours, and 50% inhibition of acid secretion lasts about 2 hours after an oral dose (Figure 15–11). The effects of the drug are gone after 5 hours. The relatively short biologic effect necessitates a minimum of an 8 hourly dosage schedule. It is evident from these observations that cimetidine given at these doses and intervals results in only mild to moderate inhibition of acid secretion for a short part of any 24 hour period. In spite of this, it has been difficult to prove a clinical advantage for the newer, more potent, H_2 blockers over cimetidine. The reason for this lack of improved clinical efficacy in ulcer therapy (in spite of increased potency) is presumedly because partial (rather than complete) suppression of gastric acid secretion is all that is necessary for the healing of most gastroduodenal ulcers.[72]

Cimetidine has few significant side effects in dogs and cats other than microsomal enzyme inhibition and perhaps reduced hepatic blood flow, both of which can lead to adverse drug interactions.[72,80] High doses of cimetidine in mice have been shown to reduce the intestinal absorption of glucose and amino acids and to alter brush border enzyme levels.[81]

Ranitidine (Zantac, Glaxo) at a dose of 1.0 mg/kg inhibits acid secretion to a greater extent than cimetidine in dogs.[79] Inhibition peaks at about 90%, and 50% inhibition lasts 4 hours (Figure 15–11). The longer biologic effect leads to a recommendation that the drug be given only twice daily. At that schedule 50% acid secretion inhibition is in effect for only 8 out of 24 hours. Continuous infusion of ranitidine at a rate of 16.0 µg/kg per minute in dogs reduces acid secretion 70% to 80% and pepsin secretion 40%.[82] When administered at a dose of 1 mg/kg, ranitidine is 6 to 10 times more potent than cimetidine in inhibiting acid secretion stimulated by histamine, pentagastrin, or bethanechol. Another advantage of ranitidine over cimetidine is less inhibition of miscrosomal enzymes resulting in less potential problems with drug interactions. In addition, it may have prokinetic properties in dogs.[83] Both cimetidine and ranitidine are safe for use in dogs and cats and have been utilized extensively in the treatment of gastric ulcers of a variety of causes.

Famotidine (Pepcid, Merck) is a newer H_2-receptor antagonist that has been promoted as being more effective than both cimetidine and ranitidine. However, studies in dogs have suggested that famotidine is of similar potency to ranitidine (Figure 15–12).[84, 85] Little is known of the side effects of famotidine in small animals.

Recently, nizatidine (Axid, Eli Lilly), a new H_2-receptor antagonist, has been shown to have anticholinesterase activity and to enhance gastrointestinal motility significantly in dogs.[86] Other H_2-receptor blockers, with the possible exception of ranitidine, have negligible prokinetic properties, suggesting that nizatidine may be advantageous in patients with gastric ulcers that have concurrent gastric motility abnormalities.

Omeprazole. Omeprazole (Prilosec; Losec, Merck) is a substituted benzimidazole that inhibits H^+/K^+ ATPase (the proton pump) at the apical border of oxyntic cells, reducing hydrogen ion secretion. Omeprazole inhibits acid secretion no matter what secretagogues are present, and in dogs its potency is 5 to 10 times greater than that of cimetidine.[87] A single daily dose can result in virtual antacidity. The drug does not affect other gastrointestinal secretion in dogs.[88] Omeprazole is a weak base that is lipophilic at physiologic pH. Once the drug enters oxyntic cell canaliculi into which hydrogen ions are being secreted, it becomes trapped in its active (protonated) form within the cell. When not in an acidic environment, the drug does not accumulate and remains inactive.

Omeprazole may prove to be useful in diseases requiring profound inhibition of acid secretion. For instance, in humans and dogs it has been shown to be superior to H_2 blockers for the treatment of severe reflux esophagitis and the occasional indolent gastroduodenal ulceration.[27,89] The drug is safe in dogs and probably in cats, although there has as yet been little clinical experience with the drug in cats. Omeprazole inhibits microsomal enzymes to a similar extent as cimetidine.[72] Therefore, when using omeprazole in multidrug therapeutic protocols, the potential for drug interactions must be evaluated carefully.

ANTACIDS. Gastric acid can be transiently neutralized with antacids. These drugs must be given at least six times per day to have any benefit in the treatment of gastric ulcers, an administration schedule that makes them impractical in small animal medicine. Infrequent administration may actually result in greater than normal rates of acid secretion ("acid rebound"), potentially exacerbating ulcer disease. The clinical significance of acid rebound has been challenged in recent years, however.[90] Acid rebound is due in part to hypergastrinemia stimulated by neutralization of gastric contents. Hypergastrinemia also occurs with H_2 blockers and omeprazole, but because of their longer duration of action there is little time for the hypergastrinemia to actually stimulate acid secretion. In contrast, the buffering capacity of the antacid is rapidly consumed, leaving the mucosa exposed to the greater acid secretion. Acid rebound may also result from direct stimulation of the oxyntic cell by calcium-containing antacids.[90]

Antacids vary in the cations and anions they contain (Table

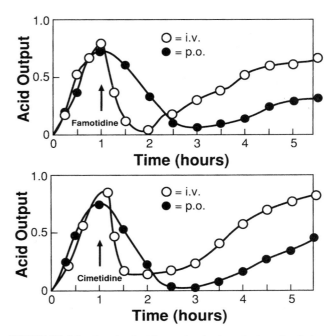

FIGURE 15–12. Graph of acid secretion in dogs during stimulation by histamine and inhibition by cimetidine or famotidine. Drugs were given orally (PO) or intravenously (I V).

15–5). Each has a different buffering capacity and unique side effects. The acid-neutralizing capabilities of common antacids have been tabulated in a recent review.[69] Common cations of antacids include aluminum, calcium, and/or magnesium. Aluminum- or magnesium-containing antacids are thought to be the most efficacious.[80] Calcium-containing antacids tend to promote constipation whereas magnesium-containing antacids encourage looser stools. Aluminum reduces gastric motility and delays gastric emptying. Aluminum also interacts with dietary phosphorus, resulting in both increased fecal excretion and reduced intestinal absorption of phosphate.[91] Hypophosphatemia and accumulation of aluminum are potential sequelae with long-term usage. Administration of excess calcium antacids may predispose to renal calculi. Absorbable antacids such as sodium bicarbonate can result in alkalosis. Milk is not an antacid.

CONTROL OF GASTRIC HEMORRHAGE. Control of gastric bleeding from gastric ulcers is usually readily achieved by measures such as fasting and, if necessary, the use of inhibitors of

Table 15–5

ANTACID COMPOSITION AND SIDE EFFECTS

ANTACID	COMPOSITION		
	Aluminum*	Magnesium**	Calcium*
Amphojel	+		
Aludrox	+	+	
Basaljel	+		
Camalox	+	+	+
Gaviscon	+	+	
Gelusil	+	+	
Maalox	+	+	
Milk of magnesia		+	
Riopan	—	—	—

*Aluminum and calcium have constipating effect.
**Magnesium has a laxative effect.

gastric acid secretion and blood transfusion. If hemorrhage continues, gastric lavage with ice water has been recommended but has been shown to be ineffective in dogs and may actually prolong bleeding.[92] Alternatively, visceral cooling by intraperitioneal injection of cold saline has been used experimentally to control gastric bleeding in dogs.[93] In addition, the potent vasoconstrictor, norepinephrine, has been given intragastrically (8 mg free base in 500 mL saline) or intraperitoneally (8 mg free base in 100 mL saline) to successfully prevent the death by exsanguination of dogs with experimental gastric bleeding.[94] Norepinephrine briefly reduces portal blood flow to one-third of normal and causes portal blood pressure to double for 5 minutes, after which it decreases to normal. Systolic and diastolic blood pressure change little because catecholamines given intraperitoneally are rapidly removed from the portal circulation by the liver.

Injection therapy using a sclerotherapy needle under endoscopic guidance has been shown to be effective at controlling hemorrhage from experimental gastric ulcers in dogs.[95] Epinephrine (1:10,000; 1–2 mL in each quadrant of the ulcer) rapidly reduces but does not halt the hemorrhage whereas absolute ethanol (0.1–1 mL in the ulcer) is slow to control hemorrhage but eventually induces definitive vessel thrombosis. Unfortunately, the ethanol creates transmural gastric injury and injecting the ulcer bed can lead to peritoneal injection of the sclerosing solution.[95] If medical management fails to control gastrointestinal bleeding, a partial or complete gastrectomy should be performed.

ADJUNCTIVE MEDICAL THERAPY. Antiemetics are rarely necessary in animals with gastric ulcers because vomiting is usually not persistent. If these drugs are necessary, the same drugs used for the treatment of vomiting due to acute gastritis are suitable (see Chapter 14). Prokinetic drugs such as metoclopramide and cisapride (see later and Chapter 14) are occasionally helpful if the patient has a concurrent gastric motility abnormality resulting in delayed gastric emptying. Locally acting protectants, such as sucralfate or colloidal bismuth subcitrate, are indicated. These drugs are discussed fully in Chapter 14. Bismuth, in particular, has been shown in humans to be as effective as the H_2 antagonists but to be less expensive and offer a lower rate of relapse, perhaps because of its effectiveness against *H. pylori*.[96] Antibiotics are usually not necessary in the treatment of gastric ulcers unless there is evidence of a microbial cause (such as *H. pylori* infection; see earlier) or abdominal perforation is suspected.

If gastric perforation occurs, treatment must be rapid to save the animal (see Chapter 26). The patient should be placed on fluids to provide cardiovascular support and broad-spectrum antibiotics to attend to the abdominal contamination. A suitable combination of antibiotics is metronidazole (for anaerobes including *Bacteroides fragilis* that commonly lead to abdominal abscessation if not treated), gentamicin (for gram negative aerobes that lead to life-threatening sepsis), and a penicillin derivative to cover the gram positive aerobes. As soon as the patient is stable cardiovascularly, a celiotomy is indicated to repair the lesion and lavage the abdomen.

SURGERY. Partial gastrectomy is necessary for resection of indolent peptic ulcers or neoplastic ulcers. Surgery is also indicated for the removal of pancreatic gastrinomas.

Prognosis

The prognosis for patients with peptic ulcers and benign gastric neoplasms is good. The prognosis for gastric ulcers secondary to kidney or liver failure is poor. Similarly, because of early metastatic spread, the prognosis for animals affected with gastric carcinoma or pancreatic gastrinoma is poor.

DELAYED GASTRIC EMPTYING

Clinical Synopsis

Diagnostic Features

- Vomiting of food at times more than 12 hours after ingestion
- Abdominal distention and tympany may be present
- Gastric retention apparent on survey radiographs
- Abnormal gastric emptying studies (e.g., BIPS)
- Endoscopy or celiotomy may reveal gastric-outlet obstruction
- Absence of outlet obstruction implies gastric motility disorder

Standard Treatment

- Attention to primary cause
- Prokinetics (metoclopramide 0.2–0.4 mg/kg PO administered immediately before meals, or cisapride or erythromycin; see text)
- Pyloromyotomy or pyloroplasty may be required

Abnormal retention of food in the stomach can be caused by gastric-outlet obstruction, gastric motility disorders, or a combination of both. Common causes of gastric-outlet obstructions and motility disorders are listed in Table 15–6. Vomiting of large volumes of food greater than 12 hours after ingestion is pathognomonic for delayed gastric emptying and should prompt the clinician to consider the differential diagnoses discussed here. It is important to note that few of these diagnoses are likely to respond to routine symptomatic management for vomiting. Therefore, whenever an animal presents with the clinical signs of delayed gastric emptying, a diagnostic workup to identify the primary cause of the problem is indicated

Clinical Signs

The most prevalent clinical sign of delayed gastric emptying is vomiting. As already stated, the distinguishing feature of the vomiting is that it often occurs long after ingestion at a time when the stomach of a normal animal would have been near empty. Not uncommonly, vomition of food consumed the previous day is observed, an occurrence that is diagnostic for delayed gastric emptying. Occasionally, affected animals will vomit explosively large volumes of liquidized food with few of the usual prodromal signs of vomiting such as salivation and retching (so-called "projectile vomiting"). The food in the vomitus usually appears digested but occasionally will be undigested in spite of a prolonged residence in the stomach. The latter is highly suggestive of lack of trituration of food as a result of poor gastric motility, but the clinician should recheck the history to ensure the animal is indeed vomiting and not regurgitating. Occasionally the vomitus has a fecal odor, a finding that also occurs in animals with intestinal obstruction.

Animals with delayed gastric emptying may also show abdominal discomfort and distension due to the dilated stomach. Anorexia and depression will occur if the delayed gastric emptying is due to an inflammatory or neoplastic

Table 15–6

CAUSES OF DELAYED GASTRIC EMPTYING

Gastric Outflow Obstruction
  Antral polyps
  Chronic hypertrophic gastritis
  Chronic hypertrophic pyloric gastropathy (pyloric stenosis)
  External compression (adhesions, neoplasia, pancreatic abscesses)
  Eosinophilic granuloma
  Foreign bodies
  Gastric neoplasia
  Granulomatous gastritis (idiopathic, fungal)
  Peripyloric masses (e.g., pancreatic abscesses, abdominal masses)
  Pyloric fibrosis

Acute and Subacute Gastric Motility Abnormalities
  Acidosis
  Acute gastroenteritis
  Acute pancreatitis
  Gastric overdistension (e.g., from gluttony)
  Hypercalcemia
  Hypocalcemia
  Hypokalemia
  Nausea from any cause
  Pain
  Peritonitis
  Stress
  Trauma (especially to abdomen or CNS)
  Surgery (abdomen; spine)
  Drugs (anticholinergics, beta-adrenergic agonists, narcotics)

Chronic Gastric Motility Abnormalities
  Constipation
  Diabetes mellitus?
  Dysautonomia
  Gastric dilatation-volvulus
  Gastric ulceration
  Hypoadrenocorticism
  Hypothyroidism?
  Inflammatory bowel disease
  Liver failure
  Chronic gastritis
  Gastric neoplasia
  Gastric arrhythmia
  Gastric bradyarrhythmia
  Gastric tachyarrhythmia
  Malabsorption
  Pylorospasm?
  Uremia

---

lesion but is atypical of the other causes of gastric retention except during periods of marked gastric distension just prior to vomiting. Affected animals may or may not lose weight. Dogs with gastric-outlet obstruction due to gastric adenocarcinoma often have melena or hematemesis.

Laboratory Findings

The laboratory changes in animals with delayed gastric emptying are usually mild and nonspecific. Patients with the problem may show lipemia persisting more than 12 hours after feeding. Alkalosis, particularly with paradoxical aciduria, is compatible with pyloric obstruction. Anemia is not uncommon with gastric adenocarcinoma. Hypokalemia may be observed and should be corrected before further diagnostic steps are pursued because it may be the cause of gastric retention or, conversely, may be a result of the vomiting. If hyper- or hypocalcemia are present, these electrolyte abnormalities should be actively pursued diagnostically because they are likely to be responsible for the gastric retention. Occasionally,

specific causes of delayed gastric emptying, such as renal failure or pancreatitis, will be revealed by the serum chemistry profile

Assessment of Gastric Emptying

Gastric emptying studies to confirm delayed gastric emptying are useful if the history and clinical signs are suggestive but not diagnostic of this problem. They are also of value if the clinician wishes to quantify the emptying rate to allow objective measurement of the effects of different therapeutic options. Gastric emptying studies are usually unnecessary if the history establishes beyond doubt that gastric emptying is delayed or suggests the gastric emptying is likely to be a transient phenomenon as a result of a readily reversible cause such as postoperative ileus or acute gastroenteritis

Radiographic studies are the most widespread means of confirming delayed gastric emptying (see Chapter 6 also).[97–100] Survey films of the abdomen often show retention of fluid and food in the stomach at a time it should be empty.

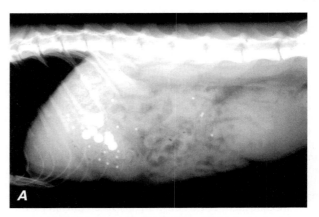

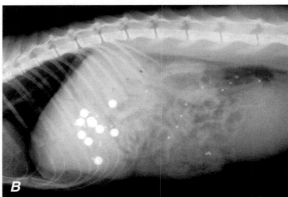

FIGURE 15–13. Lateral abdominal radiographs of a 6-month-old Persian cat with inflammatory bowel disease. To assess gastric emptying rate and small-bowel transit time, BIPS were fed to the cat in a 10th of a can of Hills Presciption Diet d/d and radiographs taken after 4 hours *(A)* and 7 hours *(B)*. Approximately 15% and 45% of the small BIPS have left the stomach after 4 and 7 hours, respectively. Only 3% of small BIPS have entered the large bowel after 7 hours (confirmed with a VD radiograph not shown). This indicates a slower than average gastric emptying and small-bowel transit rate, a not uncommon observation in animals with malabsorption. None of the large BIPS have left the stomach by 7 hours. This is not considered abnormal because the large BIPS are often retained until the stomach is empty and then rapidly ejected into the small bowel in the interdigestive period.

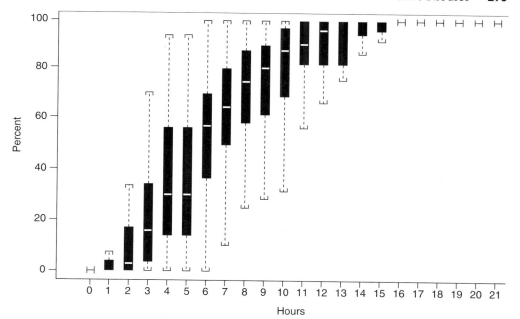

FIGURE 15-14. Normal gastric emptying rate of small BIPS when fed to dogs in a 1/4 can of Hills Prescription Diet d/d per 10 kg body weight. The white lines represent the median gastric emptying percentage. The black bars are the upper to lower quartile. The dotted lines and brackets represent the 95% confidence interval. (Courtesy Dr. Frazer Allan)

Radiopaque markers, such as barium-impregnated polyspheres (BIPS, Ken Bowman Assoc., Diamond Bar, CA; Arnolds, Shrewsbury, U.K.), are a convenient method to quantify gastric emptying in dogs and cats.[99,100] The BIPS are administered in food (usually Prescription Diet d/d in sufficient quantities to meet 25% of the animal's daily caloric needs) and two to four abdominal radiographs are taken at convenient intervals over the next 12 to 24 hours (Figure 15–13). The percentage of BIPS that have left the stomach is calculated and compared to the standard gastric emptying curves provided in the packaging leaflet by the manufacturer (Figure 15–14). BIPS have been used successfully in dogs and cats at the Massey University Veterinary Clinic to detect delayed gastric emptying from a variety of causes, including uremia, pancreatitis, and pyloric fibrosis.[100]

Gastric emptying studies can also be performed with barium suspensions but suffer several disadvantages in comparison to BIPS. The studies are not quantitative and mimic the emptying of liquid rather than that of food. The qualitative nature of the liquid barium study introduces subjectivity into the assessment of gastric emptying rate. As a result liquid gastrograms will only detect markedly delayed gastric emptying rates (Figures 15–15 and 15–16) and will often be normal even in the presence of clinically significant gastric retention (Figure 15–17). The failure of barium suspensions to estimate the emptying rate of food is a serious disadvantage because delayed gastric emptying of food is more prevalent than gastric retention of liquids.

To overcome this problem, liquid barium can be mixed with food prior to administration. Unfortunately, liquid barium rapidly dissociates from food, potentially producing misleading results.[101] Furthermore, as with liquid gastrograms, barium-coated food studies are not quantitative and they have shown marked variability in normal animals.[101,102] In dogs, the stomach is not completely emptied of food until 5 to 15 hours after feeding, whereas the emptying of liquid contrast is completed within 2 hours.[103] In two other studies of dogs fed kibble, the mean complete emptying time was 7.0 hours in one study and 10.9 hours in another.[101,102] In cats fed canned food, the mean gastric emptying time was deter-

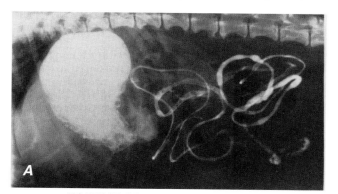

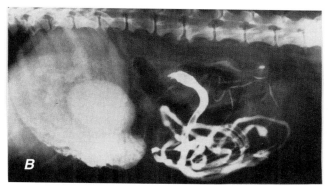

FIGURE 15-15. Lateral radiographs of abdomen of 11-year-old Dalmatian presented with clinical signs of postprandial vomiting and abdominal distention. At the time of the study the animal had received no drugs and had undergone no surgery. There was no history of an episode of acute dilation. The dog was not excited at the time of the study. Fluoroscopy after the administration of positive-contrast medium revealed no gastric motility. Film taken at 15 minutes (A) shows that contrast that has left the stomach moves normally through the small bowel. The film taken at 2.5 hours (B) shows further distention of the stomach and diminution of the contrast's density. This results from gastric secretions accumulating in the stomach. Gastric retention of contents with subsequent distention is a potent stimulus for gastric secretion. Diagnosis in this case was chronic gastric atony.

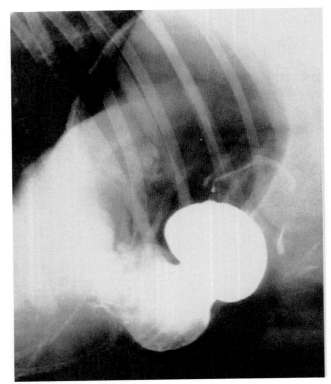

FIGURE 15–16. Lateral (right-side down) radiograph taken of dog with clinical signs of gastric-outlet obstruction. Liquid positive-contrast medium was administered, and radiographs were taken 60 minutes later. The distended antrum shows a wave of peristaltic contraction, and examination under fluoroscopic control showed gastric motility to be normal. A minimal amount of contrast is seen entering the duodenum. Subsequent radiographs showed persistence of these findings. It is essential to follow these abnormalities with a sequence of radiographs. A diagnosis of pyloric stenosis was confirmed during surgery. Treatment with pyloromyotomy corrected the problem.

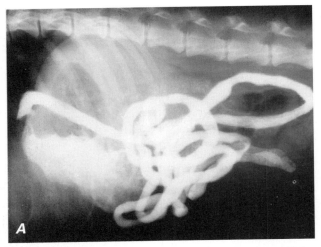

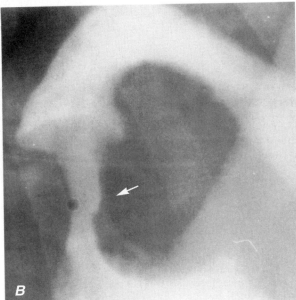

FIGURE 15–17. Lateral radiographs taken of 9-month-old Doberman showing clinical signs of gastric-outlet obstruction. Liquid positive-contrast medium was administered (A) The 15-minute film shows considerable emptying into the small intestine. The wall of the pyloric canal is thickened and the lumen is narrow. (B) The spot film shows magnification of the pyloric canal (arrow). Such cases should be examined under fluoroscopic control because a similar appearance is possible in normal dogs. During an exploratory laparotomy the pyloric muscles were hypertrophied and a pyloromyotomy was performed. Complete remission of clinical signs followed. Diagnosis was pyloric stenosis.

mined to be 11.6 hours.[104] Gastric retention of large quantities of barium-coated food for 8 to 10 hours supports the clinical diagnosis of delayed gastric emptying.

Gastric emptying studies can also be performed by scintigraphy. This method uses radioactive tracers mixed with food. It is the technique of choice but has not received widespread usage because of expense, limited availability, and the logistical concerns associated with the administration of radioisotopes. Double-labeling scintigraphic techniques can be used to allow simultaneous assessment of the emptying of solids and liquids.[105] Scintigraphic studies have indicated that liquid diets empty with a half-time of 1.0 to 1.5 hours in normal dogs.[106] Nearly complete emptying (95%) is seen in 2.5 hours. The 50% emptying time of dry cereal diets ranges from 2.9 hours[107] to 4.9 hours in dogs.[108] Scintigraphic procedures have been used successfully to detect delayed gastric emptying from a variety of causes in dogs at the UCD VMTH.

Abdominal ultrasonography has been found to be a useful method for the assessment of gastric emptying of humans. Gastric antral volume is measured and used to estimate gastric emptying.[109] A variety of other less practical techniques can be used to assess gastric emptying. These techniques include dye dilution methods, CT and MRI scans, and measurement of blood concentrations of intestinally absorbed drugs. Because of complexity, expense, or invasiveness these techniques have not been applied to clinical veterinary medicine.

Diagnosis

If chronic delayed emptying is confirmed, further diagnostic procedures are necessary to determine the cause. Ultimately inspection and biopsy of the stomach by endoscopy or celiotomy is usually required but, in the interim, diagnostic imaging techniques are helpful in assessing gastric motility and refining the list of likely diagnoses. Ultrasonography, in

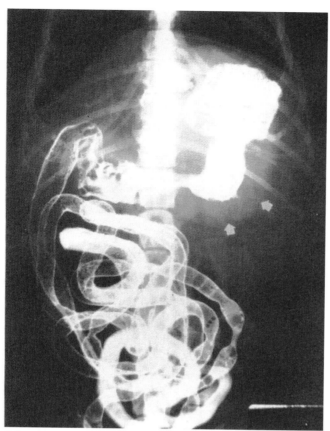

FIGURE 15–18. Dorsoventral radiograph of 9-year-old Keeshound with clinical signs of intermittent vomiting over a period of 6 to 8 months. Positive-contrast medium was administered, and the distal part of stomach shows a marked thickening of the wall (arrows). An ulcer crater evident in the thick part is suggestive of a tumor. There is an absence of any rugal pattern over the area involved. The narrowing of the body and antrum of the stomach was a consistent finding on several films, suggesting it was not a wave of peristaltic contraction. Diagnosis of scirrhous carcinoma was made on histologic examination of biopsy tissue.

particular, is valuable because it is a noninvasive method of evaluating motility (by determining if the frequency of antral contractions is normal). Furthermore, the stomach can be evaluated ultrasonographically for foreign bodies and masses obstructing gastric outflow or thickenings of the gastric wall suggestive of infiltrative diseases. In addition, ultrasound-guided biopsy or fine needle aspiration of gastric masses will occasionally provide a definitive diagnosis. Liquid gastrograms will occasionally identify radiolucent foreign bodies, gastric masses, or ulcers (Figure 15–18). Fluoroscopic examination of animals given barium suspensions or barium-coated food can be used to evaluate gastric motility.

Absence of antral motility supports a diagnosis of gastric retention due to a gastric motility abnormality but does not establish if the hypomotility is due to a primary motility disorder or is secondary to another gastric disease. Therefore, endoscopy or celiotomy must be performed to obtain gastric biopsy samples and to definitively rule out subtle gastric outlet problems that may have been missed by the imaging procedures.

The decision whether to opt for endoscopic or surgical examination of the stomach is based on a number of consid-

erations including the most likely diagnosis and the owner's attitude about invasive procedures such as celiotomy. In general, endoscopy and celiotomy have similar diagnostic accuracy for most diseases causing gastric retention with the exception of disorders located in the gastric submucosal or muscle layers. However, for a number of reasons, celiotomy is the technique of choice in most animals with gastric retention. In contrast to endoscopic pinch biopsy samples, surgical biopsy specimens include the full thickness of the stomach wall. This is advantageous because it allows examination of the gastric muscle and nervous plexuses, a potential site of lesions in gastric motility abnormalities. Furthermore, celiotomy is often a "one-step procedure" for both the diagnosis and treatment of delayed gastric emptying resulting from such diseases as pyloric stenosis. Moreover, celiotomy allows the placement of a jejunostomy tube in animals in need of nutritional support. The authors select endoscopy in preference to celiotomy if the history, clinical signs, laboratory findings, or results of imaging procedures suggest the probable cause of the gastric retention is inflammatory bowel disease, chronic gastritis, or advanced gastric adenocarcinoma. Endoscopy is usually an effective method of diagnosis in these diseases and surgical treatment is rarely indicated.

Electrogastrograms are sometimes of value in the diagnosis of delayed gastric emptying. Electrogastrograms differentiate aberrant gastric motility patterns such as tachygastria, bradygastria, and gastric dysrhythmia. This technique is not widely available.

Management of Delayed Gastric Emptying

The treatment of delayed gastric emptying depends heavily on diagnosis of the primary cause. The treatment options available for the specific therapy of the diseases causing gastric retention are discussed in the disease-specific sections here. The following section deals with some general management strategies of value for delayed gastric emptying.

NUTRITIONAL MANAGEMENT. The nutritional management of delayed gastric emptying involves frequent feeding of low-fat diets and, if necessary, liquidizing the diet. In addition, hyperosmolar diets and gel-forming fibers should be avoided (see Chapter 38).

PROKINETIC DRUGS. Drugs that enhance gastrointestinal motility are valuable in the treatment of delayed gastric emptying resulting from motility abnormalities but are of limited effectiveness and may be contraindicated in animals with gastric-outlet obstructions. A variety of prokinetic drugs are now available. Metoclopramide has both antiemetic and prokinetic properties and is discussed in detail in Chapter 14. Domperidone is very similar to metoclopramide but has fewer CNS side effects.

Cisapride (Prepulsid; Janssen) is a newly available prokinetic drug. It is a benzamide that facilitates cholinergic transmission in the enteric nervous system. Cisapride accelerates gastric emptying in dogs by stimulating pyloric and duodenal contractions and enhancing antro-pyloro-duodenal coordination.[110] There are indications that cisapride is more effective than metoclopramide and domperidone in encouraging gastric emptying of solids in dogs.[70,105,110] The ideal dose of cisapride for use in dogs with delayed gastric emptying has not been determined, but in healthy dogs doses from 0.1 to 5.0 mg/kg have been shown to accelerate gastric emptying.[70,105] In the authors' hands, cisapride at a dose of 0.25 to 0.5 mg/kg PO q 8 hours has given good results in dogs with delayed gastric emptying. In cats, a dose of 2.5 to 5 mg PO q 8 hours has been suggested.[70]

Recently, the antibiotic erythromycin has been shown to be a valuable prokinetic in dogs when used in low doses.[110–112] In some but not all studies, erythromycin has been found to mimic the effects of the hormone motilin.[110,111] It stimulates smooth muscle motilin receptors that are located throughout the gastrointestinal tract of mammals.[113] In addition, erythromycin acts on presynaptic cholinergic neurons to stimulate gastric, pyloric, and duodenal contractions.[110] Erythromycin is beneficial in humans with idiopathic gastroparesis and gastroparesis due to diabetes mellitus.[114,115] The role of erythromycin in the treatment of the differing causes of delayed gastric emptying in dogs and cats needs investigation. The dose required in clinically affected dogs remains to be determined, but in normal dogs 1 to 7 mg/kg IV induces significant propulsive activity in the stomach and small intestine. The higher dose is necessary to induce propulsive activity in postprandial dogs whereas the lower dose is sufficient in fasted dogs. Too high a dose promotes vomiting rather than accelerated gastric emptying. The authors currently use a postprandial dose of 5 mg/kg q 8 hours PO in dogs with delayed gastric emptying due to gastric motility abnormalities. A potential problem with erythromycin is its variable absorption when given with food.[116]

ENDOSCOPIC MANAGEMENT. Through-the-endoscopic balloon dilatation has recently been used successfully in humans to treat gastric-outlet obstructions resulting from idiopathic ulceration, anastomotic strictures, and NSAIDs-induced pyloric damage.[117] This technique may find application in similar situations in veterinary medicine.

SURGICAL PROCEDURES. Pyloromyotomy or pyloroplasty procedures of various types are sometimes required to treat gastric retention. Their effectiveness in motility disorders have been questioned but they are useful in the treatment of pyloric outlet obstruction. These procedures are discussed here in the section on antral pyloric hypertrophy syndrome.

ANTRAL PYLORIC HYPERTROPHY SYNDROME (PYLORIC STENOSIS)

Clinical Synopsis

Diagnostic Features

- Chronic vomiting, especially in brachycephalic dogs
- Clinical and radiographic signs of delayed gastric emptying (see earlier)
- Contrast radiography or endoscopy may reveal gastric-outlet obstruction
- Celiotomy confirms gastric-outlet obstruction due to pyloric muscular hypertrophy, gastric mucosal hyperplasia, or both

Standard Treatment

- Pyloromyotomy* for selective pyloric muscular hypertrophy
- Pyloroplasty if combined muscular and mucosal thickening
- Gastroduodenal anastomosis for severely affected patients

---

*Selective pyloric muscular hypertrophy is rare in comparison to the combined disorder, and pyloromyotomy is ineffective if mucosal hyperplasia is present.

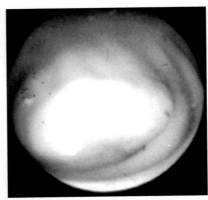

FIGURE 15–19. Antral pyloric hypertrophy syndrome. The pyloric stenosis is due to muscular hypertrophy. Note the protuberant, thickened pylorus and compare to Figure 15–5 in which the pyloric stenosis is due to mucosal hypertrophy. (Courtesy of Dr. Brent Jones)

Stenosis of the pyloric canal is one of the more common causes of gastric-outlet obstruction.[70] The narrowing can be caused by hypertrophy of the circular muscle of the pylorus (Figure 15–19), by hyperplasia of the antropyloric mucosa (Figure 15–5), or by a combination of both muscular and mucosal thickening. Selective hypertrophy of the pyloric muscle is the least common form of the disease and is usually seen as a congenital lesion in boxers and Boston terriers.[13,14,118,119] In these young animals the disease is often referred to as congenital pyloric stenosis. Most adult dogs with antral pyloric hypertrophy syndrome are affected by either selective mucosal hypertrophy or by a combination of muscular and mucosal hypertrophy.[118,119] The hypertrophic mucosa may be focal (a polyp or single mucosal fold), multifocal (multiple polyps or folds), or generalized (involving the entire pyloric antrum).[119] The adult syndrome has been variously termed acquired antral pyloric hypertrophy, chronic hypertrophic pyloric gastropathy, acquired pyloric stenosis, hypertrophic gastritis, and multiple polyps.[36,37,119,120] In this chapter we refer to the congenital and adult forms of the disease as congenital or adult-onset antral pyloric hypertrophy syndrome (APHS) in recognition of the bimodal age of onset, the involvement of the antrum in addition to the pylorus, the hypertrophic nature of the lesions, and the probability of nonspecific etiology. Hypertrophic gastritis occurring independently of antral pyloric hypertrophy (for example, in the gastric body) is discussed elsewhere in this chapter.

Etiopathogenesis

The cause(s) of APHS is unknown, but excessive secretion of gastrin has been implicated. Gastrin has potent trophic effects on gastric smooth muscle as well as on the mucosa of the gastric body. Gastrin injections in bitches during pregnancy cause more than one-fourth of the pups to be born with pyloric stenosis.[121] The pyloric circular muscle of affected pups is hypertrophied and appears identical to that seen in the spontaneous congenital disease. Similarly, in human infants with congenital hypertrophic pyloric stenosis there is an increase in serum gastrin levels that persists after surgical correction of the stenosis.[122] It should be noted, however, that in some congenital cases of "pyloric stenosis" in cats and dogs no pyloric thickening has been identified, suggesting that functional rather than anatomic abnormalities underlie the gastric-outlet obstruction in some animals. Recent studies in children with pyloric stenosis have shown a marked loss of peptide immunoreactivity in the intrinsic nerves of the pyloric muscle.[123] Associated with this loss are low levels of nitric oxide synthase.[124] These abnormalities in innervation may result in a pylorus that is unable to relax sufficiently for normal function (see also "pylorospasm" later).

Whether the pathogenesis of adult-onset APHS is different from that of the congenital form of the disease is unknown. It is possible that some dogs with adult-onset APHS are affected initially by subclinical congenital pyloric stenosis, the clinical signs of which slowly worsen over time until veterinary attention is finally sought in adulthood. Mild congenital pyloric stenosis or dysfunction could lead to gastric retention that in turn would stimulate chronic hypergastrinemia (Figure 15–20). Gastrin's trophic effects on pyloric musculature would eventually exacerbate the disease by encouraging pyloric muscular hypertrophy. However, hypergastrinemia is unlikely to explain the antral mucosal hypertrophy characteristic of the adult form of the disease because gastrin is primarily trophic to the mucosa of the corpus and not the antral mucosa.[20] It is possible, however, that the antral mucosal hypertrophy is simply a result of mucosal irritation from chronic retention of indigestible material that cannot be eliminated in the normal manner. Thus, it would seem credible that at least some cases of adult-onset APHS are a result of a congenital rather than acquired lesion.

Prevalence and Signalment in Dogs

The prevalence of APHS in dogs at the UC Davis VMTH is 6.5 cases per 10,000. A wide range of ages can be affected. In a recent review of the records of UC Davis, approximately 30% of the cases of APHS were in dogs under 1 year of age. Of these animals, some pups began to vomit soon after weaning but most began between 6 to 12 months of age. An additional 33% of the dogs with APHS were 4 to 7 years old. In contrast, in a Dutch study, the median ages of dogs affected with pyloric muscular or mucosal hypertrophy were 5.6 and 4.2 years, respectively.[120]

There is a breed tendency for pyloric muscular hypertrophy in boxers and Boston terriers.[118,120] The prevalence of APHS in these breeds at UC Davis is 10 times higher than expected. Small breeds, such as Lhasa apso, Maltese, Pekingese, and Shih tzu, appear to be frequently affected by adult-onset APHS.[15,119] Male dogs are also predisposed.[15,120,125] Cats with "pyloric stenosis"

have been reported, but appear to be affected more by a functional rather than anatomic disease of the pylorus (see later).

Clinical Signs

The clinical signs of APHS are those of delayed gastric emptying (see earlier). Vomiting, anorexia, and weight loss are common. The vomiting often occurs many hours after eating, usually contains food, and may be projectile. In one study, projectile vomiting was seen in 25% of affected patients.[120] It is important to note, however, that projectile vomiting is not pathognomonic for APHS. Some dogs and cats with pyloric stenosis regurgitate in addition to vomiting.[149]

Diagnosis

APHS should be suspected in any dog with delayed gastric emptying but particularly if it is a male and belongs to one of the breeds of predilection. In comparison to some of the other causes of gastric outlet obstruction, such as gastric neoplasia, affected dogs are often relatively well. Laboratory findings are usually unremarkable, but hypokalemia, hypochloremia, metabolic alkalosis, and paradoxical aciduria were frequently observed in one study of APHS.[15] These abnormalities are consistent with vomiting due to a pyloric obstruction (see Chapter 39). As discussed earlier, contrast radiography can be used to confirm delayed gastric emptying and in dogs with APHS will often reveal pyloric thickening, an abrupt narrowing of the pyloric canal (the "beak" sign), or an elongated narrow streak of contrast material leaking through the enlarged pylorus. Fluoroscopy may reveal gastric hypermotility rather than the hypomotility characteristic of many gastric motility abnormalities.[15,119]

Endoscopy may demonstrate hyperplastic pyloric mucosa, often with small scattered erosions (Figure 15–5).[126] Alternatively, a protuberant muscular pylorus that is difficult to intubate with the endoscope may be apparent. If just the muscle layers of the pylorus are thickened, the endoscopic changes can be quite subtle and can be missed by inexperienced endoscopists. At surgery, the pylorus often feels thickened, and gastrostomy may reveal abnormal mucosal folds in the pylorus and antrum.

Histologically, the mucosa may be normal or may be thickened with erosions, edema, and hyperplastic and/or cystic changes in the gastric glands.[15,126] Foci of ulceration and infiltration with lymphocytes and plasma cells may be apparent. Surgical biopsy may reveal hypertrophy of pyloric muscle. Endoscopic biopsy specimens are of sufficient quality to detect mucosal changes characteristic of the disease, but the changes are relatively subtle.[126] The most consistent microscopic finding in endoscopic biopsy samples is a more pronounced papillary and branching pattern of the surface foveolae (gastric pits) and the presence of more isolated segments of foveolae in the lamina propria.[126] The biopsy specimens should be examined carefully for intraepithelial Campylobacter-like organisms, which have been recently reported in association with antral hyperplastic gastritis in a dog.[21]

Treatment

The treatment of APHS is surgical.[13,14,119,127] When muscular hypertrophy of the pylorus is the predominant lesion,

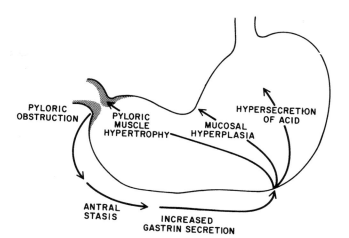

FIGURE 15–20. Schematic of stomach with effects of abnormal retention of contents. Chronic distention of antrum stimulates gastrin release, which has trophic effects on pyloric muscles and gastric mucosa. Gastrin is also the most potent stimulus for acid secretion. The events can progress to produce gastric-outlet obstruction.

good results have been reported with simple pyloromyotomy procedures such as the Fredet-Ramstedt procedure.[15,120] More extensive pyloroplasty procedures are indicated if diagnostic evaluations or palpation through the incised muscularis (after pyloromyotomy) suggest the pyloric muscular hypertrophy is complicated by hypertrophic gastritis.[15,120] These procedures involve incisions through the mucosa (rather than just the muscularis) and allow visual inspection of the antral mucosa and resection and biopsy of thickened folds. Pyloroplasty procedures that have been used successfully include the Heineke-Mikulicz pyloroplasty and the Y-U antral flap advancement.[15,119,125,127,128] With more extensive disease, the pylorus is sometimes resected and a gastroduodenostomy performed. Gastroduodenal anastomoses (such as Billroth I gastroduodenostomy) are the preferred technique of some surgeons no matter what the type of APHS diagnosed.[13,14] The prognosis is excellent but serious postoperative complications (particularly following gastroduodenal anastomosis) can occur. It is worthy of note that, in spite of good clinical results following these surgical procedures, it has been difficult to demonstrate objectively improved gastric emptying rates for food.[129-131] Temporary losses of gastrointestinal motility following these surgeries can be treated with beneficial results by metoclopramide.[132]

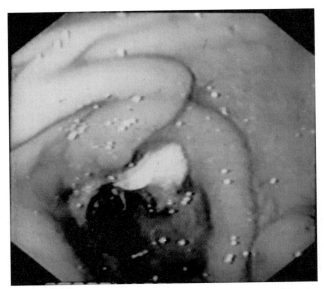

FIGURE 15–21. Endoscopic picture of a bone wedged in the pylorus. The cut end of a lamb's femur can be seen protruding into the stomach.

MISCELLANEOUS CAUSES OF GASTRIC-OUTLET OBSTRUCTION

Intraluminal foreign bodies lodged in the pylorus can produce gastric retention (Figure 15–21). The gastric outlet can be obstructed by antral polyps (see Chapter 27). Granulomatous gastritis (see earlier) and gastric neoplasia (see Chapter 27) are infrequent causes of gastric outflow obstruction. In addition, we have observed pyloric stenosis from scar tissue formed following acute pancreatitis, and from intramural pyloric fibrosis associated with the use of NSAIDs.

GASTRIC MOTILITY DISORDERS SECONDARY TO OTHER DISEASES

Disorders causing gastrointestinal motility abnormalities are a frequent cause of delayed gastric emptying (Table 15–6). Many of these disorders are acute or subacute conditions such as stress, acute pancreatitis, peritonitis, and gastroenteritis that transiently reduce motility throughout the gastrointestinal tract via sympathetic or vagal nonadrenergic inhibitory fibers.[133,134] Trauma and surgery of the abdomen and spine often cause transient gastric atony. Large losses of potassium through vomiting reduce motility, contributing to gastric retention. Motility does not return to normal until the potassium deficits are replaced. Gastric overdistension (for example, from gluttony) results in reflex constriction of the pylorus and relaxation of the stomach, delaying gastric emptying and protecting the duodenum from gastric dumping.[135,136]

Chronic gastric emptying dysfunction can result from a variety of disorders (Table 15–6) including gastric dilatation-volvulus (see Chapter 16) and chronic inflammatory conditions, such as chronic gastritis. Gastric ulceration reduces antral motility, and it also disrupts the interdigestive MMC so that emptying is inhibited in the fed and unfed state.[70,137] Cats and dogs with dysautonomia also have delayed gastric emptying. High-fat meals and malabsorption of small intestinal nutrients delay gastric emptying.[138,139] The malabsorbed nutrients are likely to stimulate ileal receptors that trigger the delayed gastric emptying (the "ileal brake"; see Chapter 12). The ileal brake may be the mechanism by which some animals with inflammatory bowel disease have slower than average gastric emptying.[140] Endocrinopathies, such as hypothyroidism, diabetes mellitus, hypo- and hyperparathyroidism (via hypo-/and hypercalcemia), and hypoadrenocorticism are likely to delay gastric emptying in dogs and possibly cats.[70,141] Acidosis has been shown to depress the contractility of gastrointestinal muscle in laboratory animals[142] and acidemia is likely to do the same in dogs and cats. Uremia delays gastric emptying in dogs and cats[100] and hepatic failure is likely to do the same. Furthermore, constipation has recently been demonstrated to delay gastric emptying in humans.[143]

Gastric motility can also be altered by gastric surgery. On most occasions the changes are transient (surgical ileus), but chronic problems can occur as a result of surgical interruption of gastric parasympathetic innervation or extensive muscle damage. Surgical incision of the stomach during gastrotomy should be parallel to longitudinal muscle fibers in order to minimize the loss of normal motility.[144] Longitudinal muscles propagate the electrical control activity or pacemaker potential.[145] Transverse section of these muscles results in loss of the propagation of contractile activity. With good suturing techniques, normal motility is usually regained within 2 weeks. Propagation of contractile activity over the stomach can be permanently lost as a result of poor surgical technique, resulting in abnormal gastric emptying of solids. Gastric emptying of liquids is not affected unless surgery involves the fundus. Surgical procedures around the cardia can remove the center where electrical control activity originates.[146] With its loss, a new center of activity arises in a region just distal to the site of resection. The new pacemaker beats more slowly, retarding gastric emptying. Damage to the vagal innervation of the proximal part of the stomach produces a persistent loss of motility in the fundus and body and a transient loss of motility in the antrum (lasting 3 weeks).[147] The vagal damage compromises receptive relaxation resulting in accelerated emptying of liquids. In contrast the decreased motility in the body and antrum slows the gastric emptying of food. Parasympathetic denervation of both the distal and proximal stomach produces more severe gastric retention.

Treatment of delayed gastric emptying due to these conditions depends heavily on treatment of the primary cause. Adjunctive therapy includes the prokinetic drugs and surgical procedures discussed earlier.

IDIOPATHIC (PRIMARY) GASTRIC MOTILITY DISORDERS

Chronic delayed gastric emptying due to gastric motility dysfunction in the absence of the diseases described here is occasionally recognized in the authors' practices and by others.[70,120] Because of the difficulties involved in detecting gastric motility abnormalities, these diseases are usually diagnoses of exclusion. Several such chronic idiopathic gastric motility abnormalities have been described.

"Pylorospasm"

"Pylorospasm" is a diagnosis that has been applied to animals with delayed gastric emptying, normal antral contractions, and radiographic evidence suggestive of abnormal contraction of the pyloric sphincter. Specifically, the identification of intermittent periods when positive contrast medium cannot be seen in the pyloric canal was considered indicative that a pyloric spasm had occluded the lumen and was responsible for delayed gastric emptying. However, the diagnosis of pylorospasm has been called into question by recent physiological observations suggesting the antrum, pylorus, and duodenum act together to control the emptying of solids from the stomach (see Chapter 12).[148] Furthermore, phasic contraction and relaxation of the pylorus is a normal phenomenon that is carefully coordinated with antral and duodenal muscular activity to facilitate both antral grinding and gastric emptying (see Chapter 12). Thus, it seems likely that the primary abnormality in animals with pylorospasm is not solitary spasm of the pylorus but instead a lack of coordination between antral, pyloric, and duodenal motility leading to delayed gastric emptying.

Pylorospasm should be carefully differentiated from APHS and should be considered distinct from gastric motility disorders such as bradygastria and tachygastria. Historically, pylorospasm is reputed to respond to anticholinergics, although modern prokinetics such as cisapride may be of more value

Pyloric Dysfunction in Cats

Pyloric "stenosis" or, more correctly, pyloric dysfunction has also been reported in cats, almost all of which were Siamese.[149-151] The pylorus did not appear abnormal and no evidence of stenosis or muscular hypertrophy was observed. Despite lack of evidence for abnormal gastric motility, gastric emptying time was abnormal, and was corrected by pyloromyotomy or pyloroplasty.

Gastric Dysrhythmias

Gastric emptying may be delayed by gastric dysrhythmias, which can be an abnormally slow rhythm (bradygastria), an abnormally fast rhythm (tachygastria), or an irregular rhythm (arrhythmia).[70,152,153] Bradygastria is thought to result from a dysfunction of the gastric pacemaker resulting in the infrequent (less than three per minute) aboral spread of slow waves. Tachygastria and arrhythmia originate from an ectopic pacemaker in the distal antrum resulting in propagation of electrical activity from the antrum through the body of the stomach. The reversed direction of motor activity prevents normal gastric emptying. The contractions accompanying tachygastria are weak or absent. Arrhythmias have been observed during fasting in as many as 50% of healthy dogs.[70] The gastric electrical activity of the majority of dogs with fasting arrhythmias normalizes once the dogs are fed.[70] Dysrhythmias in dogs can be spontaneous or induced by anticholinergics, epinephrine, glucagon, or prostaglandins.[70]

The clinical signs in dogs with gastric dysrhythmias are variable. Some dogs appear clinically normal whereas others show abdominal discomfort, vomiting, and gastric stasis. Definitive diagnosis of gastric dysrhythmia is difficult in the clinical setting because recordings of gastric electrical activity (electrogastrograms or EGG) are required.

Treatment of idiopathic gastric motility abnormalities should initially be by dietary and medical means (metoclopramide, cisapride, erythromycin; see earlier). If these therapies fail, pyloroplasty procedures may afford some relief but the prognosis is guarded.[120]

GASTRIC NEOPLASIA

Gastric-outlet obstruction and motility deficits are seen occasionally as a result of primary and metastatic neoplasms. Gastric neoplasia is discussed in Chapter 27.

ACCELERATED GASTRIC EMPTYING

Rapid gastric emptying can result in duodenal ulceration and intestinal overload that results in maldigestion and osmotic diarrhea. Humans with rapid gastric emptying can also suffer from the so-called dumping syndrome characterized by tachycardia, postprandial abdominal pain, nausea, vomiting, diarrhea, and weakness. These signs usually occur within 10 to 30 minutes of meals but can be delayed by up to several hours. There is considerable variability in the response of individuals to the same volume of hypertonic material infused experimentally into the duodenum, implying the rate of gastric emptying is not the only parameter dictating the occurrence of the dumping syndrome.[154] The pathogenesis of the dumping syndrome has been attributed to massive fluid shifts from the duodenal interstitium into the hyperosmolar lumen. However, it has recently been demonstrated that peripheral vasodilation (more so than hypovolemia) is an integral feature of dumping and it has been suggested that intestinal hypermotility stimulated by high duodenal solute concentration may explain the gastrointestinal signs.[154]

Accelerated gastric emptying is infrequent in dogs and cats but is most often a result of gastric surgical procedures such as vagotomy with pyloroplasty, gastroenterostomy, and partial gastrectomy. Very rapid emptying and intestinal transit has been observed in a dog with myenteric ganglionitis.[155] Hyperthyroidism is associated with increased gastric myoelectrical activity in humans[70] and has been shown to speed orocolic transit time in cats.[156] Diseases affecting the duodenal mucosa should result theoretically in rapid gastric emptying. As described in Chapter 12, the rate of gastric emptying is partially controlled by hormones released from the duodenal mucosa and partially by the enterogastric reflex. Function in one or both of these feedback systems can be impaired in chronic mucosal diseases. Similarly, exocrine pancreatic insufficiency should result theoretically in accelerated gastric emptying because maldigestion reduces the amount of the fatty acids in the upper small intestine and fatty acids produce more inhibition of gastric emptying than do triglycerides.[70]

The clinical signs of gastric dumping can be minimized by frequent feeding of meals of low osmolality. As discussed in Chapter 38, diets with a high soluble fiber content may be useful in the management of dumping. Feeding dry food and avoiding drinking fluids with the meal may also be helpful.

REFERENCES

1. Hottendorf GH, Hirth RS. Lesions of spontaneous subclinical disease in beagle dogs. Vet Pathol 11:240–258, 1974.
2. Rubin CE. Histologic classification of chronic gastritis: An iconoclastic view. Gastroenterology 102:360–361, 1992.
3. Correa P, Yardley JH. Grading and classification of chronic gastritis: One American response to the Sydney system. Gastroenterology 102:355–359, 1992.
4. van der Gaag I, Happe RP. Follow-up studies by peroral gastric biopsies and necropsy in vomiting dogs. Can J Vet Res 53:468–472, 1989.
5. Brunschwig A, vanProhaska J, Clarke TH, et al. A secretory depressant in gastric juice of patients with pernicious anemia. J Clin Invest 18:415–422, 1939.
6. Smith WO, Joel W, Wolf S. Experimental atrophic gastritis associated with inhibition of parietal cells. Trans Assoc Am Phy 71:306–311, 1958.
7. Hennes AR, Sevelius H, Lewellyn T, et al. Atrophic gastritis in dogs. Arch Pathol 73:281–287, 1962.
8. Krohn KJE, Finlayson NDC. Inter-relations of humoral and cellular immune responses in experimental canine gastritis. Clin Exp Immunol 14:237–245, 1973.
9. Cheli R, Perasso A, Giacosa A. Gastritis. Springer-Verlag, New York, 1987.
10. Fukuma K, Sakaguchi S, Kuribayashi K, et al. Immunologic and clinical studies on murine experimental autoimmune gastritis induced by neonatal thymectomy. Gastroenterology 94:274–283, 1988.
11. Siegal J. Gastrointestinal ulcer—Arthus reaction! Ann Allergy 32:127–130, 1974.
12. Davenport HW. Prevention and suppression by azathioprine of venom-induced protein-losing gastropathy in dogs. Proc Nat Acad Sci (USA) 73:968–970, 1976.
13. Matthiesen DT, Walter MC. Surgical treatment of chronic hypertrophic pyloric gastropathy in 45 dogs. J Am Anim Hosp Assoc 22:241–247, 1986.
14. Sikes RI, Birchard S, Patnaik A, et al. Chronic hypertrophic pyloric gastropathy: A review of 16 cases. J Am Anim Hosp Assoc 22:99–104, 1986.
15. Bellenger CR, Maddison JE, MacPherson GC, et al. Chronic hypertrophic pyloric gastropathy in 14 dogs. Aust Vet J 67:317–320, 1990.
16. Slappendel RJ, van der Gaag I, van Ness JJ, et al. Familial stomatocytosis-hypertrophic gastritis (FSHG), a newly recognised disease in the dog (Drentse patrijshond). Vet Q 13:30–40, 1991.
17. Jubb KVF, Kennedy PC. Pathology of Domestic Animals, Vol 2. Academic Press, New York, 1970.
18. Twedt DC, Magne ML. Chronic gastritis. In: Kirk RW (ed) Current Veterinary Therapy X. WB Saunders, Philadelphia, 852–856, 1989.
19. Vanderlindesipman JS, Boersema JH, Berrocal A. 3 cases of hypertrophic gastritis associated with Ollulanus tricuspis in the cat. Tijdschrift Voor Diergeneeskunde 117:727–729, 1992.
20. Walsh JH. Gastrointestinal hormones. In: Johnson LR (ed) Physiology of the Gastrointestinal Tract, 2nd ed. Raven Press, New York, 181–253, 1987.
21. Leblanc B, Fox JG, Le Net JL, et al. Hyperplastic gastritis with intraepithelial Campylobacter-like organisms in a beagle dog. Vet Path 30:391–394, 1993.
22. Van der Gaag I, Happe RP, Wolvekamp W Th C. A boxer dog with chronic hypertrophic gastritis resembling Menetrier's disease in man. Vet Pathol 13:172–185, 1976.
23. Van Kruiningen HJ. Giant hypertrophic gastritis of basenji dogs. Vet Pathol 14:19–28, 1977.
24. Hansen OH, Jensen KB, Larsen JK, et al. Gastric mucosal cell proliferation and immunoglobulin containing cells in Menetrier's disease. Digestion 16:293–298, 1977.
25. Isenberg JI. Gastric secretory testing. In: Sleisenger MH, Fordtran JS (eds) Gastrointestinal Disease. WB Saunders, Philadelphia, 1973.
26. Mavligit GM. Immunologic effects of cimetidine: Potential uses. Pharmacotherapy 7:120S–124S, 1987.
27. Stanton ME, Bright RM. Gastroduodenal ulceration in dogs. J Vet Int Med 3:238–244, 1989.
28. Hayden DW, Fleischman RW. Scirrhous eosinophilic gastritis in dogs with gastric arteritis. Vet Pathol 14:441–448, 1977.
29. Narama I, Kuroda J, Nagatani M, et al. Superficial eosinophilic gastritis in laboratory beagle dogs attributable probably to diet. Jpn J Vet Sci 52:581–589, 1990.
30. McLeod CG, Langlinais PC, Brown JC. Ulcerative histiocytic gastritis and amyloidosis in a dog. Vet Path 18:117–120, 1981.
31. van der Gaag I, van Niel MHF, Belshaw BE, et al. Gastric granulomatous cryptococcosis mimicking gastric carcinoma in a dog. Vet Q 13:185–189, 1991.
32. Weber AF, Hasa O, Sautter JH. Some observations concerning the presence of spirillia in the fundic glands of dogs and cats. Am J Vet Res 19:677–680, 1958.
33. Blaser MJ. Gastric campylobacter-like organisms, gastritis, and peptic ulcer disease. Gastroenterology 93:371–383, 1987.
34. Henry GA, Long PH, Burns JL, et al. Gastric spirillosis in beagles. Am J Vet Res 48:831–836, 1987.
35. Lee A, Hazell SL, O'Rourke J, et al. Isolation of a spiral-shaped bacterium from the cat stomach. Infect Immunol 56:2843–2850, 1988.
36. Paster BJ, Lee A, Fox JG, et al. Phylogeny of Helicobacter felis sp. nov., Helicobacter mustelae, and related bacteria. Int J Syst Bacteriol 41:31–38, 1991.
37. Geyer C, Colbatzky F, Lechner J, et al. Occurrence of spiral-shaped bacteria in gastric biopsies of dogs and cats. Vet Rec 133:18–19, 1993.
38. Lee A, Krakowka S, Fox JG, et al. Role of Helicobacter felis in chronic canine gastritis. Vet Pathol 29:487–494, 1992.
39. Feinstein RE, Olsson E. Chronic gastroenterocolitis in nine cats. J Vet Diagn Invest 4:293–298, 1992.
40. Lichtenberger LM. Mechanisms of gastric mucosal protection. Proc ACVIM, Washington DC, 74–79, May 1993.
41. Heresbach D, Raoul JL, Bretagne JF, et al. Helicobacter pylori: A risk and severity factor of non-steroidal anti-inflammatory drug induced gastropathy. Gut 33:1608–1611, 1992.
42. Smith JL, Garner BM. Medical and surgical management of peptic ulcer disease. Curr Opin G 9:909–916, 1993.
43. Lavelle JP, Landas S, Mitros FA, et al. Acute gastritis associated with spiral organisms from cats. Dig Dis Sci 39:744–750, 1994.
44. Radin MJ, Eaton KA, Krakowka S, et al. Helicobacter pylori gastric infection in gnotobiotic beagle dogs. Infect Immun 58:2606–2612, 1990.
45. Hargis AM, Prieur DJ, Gaillard ET. Chlamydial infection of the gastric mucosa in twelve cats. Vet Pathol 20:170–178, 1983.
46. Barsanti JA, Attleberger MH, Henderson RA. Phycomycosis in a dog. J Am Vet Med Assoc 167:293–297, 1975.
47. Miller RI. Gastrointestinal phycomycosis in 63 dogs. J Am Vet Med Assoc 186:473–478, 1985.
48. Hargis AM, Prieur DJ, Blanchard JL. Prevalence, lesions, and differential diagnosis of Ollulanus tricuspis infection in cats. Vet Pathol 20:71–79, 1983.
49. Reindel JF, Trapp AL, Armstrong PJ, et al. Recurrent plasmacytic stomatitis-pharyngitis in a cat with esophagitis, fibrosing gastritis, and gastric nematodiasis. J Am Vet Med Assoc 190:65–67, 1987.
50. Wilson RB, Presnell JC. Chronic gastritis due to Ollulanus tricuspis infection in a cat. J Am Anim Hosp Assoc 26:137–139, 1990.
51. Guy PA. Ollulanus tricuspis in domestic cats—prevalence and methods of post-mortem diagnosis. NZ Vet J 32:81–84, 1984.
52. Bell AG. Ollulanus tricuspis in a cat colony. NZ Vet J 32:85–87, 1984.
53. Burrows CF. Infection with the stomach worm Physaloptera as a cause of chronic vomiting in the dog. J Am Anim Hosp Assoc 19:947–950, 1983.
54. Santen DR, Chastain CB, Schmidt DA. Efficacy of pyrantel pamoate against Physaloptera in a cat. J Am Anim Hosp Assoc 29:53–55, 1993.
55. Clark JA. Physaloptera stomach worms associated with chronic vomition in a dog in western Canada. Can Vet J 31:840, 1990.
56. Todd AC, Crowley J, Scholl P, et al. Critical tests with pyrantel pamoate against parasites in dogs from Wisconsin. VM/SAC 70:936–939, 1975.
57. Kirkpatrick CE, Lok JB, Goldschmidt MH, et al. Gastric gnathostomiasis in a cat. J Am Vet Med Assoc 190:1437–1439, 1987.
58. Mense MG, Gardiner CH, Moeller RB, et al. Chronic emesis caused by a nematode-induced gastric nodule in a cat. J Am Vet Med Assoc 201:597–598, 1992.
59. Curtsinger DK, Carpenter JL, Turner JL. Gastritis caused by Aonchotheca putprii in a domestic cat. J Am Vet Med Assoc 203:1153–1154, 1993.
60. Happe RP, Van Den Broyn WE. Duodenogastric reflux in the dog, a clinicopathical study. Res Vet Sci 33:280–286, 1982.
61. Ritchie WP. Alkaline reflux gastritis: A critical reappraisal. Gut 25:975–987, 1984.
62. Heading RC. Duodenogastric reflux. Gut 24:507–509, 1983.
63. Seino Y, Matsukura S, Inoue Y, et al. Hypogastrinemia in hypothyroidism. Am J Dig Dis 23:189–191, 1978.
64. DeNovo RC. Characteristics of gastric mucosal healing. Proc ACVIM, Washington DC 82–84, May 1993.

65. Schaudies RP. Epidermal growth factor. Proc ACVIM, Washington DC, 80–81, May 1993.
66. Lemoine NR, Leung HY, Gullick WJ. Growth factors in the gastrointestinal tract. Gut 33:1297–1300, 1992.
67. Brzozowskii T, Konturek SJ, Majka J, et al. Epidermal growth factor, polyamines, and prostaglandins in healing of stress-induced gastric lesions in rats. Dig Dis Sci 38:276–283, 1993.
68. Marcuard SP, Silverman JF, Finley JL. Ornithine decarboxylase activity during gastric ulcer healing in dogs. Dig Dis Sci 37:1015–1019, 1992.
69. Moreland KJ. Ulcer disease of the upper gastrointestinal tract in small animals: Pathophysiology, diagnosis, and management. Comp Contin Ed Pract Vet 10:262–272, 1988.
70. Hall JA, Twedt DC, Burrows CF. Gastric motility in dogs. II. Disorders of gastric motility. 12:247–261, 1990.
71. Wolfe NM, Soll AH. The physiology of gastric acid secretion. N Eng J Med 319:1707–1715, 1988.
72. Papich MG. Antiulcer therapy. Vet Clin N Am 23:497–512, 1993.
73. Sagge MR, Butler ML. Reassessment of the management of benign gastric ulcer with achlorhydria. Clin Gastroenterol 3:13–15, 1981.
74. Feldman M. Inhibition of gastric acid secretion by selective and nonselective anticholinergics. Gastroenterology 86:361–366, 1984.
75. Klempa I, Holle F, Bruckner W, et al. The effect of selective proximal vagotomy and pyloroplasty on gastric secretion and motility in the dog. Arch Surg 103:713–719, 1971.
76. Robert A, Schultz JR, Nezamis JE, et al. Gastric antisecretory and antiulcer properties of PGE$_2$, 15-methyl PGE$_2$, and 16, 16-Dimethyl PGE$_2$. Gastroenterology 70:359–370, 1976.
77. Reinhart WH, Muller O, Halter F. Influence of long-term 16, 16-dimethyl prostaglandin E$_2$ treatment on the rat gastrointestinal mucosa. Gastroenterology 85:1003–1010, 1983.
78. Murtaugh RJ, Matz ME, Labato MA, et al. Use of synthetic prostaglandin E$_1$ (Misoprostol) for prevention of aspirin-induced gastroduodenal ulceration in arthritic dogs. J Am Vet Med Assoc 202:251–256, 1993.
79. Daly MJ, Humphray JM, Stables R. Inhibition of gastric acid secretion in the dog by the H$_2$-receptor antagonists, ranitidine, cimetidine, and metiamide. Gut 21:408–412, 1980.
80. Forrester SD, Merton Boothe D, Willard MD. Clinical pharmacology of antiemetic and antiulcer drugs. Sem Vet Med Surg 4:194–201, 1989.
81. Gill M, Sanyal S, Sareen ML. Effect of cimetidine on intestinal absorption and digestive functions in mice. Indian J Med Res 92:109–114, 1990.
82. Frislid K, Guldvog I, Berstad A. Kinetics of the inhibition of food-stimulated secretion by ranitidine in dogs. Eur Surg Res 17:360–365, 1985.
83. Mizumoto A, Fujimura M, Iwanaga Y, et al. Anticholinesterase activity of histamine H$_2$-receptor antagonists in the dog: Their possible role in gastric motor activity. J Gastrointest Motil 2:273–280, 1990.
84. Takagi T, Takeda M, Maeno H. Effect of a new potent H$_2$-blocker, 3[-2(diaminomethylene) amino]-4-thiazolyl]methyl]-thio]-N^2- sulfamoylpropionamidine (YM-11170) on gastric acid secretion induced by histamine and food in conscious dogs. Arch Int Pharmacodyn 256:49–58, 1982.
85. Katz LB, Tobia AJ, Shriver DA. Effects of ORF 17583, other histamine H$_2$-receptor antagonists, and omeprazole on gastric acid secretory states in rats and dogs. J Pharmacol Exp Ther 242:437–442, 1987.
86. Ueki S, Seiki M, Yoneta T, et al. Gastroprokinetic activity of nizatidine, a new H$_2$-receptor antagonist, and its possible mechanism of action in dogs and rats. J Pharmacol Expl Ther 264:152–157, 1993.
87. Larsson H, Carlsson E, Junggren U, et al. Inhibition of gastric acid secretion by omeprazole in the dog and rat. Gastroenterology 85:900–907, 1983.
88. Konturek SJ, Cieszkowski M, Kwiecien N, et al. Effects of omeprazole, a substituted benzimidazole, on gastrointestinal secretions, serum gastrin, and gastric mucosal blood flow in dogs. Gastroenterology 86:71–77, 1984.
89. Jenkins CC, DeNovo RC. Omeprazole: A potent antiulcer drug. Comp Contin Educ Pract Vet 13:1578–1582, 1991.
90. Holtermuller KH. Acid rebound: Fact or fiction. Hepato-gastroenterol 29:135–137, 1982.
91. Spencer H, Lender M. Adverse effects of aluminum-containing antacids on mineral metabolism. Gastroenterology 76:603–606, 1979.
92. Gilbert DA, Saunders DR. Iced saline lavage does not slow bleeding from experimental canine gastric ulcers. Dig Dis Sci 26:1065–1068, 1981.
93. LeKagul S, Smyth NP, Brooks MH, et al. The control of upper gastrointestinal hemorrhage in the dog by intraperitioneal cooling. J Surg Res 10:423–431, 1970.
94. LeVeen HH, Falk G, Diaz C, et al. Control of gastrointestinal bleeding. Am J Surg 123:154–159, 1972.
95. Rutgeerts P, Geboes K, Vantrappen G. Experimental studies of injection therapy for severe nonvariceal bleeding in dogs. Gastroenterology 97:610–621, 1989.
96. Gorbach SL. Bismuth therapy in gastrointestinal diseases. Gastroenterology 99:863–875, 1990.
97. Jakovljevic S. Gastric radiology and gastroscopy. Vet Ann 28:172–182, 1988.
98. Evans SM. Double versus single contrast gastrography in the dog and cat. Vet Radiol 24:6–10, 1983.
99. Hall JA, Willer RL, Seim HB, et al. Gastric emptying of nondigestible radiopaque markers after circumcostal gastropexy in clinically normal dogs and dogs with gastric dilatation-volvulus. Am J Vet Res 53:1961–1965, 1992.
100. Allan FJ, Guilford WG. Radiopaque markers: Preliminary clinical observations [abstract]. J Vet Int Med 8:151, 1994.
101. Miyabayashi T, Morgan JP. Gastric emptying in the normal dog. Vet Radiol 25:187–191, 1984.
102. Burns J, Fox SM. The use of a barium meal to evaluate total gastric emptying time in the dog. Vet Radiol 27:169–172, 1986.
103. Miyabayashi T, Morgan JP, Atilola MAO, et al. Small intestinal emptying time in normal beagle dogs. Vet Radiol 27:164–168, 1986.
104. Steyn PF, Twedt DC. Gastric emptying in the normal cat: A radiographic study. J Am Anim Hosp Assoc 30:78–80, 1994.
105. Gue M, Fioramonti J, Bueno L. A simple double radiolabeled technique to evaluate gastric emptying of canned food meal in dogs. Application to pharmacological tests. Gastroenterol Clin Biol 12:425–430, 1988.
106. Van den Brom WE, Happe RP. Gastric emptying of a radionuclide-labeled test meal in healthy dogs: A new mathematical analysis and reference values. Am J Vet Res 47:2170–2174, 1986.
107. Burrows CF, Bright RM, Spencer CF. Influence of dietary composition on gastric emptying and motility in dogs: Potential involvement in acute gastric dilatation. Am J Vet Res 46:2609–2612, 1985.
108. Hornof WJ, Koblik PD, Strombeck DR, et al. Scintigraphic evaluation of solid-phase gastric emptying in the dog. Vet Radiol 30:242–248, 1989.
109. Bolondi L, Bortolotti M, Santi V, et al. Measurement of gastric emptying time by real-time ultrasonography. Gastroenterology 99:752–759, 1985.
110. Sarna SK, Otterson MF. Gastroduodenal motility. Curr Opin G 9:922–929, 1993.
111. Itoh Z, Nakaya M, Suzuki T, et al. Erythromycin mimics exogenous motilin in gastrointestinal contractile activity in the dog. Am J Physiol 247:G688–G694, 1984.
112. Weber FH, Richards RD, McCallum RW. Erythromycin: A motilin agonist and gastrointestinal prokinetic agent. Am J Gastroenterol 88:485–490, 1993.
113. Camilleri M. The current role of erythromycin in the clinical management of gastric emptying disorders. Am J Gastroenterol 88:169–170, 1993.
114. Janssens J, Peeters TL, Vantrappen G, et al. Improvement of gastric emptying in diabetic gastroparesis by erythromycin: Preliminary observations. N Eng J Med 322:1028–1031, 1990.
115. Richards RD, Davenport K, McCallum RW. The treatment of idiopathic and diabetic gastroparesis with acute intravenous and chronic oral erythromycin. Am J Gastroenterol 88:203–207, 1993.
116. Eriksson A, Rauramaa V, Happonen I, et al. Feeding reduced the absorption of erythromycin in the dog. Acta Vet Scand 31:497–499, 1990.
117. Kozarek RA, Botoman VA, Patterson DJ. Long term follow-up in patients who have undergone balloon dilatation for gastric outlet obstruction. Gastrointest Endosc 36:558–561, 1990.
118. DeNovo RC. Antral pyloric hypertrophy syndrome. In: Kirk RW (ed) Current Veterinary Therapy X. WB Saunders, Philadelphia, 918–921, 1989.
119. Walter MC, Matthiesen DT. Acquired antral pyloric hypertrophy in the dog. Vet Clin N Am 23:547–554, 1993.
120. Peeters ME. Pyloric stenosis in the dog: Developments in the surgical treatment and a retrospective study in 47 patients. Eur J Compan Anim Pract 2:37–40, 1991.
121. Dodge JA, Karim AA. Induction of pyloric hypertrophy by pentagastrin. Gut 17:280–284, 1976.
122. Moazam F, Rodgers, BM, Talbert JL, et al. Fasting and postprandial serum gastrin levels in infants with congenital hypertrophic pyloric stenosis. Ann Surg 188:623–625, 1978.
123. Wattchow DA, Cass DT, Furness JB, et al. Abnormalities of peptide-containing nerve fibers in infantile hypertrophic pyloric stenosis. Gastroenterology 92:443–448, 1987.
124. Vanderwinden JM, Mailleux P, Schiffmann SN, et al. Nitric oxide synthase activity in infantile hypertrophic pyloric stenosis. N Engl J Med 327:511–515, 1992.
125. Walter MC, Matthiesen DT. Gastric outflow surgical problems. Prob Vet Med 1:196–214, 1989.
126. Leib MS, Saunders GK, Moon ML, et al. Endoscopic diagnosis of chronic hypertrophic pyloric gastropathy in dogs. J Vet Int Med 7:335–341, 1993.
127. Walter MC, Matthiesen DT, Stone EA. Pylorectomy and gastroduodenostomy in the dog: Technique and clinical results in 28 cases. J Am Vet Med Assoc 187:909–914, 1985.
128. Bright RM, Richardson DC, Stanton ME. Y-U antral flap advancement pyloroplasty in dogs. Comp Contin Ed Pract Vet 10:139–141, 1988.
129. Meyer JH, Thomson JB, Cohen MB, et al. Sieving of solid food by the canine stomach and sieving after gastric surgery. Gastroenterology 76:804–813, 1979.
130. Fox SM, Burns J. The effect of pyloric surgery on gastric emptying in the dog: Comparison of three techniques. J Am Anim Hosp Assoc 22:783–788, 1986.
131. Papageorges M. Does pyloroplasty accelerate gastric emptying? J Am Anim Hosp Assoc 23:248, 1987.

132. Stanton ME, Bright RM, Toal R, et al. The use of metoclopramide after Y-U pyloroplasty in dogs [abstract]. Vet Surg 16:103, 1987.

133. Glise H, Abrahamsson H. Reflex vagal inhibition of gastric motility by intestinal nociceptive stimulation in the cat. Scand J Gastroenterol 15:769–774, 1980.

134. Gue M, Peeters T, Depoortere I, et al. Stress-induced changes in gastric emptying, postprandial motility, and plasma gut hormone levels in dogs. Gastroenterology 97:1101–1107, 1989.

135. Schulze-Delrieu K. Intrinsic reflexes between the esophagus and stomach. Gastroenterology 91:1568–1569, 1986.

136. DePonti F, Azpiroz F, Malagelada JR. Reflex gastric relaxation in response to distention of the duodenum. Am J Physiol 252:G595–G601, 1987.

137. Malbert CH, Hara S, Ruckenbusch Y. Early myoelectrical activity changes during gastric or duodenal ulceration in dogs. Dig Dis Sci 32:737–742, 1987.

138. Welch I, Cunningham KM, Reed NW. Regulation of gastric emptying by ileal nutrients in humans. Gastroenterology 94:401–404, 1988.

139. Keinke O, Ehrlein HJ. Effect of oleic acid on canine gastroduodenal motility, pyloric diameter and gastric emptying. Q J Exp Physiol 68:675–686, 1983.

140. Guilford WG. Unpublished observations, 1994.

141. Kowalewski K, Kolodej A. Myoelectrical and mechanical activity of stomach and intestine in hypothyroid dogs. Am J Dig Dis 22:235–240, 1977.

142. Schulze-Delrieu K, Lipsien G. Depression of mechanical and electrical activity in muscle strips of opossum stomach and esophagus by acidosis. Gastroenterology 82:720–725, 1982.

143. Tjeerdsma HC, Smout AJPM, Akkermans LMA. Voluntary suppression of defecation delays gastric emptying. Dig Dis Sci 38:832–836, 1993.

144. Cannon WB. The Mechanical Factors of Digestion. New York, Longmans, 1911.

145. Bedi BS, Kelly KA, Holley KE. Pathways of propagation of the canine gastric pacesetter potential. Gastroenterology 63:288–296, 1972.

146. Kelly KA, Code CF. Canine gastric pacemaker. Am J Physiol 220:112–118, 1971.

147. Klempa I, Holle F, Bruckner W, et al. The effect of selective proximal vagotomy and pyloroplasty on gastric secretion and motility in the dog. Arch Surg 102:713–719, 1971.

148. Edwards DAW, Rowlands EN. Physiology of the gastroduodenal junction. In: Code CF (ed) Handbook of Physiology, Sect. 6, Alimentary Canal, Vol. 4 American Physiological Society, Washington, DC, 1985–2000, 1968.

149. Pearson H, Gaskell CJ, et al. Pyloric and oesophageal dysfunction in the cat. J Sm Anim Pract 15:487–501, 1974.

150. Twaddle AA. Pyloric stenosis in three cats and its correction by pyloroplasty. NZ Vet J 18:15–17, 1970.

151. Twaddle AA. Congenital pyloric stenosis in two kittens corrected by pyloroplasty. NZ Vet J 19:26–27, 1971.

152. Kim CH, Zinsmeister AR, Malagelada JR. Mechanisms of canine gastric dysrhythmia. Gastroenterology 92:993–999, 1987.

153. Kim CH, Azpiroz F, Malagelada JR. Characteristics of spontaneous and drug-induced gastric dysrhthmias in a chronic canine model. Gastroenterology 90:421–427, 1986.

154. Snook JA, Wells AD, Prytherch DR, et al. Studies on the pathogenesis of the early dumping syndrome induced by intraduodenal instillation of hypertonic glucose. Gut 30:1716–1720, 1989.

155. Willard MD, Mullaney T, Karasek S, et al. Diarrhea associated with myenteric ganglionitis in a dog. J Am Vet Med Assoc 193:346–348, 1988.

156. Papasouliotis K, Muir P, Gruffydd-Jones TJ, et al. Decreased orocecal transit time as measured by the exhalation of breath hydrogen in hyperthyroid cats. Res Vet Sci 55:115–118, 1993.

16 Gastric Dilatation, Gastric Dilatation-Volvulus, and Chronic Gastric Volvulus

W. GRANT GUILFORD

GASTRIC DILATATION

Clinical Synopsis

Diagnostic Features

- Abdominal enlargement but minimal tympany
- No evidence of marked cardiovascular compromise
- Radiographs including a right lateral view do *not* demonstrate any volvulus

Management

- Orogastric intubation and lavage
- Emetics

Prevalence and Signalment

Overdistension of the stomach without concomitant volvulus occurs occasionally in dogs of all sizes and ages. It is most common in young dogs but is occasionally seen in adults.

Etiology and Pathogenesis

Gluttony is the most common cause of gastric dilatation. In most cases, overdilatation is relieved by vomiting and eructation. In some cases, overdistension of the stomach results in gastric atony, and the dilatation becomes persistent. In this eventuality, fermentation of food results in the generation of considerable amounts of gas, exacerbating the gastric distension. Gastric dilatation in large-breed dogs may occur for the same reasons as gastric dilatation-volvulus (see later).

Clinical Findings

The history often reveals access to trash or appetizing food. Gastric overdistension results in abdominal enlargement, depression, discomfort, eructation, and intermittent, largely ineffectual retching and vomiting. Palpation of the abdomen may reveal an enlarged and doughy stomach due to impacted ingesta. Affected dogs are usually hemodynamically stable and rarely have a drum-tight, tympanic abdomen. In large-breed dogs, gastric dilatation can lead to gastric volvulus, resulting in progression of abdominal fullness to tympany and rapid deterioration of condition. Tympany, particularly in large-breed dogs, should raise strong suspicion of gastric dilatation-volvulus rather than simple dilatation.

Diagnosis

Diagnosis of gastric dilatation relies on an appropriate history and clinical signs. Radiographs, including a view taken of the patient in right lateral recumbency, are recommended to rule out the possibility of accompanying volvulus.

Management and Prognosis

Passing a stomach tube can relieve accumulated gas and fluid. If the dilatation is due to impacted ingesta, however, this procedure may not be successful. Use of an emetic agent such as apomorphine usually succeeds in relieving the distension. The dose can be titrated by placing an apomorphine tablet in the subconjunctival sac and removing it as soon as nausea and retching begin. Emetics should not be used if there is any suspicion of ingestion of caustic or sharp materials or if the animal appears hypovolemic or mentally depressed to the point where it is unlikely to be able to protect its airway. If these measures fail, gastric decompression may require anesthesia (with tracheal intubation), passage of a large-bore stomach tube, and gastric lavage with warm water. On rare occasions, gastrostomy is necessary to remove impacted material.

The prognosis is good but recurrent gastric dilatation or dilatation and volvulus can occur. The latter is particularly likely in large-breed dogs. Therefore, prophylactic gastropexy should be considered in large-breed dogs affected by gastric dilatation unless there is a clear history of gluttony preceding the attack.

GASTRIC DILATATION-VOLVULUS

Clinical Synopsis

Diagnostic Features

- Acute onset of abdominal tympany due to gastric dilatation
- Right lateral radiograph demonstrating gastric volvulus

Treatment

- Lactated Ringer's (LRS) bolus 45 mL/kg over first 15 to 30 minutes
- Slow gastric decompression by orogastric intubation or trocarization
- Additional LRS volume replacement up to a total of 90 mL/kg (as dictated by cardiovascular status and PCV/TP) over the next 1 to 2 hours
- Maintenance LRS (3–10 mL/kg/hour) supplemented by potassium chloride (20 mEq/L)
- Intravenous broad-spectrum antibiotics
- Ranitidine (1–2 mg/kg q 8–12 hours IV IM PO) or cimetidine (4–5 mg/kg q 8 hours IV IM PO)
- Surgical correction (once patient is stable) followed by gastropexy to prevent recurrence
- When indicated (see text), supplemental therapy may include dextran 70, plasma, blood, sodium bicarbonate, corticosteroids, antiarrhythmics, heparin, metoclopramide, sucralfate, dopamine or dobutamine, oxygen free-radical scavengers, enteral or parenteral nutrition.

Monitoring

- Close postoperative monitoring is essential for successful treatment
- Depending on the dog's condition monitoring may include some or all of repeated physical examinations; blood gases; serum electrolyte, glucose, BUN, ALT, and bilirubin concentrations; PCV/TP and/or CBC; urinalysis; blood pressure, CVP, and ECG; clotting times.

Prevalence and Signalment

The prevalence of acute gastric dilatation-volvulus (GDV) in the general canine population is relatively low. In a 7 year period at the VMTH at Davis, 13 cases of GDV were recorded per 10,000 patients. A similar prevalence is observed at the Massey University Veterinary Clinic. The incidence is higher in emergency clinics and in some rural clinics. For instance, 3% of dogs presented to a rural German clinic had gastric dilatation or GDV.[1] Furthermore, within predisposed breeds, GDV is an important cause of morbidity and mortality. For example, 3.3% of the Great Danes presented to one clinic were afflicted with GDV.

Acute GDV is most common in large-breed, deep-chested dogs such as the Great Dane, German shepherd, Saint Bernard, Irish setter, and Doberman pinscher.[1,2] GDV has occasionally been reported in cats and in smaller breeds of dogs such as dachshunds, bassets, English bulldogs, terriers, miniature poodles and pekingese. GDV can occur in dogs of any age. A range of 2 months to 15 years with a mean of 5.2 ± 2.9 years was reported in one study.[2] In a recent large study (391 dogs) of gastric dilatation and GDV, the mean age was 7.2 years.[1] No sex predisposition has been established.

Predisposing Causes of Gastric Dilatation-Volvulus

INTRODUCTION. A singular cause of GDV has not been identified. More than likely, the disease results from an additive interaction between risk factors, which in combination eventually result in GDV (Figure 16–1). GDV may have any of a number of precipitating causes provided the appropriate foundation of predisposing causes is in place. Which predisposing causes are essential to the development of GDV and which are not remains to be established. It is important to note that some apparent risk factors may simply reflect techniques common in the management of large dogs rather than being true predisposing causes. Certainly, two events must occur before GDV will develop. There must be overdistension of the stomach with gas and fluid, and volvulus must occur. It is probable that either of these two events can precipitate GDV. That is, volvulus can cause dilatation, just as dilatation can cause volvulus.

DILATATION OF THE STOMACH. Gastric overdistension can lead to volvulus and thus GDV. Dilatation causes the greater curvature of the stomach to move ventrally, causing the pylorus to move dorsally and to the left. Gastric movement displaces the spleen by way of the gastrosplenic ligament. Once displaced, the spleen engorges and may inhibit spontaneous reversibility of the gastric torsion. Stomach dilatation can result from accumulation of gas, fluid, or food. Gastric gas is derived from aerophagia, fermentation, and acidification of bicarbonate. Gastric fluid is derived from ingesta, gastric secretions, and exudation of extracellular fluid secondary to increased hydrostatic pressure from venous obstruction and to increased mucosal permeability.

GASTRIC VOLVULUS. Gastric volvulus is usually considered a consequence of gastric dilatation. There is little evidence to refute the suggestion, however, that volvulus could precede dilatation.[3] Dogs with gastric volvulus without dilatation have been observed at the UCD VMTH and have been reported by others.[4] These dogs commonly have a history of recurrent bouts of mild gastric distension. This syndrome is described as chronic volvulus (see later). Gastric volvulus compromises gastric emptying of gas and ingesta and can progress to dilatation and GDV. The cause(s) of gastric volvulus is unknown.

CONFORMATION. Deep-chested body conformation predisposes dogs to the development of GDV, perhaps through increasing the likelihood of volvulus, or by altering anatomic relationships at the gastroesophageal sphincter and thus impairing eructation.

LAXITY OF THE GASTRIC LIGAMENTS. Laxity of hepatoduodenal and hepatogastric ligaments may increase the likelihood of volvulus. Stomachs with apparently normal ligamentous attachments, however, can be readily displaced at surgery into a volvulus position. Thus it appears there is sufficient laxity in normal gastric and duodenal ligaments to permit rotational instability.

POSTPRANDIAL EXERCISE. Vigorous exercise by dogs with a stomach distended by food or water may physically displace the stomach and increase the likelihood of volvulus. However, in a recent large study, the onset of clinical signs varied from 1 to 40 hours (average 7 hours) after the dogs were last fed.[1]

COMPOSITION OF DIET. GDV has been considered a disease of domestication, because the incidence is thought to be greater in dogs fed commercial dog foods than in dogs fed "natural" diets. However, a direct causal relationship between the type of food eaten and the development of GDV has not been proven in spite of the well-known effects of diet on gastric emptying and intestinal gas production (see Chapter 39). GDV has been reported in dogs eating meat, soy, or cereal-based diets, and in dogs fed free-choice or single daily meals. In a recent study, 39.6% of dogs with GDV or gastric dilatation were fed dry food, 26.3% were fed canned food, and 25.3% were fed fresh meat, rice, and meat by-products (in 8.7% of cases, diet was unknown).[1] The swelling of dry food in the stomach has been proposed as a cause of GDV. The in-

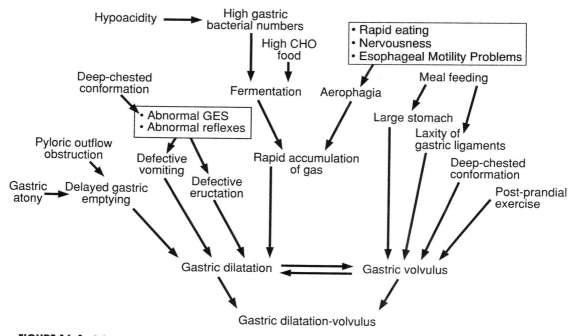

FIGURE 16-1. Schematic representation of the interaction of the predisposing causes of gastric dilatation-volvulus.

hospital incidence of GDV at the UCD VMTH declined when dry food was dampened prior to feeding.

INTAKE OF LARGE VOLUME OF INGESTA. Rapid intake of a large volume of food or water causes gastric dilation and may precipitate GDV. The stomachs of dogs fed dry dog food once per day eventually become significantly larger than the stomachs of dogs fed dry dog food three times per day, and dogs fed meat and bone rations. Thus, chronic intake of large volumes of dry food leads to gastric hypertrophy.[5] A similar phenomenon is well documented in laboratory rodents. Large volumes of food take longer to empty than smaller volumes of food, resulting in a more prolonged period in which food is available for fermentation. Damage to the stomach by overdilatation resulting in deranged myoelectrical activity and impaired gastric emptying, has also been hypothesized.[5]

INCREASED PRODUCTION OR INTAKE OF GASTRIC GAS. GDV is associated with abnormal retention of gas in both the fed and unfed stomach. The gas has been suggested to be swallowed air, to result from the reaction of gastric acid with secretions containing bicarbonate, or to be derived from bacterial fermentation. Gastric gas analyses have been somewhat variable. In general the gastric gas composition has been found to be similar to that of atmospheric gas with the exception of an elevated carbon dioxide concentration. In one study the carbon dioxide concentration reached 10%.[6] The most likely source of the carbon dioxide is the interaction of gastric bicarbonate and acid. The gastric bicarbonate is thought to derive from saliva or from leakage of extracellular fluid. However, another possible source of the carbon dioxide is bacterial fermentation of food.[7] Other gaseous products of bacterial fermentation have been found in one study[7] but not in another.[6]

Air is swallowed during drinking and eating, the amounts increasing with rapid eating and the gulping of liquids. Aerophagia may also occur in nervous, excited, or dyspneic animals. Marked aerophagia as a result of hyperventilation or greedy eating has been reported in association with a series of cases of GDV.[3] Aerophagia caused by esophageal motility abnormalities has been observed in 60% of dogs with recur-

rent GDV.[8] Furthermore, an association between respiratory difficulty and gastric dilatation was noted in one human study.[9] In normal dogs, swallowed air does not accumulate but escapes by eructation. Thus, aerophagia in association with defective eructation could result in GDV. The esophagus can generate sufficiently high peristaltic pressure to force swallowed air through the gastroesphageal junction into the gas-distended stomach, but aerophagia by itself would be unlikely to produce the very high intragastric pressures recorded in the stomachs of some dogs with GDV.

Gas-producing bacteria, in particular clostridia, have been suggested as the origin of the gastric gas in GDV.[7] Gas is not produced by fermentation in the normal empty stomach because bacteria numbers are kept very low by gastric acidity.[20] During feeding, bacterial numbers increase to 10^5 per gram of contents. The sources of the bacteria are the oral cavity and diet. Increased numbers of gas-producing bacteria in the stomach could predispose to GDV. Gas-producing clostridia were found in the gastric content of dogs with GDV in one study,[7] but not in another.[6]

In summary, it is probable that the proportion of gas derived from aerophagia, gastric bicarbonate, and bacterial fermentation varies considerably among different dogs with GDV, depending on such factors as the dog's temperament, the type and quantity of food in the stomach at the time of the volvulus, and the duration of the volvulus.

DEFECTIVE ERUCTATION. It is probable that impaired eructation predisposes to GDV. The eructation reflex is initiated by gaseous distension of the cardia. It is mediated by receptors in the cardia and vagal afferents to the brain. The motor response is a reduction in pressure to less than that in the stomach so gas can escape. Defective eructation could therefore result from an anatomically or functionally abnormal gastroesophageal junction or a defect in the eructation reflex.

The correlation of GDV with animal size suggests an anatomic factor may contribute to the problem. Many dogs of the larger breeds have relatively deep chests, altering anatomic relations between the stomach, esophagus, gastroesophageal junction, and diaphragm. Anatomic arrangements of this area are designed to prevent gastroesophageal reflux. The antireflux mechanisms include the oblique angle at which the esophagus enters the stomach, fundic pressure, the diaphragmatic crura, the intra-abdominal esophagus, and the gastroesophageal sphincter (GES) muscle. Any exaggeration of these antireflux mechanisms could prevent normal eructation of gastric gas. For instance, surgical wrapping of the gastric fundus around two-thirds of the intra-abdominal segment of esophagus (fundoplication) does not interfere with eating but does prevent vomiting, and gastric dilatation is a continuous problem.[11] The gastroesophageal junction remains patent, but a one-way valve is formed. Furthermore, elimination of the valve of His by fundectomy has helped two dogs with recurrent gastric dilatation treated at the VMTH at Davis.

Although dogs with GDV appear to have deranged eructation it is unlikely GES dysfunction alone is an adequate explanation.[12] Dogs recovered from GDV have normal gastroesophageal pressures in the fasting and postprandial state.[12] High levels of some hormones, such as gastrin, elevate GES pressure. Plasma gastrin levels are high in dogs with acute GDV and in dogs 3 to 6 months after recovery from GDV,[13] raising the possibility that high gastrin levels predispose dogs to GDV by raising GES pressure. This would seem unlikely, however, because it is uncertain whether gastrin is physiologically important to GES function.[14] Furthermore, the augmented GES pressure following feeding or use of drugs such as metoclopramide or cisapride does not impair eructation.[15–17] Moreover, dogs 9 to 60 months after recovery from GDV do not have elevated gastrin levels.[12] Collectively, these observations suggest that the gastrin elevations observed in GDV are a result of GDV rather than a cause. It is likely the elevated plasma gastrin in the postoperative period is due to chronic gastric distension resulting from GDV-induced gastric emptying dysfunction

Failure of eructation in dogs with GDV could also result from disruption of the neural reflex for eructation. Eructation is abolished by vagotomy. One reason for this is that vagotomy of the caudal canine esophagus abolishes the animal's ability to retract its intra-abdominal esophageal segment into the thorax.[18] This is necessary prior to vomiting and presumably prior to eructation. Thus, failure of the dogs that develop GDV to eructate gas could be partly due to a loss of normal vagal innervation to the caudal esophagus.[15] Support for this possibility is provided by the observation that esophageal motility abnormalities are common in GDV.[8]

Failure of eructation could also result from inadequate distension of the cardia by gas. In normal dogs, distension of the cardia is a prerequisite for the reduction in GES pressure that precedes eructation. Distension of the cardia is caused readily by relatively small amounts of gas when compared with similar amounts of liquid (Figure 16–2). The stomach normally rotates during filling. With increasing distension, the rotation limits the freedom for the cardia to be distended by intragastric gas. Body position also influences the location of gas in the stomach. Eructation is least frequent in dogs lying in a left lateral position. The frequency is up to twice as great in dogs lying in a supine or right lateral position, and the eructation frequency is five times greater in standing dogs.[19] Normal gastric motility may also be important to eructation. When body position determines that gas is not in the gastric cardia, gastric motility moves the gas to the cardia so it can be eructated. Without such motility, gas eructation would not be evident in dogs lying in a left lateral position.

Eructation is also abolished by damage to the distensibility and sensory function of the cardia.[17] Acute GDV from any cause may overdistend and damage the gastric cardia to a degree that eructation is impaired even after clinical recovery. Such damage may partly explain why the recurrence rate of GDV is high.

DELAYED GASTRIC EMPTYING. It is probable that delayed gastric emptying contributes to the pathophysiology of GDV, but there is only limited evidence to suggest that delayed gastric emptying is an important *cause* of GDV. Once gastric volvulus occurs, compression of the duodenum results and is likely to inhibit gastric emptying, predisposing to further dilatation. In addition, delayed gastric emptying of solids (but not liquids) is an important complication of GDV.[20–22]

GDV has been observed in dogs immediately following trauma, spinal surgery, and major abdominal surgery. It is possible that delayed gastric emptying secondary to ileus precipitates these cases of GDV, but it is likely that eructation is also inhibited. General anesthesia can cause gastric dilatation, a phenomenon that may also be mediated by gastric atony. Gastrin in pharmacologic doses can inhibit gastric emptying. As noted earlier, elevated gastrin levels have been detected in the plasma of dogs shortly after GDV, but it is unlikely that high gastrin levels precede GDV.[12]

Pathophysiology: Gastric[24,25]

GASTRIC PATHOLOGY. The accumulation of gastric gas and fluid in GDV results in intragastric pressures that usually range from 9 to 62 mm Hg with a mean of 23 mm Hg.[26] Pressures as high as 80 mm Hg have been recorded, however.[27] Pressures of 30 mm Hg are sufficient to distend the stomach to a volume of approximately 3 L in dogs of 20 to 30 kg body weight.[28] The degree of gastric volvulus in GDV varies from 90° to 360° with a clockwise rotation of 180° being most common.[1] These perturbations cause gastric pathology that ranges from mild edema and hemorrhage in one or more tissue layers to full thickness necrosis and perforation. In spontaneous GDV, serosal hemorrhage, mucosal hemorrhage, and necrosis are frequently observed, and full thickness necrosis and perforation occasionally occur. Infarction and necrosis most often occur along the greater curvature near to the gastric vessels. Avulsion of the short gastric vessels and the epiploic branch of the left gastroepiploic artery can occur. In experimentally induced GDV, pathologic changes in the

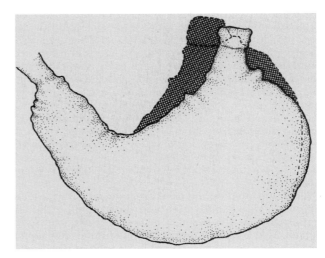

FIGURE 16–2. Comparison of distension of gastric cardia by saline (unshaded) with distension by saline and air (shaded).

stomach are also most common in the fundus and body. Mucosal necrosis and ulceration is less consistent in experimental models than in spontaneous GDV.[29–31]

Prominent histologic changes in the stomach consist of submucosal edema and hemorrhage, acute myonecrosis of the longitudinal muscle layer, and neutrophil infiltration, hemorrhage, and edema in the serosa.[31–33] The histopathologic changes are minimal at the end of 2.5 hours of experimental GDV, but are pronounced 4 hours after the deflation and derotation of the stomach (resuscitation).[31] Gross submucosal edema develops within minutes of resuscitation. Seven days after GDV, prominent histologic lesions in the stomach include subserosal fibrosis and chronic inflammation of the muscularis.[32] It is probable that the gastric pathology results from a combination of ischemia, reperfusion injury, and gastric acid injury.

PATHOMECHANISM OF GASTRIC ISCHEMIA AND EDEMA. Experimental GDV causes a marked reduction in gastric blood flow[33] with a 92% decline of gastric surface oxygen tension.[34] The ischemia is likely to be particularly catastrophic for the gastric mucosa, which requires 80% of the total gastric blood flow in order to sustain its metabolic requirements. The origin of the gastric ischemia is probably multifactorial, resulting from gastric volvulus, dilatation, infarction and edema, reduced cardiac output, and perhaps from increased sympathetic tone.

Gastric volvulus (360°) impairs gastric blood flow by obstructing gastric venous outflow.[35] Gastric blood flow is also reduced by elevated gastric pressure. It has been suggested that canine gastric mucosal blood flow is not impaired until intragastric pressures reach very high levels.[36] Blood flow was assessed by indirect methods in this study, however, and it is probable that significant blood flow reductions occur at the pressures commonly encountered in GDV. Support for this contention is provided by the observation that in cats increasing intragastric pressures above 8 mm Hg produces graded decreases in gastric mucosal and muscularis blood flow.[37] Furthermore, in the canine intestine, experimentally elevated pressures at or above 30 to 60 mm Hg result in stepwise decreases in intestinal blood flow.[38] At a pressure of 30 mm Hg, blood flow to the mucosa and muscularis is markedly impaired but that to the serosa and submucosa is maintained even at pressures as high as 90 mm Hg. It is likely that decreased mucosal and muscularis blood flow but preserved serosal and submucosal blood flow also occurs in the stomachs of dogs affected by GDV.

Infarction of microvasculature is a common complication of ischemia. The infarction is a result of neutrophil accumulation in the microvasculature and/or thrombosis developing secondarily to vascular pooling and damage to vessel walls. Infarction is likely to contribute to the tissue damage in GDV. Marginated neutrophils are common in the microvasculature of dogs with experimental GDV.[31] The gastric and splenic veins are occasionally thrombosed in GDV, and rare microthrombi are noted in the gastrointestinal tissues.

Gastric edema also reduces gastric blood flow. Increased tissue hydrostatic pressure, resulting from interstitial edema, decreases capillary flow. The gastric edema develops after deflation, presumably as a result of increased capillary permeability and hydrostatic pressure. Increased capillary permeability is a complication of ischemia, and is exacerbated by reperfusion injury of the endothelium. Increased capillary hydrostatic pressure is initially due to venous obstruction and, after resuscitation, to visceral hyperperfusion. The visceral hyperperfusion is a result of volume repletion in association with profound local vasodilation in the previously ischemic vascular beds. The transudation of fluid into the gastric wall

may be compounded by decreases in oncotic pressure resulting from the administration of large volumes of intravenous fluids at the time of resuscitation.

Increased sympathetic tone resulting from acute stress is likely to further compromise gastric blood flow. Importantly, ischemia resulting from sympathetic activity, gastric edema, and gastric infarction is likely to persist long after surgical correction of the GDV, and may explain the not uncommon development of postoperative gastric necrosis.

RELATIONSHIP OF GASTRIC ACID TO GASTRIC ULCERATION. The presence of gastric acid is required for the development of gastric ulceration in models of gastric ischemia[39] and gastric dilatation.[40,41] Gastric acid is able to penetrate the mucosal barrier because reduced mucosal circulation compromises epithelial integrity. The reduced flow also allows hydrogen ions to accumulate, eventually leading to acid-induced mucosal necrosis and ulceration. A potential role for gastric acid in GDV-induced gastric ulceration is implied by the observation of a correlation between low plasma bicarbonate concentration and gastric ulceration following gastric dilatation.[30] Experiments in rats have implicated gastric acid (more so than oxygen radicals) in the damage to the superficial gastric mucosa that occurs during gastric ischemia (i.e., prior to reperfusion).[42]

PATHOMECHANISM OF DISORDERED GASTRIC MOTILITY. Disordered gastric motility and delayed gastric emptying have been reported following GDV.[21,43,44] The disordered motility consists of intermittent gastric tachyarrhythmias, decreased electrical-mechanical coupling, and decreased contractile amplitude.[43] The disordered motility was transient (9 days) in experimental models but appeared more persistent during recovery from spontaneous GDV.[44] If GDV is not corrected within approximately 4 hours, the atony or deranged motility become irreversible. The cause of the disordered motility appears to be gastric ischemia and overdistension. Acute myonecrosis of the gastric longitudinal muscle layer is a consistent early lesion in experimental GDV. The proximity of the myonecrosis to the cells of Cajal (the putative source of the basal electrical rhythm) suggests this lesion may be one cause of the disordered motility. Direct ischemic damage to the myenteric plexus is another proposed cause of the gastric dysrhythmias.

Pathophysiology: Cardiovascular

CARDIOVASCULAR DYSFUNCTION AND PATHOLOGY. Experimental models of gastric dilatation and GDV produce immediate decreases in cardiac output (40%–89% decline), systemic mean arterial pressure (5%–50%), pulmonary artery mean blood pressure (20%), and wedge pressure (3 mm Hg) (Figure 16–3).[26,27,31,33,34,45–47] Coronary artery flow decreases (50%), as does myocardial oxygen consumption (50%).[27] Total peripheral resistance and heart rate increase during GDV and decline during resuscitation.[34,45,47] Intra-abdominal caudal vena caval pressure increases in proportion to the intragastric pressure.[45,47,48] Portal pressure increases two- to threefold.[33,46] Central venous pressure remains unchanged in some studies,[34,47] and declines in others.[45] GDV causes a rapid decrease in the surface oxygen tension of the stomach (92% decline), duodenum (80%), jejunum (45%), liver (45%), and pancreas (45%).[34] The reduced surface oxygen tension implies a profound reduction in local blood flow that has been confirmed in the stomach, jejunum, pancreas, kidney lungs, and cerebrum by use of microspheres.[33] The severity of abdominal organ ischemia is variable in individual dogs, but is sufficient to cause damage to most tissues.

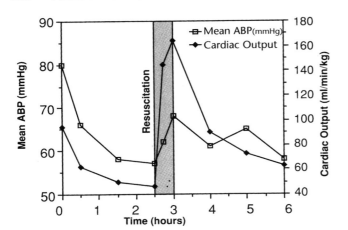

FIGURE 16-3. Mean arterial blood pressure and cardiac output before, during, and after acute GDV.

After deflation and derotation of the stomach, the cardiac output improves transiently but does not return to normal.[26,27,45] If crystalloid fluid administration (90 mL/kg) accompanies the gastric deflation and derotation (resuscitation), the cardiac output rises transiently to 50% above baseline but within 1.5 hours declines again to below baseline. The surface oxygen tension of all abdominal organs except the liver returns to near-normal values after resuscitation. Similarly, the blood flows of most organs return transiently to normal after resuscitation.[33] The persistently low surface oxygen tension of the liver suggests the oxygen demands of the liver outstrip oxygen delivery even after resuscitation of the GDV patient.

PATHOMECHANISM OF THE CIRCULATORY CHANGES. The distended stomach interferes with splanchnic circulation by directly compressing adjacent large veins and by compressing distant veins and vascular beds by way of increased intra-abdominal pressure. The dilated stomach occludes or partially occludes the caudal vena cava at a level that varies from the T12 to L4 vertebrae.[47,49] The caudal vena caval compression reduces venous return to the heart. Collateral flow through the ventral sinuses and azygous veins partially compensates for the reduced caudal vena caval flow.[49] Blood flow through the portal vein is also reduced. This appears to be due to gastric dilatation rather than gastric volvulus.[35] The liver becomes congested in 50% of dogs during experimental GDV, implying that in some dogs posthepatic portal hypertension occurs, perhaps due to compression of the hepatic veins against the diaphragm by forward displacement of the liver.[28] Hypertension in the caudal vena cava and portal vein reduces splanchnic blood flow. Portal hypertension promotes the pooling of blood in the splanchnic viscera and the movement of plasma fluid into the gastrointestinal tract. Persistently increased venous sympathetic tone probably perpetuates the vascular pooling.

Experimentally elevated intra-abdominal pressure produces some, but not all, of the circulatory changes seen with elevated intragastric pressure. Increased intra-abdominal pressure, created by the inflation of a large-volume intra-abdominal bag to pressures of 20 to 40 mm Hg, markedly decreases cardiac output and absolute blood flow to both abdominal and thoracic viscera.[48] At intra-abdominal pressures of 40 mm Hg, the blood flow to the abdominal organs (except the kidney and adrenal) decreases to 20% to 40% of baseline. This decline in blood flow is greater than could be

accounted for by the decline in cardiac output, suggesting a direct pressure effect on local abdominal organ blood flow. One important difference between this model and GDV is that overall venous return and systemic blood pressure did not appear to be impaired. Decreased venous return and blood pressure, as seen in GDV, would be expected to further reduce the visceral blood flow.

After gastric decompression (and improved venous return), cardiac output may continue to be compromised in some dogs by release of sequestered circulating cardiodepressant substances.[50] Myocardial depressant factor is the best described cardioinhibitory factor. It is a polypeptide thought to originate from protease activation in the ischemic pancreas. Together with endotoxin, it is thought to cause negative inotropy, splanchnic vasoconstriction, and reticuloendothelial system depression.

Tachycardia, elevated total peripheral resistance, and perhaps in some dogs increased ventricular contractility[26] provide partial compensation for the reduced systemic blood flow and perfusion pressure during GDV. These compensatory responses are likely to be mediated by increased sympathetic tone in response to both decreased blood pressure[26] and acute gastric distension,[51] and in response to release of cardiostimulatory substances such as catecholamines.[50] Increased contractility, however, raises myocardial oxygen demand and exacerbates the myocardial ischemia resulting from decreased coronary blood flow. The coronary blood flow is decreased because of tachycardia and decreased aortic blood pressure.[27] Cardiac arrhythmias and subendocardial necrosis develop as a result of cardiac ischemia and are probably exacerbated by increased sympathetic tone, raised serum catecholamine levels, and electrolyte and acid-base disturbances.[2,27,52]

PATHOMECHANISM OF SHOCK. Shock is defined as inadequate tissue perfusion.[53,54] In GDV the cause of shock is multifactorial. It is initiated by hypovolemia secondary to vascular pooling and is compounded by varying degrees of endotoxic and septic shock. Decreased cardiac output, blood volume, and arterial pressure lead to inadequate organ perfusion. Prolonged poor tissue perfusion with resultant insufficient tissue oxygenation eventually leads to the development of irreversible shock, signaled by the failure of any treatment to restore blood pressure and cardiac output. Shock becomes irreversible when tissue hypoperfusion persists for several hours in hemorrhagic shock models. Irreversibility is directly related to the extent of the tissue oxygen debt and is also related to the amount of endotoxin entering the circulation. Plasma endotoxin levels increase significantly during GDV.[33] Endotoxic and septic shock develop as a result of portal venous occlusion and loss of the mucosal barrier. Experimental obstruction of a dog's portal vein for as little as 30 minutes results in death within 24 hours. Endotoxin enters the circulation by way of the peritoneal surface or lymphatics. The restriction of portal blood flow prevents removal of the toxin by the reticuloendothelial system of the liver.[55]

Endotoxin release and tissue hypoxia in the splanchnic viscera both activate a series of interacting cascades. These include the arachidonic acid and complement cascades, and the fibrinolytic and kallikrein-kinin systems. Platelets, granulocytes, and macrophages marginate and release a variety of vasoactive and cytotoxic substances that result in microvasculature injury and leakage. Complement and cytokines such as interleukin and cachectin appear to be very important mediators of endotoxic and gram negative sepsis. Tissue proteases produce peptides with myocardial depressant and vasoactive properties, such as myocardial depressant factor. In combination with acid-base and electrolyte derangements, the aforementioned mediators perpetuate the inadequate tissue blood flow and eventually precipitate vascular collapse and death.

PATHOMECHANISM OF DISSEMINATED INTRAVASCULAR COAGULATION. Disseminated intravascular coagulation complicates GDV in 10% to 40% of cases.[3,56,57] Widespread activation of the coagulation cascade results from a combination of factors including vascular sludging, endothelial damage, platelet activation, acidosis, and activation of Hageman factor by endotoxin, kallikrein, and pancreatic proteases. Abnormal hemostatic profiles are more common in dogs with GDV complicated by gastric necrosis.[57]

Pathophysiology: Respiratory

Acute gastric distention applies pressure on the diaphragm and thorax, restricting pulmonary function and reducing tidal volume. There is an increase in inspiratory and expiratory resistance and a marked decrease in lung compliance.[9] Compensation is made by increasing respiratory rate, but as dilatation worsens normal minute volumes cannot be maintained. Histologic changes in lungs of dogs with GDV include leukostasis, atelectasis, congestion, and edema.[33] These lesions are consistent with endotoxemia.[33]

The result of respiratory impairment is decreased blood oxygen tension, with the fall greatest in the caudal vena cava.[45] The hypoxemia associated with the circulatory changes accelerates tissue death from hypoxia.

Pathophysiology: Abdominal Organs

HEPATIC PATHOPHYSIOLOGY. Mild to severe elevations in the serum concentration of ALT occur in spontaneous and experimental GDV.[29,31,58,59] The ALT activity in the serum of dogs with experimental GDV increases immediately after resuscitation, and within four hours can reach concentrations as high as 11,000 U/L (Figure 16–4).[31] This sudden rise in plasma liver enzyme activity may be due to the flushing of pooled hepatic venous blood into systemic circulation, or it may result from reperfusion-induced acute necrosis. The SAP concentration increases in most dogs to 200 to 300 U/L during experimental GDV, whereas the bilirubin changes little.[31]

Sixty percent of dogs with GDV presented to the UCD VMTH have gross or histologic evidence of hepatic pathology.[58] On most occasions the liver damage is mild to moderate in severity and potentially reversible. However, in approximately 6% of dogs with GDV-associated hepatopathy, the damage is severe and may be sufficient to directly result in death.[58] Hepatic volvulus in association with GDV has occasionally been reported.[3]

Congestion, hemorrhage, and/or necrosis are the most frequent histopathologic abnormalities in the livers of dogs dying acutely from GDV. Histologic examination of the liver of dogs subjected to experimental GDV shows minimal changes at the conclusion of 2.5 hours of GDV. However, liver biopsies taken following reperfusion show congestion, neutrophil infiltration, and moderate to severe hepatic necrosis.[31,33] The hepatic pathology is probably caused by endotoxin absorption, venous occlusion, and ischemia-reperfusion injury to the hepatic microvasculature and parenchyma.[31,33]

PANCREATIC PATHOPHYSIOLOGY. Experimental GDV results in mild increases in the serum concentration of lipase and to a lesser extent amylase. These changes are associated with mild pancreatic edema and scattered pancreatic necrosis of individual acinar cells.[31,33] Ischemia-induced acute pancreati-

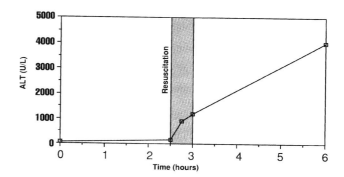

FIGURE 16-4. Mean serum activity of ALT before, during, and after acute GDV.

tis is thought to be relatively common in spontaneous GDV. Gross pathologic evidence of mild to moderate pancreatitis is noted in 40% of dogs dying from GDV at the UCD VMTH.

RENAL PATHOPHYSIOLOGY. Slight increases in BUN and creatinine occur during experimental GDV.[29,31,60] Histopathologic changes are minimal,[33] implying the azotemia is predominantly prerenal. Renal failure does occur in a significant number of cases of spontaneous GDV, however. In one series, renal failure was cited as a postoperative complication in 17% of dogs.[3]

SPLENIC PATHOPHYSIOLOGY. The spleen is frequently damaged by GDV.[1] Rotation of the stomach displaces the spleen by way of the gastrosplenic ligament. Splenic congestion develops because splenic venous drainage is impaired. The spleen can also rotate on its own pedicle. Splenic rupture, necrosis, and thrombosis, or avulsion of splenic vessels frequently complicate GDV.

INTESTINAL PATHOPHYSIOLOGY. Experimental GDV can cause extensive edema, hemorrhage, neutrophil infiltration, and necrosis of the longitudinal muscle layer of the duodenum and jejunum.[31] Changes in the serosa are similar. The cause of the pathology in the muscularis and serosa is unclear. In some dogs, extensive sloughing of the small intestinal epithelium also occurs.[33] The intestinal epithelial lesions are seen in the dogs with the lowest cardiac outputs, mean blood pressures, and surface oxygen tensions, implying the mucosal lesions result from intestinal hypoperfusion.[34] Occasionally the large bowel is affected by serositis.[33] As was noted in the stomach and liver, the damage in the small intestine is more severe after reperfusion than at the end of GDV. The frequency of these lesions in spontaneous GDV is unknown.

Pathophysiology: Reperfusion Injury

The majority of the damage to transiently ischemic tissues occurs not during the period of ischemia, but rather when the ischemia is relieved and the tissues reperfused.[61] A number of investigators have demonstrated the central role of oxygen free radicals in the pathogenesis of the so-called reperfusion injuries of visceral tissues.[42,61–64] In a recent study in rats, it has been estimated that oxyradicals account for 50% of the more permanent ischemic injury to the deeper gastric mucosa with the majority of the injury occurring within the first 5 minutes of reperfusion.[42]

Oxygen-derived free radicals damage tissues by a wide variety of means including the initiation of microvascular damage by causing lipid peroxidation of endothelial cell membranes. The major sources of reperfusion-induced free radicals appear to be the tissue enzyme xanthine oxidase and neutrophil enzymes such as NADPH oxidase myeloperoxidase. Xanthine oxidase is derived from the proteolysis of xanthine dehydrogenase by a calcium-dependent enzyme. Xanthine dehydrogenase is present in high concentration in many tissues, including the liver and the mucosa of the gastrointestinal tract. Neutrophils rapidly accumulate in tissues subjected to ischemia and reperfusion. Strong evidence suggests that scavenging of free radicals or pharmacologic inhibition of free radical formation will reduce the ischemia-reperfusion related tissue damage that occurs in the stomach and other portions of the digestive tract.[39,42,61-66]

Phospholipase A_2 may also be involved in reperfusion injury.[64] Circulating phospholipase A_2 activity increases significantly after intestinal ischemia and reperfusion. This enzyme is capable of releasing toxic lysophospholipids and stimulating the arachidonic acid cascade, both of which can contribute to the chemotaxis of neutrophils. Phospholipase A_2 inhibitors reduce intestinal ischemia-reperfusion injury in rats.[64]

Gastric dilatation-volvulus results in ischemia of the stomach and associated visceral organs. Circulatory volume replacement and surgical correction of the dilatation and volvulus results in reperfusion of the ischemic tissues. Thus, it would seem likely the pathogenesis of GDV involves tissue damage due to reperfusion injury and, in particular, oxygen-derived free radicals. Experimental support for this concept, however, remains indirect. Tissue damage in GDV has been shown to be worse after 4 hours of reperfusion than at the end of ischemia.[31] Evidence of lipid peroxidation is present in the liver, pancreas, and intestine of dogs subjected to experimental GDV.[46] Two studies, however, have failed to detect evidence of lipid peroxidative damage in gastric tissues.[3,46] Administration of allopurinol, a specific inhibitor of xanthine oxidase, to dogs subjected to experimental GDV causes a trend toward decreased lipid peroxidation[46] and gastric edema[31] and significantly reduces hepatic necrosis.[31] Furthermore, survival of dogs with GDV appears to be improved by administration of a free-radical scavenger or desferrioxamine (an hydroxyl radical inhibitor).[46,67] The recent observation that gradual reintroduction of oxygen reduces reperfusion injury in the cat stomach[39] may have future bearing on the decompression management of dogs with GDV.

Pathophysiology: Clinical Pathologic Changes

PACKED CELL VOLUME, TOTAL PROTEIN, AND ALBUMIN. Packed cell volume (PCV) rises transiently immediately after initiation of experimental GDV[31] or raised intra-abdominal pressure.[48] Blood volume, however, remains unchanged during the first 30 minutes of gastric dilatation.[68] The increased PCV thus appears to reflect a release of sequestered red blood cells, the origin of which is uncertain. Subsequently, loss of plasma fluid into the gut and abdominal cavity further raises PCV and, to a lesser extent, total protein.[29] If crystalloid fluids (90 mL/kg) are rapidly administered at resuscitation, mean PCV, total protein, and serum albumin concentrations are transiently reduced to 20%, 2.8 g/dl, and 1 g/dl, respectively.[31] In some dogs, anemia and hypoproteinemia develop in the postoperative period, presumably due to loss of plasma or blood from ruptured abdominal vessels or damaged gastrointestinal mucosa. Reduced PCV significantly decreases the oxygen-carrying capacity of the blood, a detrimental effect partially offset by improved perfusion due to decreased blood viscosity. The PCV that produces an ideal balance between viscosity and oxygen-carrying capacity in dogs is 30% to 40%,[69] and it is desirable to maintain the PCV above 20% to 25%.[53] Reductions of serum albumin to 1 g/dl markedly reduce plasma oncotic pressure to the point where tissue edema is likely.

POTASSIUM. Serum potassium content gradually increases during experimental GDV,[29,31,60] and rises, rapidly (Figure 16-5) but transiently, immediately after gastric decompression.[31,60] In some dogs, the postdecompression rise in serum concentration is as great as 1.5 mEq/L within 15 minutes. Potassium is released from degenerating cells, where its concentration is 30 times that in extracellular fluid. During the first 1 to 2 minutes after decompression of the experimentally distended intestine, potassium concentration in the venous effluent rises rapidly by 1 mEq/L and then declines to normal levels.[38] Hyperkalemia is rarely detected in spontaneous GDV, probably because of its transient nature in many dogs. In contrast, hypokalemia is more commonly noted, particularly in the postoperative period.[2] The hypokalemia probably results from decreased intake of potassium in association with increased loss in vomitus and sequestered gastric fluid. Furthermore, metabolic alkalosis and/or hypovolemia-induced hyperaldostronemia can compound the hypokalemia.

PHOSPHORUS. Serum phosphorus concentrations rise as much as threefold during experimental GDV.[29,31,60] Phosphorus is released from degenerating cells and by the breakdown of adenosine triphosphate during hypoxia. Decreased glomerular filtration may also contribute to the rise in serum phosphorus.

SODIUM, CHLORIDE, AND CALCIUM. Serum levels of sodium and chloride remain little changed in experimental GDV, but occasionally they are increased or decreased in clinical cases. The variability is due to the opposing effects of hemoconcentration caused by free water loss and loss of electrolytes in vomitus or sequestered gastric fluid. Serum calcium levels usually remain within the normal range.

GLUCOSE. Serum glucose concentrations rise during experimental GDV,[20,60] and transiently decrease at the time of resuscitation.[31] The mean drop in glucose concentration in one study was 40 mg/dl. The glucose concentration of the worst affected dogs dropped to 15 to 50 mg/dl. The cause of the decreased glucose may have been a combination of hemodilution, sudden tissue demand, and endotoxin release.

CREATINE PHOSPHOKINASE. Serum creatine phosphokinase rises during experimental GDV.[29] The rise has been attributed to ischemic damage to caudal skeletal muscle mass.

BLOOD GAS AND ACID-BASE CHANGES. Metabolic acidosis develops during experimental GDV. Serum lactate concentra-

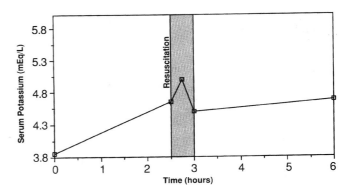

FIGURE 16-5. Mean serum potassium concentrations before, during, and after acute GDV.

tions[29,31] and base deficits[30,31] increase during GDV, resuscitation, and the ensuing shock. Blood pH and serum bicarbonate concentration decrease during experimental GDV, particularly at the point of resuscitation, or during ensuing shock.[31] Lactic acidosis develops as a consequence of anaerobic tissue metabolism. The worsened acid-base status during resuscitation presumably reflects washout of accumulated hydrogen ions. During the first 1 to 2 minutes after decompression of the experimentally distended intestine, pH in venous effluent decreases by 0.1 units.[38]

Venous PO_2 declines during experimental GDV and rapidly increases at resuscitation. Changes are closely correlated to cardiac output. During the latter stages of GDV, tissue oxygen uptake (cardiac index × AV oxygen content difference) increases by approximately 20%; oxygen delivery (cardiac index × arterial oxygen content) decreases by approximately 50%.[34] During resuscitation, the tissue oxygen uptake remains at 20% above baseline and the oxygen delivery increases by approximately 15%. Four hours after resuscitation, the tissue oxygen uptake is further increased to 30% above normal, whereas the oxygen delivery declines to approximately 50% of normal. Tissue oxygen uptake reflects the sum of all oxidative metabolic reactions. It can be rate limited by circulation and increased by sepsis and various forms of tissue damage. Increased tissue oxygen uptake does not indicate an adequate circulatory supply of oxygen because increased requirements can outstrip supply.[54] Thus, it appears that at no stage during experimental GDV are increases in whole body tissue oxygen demands matched by adequate increase in oxygen delivery. Surface oxygen recordings suggest that much of this oxygen deficit may occur in the liver.

Pathophysiology Summary

Gastric dilatation and/or volvulus traps gastric ingesta and gas in the stomach. Further gas and fluid accumulate, eventually leading to extremely elevated intragastric pressure and gastric dilatation-volvulus. Gastric blood flow is impeded, initially by the volvulus and raised intragastric pressure, and subsequently by gastric wall edema, thrombosis, and perhaps sympathetic mediated vasoconstriction. Gastric ischemia, in association with gastric acid, leads to gastric ulceration and necrosis, and occasionally perforation and peritonitis. The gastric displacement malpositions the spleen, resulting in splenic congestion and progressing, at times, to splenic thrombosis and necrosis.

The gastric dilatation reduces tidal volume, obstructs venous return, and compresses the splanchnic viscera, resulting in impaired respiration, acidosis, decreased cardiac output, poor perfusion of the visceral organs, vascular pooling, and shock. Ischemia of the splanchnic viscera, probably exacerbated by endotoxin release, results in hepatic, pancreatic, and intestinal necrosis. Sepsis and DIC commonly result. If GDV is untreated, the respiratory compromise, visceral damage, shock, sepsis, and/or peritonitis are eventually fatal.

Resuscitation of dogs with GDV by sudden gastric deflation and derotation and by the rapid administration of large volumes of crystalloid fluids is a period of profound cardiovascular and metabolic stress, resulting from some or all of a decrease in peripheral resistance, hyperkalemia, hypoglycemia, metabolic acidosis, hemodilution, liberation of cardiodepressant substances, and probably reperfusion injury and endotoxin release. Surviving dogs may be affected by gastric motility abnormalities.

Clinical Findings

The clinical signs of GDV are characteristic. The most consistent historical findings are acute onset of depression in association with retching but not vomiting. Excessive salivation may be seen. Affected dogs are usually reluctant to stand and walk. Some are found in lateral recumbency or moribund. Abdominal tympany is usually evident and easily confirmed by palpation. Cardiovascular failure is identified by rapid weak pulse, poor capillary refill time, and pale mucous membranes. Caudal venous distension may be apparent. Respirations are rapid, shallow, and dyspneic. Dehydration is usually not seen.

Laboratory Findings

Laboratory evaluation usually shows hemoconcentration. Metabolic acidosis and hypokalemia are common abnormalities, but metabolic alkalosis, respiratory acidosis, respiratory alkalosis, hyperkalemia, hypochloremia, and hypernatremia can also be seen.[2] Mild increases in blood urea nitrogen and creatinine, and slight to moderate increases in plasma lactate, ALT, CPK, and phosphorus levels are often observed. Lipase and venous oxygen content are sometimes elevated.

Radiographic Findings

Following fluid therapy and decompression, radiographs should be taken to determine whether gastric volvulus persists. The right lateral recumbent position provides the radiographic view of choice.[70] Residual gastric dilatation is readily identified radiographically by finding a large gas- and fluid-filled stomach (Figure 16–6.) Volvulus is identified by a soft tissue fold that appears to compartmentalize the stomach (Figure 16–7). A key finding in the right lateral recumbent view is the observation of a gas-filled pylorus located dorsal to the fundus of the stomach.[71] Radiography may also identify splenic torsion, abdominal fluid suggestive of peritonitis or hemorrhage, free abdominal gas suggestive of perforation, and megaesophagus. The megaesophagus usually resolves

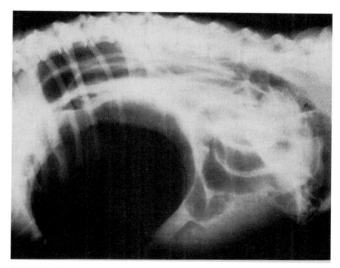

FIGURE 16–6. Lateral radiograph of an 8-year-old Walker hound presented with marked abdominal distension. The film shows gastric gaseous distension. The pylorus is situated in its proper location. There is no evidence of torsion.

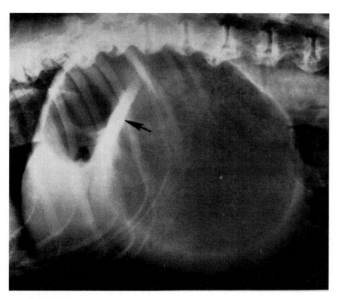

FIGURE 16–7. Lateral radiographs of abdomen of a Saint Bernard presented with clinical signs of acute abdominal distension. The stomach is distended with gas. A pillar of soft tissue (arrow) suggests pyloric displacement. The esophagus is distended with contents, suggesting the gastroesophageal junction is blocked. The spleen is not identified because of rotation. The transverse colon is displaced caudally. No peritoneal fluid is evident. The spondylosis deformans has no significance for the current problem. Diagnosis is acute gastric dilatation with volvulus.

spontaneously, but the other conditions require immediate surgery.

Diagnosis

GDV is diagnosed on clinical findings and confirmed by successful gastric decompression and subsequent radiographic demonstration of gastric volvulus. Diagnostic evaluations such as a PCV/TP, a CBC, a venous blood gas analysis, an electrolyte panel, a serum chemistry analysis, a urinalysis, and cardiovascular monitoring should be instituted as soon as possible to help tailor therapy and identify likely complications of GDV.

Treatment

Management begins with rapid fluid therapy, followed by controlled decompression of the gastric dilatation. Supplemental therapy of probable benefit administered at or prior to decompression includes corticosteroids, H_2 blockers, antibiotics, and perhaps oxygen-derived free radical inhibitors or scavengers. After decompression of the stomach and stabilization of the clinical condition of the dog, the stomach is repositioned and a gastropexy is performed. Subsequently, therapy may be required for various complications, including electrolyte imbalances, cardiac arrhythmias, and DIC.

FLUID THERAPY. Intravenous fluid therapy should begin prior to gastric decompression[59] because of the risk of cardiovascular collapse due to the sudden fall in total peripheral resistance and the release of sequestered cardioinhibitory factors that accompany decompression. Those dogs exhibiting extreme respiratory comprise should be partially decompressed by way of a percutaneously placed needle while intravenous catheterization is in progress. Experimental data suggests that 45 mL/kg of a polyionic crystalloid fluid, such as lactated Ringer's solution, administered intravenously over a 15 minute period beginning just prior to decompression, is sufficient to return the cardiac output to normal in dogs with GDV.[31] To avoid excessive hemodilution (serum total protein below 3.5 g/dl) the fluid rate should then be slowed. The alleviation of peripheral vasoconstriction and restoration of acceptable pulse quality determines the end point of volume replacement therapy for a particular dog. Central venous pressure assessment provides another guide, with fluid given until the CVP increases. Most dogs require 90 mL/kg in the first 1 to 2 hours of therapy.

The cardiovascular and hydration status of the dog dictates the fluid administration rate required after initial volume replacement. A rate of 10 mL/kg/hour is usually appropriate for the immediate postdecompression period. After several hours, the rate can usually be reduced to between 3 to 5 mL/kg/hour.

The composition of the fluid administered should be tailored to the dog's individual requirements as determined by repeated electrolyte, acid-base, glucose, and PCV/TP assessments. Supplemental potassium administration is commonly required (see Chapter 39). Because acidosis is not a predictable finding in GDV and bicarbonate administration has the potential to cause significant adverse effects, bicarbonate should only be administered if blood gas data suggests a severe acidemia (pH below 7.2). Bicarbonate administration is described in Chapter 39. Supplementation of fluids with 5% dextrose may be necessary because of the hypoglycemia that can occur during resuscitation of dogs with GDV.

Colloidal fluids such as plasma or dextran 70 are necessary if total protein levels decline below 3.5 g/dl and perhaps should be used routinely in GDV. Colloidal fluids will decrease fluid transudation from the vasculature and will support cardiac output for more prolonged periods than crystalloids.[72] A suitable initial dose of plasma is 20 mL/kg administered over 1 to 2 hours. Dextran is usually administered at rates not exceeding 5 mL/kg/hour and daily doses less than 20 mL/kg. A lack of response to colloids suggests the shock is irreversible. If PCV declines below 25, whole blood therapy is recommended prior to anesthesia and surgery.

GASTRIC DECOMPRESSION. Decompression of the dilated stomach is achieved by passage of a stomach tube or, more preferably, by trocarization. Because of the cardiovascular changes and reperfusion injury that accompany decompression, sudden decompression is less desirable than a slower release of pressure.[39] Trocarization is less stressful to most dogs than stomach tubing. In addition, it facilitates slow decompression, and is rarely associated with peritonitis. Trocarization of the stomach is achieved with a 16 to 18 gauge 1.5 to 2 inch needle. Following partial decompression by trocarization, attempts are again made to pass a large-bore stomach tube to complete gastric deflation. When a large-diameter tube can be passed, the contents of the stomach should be removed by lavage. If the stomach tube will not pass into the stomach, 90° to 180° rotation of the tube or placement of the dog in a sitting position may facilitate passage of the tube. Excessive force must not be used during attempts to pass the tube because rupture of the gastroesophageal junction may occur. Inability to pass a stomach tube is not diagnostic for volvulus, and passage of the tube does not rule it out.

Gastric decompression can also be achieved by gastrostomy. The procedure is usually performed under local anesthesia caudal to the right costal arch.[73] The introduction of decompression by gastrostomy (in association with effective stabilization prior to surgical correction of volvulus) reportedly reduced mortality at one institution from 68% to 33%. The gastrostomy fixes the stomach to the abdominal wall and does not return a rotated stomach to its normal position. This temporary procedure is primarily indicated in patients judged unfit for anesthesia for several days (e.g., with concurrent pneumonia) or if gastric decompression cannot be achieved by stomach tube or trocarization.

Following gastric decompression, spontaneous repositioning of the stomach can occur. In many dogs, however, surgical correction of the volvulus is required. Controversy surrounds the most appropriate time to operate on dogs that have been decompressed. Because gastric blood flow is compromised by marked gastric volvulus,[35] and because full thickness gastric necrosis and delayed onset arrhythmias are not uncommon in GDV, it is my preference to operate on dogs with persistent gastric volvulus as soon as the dog's clinical condition and hemodynamic, electrolyte, and acid-base status have been stabilized by appropriate decompression and fluid therapy. This is usually accomplished within 1 to 2 hours of admission. Others prefer more prolonged periods of stabilization, and periods as long as 48 hours have been used without apparent adverse effect. If gastric material is noted to contain digested blood (coffee grounds), celiotomy should not be delayed longer than the initial stabilization period of 1 to 2 hours because severe gastric ulceration is likely, and perforation may follow. Similarly, if radiographic evidence of perforation and peritonitis are detected, surgery should not be delayed. During prolonged periods of stabilization, decompression can be maintained by nasogastric tubes, pharyngostomy tubes, or gastrostomy.

ANTIBIOTICS. Antibiotics are routinely administered to dogs with GDV because they are predisposed to sepsis. The sepsis can develop from portal hypertension, shock, and/or mucosal damage. Blood cultures may be necessary to determine effective antibiotic therapy because a wide variety of bacteria can gain access to the bloodstream from the bowel. The antibiotic(s) chosen should be rapidly effective against gram positive and gram negative anaerobes and aerobes. Suitable antibiotics in less severely affected dogs are second-generation cephalosporins, trimethoprim-sulfa combinations, and ampicillin. More severely affected dogs should receive ampicillin (10–20 mg/kg IV) and gentamicin (2.2 mg/kg SC q 8 hours), particularly if shock or marked gastrointestinal necrosis is evident. Although highly effective against life-threatening gram negatives, gentamicin is particularly nephrotoxic in the face of hypovolemia. Thus, it must not be administered until after the initial intravenous fluid bolus. Amikacin (5.0 mg/kg SC q 8 hours) can be substituted for the gentamicin, and at this dose may be less nephrotoxic than gentamicin.

CORTICOSTEROIDS. Corticosteroids are used routinely in managing shock. No controlled studies have shown that steroids increase long-term survival rates in animals in shock,[74] but the many theoretically beneficial effects ascribed to glucocorticoids has resulted in their continued use. Beneficial effects of glucocorticoid administration, particularly relevant to GDV, include reduced absorption of intestinal endotoxin during intestinal ischemia, inhibition of phospholipase A_2, reduced leukocyte margination and diapedesis, decreased capillary permeability, and improved capillary flow. Administration of prednisolone succinate (6.6 mg/kg IV) 30 minutes prior to deflation of the dilated stomach tended to reduce the severity of gastric lesions in one experimental study of gastric dilatation.[30] A large number of adverse effects of

corticosteroids have also been reported. Fortunately, the majority of these adverse effects result from long-term usage rather than the short-term, high-dose therapy reportedly beneficial in shock. Adverse effects of corticosteroids of concern in GDV include promotion of acute pancreatitis and potentiation of sepsis. Doses commonly employed for the therapy of shock include prednisolone sodium succinate (30 mg/kg IV) and dexamethasone sodium phosphate (6–15 mg/kg IV).

NONSTEROIDAL ANTI-INFLAMMATORY DRUGS. Nonsteroidal anti-inflammatory drugs, such as flunixin meglumine, have shown beneficial effects in the treatment of endotoxic shock and other forms of shock in dogs.[33,75] Flunixin meglumine (2.2 mg/kg IV) was not found to be beneficial in one small study of surgically induced GDV, however.[33] The theoretical beneficial effects of flunixin are offset by the rapidity (24 hours) with which the drug can induce gastric ulceration in dogs when used alone,[75] and especially when used in conjunction with glucocorticoids.[76] Furthermore, nonsteroidal anti-inflammatory agents markedly potentiate ischemic renal damage resulting from hypotension. If flunixin meglumine is used, it should probably be restricted to a single injection, administered after volume replacement at the time of gastric decompression (prior to peak endotoxemia). Reportedly effective doses range from 0.25 to 2.2 mg/kg IV.

MISCELLANEOUS PHARMACOLOGIC THERAPY. Administration of H_2 blockers such as ranitidine (1–2 mg/kg q 8–12 hours IV, IM, PO) and cimetidine (4–5 mg/kg q 8 hours IV, IM, PO) may ameliorate gastric ulceration. Ranitidine is preferred over cimetidine because ranitidine is a more potent inhibitor of gastric secretion and does not depress hepatic microsomal mixed-function oxidase function to the same degree as cimetidine. Sucralfate (0.5–1 g q 8 hours PO) may also facilitate healing of gastric ulcers.

Oxygen-derived free radical inhibitors and scavengers such as allopurinol, dimethylsulfoxide (DMSO), desferrioxamine, mannitol, and superoxide dismutase have been demonstrated experimentally to protect a number of organs against reperfusion injury, including those commonly affected by GDV such as liver, pancreas, heart, and gastrointestinal tract mucosa. Allopurinol is unlikely to be of great clinical benefit because the drug must be given well prior to reperfusion for maximum benefit. DMSO (25% solution administered at 2.0 mL/kg) did not result in significant improvement in survival in a small study of dogs undergoing experimental GDV.[67] A larger study is required, however, before a beneficial role for DMSO is discounted. Deferoxamine (50 mg/kg IV) administered immediately before reperfusion appeared to improve survival in the same study of experimental GDV.[67] Support for this finding is provided by the observation that desferrioxamine mesylate (25 mg/kg IM) given 30 minutes after initial bleeding of hypovolemic dogs increases survival from 10% to 50% and markedly decreases degenerative changes in the liver.[77] Caution is necessary, however, because high doses of desferrioxamine may actually potentiate oxidant damage.[78] Furthermore, this agent can induce cerebral and ocular toxicity in humans.[79] Future research may clarify the role of these and other antioxidant drugs, such as mannitol, in the therapy of GDV. It is important to note, however, that if these drugs are used, they must be administered prior to or very early (first few minutes) in reperfusion to be effective.

Blood pressure support is best provided by adequate crystalloid and colloidal fluid therapy. If additional support is required, dopamine (5–10 μg/kg/minute or dobutamine (5–20 μg/kg/minute) continuous infusions may be utilized. Overdosage of these agents can induce tachycardia and cardiac arrhythmias.

ANESTHESIA. Anesthetic regimens chosen should be minimally cardiovascular depressant. Balanced anesthesia, incorporating narcotics and muscle relaxants to lower the requirements for inhalation anesthetics, is the preferred technique but requires ventilatory support. In lieu of balanced anesthesia, mask induction with isoflurane is suitable. Isoflurane reportedly does not depress cardiovascular function during GDV. If premedication is required, low doses of meperidine (4 mg/kg SC) or oxymorphone (0.02–0.05 mg/kg SC) may be used. If intravenous induction is deemed necessary, low-dose ketamine (2.5 mg/kg IV) combined with valium (0.5 mg/kg IV) may be given, and the dogs maintained with minimal concentrations of inhalation agents. In theory, nitrous oxide should be avoided to prevent exacerbation of gastric dilatation by accumulation of intragastric nitrous oxide.

SURGERY. Surgical intervention in GDV has two roles. The first is therapeutic and the second preventative. For therapeutic purposes, residual gas, fluid, and ingesta are removed, the stomach is repositioned, and any areas of gastric necrosis are resected. Partial gastrectomy is required in 10% of dogs with GDV.[80] If gastric rupture is observed at surgery, euthanasia should be considered because the prognosis is very poor.

Recurrence rates of GDV treated without surgical gastropexy are often as high as 75% to 80%.[81,82] Therefore, in order to prevent recurrence, all dogs presented with GDV should undergo surgical gastropexy. A number of techniques are in use including fundopexy, circumcostal gastropexy, muscular flap gastropexy, incisional gastropexy, belt loop gastropexy, median gastropexy, and tube gastropexy. The fundopexy, circumcostal, incisional, and muscular flap gastropexy techniques result in lower rates of recurrence (0%–3.3%) than the tube gastrostomy (3%–11%) technique.[83] Gastrostomy tube failure is a common occurrence following tube gastrostomy. It is usually due to rupture of the balloon of the Foley-like catheters and can result in peritonitis. Tube gastrostomy can also induce persistent dysrhythmia in dogs.[44] Advantages of the tube gastrostomy, however, include short operation time, the ability to maintain gastric decompression postoperatively, and the ability to provide supplemental nutrition. For these reasons, my preference is to use tube fixation in critically ill dogs in which the benefits of shorter operation time, continued decompression, and enteral nutrition outweigh the disadvantages of this technique. The gastrostomy catheter is usually removed after five to seven days but may be kept longer if required. The recently described median gastropexy is rapid to perform and has a recurrence rate of approximately 7%.[82]

Other surgical methods for reducing the recurrence rate of GDV have included splenectomy and procedures to accelerate gastric emptying. Splenectomy does not prevent recurrences but may be required for other reasons, such as splenic infarction. Little evidence supports the prophylactic use of procedures aimed at increasing gastric emptying, such as pyloromyotomy and pyloroplasty.[3,83–85]

Recurrence of acute gastric dilatation (without volvulus) can occur in spite of successful gastropexy. Gastric fixation prevents gastric volvulus, but does not necessarily prevent gastric dilatation. There appear to be a number of causes for recurrent gastric dilatation following gastropexy. The dilatation may be precipitated by aerophagia.[3] Incorrectly performed gastropexy procedures can result in iatrogenic gastric torsion. Adhesions induced by the gastropexy procedure can inhibit gastric outflow.[86] On most occasions, however, no physical obstruction to gastric emptying can be found and defective eructation, or a gastric motility problem causing delayed gastric emptying, is presumed.[83] Recurrences of gastric dilatation due to functional abnormalities of gastric emp-

tying can be minimized by frequent feeding of low-carbohydrate, low-fat, high-protein meals, and the use of prokinetic drugs such as metoclopramide. Antifoaming agents have met with mixed success. Beta-adrenergic drugs increase eructation frequency in dogs and therefore may be of value in some cases.[17]

NUTRITION. Oral nutrition is begun after 24 to 48 hours. Small quantities of bland, low-fat, easily digestible diets fed three to four times per day are usually selected. If vomiting ensues, feeding is stopped for a further 24 to 36 hours and tried again. Patients recovering from GDV should not be allowed to go without food for more than 3 days before enteral or parenteral nutrition is commenced.

Management of Complications

MONITORING. Complications are common during recovery from GDV, necessitating close monitoring (Table 16–1).[85] Physical examinations should be repeated frequently, paying particular attention to attitude, hydration status, body temperature, cardiovascular function, and mucous membrane appearance. In addition, depending on the condition of the dog, some or all of the following monitoring procedures may be useful. Repeated measures of body weight, PCV/TP, electrolyte and acid-base status help assess the adequacy of fluid therapy. Electrocardiograms and measurement of CVP and arterial blood pressure facilitate detection of serious arrhythmias and cardiovascular compromise. Repeated evaluation of complete blood counts, venous oxygen content, and blood glucose concentration aid discovery of sepsis. Measurement of clotting times (APTT, OSPT, ACT), bleeding times, platelet counts, and fibrinogen help reveal DIC. A serum chemistry profile and urinalysis help identify damage to liver and kidney. If gastric necrosis, peritonitis, or abdominal hem-

Table 16–1

COMPLICATIONS OF GASTRIC DILATATION-VOLVULUS

Hematologic
Blood loss anemia
Electrolyte and acid-base imbalances
Hypoproteinemia

Gastrointestinal
Esophageal perforation and mediastinitis
Gastric atony
Gastric necrosis and melena
Gastric rupture and peritonitis
Hepatopathy
Intestinal volvulus
Intussusception
Pancreatitis
Paralytic ileus
Vomiting

Cardiovascular
Cardiac arrhythmias
Shock

Respiratory
Bronchopneumonia
Pneumothorax (most commonly after circumcostal gastropexy)
Pulmonary thromboembolism

Miscellaneous
Cerebral damage
DIC
Endotoxemia/sepsis
Renal failure
Splenic hemorrhage or infarction

orrhage is suspected, abdominocentesis may be performed. In addition, a scintigraphic technique has recently been developed to detect gastric wall ischemia in dogs.[87]

CARDIAC ARRHYTHMIAS. Cardiac arrhythmias occur in 40% to 50% of dogs with GDV.[88] The cardiac arrhythmias associated with GDV usually begin between 12 and 36 hours after the onset of GDV but can exist at presentation or have an onset as delayed as 72 hours after presentation. They consist primarily of premature ventricular contractions and paroxysmal or persistent ventricular tachycardia.[27,88] These cardiac arrhythmias are often resistant to therapy. Correction of acid-base and electrolyte abnormalities, especially potassium depletion, appears to improve the responsiveness of the arrhythmias. Thus, the first step in arrhythmia management is appropriate fluid therapy. Even in the face of normokalemia, it is advisable to provide supplemental potassium (20–30 mEq/L of maintenance fluids) to replete intracellular potassium.

Antiarrhythmic drugs should not be used indiscriminantly. Ventricular tachycardia with heart rates greater than 140 to 150 beats per minute requires therapy. Premature ventricular contractions need only be treated if they are multifocal, demonstrate the "R on T" phenomenon, or are associated with clinical evidence of hypoperfusion. Lidocaine hydrochloride is the usual therapy (2–4 mg/kg IV as a slow initial bolus, followed by a continuous infusion of 50–100 μg/kg/minute for several days). If necessary, antiarrhythmic therapy can be supplemented and continued with procainamide hydrochloride (12–20 mg/kg IM q 6 hours, followed by 12–20 mg/kg PO q 6 hours). Procainamide may also be administered slowly IV (12–20 mg/kg over 15–20 minutes), followed by a constant rate infusion of 10 to 40 μg/kg/minute. If supraventricular arrhythmias are noted, quinidine sulfate may be useful (6–8 mg/kg IM q 6 hours, or 6–16 mg/kg PO q 6 hours). Verapamil (0.1 mg/kg slowly IV followed by 1 mg/kg PO q 8 hours) has also been reported to be useful for the treatment of GDV-induced arrhythmias.[89]

Great care must be exercised in the use of the antiarrhythmic agents. Many GDV patients have significant hepatic and/or renal dysfunction. Lidocaine, procainamide, and quinidine are all metabolized by the liver and excreted by the kidneys. Therefore, the potential for toxicity is high. Although some of the toxicities of these drugs are reasonably characteristic (for instance, the tremors and seizures of lidocaine overdosage), other signs of drug toxicity (such as vomiting, diarrhea, and, paradoxically, cardiac arrhythmias) may be wrongly attributed to complications of GDV and lead to continued, or even increased, dosage of the antiarrhythmics. Furthermore, lidocaine may affect septic patients detrimentally,[90] although it appears to reduce gastric mucosal injury following gastric dilatation.[30]

GASTROINTESTINAL MOTILITY ABNORMALITIES AND VOMITING. The gastric dysrhythmias resulting from GDV will usually resolve without therapy. Transient paralytic ileus occurs in as many as 30% of patients. Both ileus and delayed gastric emptying may be treated with metoclopramide (0.2–0.4 mg/kg q 6 hours IV, SC, PO) without significantly reducing eructation frequency.[16,91] Vomiting usually resolves spontaneously. If vomiting persists, metoclopramide and ranitidine or cimetidine may be beneficial.

DISSEMINATED INTRAVASCULAR COAGULATION. Disseminated intravascular coagulation (DIC) occurs in 10% to 40% of dogs with GDV.[3,57] DIC is treated with plasma in association with heparin (50–150 units/kg, SC q 8 hours), administered in quantities sufficient to prolong clotting times to 1.5 to 2 times normal. If the underlying cause of the DIC has not been managed, therapy will be unsuccessful.

Prognosis

The mortality associated with canine GDV is 23% to 60%.[1,3,82,92] The mortality is as high as 63% to 80% when partial gastrectomy is required.[3,80] In one study, the mortality rate was higher in patients presenting with clinically apparent compromised cardiovascular function and/or with depressed mentation. Thus, pulse rates greater than 180 per minute, weak or arrhythmic pulses, pale or cyanotic mucous membranes, and capillary refill times greater than 1 second at presentation were associated with mortalities greater than 55%.[3] In the same study, mortality was not found to be different in dogs decompressed early versus those whose compression was delayed. The presence of marked coagulation abnormalities also suggests a poorer prognosis. Most dogs that die in the postoperative period do so within the first 4 days.

CHRONIC GASTRIC VOLVULUS

Clinical Synopsis

Diagnostic Features

- Historical reports of chronic self-relieving mild to moderate gastric distension, anorexia, and/or vomiting
- Absence of gastric tympany or evidence of shock
- Radiographic evidence of a torsed stomach

Treatment

- Gastropexy

Prevalence and Signalment

Dogs with gastric volvulus but without concomitant gastric dilatation have been occasionally observed at the UCD VMTH and have been reported by others.[1,4,93–95] The disorder appears most common in deep-chested breeds. No age or sex predilection has been recognized.

Etiology and Pathogenesis

The cause of the gastric volvulus is unknown. The intermittent gastric dilatation is presumably a reflection of impaired ability to eructate, and, perhaps, delayed emptying of solids. Gastric emptying of liquids has been normal in the few dogs in which emptying studies have been performed.

Clinical Findings and Diagnosis

Dogs with chronic gastric volvulus usually have a history of weeks to months of recurrent bouts of mild gastric distension. The distension most often resolves spontaneously but on some occasions requires orogastric intubation. Anorexia, vomiting, borborygmi, eructation, and weight loss have also been reported.[4] Physical examination is usually unremarkable. Diagnosis depends on radiographic or surgical demonstration of gastric volvulus in the absence of gastric dilatation. Laboratory tests are usually normal although evidence of hepatopathy may be observed because chronic volvulus is frequently associated with chronic passive congestion of the liver, periportal fibrosis, and bile duct proliferation.[58] The cause for the cholestasis in chronic volvulus may be chronic obstruction of the common bile duct by gastric displacement.

Treatment and Prognosis

Resolution of the majority of clinical signs usually follows gastropexy. The prognosis is good.

REFERENCES

1. Nagel ML, Neumann W. Magendilatation-volvulus-syndrom beim hund. Derpraktische Tierarzt 9:871–876, 1992.
2. Muir WW. Acid base and electrolyte disturbances in dogs with gastric dilatation-volvulus. J Am Vet Med Assoc 181:229–231, 1982.
3. Van Sluijs FJ. Gastric-dilatation volvulus in the dog. Thesis, Dept. Small Animal Medicine and Surgery, University of Utrecht, 1987.
4. Leib MS, Monroe WE, Martin RA. Suspected chronic gastric volvulus in a dog with normal gastric emptying of liquids. J Am Vet Med Assoc 191:699–700, 1987.
5. Van Kruiningen HJ, Wojan LD, Stake PE, et al. The influence of diet and feeding frequency on gastric function in the dog. J Am Anim Hosp Assoc 23:145–152, 1987.
6. Caywood D, Teague HD, Jackson DA, et al. Gastric analysis in the canine gastric dilatation volvulus syndrome. J Am Anim Hosp Assoc 13:459–462, 1977.
7. Van Kruiningen HJ, Gregoire K, Meuten DJ. Acute gastric dilatation: A review of comparative aspects, by species, and a study in dogs and monkeys. J Am Anim Hosp Assoc 10:294–324, 1974.
8. Van Sluijs FJ, Wolvekamp WTC. Abnormal esophageal motility in dogs with recurrent gastric dilatation-volvulus (abstract). Proc Eur Col Vet Surg, 250, 1993.
9. Byrne JJ, Cahill JM. Acute gastric dilatation. Am J Surg 101:301–309, 1961.
10. Draser BS, Hill MJ. Human Intestinal Flora. Academic Press, London, 1974.
11. Rasche R, Butterfield WC. Bloating and the inability to vomit after the Belsey hiatal hernia repair. J Thorac Cardiovasc Surg 65:646–648, 1973.
12. Hall JA, Twedt DC, Curtis CR. Relationship of plasma gastrin immunoreactivity and gastroesophageal sphincter pressure in clinically normal dogs and in dogs with previous gastric dilatation- volvulus. Am J Vet Res 50:1228–1232, 1989.
13. Leib MS, Wingfield WE, Twedt DC, et al. Plasma gastrin immunoreactivity in dogs with acute gastric dilatation-volvulus. J Am Vet Med Assoc 185:205–208, 1984.
14. Strombeck DR, Harrold D. Effect of gastrin, histamine, serotonin, and adrenergic amines on gastroesophageal sphincter pressure in the dog. Am J Vet Res 46:1684–1690, 1985.
15. Strombeck DR, Harrold D, Ferrier W. Eructation of gas through the gastroesophageal sphincter before and after truncal vagotomy in dogs. Am J Vet Res 48:207–210, 1987.
16. Strombeck DR, Turner WD, Harrold D. Eructation of gas through the gastroesophageal sphincter before and after gastric fundectomy in dogs. Am J Vet Res 49:87–89, 1988.
17. Strombeck DR, Griffin DW, Harrold D. Eructation of gas through the gastroesophageal sphincter before and after limiting distention of the gastric cardia or infusion of a β-adrenergic amine in dogs. Am J Vet Res 50:751–753, 1989.
18. Edwards MH. Selective vagotomy of the canine esophagus—a model for the treatment of hiatal hernia. Thorax 311:185–189, 1976.
19. Little AF, Martin CJ, Dent J, et al. Postural suppression of transient lower esophageal relaxations and gastroesophageal reflux in the dog. Gastroenterology 90:1522–1525, 1986.
20. Allan FJ, Guilford WG, Gastric emptying of solid radiopaque markers in dogs. Unpublished observations, 1993.
21. Hall JA, Willer RL, Seim HB, et al. Gastric emptying of nondigestible radiopaque markers after circumcostal gastropexy in clinically normal dogs and dogs with gastric dilatation-volvulus. Am J Vet Res 53:1961–1965, 1992.
22. VanSluijs FJ, van den Brom WE. Gastric emptying of a radionuclide-labeled test meal after surgical correction of gastric dilatation-volvulus in dogs. Am J Vet Res 50:433–435, 1988.
23. Thomas RE. Gastric dilatation and torsion in miniature breeds of dogs—three case reports. J Sm Anim Pract 23:271–277, 1982.
24. Wingfield WE, Cornelius LM. DeYoung DW. Pathophysiology of the gastric dilatation-torsion complex in the dog. J Sm Anim Pract 15:735–739, 1974.
25. Wingfield WE, Betts CW, Rawlings CA. Pathophysiology associated with

26. Orton EC, Muir WW. Hemodynamics in experimental gastric dilatation-volvulus in dogs. Am J Vet Res 44:1512–1515, 1983.
27. Horne WA, Gilmore DR, Dietze AE, et al. Effects of gastric distention-volvulus on coronary blood flow and myocardial oxygen consumption in the dog. Am J Vet Res 46:98–104, 1985.
28. Guilford WG, Komtebedde J, Haskins SC, et al. Unpublished observations, 1989.
29. Merkley DF, Howard DR, Krehbiel JD, et al. Experimentally induced acute gastric dilatation in the dog: Clinicopathologic findings. J Am Anim Hosp Assoc 12:149–153, 1976.
30. Pfeiffer CJ, Keith JC, April M. Topographic localization of gastric lesions and key role of plasma bicarbonate concentration in dogs with experimentally induced gastric dilatation. Am J Vet Res 48:262–267, 1987.
31. Guilford WG. Influence of allopurinol on the pathophysiology of surgically-induced gastric dilatation-volvulus in dogs. In: Experimental Studies of Gastrointestinal Ischemia-Reperfusion Injury and Food Sensitivity in Dogs. PhD thesis, University of California, Davis, 49–76, 1993.
32. Wheaton LG, Thacker HL, Caldwell S. Intravenous fluorescein as an indicator of gastric viability in gastric dilatation-volvulus. J Am Anim Hosp Assoc 22:197–204, 1986.
33. Davidson JR, Lantz GC, Salisbury SK, et al. Effects of flunixin meglumine on dogs with experimental gastric dilatation-volvulus. Vet Surg 21:113–120, 1992.
34. Komtebedde J, Guilford WG, Haskins SC, et al. Evaluation of systemic and splanchnic visceral oxygen variables in dogs with surgically induced gastric dilatation-volvulus. Vet Crit Care 1:5–13, 1991.
35. Lantz GC, Bottoms GD, Carlton WW, et al. The effect of 360 gastric volvulus on the blood supply of the nondistended normal dog stomach. Vet Surg 13:189–196, 1984.
36. Durbin RP, Moody FG. Water movement through a transporting epithelial membrane: The gastric mucosa. Symp Soc Exp Biol 19:299–306, 1965.
37. Varhaug JE, Svanes K, Lysen LJ, et al. The effect of intragastric pressure on gastric blood flow after partial devascularization of the stomach in cats. Eur J Surg Res 12:415–427, 1980.
38. Boley SJ, Girdhar PA, Warren AR, et al. Pathophysiologic effects of bowel distension on intestinal blood flow. Am J Surg 117:228–234, 1969.
39. Perry MA, Wadhwa SS. Gradual reintroduction of oxygen reduces reperfusion injury in cat stomach. Am J Physiol 254:G366–G372, 1988.
40. Bulkley G, Goldman H, Silen W. Pressure injury to the gastric mucosa. Am J Surg 117:193–203, 1969.
41. Alphin RS, MD, Gregory RL. Role of intragastric pressure, pH, and pepsin in gastric ulceration in the rat. Gastroenterology 73:495–500, 1977.
42. Andrews FJ, Malcontenti C, O'Brien PE. Sequence of gastric mucosal injury following ischemia and reperfusion. Role of reactive oxygen metabolites. Dig Dis Sci 37:1356–1361, 1992.
43. Hall JA, Solie TN, Seim HB, et al. Acute gastric dilatation alters gastric electromechanical activity in the dog. Gastroenterology 95:869, 1988.
44. Stampley AR, Burrows CF, Ellison GW, et al. Gastric myoelectric activity after experimental gastric dilatation-volvulus and tube gastrostomy in dogs. Vet Surg 21:10–14, 1992.
45. Merkley DF, Howard DR, Eyster GE, et al. Experimentally induced acute gastric dilatation in the dog: Cardiopulmonary effects. J Am Anim Hosp Assoc 12:143–148, 1976.
46. Badylak SF, Lantz GC, Jeffries M. Prevention of reperfusion injury in surgically induced gastric dilatation-volvulus in dogs. Am J Vet Res 51:294–299, 1990.
47. Engler HS, Kennedy TE, Ellison LT, et al. Hemodynamics of experimental acute gastric dilatation. Am J Surg 113:194–197, 1967.
48. Caldwell CB, Ricotta JJ. Changes in visceral blood flow with elevated intraabdominal pressure. J Surg Res 43:14–20, 1987.
49. Wingfield WE, Cornelius LM, Ackerman N, et al. Experimental acute gastric dilation and torsion in the dog. II. Venous angiographic alterations seen in gastric dilatation. J Sm Anim Pract 15:55–60, 1974.
50. Orton CE, Muir WW. Isovolumetric indices and humoral cardioactive substance bioassay during clinical and experimentally induced gastric dilatation-volvulus in dogs. Am J Vet Res 44:1516–1520, 1983.
51. Longhurst JC, Spilker HL, Ordway GA. Cardiovascular reflexes elicited by passive gastric distension in anesthetized cats. Am J Physiol 240:H539–H545, 1981.
52. Muir WW, Weisbrode SE. Myocardial ischemia in dogs with gastric dilatation-volvulus. J Am Vet Med Assoc 181:363–366, 1982.
53. Mitchell AR. What is shock? J Sm Anim Pract 26:719–738, 1985.
54. Shoemaker WC. Circulatory mechanisms of shock and their mediators. Crit Care Med 15:787–794, 1987.
55. Saba TM. Reticuloendothelial systemic host defense after surgery and traumatic shock. Circ Shock 2:91–108, 1975.
56. Lees GE, Leighton RL, Hart R. Management of gastric dilatation-volvulus and disseminated intravascular coagulation in a dog: A case report. J Am Anim Hosp Assoc 13:463–469, 1977.
57. Millis DL, Hauptman JG, Fulton RB. Abnormal hemostatic profiles and gastric necrosis in canine gastric dilatation-volvulus. Vet Surg 22:93–97, 1993.

58. Guilford WG. A retrospective study of the association between gastric dilatation-volvulus and hepatic disease. In: Ischemia-Reperfusion Injury and Food Sensitivity in Dogs. PhD thesis, University of California, Davis, 77–86, 1993.
59. Kirby R. Gastric dilatation-volvulus complex; retrospective review of factors important to survival. Unpublished data, University of Pennsylvania, 1988.
60. Wingfield WE, Cornelius LM, DeYoung DW. Experimental acute gastric dilatation and torsion in the dog. I. Changes in biochemical and acid-base parameters. J Sm Anim Pract 15:41–53, 1974.
61. Granger DN, Rutili G, McCord JM. Superoxide radicals in feline intestinal ischemia. Gastroenterology 81:22–29, 1981.
62. Sanfey H, Buckley GB, Cameron JL. The role of oxygen-derived free radicals in the pathogenesis of acute pancreatitis. Ann Surg 200:405–413, 1984.
63. Parks DA, Granger DN. Ischemia reperfusion injury: A radical view. Hepatology 8:680–682, 1988.
64. Schoenberg MH, Beger HG. Reperfusion injury after intestinal ischemia. Crit Care Med 21:1376–1386, 1993.
65. McCord JM. Oxygen derived free radicals in postischemic tissue injury. N Eng J Med 312:159–163, 1985.
66. Parks DA, Buckley GB, Granger DN, et al. Ischemic injury in the cat small intestine: Role of superoxide radicals. Gastroenterology 82:9–15, 1982.
67. Lantz GC, Badylak SF. Treatment of reperfusion injury in dogs with experimentally induced gastric dilatation volvulus. Am J Vet Res 53:1594–1598, 1992.
68. Williams JS. Hemodynamic alterations in acute gastric dilatation in the dog. Surg Forum 16:335–336, 1965.
69. Bryan-Brown CW. Blood flow to organs: Parameters for function and survival in critical illness. Crit Care Med 16:170–178, 1988.
70. Hathcock JT. Radiographic view of choice for the diagnosis of gastric volvulus: The right lateral recumbent view. J Am Anim Hosp Assoc 20:967–969, 1984.
71. Kneller SK. Radiographic interpretation of the gastric dilatation-volvulus complex in the dog. J Am Anim Hosp Assoc 12:154–157, 1976.
72. Allen DA, Schertel ER, Muir et al. Hypertonic saline/dextran resuscitation of dogs with experimentally induced gastric dilatation-volvulus shock. Am J Vet Res 52:92–96, 1991.
73. Pass MA, Johnston DR. Treatment of gastric dilatation-torsion in the dog. Gastric decompression by gastrotomy under local analgesia. J Sm Anim Pract 14:1131–1142, 1973.
74. Reichgott MJ, Melmon KL. Should corticosteroids be used in shock? Med Clin N Am 57:1211–1223, 1973.
75. Stegelmeier BL, Bottoms GD, Denicola DB, et al. Effects of flunixin meglumine in dogs following experimentally induced endotoxemia. Cornell Vet 78:221–230, 1988.
76. Dow SW, Rosychuk RAW, McChesney AE, et al. Adverse effects of flunixin meglumine and flunixin plus prednisone on the gastrointestinal tract of dogs. Am J Vet Res 51:1131–1138, 1990.
77. Sanan S, Sharma G, Singh B, et al. Evaluation of desferrioxamine mesylate on survival and prevention of histopathological changes in the liver, in hemorrhagic shock: An experimental study in dogs. Resuscitation 17:63–75, 1989.
78. Davies MJ, Donkor R, Dunstar CA, et al. Desferrioxamine and superoxide free radicals. Formation of an enzyme damaging nitroxide. Biochem J 240:725–729, 1987.
79. Blake DR, Winyard P, Lunec J, et al. Cerebral and ocular toxicity induced by desferrioxamine. Q J Med 219:345–355, 1985.
80. Matthieson DT. Partial gastrectomy as treatment of gastric volvulus. Results in 30 dogs. Vet Surg 14:185–193, 1985.
81. Dann JR. Medical and surgical treatment of canine acute gastric dilatation. J Am Anim Hosp Assoc 12:17–22, 1976.
82. Meyer-lindenberg A, Harder A, Fehr M, et al. Treatment of gastric dilatation-volvulus and a rapid method for prevention of relapse in dogs: 134 cases (1988–1991). J Am Vet Med Assoc 203:1303–1307, 1993.
83. Ellison GW. Gastric dilatation-volvulus. Surgical prevention. Vet Clin N Am 23:513–530, 1993.
84. Greenfield CL, Walshaw R, Thomas MW. Significance of the Heineke-Mikulicz pyloroplasty in the treatment of gastric dilatation-volvulus. Vet Surg 18:22–26, 1989.
85. Whitney WO. Complications associated with the medical and surgical management of gastric dilatation-volvulus in the dog. Prob Vet Med 1:268–280, 1989.
86. Jennings PB, Mathey WS, Ehler WJ. Intermittent gastric dilatation after gastropexy in a dog. J Am Vet Med Assoc 200:1707–1708, 1992.
87. Berardi C, Wheaton LG, Twardock AR, et al. Use of nuclear imaging technique to detect gastric wall ischemia. Am J Vet Res 52:1089–1096,1991.
88. Muir WW, Lipowitz AJ. Cardiac dysrhythmias associated with gastric dilatation-volvulus in the dog. J Am Vet Med Assoc 172:683–689, 1978.
89. Dierkes A. Comparative study of verapamil and lidocaine for preventing and treating cardiac arrhythmia in dogs. Dissertation, Tierarztliche Hochschule, Hanover, Germany, 1–120, 1990.
90. Hardie EM, Rawlings CA, Shotts EB, et al. Lidocaine treatment of dogs with Escherichia coli septicemia Am J Vet Res 49:77–81, 1988.
91. Graves GM, Becht JL, Rawlings CA. Metoclopramide reversal of decreased gastrointestinal myoelectric and contractile activity in a model of canine postoperative ileus. Vet Surg 18:27–33, 1989.
92. Wingfield WE, Betts CW, Greene RW. Operative techniques and recurrence rates associated with gastric volvulus in the dog. J Sm Anim Pract 16:427–432, 1975.
93. Leib MS, Blass CE. Acute gastric dilatation in the dog: Various clinical presentations. Comp Contin Educ Pract Vet 4:677–682, 1984.
94. Boothe HW, Ackerman N. Partial gastric torsion in two dogs. J Am Anim Hosp Assoc 12:27–30, 1976.
95. Frendin J, Funkquist B, Stavenborn M. Gastric displacement in dogs without clinical signs of acute dilatation. J Sm Anim Pract 29:775–779, 1988.

17 Small and Large Intestine: Normal Structure and Function

DONALD R. STROMBECK

INTRODUCTION

The alimentary tract caudal to the stomach is divided into the small and large intestines, which differ in function and in diameter of their lumen. In the dog and cat, the anatomic difference is small. The intestinal tract digests and absorbs food. Important motility functions aid in digestion and absorption processes and in moving the contents aborally. Integration of gastrointestinal functions is mediated by hormones and the nervous system.

The intestines contain the most complex ecosystem in the body, with a bacterial microflora consisting of many different members. The intestine possesses an immune system to protect the animal against invasion by bacterial opportunists of pathogens and against the absorption of antigenic substances.

Within the intestinal tract, function differs between the small and large intestines. The small intestine absorbs primarily nutrients and moves its contents continuously in an aboral direction. The large intestine serves as a reservoir, holding its contents for longer periods, and it absorbs primarily fluids and electrolytes. Within the small intestine, function is regionalized further, for example with the special ileal mechanisms for bile acid and cyanocobalamin absorption.

GROSS STRUCTURE[1–3]

Small Intestine (Figure 17-1)

The small intestine is divided arbitrarily into the duodenum, jejunum, and ileum. No definite anatomic dissimilarity permits a differentiation of one segment from another; the functional differences are not translated into differences in gross structure. The small intestine is 1.80 to 4.80 m long in the dog and about 1.30 m long in the cat.

The duodenum is the most cranial part of the small intestine. Beginning at the pylorus, it constitutes about 10% of the length of the entire small bowel. The first part begins at the right of the median plane and passes dorsally and to the right at the level of the ninth intercostal space. The duodenum is immobilized at this site by the hepatoduodenal ligament, connecting it to the liver, and by the mesentery containing the pancreas, to which it is closely related. The duodenum turns caudally at the cranial flexure and becomes the descending duodenum, which lies against the right dorsolateral abdominal wall and is not covered by the greater omentum. It is also related to the ventral caudal aspects of the right kidney. At the level of the fifth and sixth lumbar vertebrae, the duodenum forms the caudal flexure, which consists of the organ moving from right to left around the cecum and root of the mesentery. From this point forward, the duodenum passes as an ascending segment that lies between the cecum, ascending colon, and root of the mesentery, on the right, and the descending colon and left kidney, on the left. There are mesenteric attachments between the ascending duodenum and the colon in the duodenocolic fold. The transition from duodenum to jejunum occurs at the duodenojejunal flexure, located to the left of the root of the mesentery, from which the jejunum passes ventrally and caudally.

The jejunum and ileum account for approximately 90% of the total length of the small intestine. The jejunum is not fixed other than by long mesentery that contains vessels and nerves supplying the intestine. Thus, the jejunum is distributed throughout the abdominal cavity. It is displaced dorsally

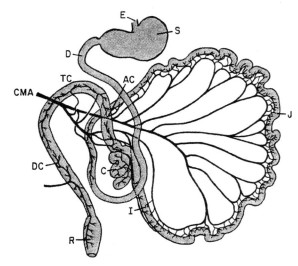

FIGURE 17-1. Anatomy of the small and large intestine. AC = ascending colon, C = cecum, CMA = cranial mesenteric artery, DC = descending colon, E = esophagus, I = ileum, J = jejunum, R = rectum, S = stomach, TC = transverse colon.

and to the right when the stomach becomes distended. The ventral and lateral surfaces of the jejunal mass are covered by omentum. The jejunum can be palpated throughout its length. Accomplishing that with some deep-chested breeds depends on elevating the cranial part of the animal. The ileum, the most caudal part of the small intestine, is the segment connected to the cecum by the ileocecal fold, supplied by vessels that pass to it from the cecum and colon. The ileum enters the proximal end of the ascending colon at the ileal orifice, located at the level of the first or second lumbar vertebra. A distinct anatomic sphincter is found, the ileocecal sphincter.

Large Intestine (Figures 17-1, 17-2)

The large intestine is relatively short in the dog and cat because its only purposes are to absorb salt and water and to serve as a reservoir, in contrast to the large colon of herbivores, required to digest and absorb polysaccharides. Together, the large intestine and rectum are 10% to 20% as long as the small intestine, measuring 0.2 to 0.6 m in the dog and 0.2 m in the cat.

The cecum is 0.08 to 0.3 m long in the dog and 0.02 to 0.04 m long in the cat. The cecum is associated with the ileum and ascending colon and related to the second to fourth lumbar vertebrae on the right side of the median plane. The cecum is related also to the ventral surface of the right kidney and the descending duodenum, which contains the pancreas in its mesentery.

The large intestine begins as a short segment designated as the ascending colon. It has the same spatial arrangement as the cecum. The next aborad part is a short segment of transverse colon. It exists as a flexure connecting the ascending colon to the most terminal part, the descending colon. The transverse colon passes around the root of the mesentery, caudally adjacent to the stomach, and from right to left at the level of the twelfth thoracic vertebra. The descending colon extends to the pelvic inlet, where the rectum begins. It lies to the left of the median plane and is related to the ascending duodenum by connections through the duodenocolic fold. The large intestine is palpable on physical examination. The cranial parts may not be reached in deep-chested breeds.

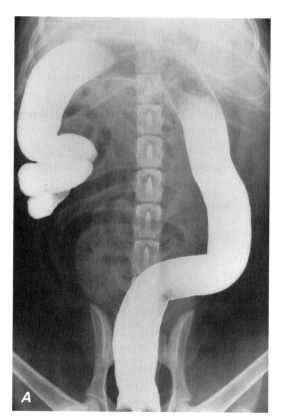

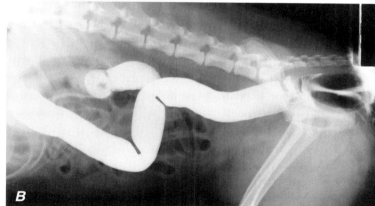

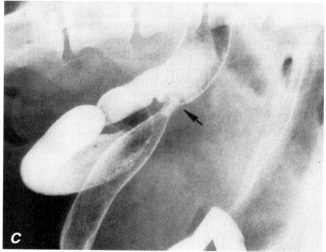

FIGURE 17–2 *(A)* Dorsoventral and *(B)* lateral radiographs of a normal colon in a 1-year-old cocker spaniel after a barium enema. The bowel was evidently well prepared because no filling defects are seen. Gas in the transverse colon will move with positioning. The lateral view shows a stricture in the rectum, a response due to the end of the enema tube. The cecum is filled and excess pressure is not exerted, so no contrast has entered the small intestine. The location of the colon is normal, and the tendency toward a redundant colon is great. *(C)* Lateral radiograph of a dog following a barium enema, showing a normal ileocecal valve.

Blood Supply and Lymphatics

The major blood supply to the small intestine is provided through the cranial mesenteric artery. The cranial part of the duodenum is supplied by branches of the celiac artery. Blood flow to the large intestine is via both the cranial and caudal mesenteric vessels. Mesenteric vessels to the small intestine form anastomosing arcades. If blood flow in a set of mesenteric vessels is obstructed, there is collateral flow through the vessels anastomosing with adjacent segments so the tissue can survive.[4] Venous flow from the intestines is into the portal vein. Lymphatic drainage is through one of the large number of lymph nodes that are scattered throughout the mesentery that contains the intestine.

Innervation

The efferent nerves to the intestines are parasympathetic and sympathetic fibers of the autonomic nervous system. The parasympathetics are important for regulation of normal function. The vagus supplies these fibers to the small intestine and to the first part of the large intestine. Parasympathetic fibers to the remainder of the large bowel arise from nuclei in the sacral cord and pass to the organ by way of pelvic nerves. Sympathetics play a minor role in normal intestinal function. They pass to the organ from a number of sympathetic ganglia, scattered through abdominal cavity, that receive fibers from the paravertebral sympathetic trunk.

Function in the intestines depends on the reception and transmission of information regarding intraluminal events in the gut. Afferent fibers in both parasympathetic and sympathetic nerve trunks relay that information to central or peripheral synapses for evocation of the reflexes.

MICROSCOPIC STRUCTURE[5,6]

Small Intestine

The intestines are similar to the esophagus and stomach in possessing mucosal, submucosal, and muscle layers (Figure 17–3). The mucosal layer, involved with secretory and absorptive functions, provides a barrier between the outside environment and the interior of the body. A submucosal layer, interposed between the mucosal and muscularis layers, provides support and contains blood vessels, lymphatics, and nerves. The outer muscular layers provide motility to intestinal contents at a slow rate in the aboral direction.

MUCOSA. The intestinal mucosa consists of a single layer of cells overlying a layer of loose connective tissue, vessels, and nerves. The structures beneath the surface cells form the lamina propria. The mucosa is thrown up into folds as illustrated in Figure 17–4. The surface mucosal cells are primarily epithelial cells, with a number of mucus-secreting goblet cells scattered throughout. Occasional argentaffin or enterochromaffin cells (endocrine secreting) are found in the basal part of the epithelium.

Epithelial Cells. The epithelial cells of the intestinal mucosa are basically the same in fine structure as the transporting epithelial cells of the tubules in the kidney, salivary ducts, and gallbladder. The luminal surface consists of a brush border made up of numerous microvilli (Figure 17–5). The surface of the brush border is covered with a polysaccharide, glycocalyx, synthesized by the cell and secreted onto its surface. The function of this carbohydrate layer is not known.

It may function similarly to an ion exchange resin by attracting and concentrating substances at the cell surface in order to facilitate absorption. The glycocalyx may also trap and retain brush border enzymes to enable digestion at the site of absorption on the cell surface. The glycocalyx may also protect the cell. Loss of the glycocalyx during bowel ischemia increases susceptibility of cells to destruction by proteases within the lumen.

The microvilli increase the area of mucosa available for digestion and absorption. Microvillous membranes possess special mechanisms for transporting monosaccharides and amino acids. They are also capable of absorbing material by pinocytosis. The brush border contains enzymes to digest disaccharides, oligosaccharides, and some small peptides. These enzymes exert most of their activity while remaining on the brush border or, at least, within the environment of the glycocalyx. Although electron micrographs do not make it apparent, the microvilli form a dynamic structure that is constantly changing morphologically in the living cell.

The epithelial cell is concerned also with the absorption and secretion of electrolytes and water. Sodium transport is more important than the transport of other electrolytes and is thought to involve membrane ATPase, an enzyme that histochemistry has shown to be located on cell membranes. Adenylate cyclase, an enzyme that generates the nucleotide cyclic AMP, is thought to be involved in secretion of fluid by the epithelial cell. This enzyme is found primarily on the membranes of the lateral and basal cell surfaces.

The brush border also contains proteins that bind a variety of substances to be absorbed, such as calcium, iron, and vitamin B_{12}.

All epithelial surface membranes are semipermeable, permitting diffusion of small monovalent ions. The surface area of cell membranes is mostly lipid, which permits lipid-soluble substances to diffuse across the membrane.

Intracellular design of the epithelial cell reflects its functions. Below the brush border a mesh of filaments forms the terminal web, with the function of providing skeletal support for the cell. The epithelial cell does not synthesize protein for export. Consequently, the structure that synthesizes protein, the rough endoplasmic reticulum, is found only in amounts necessary to meet the cell's own needs. The Golgi apparatus is not well developed because there is little need for the packaging of substances for export. Intracellular transport of nutrients is important, however, and is accomplished by an extensive system of canals provided by the smooth endoplasmic reticulum. Many mitochondria are found to provide the energy required for transport processes. Mitochondria are

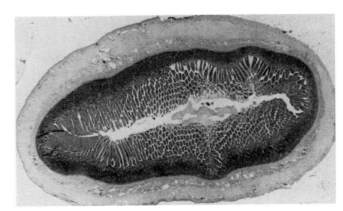

FIGURE 17–3. Cross section of the small intestine, showing inner layers of mucosa and submucosa and two outer layers of smooth muscle.

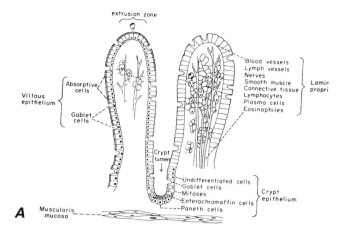

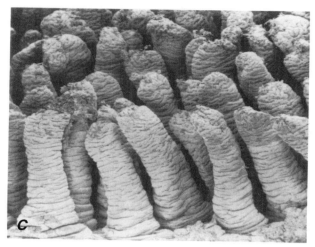

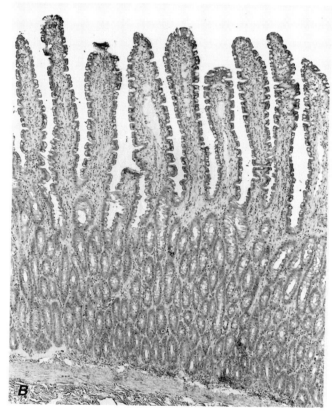

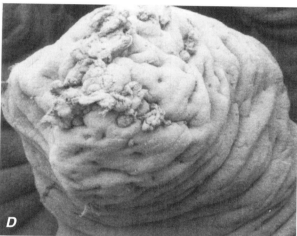

FIGURE 17-4. *(A)* Schematic diagram of two sectioned villi and a crypt to illustrate the histologic organization of the small intestinal mucosa. (From Trier JS, Handbook of Physiology, Sec. 6, Vol. 3, Chap. 63, 1127; by permission of the American Physiological Society.) *(B)* Photomicrograph of canine jejunum. *(C)* Scanning electron micrograph of canine jejunum. ×65. *(D)* Scanning electron micrograph of canine jejunum. ×530. Mucous or goblet cells can be identified either as rounded protuberances if they contain numerous mucigen droplets or a small depression if they have discharged their mucus. Debris at the very tip of the villus probably represents cells being shed into the lumen of the intestine.

found most abundantly in the epithelial cells that have the major function of absorbing or secreting electrolytes and water. Intestinal epithelial cells possess many lysosomes, which contain large numbers of enzymes able to degrade the many substances absorbed. Lysosomes fuse with vesicles containing material absorbed by pinocytosis and release enzymes into a common vesicle known as a phagolysosome. A protective function of the cell is the degradation of foreign material to prevent it from making its way into the body.

Goblet Cells. Surface mucosal cells that secrete mucus are called goblet cells. They are interspersed between epithelial cells, increasing in relative numbers distally in the intestinal tract. The luminal border of the goblet cell contains few microvilli. The appearance of the cell is marked by engorgement with mucin, packaged in granules ready for release. The rough endoplasmic reticulum and the Golgi apparatus are well developed in order to synthesize and package mucin

for export. Because energy needs are not great, few mitochondria are found.

Immature Crypt Cells. The epithelial cells on the villi differ from those in the crypts of Lieberkuhn. Cells of the villi are fully differentiated, so they synthesize and secrete enzymes and perform absorptive functions. Mature villous cells develop from immature or stem cells in the crypts by moving up the side of the villous in a sheet. During migration, the cells mature and acquire the highly developed function of the villous cell. Migration requires about two days. The cells are fully mature when the migration is one-third to one-half completed. Cells in the crypts are morphologically immature. They have undeveloped brush borders, and the intracellular appearance resembles that of secretory cells more than absorptive cells. Secretion of intestinal fluid may be a normal function of crypt cells. The primary function of crypt cells is to replenish mature villus epithelial cells.

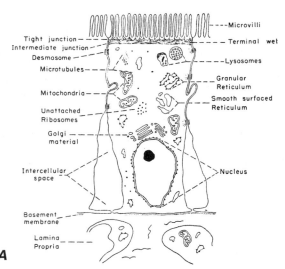

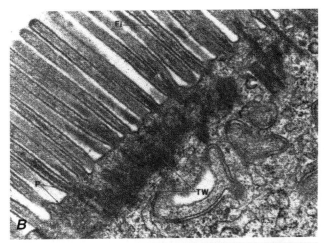

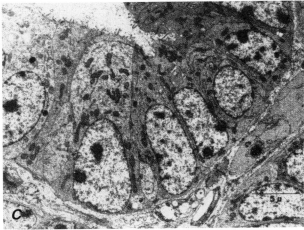

FIGURE 17-5. *(A)* Schematic diagram of an intestinal absorptive cell. (From Trier JS, Handbook of Physiology, Sec. 6, Vol. 3, Chap. 63, 1133; by permission of the American Physiological Society.) *(B)* Electron micrograph of canine duodenal epithelial cell showing microvilli. Fi = filaments of microvillus, TW = terminal web, P = plasmalemma. ×25,700. *(C)* Electron micrograph of canine duodenal epithelium. ×2550.

Endocrine-Paracrine-Secreting Cells.[7] Amine-precursor-uptake decarboxylase (APUD) and peptide-hormone-producing cells are found in the mucosal surface layer, interspersed between epithelial cells. As many as 15 types of endocrine-paracrine cells have been identified in the gastrointestinal tract. Most produce active peptides and some also biogenic amines. APUD cells synthesize and secrete biogenic amines (e.g., serotonin) and biologically active peptides (e.g., vasoactive intestinal peptide). The argentaffin cell is an APUD cell containing biogenic amines stored in abundance in secretory granules. APUD cells have a broad base that borders on the basement membrane and an apex that may not reach and border on the intestinal lumen. Thus, the cell is designed to secrete a product into the circulation rather than into the lumen of the gut. The peptide endocrines produced in many different cells were isolated and characterized before it was determined where they are produced. Some are true endocrine hormones released to the circulation, which carries the hormone to its target organ. Others, such as somatostatin, are paracrines; the hormone is released to act locally on an adjacent cell. The secretions of all the endo-paracrine cells are important in integrating functions within the alimentary canal.

Intercellular Association (Figure 17-6). The mucosal surface epithelium is remarkably competent in preventing particulate matter and large molecules from penetrating into the body from the gut. The mucosa is a semipermeable barrier to the movement of electrolytes. It prevents the loss of extracellular fluid into the lumen of the gut and regulates the rate of absorption of fluid from the gut. The semipermeable membrane consists of both the brush border and junctions between cells. These latter intercellular connections have been called tight junctions because morphologically they appear to form a tight barrier to the movement of fluid and ions. These junctions are not tight, however; they actually form the most permeable area of the mucosal surface. Thus, passive diffusional fluxes of ions and water across the mucosa are greatest through the so-called tight junctions.

The lateral basal cell membranes transport sodium from inside the cell to the lateral intercellular space. Water follows osmotically, markedly dilating the space during active sodium transport. Hydrostatic pressure increases in the space, and fluid leaves, following pressure gradients. By this means fluid is transported from the lumen of the gut into the circulation. The leaky tight junctions permit diffusion of fluid from the dilated intercellular space back into the intestinal lumen. The junctions are less leaky in the ileum and large intestine, making absorption of fluid more efficient there because there is less back diffusion.

Basement Membrane. The basement membrane is a glycoprotein on which the mucosal cells abut. Although its morphologic appearance does not support it, the basement membrane is readily permeable to the movement of macromolecules and some blood cells.

MUCOSAL CIRCULATION.[8,9] Blood flow to the villus is provided by an arteriole that passes through the lamina propria to the end of the villus (Figure 17-7). It runs unbranched to the villus tip, where it arborizes, producing a fountain of vessels that form a dense subepithelial capillary network. Drainage from the capillaries is by veins that begin in the upper part of the villus in the dog and the lower part in the cat. The crypt epithelial cells are supplied by arterial vessels that are separate from those entering the villi. Control over the vascular beds is different in the two different regions, and blood flow can be increased selectively in one while

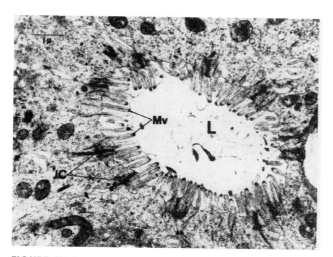

FIGURE 17-6. Electron micrograph of intestinal epithelial cells, showing the so-called tight junctions, which are in fact quite leaky to the movement of water and monovalent ions. L = lumen of intestinal gland, Mv = microvilli, JC = junctional complex. ×8770.

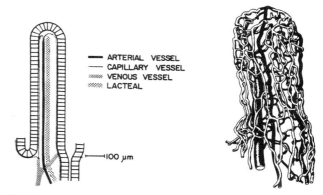

FIGURE 17-7. Schematic drawing of vascular network of villus. Arterial vessel (black) runs unbranched to tip of villus, where it arborizes into a capillary network that drains into a venous vessel (gray). (Lundgren D. Gut 15:1005, 1974; by permission.)

decreased in the other. Capillaries in the intestinal lamina propria have many large fenestrations.[10] These pores enable a considerable amount of plasma proteins to move from the vessels into the interstitial space. This results in a serum albumin space three times that in most tissues of the body, which may be important in some abnormal situations that produce a diarrhea.[11] It also illustrates how a protein-losing enteropathy can easily occur when the one-cell epithelial barrier is defective. Fluid lost from the interstitium of the intestine is richer in plasma proteins than fluid from other tissues.

A lymphatic vessel, the lacteal, is situated in the lamina propria in the center of the villus. This is the avenue for absorption of most of the triglycerides, which are transported from the gut as chylomicrons.

RENEWAL OF MUCOSAL SURFACE.[12–14] Mucosal epithelial cells normally desquamate from the tips of the villi and are replaced by cells migrating from replicating crypt stem cells. The number of cells on any one villus is determined by the rate of production of new cells and the rate of loss of mature cells. The rate of cell division is controlled by humoral factors.[15,16] Excessive amounts of any hormone with trophic effects, such as gastrin, produce mucosal hyperplasia. The trophic effects depend on permissive effects of adrenal corticosteroids and possibly other hormones. Some peptide hormones such as epidermal growth factor and transforming growth factor alpha can modulate proliferation and differentiation of mucosal epithelial cells.

A number of factors cause cell turnover to increase and can lead to mucosal atrophy. Physical or chemical trauma increase cell loss; normal bacterial microflora cut the average cell life to half of what it would be if no microorganisms were present. Increased bacterial numbers cause villus atrophy. Protozoal infection increases epithelial cell turnover.[17] Dietary changes and changes in the composition of the microflora can speed mucosal cell loss. Drugs that interfere with cell division or the cells' metabolic functions and fasting during parenteral nutrition prevent normal cell renewal, and the mucosa atrophies. Anticancer drugs and some antibiotics can have an antimetabolic effect. Because vitamin B_{12} and folic acid are essential for cell renewal, a deficiency of either results in mucosal atrophy.

The balance between rates of renewal and loss determines villus size. Growth exceeding loss causes villus hypertrophy.

When rate of loss exceeds growth, the villi atrophy. The migration time of crypt cells is considerably shorter when the villi are atrophied, which suggests the villous cells are not completely mature. Maintenance of mucosal renewal and integrity is essential to the mucosal barrier protecting the body from the deleterious agents in the intestinal lumen. The barrier's function includes preventing luminal bacteria and endotoxins from reaching systemic organs and tissues. The systemic spread of bacteria from the intestine to systemic organs, bacterial translocation, is prevented by enteral feeding, dietary fiber, and possibly by dietary glutamine.

SUBMUCOSA. The submucosa is separated from the mucosa by the muscularis mucosa. The submucosa contains blood vessels, lymphatics, and nerves in a loosely arranged bed of connective tissue. The submucosa also contains glands, although in the cat and dog the glands are restricted to the first few centimeters of the duodenum. The Brunner's glands are characterized by acini of cuboidal mucus-secreting cells that produce an alkaline watery mucoid fluid.

MUSCULARIS.[18,19] The wall of the intestine contains an outer thinner layer of longitudinal smooth muscle and a thicker inner layer of circular muscle. The intestinal smooth muscle is similar in structure to that found elsewhere in the body. The muscle cells appear different from skeletal muscle cells because no myosin filaments are seen, even though myosin is present. The actin filaments are probably linked in series by aggregates of myosin that connect their ends. The smooth muscle cells have a definite sarcolemma, and there is intercellular continuity between elements of adjacent cells. Intestinal smooth muscle has the property of propagating electrical activity through a number of its cells. Cell-to-cell transmission of this activity occurs through the nexus, which is a region of fusion of plasma membranes. This allows the layers of smooth muscle to function as a syncytium

NEURAL PLEXUSES.[18,19] Neural control of intestinal function is mediated via nerves that synapse in a number of different ganglia in the wall of the intestine (Figure 17-8). The ganglia, with their afferent fibers, are organized into plexuses. One such center is located in the subserous plexus at the attachment of the mesentery. It is a point of transmission between the mesenteric nerve bundles and the plexuses that lie deep within the intestinal wall. The myenteric plexus, one of the internal plexuses, is located between the circular and longitudinal muscle layers. Another group of neural ganglia are found in the submucous plexuses scattered throughout the submucosa. Extensions of the submucous plexuses into the mucosa have been termed mucosal plexuses. There

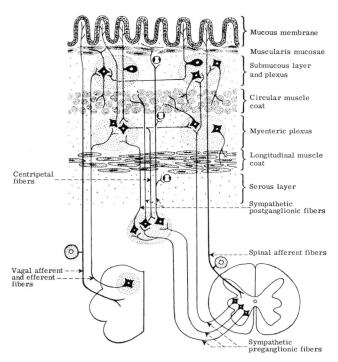

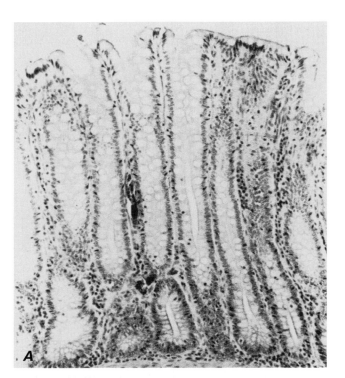

FIGURE 17-8. Schematic of extrinsic and intrinsic nerve fibers in the enteric plexus. (From Schofield GC, Handbook of Physiology, Sec. 6, Vol. 4, Chap. 80, 1611, 1968; by permission of the American Physiological Society.)

are communicating fibers between ganglia in the same layer of intestine and between those at different levels. Most of the fibers to and from the plexuses are afferents and parasympathetics. Some sympathetic fibers synapse on the ganglia and modulate neural activity.

Colonic Microscopic Structure

The surface of the mucosa of the colon is flat and contains no villi (Figure 17–9). Straight tubular glands extend from the surface through the entire thickness of the mucosa, reaching the muscularis mucosa. These glands, called crypts of Lieberkuhn, contain both mucous and epithelial cells near the surface and primarily mucous cells in the deepest parts of the gland. The surface is lined with mostly epithelial cells. Crypt cells multiply and differentiate as they migrate up the gland walls to replace surface epithelial cells. The tubular glands are packed close together, leaving room for only a minimal amount of lamina propria. The remainder of the wall of the colon is histologically similar to the wall of the small intestine.

FUNCTION

Motility: Small Intestine[20-23]

The small intestine contains smooth muscle that performs two basic functions. It mixes and slows the passage of contents through the tube, thus ensuring completeness of digestion and absorption. It functions also to move contents continuously in the aboral direction. The type of motility that

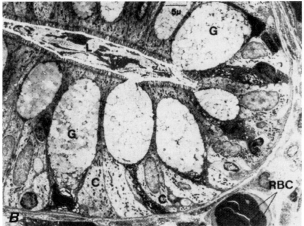

FIGURE 17-9. *(A)* Photomicrograph of normal canine colon. *(B)* Electron micrograph of normal canine colon. L = lumen of intestinal gland, G = goblet or mucus cell, C = columnar cell. ×1088.

slows the movement is rhythmic segmentation which contributes to resistance in the intestinal conduit. The other type of motility, functioning to move the contents in the aboral direction, is called peristalsis. Several other types of movement have been described, such as pendulous movements and peristaltic rushes. Such phenomena result when the balance between segmentation and peristalsis is altered so that the contents move rapidly through more than a few centimeters of intestine. The movement of contents through the small intestine is thus the net effect of the braking action of segmentation and the accelerator effect of peristalsis. The mixing of intestinal contents is a function of both segmentation and longitudinal contractions.[24]

RHYTHMIC SEGMENTATION.[20,25] Rhythmic segmentation is a type of intestinal motility characterized by random contractions of the circular muscles. This motility is minimal when the intestine is empty, yet is able to maintain pressures 6 mm Hg above atmosphere.[26] The strength of the contraction increases when stimulated by distension from food entering the intestine. The increase in activity is mediated by reflexes that have pathways through the intrinsic plexuses (Figure 17–8). The locally initiated increased motility is augmented by incoming vagal nerve activity that increases during the feeding state. Rhythmic segmentation performs two functions. One is to mix food with digestive enzymes and to bring nutrients into contact with mucosal absorptive surfaces. The other function is to increase resistance to the passage of nutrients through the intestine, giving digestion and absorption processes time for completion. The unstimulated intestine is a flaccid tube that offers little resistance to the flow of liquid contents through its lumen. Resistance to flow is increased by reducing the lumen of the tube, as illustrated in Figure 17–10. Thus, an intestine with strong contractions of rhythmic segmentation is one with considerable motility (hypermotile) whereas the flaccid bowel has little motility (hypomotile). The rate of the muscle contractions that produce rhythmic segmentation, fairly constant for each level in the small intestine, is determined by electrical control activity, a basic property of muscle in the longitudinal layer. The rate is higher in the duodenum (18 to 19 contractions per minute) than in the ileum (8 to 10 per minute). Thus, motor activity decreases in the aboral direction.

The level of excitability, produced by activity over nerves to the muscles or by hormones, determines the strength of these contractions. In general, animals with diarrhea have a decrease in the strength of normal segmentation, so the bowel is in a flaccid (hypomotile) state, offering little resistance to the flow of contents through it. The rate of contractions, however, is not markedly affected.

PERISTALSIS.[20,21,25] Peristalsis is the second important type of motility. A peristaltic wave can be described as a ring of constriction that moves aboral over a short segment of intestine. In each very short section of intestine, peristaltic waves develop at the same frequency as rhythmic segmentation contractions, both rates determined by the electrical-control activity. Therefore, the rate of generation of peristaltic waves is different in each level of the intestinal tract. The rate of development of peristaltic waves is greatest in the duodenum, and the decreasing rate in the aboral segments is responsible for the movement of the contents in the proper direction. Each wave is about 5 cm long in the duodenum and becomes shorter in the caudal small intestine. The length of each wave is determined by the length of intestine that has the same frequency of electrical-control activity.

Propulsive activity is found during both fed and unfed states. In the unfed state propulsive activity is periodic with intervals of no activity lasting an hour between propulsive waves. The peristaltic waves during unfed states constitute the interdigestive migrating motility complex (IDMC), which provides the interdigestive housekeeping activity for keeping the intestine cleared of bacteria and debris. Myoelectrical measurements show three different patterns that correspond to a phase 1 of no motility, a phase 2 of propulsive activity that is similar to peristaltic waves seen with feeding, and a phase 3 of maximum propulsive activity when the housekeeping function is operating. At any point in the intestine the hour of phase 1 inactivity is followed by first 15 to 40 minutes of phase 2 activity and then 4 to 8 minutes of phase 3 intense contractile activity. The interval between each cycle and the time for migration from the upper to lower small bowel is 2 to 3 hours. The IDMC cycle of activity is disrupted by feeding.

The migrating motility complex (MMC) changes from the cyclic pattern seen with the IDMC to the fed pattern of phase

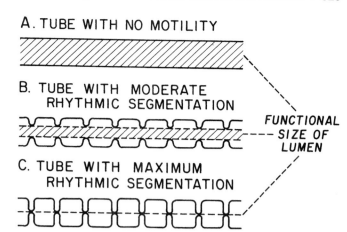

A. TUBE WITH NO MOTILITY

B. TUBE WITH MODERATE RHYTHMIC SEGMENTATION

FUNCTIONAL SIZE OF LUMEN

C. TUBE WITH MAXIMUM RHYTHMIC SEGMENTATION

FIGURE 17–10. Schematic of intestine with varying degrees of resistance to flow of chyme. Rate of peristaltic flow in intestine is determined by resistance in tube. Flow is directly proportional to radius of tube:

$$\frac{\Delta P \pi r^4}{8Ln}$$

Resistance is inversely related to radius of tube:

$$R = \frac{\Delta P}{F} = \frac{8Ln}{\pi r^4}$$

Resistance to flow is produced by rhythmic segmentation stimulated by food, distending the intestine.

2 contractions after consumption of a meal. The physical and chemical composition of the food determines the length of time before the IDMC pattern returns. Dogs fed milk develop the fed pattern for 2.5 to 4 hours. The type of nutrient is important in that isocaloric amounts of peptides, glucose, and medium chain triglycerides cause fed patterns of 2.8, 4.8, and 7.5 hours, respectively. It is evident that propulsion of intestinal contents by the MMC is well regulated by events in the intestinal lumen. Propulsion is augmented both by food's stimulating a local reflex and by extrinsic nerve fiber activity in the vagi. When segmentation and and resistance to flow are reduced in the flaccid intestine, very little peristaltic activity is needed to propel liquid contents over a long span with relative ease. In animals with diarrhea, the rate of peristaltic activity need not be increased to contribute to the problem. A number of problems can induce frequent MMC, however, and that contributes to diarrhea. Intestinal parasites, intestinal bacterial overgrowth, bacterial infection, and ricinoleic acid stimulate MMC that can propel fluid rapidly through the unfed intestine.

Regulation of Motility[21,25]

SLOW-WAVE OR ELECTRICAL-CONTROL ACTIVITY. The frequency of rhythmic segmentation contractions and peristaltic waves is determined by the slow-wave, electrical-control activity, or basic electrical rhythm, which is a property of the smooth muscle that has been stripped of all its nerves (Chapter 1). Slow waves are influenced by hormones, neural activity, feeding, and disease states. In the small intestine, however, hormones and neural activity have little effect on this activity. The generation of intestinal slow waves is not well understood but is most likely the result of membrane properties and changes in intracellular and extracellular electrolytes. Slow-wave activity is known to be sensitive to low extracellular potassium levels,[27] and loss of normal intestinal motility is often associated with hypokalemia. In these cases, normal intestinal motility is not regained until potassium deficits are corrected. Slow-wave activity also disappears during vomiting when retrograde intestinal contractions are seen.

ELECTRICAL-RESPONSE ACTIVITY. Slow-wave activity governs the rate of the muscle contraction that causes segmentation or peristaltic movement; it does not initiate the contraction. Stimulation of the intestinal smooth muscle to contract comes from the electrical-response activity or spike potentials, which are generated by a number of different means. This activity is initiated by stimuli that arise from within the intestine or from without, such as by distension of the intestine with food and by psychic stimuli generated during the feeding process. The afferent impulses are carried to synapses in the intrinsic plexuses of the control nuclei of the vagus, where they initiate the stimulus for electrical-response activity. In addition to activity in the extrinsic nerves, electrical-response activity is stimulated by hormones. The strength of smooth muscle contractions is variable, determined by the amount of neural or humoral stimulation. Thus, the rate of muscular contraction is normally constant and predetermined, whereas the strength of contractions in segmentation and peristalsis is variable, modulated by neural and humoral controls. Both contractions are phasic because they are determined by slow-wave activity, which is phasic. Propagated waves of contraction only occur over short distances; then timing and velocity of propagation are determined by the slow wave in any segment of intestine.

CHOLINERGIC CONTROLS.[21] The intrinsic nervous system mediates stimulation of spike potentials. The release of acetylcholine at the ganglionic synapse and motor end plate stimulates motility, as shown in Figure 17–11. Following release, acetylcholine binds to muscarinic cholinergic receptors on the muscle. Muscle contraction is blocked by atropine, which also binds to the receptors. Nicotinic cholinergic receptors are found in the ganglia and in the muscle and plate. High levels of nicotine and hexamethonium block acetylcholine's effect at these sites. Parasympathetic fibers in the vagus and pelvic nerves mediate release of acetylcholine.

ADRENERGIC CONTROL.[21,28] Adrenergic nerve activity stimulates release of a second type of neurotransmitter to alter intestinal motility. Alpha-adrenergic receptors are found on the postganglionic nerves of the myenteric plexus. The stimulation of adrenergic fibers to release norepinephrine inhibits activity in the cholinergic fibers to which it binds, thus inhibiting intestinal motility . Stimulation of vagal adrenergic fibers inhibits intestinal motility. Beta-adrenergic receptors are also found on intestinal smooth muscle cells. Epinephrine acting on these sites inhibits intestinal motility. The adrenergic receptors do not play a role in the normal motor functions of the intestine.

SEROTONERGIC CONTROL.[20,21] Receptors for serotonin are found on intestinal smooth muscle cells and on the intrinsic nerves. This biogenic amine is thought to be an important neurotransmitter for peristalsis. Infusion of serotonin produces an initial tonic contraction of intestinal smooth muscle, followed by phasic contraction.[29] Serotonin is released from the intestine during stimulation by distention, which suggests it plays a physiologic role. Large amounts of serotonin are released from some carcinoid tumors, causing diarrhea as a major clinical sign.[30] Inhibition of serotonin synthesis inhibits the diarrhea, suggesting serotonin is a neurotransmitter for peristalsis. Serotonin also affects absorption and secretion of fluid in the intestine, however, which may be the basis for the diarrhea. There is no evidence that

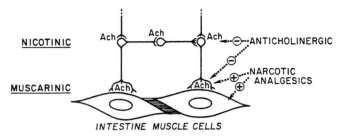

FIGURE 17–11. Schematic of nerve muscle unit with ganglionic synapses. Primary neurotransmitter is acetylcholine (Ach), and transmission is blocked (-) by anticholinergics. Two types of receptors are found, nicotinic and muscarinic. Narcotic analgesics stimulate smooth muscle contraction by acting at the synapse and directly on the muscle.

antiserotonin drugs reduce peristalsis and would be effective in treating diarrhea.

CONTROL OF MOTILITY BY OTHER HUMORAL AGENTS. Other chemicals affect smooth muscle contractility, but it is uncertain whether they play a physiologic role in motor function of the intestine.[31] Some of the gut peptide hormones, such as cholecystokinin, stimulate muscle contraction (Table 1–4). Intestinal smooth muscle possesses receptors for these hormones, and their interaction is thought to be physiologically important. Other chemicals, such as histamine, have an effect on smooth muscle contraction throughout the body. It has not been shown that histamine is either a neurotransmitter or plays a physiologic role. A number of basic peptides have properties similar to this property of histamine. Prostaglandins have potent effects to stimulate smooth muscle contraction, but it is not known whether they contribute to normal function. The circulating levels of prostaglandins are increased in some diseases with a diarrhea. In addition to their effects on motility, prostaglandins increase blood flow and stimulate the secretion of fluid in the intestine. Thus, it is difficult to determine whether diarrhea is caused by augmented intestinal propulsion or by secretion of intestinal fluid.

Other neurotransmitters are released by neural activity to the intestinal muscles. Some nerve activity is inhibitory, and the fibers are neither cholinergic nor adrenergic. These nerves have been designated as purinergic, and the neurotransmitter may be VIP or a purine metabolite such as ATP.[32] Recent studies show nitric oxide to be an important mediator for nonadrenergic noncholinergic neural inhibition of gastrointestinal smooth muscle. Nitric oxide mediates muscle relaxation by stimulating 5'–cyclic guanosine monophosphate production. There is also evidence that postganglionic noncholinergic nerves stimulate intestinal contractions.

In summary, it is evident that a great number of chemicals can affect the contractility of intestinal smooth muscle. The most important neurotransmitter for normal function is acetylcholine, for which there are receptors on both neural elements and muscle fibers. The many other chemicals found in the intestine that have effects on smooth muscle function indicate how complex regulation of intestinal motility could be and probably is.

Long Intestinal Reflexes

Local events in the intestinal tract dictate patterns of motility within that region. Events in one part of the alimentary tract also influence motility in other regions, via long intestinal reflexes. The general purpose of these reflexes is to prepare the way for events that will soon follow. The gastrocolic reflex is a long reflex in which receptors in the stomach are stimulated to produce a motor response in the colon. The stimulus is food in the stomach; the response is an increase in the type of colon activity that evacuates the colon. The effect is mediated through a reflex with afferent fibers that synapse in the central nervous system and with efferents in parasympathetic fibers. Another reflex, the ileal brake, inhibits gastric and jejunal motility by PYY, a peptide released from ileal mucosa. PYY release is stimulated by luminal nutrients and its action to inhibit upper gastrointestinal motility is mediated by local release of nitric oxide. A colonic brake may function similarly when nutrients bathe the mucosa of the colon. The intestino-intestinal inhibitory reflex is another that causes a loss of motility when a stimulus is applied to the intestine. The reflex is not readily apparent under normal conditions. Its effect can be mediated by sympathetic fibers that, when stimulated, can cause a loss of motility throughout the entire small intestine. Intrinsic neural pathways are responsible for some of these reflexes.[33] The stimulus can be acute distension of one part such as that produced by an intestinal obstruction. Trauma or extensive manipulation of the intestines during abdominal surgery can also stimulate the reflex. In association with electrolyte changes, this reflex produces the pathologic situation found in paralytic ileus. Experimental stimulation of the reflex by itself does not produce ileus, however.[34] When a segment of intestine loses motility and becomes a flaccid tube, fluid and gas accumulate. Because there are no restrictions to the rapid movement of fluid through hypomotile loops of intestine, diarrhea appears. For intestinal contents to move rapidly through the intestine, the conduit's resistance must decrease. Temporary loss of resistance is required for a peristaltic rush to occur. Thus, segmentation ceases as an essential part of mass peristaltic movements, and this cessation is mediated by long intestinal reflexes.

Small intestinal motility is coordinated after feeding so that solid particles and fluid move at the same rate unless the volume of fluid increases greatly, in which case fluid moves faster.[35] Non-nutrient components of the diet also influence the rate of transit. The addition of fiber in the form of bran, guar gum, or cellulose increases small intestinal transit time 28%, 51%, and 900%, respectively.[36]

Ileocecal Junction[37,38]

A well-defined anatomic sphincter is found surrounding the ileocecal orifice. It is not certain whether the muscles in this structure create a functional sphincter. Experimental studies show that ileal contents are rapidly evacuated into the colon during stimulation of the gastroileal reflex. This reflex, stimulated by food entering the stomach, serves to prepare the way for food that will soon enter the small intestine. It is not known whether this reflex functions to "open" the sphincter. The structure possesses all the requirements for a sphincter in that manometric measurements reveal intraluminal pressure is higher in the sphincter than in adjacent structures.[39] The sphincteric pressure decreases in response to appropriate stimulation, which, in this case, is distension by contents in the ileum. The pressure in the sphincter increases when intraluminal pressure increases in the colon. Thus, the sphincter opens to allow contents to pass through in the proper direction, and it prevents the reflux of colonic contents into the ileum. Its most important function is to prevent colonic reflux because that would contaminate the small intestine with a fecal type of bacterial flora.[40] Motility in the

ileum is more important in controlling the movement of contents from the ileum to the colon than is the sphincter.[41]

The control of function in the ileocecal sphincter is not clearly understood. In general, increased vagal activity causes the sphincter muscles to contract, and anticholinergics block this response. Paradoxically, stimulation of sympathetics also causes contraction in the sphincter. Catecholamines, acting on alpha-adrenergic receptors on muscle cells, appear to mediate the contraction. This action is in contrast to sympathetic effects on intestinal smooth muscle. It is not known how sphincter pressure decreases when the ileum is distended. Noncholinergic, nonadrenergic fibers promoting relaxation of the gastric fundus may similarly control ileocecal sphincter function. The therapeutic use of anticholinergics to treat diarrheas decreases the ability of the sphincter to generate and maintain a high-pressure zone and prevent reflux of colonic contents. Drugs that increase motility in the sphincter, such as narcotic analgesics, reduce the possibility of reflux.

Structural and Functional Features of the Colon

The structure and functions of the colon are essentially the same as those of the small intestine, with a few exceptions. The colon serves as a reservoir and completes the absorption of fluid and electrolytes. The reservoir function is similar to that of the stomach; that is, contents are retained and released slowly at the proper time. Food is not retained in the small intestine but is transported at a programmed rate. Although the colon is anatomically more similar to the small intestine, it is physiologically more like the stomach because they both consist of two functionally distinct regions

Motility: Colon[42,43]

The types of motor activity are similar in the large and small intestines. Rhythmic segmentation and propulsive movements are found in both. Segmentation retards the passage of and mixes colonic contents so absorption is completed. The rate of segmentation is determined by the electrical-control or slow-wave activity of the colonic smooth muscle. The rate of slow-wave activity is less than 5 cycles per minute, consistent with the motor activity of the colon being at the lowest end of the gradient of slow-wave activity.

Three patterns of motility are recognized in the colon. The cranial colon shows antiperistalsis where over a period of 2 to 8 minutes rings of contraction move cephalad rather than caudal at a frequency of contractions of about 5 per minute. The activity is followed by rest intervals to 15 minutes. The retrograde peristalsis mixes food and prevents its passage until absorption complete. Colonic contents can be for relatively long periods of time in the cranial colon. The rings of contraction are equivalent to segmentation, which also retards the movement of contents. The middle of the colon shows coordinated peristalsis where tonic contraction rings move caudally. Colonic contents stimulate the contractions by distention; the contractions slow the passage of contents but also propel the contents toward the rectum. The caudal colon shows strong contractions that move caudally and empty the colon.

Occasionally colonic contents are seen to move rapidly over a relatively long distance; the phenomenon is called mass movements. Before peristalsis can move colonic contents in a mass movement, segmentation must disappear over the segment traversed. With segmentation eliminated, only small forces are needed to propel liquid contents.

Colonic motor functions are determined by slow waves or electrical-control activity. Besides determining the rate of contractions, slow waves are essential for spike potentials to initiate muscle contractions (Chapter 1). In contrast to the situation in the stomach and small intestine, wave activity is generated by the circular rather than the longitudinal muscle layer. Slow waves are generated at a site in a more caudal part of the most proximal one-third of the colon. A pacemaker generates slow waves at a frequency of about 6 cycles per minute. The slow waves move cephalad toward the cranial end of the colon, which has a slow-wave frequency of 4.5 cycles per minute. Because frequency of slow waves determines the rate of muscle contractions, there is a reversed gradient of motor activity between the ileocecal valve and the colonic pacemaker. The reversed gradient moves contents in the cephalad direction. This type of gradient can be produced experimentally in the small intestine by surgically reversing a small section. This results in a segment of bowel with a functional obstruction, through which the intraluminal contents are not propelled. The reversed gradient exists over the cranial third of the colon. There is virtually no gradient for slow-wave activity over the caudal half except in the most caudal 10%.

The frequency of colonic slow-wave activity is influenced by electrolyte concentrations in interstitial fluid. Hyperkalemia reduces the frequency and amplitude of slow-wave activity. Hypokalemia also reduces the amplitude.

Cholinergic agonists produce spike bursts on each wave of slow-wave activity. They prolong the duration of its activity but have no effect on its frequency. Serotonin and morphine have similar effects on the first two parameters, but they reduce the frequency.

Most observations on colonic motility are from studies in the cat. Similar studies in the dog show no major differences between the two species. When diarrhea develops as the result of natural disease or is produced by drugs, multiple pacemakers appear in the cranial part of the colon, and the integrated and reversed gradient is lost.

The colon exhibits a second type of electrical activity, characterized by a prolonged burst of spikes or electrical-response activity. This is unrelated to the slow-wave activity and its regular pattern of intermittent spike potentials. The prolonged bursts of spikes originate in the middle of the colon and progress in the caudal direction, and for this reason have been called the migrating spike burst. This activity is responsible for mass peristaltic movements. Migrating spike bursts are associated with prolonged and powerful contractions of the circular muscle layer.

The patterns of motility in the colon follow the electromyographic activity. The predominant activity in the cranial part is segmentation and retrograde peristalsis. Rings of contraction contribute to resistance in the tube, so that liquid contents entering the colon are unable to pass through rapidly. The retrograde peristalsis contributes to the reservoir function by retaining the contents so that water and electrolyte absorption can be thorough. There is virtually no gradient of electrical-control activity in the caudal part of the colon. Segmentation is the dominant form of activity. It moves the contents back and forth over very short distances and slowly moves contents toward the rectum. The migrating spike burst, which is independent of slow-wave activity, stimulates mass movements, which in turn move the colonic contents rapidly over long distances. During mass movements the segmentation contractions disappear in the segment receiving the contents.

Both extracolonic and intracolonic factors regulate colonic motility. The primary intracolonic stimulus for motility in the normal animal is distension by contents entering from the ileum. Distension stimulates segmentation via reflexes mediated through nerves in the intrinsic nervous system, slowing the passage of contents through the colon. With a low-residue diet, the small quantities of bulk entering the colon may be insufficient to stimulate normal segmentation. When that causes diarrhea, fiber added to the diet gives favorable results.

Distension of the colon also stimulates propulsive activity. The amount of undigested matter in the colon determines the degree of distension in the normal state. The amount of residue is optimum in most diets, so that colonic contents are adequately processed before being defecated. Excessive residue, as in some commercial foods, results in more frequent bowel movements. Constipation can be a problem with a normal residue diet when propulsive activity is insufficient to move colonic contents caudal at the proper rate. Added fiber frequently corrects the problem, with bowel movements returning to normal.

The extrinsic neural and humoral regulation of colonic motility is poorly understood. In general, parasympathetic activity stimulates segmentation motility; sympathetic activity produces inhibition. Sympathetic denervation increases intraluminal colonic pressure. The primary inhibitory neural pathways are noncholinergic and nonadrenergic with inhibition mediated by a substance such as ATP, VIP, or gamma-aminobutyric acid. In general, the inhibition is mediated by the synthesis and release of nitric oxide.

Reflexes coordinating colonic motility, especially movement of contents over relatively long distances, can be stimulated in one part of the colon and produce an effect in another. Regulation of the reflexes occurs on three levels, via neural activity, through prevertebral ganglia, lumbosacral spinal centers, and centers in the brain. The reflexes through prevertebral ganglia are complicated in that the nerve processes contain a number of peptides and other chemicals that can act as neurotransmitters. They include VIP, enkephalins, substance P, somatostatin, CCK, and bombesin.

The effects of drugs on colonic function are not well understood. Cholinergic agents usually stimulate contraction of the right side of the colon and inhibit the motility in the distal colon, which together evacuate the colon. Anticholinergics have more unpredictable effects on colonic motility. Any depression of motility is slight and brief. Beta-adrenergic drugs inhibit motility. Morphine and prostaglandins stimulate colonic muscle contraction.

In summary, rhythmic segmentation, an important motor function of the colon, is stimulated by local events through the intrinsic nervous system. The extrinsic neural control is primarily inhibitory and is the important mechanism for reducing segmentation activity. It is only after resistance is removed from the colonic conduit that propulsive activity is able to move contents in the caudal direction. These concepts are important to understanding what type of drug to use for treating an animal with diarrhea. No drug should be used that can reduce segmentation motility even further. Thus, if anticholinergics can reduce segmentation, they should not be used. Drugs such as narcotic analgesics increase segmentation.

An old concept holds that diarrhea reflects a hypermotile state and that constipation results from a hypomotile state. Intraluminal pressure measurements of the colon show that just the opposite is true. The colon that possesses no segmentation type of motility is a flaccid tube in which intraluminal pressure is low. As a consequence there is no resistance to rapid flow through its lumen. The flow is, in large part, due to gravity, which is determined by body position. Gravitational effects are reduced when an animal is confined to a hospital cage. The clinician is presented with many chronic diarrheas that are not severe, but are frustrating, because response to cage rest is followed by relapse upon discharge from the hospital; bowel movements are normal in the hospital but become abnormal as soon as normal activity is resumed. Part of the cause for the favorable responses to the cage rest is undoubtedly reduction in the effects of gravity. With a mild food intolerance, cage rest may be the single change in management necessary for full compensation and the production of normal feces. With strong segmentation contractions, manometric pressure within the colonic lumen is great, and colonic transit is delayed, producing constipation.

Evaluation of Intestinal Motility[44]

Motility in the small and large intestine can be evaluated by determining the transit time, or the time it takes for a marker to pass through the intestines. Studies of intestinal motility have used a wide variety of markers in normal animals, abnormal animals, and animals treated with drugs. Transit times are usually estimated from the rate of barium movement in an upper GI study. In humans, barium studies suggest that small intestinal transit is more rapid in the diarrheic state, but that is not true if the barium is given with a test meal. A number of other techniques have shown that small intestinal transit time is not altered in patients with diarrhea that arises from many different causes. In fact, it is possible to increase the rate of small intestinal transit with some drugs, such as metoclopramide, without necessarily causing diarrhea. Diarrhea caused by increased secretion of intestinal fluid following administration of prostaglandins is not associated with a faster small intestinal transit. Clinical and experimental studies both show that rapid transit of contents through the colon is the consistent feature of diarrheas, rather than an alteration in small intestinal transit. Colonic transit increases with small-bowel problems when the reserved gradient is lost. Diarrhea is defined partly by changes in fecal weight, which is determined largely by colonic function. Fecal weights are greater after colonic resection, but not after small intestinal resection. In summary, transit times are difficult to measure, and the abnormalities most important in producing diarrhea are found in the large intestine.

Stress and emotions are recognized as factors in the development of colonic problems based on abnormal motility. Psychogenic influences in humans can produce a chronic state that alternates between diarrhea and constipation. A similar type of problem has not been proven in small animals.

DIGESTION AND ABSORPTION

Digestion

The pancreas, intestinal mucosa, and biliary system contribute secretions for the intestinal digestion and absorption of a meal. The pancreas secretes enzymes that are important for the digestion of starch, protein, and lipids (Figure 17–12). Some enzymes are synthesized in an active form, including an alpha-amylase, lipase, ribonuclease, deoxyri-

Starch	-	α-amylase
Lipids	-	lipase
		phospholipase
Proteins	-	trypsin
		chymotrypsin
		carboxypeptidase
		elastase
		collagenase
		leucine aminopeptidase
		ribonuclease
		deoxyribonuclease

FIGURE 17–12. Enzymes secreted by the pancreas and the substrates they act on.

bonuclease, collagenase, and leucine aminopeptidase. Enzymes synthesized as inactive precursors are the proteases trypsin, chymotrypsin, carboxypeptidase and elastase, and the lipase phospholipase A. The pancreas also secretes an alkaline fluid to provide a medium for optimum enzyme activity. Intestinal mucosal cells synthesize and secrete substances into the lumen of the gut and the circulation. Secretions into the lumen consist of mucosal brush border digestive enzyme (disaccharidases and peptidases), secretory immunoglobulins, and fluids resembling extracellular fluid. Small intestinal secretions are important because their loss causes major clinical signs of disease. The chemicals secreted into the circulation are peptide endocrines, biogenic amines, and prostaglandins, all which are suggested to participate in the regulating of gastrointestinal function. Bile acids are secreted by the liver and evacuated through the biliary system. They are required for normal lipid digestion and absorption.

DIGESTION OF CARBOHYDRATES.[45–48] Carbohydrate in the form of starch is usually the major constituent of diets for small animals. Some diets contain disaccharides, such as sucrose and lactose. Sucrose is not a usual dietary ingredient unless the animal is fed semimoist dog foods or human foods. Lactose is the major source of carbohydrate in animals that subsist on milk.

One component of starch is amylose, a straight chain polymer repeating units of glucose connected by alpha-1,4 bonds. Amylopectin, the major component of starch, has the same basic structure as amylose except that some chains of glucose are attached to others by alpha-1,6 linkages. Pancreatic alpha-amylase rapidly acts on starch at most alpha 1,4 bonds to

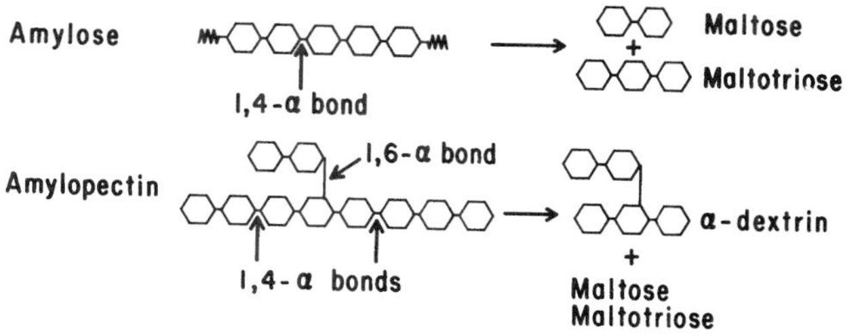

FIGURE 17–13. Schematic showing the sites of action of pancreatic amylase at the 1,4-alpha bonds of amylose and amylopectin to produce maltose, maltotriose, and alpha-dextrin. Amylase does not act at 1,6-alpha bonds.

hydrolyze it into smaller units (Figure 17–13). Very little glucose is produced. Amylase action produces maltose, a disaccharide of glucose, and maltotriose, a three-unit carbohydrate. These same carbohydrates are produced from amylopectin hydrolysis, which also produces alpha-limit dextrins that are composites of glucose, connected by both the alpha-1,4 and alpha-1,6 linkage. Oligosaccharides are also produced.

Amylase is a protein that can be rapidly and irreversibly denatured by the low pH of acid chyme, but that possibility is prevented by pancreatic secretion of a bicarbonate-rich fluid. The level of carbohydrate in the diet determines the amount of amylase secreted. High- starch diets increase amylase secretion, and glucose substituted for starch further increases the amount secreted. This adaptation can be seen within 4 to 5 days of a diet change. The pancreas produces no known inhibitors of amylase.

Complete hydrolysis of carbohydrates to glucose is necessary for absorption. Final hydrolysis is achieved by brush border enzymes of the mucosal epithelial cell. The enzymes are part of the outer membrane surface and may extend into the glycocalyx.[49] The enzymes are not released into the intestinal contents until the cell desquamates and degenerates. Thus, the enzymes are released without being secreted. Brush border enzymes are designated by their activities as maltase, sucrase, alpha-dextranase (isomaltase), and lactase.[50] There are at least two forms of each enzyme. Some maltases are not specific in activity; these hydrolyze sucrose and alpha-limit dextrins as well as maltose.

The levels of carbohydrate-digesting enzymes in the brush border vary with age, diet, and disease (Table 17–1). The concentrations of enzyme activity generally reflect an animal's needs. Young animals receiving lactose as the only source of carbohydrates have high levels of lactase. At weaning, lactase activity decreases, and concentrations of maltase and sucrase increase to reflect the carbohydrate composition of the diet. When a diet is changed, at least 2 days are required for the activity of these enzymes to adapt to new levels. This is the time the cells require to migrate from the crypts to the villus. The enzymes not only respond to dietary levels of carbohydrates but also respond to the amount of undigested carbohydrates in the lumen of the intestine. A decrease in the secretion of pancreatic enzymes causes an increase in the levels of brush border enzymes in order to digest carbohydrates,[51] an adaption expected with chronic pancreatic exocrine deficiency. Disaccharidase activity increases in intestinal contents following cholecystokinin-induced release of enzymes.[52] This is the only recognized means of stimulating enzyme release from the brush border.

Alteration of the mucosal brush border by disease results in a loss of its enzyme activity that often produces diarrhea. Enteritis due to infectious or toxic agents, overgrowth of the intestinal microflora, and bacterial enterotoxins result in a loss of enzyme.[53] Brush border enzyme activity is essential for completion of carbohydrate digestion and absorption, without which malabsorption appears and can cause diarrhea.

Bile salts that have been deconjugated by the large numbers of bacteria produce the damaging effects of bacterial overgrowth—distortion and denudation of microvilli. Following this type of insult, it takes 2 to 7 days for enzyme levels to return to normal.[54]

Diarrhea of unknown etiology is often managed with a high-carbohydrate diet, primarily starch. With problems not involving the small intestine and not reducing disaccharidase activity, animals can adapt to greater amounts of carbohydrates and continue to digest nutrients completely. Levels of brush border disaccharidases decrease during fasting. Resumption of the feeding of carbohydrates should be gradual to allow enzyme activity to return.

DIGESTION OF PROTEINS.[47,48,55–58] Proteins must be hydrolyzed to amino acids and peptides before absorption is possible. Protein digestion and absorption are completed in the cranial half of the small intestine. Consequently, the caudal half represents a large reserve of mucosal enzyme activity and absorptive surface. Digestion of proteins begins in the stomach, due to the action of pepsin, and is continued in the small intestine by pancreatic trypsin, chymotrypsin, elastase, and carboxypeptidase. The products of digestion are mostly small peptides (containing two to six amino acids) and a few amino acids. The pancreatic enzymes are more important than pepsin for protein digestion. Even when there is no pancreatic enzyme activity, half to two-thirds of the dietary protein is absorbed.

The most important pancreatic proteases are endopeptidases, which split bonds within the peptide chain (Figure 17–14). These include the trypsins, which break bonds at the site of a basic amino acid, and elastase, which acts at the site of a nonpolar amino acid. Trypsin is secreted as an inactive precursor, trypsinogen, which is prevented from being activated in the pancreas by pancreatic trypsin inhibitors. Enzymatically active trypsin is produced by the action of the intestinal enzyme enterokinase, which splits a hexapeptide from the amino-terminal end of trypsinogen. Once activated, trypsin rapidly activates more trypsin and also activates chymotrypsin, elastase, carboxypeptidase, and phospholipase. The carboxypeptidases split amino acids from either the carboxyl or the amino end.

The rates of secretion and disappearance of the proteases determine the level of protease activity in the intestine. The rate of synthesis and secretion of pancreatic proteases parallels the level of protein in the diet. Deficiencies in amino acids can result in decreased pancreatic proteases. Protease inhibitors added to the diet stimulate an increase in pancreatic proteases, as is seen by feeding a high-protein diet. A high-protein diet stimulates both the synthesis and transport of zymogen from the acinar cell to the duct. The level of activity of proteases in the intestine is also determined by the synthesis and secretion of adequate amounts of enterokinase. Duodenal mucosal disease can reduce the luminal activity of this protease-activating enzyme.

Protein digestion is completed at the brush border and within the epithelial cell. Small peptides can be completely hydrolyzed at the brush border. They can also be absorbed by the epithelial cell and hydrolyzed within. Small amounts of proteins can be absorbed unaltered and can be resistant to protease activity outside or inside the cell. Very little peptidase activity is found in the lumen of the intestine. About 80% is found within the cell in the cytoplasm in a soluble form. The remainder is bound to the brush border membranes. The intracellular peptidases are similar to those found in other organs of the body. The functions of the

Table 17–1

BRUSH BORDER CARBOHYDRASE ACTIVITIES IN DOGS

DISACCHARIDASE	ACTIVITY*
Maltase	0.238 ± 0.13
Sucrase	0.057 ± 0.02
Lactase	0.026 ± 0.01
Amyloglucosidase	0.049 ± 0.03

*Nanomoles of disaccharide hydrolyzed/mg protein/minute. Data from reference 50.

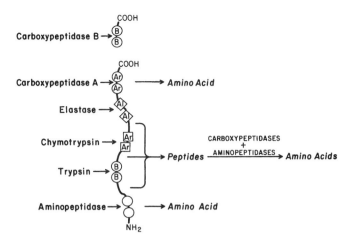

FIGURE 17-14. Schematic showing the sites of action of pancreatic proteases. B = basic amino acid, Ar = aromatic amino acid, Al = aliphatic amino acid.

brush border and cytoplasmic enzymes are probably complementary. Large amounts of different peptidases are found, each with the ability to hydrolyze a number of different peptides. The rate of hydrolysis varies for each peptide, suggesting that each peptidase has some degree of specificity. The enzymes found, designated according to the activity they show, are called dipeptidases, tripeptidases, oligopeptidases, and leucylnaphthylamidase.

The regulation of epithelial cell peptidase activity is not understood as well as that for carbohydrate digestion. High-protein diets increase brush border peptidase activity, but effects on intracellular peptidases are variable and depend on the type of protein.[59] Starvation decreases enzyme activity in the brush border but increases that in the cell.[60] Although brush border enzymes are lost with extensive mucosal disease, clinical signs of protein malabsorption seldom follow. Thus, the importance of brush border enzymes is questionable. If pancreatic enzymes can carry digestion to the level of small peptides, and if peptides can be absorbed and hydrolyzed within epithelial cells, the brush border enzymes are not needed. A deficiency of one mucosal peptidase, enterokinase, causes protein malabsorption. This enzyme is released to activate trypsin from trypsinogen

DIGESTION OF LIPIDS.[47,61–65] Digestion of lipids requires pancreatic lipase and bile acids. Lipase hydrolyzes fatty acids from the outer ester bonds of triglyceride molecules (Figure 17–15), leaving a monoglyceride with the fatty acid esterified to the middle carbon. In that state, long chain fatty acids and monoglycerides, normally relatively water insoluble, become very soluble, following interaction with bile acids to form micelles. Lipase hydrolysis is necessary for absorption because triglycerides and diglycerides are not solubilized by bile acids. The emulsification properties of bile acids increase the effectiveness of lipase by increasing the surface area of the oil-water interface. Bile acids also trap free fatty acids in emulsified fats, which ensures that resynthesis of triglycerides does not occur before absorption. Like many enzymes, lipase catalyzes both directions of the chemical process, hydrolysis and esterification.

Pancreatic lipase is very unstable and is susceptible to rapid and irreversible inactivation. Lipase is secreted in its active form, but it requires bile salts and a lipase cofactor for full enzyme activity. Lipase has a pH optimum of 8.0, which bile acids reduce to 6.0, making the enzyme more effective at the

pH of duodenal contents. A fat-rich diet increases pancreatic lipase secretion, with unsaturated fatty acids the most potent stimulus. High-protein diets also stimulate synthesis and secretion of lipase. High-carbohydrate diets decrease lipase production. No inhibitors of lipase have been found in animals.

The pancreas secretes phospholipases as precursors that require activation by trypsin. Calcium is necessary for optimum activity. Phospholipase A splits the fatty acid from the beta position in lecithin, cephalin, phosphatidyl ethanolamine, and the plasminogens containing choline and ethanolamine. Removal of this fatty acid from lecithin produces a toxic compound, lysolecithin, which enters into cell membranes and results in lysis of the cell. Another phospholipase splits fatty acids from the A position in lysolecithin. Lysolecithin, produced in the intestine by phospholipase activity on phospholipids in bile and the diet, does not damage mucosal epithelial cells. No natural inhibitors of phospholipase have been identified.

Bile acid molecules have polar and nonpolar regions. The nonpolar areas combine with monoglycerides and fatty acids to form micelles, small particles 40Å to 50Å in diameter. The polar regions cover the surface of the micelle, with nonpolar lipids and bile acids in the center (Figure 17–15). The lipid interior also contains fat-soluble vitamins and water-insoluble steroids, such as cholesterol. The formation of micelles is a physical-chemical reaction that proceeds spontaneously when the concentration of bile acids, monoglycerides, and fatty acids is optimum. A micellar solution is clear and waterlike, in contrast to an emulsion of fats. The smallest particle that can be produced by emulsification is about 100 times the diameter of a micelle. The formation of micelles increases the amount of fatty acids in solution by 1000 times. Small

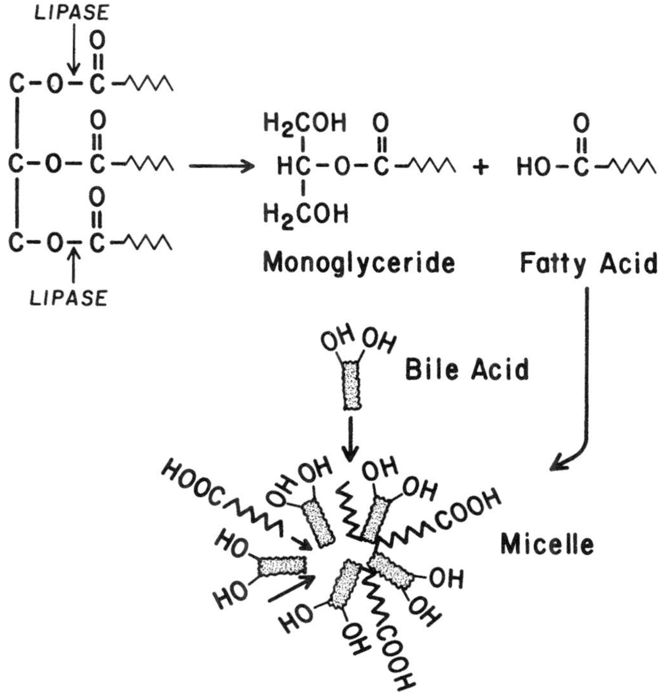

FIGURE 17-15. Schematic showing the digestion of triglycerides by pancreatic lipase and the formation of micelles. Lipase acts on the outer two ester bonds to form monoglycerides and fatty acids. Micelles are formed spontaneously when monoglycerides, fatty acids, and bile acids are present. Micelles are water soluble because the polar groups of their constituents are on the surface of the sphere, with the hydrophobic part of the molecules in the interior.

emulsified fat particles pass through the lipid part of the membrane, but their diffusion coefficient is one-eighth of micelles, which pass through the cell membrane much more readily.

The brush border contains enzymes with esterase activity for cholesterol and vitamin A esters, but the significance is unknown because there are pancreatic enzymes with this activity. The brush border also contains sphingomyelinase and phospholipase A activity.

Dietary fat levels vary in commercial pet foods, with canned preparations containing more fat than dry foods. All meat diets are also high in fat. Fat absorption is usually nearly complete, so that less than 5% of the dietary fat is excreted in the feces. The essential requirements for normal fat excretion are adequate bile and lipase secretions and normal surface area of the small intestinal mucosa. Surprisingly, the complete loss of either lipase activity or bile acids does not result in complete fat malabsorption. At least 50% of dietary fats can be absorbed in the absence of bile to form micelles. The same amount is absorbed with a loss of all pancreatic enzymes. Thus, although lipase and bile are not necessary for lipid absorption, they are essential for normal digestion and absorption. With progressive reductions in pancreatic enzyme activity, lipid malabsorption may be apparent before that of other nutrients. Lipid assimilation is slower than that of other nutrients and requires most of the small intestine. Inadequate lipase activity delays lipid digestion and presents more lipid to the terminal small intestine for digestion. The terminal jejunum and ileum do not have the capacity to absorb increased amounts of lipids.

DETERMINANTS OF INTRALUMINAL ENZYME ACTIVITY. Adequate intraluminal pancreatic enzyme activity is required to satisfy digestive needs. With time, this activity disappears, although not before digestion is complete. The pH of the medium into which the enzymes are secreted, enzyme inhibitors, and the activity of bacterial proteases determine the rate of disappearance of enzyme activity. At a low pH trypsin is more stable than amylase or lipase but is rapidly degraded by pepsin. Both trypsin and chymotrypsin activities diminish during their transit through the intestines, with trypsin disappearing more rapidly. Some of the loss of activity may be due to inhibitors found in pancreatic secretions. Although these inhibitors reduce the activity of most proteases found in the intestine, most of the inhibitors are rapidly degraded. Bacterial lysosomal proteases destroy inhibitors that are resistant to tryptic digestion by pancreatic proteases. Disappearance of intestinal pancreatic enzyme activity is due primarily to digestion by proteases from the pancreas, bacteria, and mucosal cell lysosomes. Bacterial overgrowth of the small intestine causes a faster enzyme destruction, resulting in maldigestion and malabsorption. Effects of colonic bacteria to inactivate digestive enzymes are apparent in fecal digestion tests where aged fecal samples show no proteolytic activity, but a fresh sample repeated on the same individual shows normal proteolytic activity.

As would be expected, the synthesis and secretion of pancreatic enzymes are reduced in a patient having chronic pancreatitis or recovering from acute pancreatitis.

Secretion

FLUID AND ELECTROLYTE SECRETION: PANCREATIC.[66,67] Both the acinar cells and the cells lining the ducts derive the fluid and electrolyte component of pancreatic secretion from extracellular fluid. At low rates of secretion, pancreatic juice is similar to plasma in electrolyte composition. The bicarbon-

ate content is a little higher than in plasma, and chloride content is lower. The concentration of sodium is 10 to 12 mEq/L greater in pancreatic secretion than in plasma, the result of a lower protein content in pancreatic juice because the osmolality is the same for both fluids. Upon stimulation of fluid secretion, the concentration of bicarbonate increases and that of chloride decreases with their sum remaining fairly constant at any rate of secretion (Figure 17–16). Bicarbonate can increase to 150 mEq/L, in which case it makes up almost the total anions in the secretion. Other electrolytes in pancreatic secretion are small amounts of calcium and magnesium at lower concentrations than in plasma. Thus, the pancreas responds to stimulation with a isosmotic secretion that is like plasma, except it is rich in bicarbonate.

The fluid secreted by acinar cells is like extracellular fluid in ionic composition. It is produced by the active transport of sodium ions across the acinar cell (Figure 17–17). The movement of water that accompanies it carries all the other ions passively by "solvent drag." This activity maintains zero concentration gradients for all ions across the acinar cell, and thus electrical neutrality. As this primary secretion of fluid passes through the ducts, it is modified by the addition of duct cell secretions. The ducts actively secrete bicarbonate into the fluid and cause the stimulated secretion to be bicarbonate rich. Sodium is also secreted by a process that may be active. The ducts are permeable to both bicarbonate and chloride, however, so that the ions can readily diffuse across the duct epithelium, and pancreatic secretions can equilibrate with interstitial fluid. At low rates of secretion when little bicarbonate and fluid are secreted, less fluid moves slowly through a duct that is permeable to anions. Under these conditions chloride and bicarbonate readily diffuse across duct membranes and equilibrate with the interstitial fluids; the final product of secretion becomes more like plasma. At high rates of secretion after stimulation by secretin, large amounts of bicarbonate are secreted, and because the fluid moves through the ducts rapidly, little bicarbonate diffuses across the permeable membranes to equilibrate with the plasma and interstitial fluid. In this case the final product of secretion is rich in bicarbonate.

Epithelial cells that produce and transport bicarbonate contain large amounts of carbonic anhydrase. In the pan-

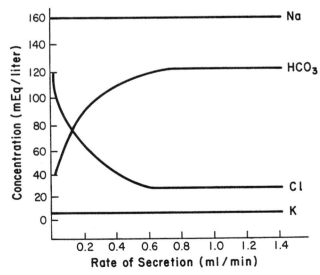

FIGURE 17-16. Graph showing the ionic composition of pancreatic secretions at different rates. The bicarbonate content increases when the pancreas is stimulated to secrete. The chloride concentration varies inversely with that of bicarbonate.

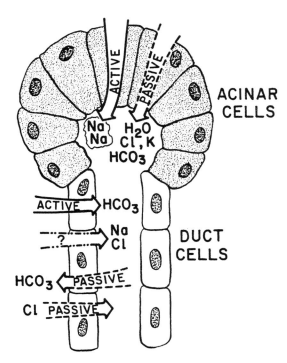

FIGURE 17-17. Schematic of pancreatic acinar cell and secretory duct. Active secretion of sodium by the acinar cells and bicarbonate by the duct cells produces the final secretion. Passive movement of ions through the semipermeable membranes of the ducts modifies the secretion.

creas this enzyme is found only in the ductal epithelium, where it catalyzes the reversible reactions in which carbon dioxide is hydrated to form carbonic acid (Figure 17–18). Inhibitors of carbonic anhydrase have been used to study pancreatic secretion. They have a general effect of inhibiting the production and transport of bicarbonate. It has been shown, however, that in the pancreas one carbonic anhydrase inhibitor, acetazolamide, interferes with both chloride and enzyme secretion as well as with bicarbonate secretion. Other studies have shown that if carbon dioxide is not present in the bathing medium of in vitro pancreatic tissue, very little bicarbonate is produced. Thus, some of the bicarbonate is derived from plasma carbon dioxide as well as from plasma bicarbonate. In clinical cases, the pancreas's secretion of bicarbonate is increased by metabolic alkalosis and impaired by metabolic or respiratory acidosis.

The volume and bicarbonate concentration of pancreatic juice changes with pancreatic disease. The volume of secretion is reduced in humans with most types of pancreatic disease except in those recovering from acute pancreatitis, in which case secretion rates are abnormally high although the total output of bicarbonate is normal. The capacity to secrete bicarbonate is reduced in chronic pancreatitis, pancreatic atrophy, and pancreatic carcinomas. In humans with chronic pancreatitis, the capacity to secrete bicarbonate is reduced more than the capacity to secrete enzymes. In humans recovering from acute pancreatitis, enzyme secretion is reduced while volume and bicarbonate secretions are normal or increased. Similar changes are found in small animals with pancreatic disease.[68]

Calcium and magnesium, normally at a lower concentration in pancreatic juice than in plasma, are part of the secretion of the acinar cell, with the amount secreted in proportion to the amount of amylase secreted.

CONTROL OF PANCREATIC SECRETION.[69-72] The autonomic nervous system and a number of endocrines control pancreatic secretion (Figure 17–19). It is stimulated, and in some cases inhibited, by events that occur in the initial stages of feeding as well as by the well-known events that occur when food enters the intestine. The regulation of pancreatic secretion has been divided into cephalic, gastric, and intestinal phases.

The cephalic phase is the initial step, and its effects are mediated primarily though the autonomic nervous system. This phase is stimulated by such psychologic factors as the anticipation of food, which is reinforced by the oral events in eating. The motor pathway is in parasympathetic fibers in the vagi; the pancreatic response is a small volume of secretion, rich in enzymes. Stimulation of the cephalic phase initiates the synthesis of new enzymes in preparation for the food that will soon enter the intestine and require their activity for digestion. The pancreas does not contain a large store of enzymes, and production must begin early in order to supply some of the needs necessary to digest a meal. Vagal impulses have little effect in stimulating the secretion of water and electrolytes, One component of the cephalic phase is controlled by a pathway that is partly neural and partly humoral. Stimulation of the cephalic phase causes the vagally mediated release of gastrin from the gastric mucosa. Gastrin, a peptide hormone structurally similar to cholecystokinin (CCK), stimulates pancreatic secretion. Thus, this hormone participates in stimulation of the small-volume and enzyme-rich secretion in the cephalic phase.

The gastric phase of pancreatic secretion, stimulated by events in the stomach, is mediated both neurally and humorally. One entirely neural pathway is a vagovagal reflex (gastropancreatic reflex), in which stimulation of the body of the stomach sends information to the brain via vagal afferents, and, after central synaptic transmission, a motor response is sent to the pancreas via vagal parasympathetics. Vagotomy abolishes the reflex. The second compo-

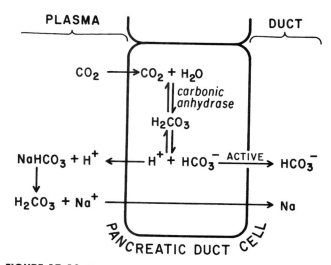

FIGURE 17-18. Pancreatic duct cell that forms bicarbonate from carbonic acid and secretes it via an active process into the duct. The reaction requires the catalytic enzyme carbonic anhydrase to provide a sufficient amount of bicarbonate for secretion.

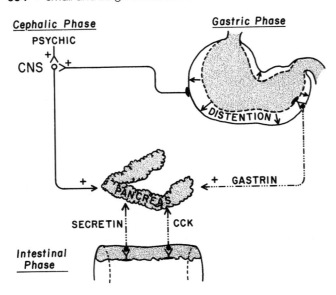

FIGURE 17-19. Regulation of pancreatic secretion. The cephalic phase primarily stimulates the secretion of enzymes by a cholinergic neural pathway. Distention and food in the stomach stimulates a neural pathway through the CNS and the release of gastrin to cause the pancreas to secrete enzymes. When acid chyme enters the intestine, secretion and CCK are released to stimulate the pancreas.

nent of the gastric phase involves a humoral response mediated by gastrin, a hormone released by chemical and mechanical stimulation of the antrum of the stomach. These stimuli evoke a local cholinergic pathway and release gastrin. That response is well documented, but it is less certain whether stimulation of the antrum initiates another vagovagal reflex to either directly stimulate the pancreas via nerve fibers or indirectly stimulate the organ via gastrin release. The response of the pancreas to either direct neural or indirect gastrin stimulation is, again, a small volume of enzyme-rich juice.

The intestinal phase of pancreatic secretion, stimulated by events in the small intestine. is hormonally mediated. There may be short neural pathways in the wall of the intestine that are involved in the release of the hormones. The hormones synthesized primarily to stimulate pancreatic secretion are CCK and secretin. Less potent stimulators of pancreatic secretion are gastrin and vasoactive intestinal peptide (VIP). All four hormones are synthesized and released from the intestinal mucosa even though the primary site of gastrin production is in the antrum of the stomach. Intraluminal ionized calcium appears to be a universal stimulant of hormone release. Classically, it has considered that acid pH releases secretin and that digestive products release CCK. Acid pH in the duodenum is the single important factor that stimulates the release of secretin. Below pH 3.0, the amount of bicarbonate that is secreted is independent of the pH of the chyme entering the duodenum. Between pH 3.0 and 4.5, the amount of bicarbonate secreted is proportional to the pH of chyme in the duodenum. The secretory response is also a function of both the rate of entry of titrable acid into

the intestine and the length of small intestine that is acidified. The threshold below which the release of secretin is stimulated is pH 4.5. The amount of secretin in the duodenal mucosa follows a gradient that decreases aborally. Fatty acids also stimulate the release of secretin and bicarbonate secretion. The half-life of secretin is less than 3 minutes and the kidney is the major site of its degradation.[73,74]

The amino acid L-isomers of tryptophan, phenylalanine, valine, and possibly methionine stimulate the release of CCK. Acid pH and fatty acids of the aliphatic series, with carbon chains greater than 10, also release CCK. Fatty acids such as oleate are a potent stimulator of CCK release and pancreatic enzyme secretion, even more so than amino acids. Acid pH is a weak stimulus of CCK release. The release of duodenal gastrin is stimulated by neutral or alkaline pH and inhibited by acid pH. Both D- and L-isomers of amino acids of the sarcosine series (glycine, alanine, serine, etc) also release duodenal gastrin. Short chain aliphatic alcohols and fatty acids (C2 and C3) are weak stimulators of gastrin release. The physiologic effect of VIP on pancreatic secretion most closely resembles that of secretin but with less potency. Vagal stimulation is the normal stimulus for VIP release.

The effects of these hormones are selective stimulation, on one hand, of the secretion of a large volume of fluid rich in bicarbonate and, on the other, of a secretion rich in enzymes. Secretin and VIP primarily stimulate fluid secretion. Other hormones similar to VIP, glucagon and gastric inhibitory peptide (GIP), have variable effects. The amino acid sequences of these peptides are similar; the terminal three amino acids at the end of the peptide, which are essential for physiologic activity, are the same for secretin and VIP. Secretin is the hormone designed for maximum stimulation. VIP has about 20% of the potency of secretin. Because these structurally similar hormones stimulate secretion, they both bind to the receptor site on pancreatic secretory cells. When bound to the cell, VIP prevents the binding of secretin, thus competitively inhibiting the action of secretin. Glucose in the lumen of the intestine also inhibits the maximum secretory response to the infusion of secretin. Glucose in the small intestine causes the release of glucagon, and the blunting of the secretin response may be the competitive inhibition of secretin by glucagon. Small doses of glucagon inhibit the pancreatic secretion stimulated by secretin and CCK, but have no effect on basal secretion.

Gastrin and CCK constitute another family of gastrointestinal hormones. All forms of gastrin and CCK have the same five amino acids at the terminal end that are essential for activity. Thus, it is expected their functions will overlap. Gastrin stimulates pancreatic secretion as well as gastric secretion. Although CCK's major function is to stimulate the pancreas, it also stimulates gastric secretion. Thus, CCK is a partial agonist of gastric secretion and a full agonist of pancreatic secretion. When CCK is infused in a dog stimulated to maximum gastric secretion, the rate of secretion falls. This illustrates how structurally similar CCK, a partial agonist for gastric secretion, competitively displaces gastrin from the receptor sites on the partial cells; the weaker stimulus is unable to promote the maximum secretory capacity of the cells. However, at low levels of gastrin-stimulated gastric secretion, CCK acts as a partial agonist and will augment secretion by binding to any free receptor sites.

Each end organ in the digestive tract has two receptor sites, one for the gastrin family of hormones and one for the secretin family. Pairs of hormones within a family may interact by augmenting (CCK on low rates of gastric secretion) or by inhibiting, either competitively (VIP on secretin-stimulated pancreatic secretion) or noncompetitively, the primary action of one member of the pair. There also is some potentiation between hormones bound to the two receptor sites. For example, CCK augments the low fluid and bicarbonate response of the pancreas stimulated by small amounts of secretin. Gastrin and cholinergic stimuli have the same effect. Secretin and VIP have a similar effect of potentiating low rates of enzyme secretion stimulated by CCK.

The pancreas is a rich source of somatostatin and pancreatic polypeptide. Plasma levels of both increase after feeding, and the hormones are potent inhibitors of pancreatic secretion. Somatostatin and VIP inhibit pancreatic enzyme and bicarbonate secretions following either neural- or hormone-mediated stimulation. Because the hormones are released from cells in the pancreas to act on other cells in the pancreas, the concentrations of these hormones on their target cell would be much greater than in plasma. Peptide YY, found in highest concentration in the ileum and colon, is another inhibitor of pancreatic secretion. Fatty acids are potent stimulators of peptide YY release, especially in the distal small intestine. Cholinergic mechanisms are involved with vagally mediated pancreatic secretion and the release of many humoral agents. Anticholinergic drugs inhibit vagally mediated secretion and the release of intestinal hormones that stimulate secretion, but they have no effect on the action of the hormone on the secretory cell. Acids or food products in the intestine stimulate receptors for neural pathways to the hormone cells in the mucosa. Anticholinergics (such as atropine) usually block hormone release, and local anesthetics applied to the mucosa also prevent their release. Thus, anticholinergics can inhibit pancreatic secretion by acting both directly on the vagally mediated pathways of stimulation and indirectly on the neurally mediated release of hormones that stimulate secretion

Blood flow increases within an organ that is actively secreting digestive juices. The increased flow is necessary not only to meet the metabolic requirements for transport but also to provide the fluid and electrolytes in the secretion. Pancreatic blood flow increases when either the vagal parasympathetics or the hormones CCK and secretin stimulate the organ. The vagal effects may be the result of kallikrein-induced kinin formation, similar to the events that occur in the salivary glands during neural stimulation. It is also possible that vagal vasodilator fibers exist to produce the effect. All of the hormones discussed in this section have vasodilator properties, and in the case of VIP the property is very potent, as the name of the hormone implies. VIP can cause vasodilation to the point that a large volume of fluid is secreted into the intestinal tract. This occurs in some pathologic situations caused by a VIP-secreting tumor. Nitric oxide may be the final vasodilating mediator for neural stimulation and many circulating chemicals that increase mucosal blood flow. Substances such as acetylcholine, bradykinin, and gastrin increase mucosal blood flow by stimulating nitric oxide synthesis.

The sympathetic nervous system does not play a role in the control of normal pancreatic function. Cutting the sympathetics to the pancreas increases secretion, and stimulation causes vasoconstriction and a concomitant decrease in secretory rates. The sympathetic nerves have an important effect on the pancreas whenever they are intensely stimulated, such as during shock. The pancreas releases proteases and toxic peptides into the circulation during shock and during acute pancreatitis. Pancreatic ischemia as a result of intense sympathetic activity is either the cause or is a severe complication contributing to the problem.

INTRALUMINAL DIGESTION. Factors that determine how chemical reactions proceed dictate the hydrolysis of carbohydrates, proteins, and lipids into subunits that can be absorbed. Most of these reactions are catalyzed by enzymes with activities that are optimum at a certain pH and at a specific temperature. The optimum pH for enzymes acting in the small intestine is in the range of 7 to 8, normally provided by pancreatic secretion of bicarbonate. That may not be the case, however, in several situations. When acid contents from the stomach rapidly enter the duodenum at a rate exceeding the capacity of pancreatic secretions to neutralize them, the intestinal medium is at a pH in which the pancreatic enzymes are inactive. This situation can result from gastric surgery, which may lead to an increase in the rate of stomach emptying. Inadequate neutralization of gastric chyme is also a problem in an animal with pancreatic insufficiency that reduces the ability to secrete bicarbonate. In this case, pH cannot be maintained close to optimum levels until the secretion of intestinal fluid buffers the acid chyme entering from the stomach. Buffering may not happen until after the enzymes have been inactivated or after the nutrients have passed their major absorptive sites. Some of the enzymes require specific ions that act as cofactors. Deficiencies of cofactors have not been recognized as a cause of clinical problems. In general, isotonic conditions should prevail for maximum activity. As in any enzymatic reactions, the amount of enzyme and the amount of substrate determine the amount of products from hydrolytic activity. All of the chemical reactions proceed at a given rate, varying with the conditions described, and so the nutrients must remain in the intestine for a given time before digestion is complete.

Starch digestion and absorption was at one time thought to be more complete than that for protein and lipids. Starch assimilation, however, can be incomplete even when a low starch diet is fed.[75] The source of dietary starch is one factor determining variability in assimilation (Figure 17–20). Sources of starch such as rice are digested more completely than other sources of starch.[76] Digestibility also varies between different strains of one grain, and processing has an additional important effect (Table 17–2).[77] Commercially prepared diets contain modified food starches added for non-nutrient purposes, and they may be digested less efficiently.[78] Protein digestion is not as important as carbohydrate digestion because the protein content of the diet is much less, and peptides are absorbed as efficiently as amino acids. Because digestion of lipids is slower, a delay in intestinal transit is more important for optimum fat assimilation than for the other nutrients. In general, absorption, not digestion, is the rate-limiting step in the assimilation of nutrients in the alimentary canal.

INTESTINAL SECRETION OF FLUID AND ELECTROLYTES.[79–81] Under certain normal and abnormal conditions, fluid and electrolytes are secreted in the small and large intestine. Abnormal secretion of fluid by the small and large intestine is a significant cause of diarrhea. Understanding the pathophysiology and management of diarrhea due to hypersecretion of intestinal fluid depends on knowledge of how the normal mechanisms operate because they are suggested to be functioning at an uncontrolled rate.

Under normal conditions, fluid is secreted into the intestine upon the delivery of hypertonic contents into that segment. The contents of the intestine also become hypertonic as digestion proceeds in order to reduce large molecules to their subunits. This greatly increases the number of osmotically active particles, generating a force to draw fluid into the lumen.

The mucosa of the small intestine is the membrane most permeable to water and ion movement of any body surface facing the external environment. This is the site for greatest potential loss of fluid from the body. Within the small intestine the mucosa of the duodenum is the most permeable.

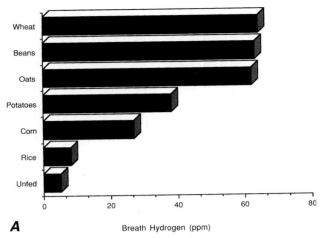

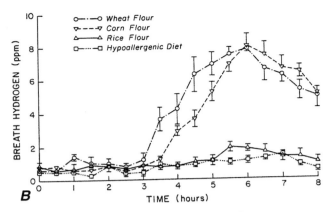

FIGURE 17-20. *(A)* Breath hydrogen concentration (humans) after ingestion of 100 g of carbohydrate in various forms. Adapted from reference 76. *(B)* Breath hydrogen concentration (dogs) after ingestion of various forms of carbohydrate added to a hypoallergenic diet. Adapted from reference 130.

The jejunum is 10 times as permeable to water movement as the stomach. Rates of flux for sodium in the stomach are virtually zero compared with the high flux rates in the small intestine. The mucosa becomes less permeable in the caudal direction, making the ileum least permeable. The large intestine is relatively impermeable to fluid and sodium movement. Fluid moves across the mucosa through cells and through tight junctions between cells. Tight junctions are more permeable to fluid and ion movement than cell membranes. Fluid moves across the mucosa by diffusion, and chemicals that plug channels in the tight junctions dramatically reduce passive diffusional fluxes across the cell. As much as 8 to 10 L of fluid move in and out of the intestine daily in a 20 kg animal. The diffusional fluxes in and out are equal, so that during fasting the intestine remains empty. With the extracellular fluid volume representing 25% of the body weight, the diffusional fluxes account for the daily movement of a volume double that of the total extracellular fluid volume. Although large bidirectional fluxes of fluid are a normal feature of an epithelial surface, it is apparent that any shift in the forces that maintain the balance can cause large movements of extracellular fluid into the intestinal tract, which is essentially outside of the body. A number of factors determine the permeability of the mucosa as well as regulate the fluxes.

The number and size of a membrane's pores determine its permeability. The pores for water, ions, and polar molecules are suggested to be water-filled pores. The pores for lipid-soluble substances are thought to be in the lipid layers of the membrane. The overall permeability of the epithelial surface is a composite of properties of all its cell membranes. This includes characteristics of the cell's basal and apical surface and its intercellular junctions. Permeability to passive movement of water and ions is in the so-called tight junction. The chemical environment immediately adjacent to the membrane also determines the passive movement of water and ions. The lipid surface of the cell membrane causes a layer of water to be oriented along its surface; the water is so structured that ions are excluded. Physical chemical forces produce this barrier, the "unstirred" water layer, which makes a membrane less permeable to water and ion movement. The concept of different types of pores is a simplified functional concept that has no anatomic counterpart.

Figure 17–21 depicts the direction and magnitude of the passive diffusional fluxes across the intestinal mucosa. Fluid is shown moving from the intestine into the circulation, representing the absorption of all other fluid entering the intestinal tract each day. This fluid is contributed by the diet and secretions of salivary, gastric, pancreatic, and intestinal juices, constituting 2 to 2.5 L of fluid that the intestine in a 20 kg animal must absorb. Active energy-dependent transport processes absorb this fluid at constant rates unless the mucosa is damaged. Another flux, shown in Figure 17–21, represents secretion of fluid into the intestine.

Secretions of intestinal fluid are similar in composition to secretions of extracellular fluid. Osmolality and sodium concentration are the same as those of extracellular fluid. The concentration of bicarbonate is low in secretions from the cranial small intestine and high in secretions from the caudal part. This difference results in a pH as low as 6.3 cranially and as high as 7.8 in the ileum. The mechanism for modification of bicarbonate is unknown. The primary secretion of intestinal fluid may be similar in composition to extracellular fluid, which is then modified by the appropriate secretion and absorption of hydrogen and bicarbonate ions. Experimental studies supporting that scheme show that fluid secreted at low rates is modified maximally, so that bicarbonate levels are very low in the cranial small intestine and very high in the caudal part.[82] However, in the fluid secreted at maximal rates the concentration of bicarbonate in each region changes and approaches bicarbonate levels in plasma.

The concentration of potassium in intestinal secretions is 10 to 15 mEq/L, which also differs from the concentration in extracellular fluid. Losses of small intestinal secretions deplete total body potassium. Potassium levels are high in intestinal secretions because of the permeability of epithelial membranes for potassium and because of the electrical potential gradient across the mucosa. The potential is created by the differential transport of ions in the transport processes.

The mechanisms for intestinal fluid secretion and their regulation are incompletely understood. The secretion of fluid is suggested to be due to an active secretory mechanism in the epithelial cell. In addition, however, fluid can move into the intestine as a result of changes in the forces that determine the passive fluxes. The secretion of intestinal fluid is undoubtedly an effect of both active and passive secretory processes.

Table 17–2

FACTORS AFFECTING STARCH DIGESTIBILITY

FOOD FORM	FIBER (TYPE)
Particle size	Antinutrients
Starch source	Phytate
Amylose content	Lectins
Amylopectin content	Tannins
Degree of gelatinization	Saponins
Cooking process	Enzyme inhibitors
Starch-nutrient interactions	

Adapted from reference 77.

Many different neurohumoral chemicals, endogenous substances such as bile acids, and a number of bacterial toxins stimulate secretion of fluid in the intestine. Although there are variations between the effects of each on different species of animals and on different sites in the intestine, a general scheme can be described for the transport mechanisms they affect (Figure 17–22). Common to all of the stimulants is a property for increasing intracellular calcium by promoting either calcium entry into cells or calcium release from intracellular stores. The increased calcium stimulates prostaglandin formation following increased phospholipase and cyclooxygenase activities. Phosphatidylinositol formation, in addition to promoting prostaglandin formation, can

Factors that determine magnitude of fluxes when permeability of membranes is normal:

A&B
1. Capillary and interstitial fluid
   a. Hydrostatic pressure
   b. Colloid osmotic pressure
2. Intestinal lumen contents
   a. Osmotic pressure

C
1. Active transport of sodium
2. Active transport of sugars and amino acids

D
1. Activation of latent secretory process by enterotoxins

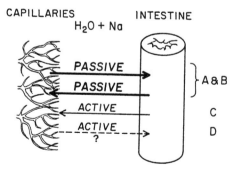

FIGURE 17–21. Direction and magnitude of passive and active movement of fluid across the intestinal mucosa. The passive fluxes account for the movements of fluid volumes that are four times the volume of fluxes absorbed by the active processes. The passive fluxes are determined by the balance of physical forces on either side of the mucosal surface. The direction and magnitude of the passive fluxes are determined by the osmolality of intestinal contents, the plasma and interstitial fluid oncotic pressures, and the hydrostatic pressures in the capillary and interstitial fluids. The secretory flux is not evident in the normal state and the basis of its generation is not known.

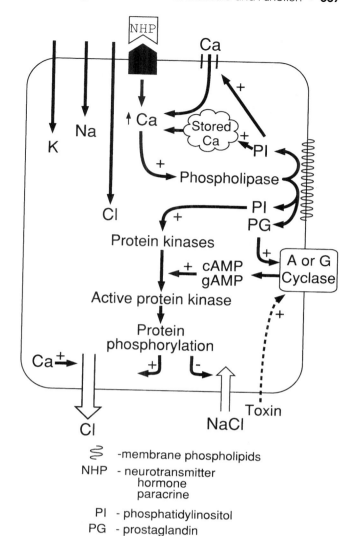

FIGURE 17–22. Schematic showing mechanisms for secretion of fluid in the small intestine.

increase membrane permeability for calcium, mobilize calcium from intracellular stores by inositol triphosphate formed from phosphatidylinositol, and activate protein kinases that may be involved with ion transport.

Prostaglandins stimulate cyclic AMP formation that promotes cellular uptake of chloride by a sodium- and potassium-dependent process. The increase in uptake may be caused by increased permeability of the cells' basolateral membranes. Prostaglandins also decrease the resistance of brush border or apical membranes so that the membranes become more permeable to chloride movement.

Increased intracellular calcium has the general effects of reducing absorption of sodium and chloride, increasing chloride secretion by increasing apical membrane permeability for chloride, and increasing efflux of potassium from cells. Some of these effects are not associated with changes in prostaglandins or cyclic AMP. Intracellular calcium concentrations also determine calcium-calmodulin levels, which regulate absorption of sodium and chloride and secretion of potassium but not chloride.

Secretion of intestinal fluid stimulated by bacterial enterotoxins has been studied to gain most of the understanding of

Table 17–3

CHEMICALS STIMULATING INTESTINAL SECRETION

Acetylcholine	GIP
Adenosine	Glucagon
ATP	Histamine
Bombesin	Neurotensin
Bradykinin	Motilin
Calcitonin	Prostaglandins
Cholecystokinin	Secretin
Gastrin	Serotonin
	Substance P
	VIP

secretory mechanisms. Toxins stimulate normal cellular mechanisms to secrete abnormal amounts of fluid. Following exposure, enterotoxins bind to brush border surfaces and secretion of fluid begins within 15 to 60 minutes. The initiation of secretion is associated with activation of the enzyme adenylate cyclase, which is located on the basal cell membranes. Some heat-stable enterotoxins stimulate the brush border enzyme guanylate cyclase to increase intracellular cyclic GMP levels. Adenylate cyclase activity increases intracellular cyclic AMP levels, which, associated with the concurrent secretion of fluid, suggests that cyclic AMP stimulates a secretory mechanism. The secreted fluid is chloride rich in the cranial small intestine and bicarbonate rich in the caudal small intestine. The mechanism of toxin action is suggested to result in the secretion of anion and the inhibition of sodium absorption. This conclusion is based on studies of in vitro preparations of intestinal mucosa in which electrical parameters and ion fluxes were measured. Inhibition of phosphodiesterase activity also increases intracellular concentrations of cyclic AMP. Theophylline inhibits this enzyme and produces the same changes in ion fluxes and electrical parameters as enterotoxins in the in vitro preparation. However, when this drug is placed in the intestine it does not duplicate the massive secretory effects of enterotoxin in the in vivo animal models. The movement of ions in in vitro tissues represents micro amounts, and it has not been shown that these these small changes in ion movements across an isolated sheet of cells represent what happens to cause massive secretion in in vivo loops in the intact animal.

During secretion passive ion fluxes across the membranes change in both directions. The permeability changes seen with enterotoxin-induced secretion are for ions only because the permeability for small nonelectrolytes does not change. No significant structural alterations are evident by light or electron microscopy. Thus, unexplained permeability changes contribute to secretion in addition to changes in activity of biochemical mechanisms for anion secretion. The best understood active ion transport process in the intestine, that for glucose-dependent sodium transport, is not affected by enterotoxins.

Physical forces that determine passive movement across the intestinal mucosa influence the secretion of intestinal fluid. The bidirectional fluxes of fluid depend on Starling forces on the basal side of the epithelial cell. Effective intracapillary hydrostatic pressure is an important determinant of fluid secretion. Intra-arterial infusion of hormonal vasodilators, such as vasoactive intestinal peptide, glucagon, and prostaglandins, increases capillary pressure and produces secretion of fluid approximating that seen with enterotoxins.[83,84] Interstitial space changes disrupt the balance of the forces that maintain a steady state in the bidirectional fluxes between blood and intestinal lumen. Bacterial enterotoxin changes the gel-like structure in this space, so that increased amounts of plasma proteins escape into the interstitial space.[11] Toxin also changes the amount of structured water within the tissue, altering diffusion fluxes across the mucosa.[85] These physical and chemical changes in mucosal tissues that produce secretion may regulate normal secretion as well as represent a pathologic mechanism.

Intestinal fluid is secreted as a normal response to hypertonic solutions within the intestine. The osmotic stimulus draws interstitial fluid into the lumen. It also causes release of vasoactive peptides and biogenic amines, increasing capillary blood flow. These events can be exaggerated in pathologic situations.

The regulation of normal intestinal secretion is poorly understood and probably involves an interaction of numerous factors. Relatively large volumes of secretion are normally produced during assimilation of a meal. Stimulation of that secretion is due to intraluminal factors, including bile acids and fatty acids that result from digestion, humoral factors (Table 17–3), and local paracrine/neural factors. To some degree the secretion of intestinal fluid may not actually be regulated but rather results from properties of the normal mucosa and the balance between physical, chemical, and electrical properties of the mucosa and the contents of the intestinal lumen.

SECRETORY IMMUNOGLUBLINS.[86,87] The mucosa secretes immunoglobulins, which adhere to and protect the brush border surface (Chapter 3). The predominant immunoglobulin is of the IgA type, with some of the others also secreted. Plasma cells that have been transformed from sensitized beta-lymphocytes synthesize IgA. Following secretion into the lamina propria, IgA is transported through the epithelial cell and transferred to the surface of the brush border. It is attached to the brush border surface by a peptide, called secretory piece, that epithelial cells synthesize.

MUCUS SECRETION.[88–90] Goblet cells secrete mucus in a gelatinous form. Secreted mucus spreads out and fuses with secretions of neighboring cells to form a continuous protective layer over the mucosal surface. This layer protects and stabilizes the microenvironment of the mucosa. The mucus layer traps microorganisms in the lumen of the small intestine. Peristalsis moves the layer caudal, reducing the numbers of bacteria in the small intestine. This also prevents colonization by foreign bacteria that are normally only transient. Mucus acts as a lubricant, and the amount secreted increases in the regions of the intestine where the contents are normally more solidified. Some mucins bind bacterial enterotoxins and inhibit their effects.[91] The mucosa responds to a toxin's presence by secreting copious amounts of mucus, a purposeful response in view of mucin's toxin-inactivating properties.

Mucus consists of a number of different substances or fluids with a high viscosity and contains significant amounts of bound carbohydrates, especially amino sugars. Glycoprotein, one type of mucin, consists of a core of protein with chains of carbohydrates attached. Chains consisting of neutral oligosaccharides produce neutral glycoproteins. Chains of sialic acid produce acid glycoproteins. Mucopolysaccharides are polymers of monosaccharides, of which some are amino sugars. They are neutral unless they contain uronic acid or sulfate esters, which give them acid properties. The mucopolysaccharides can be linked to a peptide or protein.

SECRETION BY ENDOCRINE CELLS. The hormones secreted by intestinal endocrine cells include peptides, such as secretin, cholecystokinin, enteroglucagon, vasoactive intestinal peptide, gastrin, and gastric inhibitory peptide; lipids, such as prostaglandins; and vasoactive amines, such as histamine, serotonin, kinins, and so on. The physiologic role of these chemicals is discussed in Chapter 1.

Absorption in Small and Large Intestines

Fluid and nutrients entering the small intestine are efficiently absorbed, allowing less than 5% to pass into the large intestine. Mechanisms are present to absorb digested nutrients, vitamins, and electrolytes. Small intestinal absorption of water is largely a function of glucose and sodium absorption. Digested nutrients are absorbed in the small intestine. Some that pass into the large intestine can be fermented to products that can be absorbed. Fluid is absorbed in both the small and large intestines; with malabsorption of fluid in the small intestine, the colon has a reserve capacity for accommodating and absorbing additional fluid.

ABSORPTION OF CARBOHYDRATES.[48,92–94] Carbohydrates must be in the form of a monosaccharide before absorption is possible (Figure 17–23). Monosaccharides are water-soluble molecules that are too large to move readily across cell membranes through the transport channels for water-soluble substances. The sugars glucose and galactose require a special mechanism to enter the epithelial cell. They bind to a brush border protein, which is suggested to function as a carrier that can translocate across the membrane and carry glucose to its intracellular surface, where it is released into the cytoplasm. Sodium ions determine the activity of this carrier. When a sodium-free glucose solution is administered it is likely that the passive serosal-to-lumen flux of sodium through the leaky tight junctions is large enough to provide a ready source of sodium for facilitating glucose absorption. Thus, sodium determines the absorption of glucose, but this mechanism is also a means for sodium absorption. Glucose transport is an energy-dependent process. The mechanism is able to move glucose up a concentration gradient, so that glucose can be absorbed from the intestine when intraluminal concentrations fall at the end of the absorptive process. Most of the glucose is delivered to the circulation in intact form. Some can be used for energy in the epithelial cell, resulting in the delivery to the circulation of metabolic intermediates such as lactate.

The electrochemical gradient for sodium determines hexose transport across the brush border. Sodium interacts with the transporting protein and enters the epithelial cell because of the gradient that results when low intracellular sodium levels and a negative electrical field attract a positively charged ion. Glucose interacts with the sodium transport and is carried into the cell with sodium. The energy driving the sodium and glucose entry across the brush border is a derivative of ATP consumed by an ATPase on the basolateral cell membranes. Sodium and potassium stimulate the ATPase to transport sodium from the cell and, in exchange, to move potassium into the cell. Potassium does not accumulate excessively because it leaks from the cell continuously. The transport of sodium from the cell by the ATPase maintains very low intracellular concentrations of sodium, providing the chemical gradient for sodium to move from the lumen and across the brush border. A process of facilitated diffusion transports glucose from cells across basolateral membranes. The mechanism is not dependent on cotransport with sodium or any other ion, and an ATPase is not involved.

The carrier-mediated membrane transport of sugars is specific for glucose and galactose. The grouping at carbon-2 of a

Carbohydrate Digestion and Absorption

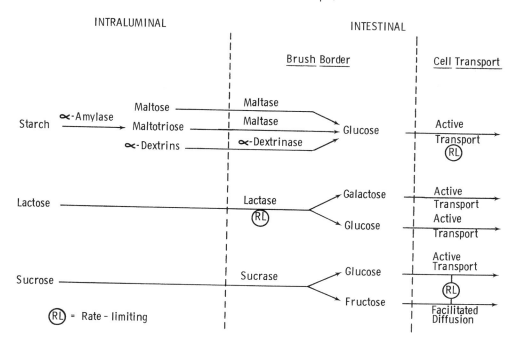

FIGURE 17–23. Digestion of carbohydrates by brush border enzymes and mode of absorption of monosaccharides into the epithelial cell.

monosaccharide is most important in determining whether the sugar can be transported. If the hydroxyl at that site is altered to form the epimere of glucose or if it is substituted the transport process is lost. Also important for the binding between sugar and carrier are the configurations at carbons 3, 4, and 6. Substitutions can be made on carbon-1 with the least effect on transport.

The other common monosaccharide in the diet, fructose, is a product of sucrose hydrolysis. Fructose moves across the brush border by diffusion, which is suggested to be facilitated by a special mechanism. Because the process is not energy dependent, fructose cannot be absorbed against a gradient. The rate of fructose absorption is only 60% to 70% that of glucose. Fructose can be converted to glucose in the mucosal epithelial cell.

In a normal meal, most of the glucose is absorbed in the cranial half of the jejunum. Because glucose can be absorbed throughout the entire length of small intestine, the caudal half represents a reserve absorptive area. When mucosal disease develops, more than half of the area must be lost before sugar malabsorption becomes a problem.

PROTEIN ABSORPTION.[48,58,94,95] The absorption of proteins involves mechanisms for the absorption of amino acids and for the absorption of peptides and proteins. Amino acids are transported across the brush border membranes after combining with a carrier in the same manner as that for glucose. Sodium is required for this interaction. The amino acids are transported through the cytoplasm and actively extruded into the lateral intercellular space. The process requires energy, and amino acids are moved up a concentration gradient so that all the amino acids in the intestinal lumen can be absorbed effectively. Glucose and galactose compete with amino acids for transport. It is thought that the competition is for energy rather than for binding to a carrier common for their transport. Amino acids, with the exception of glutamine, are not metabolized during absorption.

There are different mechanisms for transporting different types of amino acids. The L-isomers are actively transported, whereas the D-isomers are absorbed by passive diffusion. Active transport is facilitated when the alpha-carbon is bonded to (1) a free carboxyl group; (2) a free amino group; (3) a nonpolar R-group; or (4) hydrogen (Figure 17–24). The neutral amino acids containing one amino and one carboxyl group are transported by active sodium-dependent carrier mechanisms that operate very rapidly and efficiently. Dibasic amino acids, such as lysine, arginine, ornithine, and cystine, are transported by an active and partially sodium-dependent mechanism. These amino acids are absorbed rapidly, although only 10% as fast as the neutral ones. A third mechanism transports glycine and the amino acids proline and hydroxyproline. This mechanism is active and may be sodium dependent, but the rate of transport is slow. A fourth carrier system is necessary for transport of the dicarboxylic acids, glutamic acid and aspartic acid. This mechanism operates rapidly, is probably active, and is partially sodium dependent.

Special mechanisms at the basolateral membrane transport amino acids from epithelial cells. Transport is via a sodium-independent process that has no special energy requirements. The sodium gradient, which is established and maintained by an ATPase at the basolateral membrane, promotes amino acid uptake at the brush border. Thus, the mechanism is similar to that for hexose transport, where an energy-dependent process maintains sodium at very low intracellular levels.

Glutamine and glutamate are important sources of energy for intestinal epithelial cells. These amino acids can be

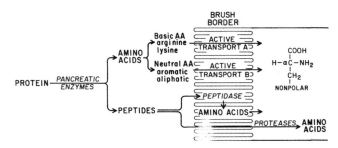

FIGURE 17–24. Digestion and absorption of dietary protein. Peptide absorption and the intracellular digestion route absorb more efficiently. Amino acid absorption is carried out by two different active transport processes, one for basic and one for neutral amino acids.

removed from the circulation as well as be absorbed from the intestine. For uptake from the circulation the basolateral membrane has a sodium-dependent mechanism similar to that for other amino acids transported across the brush border.

The carrier mechanisms for the absorption of amino acids are identical in the intestine and proximal tubule of the kidneys. An occasional animal is born without one of these mechanisms. In humans, a deficiency of the mechanism to absorb neutral amino acids results in a clinical syndrome called Hartnup disease. Deficiency develops for seven of the eight essential amino acids because they are not properly absorbed. The syndrome has not been recognized clinically in small animals, probably because they do not survive long after birth. The carrier mechanism to absorb dibasic amino acids is sometimes deficient in animals. Lysine is the only essential amino acid absorbed by this carrier, but that amino acid is also absorbed by passive diffusion and as a part of absorbed peptides, so no nutritional deficiency is apparent. Because this transport mechanism also recovers amino acids from the glomerular filtrate as it passes through the proximal tubule, a deficiency results in cystinuria from the failure of cystine reabsorption. This deficiency leads to the formation of cystine stones, which are seen occasionally in small animals.

Peptides are absorbed via mechanisms other than those for the amino acids. They are absorbed by the intestinal mucosa to provide an important means for protein assimilation. Peptides larger than three amino acids are not absorbed. Those of two and three amino acids are transported across the brush border by a sodium-independent mechanism. A proton gradient where the peptides are transported by a membrane carrier that carries hydrogen ions into the cell may drive peptide transport.[96] The observation of negative electrical potential inside the cell supports the idea that such a gradient exists. The proton gradient is thought to be established and maintained by an ATPase-driven transport of hydrogen ions across the basolateral membranes.

Absorption of amino acids is frequently more rapid from a solution of di- or tripeptides than from an equivalent solution of amino acids. There is little competition between amino acids for a common carrier when the dietary nitrogen is absorbed largely in the form of peptides. There is also no competition for absorption between amino acids and peptides, although there is between peptides. The specificity of the mechanisms for uptake does not appear to be great because very dissimilar peptides inhibit each other's uptake. There may be more than one type of carrier with a specificity that is greater for one type of peptide. Peptides must have an unaltered amino and carboxyl terminal in order to have normal affinity for transport. They must contain L-isomers of amino acids to be absorbed. Peptides that are relatively nonpolar are absorbed more readily; once inside epithelial cells, peptides are hydrolyzed to amino acids.

Peptides are readily absorbed in the cranial part of the jejunum. There is evidence that peptide absorption is equally efficient in the ileum of some species but poor in others. Amino acids are absorbed throughout the small intestine, although more readily from the cranial part. The absorption of dietary protein, like that of carbohydrates, is essentially completed in the first half of the small intestine. The remainder of the small intestine represents a reserve.

Because protein malnutrition does not develop with a deficiency of the amino acid transport systems, peptide absorption must be an important means for absorption of protein. When gluten-induced enteropathy reduces the mucosal surface area, the number of amino acid carriers is reduced. The absorption of peptides, however, is not reduced as severely as that of amino acids. The same reduction in mucosal surface area is evident in patients with chronic overgrowth of the intestinal microflora. Villous changes can be seen with pancreatic enzyme deficiencies that cause secondary bacterial overgrowth. The differential absorption rate of amino acids and peptides has therapeutic implications. Elemental diets are frequently used to treat chronic intestinal mucosal disease and enzyme deficiencies. These diets contain amino acids as their nitrogen source. Because it is evident that peptides are absorbed more readily than amino acids, peptides are a better source of nitrogen in elemental diets fed to patients with mucosal disease or enzyme deficiency. Peptides are absorbed more readily than amino acids in animals with no pancreatic enzymes.[97] Thus, elemental diets containing oligopeptides are nutritionally and economically more advantageous than diets containing a mixture of amino acids.

Proteins can be absorbed intact from the small intestine.[98] They bind to brush border receptors and are absorbed by pinocytosis. Once inside the cell, cytoplasmic and lysosomal proteases degrade most proteins to amino acid. Some proteins are not degraded and leave the cell to enter the portal circulation, as has been shown to be the case with serum albumin placed in the small intestine. Following absorption, these foreign antigens can sensitize the animal. This causes immune reactions at a time of reexposure to and absorption of the antigen. A great number of foreign proteins are absorbed and remain immunologically competent after passage through the mucosal epithelial cell. They are normally removed by the monocyte phagocytic system of the liver. Failure of this removal results in the production of many antibodies against antigens absorbed from the gut. Bacterial enterotoxins can also be absorbed intact. They are quite resistant to digestion by cytoplasmic proteases but are susceptible to digestion by acid lysosomal proteases.[99]

ABSORPTION OF LIPIDS.[65,100–102] For fat absorption to be normal, micelles are formed. They contain bile acids, fatty acids, and monoglycerides, with a small amount of lipid-soluble vitamins and cholesterol. The intact micelle moves from the lumen of the gut into the lipid part of the brush border membrane (Figure 17–25). This movement is due to passive diffusion. Within the membrane the micelle breaks up and bile acids move back out of the membrane into the lumen of the intestine. The free fatty acids and monoglycerides released from the micelle diffuse either into the cell or back into the lumen of the gut. After movement into the cell the endoplasmic reticulum rapidly esterifies them to form triglycerides. This process traps lipid digestion products in the cell because triglycerides cannot back-diffuse across the cell mem-

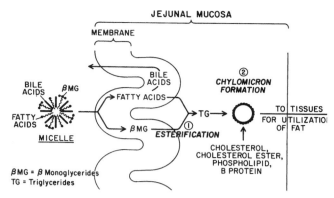

FIGURE 17–25. Absorption of dietary fat in the intestine. Micelles enter the brush border membranes, where they break up and release their constituents. Fatty acids and monoglycerides enter the cell, and bile acids return to the lumen of the intestine. The components entering the cell are reesterified by triglycerides, after which they are formed into chylomicrons by the addition of a lipoprotein coating that also contains lipids. After transport from the cell the chylomicrons enter the lymphatics. Bile acids are absorbed by the ileum and recycled for use twice each meal.

brane. The removal of fatty acids and monoglycerides by reesterification maintains a gradient of high levels outside the cell and low levels inside, which is the force for passive movement into the cell. Triglycerides are absorbed incompletely only if their fatty acid composition is unusual (containing a high percentage of saturated or long chain fatty acids).

The length of the carbon chain in fatty acids determines its mode and pathway of absorption. Fatty acids with carbon chains of 10 or less are sufficiently polar to have some degree of water solubility. When triglycerides containing short chain fatty acids are hydrolyzed, the water-soluble products are absorbed through the brush border membranes without being incorporated into micelles. Short chain fatty acids diffuse rapidly into the cell, and, if not reesterified, they are transported from the intestine by the portal circulation. Triglycerides that contain medium or short chain fatty acids are absorbed to some degree without being hydrolyzed. Thus, less lipase activity is required for their assimilation. As described, the barrier to absorption through the cell membrane consists of the lipid membrane with the unstirred layer of water attracted to it. The lipid layer is a barrier to movement of polar fatty substances such as medium and short chain fatty acids; the unstirred water layer is a barrier to movement of long chain fatty acids, which are relatively nonpolar.

Monoglycerides and fatty acids are resynthesized to triglycerides inside the cell. They are formed by the direct acylation of monoglycerides, which accounts for about 80% of the lipids that appear in the chylomicrons. The other 20% of triglycerides transported from the cell are formed from glycerol synthesized through the glycerophosphate and dihydroxyacetone phosphate pathways. That is important when little monoglyceride remains to provide a framework for direct acylation. Glycerol released during the intraluminal hydrolysis of triglycerides is water soluble and enters the cell much more rapidly than the monoglycerides and fatty acids. There, it is metabolized for energy or it can enter the circulation. Either way, it is lost for the resynthesis of triglycerides because not all the units needed for resynthesis are present within the cell at the same time. Long chain fatty acids in epithelial cells promote the synthesis of triglycerides. The enzymes catalyzing this action are concentrated in the cranial small intestine, where most fat absorption takes place. These enzymes are found in the endoplasmic reticulum. Increasing the fat content of the diet augments their activity. The enzymes require adrenocorticosteroid hormones to maintain their levels of activity. Adrenal insuffiency can cause malabsorption of fat, the result of a decreased ability to esterify fats in the cell. The levels of reesterifying enzymes are reduced during starvation. This situation illustrates the importance of using low-fat diets when feeding is resumed after a long fast. Lipases are found in the cell, and their action is primarily on triglycerides made up of medium chain fatty acids. These lipids are preferentially hydrolyzed and not resynthesized, so their components are transferred to the portal circulation.

In contrast to the relatively rapid absorption and appearance of triglycerides in the lymph, cholesterol, which enters the cell in the micelle, distributes throughout the cell and leaves slowly, with a half-life of about 12 hours. Half of the cholesterol that enters the cell is lost when normal desquamation occurs. Cholesterol can also be synthesized by the cell, with the rate unaffected by fasting or feeding. Bile, however, inhibits cholesterologenesis. Dietary cholesterol can be esterified with fatty acids. Some cholesterol ester hydrolases are present that break this bond, and others are found that promote synthesis of the ester. Cholesterol is absorbed more readily into the cell when it is not esterified. Most of the cholesterol that leaves the cell to enter the lymph is esterified.

Lipids are transported from the intestine within chylomicrons, which consist of a core of triglyceride, cholesterol ester, and free cholesterol surrounded by a coating of phospholipid, cholesterol, and protein. Chylomicrons are produced only after a meal. The chylomicrons are formed in the endoplasmic reticulum and can be stored in the Golgi apparatus. They are subsequently released into the intercellular spaces by exocytosis. During fasting periods, smaller fat-containing particles are found in the mucosal cell and lymph. Designated as very low density lipoproteins, they contain triglycerides and cholesterol. During fat absorption these particles take up more triglyceride and expand to form the larger chylomicrons. Synthesis of a protein to produce beta-lipoproteins is essential for chylomicrons to leave the epithelial cell. If synthesis of this protein is deficient or depressed, triglycerides accumulate in the cell, with fat malabsorption following. A deficiency of this lipoprotein is recognized in some humans. A reduction in protein synthesis is a feature of other mucosal diseases, such as gluten-induced enteropathy. In this case, the deficiency results in a decreased esterification of triglycerides, as well as reduced lipid transport from the cell. Any drugs that inhibit protein synthesis have this effect. Diets rich in triglycerides that contain medium chain fatty acids bypass both of these defects, because the shorter chain fatty acids need not be reesterified or incorporated into chylomicrons and are transported into the portal circulation.

Lipids are digested and absorbed primarily by chemical processes instead of regulated physiologic functions. Lipase activity is normally in great excess, so the rate of digestion is not a rate-limiting step in fat assimilation. Micelle formation has been suggested to be rate limiting, but lipase activity and bile acids are normally abundant so that micelles can be readily formed. Under some circumstances solubilization of lipolytic products by micelles may be reduced, giving micellar formation the appearance of being a rate-limiting step. Uptake across the brush border is probably the most important step determining lipid assimilation in the jejunum. The unstirred water layer is the major barrier for uptake of large molecular structures such as micelles, and the lipid membrane is the major barrier against diffusion by smaller molecules. Limits may also exist for intracellular reesterification of lipids and their incorporation into chylomicrons. Reesterification usually is not limiting for lipid assimilation. Chylomicron formation can be limiting for fat assimilation in the ileum. The ileum is not prepared to absorb large amounts of lipids. When dietary fats are excessive and escape assimilation in the jejunum, the ileum may not be able to synthesize lipoproteins fast enough for their transport from the epithelial cell. Thus, the rate-limiting step for fat assimilation is not the same for different regions of the small intestine. The size of the surface area of the mucosa becomes important when it is reduced by disease, and under such circumstances surface area size becomes a rate-limiting step. Disease of the epithelial cell is seldom recognized as a factor unless the total number of cells is reduced.

Following absorption, chylomicrons are transported through lymphatics, and their obstruction can cause malabsorption. Lymphangiectasia, caused by obstruction, usually results from occlusion of lymph channels by granulomatous processes. Management of lymphangiectasia includes feeding triglycerides containing medium to short chain fatty acids, which are absorbed through the portal circulation.

Bile acids are essential for micellar formation. An enterohepatic circulation sustains levels of bile acids in the intestine.[103] The recirculation of bile acid involves release of bile into the intestine from the gallbladder and biliary system, absorption from the small intestine, and uptake from the blood by the liver, followed by resecretion into the biliary system. This process must be efficient and rapid because the entire pool of bile acids in the body is small and must be recycled two or three times during a single meal. Most bile acids are absorbed in the ileum by an active energy-requiring and sodium-dependent mechanism.

Bile acids are transported up a concentration gradient, a process inhibited by the same drugs that inhibit sodium transport. A loss of this function of the ileum results in bile acid deficiency and fat malabsorption because the synthesis of new bile acids by the liver cannot increase enough to supply the animal's needs. Some absorption of bile acids occurs via passive diffusion, depending on the species of animal and the type of bile acid. If the pKa of a bile acid is low, it is in its ionized form at neutral pHs. Taurocholate has a low pKa and is quite lipid insoluble because it is ionized. Consequently, it does not readily cross lipid cell membranes by diffusion. Little taurocholate is absorbed from the jejunum of the dog.[104] Bacteria can deconjugate bile acids in the intestine, removing the amino acid; the products formed have a pKa greater than that of the conjugated form. Thus, the unconjugated bile acid is unionized near neutral pH, is lipid soluble, and can cross cell membranes readily. Bacterial overgrowth of the intestinal microflora can deconjugate an excessive amount of bile acids. This activity results in rapid absorption of bile acids from the intestine, which leads to a bile acid deficiency and malabsorption of lipids. In summary, the absorption of fats depends on adequate concentrations of bile acids in the intestine. This is influenced by reabsorption of bile acids in the ileum and by a minimum amount of deconjugation, which is achieved by control of the bacterial numbers in the intestine.

Gastric functions determine lipid assimilation. Gastric motility is essential for trituration of food in order to release nutrients sequestered within particles. Reducing gastric motility by vagotomy and antrectomy in dogs impairs particle size reduction, and less dietary fat is absorbed from a solid but not a liquid diet.[105] The nature of the diet also determines lipid assimilation. Fat assimilation is 97% complete in dogs fed a meat-based diet with a fat content of 35% of dry matter.

When fed a cereal-based diet with a fat content of 11% of dry matter, assimilation is only 90% complete. Less fat is digested and absorbed when dogs are fed a cereal diet with a poorer digestibility.[106] Differences in lipid assimilation also develop when the relative amounts of saturated to unsaturated fats increase; then lipid absorption increases.[107]

FIBER REGULATION OF ASSIMILATION.[108] Dietary factors other than carbohydrate, protein, and lipid content affect overall digestion and absorption of all nutrients. Diets that delay gastric emptying enhance assimilation. High-fat diets as described earlier slow gastric emptying; fibers such as pectin and guar gum have the same effect by increasing viscosity of gastric contents. Similar effects are suggested for small intestinal transit time, but no reliable conclusions can be made. Dietary fiber reduces activities of pancreatic digestive enzymes. Fiber that binds and increases fecal excretion of bile acids can reduce fat assimilation. Absorption of all nutrients is reduced by fiber that maintains luminal contents at such a high viscosity that contact is reduced between nutrients and the brush border. The mucosal surface area determines overall absorptive capacities. Fiber in the diet reduces villus numbers and surface area; feeding cereal-based high-fiber diets does not result in the optimum mucosal area for absorption that is found with meat-based low-residue diets.

Fiber is an important undigestable component of cell walls in unrefined foods. That fiber as well as fiber added to refined foods limits the digestibility of refined foods. Cell wall fiber prevents release of carbohydrates, proteins, and lipids until digestion of the fiber by colonic bacteria. Evaluation of digestibility of carbohydrates is made by the glycemic response, the degree of hyperglycemia that the carbohydrate produces after feeding. In addition to the type of food, the form of the food ingested determines the glycemic response. For example, consuming whole rice results in flattened glucose and insulin responses, whereas consuming ground rice results in plasma increases for both glucose and insulin.

Increasing dietary fiber increases fecal excretion of nitrogen. The effect is caused primarily by an increase in growth for colonic bacteria. The increased bacterial mass is promoted by an increase in flow of unassimilated nutrients (fiber, carbohydrate, protein, and lipids) from the small intestine. The nitrogen entering the colon sustains bacterial growth, but the amount escaping assimilation in the small intestine is not sufficient to result in a nitrogen imbalance. Relatively small amounts escape digestion and absorption because of additional fiber in the diet.

High dietary fiber, either as part of natural foods in the diet or as fiber added to the diet, increases fecal fat. Fat in a higher fiber cereal-based diet is not as completely assimilated as fat in lower fiber meat-based diets. Both lipid digestion and absorption are impaired. In addition, as described earlier, fiber promotes fecal losses or bile acids; reduced bile acid availability results in greater lipid malassimilation.

COLONIC DIGESTION AND ABSORPTION.[109,110] Digestion and absorption are important to normal colonic physiology. Colonic bacteria metabolize carbohydrates, proteins, and lipids to produce a number of products that are excreted or absorbed. Bacteria metabolize carbohydrates to short chain fatty acids (acetic, propionic, and butyric acids) and gases (hydrogen, methane, and carbon dioxide). About 95% to 99% of the fatty acids are rapidly absorbed. Colonic mucosal cells metabolize some butyrate; the liver clears the remaining butyrate and propionate. Peripheral tissues take up and metabolize acetate. The carbohydrates entering the colon include nonstarch polysaccharides (dietary fiber), starch (which can amount to 10% to 20% of total dietary starch), and small amounts of sugars (such as lactose) and oligosac-

charides (such as raffinose and stachyose). Dietary fiber is metabolized or fermented to different degrees, depending on its source and structure. Lignification of cell walls reduces fermentation, as for example with bran. Increases in water solubility enhance digestibility. Other factors determining digestibility of polysaccharides include particle size, molecular structure, effect of food processing, the type of gut microflora, and transit time.

Unassimilated starch may represent the most important substrate for bacterial fermentation in the colon. Starch can escape digestion for a number of reasons. It may appear in the diet as ungelatinized starch granules, or because the diet contains alpha-amylase inhibitors, or because of reduced availability in complexes with other foods such as fat or protein, or because the starch is not released from unmilled grains. Fermentation of polysaccharides allows the colon to salvage carbohydrates escaping assimilation in the small intestine. That salvage may not add significantly to the animal's nutritional needs, but it does remove substances that contribute to increased fecal volume that in some cases results in diarrhea. The absorption of short chain fatty acids is by nonionic diffusion and it promotes sodium and water absorption probably by Na^+-H^+ exchange. Loss of that substrate could inhibit sodium absorption to the degree that diarrhea follows.

Short chain fatty acids provide an important source of energy for colonic epithelial cells. Of the fatty acids butyrate is the most important, affecting both colonocyte morphology and function. Deprivation of short chain fatty acids leads to colonic mucosal atrophy characterized by reductions in mucosal blood flow, mucus release, and cell renewal (eventually progressing to colitis), and results in reduced absorption of fluid and sodium. Normal colonic structure and function require luminal unabsorbed starch and/or nonstarch polysaccharide that can be fermented to short chain fatty acids.

ABSORPTION OF WATER AND ELECTROLYTES.[111-115] The absorption of water in the small and large intestine is a passive process that follows the transport of solutes across the cell. The net movement of fluid from the mucosal to the serosal border of the cell can be conceived of as the difference between the two bidirectional fluxes found across the cell. This movement of fluid, dependent on energy, is determined by the transport of nonelectrolyte solutes and sodium. A number of different factors, such as the leakiness of the membrane and regulation of the circulation, influence the efficiency of transport.

Solute-Mediated Fluid Transfer. The absorption of fluid is related directly to the absorption of a solute. The absorption of fluid in the jejunum results from the transport of sodium that can be coupled to the transport of a monosaccharide or amino acid. Sodium is the essential solute for fluid absorption in the distal ileum and the colon. During glucose absorption, movement across the brush border depends on an interaction between an actively transported monosaccharide and sodium (Figure 17–26). Glucose and glutamine supply energy. Some actively transported hexoses are metabolized by epithelial cells. Galactose is actively transported with sodium, but galactose is not metabolized, and so transport ceases until the cell is provided with sources of energy.

Fructose is not coupled with sodium during its transport by a special carrier into epithelial cells. When fructose is the only sugar present, sodium still influxes into the cells but flux is less than with glucose. Fructose uptake carries water passively by solvent drag, where the osmotic force generated by movement of solute particles moves the water. Fructose also supports sodium transport by another mechanism because it can be converted to glucose and become a source of energy. Thus, during hexose transport sodium can enter the cell

MODEL OF THREE COMPONENTS OF SODIUM TRANSPORT

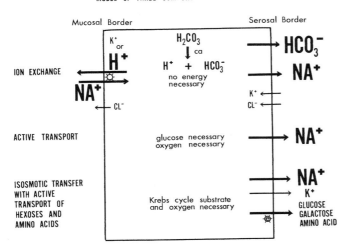

FIGURE 17-26. Schematic of intestinal epithelial cell, showing the three mechanisms for the nonpassive movement of sodium from the lumen of the gut into the circulation.

through more than one process. In one, sodium is coupled with an actively transported sugar, and in another, it requires no accompanying nonelectrolyte. After feeding, the cotransport with hexoses and amino acids is responsible for 56% of the sodium absorbed by mucosal cells.

Nonelectrolyte-dependent sodium entry into epithelial cells provides a second important means for fluid absorption. Sodium can couple with chloride and move across brush borders by diffusion. Sodium moves down an electrochemical gradient through membranes that are semipermeable to sodium diffusion. After feeding, this flux is responsible for absorption of 37% of the total sodium; in the unfed state it represents 85% of the total sodium absorbed.

A third and minor mechanism for fluid absorption is a sodium-hydrogen ion exchange. The exchange operates in association with an exchange mechanism for chloride and bicarbonate ions. The cation exchanges are responsible for 10% to 15% of the sodium that enters mucosal cells. In the jejunum sodium-hydrogen ion exchange causes luminal fluid to be slightly acid (Figure 17–26). However, secretions in the ileum and colon are slightly alkaline because there is a very active bicarbonate-chloride exchange process. The secretion of large amounts of bicarbonate in these regions negates the effect of hydrogen ions secreted by the sodium-hydrogen ion exchange process. If, however, chloride is replaced by a large anion, such as sulfate, that the bicarbonate cannot exchange with, ileal contents become acid from the ongoing sodium-hydrogen exchange. Carbonic anhydrase inhibitors reduce net sodium absorption in the ileum, which illustrates the importance of the exchange mechanism to the transport of sodium in this region of the intestine.

During the absorption of glucose or galactose, large intracellular concentrations can be produced. Glucose leaves the cell across the basal borders via facilitated diffusion, following the concentration gradient created by high levels inside the cell and low levels outside. Water moves with the glucose due to osmotic attraction. Ions in the water are carried along. This movement of ions across the cell is called solvent drag. The sugar osmotically drags the solvent, and the ions within the solvent are not selectively separated out.

In contrast to the passive movement of glucose, sodium is transported from the cell by a special mechanism. The basal

lateral membranes contain transport mechanisms that actively move sodium from a low concentration in the cell to a high one in the intercellular space. Water follows osmotically into the space, causing it to enlarge, a change that is morphologically evident in mucosa which is actively transporting fluid. Hydrostatic pressure increases in the intercellular space. The fluid flows out into the interstitial space and is carried away by the microcirculation. The membrane transport mechanism is specific for sodium and requires energy supplied by glucose. This area of the cell membrane is a rich source of Na-K-dependent ATPase, an enzyme stimulated by sodium and potassium. The enzyme splits ATP and releases high levels of energy. In most species this enzyme is inhibited by cardiac glycosides, chemicals that also inhibit active sodium transport. Hence, the ATPase is either the sodium pump or provides energy for it. An electrical charge is generated across some tissues when its cells actively transport sodium. The electrical charge occurs when the transport does not involve a cation- or anion-exchange process or a tightly coupled accompaniment of an anion. The electrical charge results from a transport of sodium that is not associated with an equal and simultaneous movement of anions. The result is a slight excess of positive sodium ions on the serosal border and a slight excess of anions left behind on the luminal border, creating a measurable potential difference across the cell.

The leakiness of the tight junctions determines whether the epithelial surface maintains gradients for both ion concentrations and electrical potentials across cell membranes. These junctions are very leaky in the duodenum and jejunum, and fluid that is transported into the intercellular space is able to diffuse freely, through the leaky junctions between cells, back into the lumen of the gut. Thus, any differences in ion concentrations between the two sides of the cell become equalized. This equalization is unimportant in the jejunum because the primary force for the absorption of fluid there is glucose and amino acid transport. The direction of glucose movement is always toward the serosal side of the cell, so the flow to move sodium by solvent drag is always in that direction.

The glucose- and amino acid-mediated absorption of sodium is most important in the jejunum. In the distal ileum and colon, absorption of sodium is not coupled to transport of other solutes. The cell-to-cell junctions in these tissues are tight and relatively nonleaky, allowing the tissues to create high concentrations of sodium on the serosal side of the cell from low luminal levels. If the junctions were leaky, it would make the absorption of sodium a very inefficient process because much of it would leak back before it had a chance to leave the intercellular space.

Apical membranes of colonic epithelial cells are less permeable than those of the small intestine to the entry of sodium. In the colon, sodium entry is the rate-limiting step for absorption. Sodium entry is driven by an electrochemical gradient, where sodium moves by diffusion from a high concentration in the lumen to a very low concentration intracellularly. The colonic epithelial cell generates a greater electrical potential difference across its membranes than small intestinal cells do, and that electrical activity also promotes diffusion across apical membranes. Entry across those membranes occurs through pores; movement through the pores is inhibited by amiloride and high luminal sodium concentrations and is promoted by aldosterone and high luminal anion concentrations. An ATPase driven by sodium and potassium, with their exchange promoted across the basolateral membrane, transports sodium from colonic epithelial cells. Glucocorticoids and mineralocorticoids stimulate the transport. Sodium does not leak back into the cell because the basolateral membranes are highly impermeable to sodium diffusion. The permeability is greater for potassium, which allows its diffusion from the cell.

About 2.7 L of fluid must be absorbed each day in a 20 kg animal. Half of this is absorbed in the jejunum, and 75% of the remaining 1350 ml is absorbed in the ileum. About 350 ml remains to enter the colon, where up to 90% can be absorbed.

The movements of potassium, bicarbonate, and chloride as described can be summarized as follows. Potassium movements are entirely passive throughout the small intestine. Their movement follows concentration and electrical gradients. Thus, some potassium will move from the lumen to the cell when concentrations in the lumen are high. Most of the potassium is absorbed by solvent drag, in the jejunum as a result of glucose and amino acid transport, and in the ileum as a result of sodium transport. Regardless of whether there is net absorption of potassium or whether the fluxes are in steady state, the concentration of the ion is higher in intestinal contents than in plasma water. The electrical potential difference, with the lumen negative, attracts potassium, a cation with a positive charge that is attracted to a negatively charged site. Thus, loss of fluid from any site in the gastrointestinal tract is accompanied by a greater potassium loss than water loss, leaving the animal more depleted in potassium than in water. The potential difference across the small intestine is small, so that the levels of potassium are not excessively greater in small intestinal secretion than in body fluids. The potential difference across the large intestine is greater than in the small intestine; it can be as great as 30 to 50 mv. This greater potential causes the secretion of large amounts of potassium into the colon. The secretion of potassium can produce concentrations that approach 100 mEq/L. Because the potential difference cannot account for an amount that great, the entire amount secreted requires an additional mechanism. Either sodium and water absorption is more complete at a site that is relatively impermeable to potassium and distal to the location for high potassium permeability, or a mechanism exists for active secretion of potassium. The active component may be represented by ATPase activity, driven by sodium and potassium at the basolateral membrane; that activity would lead to their loading of cells with potassium and would promote diffusion across the apical border. The active component may also be an apical membrane potassium conductance regulated by intracellular cyclic AMP and calcium levels, with increases in conductance promoting potassium secretion.

The anions chloride and bicarbonate are passively absorbed in the jejunum by solvent drag, created by glucose and amino acid absorption. The chloride for the bicarbonate-exchange mechanism is present in the jejunum, but its effects are dwarfed by the large amount of fluid and ions moved via solvent drag. The mechanism is not apparent in the fed state. Chloride and bicarbonate are not absorbed by passive forces via solvent drag in the ileum. Thus, the effects of the chloride-bicarbonate exchange mechanism are evident in the ileal contents, which are high in bicarbonate and low in chloride. The low concentration of bicarbonate in the jejunum does not imply the ion is actively transported from a region of low concentration to one of high concentration, fulfilling the criteria for active transport. Bicarbonate is low in the jejunum because hydrogen ions secreted in the exchange process react with bicarbonate to form carbonic acid and the evolution of carbon dioxide. Bicarbonate is lost in the carbon dioxide that is absorbed. The chloride-bicarbonate exchange process operates in the colon so that the colonic contents are normally alkaline.

In summary, the fluid entering the colon from the ileum contains sodium at a level the same as that in plasma water. Thus, the colon normally absorbs up to 40 mEq sodium in the 20 kg animal, in addition to 300 ml water. An equivalent amount of chloride is absorbed. Bicarbonate and potassium are secreted. The large electrical potential difference is the result of an active sodium-transport process through a tissue that has a relatively impermeable tight junction. The anion movements are the result of the exchange mechanism, and potassium secretion is passive.

Regulation of Fluid Absorption. The absorption of fluid, just like that of secretion, is influenced by forces determined by the circulation (Figure 17–21). The colloid osmotic pressure of the plasma and interstitial fluid, hydrostatic pressure in the capillaries and interstitial fluid, and osmotic forces in the lumen of the intestine determine the absorption of fluid and electrolytes. In the normal state the fluid entering the small intestine is isosmotic, so that osmolality is not a factor affecting absorption. Changes in pressure in the lumen of the gut have no effect on the absorption of fluid unless the pressure is so great that circulation of the tissue is compromised. Increases up to a pressure of 40 cm of water have no effect. Most of the changes that can occur to alter the physical forces are found on the serosal side of the cell. Small changes in pressure on the cell's serosal side markedly affect fluid absorption. Increases of less than 5 cm of water decrease absorption, and greater increases can result in secretion of fluid. That result can be readily demonstrated in in vitro preparations of intestinal mucosa.[116] It can also be shown in dogs by infusing large amounts of saline to increase hydrostatic pressure in the microcirculation of the mucosa. Such a procedure depresses the absorption of fluid.[117] Obstructing either lymphatic or venous drainage can also produce hydrostatic pressure increases. Lymphangiectasia is recognized in clinical cases, and the diarrhea that results is due in part to an impairment of fluid absorption. With increased venous pressure, there is a good capacity for compensation before absorption is severely impaired. The colloid osmotic pressure falls in the interstitial fluid as the hydrostatic pressure increases, and this response has a dilutional effect, which ends in promoting fluxes of fluid into the capillary and lymphatics.[118] Portal hypertension increases interstitial hydrostatic pressure, as seen in problems that range from cardiac disease to hepatic disease. In an attempt to reduce the intracapillary pressure there is a reflex change in arteriolar resistance in the microcirculation, but the net effect of increased pressure remains, and the absorption of fluid is inhibited. As would be expected, an increased plasma colloid osmotic pressure increases the absorption of fluid from the intestine. The epithelium is a leaky membrane that permits ready movement of fluids in either direction in response to osmotic gradients.

Fluid absorption is probably not affected by osmotic forces in clinical cases unless measurable changes in colloid osmotic pressure can be demonstrated. Dogs made acutely hypoalbuminemic by plasmapheresis develop diarrhea.[119] Diarrhea can begin when albumin is at or below 2.0 g per deciliter. Plasma proteins are lost at an excessive rate in many animals with gastrointestinal problems. Reductions in plasma oncotic pressure follow and may contribute to difficulties in management of a diarrhea.

It is evident that blood flow has an effect on the absorption of many substances from the lumen of the intestine.[112] When blood flow is reduced below a normal resting rate, the absorption of most substances decreases. When the rate is increased, the absorption increases for lipid solutes and small un-ionized water-soluble solutes. The absorption of larger

Table 17–4

CHEMICALS STIMULATING INTESTINAL ABSORPTION	
Aldosterone	Insulin
Angiotensin	Neuropeptide Y
Catecholamines	Nitric oxide
Enkephalins	Somatostatin
Glucocorticoids	Vasopressin

solutes is unaffected by blood flow. The mucosal absorption of solutes is a function of their rate of transfer across the epithelial surface and the rate of removal from the lamina propria by the circulation. The absorption of solutes that can pass across the barrier with relatives ease will be very dependent on blood flow. The rate-limiting process is the crossing of the barrier by substances that require a special mechanism to cross the cell. Blood flow is not an important factor in determining their rate of absorption. Where fluid flux rates are relatively high as in the jejunum, a substance promoting nitric oxide formation (and hence increasing mucosal circulation), L-arginine, stimulates fluid absorption and helps protect the mucosa. Glutamine enrichment of the diet also increases mucosal blood flow, which may in part explain this amino acid's protective effect on the intestinal mucosa. (Short chain fatty acids have a similar effect.) The clinical importance of circulation on absorption relates mostly to states in which interstitial hydrostatic pressure is increased or colloid osmotic pressure is decreased, in which case fluid absorption is affected regardless of the solute that moves it.

Absorptive mechanisms in epithelial cells operate at fixed rates once they are stimulated with a goal of complete absorption for a solute. Epithelial cell absorption may be regulated by neural and endocrine/paraendocrine mechanisms.[120] Chemicals released following stimulation of neural pathways, endocrines, and paracrines can influence epithelial cell function (Table 17–4). Studies done mostly on isolated tissues or cells show that many different chemicals have an effect on epithelial cell transport. The importance of any one chemical is not known. The knowledge that these chemicals can affect transport holds promise; drugs that alter electrolyte transport may be developed as a management for diarrhea.

Absorption of Iron.[121,122] The absorption of iron is regulated, which is important because iron has no avenue of excretion from the body. The amount in the diet is almost always adequate. Because the rate of iron absorption is small, it is currently recommended that 10 mg of iron be consumed with each 1000 calories of food in order to maintain normal iron stores. In general, only 50% of the iron is released from food during its digestion. The percentage is less for cereals and vegetables, and greater for most digested animal proteins.

After digestion releases the iron, the absorption rate remains optimum as long as the iron remains in solution. The ferrous form of iron is absorbed better than the ferric form. Chelation with a large mucopolysaccharide secreted in the stomach and with ascorbate, citrate, some hexoses, and certain amino acids maintains iron in a soluble form. The iron remains in this form until the complex comes in contact with the brush border membrane. Iron that fails to be chelated is changed at the higher pH of the small intestine and precipitates as ferric hydroxide. Bile, possibly as a result of its ascorbate content, facilitates iron absorption. Acid secretion in the stomach is important for maintaining iron as soluble as possible, especially the ferric form. Acid assists in the formation of soluble iron chelates of ascorbic acid. Not all forms of iron are effectively prepared by acid for optimal absorption. The iron in egg is not effectively released by acid in the stomach. Acid reduces rather than enhances the absorption of iron in hemoglobin because acid renders heme insoluble. Heme is absorbed intact by the small intestinal mucosa, however, after which iron is released within the cell. Phosphates and carbonates form salts with iron that are relatively insoluble. Pancreatic bicarbonate reduces iron absorption; pancreatic exocrine deficiency promotes iron uptake.

Iron is absorbed mainly in the duodenum and the first part of the jejunum. The transport of iron from the cell to the circulation requires a special system found in this cranial region of the gut. This system is the rate-limiting step in the absorptive process. Less iron is able to enter the mucosal cell at more caudal sites because less survives in soluble form as the pH of gut contents increases. Ferrous iron is transported across the brush border by an active ATP energy-requiring process (Figure 17–27). It is either stored in a ferrous iron pool or transported out of the cell. The cell synthesizes a number of iron-binding proteins, and ferrous iron entering the cell is bound to it to form a complex, the most well known being ferritin. If no binding protein is present, the ferrous iron is transported across the serosal border and, upon reaching the circulation, binds to a plasma-transporting protein called transferritin.

Events that take place in the immature epithelial cells before they migrate out of the crypt determine the rate of absorption of iron by villous epithelial cells. If stores of iron are low in the body, little plasma ferrous iron enters the crypt cells, and as a result, there is little stimulation to synthesize iron-binding proteins. When the cell migrates to the villus, there is little or no protein to bind iron entering the cell. Consequently, most of the iron is transferred to the circula-

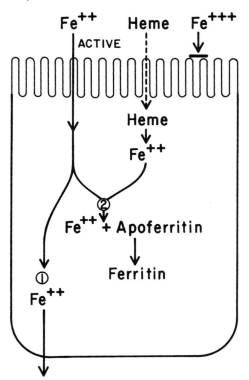

FIGURE 17–27. The absorption of iron in the small intestine. Only the ferrous form enters the cell, due to an active transport mechanism. Iron passes through the cell and is absorbed unless apoferritin is present to sequester it. The amount of apoferritin in the cell determines the regulation of absorption.

tion. However, with a large store of iron in the body, iron entering crypt cells stimulates iron-binding protein synthesis. This subsequently results in the binding of most of the absorbed ferrous iron in cells at the villus site. The iron is not released to the circulation, and it is lost into the lumen of the gut when the cell desquamates. The release of iron from heme in the cell is also regulated. Excessive ferrous iron in the absorptive cell inhibits the enzyme that hydrolyzes heme, and no additional iron is released.

ABSORPTION OF CALCIUM.[123,124] Calcium absorption, like iron absorption, depends on digestive processes in the stomach and small intestine. Special mechanisms are present to absorb calcium that are more sophisticated than those for iron absorption. Iron and calcium are both divalent cations less readily absorbed than a monovalent cation such as sodium. Because calcium is the most abundant cation in the body, there must be special mechanisms to ensure that adequate amounts are absorbed. In contrast, the needs for iron are small, and its absorptive mechanism is designed to prevent iron overload by limiting the rate of absorption instead of facilitating it.

Calcium absorption is directly related to the amount that is soluble and ionized in the small intestine. Many calcium salts, such as those of phosphate and carbonate, are quite insoluble at neutral pH. Digestion of foods at the acid pH of the stomach increases the amount of soluble calcium. Amino acids such as arginine, lysine, and tryptophan enhance calcium absorption, as do the antibiotics penicillin, neomycin, and chloramphenicol. Calcium absorption is depressed by corticosteroids, thyroid hormone, estrogens, excessive unabsorbed fatty acids, diets rich in oxalates or organic phosphates, excessive antacid administration, and achlorhydria. The type of organic phosphate is hexaphosphoinositol, which is found in bran.

The net absorption of calcium is the difference between the flux of calcium from the lumen to the blood and the flux in the opposite direction. The lumen-to-plasma flux is highest in the duodenum, which enables this part of the small intestine to be the most efficient in absorbing calcium. The plasma-to-lumen flux of calcium is about the same in the duodenum and ileum. When calcium is not present in the lumen, the secretory (plasma-to-lumen) flux becomes apparent. In the duodenum, this is reabsorbed. It is not reabsorbed in the ileum, however, and the net secretion of calcium represents a calcium loss from the body that is continuous when dietary calcium is low. Even though the control mechanisms are activated to absorb and conserve calcium more efficiently, there is still a negative calcium balance.[125] The nature of the calcium transport mechanisms in the intestinal mucosa is not well understood. In the duodenum, calcium is transported by a carrier-mediated energy-dependent process. Hormones and vitamin D can regulate the efficiency of this transport system. Because this mechanism is located only in the duodenum, through which chyme passes fairly rapidly, it is the limiting factor in the overall absorption of calcium. Most of the calcium is absorbed in the remainder of the small intestine by passive or facilitated diffusion.

Vitamins and hormones regulate calcium absorption (Figure 17–28). Vitamin D is not biologically active on calcium absorption until after it has been hydroxylated, first in the liver, forming 25-hydroxycholecalciferol, and later in the renal cortex, forming 1,25-dihydroxycholecalciferol, which is the active chemical that regulates intestinal absorption of calcium. The kidney can also convert the hydroxylated form produced in the liver to 21,25-dihydroxycholecalciferol, an inactive form. Levels of serum calcium and parathyroid hormone determine whether the form produced will be inactive

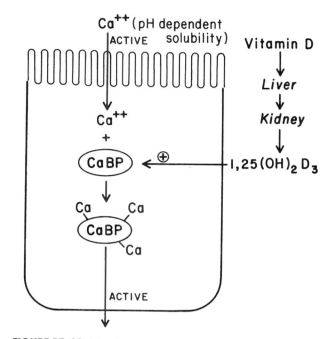

FIGURE 17–28. The absorption of calcium in the small intestine. Calcium absorption is regulated by vitamin D absorption and metabolism.

or active, Reductions in serum calcium cause release of parathormone, which stimulates synthesis and release of the active form. Thus, this arm of the regulation of intestinal calcium depends on normal renal function, normal parathyroid function, and absorption of vitamin D. Serum levels of phosphate determine the secretion of 1,25-dihydroxycholecalciferol. Low phosphate levels stimulate its synthesis and release, causing an increased absorption of phosphate in the intestine and probably in the renal tubule. Parathormone is primarily a regulator of calcium ions, but it causes an increased absorption of intestinal phosphate by the vitamin D derivative, increasing serum levels. Thyrocalcitonin has no effect on the absorption of calcium from the intestine.

The effect of 1,25-dihydroxycholecalciferol is to stimulate the synthesis of a calcium-binding protein in the intestinal epithelial cell. Synthesis occurs primarily in the duodenal mucosa, where an active transport process is involved. It is suggested that the binding protein functions as a carrier.

Cushing syndrome or prolonged administration of corticosteroids can cause bone demineralization. Corticosteroids cause decreased calcium absorption in the intestine. It is not known whether this effect is one directly on the mucosal cell or whether the steroids interfere with vitamin D metabolism. A failure to absorb calcium properly from the intestine cannot be critically evaluated by measuring serum calcium levels. Bone changes become apparent, however, alerting the clinician to a problem. Calcium malabsorption is a possibility when there is fat malabsorption for any reason and when chronic renal disease has progressed to the extent that the metabolism of vitamin D to its active form is no longer adequate to meet the animal's needs.

ABSORPTION OF MAGNESIUM. Magnesium is an important divalent cation necessary for the functioning of enzyme systems in the body. Little is known about its metabolism. There are no known special mechanisms for absorption of this ion, which occurs primarily in the cranial part of the jejunum. Magnesium salts are relatively water soluble, and malabsorption does not engender clinical signs until it becomes a very severe problem.

ABSORPTION OF VITAMINS.[126,127] Fat-soluble vitamins are absorbed with dietary lipids, and no deficiencies are seen unless fat malabsorption occurs. Water-soluble vitamins are absorbed by processes of simple diffusion, with several exceptions. The assimilation of vitamin B_{12} and folic acid by the intestinal mucosa is important clinically and involves processes that are more complicated.

Absorption of Vitamin B_{12}. It is estimated that a year's supply of vitamin B_{12} is stored in the body, so its malabsorption must persist for some time before signs of deficiency appear. Vitamin B_{12} is necessary for the production of normal erythrocytes. A deficiency causes megaloblastic erythropoiesis. The source of all vitamin B_{12} to small animals is in the diet. Intestinal bacteria synthesize the vitamin, but only in the colon, where it cannot be absorbed. Dietary vitamin B_{12} is found only in animal protein or in food in which it has been synthesized by contaminating microorganisms. The vitamin is released from food during digestion in the stomach, after which it binds to a glycoprotein, called intrinsic factor, that the stomach secretes. Recent studies report its presence in pancreatic secretions of dogs.[128] The amount of B_{12} normally present in the diet is less than 5 µg per day. Binding to intrinsic factor is necessary for absorption of 20% of this intake. The complex of vitamin B_{12} and intrinsic factor passes through the small intestine to the ileum. The intrinsic factor not only resists proteolytic destruction of B_{12} by bacterial or pancreatic enzymes but also minimizes the utilization of B_{12} by bacteria within the lumen. The mucosa of the ileum contains receptor sites on the surface of the microvilli that bind the complex. After the binding the B_{12} is released and crosses the cell membrane by an active transport process. The vitamin is transported through the cell and released to the circulation, where it binds to one of two carrier proteins, transcobalamin. There is a definite rate-limiting step in the absorption of B_{12}, but it is not known whether it is in its attachment to the ileum or in the transport mechanism. Bile's vitamin B_{12} content is high and most of the vitamin is reabsorbed in the ileum. Loss of the ileal function to absorb vitamin B_{12} represents a means for continued loss of the vitamin from the body.

There are clinical situations of reduced absorption of vitamin B_{12}. A deficiency of intrinsic factor, causing B_{12} malabsorption, is possible. Intrinsic factor deficiency develops in humans with atrophic gastritis, but has not been reported as a problem in small animals. It can be a problem in animals with partial gastrectomy or possibly with pancreatic diseases. Abnormalities in the small intestine influence vitamin B_{12} absorption. Increased numbers of intestinal bacteria consume vitamin B_{12}; microflora can increase to the point where they use most of the vitamin, leaving little for absorption in the ileum.[129] Such overgrowth occurs in regions of the small intestine cranial to a partial obstruction. In humans, intestinal parasites can consume B_{12} to the point of creating a deficiency. That situation has not been recognized in small animals. A deficiency of pancreatic secretions can also impair vitamin B_{12} absorption. The malabsorption that follows the enzyme deficiency is accompanied by an overgrowth of the microflora of the intestine, which use B_{12} and leave less for absorption. Malabsorption also lowers the pH of the intestinal contents through the bacterial flora's fermentation of unabsorbed oligosaccharides. Pancreatic disease results in a deficiency of pancreatic bicarbonate secretion, augmenting the acidity of intestinal contents. Mucosal binding of the B_{12} intrinsic factor complex is inhibited at a pH of less than 6.5. Malabsorption can also reduce calcium concentrations by precipitation of calcium with fatty acids. Calcium must be present for normal binding of the B_{12} intrinsic factor complex to the ileal mucosa. Lastly, severe chronic disease of the ileum can result in vitamin B_{12} deficiency. Ileitis or regional enteritis is not uncommon in humans but has seldom been reported in small animals. Vitamin B_{12} absorption tests are conducted in humans but are rarely done in animals. In general, vitamin B_{12} deficiency is seldom recognized in animals.

Absorption of Folic Acid. Folic acid has a much shorter biologic half-life than vitamin B_{12} so a deficiency can be seen within a month after intake ceases. Folates are necessary for synthetic reactions that involve methionine, purines, and pyrimidines. Deficiency results in megaloblastic changes in the bone marrow. Folic acid (pteroylglutamic acid) consists of three components. A pteridine ring and para-aminobenzoic acid (making up pteroic acid) are connected to glutamic acid. The natural form of folate in the diet consists of folic acid with a number of additional moieties of glutamic acid. The monoglutamate form is found in plasma. The diet contains up to 300 µg of folate per 100 calories, and the vitamin is widely distributed in foods. Folate is absorbed from the cranial part of the small intestine, and the capacity for absorption is in excess of the daily needs. The epithelial cell absorbs the natural form, polyglutamates, after which a lysosomal glutamyl peptidase reduces the glutamyl peptide chain to a mono- or diglutamate. The reduced form of these products is subsequently methylated in the cell to form methyltetrahydrofolate. The nature of the mechanism for transport of folate is unknown. Interference with the intracellular metabolic transformations inhibits its absorption.

Occasionally, a small animal patient is seen that has a chronic bowel problem and evidence for a megaloblastic anemia. The important site of folate absorption is in the jejunum, pathology of which can cause a deficiency of absorption. Resection of a large part of small intestine and gluten-induced enteropathy lead to folate malabsorption in humans. Extensive intramural disease of the intestinal mucosa produces the same results. Bacteria produce folate that can be absorbed and supply the body's needs. Bacteria also consume folate, to the extent that low plasma folate deficiencies can develop with bacterial overgrowth of the jejunum.[129] Drugs are known to interfere with folate absorption. Diphenylhydantoin is the only one of these that is frequently used in small animal medicine. In summary, megaloblastic anemia associated with chronic gastrointestinal disease should be considered as a possible result of a deficiency of folate absorption.

REFERENCES

1. Miller ME, Christensen GC, Evans HE. Anatomy of the Dog. WB Saunders, Philadelphia, 1964.
2. Nickel R, Schummer A, Seiferle E, et al. The Viscera of Domestic Animals. Springer-Verlag, New York, 1973.
3. Dyce KM, Sack WO, Wensing CJG. Textbook of Veterinary Anatomy. WB Saunders, Philadelphia, 1987.
4. Bonakdarpour A, Ming S, Lynch PR, et al. Superior mesenteric artery occlusion in dogs: A model to produce the spectrum of intestinal ischemia. J Surg Res 19:251–257, 1975.
5. Creamer B. Intestinal structure in relation to absorption. In: Smyth DH (ed) Biomembranes, Vol. 4A, Intestinal Absorption. Plenum Press, New York, 1–42, 1974.
6. Madera JL, Trier JS. Functional morphology of the mucosa of the small intestine. In: Johnson LR (ed) Physiology of the Gastrointestinal Tract. Raven Press, New York, 1209–1249, 1987.
7. Solcia E, Capella C, Buffa R, et al. Endocrine cells of the digestive system. In: Johnson LR (ed) Physiology of the Gastrointestinal Tract. Raven Press, New York, 111–130, 1987.
8. Lundgren O. The circulation of the small bowel mucosa. Gut 15:1005–1013, 1974.
9. Granger DN, Kvietys PR, Perry MA, et al. The microcirculation and intesti-

nal transport. In Johnson LR (ed) Physiology of the Gastrointestinal Tract. Raven Press, New York, 1671–1697, 1987.

10. Casley-Smith JR. Endothelial fenestrae in intestinal villi: Differences between the arterial and venous ends of capillaries. Microvasc Res 3:49–68, 1971.

11. Strombeck DR. Effect of *Vibrio cholera* toxin on vascular and extravascular spaces of rat intestine. Proc Soc Exp Biol Med 141:70–75, 1972.

12. Eastwood GL. Gastrointestinal epithelial renewal. Gastroenterology 72:962–975, 1977.

13. Lipkin M. Proliferation and differentiation of normal and diseased gastrointestinal cells. In: Johnson LR (ed) Physiology of the Gastrointestinal Tract. Raven Press, New York, 255–285, 1987.

14. Johnson LR. Regulation of gastrointestinal growth. In: Johnson LR (ed) Physiology of the Gastrointestinal Tract. Raven Press, New York, 301–333, 1987.

15. Barrowman JA. The trophic action of gastrointestinal hormones. Digestion 12:92–104, 1975.

16. Hughes CA, Bates T, Dowling RH. Cholecystokinin and secretin prevent the intestinal mucosal hypoplasia of total parenteral nutrition in the dog. Gastroenterology 75:34–41, 1978.

17. MacDonald TT, Ferguson A. Small intestinal epithelial cell kinetics and protozoal infection in mice. Gastroenterology 74:496–500, 1978.

18. Schofield GC. Anatomy of muscular and neural tissues in the alimentary canal. In: Code CF (ed) Handbook of Physiology, Sec. 6, Alimentary Canal, Vol. 4. American Physiology Society Washington, DC, 1579–1627, 1968.

19. Gabella G. Structure of muscles and nerves in the gastrointestinal tract. In: Johnson LR (ed) Physiology of the Gastrointestinal Tract. Raven Press, New York, 335–381, 1987.

20. Hightower NC. Motor action of the small bowel. In: Code CF (ed) Handbook of Physiology, Sec. 6, Alimentary Canal, Vol. 4. American Physiology Society, Washington DC, 2001–2024, 1968.

21. Weisbrodt NW. Motility of the small intestine. In: Johnson LR (ed) Physiology of the Gastrointestinal Tract. Raven Press, New York, 631–663, 1987.

22. Ehrlein HJ, Schemann M, Siegle M-L. Motor patterns of small intestine determined by closely spaced extraluminal transducers and videofluoroscopy. Am J Physiol 353:G359–G367, 1987.

23. Schemann M, Ehrlein H-J. Postprandial patterns of canine jejunal motility and transit of luminal content. Gastroenterology 90:991–1000, 1986.

24. Melville J, Macagno E, Christensen J. Longitudinal contractions in the duodenum: Their fluid-mechanical function. Am J Physiol 228:1887–1892, 1975.

25. Bortoff A. Myogenic control of intestinal motility. Physiol Rev 56:418–434, 1976.

26. Tasaka K, Farrar JT. Intraluminal pressure of the small intestine of the unanesthetized dog. Pflug Arch 364:35–44, 1976.

27. Job DD, Bloomquist WE, Bridgeforth J. Correlations between electrolyte content and spontaneous electrical activity in intestinal muscle. Am J Physiol 226:1502–1509, 1974.

28. Celander O. Are there any centrally controlled sympathetic inhibitory fibers to the musculature of the intestine? Acta Physiol Scand 47:299–309, 1959.

29. Burks TF, Jaquette DL, Grubb MN. Motility responses of dog and monkey isolated perfused intestine to morphine, 5-hydroxytryptamine and cholinergic stimulants. Comp Gen Pharmacol 5:213–216, 1974.

30. Sjoerdsma A, Lovenberg W, Engelman K, et al. Serotonin now: Clinical implications of inhibiting its synthesis with parachlorophenylalanine. Ann Int Med 73:607–629, 1970.

31. Schemann M, Ehrlein H-J. Effects of neurohormonal agents on jejunal contraction spread and transit in the fed dog. Gastroenterology 90:1950–1955, 1986.

32. Burnstock G. Purinergic nerves. Pharmacol Rev 24:509–581, 1972.

33. Frantzides CT, Sarna SK, Matsumoto T, et al. An intrinsic neural pathway for long intestino-intestinal inhibitory reflexes. Gastroenterology 92:594–603, 1987.

34. Mishra NK, Appert HE, Howard JM. Studies of paralytic ileus. Effects of intraperitoneal injury on motility of the canine small intestine. Am J Surg 129:559–563, 1975.

35. Williams NS, Meyer JH, Jehn D, et al. Canine intestinal transit and digestion of radiolabeled liver particles. Gastroenterology 86:1451–1459, 1984.

36. Bueno L, Praddaude F, Fioramonti J, et al. Effect of dietary fiber on gastrointestinal motility and jejunal transit time in dogs. Gastroenterology 80:701–707, 1981.

37. Quigley EMM, Phillips SF, Cranley B, et al. Tone of canine ileocolonic junction: Topography and response to phasic contractions. Am J Physiol 249:G350–G357, 1985.

38. Spiller RC, Brown ML, Phillips SF, et al. Scintigraphic measurements of canine ileocolonic transit. Gastroenterology 91:1213–1220, 1986.

39. Kelly ML, Jr, Gordon EA, Deweese JA. Pressure responses of canine ileocolonic junctional zone to intestinal distention. Am J Physiol 211:614–618, 1966.

40. Kumar D, Phillips SF, Brown ML. Reflux from ileum to colon in the dog. Dig Dis Sci 33:345–352, 1988.

41. Holgate AM, Read NW. Effect of ileal infusion of intralipid on gastrointestinal transit, ileal flow rate, and carbohydrate absorption in humans after ingestion of a liquid meal. Gastroenterology 88:1005–1011, 1985.

42. Christensen J. Motility of the colon. In: Johnson LR (ed) Physiology of the Gastrointestinal Tract. Raven Press, New York, 665–693, 1987.

43. Connell AM. Motor action of the large bowel. In: Code CF (ed) Handbook of Physiology, Sec. 6, Alimentary Canal, Vol. 4. American Physiology Society, Washington, DC 2075–2091, 1968.

44. Waller SL. Differential measurement of small and large bowel transit times in constipation and diarrhea: A new approach. Gut 16:372–378, 1975.

45. Gray GM. Carbohydrate digestion and absorption. Gastroenterology 58:96–107, 1970.

46. Semenza G. Pancreatic amylase In: Code CF (ed) Handbook of Physiology, Sec. 6, Alimentary Canal, Vol. 5. American Physiology Society, Washington, DC, 2637–2645, 1968.

47. Wormsley KG, Goldberg DM. The interrelationships of the pancreatic enzymes. Gut 13:398–412, 1972.

48. Alpers DH. Digestion and absorption of carbohydrates and proteins. In: Johnson LR (ed) Physiology of the Gastrointestinal Tract. Raven Press, New York, 1469–1487, 1987.

49. Johnson CF. Disaccharidase localization in hamster intestine brush borders. Science 155:1670–1672, 1967.

50. Noon KF, Rogul M, Brendle JJ, et al. Detection and definition of canine intestinal carbohydrases using a standardized method. Am J Vet Res 38:1063–1067, 1977.

51. Caspary WF, Winckler K, Lankish PG, et al. Influence of exocrine and endocrine pancreatic function on intestinal brush border enzymatic activities. Gut 16:89–92, 1975.

52. Dyck WP, Bonnett D, Lasatter J, et al. Hormonal stimulation of intestinal disaccharidase release in the dog. Gastroenterology 66:533–538, 1974.

53. Newcomer AD. Disaccharidase deficiencies. Mayo Clin Proc 48:648–652, 1973.

54. Gracey M, Houghton M, Thomas J. Deoxycholate depresses small intestinal enzyme activity. Gut 16:53–56, 1975.

55. Gray GM, Cooper HL. Protein digestion and absorption. Gastroenterology 61:535–544, 1971.

56. Keller PJ. Pancreatic proteolytic enzymes. In: Code CF (ed) Handbook of Physiology, Sec. 6, Alimentary Canal, Vol. 5. American Physiology Society, Washington, DC, 2605–2628, 1968.

57. Kim YS, Freeman HJ. Digestion and absorption of proteins. Ann Rev Med 29:99–116, 1978.

58. Wiseman G. Absorption of protein digestion products. In: Smyth DH (ed) Biomembranes, Vol.4A, Intestinal Absorption. Plenum Press, New York, 363–481, 1974.

59. Nicholson JA, Mccarthy DM, Kim YS. The responses of rat intestinal brush border and cytosol peptide hydrolase activities to variation in dietary protein content. J Clin Invest 54:890–898, 1974.

60. Kim YS, McCarthy DM, Lane W, et al. Alterations in the levels of peptide hydrolases and other enzymes in the brush border and cytosol fractions of rat small intestinal mucosa during starvation and refeeding. Biochem Biophys Acta 321:262–273, 1973.

61. Desnuelle P. Pancreatic lipase. In: Code CF (ed) Handbook of Physiology, Sec. 6, Alimentary Canal, Vol. 5. American Physiology Society, Washington, DC, 2629–2636, 1968.

62. Hofmann AF, Borgstrom B. The physico-chemical state of lipids in intestinal content during their digestion and absorption. Fed Proc 21:43–50, 1962.

63. Hofmann AF, Small DM. Detergent properties of bile salts: Correlation with physiological function. Ann Rev Med 18:333–376, 1967.

64. Mattson FH, Volpenhein, RA. The digestion and absorption of triglycerides. J Biol Chem 239:2772–2777, 1964.

65. Shiau Y-F. Lipid digestion and absorption. In: Johnson LR (ed) Physiology of the Gastrointestinal Tract. Raven Press, New York, 1527–1556, 1987.

66. Janowitz HD. Pancreatic secretion of fluid and electrolytes. In: Code CF (ed) Handbook of Physiology Sec. 6, Alimentary Canal, Vol. 2. American Physiology Society, Washington, DC, 925–933, 1968.

67. Schulz I. Electrolyte and fluid secretion in the exocrine pancreas. In: Johnson LR (ed) Physiology of the Gastrointestinal Tract. Raven Press, New York, 1147–1171, 1987.

68. Strombeck DR, Wheeldon R, Harrold D. Model of chronic pancreatitis in the dog. Am J Vet Res. 45:131–136, 1984.

69. Harper AA. The control of pancreatic secretion. Gut 13:308–317, 1972.

70. Rayford, PL, Miller TA, and Thompson JC. Secretin, cholecystokinin, and newer gastrointestinal hormones. N Eng J Med 295:1093–1101, 1157–1164, 1976.

71. Singh, M, Webster PD. Neurohormonal control of pancreatic secretion — a review. Gastroenterology 74:294–309, 1978.

72. Solomon TE. Control of exocrine pancreatic secretion. In: Johnson LR (ed) Physiology of the Gastrointestinal Tract. Raven Press, New York, 1173–1207, 1987.

73. Curtis PJ, Fender HR, Rayford PL, et al. Disappearance half-time of endogenous and exogenous secretin in dogs. Gut 17:595–599, 1976.

74. Curtis PJ, Fender HR, Rayford PL, et al. Catabolism of secretin by the liver and kidney. Surgery 80:259–265, 1976.

75. Flourie B, Leblond A, Florent Ch, et al. Starch malabsorption and breath gas excretion in healthy humans consuming low- and high-starch diets. Gastroenterology 95:356–363, 1988.

76. Levitt MD, Hirsh P, Fetzer CA, et al. H_2 excretion after ingestion of complex carbohydrates. Gastroenterology 92:383–389, 1987.

77. Jenkins DJA, Jenkins AL, Wolever TMS, et al. Simple and complex carbohydrates. Nutr Rev 44:44–49, 1986.

78. Warzburg OB. Nutritional aspects and safety of modified food starches. Nutr Rev 44:74–79, 1986.

79. Hendrix TR, Bayless TM. Digestion: Intestinal secretion. Ann Rev Physiol 32:139–164, 1970.

80. Banwell JG, Sherr H. Effect of bacterial enterotoxins on the gastrointestinal tract. Gastroenterology 65:467–497, 1973.

81. Donowitz M, Welsh MJ. Regulation of mammalian small intestinal electrolyte secretion. In: Johnson LR (ed) Physiology of the Gastrointestinal Tract. Raven Press, New York, 1351–1388, 1987.

82. Strombeck DR. The production of intestinal fluid by cholera toxin in the rat. Proc Soc Exp Biol Med 140:297–303, 1972.

83. Barbezat GO, Grossman MI. Intestinal secretion: Stimulation by peptides. Science 174:422–424, 1971.

84. Pierce NF, Carpenter CCJ, Elliott HL, et al. Effects of prostaglandins, theophylline, and cholera exotoxin upon transmucosal water and electrolyte movement in the canine jejunum. Gastroenterology 60:22–32, 1971

85. Udall JN, Alverez LA, Nichols BL, et al. The effects of cholera enterotoxin on intestinal tissue water as measured by nuclear magnetic resonance (NMR) spectroscopy. Physiol Chem Phys 7:533–539, 1975.

86. Brown WR. Relationships between immunoglobulins and the intestinal epithelium. Gastroenterology 75:129–138, 1978.

87. Kagnoff MF. Immunology of the digestive system. In: Johnson LR (ed) Physiology of the Gastrointestinal Tract. Raven Press, New York, 1699–1728, 1987.

88. Horowitz MI. Mucopolysaccharides and glycoproteins of the alimentary tract. In: Code CF (ed) Handbook of Physiology, Sec. 6, Alimentary Canal, Vol. 2. American Physiology Society, Washington, DC, 1063–1085, 1967.

89. Schrager J. The chemical composition and function of gastrointestinal mucus. Gut 11:450–456, 1970.

90. Neutra MR, Forstner JF. Gastrointestinal mucus: Synthesis, secretion, and function In: Johnson LR (ed) Physiology of the Gastrointestinal Tract. Raven Press, New York, 975–1009, 1978.

91. Strombeck DR, Harrold D. Binding of cholera toxin to mucins and inhibition by gastric mucin. Infect Immun 10:1266–1272, 1974.

92. Crane RK. Absorption of sugars. In: Code CF (ed) Handbook of Physiology, Sec. 6, Alimentary Canal, Vol. 4. American Physiology Society, Washington, DC, 1323–1351, 1967.

93. Crane RK. Intestinal absorption of glucose. In: Smyth DH (ed) Biomembranes, Vol. 4A. Intestinal Absorption. Plenum Press, New York, 541–553, 1974.

94. Hopfer U. Membrane transport mechanisms for hexoses and amino acids in the small intestine. In: Johnson LR (ed) Physiology of the Gastrointestinal Tract. Raven Press, New York, 1499–1526, 1987.

95. Walker WA, Isselbacher KJ. Uptake and transport of macromolecules by the intestine. Possible role in clinical disorders. Gastroenterology 67:531–550, 1974.

96. Ganapathy V, Leibach FH. Is intestinal peptide transport energized by a proton gradient? Am J Physiol 249:G153–G160, 1985.

97. Imondi AR, Stradley RP. Utilization of enzymatically hydrolyzed soybean protein and crystalline amino acid diets by rats with exocrine pancreatic insufficiency. J Nutr 104:793–801, 1974.

98. Gardner MLG. Gastrointestinal absorption of intact proteins. Ann Rev Nutr 8:329–350, 1988.

99. Strombeck DR, Harold D. Comparison of the rate of absorption and proteolysis of (14C) choleragen and (14C) bovine serum albumin in the rat jejunum. Infect Immun 12:1450–1456, 1975.

100. Borgstrom B. Fat digestion and absorption. In: Smyth DH (ed) Biomembranes, Vol. 4B, Intestinal Absorption. Plenum Press, London, 556–620, 1974.

101. Brindley DN. The intracellular phrase of fat absorption. In: Smyth DH (ed) Biomembranes, Vol. 4B, Intestinal Absorption. Plenum Press, London, 621–671, 1974.

102. Jackson MJ. Transport of short chain fatty acids. In: Smyth DH (ed) Biomembranes, Vol. 4B, Intestinal Absorption. Plenum Press, London, 673–709, 1974.

103. Erlinger S. Physiology of bile secretion and enterohepatic circulation. In: Johnson LR (ed) Physiology of the Gastrointestinal Tract. Raven Press, New York, 1557–1580, 1987.

104. Playout MR, Lack L, Weiner IM. Effect of intestinal resection on bile salt absorption in dogs. Am J Physiol 208:363–369, 1965.

105. Doty JE, Meyer JH. Vagotomy and antrectomy impairs canine fat absorption from solid but not liquid dietary sources. Gastroenterology 94:50–56, 1988.

106. Merritt AM, Burrows, CF, Cowgill, L, et al. Fecal fat and trypsin in dogs fed a meat-base or cereal-base diet. JAVMA 174:59–61, 1979.

107. Thomson ABR, Keelan M, Clandinin MT, et al. Dietary fat selectively alerts transport properties of rat jejunum. J Clin Invest 77:279–288,1986.

108. Vahouny GV. Effects of dietary fiber on digestion and absorption. In Johnson LR (ed) Physiology of the Gastrointestinal Tract. Raven Press, New York, 1623–1648, 1987.

109. Cummings JH, Englyst HN, Wiggins HS. The role of carbohydrates in lower gut function. Nutr Rev 44:50–54, 1986.

110. Herschel DA, Argenzio RA, Southworth M, et al. Absorption of volatile fatty acid, Na, and H_2O by the colon of the dog. Am J Vet Res 42:1118–1124, 1981.

111. Edmonds CJ. Salts and water. In Smyth DH (ed) Biomembranes, Vol. 4A, Intestinal Absorption. Plenum Press, New York, 711–759, 1974.

112. Svanvik J. Mucosal blood circulation and its influence on passive absorption in the small intestine. Acta Physiol Scand Suppl 385:1–44, 1973.

113. Wright EM. The passive permeability of the small intestine. In: Smyth DH (ed) Biomembranes, Vol. 4A, Intestinal Absorption Plenum Press, New York, 159–198, 1974.

114. Powell DW. Intestinal water and electrolyte transport. In: Johnson LR (ed) Physiology of the Gastrointestinal Tract. Raven Press, New York, 1267–1305, 1987.

115. Armstrong WM. Cellular mechanisms of ion transport in the small intestine. In: Johnson LR (ed) Physiology of the Gastrointestinal Tract. Raven Press, New York, 1251–1265, 1987.

116. Hakin AA, Lifson N. Effects of pressure on water and solute transport by dog intestinal mucosa in vitro. Am J Physiol 216–284, 1969.

117. Mailman D, Jordan K. The effect of saline and hyperoncotic dextran infusion on canine ileal salt and water absorption and regional blood flow. J Physiol 252:97–113, 1975.

118. Johnson PC, Richardson DR. The influence of venous pressure on filtration forces in the intestine. Microvas Res 7:296–306, 1974

119. Starling EH. On the absorption of fluids from the connective tissue spaces. J Physiol 19:312–326, 1986.

120. Cooke HJ. Neural and humoral regulation of small intestinal electrolyte transport. In: Johnson LR (ed) Physiology of the Gastrointestinal Tract. Raven Press, New York, 1307–1350, 1987.

121. Callender, ST. Iron absorption. In: Smyth DH (ed) Biomembranes, Vol. 4B, Intestinal Absorption. Plenum Press, London, 761–791, 1974.

122. Conrad ME. Iron absorption. In: Johnson LR (ed) Physiology of the Gastrointestinal Tract. Raven Press, New York, 1437–1453, 1987.

123. Harrison HE, Harrison HC. Calcium. In: Smyth DH (ed) Biomembranes, Vol. 4B, Intestinal Absorption. Plenum Press, London, 793–846, 1975.

124. Bronner F. Calcium absorption. In: Johnson LR (ed) Physiology of the Gastrointestinal Tract. Raven Press, New York, 1419–1435, 1987.

125. Younoszai MK, Schedl HP. Intestinal calcium transport; comparison of duodenum and ileum in vivo in the rat. Gastroenterology 62:565–571, 1972.

126. Matthews DM. Absorption of water-soluble vitamins. In: Smyth DH (ed) Biomembranes, Vol. 4B, Intestinal Absorption. Plenum Press, London, 847–915, 1974.

127. Rose RC. Intestinal absorption of water-soluble vitamins. In: Johnson LR (ed) Physiology of the Gastrointestinal Tract. Raven Press, New York, 1581–1596, 1987.

128. Batt RM, Horadagoda NU. Role of gastric and pancreatic intrinsic factors in the physiologic absorption of cobalamin in the dog. Gastroenterology 90:1339, 1986.

129. Batt RM, Morgan JO. Role of serum folate and vitamin B_{12} concentrations in the differentiation of small intestinal abnormalities in the dog. Res Vet Sci 32:17–22, 1982.

130. Washabau RJ, Strombeck DR, Buffington CA, et al. Evaluation of intestinal carbohydrate malabsorption in the dog by pulmonary hydrogen gas excretion. Am J Vet Res 47:1402–1406, 1986.

18

Classification, Pathophysiology, and Symptomatic Treatment of Diarrheal Diseases

W. GRANT GUILFORD AND DONALD R. STROMBECK

DIARRHEA AND THE SIGNS OF INTESTINAL DISEASE

Diarrhea, the most consistent manifestation of intestinal disease, is defined as a change in the frequency, consistency, or volume of bowel movements (Table 18–1). Stool weight and frequency are easy to measure, but an objective method for quantifying stool consistency has yet to be developed. Increased stool frequency can result from diseases that cause tenesmus or from derangements that cause larger fecal volume. Larger fecal volume is usually due to a greater content of fecal water or to greater amounts of undigested and unabsorbed nutrients such as fiber. In normal animals, the fiber content of the diet determines stool volume. Fecal water content will increase when an intestinal problem causes increased secretion or decreased absorption of fluid. The consistency (fluidity) of bowel movements is primarily determined by fecal water content but is also influenced by the physical and chemical properties of the stool matrix. Water content is 60% to 80% in normal bowel movements and 70% to 90% in unformed and watery feces. Thus, small changes in fecal water content transform normal bowel movements to liquid feces.

About 2.5 L of fluid enter the duodenal lumen each day in a 20 kg dog. The sources of the fluid are shown in Table 18–2. The amount absorbed in each region is shown in Table 18–3. The greatest volume of fluid is absorbed in the proximal small intestine, but the efficiency of the absorptive process increases in the more caudal regions of the bowel. For instance, the jejunum absorbs approximately four times as much fluid as the large intestine, but it is only half as efficient (Table 18–3). The colon has a capacity to absorb more than three times the water it normally absorbs. Thus, the volume of fluid entering the colon from the ileum must be large to exceed the colon's reserve absorptive capacity and cause diarrhea. In contrast, only minor abnormalities affecting either the colon's reservoir function or its absorptive capacity have profound effects on fecal properties. For example, a decrease in colonic water absorption from 300 mL to 290 mL, changing the volume of the stool from 50 to 60 mL, represents a 20% increase in fecal water and will cause diarrhea even though colonic absorption has been reduced only slightly.

The problem of diarrhea should be differentiated from the problem of fecal incontinence, which is the inability to retain feces until defecation is appropriate. Diarrhea challenges the continence mechanisms, but animals with diarrhea need not develop fecal incontinence. Similarly, animals with fecal incontinence need not have diarrhea.

Intestinal disease can cause many clinical signs in addition to, or instead of, diarrhea. Bowel movements may show other abnormalities, such as the appearance of blood, mucus, malassimilated nutrients, and melena. Colonic and rectal problems are often associated with tenesmus or dyschezia. The production and accumulation of abnormal amounts of gas can produce abdominal distention, borborygmus, eructation, flatus, discomfort, and pain. Halitosis is often recognized. Salivation, shivering, and hiding may be seen when smooth muscles of the intestine are stretched or in spasms. Appetite varies from complete anorexia to polyphagia. Water consumption frequently increases. Weight loss appears as a result of disrupted nutritional homeostasis. Thus, diseases of the intestinal tract can have a number of manifestations and the absence of diarrhea does not preclude intestinal disease. The diagnostic approaches to diarrhea and the other manifestations of intestinal disease are outlined in Chapter 5.

CLASSIFICATION OF DIARRHEAL DISEASES

Diseases resulting in diarrhea can be classified by duration, anatomic site, pathophysiology, pathologic appearance, and, when possible, by cause. Classifying diarrheal disorders as acute or chronic and large or small bowel helps the clinician determine appropriate diagnostic and therapeutic regimens. Classifi-

Table 18–1

DEFINITION OF DIARRHEA*

Increased frequency of defecation
  and/or
Increased fluidity or loose consistency of stools
  and/or
Increased fecal volume
  —increased water content (10%–20%)
  —or increased fecal solids

*Note: By this definition the frequent passage of bulky but well-formed stools should still be considered diarrhea.

Table 18–2

VOLUME AND SOURCES OF FLUID ENTERING
GUT PER DAY*

Diet: 600 mL
Saliva: 300 mL
Gastric: 600 mL
Bile: 300 mL
Pancreatic: 600 mL
Small intestine: 300 mL
Total: 2700 mL

*Figures from a 20 kg dog.

cation according to pathophysiology helps the clinician grasp the underlying similarities of many diarrheal diseases of widely disparate cause, which in turn suggests common therapeutic approaches. A scheme to describe the pathophysiology of diarrhea is found in Table 18–4. Classification according to pathologic appearance groups disorders that are likely to have similar pathophysiology and may, in some cases, have similar cause. Categorization according to cause is the most useful classification system for the clinician, but, unfortunately, the causes of many diarrheal diseases are unknown.

PATHOPHYSIOLOGY OF DIARRHEA[1]

Introduction

Diarrhea can result from a number of different pathophysiologic processes (Table 18–4 and 18–5; Figures 18–1, 18–2, and 18–3). Accumulation of osmotically active particles in the intestinal tract, breakdown of the intestinal permeability barrier, stimulation of intestinal secretory mechanisms, and alterations of intestinal motility can all result in diarrhea. Of these pathomechanisms, osmotic diarrheal diseases and diarrhea resulting from deranged permeability are thought to be the most common causes of diarrhea in dogs and in cats. It is important to note that more than one pathophysiologic process may be operative simultaneously in many patients with diarrhea.

Osmotic Diarrhea

PATHOPHYSIOLOGY OF OSMOTIC DIARRHEA. The number of osmotically active particles in the feces determines fecal water content. Increases in unabsorbed solutes elevate fecal water content (Figure 18–2) and can lead to osmotic diarrhea. The proximal small bowel is highly permeable to water and NaCl. When hyperosmolar chyme enters the duodenum, water flows across the duodenal mucosa and rapidly reduces the osmolality of the fluid to that of plasma. Sodium diffuses down a concentration gradient from the plasma into the diluted intestinal fluid. The passage of sodium into the intestinal fluid continues to draw more water into the intestinal lumen, in spite of the rapid equilibration of plasma and duodenal osmolality. The ileum and large bowel have low permeability to water and sodium, and active transport systems for the absorption of NaCl against steep electrochemical gradients. As a result, NaCl and water are absorbed as the intestinal fluid traverses the ileum and colon. However, in the presence of large amounts of nonabsorbable solute, the intestinal fluid volume does not return to normal, and diarrhea results.

Table 18–3

VOLUME AND SOURCES OF FLUID ABSORBED
FROM THE GUT PER DAY*

Jejunum: 1350 mL (50% of 2700 mL)
Ileum: 1000 mL (75% of 1350 mL)
Colon: 315 mL (90% of 350 mL)

*Figures from a 20 kg dog. Note that the absorptive processes are more efficient in the caudal intestine. Greater than 98% of all the fluid entering the intestine is normally absorbed.

CAUSES OF OSMOTIC DIARRHEA. Osmotic diarrhea can result from overeating, sudden diet changes, ingestion of excessive amounts of osmotic laxatives, gastric dumping, maldigestion, or malabsorption. Overeating causes diarrhea by overloading the intestinal tract with poorly absorbable nutrients, usually carbohydrates or divalent and trivalent ions such as phosphate or sulfate. Sudden change to a new diet containing a nutrient not previously fed in significant amounts results in diarrhea because of saturation of digestive and absorptive mechanisms for the novel nutrient. After several days have elapsed, adaption to the diet due to an increase in secretion of pancreatic and intestinal digestive enzymes may resolve the diarrhea. The rationale for making dietary changes gradually is based on the need for such adaptation to a new diet.

Many laxatives contain poorly absorbable ions such as magnesium, sulfate, or phosphate and will induce diarrhea if ingested in excessive quantities. Increased rate of delivery of food from the stomach to the small intestine (dumping) can cause osmotic overload. Maldigestion results in the accumulation of nutrients inadequately prepared for absorption. These accumulated molecules lead to osmotic and secretory diarrhea. Ineffective absorption of adequately digested nutrients (malabsorption) can also lead to osmotic diarrhea. Many

Table 18–4a

PATHOGENESIS OF DIARRHEA*

1. High volume input to colon with normal colonic absorption
2. Normal volume input to colon with decreased colonic absorption
3. Abnormal small and large intestine
4. Normal volume input to colon with normal colonic absorption

*General concepts of pathophysiology of diarrhea. Situation numbers 1 and 3 reflect diseases of the small intestine. Situation numbers 2, 3, and 4 reflect diseases of the large intestine. Number 4 occurs when the pathology involves the most caudal part of the large intestine or the rectum.

Table 18–4b

PATHOGENESIS OF DIARRHEA: CHANGES IN THE
SMALL AND LARGE INTESTINE THAT CAN CAUSE
DIARRHEA

Small Intestine
1. Decreased absorption of fluid and electrolytes
2. Incomplete absorption of nutrients (fats and carbohydrates)
3. Increased secretion of fluid and electrolytes
Large Intestine
1. Decreased absorption of fluid and electrolytes
2. Secretion of fluid and electrolytes
3. Failure of reservoir function

Table 18–5

ETIOPATHOGENESIS OF DIARRHEA

I. Osmotic diarrheas
  A. Dietary overload
  B. Malabsorption
    1. Pancreatic enzyme deficiency
      a. Absence of acinar tissue
        congenital: juvenile atrophy
        acquired: chronic relapsing pancreatitis; pancreatic
          interstitial fibrosis
      b. Obstruction of pancreatic ducts: neoplasms
    2. Bile deficiency
      a. Extrahepatic biliary obstruction
      b. Intrahepatic disease
      c. Chronic ileitis
    3. Duodenal mucosal disease
      a. Loss of regulation of secretin and PCZ release
      b. Loss of enterokinase secretin
      c. Loss of regulation of gastric emptying
    4. Small intestinal mucosal disease
      a. Loss of brush border enzymes
      b. Loss of transport mechanisms
      c. Absence of lipid transport lipoproteins
    5. Small intestinal intramural disease
      a. Physical obstacles to absorption
        i. Cellular infiltration of lamina propria
        ii. Fluid accumulation in lamina propria
      b. i. Loss of villous circulation
        ii. Loss of lymphatic circulation
        iii. Systemic circulatory disease
II. Abnormal electrolyte and water transport with normal mucosal
    permeability
  A. Secretion stimulated by bacterial enterotoxins and endotoxins
  B. Inhibition of absorption by unconjugated bile acids
  C. Inhibition of absorption by hydroxylated fatty acids
  D. Secretion stimulated by endocrines
III. Diarrheas caused by abnormal mucosal permeability
  A. Abnormal permeability to fluid and electrolytes (increased)
    1. Invasive bacteria
    2. Secondary to malabsorption or enterotoxins
  B. Abnormal permeability to plasma proteins: protein-losing
    enteropathy
    1. Abnormal metabolism or turnover of mucosal cells
    2. Mucosal ulceration by viral, bacterial, or parasitic agents
    3. Lymphatic obstruction
      a. Congenital absence: lymphangiectasia
      b. Obstruction by inflammation, neoplasia, or fibrosis
      c. Obstruction secondary to circulatory disease
  C. Abnormal permeability to fluid and electrolytes (decreased)
IV. Diarrheas as a result of changes in intestinal transit time
  A. Transit too slow: stagnant loop syndrome, ileus
  B. Transit too fast
    1. Absence of segmentation with normal peristalsis
    2. Spasms

---

the fermentation of malabsorbed carbohydrates to volatile fatty acids.

Secretory Diarrhea

PATHOPHYSIOLOGY OF SECRETORY DIARRHEA.[2] The intestine is capable of secreting vast quantities of fluid. The enterocytes in the intestinal crypts are thought to be the predominant source of this fluid, whereas those on the villi tips are the primary site of fluid absorption. In normal intestine, the magnitude of intestinal fluid and ion absorption exceeds that of intestinal secretion. In abnormal intestine, secretion can exceed resorption resulting in secretory diarrhea. Net intestinal ion secretion can result from either the stimulation of secretion to a greater than normal level (active secretion) or from an inhibition of intestinal absorption (passive secretion). Current evidence suggests that many mediators of active intestinal ion secretion also simultaneously inhibit intestinal ion absorption.[3] It is difficult to ascertain which of these processes dominates the activity of individual secretagogues. The intracellular second messages that are generated by secretagogues include cyclic AMP, cyclic GMP, calmodulin, calcium, and phospholipids.[1] These second messengers go on to stimulate active chloride secretion and may inhibit sodium absorption. Some secretagogues increase secretion by virtue of increasing the leakiness of the intestinal tight junctions.

As a result of intestinal secretion, the intestinal lumen will contain increased quantities of monovalent ions and water. It is important to note that marked secretory diarrhea can be present even though the mucosa has normal histologic features and that permeability and many transport processes, such as that for glucose absorption, may still be intact.

CAUSES OF SECRETORY DIARRHEA. A large number and variety of secretory agents and disease processes influence intestinal secretion (Table 18–6). These include various neuropeptides of the enteric nervous system, cholinergic agonists, gastrointestinal hormones, bacterial enterotoxins, deconjugated bile acids, and hydroxy fatty acids (see Chapter 17).

Enterotoxigenic bacteria attach to, but do not penetrate, the mucosal surface and produce secretory diarrhea by releasing an enterotoxin. The enterotoxin binds to the epithelial cell and stimulates the formation of second messengers such as cyclic AMP. Many organisms produce enterotoxins, including *Escherichia coli, Clostridium perfringens, Campy-*

disease processes can cause malabsorption and maldigestion (see Chapter 19).

CLINICAL APPEARANCE OF OSMOTIC DIARRHEA. Clinically, osmotic diarrhea is characterized by large volumes of watery diarrhea that resolves when food is withheld for 24 to 48 hours. Cessation of diarrhea following fasting does not rule out a secretory component to the diarrhea, however. For instance, diarrhea resulting from malabsorbed secretagogues such as fatty acids or bile acids will also stop or decrease when feeding is ceased. Analysis of fecal electrolytes from patients with osmotic diarrhea should show an osmolar gap, but as discussed in Chapter 6, fecal osmolar gaps must be interpreted with caution in dogs and cats until additional validation of the technique is performed. Fecal pH is usually low (< 7) in osmotic diarrhea because of

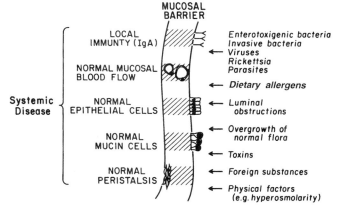

FIGURE 18-1. Diagram of causes of acute diarrhea and factors in the intestinal mucosa to prevent pathology and clinical signs from developing.

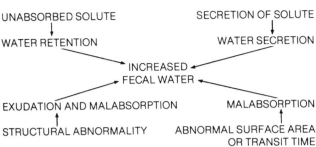

FIGURE 18-2. Pathogenesis of increased fecal water content, leading to diarrhea.

lobacter species, *Salmonella typhimurium, Staphylococcus aureus, Klebsiella pneumoniae,* and *Yersinia enterocolitica.* The importance of enterotoxigenic organisms in producing disease in small animals is unknown. Enterotoxigenic diarrhea is discussed in more detail in Chapter 21.

Decreased small intestinal absorption of deconjugated dihydroxy bile acids, such as deoxycholic and chenodeoxycholic acid, stimulates colonic secretion of fluid. The deconjugated bile acids cause secretion, at least partly, by increasing the leakiness of the tight junctions. Hydroxylated fatty acids are capable of inciting diarrhea in both the large and small intestine. The pathomechanism may be partly due to increased transcellular permeability and hence passive secretion. Vasoactive intestinal polypeptide and serotonin are responsible for profuse secretory diarrhea in humans with pancreatic cholera and the carcinoid syndrome, respectively. Prostaglandin E_2, substance P, HETE, HPETE, and bradykinin can be increased in inflamed tissues and are capable of stimulating intestinal secretion. Cardiac glycosides increase intestinal secretion, as do certain laxatives such as bisacodyl. Elevated venous pressure, lymphatic obstruction, hypoalbuminemia, and increases in epithelial permeability all alter fluid dynamics in the mucosa and can result in decreased absorption and a passive secretory diarrhea. Any disease process, such as coronavirus infection, that preferentially damages villus tips will reduce intestinal absorption.

CLINICAL APPEARANCE OF SECRETORY DIARRHEA. Secretory diarrhea is characterized clinically by large volumes of watery diarrhea, the absence of a fecal osmolar gap, high fecal pH (> 7), persistence of the diarrhea during fasting, and the absence of inflammatory cells, blood, or fat in the feces. It is not uncommon for patients to present with secretory diarrhea in association with osmotic diarrhea, blurring the clinical differentiation of these two conditions (see earlier).

Diarrhea Resulting from Increased Permeability

STRUCTURE OF THE INTESTINAL PERMEABILITY BARRIER. The mucosa of the small and large intestine forms a semipermeable barrier that controls the transmucosal movement of fluid and electrolytes and restricts the absorption or loss of larger molecules. Important epithelial components of the barrier include the mucus layer, the glycocalyx, the epithelial cells, and the tight junctions situated at the apical borders of the epithelial cells. The tight junctions appear to have a very important role in maintaining intestinal epithelial permeability. At the tight junctions, the lateral plasma membranes of adjacent cells come into close apposition with each other, forming a series of punc-

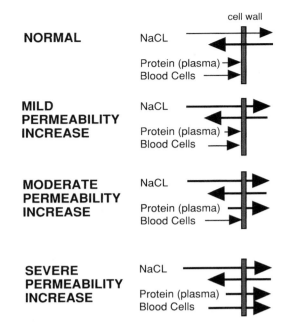

FIGURE 18-3. Effects of permeability changes on fluid and macromolecule loss into intestine.

tate membrane fusions linked by strands of what appear to be proteins. Tight junction morphology correlates with the permeability characteristics of the membrane. Thus, the paracellular permeability decreases as the junctional strand count increases.[4] Moreover, recent evidence suggests that tight junction permeability can be regulated by a perijunctional ring of actin and myosin, raising the possibility that transjunctional mucosal permeability can be finely regulated on a minute-by-minute basis.[5] The suggested importance of tight junctions in regulating intestinal permeability is compatible with recent concepts of intestinal absorption and secretion, in which the absorptive cell is believed to concentrate Na and Cl in the basolateral space, from whence it diffuses into the lamina propria. The tight junction is thus in a position to regulate the back leakage of fluid and electrolytes from the basolateral space into the lumen of the intestine. Tight junctions in the upper small intestine are known to be permeable to fluid, electrolytes, and other small solutes. The result is a predominance of passive fluid fluxes across the small intestine. In contrast, the tight junctions of the colon are impermeable to fluid and electrolytes,

Table 18-6

PUTATIVE CAUSES OF SECRETORY DIARRHEA

Enterotoxins
APUD neoplasms
Laxatives (castor oil, dioctyl sodium sulfosuccinate, Bisacodyl)
Cardiac glycosides
Bile acid malabsorption
Fatty acid malabsorption
Congenital defects
Intestinal inflammation
Intestinal lymphoma
Giardiasis
Hyperthyroidism
Malignant carcinoid syndrome?
Medullary carcinoma of the thyroid
Mechanical irritation
Circulatory defects

allowing the active transport of electrolytes against concentration gradients.

The capillaries and lymphatics of the mucosa have important functions in maintaining normal permeability. One of these functions is the conservation of plasma protein and another is the removal of absorbed fluid, preventing increased mucosal interstitial hydrostatic pressure. Additional components of the intestinal permeability barrier include the cellular and humoral immune system in the lamina propria and the mononuclear-phagocyte system in the liver. Defects in these systems permit an excessive amount of macromolecules to enter the body.

PATHOPHYSIOLOGY OF DIARRHEA RESULTING FROM INCREASED INTESTINAL PERMEABILITY.   The intestinal permeability barrier has a number of different functions. One of these functions is to act as a semipermeable membrane that retains electrolytes absorbed by active or facilitated diffusion against concentration gradients. The effective retention of these electrolytes creates an osmotic gradient by which water can be absorbed from the intestinal lumen. If intestinal permeability increases, absorbed electrolytes flow back into the bowel, no concentration gradient develops, and fecal water concentration will increase. Therefore, mild increases in permeability result in reduced absorption of ions and water and lead to a net intestinal fluid loss. Mild permeability increases are thus sometimes referred to as a cause of "passive" secretory diarrhea.

If the epithelial permeability barrier becomes further deranged, plasma proteins, such as albumin, that reside in the interstitium of the lamina propria may be lost into the lumen of the bowel. If the permeability failure extends to involve the mucosal blood vessels, additional plasma proteins and eventually red blood cells may be lost (Figure 18–3). The loss of red blood cells requires a greater than 10,000-fold increase in pore size.

Another function of the mucosal permeability barrier is to prevent the unrestrained absorption of macromolecules from the lumen, thus helping maintain oral tolerance (see Chapter 3). The barrier to the absorption of macromolecules includes not only the physical barrier provided by the epithelial cell, which possesses some ability to degrade proteins, but also the cellular and humoral immune system in the lamina propria and the mononuclear-phagocyte system in the liver. Defects in any one of the three permit an excessive amount of macromolecules to enter the body. As discussed in Chapter 3, the permeability to macromolecules is an age-related phenomenon, with intestinal "closure" occurring in most domestic species within several days of birth, but in carnivores being delayed for as long as 10 to 12 days.[6] Furthermore, closure is never complete; adult animals absorb up to 2% of dietary protein intact, presumably largely through the intestinal M cells.

CAUSES OF INCREASED INTESTINAL PERMEABILITY.   Abnormalities that increase intestinal epithelial permeability include epithelial erosion or ulceration, mucosal inflammation, cellular infiltration of the lamina propria by neoplastic cells, and circulatory diseases that result in ischemia or lymphatic hypertension.

The most obvious cause of increased epithelial permeability is destruction of the enterocyte. The resultant erosions or ulcerations freely ooze interstitial fluid or blood. Gastrointestinal erosions and ulcerations may result from a wide variety of conditions including severe mucosal inflammation, intestinal neoplasia, mucosal ischemia, invasive infectious agents, toxins, anti-inflammatory medications, uremia, mastocytosis, hepatic insufficiency, gastrinomas, stress, and perhaps inadequate mucosal bicarbonate or mucus secretion.[7]

Mucosal inflammation is known to increase intestinal

epithelial permeability. The latter is a well-recognized complication of chronic inflammatory bowel disease, gluten-induced enteropathy, and soy and milk protein intolerance. The pathomechanisms of the increased epithelial permeability are unclear, but proposals include epithelial denudation or, in less severe cases, the development of a less differentiated epithelium as a result of increased cell turnover.[8] Furthermore, gamma interferon increases epithelial tight junction permeability, as does increased mucosal fibrinolytic activity.

Circulatory disorders result in increased permeability due to increased hydrostatic pressure, which increases pore size. Additional factors known to increase mucosal epithelial permeability include exposure of the mucosa to bile salts, lysolecithin, and hyperosmolar solutions, and treatment with nonsteroidal anti-inflammatory agents[9] and cytotoxic drugs such as 5-fluorouracil.[6,10,11] Surgical trauma to the intestine, intestinal ischemia, protein malnutrition, systemic anaphylaxis, and parasite infections also increase epithelial permeability.[6]

The permeability of intestinal capillaries is increased by a variety of pathologic interventions, including ischemia, exposure to E. coli endotoxin, histamine, and bradykinin.[12] The majority of these conditions increase capillary permeability by increasing the diameter of large-size capillary pores resulting in increased protein leakage into the interstitium.

CLINICAL APPEARANCE OF DIARRHEA RESULTING FROM INCREASED PERMEABILITY.   Diarrhea resulting from permeability disorders does not completely abate when food is withheld. Severe increases in permeability are characterized by hypoproteinemia, melena, dysentery, hematochezia, and sometimes by evidence of gastrointestinal inflammation such as tenesmus or increased fecal leukocyte concentration.

Diarrhea Resulting from Deranged Motility

PATHOPHYSIOLOGY OF DERANGED MOTILITY.   Disordered intestinal motility contributes to the pathogenesis of many diarrheal diseases and may be the primary pathomechanism in some cases (Tables 18–5 and 18–7). It can be difficult to establish whether a motility abnormality is the cause of diarrhea or simply a secondary consequence of a primary disease process, such as inflammation.

Motility changes that speed intestinal transit cause diarrhea. These changes result in decreased intestinal fluid absorption, presumably due to decreased contact time between the enterocyte and the luminal content. Accelerated intestinal passage can result from two different types of motility abnormalities: decreased segmentation contractions or increased peristaltic contractions. The most common cause is a decreased frequency of segmental contractions, which reduces the resistance of the intestinal tract to the flow of ingesta. Increased frequency of peristaltic contractions was initially thought to be a very important cause of diarrhea, but it now appears that few cases of diarrhea result from increased peristaltic activity. In contrast, reduced or deranged peristaltic activity may lead to diarrhea by predisposing the intestinal tract to bacterial overgrowth.

CAUSES OF DERANGED INTESTINAL MOTILITY.   Deranged intestinal motility in association with diarrhea has been documented in hookworm infections of dogs,[13] canine dysautonomia, a small percentage of cases of feline dysautonomia, canine pseudo-obstruction syndrome, and feline colitis (Table 18–7). In parasite infections, violent intestinal contractions have been reported as part of the "self-cure"

Table 18–7

DIARRHEAL DISEASES IN WHICH DERANGED MOTILITY MAY PLAY A ROLE

Irritable bowel syndrome
APUD tumors
Hyperthyroidism
Bile acid malabsorption
Myenteric ganglionitis
Dysautonomia
Infectious gastroenteritis
Gastrointestinal parasitism
Gastrointestinal neoplasia
Pseudo-obstruction syndrome
Colitis
Bacterial overgrowth

response resulting from mast cell degranulation. In a dog with myenteric ganglionitis, the transit time of barium from the stomach to the colon was very rapid (3 minutes), strongly suggesting a motility defect, perhaps decreased segmental contractions.[14]

With colitis, deranged motility due to the inflammatory process compromises the reservoir function of the large bowel. In cats and, to a lesser extent, dogs the cranial half of the large intestine has a gradient of motility that is normally reversed, so propulsive activity retains contents until absorption is nearly complete. This gradient is lost during colitis[15] and perhaps with other causes of diarrhea. Colonic inflammation also decreases segmentation motility, contributing to an accelerated transit of material through the cranial colon. The pathogenesis of the motility disturbances is not clear but probably results either from a direct effect of the mediators such as PGE_2 or leukotrienes on smooth muscle function or from an indirect effect of these mediators on the enteric nervous system. The importance of deranged motility due to irritable bowel syndrome in animals has yet to be established (see Chapter 28).

CLINICAL APPEARANCE OF DIARRHEA RESULTING FROM MOTILITY DISTURBANCE. In view of the difficulty in definitively diagnosing motility derangements as the cause of diarrhea, there is no well-recognized clinical picture associated with motility diarrheas. Humans suspected of having "motility" diarrhea reportedly have voluminous diarrhea that is reduced by fasting. In addition they have a fecal electrolyte pattern with no osmolar gap during the unfed state, and a slight osmolar gap with mild steatorrhea following eating.[3] Hypomotility in association with bacterial overgrowth may generate the clinical-laboratory features characteristic of bacterial overgrowth (see Chapter 19).

CAUSES OF ACUTE GASTROINTESTINAL DISEASES

The acute onset of diarrhea is a very common problem that has a wide range of possible causes, many of which are infectious, parasitic, or toxic in nature (Table 18–5). The specific cause of acute diarrhea in an individual animal is seldom identified because the transient nature of the clinical signs precludes extensive diagnostic evaluation.

Acute diarrhea often occurs as a result of a dietary change. This may be due to a transient malassimilation as a result of insufficient time for pancreatic secretion and intestinal brush border activity to adjust to the dominant nutrients in the new

diet. Alternatively, the diarrhea may result from a specific food intolerance.

Animals with an acute onset of vomiting and diarrhea are frequently suspected of inadvertent or malicious poisoning. The likelihood of toxicity is considerably greater in an animal with access to an unknown environment rather than an animal restricted to its own property. However, even within the closeted environment of the indoor pet, the list of potential toxins that can result in acute gastrointestinal upset is extensive.[16-18] Acute vomiting and diarrhea due to poisoning should be particularly suspected in patients with concurrent clinical signs of other body systems. For instance, generalized parasympathetic overactivity manifest as hypersalivation, vomiting, diarrhea, and pinpoint pupils is suggestive of organophosphate or carbamate toxicity. Table 18–8 lists cross-referenced associations of clinical signs from different body systems that may help determine the toxin involved.

Acute diarrhea can also be produced by infectious agents. Examples of viruses causing diarrhea are canine distemper virus, affecting a number of organ systems, and feline panleukopenia virus, affecting only the gastrointestinal tract. Rickettsial agents are responsible for the diarrhea of salmon poisoning. Enteric bacterial pathogens such as *Salmonella* spp, *Clostridium perfringens*, *Campylobacter* spp, and *Yersinia enterocolitica* can cause diarrhea. In general, enteropathogenic bacteria are not frequent causes of diarrhea in dogs and cats and much of their importance lies in their zoonotic potential. Parasites such as ascarids, hookworms, whipworms, *Cryptosporidia*, and *Coccidia* may also cause diarrhea.

DIAGNOSTIC APPROACH TO ACUTE GASTROINTESTINAL DISEASES

The diagnosis of acute gastrointestinal diseases should use the problem-oriented approach. The diagnostic approaches to the common manifestations of acute gastrointestinal diseases such as the problems of vomiting, diarrhea, and acute abdomen are described in Chapter 5. The diagnostic evaluation of most patients with acute gastrointestinal problems is largely restricted to a history and physical examination. Unless warning signs of serious disease are present, any further diagnostic endeavors are usually delayed until the response to a therapeutic trial has been evaluated.

The patient's signalment, vaccination history, anthelmintic history, and the nature of the environment is determined. Young animals are more prone to nutritional, microbial, and parasitic causes of diarrhea. Certain breed predispositions are apparent (Table 5–3). A dog or cat developing diarrhea following placement in a boarding kennel is likely to have an infectious enteritis. An animal with complete freedom in an unknown environment is more likely to develop infectious, toxic, and traumatic disorders. The animal's diet should be determined. Adverse reactions to food are a prominent cause of diarrhea and the history is a rapid way to identify responsible nutrients. Ingestion of salmon or trout in certain areas raises the likelihood of salmon poisoning. Evidence of multisystemic disease increases the index of suspicion for distemper or toxicities (see Table 18–8).

Particularly important parts of the physical examination are the assessment of the animal's attitude, cardiovascular status, and degree of dehydration; oral examination; abdominal palpation; and rectal examination. Fever in association with acute gastrointestinal disease is suggestive of severe mucosal breakdown such as can occur with enteroinvasive organisms.

The clinical examination rarely definitively determines the

Table 18–8

TOXICITIES THAT CAN CAUSE VOMITING AND DIARRHEA CATEGORIZED ACCORDING TO LIKELY CONCURRENT CLINICAL SIGNS

Vomiting and/or Diarrhea with Stomatitis

Acids and alkalis	Paraquat
Aldehydes	Petroleum distillates
Caustic products	Phenols
Detergents	Philodendron
Diffenbachia	Thallium
Mercury	

Vomiting and/or Diarrhea with Cardiac Arrhythmias

Foxgloves	Organophosphates
Lily of the valley	Thallium
Oleander	Yew (Taxus spp.)

Vomiting and/or Diarrhea with Hepatotoxicity

Aflatoxins	Blue-green algae
Amanita spp. mushrooms	Phosphorus

Vomiting and/or Diarrhea with Respiratory Toxicity

ANTU
Organophosphates
Paraquat

Vomiting and/or Diarrhea with Nephrotoxicity

Amanita spp. mushrooms	Mock orange
Amaryllis bulbs	Organophosphates
Arsenic	Phosphorus
Azalea	Rhododendron
Castor bean	Mercury
Daffodil bulbs	Nightshades
English ivy	Lead
Horse chestnut	Paraquat
Iris bulbs	Phenols
Jasmine	Thallium

Vomiting and/or Diarrhea with CNS Signs

Chlordane	Organophosphates
Ethylene glycol	Phenols
Lead	Mercury
Organochlorines	Metaldehyde

Vomiting and/or Diarrhea with Generalized Parasympathetic Stimulation

Amanita spp. mushrooms
Carbamates
Organophosphates

cause of acute vomiting or diarrhea but usually unearths likely possibilities. Moreover, the physical examination is the prime guide to the severity of the patient's condition. Warning signs of serious disease include depression, anorexia, weight loss, weakness, dehydration, hyperpnea, pale, congested, or discolored mucous membranes, slow capillary refill, weak rapid pulse, fever, melena, and abdominal organomegaly, pain, masses, or effusions.

By the conclusion of the clinical examination the veterinarian should be able to locate the site of the disorder (e.g., large- or small-bowel diarrhea) and assess the degree of severity. If the cause of the gastrointestinal dysfunction is not apparent following the clinical examination and warning signs of serious disease are present, the clinician is obligated to recommend supportive therapy and a diagnostic workup to determine safe and effective therapy. In the absence of warning signs, symptomatic therapy and treatment trials are permissible. Toxicologic analyses may be indicated depending on the likelihood of exposure.

LABORATORY FINDINGS AND DIAGNOSIS OF ACUTE GASTROINTESTINAL DISEASES

Microscopic examination of a fecal smear or rectal scrape is a useful diagnostic evaluation in patients with acute diarrhea. This inexpensive procedure will occasionally reveal parasitic ova and protozoa or abnormal bacterial flora (e.g., excessive numbers of *Clostridium perfringens* spores). Stained rectal scrapes may disclose inflammatory cells, suggestive of a colitis or enterocolitis. Only heavy parasitic infestations are identified on direct smears. Therefore, examination for intestinal parasites by fecal flotation is necessary, but even this concentration technique has questionable reliability when the patient's feces are very watery.

If bacterial pathogens are suspected (see Chapters 5 and 6) feces may be cultured. Routinely identification of enteropathogenic *E. coli* is not performed because serotyping and various other refined subtyping procedures are required. The serotyping systems are generally based on recognition of somatic (O), flagellar (H), and capsular (K) antigens. Over 150 somatic (O) antigens and more than 40 flagellar (H) antigens have been recognized. Tests of feces for clostridial or coliform enterotoxins may also be of value in select cases as may virus identification procedures.

If the history and physical examination reveal evidence of gastrointestinal obstruction, systemic problems, or serious disease, additional diagnostic evaluations such as a hemogram, blood chemistry panel, urinalysis, blood gas analysis, and/or survey abdominal radiographs may be required. These diagnostic procedures provide information that greatly helps differential diagnosis and case management.

Gastrointestinal biopsy is rarely of use in identifying the cause of acute diarrhea. Enterotoxin stimulates epithelial cells to secrete fluid without changing their appearance. After 24 hours secondary changes may begin to appear but these are nonspecific. Invasion by a pathogen produces an enteritis that cannot be differentiated histologically from enteritis due to opportunistic invasion by a member of the normal microflora. However, biopsy helps differentiate bacterial infection from idiopathic inflammatory bowel disease because the former is more likely to be associated with suppuration than the latter. Causal organisms are seldom identified by biopsy. Exceptions include the attachment to the mucosa of enteroadherent bacteria and the invasion of the mucosa by fungal agents (Figure 18–4) or protozoa. Postmortem changes in the intestine are rapid, being accelerated by the bacteria and proteases in the intestinal lumen. Consequently, even at necropsy it is often difficult to determine how the mucosa appeared at the time of death.

SYMPTOMATIC THERAPY OF ACUTE DIARRHEA

As with any medical problem, the therapy of a patient with acute diarrhea is best based on a knowledge of cause. Unfortunately, however, the causes of diarrheal diseases are often never ascertained, either because of the elusive nature of the disease process or because minimal diagnostic effort is expended in view of financial constraints or anticipated brevity of the diarrhea. As a result, the symptomatic therapy of diarrhea is commonplace in veterinary practice. Symptomatic therapy is also of importance in the adjunctive treat-

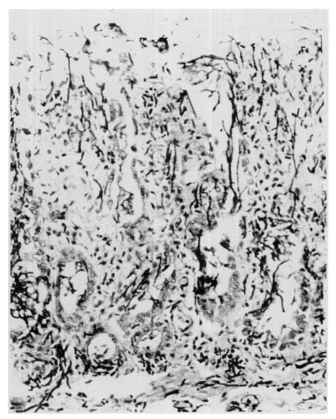

FIGURE 18–4. Jejunum from cat stained with PAS to show mycotic organisms causing enteritis. Branching septate hyphae are typical of aspergillosis. The animal was immunosuppressed as shown by severe hypoplasia of lymphoid tissues and bone marrow; the cause is unknown.

ment of patients with diarrhea in whom the primary cause is known.

The most critical aspects of the symptomatic treatment of acute diarrhea are bowel rest and the maintenance of fluid and electrolyte homeostasis. Of additional concern in some patients is the prevention or treatment of septicemia. Furthermore, the patient may benefit from agents that alter the motility of the gut or act as mucosal protectives.

The symptomatic treatment of diarrhea is still largely empirical. Many methods are used that are time honored but not scientifically validated. Most animals recover from diarrhea whether or not they are treated. The high incidence of spontaneous remission reinforces the mistaken belief that certain inappropriate therapies, such as anticholinergic agents and oral aminoglycosides, are effective. In many cases it is more appropriate to conclude that the patient recovered in spite of the therapy.

Fluid Therapy

The administration of fluids, of sufficient volume and appropriate composition to correct preexisting fluid, electrolyte, and acid-base derangements and to satisfy ongoing requirements, is the single most important consideration in the therapy of any patient with diarrhea. Decisions must be made regarding the route of administration, the quantity of fluid to be delivered, the composition of the fluid, and the

rate of delivery. These considerations are addressed in detail in Chapter 39.

The preferred method of administration of fluids to markedly dehydrated animals is the intravenous route unless the patient is intractable. If venous collapse in a hypovolemic animal prevents percutaneous placement of an intravenous catheter, a venous cut-down should be performed or alternatively the intramedullary route used to administer the fluids. The subcutaneous route is contraindicated in this situation because the vasoconstricted cutaneous vascular beds will not take up the fluid for many hours if at all.

The fluid, electrolyte, and acid-base derangements occurring in patients with gastrointestinal diseases are quite variable. As a result, the composition of the fluid administered is best judged by the serum electrolyte, total protein, and glucose concentration, and by the hematocrit. Choices include lactated Ringer's solution and 0.45% or 0.9% sodium chloride with added potassium chloride, sodium bicarbonate, or dextrose; dextrans; plasma; and blood. In most patients with diarrhea, an appropriate *replacement* fluid is lactated Ringer's solution supplemented with an additional 10 to 15 mEq of potassium chloride per liter. The volume administered depends on the patient's body weight and estimated degree of dehydration (5%–12%). For most patients with uncomplicated diarrheal disease, replacement of preexisting fluid losses can be achieved within 6 to 12 hours. Additional fluid is required to replace the patient's maintenance requirements (50–70 mL/kg/day) and ongoing additional losses. The latter are estimated from the volume of diarrhea or vomitus passed by the patient.

Cooperative patients that are not markedly dehydrated may be treated with glucose-containing oral rehydration solutions (e.g., Enterolyte; Beecham) or food-based oral rehydration syndromes (see Chapter 38). During many diarrheal processes, including secretory diarrhea, it appears that the sodium-organic solute (glucose or neutral amino acid) absorption mechanism it still active.[1]

Dietary Management

Dogs and cats with acute diarrhea are usually fasted for 12 to 48 hours and then offered a hypoallergenic low-fat diet fed frequently and in small quantities for 3 to 7 days (see Chapter 38).

The period of fasting has been considered necessary to provide "bowel rest." Specifically, the absence of nutrients in the intestinal tract reduces gastrointestinal secretions, minimizes the amount of osmotically active particles in the bowel, decreases the numbers of intestinal bacteria, and lessens the desquamation of mucosal epithelial cells. In addition, withholding food reduces the chances that dietary antigens will be absorbed intact through the inflamed mucosa, which can sensitize the animal to subsequent contact with the same diet. Furthermore, most diarrheal diseases reduce the activity of small intestinal brush border enzymes. In particular, the loss of disaccharidases results in difficulty in assimilating certain carbohydrates such as lactose. Recently, however, the long-held belief in the value of bowel rest for treatment of diarrhea has been challenged by the concept of feeding-through-diarrhea. Feeding-through-diarrhea maintains greater mucosal barrier integrity and helps minimize malnutrition, usually without prolonging the duration of diarrhea. Caution is required, however, before the tried-and-true "no food per os" recommendation is abandoned in dogs and cats with diarrhea because feeding-through is likely to be less successful in the osmotic diarrheal diseases that most commonly affect dogs and cats (see Chapter 38).

The return to feeding should follow a number of important principles (see Chapter 38). The food selected should be given in small amounts at frequent intervals so that osmotic overload is not problem. The diet should contain nutrients that are easily digested and absorbed. Dietary fat is kept to a minimum because fat undergoes a complex digestion and absorption process that is easily disrupted by gastroenteritis. Furthermore, malabsorbed fatty acids and bile acids promote secretory diarrhea in the large bowel. The diet should be hypoallergenic, to minimize the likelihood of sensitization during the recovery phase. Because most antigens are proteins, the type and amount of protein to incorporate in the diet should be carefully considered (see Chapters 24 and 38). Lastly, the diet must be palatable because the appetites of animals with diarrhea are often capricious.

Suitable diets for the management of diarrhea are described in Chapter 38. Briefly, homemade diets are usually formulated from highly digestible carbohydrate and protein sources. The protein source should be lean and not part of the usual diet of the patient. Suitable choices are cottage cheese, lean meats, poultry, fish, eggs, and tofu. The most convenient carbohydrate source for dogs is boiled white rice. In cats, carbohydrate is often omitted from the diet for the first week or two of therapy, but baby rice cereal is a suitable carbohydrate source if required. The usual ratio of protein source to cooked rice is 1 to 2 (dogs) or 1 to 1 (cats). Vitamins and minerals are added if long-term use of the diet is anticipated. The addition of fiber is indicated if large-bowel diarrhea is present. Suitable selected-protein commercial diets are also now widely available. The controlled diet is usually fed for approximately 7 days. If the diarrhea resolves, the controlled diet can be gradually changed back to the patient's regular diet over a period of 2 to 3 days.

Antibiotics[19-25]

ADVERSE EFFECTS OF ANTIBIOTIC ADMINISTRATION. Antibiotics have a number of predictable adverse effects on the gastrointestinal tract (Table 18–9) and if injudiciously used will complicate recovery from diarrhea.[26] Of particular concern is the adverse effects on the normal flora that can predispose the patient to diarrhea, infection with virulent pathogens, and sepsis. In the large intestine, antibiotic administration results in a slight transient reduction of the total numbers of bacteria. Within 1 to 2 days, bacterial numbers return to their previous level in spite of continued administration of the antibacterial agent. Although the total numbers of bacteria in the large bowel are little affected by antibiotics, fecal bacterial composition can be markedly altered. Bacteria that develop resistance to antibiotics slowly, such as the gram positive anaerobes, may be depressed for prolonged periods of time following the administration of antibiotics with efficiency against anaerobic bacteria. In contrast, coliform numbers can usually be significantly lowered only on a transient basis because they rapidly develop antibiotic resistance. Antibiotic resistance possessed by one group of coliforms can be readily transferred to another within 24 to 48 hours. Within several days, the numbers of coliforms return to normal and, in the presence of a depressed anaerobic population, these potentially more virulent gram negative organisms may proliferate in excessive numbers, predisposing the animal to sepsis. For example, in guinea pigs, erythromycin suppresses anaerobes and causes intestinal coliforms to increase from 10^2 bacteria per gram of feces to 10^7 per gram, resulting in death within

10 to 14 days. Overgrowth by yeasts and fungi may also occur following prolonged antibiotic administration.[27]

The animal with diarrhea is particularly vulnerable to the adverse effects of antibiotics on the composition of bacterial flora. Dogs with diarrhea have a decreased number of *Lactobacilli* spp. and increased numbers of *Bacteroides* spp. and members of the *Enterobacteriaceae.*[28] Overall, the total numbers of colonic anaerobes is reduced in the feces during diarrhea because these organisms normally require stasis, and the low oxygen environment it provides, for their growth.[29] Pathologic processes such as malassimilation markedly alter the intestinal milieu, leading to derangements in the composition of bacteria. In this situation, a pathogenic opportunist such as *Salmonella* can colonize the bowel, whereas it may have been previously excluded by the resistance of the normal flora. Use of antibiotics further deranges the normal flora and, if poorly chosen, may not inhibit the growth of bacteria such as *Salmonella,* further predisposing the animal to colonization by pathogens. Normal intestinal function does not return until the microbial population of the gut returns to normal

Additional adverse effects of antibiotics include various side effects such as anorexia, vomiting, and iatrogenic diarrhea that can confuse the clinical picture and delay recovery. Gastrointestinal upset is most commonly seen in dogs and cats as a result of treatment with neomycin, tetracycline, erythromycin, metronidazole, penicillins, clindamycin, or chloramphenicol. The cause of antibiotic-associated diarrhea can be due to a direct adverse effect on the mucosa by the antibiotic or, alternatively, a result of derangement of normal flora. Humans who develop antibiotic-associated diarrhea have markedly impaired colonic fermentation while receiving antibiotics in comparison to those who do not develop diarrhea during antibiotic usage.[30] It is likely that the resultant lack of volatile fatty acids impairs the ability of the colon to absorb water and electrolytes and predisposes the patient to diarrhea.[30] In humans, the diarrhea from neomycin administration is due to a malabsorption syndrome associated with only a mild morphologic defect. The malabsorption results from direct precipitation of micellar fatty acids and monoglycerides or from alteration of microbial flora in favor of species such as *Bacteroides* spp. and *Clostridia* spp. that secrete amidases capable of deconjugating bile salts. Neomycin also appears to interfere with pancreatic lipase activity and decrease bile acid resorption.[31] The diarrhea resulting from tetracyclines results from changes in the intestinal microflora and possibly from an irritative effect.

Aminoglycosides have well-recognized renal toxicity, vestibular toxicity, and ototoxicity. The renal toxicity of aminoglycosides is enhanced by youth, dehydration, overdosage, and concurrent administration of certain drugs such as some cephalosporins and nonsteroidal anti-inflammatory drugs. These predisposing conditions occur frequently in diarrheal diseases. Oral aminoglycosides are often administered in quantities that far exceed the recommended par-

Table 18–9

HARMFUL EFFECTS OF ANTIBIOTICS

Overgrowth of fungi and minor organisms of normal flora
Diarrhea due to neomycin, tetracycline, ampicillin
Produces resistant bacteria
Increases susceptibility to infection by pathogen
Prolongs carrier state in salmonellosis
Interferes with nutrition
Systemic toxicity of aminoglycosides

enteral doses. In normal animals the aminoglycoside is not absorbed, and no systemic toxicity results. In animals with a disrupted intestinal mucosal barrier, however, the absorption of oral aminoglycosides can be increased. In particular, toxic systemic levels can result if repeated oral administration is continued in an animal with decreased glomerular filtration from renal disease or dehydration.[31] Oral aminoglycoside preparations should never be given to dehydrated patients with evidence of a disrupted mucosal barrier.

The indiscriminate usage of antibiotics in small animal patients has serious public health implications. R-factor transfer of antibiotic resistance has been demonstrated in the dog, and there is good reason to believe antibiotic-resistant bacteria could be transferred from pet to owner, leading to the possibility of antibiotic-nonresponsive gastrointestinal infections in humans.[32]

INDICATIONS FOR ANTIBIOTIC THERAPY. Antibiotic usage for the treatment of diarrhea is justified only in a select group of circumstances (Table 18–10). The most frequent indication is suspicion that bacteria have invaded the intestinal mucosa, where they could be a potential cause of bacteremia or septicemia. Evidence of mucosal invasion includes hemorrhagic diarrhea (dysentery) and evidence of sepsis such as fever, depression, degenerative left-shifted leukograms, or positive blood cultures. The presence of occasional streaks of fresh blood on the stool is not an indication for antibiotic therapy.

Antibiotic therapy is aimed at eliminating bacteria that have penetrated the mucosa, are circulating in the bloodstream, or have distributed to other organs such as the liver. It is not aimed at "sterilizing" the bowel, a virtually impossible task. Therefore, under these circumstances, parenteral administration of antibiotics is by far the most suitable initial route. Subsequent antibiotics may be administered orally, but the antibiotic should be capable of systemic distribution.

Antibiotic administration is also indicated if a known pathogen is cultured from the feces of the patient or if firm evidence of a bacterial etiology is obtained by fecal smears (e.g., high numbers of clostridial spores), assays for fecal enterotoxins, quantitative culture of duodenal fluid (bacterial overgrowth), or intestinal biopsy (e.g., enteroadherent bacteria).[25] Even in the face of a positive fecal culture, if the animal is not showing evidence of sepsis, the provision of antibiotic therapy may not result in more rapid recovery than the provision of supportive care alone. Animals have a large variety of natural defenses against bacterial pathogens, not the least of which is floral resistance. Thus, most bacterial enteritis conditions will resolve without the requirement for antibiotic intervention. Factors that influence the decision whether to treat with antibiotics include the type of bacteria cultured, the nature of the clinical signs, and the likelihood of a public health risk from the particular bacteria cultured. Prophylactic antibiotic therapy is also appropriate if an animal presents with a profound neutropenia, a common complication of parvovirus infection.

Table 18–10

INDICATIONS FOR ANTIBIOTICS IN THE TREATMENT OF DIARRHEA

Acute hemorrhagic diarrhea
Culture of a known pathogen
Evidence of sepsis
Biopsy showing enteroadherent bacteria
Presence of profound neutropenia (< 1000/µL)
Small intestinal bacterial overgrowth

Table 18–11

COMPARISON OF ANTIMICROBIAL DRUGS ACTIVE AGAINST ANAEROBIC BACTERIA

DRUG	EFFECTS ON NORMAL FLORA	BACTERICIDAL ACTIVITY
Penicillin G	Minimal	Very good
Ampicillin	Major	Very good
Amoxicillin	Major	Very good
Trimethoprim-sulfa	Minimal	Very good
Metronidazole	Minimal to moderate	?
Fluoroquinolones	Minimal	Very good
Gentamicin	Minimal	Very good
Lincomycin	Major	Little
Chloramphenicol	Minimal	None
Tetracycline	Minimal	None
Erythromycin	Minimal-moderate	None
Vancomycin	? Minimal	Very good
Clindamycin	Moderate	Moderate

Routine usage of antibiotics in nonhemorrhagic diarrhea is not warranted, in view of the rarity with which enteric pathogens are cultured, the self-limiting nature of many bacterial infections, and the potential adverse effects of antibiotic therapy. Antibiotics of any form are seldom required for longer than 5 days in the treatment of acute diarrhea.

CHOICE OF ANTIBIOTIC. The effectiveness of selected antibiotics against gastrointestinal bacteria is shown in Table 18–11. Bactericidal antibiotics capable of parenteral administration are recommended in the initial treatment of patients with acute, severe hemorrhagic diarrhea, and for patients whose bacterial-mediated diarrheal process is complicated by vomiting. Nonabsorbable oral antibiotics should not be used because of the potential for toxicity if the mucosal barrier is disrupted and because, as mentioned earlier, the aim of antibiotic therapy is to kill invading bacteria, not "sterilize" the bowel lumen.

The antibiotic should be chosen with consideration as to the spectrum of activity and the concentration of the antibiotic achieved within the bowel lumen, two factors that are prime determinants of the disruptive nature of the antibiotics on normal flora (Table 18–11). Ampicillin, and, to a lesser extent, amoxicillin are broad-spectrum antibiotics that are highly disruptive of normal flora. These antibiotics should thus be avoided for the treatment of gram negative bacterial pathogens and should not be used as single agents in neutropenic animals because they predispose to gram negative intestinal overgrowth. Colonization of the gastrointestinal tract with gram negative pathogens often precedes bacteremia.[33]

A more suitable antibiotic in these situations is a trimethoprim sulfa combination because these drugs have broad-spectrum activity against invading aerobic and anaerobic bacteria but minimally disrupt intestinal flora. Trimethoprim-sulfa may not adequately inhibit some aerobes such as *Pseudomonas*, however, and if used for prolonged periods at high doses may result in anemia. In addition, other side effects such as immune-mediated polyarthritis and keratoconjunctivitis are now and then observed. On occasion, it may be advantageous to use ampicillin or amoxicillin precisely because of their effectiveness against anaerobic flora in the intestinal lumen. For instance, these drugs are indicated in the treatment of patients with clostridial overgrowths, such as those seen in intestinal obstruction. There is some suggestion that orally administered ampicillin may be more effective than orally administered amoxicillin in this regard because ampicillin is less completely absorbed that amoxicillin and so attains higher luminal concentrations.

Metronidazole is an antimicrobial drug with a very broad spectrum of activity against anaerobic bacteria including *Bacteroides fragilis*, a beta lactamase–producing bacterium that is often resistant to penicillins. The importance of *Bacteroides fragilis* infections in small animal enteric disease is unknown, and the primary role of metronidazole is in the treatment of inflammatory bowel disease, anaerobic small intestinal bacterial overgrowth, and peritonitis secondary to bowel perforation. Metronidazole has been superseded by albendazole and fenbendazole as the drug of choice for the treatment of giardiasis.

Tetracycline antibiotics have found a role in the therapy of small intestinal bacterial overgrowth. Not infrequently, tetracyclines result in anorexia, vomiting, and diarrhea, particularly in cats. Doxycycline is a unique antibiotic in that it is excreted directly through the mucosa of the gastrointestinal tract. It has been recommended for the treatment of coliform diarrheas in humans and has a broad spectrum of activity that includes anaerobes. The drug is excreted in the feces as an inactive conjugate and for this reason has minimal effect on the intestinal microflora.

Tylosin is an antibacterial agent similar to erythromycin whose use in small animals is virtually confined to the therapy of inflammatory bowel disease. Lincomycin and erythromycin have limited value in the treatment of diarrheal disease because of disruptive effects on microflora, needless expense, and, particularly in the case of erythromycin, a high incidence of drug-induced vomiting. Erythromycin is primarily indicated for the treatment of *Campylobacter*.[29] Chloramphenicol is considered the drug of choice by some for the therapy of *Salmonella*.[29]

Clindamycin is highly effective against many gram positive aerobes and most species of anaerobes, including *Bacteroides fragilis*. Clindamycin inhibits growth of sensitive organisms for up 2 weeks after its discontinuation. At high doses (25–50 mg/kg PO daily) intended for the treatment of toxoplasmosis, clindamycin includes watery diarrhea in cats.[34] A few cats receiving these doses of clindamycin also vomit.[34] The drug has been associated with pseudomembranous colitis in humans and dogs.

Cephalosporins (first generation) are increasingly used for veterinary patients. They are very effective against *Klebsiella* infections and have application in the treatment of sepsis and small intestinal overgrowth by *Staphylococcal*, *Clostridial*, coliform, and *Proteus* species.

Another class of antibiotics that is likely to be of prime importance in the treatment of enteric infections is the fluoroquinolones. Fluoroquinolones are derivatives of nalidixic acid. Fluoroquinolones such as norfloxacin (Noroxin; Merck, Sharp, & Dome) and enrofloxacin (Baytril; Bayer) are very effective at reducing the aerobic bacterial flora of feces, generally without causing resistant organisms to appear or affecting the anaerobic flora.[33] The prime advantages of these drugs are the ability to be given orally and a potent gram negative spectrum in combination with a very slow acquisition of resistance, perhaps through inhibition of plasmid transfer.[33] They have been found to be effective in the therapy of a variety of intestinal pathogens in humans, including *Campylobacter*. A superior effect to trimethoprimsulfa combinations has not been convincingly demonstrated. Fluoroquinolones are also particularly useful in the prophylactic therapy of neutropenic patients. Side effects are rare, but if used at high doses for prolonged periods the drugs may produce cartilage erosions in young animals.

Animals with fecal cultures positive for bacterial pathogens may be treated according to the sensitivity pattern of the cultured bacterium. However, the in vivo response to the antibiotic often does not reflect the in vitro sensitivity pattern. An alternative approach is to use antibiotics considered by various authorities as "first choice therapeutics" for the particular pathogen (Chapter 21). These recommendations have been made on an empirical basis and should be followed only after careful assessment of the particular antibiotic in the individual under treatment.

Animals with positive blood cultures should be treated according to the sensitivity pattern of the cultured bacterium. If blood culture results are unavailable from a patient with suspected sepsis and the animal's condition is adjudged critical, combinations of parenteral penicillins and amikacin (2–5 mg/kg q 8 hours SQ or IV or gentamicin (2.2 mg/kg q 8 hours SQ or IV) can be used. Both of these aminoglycosides should be used only after rehydration of the patient, and the duration of administration should be limited to 5 days.

Probiotics

Probiotics are defined as live microbial feed supplements that improve the host animal's microbial balance.[35] Although appealing in concept, there is as yet little objective evidence to establish a role for probiotics in the treatment of diarrhea in dogs and cats. As discussed in Chapter 38, yogurt is frequently used in small animal practice as a probiotic for the

Table 18–12

DOSES OF ANTIBIOTICS FOR THE TREATMENT OF
BACTERIAL-MEDIATED DIARRHEAS

DRUG	DOSE	COMMENT
Ampicillin	10–20 mg/kg q 6–8 hours IV, SC, PO	Anaerobic infections
		Sepsis (use with aminoglycoside)
Cephalothin	22–44 mg/kg q 6–8 hours IM, IV	Sepsis
Enrofloxacin	3–5 mg/kg q 12 hours PO	Most gram negative enteropathogens
Erythromycin	10 mg/kg q 8 hours PO	Campylobacter only
Gentamicin	2.2 mg/kg q 8 hours SC, IV	Sepsis only
Chloramphenicol	50 mg/kg q 8 hours PO, IV, SC	Minimize use; care in cats
Tetracyclines	20 mg/kg q 8 hours PO	Bacterial overgrowth
Trimethoprim-sulfa	15 mg/kg q 12 hours PO, IV, SC	General first choice in dogs; care in cats
Metronidazole	10–15 mg/kg q 8–12 hours PO	IBD, anaerobes
Norfloxacin	3–7 mg/kg q 12 hours PO	Most gram negative enteropathogens

treatment of diarrhea but, in spite of ardent anecdotal support, little objective evidence sustains this practice. Similarly, *Lactobacillus acidophilus* cultures have no proven benefits in the therapy of diarrhea in people.[36] Nevertheless, the field of probiotics is an active area of research and recent developments using bacteria that are part of the dominant anaerobic flora of the host, such as *Bifidobacterium* spp, show considerably more promise than *Lactobacillus* spp.[35]

Motility Modifiers

Intestinal transit time is largely determined by the ratio between peristalsis (the driving force for moving intestinal contents aborally) and segmentation contractions (which narrow the bowel lumen and increase the resistance to flow). Theoretically, therefore, motility modifiers could reduce diarrhea by decreasing peristaltic contractions or by increasing segmentation contractions. In actuality, reducing peristaltic activity by drugs such as anticholinergics is of little value for the treatment of diarrhea and, in fact, is generally considered contraindicated. The reason for this apparent paradox is that, contrary to popular belief, increased peristaltic activity is usually not the primary reason for the rapid transit of bowel content during acute diarrhea. In fact, during diarrhea the intestinal tract is usually relatively flaccid and both peristaltic and segmentation contractions are reduced. The lack of segmentation contractions means that resistance to flow is minimal and very little peristaltic activity is needed to propel liquid contents over a long span with relative ease. Anticholinergics reduce but in of themselves do not abolish peristalsis and they also reduce segmentation contractions.[37] As long as some peristaltic activity is present, no matter how weak, it can propel liquid contents through a flaccid tube and diarrhea will occur. In some situations, however, anticholinergics in association with other perturbations such as hypokalemia do precipitate a complete lack of motility in the bowel. This is undesirable because it results in functional bowel obstruction (adynamic ileus). On the positive side, anticholinergics reduce gastric secretions (including that of protein exudation induced by histamine), but unfortunately intestinal secretions are little affected (Table 18–13). In summary, for many years pharmacologists have recognized that anticholinergic drugs are "contrary to the mode of action of useful antidiarrheal agents."[4] Furthermore, they have been found to be disappointing agents when used for that purpose in clinical trials. The Food and Drug Administration (FDA) has restricted the claims that can be made for them and has questioned their effectiveness (Table 18–14). Because of their questionable effectiveness and potential to produce adverse effects, such as adynamic ileus, it is our belief that anticholinergics should not be used for the treatment of diarrhea.

Increasing the resistance to flow of ingesta through the

Table 18–13

PHARMACOLOGIC EFFECTS OF ANTICHOLINERGICS ON THE BOWEL*

Decrease tone and propulsion
Decrease motility caused by opiates and serotonin
High doses decrease motility due to emotional stimuli
Some tone and movement are resistant to anticholinergics
May promote ileus
Decrease gastrointestinal secretions

*The net effect is to reduce motility. The intestine in an animal with diarrhea is already hypomotile.

Table 18–14

FDA CLASSIFICATION OF EFFECTIVENESS OF DRUGS AS ADJUNCTIVE THERAPY IN TREATMENT OF ACUTE ENTEROCOLITIS, FUNCTIONAL GASTROINTESTINAL DISORDERS, AND DIARRHEA[a]

Effective
 Diban[b]: powdered opium, atropine
 Donnagel-PG[b]: powdered opium, atropine, hyoscyamine, kaolin, pectin
 Lomotil[c]: diphenoxylate, atropine
 Parapectolin[d]: paregoric, pectin, kaolin
 Imodium[e]: loperamide
Probably Effective
 Pathilon[f]: tridihexethyl chloride
 Pro-Banthine[c]: propantheline bromide
Possibly Effective
 Darbazine (Combid)[g]: prochlorperazine maleate, isopropamide iodide
 Bentyl[h]: dicyclomine hydrochloride
 Cantil[h]: mepenzolate bromide
 Librax[i]: chlordiazepoxide hydrochloride, clidinium bromide
 Quarzan[i]: clidinium bromide

[a]From literature in advertisements, drug inserts, and PDR
[b]Robins Co., Richmond, VA
[c]Searle Co., Chicago, IL
[d]Rorer, Wm. H., Fort Washington, PA
[e]Ortho Pharm, Raritan, NJ
[f]Lederle Lab, Pearl River, NY
[g]Smith, Kline and French, Philadelphia, PA
[h]Merrell-National Lab, Cincinnati, OH
[i]Roche Lab, Nutley, NJ

intestine by administering drugs that promote segmental contractions is a more sensible method of prolonging intestinal transit time. In contrast to anticholinergics, numerous publications have demonstrated objectively that drugs with this attribute (such as the opioids) effectively slow intestinal transit and reduce diarrhea.[37–46] Furthermore, opioids do not predispose the patient to adynamic ileus, a disorder that can delay the patient's recovery. Opioids increase the amplitude of rhythmic segmentation and decrease the propulsive contractions (Table 18–15).[37] They directly affect the intestinal smooth muscle,[47,48] producing both tonic and phasic contractions of the circular muscle; they also act centrally and on synapses to augment segmentation. Opioids either have no effect on longitudinal intestinal muscle in the dog or they cause relaxation.[49,50] The net effect is to markedly inhibit the flow of intestinal contents, delay gastric emptying, and increase tone in the ileocolic valve and anal sphincter.[37] Effective opioids include morphine, meperidine, paregoric, diphenoxylate, and loperamide. Suggested doses of a selected number of these opioids are listed in Table 18–16.

Some opioids, in particular loperamide and to a lesser extent diphenoxylate, also increase fluid and water absorption possibly by a calcium channel blocking effect[51] or by inhibition of the intrinsic calcium binding protein calmodulin.[1,51] In addition, loperamide and diphenoxylate inhibit the activity of certain secretagogues, including *E. coli* enterotoxin, VIP, bile acids, and prostaglandin E_2.[62] Loperamide has a faster onset of action than diphenoxylate and fewer side effects. It is available as a liquid, which facilitates its usage in small patients. We have used loperamide without clinical evidence of toxicity in cats. It is worthy of note that atropine is added in small quantities to diphenoxylate to minimize its abuse as a narcotic in humans. The atropine in this preparation (Lomotil) has no pharmacologic effect on the gastrointestinal tract.

Notwithstanding the comments just made, opioids are not

Table 18–15

OPIOIDS: PHARMACOLOGIC ACTIONS

Stomach
1. Contracts antrum
2. Decreases antral propulsion
Net effect: Delays gastric emptying
Small and Large Intestines
1. Increases tone and segmentation
2. Decreases propulsion
3. Contracts ileocecal and anal sphincters
Net effect: Increases transit time

a panacea for the treatment of diarrhea. In humans, they tend to be more effective at shortening the duration of diarrhea rather than greatly reducing stool volume, and they are ineffective in some disorders, such as idiopathic juvenile diarrhea of children.[46] The major disadvantage to using these drugs is that they are narcotics, and most produce depression of the central nervous system if used in inappropriate doses. Furthermore, there is good reason to believe that opioids are contraindicated in diarrhea resulting from infection with invasive bacteria.[32] In these cases, diarrhea forms an important protective role that probably hastens the elimination of the organism. Slowing intestinal transit may prolong the residence time of the bacteria in the bowel, leading to greater opportunity for proliferation of the organism, invasion of the mucosa, and the absorption of toxic products. It is our preference not to use these drugs in patients with suspected enteroinvasive disease (dysentery), except on occasions when intravenous fluid therapy cannot keep up with diarrheal fluid loss.

Locally Acting Drugs[37,53]

Long before either antibiotics or motility modifiers were available for the treatment of diarrhea, a wide variety of intestinal protectives and adsorbents were used. As with many pharmaceuticals that have been used empirically for centuries, few controlled studies have been conducted to prove their effectiveness. A number of these substances are classified as protectives because of their adsorbent properties.

Kaolin, hydrated aluminum silicate, is frequently used to treat diarrhea in spite of minimal effectiveness. The product is thought to have modest beneficial properties by binding toxins and bacteria and has been shown to reduce systemic levels of endotoxin in a rat model of colitis.[54] It may improve the consistency of the stool through its adsorbent properties, but it is unlikely to shorten the course of the diarrhea. It may also act as a coagulant in the intestine and thus may reduce gastrointestinal hemorrhage.[29] Kaolin may reduce the absorp-

Table 18–16

SUGGESTED DOSES OF OPIOIDS FOR THE TREATMENT OF DIARRHEA*

DRUG	DOSE
Camphorated opium tincture? (Paregoric)	0.05–0.06 mg/kg PO q 8 hours (D,C)
Diphenoxylate (Lomotil)	0.1 mg/kg PO q 8 hours (D)
Loperamide (Imodium)	0.1–0.2 mg/kg PO q 8 hours (D,C)

(D) = dog, (C) = cat
*Most opioids are not licensed for use in the dog or cat.

tion of some antibiotics from the bowel. Its routine use in diarrheal diseases is not encouraged.

Pectin is a common component of diarrhea medications. It is a carbohydrate, polygalacturonic acid, found in apples and rinds of citrus fruits. The action of pectin is unknown, but it is suspected to be an adsorbent with protective properties. In addition, the provision of volatile fatty acids to the colon by fermentation of pectin may stimulate water and electrolyte absorption and discourage growth of pathogens (see Chapter 38). In large quantities, however, the administration of this highly fermentable fiber induces diarrhea.

Activated charcoal has been used for many years to absorb toxic substances. It is still incorporated into universal-type antidotes for treating the ingestion of toxic substances. It has also been used to bind gas in the intestine in managing excessive flatus, although it is questionable whether activated charcoal significantly reduces the content of intestinal gas. It is also thought to bind bacterial toxins. There have been no controlled studies to evaluate its efficacy. The drug is messy to use and is better administered as a powder than a tablet. The primary indication remains the treatment of toxicosis. The recommended dose is 0.7 to 1.4 g/kg administered once.[53]

Bismuth subcarbonate and magnesium trisilicate adsorb gases, toxins, and bacteria. As an additional property they supposedly coat and protect the ulcerated mucosal surface.

Bismuth subsalicylate is an effective agent for the treatment and prevention of enterotoxigenic diarrhea. In humans, the diarrhea, nausea, and abdominal pain associated with infective diarrhea are reduced by bismuth subsalicylate therapy.[55] The drug has a number of beneficial effects including modest antibacterial effects on enteropathogens such as *E. coli*, *Salmonella*, and *Campylobacter jejuni*.[55] In addition, the salicylate moiety is thought to decrease intestinal secretion by interfering with prostaglandin production and by a more direct, but undefined, inhibitory effect on the generation of cyclic AMP by the enterotoxin. Contrary to popular belief, the salicylate component of bismuth subsalicylate is unlikely to cause gastric erosions because, unlike aspirin (acetosalicylic acid), the salicylate salt of bismuth is only weakly acidic.[55] In fact, bismuth subsalicylate has protective effects against gastric erosions.[55] However, salicylate intoxication can result from overdosage of this drug, particularly in cats. A safe dose of bismuth subsalicylate (Pepto-Bismol; Peptosyl) in dogs and cats is 0.25 mL/kg q 4 to 6 hours.[56] Doses greater than 7 mL/kg/day could produce toxicity.[56] It is a useful and practical therapy for acute nonspecific diarrhea. Palatability of Pepto-Bismol may be improved by refrigeration. Another useful product for the therapy of nonspecific acute diarrhea is a combination of bismuth subsalicylate with paregoric (Corrective mixture; Beecham Laboratories). This product combines the antisecretory effects of the salicylate with the improved intestinal motility of an opioid. The dose is 0.25 mL/kg PO initially, followed by half the original dose every 4 hours.[23] The administration of this mixture is at present confined to dogs.

Astringents have been used to treat diarrhea. Tannic acid, the best example, acts by precipitating proteins on the mucosal surface, forming a protective coating presumably without entering and damaging the cell. This activity decrease cell permeability and has a constipating effect. Tannic acid also forms insoluble complexes with heavy metal ions, alkaloids, and glycosides that could contribute to diarrhea. Tannic acid is now known to be hepatotoxic, causing severe centrolobular necrosis when appreciable amounts are absorbed.

Antacids have been used as antidiarrheal agents. All aluminum antacid compounds have a constipating effect. Aluminum hydroxide inhibits motility in the stomach, delaying gastric emptying.[57] Parts of its constipating effects may be due to a very slow delivery of solutes to the intestinal mucosa, permitting more complete absorption. In addition, aluminum antacids have adsorptive and binding properties. Part of aluminum's constipating effects is due to precipitation of poorly absorbed soluble anions, such as phosphates, which can cause osmotic diarrhea.

Calcium antacids are also constipating and have been used occasionally to treat chronic diarrhea. They may have absorptive properties, and they form insoluble salts with anions such as phosphate. It is not known whether high concentrations of calcium have any effects on intestinal motility. Excessive administration of calcium to treat a chronic diarrhea can produce hypercalcemia and renal hypercalciuria, which can progress to nephrocalcinosis and renal failure. In contrast to calcium, magnesium salts are cathartic because they are soluble and poorly absorbed. Magnesium may also be cathartic, due to direct effects on smooth muscle function.

Barium sulfate has been used empirically to treat chronic diarrhea. The use is based on observations that diarrhea sometimes improves after barium sulfate has been given to conduct gastrointestinal radiographic studies. There have been no controlled studies to evaluate the usefulness of barium sulfate for treating diarrhea. The method by which barium sulfate might be beneficial, if any, is undetermined. Paradoxically, barium ions stimulate the release of acetylcholine from nerve synapses in intrinsic ganglia, and when a soluble barium salt is given orally it intensely stimulates all types of muscles in the body causing vomiting, severe diarrhea, and colic.

Future Therapeutics

Alpha-2-adrenergic receptors are present on enterocytes and are involved in enterocyte fluid and electrolyte transport.[58] Alpha-2-receptor agonists enhance absorption and inhibit secretion of electrolytes in the small intestine. Clonidine is an example of an alpha-2-agonist that has been used successfully to treat experimental secretory diarrheas in rats and diabetic diarrhea and secretory diarrhea due to bronchogenic adenocarcinoma in humans.[51] The role of these agents in diarrhea therapy has yet to be defined, and their use may be limited by their sedative and hypotensive properties. Lidamidine is an alpha-2-agonist structurally similar to clonidine, but it has fewer such side effects.

Intestinal inflammation promotes the formation of prostaglandins of the E and F type, kinins, and lipoxygenase products (5-HPETE, 5-HETE); all are substances with a potent secretory effect on intestinal epithelium. Prostaglandins stimulate chloride secretion and inhibit sodium absorption. Nonsteroidal anti-inflammatory drugs that inhibit prostaglandin synthesis are beneficial in managing some secretory types of diarrhea. In contrast, prostaglandins are also cytoprotective in the gastrointestinal tract, and inhibitors of prostaglandin synthesis can produce erosion and ulceration of the mucosal epithelium. Because of the potential mucosal damage produced by NSAIDs, inhibitors of prostaglandin synthesis should not be used indiscriminantly for treating acute diarrhea. However, some agents such as bismuth subsalicylate appear to have a beneficial effect with minimal toxicity.

Lipoxygenase products and not prostaglandins are the mediators for inflammation in chronic colitis and possibly chronic inflammatory bowel disease. Drugs that inhibit leukotreine formation, such as 5-aminosalicylic acid and sulfasalazine, are effective in managing chronic colitis (see Chapter 25). Sulfasalazine, which inhibits both prostaglandin and leukotreine synthesis, and has a multiplicity of other potentially beneficial actions,[59] is effective whereas nonsteroidal anti-inflammatory drugs such as indomethacin and aspirin, which inhibit only prostaglandin synthesis, are ineffective.

Somatostatin is a potent inhibitor of intestinal motility, splanchnic blood flow, enteric hormone release, and pancreatic, gastric, and intestinal secretion. A potent somatostatin analogue (Octreotide) is now available and may be useful for the therapy of diarrhea resulting from endocrine tumors. In humans somatostatin or its analogues have been successful in treating diarrhea from a number of different causes including VIPomas, carcinoid tumors, intestinal resection, and cryptosporidiosis.[51] Additional potential therapeutic indications for Octreotide include bleeding varices, the dumping syndrome, and acute pancreatitis.[60]

Calcium appears to have a role in regulating active intestinal ion secretion and has important effects on intestinal motility and mucosal proliferation. Calcium channel blockers have shown promise in the treatment of diarrhea mediated by experimental infusion of substance P in dogs and of *Escherichia coli* enterotoxin-stimulated diarrhea in mice.[51] Nifedipine and verapamil have shown some beneficial effects in the therapy of irritable bowel syndrome in humans. Loperamide has calcium channel blocking properties; the drug inhibits intestinal secretion that is stimulated by agents which increase membrane permeability for calcium.[51]

Lithium salts change intestinal fluid and electrolyte dynamics in an unknown manner and reduce some forms of diarrhea in humans.[51] Constipation and water retention are well-described side effects of oral lithium therapy.

Calmodulin antagonists inhibit intestinal secretion of fluid stimulated by VIP, cholera toxin, *E. coli* enterotoxin, cyclic AMP, and PGE_2. These drugs are thought to reduce intestinal secretion by inhibition of calmodulin-activated cyclic nucleotide phosphodiesterase and adenylate/guanylate cyclase mechanisms. In one study, zaldaride maleate, a calmodulin inhibitor, has been shown to decrease the severity and duration of traveler's diarrhea (bacterial enteric infection) in humans.[61] Phenothiazines have an antidiarrheal action, which in part appears to be due to inhibition of calmodulin. For instance, chlorpromazine is thought to reduce diarrhea due to cholera in humans,[61] and has been shown to inhibit *E. coli* enterotoxin-induced secretion.[62]

Cholestyramine is an ion exchange resin that binds bile acids and enterotoxins. It has been shown to shorten the course of acute diarrhea in humans [46] and is the treatment of choice for bile acid malabsorption. We have found the drug useful in ameliorating the severity of diarrhea when fat (and hence bile acid) malabsorption is occurring. Caution with its use is required because it can cause hyperchloremic acidosis in humans and hastens the excretion of taurine from cats.

Other interesting antidiarrheal agents include berberine, an alkaloid from the plant *Berberis aristata*, organic acids such as nicotonic acid and glutamic acid, and chloride channel blockers such as some anthracene derivatives.[51]

IDIOPATHIC JUVENILE DIARRHEA IN CATS

Young cats occasionally develop intractable idiopathic chronic diarrhea. Fortunately, many affected cats recover spontaneously at approximately 1 year of age. The cats are usually bright and alert and still eat well. The diarrhea is most often watery and voluminous. Clinical signs of large-bowel inflammation are occasionally present but are usually low grade.

Etiopathogenesis

Little is known about the etiology or pathogenesis of the disorder but it is highly likely that it is multifactorial. Young animals are predisposed to diarrhea in comparison to adults, for a number of reasons. Early in life, the digestive and absorptive functions of the small intestine are not fully matured. Furthermore, the neonatal colon cannot compensate well for failure of the small intestine to absorb water and electrolytes. It has been suggested that the reason for this is inadequate volatile fatty acid production in these young animals as a result of poorly established colonic flora and fermentation processes.[63] For these reasons (and others such as lack of selectivity) young cats are predisposed to nutritional diarrhea. This predisposition is exacerbated by poor feeding practices by owners (for instance, the feeding of excessive cow's milk). In addition, young cats are more susceptible to parasitism such as cryptosporidia and giardia. Cryptospordiosis, in particular, may be important in the syndrome of juvenile feline diarrhea because cryptosporidiosis is difficult to diagnose and treat and would be expected to undergo spontaneous resolution as the cat matures in an analogous fashion to idiopathic juvenile feline diarrhea. Small intestinal bacterial overgrowth may be important in some affected cats because many have been treated inappropriately with antibiotics.

Diagnosis

As with adult animals, juvenile cats can develop diarrhea from a multitude of primary diseases of the gastrointestinal tract or diseases of other organs, and the diagnostic approach to diarrhea is similar in both juvenile and adult cats. For refractory cases of diarrhea the minimum laboratory database should include a CBC, a serum chemistry profile with electrolyte levels, a urinalysis, three zinc sulfate fecal flotations for giardia, and an acid-fast stain of a fecal smear for cryptosporidia. Young cats with diarrhea in association with a peripheral eosinophilia usually have eosinophilic gastroenteritis but parasitism is also possible. Panhypoproteinemia (low serum albumin and globulin) characterizes protein-losing enteropathies. Panhypoproteinemia is uncommon in juvenile cats with diarrhea but is occasionally seen with severe inflammatory bowel disease or severe subacute enteropathy secondary to nonfatal panleukopenia. Serologic tests for feline leukemia, feline immunodeficiency virus, and feline infectious peritonitis (FIP) may also be warranted because these diseases can be associated with chronic enteropathies. The FIP titer must be interpreted carefully. In cats with small-bowel diarrhea, a Sudan stain of fresh feces for fat can be worthwhile. Large quantities of undigested fats raise the unlikely possibility of exocrine pancreatic insufficiency that can be confirmed by azocasein hydrolysis or radial enzyme diffusion tests but, as yet, not by serum trypsin-like immunoreactivity testing. If large-bowel diarrhea is suspected, a stained fecal smear and/or rectal scraping should be examined and may reveal inflammatory cells suggestive of colitis or fungi such as *Histoplasma*. Large amounts of neutrophils in a fecal smear or evidence of contagion are indications for fecal culture, which is otherwise usually a low-yield procedure.

If no diagnosis is apparent after performance of these initial laboratory tests and no warning signs of serious disease are apparent, it is customary to discharge the cat on a controlled diet for 2 to 3 weeks to determine if the diarrhea is food responsive. The diet should contain a single protein source that the cat has not been fed in the last 6 months

If the diarrhea fails to respond to the controlled diet, further tests are indicated. Because of the high incidence of inflammatory bowel disease (even in very young cats), upper gastrointestinal biopsy is usually the next diagnostic procedure of choice. In cats with idiopathic juvenile diarrhea, biopsy specimens of the small and large bowel are normal, although some cats may have a slight increase in lymphocyte and plasma cell numbers in the lamina propria.

Symptomatic Therapy

Young cats with diarrhea should be held off food for 1 to 2 days and then provided a highly digestible, selected protein diet such as boiled chicken. For long-term use, the chicken should be diced into human infant rice cereal made up in chicken stock and balanced with the appropriate vitamins and minerals (see Chapter 38). The addition of a small quantity of a fermentable fiber is also of value. Commercially available selected protein diets are also useful. In our hands, the diet with the best track record in idiopathic juvenile diarrhea is Iams dry kitten food. Frequent small feedings are advantageous.

Opioids such as Imodium (loperamide, 0.1–0.2 mg/kg q 8 hours PO) can reduce the severity of the diarrhea but do not offer a cure. Bismuth subsalicylate (Pepto Bismol) is useful (0.5–1 mL/kg q 12 hours for 2–3 days) because the drug has antibacterial and antisecretory properties. In our experience, antibiotics should be avoided in the treatment of idiopathic juvenile feline diarrhea because they are rarely effective and are likely to further upset the bowel flora of affected cats. However, antibiotics are indicated if the diarrhea is hemorrhagic, a known pathogen has been cultured from the feces, or there is evidence of bacterial overgrowth or sepsis. Fluoroquinolones are a good choice of antibiotic for the treatment of hemorrhagic diarrhea because they are very effective against enteric pathogens. If anaerobic small intestinal bacterial overgrowth is suspected, metronidazole (10–20 mg/kg PO q 12 hours for 7–10 days) is useful. Metronidazole is also useful in cats for the treatment of giardiasis, although albendazole (25 mg/kg PO q 12 hours for 5 days) is also successful. In young cats with acute large-bowel diarrhea an oral sulphonamide is sometimes useful because of the possibility of coccidiosis. Oral aminoglycosides, such as neomycin, should *not* be used for the treatment of diarrhea. However, if cryptosporidiosis is diagnosed, the oral aminoglycoside paromomycin (Humatin; Parke-Davis) at a dose of 125 to 165 mg/kg PO q 12 hours for 5 days appears to be more successful than previously recommended therapies.[64] Symptomatic therapy of juvenile feline diarrhea with glucocorticoids is discouraged unless a diagnosis of inflammatory bowel disease has been made.

REFERENCES

1. Ooms L, Degryse A. Pathogenesis and pharmacology of diarrhea. Vet Res Commun 10:355–397, 1986.
2. Ewe K. Intestinal transport in constipation and diarrhea. Pharmacology 36:73S–84S, 1988.
3. Fine KD, Krejs GJ, Fordtran JS. Diarrhea. In: Sleisenger MH, Fordtran JS (eds) Gastrointestinal Disease. Pathophysiology, Diagnosis, and Management, 4th ed. WB Saunders, Philadelphia, 290–316, 1989.

4. Madara JL, Trier JS. Functional morphology of the mucosa of the small intestine. In: Johnson LR (ed) Physiology of the Gastrointestinal Tract, 2nd ed. Raven Press, New York, 1209–1249, 1987.

5. Madara JL, Moore R, Carlson S. Alteration of intestinal tight junction structure and permeability by cytoskeletal contraction. Am J Physiol 253:C854–C861, 1987.

6. Vellenga L, Mouwen JMVN, van Dijk JE, et al. Biological and pathological aspects of the mammalian small intestinal permeability to macromolecules. Vet Q 7:322–332, 1985.

7. Moreland KJ. Ulcer disease of the upper gastrointestinal tract in small animals: Pathophysiology, diagnosis, and management. Comp Contin Ed Pract Vet 10:1265–1280, 1988.

8. Ramage JK, Hunt RH, Perdue MH. Changes in intestinal permeability and epithelial differentiation during inflammation in the rat. Gut 29:57–61, 1988.

9. Bjarnason I, Williams P, So A. Intestinal permeability and inflammation in rheumatoid arthritis: Effects of non-steroidal anti-inflammatory drugs. Lancet 1171–1174, November 1984.

10. Ecknauer R, Buck B, Breitig D. An experimental model for measuring intestinal permeability. Digestion 26:24–32, 1983.

11. Siber GR, Mayer RJ, Levin MJ. Increased gastrointestinal absorption of large molecules in patients after 5-fluorouracil therapy for metastatic colon carcinoma. Cancer Res 40:3430–3436, 1980.

12. Granger DN, Kvietys PR, Perry MA, et al. The microcirculation and intestinal transport. In: Johnson LR (ed) Physiology of the Gastrointestinal Tract, 2nd ed Raven Press, New York, 1671–1697, 1987.

13. Burrows CF, Greiner EC, Tooker J, et al. Hookworm infection disrupts canine jejunal myoelectric activity[abstract]. Am Col Vet Int Med Proc, 741, 1988.

14. Willard MD, Mullaney T, Karasek S, et al. Diarrhea associated with myenteric ganglionitis in a dog. J Am Vet Med Assoc 193:346–348, 1988.

15. MacPherson BR, Shearin NL, Pfeiffer, CJ. Experimental diffuse colitis in cats: Observations on motor changes. J Surg Res 25:42–49, 1978.

16. Osweiller GD. A brief guide to clinical signs of toxicosis in small animals. In: Kirk RW (ed) Current Veterinary Therapy IX. WB Saunders, Philadelphia, 132–135, 1986.

17. Osweiller GD, Household and commercial products. In: Kirk RW (ed) Current Veterinary Therapy IX. WB Saunders, Philadelphia, 193–196, 1986.

18. Ruhr LP. Ornamental toxic plants. In: Kirk RW (ed) Current Veterinary Therapy IX. WB Saunders, Philadelphia 216–220, 1985.

19. Drasar BS, Hill J. Human intestinal flora. Academic Press, London, 1974.

20. Goodman JS. Infections by anaerobic bacteria of the bowel. Adv Int Med 21:129–147, 1976.

21. Kikuchi T, Oikawa T, Inoue K, et al. The effect of antibiotics against the intestinal bacterial flora. In: Heneghan JB (ed) Germ Free Research Academic Press, New York, 355–359, 1973.

22. Nichols RL, Condon RE. Role of the endogenous gastrointestinal microflora in postoperative wound sepsis. Surg Ann 7:279–293, 1975.

23. DeNovo RC. Therapeutics of gastrointestinal diseases. In: Kirk RW (ed) Current Veterinary Therapy IX. WB Saunders, Philadelphia, 862–872, 1986.

24. Davenport D. Antimicrobial therapy for gastrointestinal, pancreatic, and hepatic disorders. Prob Vet Sci 2:374–393, 1990.

25. Jergens AE. Rational use of antimicrobials for gastrointestinal disease in small animals. J Am Anim Hosp Assoc 30:123–131, 1994.

26. Leight DA, Simmons K. Effect of clindamycin and lincomycin therapy on fecal flora. J Clin Path 31:439–443, 1978.

27. Hirsch DC. Microflora, mucosa, and immunity. In:Anderson NV (ed) Veterinary Gastroenterology 199–219, 1980.

28. Ishikawa H, Baba E, Matsumoto H. Studies on bacterial flora of the alimentary tract. dogs. III. Fecal flora in clinical and experimental cases of diarrhea. Jap J Vet Sci 44:343–347,1982.

29. Greene CE. Gastrointestinal, intra-abdominal, and hepatobiliary infections. In: Green CE (ed) Clinical Microbiology and Infectious Diseases of the Dog and Cat. WB Saunders, Philadelphia, 247–268, 1984.

30. Clausen MR, Bonnen H, Tvede M, et al. Colonic fermentation to short-chain fatty acids is decreased in antibiotic-associated diarrhea. Gastroenterology 101:1497–1504, 1991.

31. Sande MA, Mandell GL. Antimicrobial Agents: The Aminoglycosides. In: Goodman Gilman A, Goodman LS, Gilman A, et al. (eds) The Pharmacologic Basis of Therapeutics, 7th ed. Macmillan, New York, 1150–1169, 1985.

32. English PB, Prescott CW. Antimicrobial therapy in the dog. I. Related to body system or organ infected. J Sm Anim Pract 24:277–292, 1983.

33. Wolfson JS, Hooper DC. Norfloxacin: A new targeted fluoroquinolone antimicrobial agent. Ann Int Med 108:238–251, 1988.

34. Green CE, Lappin MR, Marks A. Effect of clindamycin on clinical, hematological, and biochemical parameters in clinically healthy cats. J Anim Hosp Assoc 28:323–326, 1992.

35. Bouhnik Y, Pochart P, Marteau P, et al. Fecal recovery in humans of viable *Bifidobacterium* spp. ingested in fermented milk. Gastroenterology 102:875–878, 1992.

36. de Dios Pozo-Olando J, Warram JH, Gomez RG, et al. Effect of a lactobacilli preparation on traveler's diarrhea. Gastroenterology 74:829–830,1978.

37. Goodman LA, Gilman A. The Pharmacological Basis of Therapeutics. Macmillan, New York, 1975.

38. Connell AM. The motility of the pelvic colon. II. Paradoxical motility in diarrhea and constipation. Gut 3:342–348, 1962.

39. Ludwick JR, Wiley JN, Bass P. Extraluminal contractile force and electrical activity of reversed canine duodenum. Gastroenterology 54:41–51, 1968.

40. Plant OH, Miller GH. Effects of morphine and some other opium alkaloids on the muscular activity of the alimentary canal. I. Action on the small intestine in unanesthetized dogs and man. J Pharmacol Exp Ther 27:361–383, 1926.

41. Templeton RD, Alder HF. The influence of morphine on transportation in the colon of the dog. Am J Physiol 131:428–431, 1940.

42. Vaughan Williams EM, Streeten DHP. The action of morphine, pethidine, and amidone upon the intestinal motility of conscious dogs. Brit J Pharmacol Chem Ther 5:584–603, 1950.

43. Bass P, Kennedy JA, Wiley JN, et al. CI-750, a novel antidiarrheal agent. J Pharmacol Exp Ther 186:183–198, 1973.

44. Burks TF. Gastrointestinal pharmacology. Ann Rev Pharmacol Toxic 16:15–31, 1976.

45. Tijtgat GN, Meuwissen SGM, Hubregtse K. Loperamide in the symptomatic control of chronic diarrhea. Ann Clin Res 7:325–330, 1975

46. Snyder JD, Molla AM, Cash RA. Home-based therapy for diarrhea. J Pediatr Gastroenterol Nutr 11:438–447, 1990.

47. Burks TF. Vascularly perfused isolated intestine. In: Proc 4th Int Symp: Gastrointestinal motility. Mitchell, Vancouver, 305–312, 1974.

48. Stewart JJ, Weisbrodt NW, Burks TF. Central and peripheral actions of morphine on intestinal transit. J Pharmacol Exp Ther 205:547–555, 1978.

49. Bass P, Wiley JN. Electrical and extraluminal contractile force activity of the dog. Am J Dig Dis 10:183–200, 1965.

50. Rinaldo JA, Orinion EA, Simpelo RV, et al. Differential response of longitudinal and circular muscles of intact canine colon to morphine and bethanecol. Gastroenterology 60:438–444, 1971.

51. Fedorak RN, Field M. Antidiarrheal therapy. Prospects for new agents. Dig Dis Sci 32:195–205, 1987.

52. DuPont HL, Hornick RB, Adverse effect of Lomotil therapy in shigellosis. J Am Med Assoc 226:1525–1528, 1973.

53. Wilcke JR. The use of adsorbents to treat gastrointestinal problems in small animals. Sem Vet Med Surg 2:266–273, 1987.

54. Gardiner KR, Anderson NH, McCaigue MD, et al. Adsorbents as antiendotoxin agents in experimental colitis. Gut 34:51–55, 1993.

55. Gorbach SL. Bismuth therapy in gastrointestinal diseases. Gastroenterology 99:863–875, 1990.

56. Papich MG, Davis CA, Davis LE. Absorption of salicylate from an antidiarrheal preparation in dogs and cats. J Am Anim Hosp Assoc 23:221–226, 1987.

57. Hurwitz A, Robinson RG, Vats TS, et al. Effects of antacids on the gastric emptying. Gastroenterology 71:268–273, 1976.

58. Dijoseph JF, Taylor JA, Mir GN, et al. Alpha-2 receptors in the gastrointestinal system: A new therapeutic approach. Life Sci 35:1013–1042, 1984.

59. Gaginella TS, Walsh RE. Sulfasalazine; Multiplicity of action. Dig Dis Sci 37:801–812, 1992.

60. Burroughs AK, Malagelada R. Potential indications for octreotide in gastroenterology: Summary of workshop. Digestion 54 (suppl 1):59–67, 1993

61. DuPont HL, Ericsson CD, Mathewson JJ, et al. Zaldaride maleate, an intestinal calmodulin inhibitor in the therapy of travellers diarrhea. Gastroenterology 104:709–715, 1993.

62. Gupta S, Yadava JNS. Comparative efficacy of various antidiarrhoeal drugs against *E. coli* enterotoxins induced diarrhoea in animal models. Indian Vet J 14:1–16, 1990.

63. Argenzio R, Moon H, Kemeny L, et al. Colonic compensation in transmissible gastroenteritis of swine. Gastroenterology 86:1501–1509, 1984.

64. Barr SC. Personal communication, 1993.

19

Malabsorption, Small Intestinal Bacterial Overgrowth, and Protein-Losing Enteropathy

DAVID A. WILLIAMS

INTRODUCTION

Diseases in which digestion of food and/or subsequent net absorption of nutrients are defective are traditionally classified as either primary failure to digest (maldigestion) or primary failure to absorb (malabsorption). Both of these classifications are sometimes grouped under the umbrella term *malassimilation*. This classification is misleading, however, because the digestive and absorptive processes are inextricably linked, and failure of absorption is an inevitable consequence of defective digestion. Most patients with exocrine pancreatic insuffiency EPI have associated abnormalities of small intestinal function (see Chapter 20), and most diseases affecting the small intestine will inevitably impair the terminal processes of digestion that take place at the luminal surface of the intestinal mucosa. It is therefore preferable to use the term *malabsorption* as a global one to encompass all aspects of impaired digestion and absorption.[1]

Utilizing this broad definition of malabsorption, it is useful to categorize diseases by the site of the primary abnormality into premucosal (intraluminal), mucosal, or postmucosal (hemolymphatic) defects (Table 19–1).[2] Associated pathophysiologic mechanisms can also be categorized as to whether premucosal, mucosal, or postmucosal phases of absorption are compromised (Table 19–2).[1] It is important to recognize, however, that additional factors (such as defective gastrointestinal motility or immunologic function) may also be involved, and that intraluminal, mucosal, and hemolymphatic abnormalities often coexist.

Depending on the mechanisms in play, one or many nutrients may be malabsorbed, resulting in a variety of potential clinical consequences (Table 19–3). With longstanding disease there may be a spectrum of abnormalities including weight loss, diarrhea, muscle wasting, coagulopathy, skin and hair coat changes, anemia, and hypoproteinemia. Although documented reports of specific deficiencies are rare, vitamin K deficient bleeding has been reported in two cats with malabsorption syndrome due to lymphocytic-plasmacytic enteritis,[3] and a cat with EPI.[4]

Malabsorption of fat causes increased absorption of dietary oxalate. Absorption of oxalate is normally limited by precipitation with calcium as an insoluble salt. Fat malabsorption results in chelation of dietary calcium with unabsorbed fatty acids such that less calcium is available for precipitation with oxalate. Consequently, oxalate remains in a soluble form that is subsequently absorbed in the colon,[5] and this is facilitated

by the effects of bile acids and fatty acids in increasing the permeability of the colonic mucosa.[6] The hyperoxaluria may lead to oxalate crystalluria or even urolithiasis in some patients. Hyperoxaluria in human patients may be reduced by treatment with oral calcium and aluminum salts.[7]

DEFECTS OF PREMUCOSAL FUNCTION (INTRALUMINAL MALABSORPTION)

Exocrine Pancreatic Insufficiency

Progressive loss of pancreatic acinar cells ultimately leads to malabsorption due to inadequate production of digestive enzymes (Table 19–4). The functional reserve of the pancreas is considerable, however, and signs of EPI do not occur until a large proportion of the gland has been destroyed. The most common cause of EPI in the dog is pancreatic acinar atrophy. Pancreatic insufficiency is caused less commonly by chronic pancreatitis, and rarely by pancreatic neoplasia (see Chapter 20). EPI is rela-

Table 19–1

A CLASSIFICATION OF MALABSORPTIVE DISORDERS

LOCATION OF PRIMARY ABNORMALITY	REPRESENTATIVE DISEASES
Premucosal defect (intraluminal defect)	Exocrine pancreatic insufficiency
	Small intestinal bacterial overgrowth
Mucosal defect	Inflammatory bowel diseases
	Infectious enteropathies (parasitic, fungal, bacterial, others?)
	Dietary sensitivities
	Villous atrophy
	Neoplastic infiltration
	Intestinal resection
	Brush border enzyme deficiencies (congenital)
Postmucosal defect (hemolymphatic defect)	Primary (congenital) intestinal lymphangiectasia
	Secondary (acquired) intestinal lymphangiectasia

Table 19–2

PATHOPHYSIOLOGIC MECHANISMS OF MALABSORPTION

PHASE OF ABSORPTIVE PROCESS	PATHOPHYSIOLOGIC MECHANISM (EXAMPLE OF DISEASE PROCESS)
Premucosal (luminal)	Defective substrate hydrolysis
	Enzyme deficiency (exocrine pancreatic insufficiency)
	Enzyme inactivation (gastric acid hypersecretion)
	Rapid intestinal transit (hyperthyroidism)
	Defective solubilization of fat
	Decreased bile salt secretion (biliary obstruction)
	Bile salt deconjugation (bacterial overgrowth)
	Bile salt loss (resection or disease of terminal ileum)
	Impaired release of pancreatic secretogogue (severe small intestinal disease)
	Intrinsic factor deficiency (exocrine pancreatic insufficiency)
	Bacterial competition for cobalamin (bacterial overgrowth)
Mucosal	Brush border enzyme deficiency
	Congenital defects (enteropeptidase, lactase: humans)
	Acquired defect secondary to diffuse enteropathies
	Brush border transport deficiency
	Selective defects (inherited selective cobalamin malabsorption)
	Generalized defects (inflammatory bowel diseases, infectious enteropathies, dietary sensitivities, villous atrophy, intestinal resection)
	Enterocyte processing defects (abetalipoproteinemia: humans)
	Disruption of lamina propria
Postmucosal (hemolymphatic)	Lymphatic obstruction
	Primary lymphangiectasia
	Secondary (acquired) lymphatic obstruction (neoplasia, infiltrative infectious or inflammatory disease)
	Vascular failure (intestinal ischemia, intestinal vasculitis, portal hypertension)

tively uncommon in cats, in which it occurs most frequently as a consequence of chronic pancreatitis. Although not yet documented, it is likely that congenital abnormalities of pancreatic exocrine function such as pancreatic hypoplasia, isolated deficiencies of individual pancreatic enzymes, and deficiency of enteropeptidase or colipase also occur.[8–11] Secretion of pancreatic enzymes may be diminished in some patients with severe small intestinal disease in which liberation of the pancreatic secretory hormones secretin and cholecystokinin may be compromised, although this is probably rare.[12] Activity of pancreatic lipase may also be compromised by deficiency of bile acids (see later). The etiology, pathophysiology, diagnosis, and treatment of the primary causes of EPI are discussed in detail in Chapter 20.

INACTIVATION OF PANCREATIC DIGESTIVE ENZYMES. When hypersecretion of gastric acid is extreme (specifically in Zollinger-Ellison syndrome, in which there is hypergastrinemia due to a gastrin-secreting tumor), the small intestinal intraluminal pH can become acid as the normal acid-neutralizing mechanisms are overwhelmed. At acid pH pancreatic proteases become reversibly inactivated, and pancreatic lipase is irreversibly denatured. Because pancreatic lipase is particularly important in fat absorption, its inactivation results in fat malabsorption, steatorrhea, diarrhea, and weight loss. Tests for gastric hypersecretion of gastric acid are described in Chapter 6. Therapy to inhibit gastric acid secretion will normalize pancreatic digestive enzyme activity.

Bile Salt Insufficiency

DEFICIENT BILE SALT SECRETION. Normal digestion and absorption of dietary fat depends on adequate secretion of bile. Bile acids participate in emulsification of fat, in activation, with colipase, of pancreatic lipase, and in formation of

micelles that facilitate transfer of the products of fat digestion to the intestinal mucosa.[13] Absence of bile salts does not completely block fat absorption, however; significant absorption of lipid is thought to occur instead from liquid crystalline vesicular structures with multilamellar and unilamellar forms, perhaps leading to as much as approximately 50% of normal fat absorption.[13] Steatorrhea is generally more dramatic in the absence of pancreatic lipase than when bile salts are deficient. Nonetheless, intrahepatic and extrahepatic biliary obstruction secondary to any cause will cause mild to moderate fat malabsorption.[1]

Cholecystitis, and cholangiohepatitis, and cholelithiasis may all cause biliary obstruction. Complete bile duct obstruction is most frequently caused by neoplasms of the pancreas, lymph nodes, or intestine. Bile duct obstruction can also be a complication of acute pancreatitis, perforated gastric or duodenal ulcer, and abscesses. Occasionally, intestinal parasites or migrating foreign bodies enter and obstruct the lumen of the duct.

Complete obstruction of the biliary tract results not only in systemic icterus due to hyperbilirubinemia, but also in pale feces (acholic feces) because of the lack of bile pigments in the gut lumen. Fecal color is due mainly to products of bile pigment metabolism. Bilirubin secreted in bile is metabolized by intestinal bacteria to form stercobilinogen (urobilinogen), which is further oxidized to the brown pigment of feces, stercobilin (urobilin). Only small amounts of bile are needed to produce brown feces, however; thus, acholic feces are only produced when the bile duct is almost totally obstructed. Although stool color can provide clues to the patency of the biliary tree, it should be noted that fecal color also varies with the diet. Light-colored feces are produced when milk proteins are the only source of nitrogen. Antibiotic therapy can change the intestinal microflora that metabolizes bile pigments, leading to lighter-colored feces. Similarly, when diar-

Table 19–3

CLINICAL SEQUELAE TO NUTRIENT MALABSORPTION

NUTRIENT	CLINICAL SIGNS/ LABORATORY ABNORMALITIES
Fat	Diarrhea, weight loss/steatorrhea (increased oxalate absorption)
Protein	Weight loss, muscle wasting, edema/hypoalbuminemia
Carbohydrate	Weight loss, diarrhea, flatulence, borborygmi/positive hydrogen breath test
Cobalamin	Anorexia/subnormal serum cobalamin
Folate	Diarrhea?, anemia?/subnormal serum folate
Vitamin K	Coagulopathy/prolonged prothrombin/activated partial thromboplastin times
Vitamin A	Hyperkeratosis?, night blindness?, impaired immunologic function?
Vitamin D	Osteomalacia?
Vitamin E	Retinal degeneration, myopathy, myelopathy/oxidant-induced hemolysis
Calcium	Tetany (very rare)/hypocalcemia
Zinc	Anorexia?, zinc responsive dermatitis?/subnormal serum zinc
Iron	Anemia/microcytic, hypochromic erythrocytes

rhea is profuse and watery the flushing of large numbers of bacteria from the gut combined with rapid transit time leads to reduced bile pigment metabolism.

Reduced hepatic bile salt synthesis may sometimes occur with hepatocellular liver disease in the absence of jaundice, also leading to fat malabsorption secondary to reduced secretion by hepatocytes.[1] Reduced extraction of bile acids from portal blood by hepatocytes may also contribute to reduced bile acid secretion in hepatocellular disease; the total body bile acid pool can be normal, even though intestinal concentrations are deficient. Abnormalities in fat absorption in hepatocellular disease are usually subtle under these circumstances, however, more commonly manifesting as reduced absorption of fat soluble vitamins (vitamins K and E) rather than overt steatorrhea.

Bile acids have also been reported to play a role in the activation of trypsinogen by enteropeptidase;[14] failure of activation of trypsinogen to trypsin results in failure of activation of other pancreatic proteases and phospholipases.

BILE SALT DECONJUGATION. Fat malabsorption in patients with small intestinal bacterial overgrowth is related in large part to bacterial changes in bile salts. Conjugated bile acids exist as fully ionized, water soluble bile salts at neutral pH. In this form they participate in micelle formation, and remain free in the lumen of the upper small intestine because they are not absorbed across the intestinal mucosa until they contact specific receptors in the ileum. Bacteria in the gut lumen, particularly obligate anaerobic bacteria, can deconjugate bile acids to form protonated (nonionized, lipid soluble) free bile acids that are readily absorbed by passive means along the entire length of the small intestine, rendering them relatively ineffective or unavailable to participate in micelle formation.[15] Diagnosis of small intestinal bacterial overgrowth is discussed later in this chapter and in Chapter 6; antibiotic therapy will restore normal bile salt activity.

Deconjugated bile acids also have pronounced effects on fluid and electrolyte absorption in the intestine, particularly the colon. Although these effects can occur with all bile acids, the nonpolar deconjugated forms are far more potent, perhaps because they enter enterocyte membranes more readily. Deconjugated bile acids have some additional effects in the small intestine including inhibition of brush border enzyme activities and absorption of monosaccharides.[16,17] Thus, absorption of all nutrients can be inhibited in the presence of excess deconjugated bile acids.

BILE SALT PRECIPITATION. Some drugs, including neomycin, cause precipitation of bile salts so that they are ineffective in micelle formation. Glycine-conjugated bile acids also precipitate out of solution when the pH falls below 5.0. In addition, fatty acids are protonated when the pH is less than 6.0, and have poor solubility in bile salt micelles, an additional factor contributing to fat malabsorption in gastric acid hypersecretory states.[13]

BILE SALT BINDING. Cholestyramine is a drug that specifically binds bile salts, and it is used to inhibit bile salt–mediated diarrhea. However, it renders bile salts ineffective in fat absorption, and when used in excess results in steatorrhea.

BILE SALT LOSS. Conjugated bile salts are normally reabsorbed by a highly efficient and specific active transport mechanism located in the ileum, by which route they undergo enterohepatic circulation. The adequacy of this enterohepatic circulation is very important in maintaining intestinal bile acid concentration because the total bile acid pool is very small; the bile acid pool passes through the enterohepatic circulation two or three times during a single meal, thereby maintaining adequate intraluminal bile acid concentrations.

When there is severe ileal disease or following ileal resection, bile acid reabsorption fails, which results in bile acid–mediated diarrhea. Villus atrophy confined to the ileum, resulting in a primary bile acid malabsorption and chronic watery diarrhea, has been reported in humans.[18] In these circumstances bile acid binding agents such as cholestyramine will improve the bile acid–mediated diarrhea. However, bile acid malabsorption may eventually lead to progressive depletion of the circulating bile acid pool because there is limited scope for increased de novo synthesis of bile acids by hepatocytes to compensate for increased fecal loss. Eventually the intraluminal concentration

Table 19–4

FACTORS THAT MAY DECREASE PANCREATIC ENZYME ACTIVITY IN THE LUMEN OF THE SMALL INTESTINE

Decreased synthesis (reduced functional acinar cell mass)	Pancreatic acinar atrophy
	Chronic pancreatitis
	Pancreatic or extrapancreatic neoplasia
	Congenital enzyme deficiency
Decreased secretion (reduced pancreatic stimulation)	Decreased secretagogue release with severe enteropathies
Decreased zymogen activation	Enteropeptidase (enterokinase) deficiency
Decreased enzyme cofactors	Bile salt deficiency
	Colipase deficiency
Increased enzyme degradation	Small intestinal bacterial overgrowth
Enzyme inactivation or denaturation	Gastric acid hypersecretion

of bile acids falls so that the critical micellar concentration is not reached, leading to failure of normal fat absorption.[19] In these circumstances supplementation with oral bile acids will ameliorate steatorrhea and diarrhea.[20]

Diagnosis and Therapy of Deficient Bile Secretion

A specific diagnosis of maldigestion of lipids due to deficient bile secretion is rarely made, because the clinical signs of the primary disorder usually overshadow the more subtle signs of the maldigestion.[19] Thus, animals with biliary tract obstruction present with icterus or hyperbilirubinemia, rather than because of steatorrhea per se. Patients with hepatocellular liver disease of sufficient severity to cause significant failure of bile acid secretory capacity usually have other laboratory evidence of liver disease (elevated liver enzymes, icterus, etc.).

The therapy of bile deficiency is usually directed at the primary cause of the disorder. When this is not possible then oral supplementation with bile salts may be helpful, and in some cases where diarrhea is the major clinical problem, feeding a low-fat diet can be helpful in controlling clinical signs.[19]

SMALL INTESTINAL BACTERIAL OVERGROWTH

Clinical Synopsis

Diagnostic Features

- Intermittent "small-bowel" type diarrhea with or without weight loss
- Greater than 10^5 bacteria per mL of duodenal fluid (dog)
- Normal trypsinlike immunoreactivity test (unless coexistent EPI)
- Increased breath hydrogen concentration (80% of patients)
- Increased serum folate concentration (50% of patients)
- Decreased serum cobalamin (25% of patients)
- Steatorrhea (10% of patients, usually minimal to mild)

Standard Treatment

- Correct underlying cause, if known
- Oxytetracycline, 10 to 20 mg/kg q 12 hours for 1–2 months. Repeat for 10 to 14 day courses if signs recur.

Follow-up

- Repeated antibiotic therapy during clinical exacerbations

DEFINITION. Small intestinal bacterial overgrowth (SIBO) describes the proliferation of abnormal numbers of bacteria in the lumen of the upper small intestine. The abnormal microflora usually includes species that are normal inhabitants of that area, but may also include species not normally present in upper small intestine.

It is generally accepted that in normal dogs no more than 10^4 to 10^5 bacteria per mL of juice are present in the lumen of the upper small intestine.[21–24] Species most commonly isolated include *E. coli*, enterococci, and lactobacilli; obligate anaerobic species are rare in the proximal small intestine of the dog. In marked contrast cats may have up to 10^5 to 10^8 bacterial per mL of juice, and this microflora commonly includes obligate anaerobic bacteria such as *Bacteroides, Eubacteria,* and *Fusobacteria; Pasteurella* species were the most common aerobic bacteria isolated.[25]

ETIOLOGY. Normal physiologic processes, including secretion of gastric acid, intestinal propulsive movements, and secretion of antibacterial factors in pancreatic juice, function to regulate bacterial numbers within the small intestine. Gastric acid kills many ingested bacteria and inhibits seeding of the duodenum with microbes. Even when acid secretion is inhibited, however, if intestinal motility is normal then the cleansing action of normal intestinal motility effectively limits bacterial proliferation.[22] In contrast, even when acid secretion is normal, if intestinal propulsive activity is disrupted, then SIBO develops.[22] Subsequently, factors such as host malnutrition may be important in favoring persistence of the abnormal microflora by affecting factors such as local immunity and mucus secretion.

When SIBO develops, the factors that determine what species of bacteria subsequently proliferate and to what total population are less well understood, but complex interactions between bacteria within the gut lumen are certainly important. These microbial interactions include competition for available nutrients, alteration of intraluminal pH or redox potential, production of toxic metabolites, enzyme sharing, and transfer of antibiotic resistance.[15,26]

In human beings SIBO most commonly occurs when there are abnormalities that result in impairment of normal motility. This most commonly happens with anatomic changes such as may occur with obstruction secondary to gastrointestinal neoplasms or after surgical manipulations such as bypass operations, and with functional motor changes secondary to diseases such as diabetic autonomic neuropathy or idiopathic pseudo-obstruction;[15] similar circumstances can clearly arise in veterinary patients.[27] In dogs, SIBO has been documented as an idiopathic abnormality in patients with gastrointestinal signs,[21] in association with exocrine pancreatic insufficiency[28,29] and degenerative myelopathy,[30] and also as a subclinical finding in apparently healthy beagles[31] and German shepherd dogs.[32] In a university referral practice setting in the United Kingdom, about 50% of cases with chronic small intestinal disease were shown to have associated SIBO.[33] There are no reports of SIBO in cats.

PATHOPHYSIOLOGY. The pathophysiology of SIBO is very complex and involves both intraluminal effects of proliferating bacteria and direct damage to enterocytes themselves. Potential mechanisms at play include direct injurious effects on brush border enzymes and carrier proteins, secretion of enterotoxins, deconjugation of bile acids, hydroxylation of fatty acids, and competition for nutrients.

INTRALUMINAL EFFECTS. Many species of bacteria, particularly gram negative aerobes and obligate anaerobes, compete very effectively with the host for intraluminal supplies of cobalamin, preventing its uptake by enterocytes.[34] Although other species of bacteria may synthesize cobalamin, they retain it internally and so it is not available for absorption by the host. Although intrinsic factor inhibits uptake of cobalamin by aerobic microbes, it is ineffective against uptake by gram negative anaerobes such as *Bacteroides* spp. Over time, this malabsorption of cobalamin leads to subnormal serum concentrations of the vitamin as body stores are depleted; thus, subnormal serum cobalamin concentration provides some evidence in support of suspected SIBO (see Chapter 6).

In contrast to the situation with cobalamin, enteric bacteria synthesize and secrete some other vitamins, including folate and vitamin K. In the case of folate, this does not usually benefit the host unless coprophagy is part of normal ingestive behavior as in rats and rabbits because specific folate carriers are only present in the upper small intestine. However, in SIBO the folate is available for absorption because it is produced in the upper small intestine.[35,36] Thus, folate absorption is promoted in SIBO, and serum concentrations of this vitamin tend to increase over time, providing evidence in support of suspected SIBO (see Chapter 6).

Toxic products that may appear in the gut lumen as a result of bacterial metabolic activity include bacterial enzymes (proteases and glycosidases), unconjugated bile acids, ethanol, enterotoxins, endotoxin, and peptidoglycan-polysaccharide polymers.[37,38] These agents may not only be toxic to the enterocytes locally, but may be absorbed into the portal blood and lead to hepatotoxicity.[39] The mechanisms of toxic damage to enterocytes are not well understood, but many bacteria, particularly obligate anaerobic bacteria, are particularly effective at producing enzymes that damage exposed brush border enzymes.[28,40,41,] This type of damage is accelerated by malnutrition, which may impair enterocyte ability to synthesize new brush border proteins and mucin.[28,40]

Deconjugation of bile acids allows them to be reabsorbed from the gut lumen, rendering them unavailable for participation in normal fat absorption (see earlier). Although this contributes to fat malabsorption in SIBO, it is not the sole mechanism because fat absorption is less impaired in rats with ligated bile ducts (presumably with zero intraluminal bile acids) than in rats with SIBO.[15] Malabsorption of fat is also related to tonic damage to enterocytes, for example by exposure to high concentrations of deconjugated bile acid that impair normal absorptive processes.[15]

Malabsorbed fatty acids in patients with SIBO are available for hydroxylation by the abnormal intraluminal microflora.[42] These hydroxy fatty acids are then available, along with other agents such as organic acids and sugars (products of bacterial fermentation of other malabsorbed substances), to stimulate secretion of water and electrolytes into the bowel lumen, contributing to diarrhea.

MORPHOLOGIC CHANGES.[43] Bacterial overgrowth often does not cause morphologic changes in the mucosa that are apparent by light microscopy.[28,41,44] Occasionally there may be a patchy mild lymphocytic-plasmacytic inflammatory infiltrate with some degree of villous blunting or shortening.[28,45] Similar changes are reported in human patients and experimental rats with SIBO. [15,46,47] These changes may be more marked in the face of severe malnutrition.[28]

BIOCHEMICAL CHANGES. Bacterial overgrowth commonly causes changes in activities of brush border enzymes. Obligate anaerobic bacteria in particular are very effective at degrading or releasing exposed brush border enzymes, an effect that is accelerated in the face of malnutrition such as occurs with untreated EPI (Figure 19–1).[28,48] The activities of the disaccharidases maltase, sucrase, and lactase, or the peptidase leucyl-2-naphthylamidase were surprisingly little affected in a series of 10 German shepherd dogs with relatively mild diarrhea and weight loss due to an idiopathic enteropathy associated with predominantly aerobic bacterial overgrowth.[41] However, the activity of intestinal gamma-glutamyltransferase activity was increased and that of alkaline phosphatase was reduced in these dogs.[41] In contrast, in a group of 7 German shepherd dogs with an enteropathy associated with anaerobic overgrowth, although there was no change in brush border enzyme specific activities, there was a marked reduction in brush border density, indicative of a fall in the glycoprotein to lipid ratio of the brush border.[41,48] These changes reverse in response to antibiotic therapy.[44] Clearly many factors influence the pathophysiologic and clinical consequences of SIBO, including the type of bacteria and the nutritional state of the host.

The mechanisms by which bacterial overgrowth cause these biochemical abnormalities are unclear, but potential contributory factors include direct attack of exposed glycoproteins by bacterial proteases and glycosidases, the effects of bacterial enterotoxins, deconjugated bile acids, and malnutrition.[40,49]

Bacteria produce many short chain fatty acids (acetic, propionic, butyric, and others) by their fermentative actions, contributing to increased intraluminal osmolality and reduced intraluminal pH.[50] Medium and long chain fatty acids directly inhibit fluid absorption in both the small and large intestine. Fatty acids with a chain length greater than seven carbons have an inhibitory effect on absorption, and this inhibitory effect is greater with increasing chain length.[51] Intraluminal fatty acids may undergo hydroxylation by intestinal bacteria, producing hydroxy fatty acids such as hydroxystearic acid and ricinoleic (12-hydroxyoleic) acid that are even more potent inhibitors of fluid absorption and may actually stimulate fluid secretion. Furthermore, deconjugated bile acids and fatty acids may act synergistically to stimulate intestinal secretion of fluid, their net effects being modified in some cases by other factors, including the concentration of conjugated bile acids.[52]

Morphologic studies reveal that fatty acids cause structural changes characterized by villus shortening, increased cell exfoliation, and brush border damage.[53] These changes may reflect detergent properties of fatty acids, which are able to solubilize components of the cell membrane and thereby damage enterocytes.[53] Fatty acids may also exert effects on gastrointestinal function through changes in intestinal motility.[54,55]

Additional biochemical or functional abnormalities that have been reported in association with SIBO include diminished transport of monosaccharides, amino acids, and fatty acids as well as reduced activities of disaccharidases and peptidase, and also protein-losing enteropathy,[15,28,46,56] enteric blood loss, and decreased enteropeptidase concentration.[27,46]

MALABSORPTION IN SIBO. Via a combination of primary intraluminal and secondary mucosal mechanisms, SIBO leads to failure of absorption of fat, fat soluble vitamins, carbohydrate, and protein. Bacterial competition for some nutrients, decreased brush border enzyme activities, and damage to carrier proteins are probably of major importance in the failure of these absorptive processes. In addition, there is an antibiotic-responsive protein-losing enteropathy that contributes to progressive protein depletion, muscle wasting, and eventual hypoproteinemia.[56]

Unabsorbed peptides and amino acids are metabolized by intestinal bacteria. Many are deaminated, and the ammonia formed is absorbed and converted to urea, so that this nitrogen is lost to the animal. Other bacterial metabolites are also absorbed and metabolized to compounds that are eventually excreted in the urine, where they provide evidence for bacterial metabolism of malabsorbed protein (see urinary nitrosonaphthol and indican tests, Chapter 6).

CLINICAL FINDINGS. Bacterial overgrowth in dogs results in chronic intermittent diarrhea, with or without weight loss. Additional clinical signs related to the predisposing cause for the overgrowth may be seen (for example, vomiting secondary to chronic partial obstruction), and with chronic SIBO, signs related to progressive nutrient deficiency (for example, anorexia secondary to cobalamin deficiency) may develop. Steatorrhea may be present but is usually mild and rarely if ever severe enough to be unequivocally diagnosed by examination of Sudan-stained fecal samples. Bacterial overgrowth in many instances is a subclinical finding, although functional disturbances can be found if factors such as serum cobalamin, folate, and tocopherol, or intestinal permeability are examined.[28,30,31,46]

DIAGNOSIS OF SIBO. The sine qua non for the diagnosis of SIBO is a properly collected and appropriately cultured aspirate from the proximal small intestine.[15] The aspirate should be collected by peroral intubation or direct needle puncture under anaerobic conditions, and diluted serially to allow quantitative culture on a variety of selective media (see Chapter 6).[57] This is technically difficult, time consuming, and expensive, and rarely feasible outside of referral settings. Even this approach may miss SIBO in some individuals due to pockets of overgrowth away from the point of sampling.

Numerous noninvasive, indirect laboratory tests have been evaluated for the diagnosis of SIBO in human beings, including assay of serum cobalamin and folate,[58] assay of serum unconjugated bile acids[59] or urinary indican (or other products of bacterial metabolism within the intestine),[60] and a variety of breath tests (^{14}C-xylose,[14]C-bile acid, lactulose-hydrogen, glucose-hydrogen) designed to detect microbial activity within the upper small intestine (see Chapter 6).[15] Of these, the various breath tests, particularly the ^{14}C-xylose breath test, appear to be the most sensitive and specific, but although technically feasible are generally not available in veterinary practice.[33,61–64] Intestinal permeability was increased in beagles with SIBO compared to those without SIBO, and was particularly elevated in dogs with anaerobic overgrowth.[31] Increased intestinal permeability is not a specific abnormality associated only with SIBO, however.[65]

Assays of serum cobalamin and folate appear to be the most helpful aids to diagnosis of SIBO in the dog presently available for use by veterinarians in general practice, although they undoubtedly have poor sensitivity (that is, many affected dogs do not have abnormal test results). If pancreatic function is normal (that is, serum trypsinlike immunoreactivity, TLI, is normal), then finding a decreased serum cobalamin or increased serum folate is supportive of SIBO. If both of these abnormalities are found, then this is strong evidence in support of SIBO, but this combination is uncommon.[21] In patients with SIBO, elevated folate alone is seen in about 50% of cases, and decreased cobalamin alone in about 25% of cases.[66] The value and limitations of serum cobalamin and folate assays in diagnosis of SIBO is discussed in more detail in Chapter 6.

In the future, assay of deconjugated bile acids in serum may provide evidence of the presence of SIBO. In normal patients serum bile acids are largely conjugated (the form of bile acids specifically absorbed in the ileum) but when there is SIBO the intraluminal bacteria may deconjugate the bile acids allowing them to be nonspecifically absorbed along the small intestine. Deconjugated bile acids may be detected both in duodenal aspirates and serum of human patients with SIBO.[59,67–73] At present, evaluation of this approach in canine patients is limited by technical complexities associated with selective assay of deconjugated bile acids.

TREATMENT OF SIBO. Elimination of SIBO is most likely to be successful if the underlying primary cause is known and can be corrected, such as in the case of surgical resection of mechanical obstructions. Antibiotic administration in such cases is probably not required in order to eliminate the overgrowth, but may well be given for other reasons. Specific antibiotic therapy for many animals, such as those patients with SIBO associated with EPI, is probably not required in most cases; those patients usually have subclinical SIBO and therapy with pancreatic enzyme replacement alone will resolve clinical signs (although it rarely rectifies cobalamin malabsorption; see Chapter 20). In an unpublished study the author noted no difference in the rate of return to normal body weight when a group of affected animals were treated with enzyme replacement in combination with antibiotic therapy (oxytetracycline) for 1 month, compared to treatment with enzymes alone, even though SIBO almost certainly persisted.[29] In some patients with EPI, however, SIBO is clinically significant and recovery is not complete until antibiotic therapy is given.[28]

In most dogs with SIBO the overgrowth consists of a broad spectrum of aerobic and anaerobic bacteria, and therefore broad-spectrum antibiotic therapy is appropriate; oral oxytetracycline (10–20 mg/kg q 8–12 hours for 28 days) has been

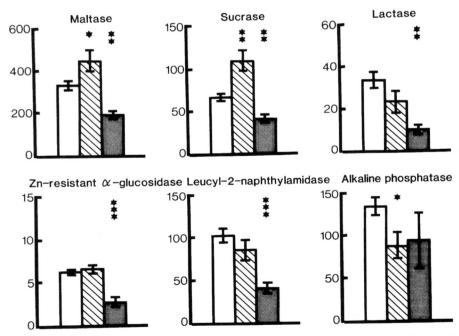

FIGURE 19–1. Activities of jejunal brush border enzymes in normal dogs (open bars) and dogs with exocrine pancreatic insufficiency with (stippled bars) and without (striped bars) anaerobic small intestinal bacterial overgrowth. In the face of malnutrition, as may occur with exocrine pancreatic insufficiency, obligate anaerobic bacteria are very effective at degrading or releasing exposed brush border enzymes, leading to markedly reduced activities. (Reproduced from Williams DA, et al: Bacterial overgrowth in the duodenum of dogs with exocrine pancreatic insufficiency. J Am Vet Med Assoc 191:201–206, 1987.)

found to be effective in improving clinical signs and reducing bacterial counts, often eliminating growth of *Clostridia*.[28,44] The appropriate duration for therapy is not known, but an initial course of treatment for 1 month is often prescribed. If there are recurrences of clinical signs, then subsequent shorter courses of treatment may prove to be effective.[46] Oral tylosin (15 mg/kg q 12 hours for 7 days) has also been shown to be effective in eliminating SIBO in dogs with EPI.[29] Metronidazole is perhaps a logical choice in the cat given the reported anaerobic nature of the upper small intestinal microflora in that species.[25]

Additional supportive therapy for patients with SIBO may be required. Nutritional support is of prime importance, and particular attention must be given to ensure that vitamin status is adequate. Cobalamin deficiency, if present, may require parenteral therapy (100–250 µg SC or IM q 7 days for 8 weeks) in order to normalize serum concentrations. The prognosis is difficult to predict; in some cases return to normal is rapid and repeat therapy is not required.[28] In other instances there is apparent full recovery after rather prolonged antibiotic therapy.[45] Recurrence of signs soon after therapy is discontinued probably reflects inability to correct the underlying cause for development of overgrowth. Failure to respond at all suggests either antibiotic resistance (unlikely in most circumstances) or that factors related to the underlying predisposing cause for the development of SIBO are sufficient to cause clinical signs alone, irrespective of the presence of overgrowth.

DEFECTS OF MUCOSAL FUNCTION (MUCOSAL MALABSORPTION)

It is important to remember that mucosal disease of the small intestine results in failure of digestion as well as defective absorption. The mechanisms are multifactorial, but probably most commonly involve reduced synthesis or increased degradation of brush border carbohydrases and peptidases that complete the process of digestion. Normal digestion and absorption is also compromised by reduction in villous or microvillous surface area, as well by damage to membrane carrier proteins even when the surface area available for absorption is not reduced. Additional factors that may play a role include interference with normal reflex mechanisms that initiate and coordinate secretion of pancreatic enzymes, bile, and regulate gastric emptying.

Clinical Synopsis

Diagnostic Features

- "Small-bowel" type diarrhea with weight loss
- Steatorrhea may be present
- Serum cobalamin, folate, and fat soluble vitamin concentrations may be subnormal
- Breath hydrogen test results may be abnormal reflecting carbohydrate malabsorption
- Xylose absorption test results often normal (reflecting poor test sensitivity)

Standard Treatment

- Depends to a large extent on cause; treat for specific infectious etiologies (e.g., histoplasmosis)
- Low-fat diets with easily assimilated carbohydrate and protein

- Low-fiber highly digestible diets
- Elimination or hypoallergenic diets (for dietary sensitivity)
- Prednisolone is effective in many patients with idiopathic inflammatory bowel disease or villous atrophy
- Additional immunosuppressive therapy (azathioprine, chlorambucil) is required in some patients

Follow-up

- Depends on cause

Etiology and Pathophysiology of Mucosal Malabsorption (Tables 19-1 and 19-2)

The most common cause of chronic malabsorption in the dog and cat is idiopathic chronic inflammatory bowel disease, which can be characterized according to the inflammatory cell components present as lymphocytic, lymphocytic-plasmacytic, eosinophilic, and so on. In a small minority of cases underlying or associated dietary sensitivity or SIBO can be identified.[45,48,74] Occasionally villous atrophy with a minimal inflammatory component is seen. Diffuse neoplastic infiltration may be seen with intestinal lymphosarcoma. In some geographic areas a variety of fungal and other infectious enteropathies such as histoplasmosis or phycomycosis may be encountered; parasitic enteropathies such as that caused by giardiasis are widely recognized as common causes of malabsorption in many locations. Finally, resection of large amounts of intestine may lead to significant nutrient malabsorption.

LOSS OF BRUSH BORDER ENZYMES. Brush border enzymes may become deficient secondary to either acute or chronic mucosal disease.[75] Severe infectious enteritis may lead to massive loss of disaccharidases until new mature enterocytes migrate from the crypts. Toxic drugs and other agents (e.g., neomycin and kanamycin) have a similar effect and also reduce crypt cell replication.[1] Reduced disaccharidase (maltase, sucrase, and lactase) activities may be seen as a component of the injury associated with numerous chronic clinical entities of dogs including eosinophilic enteritis, neutrophilic enteritis with villus atrophy, histiocytic enteritis with villus atrophy, lymphosarcoma with villus atrophy, lymphangiectasia, idiopathic villus atrophy unaccompanied by inflammation, and SIBO in dogs with EPI.[28,75,76]

Reduced enzyme activities may be caused by accelerated destruction as a result of intraluminal events as in SIBO, by reduced synthesis by the enterocytes themselves, or as a consequence of accelerated enterocyte turnover (migration up the villus) such that the villi possess fewer mature epithelial cells with a normal complement of brush border enzymes by the time enterocytes are sloughed from the villous tips. Chronic iron deficiency in growing dogs has been reported to reduce disaccharidase activities,[77] as has parasite infestation in rats.[78] Congenital deficiencies of specific brush border enzymes are well documented in human beings, but not in domestic species.[79]

Unabsorbed sugars in the colon contribute to osmotic retention of water in the gut lumen and hence to diarrhea. However, much of the sugar is metabolized by colonic bacteria, reducing the severity of the diarrhea.[80] Lactase activity is particularly susceptible to damage in many acquired enteropathies, explaining the poor tolerance of milk products exhibited by many affected patients. Normal dogs can tolerate lactose ingestion of 1 g/kg/day; diarrhea develops when more than 1.5 g/kg/day of lactose is fed.[81]

In contrast to the situation with lactase and lactose, activities of maltase generally remain sufficient to digest a normal intake of starch even in the face of severe enteropathies. Dietary restriction of carbohydrates other than lactose is not usually necessary. When diarrhea is managed using diets containing cottage cheese, it should be noted that this contains about 10% of the lactose of whole milk based on the ratio of lactose to protein. Also, lactose in fermented dairy produce such as yogurt may have been degraded by bacteria during the process of fermentation.

Mucosal damage also results in a loss of brush border peptidases. These losses are generally not critical because peptides are digested more readily than oligosaccharides and some dipeptides and tripeptides are absorbed intact. Nitrogen deficiency associated with chronic small intestinal disease is usually a reflection of anorexia and protein-losing enteropathy.

LOSS OF MUCOSAL ABSORPTIVE AREA. A reduction in mucosal surface area is an important cause of malabsorption in both acute and chronic conditions. Bacterial toxins and metabolites, bile acid metabolites, parasites, and dietary or bacterial antigens may all contribute to this decrease in mucosal surface area. Some changes are due to direct toxic effects on the intestinal mucosa, and others are mediated by the local immune response, which may itself be a primary cause of the intestinal disease in some patients. Crypt hypertrophy may be evident in association with villous atrophy. Microvilli may also be abnormal, further aggravating digestive and absorptive dysfunction.

SELECTIVE LOSS OF TRANSPORT MECHANISMS. Lack of specific transport mechanisms for individual nutrients have been reported in patients with normal villous architecture. Congenital absence of special transport mechanisms for hexoses, amino acids, or certain vitamins and minerals result in their malabsorption, and sometimes in specific deficiency states.[1,82,83]

ENTEROCYTE PROCESSING DEFECTS. Intracellular defects are common causes of malabsorption. Malabsorption from mucosal disease is usually caused by abnormalities at the rate-limiting steps of absorption, which occur for most nutrients at the mucosal surface. After sugars enter the cell no special mechanisms are required for their transport into the circulation. Sugars also do not require metabolic transformation to leave the cell. Proteins require further degradation if they enter the cell as peptides, but intracellular digestion is not rate limiting and is not significantly affected by most mucosal diseases. Lipids require metabolic transformation before they can leave mucosal cells but, as with proteins, the rate-limiting step in lipid assimilation is diffusion across the brush border.[13,84] Lipids do require reesterification prior to incorporation into chylomicrons, a process that depends on the synthesis of a beta lipoprotein; congenital abetalipoproteinemia in human beings leads to a characteristic accumulation of triglycerides in enterocytes.[1] The severe fat malabsorption subsequently leads to tocopherol malabsorption and neurologic problems related to deficiency of this vitamin.

DISRUPTION OF THE LAMINA PROPRIA. The structure of the lamina propria is important for optimum absorption of fluid and nutrients. This part of the mucosa contains a loose array of blood vessels and connective tissue. The vessels lie immediately adjacent to the basal border of the mucosal cells, making the path short for absorbed particles to enter the circulation. Pathology in the lamina propria affecting absorption includes cellular infiltration, fibrosis, and accumulation of fluid. The types of cells infiltrating the lamina propria include lymphocytes, plasma cells, histiocytes, macrophages, eosinophils, neutrophils, mast cells, and basophils. Signs of inflammation may be evident, or the lamina propria may be extensively infiltrated with neoplastic lymphocytes without evidence of inflammation. A case of fucosidosis, a lysosomal storage disease of English Springer spaniels, has been reported in which malabsorption was attributed to infiltration of the lamina with vacuolated macrophages.[85] Infiltrating cells probably create a

barrier between the normal-appearing mucosal surface and the capillaries, interfering with normal diffusion of absorbed fluid and solutes. With the exception of very rare severe infiltrative disorders such as intestinal lymphomas, this mechanism is probably of secondary importance to other mechanisms outlined earlier.

Laboratory Findings and Diagnosis of Mucosal Malabsorption

The approach to the diagnosis of malabsorption is described in Chapter 6. Fecal fat output is the only reliable screening test for malabsorption of fat, but is often mild or not present in patients with small intestinal disease. Plasma turbidity and fecal Sudan stain lipid absorption tests are too unreliable to be recommended as screening tests for steatorrhea. Breath hydrogen testing is a good screening test for carbohydrate malabsorption but does not distinguish patients with malabsorption resulting from disaccharidase deficiencies or generalized mucosal disease from those with SIBO or rapid transit time. The xylose absorption test has poor sensitivity for canine and feline small intestinal disease. Serum cobalamin and folate assays are simple to perform and abnormal test results not only confirm that there is malabsorption but provide clues to its location and to the site of malabsorption. These tests also have limited sensitivity, but they are superior to the xylose absorption test.

Small animal patients with mucosal malabsorption seldom have radiographically identifiable changes in the small intestine. Positive-contrast radiographic studies are occasionally performed to rule out adynamic ileus or mechanical obstructions that may predispose to SIBO and malabsorption. Simple positive-contrast studies of the intestinal tract occasionally identify mucosal morphologic abnormalities in patients with intestinal lymphosarcoma or severe eosinophilic enteritis, for example, but they do not differentiate these diseases. Enteroclysis is a more sensitive method for detection of intestinal mucosal abnormalities (see Chapter 6), but is considerably more complex to perform and suffers from a similar lack of specificity.

Examination of biopsy material from the intestine is often the only means of characterizing small intestinal disease, although normal mucosal morphology does not rule out malabsorption; by definition a test of absorptive function is required to make a diagnosis of malabsorption. In many cases no definitive diagnosis is possible, although there is usually sufficient histopathologic or gut function test information to direct the course of treatment. Assessment of the biopsy includes evaluation of (1) absorptive surface area, (2) the type and severity of cellular infiltration, and (3) the hemolymphatic drainage of the mucosa. Most of the commonly seen changes (mild villous atrophy and infiltration by lymphocytes, plasma cells, or eosinophils) are nonspecific, but do indicate the presence of small intestinal disease. Specific diagnosis of dietary sensitivity, for example, requires documentation of changes in intestinal biopsies in combination with well-controlled challenge testing.[74]

Management of Mucosal Malabsorption

The management of malabsorption depends on the primary cause. See the chapters on infectious and parasitic intestinal diseases, inflammatory bowel disease, intestinal obstruction, adverse reactions to food, gastrointestinal neoplasia, and exocrine pancreatic insufficiency. The management of bacterial overgrowth was discussed earlier; therapy of protein-losing enteropathies is discussed later. Whatever the underlying cause, attention should be given to correction of vitamin, mineral, and protein-calorie malnutrition. The relationship between the severity and nature of histologic abnormalities and results of function tests and subsequent response to therapy are not clear. Some patients have apparently self-limiting disease; others have chronic signs that respond only partially to treatment or respond but relapse when treatment is discontinued.

DEFECTS OF POSTMUCOSAL FUNCTION (POSTMUCOSAL MALABSORPTION)

Lymphatic Obstruction

Obstruction of the lymphatic system, either as a primary defect or secondary to pressure changes in the vasculature into which the lymphatic vessels drain (as in heart failure), leads not only to impaired absorption of chylomicrons (and hence steatorrhea), lymphocytes, and extracellular fluid proteins present in lymph, but also in some case to accelerated loss of the latter into the gut lumen. If severe, protein-losing enteropathy can lead to such massive loss of plasma protein that the limited capacity for compensatory increased synthesis of albumin and other protein is insufficient and panhypoproteinemia ensues. Diagnosis and management of these lymphatic disorders are discussed further in the section on protein-losing enteropathy later in this chapter.

Vascular Disease

Chronic portal venous hypertension secondary to chronic liver disease (cirrhosis) or intestinal vasculitis, thrombosis, or neoplastic infiltration may lead to nutrient malabsorption and perhaps enteric protein loss.[86] Intestinal ischemia secondary to vascular insufficiency may also cause fat malabsorption. This is thought to reflect impaired absorptive function rather than impaired postmucosal removal in most cases; however, the rate of removal of rapidly transported nutrients may be blood flow dependent in some cases.[1] Diagnosis and management of these vascular disorders are discussed in the sections on protein-losing enteropathy.

PROTEIN-LOSING ENTEROPATHY[75,87–92]

Clinical Synopsis

Diagnostic Features

- Mild "small-bowel" type diarrhea or no diarrhea
- Panhypoproteinemia and lymphopenia
- Hypocholesterolemia and hypocalcemia
- Malabsorption of fat, fat soluble vitamins, and other nutrients possible
- Normal pancreatic function

Standard Treatment

- Low-fat high-quality protein diet
- Medium chain triglyceride oil if underweight (1–2 mL/kg per day)

- Prednisolone 1 to 2 mg/kg q 12 hours PO for 1 to 2 weeks; tapered to eventual alternate day therapy

Follow-up

- Lifelong therapy may be required in some cases
- Monitor body weight and serum albumin
- Adjust diet accordingly

Excessive loss of plasma and other protein-containing tissues into the gastrointestinal tract is referred to as protein-losing enteropathy. Protein-losing enteropathy occurs in association with numerous gastrointestinal and systemic disorders including idiopathic inflammatory enteropathies such as lymphocytic-plasmacytic, eosinophilic, or granulomatous gastroenteritis, gastrointestinal neoplasia, foreign bodies, intussuceptions, SIBO (see earlier), parasitic and fungal enteropathies, acute infectious (viral or bacterial) enteritis, nonspecific enteritis, intestinal lymphangiectasia, immune-mediated and allergic diseases (Table 19–5).

Plasma proteins normally turn over with half-lives that vary from 8 to 10 days. Albumin is synthesized by the liver, and this function accounts for about 25% of all protein the liver produces. The liver is able to increase the rate of synthesis slightly (no more than twofold) in the face of increased loss of albumin, provided the required nutrients are provided. The most important site of albumin degradation is unknown. Degradation by the liver and intestine are each believed to account for about 10% of the total turnover.[93,94] The rate of catabolism appears to be constant at other sites, although catabolism may decrease in the face of increased renal or intestinal loss.

The mechanism for protein loss in protein-losing enteropathy may be related to inflammation or erosion affecting the normal barrier function of the gut, or to acquired or congenital abnormalities in intestinal lymphatic or vascular drainage.[56,87,95–100] Protein-losing enteropathy often arises as a consequence of disruption of mucosal and postmucosal absorptive mechanisms. The mucosa of the small and large intestines forms a semipermeable barrier that controls the transmucosal movement of fluid and electrolytes and restricts that of larger molecules, including proteins, whether they are in the intestinal lumen or on the capillary side of the cell. However, the intestinal mucosa provides only a tenuous barrier to the loss of plasma proteins from the body.[101]

The source of the enteric protein loss in protein-losing enteropathy is either the mucosal vasculature or the mucosal interstitial space. Normally, one-third to one-half of plasma proteins are found inside the vascular compartment, with the remainder in extravascular spaces. Capillaries in intestinal mucosa have large fenestrations that readily permit macromolecules to move into the interstitial space. In addition, the gel in the interstitial space accommodates large amounts of plasma protein. Alteration of the mucosal epithelial barrier by disease results in loss of these plasma proteins into the intestinal lumen. Thus, when plasma proteins are lost into the intestinal tract, both albumin and globulins are lost at an equal rate. The resultant hypoalbuminemia and hypoglobulinemia (panhypoproteinemia) is characteristic of protein-losing enteropathies and helps differentiate them from the hypoproteinemia of glomerular and hepatic disease, which is usually characterized by hypoalbuminemia alone.

Protein can be lost into the gastric and intestinal lumina without evidence of any morphologic damage to the mucosa. Permeability through the tight junctions is probably increased, and protein loss has been shown to occur by that intercellular route in experimental situations.[102] The pathogenesis of the increased permeability is not well understood.

Protein-losing gastroenteropathy can be produced in experimental animals by X-irradiation or intraperitoneal injection of 5-fluorouracil. Increases in the fibrinolytic activity of intestinal tissue are found in experimental and some naturally occurring protein-losing gastroenteropathies.[103] Protein loss is reduced in both situations by an antiplasmin agent, trans-4-aminomethyl cyclohexane carboxylic acid, suggesting that fibrinolytic activity of the enzyme plasmin plays an important role in enhancing mucosal permeability to protein movement. Additional factors of potential importance in gastroenteric protein loss include increased degradation of plasma proteins by inflammatory cells in the lamina propria and by proteases within epithelial cells, as well as frank hemorrhage or oozing of tissue fluids across ulcerated mucosal surfaces.

Lymphatic stasis results in lymphatic hypertension, which causes interstitial fluid to leak out into the abdominal cavity and into the lumen of the intestine. The protein-rich fluid passes into the intestine by a paracellular route through widened tight junctions.[104] Lymphatic obstruction also causes a loss of lymphocytes into the intestinal lumen. Thymus-dependent lymphocytes are sensitized in Peyer's patches. They leave the intestine by way of the lymphatics and are transformed into lymphoblasts, which, after passing through lymph nodes and the circulation, return to the lamina propria of the intestine, where they are transformed into plasma cells. Lymphangiectasia prevents the T lymphocytes from leaving the intestine, and they are lost into the lumen. Lymphangiectasia is therefore characterized by lymphopenia as well as hypoproteinemia. The loss of a large number of long-living T lymphocytes leaves the animal with deficient cell-mediated immune responses. Although lymphopenia is one criterion that can be used to help differentiate lymphangiectasia from other causes of protein-losing gastroenteropathy, it is not specific because lymphopenia ia a common abnormality in stressed animals.

The most important protein-losing gastroenteropathies are associated with chronic inflammatory diseases and circulatory diseases such as lymphangiectasia (Table 19–5). When severe panhypoproteinemia is present, underlying hemolymphatic disease or circulatory diseases are usually responsible, rather than chronic inflammatory diseases. Conversely, when loss of plasma proteins is by protein-losing gastroenteropathy due to inflammation, there are often associated clinical signs of gastrointestinal disease such as vomiting, anorexia, or diarrhea that suggest an underlying problem in the gastrointestinal tract.

Protein-losing enteropathy is one mechanism contributing to weight loss in gastrointestinal disease. In some cases there is severe loss of proteins such that compensatory increased synthesis cannot maintain plasma protein concentrations. Hypoalbuminemia and hypoglobulinemia may follow, and hypoalbuminemia may be sufficiently severe to cause ascites, edema, or rarely hydrothorax.[87]

PRIMARY INTESTINAL LYMPHANGIECTASIA.[89–91] This congenital intestinal disorder arises as a consequence of an idiopathic abnormality of lymphatic drainage.[89] It is characterized histologically by a ballooning dilation of the lacteals in the villi and distension of the submucosal lymphatic vessels. The disorder is a prominent feature of the enteropathy associated with protein-losing enteropathy in the Lundehund,[105] but the disease is not confined to this breed. Total lymph flow is reduced because the numbers of lymphatic vessels are insufficient to remove interstitial fluid. In some canine patients the lymphatic abnormalities are not confined to the gastrointestinal tract,[96] probably indicating diffuse developmental defects in the lymphatic system.

SECONDARY INTESTINAL LYMPHANGIECTASIA. The lymphatic stasis that apparently develops in adult animals is usually associated with obstructive lesions developing throughout the lymphatics. Lipogranulomatous lesions within and around the lymphatics are commonly observed,[97,106] and may even be present in other organs such as the liver.[107] It is possible that such apparently acquired lymphangiectasia develops in dogs with congenitally compromised lymphatic systems that allow leakage of lymph, to which a granulomatous response develops, further aggravating the lymphatic abnormality.

Lymphatic stasis can also arise from venous hypertension at the site where lymphatics enter the venous circulation, as happens in congestive heart failure. Lymphangiectasia can be produced experimentally by complete occlusion of all mesenteric lymphatics, but experimental obstruction of the thoracic duct does not induce the disease.[108,109]

Table 19–5

SOME DISORDERS ASSOCIATED WITH PROTEIN-LOSING GASTROENTEROPATHY

Gastrointestinal ulceration	Gastric carcinoma and lymphoma
	Ulcerative gastritis/enteritis
	Chronic foreign body
	Intussusception
	Parasitic gastroenteritis (hookworms, whipworms)
	Intestinal neoplasia
	Drugs/toxins
Gastrointestinal inflammation	Lymphocytic-plasmacytic gastritis/enteritis
	Eosinophilic gastritis/enteritis
	Granulomatous enteritis
	Histoplasmosis
	Phycomycosis
	Acute viral/bacterial enteritis
Disorders of intestinal hemolymphatic system	Primary intestinal lymphangiectasia
	Neoplastic lymphatic infiltration
	Granulomatous lymphatic infiltration
	Congestive heart failure
	Vasculitis
Disorders without ulceration or inflammation	Small intestinal bacterial overgrowth
	Systemic lupus erythematosus
	Gastrointestinal parasitism (giardiasis)
	Portal hypertension

CLINICAL SIGNS OF PROTEIN-LOSING ENTEROPATHIES Animals with protein-losing enteropathies usually exhibit signs of weight loss (muscle wasting and decreased body fat). There may be vomiting and diarrhea, but these signs are by no means always seen. Failure to exhibit diarrhea or other characteristic signs of gastrointestinal disease does not eliminate the possibility of protein-losing enteropathy.

Signs related to the underlying disease responsible for protein-losing enteropathy may be present, and physical examination may reveal evidence of thickened bowel loops, an abdominal mass, or cardiac abnormalities. If hypoalbuminemia is severe, it may be responsible for the sole presenting signs (edema, ascites, or dyspnea due to pleural effusion). Edema and ascites are generally present when the serum albumin concentration decreases to 1.0 g/dl, and may occur at higher albumin values if there is concomitant capillary hypertension from such causes as congestive heart disease, in which case the ascites fluid will have a higher protein content. Ascites can also develop because of lymphatic hypertension, resulting in the accumulation of an ultrafiltrate of lymphatic or interstitial fluid. The intestinal serosa and muscle layers effectively exclude movement of protein molecules from the interstitial space so the ascitic fluid is virtually free of protein. The fluid does contain fats, however; they are solubilized in micelles so the fluid is clear and colorless.

DIAGNOSIS. Unless a specific diagnosis is made based on history, physical examination, or results of a complete blood count, serum biochemical profile, urinalysis, or fecal examination for parasites, diagnosis is at present most commonly made by elimination of liver disease (serum bile acids) and protein-losing nephropathy (urinalysis and, if necessary, urine protein to creatinine ratio) as causes of hypoalbuminemia.[75,88,90] If hypoglobulinemia accompanies hypoalbuminema then protein-losing enteropathy is nearly always the cause of hypoalbuminema because hypoglobulinemia is very rarely seen with protein-losing nephropathy. However, not all patients with protein-losing enteropathy will have hypoglobulinema. For example, in histoplasmosis the systemic infection may lead to a significant increase in globulin production as part of the inflammatory response. Serum cobalamin and folate concentrations or results of breath hydrogen testing or testing of intestinal permeability (see Chapter 6) may provide additional evidence for gastrointestinal disease.

The protein-losing enteropathy reported in Basenji dogs is unusual in that it is characterized by hyperglobulinemia and hypoalbuminemia.[110] A recently reported protein-losing enteropathy in soft-coated Wheaten terriers is also unusual in that it appears to be accompanied by coexistent protein-losing nephropathy.[111] In many cases there is protein loss from the gastric mucosa, as well as from the intestinal mucosa, and so the term *protein-losing gastroenteropathy* may be a more accurate one.

Hypocalcemia is sometimes present. This finding is primarily a reflection of decreased serum albumin, but calcium absorption may be reduced because excess unabsorbed free fatty acids bind dietary calcium to form insoluble salts. Vitamin D malabsorption may also play a role in the hypocalcemia, but the intestinal absorption of calcium has been reported to be normal in humans with lymphangiectasia.[112] Hypocholesterolemia is common in dogs with lymphangiectasia, and presumably results from the fat malabsorption associated with failure of chylomicron transport.[107]

The classical gold standard for diagnosis of protein-losing enteropathy is to quantitate loss of radioactive (^{51}Cr-labeled) albumin into the gastrointestinal tract.[113,114] Although albumin lost into the GI tract may be degraded by digestive enzymes and constituent amino acids reabsorbed, the chromium label is not reabsorbed and is excreted in feces. Thus, following administration of isotope to label albumin in vivo, quantitation of radioactivity in feces collected over several days provides an index of gastrointestinal protein loss. Obvious technical constraints (separating urine from feces, prolonged hospitalization in a metabolism cage in a facility approved for radioisotope use), safety concerns related to exposure to radioisotope, aesthetic considerations related to handling large volumes of feces, and expense have all limited the application of this approach.

Assay of alpha-1-protease inhibitor (α_1-PI) in a single sample of feces has been shown to be a reliable method to detect protein-losing enteropathy in human patients.[115–119] This plasma protease inhibitor has a molecular weight similar to that of albumin, and is present in the vascular space, in the intercellular space, and in lymph (Table 20–3, Figure 20–2). It is therefore lost into the gastrointestinal tract when there is leakage from these sites in disease states. Unlike albumin, however, α1-PI is not degraded by enzymes when it is lost into the gut lumen by virtue of its broad-spectrum inhibition of digestive proteases (see Chapter 20); it is therefore passed in feces essentially intact, and can be detected using immunoassay methods.[120]

There are substantial species differences in the antigenic determinants of α_1-PI, and specific immunologic methods usually need to be developed for each species. A commercially available kit for human α_1-PI unfortunately does not detect canine α_1-PI.[98] Preliminary investigation of a radial immunodiffusion assay for canine α_1-PI showed concentrations in feces to be increased in dogs with protein-losing enteropathy[121] and prompted development of a more sensitive and accurate immunoassay.[122] Assay of canine α_1-PI is currently being used in the author's laboratory to study the fate of α_1-PI lost into the lumen of the canine gastrointestinal tract. The method shows promise as new test for the diagnosis of protein-losing enteropathy in dogs and for indirect quantitation of enteric protein loss.

Ideally the presence of suspected gastroenteropathy is confirmed by identification of the underlying cause and/or by gastrointestinal biopsy. With lymhangiectasia, the mucosa may appear more granular on endoscopic examination, and patches of white, lipid-filled dilated villi may be visible. Although endoscopic examination and biopsy may provide diagnostic information, in some cases full thickness intestinal biopsy may be required to demonstrate the presence of disease. Certainly, full thickness biopsy is required to document submucosal lymphatic obstruction in patients with primary or secondary intestinal lymphangiectasia. The villi enlarge, and structures of the lamina propria are displaced by the dilated lymphatics. Because chylomicrons are not transported normally from the villi, those not lost into the gut lumen (causing steatorrhea) are removed by macrophages, which therefore have a foamy appearance. Granulomas can usually be found with acquired lymphangiectasia. Lymphedema is found only if the mucosa is in the absorptive state.[123] Mild diffuse accumulations of plasma cells and lymphocytes are also often seen.

The risk of dehiscence of full thickness biopsies in debilitated hypoalbuminemic animals is minimized if nonabsorbable suture material is used, and this complication is rare. Risk of hypotension and other anesthetic problems can be minimized by plasma transfusion prior to induction of anesthesia. During exploratory laparotomy the major intestinal lymphatics of patients with lymphangiectasia will often be abnormally dilated and prominent.

It should be remembered that dilated lacteals are also occasionally seen in association with lymphocytic-plasmacytic enteritis and other enteropathies, and that this acquired change may be restricted to mucosal lymphatic vessels and is therefore not a true lymphangiectasia.

In many cases the diagnosis is presumptive because either patients are poor candidates for anesthesia and intestinal biopsy because of malnutrition and hypoproteinemia, or the expense of plasma transfusion and exploratory surgery or endoscopy is prohibitive.

TREATMENT. Recovery from acute protein-losing enteropathies associated with infectious and parasitic enteropathies is rapid following specific treatment (parasitic enteropathies) and often self-limiting (viral enteritis) providing supportive care is provided.

Treatment of chronic protein-losing enteropathies is directed at the underlying disease, if identified. Surgical removal of localized gastric or enteric chronic inflammatory, ulcerative, or neoplastic lesions can successfully halt enteric protein loss. In many instances the underlying abnormality cannot be corrected; however, in such patients nonspecific treatment, including feeding a high-quality protein low-fat content diet (to minimize distension of intestinal lymphatic vessels) is helpful. In some instances feeding a single source of carbohydrate and a single source of protein (such as a rice and low-fat cottage cheese–based diet) is beneficial.

Dietary triglycerides containing long chain fatty acids must be minimized because absorption of long chain triglyceride is a major stimulus for intestinal lymph flow. After digestion and absorption, these fatty acids are reesterified and incorporated into chylomicrons that must be transported out of the gut through the intestinal lymphatics. Restriction of dietary long chain triglyceride reduces lymphatic distension and thereby reduces gastrointestinal protein loss and lipid exudation into the perilymphatic tissues.

The calorie content of the diet may be increased by supplementation with medium chain triglyceride oil (Mead Johnson; Evansville, IN) at a dose of 1 to 2 mL/kg per day. Medium chain triglycerides are readily hydrolyzed by pancreatic lipase, but a considerable proportion of medium chain triglyceride is absorbed intact without prior lipolysis. Medium chain fatty acids are not dependent on micellarization for absorption, and once absorbed they need not be reesterified, but instead rapidly enter the portal circulation, thus bypassing the lymphatics and minimizing lymphatic distension.[124] Unfortunately, medium chain triglyceride oil does not provide the essential fatty acids; these can be provided adding a small amount of vegetable oil to the diet. Furthermore, medium chain triglyceride oil is expensive, and not particularly palatable to some animals. An alternative to medium chain triglyceride oil is a powdered elemental diet mix (Portagen; Mead Johnson, Evansville, IN) (1½ cups added to water to make a 1 quart mixture that contains 1 calorie/mL).[98]

Glucocorticoid therapy (to inhibit inflammation, exert an immunosuppressive effect, and to promote enterocyte function) is also often given and appears effective provided that specific infectious or obstructive enteropathies are not present. In patients that respond poorly to glucocorticoids or in which adverse side effects of therapy are unacceptable, immunosuppressive agents such as azathioprine or chlorambucil may be effective.

Plasma administration is usually of no long-term value because alleviation of hypoproteinemia is only transient. Plasma transfusion is of value immediately prior to general anesthesia, however, in order to minimize risk of hypotension when vascular compensatory mechanisms are inhibited.

Enhanced intestinal fibrinolytic activity has been reported in mucosal biopsies from some human patients with refractory protein-losing enteropathy. Although controversial, some human patients may respond to antifibrinolytic therapy with agents such as trans-4-aminomethyl cyclohexane carboxylic acid.[125–128] There are no reports of this approach to therapy in canine or feline patients with protein-losing enteropathy.

Unfortunately, there are few reports of long-term follow-up of dogs or cats with protein-losing enteropathy. The effectiveness of the therapeutic measures cited here has not been documented and is largely anecdotal. It is hoped that availability of an assay for canine α_1-PI will facilitate objective evaluation of different therapeutic options. In general, however, the prognosis for protein-losing enteropathies of inflammatory origin is guarded. Many patients with severe inflammatory bowel disease will eventually respond, but the therapy is often protracted and may need to be lifelong. Lymphangiectasia also carries a guarded prognosis. Response to therapy is unpredictable, and depends to a large extent on the severity of the disease process at presentation. Patients that are inappetant and severely malnourished at presentation should receive a poor prognosis.

As with protein-losing nephropathy, there may be significant loss of antithrombin III (which has a similar molecular weight to albumin and α_1-PI) and this, together with vascular damage resulting from the presence of immune complexes, may dispose to pulmonary thromboembolism.[88,129]

REFERENCES

1. Riley SA, Turnberg LA. Maldigestion and malabsorption. In: Sleisenger MH, Fordtran JS (eds) Gastrointestinal Disease: Pathophysiology/Diagnosis/Management. WB Saunders, Philadelphia, 1009–1027, 1993.
2. Klein S, Jeejeebhoy KN. Long-term nutritional management of patients with maldigestion and malabsorption. In: Sleisenger MH, Fordtran JS. Gastrointestinal Disease: Pathophysiology/Diagnosis/Management. WB Saunders, Philadelphia, 2048–2062, 1993.
3. Edwards DF, Russell RG. Probable vitamin K-deficient bleeding in two cats with malabsorption syndrome secondary to lymphocytic-plasmacytic enteritis. J Vet Int Med 1:97–101, 1987.
4. Perry LA, Williams DA, Pidgeon G, et al. Exocrine pancreatic insufficiency with associated coagulopathy in a cat J Am Anim Hosp Assoc 27:109–114, 1991.
5. Dobbins J, Binder HJ. The colon: The site of oxalate absorption in patients with hyperoxaluria and steatorrhea. Gastroenterology 70:879, 1976.
6. Dobbins JW, Binder JJ. Effect of bile salts and fatty acids on the colonic absorption of oxalate. Gastroenterology 70:1096–1100, 1976.
7. Earnest DL, Gancher S, Admirand WH. Treatment of enteric hyperoxaluria with calcium and aluminum. Gastroenterology 70:881, 1976.
8. Lerner A, Lebenthal E. Hereditary diseases of the pancreas. In: Go VLW, DiMagno EP, Gardner JD, et al. (eds) The Pancreas: Biology, Pathobiology and Disease. Raven Press, New York, 1083–1094, 1993.
9. Boari A, Williams DA, Famigli-Bergamini P. Observations on exocrine pancreatic insufficiency in a family of English setter dogs. J Sm Anim Pract 35:247–250, 1994.
10. Ligumsky M, Granot E, Branski D, et al. Isolated lipase and colipase deficiency in two brothers. Gut 31:1416–1418, 1990.
11. Borgström, B. Luminal digestion of fats. In: Go VLW, DiMagno EP, Gardner JD, et al. (eds) The Pancreas: Biology, Pathobiology and Disease. Raven Press, New York, 475–488, 1993.
12. Lebenthal E, Antonowicz I, Schwachman H. Enterokinase and trypsin activities in pancreatic insufficiency and diseases of the small intestine. Gastroenterology 70:508–512, 1976.
13. Turnberg LA, Riley SA. Digestion and absorption of nutrients and vitamins. In: Sleisenger MH, Fordtran JS (eds) Gastrointestinal Disease: Pathophysiology/Diagnosis/Management. WB Saunders, Philadelphia, 977–1008, 1993.
14. Hadorn B, Hess J, Troesch V, et al. Role of bile acids in the activation of trypsinogen by enterokinase: Disturbance of trypsinogen activation in patients with intrahepatic biliary atresia. Gastroenterology 66:548–555, 1974.
15. Toskes PP, Donaldson RM. Enteric bacterial flora and bacterial overgrowth syndrome. In: Sleisenger MH, Fordtran JS (eds) Gastrointestinal Disease: Pathophysiology/Diagnosis/Management. WB Saunders, Philadelphia, 1106–1118, 1993.

16. Gracey M, Papadimitriou J, Burke V, et al. Effects on small intestinal function and structure induced by feeding a deconjugated bile salt. Gut 14:519–528, 1973.
17. Gracey M, Houghton M, Thomas J. Deoxycholate depresses small intestinal enzyme activity. Gut 16:53–56, 1975.
18. Popovic OS, Kostic KM, Milovic VB. Primary bile acid malabsorption. Gastroenterology 92:1851–1858, 1987.
19. Simpson JW, van den Broek A. Deficiency of bile salts causing steatorrhea and weight loss in two dogs. J Sm Anim Pract 30:567–569, 1989.
20. Little KH, Schiller LR, Bilhartz LE, et al. Treatment of severe steatorrhea with ox bile in an ileectomy patient with residual colon. Dig Dis Sci 37:929–933, 1992.
21. Batt RM, Needham JR, Carter MW. Bacterial overgrowth associated with a naturally occurring enteropathy in the German shepherd dog. Res Vet Sci 35:42–46, 1983.
22. Greenlee HB, Gelbart SM, DeOrio AJ, et al. The influence of gastric surgery on the intestinal flora. Am J Clin Nutr 30:1826–1833, 1977.
23. Ihász M, Gyarmati I, Vutskits Z, et al. Effect of truncal vagotomy on the bacterial flora in the duodenal juice of dogs. Acta Sci Hung 17:215–221, 1976.
24. Gelbart SM, Larson CH, Paez JE, et al. Effect of deworming medication on the microbial flora of the upper gastrointestinal tract of dogs. Lab Anim Sci 26:640–643, 1976.
25. Johnston K, Lamport A, Batt RM. An unexpected bacterial flora in the proximal small intestine of normal cats. Vet Rec 132:362–363, 1933.
26. Willard MD, Simpson RB, Delles EK, et al. Effects of dietary supplementation of fructo-oligosaccharides on small intestinal bacterial overgrowth in dogs. Am J Vet Res 55:654–659, 1994.
27. Leib MS. Stagnant loop syndrome in the dog and cat. Sem Vet Med Surg 2:257–265, 1987.
28. Williams DA, Batt RM, McLean L. Bacterial overgrowth in the duodenum of dogs with exocrine pancreatic insufficiency. J Am Vet Med Assoc 191:201–206, 1987.
29. Westermarck E, Myllys V, Aho M. Effect of treatment on the jejunal and colonic bacterial flora of dogs with exocrine pancreatic insufficiency. Pancreas 8:559–562, 1993.
30. Williams DA, Batt RM, Sharp NJH. Degenerative myelopathy in German shepherd dogs: An association with mucosal biochemical changes and bacterial overgrowth in the small intestine. Clin Sci 66:25, 1984.
31. Batt RM, Hall EJ, McLean L, et al. Small intestinal bacterial overgrowth and enhanced intestinal permeability in healthy beagles. Am J Vet Res 53:1935–1940, 1992.
32. Willard MD, Simpson RB, Fossum TW, et al. Characterization of naturally developing small intestinal bacterial overgrowth in 16 German shepherd dogs. J Am Vet Med Assoc 204:1201–1206, 1994.
33. Rutgers HC, Lamport A, Simpson KW, et al. Bacterial overgrowth in dogs with chronic intestinal disease. J Vet Int Med 7:133,1993.
34. Welkos SL, Toskes PP, Baer H, et al. Importance of aerobic bacterial in the cobalamin malabsorption of the experimental blind loop syndrome. Gastroenterology 80:313–320, 1981.
35. Bernstein LH, Gutstein S, Efron G, et al. Experimental production of elevated serum folate in dogs with intestinal blind loops: Relationship of serum levels to location of the blind loop. Gastroenterology 63:815–819, 1972.
36. Bernstein LH, Gutstein S, Efron G, et al. Experimental production of elevated serum folate in dogs with intestinal blind loops. II. Nature of bacterially produced folate coenzymes in blind loop fluid. Am J Clin Nutr 28:925–929, 1975
37. Klipstein FA, Schenk EA. Enterotoxigenic intestinal bacteria in tropic sprue. II. Effect of the bacteria and their enterotoxins on intestinal structure. Gastroenterology. 68:642–655, 1975
38. Lichtman SN, Sartor RB, Keku J, et al. Hepatic inflammation in rats with experimental small intestinal bacterial overgrowth. Gastroenterology. 98:414–421, 1990.
39. Nolan JP. Intestinal endotoxins as mediators of hepatic injury—an idea whose time has come again. Hepatology 10:887–891, 1989.
40. Sherman P, Wesley A, Forstner G. Sequential disaccharidase loss in rat intestinal blind loops: Impacts of malnutrition. Am J Physiol 248:G26–G632, 1985.
41. Batt RM, McLean L. Comparison of the biochemical changes in the jejunal mucosa of dogs with aerobic and anaerobic bacterial overgrowth. Gastroenterology. 93:986–993, 1987.
42. Kim YS, Spritz N. Metabolism of hydroxy fatty acids in dogs with steatorrhea secondary to experimentally produced intestinal blind loops. J Lipid Res 9:487–491, 1968.
43. Abrams GD. Microbial effects on mucosal structure and function. Am J Clin Nutr 30:1880–1886, 1977.
44. Batt RM, McLean L, Riley JE. Response of the jejunal mucosa of dogs with aerobic and anaerobic bacterial overgrowth to antibiotic therapy. Gut 29:473–482, 1988.
45. Rutgers HC, Batt RM, Kelly DF. Lymphocytic-plasmacytic enteritis associated with bacterial overgrowth in a dog. J Am Vet Med Assoc 192:1739–1742, 1988.
46. Banwell JG, Kistler LA, Giannella RA, et al. Small intestinal bacterial overgrowth syndrome. Gastroenterology 80:834–845, 1981.
47. Toskes PP, Giannella RA, Jervis, HR, et al. Small intestinal mucosal injury in the experimental blind loop syndrome. Light and electron-microscopic and histochemical studies. Gastroenterology 68:1193–1203, 1975.
48. Batt RM, Hall EJ. Chronic enteropathies in the dog. J Sm Anim. Pract 30:3–12, 1989.
49. Sherman P, Forstner J, Roomi N, et al. Mucin depletion in the intestine of malnourished rats. Am J Physiol 248:G418–G423, 1985.
50. Prizont R, Whitehead JS, Kim YS. short chain fatty acids in rats with jejunal blind loops. I. Analysis of SCFA in small intestine, cecum, feces, and plasma. Gastroenterology. 69:1254–1264, 1975.
51. Ammon HV, Phillips SF. Inhibition of ileal water absorption by intraluminal fatty acids. Influence of chain length, hydroxylation and conjugation of fatty acids. J Clin Invest 53:205–210, 1974.
52. Lamabadusuriya SP, Guiraldes E, Harries JT. Influence of mixtures of taurocholate, fatty acids, and monolein on the toxic effects of deoxycholate in rat jejunum in vivo. Gastroenterology 69:463–469, 1975.
53. Cline WS, Lorenzon V, Benz L, el al. The effects of sodium ricinoleate on small intestinal function and structure. J Clin Invest 53:380–390, 1976.
54. Stewart JJ, Bass P. Effects of ricinoleic and oleic acids on the digestive contractile activity of the canine small and large bowel. Gastroenterology 70:371–376, 1976.
55. Gaginella TS, Stewart JJ, Gullikson GW, el al. Inhibition of small intestinal mucosal and smooth muscle cell function by ricinoleic acid and other surfactants. Life Sic 16:1595–1606, 1975.
56. King CE, Toskes PP. Protein-losing enteropathy in the human and experimental rat blind loop syndrome. Gastroenterology 80:504–509, 1981.
57. Davenport DJ, Ludlow CL, Hunt J, et al Effect of sampling method on quantitative duodenal cultures in dogs: Endoscopy vs. permucosal aspiration. J Vet Int Med 8:152, 1994.
58. Batt RM, Morgan JO. Role of serum folate and vitamin B_{12} concentrations in the differentiation of small intestinal abnormalities in the dog. Res Vet Sci 32:17–22, 1982.
59. Bolt, MJG, Stellaard F, Paumgartner G. Serum unconjugated bile acids in patients with small bowel bacterial overgrowth. Clin Chim Acta 181:87–102, 1989.
60. Burrows CF, Jezyk PF. Nitrosonaphthol test for screening of small intestinal diarrheal disease in the dog. J Am Vet Med Assoc 183:318–322,
61. Dill-Macky E, Williams DA. Breath[14]CO_2 output following oral administration of ^{14}C-D-xylose to healthy dogs. J Vet Int Med 3:132, 1989.
62. Washabau RJ, Strombeck DR, Buffington CA, et al. Use of pulmonary hydrogen gas excretion to detect carbohydrate malabsorption in dogs. J Am Vet Med Assoc 189:674–679, 1986.
63. Washabau RJ, Strombeck DR, Buffington CA, et al Evaluation of intestinal carbohydrate malabsorption in the dog by pulmonary hydrogen gas excretion. Am J Vet Res 47:1402–406, 1986.
64. Ludlow CL, Bruyette DS, Davenport DJ, et al. Relationship between breath hydrogen fraction and calculated breath hydrogen excretion in healthy dogs. J Vet Int Med 8:152, 1994.
65. Hall EJ, Batt RM. Differential sugar absorption for the assessment of canine intestinal permeability: the cellobiose/mannitol test in gluten-sensitive enteropathy of Irish setters. Res Vet Sci 51:83–87, 1991.
66. Batt RM, Rutgers HC. Unpublished observations.
67. Campbell CB, Cowan AE, Harper J. Duodenal bacterial flora and bile salt patterns in patients with gastrointestinal disease. Aust NZ J Med 3:339–348, 1973.
68. Setchell KDR, Harrison DL, Gilbert JM, et al. Serum unconjugated bile acids: Qualitatine and quantitative profiles in ileal resection and bacterial overgrowth. Clin Chim Acta 152:297–306, 1985.
69. Tangerman A, van Schaik A, van der Hoek E W. Analysis of conjugated and unconjugated bile acids in serum and jejunal fluid of normal subjects. Clin Chim Acta 159:123–132, 1986
70. Henriksson ÅEK Blomquist L, Nord C-E, et al. Small intestinal bacterial overgrowth in patients with rheumatoid arthritis. Ann Rheum Dis 52:503–510, 1993.
71. Salemans JMJI, Nagengast FM, Tangerman A, et al. Postprandial conjugated and unconjugated serum bile acid levels after proctocolectomy with ileal pouch-anal anastomosis. Scand J Gastroenterol 28:786–790, 1993
72. Einarsson K, Bergström M, Eklöf R, et al. Comparison of the proportion of unconjugated to total serum cholic acid and the [14C]-xylose breath test in parents with suspected small intestinal bacterial overgrowth. Scand J Clin Lab Invest 52:425–430, 1992.
73. Masclee A, Tangerman A, van Schaik A, et al. Unconjugated serum bile acid as a marker of small intestinal bacterial overgrowth. Eur J Clin Invest 19:384–389, 1989
74. Hall EJ. Gastrointestinal aspects of food allergy: A review. J Sm Anim Pract 35:145–152, 1994.
75. Hill FWG, Kelly DF. Naturally occurring intestinal malabsortion in the dog. Dig Dis 197:649–665, 1974.
76. Batt RM, Bush BM, Peters TJ. Subcellular biochemical studies of a naturally occurring enteropathy in the dog resembling chronic tropical sprue in human beings. Am J Vet Res 44:1492–1496, 1983.

77. Hoffbrand AV, Broitman SA. Effect of chronic nutritional iron deficiency on the small intestinal disaccharidase activities of growing dogs. Proc Soc Exp Biol Med 130:595–598,1969.

78. Symons LEA, Fairbarin D. Pathology, absorption, transport and activity of digestive enzymes in rat jejunum parasitized by the nematode, Nippostrongylus brasiliensis. Fed Proc 21:913–918, 1962.

79. Alpers DH, Seetharam B. Pathophysiology of diseases involving intestinal brush border proteins. N Engl J Med 296:1047–1050, 1977

80. Bond JH, Levitt MD. Quantitative measurement of lactose absorption. Gastroenterology 70:1058– 1062, 1976.

81. Mundt HC, Meyer H. Pathogenesis of lactose-induced diarrhea and its prevention by enzymatic splitting of lactoset. In: Burger, IH, Rivers JPW (eds) Nutrition of the Dog and Cat. Cambridge University Press, Cambridge, 267–274, 1989.

82. Traber MG, Sokol RJ, Burton GW, et al. Impaired ability of patients with familial isolated vitamin E deficiency to incorporate alpha-tocopherol into lipoproteins secreted by the liver. J Clin Invest 85:397–407, 1990.

83. Fyfe JC, Ramanujam KS, Ramaswamy K, et al. Defective brush-border expression of intrinsic factor-cobalamin receptor in canine inherited intestinal cobalamin malabsorption. J Biol Chem 266,(7):4489–4494 1991.

84. Gangl A Ockner RK. Intestinal metabolism of lipids and lipoproteins. Gastroenterology. 68:167–186, 1975.

85. Freind SCE, Barr SC, Embury D. Fucosidosis in an English Springer spaniel presenting as malabsorption syndrome. Aust Vet J 62:415–420, 1985.

86. Sarfeh LH, Aaronson S, Lombino D, et al. Selective impairment of nutrient absorption from intestines with chronic venous hypertension. Surgery 99:166–169, 1986.

87. Tams TR, Twedt DC. Canine protein-losing gastroenteropathy syndrome. Comp Cont Ed Prac Vet 3:105–114, 1981.

88. Finco DR, Duncan JR, Schall WD, et al. Chronic enteric disease and hypoproteinemia in 9 dogs. J Am Vet Med Assoc 163 (3):262–271, 1973.

89. Mattheeuws D, De Rick A, Thoonen H, et al. Intestinal lymphangiectasia in a dog. Small Anim Pract 15:757–761, 1974.

90. Waldmann TA. Protein-losing gastroenteropathies. In: Bockus HL (ed) Gastroenterology. WB Saunders, Philadelphia, 1976.

91. Sherding RG. Canine intestinal lymphangiectasia. Proc ACVIM, 406–408, 1988.

92. Williams DA. Protein-losing enteropathy. Proc 11th Ann Vet Med Forum ACVIM, 425–428, 1993.

93. Katz J Rosenfeld S Sellers AL. Sites of plasma albumin catabolism in the rat. Am J Physiol 200:1301–1306, 1961.

94. Brasitus TA. Protein-losing gastroenteropathy. In: Sleisenger MH, Fordtran JS (eds) Gastrointestinal Disease: Pathophysiology/Diagnosis/Management. WB Saunders, Philadelphia, 1027–1035, 1993.

95. Van Kruiningen HJ, Lees GE, Hayden DW, et al. Lipogranulomatous lymphangitis in canine intestinal lymphangiectasia. Vet Pathol 21:377–383, 1984.

96. Fossum TW, Sherding RG, Zack PM, et al. Intestinal lymphangiectasia associated with chylothorax in two dogs. J Am Vet Med Assoc 190(1):61–64, 1987

97. Meschter CL, Rakich PM, Tyler DE. Intestinal lymphangiectasia with lipogranulomatous lymphangitis in a dog. J Am Vet Med Assoc 190,(4):427–430, 1987.

98. Fossum TW. Protein-losing enteropathy. Semin Vet Med Surg 4:219–225, 1989.

99. Kobayashi K. Asakura H, Shinozawa T, et al. Protein-losing enteropathy in systemic lupus erythematosus. Observations by magnifying endoscopy. Dig Dis Sci 34:1924–1928, 1989.

100. Bai JC, Sambuelli A, Sugai E, et al. Gluten challenge in patients with celiac disease: Evaluation of a₁-antitrypsin clearance. Am J Gastroenterol 86:312–316, 1991.

101. Tidball CS. The nature of the intestinal epithelial barrier. Am J Dig Dis 16:745–767, 1971.

102. Munor DR. Route of protein losing during a model protein-losing gastropathy in dogs. Gastroenterology 66:960–972, 1974.

103. Kondo M, Nakanishi K, Banba T, et al. Experimental protein-losing gastroenteropathy. Role of tissue plasminogen activator. Gastroenterology. 71:631–634, 1976.

104. Kaup FJ, Drommer W, Kersten U, et al. Ultrastrukturelle untersuchungen bei einem Fall von intestinaler Lymphangiektasie. Kleintierpraxis 33:81–86, 1988.

105. Flesjå K, Yri T. Protein-losing enteropathy in the Lundehund. J Sm Anim Pract 18:11–23, 1977.

106. Van Kruiningen HJ, Lees GE, Hayden: Lipoganulomatous lymphangitis in canine intestinal lymphangiectasia. Vet Pathol 21:377, 1984.

107. Burns MG. Intestinal lymphangiectasia in the dog: A case report and review. J Am Anim Hosp Assoc 18:97–105, 1982.

108. Bank S, Fisher G, Marks IN, et al. The lymphatics of the intestinal mucosa. A clinical and experimental study. Am J Dig Dis 12:619, 1967.

109. Danese CA, Georgulas-Penesis M, Kark A. Studies of the effects of blockage of intestinal lymphatics. Am J Gastroenterol 57:541–546, 1972.

110. Breitschwerdt EB, Halliwell WH, Foley CW, et al. A heredity diarrhetic syndrome in the Basenji characterized by malabsorption, protein-losing enteropathy, and hypergammaglobulinemia. J Am Anim Hosp Assoc 16:551–560, 1980.

111. Littman MP, Giger U. Familial protein-losing enteropathy (PLE) and/or protein-losing nephropathy (PLN) in soft-coated Wheaten terriers (SCWT). J Vet Int Med 4 (2):133, 1990

112. Nicolaidou K, Ladefoged K, Hylander E, et al. Endogenous faecal calcium in chronic malabsorption syndromes and in intestinal malabsorption. Scand J Gastroenterol 15:587–592, 1980.

113. Waldmann TA. Protein-losing enteropathy. Gastroenterology 50:422–433, 1966.

114. Barton CL, Smith C, Troy G, et al. The diagnosis and clinicopathology features of canine protein-losing enteropathy. J Am Anim Hosp Assoc 14:85–91, 1978.

115. Crossley JR, Elliott RB. Simple method for diagnosing protein-losing enteropathies. Br Med J 1:428–429, 1977.

116. Bernier JJ, Florent CH, Desmazures CH, et al. Diagnosis of protein-losing enteropathy by gastro-intestinal clearance of alpha₁-antitrypsin. Lancet 2:763–764, 1978.

117. Florent C, L'Hirondel C, et al. Intestinal clearance of a₁-antitrypsin: A sensitive method for the detection of protein-losing enteropathy. Gastroenterology 81:777–780, 1981.

118. Karbach U, Ewe Bodenstein H. Alpha₁-antitrypsin, a reliable endogenous marker for intestinal protein loss and its application in patients with Crohn's disease. Gut 24:718–723,1983.

119. Thomas DW, Sinatra FR, Merritt RJ. Random fecal alpha₁-antitrypsin concentration in children with gastrointestinal disease. Gastroenterology 80:776–782,1981.

120. Brouwer J, Smekens F. Determination of a₁-antitrypsin in fecal extracts by enzyme immunoassay. Clin Chim Acta 189:173–180,1990.

121. Williams DA. Evaluation of fecal alpha₁-protease inhibitor(a₁-PI) concentration as a test for canine protein-losing enteropathy (PLE). J Vet Int Med 5:133, 1991.

122. Melgarejo T, Asem EK, Williams DA. Enzyme-Linked immunoadsorbant assay for canine alpha 1-protease inhibitor(a₁-PI). J Vet Int Med 7:133, 1933.

123. Wilk P, Karipineni R, Dreiling DA, et al. Studies of the effects of blockage of intestinal lymphatics. Am J Gastroenterol 63:400–403, 1975.

124. Kalser MH. Medium chain triglycerides. Adv Intern Med 17:301–322, 1971.

125. Mine K, Matsubayashi S, Nakai Y, et al. Intestinal lymphangiectasia markedly improved with antiplasmin therapy. Gastroenterology 96:1596–1599, 1989.

126. Cohen SA, Diuguid DL, Whitlock RT, et al. Intestinal lymphangiectasia and antiplasmin therapy [letter]. Gastroenterology 102:2193, 1992.

127. Kondo M, Bamba T, Hosokawa K, et al. Tissue plasminogen activator in the pathogenesis of protein-losing gastroenteropathy. Gastroenterology 70:1045–1047, 1976.

128. Henry DA, O'Connell DL. Effect of fibrinolytic inhibitors on mortality from upper gastrointestinal haemorrhage. Br Med J 298:1142–1146, 1989.

129. Conlan MG, Haire WD, Burnett DA. Prothrombotic abnormalities in inflammatory bowel disease. Dig Dis Sci 34:1089–1093, 1989.

20

The Pancreas

DAVID A. WILLIAMS

INTRODUCTION

Secretion of digestive enzymes is the major, but not the only, function of the exocrine pancreas (Table 20–1).[1] Pancreatic juice also contains bicarbonate, which contributes to the neutralization of gastric acid,[2] colipase, which facilitates the action of pancreatic lipase,[3-6] and factors necessary for the absorption of cobalamin (vitamin B_{12})[7-11] and zinc.[12,13] Pancreatic secretions inhibit bacterial proliferation in the proximal small intestine, contribute to the normal degradation of exposed brush border enzymes,[14-17] and, together with biliary secretions, exert a trophic effect on the mucosa.[14,17-20] Finally, the pancreas protects itself against autodigestion by several mechanisms, including the synthesis of a specific enzyme inhibitor that is stored and secreted together with the digestive enzymes.[21-23]

ANATOMY

The pancreas of dogs and cats consists primarily of right and left lobes with a small central body where the lobes join together (Figure 20–1).[24,25] It develops from ventral and dorsal budlike primordia that arise from the embryonic small intestine, and therefore represents an extension of the glandular mucosa of the duodenum, to which it remains connected by secretory ducts.[25] Because either the dorsal or ventral primordium or their associated ducts may involute during development, there is marked species, and to a lesser extent individual, variation in the origin of the gland and the pattern of its duct system.[24,25] Although the areas of pancreas derived from the two primordia resemble one another histologically, that tissue derived from the ventral pancreatic bud, which contributes primarily to the right lobe, contains most of the pancreatic polypeptide-producing cells. In contrast, glucagon-secreting cells predominate in the tissue that develops from the dorsal bud, which contributes primarily to the left lobe.[26,27]

In the dog, both primordia usually persist and fuse, and the two original ducts are retained. The duct of the ventral primordium is the pancreatic duct (Wirsung's duct) and opens adjacent to the bile duct on the major duodenal papilla. The duct of the dorsal primordium is the accessory pancreatic duct (Santorini's duct) and opens on the minor duodenal papilla a few centimeters distal to the major duodenal papilla.

These two duct systems usually intercommunicate within the gland.[24] In some dogs only the accessory pancreatic duct (the larger of the two) is present, and all pancreatic juice enters the duodenum through the minor duodenal papilla.[24,25] In the majority of cats only the duct of the ventral primordium, the pancreatic duct, persists, and it fuses with the bile duct before opening on the major duodenal papilla.[25,28] However, in approximately 20% of cats the accessory pancreatic duct is also present.[25]

The color of the pancreas varies from pale pink to dark red depending on the amount of blood it contains; it is particularly dark in color following a meal.[1,25] Anatomically the pancreas is closely associated with the stomach, liver, and duodenum (Figure 20–1). The body lies in the bend of the cranial part of the duodenum where it is crossed dorsally by the portal vein on its way to the liver.[25] The right lobe lies in the mesoduodenum and accompanies the descending duodenum, in some cases extending to the cecum. The left lobe lies in the deep wall of the greater omentum and accompanies the pyloric part of the stomach to the left where it also makes contact with the liver, transverse colon, and sometimes the left kidney and spleen. Additional accessory pancreatic tissue may be present sporadically in some individuals.[24,25]

Each pancreatic lobule is composed primarily of cells that synthesize the digestive enzymes and store them in zymogen granules (acinar cells), and a smaller number of cells that make up the branching duct system (intralobular, interlobular, and main pancreatic ducts).[29,30] The cells comprising the initial part of the intralobular, or intercalated, ducts are termed centroacinar cells where they line the tubular segments of the gland into which acinar cells secrete.[31] These centroacinar cells are the major site of pancreatic bicarbonate and fluid secretion.[2] The pancreas also contains endocrine tissue, the islets of Langer-

Table 20–1

FUNCTIONS OF THE EXOCRINE PANCREAS

Secretion of digestive enzymes
Secretion of colipase
Secretion of bicarbonate
Facilitation of cobalamin and zinc absorption
Secretion of antibacterial factors
Modulation of intestinal mucosal function
Protection against autodigestion

381

382 • The Pancreas

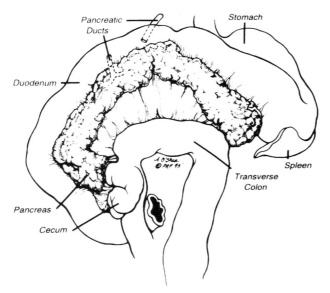

FIGURE 20–1. Anatomical associations of the canine pancreas.

hans, but this accounts for only 1% to 2% of the gland, whereas the exocrine tissue together with associated vessels and nerves accounts for more than 98% of the pancreatic mass.[27]

The pancreas is well supplied with blood by branches of the celiac and cranial mesenteric arteries.[24] The main vessels to the right lobe are the cranial and caudal pancreaticoduodenal arteries that anastomose within the gland and arise from the celiac and cranial mesenteric arteries respectively. The left lobe is supplied predominantly by the pancreatic branch of the splenic artery arising from the celiac artery. Small branches from the common hepatic and gastroduodenal arteries as well as direct branches from the celiac artery may also supply portions of the gland. Satellite veins corresponding to the caudal and cranial pancreaticoduodenal arteries, and other veins terminating in the splenic vein, drain the right and left lobes, respectively, and enter the portal vein leading to the liver.[24]

Morphologic studies have demonstrated that in many species, including dogs and cats, an islet-acinar portal system communicates between the endocrine islet tissue and the exocrine acinar tissue.[26,27,32] Pancreatic intralobular arteries give branches that divide to form capillary glomeruli within the islets. Numerous efferent vessels, insuloacinar portal vessels, emerge from the glomeruli and enter the surrounding exocrine tissue capillary beds, from which vessels emerge and coalesce into venules. It is believed that essentially all of the blood leaving the islets goes into acinar capillaries before leaving the pancreas, and that the acinar cells, particularly those surrounding the islets, are therefore exposed to high concentrations of islet hormones. This is thought to be an important mechanism by which insulin, and perhaps other peptides, may exert a regulatory role on the exocrine pancreas.[27]

Although the pancreas is not supplied by well-defined extrinsic nerves, it is richly supplied with myelinated and unmyelinated nerve fibers, and nerve trunks and intrapancreatic ganglia are often scattered throughout the tissue.[33] These neurons are either derived from the vagus and splanchnic nerves and reach the organ by following branches of the celiac and cranial mesenteric arteries, or are intrinsic to the gland. In addition to the traditional cholinergic (parasympathetic) and adrenergic (sympathetic) transmitters,

it is apparent that serotonin, dopamine, and a variety of regulatory peptides including vasoactive intestinal polypeptide (VIP), gastrin-releasing peptide (GRP), substance P, neuropeptide Y, and enkephalin-related peptides are also present in these nerve fibers and play a role in the regulation of pancreatic function.[33]

BIOCHEMISTRY AND PHYSIOLOGY

Digestive Enzymes

The acinar cells secrete a fluid rich in enzymes that degrades proteins, lipids, and polysaccharides (Table 20–2).[23] Trypsins, chymotrypsins, and elastases are endopeptidases that cleave peptide bonds at specific sites within polypeptide chains; the carboxypeptidases are exopeptidases that cleave specific carboxyl-terminal residues.[23] Alpha-amylase hydrolyzes 4-glycosidic bonds in starches, phospholipase A_2 hydrolyzes fatty acid esters at the 2-position of some membrane phospholipids, and lipase, in the presence of the coenzyme colipase, hydrolyzes ester bonds in the 1 and 3 positions of triglycerides.[23]

This protein-rich secretion is diluted and carried along the duct system by the profuse, watery, bicarbonate-rich secretion of the centroacinar and duct cells.[2] Although this bicarbonate contributes to the neutralization of gastric acid emptied into the duodenum, it is probably not indispensable for the maintenance of a neutral pH. Secretion of bicarbonate and absorption of hydrogen ions by the intestinal mucosa itself provide the duodenum with a tremendous capacity to dispose of acid to which it is exposed, even in the absence of alkaline biliary and pancreatic secretions.[34,35]

Defenses Against Autodigestion

Several mechanisms exist that discourage autodigestion of the pancreas by the enzymes it secretes.[20,23] Firstly, proteolytic and phospholipolytic enzymes are synthesized, stored, and secreted by the pancreas in the form of catalytically inactive zymogens (indicated by the addition of the prefix *pro-* or the suffix *-ogen* to the enzymes name (Table 20–2). These zymogens are activated by enzymatic cleavage of a small peptide, the activation peptide, from the amino terminal of the polypeptide chain (Figure 20–2).[23] Enzymes from several sources, including some lysosomal proteases, are capable of

Table 20–2

MAJOR SECRETORY PROTEINS OF THE EXOCRINE PANCREAS OF THE DOG

Enzymes secreted as inactive zymogens
  Trypsinogens [1 (anionic), 2 and 3 (cationic)]   trypsins
  Chymotrypsinogens (1, 2, and 3)   chymotrypsins
  Proelastases (1 and 2)   elastases
  Procarboxypeptidases (A_1, A_2, A_3, and B)   carboxypeptidases
  Prophospholipase A_2 phospholipase A_2
Coenzyme
  Procolipase   colipase
Enzymes
  Alpha-amylase
  Lipase
Inhibitor
  Pancreatic secretory trypsin inhibitor

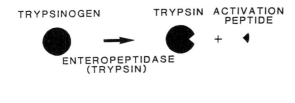

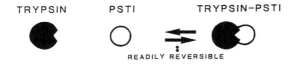

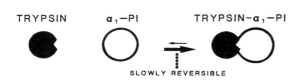

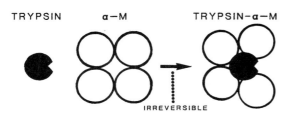

FIGURE 20-2. Diagrammatic representations of zymogen activation (trypsinogen) and the binding of proteases (trypsin) by major inhibitors. PSII = pancreatic secretory inhibitor, α_1 = alpha$_1$, and α–M = alpha-macroglobulin. (From Williams DA: Exocrine pancreatic disease. *In* Ettinger SJ, Feldman EC: Textbook of Veterinary Internal Medicine. 4th ed. Philadelphia, WB Saunders Company, 1995, p. 1373.)

activating pancreatic zymogens, but ordinarily activation of zymogens does not occur until they are secreted into the small intestine. The enzyme enteropeptidase (enterokinase), which is synthesized by the enterocytes lining the duodenal mucosa, is particularly effective at cleaving the activation peptides from trypsinogens to form trypsins. Active trypsins subsequently cleave the activation peptides from other digestive zymogens (Figure 20–3). Enteropeptidase therefore plays a crucial role in the activation of digestive enzymes.[23]

Secondly, from the moment synthesis of digestive enzymes begins, they are segregated, along with potentially damaging lysosomal enzymes, into the lumen of the rough endoplasmic reticulum.[36] This is part of the cisternal space of the acinar cell, a compartment separate from the cell cytosol, which contains other enzymes with the potential to activate the zymogens. Biochemical studies have demonstrated that this segregation is due to the presence of a transient peptide extension on the amino terminal of the enzymes as they are translated from mRNA on the ribosomes. This extension, the signal sequence or signal peptide, serves only to route the protein being synthesized into the cisternal space, and its presence is indicated by the addition of the prefix *pre-* to the name of the enzyme of zymogen (e.g., preamylase, prepro-

elastase, pretrypsinogen).[37] The signal peptide is removed by the action of a signal peptidase located on the inside surface of lumen of the rough endoplasmic reticulum while the remainder of the peptide is being synthesized, so complete polypeptide chains representing the enzyme or zymogen with its signal peptide extension, such as preamylase, never actually exist in vivo.[37] Segregation of enzymes in the cisternal space is continued as they are processed through the Golgi apparatus, where lysosomal enzymes are selectively routed to lysosomes, and digestive enzymes are incorporated into condensing vacuoles and ultimately zymogen granules, in which they are stored prior to secretion (Figure 20–4).[36]

Finally, the acinar cells contain a specific trypsin inhibitor that is synthesized, segregated, stored, and secreted along with the digestive enzymes.[21-23] This low molecular weight pancreatic secretory trypsin inhibitor (PSTI) is distinct from the much larger plasma protease inhibitors (Table 20–3). It is believed that PSTI immediately inhibits any trypsin activity produced should there be activation of trace amounts of trypsinogen within the acinar cell of duct system, and therefore blocks further intrapancreatic activation of the digestive enzymes (Figure 20–2).[23]

Regulation of Pancreatic Secretion

The exocrine pancreas secretes juice into the duodenum both in the absence of food (basal or interdigestive secretion) and in response to a meal. The basal rate secretion in dogs is about 2% (bicarbonate) or 10% (enzymes) of the maximal secretory rate in response to a meal,[2] but increases transiently in association with the cyclic interdigestive contractile activity of the upper gastrointestinal tract.[38,39] The response following feeding is biphasic: an initial phase that peaks at 1 to 2 hours and is rich in enzymes, and a second more voluminous phase that peaks at 8 to 11 hours and is rich in bicarbonate.[2,39]

Pancreatic secretion related to feeding occurs as a response cephalic stimulation, such as the anticipation and smell of food, as well as gastric and intestinal stimulation due to the presence of food in the stomach and small intestine.[38,39] The response to these stimuli is mediated by a complex interplay of excitatory and inhibitory nervous and hormonal mechanisms; in dogs and cats the endocrine mechanisms are probably of particular importance.[39] Secretin and cholecystokinin, released into the blood from the proximal small intestine when acid and partly digested food are emptied from the stomach into the duodenum, stimulate the secretion of bicarbonate-rich and enzyme-rich components of pancreatic juice, respectively.[2,38,39]

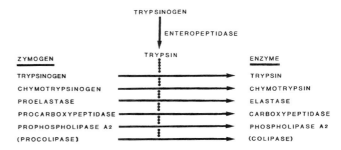

FIGURE 20-3. Activation of pancreatic proteases and phospholipase. (From Williams DA: Exocrine pancreatic disease. *In* Ettinger SJ, Feldman EC: Textbook of Veterinary Internal Medicine. 4th ed. Philadelphia, WB Saunders Company, 195, p. 1373.)

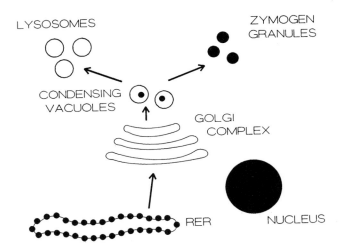

FIGURE 20-4. Normal intracellular routing of digestive and lysosomal enzymes by the pancreatic acinar cell. (From Williams DA: Exocrine pancreatic disease. *In* Ettinger SJ, Feldman EC: Textbook of Veterinary Internal Medicine. 4th ed. Philadelphia, WB Saunders Company, 1995, p. 1374.)

Pancreatic Enzymes in the Blood

Amylase, lipase, and the zymogens of pancreatic proteases and phospholipase A_2 are present at low concentrations in the plasma of normal healthy animals. These pancreatic proteins are believed to leak directly from the gland into the bloodstream, from which they are cleared by glomerular filtration, with subsequent variable degradation by renal tubular epithelial cells.[40-42] Detectable amounts of intact pancreatic digestive enzyme are not absorbed from the intestinal lumen, and reports of a significant "enteropancreatic" circulation of these enzymes are now discounted.[43] If there was such a circulation then pancreatic proteases would be present in blood in active forms, whereas only inactive zymogens are detectable in serum from normal mammals.[40-42,44,45]

Clinical Synopsis

Diagnostic Features

- Acute onset of anorexia, depression, vomiting
- Abdominal pain, abdominal mass, fever, dehydration, and dyspnea may be present
- Coagulopathy, pulmonary edema, cardiac arrhythmias, and shock are poor prognostic signs
- Serum amylase, lipase, and trypsin-like immunoreactivity are often, but not always, increased
- Increased serum amylase and lipase are not specific markers for pancreatitis
- Liver enzyme activities and bilirubin may be markedly increased
- Ultrasound is useful for confirming the diagnosis

Standard Treatment

- Withhold oral food and water for 3 to 5 days
- Maintain normal fluid and electrolyte balance
- Plasma transfusion can be life-saving in critical patients
- Correct any drug or toxin exposure that may have precipitated disease
- Antibiotic therapy (trimethoprim-sulpha, fluquinolone) often given, but infection rarely present
- Surgical intervention rarely helpful
- Gradually reintroduce a low-fat moderate protein content diet
- Avoid high fat content diets and obesity

Follow-up

- Complete recovery is possible
- Feed low-fat diet to patients with recurrent disease

PANCREATITIS

Inflammatory disease of the human pancreas is usually divided into acute and chronic types based on a combination of clinical and pathologic criteria that may be loosely applied to cats and dogs (Table 20-4).[46-48] Acute pancreatitis (Table 20-5) may be defined as inflammation of the pancreas with a sudden onset. Recurrent acute disease refers to repeated bouts of inflammation with little or no permanent pathologic changes. Chronic pancreatitis is a continuing inflammatory disease characterized by irreversible morphologic change and possibly leading to permanent impairment of function. Both acute and chronic pancreatitis may be further subdivided based on the etiology, if known, and the degree of severity. Diagnostic limitations often preclude the strict application of these criteria in veterinary medicine, and the true prevalence of each is not known, but acute and recurrent acute disease are more commonly diagnosed than chronic pancreatitis.

Complications of both types may include pseudocyst (a collection of sterile pancreatic juice enclosed by fibrous or granulation tissue), abscess (a circumscribed collection of pus containing little or no pancreatic necrosis, from which bacteria can usually be cultured), or infected necrosis.[48] Use of these clearly defined terms renders older ambiguous terms such as *phlegmon* or *infected pseudocyst* redundant, and their use is discouraged.[48] Acquisition of knowledge about naturally occurring pancreatitis in dogs and cats has been hindered by the lack of specific laboratory tests, the inaccessibility of the gland, and reluctance to biopsy pancreatic tissue. When examined at exploratory laparotomy or necropsy, affected pancreas is often edematous, swollen, and soft, and there may be fibrinous adhesions to adjacent organs.[28] Acute fluid collections (often bloodstained and containing fat droplets, but lacking a wall of granulation or fibrous tissue) may be seen in or near the pancreas or throughout the peritoneal cavity, particularly in cats. Severely affected areas of pancreas may be liquified, secondary infection with enteric organisms may produce abscesses or infected necrosis, and pseudocysts may form.[28,49,50] Hemorrhages may be present in the omentum and in the pancreas, and there are often chalky areas of fat necrosis both adjacent to the pancreas and also in fat as far away as the anterior mediastinum. Histologically there is extensive multifocal infiltration by neutrophils, and varying degrees of hemorrhage, necrosis, edema, and vessel thrombosis.[28]

If an initial acute episode is not fatal, there may be complete resolution, or alternatively the inflammatory process

Table 20–3

MAJOR PROTEASE INHIBITORS IN CANINE PANCREAS AND PLASMA			
INHIBITOR	PANCREATIC SECRETORY TRYPSIN INHIBITOR (PSTI)	α_1-PROTEASE INHIBITOR (α_1-ANTITRYPSIN) (α_1-PI)	α-MACROGLOBULINS (α-M_1 AND α-M_2)
Principal locations	Pancreas, pancreatic juice	Plasma, intercellular space	Plasma
Approximate molecular weight	6000	58,000	750,000
Specificity	Trypsin only	Broad spectrum (serine proteases)	Broad spectrum (serine and other proteases)
Inhibition	Temporary (slowly degraded by trypsin)	Transient (transfers enzyme to α-M)	Irreversible (permanent trap for captured enzyme)
Function	Inhibits intrapancreatic autoactivation of trypsin	Readily diffusible inhibitor present in the intercellular space	Traps proteases prior to removal by monocyte-macrophage system

may smolder continuously and asymptomatically. Extensive destruction of pancreatic tissue may reduce the gland to a few distorted lobules adjacent to where the ducts enter the duodenum (Figure 20–5).[28]

Although reports have described acute necrotizing pancreatitis in cats similar to that seen in dogs[51,52] as well as a histologically distinct suppurative form,[51] chronic mild interstitial pancreatitis characterized by inflammation of interstitial tissue apparently spreading from the ducts is the type of pancreatic inflammation most commonly reported in cats.[28,53,54] This latter type of pancreatitis is often accompanied by cholangiohepatitis, and sometimes by interstitial nephritis, either of which may be of greater clinical significance than the pancreatitis.

PATHOPHYSIOLOGY

Numerous experimental procedures lead to the development of pancreatitis (Table 20–5), but these models often cause extremely severe pancreatitis, and their relevance to spontaneous disease is unknown.[55] Alternative models based on dietary manipulation or hyperstimulation of the pancreas have recently been developed. These newer models induce a mild to moderate inflammation that probably corresponds

Table 20–4

A CLASSIFICATION OF PANCREATITIS

Acute
  Etiology: various
  Severity: mild
    no multisystem failure
    uncomplicated recovery
  Severity: severe
    multisystem failure
    complication (e.g., pseudocyst, abscess)
Chronic
  Etiology: various
  Severity: mild
    minimal morphologic change
    subclinical loss of exocrine or exocrine function
  Severity: severe
    severe morphologic damage
    clinical exocrine pancreatic insufficiency or diabetes mellitus

more closely to the natural disease, and information obtained from these models has shed new light on the pathophysiology of pancreatitis.[56–59]

It is generally believed that pancreatitis develops when there is activation of digestive enzymes within the gland with resultant pancreatic autodigestion. The site of initiation of enzyme activation has been assumed to be the intercellular space or duct system, but recent studies of both diet-induced and hyperstimulation-induced pancreatitis have indicated a potential common acinar intracellular basis for abnormal zymogen activation.[55,56,60] Using these models it has been shown that prior to the development of overt pancreatitis abnormal fusion of lysosomes and zymogen granules occurs, probably due to failure of normal secretory processes (Figure 20–6).[56] It is known that lysosomal proteases, such as cathepsin B, are capable of activating trypsinogen,[55,61] and that the trypsin inhibitor present in zymogen granules is ineffective at the acid pH present in lysosomes.[23,62] Failure of the normal subcellular mechanism for effective segregation of zymogens and lysosomal proteases may well explain development or progression of spontaneous and experimental pancreatitis due to a variety of otherwise dissimilar causes.[23,55,61,62]

Whatever the underlying mechanism by which enzyme activation is initiated, unopposed free radicals may be important in the progression of pancreatitis.[63] These radicals can damage cell membranes directly by peroxidation of lipids within the membrane. Under normal circumstances, the small amounts of free radicals that form in all cells are detoxified by scavenger enzymes such as superoxide dismutase and catalase. Under some pathologic conditions the capacity of the defense mechanisms is exceeded and tissue injury ensues. An important aspect of this injury is thought to be increased capillary permeability due to endothelial cell membrane damage, with resultant pancreatic edema.[64] Similar changes in duct cell permeability may also trigger other pathophysiologic mechanisms and thereby exacerbate pancreatitis.[58] Perfusion of the pancreas with free radical scavengers ameliorated the severity of pancreatitis induced by experimental ischemia, duct obstruction, and free fatty acid infusion in a canine model.[63–68]

Once intracellular and intraductal activation of trypsinogens to trypsins takes place, further activation of all zymogens, particularly proelastase and prophospholipase, will amplify pancreatic damage. Experimental and clinical studies indicate that activation of progressively larger amounts of protease and phospholipase within the gland is associated with transforma-

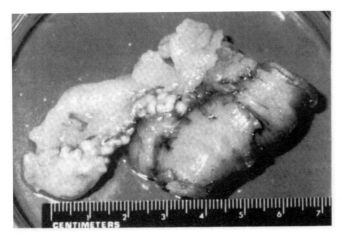

FIGURE 20-5. Chronic pancreatitis observed at necropsy of an old dog with a history of several bouts of severe acute pancreatitis. Acinar cells were restricted to a few residual nodular areas of relatively normal-looking tissue. The pancreatic pathology was not associated with any clinical signs at the time of euthanasia, although the serum concentration of trypsin-like immunoreactivity was subnormal. (From Williams DA: Exocrine pancreatic insufficiency. Waltham Int. Focus 2:9, 1992.)

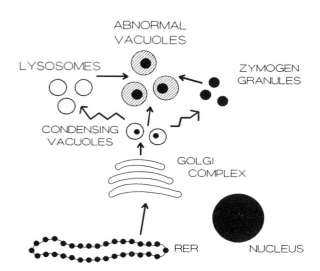

FIGURE 20-6. Abnormal intracellular routing of digestive enzymes destined for secretion results in mixing of zymogens and lysosomal proteases in abnormal intracellular vacuoles. Subsequent activation of zymogens by lysosomal proteases is currently considered to initiate development of pancreatitis. (From Williams DA: Exocrine pancreatic disease. *In* Ettinger SJ, Feldman EC: Textbook of Veterinary Internal Medicine. 4th ed. Philadelphia, WB Saunders Company, 1995, p. 1375.)

tion of mild edematous pancreatic inflammation to hemorrhagic or necrotic pancreatitis with multisystem involvement and consumption of plasma protease inhibitors (Figure 20–7 and Table 20–6)[69–86]

The plasma protease inhibitors alpha-macroglobulins and alpha₁-protease inhibitor (Table 20–3 and Figure 20–2) are vital in protecting against the otherwise fatal effects of proteolytic enzymes in the vascular space.[22,74,80–83] Alpha-macroglobulins are particularly important in this regard. Dogs tolerate intravenous injection of trypsin or chymotrypsin without showing adverse effects providing that free alpha-macroglobulins are available to bind the active proteases. Once alpha-macroglobulins are no longer available, however, dogs die rapidly from acute disseminated intravascular coagulation and shock as the free proteases activate the kinin, coagulation, fibrinolytic, and complement cascade systems (Figure 20–7).[74,80,81]

Binding of proteases by alpha-macroglobulin results in a change in conformation that allows the complex to be recognized and rapidly cleared from the plasma by the monocyte-macrophage system.[80,87] This removal is important because alpha-macroglobulin-bound proteases retain catalytic activity, particularly against low molecular weight substrates (Figure 20–2);[23,80] normal functioning of the monocyte-macrophage system is an important factor determining survival in experimental pancreatitis.[88,89]

Table 20–5

EXPERIMENTAL MODELS OF PANCREATITIS

Pancreatic duct obstruction
Intraductal bile injection
Intraductal enzyme injection
Intraductal fatty acid injection
Duodenal reflux (closed duodenal loop)
Pancreatic ischemia
Diet induced (ethionine supplemented, choline deficient)
Hyperstimulation induced (cholecystokinin, caerulein,
    carbamylcholine, scorpion venom)
Endotoxin injection (intravenous)

In experimental studies 80% of plasma alpha₁-protease inhibitor is still available to bind proteases when alpha-macroglobulins are saturated with trypsin, but the available alpha₁-protease inhibitor is not life saving.[74] The primary function of alpha₁-protease inhibitor is to inhibit neutrophil elastase during inflammation.[90] Although pancreatic proteases do bind to alpha₁-protease inhibitor and are effectively inhibited, the binding is reversible (Figure. 20–2).[74] In pancreatitis alpha₁-protease inhibitor probably serves as a transient inhibitor and an intermediary in the transport of protease to the protective alpha-macroglobulins, particularly in the extravascular spaces into which large alpha-macroglobulin molecules cannot permeate.[80]

ETIOLOGY

The inciting cause of spontaneous canine and feline pancreatitis is usually unknown. It has been suggested that dogs older than 7 years of age and neutered dogs, as well as terrier breeds, may be at increased risk, but the evidence for this is inconclusive because many cases in that study lacked a definitive diagnosis of pancreatitis.[91] Based on causes documented in human patients, experimental studies, and clinical observations the following potential factors should be considered.[20,60,91–93]

Nutrition/Hyperlipoproteinemia

The exocrine pancreas is highly responsive to changes in nutritional substrates present in the diet, and it has been reported that pancreatitis is more prevalent in obese animals.[94–98] There is evidence that low-protein high-fat diets induce pancreatitis and that pancreatitis is more severe when induced in dogs being fed a high-fat diet, and less severe when induced in lean dogs.[60,94–98] Malnutrition has also been

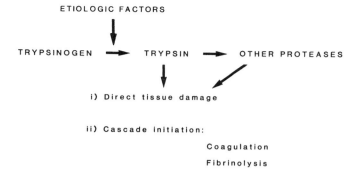

ETIOLOGIC FACTORS

TRYPSINOGEN ⟶ TRYPSIN ⟶ OTHER PROTEASES

i) Direct tissue damage

ii) Cascade initiation:

Coagulation

Fibrinolysis

Complement

Kallikrein-kinin

FIGURE 20-7. Local and systemic effects of trypsin in pancreatitis. (From Williams DA: Exocrine pancreatic disease. *In* Ettinger SJ, Feldman EC: Textbook of Veterinary Internal Medicine. 4th ed. Philadelphia, WB Saunders Company, 1995, p. 1376.)

reported to cause pancreatic inflammation and atrophy in human patients, and pancreatitis has been observed after refeeding following a prolonged fast, particularly in extremely malnourished individuals.[68] Supplementation of the diet with the amino acid analogue ethionine induces pancreatitis in several species, including dogs and cats.[99–102]

Hyperlipoproteinemia, often grossly apparent, is common in dogs with acute pancreatitis, and may develop secondary to pancreatitis as a result of abdominal fat necrosis, or may be a cause of the disease.[103] Some familial hyperlipoproteinemias of human beings are associated with frequent episodes of pancreatitis that respond to control of serum triglyceride levels,[68,104] and the clinical impression of a high prevalence of pancreatitis in the miniature schnauzer dog in the United States may be related to underlying idiopathic hyperlipoproteinemia.[103,105] There is also anecdotal evidence that pancreatitis in dogs often develops following a fatty meal.[20] It is not known why hyperlipidemia might cause pancreatitis, but it has been suggested that toxic fatty acids are generated within the pancreas by the action of lipase on abnormally high concentrations of triglycerides in pancreatic capillaries.[68,104,106,107]

Table 20-6

THE ROLE OF ENZYMES IN THE PATHOPHYSIOLOGY OF PANCREATITIS

ENZYME	PATHOPHYSIOLOGIC ACTION
Trypsin	Activation of other proteases; coagulation and fibrinolysis (disseminated intravascular coagulation)
Phospholipase A_2	Hydrolysis of cell membrane phospholipids; pulmonary surfactant degradation; demyelination (cell necrosis and liberation of toxic substances such as myocardial depressant factor; respiratory distress; neurologic signs: pancreatic encephalopathy)
Elastase	Degradation of elastin in blood vessel walls (hemorrhage, edema, respiratory distress)
Chymotrypsin	Activation of xanthine oxidase and subsequent generation of oxygen-derived free radicals (membrane damage)
Kallikrein	Kinin generation from kininogens
Kinins	Vasodilation, pancreatic edema (hypotension, shock)
Complement	Cell membrane damage, aggregation of leucocytes (local inflammation)
Lipase	Fat hydrolysis (local fat necrosis, hypocalcemia)

Drugs/Toxins/Hypercalcemia

A number of drugs may cause pancreatitis, although absolute proof of a causal relationship is often unavailable. Suspect drugs commonly used in veterinary medicine include thiazide diuretics, furosemide, azathioprine, L-asparaginase, sulfonamides, and tetracycline.[68,108–112] Corticosteroids have also been implicated, but considerable controversy exists about the supposed association of pancreatitis with the use of these drugs. High doses of glucocorticoids in association with spinal trauma (intervertebral disc disease and surgery) do seem to predispose to pancreatitis.[113] Corticosteroids may affect the pancreas in several ways including sensitization of the pancreas to cholecystokinin-mediated stimulation,[114] promotion of pancreatic duct hyperplasia,[115] and inhibition of clearance of enzyme-alpha-macroglobulin complexes by the monocyte-macrophage system.[20] However, the evidence that steroids alone induce pancreatitis is weak.[108] It is probably wise to discontinue use of these drugs in patients with pancreatitis.

Administration of cholinesterase inhibitor insecticides and cholinergic agonists has been associated with the development of pancreatitis, probably by causing hyperstimulation of the gland.[51,116–123] Scorpion stings are frequent causes of pancreatitis in human beings in Trinidad, and experimental administration of scorpion venom to dogs also elicits pancreatitis via a hyperstimulation-type mechanism.[92,116] Hyperstimulation may also explain the possible association of pancreatitis with hypercalcemia due to hyperparathyroidism and other causes.[60,92,124–129]

Duct Obstruction

Experimental obstruction of the pancreatic ducts produces only minimal inflammation unless the gland is simultaneously stimulated to secrete. The pathology following duct obstruction is characterized by pancreatic edema, chronic inflammation, atrophy, and fibrosis in most species, a notable exception being the opossum, which develops a severe hemorrhagic pancreatitis.[56,92] Clinical conditions that may lead to partial or complete obstruction of the pancreatic ducts include biliary calculi, sphincter spasm, edema of the duct or duodenal wall, tumor, parasites, trauma, and surgical interference.[92,130] Biliary calculi are a major cause of pancreatitis in humans, but this has not been reported in dogs and cats, presumably because of the low prevalence of gallstones in these species, and in dogs, the separation of the pancreatic and bile ducts. Coexistent chronic interstitial pancreatitis and cholangiohepatitis have been observed in cats, and although the relationship between the changes in the two organs is not clear, the convergence of the feline biliary and pancreatic ducts may be a factor.[28,51,53,54,131] Reduced distensibility of the pancreas following chronic pancreatitis may result in increased interstitial pressure during secretion, mimicking partial obstruction.[132] Congenital anomalies of the pancreatic duct system may predispose to pancreatitis in humans, and this may occur in other species as well.[92]

Duodenal/Biliary Reflux, Pancreatic Trauma, and Pancreatic Ischemia/Reperfusion

Reflux of duodenal juice into the pancreatic ducts secondary to surgical creation of a closed duodenal loop causes severe acute pancreatitis.[92,133] Enteropeptidase, activated pancreatic enzymes, bacteria, and bile present in the duodenal juice may all contribute to development of pancreatitis, and biliary reflux in cats with infected bile may be particularly important in establishing pancreatitis in that species.[58,134] Under normal circumstances duodenal reflux is probably minimal because the duct opening is surrounded by a specialized compact, smooth mucosa over the duodenal papilla, and is equipped with an independent sphincter muscle.[135] This antireflux mechanism may fail intermittently when duodenal pressure transiently exceeds pancreatic duct pressure, such as may occur postprandially, with vomiting, or after trauma to the duodenum.[136]

Surgical manipulation, automobile accidents, and falling from high buildings are potential causes of pancreatic trauma, but reports of pancreatitis following such insults are rare, and in most cases of abdominal trauma injury to the pancreas is probably mild or unrecognized.[137,138] Although much has been made of the supposed sensitivity of the pancreas to surgical manipulation, pancreatitis is a very rare complication of pancreatic biopsy using either wedge resection or needle core techniques, and is also uncommon following resection of pancreatic neoplasms.[92,139–144]

Experimental and clinical reports have indicated ischemia to be important in the pathogenesis of pancreatitis, either as a primary cause or as an exacerbating influence.[145–150] Pancreatic ischemia may develop during shock, secondary to hypotension during general anesthesia, as well as during temporary occlusion of venous outflow during surgical manipulations in the anterior abdomen, and may explain some instances of postoperative pancreatitis in which surgery involved areas remote from the pancreas.[92]

Miscellaneous

Bacterial, viral, mycoplasmal, and parasitic infections may be associated with pancreatitis, although this is usually recognized as part of a more generalized disease.[92,151–156] It is not known if infection plays a role in the development of isolated pancreatitis in some instances, but concomitant bacterial infection does increase the severity of experimental pancreatitis, endotoxin administration can induce pancreatitis in experimental studies, and infection, possibly as a result of bacterial translocation from the gut, is the major cause of mortality in human patients with severe pancreatitis.[134,157–160] In one report, 11 of 23 patients with septic peritonitis had evidence of coexistent pancreatitis, but this did not appear to affect outcome.[156]

Morphologic changes in the pancreas have been associated with renal failure in a number of species.[161] Uremic pancreatitis may contribute to clinical signs of depression and anorexia in end-stage renal disease, although severe acute pancreatitis is clearly not a common complication of renal failure in dogs and cats. It is likely that renal failure secondary to acute pancreatitis is encountered more frequently.[161]

Finally, acute pancreatitis has been observed in patients with liver disease.[162,163] Possible explanations include vascular compromise secondary to coagulation abnormalities, accumulation of toxins (endotoxins, bile acids) secondary to impaired liver function, response to the same initial common cause (viral infection), reaction to drugs given in an attempt to manage the hepatic failure, or coincidence.[162,163]

DIAGNOSIS

History and Clinical Signs

Dogs with acute pancreatitis are usually presented because of depression, anorexia, vomiting, and in some cases, diar-

rhea. Severe acute disease may be associated with shock and collapse; other cases may have a history of less dramatic signs extending over several weeks. Some dogs demonstrate abdominal pain by assuming a prayer position with the forelimbs outstretched, the sternum on the floor, and the hindlimbs raised. Signs of pain may be elicited by abdominal palpation, although some animals do not react even though they have severe acute pancreatitis. An anterior abdominal mass is palpable in some cases, and occasionally there is mild ascites. Most affected animals are mildly to moderately dehydrated and febrile. Uncommon systemic complications of pancreatitis that may be apparent on physical examination include jaundice, respiratory distress, bleeding disorders, and cardiac arrhythmias.[49,124,164–167] Although dogs of any age may develop pancreatitis, affected animals are usually middle aged or older, sometimes obese, and the onset of signs may have followed ingestion of a large amount of fatty food.[94,103,124,164–168] The clinical signs of chronic pancreatitis are poorly documented, but are probably extremely variable and nonspecific.

Clinical signs of pancreatitis in cats are not well defined. In an experimental study, fever, tachycardia, and variable signs of abdominal pain were observed with only rare episodes of vomiting.[169] A survey of 40 cases of fatal pancreatitis in the cat revealed that nearly all were severely lethargic and anorexic, and that more than 50% were dehydrated or hypothermic. Vomiting was noted in 35% of cases, and 25% of the patients demonstrated abdominal pain or had a palpable abdominal mass.[51]

Radiographic Signs

Radiographic signs reported with pancreatitis include increased density, diminished contrast and granularity in the right cranial abdomen, displacement of the stomach to the left, widening of the angle between the pyloric antrum and the proximal duodenum, displacement of the descending duodenum to the right, presence of a mass medial to the descending duodenum, static gas pattern in or thickened walls of the descending duodenum, static gas pattern in or caudal displacement of the transverse colon, gastric distension suggestive of gastric-outlet obstruction, and delayed passage of barium through the stomach and duodenum with corrugation of the duodenal wall indicating abnormal peristalsis (Figure 20–8).[137,165,166,170–172] Unfortunately, definitive radiographic evidence of pancreatitis is usually not present, the most common finding being a somewhat subjective loss of visceral detail ("ground glass appearance") in the anterior abdomen.

Ultrasonic imaging is used increasingly to identify patients with pancreatitis. Nonhomogeneous masses and loss of echodensity have been noted in dogs and cats with experimental and spontaneous pancreatitis (Figure 20–9). Ultrasonography may reveal cystic masses when there are pancreatic pseudocysts or abscesses, and increased echodensity when there are areas of fibrosis.[49,173–177] Computed tomography is presently the most useful modality for visualizing the pancreas and associated pathology in human patients. Serial examinations are particularly useful for identification and management of complications such as pancreatic abscess in patients that are not responding well to conservative therapeutic measures.[178,179]

Laboratory Aids to Diagnosis

Leucocytosis is a common hematologic finding in acute pancreatitis. The packed cell volume may be increased as a

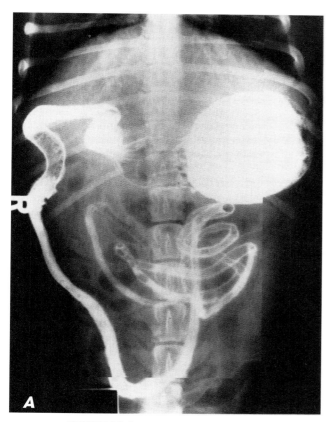 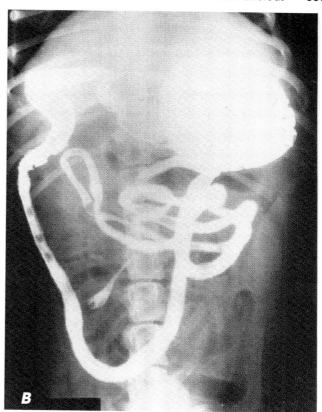

FIGURE 20–8. Dorsoventral radiographs taken of a dog with acute pancreatitis. Positive contrast medium was given and films taken at 10 *(A)* and 30 *(B)* minutes show the descending part of the duodenum to be in a fixed position. The duodenum also shows irregularities along the visceral border.

result of dehydration, although in some cases, particularly in cats, anemia is observed following rehydration.[51,24,169,180–182]

Azotemia is frequently present, and usually reflects dehydration, but sometimes there may be acute renal failure secondary to hypovolemia, or to other mechanisms such as circulating vasotoxic agents and plugging of the renal microvasculature by either fat deposits or microthrombi from the sites of disseminated intravascular coagulation.[124,169,180–185]

Liver enzyme activities are often increased, reflecting hepatocellular injury as a result of either hepatic ischemia or exposure of the liver to high concentrations of toxic products delivered from the pancreas in portal blood.[51,124,186–188] In some cases, particularly in cats, there is hyperbilirubinemia and sometimes clinically apparent icterus, which may indicate severe hepatocellular damage and/or intrahepatic and extrahepatic obstruction to bile flow.

Hyperglycemia is common in dogs and cats with necrotizing pancreatitis, probably as a result of hyperglucagonemia and stress-related increases in the concentrations of catecholamines and cortisol. In contrast, cats with suppurative pancreatitis often develop hypoglycemia.[51] Some animals become diabetic following recovery from episodes of acute pancreatitis.[51,94,125,164,168]

Hypocalcemia has often been reported, but is usually mild to moderate and rarely associated with clinical signs of tetany.[51,124,164,169,180–182] Although rare, rhabdomyolysis has been associated with severe, prolonged hypocalcemia in human patients.[189] The mechanism leading to development of hypocalcemia is not clear, but deposition of calcium as soaps

following excessive breakdown of fat by released pancreatic lipase is one potential explanation.[84,124,165]

Hypercholesterolemia and hypertriglyceridemia are very common and hyperlipemia is often grossly apparent even though food has not been ingested for many hours.[51,84,124,165] Extreme hyperlipemia may prevent accurate determination of other serum biochemical values. Analysis of plasma lipids has not revealed any clear-cut pattern characteristic of acute pancreatitis.[190]

Serum concentrations of pancreatic enzymes and zymogens are often elevated in animals with pancreatitis.[169,180–182, 191–195] Clinical and experimental observations have primarily involved amylase and lipase, but phospholipase A2 and trypsinlike immunoreactivity (TLI) have also been investigated.[69,72,79,169,181,182,191–197] Numerous different assay methods exist, including conventional catalytic assays and newer highly specific immunoassays (Figure 20–10), and it is important that a method appropriate for each species be utilized. Canine amylase can be reliably assayed by amyloclastic methods, but saccharogenic methods will give falsely high values because of the presence of maltase and glucoamylase in canine serum.[198,199] Immunoassays are generally only applicable to the species for which they were developed.

Increased concentrations of circulating pancreatic enzymes also arise secondary to reduced clearance from the plasma, as happens in renal failure.[161,200] Because azotemia is common in acute pancreatitis it is sometimes difficult to determine whether increased levels of pancreatic enzymes are due to pancreatic inflammation or renal disease.

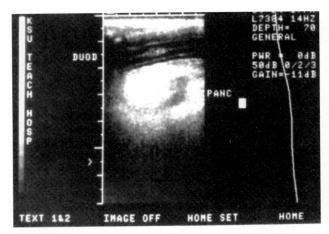

FIGURE 20–9. Ultrasonographic examination of the abdomen in pancreatitis may reveal areas of pancreas with loss of normal echodensity (PANC) adjacent to areas of increased density, reflecting patchy areas of edema, hemorrhage, inflammation, and fibrosis. (From Williams DA: Exocrine pancreatic disease. *In* Ettinger SJ, Feldman EC: Textbook of Veterinary Internal Medicine. 4th ed. Philadelphia, WB Saunders Company, 1995, p. 1378.)

Increases more than two to three times above the upper limit of normal are unlikely to result from renal dysfunction alone, although there are exceptions.[161,193]

Unlike trypsin, which is pancreas specific, amylase, lipase, and phospholipase originate from both pancreatic and extrapancreatic sources, including gastric and small intestinal mucosa, and serum activities of these extrapancreatic enzymes may increase in dogs with hepatic or neoplastic disease.[192,195,200–204] Lipase activity has been reported to be a more reliable marker for the diagnosis of pancreatitis than amylase.[201] However, dexamethasone administration has been shown to increase canine serum lipase activity up to fivefold without histologic evidence of pancreatitis, whereas decreases in amylase activity occur.[205] Moderate elevations of serum lipase in dogs receiving dexamethasone or other glucocorticoids should therefore not be taken as strong evidence for pancreatitis unless amylase is also increased.[205a]

Attempts to identify a pancreas-specific isoenzyme of canine amylase, as has been possible in human beings, have produced contradictory findings.[192,203,206–208] The persistence of all four canine isoenzymes both in dogs with acinar atrophy and in pancreatectomized dogs would seem to indicate that no such isoform exists in this species.[203,204] Furthermore, urinary amylase activity does not appear to be a useful marker for pancreatitis in dogs, perhaps reflecting tubular degradation or formation of nonfiltered polymers or complexes with other serum proteins.[209,210]

Experimental studies indicate that during the course of canine acute pancreatitis, the changes that occur in serum levels of different pancreatic enzymes are roughly parallel except that the proportional increase in serum TLI is greater and tends to develop and resolve sooner than with lipase and amylase, perhaps reflecting its shorter half-life.[195,196,211,212] In a model of chronic pancreatitis, however, in which dogs with mild or marked disease were followed for 12 months, serum TLI increased in inflammatory stages of the model in both groups, but subsequently decreased to values significantly lower than initial control values in those dogs with marked fibrosis and duct dilation.[213] Serum TLI remained elevated for the duration of the study in those dogs with milder smol-

dering pancreatitis, and in neither group were significant changes in serum amylase noted at any time.[213] In dogs with spontaneous disease it has also been stated that there may be elevations of one enzyme accompanied by minimal increases in another.[124,194,201] Definitive studies investigating serum levels of pancreatic enzymes in cases of spontaneously occurring pancreatitis are lacking. It is possible that in some patients nonpancreatic release of some enzymes (e.g., gastric lipase) are erroneously taken as evidence to support a diagnosis of pancreatitis. Conversely, persistently normal activities are seen in some cases of documented pancreatitis.[124,194,201] By the time some clinical cases are investigated it may be that depletion of stored enzymes combined with disruption of synthesis of new enzymes results in lowered serum levels.[214,215] This may also explain the lack of correlation between the magnitude of the increases in enzyme activities and the clinically perceived severity of disease and eventual outcome.

Reports of acute pancreatitis in cats are few, but elevations of serum amylase and lipase are less than in dogs, as are normal activities of these enzymes.[51,52,168,169] An experimental study demonstrated that although serum lipase increased significantly in cats following induction of pancreatitis, amylase activity never increased above normal, but rather decreased to 60% to 80% of initial values during the course of the disease.[169] Preliminary studies with an immunoassay for feline TLI have shown that normal serum TLI concentrations in cats are higher than in dogs, and that serum TLI was above normal in two cats with acute pancreatitis.[216a]

Methemalbumin is formed in humans with hemorrhagic pancreatitis as pancreatic enzymes degrade hemoglobin with subsequent binding of oxidized heme (hemin) to albumin.[217] Hemin does not bind to canine albumin, however, but rather to a variety of different serum proteins, so true methemalbuminemia cannot exist in dogs.[217] Although these protein-bound forms of hemin may also be formed in other conditions, such as hemolytic dyscrasias and intestinal infarctions, their presence in patients with other evidence of pancreatitis is highly suggestive of the hemorrhagic form of the disease and their concentration may be of prognostic value.[217] Serum concentrations of inflammatory mediators (neutrophil elastase, kallikreins, complement factors, C-reactive protein, interleukin-8), although not specific for pancreatitis, have similarly been investigated as possible markers to indicate the severity of pancreatitis.[218,219]

Trypsin complexed with plasma alpha$_1$-protease inhibitor (Figure 20–2) and trypsinogen activation peptides (TAP; Figure 20–2, Table 20–7) are not normally present in plasma or urine. They are only produced and released as a result of pancreatic inflammation and are thus specific markers for pancre-

IMMUNOLOGIC ASSAY   CATALYTIC ASSAY

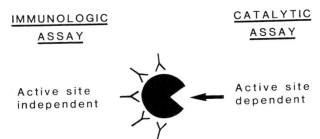

Active site independent   Active site dependent

FIGURE 20–10. Assay of pancreatic enzymes and zymogens in serum. Catalytic assays detect degradation of specific substrates exposed to the active site of the molecule, and therefore measure activity. Immunoassays detect antigenic sites over the surface of the molecule and therefore measure enzyme or zymogen concentration. (From Williams DA: Exocrine pancreatic disease. *In* Ettinger SJ, Feldman EC: Textbook of Veterinary Internal Medicine. 4th ed. Philadelphia, WB Saunders Company, 1995, p. 1378.)

atitis.[71,73,80,83,85,86,116,220–222] In human patients, the concentration of these markers correlates well with the severity and clinical course of the disease.[42,69,70–73,80–83,85,86,116,220–222] Technical complexities presently limit the usefulness of assays of species-specific trypsin-alpha1-protease inhibitor complex, but assays for the Asp-Asp-Asp-Asp-Lys peptide sequence common to TAP in all vertebrates (Table 20–6) may prove to be of practical value.[223]

Clearly there is no widely available ideal test or combination of tests for the diagnosis of acute pancreatitis, in the absence of direct examination of pancreatic tissue, the diagnosis can only be tentative. Nonetheless, careful evaluation of the entire clinical picture, particularly if supported by ultrasonographic pancreatic abnormalities, will in many instances give a high degree of confidence in the presumptive diagnosis. If gross or histopathologic confirmation of the diagnosis is required, or the possibility of other abdominal disease needs to be eliminated, it is important that attention be given to stabilization of fluid and electrolyte status prior to general anesthesia and surgical exploration of the abdomen.

TREATMENT

The treatment of acute pancreatitis involves maintenance of fluid and electrolyte balance while withholding food and water, thereby allowing the pancreas to rest and recover from the inflammatory episode.[93,224–226] If drug-induced pancreatitis is suspected, any incriminated agents should be withdrawn and replaced by an unrelated alternative drug if necessary. Other potential etiologic factors (see earlier) should similarly be investigated, and if possible rectified. Mild cases of pancreatitis are probably self-limiting and may spontaneously improve after 1 or 2 days of basic supportive therapy. Other patients require aggressive fluid therapy over several days to treat severe dehydration and ongoing fluid electrolyte loss due to vomiting and diarrhea. Many animals become hypokalemic during such therapy and serum potassium should be monitored and supplemented as needed by addition of potassium chloride to the IV fluids. Serum creatinine or BUN should also be followed to monitor renal function. Although metabolic acidosis is probably common in acute pancreatitis, this may not always be the case, and vomiting patients may be alkalotic. Blind correction of suspected acid-base abnormalities should therefore not be attempted unless documented by appropriate testing.[225] Excessive bicarbonate administration may precipitate signs of hypocalcemia in individuals with borderline low calcium levels.

It is common practice to give parenteral antibiotics during this supportive period, particularly when toxic changes are evident in the hemogram or when the patient is febrile.[224,225]

Trimethoprim-sulphadiazine and enrofloxacin penetrate well into canine pancreas and are effective against many common pathogens isolated from human patients with pancreatitis.[227]

If abdominal pain is severe, then analgesic therapy (meperidine hydrochloride, 1–5 mg/kg IM or SC q 1–6 hours, or butorphanol tartrate, 0.1–1.0 mg/kg SC q 1–6 hours) should be given to provide relief.[52,228] Hyperglycemia is often mild and transient, but in some cases frank diabetes mellitus may develop and require treatment with insulin. Respiratory distress, neurologic problems, cardiac abnormalities, bleeding disorders, and acute renal failure are all poor prognostic signs.

Recent observations have indicated that in severe pancreatitis there is marked consumption of plasma protease inhibitors as activated pancreatic proteases are cleared from the circulation, and that saturation of available alpha-macroglobulins is rapidly followed by acute disseminated intravascular coagulation, shock, and death.[69,72,73,80–83,229–232] Transfusion of plasma or whole blood to replace alpha-macroglobulins may be life saving in these circumstances, and has the additional benefit of maintaining plasma albumin concentrations.[231,233] Albumin is probably beneficial in pancreatitis because of its oncotic properties that not only help maintain blood volume and prevent pancreatic ischemia, but also limit pancreatic edema formation.[145] Albumin also binds detergents such as free fatty acids and lysolecithin, produced in pancreatitis by the catalytic actions of lipase and phospholipase A_2, that otherwise may disrupt cell membranes.[234]

Low molecular weight dextrans have also been used to expand plasma volume, but they may aggravate bleeding tendencies, contain no protease inhibitor, and provide no major advantages over plasma administration.[224,225] A hypertonic saline-dextran 70 combination was effective in maintaining cardiac function while avoiding massive fluid administration and avoiding pulmonary hypertension and edema that can accompany therapy with lactated Ringer's solution alone.[235] Hyperoncotic ultrahigh molecular weight dextran solutions have recently been shown to reduce trypsinogen activation, prevent acinar necrosis, and lower mortality in rodent pancreatitis, perhaps by promoting pancreatic microcirculation.[236]

Plasma beta-endorphin increases in intraductal bile/trypsin-induced pancreatitis in dogs;[237,238] the opiate antagonist naloxone (2 mg/kg/hour IV) is effective in protecting against cardiovascular collapse in this model of pancreatitis, as has been reported in some models of hemorrhagic and endotoxic shock.[237]

The use of corticosteroids in pancreatitis has been recommended because they stabilize lysosomal membranes, reduce inflammation, and alleviate shock, but they have not been

Table 20–7

AMINO ACID SEQUENCES OF TRYPSINOGEN ACTIVATION PEPTIDES FROM A VARIETY OF SPECIES

SPECIES								
Dog: cationic trypsin	Phe-	Pro-	Ile-	Asp-	Asp-	Asp-	Asp-	Lys-
Dog: anionic trypsin	Thr-	Pro-	Thr-	Asp-	Asp-	Asp-	Asp-	Lys-
Cat	Phe-	Pro-	Ile-	Asp-	Asp-	Asp-	Asp-	Lys
Cow			Val-	Asp-	Asp-	Asp-	Asp-	Lys-
Goat			Val-	Asp-	Asp-	Asp-	Asp-	Lys-
Pig	Phe-	Pro-	Thr-	Asp-	Asp-	Asp-	Asp-	Lys-
Horse	Ser-	Ser-	Thr-	Asp-	Asp-	Asp-	Asp-	Lys-
Dogfish		Ala	Pro-	Asp-	Asp-	Asp-	Asp-	Lys-

shown to be of value in experimental studies.[239] They should be given only on a short-term basis to animals in shock associated with fulminating pancreatitis, and then in concert with fluids and plasma as described earlier.[225] Longer periods of administration may impair removal of alpha-macroglobulin-bound proteases from the plasma by the monocyte-macrophage system, with resultant complications due to systemic effects of circulating uninhibited enzymes.[88,89]

Nasogastric suctioning of gastric secretions and use of antacids or cimetidine have been recommended in order to indirectly inhibit pancreatic secretion;[224] however, none of these methods has been consistently shown to be effective, and their value has largely been discounted.[93] Attempts to rest the pancreas using direct inhibitors of secretion such as atropine, acetazolamide, glucagon, and calcitonin have not proved to be effective.[224,226,239–243] Indeed, stimulation with high-dose intravenous secretin was beneficial in a rat model of pancreatitis, resulting in less severe histopathologic damage reestablishment of pancreatic juice flow, and partial restoration of protein output.[244]

Somatostatin and its analogues may reduce complications and improve survival in human patients, but there is not yet sufficient evidence to recommend its routine use.[245,246] Infusion of dopamine at a dose that stimulates both dopaminergic and beta-adrenergic receptors (5 µg/kg/minute, IV) is helpful in reducing severity and progression of some feline models of pancreatitis;[58,247] it is thought that the beneficial effect of dopamine is related to reduction of microvascular permeability that is otherwise promoted by a variety of vasoactive substances such as bradykinin and prostaglandins, rather than to promotion of pancreatic blood flow.[58] Pancreatic gamma irradiation is an effective if impractical method that reduces pancreatic secretion and lessens the severity of experimental pancreatitis.[248]

Administration of a variety of naturally occurring and synthetic enzyme inhibitors with selective actions against individual pancreatic digestive enzymes has shown promise in experimental studies, but their value remains to be demonstrated in clinical trials.[224,238,249–251] Future clinical and experimental trials will probably be directed at the use of agents to modify intracellular events that are currently believed to be important in the pathobiology of pancreatitis, including free radical scavengers, enzyme synthesis and transport inhibitors, and factors that may stabilize lysosomal and other membranes.[251–253]

The use of peritoneal dialysis to remove toxic material accumulated in the peritoneal cavity is beneficial experimentally, and is thought by many to be useful in human patients.[224] Although impractical in some veterinary hospitals, peritoneal dialysis may be of value in some cases. Certainly in those patients in which acute pancreatitis is confirmed at exploratory laparotomy, removal of as much free fluid as possible by abdominal lavage is advisable. In some cases pancreatitis may be localized to one lobe of the gland, and surgical resection of the affected area may be followed by complete recovery.[175,254]

Utilization of ultrasonographic imaging has contributed to increased recognition of pancreatic masses (pseudocyst, abscess).[49,175,176,255] These lesions are sterile pseudocysts in most cases, but there are no reports of a large series of cases in which bacteriologic studies were done. It is not clear whether these cases are best managed conservatively with supportive therapy, or if surgical intervention to debride necrotic tissue and allow drainage of affected areas facilitates recovery. In one study of 7 dogs with pancreatic masses, 1 patient recovered spontaneously but the remaining 6 dogs died within 9 days of necrosectomy and biliary decompression.[176] Three of 6 dogs

with pancreatic masses recovered after open abdominal drainage and intensive care in another report.[175] Bile duct obstruction accompanying pancreatitis has also been increasingly recognized through the use of ultrasonography. Cholecystoduodenostomy was followed by recovery in 6 dogs with fibrotic obstructive masses.[255] Given these mixed results and the risks, difficulties, and expense associated with anesthesia, surgery, and postoperative care, it is probably wise to avoid surgical intervention unless there is clear evidence of an enlarging mass and/or sepsis in a patient that is not responding well to medical therapy. Many patients that develop obstructive jaundice in association with acute pancreatitis recover spontaneously over 2 or 3 weeks with conventional supportive care alone.[256]

Small amounts of water should be offered after the patient has stopped vomiting. If there is no recurrence of clinical signs, food may be gradually reintroduced. The diet should have a high carbohydrate content (rice, pasta, potatoes) because protein and fat are more potent stimulants of pancreatic secretion and may therefore be more likely to promote a relapse. If there is continued improvement, gradual introduction of a low-fat maintenance diet should be attempted. Another period of food deprivation should be instituted if signs of pancreatitis recur.[166,225] Although the prognosis is poor for those patients that repeatedly cannot tolerate food, total parenteral nutrition may be beneficial by sustaining such patients while the digestive system is rested for 7 to 10 days.[226]

In many patients a single episode of pancreatitis occurs, and all that is necessary in the way of long-term therapy is to avoid feeding meals with an excessively high-fat content. In other patients repeated bouts of pancreatitis occur, and it may be beneficial to feed a moderately or severely fat-restricted diet permanently. In spite of this, some animals experience recurrent disease.[166,225]

Oral pancreatic enzyme supplements may decrease the pain that accompanies chronic pancreatitis in human beings, probably by feedback inhibition of endogenous pancreatic enzyme secretion.[257] It is not known if they are of similar value in dogs or cats, but there is evidence for inhibition of pancreatic secretion mediated by intraluminal pancreatic enzymes in dogs.[258,259] However, there is also evidence in human beings that pancreatic enzyme extracts given at clinical dosages and with food do not inhibit, but rather stimulate pancreatic secretion.[260] Despite these contradictory observations, a trial period of enzyme therapy may be warranted in individuals with chronic or recurrent signs attributable to pancreatitis.

PROGNOSIS

Pancreatitis is an unpredictable disease of widely varying severity, and it is difficult to give a prognosis even when a diagnosis is definitively established.[223] Life-threatening signs accompanying acute fulminating pancreatitis are usually followed by death in spite of supportive measures, but some dogs recover fully following an isolated severe episode. In other cases, relatively mild or moderate chronic or recurrent pancreatitis persists despite all therapy, and either the patient dies in an acute severe exacerbation of the disease or is euthanatized because of failure to recover and/or the expense of long-term supportive care. Most patients with uncomplicated pancreatitis probably recover spontaneously after a single episode and do well as long as high-fat foods are avoided.

EXOCRINE PANCREATIC INSUFFICIENCY

Progressive loss of pancreatic acinar cells ultimately leads to malabsorption due to inadequate production of digestive enzymes. The functional reserve of the pancreas is considerable, however, and signs of exocrine pancreatic insufficiency (EPI) do not occur until a large proportion of the gland has been destroyed. Steatorrhea and azotorrhea do not develop in humans until more than 90% of the secretory capacity of the pancreas has been lost.[261] Similarly, in dogs with EPI both the amylase secretory capacity and the serum concentration of trypsinlike immunoreactivity are reduced to less than 15% of normal. The most common cause of EPI in the dog is pancreatic acinar atrophy (Figure 20–11). Pancreatic insufficiency is caused less commonly by chronic pancreatitis and rarely by pancreatic neoplasia.[94,164,262–267] Although not yet documented, it is likely that congenital abnormalities of canine pancreatic exocrine function such as pancreatic hypoplasia, isolated deficiencies of individual pancreatic enzymes, and deficiency of enteropeptidase also occur.[268]

Clinical Synopsis

Diagnostic Features

- Weight loss
- "Small-bowel" type diarrhea
- Subnormal serum trypsinlike immunoreactivity
- Subnormal fecal proteolytic activity
- Abnormal breath hydrogen test
- Xylose absorption test results often abnormal

Standard Treatment

- Pancreatic enzyme replacement therapy: 2 teaspoonsful/20 kg body weight with each meal
- Oral tetracycline to treat small intestinal bacterial overgrowth if poor response to enzyme replacement alone
- Low-fiber diet may be beneficial
- Parenteral cobalamin supplementation often required (especially in cats)

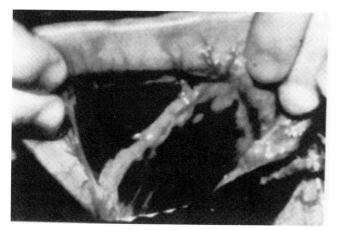

FIGURE 20–11. The duodenal limb of the pancreas of a dog with pancreatic acinar atrophy. Residual tissue contains islet (endocrine) cells and blood vessels, and so diabetes mellitus is not a feature of this disease. (From Williams DA: Exocrine pancreatic insufficiency. Waltham Int. Focus 2:9, 1992.)

- High oral doses of fat soluble vitamins may be required (especially vitamins K and E)
- Oral prednisolone may be helpful in patients that do not respond to the above therapy
- Oral H_2-receptor antagonists rarely if ever improve clinical response to enzyme replacement

Follow-up

- Lifelong therapy almost always required

Although pancreatic enzymes perform essential digestive functions, alternative pathways of digestion for some nutrients do exist. Following experimental exclusion of pancreatic secretion from the intestine, dogs can still absorb up to 63% of ingested protein and 84% of ingested fat.[269–271] This residual enzyme activity probably originates from lingual and/or gastric lipases and gastric pepsins, from intestinal mucosal esterases and peptidases, and, in young animals, from bile salt–activated lipase in milk.[202,268,272,273,274] Nonetheless, when exocrine pancreatic function is severely impaired, these alternative routes of digestion are inadequate, and clinical signs of malabsorption occur.

ETIOLOGY

Pancreatic Acinar Atrophy (PAA)

Atrophy of pancreatic acinar cells without concomitant inflammation occurs in a variety of experimental circumstances as outlined here. Spontaneous development of PAA in previously healthy adult animals appears to be uniquely common in the dog, although similar conditions occur sporadically in other species.[275–280]

The underlying cause of canine PAA is unknown, but numerous nutritional deficiencies, such as amino acid imbalance and copper deficiency in the rat and protein-calorie malnutrition in humans, cause atrophy of exocrine tissue.[116,281–286] The etiology of canine PAA is unknown, but the possibility of a nutritional imbalance, acquired perhaps as a consequence of an underlying small intestinal mucosal abnormality, is an attractive theory for the development of PAA in dogs. Although preexisting small intestinal disease in dogs with PAA has not been documented, it is has been observed that affected dogs often have a history of gastrointestinal disturbances long before the development of severe weight loss.[287,288] Alternative potential explanations for development of PAA include (1) pancreatic duct obstruction, (2) a primary congenital abnormality in the pancreas itself, (3) toxicosis, (4) ischemia, (5) viral infection, (6) immune-mediated disease, and (7) defective secretory and/or trophic stimuli. There is little evidence to support the role of any of these etiologies in naturally occurring canine PAA.[287, 288a] Antipancreatic antibodies have recently been described in both normal dogs and dogs with EPI;[289] their significance is not clear.

Although PAA may occur at any age in a wide variety of breeds, a high prevalence in German shepherd and collie dogs is recognized.[287,288,290–296] Investigations of family histories have suggested that predisposition to development of the disease is inherited in an autosomal recessive fashion in the German shepherd dog.[293,297]

The pancreatic atrophy of CBA/J in mice is the only naturally occurring disorder that resembles canine PAA.[279] Morphologic study of pancreas from affected mice has implicated destabilization zymogen granules as one of the earliest ultrastructural abnormalities; biochemical studies indicate that premature activation of trypsinogen and chymotrypsinogens occurs within zymogen granules.[277,279] Progressive ultrastructural abnormalities of zymogen granules similarly preceded (by almost 2 years) development of overt PAA in a young German shepherd dog (Figure 20–12).[297] These observations illustrate that the variable inflammatory response observed in canine PAA may arise secondary to an earlier and more subtle underlying abnormality in the acinar cells themselves.[265,266,288,290]

Chronic Pancreatitis

Although chronic pancreatitis resulting in progressive destruction of pancreatic tissue is a common cause of EPI in adult human beings, it is a rare cause of EPI in dogs.[94,164,263,266,288,291] Animals with EPI and coexistent diabetes mellitus probably fall into this category, because inflammation

is likely to damage both endocrine and exocrine tissue, in contrast to the selective acinar cell damage in PAA.[298,299] Exocrine pancreatic insufficiency is much less commonly diagnosed in cats that in dogs, but chronic pancreatitis has been the underlying cause in the majority of the few cases reported.[103,262,300–303]

Hereditary, Congenital, and Miscellaneous Causes of EPI

Cystic fibrosis and Schwachman-Diamond syndrome are the most common causes of EPI in children, but these disorders differ from canine and feline EPI in that there are also abnormalities of organs other than the pancreas.[268] Other extremely rare causes of EPI in children include congenital deficiencies of individual pancreatic digestive enzymes or of intestinal enteropeptidase, but these have not been described in dogs or cats.[304] Occasionally young dogs are seen that have

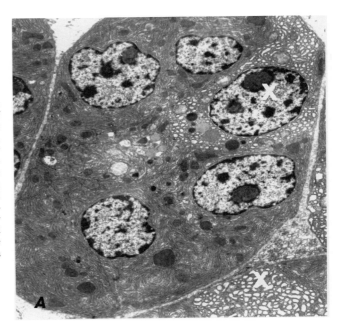

FIGURE 20–12. *(A)* Electron microscopic appearance of a pancreatic biopsy specimen taken at 6 weeks of age from a dog that developed clinical signs of EPI due to pancreatic acinar atrophy at 2 years of age. Early stages of acinar atrophy are apparent; in a few acinar cells (X) the rough endoplasmic reticulum is slightly dilated and organization is tubular. (Reproduced from Westermarck E, et al: Sequential study of pancreatic structure and function during development of pancreatic acinar atrophy in a German shepherd dog. Am J Vet Res 54:1088–1094, 1993.) *(B)* Electron microscopic appearance of a pancreatic biopsy specimen taken at 22 months of age from same dog illustrated in Figure 20–12A. A cell with early stage atrophy (1) contains parallel stacks of rough endoplasmic reticulum that are slightly dilated, and zymogen granules that are larger than in an apparently normal cell (N). A cell with later stage atrophy (3) has more dilated and tubular rough endoplasmic reticulum and extensive fusion of zymogen granules. Another cell has end stage atrophy (4) and is frankly necrotic. (Reproduced from Westermarck E, et al: Sequential study of pancreatic structure and function during development of pancreatic acinar atrophy in a German shepherd dog. Am J Vet Res 54:1088–1094, 1993.)

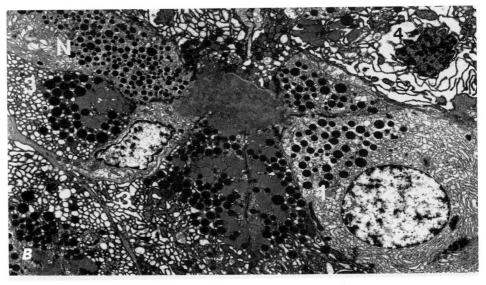

signs of EPI and sometimes diabetes mellitus from a very early age, and congenital pancreatic hypoplasia or aplasia may be the underlying cause.[28,305] There are also sporadic reports of apparently reversible EPI in association with subtotal acinar atrophy and mild inflammation that is not easily classified but may reflect subclinical PAA.[306]

Finally, EPI has been reported as a complication of proximal duodenal resection and cholecystoduodenostomy in cats. This may reflect the absence of dual pancreatic ducts in this species, with blockage of pancreatic secretion occurring as a result of damage to the major duodenal papilla.[307]

PATHOPHYSIOLOGY

Nutrient malabsorption in canine EPI does not arise simply as a consequence of failure of intraluminal digestion. Morphologic changes in the small intestine of some dogs with EPI have been reported, and studies of naturally occurring and experimental EPI in several species have revealed abnormal activities of mucosal enzymes and impaired function as indicated by abnormal transport of sugars, amino acids, and fatty acids.[264,290,308–320] The cause of this mucosal pathology is unknown, but the absence of the trophic influence of pancreatic secretions, bacterial overgrowth in the small intestine, and endocrine and nutritional factors may all be contributory.[17–19,321–325]

Small Intestinal Mucosa

EPI in several species is associated with increased activities of jejunal brush border maltase and sucrase (Figure 20–13), as well as an increase in the proportion of microvillar membrane proteins of large relative molecular mass (> 220 kDa).[17,320,326,327] These changes are attributed to reduced degradation of exposed brush border proteins as a consequence of decreased pancreatic protease activity within the gut lumen (Figure 20–14).[15,16,314,315] This explanation is supported by the reversal of the abnormalities in EPI after treatment with pancreatic enzymes.[16,320,328,329] The abnormal accumulation of these and other proteins on the surface of the brush border membrane may interfere with normal absorption.

In contrast to the increased activities of maltase and sucrase, the activity of brush border peptidase (leucyl-2-naphthylamidase) is unchanged; that of alkaline phosphatase is decreased in dogs with EPI (Figure 20–13).[327–329] These proteins are relatively resistant to degradation by intraluminal proteases.[328,330–335]

Protein synthesis by jejunal mucosa is decreased in dogs with EPI, but increases to normal following treatment.[328,336] Jejunal alkaline phosphatase activity also normalizes following treatment, suggesting the activity of this enzyme particularly depends on the rate of protein synthesis (Figure 20–14). The mechanism for the defect in protein synthesis is not known, but contributory factors may include malnutrition and intraluminal or humoral factors. Intraluminal pancreatic secretions and the products of digestion exert a trophic effect on the small intestine,[18,19] and both are deficient in untreated dogs. Hormones and other regulatory peptides including gastrin, enteroglucagon, glucagon, insulin, glucagon, and epidermal growth factor may mediate these trophic effects.[324,325] Disturbances of glucose homeostasis are common in dogs with EPI, and in these dogs insulinopenia may be an additional factor affecting intestinal mucosal function. Insulin receptors are present both on basolateral and brush border membranes of enterocytes, and insulin has a stimulatory effect on DNA synthesis in the gastrointestinal tract.

Small Intestinal Microflora

Bacterial overgrowth in the lumen of the small intestine is common in canine EPI.[17,343,344] Changes in the intestinal microflora may arise secondary to loss of the antibacterial properties of pancreatic juice,[14] or as a consequence of as yet undefined abnormalities of intestinal immunity or motility. Achlorhydria may also predispose to bacterial overgrowth, but is not a feature of canine EPI.[321,345,346]

The pathologic changes associated with bacterial overgrowth depend on the type of bacteria involved and probably the chronicity of the overgrowth. In those dogs with increases in aerobic and facultative anaerobic bacteria, changes are similar to those observed in dogs with EPI that do not have bacterial overgrowth.[17] In these dogs activities of brush border enzymes other than alkaline phosphatase are either normal or increased (Figure 20–13). In contrast, when the overgrowth includes obligate anaerobic bacteria there is often an associated decrease in many enzyme activities (Figure 20–13), and in some cases, partial villous atrophy (Figure 20–15).[17,320] These findings are consistent with the known ability of some strains of obligate anaerobic bacteria to produce enzymes that release or destroy exposed brush border enzymes.[181,323,347–349] Even when bacterial overgrowth does not include large numbers of obligate anaerobes, the abnormal microflora may be of clinical significance because bacteria may indirectly impair absorption by competing for nutrients and by changing intraluminal factors such as the concentration of conjugated bile salts.[321,349]

Pancreatic Regulatory Peptides

Histopathologic examination of pancreas from dogs with PAA reveals almost total atrophy of acinar tissue, but plentiful disorganized islet tissue, accompanied by numerous ganglia and patent exocrine ducts.[265,290] Immunohistochemical staining of PAA pancreas shows many insulin-, glucagon-, somatostatin-, and pancreatic polypeptide-immunoreactive cells scattered haphazardly throughout residual islet tissue.[20,329] This differs from the more organized arrangement of cells in healthy canine pancreas, in which a central core of insulin- and scattered somatostatin-immunoreactive cells is surrounded by a halo of glucagon- (left lobe) or pancreatic polypeptide- (right lobe), immunoreactive cells.[350,351] In addition, enkephalin- and vasoactive intestinal polypeptide (VIP)-immunoreactive nerve fibers are extremely profuse in PAA islet tissue, accompanied by numerous enkephalin- and VIP-immunoreactive nerve cell bodies; whereas in normal pancreas, enkephalin-immunoreactive fibers are very rare. VIP-immunoreactive innervation is moderate in acinar tissue but rarely present in islets.[329,350] A similar remarkable increase in VIP-immunoreactive fibers is reported in cats with experimental chronic pancreatitis.[130] Enkephalinlike immunoreactivity in PAA pancreas is probably due to a precursor immunochemically related to proenkephalin.[352]

Disturbance of the morphologic relationships between cells in islet pancreatic tissue may impair intra-islet and/or entero-islet homeostatic mechanisms and might account for subnormal basal plasma insulin concentrations in dogs with PAA.[353] The neuronal regulatory peptide abnormalities may represent a primary defect in canine PAA, or they may occur secondary

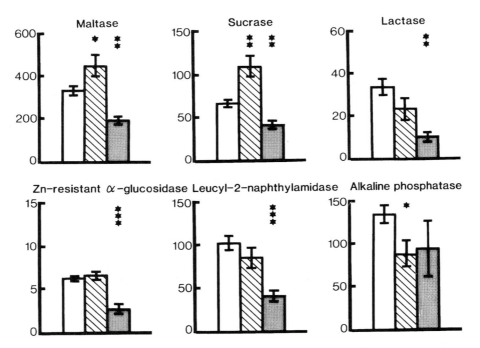

FIGURE 20-13. Specific activities of brush border enzymes in canine EPI. Enzyme activities (mU/mg) are expressed as mean ± SE. The open bars indicate activities in healthy control dogs, the stippled bars activities in dogs with EPI that did not have overgrowth of obligate anaerobic bacteria in the small intestine, and the striped bars activities in a group of dogs with EPI accompanied by duodenal overgrowth of obligate anaerobic bacteria. *$p < 0.05$; **$p < 0.01$; ***$p < 0.001$ compared to control values. (Reproduced from Williams DA, et al: Bacterial overgrowth in the duodenum of dogs with exocrine pancreatic insufficiency. JAVMA 191:201–206, 1987.)

to the atrophy of acinar tissue, perhaps arising as a result of neuronal overgrowth in response to loss of target tissue.

Glucose Intolerance

In patients with EPI secondary to pancreatitis there may be frank diabetes mellitus secondary to islet cell destruction. Oral and intravenous glucose tolerance are also abnormal in untreated dogs with PAA, although diabetes mellitus has not been reported in these dogs.[353–355]

The "incretin" effect is reduced in dogs with experimental pancreatic atrophy.[356] "Incretin" refers to insulinotropic factors released from the gut that are responsible for the augmentation of insulin secretion in response to orally administered glucose compared to that stimulated by the same dosage of intravenously administered glucose.[357] Gastric inhibitory polypeptide (GIP) is probably an important factor contributing to "incretin" activity, and feeding does not stimulate GIP release from the small bowel of dogs with PAA unless pancreatic enzymes are added to the food.[357–359] Similar observations have been made in children with cystic fibrosis, and the failure of GIP secretion appears to arise because products of digestion (glucose, amino acids, fatty acids) are the stimuli for GIP release rather than the act of feeding or the undigested constituents of food itself.[357,359] The relationship of plasma GIP responses to oral glucose intolerance in canine PAA, and whether oral glucose tolerance returns to normal following treatment, has not been reported.

Intravenous glucose tolerance in untreated dogs with PAA is associated with subnormal resting and stimulated insulin concentration,[329,353] abnormalities presumably independent of "incretin." Similar abnormalities have been reported in dogs with experimental pancreatic atrophy.[356,360] Treatment of PAA is followed by normalization of intravenous glucose tolerance, although basal plasma insulin concentrations remain subnormal.[329,353]

It is probable that the abnormalities in glucose homeostasis are related at least in part to metabolic changes associated with the catabolic and undernourished state of many untreated dogs with EPI.[68,361–363] Withholding food from dogs for a period of 2 weeks produces a decrease in circulating insulin concentrations, and severely undernourished dogs develop markedly subnormal insulin responses to glucose.[68,364] This probably represents an adaptation to reduced food intake because lower insulin levels facilitate enhanced lipolysis leading to increased concentrations of plasma free fatty acids that are available as an energy source.[364]

Nutritional Status

Many dogs with EPI have been suffering from malabsorption for a considerable period of time before a diagnosis is made. Thus, the clinical and pathophysiologic features associated with EPI may in some instances be due to malnutrition rather than EPI per se.

Protein-Calorie Malnutrition

Cachexia may perversely affect intestinal function in a variety of ways. Changes in small intestinal mucosal enzyme activ-

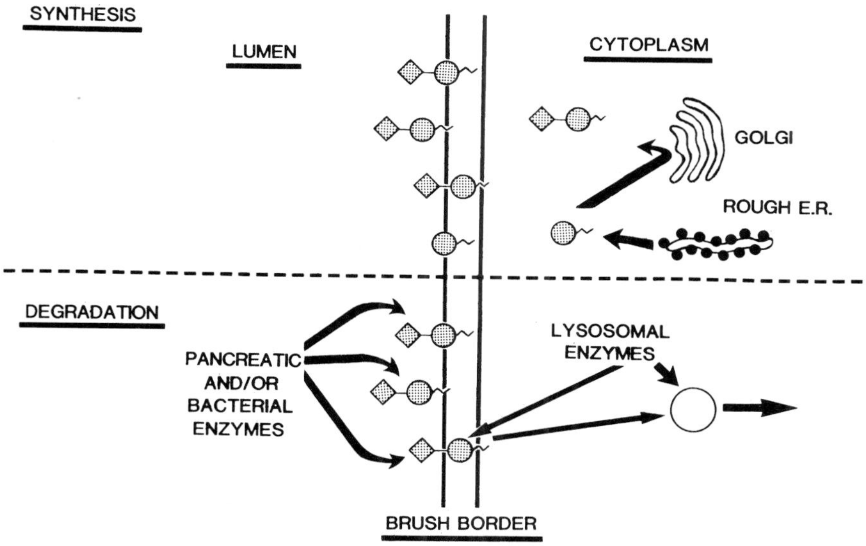

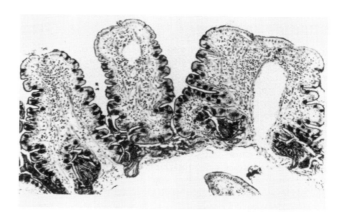

FIGURE 20-14. Factors influencing activities of jejunal brush border enzymes. The importance of degradation by intraluminal proteases depends at least in part on the location of the enzyme in the membrane, and hence its susceptibility to proteolytic attack. (Modified from Alpers DH and Seetharam B: Pathophysiology of diseases involving intestinal brush-border proteins. N Engl J Med 296:1047, 1977.)

ities have been observed in severely malnourished children, and may be a direct effect of nutrient deficiency impairing protein synthesis.[18,19,322,365] Severe protein-calorie malnutrition may also affect the normal immune response, and this in turn may contribute to development of changes in the intestinal microflora.[321,366] Furthermore, malnutrition in rats impairs the capacity to maintain protective mucosal mucin content, and accelerates the development of brush border enzyme deficiency in intraluminal bacterial overgrowth.[323,367] In addition to its effects on the intestine, protein-calorie malnutrition per se may contribute to EPI, perhaps through impairment of pancreatic protein synthesis, and this may worsen already impaired exocrine pancreatic function.[68,368] Metabolic changes associated with increased catabolism also affect glucose homeostasis, as discussed earlier.

Trace Elements

Absorption of trace elements in EPI may be promoted or inhibited secondary to either loss of specific factors affecting absorption or to a change in intraluminal pH.[12,369–371] Trace element deficiencies may potentially exacerbate exocrine dysfunction by impairing activities of metalloenzymes important in defenses against free radical injury.[68] Although trace element deficiencies have been reported in human patients with EPI,[372] deficiencies have not been documented in dogs. Serum copper and zinc have been shown to be normal in dogs with EPI, but other trace elements have not been investigated.[329]

Vitamins

Malabsorption of cobalamin (vitamin B_{12}) is well documented in association with EPI in human patients, and mildly to severely subnormal serum cobalamin levels are commonly observed in dogs and cats with EPI.[296,302,329,373–375] Cobalamin absorption is a complex process that involves binding of the vitamin by salivary and/or gastric R proteins with subsequent release from these proteins by pancreatic proteases. Cobal-

amin must then bind to intrinsic factor in order to be absorbed. Clearly, deficiencies of pancreatic proteases as well as pancreatic intrinsic factor would adversely affect cobalamin absorption.[7,11,375–377] Overgrowth of cobalamin-binding bacteria in the proximal small bowel may also be a contributory factor.[17,321,375] Because serum cobalamin concentrations usually do not normalize following treatment with oral pancreatic enzymes (Figure 20–16), cobalamin malabsorption is probably not solely due to lack of pancreatic enzymes in the gut lumen.[329,375,378,379] In experimental canine EPI, exogenous canine pancreatic juice, but not bovine pancreatic enzyme extract, enhances colbalamin absorption,[375] perhaps reflecting the intrinsic factor content of canine pancreatic juice. Cobalamin is essential for DNA synthesis, and severely subnormal serum cobalamin concentrations may adversely affect the normal proliferation of crypt cells in the intestinal mucosa, and hence the specific activities of jejunal mucosal enzymes.[380,381] It is therefore possible that intestinal dysfunc-

FIGURE 20-15. Partial villous atrophy in a jejunal biopsy specimen from a dog with exocrine pancreatic insufficiency due to pancreatic acinar atrophy. Villi are short and stumpy with a broadened plateau at the extrusion zone, and there is evidence of folding or fusion of villi. (From Williams DA, et al: Bacterial overgrowth in the duodenum of dogs with exocrine pancreatic insufficiency. JAVMA 191:201, 1987.)

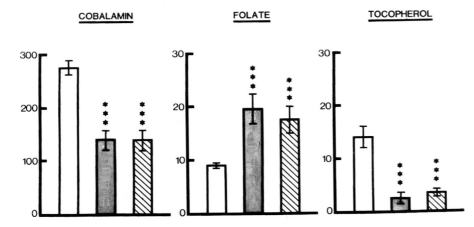

FIGURE 20–16. Serum cobalamin (ng/L), folate (μg/L), and tocopherol (mg/L) in dogs with EPI. Results are presented as mean ± SE. The open bars indicate control values, the stippled bars values in dogs with EPI before treatment, and the striped bars the values in the same group of dogs after treatment. ***p < 0.001 compared to control values. (Reproduced with permission from Williams DA: Exocrine pancreatic insufficiency. *In* Anderson NV, ed. Veterinary Gastroenterology, Philadelphia, Lea & Febiger, 1992, pp. 283–294.)

tion due to persistent cobalamin deficiency may be a contributory factor in those cases with suboptimal response to enzyme replacement therapy. Cobalamin deficiency might also be responsible for the anorexia reported in a minority of dogs with EPI[382] because anorexia is the major clinical sign noted in inherited selective cobalamin deficiency in the dog.[383]

Serum folate concentrations are often increased in dogs with EPI both before and after treatment (Figure 20–16).[296,329,373,379] Intraluminal bacteria commonly synthesize and release folate, and overgrowth of such bacteria in the proximal small intestine may elevate serum concentrations of this vitamin.[384] Bacterial overgrowth is common in dogs with EPI and because it does not resolve in response to enzyme therapy, this may explain the persistent elevations of serum folate seen in some dogs. Alternatively, folate absorption may be promoted due to decreased duodenal pH occurring as a result of reduced pancreatic bicarbonate secretion.[385] This is perhaps a less likely explanation, however, because pancreatic bicarbonate secretion is relatively well preserved in canine PAA and the duodenum itself has significant ability to neutralize acid.[34,290] The elevations of serum folate associated with canine EPI are probably of no functional significance.

Serum tocopherol (vitamin E) concentrations are often severely subnormal in canine EPI,[386] which is not surprising given the severe fat malabsorption that occurs. Overgrowth of small intestinal bacteria may contribute to deficiencies of fat soluble vitamins by deconjugating bile acids and exacerbating fat malabsorption. Serum tocopherol concentrations do not increase in response to treatment (Figure 20–16),[386] perhaps because treatment does not return fat absorption to normal or because intraluminal bacterial overgrowth persists.[344,387]

Tocopherol deficiency decreases the proliferative response of canine lymphocytes to mitogenic stimulants and if this reflects an in vivo defect in immune function, tocopherol deficiency may be an additional factor predisposing to overgrowth of intestinal bacteria in dogs with EPI. Tocopherol deficiency may cause pathologic change in erythrocyte membranes, smooth muscle, central nervous system, skeletal muscle, and retina,[388–393] and although not yet reported similar changes may accompany chronic untreated tocopherol deficiency in dogs with EPI.

Subnormal serum concentrations of vitamin A have also been observed in dogs with EPI, but no associated signs of deficiency have been reported.[94] Vitamin K–responsive coagulopathy has been reported in a cat with EPI.[302] The potential for selective chronic nutrient deficiencies in canine and feline EPI deserves further investigation.

DIAGNOSIS

History

Animals with EPI usually have a history of weight loss in the face of a normal or increased appetite. Polyphagia is often severe and owners may complain that dogs ravenously devour all food offered to them as well as scavenge from waste bins. This is by no means always the case, however, and some dogs may even have periods of inappetence. Coprophagia and pica are also common, probably as manifestations of polyphagia, but also perhaps as a consequence of specific nutritional deficiencies. Water intake may also increase in some dogs, and in chronic pancreatitis there may be polyuria and polydipsia due to diabetes mellitus.[94,103,164,262–264,266,291,368,378,382,394]

Diarrhea often accompanies EPI, but can be very variable in character. Most owners report frequent passage of large volumes of semiformed feces, although some patients have intermittent or continuous explosive watery diarrhea; in other instances, diarrhea is infrequent and not considered a problem. Diarrhea generally improves or resolves in response to fasting. Introduction of a low-fat diet may also decrease or eliminate diarrhea. There may be a history of vomiting, and commonly there is marked borborygmus and flatulence. Owners sometimes report the affected dogs appear to be suffering from episodes of abdominal discomfort.[94,103,164,262–266,288,290,291,368,382,395]

In some dogs there has been a protracted history of gastrointestinal disturbances prior to the final diagnosis of EPI, the significance of which is not clear, but may merely represent initial failure to diagnose EPI.[264,368] Unless signs of vomiting, diarrhea, borborygmus, or flatulence are severe many owners may not seek veterinary advice until weight loss is marked, and even when animals are presented early, the diagnosis may be missed because the classic signs have not yet appeared. Appropriate testing in such early cases will allow the diagnosis of EPI to be made before severe deterioration of body condition occurs.

Pancreatic acinar atrophy is very prevalent in young German shepherd dogs; thus, EPI is often initially suspected because of the age and breed of the affected dog.[296] It must be emphasized, however, that even in young German shepherd dogs small intestinal disease is more prevalent that EPI, and PAA may occur in a wide variety of breeds at any age.[295,296] Chronic pancreatitis is probably more common in older dogs, but the true prevalence of EPI due to chronic pancreatitis is not known. Whatever the underlying pathology, results based on radioimmunoassay of serum trypsin-like immunoreactivity indicate that in the United States numerous breeds are affected, and only approximately 40% are German shepherd dogs.[295]

Clinical Signs

Mild to marked weight loss is usually seen in association with EPI. Some dogs are very emaciated at presentation with severe muscle wasting and no palpable body fat, and in extreme cases dogs may be physically weak owing to loss of muscle mass. The hair coat is often in poor condition and some animals may give off a foul odor because of soiling of the coat with fatty fecal material and passage of excessive flatus.[94,103,164,262–266,288,290,291,368,382,396] Greasy soiling of the haircoat is particularly noticeable in cats when steatorrhea is marked.[280]

Diagnosis

The history and clinical signs of EPI are nonspecific, vary in severity, and do not distinguish the condition from other causes of malabsorption. Although replacement therapy with oral pancreatic enzymes is generally successful, response to treatment is not a reliable diagnostic approach. Not all dogs with EPI respond to treatment, and dogs with self-limiting small intestinal disease might improve spontaneously, giving the false impression of a response to enzyme supplementation. Furthermore, veterinarians often advise a change in diet when treating dogs with EPI, and this in itself can lead to clinical improvement in some dogs with small intestinal disease. It also appears that pancreatic extracts might have a favorable effect in the treatment of malabsorption due to causes other than EPI.[397]

In dogs with PAA, extreme atrophy of the pancreas is readily observed on gross inspection at either exploratory laparotomy or laparoscopy. In dogs with chronic pancreatitis it may be impossible to gauge accurately the amount of residual exocrine pancreatic tissue because of severe adhesions and fibrosis. These procedures involve unnecessary anesthetic and surgical risks and their use for diagnostic purposes cannot be recommended given the availability of reliable noninvasive tests.

Pancreatic juice secreted into the gut lumen can be collected following peroral intubation of the canine duodenum, and the enzyme activity of this intestinal juice can then be assayed in vitro.[290] This technique has been used to investigate secretion of pancreatic amylase and bicarbonate by dogs with EPI in response to stimulation with exogenous secretin and cholecystokinin. The value of this test as a diagnostic aid has not been assessed;[290] moreover, obvious technical difficulties would limit whatever clinical application it might have.

Routine laboratory test results are generally not helpful in establishing the diagnosis of EPI. Serum alanine aminotransferase levels are mildly to moderately increased and may reflect hepatocyte damage secondary to increased uptake of hepatotoxic substances through an abnormally permeable small intestinal mucosa.[264,290,398] Other routine serum biochemical test results are unremarkable, except that total lipid, cholesterol, and polyunsaturated fatty acid concentrations are often reduced.[264,290,395] Dogs with EPI display a remarkable ability to maintain normal serum protein concentrations even when severely malnourished. Mild lymphopenia and eosinophilia are occasionally seen in dogs with EPI, but complete blood count results are usually within normal lim-

its, and major abnormalities should be perused as evidence of additional or alternative underlying disorders.[368,395]

Canine serum amylase, isoamylases, lipase, and phospholipase A_2 activities are generally normal or only slightly reduced in EPI, and these tests are not useful in the identification of affected dogs.[204,290,395,399] Nonpancreatic sources of these enzymes are clearly present in dogs, and although their activities may increase in inflammatory disease of the pancreas, they do not decrease proportionately as the mass of functional exocrine pancreatic tissue declines.[203,206,290]

Many laboratory tests for the diagnosis of EPI have been described, but their sensitivities and specificities are often highly questionable (see Chapter 6). The most reliable and widely used tests currently available are assay of serum trypsinlike immunoreactivity and assay of fecal proteolytic activity using a casein- or albumin-based substrate.

Serum Trypsin-like Immunoreactivity (TLI)

Trypsinogen is synthesized exclusively by the pancreas, and measurement of the serum concentration of this zymogen by species-specific radioimmunoassay (Canine TLI Assay, Diagnostic Products Corporation, 5700 West 96th Street, Los Angeles, CA 90045) provides a good indirect index of pancreatic function in the dog.[400] This immunoassay detects both trypsinogen and trypsin, hence the use of the term *trypsin-like immunoreactivity* to describe the total concentration of two immunoreactive species. Serum TLI concentration is both highly sensitive and specific for the diagnosis of canine EPI. Concentrations are dramatically reduced in dogs with EPI whereas those in dogs with small intestinal disease are not significantly different from normal (Figure 20–17).[400,401] Marked reductions in serum TLI (to less than 2 µg/L) may even precede signs of weight loss or diarrhea, at a time when results of other tests (fecal proteolytic activity, bentiromide absorption) are still within the control ranges (Figure 20–18).[297,305,401]

Utilization of this test is simple in that analysis of a single serum sample obtained after food has been withheld for several hours is all that is required. Serum TLI is very stable and samples can therefore be mailed to an appropriate laboratory of analysis. Other aspects of this test for canine EPI are discussed in detail in Chapter 6. A specific radioimmunoassay for feline TLI has recently been developed (Feline TLI assay available from Dr. David A. Williams, GI Lab-1248 Lynn Hall, Purdue University, West Lafayette, IN 47907-1248. Tel. (317) 494-0339, Fax (317) 496-1796).[216] Preliminary investigations have shown that there is no cross-reactivity between canine and feline TLI, normal serum TLI values in cats are greater than those in dogs, and serum TLI is subnormal in cats with EPI.[216, 401a]

Fecal Proteolytic Activity

Fecal proteolytic activity can be measured precisely using dyed protein substrates such as azocasein,[264,402] or by radial enzyme diffusion into agar gels containing casein substrate (Figure 6–7).[403,404] Fecal proteolytic activity as assessed by these methods is consistently low in most dogs and cats with EPI, but because both dogs and cats with normal pancreatic function occasionally pass feces with low proteolytic activity, either repeated determinations must be made (Figure 6–8),[264,301,397,402] or, in dogs, the test can be performed on a single sample collected after feeding crude soybean meal for 2 days.[400,404,405] Some dogs with EPI have normal fecal prote-

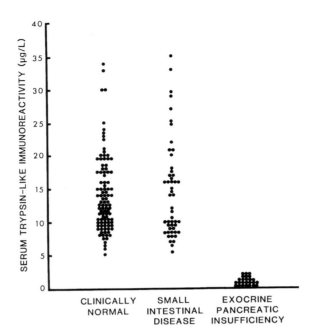

FIGURE 20–17. Serum trypsin-like immunoreactivity in 100 healthy dogs, 50 dogs with small intestinal disease and 25 dogs with exocrine pancreatic insufficiency. (From Williams DA and Batt RM: Sensitivity and specificity of radioimmunoassay of serum trypsin-like immunoreactivity for the diagnosis of canine exocrine pancreatic insufficiency. JAVMA 192:195–201, 1988.)

olytic activity as assessed by this assay, but this is rare;[400,401] it is likely that a similar situation exists in cats. Other aspects of this approach to diagnosis of EPI are discussed in Chapter 6.

Other Tests

Other tests used for diagnosis of EPI include the bentiromide test,[302,311,312,395,400,401,406–412] assay of fecal proteolytic activity using gelatin digestion, plasma turbidity after oral fat administration,[413] and microscopic examination of feces.[402,407] These tests are either relatively impractical or give significant proportions of false negative and false positive results (see Chapter 6); their use even as crude screening tests is not recommended.

TREATMENT

Enzyme Replacement

Most dogs and cats with EPI can be managed successfully by supplementing each meal with pancreatic enzymes present in commercially available dried pancreatic extracts.[414] Numerous formulations of these extracts are available (tablets, capsules, powders, granules) and their enzyme contents and bioavailabilities vary widely.[414–420] Addition of 2 teaspoons of powdered pancreatic extract per 20 kg of body weight to each meal is generally an effective starting dose. This can be mixed with a maintenance dog food immediately prior to feeding. Two meals a day are usually sufficient to promote weight gain. Dogs will generally gain 0.5 to 1.0 kg per week, and diarrhea and other clinical signs such as polyphagia and coprophagia often resolve within 4 to 5 days.

As soon as clinical improvement is apparent, owners can determine a minimum effective dose of enzyme supplement that prevents return of clinical signs. This varies slightly between batches of extract, and also from dog to dog, probably reflecting individual variation in extrapancreatic digestive reserve. Most affected dogs require at least 1 teaspoonful of enzyme supplement per meal, but lower doses may be adequate in cats and small dogs. One meal per day is sufficient in some dogs; others continue to require two. Commercial dried pancreatic extracts are expensive, and when available, substitution of 3 to 4 ounces per 20 kg of body weight of chopped raw ox or pig pancreas obtained from animals certified as healthy following appropriate postmortem inspection is a more economical alternative.[421] Pan-

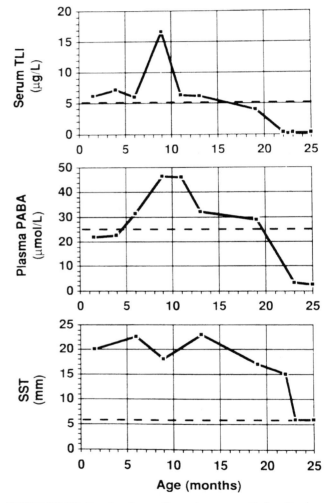

FIGURE 20–18. Results of tests of exocrine pancreatic function in a German shepherd dog between 6 weeks and 25 months of age. The dog developed clinical signs of EPI at 2 years of age. Data indicate preprandial serum trypsinlike immunoreactivity (TLI) concentration, 1-hour plasma p-amino benzoic acid concentration (PABA) after oral administration of bentiromide, and fecal proteolytic activity after soybean stimulation testing (SST) measured by radial enzyme diffusion. Dotted lines define the lower limit of control values in healthy dogs established for the TLI and bentiromide tests, and the diameter of the well that represents no activity in the SST. (Reproduced from Westermarck E, et al: Sequential study of pancreatic structure and function during development of pancreatic acinar atrophy in a German shepherd dog. Am J Vet Res 54:1088–1094, 1993.)

creas can be stored frozen at –20° C for at least 3 months without loss of enzyme activity.

Measures to Increase the Effectiveness of Enzyme Supplementation

Although administration of pancreatic enzymes with food is generally successful, only a small proportion of the oral dose of each enzyme, particularly of lipase, is delivered functionally intact to the small intestine, and fat absorption does not return to normal.[387,414–416,422,423] Pancreatic lipase is rapidly inactivated at the acid pH encountered in the stomach; trypsin and some other pancreatic proteases, although relatively acid resistant, are susceptible to degradation by gastric pepsins.[422] In human beings only 35% of trypsin and 17% of lipase ingested with a meal can be recovered intact from the duodenum.[420] Numerous attempts have been made to increase the effectiveness of enzyme supplementation. These include preincubation of enzymes with food prior to feeding, supplementation with bile salts, neutralization or inhibition of secretion of gastric acid, and use of enteric-coated preparations.[387,423,424]

Preincubation of food with enzyme powder for 30 minutes prior to feeding does not improve the effectiveness of oral enzyme treatment in promoting fat absorption in dogs with ligated pancreas ducts.[387] This is not surprising because optimal lipase activity will not be achieved unless the enzyme is in solution at the appropriate pH and temperature and in the presence of appropriate concentration of colipase and bile acids, conditions unlikely to be encountered in the feeding bowl.

Supplementation with oral bile salts has been investigated as a means of enhancing fat digestion and absorption in dogs with EPI.[387] There is no evidence, however, that intraluminal bile concentrations are subnormal in patients with EPI, and addition of bile salts to enzyme supplements does not improve fat absorption in dogs with ligated pancreatic ducts.[387] Precipitation of bile salts in individuals with abnormally low small intestinal pH may cause steatorrhea due to functional bile salt deficiency; however, supplementation with oral bile salts will not rectify such a situation.[425] In any case, drastic reductions in duodenal pH in canine EPI are unlikely, so functional bile salt deficiency is probably of no importance.

Gastric acid secretion may be reduced by administration of H_2-receptor antagonists. Cimetidine at a dosage of 300 mg/20 kg body weight given with food mixed with pancreatic enzymes does improve fat absorption in dogs with ligated pancreatic ducts, but does not decrease fecal wet or dry weight.[387] The routine use of H_2 blockers in the treatment of EPI cannot be recommended given the expense of the drug and the fact that so many patients respond well when treated with enzymes alone.[387] Oral antacids such as sodium bicarbonate or aluminum or magnesium hydroxide are inexpensive but do not increase the effectiveness of enzyme therapy either in experimental canine EPI or in human patients with chronic pancreatitis.[233,428] Indeed, it is possible that the use of antacids may be detrimental because although they may increase the quantity of pancreatic lipase reaching the small intestine, they may also inhibit gastric lipase activity.[166,426] The latter probably accounts for the considerable residual fat absorption in dogs with EPI.[6,272,427,428]

Enteric-coated preparations have been formulated in an attempt to protect orally administered enzymes from gastric acid.[414,419,422,423] In humans these preparations have generally proved to be no more effective than nonenteric-coated extracts.[420] A survey of canine patients with EPI showed enteric-coated preparations are often actually ineffective or less effective than powdered pancreatic extract.[296] This may reflect selective retention of enteric-coated particles in the stomach, or perhaps rapid intestinal transit preventing adequate enzyme release in the upper small intestine.[419,423] Similar mechanisms may explain the ineffectiveness of an uncrushed tablet formulation of pancreatic enzymes; in contrast, the same formulation was effective when crushed prior to feeding.[387] Although they are not commercially available, it is possible to formulate sustained-release preparations of pancreatic extracts that release enzymes for a prolonged period of time in a site that is favorable for their function in the dog.[429]

It is possible that in the future enzyme preparations containing acid-resistant fungal lipase may prove to be useful. An experimental study in dogs showed such a preparation to be effective.[430] Whether this or any other method of increasing enzyme delivery to the small intestine will benefit those dogs with suboptimal weight gain remains to be seen. Such animals usually do not improve after either increasing the dose of enzymes above 2 teaspoonfuls per meal or giving cimetidine, suggesting that factors other than enzyme delivery to the small intestine are involved.[20]

Dietary Modification

Clinical studies in humans and experimental studies in the dog show that fat absorption does not return to normal despite appropriate enzyme therapy.[166,387,420,423] Dogs appear to compensate by eating slightly more than usual, and as with any individual dog, it is necessary to regulate the amount of food given in order to maintain ideal body weight.

In order to overcome residual digestive deficits, the feeding of a highly digestible low-fiber diet has been advocated.[431] A nonblinded clinical study found that owners considered that their dogs generally did better (reduced flatulence and borborymi, decreased fecal volume and frequency of defecation) when fed a commercial highly digestible diet compared to previously fed home-cooked or regular maintenance diets, but there was no difference in appetite, drinking, color or consistency of feces, or in coprophagy.[432] Results of experimental studies to evaluate highly digestible diets have shown consistent reductions in fecal weight, but have not shown consistent benefit with regard to fat digestibility, probably because different studies were not comparable with regard to variables such as feeding patterns and the use of gastric acid modifiers that might affect digestibilities of different diets.[166,379] Dietary fiber does impair pancreatic enzyme activity in vitro, and high-fiber diets probably should be avoided.[433,434] Highly digestible diets may be of value in promoting caloric uptake in those dogs with EPI that do not regain normal body weight. These patients may also benefit from addition of medium chain triglycerides to the food. Some medium chain triglycerides are absorbed intact, and they are hydrolyzed more readily by gastric lipase than are long chain triglycerides,[422] their absorption is not completely independent of pancreatic enzymes, however, and they are probably not as well absorbed in EPI as commonly accepted.[435]

Vitamin Supplementation

Dogs and cats with EPI may have severely subnormal concentrations of serum cobalamin and tocopherol.[401a] Serum levels of these vitamins do not necessarily increase in response to treatment with oral pancreatic enzymes, even when the clinical response is otherwise excellent.[329,378,386] Clinical signs associated with naturally occurring deficiencies of these vitamins in the dog have not been well documented, but intestinal mucosal changes, myopathy, myelopathy, and other abnormalities of nervous tissue have been reported in other species. It therefore seems prudent to supplement with these vitamins if serum concentrations are subnormal. In the author's experience, supplementation with large oral doses of tocopherol (400–500 IU/20 kg body weight given once daily with food for 1 month) is effective in returning serum concentrations to normal. In contrast, cobalamin must be given parenterally (100–250 μg by intramuscular or subcutaneous injection once a week for several weeks) to normalize serum concentrations. Long-term monitoring of serum cobalamin concentration (every 12 months) is probably warranted in canine and feline patients with EPI.

Malabsorption of vitamin A has also been demonstrated in association with EPI[94] and one case of vitamin K responsive coagulopathy has been reported.[302] Malabsorption of fat soluble vitamins is to be expected even after treatment in view of the failure of pancreatic replacement therapy to return fat absorption to normal. Malabsorption of vitamins A, D, and K may not be as marked as malabsorption of tocopherol because the latter appears to be particularly sensitive to abnormalities in the intestinal lumen.[436] It should be noted that doses of individual vitamins in multivitamin preparations may be insufficient to normalize serum concentrations and that parenteral or very high oral doses may be required for adequate supplementation

Antibiotic Therapy

Dogs with PAA commonly have overgrowth of bacteria in the small intestine, but in most cases this is a subclinical abnormality and affected individuals respond very well to treatment with oral enzyme replacement alone even though the overgrowth often persists.[17,344,379] Bacterial overgrowth can cause malabsorption and diarrhea, however, and in those individuals that do not respond to oral enzyme supplementation alone, antibiotic therapy may be of value.[17] Oral oxytetracycline, metronidazole, or tylosin may be effective in improving the clinical response in some of these dogs.[17,344] Chronic untreated bacterial overgrowth may cause mucosal damage that is only partially reversible following even prolonged antibiotic therapy,[437] which may explain why some dogs fail to return to normal body weight. It is not clear if a predisposition to recurrent development of overgrowth exists following antibiotic therapy.

Glucocorticoid Therapy

In those few patients that respond poorly to the treatments just outlined, oral prednisolone (or prednisone) at an initial dosage of 1 to 2 mg/kg q 12 hours for 7 to 14 days is usually beneficial.[378] This may be due to resolution of coexisting lymphocytic-plasmacytic gastroenteritis or other effects of glucocorticoids on the gastrointestinal tract.[378,438] Long-term glucocorticoid administrations is generally unnecessary.[378]

PROGNOSIS

The underlying pathologic process leading to EPI is generally irreversible, and lifelong treatment is required. Nonetheless, given the expense of treatment it is reasonable to withdraw enzyme supplement for a trial period every 6 months or so and observe the patient for recurrence of clinical signs. Pancreatic acinar tissue does have some capacity to regenerate[102] and it is not inconceivable that following either pancreatitis or subtotal PAA, residual acinar tissue might regenerate sufficiently to normalize digestive function. Possible recoveries from clinically significant enzyme deficiency have been reported.[306] Provocative withdrawal of treatment seems particularly advisable in those patients with consistently borderline diagnostic pancreatic function test results or in those patients in which chronic relapsing pancreatitis is suspected. In most cases treatment will be required for life, but provided owners are willing to accept the cost of enzyme replacement, the prognosis is generally good.[296] Some dogs may fail to regain normal body weight, but these animals usually have total resolution of diarrhea and polyphagia and are quite acceptable as pets. A high prevalence of mesenteric torsion has been reported in German shepherd dogs with PAA in Finland,[439] but this has not been documented elsewhere.

Treatment of patients with diabetes mellitus and EPI due to chronic pancreatitis is likely to be troublesome and expensive. Diabetes mellitus secondary to chronic pancreatitis is potentially more difficult to regulate than simple diabetes in view of probable coexisting derangements in the secretion of glucagon and somatostatin. Moreover, anorexia and vomiting due to pancreatitis may further complicate treatment of diabetes mellitus.

NEOPLASIA OF THE EXOCRINE PANCREAS

Pancreatic adenocarcinomas may be acinar or duct cell in origin, but both are uncommon and they are particularly rare in cats. In both species they are seen in older animals. Pancreatic carcinoma may be more common in Airedale terriers than other breeds.[28,394,440–442]

Adenocarcinomas are usually highly malignant tumors, and have often metastasized to the duodenal wall, liver, and local lymph nodes, or less commonly to the lungs, at the time of presentation. Clinical signs are usually nonspecific: weight loss, anorexia, depression, and vomiting. Affected animals are often icteric due to associated obstruction of the bile ducts or widespread hepatic metastasis. Occasionally dogs will present with characteristic signs of diabetes mellitus or EPI due to obstruction of the pancreatic ducts or beta cell destruction.[200,267,440]

Abdominal tenderness due to associated pancreatitis may be present, and occasionally an anterior abdominal mass is palpable. Abdominal radiographs may suggest pancreatitis or indicate the presence of an anterior mass; thoracic radiographs may reveal pulmonary metastasis. Ultrasonographic examination may help further define pancreatic abnormalities, and cytologic examination of abdominal fluid or of material aspirated from suspect areas may reveal neoplastic cells.

There are no specific laboratory tests for pancreatic carcinoma, and results of routine tests may be misleading. Instead serum and lipase activities are seen in some dogs. Serum alkaline phosphatase and bilirubin, and to a lesser extent alanine aminotransferase, are elevated in some cases possibly reflecting an associated obstructive hepatopathy.[200,440] In most cases definitive diagnosis requires exploratory laparotomy. It is important to biopsy abnormal pancreatic tissue because chronic pancreatitis may grossly resemble pancreatic carcinoma.

Given the frequency of metastasis at the time of diagnosis, the prognosis for animals with carcinomas of the exocrine pancreas is extremely poor;[226] survival for more than a year after diagnosis has not been reported. Surgical excision of localized lesions, perhaps in combination with chemotherapy or radiation therapy, may be palliative.[226] Therapy with insulin and pancreatic enzymes may be required to treat associated diabetes mellitus and EPI.[267,440]

PANCREATIC FLUKES IN CATS

There are several reports of infection with the pancreatic fluke, *Eurytrema procyonis,* in domestic cats.[443–446] Associated pathology generally includes pancreatic atrophy and fibrosis, which may result in decreased exocrine pancreatic secretory capacity. In spite of marked loss of exocrine tissue, however, the infection is usually subclinical and is often diagnosed as an incidental finding based on observation of characteristic eggs in the feces. There is one report, however, of an infected cat with a 2 year history of weight loss and intermittent vomiting, consistent with pancreatitis perhaps progressing to clinical EPI. This cat had marked pancreatic inflammation in association with the parasites. Treatment with fenbendazole has been reported to be effective.[445]

REFERENCES

1. Bernard C. Memoir on the Pancreas and on the Role of Pancreatic Juice in Digestive Processes. Particularly in the Digestion of Neutral Fat (Henderson J, trans.). Monographs or the Physiological Society No. 42. Academic Press, New York, 1985.
2. Case RM, Argent BE. Pancreatic duct cell secretion: Control and mechanisms of transport. In: Go VLW, DiMagno EP, Gardner JD, et al. (eds) The Pancreas: Biology, Pathobiology and Disease. Raven Press, New York, 301–350, 1993.
3. Borgstrom B. Relative colipase deficiency as a cause of fat malabsorption in humans and the importance of the law of mass action for clinical medicine. Gastroenterology 86:194–204, 1984.
4. Erlanson-Albertsson C. Pancreatic colipase. Structural and physiological aspects. Biochim Biophys Acta Lipid Metab 1125:1–7, 1992.
5. Van Tilbeurgh H, Sarda L, Verger R, et al. Structure of the pancreatic lipase-procolipase complex. Nature 359:159–162, 1992.
6. Borgstöm B. Luminal digestion of fats. In: Go VLW, DiMagno EP, Gardner JD, et al. (eds) The Pancreas: Biology, Pathobiology and Disease. Raven Press, New York, 475–488, 1993.
7. Herzlich B, Herbert V. The role of the pancreas in cobalamin (vitamin B₁₂) absorption. Am J Gastroenterol 79:489–493, 1984.
8. Abels Muckerheide MM. Absorption of vitamin B₁₂ in dogs. Clin Res 18:530, 1970.
9. Abels J, Muckerheide MM, Van Kapel J, et al. A dual role for the dog pancreas in the absorption of vitamin B₁₂. Program American Society of Hematology, 17th Meeting, Atlanta, 951–974.
10. Horadagoda NU, Batt RM, Vaillant, C, et al. Identification and characterization of a pancreatic intrinsic factor in the dog. Gastroenterology 90:1464, 1986.
11. Batt RM, Horadagoda NU, McLean L, et al. Identification and characterization of a pancreatic intrinsic factor in the dog. Am J Physiol 256:G517–G523, 1989.
12. Evans GW, Grace CI, Votava HJ. A proposed mechanism for zinc absorption in the rat. Am J Physiol 228:501–505, 1975.
13. Sturniolo GC, D'Incà R, Montino MC, et al. Citric acid corrects zinc absorption deficiency in chronic pancreatitis. J Tr Elem Exp Med 3:267–271, 1990.
14. Rubinstein E, Mark Z, Haspel J, et al. Antibacterial activity of the pancreatic fluid. Gastroenterology 88:927–932, 1985.
15. Alpers DH, Tedesco FJ. The possible role of pancreatic proteases in the turnover of intestinal brush border proteins. Biochim Biophys Acta 401:28–40, 1975.
16. Kwong WKL, Seetharam B, Alpers DH. Effect of exocrine pancreatic insufficency on small intestine in the mouse. Gastroenterology 74:1277–1282, 1978.
17. Williams DA, Batt RM, McLean L. Bacterial overgrowth in the duodenum of dogs with exocrine pancreatic insufficiency. J Am Vet Med Assoc 191:201–206, 1987.
18. Williamson RCN. Intestinal adaptation: Structural, functional and cytokinetic changes. N Engl J Med 298:1393–1402, 1978.
19. Williamson RCN. Intestinal adaptation: Mechanisms of control. N Engl J Med 298:1444–1450, 1978.
20. Williams DA. Exocrine pancreatic disease. In: Ettinger SJ (ed) Textbook of Veterinary Internal Medicine. WB Saunders, Philadelphia, 1528–1544, 1989.
21. Eddeland A, Ohlsson K. Purification of canine pancreatic secretory trypsin inhibitor and interaction in vitro with complexes of trypsin-a-macroglobulin. Scan J Clin Lab Invest 36:815–820, 1976.
22. Laskowski M, Kato I. Protein inhibitors of proteinases. Ann Rev Biochem 49:593–626, 1980.
23. Rinderknecht H. Pancreatic secretory enzymes. In: Go VLW, DiMagno EP, Gardner JD, et al. (eds) The Pancreas: Biology, Pathobiology and Disease. Raven Press, New York, 219–251, 1993.
24. Evans HE, Christensen GC. The digestive apparatus and abdomen. In: Evans HE, Christensen GE (eds) Millers Anatomy of the Dog. WB Saunders, Philadelphia, 411–506, 1979.
25. Schummer A, Nickel R, Sack WO. Digestive System. Springer-Verlag, New York; Heidelberg Berlin, 21–203, 1979.
26. Williams JA, Goldfine ID. The insulin-acinus relationship. In: Go VLE (ed) The Exocrine Pancreas: Biology Pathobiology and Disease. Raven Press, New York, 347–360, 1986.
27. Williams JA, Goldfine ID. The The insulin-acinar relationship. In: Go VLW, DiMagno EP, Gardner JD, (eds) et al. The Pancreas: Biology, Pathobiology and Disease. Raven Press, New York, 789–802, 1993.
28. Jubb KVF, Kennedy PC, Palmer N. The pancreas. In: Jubb KVF, Kennedy PC, Palmer N. (eds) Pathology of Domestic Animals. Harcourt Brace Jovanovich, Orlando, 313–327, 1985.
29. Bockman DE. Anatomy of the pancreas. In: Go VLW, DiMagno EP, Gardner JD, (eds) The Pancreas:Biology, Pathobiology and Disease. Raven Press, New York, 1–8, 1993.
30. Kern HF. Fine structure of the human exocrine pancreas. In: Go VLW, DiMagno EP, Gardner JD, et al. (eds) The Pancreas: Biology, Pathobiology and Disease. Raven Press, New York, 9–19, 1993.
31. Bockman DE. Anastomosing tubular arrangement of dog exocrine pancreas. Cell Tissue Res 189:497–500, 1978.
32. Bonner-Weir S. The microvasculature of the pancreas, with emphasis on that of the islets of Langerhans: Anatomy and functional considerations. In: Go VLW, DiMagno EP, Gardner JD (eds) The Pancreas: Biology, Pathobiology and Disease. Raven Press, New York, 759–768, 1993.
33. Holst JJ. Neural regulation of pancreatic exocrine function. In: Go VLW, DiMagno EP, Gardner JD, et al. (eds) The Pancreas: Biology, Pathobiology and Disease. Raven Press, New York, 381–402, 1993.
34. Dorricott, NJ, Fiddian-Green RG, Silen W. Mechanisms of acid disposal in canine duodenum. Am J Physiol 228:269–275, 1975.
35. Ovesen L, Bendtsen F, Tage-Jensen U, et al. Intraluminal pH in the stomach, duodenum, and proximal jejunum in normal subjects and patients with exocrine pancreatic insufficiency. Gastroenterology 90:958–962, 1986.
36. Scheele GA, Kern HF. Cellular compartmentation, protein processing, and secretion in the exocrine pancreas. In: Go VLW, DiMagno EP, Gardner JD, et al. (eds) The Pancreas: Biology, Pathobiology and Disease. Raven Press, New York, 121–150, 1993.
37. Scheele GA. Biosynthesis, segregation and secretion of exportable proteins by the exocrine pancreas. Am J Physiol 238:G467–G477, 1980.
38. Chey WY. Hormonal control of pancreatic exocrine secretion. In: Go VLW, DiMagno EP, Gardner JD, et al. (eds) The Pancreas: Biology, Pathobiology and Disease. Raven Press, New York, 403–424, 1993.
39. Singer MV. Neurohormonal control of pancreatic enzyme secretion in animals. In: Go VLW, DiMagno EP, Gardner JD, et al. (eds) The Pancreas: Biology, Pathobiology and Disease. Raven Press, New York, 425–448, 1993.
40. Geokas MC, Largman C, Brodrick JW, et al. Molecular forms of immunoreactive pancreatic elastase in canine pancreatic and peripheral blood. Am J Physiol 238:G238–246, 1980.
41. Borgström A. The fate of intravenously injected trypsinogens in dogs. Scand J Gastroenterol 16:281–287, 1981.
42. Geokas MC, Reidelberger R, O'Rourke M, et al. Plasma pancreatic trypsinogens in chronic renal failure and after nephrectomy. Am J Physiol 242:177–182, 1982.
43. Levitt MD, Eckfeldt JH. Diagnosis of acute pancreatitis. In: Go VLW, DiMagno EP, Gardner JD, et al. (eds) The Pancreas: Biology, Pathophysiology and Disease. Raven Press, New York, 613–635, 1993.
44. Levitt MD, Ellis CJ, Murphy SM, et al. Study of the possible enteropancreatic circulation of pancreatic amylase in the dog. Am J Physiol 241:G54–58, 1981.

45. Florholmen J, Vonen B, Burhol PG. The "endocrine" enzyme secretion from the pancreas. Scand J Gastroenterol 21:513–515, 1986.
46. Sarner M. Pancreatitis: Definitions and Classification. In: Go VLW, DiMagno EP, Gardner JD, et al. (eds) The Pancreas: Biology, Pathobiology and Disease. Raven Press, New York, 575–580, 1993.
47. Banks PA. A new classification system for acute pancreatitis. Am J Gastroenterol 89:151–152, 1994.
48. Bradley EL. A clinically based classification system for acute pancreatitis. Arch Surg 128:586–590, 1993.
49. Rutgers HC, Herring DS, Orton EC. Pancreatic pseudocyst associated with acute pancreatitis in a dog: Ultrasonographic diagnosis. J Am Anim Hosp Assoc 21:411–416, 1985.
50. Bellenger CR, Llkiw JE, Malik R. Cystogastrostomy in the treatment of pancreatic pseudocyst/abscess in two dogs. Vet Rec 125:181–184, 1989.
51. Hill RC, Van Winkle TJ. Acute necrotizing pancreatitis and acute suppurative pancreatitis in the cat. A retrospective study of 40 cases (1976–1989). J Vet Int Med 7:25–33, 1993.
52. Schaer M, Holloway S. Diagnosing acute pancreatitis in the cat. Vet Med 1986:782–795, 1991.
53. Kelly DF, Baggot DG, Gaskell CJ. Jaundice in the cat associated with inflammation of the biliary tract and pancreas. J Sm Anim Pract 16:163–172, 1975.
54. Duffell SJ. Some aspects of pancreatic disease in the cat. J Sm Anim Pract 16:365–374, 1975.
55. Steer ML, Meldolesi J. The cell biology of experimental pancreatitis. N Engl J Med 316:144–150, 1987.
56. Steer ML, Saluja AK. Experimental acute pancreatitis: Studies of the early events that lead to cell injury. In: Go VLW, DiMagno EP, Gardner JD, et al. (eds) The Pancreas: Biology, Pathobiology and Disease. Raven Press, New York, 489–500, 1993.
57. Gorelick FS, Adler G, and Kern HF. Cerulein-induced pancreatitis. In: Go VLW, DiMagno EP, Gardner JD, et al. (eds) The Pancreas: Biology, Pathobiology and Disease. Raven Press, New York, 501–526, 1993.
58. Reber HA, Adler G, Karanjia N, et al. Permeability characteristics of the main pancreatic duct in cats: Models of acute and chronic pancreatitis. In: Go VLW, DiMagno EP, Gardner JD, et al. (eds) The Pancreas: Biology, Pathobiology and Disease. Raven Press, New York, 527–550, 1993.
59. Shorrock K, Austen BM, Hermon-Taylor J. Hyperstimulation pancreatitis in mice induced by cholecystokinin octapeptide, caerulein, and novel analogues: Effect of molecular structure on potency. Pancreas 6:40–406, 1991.
60. Simpson KW. Current concepts of the pathogenesis and pathophysiology of acute pancreatitis in the dog and cat. Comp Cont Ed Prac Vet 15:247–253, 1993.
61. Rinderknecht H. Activation of pancreatic zymogens. Normal activation, premature intrapancreatic activation, protective mechanisms against inappropriate activation. Dig Dis Sci 31:314–321, 1986.
62. Steer ML, Meldolesi J, Figarella C. Pancreatitis, the role of lysosomes. Dig Dis Sci 29:934–938, 1984.
63. Sanfey H, Bulkley GB, Cameron JL. The role of oxygen-derived free radicals in the pathogenesis of acute pancreatitis. Ann Surg 200:405–413, 1984.
64. Sanfey H, Cameron JL. Increased capillary permeability—an early lesion in acute pancreatitis. Surgery 96:485–491, 1984.
65. Sanfey H, Bulkley GB, Cameron JL. The pathogenesis of acute pancreatitis: The source and role of oxygen-derived free radicals in three different experimental models. Ann Surg 201:633–639, 1985.
66. Niederau C, Schultz, HU, Letko G. Involvement of free radicals in the pathophysiology of chronic pancreatitis: Potential of treatment with antioxidant and scavenger substances. Klin Wochenschr 69:1018–1024, 1991.
67. Schoenberg MH, Büchler M, Beger HG. The role of oxygen radicals in experimental acute pancreatitis. Free Rad Biol Med 12:515–522, 1992.
68. Pitchumoni CS, Scheele GA. Interdependence of nutrition and exocrine pancreatic function. In: Go VLW, DiMagno EP, Gardner JD, et al. (eds) The Pancreas: Biology, Pathobiology and Disease. Raven Press, New York, 449–473, 1993.
69. Borgström A, Ohlsson K. Immunoreactive trypsins in sera from dogs before and after induction of experimental pancreatitis. Hoppe-Seylers Z Physiol Chem 361:625–631, 1980.
70. Brodrick JW, Geokas MC, Largman C, et al. Molecular forms of immunoreactive pancreatic cationic trypsin in pancreatitis patient sera. Am J Physiol 237:E474–E480, 1979.
71. Borgström A, Lasson Å. Trypsin-alpha1-protease inhibitor complexes in serum and clinical course of acute pancreatitis. Scand J Gastroenterol 19:1119–1122, 1984.
72. Geokas MC, Largman C, Durie PR, et al. Immunoreactive forms of cationic trypsin in plasma and ascitic fluid of dogs with experimental pancreatitis. Am J Pathol 105:31–39, 1981.
73. Durie PR, Gaskin KJ, Ogilvie JE, et al. Serial alterations in the forms of immunoreactive pancreatic cationic trypsin in plasma from patients with acute pancreatitis. J Pediatr Gastroenterol Nutr 4:199–207, 1985.
74. Ohlsson K, Ganrot PO, Laurell CB. In vivo interaction between trypsin and some plasma proteins in relation to tolerance to intravenous infusion of trypsin in dogs. Acta Chir Scand 137:113–121, 1971.
75. Kwaan HC, Anderson MC, Gramatica L. A study of pancreatic enzymes as a factor in the pathogenesis of disseminated intravascular coagulation during acute pancreatitis. Surgery 69:663–672, 1970.
76. Nevalainen TJ. The role of phospholipase A in acute pancreatitis. Scand J Gastroenterol 15: 641–650, 1980.
77. Geokas MC, Rinderknecht H, Swanson V, et al. The role of elastase in acute hemorrhagic pancreatitis in man. Lab Invest 19:235–239, 1968.
78. Lungarella G, Gardi C, De Santi MM, et al. Pulmonary vascular injury in pancreatitis: Evidence for a major role played by pancreatic elastase. Exp Mol Pathol 42:44–59, 1985.
79. Izquierdo R, Sandberg L, Nora MO, et al. Comparative study of protease inhibitors on coagulation abnormalities in canine pancreatitis. J Surg Res 36:606–613, 1984.
80. Lasson Å. Acute pancreatitis in man. A clinical and biochemical study of pathophysiology and treatment. Scand J Gastroenterol suppl 99:1–57, 1984.
81. Lasson Å, Ohlsson K. Acute pancreatitis. The correlation between clinical course, protease inhibitors, and complement and kinin activation. Scand J Gastroenterol 19:707–710, 1984
82. Lasson Å, Ohlsson K. Protease inhibitors in acute human pancreatitis. Correlation between biochemical changes and clinical course. Scand J Gastroenterol 19:779–786, 1984.
83. Largman C, Reidelberger RD, Tsukamoto H. Correlation of trypsin-plasma inhibitor complexes with mortality in experimental pancreatitis in rats. Dig Dis Sci 31:961–969, 1986.
84. Kornegay JN. Hypocalcemia in dogs. Comp Cont Ed Prac Vet 4:103–112,1982.
85. Gudgeon AM, Heath DI. Hurley P. et al. Trypsinogen activation peptide assay in the early prediction of severity of acute pancreatitis. Lancet 335:4, 1990.
86. Schmidt J, Fernandez-Del Castillo C, Rattner DW, et al. Trypsinogen-activation peptides in experimental rat pancreatitis: Prognostic implications and histopathologic correlates. Gastroenterology 103:1009–1016,1992
87. Borth W. a_2-macroglobulin, a multifunctional binding protein with targeting characteristics. FASEB J 6:3345–3353,1992.
88. Adham NF, Song MK, Haberfelde GC. Relationship between the functional status of the reticuloendothelial system and the outcome of experimentally induced pancreatitis in young mice. Gastroenterology 84:461–469, 1983.
89. Adham NF, Song MK, Scott S, et al. The effect of reticuloendothelial system (RES) stimulation on the outcome of bile-induced pancreatitis in dogs. Gastroenterology 84:1088, 1983.
90. Weiss SJ. Tissue destruction by neutrophils. N Engl J. Med 320:365–176, 1989.
91. Cook AK, Breitschwerdt EB, Levine JF, et al. Risk factors associated with acute pancreatitis in dogs: 101 cases (1985–1990). J Am Vet Med Assoc 203:673–679, 1993.
92. Steer ML. Etiology and pathophysiology of acute pancreatitis. In Go VLW, DiMagno EP, Gardner JD, et al. (eds) The Pancreas: Biology, Pathobiology and Disease. Raven Press, New York, 581–591 1993.
93. Leach SD, Gorelick FS, Modlin IM. New perspectives on acute pancreatitis. Scand J Gastroenterol 27 (suppl) 192:29–38, 1992,
94. Coffin DL, Thordal-Christensen A. The clinical and some pathological aspects of pancreatic disease in dogs. Vet Med 48:193–198, 1953.
95. Haig THB: Cellular membranes in the etiology of acute pancreatitis. Surg Forum 20:380–382, 1969.
96. Haig THB: Pancreatic digestive enzymes: Influence of a diet that augments pancreatitis. J Surg Res 10:601–607, 1970.
97. Goodhead B. Importance of nutrition in the pathogenesis of experimental pancreatitis in the dog. Arch Surg 103:724–727, 1971.
98. Lindsay S, Entenmann C, Chaikoff IL. Pancreatitis accompanying hepatic disease in dogs fed a high fat, low protein diet. Arch Path 45:635–638, 1948.
99. Lombardi B, Estes LW, Longnecker DS. Acute hemorrhagic pancreatitis (massive necrosis) with fat necrosis induced in mice by DL-ethionine fed with a choline-deficient diet. Am J Pathol 79:465–480, 1975.
100. Koike H, Steer ML, Meldolesi J. Pancreatic effects of ethionine: Blockade of exocytosis and appearence of crinophagy and autophagy precede celluar necrosis. Am J Physiol 242:G297–G307, 1982.
101. Lopes de Almeida A, Grossman M. Experimental production of pancreatitis with ethionine. Gastroenterology, 20:544–577,1952.
102. Walker NI, Winterford CM, Williamson RM, et al. Ethionine-induced atrophy of rat pancreas involves apoptosis of acinar cells. Pancreas 8:443–449, 1993.
103. Anderson NV, Strafuss AC. Pancreatic disease in dogs and cats. J Am Vet Med Assoc 159:885–891, 1971.
104. Guzman S, Nervi F, Llanos O, et al. Impaired lipid clearance in patients with previous acute pancreatitis. Gut 26:888–891, 1985.
105. Rogers WA, Donovan EF, Kociba GJ. Idiopathic hyperlipoproteinemia in dogs. J Am Vet Med Assoc 166:1087–1091, 1975.

106. Saharia P, Margolis S, Zuidema GD, et al. Acute pancreatitis with hyperlipidemia: Studies with an isolated perfused canine pancreas. Surgery 82:60–67, 1977

107. Cameron JL, Capuzzi DM, Zuidema GD, et al. Acute pancreatitis with hyperlipemia. Evidence for a persistent defect in lipid metabolism. Am J Med 56:482–487, 1974.

108. Mallory A, Kern F. Drug-induced pancreatitis: A critical review. Gastroenterology 78:813–820, 1980.

109. Hansen JF, Carpenter RH. Fatal acute systemic anaphylaxis and hemorrhagic pancreatitis following asparaginase treatment in a dog. J Am Anim Hosp Assoc 19:977–980, 1983.

110. Moriello KA, Bowen D, Meyer DJ. Acute pancreatitis in two dogs given azathioprine and prednisone. J Am Vet Met Assoc 191(6):695–670, 1987.

111. Morrison WB. Pancreatitis associated with cytotoxic drug administration. In: Morrison WB (ed) Proceedings of the Tenth Annual Veterinary Medical Forum of the ACVIM, San Diego, 632–633, 1992.

112. Scarpelli DG. Toxicology of the pancreas. Tox App Pharm 101:543–554, 1989.

113. Moore RW, Withrow SJ. Gastrointestinal hemorrhage and pancreatitis associated with intervertebral disk disease in the dog. J Am Vet Med Assoc 180:1443–1447, 1982.

114. Otsuki M, Okabayashi Y, Nakamura T. Hydrocortisone treatment increases the sensitivity and responsiveness to cholecystokinin in rat pancreas. Am J Physiol 257:G364–G370, 1989.

115. Bourry J, Sarles H. Secretory pattern and pathological study of the pancreas of steroid-treated rats. Dig Dis Sci 23:423–428, 1978.

116. Geokas MC, Baltaxe HA, Banks PA, et al. Acute pancreatitis. Ann Intern Med 103:86–100, 1985.

117. Dressel TD, Goodale RL, Arneson MA, et al. Pancreatitis as a complication of anticholinesterase insecticide intoxication. Ann Surg 1989:199–204, 1979

118. Dressel TD, Goodale RL, Zweber B, et al. The effect of atropine and duct decompression on the evolution of Diazinon-induced acute canine pancreatitis. Ann Surg 195:424–434, 1982.

119. Oguchi Y, Frick TW, Satterberg TL, et al. Effect of the organophosphate iso-OMPA on amylase release by pancreatic lobules of dog, guinea pig, and cat. Pancreas 2(6):664–668, 1987.

120. Oguchi Y, Dressel TD, Borner JW, et al. Inhibition of acetyl- and butrylcholinesterase and amylase release from canine pancreas. Pancreas 4(4):423–428, 1989.

121. Liu S, Oguchi Y, Borner JW, et al. Increased canine pancreatic acinar cell damage after organophosphate and acetylcholine or cholecystokinin. Pancreas 5(2):177–182, 1990.

122. Kandalaft K, Liu S, Manivel C, et al. Organophosphate increases the sensitivity of human exocrine pancreas to acetylcholine. Pancreas 6(4):–403, 1991.

123. Weizman Z, Sofer S. Acute pancreatitis in children with anticholinesterase insecticide intoxication. Pediatrics 90:204–206, 1992.

124. Schaer M. A clinicopathologic survey of acute pancreatitis in 30 dogs and 5 cats. J Am Anim Hosp Assoc 15:681–687, 1979.

125. Neuman NB. Acute hemorrhagic pancreatitis associated with iatrogenic hypercalcemia in a dog J Am Vet Med Assoc 166:381–382, 1975.

126. Layer P, Hotz J, Eysselen VE, et al. Effects of acute hypercalcemia on exocrine pancreatic secretion in the cat. Gastroenterology 88:1168–1174, 1985.

127. Layer P, Hotz J, Schmitz-Moormann HP, et al. Effects or experimental chronic hypercalcemia on feline exocrine pancreatic secretion. Gastroenterology 82:309–316, 1982.

128. Frick TW, Hailemariam S, Heitz PU, et al. Acute hypercalcemia induces acinar cell necrosis and intraductal protein precipitates in the pancreas of cats and guinea pigs. Gastroenterology 98:1675–1681, 1990.

129. Frick TW, Spycher MA, Heitz PU, et al. Hypercalcaemia and pancreatic ultrastructure in cats. Eur J Surg 158:289–294, 1992.

130. De Giorgio R, Sternini C, Widdison AL, et al. Differential effects of experimentally induced chronic pancreatitis on neuropeptide immunoreactivities in the feline pancreas. Pancreas 8:700–710, 1993.

131. Hirsch VM, Doige CE. Suppurative cholangitis in cats. J Am Vet Med Assoc 182:1223–1226,1983.

132. Karanjia ND, Singh SM, Widdison AL, et al. Pancreatic ductal and interstitial pressures in cats with chronic pancreatitis. Dig Dis Sci 37:268–273, 1992.

133. Schapiro H, Britt LG, Blackwell CF, et al. Acute hemorrhagic pancreatitis in the dog. Arch Surg 107:608–612, 1973.

134. Arendt T. Bile-induced acute pancreatitis cats: Roles of bile, bacteria, and pancreatic duct pressure. Dig Dis Sci 38:39–44, 1993.

135. Keane FB, Dozois RR, Go VLW, et al. Interdigestive canine pancreatic juice composition and pancreatic reflux and pancreatic sphincter anatomy. Dig Dis Sci 26:577–584, 1981.

136. Hendricks JC, Dimagno EP, Go VLW, et al. Reflux of duodenal contents into the pancreatic duct of dogs. J Lab Clin Med 96:912–921, 1980.

137. Suter PF, Olsson SE. Traumatic hemorrhagic pancreatitis in the cat: A report with emphasis on the radiological diagnosis. J Am Vet Radiol Soc 10:4–11, 1969

138. Westermarck E, Saario E. Traumatic pancreatic injury in a cat—a case history. Acta Vet Scand 30:359–362, 1989.

139. Brandt KR, Charboneau JW, Stephens DH, et al. CT- and US-guided biopsy of the pancreas. Radiology 187:99–104, 1993.

140. Rodriguez J, Kasberg C, Nipper M, et al. CT-guided needle biopsy of the pancreas: A retrospective analysis of diagnostic accuracy. Am J Gastroenterol 87:1610–1613, 1993.

141. Dalton JRF, Hill FWG: A procedure for the examination of the liver and pancreas in dogs. J Sm Anim Pract 13:527–530, 1972.

142. Lightwood R, Reber HA, Way LW. The risk and accuracy of pancreatic biopsy. Am J Surg 132:189–194, 1976.

143. Moossa AR, Altorki N. Pancreatic biopsy. Surg Clin N Am 63:1205–1214, 1983.

144. Wilson JW, Caywood DD. Function tumors of the pancreatic beta cells. Comp Cont Ed Prac Vet 3:458–464, 1981.

145. Sanfey H, Broe PJ, Cameron JL. Experimental ischemic pancreatitis: Treatment with albumin. Am J Surg 150:297–300, 1985.

146. Bockman DE. Microvasculature of the pancreas: Relation to pancreatitis. Int J Pancreatol 12:11–21, 1992.

147. Kyogoku T, Manabe T, Tobe T. Role of ischemia in acute pancreatitis: Hemorrhagic shock converts edematous pancreatitis to hemorrhagic pancreatitis in rats. Dig Dis Sci 37:1409–1417, 1992.

148. Waldner H. Vascular mechanisms to induce acute pancreatitis. Eur Surg Res 24 (suppl) 1:62–67, 1992.

149. Furukawa M, Kimura T, Sumii T, et al. Role of local pancreatic blood flow in development of hemorrhagic pancreatitis induced by stress in rats. Pancreas 8:499–505, 1993.

150. Yotsumoto F, Ohshio G, et al. Role of pancreatic blood flow and vasoactive substances in the development of canine acute pancreatitis. J Surg Res 55:531–536, 1993.

151. Steer ML. Etiology and pathophysiology of acute pancreatitis. In: Go VLW (ed) The Exocrine Pancreas: Biology, Pathobiology and Disease. Raven Press, New York, 465–474, 1986.

152. Smart ME, Downey RS, Stockdale PHG. Toxoplasmosis in a cat associated with cholangitis and progressive pancreatitis. Can Vet J 14:313–316, 1973.

153. Sherding RG. Feline infectious peritonitis. Com Contin Ed Sm Anim Pract 1:95–101, 1979.

154. Rothenbacher H, Lindquist WD. Liver cirrhosis and pancreatitis in a cat infected with amplimerus pseudofeliseus. J Am Vet Med Assoc 143:1099–1102, 1963.

155. Dubey JP, Carpenter JL. Histologically confirmed clinical toxoplasmosis in cats: 100 cases (1952–1990). J Am Vet Med Assoc 203:1556–1566, 1993.

156. King LG. Postoperative complications and prognostic indicators in dogs and cats with septic peritonitis: 23 cases (1989–1992). J Am Vet Med Assoc 204:407–414, 1994.

157. Keynes MW. A nonpancreatic source of the proteolytic enzyme amidase and bacteriology in experimental acute pancreatitis. Ann Surg 191:187–199, 1980.

158. Isaji S, Suzuki M, Frey CF, et al. Role of bacterial infection in diet-induced acute pancreatitis in mice. Int J Pancreatol 11:49–57, 1992.

159. Hirano T, Manabe T. Protective effects of protease inhibitor and antibiotic against diet-induced pancreatitis in mice. Med Sci Res 20:283–284, 1992.

160. Gianotti L, Munda R, Alexander JW, et al. Bacterial translocation: A potential source for infection in acute pancreatitis. Pancreas 8:551–558, 1993.

161. Polzin DJ, Osborne CA, Stevens JB, et al. Serum amylase and lipase activities in dogs with chronic primary renal failure. Am J Vet Res 44:404–410, 1983.

162. Ham JM, Fitzpatrick P. Acute pancreatitis in patients with acute hepatic failure. Am J Dig Dis 18:1079–1083, 1973.

163. Akol KG, Washabau RJ, Saunders HM, et al. Acute pancreatitis in cats with hepatic lipidosis J Vet Int Med 7:205–209, 1993.

164. Holroyd JB. Canine exocrine pancreatic disease. J Sm Anim Pract 9:269–281, 1968.

165. Anderson NV. Pancreatitis in dogs. Vet Clin N Am 2:79–97, 1972.

166. Pidgeon G. Exocrine pancreatic disease in the dog and cat. Comp Anim Pract 1:67–71, 1987.

167. Lees GE, Suter PF, Johnson GC. Pulmonary edema in a dog with acute pancreatitis and cardiac disease. J Am Vet Med Assoc 172:690–696, 1978.

168. Garvey MS, Zawie DA. Feline pancreatic disease. Vet Clin N Am: Sm Anim Pract 14:1231–1246, 1984.

169. Kitchell BE, Strombeck DR, Cullen J, et al. Clinical and pathologic changes in experimentally induced acute pancreatitis in cats. Am J Vet Res 47:1170–1173, 1986.

170. Kleine LJ, Hornbuckle WE. Acute pancreatitis: The radiographic findings in 182 dogs. J Am Vet Radiol Soc 19:102–106, 1978.

171. Kleine LJ, Clinical and radiographic aspects of acute pancreatitis in the dog. Comp Cont Ed Prac Vet 2:295–299, 1980.

172. Gibbs C, Denny HR, Minter HM. Radiological features of inflammatory conditions of the canine pancreas. J Sm Anim Pract 13:531–544, 1972.

173. Nyland TG, Mulvany MH, Strombeck DR. Ultrasonic features of experimentally induced acute pancreatitis in the dog. Vet Radiol 24:260–266, 1993.

174. Murtaugh RJ, Herring DS, Jacobs RM, et al. Pancreatic ultrasonography in dogs with experimentally induced acute pancreatitis. Vet Radiol 26:27–32, 1985.

175. Salisbury SK, Lantz GC, Nelson RW, et al. Pancreatic abscess in dogs: Six cases (1978–1986). J Am Vet Med Assoc 193:1104–1108, 1988.

176. Edwards DF, Bauer MS, Walker MA, et al. Pancreatic masses in seven dogs following acute pancreatitis. J Am Anim Hosp Assoc 26:189–198, 1990.

177. Simpson KW, Shiroma JT, Biller DS, et al. D Ante mortem diagnosis of pancreatitis in four cats. J Sm Anim Pract 35:93–99, 1994.

178. Moulton JS. The radiologic assessment of acute pancreatitis and its complications. Pancreas 6 (suppl) 1:S13–S22, 1991.

179. Meyer P, Clavien PA, Robert J, et al. Role of imaging technics in the classification of acute pancreatitis. Dig Dis 10:330–334, 1992.

180. Feldman BF, Attix EA, Strombeck DR, et al. Biochemical and coagulation changes in a canine model of acute necrotizing pancreatitis. Am J Vet Res 42:805–808, 1981.

181. Mulvany, MH, Feinberg CK, Tilson DL. Clinical characterization of acute necrotizing pancreatitis. Comp Cont Ed Prac Vet 4:394–405, 1982.

182. Jacobs RM, Murtaugh RJ, DeHoff WD. Review of the clinicopathological findings of acute pancreatitis in the dog: Use of an experimental model. J Am Anim Hosp Assoc 21:795–800, 1985.

183. Goldstein DA, Llach F, Massry SG. Acute renal failure in patients with acute pancreatitis. Arch Intern Med 136:1363–1365, 1976.

184. Wells AD, Schenk WG. Effectiveness of normal saline solution, dextran 40 or dextran 75, and aprotinin (Trasyslol) on renal blood flow preservation during acute canine pancreatitis. Am J Surg 148:624–629, 1984.

185. Fabris C, Basso D, Naccarato R. Editorial: Urinary enzymes excretion in pancreatic diseases: Clinical role and pathophysiological considerations. J Clin Gastroenter 14:281–284, 1992.

186. Tuzhilin SA, Podolsky AE, Dreiling DA. Hepatic lesions in pancreatitis. Am Gastroenterol 64:108–114, 1975.

187. Andrzejewska A, Dlugosz J, Kurasz S. The ultrastructure of the liver in acute experimental pancreatitis in dogs. Exp Pathol 28:167–176, 1985.

188. Hirano T, Manabe T, Tobe T. Impaired hepatic energy metabolism in rat acute pancreatitis: Protective effects of prostaglandin E_2 and synthetic protease inhibitor ONO 3307. J Surg Res 53:238–244, 1992.

189. Nankivell BJ, Gillies AHB. Acute pancreatitis and rhabdomyolysis: A new association. Aust NZ J Med 21:414–417, 1991.

190. Whitney MS, Boon GD, Rebar AH, et al. Effects of acute pancreatitis on circulating lipids in dogs. Am J Vet Res 48:1492–1497, 1987.

191. Mia AS, Koger HD, Tierney MM. Serum values of amylase and pancreatic lipase in healthy mature dogs and dogs with experimental pancreatitis. Am J Vet Res 39:965–969, 1978.

192. Stickle JE, Carlton WW, Boon GD. Isoamylases in clinically normal dogs. Am J Vet Res 41:506–509, 1980.

193. Wagner AE, Macy DW. Nephelometric determination of serum amylase and lipase in naturally occurring azotemia in the dog. Am J Vet Res 43:697–699, 1982.

194. Westermarck E, Rimaila-Pärnänen E. Serum phospholipase A_2 in canine acute pancreatitis. Acta Vet Scand 24:477–487, 1983.

195. Simpson KW, Batt RM, McLean L, et al. Circulating concentrations of trypsin-like immunoreactivity and activities of lipase and amylase after pancreatic duct ligation in dogs. Am J Vet Res 50:629–632, 1989.

196. Hayakawa T, Sugimoto Y, Kondo T, et al. Serum trypsin in acute experimental pancreatitis in dogs. Dig Dis Sci 31:1133, 1986.

197. Kazmierczak SC, Van Lente F, Hodges ED. Diagnostic and prognostic utility of phospholipase A activity in patients with acute pancreatitis: Comparison with amylase and lipase. Clin Chem 37:356–360, 1991.

198. Rapp JP. Normal values for serum amylase and maltose in dogs and the effect of maltose in the saccharogenic method of determining amylase in serum. Am J Vet Res 23:343–350, 1962.

199. O'Donnell MD, McGeeney GF. Amylase and glucoamylase activities in canine serum. Comp Biochem Physiol (B) 50B:269–274, 1975.

200. Cornelius LM. Laboratory diagnosis of acute pancreatitis and pancreatic adenocarcinoma. Vet Clin N Am: Sm Anim Pract 6:671–678, 1976.

201. Strombeck DR, Farver T, Kaneko JJ. Serum amylase and lipase activities in the diagnosis of pancreatitis in dogs. Am J Vet Res 42:1966–1970, 1981.

202. Blum AL, Linscheer WG. Lipase in canine gastric juice. Proc Soc Exp Biol Med 135:565–568, 1970.

203. Jacobs RM, Hall RL, Rogers WA. Isoamylases in clinically normal and diseased dogs. Vet Clin Path 11:26–32, 1982.

204. Simpson KW, Simpson JW, Lake S, et al. Effect of pancreatectomy on plasma activities of amylase, isoamylase, lipase and trypsin-like immunoreactivity in dogs. Res Vet Sci 51:78–82, 1991.

205. Parent J. Effects of dexamethasone on pancreatic tissue and on serum amylase and lipase activities in dogs. J Am Vet Med Assoc 180:743–746, 1982.

205a. Williams DA, Waters CB, Adams LG, et al. Serum trypsin-like immunore-

206. Simpson JW, Doxey DL, Brown R. Serum isoamylase values in normal dogs and dogs with exocrine pancreatic insufficiency. Vet Res Commun 8:303–308, 1984.

207. Murtaugh RJ, Jacobs RM. Serum amylase and isoamylases and their origins in healthy dogs and dogs with experimentally induced acute pancreatitis. Am J Vet Res 46:742–747, 1985.

208. Williams DA, Jacobs RM, Murtaugh RJ. Comments on isoamylases [letters]. Am J Vet Res 46:1598–1599, 1985.

209. Jacobs RM. Renal disposition of amylase, lipase, and lysozyme in the dog. Vet Pathol 25:443–449, 1988.

210. Jacobs RM. Relationship of urinary amylase activity and proteinuria in the dog. Vet Pathol 26:349–350, 1989.

211. Kiriyama S, Hayakawa T, Kondo T, et al. Stimulatory effects of bombesin on plasma trypsin release and exocrine pancreatic secretion in dogs. Digestion 46:81–88, 1990.

212. Sugimoto Y, Hayakawa T, Kondo T, et al. Peritoneal absorption of pancreatic enzymes in bile-induced acute pancreatitis in dogs. J Gastroenterol Hepatol 5:493–498, 1990.

213. Hayakawa T, Kondo T, Shibata T, et al. Longitudinal changes of plasma pancreatic enzymes and hormones in experimental pancreatolithiasis in dogs. Dig Dis Sci 38:2098–2103, 1993.

214. Murayama KM, Drew JB, Nahrwold DL, et al. Acute edematous pancreatitis impairs pancreatic secretion in rats. Surgery 107 (3):302–310, 1990.

215. Niederau C, Niederau M, Lüthen R, et al. Pancreatic exocrine secretion in acute experimental pancreatitis. Gastroenterology 99:1120–1127, 1990.

216. Medinger TL, Burchfield T, Williams DA. Assay of trypsin-like immunoreactivity (TLI) in feline serum. J Vet Int Med, 7:133, 1993.

216a. Parent C, Washabau RJ, Williams DA, et al. Serum trypsin-like immunoreactivity, amylase and lipase in the diagnosis of feline acute pancreatitis. J Vet Int Med 9:194, 1995.

217. George JW. Methemalbumin: Reality and myth. Vet Clin Path 17:43–46, 1988.

218. Gross V, Schölmerich J, Leser H-G, et al. Granulocyte elastase in assessment of severity of acute pancreatitis. Comparison with acute-phase proteins C-reactive protein, a_1-antitrypsin, and protease inhibitor a^2-macroglobulin. Dig Dis Sci 35:97–105, 1990.

219. Gross V, Andreesen R, Leser H-G, et al. Interleukin-8 and neutrophil activation in acute pancreatitis. Eur J Clin Invest 22:200–203, 1992.

220. Williams DA, Moore M. Characterization of serum trypsin-like immunoassay (TLI) in dogs with naturally occurring fatal acute pancreatitis (AP) and severe chronic renal failure (CRF). Proc 6th Ann Vet Med Forum ACVIM, 739, 1988.

221. Fernández-del Castillo C, Schmidt J, Rattner, DW, et al. Generation and possible significance of trypsinogen activation peptides in experimental acute pancreatitis in the rat. Pancreas 7:263–270, 1992.

222. Karanjia ND, Widdison AL, Jehanli A, et al. Assay of trypsinogen activation in the cat experimental model of acute pancreatitis. Pancreas 8:189–195, 1993.

223. Malfertheiner P, Domínguez-Muñoz JE. Prognostic factors in acute pancreatitis. Int J Pancreatol 14:1–8, 1993.

224. Lankisch PG. Acute and chronic pancreatitis: An update on management. Drugs 28:554–564, 1984.

225. Drazner FH. Diseases of the pancreas. In: Jones BD, Liska WD (eds) Canine and Feline Gastroenterology. WB Saunders, Philadelphia, 295–344, 1986.

226. Banks PA. Medical management of acute pancreatitis and complications. In: Go VLW, Dimagno EP, Gardner JD. (eds) The Pancreas: Biology Pathobiology and Disease. Raven Press, New York, 593–613, 1993.

227. Bradley EL. Antibiotics in acute pancreatitis. Current status and future direction. Am J Surg 158:472–477, 1989.

228. Hansen B. Analgesics in cardiac, surgical, and intensive care patients. In: Kirk RW, Bonagura JD (eds) Current Veterinary Therapy XI. WB Saunders, Philadelphia, 82–87, 1992.

229. Murtaugh RJ, Jacobs RM. Serum antiprotease concentrations in dogs with spontaneous and experimentally induced acute pancreatitis. Am J Vet Res 46:80–83, 1985.

230. McMahon MJ, Bowen M, Mayer AD, et al. Relation of a_2 macroglobulin and other antiproteases to the clinical features of acute pancreatitis. Am J Surg 147:164–170, 1984.

231. Wendt P, Fritsh A, Schulz F, et al. Proteinases and inhibitors in plasma and peritoneal exudate in acute pancreatitis. Hepato-Gastroenterology 31:277–281, 1984.

232. Kimura T, Ito T, Sumii T, et al. Serum protease inhibitor captivity for elastase and the severity of pancreatitis. Pancreas 7:680–685, 1992.

233. Cuschieri A, Cumming JRG, Meehan SE, et al. Treatment of acute pancreatitis with fresh frozen plasma Br J Surg 70:710–712, 1983.

234. Kimura W, Meyer F, Hess D, et al. Comparison of different treatment modalities in experimental pancreatitis in rats. Gastroenterology 103:1916–1924, 1992.

235. Horton JW, Dunn CW, Burnweit CA, et al. Hypertonic saline-dextran

resuscitation of acute canine bile-induced pancreatitis. Am J Surg 158:48–56, 1989

236. Schmidt J, Fernandez-Del Castillo C, Rattner DW, et al. Hyperoncotic ultrahigh molecular weight dextran solutions reduce trypsinogen activation, prevent acinar necrosis, and lower mortality in rodent pancreatitis. Am J Surg 165:40–45, 1993.

237. Stake K, Hiura A, Nishiwaki H, et al. Plasma beta-endorphin and the effect of naloxone on hemodynamic changes during experimental acute pancreatitis in dogs. Surgery 168:402–406, 1989.

238. Satake K, Hiura A, Ha S, et al. Effect of a new synthetic protease inhibitor on beta-endorphin release during acute pancreatitis in dogs. Pancreas 6:441–447, 1991.

239. Attix E, Strombeck DR, Wheeldon EB, et al. Effects of an anticholinergic and a corticosteroid on acute pancreatitis in experimental dogs. Am J Vet Res 42:1668–1674, 1981.

240. Van Ooijen B, Tinga CJ, Kort WJ, et al. Effects of long-acting somatostatin analog (SMS 201–995) on eicosanoid synthesis and survival in rats with acute necrotizing pancreatitis. Dig Dis Sci 37:1434–1440, 1992.

241. Gjorup I, Roikjær O, Andersen B, et al. A double-blinded multicenter trial of somatostatin in the treatment of acute pancreatitis. Surg Gynecol Obstet 175:397–400, 1992.

242. Dyck WP, Rudick J, Hoexter B, et al. Influence of glucagon on pancreatic exocrine secretion. Gastroenterology 56:531–537, 1969.

243. Iwatsuki K, Ono H, Hashimoto K. Effects of glucagon on pancreatic secretion in the dog. Clin Exp Pharmacol Physiol 3:59–65, 1976.

244. Renner IG, Wisner JR, Lavigne BC. Partial restoration of pancreatic function by exogenous secretion in rats with ceruletide-induced acute pancreatitis. Dig Dis Sci 31(3):305–313, 1986.

245. Gullo L, Barbara L. Treatment of pancreatic pseudocysts with octreotide. Lancet 338:540–541, 1991.

246. Mckay CJ, Imrie CW, Baxter JN. Somatostatin and somatostatin analogues—are they indicated in the management of acute pancreatitis? Gut 34:1622–1626, 1993.

247. Karanjia ND, Lutrin FJ, Chang Y-B, et al. Low dose dopamine protects against hemorrhagic pancreatitis in cats. J Surg Res 48:440–443, 1990.

248. Musa BE, Ferguson HL, Nelson AW, et al. Evaluation of gamma radiation therapy in experimentally induced hemorrhagic pancreatitis in dogs. Am J Vet Res 40:927–930, 1979.

249. Balldin G, Ohlsson K. Trasylol prevents trypsin-induced shock in dogs. Hoppe-Seylers Z Physiol Chem 360:651–656, 1979.

250. Balldin G, Lasson Å, Ohlsson K. Aprotinin turn-over studies in dog and in man with severe acute pancreatitis. Hoppe-Seylers Z Physiol Chem 365:1417–1423, 1984.

251. Hermon-Taylor J, Heywood GD. A rational approach to the specific chemotherapy of pancreatitis. Scand J Gastroenterol 117:39–46, 1985.

252. Gabryelewicz A, Dlugosz J, Brzozowski J, et al. Prostacyclin: Effect on pancreatic lysosomes in acute experimental pancreatitis in dogs. Mt. Sinai J Med 50:218–224, 1983.

253. Triebling AT, Dlugosz J, Brzozowski J, et al. The renal lysosomes in acute experimental pancreatitis in dogs treated with prostacyclin (PGI$_2$). Path Res Pract 178:280–288, 1984.

254. Denny HR, Lucke JN. A case of acute pancreatic necrosis in the dog. J Sm Anim Pract 13: 565–551, 1972.

255. Matthiesen DT, Rosin E. Common bile duct obstruction secondary to chronic fibrosing pancreatitis in the dog: Treatment by use of cholecystoduodenostomy in the dog. J Am Vet Med Assoc 189:1443–1446, 1986.

256. Williams DA. Unpublished observations.

257. Slaff J, Jacobson D, Tillman CR, et al. Protease-specific suppression of pancreatic exocrine secretion. Gastroenterology 87:44–52, 1984.

258. Shiratori K, Jo YH, Lee KY, et al. Effect of pancreatic juice and trypsin on oleic acid–stimulated pancreatic secretion and plasma secretin in dogs. Gastroenterology 96:1330–1336, 1989.

259. Hosotani R, Kogire M, Inoue K, et al. The effect of exclusion of pancreatic juice on plasma cholecystokinin and pancreatic exocrine secretions in dogs. Dig Dis Sci 31:1134, 1986.

260. Mossner J, Wresky HP, Kestel W, et al. Influence of treatment with pancreatic extracts on pancreatic enzyme secretion. Gut 30:1143–1149, 1989.

261. Dimagno EP, Go VLW, Summerskill WHJ: Relations between pancreatic enzyme outputs and malabsorption in severe pancreatic insufficiency. N Engl J Med 288:813–815, 1973.

262. Holzworth J, Coffin DL. Pancreatic insufficiency and diabetes mellitus in a cat. Cornell Vet 43: 502–512, 1953.

263. Anderson NV, Low DG. Diseases of the canine pancreas: A comparative summary of 103 cases. Anim Hosp 1:189–194, 1965.

264. Hill FWG: Malabsorption syndrome in the dog: A study of thirty-eight cases. J Sm Anim Pract 13:575–594, 1972.

265. Pfister K, Rossi GL, Freudiger U, et al. Morphological studies in dogs with chronic pancreatic insufficiency. Virchows Arch[A]386:91–105, 1980.

266. Rimaila-Pärnänen E, Westermarck E. Pancreatic degenerative atrophy and chronic pancreatitis in dogs: A comparative study of 60 cases. Acta Vet Scand 23:400–406, 1982.

267. Bright JM. Pancreatic adenocarcinoma in a dog with maldigestion syndrome. J Am Vet Med Assoc 187:420–421, 1985.

268. Lerner A, Lebenthal E. Hereditary diseases of the pancreas. In: Go VLW, DiMagno EP, Gardner JD (eds) The Pancreas: Biology, Pathobiology and Disease. Raven Press, New York, 1083–1094, 1993.

269. Vermeulen C, Owens FM, Dragstedt LR. The effect of pancreatectomy on fat absorption from the intestines. Am J Physiol 138:792–796, 1943.

270. Pessoa VC, Kim KS, Ivy AC. Fat absorption in the absence of bile and pancreatic juice. Am J Physiol 174:209–218, 1953.

271. Douglas GJ, Reinauer AJ, Brooks WC, et al. The effect on digestion and absorption of excluding the pancreatic juice from the intestine. Gastroenterology 23:452–459, 1953.

272. Carrière F, Raphel V, Moreau H, et al. Dog gastric lipase: Stimulation of its secretion in vivo and cytolocalization in mucous pit cells. Gastroenterology 102:1535–1545, 1992.

273. Wang C-S, Hartsuck JA: Bile salt-activated lipase. A multiple function lipolytic enzyme. Biochim Biophys Acta Lipids. Lipid Metab 1166:1–19, 1993.

274. Carrière F, Laugier R, Barrowman JA, et al. Gastric and pancreatic lipase levels during a test meal in dogs. Scand J Gastroenterol 28:433–454, 1993.

275. Balk MW, Lang CM, White WJ, and et al. Exocrine pancreatic dysfunction in guinea pigs with diabetes mellitus. Lab Invest 32:28–32, 1975.

276. Port CD, Maschgan ER, Pond J, et al. Chronic exocrine pancreatic insufficiency in 2 Indian lions (Panthera Leo persica). J Comp Pathol 91:483–491, 1981.

277. Leiter EH, Dempsey EC, Eppig JJ. Exocrine pancreatic insufficiency syndrome in CBA/J mice:) Biochemical studies. Am J Pathol 86:31–46, 1986.

278. Hasholt J. Atrophy of the pancreas in budgerigars. Nord Vet Med 24:458–461, 1972.

279. Eppig JJ, Leiter EH. Exocrine pancreatic insufficiency syndrome in CBA/J mice: Ultrastructural study. Am J Pathol 86:17–30, 1977.

280. Williams DA. Feline exocrine pancreatic disease. Proc 12th Ann Vet Med Forum ACVIM, San Francisco, 617–619, 1994.

281. Barbezat GO, Hansen JDL. The exocrine pancreas and protein-calorie malnutrition. Pediatrics 42:77–92, 1968.

282. Levenson SM, Kan D, Gruber C, et al. Strange hemolytic anemia and pancreatic acinar atrophy and fibrosis. Fed Proc 30:1785–1802, 1971.

283. Fell BF, King TP, Davies NT. Pancreatic atrophy in copper-deficient rats: Histochemical and ultrastructural evidence of a selective effect on acinar cells. Histochem J 14:665–680, 1982.

284. Mizunuma T, Kawamura S, Kismino Y. Effects of injecting excess arginine on rat pancreas. J Nutr 114:467–471, 1984.

285. Dubick MA, Yu GSM, Majumdar APN. Morphological and biochemical changes in the pancreas of the copper-deficient female rat. J Nutr 119:1165–1172, 1989.

286. Delaney CP, McGeeney KF, Dervan P, et al. Pancreatic atrophy: A new model using serial intra-peritoneal injections of L-arginine. Scand J Gastroenterol 28:1086–1090, 1993.

287. VanKruiningen HJ. Pancreatic atrophy. In: Comparative Gastroenterology. Charles C Thomas, Springfield, IL, 42–64, 1982.

288. Hill FWG, Osborne AD, Kidder DE. Pancreatic degenerative atrophy in dogs. J Comp Pathol 81:321–330, 1971.

288a. Washabau RJ, Callan MB, Williams DA, et al. Cholecystokinin secretion is preserved in canine pancreatic insufficiency. J Vet Int Med 9:193, 1995.

289. Simpson KW, Cobb M. Anti-pancreatic antibodies in dogs with normal and diminished exocrine pancreatic function. J Vet Int Med 7:132, 1993.

290. Sateri H. Investigations on the exocrine pancreatic function in dogs suffering from chronic exocrine pancreatic insufficiency. Acta Vet Scand (suppl) 53:1–86, 1975.

291. Anderson NV, Low DG. Juvenile atrophy of the canine pancreas. Anim Hosp 1:101–109, 1965.

292. Weber V, Freudiger U. Erbanalytische untersucmungen uber die chronische exokrine pankreasinsuffizienz geim deutschen schafermund. Schweiz Arch Tierheilkd 119:157–163, 1977.

293. Westermarck E. The hereditary nature of canine pancreatic degenerative atrophy in the German shepherd dog. Acta Vet Scand 21:389–394, 1980.

294. Westermarck E, Pamilo P, Wiberg M. Pancreatic degenerative atrophy in the Collie breed: A hereditary disease. J Vet Med (A) 36:549–554, 1989.

295. Williams DA, Minnich F. Canine exocrine pancreatic insufficiency—a survey of 640 cases diagnosed by assay of serum trypsin-like immunoreactivity. J Vet Int Med 4:123, 1990.

296. Hall EJ, Bond PM, McLean C, et al. A survey of the diagnosis and treatment of canine exocrine pancreatic insufficiency. J Sm Anim Pract 32:613–619, 1991.

297. Westermarck E, Batt RM, Vaillant C, et al. Sequential study of pancreatic

structure and function during development of pancreatic acinar atrophy in a German shepherd dog. Am J Vet Res 54:1088–1094, 1993.

298. Andriulli A, Masoero G, Felder M, et al. Circulating trypsin-like immunoreactivity in chronic pancreatitis. Dig Dis Sci 26:532–537, 1981.

299. Grendell JH, Cello JP. Chronic pancreatitis. In: Sleisenger MH, Fordtran JS (eds) Gastrointestinal Disease. WB Saunders, Philadelphia, 1485–1514, 1983.

300. Hoskins JD, Turk JR, Turk MA. Feline pancreatic insufficiency. Vet Med/Sm Anim Clin 77:1745–1748, 1982.

301. Watson ADJ, Church DB, Middleton DJ, et al. Weight loss in cats which eat well. J Sm Anim Pract 22:473–482, 1981.

302. Perry LA, Williams DA, Pidgeon G, et al. Exocrine pancreatic insufficiency with associated coagulopathy in a cat. Jour Am Anim Hosp Assoc 27:109–114, 1991.

303. Williams DA. Feline Exocrine pancreatic insufficiency. In: Kirk RW, Bonagura JD (eds) Current Veterinary Therapy XII. WB Saunders, Philadelphia, 1994.

304. Lerner A, Heitlinger LA, Lebenthal E. Hereditary abnormalities of pancreatic function. In: Go VLW et al. (eds) The Exocrine Pancreas: Biology, Pathobiology and Disease. Raven Press, New York, 819–827, 1986.

305. Boari A, Williams DA, Famigli-Bergamini P. Observations on exocrine pancreatic insufficiency in a family of English setter dogs. J Sm Anim Pract 35:247–250, 1994.

306. Westermarck E, Rimaila-Pärnänen E. Two unusual cases of canine exocrine pancreatic insufficiency. J Sm Anim Pract 30:32–34, 1989.

307. Tangner CH, Turrell JM, Hobson HP. Complications associated with proximal duodenal resection and cholecystoduodenostomy in two cats. Vet Surg 11:60–64, 1982.

308. Clark CH. Pancreatic atrophy and absorption failure in a boxer. J Am Vet Med Assoc 136:174–177, 1960.

309. Kallfelz FA, Norrdin RW, Neal TM. Intestinal absorption of oleic I and triolein I in the differential diagnosis of malabsorption syndrome and pancreatic dysfunction in the dog. J Am Vet Med Assoc 153:43–46, 1968.

310. Washabau RJ, Strombeck DR, Buffington CA, et al. Use of pulmonary hydrogen gas execretion to detect carbohydrate malabsorption in dogs. J Am Vet Med Assoc 189:674–679, 1986.

311. Batt RM, Mann LC. Specificity of the BT-PABA test for the diagnosis of exocrine pancreatic insufficiency in the dog. Vet Rec 108:303–307, 1981.

312. Rogers WA, Stradley RP, Sherding RG, et al. Simultaneous evaluation of pancreatic exocrine function and intestinal absorptive function in dogs with chronic diarrhea. J Am Vet Med Assoc 177:1128–1131, 1980.

313. Balas D, Senegas-Balas F, Bertrand C, et al. Effects of pancreatic duct ligation on the hamster intestinal mucosa. Digestion 20:157–167, 1980.

314. Senegas-Balas F, Balas D, Bouisson M, et al. Effect of pancreatic duct ligation on the hamster intestinal mucosa. Digestion 21:83–91, 1981.

315. Senegas-Balas F, Bastie MJ, Balas D, et al. Histological variations of the duodenal mucosa in chronic human pancreatitis. Dig Dis Sci 27:917–922, 1982.

316. Kotler DP, Shiau YF, Levine GM. Effects of luminal contents on jejunal fatty acid esterification in the fat. Am J Physiol 238:G414–418, 1980.

317. Shiau YF, Kotler D, Levine G. Can normal small bowel morphology be equated with normal function? Gastroenterology 76:1246, 1979.

318. Milla PJ, Kilby A Rassam UB, et al. Small intestinal absorption of amino acids and a dipeptide in pancreatic insufficiency. Gut 24:818–824, 1983.

319. Morin CL, Roy CC, Lasalle R, et al. Small bowel mucosal dysfunction in patients with cystic fibrosis. J Pediatr 88:213–216, 1976.

320. Simpson KW, Morton DB, Sorensen SH, et al. Biochemical changes in the jejunal mucosa of dogs with exocrine pancreatic insufficiency following pancreatic duct ligation. Res Vet Sci 47:338–345, 1989.

321. King CE, Toskes PP. Small intestine bacterial overgrowth. Gastroenterology 76:1035–1055, 1979.

322. Romer H, Urbach R, Gomez MA, et al. Moderate and severe protein energy malnutrition in childhood: Effects on jejunal mucosal morphology and disorcclaridase activities. J Pediatr Gastroenterol Nutr 2:459–464, 1983.

323. Sherman P, Wesley A, Forstner G. Sequential disaccharidase loss in rat intestinal blind loops: Impact of malnutrition. Am J Physiol 248:G626–G632, 1985.

324. Gallo-Payet N, Hugon JS. Insulin receptors in isolated adult mouse intestinal cells: Studies in vivo and in organ culture. Endocrinology 114:1885–1892, 1984.

325. Scheving LA, Scheving LE, Tsai TH, et al. Circadian stage-dependent effects of insulin and glucogen on incorporation of 3H-thynirdine into deoxyribonucleic acid in the esophagus, stomach, duodenum, jejunem, caecum, colon, rectum and spleen of the adult female mouse. Endocrinology 111:308–315, 1982.

326. Arvanitakis C, Olsen WA. Intestinal mucosal disaccharidases in chronic pancreatitis. Am J Dig Dis 19:417–421, 1974.

327. Batt RM, Bush BM, Peters TJ. Biochemical changes in the jejunal mucosa of dogs with naturally occurring exocrine pancreatic insufficiency. Gut 20:709–715, 1979.

328. Williams DA, Batt RM, McLean L. Reversible impairment of protein synthesis may contribute to jejunal abnormalities in exocrine pancreatic insufficiency. Clin Sci 68:37P, 1985.

329. Williams DA. Studies on the diagnosis and pathophysiology of canine exocrine pancreatic insufficiency. PhD thesis, University of Liverpool, England, 1985.

330. Critchley DR, Howell KE, Eichholz A. Solubilization of brush borders of hamster small intestine and fractionation of some of the components. Biochim Biophys Acta 394:361–376, 1975.

331. Louvard D, Maroux S, Vannier C, et al. Topological studies on the hydrolases bound to the intestinal brush border membrane. Biochim Biophys Acta 375:236–248, 1975.

332. Louvard D, Semeriva M, Maroux S. The brush border intestinal aminopeptidase, a transmembrane protein as probed by macro- molecular photolabelling. J Mol Biol 106:1023–1035, 1976.

333. Jonas A, Flanagan PR, Forstner GC. Pathogenesis of mucosal injury in the blind loop syndrome. Brush border enzyme activity and glycoprotein degradation. J Clin Invest 60:1321–1330, 1977.

334. Kenny JA, Maroux S. Topology of microvillar membrane hydrolases of kidney and intestine Physiol Rev 62:91–128, 1982.

335. Eicholz A. Studies on the organization of the brush border in intestinal epithelial cells V Subfractionation of enzymatic activities of the microvillus membrane. Biochim Biophys Acta 163:101-107, 1968.

336. Williams DA, Batt RM, McLean L. Reductions in both protein synthesis and degradation may contribute to jejunal abnormalities in canine exocrine pancreatic insufficiency. Proc 3rd Ann Med Forum ACVIM, San Diego, May 1985.

337. Malo C, Menard D. Synergistic effects of insulin and thyroxine on the differentiation and proliferation of epithelial cells of suckling mouse small intestine. Biol Neonate 44:177–184, 1983.

338. Olsen WA, Korsmo H. The intestinal brush border membrane in diabetes. J Clin Invest 60:181–188, 1977.

339. Helman CA, Barbezat GO, Bank S. Jejunal monosaccharide, water, and electrolyte transport in patients with chronic pancreatitis. Gut 19:46–49, 1978.

340. Mahmood A, Patmak RM, Agarwal N. Effect of chronic alloxan diabetes and insulin administration on intestinal brush border enzymes. Experientia 34:741–742, 1978.

341. Pothier P, Hugon JS. Immediate and localized response of intestinal mucosal enzyme activities in streptozotocin-diabetic mice. Comp Biochem Physiol 72A:505–513, 1982.

342. Gourley GR, Korsmo HA, Olsen WA. Intestinal mucosa in diabetic rats: Studies of microvillus membrane composition and microviscosity. Metabolism 30:1053–1058, 1983.

343. Simpson KW, Batt RM, Jones D, et al. Effects of exocrine pancreatic insufficiency and replacement therapy on the bacterial flora of the duodenum in dogs. Am J Vet Res 51 (2): 203–206, 1990.

344. Westermarck E, Myllys V, Aho M. Effect of treatment on the jejunal and colonic bacterial flora of dogs with exocrine pancreatic insufficiency. Pancreas 8:559–562, 1993.

345. MacLaren IF, Howard JM, Serlin O. Achlorhydria associated with chronic disease of the exocrine pancreas. Surgery 59:676–680, 1966.

346. Williams DA, Batt RM, McLean L. Duodenal bacterial overgrowth may occur in canine exocrine pancreatic insufficiency but is not due to achlohydria. Sci Proc ACVIM, Washington, DC, 34, 1984.

347. Riepe SP, Goldstein J, Alpers DH. Effect of secreted bacteroides proteases on human intestinal brush border hydrolases. J Clin Invest 66:314–322, 1980.

348. Jonas A, Krishnan C, Forstner G. Pathogenesis of mucosal injury in the blind loop syndrome. Release of disaccharidases from brush border membranes by extracts of bacteria obtained from intestinal blind loops in rats. Gastroenterology 75:791–795, 1978.

349. Batt RM, McLean L. Comparison of the biochemical changes in the jejunal mucosa of dogs with aerobic and anaerobic bacterial overgrowth. Gastroenterology 93:986–993, 1987.

350. Vaillant C, Batt RM, Williams DA. Regulatory peptide abnormalities in dogs with pancreatic acinar atrophy. Regul Pept 7:304, 1983.

351. Orci L. Patterns of cellular and subcellular organization in the endocrine pancreas. J Endocrinol 102:3–11, 1984.

352. Vaillant C, Giraud A, Williams DA. Pancreatic enkephalin immunoreactivity in canine pancreatic acinar atropy. Dig Dis Sci 29:92S, 1984.

353. Williams DA, Batt RM. Reversible intravenous glucose intolerance in canine exocrine pancreatic insufficiency. Proc 4th Ann Forum. ACVIM, Washington, DC, 14–9, 1986.

354. Hill FWG, Kidder DE. The oral glucose tolerance test in canine pancreatic malabsorption. Br Vet J 128:207–214, 1972.

355. Greve T, Anderson NV. The high-dose, intravenous glucose tolerance test (H-IVGTT) in dogs. Nord Vet Med 25:436–445, 1973.

356. Schwille PO, Engelhardt W, Gumbert E, et al. Long-term pancreatic duct

occlusion impairs the entero-insular axis in the dog—failure of plasma VIP to respond as "incretin." Peptides 4:445–450, 1984.

357. Creutzfeldt W, Ebert R. The enteroinsular axis. In: Go VLW, DiMagno EP, Gardner JD (eds) The Pancreas: Biology, Pathobiology and Disease. Raven Press, New York, 769–788, 1993.

358. Creutzfeldt W. The incretin concept today. Diabetologia 16:75–85, 1979.

359. Rogers WA, O'Dorisio TM, Johnson SE, et al. Postprandial release of gastric inhibitory polypeptide (GIP) and pancreatic polypeptide in dogs with pancreatic acinar atrophy. Dig Dis Sci 28:345–349, 1983.

360. Bewick M, Miller BHR, Compton FJ, et al. Canine pancreatic endocrine function after interruption of pancreatic exocrine drainage. Transplantation 36:246–251, 1983.

361. Smith SR, Edgar PJ, Pozefsky T, et al. Insulin secretion and glucose tolerance in adults with protein-calorie malnutrition. Metabolism 24:1073–1084, 1975.

362. Dollet J, Beck B, Villaume V, et al. Progressive adaption of the endocrine pancreas during long-term protein deficiency in rats: Effects on blood glucose homeostasis and on pancreatic insulin, glucagon and somatostatin concentrations. J Nutr 115:1581–1588, 1985.

363. Heard CRC: The effects of protein-energy malnutrition on blood glucose homeostasis. Wld Rev Nutr Diet 30:107–147, 1978.

364. de Bruijne JJ, Altszuler N, Hampshire J, et al. Fat mobilization and plasma hormone levels in fasted dogs. Metabolism 30:190–194, 1981.

365. Salazar de Sousa J. Malnutrition and small intestinal mucosa. J Pediatr Gastroenterol Nutr 3:321–322, 1984.

366. Dowd PS, Heatley RV. The influence of undernutrition on immunity. Clin Sci 66:241–248, 1984.

367. Sherman P, Forstner J, Roomi N, et al. Mucin depletion in the intestine of malnourished rats. Am J Physiol 248:G418–G423, 1985.

368. Van Kruiningen HJ. Pancreatic atrophy. In: Comparative Gastroenterology. Charles C Thomas, Springfield, IL, 42–64, 1982.

369. Jamison MH, Sharma H, Braganza JM, et al. The influence of pancreatic juice on 64 Cu absorption in the rat. Br J Nutr 50:113–119, 1983.

370. Jacob RA, Sandstead HH, Solomons NW, et al. Zinc status and vitamin A transport in cystic fibrosis. Am J Clin Nutr 31:638–644, 1978.

371. Seal CJ, Heaton FW. Chemical factors affecting the intestinal absorption of zinc in vitro and in vivo. Br J Nutr 50:317–324, 1983.

372. Lebenthal E, Lerner A, Rolston DK. The pancreas in cystic fibrosis. In: Go VLW, DiMagno EP, Gardner JD (eds) The Pancreas: Biology, Pathobiology and Disease. Raven Press, New York, 1041–1081, 1993.

373. Batt RM, Morgan JO. Role of serum folate and vitamin B$_{12}$ concentrations in the differentiation of small intestinal abnormalities in the dog. Res Vet Sci 32:17–22, 1982.

374. Brugge WR, Goff JS, Allen NC, et al. Development of a dual label Schilling test for pancreatic exocrine function based on the differential absorption of cobalamin bound to intrinsic factor and R protein. Gastroenterology 78:937–949, 1980.

375. Simpson KW, Morton, DB, Batt RM. Effect of exocrine pancreatic insufficiency on cobalamin absorption in dogs. Am J. Vet Res 50:1233–1236, 1989.

376. Marcoullis G, Rothenberg SP. Intrinsic factor–mediated intestinal absorption of cobalamin in the dog. Am J Physiol 241:G294–G299, 1981.

377. Fyfe, JC. Feline intrinsic factor (IF) is pancreatic in origin and mediates ileal cobalamin (CBL) absorption. J Vet Int Med, 7:133, 1993.

378. Williams DA. Exocrine pancreatic insufficiency. Walth Int Focus 2:9–14, 1993.

379. Williams DA. The pancreas: Exocrine pancreatic insufficiency. In Anderson NV (ed) Veterinary Gastroenterology. Lea Febiger, Philadelphia, 570–594, 1992.

380. Dowling RH, Gleeson MH. Cell turnover following small bowel resection and bypass. Digestion 8:176–190, 1973.

381. Arvanitakis C. Functional and morphological abnormalities of the small intestinal mucosa in pernicious anemia—a prospective study. Acta Hepato-Gastroenterol 25:313–318, 1978.

382. Raiha M, Westermarck E. The signs of pancreatic degenerative atrophy in dogs and the role of external factors in the etiology of the disease. Acta Vet Scand 30:477–452, 1989.

383. Fyfe JC, Jezyk PF, Giger U, et al. Inherited selective malabsorption of vitamin B$_{12}$ in giant schnauzers. J Am Anim Hosp Assoc 50:533–539, 1989.

384. Bernstein LH, Gutstein S, Efron G, et al. Experimental production of elevated serum folate in dogs with intestinal blind loops: Relationship of serum levels to location of the blind loop. Gastroenterology 63:815–819, 1972.

385. Russell RM, Dhar GJ, Dutta SK, et al. Influence of intraluminal pH on folate absorption: Studies in control subjects and in patients with pancreatic insufficiency. J Lab Clin Med 93:436–438, 1979.

386. Williams DA. The pancreas: Exocrine pancreatic insufficiency. In: Anderson NV (ed) Veterinary Gastroenterology. Lea Febiger, Philadelphia, 283–294, 1992.

387. Pidgeon G, Strombeck DR. Evaluation of treatment for pancreatic exocrine insufficiency in dogs with ligated pancreatic ducts. Am J Vet Res 43:461–464, 1982.

388. Hayes KC, Rousseau JE, Hegsted DM. Plasma tocopherol concentrations and vitamin E deficiency in dogs. J Am Vet Med Assoc 157,(1):64–71, 1970.

389. Williams DA, Mannella C, Mehta JR, et al. Erythrocyte stability and membrane composition in tocopherol deficient cats. J Vet Int Med 8:154, 1994.

390. Desai ID, Calvert CC, Scott ML. A time sequence study of the relationship of peroxidation, lysosomal enzymes, and nutritional muscular dystrophy. Arch Biochem Biophys 108:60–64, 1964.

391. Machlin LJ, Filipski R, Nelson J, et al. Effects of prolonged vitamin E deficiency in the rat. J Nutr 107:1200–1208, 1977.

392. Cordes DO, Mosher AM. Brown pigmentation (lipofuscinosis) of canine intestinal muscularis. J Path Bact 92:197–206, 1966.

393. Nelson JS, Fitch CD, Fischer VW, et al. Progressive neuropathologic lesions in vitamin E deficient rhesus monkeys. J Neuropathol Exp Neurol 40:166–186, 1981.

394. Dill-Macky E. Pancreatic diseases of cats. Comp Cont Ed Prac Vet 15:589–596, 1993.

395. Freudiger U, Bigler B. The diagnosis of chronic exocrine pancreatic insufficiency by the PABA test. Kleintier-Praxis 22:73–79, 1977.

396. Boyd JW. The Interpretation of serum biochemistry test results in domestic animals. Vet Clin Path 13:7–14, 1984.

397. Nicholson A, Watson ADJ, Mercer JR. Fat malassimilation in three cats. Aust Vet J 66:110–113, 1989.

398. Walker WA, Isselbacher KJ. Uptake and transport of macromolecules by the intestine. Possible role in clinical disorders. Gastroenterology. 67:531–550, 1974.

399. Westermarck E, Lindberg LA, Sandholm M. Quantitation of serum phosphalipase A$_2$ by enzyme diffusion in lecithin agar gels. A comparative study in man and animals. Acta Vet Scand 25:229–244, 1986.

400. Williams DA, Batt RM. Sensitivity and specificity of radioimmunoassay of serum trypsin-like immunoreactivity for the diagnosis of canine exocrine pancreatic insufficiency. J Am Vet Med Assoc 192:195–201, 1988.

401a. Steiner JM, Williams DA. Validation of a radioimmunoassay for feline trypsin-like immunoreactivity (FTLI) and serum cobalamin and folate concentrations in cats with exocrine pancreatic insufficiency (EPI). J Vet Int Med 9:193,1995.

401. Williams DA, Batt RM. Exocrine pancreatic insufficiency diagnosed by radioimmunoassay of serum trypsin-like immunoreactivity in a dog with a normal BT-PABA test result. J Am Anim Hosp Assoc 22:671–674, 1986.

402. Canfield PJ, Fairburn AJ, Church DB. Effect of various diets on fecal analysis in normal dogs. Res Vet Sci 34:24–27, 1983.

403. Williams DA, Reed SD. Comparison of methods for assay of fecal proteolytic activity. Vet Clin Path 19:20–24, 1990.

404. Williams DA, Reed SD, Perry LA. Fecal proteolytic activity in clinically normal cats and in a cat with exocrine pancreatic insufficiency. J Am Vet Med Assoc 197:210–212, 1990.

405. Westermarck E, Sandholm M. Fecal hydrolase activity as determined by radial enzyme diffusion: A new method for detecting pancreatic dysfunction in the dog. Res Vet Sci 28:341–346, 1980.

406. Strombeck DR, Harrold D. Evaluation of 60-minute blood p-aminobenzoic and concentration in pancreatic function testing of dogs. J Am Vet Med Assoc 180:419–421, 1982.

407. Zimmer JF, Todd SE. Further evaluation of bentiromide in the diagnosis of canine exocrine pancreatic insufficiency. Cornell Vet 75:426–440, 1985.

408. Imondi AR, Stradley RP, Wolgemuth R. Synthetic peptides in the diagnosis of exocrine pancreatic insufficiency in animals. Gut 13:726–731, 1972.

409. Strombeck DR. New method for evaluation of chymotrypsin deficiency in dogs. J Am Vet Med Assoc 173:1319–1323, 1978.

410. Batt RM, Bush BM, Peters TJ. A new test for the diagnosis of exocrine pancreatic insufficiency in the dog. J Sm Anim Pract 20:185–192, 1979.

411. Hawkins EC, Meric SM, Washabau RJ, et al. Digestion of bentiromide and absorption of xylose in healthy cats and absorption of xylose in cats with infiltrative intestinal disease. Am J Vet Res 47:567–569, 1986.

412. Sherding RG, Stradley RP, Rogers WA, et al. Bentiromide:xylose test in healthy cats. Am J Vet Res 43:2272–2273, 1982.

413. Simpson JW, Doxey DL. Quantitative assessment of fat absorption and its diagnostic value in exocrine pancreatic insufficiency. Res Vet Sci 35:249–251, 1983.

414. Dimagno EP. Medical treatment of pancreatic insufficiency. Mayo Clin Proc 54:435–442, 1979.

415. Graham DY. Enzyme replacement therapy of exocrine pancreatic insufficiency in man. N Engl J Med 296:1314–1317, 1977.

416. Niessen KH, Konig J, Molitor M, et al. Studies on the quality of pancreatic preparations: Enzyme content, prospective bioavailability, bile acid pattern, and contamination with purines. Eur J Pediatr 141:23–29, 1983.

417. Roberts IM. Enzyme therapy for malabsorption in exocrine pancreatic insufficiency. Pancreas 4:496–503, 1989.

418. Morrow JD. Topics in clinical pharmacology: Pancreatic enzyme replacement therapy. Am J Med Sci 298:357–359, 1989.

419. Marvola M Heinamaki J, Westermarck E, et al. The fate of single-unit enteric-coated drug products in the stomach of the dog. Acta Pharm Fenn 95:59–70, 1986.

420. Dimagno EP, Layer P, Clain JE. Chronic pancreatitis. In: Go VLW , DiMagno EP, Gardner JD (eds) The Pancreas: Biology, Pathobiology and Disease. Raven Press, New York, 665–706, 1993.

421. Westermarck E. Treatment of pancreatic degenerative atrophy with raw pancreas homogenate and various enzyme preparations. J Vet Med (A) 34:728–733, 1987.

422. Grendell JH. Nutrition and absorption in diseases of the pancreas. Clin Gastrolenterol 12:551–562, 1983.

423. Dutta SK, Rubin J, Harvey J. Comparative evaluation of the therapeutic efficacy of a Ph-sensitive enteric-coated pancreatic enzyme therapy in the treatment of exocrine pancreatic insufficiency. Gastroenterology 84:476–482, 1983.

424. Dimagno EP. Controversies in the treatment of exocrine pancreatic insufficiency. Dig Dis Sci 27:481–484, 1982.

425. Zentler-Munro PL, Fitzpatrick WJF, Batten JC, et al. Effect of intrajejunal acidity on aqueous phase bile acid and lipid concentrations in pancreatic steatorrhoea due to cystic fibrosis. Gut 25:500–507, 1984.

426. Abrams CK, Hamosh M, Hubbard VS, et al. Lingual lipase in cystic fibrosis. Quantitation of enzyme activity in the upper small intestine of patients with exocrine pancreatic insufficiency. J Clin Invest 73:374–382, 1984.

427. Balasubramanian K, Zentler-Munro PL, Batten JC, et al. Increased intragastric acid-resistant lipase activity and lipolysis in pancreatic steatorrhoea due to cystic fibrosis. Pancreas 7:305–310, 1992.

428. Carrière F, Moreau H, Raphel V, et al. Purification and biochemical characterization of dog gastric lipase. Eur J Biochem 202:75–83, 1991.

429. Heinamaki J. Formulation and radiological imaging of oral solid drug products intended for the treatment of exocrine pancreatic insufficiency in dogs. Yliopistopaino, Helsinki, Finland, 1991.

430. Griffin SM, Alderson D, Farndon JR. Acid-resistant lipase as replacement therapy in chronic pancreatic exocrine insufficiency: A study in dogs. Gut 30:1012–1015, 1989.

431. Lewis LD, Morris ML, Hand MS. Small Animal Clinical Nutrition. Mark Morris Associates, Topeka, KS, 1987.

432. Westermarck E, Wiberg M, Junttila J. Role of feeding in the treatment of dogs with pancreatic degenerative atrophy. Acta Vet Scand 31:325–331, 1990.

433. Dutta SK, Hlasko J. Dietary fiber in pancreatic disease: Effect of high fiber diet on fat malabsorption in pancreatic insufficiency and in vitro study of the interaction of dietary fibers with pancreatic enzymes. Am J Clin Nutr 41:517–525, 1985.

434. Isaksson G, Lundquist I, Ihse I. Effect of dietary fiber on pancreatic enzyme activity in vitro. The importance of viscosity, pH, ionic strength, adsorption, and time of incubation. Gastroenterology 82:918–924, 1982.

435. Caliari S, Benini L, Bonfante F, et al. Pancreatic extracts are necessary for the absorption of elemental and polymeric enteral diets in severe pancreatic insufficiency. Scand J Gastroenterol 28:749–752, 1993.

436. Sokol RJ, Farrell MK, Heubi JE, et al. Comparison of vitamin E and 25-hydroxyvitamin D absorption during childhood cholestasis. Pediat 103:712–717, 1983.

437. King CE, Toskes PP. Protein-losing enteropathy in the human and experimental rat blind loop syndrome. Gastroenterology 80:504–509, 1981.

438. Batt RM Peters TJ. Effects of prednisolone on the small intestinal mucosa of the rat. Clin Sci Mol Med 50:511–523, 1976.

439. Westermarck E, Rimaila-Pärnänen E. Mesenteric torsion in dogs with exocrine pancreatic insufficiency: 21 cases (1978–1987). J Am Vet Med Assoc 195:1404–1406, 1989.

440. Anderson NV, Johnson KH. Pancreatic carcinoma in the dog. J Am Vet Med Assoc 150:286–295, 1967.

441. Banner BF, Alroy J, Kipnis RM. Acinar cell carcinoma of the pancreas in a cat. Vet Pathol 16:543–547, 1979.

442. Withrow SJ. Tumors of the gastrointestinal system: Exocrine pancreas. In: Withrow SJ, MacEwen EG (eds) Clinical Veterinary Oncology. Lippincott, Philadelphia, 192–193, 1989.

443. Fox JN, Mosley JG, Vogler GA, et al. Pancreatic function in domestic cats with pancreatic fluke infection. J Am Vet Med Assoc 178:58–60, 1981.

444. Roudebush P, Schmidt DA. Fenbendazole for treatment of pancreatic fluke infection in a cat. J Am Vet Med Assoc 180:545–546, 1982.

445. Anderson WI, Georgi ME, Car BD. Pancreatic atrophy and fibrosis associated with eurytrema procyonis in a domestic cat. Vet Rec 120:235–236, 1987.

446. Sheldon WG. Pancreatic flukes (*Eurytrema procyonis*) in domestic cats. J Am Vet Med Assoc 148:251–253, 1966.

21 Gastrointestinal Tract Infections, Parasites, and Toxicoses

W. GRANT GUILFORD AND DONALD R. STROMBECK

INTRODUCTION: PATHOGENESIS OF ACUTE GASTROENTERITIS DUE TO MICROORGANISMS[1]

Transient exposure of the gastrointestinal tract to microorganisms that are not normal members of the intestinal flora is a frequent occurrence, but clinical evidence of gastroenteritis does not often result. Transient bacteria become pathogenic only when they colonize the bowel. Colonization is prevented in normal animals by (1) the luxuriant normal microflora, not readily displaced from the mucosal surface; (2) bacterial interactions favoring growth of only the normal microflora; (3) the production of bactericidal agents by the normal flora; (4) the production of bactericidal or bacteriostatic gastrointestinal secretions such as hydrochloric acid and pancreatic and biliary juice; (5) the normal propulsive activity of the intestine that sweeps organisms in an aboral direction; (6) the complete assimilation of food ensuring a restricted nutrient supply for bacterial growth; and (7) the "antiseptic paint" of secretory immunoglobulins that prevents adherence of specific pathogens to the mucosal surface.

A change in any one of these seven homeostatic mechanisms can cause sufficient disruption of the normal flora or local immune system to allow colonization by foreign microorganisms and signs of disease. For example, diarrhea of any etiology causes profound changes in the normal microflora. In particular, diarrhea reduces the number of anaerobes in the colon because of the more rapid transit of gastrointestinal content and hence the less anaerobic environment in the colon. This change in the normal flora interferes with floral resistance to colonization by transient aerobic pathogens and can lead to the perpetuation or worsening of the diarrhea. Similarly, malnutrition changes the normal bacterial flora so that pathogens can colonize. Stress can change the flora, perhaps in part by altering intestinal motility. Furthermore, antibiotics often modify the normal flora, permitting antibiotic-resistant pathogens to colonize and cause disease. In addition, colonization can result from disruption of the mucosal IgA layer by bacteria with the ability to secrete an IgA protease that degrades secretory immunoglobulins.[2] Once colonization has occurred, microorganisms multiply and produce diarrhea by one of four means.

Enterotoxigenic Infectious Agents[3]

Some microorganisms attach to the mucosal surface and produce diarrhea by releasing an enterotoxin. Many enterotoxigenic organisms are found in the intestines of small animals and most appear to produce diarrhea by similar mechanisms to the archetypical enterotoxigenic bacteria of humans, *Vibrio cholera*. *Vibrio cholera* enterotoxin is a heat-labile protein with a molecular weight of about 80,000 daltons. Part of the toxin molecule binds to a receptor on the epithelial cell. Following its mucosal attachment a subunit of the cholera toxin diffuses through the cell to the basal lateral membrane where the toxin activates adenyl cyclase, producing cyclic AMP. The net effect of cyclic AMP on the intestinal epithelial cell is to inhibit linked sodium and chloride absorption and increase electrogenic chloride and potassium secretion by the apical membrane.[4] The composition of the secretion induced by cyclic AMP is similar to that of normal intestinal secretions. The majority of cyclic AMP's effect on the apical membrane is related to phosphorylation of protein kinases, a phosphatase, and several substrate proteins in the membrane.[4] Part of the cyclic AMP effect may be mediated by an interaction with calcium-mediated processes. Although direct activation of the cyclic AMP system is considered the major way by which cholera toxin initiates diarrhea, an interaction of the toxin with the enteric nervous system has also been proposed.[4] Humans suffering from cholera can lose copious amounts of fluid. The fluid secretion continues for the life of the villus cell, which may be for 2 to 5 days or until the secreting cells desquamate and are replaced by newly matured cells that have migrated from the crypt. Many of the secreting mucosa's absorptive mechanisms remain intact, permitting the treatment of cholera-induced fluid losses with oral fluid replacement. The administration of balanced solutions with added glucose takes advantage of the mechanisms that provide for the mutual absorption of sodium and glucose. This facilitated transport of glucose, sodium, and chloride permits more effective absorption of fluid than does the transport of sodium and chloride alone.[5]

The intestinal secretion induced by the enterotoxins produced by *Vibrio cholera*, *Salmonella*, *Campylobacter jejuni*, *Pseudomonas aeruginosa*, and *Shigella*, and the heat-labile *Escherichia coli* enterotoxin are all mediated predominantly through the cyclic AMP mechanism just described. In contrast, the intestinal secretion induced by the enterotoxins produced by *Yersinia enterocolitica* and *Klebsiella pneumoniae,* and the heat-stable *Escherichia coli* enterotoxin are mediated predominantly through cyclic GMP–dependent mechanisms.[4] The enterotoxin secreted by *Clostridium difficile* is thought to result in calcium-dependent intestinal secretion. The effects of the cyclic GMP and calcium second messenger systems on intestinal secretion are not well understood. They are thought to be similar to the effects of cyclic AMP, but the magnitude of the chloride secretory response induced by agents acting through cyclic AMP is greater than that caused by agents acting through cyclic GMP and calcium.[4] The second messengers of the enterotoxins produced by *Clostridium perfringens* and *Staphylococcus aureus* are unknown. *Entamoeba histolytica* is a protozoa that excretes an enterotoxin capable of producing secretory diarrhea. Like many enterotoxigenic bacteria, however, this organism also secretes cytotoxic products that allow mucosal invasion. More details of the enterotoxins produced by each species of microorganism are provided in the discussion of the diarrheal syndromes pertaining to each species.

The importance of enterotoxigenic pathogens in small animals is unknown, but evidence is accumulating to suggest that those such as *E. coli* and *C. perfringens* play a significant role in both acute and chronic diarrhea (see later).

Enteroadherent Infectious Agents

Certain strains of *E. coli* tightly adhere in an extensive coat to the gastrointestinal mucosa. They efface broad expanses of microvilli, inducing a distinctive lesion characterized by an irregular scalloping of the epithelial layer and producing chronic diarrhea.[6–8] The prevalence of diarrhea due to enteroadherent organisms in cats and dogs is unknown. Isolated reports of enteroadherent *E. coli* have been reported in pups and cats with diarrhea.[6,7] Enteroadherent gram positive cocci, thought to be *Streptococcus* spp., have been associated with diarrhea in dogs.[9] Heavy infections with *Giardia* may produce diarrhea by similar mechanisms to enteroadherent bacteria.[10]

Mucosal-Invading Infectious Agents

Some pathogenic microorganisms are able to attach to and penetrate mucosal epithelial cells. These so-called enteroinvasive bacteria include *Shigella, Salmonella, Campylobacter, Yersinia,* and invasive strains of *E. coli.* Collectively, diarrhea due to one or other of these enteroinvasive organisms is relatively common in cats and dogs.

Shigella is the prototype enteroinvasive bacteria of humans. *Shigella* invade epithelial cells and produce cytotoxic enterotoxins that destroy the cell. Other enteroinvasive bacteria appear to damage the mucosa in a similar manner to *Shigella.* Disruption of the mucosal surface leads to clinical signs of enterocolitis, including watery diarrhea and, as the condition progresses, dysentery. The mechanism of fluid production in invasive diarrhea may be multifactorial. As discussed in Chapter 18, damage to the epithelial surface results in an inability to resorb fluid, creating a passive intestinal secretion. Furthermore, invasive organisms increase local synthesis of prostaglandins that may mediate the diarrhea. Moreover, villus atrophy as a result of epithelial cell destruction and increased turnover may lead to malabsorption. In addition, as mentioned earlier, many invasive organisms concurrently produce enterotoxins that stimulate surviving enterocytes to

secrete fluid. And finally, if the permeability breakdown of the mucosal barrier is sufficient, the exudation of interstitial fluid, protein, and blood is unrestricted.

Bacteria are not the only microorganisms capable of producing diarrhea by mucosal invasion. Protozoa such as *Entamoeba histolytica, Balantidium coli,* and *Coccidia* also invade the epithelium or lamina propria. Furthermore, *Giardia* has occasionally been demonstrated within intestinal epithelial cells. All enteropathogenic viruses invade the intestinal epithelium. The site at which they invade markedly affects their pathologic potential. Thus, coronaviruses, rotaviruses, and reoviruses damage the mature enterocytes on the tips of the villi. The result is mild villus atrophy, malabsorption, and a passive secretory diarrhea as a result of deficient intestinal fluid absorption. In contrast, canine parvovirus and feline panleukopenia virus infect and destroy the epithelial cells in the small intestinal crypts. The consequence of this cytotropism is denudation and collapse of the villi because of failed enterocyte replication. Diarrhea results from malabsorption and from increased permeability.

Submucosal-Invading Infectious Agents

If not kept in check by the immune system, many of the mucosal-invasive infectious agents just discussed may go on to invade the submucosa. After they penetrate the submucosa they stimulate marked inflammation characterized by neutrophil accumulation and, in the latter stages, by macrophage infiltration. Septicemia often develops when submucosal invasion occurs and normal defense mechanisms are overwhelmed. Invasive strains of *E. coli* and *Salmonella* are the most important bacteria causing septicemia from an intestinal infection. Some *Salmonella* are resistant to the effects of leukocytes and can replicate in macrophages, in which they can be transported to other parts of the body. In this intracellular location, *Salmonella* are quite resistant to many antibiotics. In the presence of antibiotics the growth of the organism is often inhibited, but as soon as the antibiotics are discontinued the *Salmonella* organisms are able to multiply rapidly. This phenomenon is the basis for the carrier state that can develop after an acute attack of Salmonella enteritis. In humans, *Yersinia enterocolitica* infection may also progress from the mucosa into the submucosa to cause septicemia, as can *Balantidium coli.* Fungi such as *Absidia, Mucor, Rhizopus, Aspergillus, Histoplasma,* and *Candida* may also invade the intestinal wall. The portal of entry may be a preexisting defect or could result from the carriage of fungal spores from the lumen into the mucosa by macrophages.

BACTERIAL GASTROENTERITIS

Campylobacteriosis

Clinical Synopsis

*Diagnostic Features**

- Young animal; often recently kenneled
- Acute onset of mild, mucoid diarrhea; rarely hemorrhagic
- *Campylobacter jejuni* cultured from feces
- Rapid response to therapy

Standard Treatment

- Erythromycin: 10 to 15 mg/kg q 8 hours PO for 5 to 7 days
- Quarantine away from children
- Advise owner on hygiene

---

*Presumptive diagnosis only.

ETIOLOGY AND EPIZOOTOLOGY. Interest in *Campylobacter* has burgeoned recently and the reader is referred to several detailed articles for in-depth discussion of this pathogen.[11-13] The majority of publications concerning campylobacteriosis have focused on *Campylobacter jejuni*, but it appears that a pathogenic role for *C. upsaliensis* and *C. coli* must also be considered.[14-18] In addition, a related bacterial family, *Helicobacter*, is a cause of gastritis and peptic ulcerations in humans and perhaps animals (see Chapter 15).[19]

Campylobacter jejuni is a small, curved, motile, microaerophilic, gram negative rod. It can be isolated from the feces of a high percentage (approximately 40%) of healthy animals that have been kenneled, particularly in animal control facilities.[14,20,21] Cohabitation increases the prevalence of *Campylobacter*.[20] Isolations of *Campylobacter* from healthy noncohabiting dogs, such as household pets or dogs in veterinary practices, are relatively low,[20] although in one study reached 12%.[21] Many studies have not found a significant difference between the frequency of isolation between normal and diarrheic dogs and cats. Moreover, experimental infection of dogs and cats with *Campylobacter jejuni* has met with inconsistent results, probably due to strain differences and variations in the susceptibility of the host populations studied.[16,22-24] There seems little doubt, however, that in young dogs and cats some strains of *Campylobacter jejuni* can act as a primary enteric pathogen.[15,16] In older animals it is likely that *Campylobacter* acts more as an opportunist, producing disease only when appropriate predisposing factors lower the host's resistance. Predisposing factors include stress and concurrent infection with other enteric pathogens such as parvovirus, coronavirus, and *Giardia*.

Campylobacter can survive for days in surface water and as long as 4 weeks in feces. The duration of excretion in infected dogs and cats can be as long as 4 months. Asymptomatic carriers are frequent.[25] Contamination of food and water sources with *Campylobacter*-infected feces is the most likely mode of transmission. The incubation period is 3 to 7 days.

PATHOGENESIS. *Campylobacter jejuni* can colonize the jejunum, ileum, cecum, and colon, but histopathologic changes are largely restricted to the large bowel. *Campylobacter jejuni* produces a secretory diarrhea and less frequently invades the epithelium.[24] The organism produces an enterotoxin that has immunologic similarity to both the cholera toxin and the *E. coli* heat-labile toxin. The secretory diarrhea resulting from *Campylobacter jejuni* is mediated by cyclic AMP. *Campylobacter* also elaborate a cytotoxic enterotoxin that is presumably responsible for the epithelial damage. Bacteremia and extraintestinal colonization, particularly in the early stages of infection, has been reported.[24,26]

CLINICAL FEATURES. Clinical signs of campylobacteriosis in dogs have ranged from mild transient diarrhea to mucus-laden bloody stools with associated tenesmus, vomiting, anorexia, and depression.[11,23,24,27-29] In cats, diarrhea is sometimes profuse and watery but is most often soft and mucoid.[30] In both species, fever is usually absent, except in the severe cases. Rare fatal cases have been recorded.[17,18] Clinical signs are usually self-limiting within several days to several weeks. Young animals exposed to a kenneling situation are most likely to be affected, particularly with the more severe signs. At necropsy, the most consistent gross abnormality is mesenteric lymphadenopathy.[24] Histologic changes are usually restricted to the large bowel and can include mucosal hyperplasia, a reduction in crypt height, a change to a cuboidal epithelium, and infiltration of the lamina propria with a mild, mixed inflammatory infiltrate. A proliferative enteritis has also been attributed to *Campylobacter*.[33] Some strains produce no histologic abnormalities.

A tentative diagnosis rests on a positive fecal culture in an animal with appropriate clinical signs. The organism is fastidious and fecal samples must be submitted to the laboratory immediately or, if delay is expected, placed in appropriate transport material. As mentioned earlier, *Campylobacter jejuni* can be cultured from normal animals, and so circumspection is required before a diarrheal process is ascribed to campylobacteriosis.

PUBLIC HEALTH CONCERNS AND THERAPY. The zoonotic potential is high. It is estimated that 5% to 11% of all human diarrhea cases result from *Campylobacter jejuni*.[34] As many as 5% of these cases may have resulted from exposure to *Campylobacter*-infected dogs and cats.[35] Humans appear to be considerably more susceptible to *Campylobacter* infection than dogs and cats, and the diarrheal process is predictably more severe. In view of the high risk to humans, antibiotic therapy of animals with *Campylobacter*-associated diarrhea is warranted. Erythromycin (10–15 mg/kg PO q 8 hours), tetracycline (20 mg/kg PO q 8 hours), or tylosin (20 mg/kg q 12 hours PO) for 5 to 7 days appear to eradicate infection from dogs and cats.[11,36] Aminoglycosides, chloramphenicol, and fluoroquinilones are also usually successful. Ampicillin and trimethoprim-sulfonamides are less effective. Occasionally additional supportive therapy, such as fluids, may be required. Owners should be advised on appropriate hygienic measures. The animal should not be allowed to come in contact with children until the diarrhea has resolved (and therefore the chance of fecal contamination of the children's environment has been reduced). It is noteworthy that the prevalence of quinilone-resistant *Campylobacter* is increasing in children and has been attributed to increasing veterinary use of these drugs.[37] Most commonly used disinfectants, including hypochlorite, will kill the organism. Consideration should be given to the possibility that the source of bacteria which infected the dog might also be a potential source for human members of the family.

Clostridium difficile

Clostridium difficile is responsible for antibiotic-associated pseudomembranous colitis. This disease has been reported in humans treated with antibiotics that suppress the normal colonic flora such as clindamycin, lincomycin, ampicillin, and cephalosporins. Pseudomembranous colitis is very uncommon in dogs or cats, but has been reported in one dog treated with clindamycin.[38] Association with *C. difficile* was not established in this case. As with *C. perfringens*, positive fecal cultures of *C. difficile* must be interpreted cautiously because the organism can be recovered from up to 40% of cats and dogs attending veterinary clinics and is present in up to 10% of healthy dogs and cats.[39,40]

Clostridium difficile infection has been incriminated as a cause of chronic diarrhea in three dogs.[41] The animals had chronic watery diarrhea. *C. difficile* and *C. difficile* toxin were recovered from the dogs, and the response to metronidazole was prompt. Metronidazole administration was required on a long-term basis in two of the dogs to maintain remission. Unfortunately, no colon biopsies were taken to confirm pseudomembranous colitis, and the authors mention no attempt to rule out other metronidazole-responsive diseases such as chronic idiopathic colitis and giardiasis.

Clostridium perfringens-Associated Diarrhea

Clinical Synopsis

*Diagnostic Features**

- Acute onset of watery or hemorrhagic diarrhea or chronic intermittent large-bowel diarrhea
- Hospitalized patients predisposed
- *Clostridium perfringens* enterotoxin isolated from the feces
- Heavy, relatively pure growths of *C. perfringens* on fecal or intestinal fluid culture
- Greater than five *C. perfringens* spores per high power oil immersion field in fecal smears
- Rapid response to therapy

Standard Treatment

- Oral or intravenous fluid therapy
- Withhold food for 24 to 48 hours in acute cases
- Ampicillin 20 mg/kg q 8 hours PO, IV, SC for 3 to 5 days if hemorrhagic diarrhea
- High-fiber diets or tylosin (10–20 mg/kg q 12–24 hours PO as required) for chronic relapsing cases

*Presumptive diagnosis only.

ETIOLOGY AND EPIZOOTIOLOGY. *Clostridium perfringens* is a gram positive, anaerobic bacillus that is a normal resident of the intestinal flora of dogs and cats. The bacteria can be cultured from the feces of approximately 50% of healthy dogs and cats in moderate numbers (10^4–10^8 colony forming units per gram of feces).[42] In dogs and cats with diarrhea, the frequency of positive *C. perfringens* fecal cultures increases to 78% and 66%, respectively, and the numbers of *C. perfringens* increase to between 10^4 and 10^{10} CFU/g of feces.[42] More importantly, *C. perfringens* enterotoxin cannot be detected in nondiarrheic feces but can be detected in approximately 50% of dogs and 30% of cats with diarrhea.[42] At Colorado State University, enterotoxigenic *C. perfringens* are identified in 15% of dogs presented with gastrointestinal disease and are occasionally observed in cats.[43] These data support a primary or secondary role for *C. perfringens* in diarrhea in dogs and cats. A zoonotic potential has not been established.

ETIOPATHOGENESIS. *C. perfringens* produces an enterotoxin that is cytotoxic in addition to altering the absorptive and secretory functions in the cell.[44] The enterotoxin can result in gastroenteritis if increased quantities of the toxin are ingested on contaminated food or if overgrowth of *C. perfringens* occurs in the intestine. The latter will occasionally happen after a sudden diet change and can result in peracute hemorrhagic diarrhea and death within 24 hours. Intestinal overgrowth with *Clostridia* can occur with any disorder that results in intestinal stasis such as intestinal obstruction or adynamic ileus. Furthermore, heavy growths of *C. perfringens* are frequently recovered from the jejunal content of dogs with parvoviral enteritis.[47]

CLINICAL FEATURES. In dogs and cats, *C. perfringens* is traditionally associated with peracute mucoid or hemorrhagic gastroenteritis.[45,46] However, the spectrum of *C. perfringens*-associated disease appears to include not only the acute hemorrhagic gastroenteritis with which the bacillus is traditionally associated but also chronic intermittent diarrhea.[43] Dogs with antibiotic-responsive chronic intermittent diarrhea that were excreting excess quantities of *Clostridial* enterotoxin have been described.[43] In the chronic cases, signs may persist for months, flaring up every few weeks. The diarrhea usually has the features of large-bowel involvement including increased fecal mucus, fresh blood, and tenesmus but occasionally watery small-bowel–type diarrhea will be observed.[43] *C. perfringens* is also emerging as an important cause of outbreaks of nosocomial diarrhea in dogs.[43,48] The clinical signs of a series of dogs with nosocomial diarrhea associated with *C. perfringens* of a variety of serotypes included mild depression and soft watery diarrhea with or without frank blood, mucus, and tenesmus.[48] Dogs with diarrhea had significantly higher fecal *Clostridial* counts than did dogs without diarrhea. *C. perfringens* enterotoxin was found in the feces of 41% of diarrheic dogs but in only 7% of dogs without diarrhea.[48]

DIAGNOSIS. *Clostridium perfringens*–associated diarrhea should be suspected in dogs with excess quantities of enterotoxin in their feces, or with histopathologic evidence of a suppurative, hemorrhagic, necrotizing, mucofibrinous or catarrhal colitis or enterocolitis that responds promptly to ampicillin or metronidazole. The enterotoxin can be measured in feces with an ELISA or reverse passive latex agglutination test. Occasional false negative results can occur.[43] Furthermore, *C. perfringens* enterotoxin can be detected in some dogs with underlying disease processes such as inflammatory bowel disease and parvoviral enteritis that presumably predispose them to *Clostridial* overgrowth.[43] Thus, identifying the enterotoxin in the feces establishes the patient has increased numbers of enterotoxigenic *C. perfringens*, but it does not prove the gastrointestinal signs are due to the organism. As mentioned earlier, *C. perfringens* is a normal component of the intestinal flora. Both enterotoxigenic and nonenterotoxigenic strains exist. Therefore, fecal cultures yielding *C. perfringens* must be interpreted cautiously. Heavy pure growths of the bacillus are probably significant, particularly if culture of small intestinal fluid reveals a similar picture. Some dogs with *Clostridium perfringens*–associated diarrhea shed endospores that can be observed on fecal smears and others have a fecal smear almost exclusively composed of gram positive bacilli. The spores have a "safety pin" appearance (Figure 6–2)[43] Greater than 5 spores per high power oil immersion is considered abnormal and suggests *C. perfringens*–associated diarrhea.[43] In dogs with chronic intermittent signs, the feces should be examined for enterotoxin or spores during a clinical episode; otherwise there may be insufficient enterotoxin or spores present to allow a diagnosis.[43]

THERAPY. Acute mild cases of watery diarrhea are likely to be self-limiting and require only supportive care such as easily digestible diets and appropriate fluid therapy. Most dogs recover within 2 to 3 days to 1 one week with or without treatment. Dogs with acute hemorrhagic diarrhea should be promptly treated by withholding food and administering antibiotics. If *Clostridial* overgrowth is suspected, ampicillin (20 mg/kg q 8 hours, PO, IV, SC) or metronidazole (10–15 mg/kg q 12 hours, PO) for 5 to 7 days is recommended. Dogs with chronic relapsing signs may require a 2 to 3 week course of antibiotics to eliminate the disease. Those dogs that repeatedly relapse after discontinuation of antibiotics should be placed on high-fiber prescription diets or should have psyllium fiber (1 tablespoon per 25 kg) added to their regular diet.[43] Soluble fiber, such as psyllium, probably helps prevent the disease by increasing the colonic volatile fatty acid content. If the addition of fiber to the diet is not successful in preventing the disease, consider daily or alternate daily ampicillin, tetracycline, metronidazole, or tylosin.[43] If nosocomial *C. perfringens* is a problem, consider placing the majority of hospitalized patients on high-fiber diets such as Prescription Diet w/d (Hills Pet Products) and thoroughly disinfecting cages and floors with sporicidal disinfectants.

Escherichia coli Enteritis[4]

Clinical Synopsis

*Diagnostic Features**

- Acute onset of watery or hemorrhagic diarrhea most common
- Enteroadherent strains may cause chronic diarrhea
- Pathogenic *E. coli* subtype cultured from feces
- Enteroadherent strains may be recognized by intestinal biopsy
- Rapid response to therapy

Standard Treatment

- Oral or intravenous fluid therapy
- Withhold food for 12 to 24 hours
- Bismuth subsalicylate 0.25 mL/kg q 4 to 6 hours for 3 to 5 days
- Trimethoprim-sulfa 15 mg/kg q 12 hours for 5 to 7 days (hemorrhagic or enteroadherent forms)
- Advise owner on hygiene

*Presumptive diagnosis only.

ETIOLOGY AND EPIZOOTIOLOGY. *Escherichia coli* are a major component of the intestinal flora. There are a very large number of *E. coli* subtypes. Most are harmless, but through refined identification techniques over 100 potentially pathogenic subtypes of *E. coli* have been defined.[4,34] In humans, *E. coli* is now thought to be one of the most common causes of acute diarrhea. Enterotoxigenic *E. coli* are isolated from 40% to 70% of people with traveler's diarrhea.[34] Invasive *E. coli* are isolated in 0% to 4% of the same syndrome. The importance of *E. coli* infections in cats and dogs is unknown, but evidence is building that they may play an important role[7,8,49–54]

Potentially pathogenic strains of hemolytic *E. coli* have been isolated from dogs and cats with diarrhea.[53,54] In one study, particularly common *E. coli* serotypes in both dogs and cats were 04K6L, 06KL, 023K181, and 025K23L.[53] A relatively slow-acting heat-labile enterotoxin of *E. coli* origin has been isolated from dogs with diarrhea,[52] and enteroinvasive strains are suspected to occur occasionally. Transient gastroenteritis associated with pathogenic strains of *E. coli* have occasionally been reported in cats.[49] In an outbreak of diarrhea in a cattery, hemolytic *E. coli* with recognized pathogenic O groups were isolated from 93% of affected cats, whereas only 22% of normal cats carried pathogenic strains.[50] Recovered cats carried the pathogenic serotype for greater than 10 months after recovery. The pathogenic serotypes most commonly implicated in feline diarrhea are 06, and to a lesser extent 078, 025, 0141, and K80.[49,51] Strains of *E. coli* that secrete a *Shigella*-like toxin have been isolated from cats and neonatal humans with diarrhea responsible for widespread outbreaks of hemorrhagic colitis in people.[57]

Diarrhea resulting from enteroadherent-effacing *E. coli* has been diagnosed in two cats presented with anorexia and diarrhea.[9] Light microscopy revealed mild neutrophilic infiltration with diffuse atrophy and focal fusion of villi. An extensive layer of bacteria were demonstrated attached to the villi in association with extensive microvilli effacement. Both the colon and small intestine were affected. Enteroadherent and effacing *E. coli* have been reported in young pups with hemorrhagic diarrhea.[7]

PATHOGENESIS. Enterotoxigenic strains of *E. coli* are a cause of secretory diarrhea in many species. Some strains produce a heat-labile toxin that increases adenylate cyclase activity. Other strains of *E. coli* produce a heat-stable enterotoxin that induces secretory diarrhea through cyclic GMP–mediated mechanisms. Enterotoxigenic strains of *E. coli* depend on specific fimbrial antigens (colonization factor antigens) for adherence to the mucosa and subsequent colonization. The antigenic structure of the fimbriae determine the species specificity of the enterotoxigenic *E. coli* strains. Thus, *E. coli* bearing K88 antigen are pathogenic for piglets; those bearing K99 antigen cause diarrhea in calves and lambs. The ability to produce enterotoxins is under genetic control that can be transferred from one strain to another through plasmids. Some strains of *E. coli* produce enterotoxins but do not cause disease because the particular strain is normally restricted to the colon, which is a site where the toxin does not act.[56] They are pathogenic only when they colonize the small intestine.

Diarrhea from enteroadherent or effacing strains of *E. coli* tends to have a chronic course. The mechanism of the diarrhea appears to relate to a diffuse effacing of the microvilli, perhaps by the release of a cytotoxin.[6] Finally, several *E. coli* strains induce diarrhea by mucosal invasion. These strains are termed enteroinvasive *E. coli*.

In all species studied, immunity to most pathogenic *E. coli* and their toxins develops readily. Older dogs are resistant to colonization by enterotoxigenic *E. coli* given orally.[56] Resistance to colonization is as great in 10- to 12-week-old pups as in adult dogs. Dogs are partially resistant to *E. coli* enterotoxin placed directly in the lumen of the small intestine. With a few subsequent challenges, they become completely resistant to the toxin. Because circulating antitoxin levels do not change, the local immune system is thought to be responsible for the resistance. The immunogenicity of the enterotoxins of most enterotoxigenic bacteria argues against an important role for enterotoxigenic bacteria in chronic diarrhea. There is evidence to suggest, however, that the heat-stable enterotoxin produced by some *E. coli* strains is less immunogenic and can be a cause of persistent diarrhea. Furthermore, the enteroadherent strains of *E. coli* appear to be able to colonize the mucosa for prolonged periods of time.

CLINICAL FEATURES. Puppies and kittens within the first few weeks of life can succumb to neonatal colibacillosis.[11,49] Clinical signs shown include acute depression, weakness, hypothermia, and cyanosis and signs of CNS dysfunction immediately before death.[11] The diagnosis is confirmed by culture of *E. coli* from tissues such as the spleen and liver.

The predominate clinical sign of enterotoxigenic *E. coli* infection is watery diarrhea, and that of enteroinvasive *E. coli* is hemorrhagic "large-bowel" type diarrhea. Unfortunately, definitive diagnosis of coliform enteritis is difficult to make clinically. Laboratory changes are nonspecific and diagnosis cannot be made by routine culture of the feces because routine culture methods do not differentiate pathogenic from nonpathogenic *E. coli*. Pathogenic *E. coli* strains can be identified by animal inoculation studies, demonstration of cytotoxicity in vero cell cultures, serotyping, or DNA probes. The detection of a significant number of pathogenic *E. coli* in the feces of an animal with watery or hemorrhagic diarrhea allows a presumptive diagnosis of coliform enteritis to be made. A rapid response to antibiotics helps confirm, but by no means proves, the diagnosis.

THERAPY. Therapy of colibacillosis depends on the presenting signs. In neonatal colibacillosis, antibiotic therapy may be attempted but is rarely successful unless begun prior to all but the mildest clinical signs. All members of the litter should be treated. The most suitable antibiotics are cephalosporins or ampicillin. In older animals, colibacillosis is usually rapidly self-limiting and therapy is primarily supportive. Treatment may include oral or intravenous fluids in association with bismuth subsalicylate. In humans, antibiotic therapy has minimal influence on the course of the enterotoxigenic diarrhea, but is recommended for therapy of the enteroinvasive *E. coli* infections. It is probable that antibiotic therapy may also be required for the enteroadherent forms of *E. coli*. Antibiotics usually effective against *E. coli* are trimethoprim-sulfa, cephalosporins, chloramphenicol, aminoglycosides, tetracycline, doxycycline, ampicillin, and fluoroquinilones.[34,58] The use of orally administered autogenous vaccines in the treatment of presumptive antibiotic-resistant *E. coli* enteritis in dogs and cats has been reported.[59]

PUBLIC HEALTH ASPECTS. Most enterotoxigenic *E. coli* are species specific so it is unlikely they are public health risks. As mentioned earlier, however, enterohemorrhagic and enteroinvasive strains are potentially important public health risks.

SUMMARY. Evidence is accumulating that pathogenic serotypes of *E. coli* are a cause of diarrhea in both neonatal and adult dogs and cats, but the prevalence of diarrhea due to *E. coli* is unknown. Enterotoxigenic and enteroinvasive *E. coli* are most likely to be responsible for acute self-limiting diarrhea in animals exposed to a kennel or cattery environment. Enteroadherent *E. coli* may be responsible for chronic diarrhea.

Klebsiella pneumoniae[60]

Klebsiella produces an enterotoxin that at low doses stimulates secretion of fluid and at high doses produces morphologic changes in the mucosa. The intestinal secretion is mediated through a cyclic GMP mechanism. The importance of this bacteria in diarrheal diseases of dogs and cats is unknown. It is occasionally isolated from the feces of dogs with diarrhea.[61]

Leptospirosis

Leptospirosis is occasionally a cause of acute vomiting and diarrhea in dogs. The disease is due to infection with pathogenic serovars of *Leptospira interrogans*. Clinical signs usually include acute onset of anorexia, depression, vomiting, and clinical evidence of sepsis, such as fever. Physical examination may reveal abdominal pain or icterus. Classically, laboratory evidence of concurrent renal failure and liver disease will be found but a variety of syndromes can occur and depend somewhat on the particular serovar involved.[62] These syndromes include an acute bleeding diathesis with rapid death, renal failure without overt liver disease, and chronic hepatitis without associated renal disease.

Diagnosis is made by demonstrating a fourfold rise in serum *Leptospira* titer, by urine culture, or by detecting spirochetal organisms in urine with darkfield microscopy or tissues with the Warthin-Starry staining technique. Treatment requires fluid and antibiotic therapy. The antibiotic of choice is penicillin

(e.g., 40,000–80,000 units/kg SQ or IM q 12 hours for 10–14 days), but oxytetracycline and doxycycline are also effective. Once renal function has improved, chronic carriers may have to be treated with dihydrostreptomycin (10–15 mg/kg IM q 12 hours for 7–14 days) to eliminate the carrier state. Oliguric dogs require intensive mannitol therapy. The zoonotic risk is high and personnel handling affected dogs must take the appropriate precautions.

Salmonellosis[63–65]

Clinical Synopsis

*Diagnostic Features**

- Young animals; often recently kenneled
- Acute onset of watery or hemorrhagic diarrhea
- *Salmonella* spp. cultured from feces and/or extraintestinal tissue
- Rapid response to therapy

Standard Treatment

- Oral or intravenous fluid therapy
- Withhold food for 12 to 24 hours
- Bismuth subsalicylate (0.25–0.5 mL/kg q 4–6 hours for 3–5 days)
- Norfloxacin** (22 mg/kg PO q 12 hours for 7 days) (hemorrhagic form) or
- Trimethoprim-sulfa (15 mg/kg PO q 12 hours for 7 days) (hemorrhagic form)
- Advise owner on hygiene

---

*Presumptive diagnosis only.
**Or other fluoroquinilone (e.g., Baytril).

Etiology and Epizootiology.[11] Salmonella organisms are gram negative aerobic bacilli with a propensity for intracellular persistence. The *Salmonella* isolated most frequently from dogs and cats are various subtypes of *Salmonella enteritidis*. This species has over 1700 potentially pathogenic serotypes. As many as 53 serotypes have been isolated from dogs.[64] The most frequently isolated serotypes are *S. typhimurium* and *S. anatum*. *Salmonella krefeld* was isolated from a nosocomial outbreak at the University of California, Davis, Veterinary Medical Teaching Hospital (UCD VMTH).[66] *Salmonella* can be cultured from the feces of normal as well as diarrheic animals. The frequency of isolation from normal animals varies considerably. Isolation frequencies as great as 36% have been reported from clinically normal dogs. In cats, isolation frequencies as high as 18% have been reported.[67] Cats appear to be more resistant to salmonellosis than dogs. At the UCD VMTH, *Salmonella* are rarely cultured from the feces of healthy household pets. Positive cultures are usually found in animals debilitated by other diseases such as parvovirus, suggesting an opportunistic behavior. The frequency of *Salmonella* isolation and *Salmonella*-associated diarrhea is highest in young, stressed, or diseased cats and dogs housed in poorly sanitary, overcrowded conditions. There may be a seasonal prevalence, with peak incidence at the coldest time of the year. Obesity, glucocorticoid therapy, and antecedent or concomitant antibiotic therapy (particularly ampicillin) are additional risk factors.[11,66,68]

Salmonella are readily transmitted from carriers by fecal contamination of food and water. Wild animals and birds are a reservoir. An outbreak of salmonellosis in cats has been linked to an epidemic of salmonellosis in a population of songbirds.[69] Products of the poultry industry are the largest reservoir of *Salmonella* but farm animal products, such as blood and bonemeal, are also important. Commercial pet foods that are not cooked during processing are a potential source of the bacteria. For instance, dehydrated dog food has been found to be a source of *Salmonella*. In contrast, canned or kibbled products are cooked during processing, destroying any *Salmonella* contained in the raw materials.

Salmonella can survive for prolonged periods outside the host, particularly in aquatic environments. The infectivity of *Salmonella* varies with the strain and the size of the inoculum. The incubation period is 3 to 5 days. Shedding may continue for 3 to 6 weeks, but can be reactivated at a later date by any intercurrent stress. As with all zoonotic pathogens, consideration must be given to the possibility that the source of bacteria which infected the dog or cat might also be a source of infection for human members of the family.

PATHOGENESIS. The primary pathogenic mechanism of *Salmonella* is mucosal invasion that induces inflammation, necrosis, and increased synthesis of prostaglandins. However, cell-free lysates of *Salmonella* stimulate intestinal secretion, and it appears that cyclic AMP–mediated secretory diarrhea induced by *Salmonella* enterotoxin is involved in the pathogenesis of salmonellosis.[4] The organism preferentially localizes in the ileum and affects the colon to a lesser extent.

CLINICAL FEATURES. The clinical signs are highly variable. Most animals infected with *Salmonella* are asymptomatic. Mild to severe acute gastroenteritis may be seen. This may progress to septicemia. The septicemia can be acute and progress rapidly to collapse and death or it may be less fulminating. The more severe cases of gastroenteritis are characterized by fever, vomiting, abdominal pain, and diarrhea. The diarrhea varies from watery to mucoid, and fresh blood may be present. Some cats[70] and dogs may present with a chronic febrile illness without specific gastrointestinal signs. Hematologic abnormalities are variable, but in the acute stage a degenerative left shift is not uncommon. A fecal smear often reveals leukocytes. Diagnosis rests on appropriate clinical signs in association with positive fecal or blood culture. As with the other enteric pathogens, a positive fecal culture proves infection, but does not establish the clinical signs are a result of the *Salmonella*. Culture of the organism from blood or other body fluid is more definitive but does not detect infections limited to the mucosa. A negative culture result does not rule out salmonellosis because the organism can be difficult to isolate. Histologic changes in the intestinal mucosa vary from mild catarrhal inflammation to extensive mucosal sloughing. Invasion of the lamina propria with neutrophils and to a lesser extent macrophages are also seen. Less than 10% of infected animals die within the acute stages of salmonellosis,[11] although occasional outbreaks have been associated with mortalities as high as 61%,[71] and salmonellosis as a complication of protracted medical problems has a 50% mortality rate.[68] Recovery usually occurs within 1 week but may take 3 to 4 weeks.

THERAPY. Recommendations on antibiotic usage in the therapy of salmonellosis remain controversial. Fluoroquinolones appear to be highly effective against all aerobic bowel pathogens including *Salmonella*, but like other antibiotics can prolong the carrier state.[72] Proposed reasons for the prolongation of the carrier state by antibiotics include the inability of antibiotics to destroy organisms localized within macrophages and the development of resistant strains. Amid this uncertainty the following recommendations can be made.

Salmonella invasion limited to the superficial mucosa produces a self-limiting gastroenteritis. In such uncomplicated cases, treatment with antibiotics is unnecessary, and therapy is best restricted to supportive measures in association with advice on appropriate hygiene and/or quarantine procedures. In contrast, antibiotic therapy is indicated if the diarrhea is hemorrhagic, the patient depressed or febrile, or laboratory evidence of sepsis such as a degenerative left shift or a positive blood culture are observed. If blood culture or fecal culture results are available, therapy may be based on sensitivity patterns. Unfortunately, the sensitivity pattern of *Salmonella* organisms can be poorly predictive of in vivo response to antibiotics.[70] If blood culture results are unavailable, the antibiotics of choice are a member of the fluoroquinilones, chloramphenicol, or a trimethoprim-sulfonamide.

Salmonella resist common forms of disinfection. Activated aqueous glutaraldehyde (2%) applied for 30 minutes to an hour is usually effective and suitable for most surfaces and equipment.[11] Because of potential risks to personnel, however, glutaraldehyde should only be used in well-ventilated areas.

Shigellosis

Shigella have been infrequently isolated from the feces and mesenteric nodes of dogs.[73] *Shigella* are known to produce enterotoxins with both secretory and cytotoxic properties. The cytotoxin is responsible for the dysentery of patients with shigellosis. *Shigella* toxins are heat labile and readily degraded by proteolytic enzymes. The virulence of these organisms depends on both their invasive properties and the ability to produce the cytotoxin.[74] *Shigella* infection results in rapid production of a toxin-neutralizing antibody of the IgM class that persists for 9 to 18 months. *Shigella* are unlikely to be an important cause of disease in animals but it is possible that dogs and cats contaminated by *Shigella* from humans could act as a transient zoonotic reservoir.

Spiral-Shaped Organisms

Helix-shaped bacteria are normal inhabitants of the gastric mucosa of dogs and cats.[75-77] Their pathogenicity has not been established, but it seems likely they can cause a low-grade chronic gastritis (see Chapter 15). Furthermore, a recent report has described bloody diarrhea in a group of Persian cats with lymphocytic-plasmacytic gastroenterocolitis associated with a spiral-shaped organism.[78] The organism was observed in the gastrointestinal lumen and intracellularly in the gastric and colonic epithelium. The organism could not be cultured and its significance is unknown, but it is noteworthy that cells containing the organism were frequently undergoing degeneration, suggesting the organism was not a commensal. It also seems likely that two spiral bacteria, *Helicobacter felis* and *Gastrospirillum hominis*, are public health risks (see Chapter 15).

Staphylococcus aureus[79]

Overgrowth of the small intestine by *Staphylococcus aureus* can be caused by broad-spectrum antibiotic therapy, resulting in diarrhea of variable severity. This microorganism produces an enterotoxin that inhibits fluid absorption in the jejunum by unknown mechanisms. It also produces cytotoxic enterotoxin. *Staphylococcus aureus* is occasionally isolated from the feces of dogs with diarrhea.[61]

Streptococcus durans

Suspicion is mounting that *Streptococcus durans* may occasionally be responsible for diarrhea in dogs and other species.[9] The organism is a gram positive coccus that appears to be capable of acting as an enteroadherent pathogen (see earlier). Presumptive diagnosis is made by microscopic examination of small intestinal biopsy specimens that reveals large numbers of gram positive cocci tightly adherent to the villus surface.[9] The organism is likely to be sensitive to penicillins.

Tuberculosis

Tuberculosis is uncommon in dogs and cats. Cats are most commonly affected by *Mycobacterium bovis* whereas dogs are most commonly affected by *M. tuberculosis*. Gastrointestinal infection is more common with *M. bovis* and respiratory infection more common with *M. tuberculosis* and, as a result, cats develop intestinal localization more commonly than dogs. In cats, the clinical signs include weight loss, anemia, vomiting, diarrhea, and palpable masses in mesenteric lymph nodes, intestine, and other abdominal organs.[11,49] Some cats develop ascites. In dogs, the signs are primarily respiratory but, in a series of 5 Basset hounds infected with *Mycobacterium avium* complex, most dogs exhibited gastrointestinal signs in association with granulomatous mesenteric masses and granulomatous enterocolitis.[80] Basset hounds appear to be predisposed to avian tuberculosis, and the gastrointestinal route appears to be the portal of entry. Diagnosis of tuberculosis can be made by intradermal skin testing but this test has inconsistencies.[11] The best test site appears to be the pinna. Definitive diagnosis is usually made by demonstration of acid-fast intracellular bacteria in biopsies of lesions. Successful treatment has been reported,[11] but infected animals are a public health risk and in some situations therapy may not be appropriate.

Tyzzer Disease[11,81]

Tyzzer disease is caused by *Bacillus piliformis,* a spore-forming, gram negative, intracellular, pleomorphic bacillus. Tyzzer disease is an important disorder of laboratory rodents, but only rarely affects dogs and cats.[82–84] The disease is primarily seen in neonates of weaning age, but will occur in immunosuppressed adult animals. Most feline cases have occurred in laboratory-reared kittens. An outbreak also occurred in kittens with familial hyperlipoproteinemia.[82] Rodents or their feces may be the source of the infection. The organism proliferates in the intestinal epithelial cells producing an enterocolitis, and spreads by way of the portal system to the liver where a periportal multifocal hepatitis develops. The most consistent clinical signs are a rapid onset of depression and abdominal discomfort. Death usually occurs within 24 to 48 hours although weight loss and recurrent attacks of diarrhea extending over several weeks were reported in one affected cat.[85] Furthermore, two kittens have been reported in which the primary manifestation of the infection with *Bacillus piliformis* was a relatively mild colitis that progressed over a 5 day period to central nervous system signs and death.[86] Diarrhea is infrequent, scant, and pasty. Diagnosis is most often made at necropsy. Multiple 1 to 2 mm diameter necrotic foci are apparent in the liver, and the ileal and colonic mucosa appears thickened and congested. Histology reveals intracellular filamentous organisms, provided special stains such as

Giemsa are utilized. To date, therapy has been unsuccessful. The disease does not affect people.

Yersiniosis

Yersinia enterocolitica is a gram negative facultative coccobacillus. The bacteria induces secretory diarrhea by virtue of a cyclic GMP–mediated enterotoxin. Some subtypes of *Yersinia* are invasive and may also secrete a cytotoxic enterotoxin.[87] It is an important enteric pathogen in people, and a significant cause of diarrhea in farm animals. It is likely that *Y. enterocolitica* can also be pathogenic to dogs and cats in spite of the fact that, like most enteropathogens, *Y. enterocolitica* can be isolated from the feces of healthy dogs and cats.[88,89] Oral administration of *Y. enterocolitica* (serogroup 0:8) to puppies results in the development of bloody diarrhea 16 to 21 days after exposure.[90] Other clinical signs include lymphadenopathy, abdominal pain, erythematous lesions on the ventral abdominal skin, icterus, and posterior paralysis. Furthermore, *Y. enterocolitica* has been isolated in large numbers from two dogs with 2 week histories of large-bowel type diarrhea that responded rapidly to antibiotics.[91] Tetracyclines and trimethoprim-sulfonamides are usually effective therapy.

Perhaps the greatest importance of *Y. enterocolitica* is as a zoonosis.[89,92,93] Dogs can carry, for prolonged periods, serotypes of *Y. enterocolitica* that are pathogenic for humans.[89] In humans it is not uncommon for enteric *Y. enterocolitica* infections to lead to septicemia. Furthermore, an intractable reactive arthritis often occurs after infection with the organism.[37] Thus, *Yersinia*-infected pets are potentially a serious public health risk.

Y. enterocolitica has not yet been reported in the cat. Another species of *Yersinia,* however, *Y. pseudotuberculosis,* can result in vomiting, diarrhea, and eventually jaundice as part of a septicemic disease in cats.[49] *Y. pseudotuberculosis* is also a public health risk producing a mesenteric lymphadenitis with associated abdominal pain in people. Tetracycline, chloramphenicol, and trimethoprim-sulfa are suitable antibiotics for the therapy of *Y. pseudotuberculosis*. Therapy must be prolonged in advanced cases and the prognosis guarded.

VIRAL GASTROENTERITIS

A large number of enteric viral pathogens affect dogs and cats. The clinical signs caused by enteric viruses range from mild transient gastroenteritis, such as characterizes enteric coronavirus infection, to life-threatening necrotizing enteritis, such as can occur with canine and feline parvovirus infections. The primary pathogenic mechanism of enteric viruses is mucosal invasion followed by varying degrees of villus atrophy and denudation. As discussed earlier, viruses that affect the rapidly dividing crypt cells have more pathogenic effects than those that invade the tips of the villi. Epithelial denudation is followed by massive secondary bacterial invasion that is responsible for the mortality. The adverse interaction between virus and bacteria is illustrated by feline panleukopenia. The responsible agent (feline parvovirus) produces few signs of disease in germ-free cats[94] but a high mortality in conventionally reared cats. Understanding the role viruses play in gastroenteritis is hampered by the need for special techniques to identify viruses,[95] and the difficulty in reproducing the disease by viral inoculation. Furthermore, relatively few large-scale virus identification studies of the feces and vomitus of dogs and cats with acute gastrointestinal disease have been conducted, and no multidisciplinary surveys of viral, bacterial, and parasitic agents and their interrelationships in producing gastrointestinal disease have been reported, even though a number of mixed viral,[96–100] viral-bacterial,[47,101] and viral-parasitic[101,102] enteric infections have been reported.

Clinical signs common to the enteric viruses include acute onset of clinical signs, evidence of rapid contagion, and a predisposition for young animals. Treatment is always symptomatic, with particular attention being paid to fluid therapy and prevention of secondary bacterial invasion. Prevention of enteric viral diseases by appropriate quarantine, hygiene, and vaccination practices is of prime importance in limiting the morbidity and mortality from enteric viruses.

Canine Coronavirus Enteritis[11]

Clinical Synopsis

*Diagnostic Features**

- Young animal; often recently kenneled
- Acute onset of vomiting and soft to watery diarrhea
- Fever and leukopenia rarely seen
- Coronavirus particles in feces
- Rapid response to therapy

Standard Treatment

- Oral or intravenous fluid therapy
- Withhold food for 12 to 24 hours

*Presumptive diagnosis only.

Coronaviruses are pleomorphic, single-stranded, enveloped RNA viruses. The virus appears to be widespread in the canine population with up to 75% of dogs demonstrating serologic titers.[103] Feces are the primary source of infection. Coronoviruses are heat labile but may persist in the environment during cooler times of the year, leading to increased outbreaks in the winter months. The virus appears to affect only dogs.

Following ingestion, coronavirus localizes in the epithelial cells of the upper two-thirds of the villi. It enters the cell by pinocytosis and replicates in the cell cytoplasm. Replication occurs by budding into cytoplasmic vesicles, and eventually results in cell death, with epithelial desquamation, shortening of the villi, decreased intestinal fluid absorption (passive secretory diarrhea), and malabsorption. Rupture of the infected cell releases the progeny virions to infect other enterocytes. Mucosal immunity plays an important role in the immunity to canine coronavirus. The duration of immunity following infection is unknown, but recurrent attacks of coronavirus appear rare in pet animals either as a result of long-term immunity or boostering of host defenses through frequent subclinical reexposure.

The incubation period ranges from 1 to 4 days. Contrary to previous information, it is likely that viremia can occur.[104] Following infection, dogs shed the virus for at least 2 weeks in their feces. The disease is highly contagious and often occurs as outbreaks in susceptible populations.

Clinical signs are most common in dogs less than 1 year. Experimental and clinical evidence suggests that uncomplicated canine coronavirus induces a relatively mild, nonfatal, self-limiting gastroenteritis.[103,105–107] Fever and leukopenia are usually not seen. The diarrhea is rarely bloody. Clinical signs

usually resolve within 1 to 12 days but the diarrhea may persist on an intermittent basis for 3 to 4 weeks. Opportunistic enteric pathogens such as *Clostridium perfringens, Campylobacter*, and *Salmonella* may increase the severity of the clinical signs, although their role in this regard remains unconfirmed.

Diagnosis is made on the basis of appropriate history and clinical signs in association with isolation of the virus from the feces or the demonstration of viral particles in the feces by electron microscopy.

Therapy is symptomatic. Effective vaccination is difficult because of the existence of multiple antigenic strains and the importance of local rather than systemic immunity in the protection against the virus. The mild nature of uncomplicated coronaviral gastroenteritis suggests that vaccination should be considered only in dogs likely to suffer from concomitant infection with another pathogen. Thus, vaccination may be considered in dogs stressed by heavy work schedules, substandard nutrition or hygiene, intercurrent disease, and frequent exposure to other animals. An alternative and more sound approach is to remedy the predisposing causes. Vaccination against coronavirus infection is not recommended in the healthy household pet. During an outbreak, strict quarantine, careful hygiene, and thorough disinfection (1:30 dilution of bleach) may help limit the extent of the spread.

Feline Enteric Coronavirus[49,108]

Feline enteric coronaviruses are pleomorphic, enveloped RNA viruses. Two strains have been characterized to date, one of which has a demonstrated cytopathic effect in tissue cultures. Feline enteric coronaviruses are antigenically and morphologically similar to feline infectious peritonitis (FIP) virus. A spectrum of feline coronaviruses exists, ranging from those that produce purely enteritis and those that produce purely FIP. The major source of the infection appears to be asymptomatic carrier cats. Transfer by fomites appears possible. Kittens become infected at weaning. The virus replicates in the apical epithelial cells of the small intestinal villi. Clinical signs are usually not apparent, but some kittens develop transient mild gastroenteritis. A fatal hemorrhagic diarrhea associated with feline enteric coronavirus infection has been described but is very uncommon. Histopathologic changes are usually mild, but villus atrophy and fusion may be seen.

Presumptive diagnosis can be made by demonstrating a rising coronavirus titer (tests for FIP can be used) or by detecting virus particles in the stool using electron microscopy. Treatment is symptomatic. Prevention is difficult (because the virus is enzootic) and unnecessary in view of the mild clinical signs.

Feline Infectious Peritonitis[49]

Feline infectious peritonitis (FIP) is caused by a coronavirus antigenically and morphologically similar to feline enteric coronavirus. In addition to the classical effusive inflammatory serosal form of FIP, a second form of the disease characterized by granulomatous inflammation of parenchymous organs including the mesenteric nodes, bowel wall, liver, and pancreas may be seen. At times, the granulomatous inflammation is largely restricted to the colon producing a granulomatous colitis.[109] Diagnosis may be made by detection of pyogranulomatous inflammation on biopsy in association with a high FIP titer (>1:32,000). Alternatively, fluorescent antibody staining may be used to demonstrate

FIP in the tissues. Brief remission of granulomatous FIP may occur in a small percentage of cats treated by immunosuppressive drugs. The disease is invariably fatal.

Canine Parvovirus Enteritis[11,110]

Clinical Synopsis

Diagnostic Features

- Young dogs primarily affected
- Acute onset of hemorrhagic diarrhea (dysentery)
- Fever and leukopenia commonly seen
- Fourfold rise in serum IgG titer over a 7 to 14 day period
- Detection of serum IgM titer in an unvaccinated dog
- Positive fecal hemagglutination or ELISA test

Standard Treatment

- Intravenous fluid therapy (lactated Ringer's and 5% dextrose and KCl)
- Withhold food for 24 to 72 hours
- Trimethoprim-sulfa 15 mg/kg q 12 hours SC, PO for 5 to 10 days (if signs of moderate severity)
- Ampicillin (20 mg/kg q 8 hours IV) and gentamicin (2.2 mg/kg q 8 hours IV, SC) for maximum of 5 days (if signs severe)
- Metoclopramide 2.0 mg/kg/24 hours as a continuous IV infusion
- *Avoid* oral aminoglycosides, flunixin meglumine, glucocorticoids, anticholinergics, opioids

Follow-up

- Continue easily digestible, hypoallergenic diet for 7 to 14 days

ETIOLOGY AND EPIZOOTIOLOGY. Canine paravoviral enteritis is caused by an unenveloped DNA virus (canine parvovirus 2) that has an affinity for rapidly dividing cells. The disease first became apparent in 1978 when epizootics of severe gastroenteritis simultaneously afflicted canine populations about the world. The origin of canine parvovirus has not been determined. The virus is antigenically distinct from a non-enteropathogenic parvovirus of dogs called "minute virus of canines" (canine parvovirus 1), but bears antigenic and genomic similarity to feline parvovirus from which it may have mutated.[110,111] Recent evidence has suggested the virus is continuing to evolve, and two subtypes of canine parvovirus 2 are now recognized (CPV-2a and CPV-2b).[110] Fortunately, the antigenic differences between the subtypes are minor and current vaccines protect adequately against these new strains.[110]

Three syndromes of parvovirus infection have been reported: hemorrhagic gastroenteritis, acute myocarditis, and neonatal mortality. This discussion refers to only hemorrhagic gastroenteritis, the most common of these syndromes.

The virus appears to be widespread in the canine population with most dogs being exposed to the virus at an early age either by vaccination or contact with the street virus. Canine parvovirus can survive for approximately 5 to 7 months in feces, and contact with feces is the primary mode of infection. Fecal-contaminated fomites are important sources of spread. The virus is able to infect most Canidae. Cats are susceptible to a self-limiting inapparent infection.

Rottweilers and Doberman pinschers appear predisposed.[112,113] The severity of the clinical signs are increased by factors such as young age, crowding, concurrent parasitism (e.g., giardiasis), and the presence of other pathogens.[113] In particular, opportunistic enteric pathogens such as *Clostridium perfringens*, *E. coli*, *Campylobacter*, *Salmonella*, coronavirus, and various parasites may increase the severity of the clinical signs.

The incubation period ranges from 3 to 8 days. Shedding may begin on day 3, often before the onset of clinical signs.[110] The duration of fecal shedding following parvoviral infection is controversial. Virus is difficult to recover within 2 to 8 days after the onset of clinical signs, but feces may still contain sufficient, albeit small, quantities of virus to infect susceptible dogs for as long as 3 weeks after the onset of clinical signs. As with coronavirus, the disease is highly contagious and outbreaks often occur in susceptible populations.

PATHOGENESIS. Following ingestion the virus replicates in the lymphoid tissue of the oropharynx from where it spreads to the bloodstream in greater or lesser amounts depending on the level of immunity (Figure 21–1). This initial immune response determines the magnitude of the viremia and the severity of the ensuing clinical signs. The viremia deposits virus in rapidly dividing cells throughout the body. Cells affected include the bone marrow, the lymphopoietic tissue, and the crypt epithelium of the jejunum and ileum. Viremia is terminated by increased serum neutralizing antibody that first appears 5 to 6 days postinfection. The replication of the virus in the lymphopoietic system and bone marrow results in lymphopenia and neutropenia, respectively. The replication of the virus in the cryptal epithelial cells results in rapid collapse of the intestinal villi, epithelial necrosis, and hemorrhagic diarrhea. Normal bacterial flora, such as *C. perfringens* and *E. coli* enter the denuded mucosa and, as a result of the deficient neutrophil numbers and depressed immune response, gain rapid access to the bloodstream resulting in fulminant sepsis, endotoxemia, and death.[47,114,115] Pulmonary edema or alveolitis, similar to that observed in the human adult respiratory distress syndrome, is a common complication of fatal cases of parvoviral infection.[114] The importance of normal bacterial flora in the pathogenesis of the disease is clearly demonstrated by the observation that infection of gnotobiotic dogs with parvovirus produces an inapparent disease. The adverse effects of the normal flora are not just due to their role in the ensuing septicemia but also because they increase the rate of epithelial turnover, thus exacerbating the speed of mucosal collapse.

In animals with a partial immunity to the virus, from either previous exposure or maternally derived immunoglobulin, the initial viremia is less intense and the immunosuppression and intestinal necrosis less severe. The result is mild or even inapparent clinical signs. In fact, parvovirus were identified virologically in 10% of healthy dogs in one study.[116] The resistance to infection and the severity of the signs correlate better with coproantibody levels than with serum titers. The duration of immunity following infection is prolonged, perhaps measured in years.

In spite of the lymphopenia, thymic atrophy, lymph node necrosis, Peyer's patch atrophy, and decrease in serum gammaglobulin concentrations that accompany parvovirus infection,[117] humoral immunity seems relatively unaffected by the disease.[113] However, parvovirus infection can predispose dogs to other infectious diseases, such as candidiasis, distemper, hemobartonellosis, and distemper vaccine–associated encephalitis, implying the virus causes at least some degree of

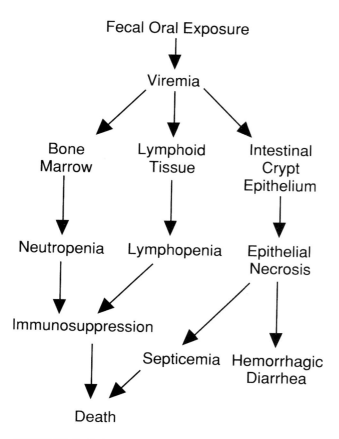

Fecal Oral Exposure

↓

Viremia

Bone Marrow → Neutropenia → Immunosuppression

Lymphoid Tissue → Lymphopenia → Immunosuppression

Intestinal Crypt Epithelium → Epithelial Necrosis → Septicemia / Hemorrhagic Diarrhea

Immunosuppression → Death

Septicemia → Death

FIGURE 21-1. Pathogenesis of canine parvoviral enteritis.

suppression of the antigen-specific immune system in addition to its adverse effects on antigen-nonspecific protection afforded by neutrophils.

CLINICAL FEATURES. Clinical signs are most common in dogs less than 1 year,[112,118] with more than 75% of cases occurring within the age bracket from 6 to 18 weeks of age.[119] Not all puppies of a litter need be clinically affected. Depression, anorexia, pyrexia, and vomiting are early clinical signs, followed by diarrhea. The vomitus is usually scant clear or bile-stained fluid. Large volumes of vomitus are unusual and should raise the suspicion of intestinal obstruction, especially intussusception. In mild cases the diarrhea is soft or watery. In severe cases the diarrhea is hemorrhagic and has a fetid smell. The same smell is associated with other causes of hemorrhagic diarrhea and is not specific for parvoviral enteritis. A rapid progression to hypothermia, septic shock, and death occurs in some dogs.

Leukopenia is present in approximately 80% of dogs at some time during illness.[112,118] Both lymphopenia and neutropenia are common, with the former slightly more common than the latter.[118] Occasionally atypical reactive lymphocytes are seen in the peripheral blood. These changes in the complete blood count should raise the index of suspicion for parvoviral enteritis, but they are not pathognomonic for the disease. For instance, leukopenia is also seen in salmonellosis. The serum chemistry profile usually shows nonspecific changes. Hypoalbuminemia and electrolyte abnormalities such as hyponatremia, hypokalemia, and hypochloremia are seen in 25% to 33% of dogs.[118] Plasma ALT is elevated in approximately 25% of dogs.[118] Acid-base abnormalities may

be seen in severely affected dogs and are usually suggestive of metabolic acidosis.

DIAGNOSIS. Antemortem diagnosis is made on the basis of appropriate history and clinical signs in association with any of the following: a fourfold rise in serum parvovirus IgG titer over a 7 to 14 day period; detection of serum IgM antibody against parvovirus in a dog that has not been vaccinated within the last 3 to 4 weeks; a positive parvovirus fecal hemagglutination or ELISA test; isolation of parvovirus from the feces; or detection of parvovirus particles in the stool using immunoelectronmicroscopy. The fecal hemagglutination and ELISA tests are simple to perform and reasonably specific but less sensitive than the other tests because of the rapidity with which viral numbers decline in the feces of affected dogs. Necropsy usually reveals fibrin-covered serosal surfaces, a congested, hemorrhagic mucosa often covered with a pseudomembrane, enlarged mesenteric nodes, thymic and Peyer's patch atrophy, and liquefaction and hyperemia of the bone marrow (Figure 21–2).[120] Histology reveals epithelial necrosis and denudation, collapse of the villi, and inflammatory infiltrates in the lamina propria. Etiologic diagnosis can be established with a high degree of certainty by routine histology, but indirect fluorescent antibody tests or in situ hybridization of tissues can be helpful in some cases.[121]

THERAPY. Supportive therapy is necessary for the treatment of most cases of parvoviral enteritis, and antibiotic administration is required for all but the most mild. For the details of supportive therapy for acute gastroenteritis see Chapter 18. Of paramount importance is the selection of an appropriate volume and composition of fluid. In most situations, lactated Ringer's solution with an additional 10 to 20 mEq of potassium chloride per liter is adequate. The use of 5% dextrose with the lactated Ringer's solution is advantageous because of the propensity of young pups to develop hypoglycemia as a result of fasting and concurrent sepsis. Lactated Ringer's with 5% dextrose can be purchased from the manufacturer or, alternatively, 100 mL of 50% dextrose can be added to a 1 L bag of lactated Ringer's to produce a similar concentration of dextrose (4.5%). The volume of fluid administered depends on the patient's body weight, estimated degree of dehydration, basal requirements, and ongoing losses. The rate of administration should be sufficiently rapid to replace the patient's fluid deficit in approximately 6 to 8 hours provided the patient's cardiovascular, respiratory, and renal systems will permit this rate. Administration of plasma or blood is occasionally required in anemic or hypoalbuminemic animals. The role of hyperimmune serum has yet to be

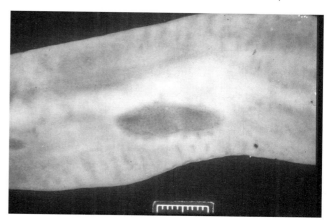

FIGURE 21-2. Lymphoid tissue (Peyer's patch) depletion in parvoviral enteritis. (Courtesy of Dr. Keith Thompson, Massey University)

defined, but administration of antiendotoxin appears to be a valuable adjunct.[115,122] Nutritional support is often required.

Antibiotic usage for the treatment of parvoviral enteritis is justified if the dog shows hemorrhagic diarrhea or evidence of sepsis such as fever, depression, degenerative left-shifted leukograms, or positive blood cultures. Our first choice antibiotic for patients with hemorrhagic diarrhea but no evidence of sepsis is trimethoprim-sulfa. This antibiotic is preferred because of a broad spectrum of activity against pathogens invading the mucosa but minimal effects on the normal flora. However, if the patient is severely depressed, shows evidence of sepsis, or has a profound neutropenia ($<1000/\mu L$), we institute a combination of parenteral ampicillin and gentamicin with the aim of broadening the spectrum of activity against gram negative and anaerobic pathogens. We do not use ampicillin as our routine first choice antibiotic, as has been recommended by others, because of the disruptive effect this antibiotic has on the normal flora and its documented ability to predispose patients to overgrowth with particularly lethal aerobic bacteria such as *Salmonella*.[66] Gentamicin should only be used after rehydration of the patient, and the duration of administration should be limited to 5 days.

An additional drug of value in the supportive therapy of dogs with parvoviral enteritis is metoclopramide. Adynamic ileus is not uncommon in the disease and predisposes the patient to bacterial overgrowth. Metoclopramide has been shown to be effective in the treatment of experimentally induced adynamic ileus in the dog and may assist a return to normal intestinal motility in parvoviral enteritis. An additional beneficial aspect of this drug is its antiemetic activity. If vomiting is persistent, therapy with a phenothiazine antiemetic may be required.

Drugs that should be avoided in the therapy of parvovirus are oral aminoglcosides, flunixin meglumine, glucocorticoids, and anticholinergics. Oral aminoglycosides disturb the normal flora, may induce diarrhea as an adverse drug reaction, and have a high risk of toxicity because of increased absorption through the denuded mucosa. Flunixin meglumine is associated with a high incidence of gastrointestinal ulceration and ischemic renal disease. It should only be used in animals with clear clinical evidence of septic or endotoxic shock and then only as a single injection after rehydration. It should not be used in association with corticosteroids because synergistic damage to the intestinal mucosa will result. The effectiveness of corticosteroids in the treatment of septic or hypovolemic shock has still not been clearly demonstrated. In addition to predictable detrimental effects on a wide range of body systems, corticosteroids may adversely affect the outcome in gram positive septic shock.[123] They have no place in the routine treatment of parvoviral enteritis. If used at all, their use should be restricted to single injections of "shock" doses administered early in the therapy of patients suffering from shock. Anticholinergics compound any adynamic ileus that may be present as a result of the disease process and are contraindicated. Opioids have potential detrimental effects when used during infective diarrheal processes and should be avoided in the treatment of parvoviral enteritis except on rare occasions when fluid therapy cannot keep up with ongoing losses. The fetid material that is defecated by many patients with parvovirus infection is likely to contain a large quantity of potentially lethal materials such as gram negative endotoxins and *Clostridial* enterotoxins. These materials are best passed from the body rather than kept in prolonged contact with the denuded mucosa by the use of potent agents such as opioids.

COMPLICATIONS. The most important complication of parvovirus infection is septicemia. Sepsis may promote the lethal complications of shock and DIC. Another complication occurring with reasonable frequency is intussusception. Patients hospitalized for parvoviral enteritis should, as a minimum, undergo a daily physical examination (including thorough abdominal palpation) to ensure that complications such as intussusceptions are not overlooked. As mentioned earlier, adynamic ileus is also common as a result of parvovirus enteritis. A complication that can occur following recovery from the acute phase of the disease is intractable diarrhea as a result of irreparable mucosal damage or persistent inflammation, perhaps a result of the deranged mucosal barrier. An association between nonregenerative anemia and parvovirous infection has also been proposed. Miscellaneous complications include pneumonia and candidiasis.

PREVENTION. Prevention is based on proper vaccination schedules in association with correct hygiene practices. The most appropriate vaccine is a modified-live preparation of parvovirus of canine origin. Most of these products break through maternal immunity earlier, produce a more rapid immunity in seronegative dogs, and result in a more long-lasting immunity than their killed counterparts. They may also induce some degree of local immunity because of replication in the bowel and subsequent transient fecal shedding. The vaccination schedule used in most veterinary practices is administration of a modified-live parvovirus vaccine of canine origin every 2 to 3 weeks from 6 to 9 weeks of age until the puppy reaches 16 weeks of age. Vaccination of pups earlier than 6 weeks of age is rarely necessary unless the pup did not receive colostrum. Modified-live virus vaccinations should be avoided in pups less than 6 weeks of age because they may cause vaccine-related morbidity. Animals not receiving colostrum should be given oral plasma (2–4 mL/kg) from a vaccinated donor if presented within the first few days of birth. If presented later, the same dose of serum may be given subcutaneously or intraperitoneally. Rottweilers should receive an additional vaccination at 18 to 20 weeks of age. If so desired, the adequacy of immunization can be established by postvaccine titers. Revaccination is usually carried out at yearly intervals.

The most common cause of a vaccine failure is inadequate quarantine or hygiene practices. No matter what the vaccination schedule, there will be a time in a pup's life when its maternal immunity will be sufficient to prevent the development of active immunity from a vaccination, but at the same time (or in the ensuing 2 weeks until the next vaccination) will be inadequate to protect the pup against serious infection by the more virulent street virus. The only way these gaps in immunity can be minimized is to reduce the likelihood of exposure of the pup to large quantities of the virus. This is achieved by careful hygiene and by restricting the pup's access to poorly cared for dogs. The immunity "gaps" cannot be filled by more frequent vaccination because intervals of less than 10 to 14 days result in "vaccine interference."[11]

During an outbreak, strict quarantine, careful hygiene, and thorough disinfection (1:30 dilution of bleach) may help limit the extent of the spread. Vaccination of unaffected dogs with modified-live vaccine of canine origin in the face of the outbreak is recommended. Protective immunity may be obtained as early as 3 to 4 days following a single vaccination even in seronegative dogs.

PROGNOSIS. In mild cases the dogs make rapid recoveries over a 2 to 3 day period. Most dogs that survive the initial 2 to 3 days of therapy will eventually go on to recover. If severely affected animals survive, recovery from the acute signs may take a week or more and diarrhea can persist for several weeks. The mortality associated with parvovirus infection has been variously reported as 16% to 35%.[112,118] Mortalities are now considerably less common than in the earlier stages of the parvovirus epidemic. The reasons for the decline in mortality is unknown but may be a result of more widespread immunity, a shift in the virulence of the organism, or perhaps improved therapeutics. Prognostic factors have proved difficult to identify. The presence of hemorrhagic diarrhea, fever, depression, or leukopenia were not found to correlate to survival.[112,118] In our experience, however, patients with septic or hypovolemic shock at presentation, fibrinous mucosal casts or severe hemorrhagic diarrhea, and pronounced neutropenia (less than 500/μl) should receive a guarded prognosis.

Feline Panleukopenia[11,49]

Feline panleukopenia is caused by a feline parvovirus. Its epidemiology, pathophysiology, clinical signs, hematologic findings, and treatment are essentially the same as that for canine parvovirus. A difference between feline and canine parvoviruses is the propensity of the feline parvovirus to produce cerebellar disease in cats infected in utero or during the early neonatal period. Cats usually develop either cerebellar or gastrointestinal signs but not both. Occasionally, however, cats positive for panleukopenia virus are affected by both cerebellar and gastrointestinal lesions.[124] As with canine parvovirus, the tissues preferentially affected in the bowel are the jejunum and ileum. Cats with panleukopenia tend to need blood more frequently than their canine counterparts because of more rapidly progressive anemia. Furthermore, earlier initiation of supplemental nutrition protocols including vitamin B complex are recommended. The prognosis is poor. Prevention is by vaccination with a modified live vaccine. Vaccination is usually begun at 8 to 9 weeks of age and a second vaccination administered at 12 weeks or older. Colostrum-deprived kittens may receive serum as described for the pup. Modified-live vaccines should not be given to kittens less than 4 weeks of age.

Miscellaneous Enteric Viral Infections

Feline leukemia (FeLV) and feline immunodeficiency viruses (FIV) have been associated with chronic gastrointestinal disease in cats. Many other types of viruses have been intermittently identified in the feces of vomitus of dogs and cats with acute gastroenteritis. These include rotaviruses, astroviruses, caliciviruses,[125-127] and reoviruses.[128] At present, the importance of many of these viruses as enteric pathogens remains to be defined.[49,96-102,131]

ASTROVIRUS. Astroviruses have been isolated from both kittens and pups with diarrhea.[99,132,133] The epithelium of the tips of the small intestinal villi appears to be the primary target.[134,135] The clinical signs associated with experimental transfer of this virus have included mild self-limiting diarrhea. Suspected clinical cases have had a more prolonged course. Inapparent infections also occur.[49]

CANINE DISTEMPER. Canine distemper produces a transient gastroenteritis characterized by vomiting and diarrhea in the early stages of the disease process. In a small number of dogs, severe enteritis is the principal manifestation. The diarrhea may be bloody and tenesmus has been observed. Leukopenia can also occur. Differentiation of this distemper variant from parvovirus is difficult because of similar clinical signs. However, if respiratory or neurologic signs become apparent, distemper should be suspected. Occasionally, gastrointestinal distemper can be differentiated from parvovirus by detection of the characteristic retinal lesions. Rarely, the diseases can be differentiated by finding intracytoplasmic distemper inclusions in red or white blood cells. In addition, distemper immunofluorescent antibody tests on conjunctival epithelium or urinary sediment may confirm distemper.[11]

FELINE IMMUNODEFICIENCY VIRUS.[49] Serologic studies of cats with FIV have revealed a significant incidence of chronic oral inflammation (50%–52%) and chronic enteritis or enterocolitis (12%–20%).[136-138] The clinical signs associated with these lesions included anorexia, chronic diarrhea, dehydration, and emaciation. The diarrhea may be persistent, and progressive intestinal thickening develops. Leukopenia is common. A high mortality was seen in the cats showing gastrointestinal signs. Histopathology shows a diffuse enterocolitis characterized by enterocyte necrosis in the glandular epithelium, villus atrophy and fusion, multiple foci of subacute ulceration, and transmural pyogranulomatous inflammation. A role for the virus in a panleukopenia-like syndrome of cats has also been proposed. The pathogenesis of these abnormalities is unknown, but it is of interest to note that gastrointestinal manifestations of the human immunodeficiency syndrome are common and have a variety of causes including *Cryptosporidium, Giardia, Coccidia, Candida,* certain viruses, and *Salmonella.* In some cats with FIV, *Yersinia pseudotuberculosis* has been isolated from the affected bowel. In addition, the type of lesions observed microscopically suggest that viral invasion, such as by enteric coronavirus, may also be involved in the pathogenesis. At present, diagnosis of FIV-associated gastrointestinal disease is made by compatible clinical-pathologic signs in association with a positive FIV titer.

FELINE LEUKEMIA. FeLV has been associated with a fatal peracute enterocolitis (panleukopenia-like syndrome).[139] It is also thought to be involved in the development of alimentary lymphosarcoma, even though many cats with alimentary lymphosarcoma have negative FeLV test.[11] FeLV can also induce a lymphocytic ileitis.[140]

ROTAVIRUS. Rotavirus has been associated with transient diarrhea in neonatal dogs[141,142] and in cats.[134,135] The prevalence of rotavirus in diarrheic stools in the United States has been reported to be very low[96] but in other countries it is higher.[143] Inapparent rotavirus infection of adult animals may be reasonably common.[96,131,143,144] Canine rotavirus have been reported to produce pathologic changes in the small intestine of dogs that are recognizable at both the light and electron microscopy level. Epithelial necrosis and mild villus atrophy were noted.[145] Diagnosis of rotavirus infections in dogs and cats can be made by a fecal ELISA test.

TOROVIRUS. A torovirus-like agent has been isolated from the fecal samples of a number of cats with the syndrome of protruding nictitating membranes and diarrhea ("haws") and may play an important role in this self-limiting syndrome.[146]

FUNGAL GASTROENTERITIS[147-149]

Low numbers of fungi are found in the normal intestinal microflora and are usually not pathogenic. However, given the right circumstances (e.g., immunosuppression) they can colonize parts of the intestine they normally do not populate, invade the mucosa, and disseminate via the bloodstream.

Candidiasis

Candida are dimorphic fungi that normally inhabit the gastrointestinal tract. They are opportunist pathogens and have been used in animal models to study how gastrointestinal fungi can become pathogenic. Fungemia can be produced by direct instillation of large amounts of yeasts into the duodenum of dogs. Gastrointestinal candidiasis can be produced by administering antibiotics along with immunosuppressive drugs. Alteration of the normal bacterial microflora by antibiotics makes overgrowth by fungi possible.

Gastrointestinal candidiasis is rare in dogs and cats.[151–153] It has been reported in the aftermath of canine parvovirus infection.[152,154] Candidal stomatitis is occasionally seen in the dog (see Chapter 9). The lesion appears as a raised white plaque or plaques on the mucosa. The diagnosis is confirmed by impression smears, biopsy, and culture. The treatment of choice for candidiasis restricted to the gastrointestinal tract is nystatin. The recommended human dose is 4.5 to 20 million units q 6 to 8 hours PO. Systemic candidiasis is best treated with ketoconazole (10 mg/kg q 12 hours) or itraconazole (2–2.5 mg/kg PO q 12 hours). Therapy should be continued for several weeks after remission.

Histoplasmosis[11,49,155–157]

Histoplasmosis is caused by a pleomorphic fungus, *Histoplasma capsulatum*. The disease is widely distributed in the world, and in the United States is endemic in the states bordering the Mississippi River. The fungus grows particularly well in soil enriched by bird or bat feces. *Histoplasma* usually enters the body through the respiratory tract. In most animals the resultant pulmonary infection is mild and self-limiting. In a small number of animals, however, the fungus disseminates to many other tissues in the body, including the gastrointestinal tract. Gastrointestinal involvement from disseminated histoplasmosis is most commonly seen in dogs but has been reported in cats.[11,156]

Gastrointestinal histoplasmosis is a chronic debilitating diarrheal disease. The diarrhea is usually profuse, intractable, and occasionally bloody when the colon is involved. The bowel wall becomes thickened by granulomatous inflammation. Malabsorption and protein-losing enteropathy are common. Physical examination or diagnostic evaluation will often reveal involvement of other tissues such as the eyes, lungs, liver, joints, bones, and spleen. A diagnosis is usually made by detection of *Histoplasma*-laden macrophages in rectal scrapes, buffy coats, bone marrow aspirates, or biopsy specimens of the colon or small intestine. Serum tests for *Hisoplasma*, such as the agar gel diffusion test, are available but can be unreliable. Traditional therapy is with amphotericin B (for 3–4 weeks) in association with ketoconazole for 4 to 6 months.[11,157] The prognosis is guarded to poor. The newer imidazoles such as itraconazole (5 mg/kg PO q 12–24 hours) and fluconazole may prove more efficacious than ketoconazole.[157]

Miscellaneous Fungi[11,158]

Disseminated aspergillosis and mucormycosis can be responsible for diarrhea in cats.[11,49,156,159] Approximately 40% of cases have intestinal involvement with both small bowel and large bowel being affected. Panleukopenia, FeLV, or antibiotic and corticosteroid administration appear important predisposing causes. In dogs, aspergillosis is rarely associated with gastrointestinal signs, but a variety of zygomycetes, including members of the genera *Mucor, Rhizopus,* and *Absidia,* have been responsible for canine intestinal zygomycosis (phycomycosis).[11] The zygomycetes are opportunist fungi that are widespread in nature. In dogs they are thought to gain entrance to the intestinal wall as a result of mucosal trauma. The affected area of bowel becomes greatly thickened and eventually

results in partial or complete intestinal obstruction. Clinical signs generally include a history of chronic diarrhea or a palpable abdominal mass. Vomiting may occur, particularly once a partial obstruction develops. Radiography, ultrasound, or exploratory celiotomy may be required to detect the mass. Diagnosis is made by intestinal biopsy. Granulomatous lesions full of branching nonseptate hyphae are characteristic. In dogs the fungi may spread to the mesenteric nodes, and in cats disseminated disease has been reported. Treatment is by surgical resection of the mass with subsequent antifungal therapy. Amphotericin B has been considered the drug of choice, but itraconazole appears to offer great promise. Itraconazole (10 mg/kg q 24 hours PO) is effective against *Aspergillus, Pythium,* and miscellaneous other enteropathogenic fungi.[160,161] The prognosis is guarded.

ALGAL GASTROENTERITIS

Acute Algal Toxicosis

Toxic algal blooms can lead to acute gastroenteritis and death in dogs that drink water containing the algae.[162] Toxic blue-green algae can elaborate an anticholinesterase that is capable of inducing vomiting, diarrhea, ataxia, and rapid death in dogs and other species.[162] Exposure of dogs to algae blooms has also been associated with hepatorenal toxicity.[163]

Prototithecosis[11,164,165]

Prototithecosis is a rare disease caused by achlorophyllous algae belonging to the genus *Prototheca*. The algae are morphologically similar to green algae and in tissues are spherical to oval in shape. They are ubiquitous in the environment and appear to be opportunist pathogens. Both dogs and cats can be affected, but in cats the infection is usually confined to the dermis and subcutis whereas in dogs the disease most often involves the gastrointestinal tract.[166] When *Prototheca* species infect the bowel they usually colonize the colon and produce a severe chronic colitis that is characterized by intermittent, protracted bloody diarrhea. The disease eventually disseminates, often causing blindness. The disseminated disease is invariably fatal. Diagnosis is usually made by biopsy of the colon, vitreous taps, or evaluation of urinary sediment, all of which may show, the organism. The algae can be readily cultured from infected tissues. Treatment of the disease in dogs is usually unsuccessful although liposome encapsulated amphotericin B has shown some promise. In cats the disease is relatively benign and excision of the skin lesions is usually curative.

RICKETTSIAL INFECTIONS

Salmon poisoning is an often fatal disease of dogs caused by the rickettsial organism *Neorickettsia helminthoeca*.[11] A second rickettsia-like organism, "Elokomin fluke fever agent," may also be involved in the disease process. This organism is probably another strain of *Neorickettsia helminthoeca*. Dogs acquire the rickettsial organism by the ingestion of fish (usually a salmon or trout) that harbor metacercaria of the canine intestinal fluke *Nanophyetus salmincola* in their tissues (in particular the kidneys). The life cycle of the fluke has an obligate requirement for a developmental stage in a particular species of freshwater snail called *Oxytremma silicula*. It is the narrow geographic distribution of this snail that has restricted the occurrence of salmon poisoning to the northern west coast of

North America.

Clinical signs of salmon poisoning include an acute onset of pyrexia, anorexia, vomiting, and diarrhea. If untreated the diarrhea becomes progressively worse and may become grossly hemorrhagic. Peripheral and mesenteric lymphadenopathy are common. Important differentials are parvovirus and distemper. Either leukopenia or leukocytosis can occur. The incubation period following the ingestion of fish is usually 5 to 7 days, although periods as long as 19 to 33 days have been reported.

The disease should be strongly suspected in dogs in endemic areas that develop acute gastroenteritis after documented or suspected access to salmonid fish. Tentative diagnosis may be made by the demonstration of operculated fluke eggs in the feces of the dogs, indirect evidence of *Neorickettsia helminthoeca* infection. Fluke eggs are most reliably demonstrated by sedimentation techniques. More definitive diagnosis can be made by aspiration cytology of enlarged lymph nodes that often reveals reactive inflammation with macrophages containing rickettsial bodies.

The rickettsial infection is best treated with tetracyclines. In profusely vomiting animals parenteral administration is preferred until vomiting is controlled (oxytetracycline 7 mg/kg q 12 hours IV for 3 days). Oral tetracycline therapy (20 mg/kg PO q 8 hours for 7 days) is successful in dogs with less profuse vomiting. Elimination of the fluke infection may be accomplished with praziquantel (Droncit) at standard cestode doses. Even though *Nanophyetes* causes few clinical signs in and of itself, eradication of the fluke is recommended because it continues to shed eggs for as long as 250 days, contributing to the contamination of more waterways. Prevention relies on restricting the access of dogs to fresh fish. Immunity following infection may be long lasting.

Other rickettsia that affect dogs produce occasional gastrointestinal signs. In ehrlichiosis these signs are generally restricted to hematochezia as a result of the bleeding tendencies that accompany rickettsial infection. Rocky Mountain spotted fever, however, can result in vomiting, diarrhea, abdominal pain, and melena.

PARASITIC INFECTIONS[167–172]

Intestinal parasites are often associated with acute diarrhea. It is not always known to what degree they contribute to clinical signs. Protozoa are normally found in the feces of some species of animals, and their numbers usually increase with the onset of diarrhea due to any cause. In this case the protozoa are a consequence and not a cause of the diarrhea. Cestodes are commonly found in dogs and cats but there is little evidence they cause clinical signs. The appearance of these worms causes aesthetic displeasure, however, and some species such as *Echinococcus, Mesocestoides,* and *Dipylidium caninum* are public health risks. The dose rates of recommended anthelmentics are given in Table 21–1. In-depth discussion of anthelmentics can be found in several publications.[173,174]

Nematode Parasites

The most important intestinal nematode parasites of dogs and cats are ascarids, hookworms, whipworms, and *Strongyloides* spp.

ASCARIDS. Ascarid infections are usually inapparent in adult dogs and cats. In puppies and kittens, however, heavy burdens of ascarids can cause ill-thrift characterized by a pot-bellied appearance, poor hair coat, and retarded growth.

Intermittent vomiting and poorly formed feces as a result of mild malabsorption and reduced villous height may also occur.[175] Migration of larval stages through the lungs can result in a pneumonitis with associated soft cough. The treatment of choice is piperazine or pyrantel pamoate. Intestinal obstruction due to the death of large quantities of worms following treatment has been recorded. *T. canis* is an important public health risk. For this reason, pups should be wormed sufficiently frequently to minimize environmental contamination with *Toxocara* eggs.[176] For puppies, worming should begin at 2 to 3 weeks of age and be repeated every 2 to 3 weeks until 3 months of age. Ascarids of cats are less likely to cause visceral larval migrans and kittens are not infected by placental transfer of larvae. Therefore, kittens can be wormed less frequently than puppies and worming need not start until 3 to 4 weeks of age.

HOOKWORMS. Hookworms (*Ancylostoma caninum* and *Uncinaria stenocephala*) are of most importance in young dogs, although *A. tubaeforme* is also a prevalent problem in cats in tropical areas. They are primarily small-bowel parasites, but will occasionally infect the large bowel if the parasite burden is sufficiently heavy. Clinical signs pertain primarily to blood loss anemia. Pyrantel pamoate, febantel, and milbemycin oxime are highly effective therapies. It is noteworthy that *Ancylostoma caninum* can infect humans and has been implicated as a cause of eosinophilic gastroenteritis in people.[177]

STRONGYLOIDES. *Strongyloides stercoralis* infection is seen most frequently in pups purchased from unsanitary kennels or pet shops. Clinical signs of strongyloidiasis include diarrhea, lethargy, listlessness, and coughing.[178] Auscultation may detect increased breath sounds, and thoracic radiology may reveal a generalized interstitial pattern overlaid with a patchy bronchoalveolar pattern.[178] The respiratory signs are a result of the migratory stages of the parasite. Rarely, fatal hyperinfections of the parasite will occur.[178] Diagnosis is best made by repeated Baermann fecal examinations.[178]

Self-cure can occur but chronic infections of the parasite in susceptible dogs can be difficult to eradicate. Thiabendazole (100–150 mg/kg PO for 3 days) is the only approved drug for use in dogs with activity against *Strongyloides.* Recently, however, it has been shown that two doses of ivermectin (200 µg/kg PO) given 2 weeks apart is a practical and effective alternative to thiabendazole.[178] Prevention aims at eradicating moist areas where the parasite larvae can persist. *Strongyloides* is a public health risk.

WHIPWORMS. *Trichuris vulpis* is an important cause of chronic enterocolitis in dogs (Figure 21–3). Whipworm infections in cats are rare. The clinical signs of whipworm infection can vary from blood-tinged mucoid feces with associated tenesmus to a profuse watery diarrhea. Diagnosis is usually made by fecal flotation. Several flotations may be required to make a diagnosis because the parasite is of low fecundity. Occasionally whipworm eggs cannot be detected in the stool and the diagnosis is made by endoscopic examination of the large bowel. The treatment of choice is fenbendazole (Panacur) at 50 mg/kg q 24 hours PO for 3 days. Mebendazole, febantel (which is metabolized to fenbendazole), and milbemycin oxime also appear to be effective.[179–181] Oxantel is commonly used for the treatment of whipworms but in our experience has not been as reliable as fenbendazole. No matter what anthelmintic treatment is selected, fecal flotations should be repeated to verify the effectiveness of therapy.

Trichuris eggs persist well in many environments, including concrete runs, a property that can lead to persistent reinfection. Adequately cleaning the environment is difficult, but flaming of concrete runs or scrubbing them with dilute sodium hypochlorite has been recommended. Feces should be collected and disposed of appropriately, but it is difficult to eradicate the parasite from grassed areas unless the owner is

Table 21-1

DOSAGES OF ANTHELMINTICS FOR SELECTED GASTROINTESTINAL PARASITES*

ANTHELMINTIC	PARASITES	DOSE
Febantel	As for fenbendazole	5–10 mg/kg q 24 hours for 1–3 days (D & C)†
Fenbendazole	All common GI nematodes and *Giardia*	50 mg/kg q 24 hours for 3 days (D & C)
Ivermectin	*Strongyloides*	200 µg/kg (D & C)‡
Mebendazole	Similar to fenbendazole	22 mg/kg q 24 hours for 3 days (D & C)§
Milbemycin oxime	As for fenbendazole but less activity against *Uncinaria stenocephala*	0.5 mg/kg (D & C)
Piperazine	Roundworms	50–100 mg/kg q 24 hours (D & C)
Pyrantel pamoate	Roundworms, hookworms, *Physaloptera*	5–10 mg/kg (D & C)

*Not all of these products are licensed for use in cats and dogs, but all seem relatively safe at the doses listed and with the precautions noted here.
†Not for use in pregnant animals; use 3 day therapy for whipworms.
‡Ivermectin is effective at this dose against hookworms, whipworms, and *Toxocara* but is not recommended for routine use because the drug is not licensed at the dosages required for activity against gastrointestinal parasites and at these doses can cause serious neurologic disturbances in collies and collie-like breeds.
§Rarely hepatotoxicity has been reported following use of mebendazole in dogs.

prepared to remove heavily contaminated topsoil. A more practical approach when reinfestation problems are suspected is to worm all dogs on the property at 8 week intervals for at least 1 year. Because the prepatent period of *Trichuris vulpsis* is approximately 10 weeks, this technique slowly reduces environmental contamination.

Coccidia[11]

Coccidia belong to an important subclass of parasites that contains many species of veterinary importance including members of *Cryptosporidia, Sarcocystidae, Hammondia, Toxoplasma, Besnoitia,* and *Cystoisospora.* The coccidia of dogs and cats that were formerly placed in the genus *Isospora* have now been placed in the genus *Cystoisospora.* The pathogenicity and life cycles of the coccidia vary considerably. Most species multiply in the epithelium of the distal small intestine.

Diagnostic characteristics of common coccidial oocysts are given in Table 21–2.[182] *Besnoitia* spp. are considered nonpathogenic and the oocysts are difficult to differentiate from *Toxoplasma gondii.* Similarly, *Hammondia hammondi* are nonpathogenic and cannot be distinguished from *T. gondii* by routine measures. For diagnostic or management purposes, *H. hammondi* oocysts in feline feces should be considered to be *T. gondii.*

CYSTOISOSPORA. *Cystoisospora* spp. are not highly pathogenic and inapparent infections are common. However, diarrhea, often with mucus or fresh blood streaks, may be seen in young animals especially if they are debilitated or have been exposed to large numbers of the parasite through poor hygiene. Moreover, it is possible that some strains of *Cystoisospora* are more pathogenic than others.[182] Diagnosis is usually made by fecal smears, which reveal large numbers of coccidial oocysts. If concentration techniques such as fecal flotation are required to detect a *Cystisospora* infection, the organism is unlikely to be present in sufficient quantities to be responsible for the patient's gastrointestinal complaint. The usual therapy is trimethoprim-sulfa (15 mg/kg PO q 12 hours for 7 days). This antibiotic may not eliminate infection but is usually associated with a marked reduction in oocyst numbers and rapid resolution of clinical signs. Chlortetracycline (25 mg/kg q 24 hours for 15 days) also appears to be useful.[183]

CRYPTOSPORIDIA. *Cryptosporidia* are extremely small (4–8 µm) coccidian parasites that have a direct fecal-oral enteric life cycle.[182] They can cause chronic and severe diarrhea in kittens, puppies, and immunosuppressed dogs and cats.[184–187] They have also been held responsible for diarrhea in adult dogs and cats without obvious evidence of immunosuppression.[188,189] As with the other coccidia, exposure of cats and dogs to the parasite appears to be widespread and asymptomatic infections are the norm.[189–192] Because of its small size, the organism is difficult to demonstrate in the feces by routine microscopy. Formol-ether sedimentation and sugar flotation are preferred over zinc sulphate flotation as a method for concentration of the organism in fecal samples.[193] Phase contrast microscopy assists identification as does immunofluorescence and modified Ziehl-Neelsen staining techniques.[193] Diagnosis is often made by intestinal biopsy, but false negatives are frequent even with this technique.[189] An unusual feature of the organism compared to other coccidia is that it only penetrates the mucosa to the level of the brush border. There is little if any host specificity and this agent is a health risk for immunosuppressed people. Treatment is difficult in immunosuppressed patients. Clindamycin and tylosin have

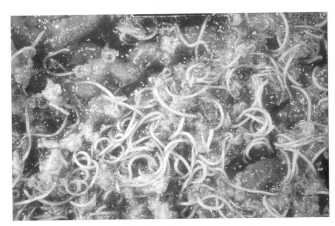

FIGURE 21-3. Heavy whipworm infection in a dog (Courtesy of Dr. Keith Thompson, Massey University)

Table 21–2

DIAGNOSTIC CHARACTERISTICS OF COCCIDIAL OOCYSTS*

OOCYST	SIZE (MM)	COCCIDIUM
Sporulated very small oocysts	< 8	*Cryptosporidium* spp.
Sporulated small oocysts or sporocysts	9–16	*Sarcocystis* spp.
Unsporulated small oocysts	10–14	*Hammondia hammondia* *Besnoitia darlingi* *Toxoplasma gondii*
Unsporulated medium-sized oocysts	20–28	*Cystoisospora rivolta*
Unsporulated large oocysts	32–53	*Cystoisospora felis*

*Data derived from reference 182.

been recommended but early results suggest that paromomycin (Humatin; Parke-Davis) at a dose of 125 to 165 mg/kg PO q 12 hours for 5 days is more successful.[194]

Sarcocystis. *Sarcocystis* is usually confined to the intestine in carnivores and is most often asymptomatic. Recently, however, a litter of pups has been described with an acute sarcocystis-like disease associated with dissemination of *Sarcocystis*-like organisms to various visceral tissues. Clinical signs included anorexia, diarrhea, mesenteric lymphadenopathy, and acute death.[195]

TOXOPLASMA. Toxoplasma are small (10–14 μm) coccidian parasites of cats that can undergo extraintestinal or enteroepithelial life cycles. In cats, they usually produce asymptomatic infections or at most transient diarrhea. FIV infected cats have a high rate of *Toxoplasma gondii*–specific IgM titers and it seems likely that active toxoplasmosis may complicate FIV infections.[137,196,197] Diarrhea secondary to reactivated toxoplasma infections has been incriminated as a cause of failure to respond to immunosuppressive drugs in cats with inflammatory bowel disease.[198] Cats shedding toxoplasma oocysts are a public health risk. Elimination of toxoplasma infections is difficult. High-dose clindamycin therapy (25 mg/kg PO q 12–24 hours for 2–3 weeks) has been recommended but produces vomiting and diarrhea in cats.[199]

Balantidium coli and Trichomonas

Balantidium coli has been detected in several dogs with acute ulcerative colitis in association with *Trichuris* infection. It is possible that the protozoa is a secondary invader. The parasite is more common in pigs. Diagnosis is made by detecting the trophozoite or cyst in feces or by colonic biopsy. Clinical signs usually resolve following treatment of the *Trichuris* infection. Metronidazole is an effective therapy for the protozoa.

Pentatrichomonas hominis, a Trichomonad parasite, has been recovered from diarrheic feces but is also found in up to 15% of normal dogs. It is unlikely to be a pathogen.[182]

Entamoeba histolytica (Amebiasis)[200]

Entamoeba histolytica is a protozoan parasite of the large bowel that is found most commonly in tropical countries but has been reported in dogs in the United States. Dogs are most likely to be infected through ingestion of water contaminated by the feces of infected humans. *E. histolytica* can produce hematochezia or a watery secretory diarrhea. Amebae possess multiple degradative enzymes, including hyaluronidase, mucinase, trypsin, pepsin, collagenase, and multiple other proteinases.[4] In addition, they can produce a cytotoxin that inhibits DNA and protein synthesis in target cells. These degradative enzymes and cytotoxins are presumably responsible for the hemorrhagic diarrhea associated with many cases of the disease. The secretory diarrhea of amebiasis is thought to be the result of either a heat-labile enterotoxin or neurohumoral substances, such as serotonin, substance P, and neurotensin, released from the amebae. Some of these changes may in part be mediated by increased mucosal prostaglandin secretion. Extraintestinal infection can occur but is rare in dogs. The diagnosis is made by observing trophozoites in smears of warm feces or in colonic biopsy specimens. The treatment of choice is metronidazole (25 mg/kg q 12 hours for 5 days).[182]

Giardiasis[11,182,201,202]

Clinical Synopsis

Diagnostic Features

- Acute or chronic small-bowel diarrhea most common
- Occasionally large-bowel diarrhea, especially in cats
- Diagnosis may require up to three zinc sulfate fecal flotations

Standard Treatment

- Intravenous fluid therapy if required
- Withhold food for 24 to 48 hours
- Dogs: Albendazole 25 mg/kg q 12 hours PO for 2 days or fenbendazole 50 mg/kg q 24 hours for 3 days
- Cats: Metronidazole 10–25 mg/kg PO q 12 hours for 5 days or albendazole 25 mg/kg q 12 hours for 5 days

ETIOLOGY AND EPIZOOTIOLOGY. *Giardia* are flagellate protozoa that can cause diarrhea in dogs and cats. There is confusion over the number of *Giardia* species and the infectivity of different species for various hosts.[182] Many authorities consider the *Giardia* from different mammals to belong to one species, *Giardia intestinalis* (otherwise known as *Giardia lamblia* or *duodenalis*), implying dogs and cats could be a source of human infection. As yet, however, little evidence supports a zoonotic role for canine and feline *Giardia*.[202]

Giardia reside as motile trophozoites in the small intestine and, to a lesser extent, the large intestine of both dogs and cats. The location of *Giardia* within the small intestine of dogs is variable. In some dogs, the entire small intestine is involved whereas in others a segmental infection of the upper or lower small intestine occurs.[203]

The life cycle of *Giardia* is direct and fecal-oral transmission occurs. Cysts can survive for weeks or months in cool, moist conditions. Contaminated waterways are a major source of infection. The latency period in dogs from ingestion to cyst excretion ranges from 5 to 12 days. In most areas the prevalence of *Giardia* in dogs and cats is less than 10% but in some regions as many as 33% of dogs are infected, many of which have no clinical signs of disease.[204–207]

PATHOGENESIS. After ingestion, *Giardia* attach themselves to the small intestinal surface where they can induce malassimilation, steatorrhea, and chronic enteritis. The pathophysiology of the malassimilation involves a number of different processes.[208] *Giardia* appear to incite a T cell–mediated increase in epithelial turnover rate, which results in cryptal hyperplasia and villus atrophy.[4] They reduce microvillus height and damage the brush border, resulting in disaccharidase deficiency. The brush border damage occurs both from a direct effect of the parasite on the mucosa and also indirectly from the local immune response of the host.[209] In addition, when present in large numbers, the protozoa may form a physical blockage to nutrient absorption by coating the mucosa. *Giardia* are able to interfere with lipase activity and glucose and amino acid transport. In addition, concurrent small intestinal bacterial overgrowth has been reported to be common in humans with giardiasis.[210] Most *Giardia* infections are self-limiting, and acquired resistance, involving both humoral and cellular mechanisms, is thought to occur.

CLINICAL FEATURES. Clinical findings vary from inapparent infections (most common) to evidence of malassimilation characterized by chronic, continuous or intermittent, soft or watery diarrhea. Mucus is occasionally seen, and steatorrhea is common. On occasion, *Giardia* are associated with signs of large-bowel dysfunction including tenesmus. The reasons for the difference in pathogenicity and clinical signs between individuals is unknown. Young animals with *Giardia* are more likely to develop diarrhea than older animals.

Diagnosis is usually made by fecal examinations including fresh smears for motile trophozoites and various flotation and staining techniques (see Chapter 6). Repeated (two to three) zinc sulfate fecal flotations are the preferred method of diagnosis.[211–213] Identification of *Giardia* cysts in feces is easier with zinc sulfate solutions than standard saturated salt flotation solutions because zinc sulfate flotation solution is less hypertonic and does not distort the fragile cysts.[202] Diagnosis can also be made by intestinal biopsy, aspiration of duodenal fluid by endoscopy, the peroral string technique, or fecal ELISA or immunofluorescence tests.[202] Administration of corticosteroids may result in increased shedding of oocysts.[213]

Therapy. In view of the potential public health risk of *Giardia*, treatment of animals with positive fecal flotations for *Giardia* is recommended regardless of whether the infection is causing diarrhea. Without therapy, dogs can remain infected with *Giardia* for as long as 6 to 36 months.[170] The recommended therapy for cats is metronidazole at a dose of 10 to 25 mg/kg q 12 hours PO for 5 to 7 days.[202,214] In dogs, treatment failures are not uncommon with metronidazole. In a study of a kennel infected with endemic giardiasis, metronidazole effected a cure rate of only 67%.[215] Treatment failures have been approached by repeating the therapy at a higher dose (50 mg/kg q 12 hours PO for 5 days) or for more prolonged periods (weeks to months). High-dose metronidazole therapy can induce serious neurological dysfunction, however, and should be avoided if at all possible. It now appears that albendazole (25 mg/kg PO q 12 hours for 2 days) or fenbendazole (50 mg/kg PO q 24 hours for 3 days) are safer and perhaps more effective than metronidazole for the treatment of canine giardiasis.[216,217] Albendazole (25 mg/kg q 12 hours PO for 5 days) may also prove useful in the treatment of feline giardiasis. Another treatment option for cats (and probably dogs) is furazolidone (4 mg/kg q 12 hours PO for 5 days).[218] Quinacrine (11 mg/kg daily for 12 days) eliminated the clinical signs but not cyst shedding in a cat. Quinacrine (6.6 mg/kg PO for 5 days) is useful, however, for the therapy of intractable canine giardiasis.[215] The high incidence of side effects of anorexia, lethargy, fever, and vomiting restrict this drug to a second choice pharmaceutical in spite of its apparent efficacy.

In catteries or kennels, control of the disease should include an effort to reduce the number of *Giardia* cysts in the environment. The recommended disinfectants are the quaternary ammonium products, but bleach (20% solution of household bleach or 1% sodium hypochlorite) and phenolic compounds are also effective.

Leishmania

Leishmania infection can cause intractable chronic colitis in dogs.[219,220] Colonoscopy reveals hyperemia and small numbers of mucosal erosions. The diagnosis is made by colonic histopathology and bone marrow aspirates that yield macrophages containing basophilic bodies (amastigotes of *Leishmania*). Treatment with multiple injections of meglumine antimoniate (Glucantime, Rhodia) at a dose of 100 mg/kg/day IM has met with success in one dog.[219] Dogs with *Leishmania* are a public health risk.

TOXIN-INDUCED ACUTE GASTROENTERITIS

A list of toxins commonly resulting in gastrointestinal signs is provided in Table 18–8. Additional information on toxin-induced gastroenteritis including specific antidotes for the various toxins may be found in several publications.[221,222] The therapy of gastrointestinal toxicities largely depends on cause, but certain guidelines for the symptomatic therapy of toxin-induced gastroenteritis may be given. The first rule of the treatment of any toxic problem is to limit further absorption. In the gastrointestinal tract, this is achieved by the judicious use of emetics, cathartics, and absorbents.

Emetic Agents

In general, emesis should be induced only if the time from ingestion of the suspected toxin to the time of examination by a veterinarian is relatively short. If the toxin was ingested on an empty stomach, most toxic materials will have completed their emptying from the stomach within 4 to 6 hours and use of emetics after this time is ineffectual. If the toxin was ingested along with food, gastric emptying may not be complete for 8 to 12 hours, suggesting that in this situation more delayed antiemetic use may still be of some value, particularly if the ingested toxin has limited absorption from the stomach. Unfortunately, because of their weight or large size, inducing vomiting will often be unsuccessful in ridding the stomach of heavy objects such as metals and large indigestible materials such as plant leaves. If emesis is unsuccessful, endoscopy or gastrotomy is indicated to remove toxic objects of this nature. The induction of emesis is contraindicated in moribund animals in case of inhalation pneumonia. It is also contraindicated in animals suspected of ingesting caustic agents or sharp metallic objects. Vomiting of caustic material may create further damage to the esophagus, which may result in esophageal stricturing. Furthermore, the violent abdominal contractions associated with vomiting may result in perforation of the stomach or esophagus.

A consistently effective emetic agent is apomorphine (Eli Lilly & Co.). Apomorphine is an opioid dopaminergic agonist that induces emesis by an effect on the chemoreceptor trigger zone. An appropriate dose in the dog and cat is 0.04

mg/kg IV or 0.08 mg/kg IM or SC. An alternative route is to place an apomorphine tablet in the conjunctival sac. The tablet is removed as soon as the patient shows evidence of nausea after which vomiting will soon follow. The advantage of this technique is the accurate titration of the apomorphine dose, thus avoiding some of the complications of excessive apomorphine, such as protracted vomiting and CNS depression. Unfortunately, it often results in conjunctivitis in the treated eye.

Syrup of ipecac (1–2 mL/kg, maximum 15 mL)[221] has been used as an emetic agent but it has several drawbacks including an efficaciousness of only 50%, a cardiotoxic effect, and a reduction of the effectiveness of activated charcoal.[221] Xylazine is an effective emetic in the cat but is less reliable in the dog. The dose of xylazine required for emesis (0.2–0.4 mg/kg IV, SC) is far below that necessary for tranquilization. At these doses bradycardia is usually not a significant problem but heart rate should be monitored. Another emetic agent of value in both dogs and cats is washing soda (sodium carbonate) crystals at a dose of approximately 40 mg/kg PO.

Gastric Lavage

Moribund animals suspected of the recent ingestion of toxins should undergo gastric lavage by stomach tube (Figure 21–4). The procedure is thought to be effective if utilized within 2 hours of ingestion.[221] Its major disadvantage is the requirement for tranquilization or anesthesia in nonmoribund patients. Ten to 15 infusion-and-drainage cycles are performed with 5 to 10 mL/kg of lavage solution instilled at each infusion. Water or activated charcoal and water are the preferred lavage solutions.

Cathartics and Absorbents

Cathartics or lavage solutions are indicated if the ingestion of the toxic material has been within 8 to 12 hours of presentation and enemas may be considered within any time period from 3 to 4 hours to several days after ingestion. Suitable cathartics include any of the osmotic laxatives, such as sodium sulfate (1 g/kg), magnesium hydroxide (Milk of Magnesia: 3 mL/kg), and magnesium sulfate (Epsom's salts: 0.5 g/kg). A suitable lavage solution is CoLyte (Reed and Carnrick) administered at 30 mL/kg by stomach tube. If the toxin is fat soluble, the cathartic may be preceded by a small quantity of mineral oil. Products such as castor oil and bisacodyl that increase the permeability of the epithelium should be avoided. Warm water enemas are the preferred enema technique. Soap should not be included because it can irritate the mucosa sufficiently to produce colitis and therefore increase mucosal permeability.

The most widely used and effective absorbent is activated charcoal. This product is usually administered in association with a cathartic. The powdered form is preferred and the recommended dose is 1 to 5 g/kg made into a slurry at a concentration of 1 g of charcoal per 10 mL of water. The slurry is administered by stomach tube and may be repeated several times a day.

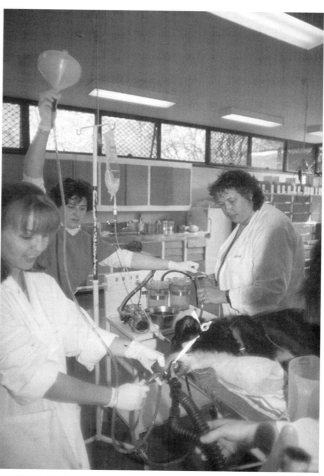

FIGURE 21-4. Gastric lavage in a dog that has recently ingested metaldehyde. The dog was anesthetized because it was undergoing seizures. A large-bore (outlet) and a small-bore (infusion) stomach tube were passed and the stomach lavaged using the pump pictured.

REFERENCES

1. Drachman RH. Acute infectious gastroenteritis. Ped Clin N Am 21:711–737, 1974.
2. Plautt AG. Microbial IgA proteases. N Eng J Med 298:1459–1463, 1978.
3. Banwell JG, Sherr H. Effect of bacterial enterotoxins on the gastrointestinal tract. Gastroenterology 65:467–497, 1973.
4. Donowitz M, Welsh MJ. Regulation of mammalian small intestinal electrolyte secretion. In: Johnson LR (ed) Physiology of the Gastrointestinal Tract, (2nd ed.) Raven Press, New York, 1351–1388, 1987.
5. Klipstein FA, Engert RF. Reversal of jejunal water secretion by glucose in rats exposed to coliform enterotoxins. Gastroenterology 75:255–262, 1978.
6. Pospischil A, Mainil JG, Baljer G, et al. Attaching and effacing bacteria in the intestines of calves and cats with diarrhea. Vet Pathol 24:330–334, 1987.
7. Janke BH, Francis DH, Collins JE, et al. Attaching and effacing *Escherichia coli* infections in calves, pigs, lambs, and dogs. J Vet Diag Invest 1:6–11, 1989.
8. Hart CA, Embaye H, Getty B, et al. Ultrastructural lesions to the canine intestinal epithelium caused by enteropathogenic *E. coli*. J Sm Anim Pract 31:591–594, 1990.
9. Jergens AE, Moore FM, Prueter JC, et al. Adherent gram-positive cocci on the intestinal villi of two dogs with gastrointestinal disease. J Am Vet Med Assoc 198:1950–1952, 1991.
10. Owens RL. Parasitic diseases. In: Sleisenger MH, Fordtran JS (eds) Gastrointestinal Disease. WB Saunders, Philadelphia, 1153–1191, 1989.
11. Greene CE. Clinical Microbiology and Infectious Diseases of the Dog and Cat. WB Saunders, Philadelphia, 1984.
12. Dillon AR, Boosinger TR, Blevins WT. Campylobacter enteritis in dogs and cats. Comp Contin Ed Pract Vet 9:1176–1182, 1987.
13. Shane SM, Montrose MS. The occurrence and significance of *Campylobacter jejuni* in man and animals. Vet Res Common 9:167–198, 1985.
14. Burnens AP, Angeloz-Wick B, Nicolet J. Comparison of *Campylobacter* carriage rates in diarrheic and healthy pet animals. J Vet Med Series (B) 39:175–180, 1992.

15. Burnens AP, Nicolet J. Detection of *Campylobacter upsaliensis* in diarrheic dogs and cats using a selective medium with Cefoperazone. Am J Res 53:48–51, 1992.

16. Diker S, Unsuren H. Clinical, hematological and pathological findings in experimental *Campylobacter* infection in dogs. Doga Turk Veterinerlik ve Hayvanc Dergisi 14:479–488, 1990.

17. Mcfarland BA, Neill SD. Profiles of toxin production by thermophilic *Campylobacter* of animal origin. Vet Micro 30:257–266, 1992.

18. Sandstedt K, Ursing J. Description of *Campylobacter upsaliensis* sp. no. previously known as the CNW group. Syst Appl Microbiol 14:39–45, 1991.

19. Krakowka AL, Fox JG, Otto G, et al. Role of *Helicobacter felis* in chronic canine gastritis. Vet Pathol 29:487–494, 1992.

20. Torre E, Tello M. Factors influencing fecal shedding of *Campylobacter* in dogs without diarrhea. Am J Vet Res 54:260–262, 1993.

21. Malik R, Love DN. The isolation of *Campylobacter jejuni/coli* from pound dogs and canine patients in a veterinary hospital. Aust Vet Pract 19:16–18, 1989.

22. Prescott JF, Karmali MA. Attempts to transmit *Campylobacter* enteritis to dogs and cats. Med Assoc J 119:1001–1002, 1978.

23. Prescott JF, Barker IK, Manninen KI, et al. *Campylobacter jejuni* colitis in gnotobiotic dogs. Can J Comp Med 45:377–383, 1981.

24. MacCartney L, Al-Mashat RR, Taylor DJ, et al. Experimental infection of dogs with *Campylobacter jejuni*. Vet Rec 122:245–249, 1988.

25. Newton CM, Newell DG, Wood M, et al. *Campylobacter* infection in a closed dog breeding colony. Vet Rec 123:152–154, 1988.

26. Blaser MJ, Reller LB. *Campylobacter* enteritis. N Eng J Med 305:1444–1452, 1981.

27. Fox JG, Moore R, Ackerman JI. *Campylobacter jejuni*–associated diarrhea in dogs. J Am Vet Med Assoc 183:1430–1433 1983.

28. Fox JG, Moore R, Ackerman JI. Canine and feline Campylobacteriosis: Epizootiology and clinical and public health features. J Am Vet Assoc 183:1420–1424, 1983.

29. Olson P, Sandstedt K. *Campylobacter* in the dogs: A clinical and experimental study. Vet Rec 121:99–101, 1987.

30. Junttila J, Crispin SM, Ophthal DV. *Campylobacter* associated epidemic in cats. Comp Anim Pract 1:16–18, 1987.

31. Murtaugh RJ, Lawrence AE. *Campylobacter jejuni*–associated enteritis. Feline Pract 14:37–42, 1984.

32. Peel RN, McIntosh AW. The dog it was that died. Lancet 2:1212, 1978.

33. Collins JE, Libal MC, Brobst D. Proliferative enteritis in two pups. J Am Vet Med Assoc 183:86–889, 1983.

34. Gorbach SL. Infectious diarrhea. In: Sleisenger MH, Fordtran JS (eds) Gastrointestinal Disease. WB Saunders, Philadelphia, 1191–1232, 1989.

35. Skirrow MB. *Campylobacter* enteritis in dogs and cats: A new zoonosis. Vet Res Commun 5:13–19, 1981.

36. Boosinger TR, Dillon AR. *Campylobacter jejuni* infections in dogs and the effect of erythromycin and tetracycline therapy on fecal shedding. J Am Anim Hosp Assoc 28:33–38, 1992.

37. Griffiths JK. Colonic infections. Curr Opin Gastroenterol 10:66–73, 1994.

38. Burrows CF. Diseases of the colon, rectum, and anus in the dog and cat. In: Anderson NV (ed) Veterinary Gastroenterology. Lea & Febiger, Philadelphia, 553–592, 1980.

39. Riley TV, Adams JE, O'Neill GL et al. Gastrointestinal carriage of *Clostridium difficile* in cats and dogs attending veterinary clinics. Epidemiol Infect 107:659–665, 1991.

40. Weber A, Kroth P, Heil G. Occurrence of *Clostridium difficile* in faeces of dogs and cats. J Vet Med Series (B) 36:568–576, 1989.

41. Berry AP, Levett PN. Chronic diarrhoea in dogs associated with *Clostridium difficile* infection. Vet Rec 118:102–103, 1986.

42. Werdeling F, Amtsberg G, Tewes S. Enterotoxin producing strains of *Clostridium perfringens* in faeces of dogs and cats. Berliner und Munchener Tierarztliche Wochenschrift 104:228–233, 1991.

43. Twedt DC. *Clostridium perfringens*–associated diarrhea in dogs. Proc Am Col Vet Int Med Forum, Washington, DC, May 1993, 121–125.

44. McDonel JL, Duncan CL. Histopathological effect of *Clostridium perfringens* enterotoxin in the rabbit ileum. Infect Immun 12:1214–1218, 1975.

45. Prescott JF, Johnson JA, Patterson JM. Haemorrhagic gastroenteritis in the dog associated with *Clostridium welchii*. Vet Rec 103:116–117, 1978.

46. El-Sanousi SM. Enterotoxaemia in cats. Vet Rec 129:334, 1991.

47. Turk J, Fales W, Miller M, et al. Enteric *Clostridium perfringens* infection associated with parvoviral enteritis in dogs: 74 cases (1987–1990). J Am Vet Med Assoc 200:991–994, 1992.

48. Kruth SA, Prescott JF, Welch MK, et al. Nosocomial diarrhea associated with enterotoxigenic *Clostridium perfringens* infection in dogs. J Am Vet Med Assoc 195:331–334, 1989.

49. Pedersen NC. Feline Infectious Diseases. American Veterinary Publications, Goleta, CA, 1988.

50. Rhoades HE, Saxena SP, Meyer RC. Serological identification of *Escherichia coli* isolated from cats and dogs. Can J Comp Med 35:218–223, 1971.

51. Wilkinson GT. Diseases of the Cat and Their Management. Blackwell Scientific, Melbourne, 1984.

52. Oslon P, Hedhammar A, Waddstrom T. Enterotoxigenic *Escherichia coli* infection in two dogs with acute diarrhea. J Am Vet Med Assoc 184:982–983, 1984.

53. Awad-Masalmeh M, Youssef U, Silber R. Properties of haemolytic *Escherichia coli* strains from dogs and cats affected by, or dead from, diarrhoea or enteritis. Virulence factors and sensitivity to antibiotics. Wiener Tierarztliche Monatsschrift 77:254–258, 1990.

54. Prada J, Baljer G, de Rycke J, et al. Characteristics of alpha-hemolytic strains of *Escherichia coli* isolated from dogs with gastroenteritis. Vet Micro 29:59–73, 1991.

55. Abaas S, Franklin A, Kuhn I, et al. Cytotoxin activity on Vero cells among *Escherichia coli* strains associated with diarrhea in cats. Am J Vet Res 50:1294–1296, 1989.

56. Sack RB, Johnson J, Pierce NF, et al. Challenge of dogs with live enterotoxigenic *Escherichia coli* and effects of repeated challenges on fluid secretion in jejunal Thiry-Vella loops. J Infect Dis 134:15–24, 1976.

57. Sack RB. Enterohemorrhagic *Escherichia coli*. N Eng J Med 317:1535-1537, 1987.

58. Moss S, Frost AJ. The resistance to chemotherapeutic agents of *Escherichia coli* in dogs and cats. Aust Vet J 61:82–84, 1984.

59. Weiss HE, Bertl F. Treatment of enteritis caused by antibiotic-resistant *Escherichia coli* in dogs and cats by orally administered autogenous vaccines. Praktische-Tierarzt 72:12–14, 1991.

60. Klipstein FA, Horowitz IR, Engert RF, et al. Effect of *Klebsiella pneumoniae* enterotoxin on intestinal transport in the rat. J Clin Invest 56:799–807, 1975.

61. Zschock M, Herbst W, Lange H, et al. Results from microbiological studies (bacteriology and electron microscopy) of diarrhoea in puppies. Tierarztliche Praxis 17:93–95, 1989.

62. Rentko VT, Clark N, Ross LA, et al. Canine leptospirosis: A retrospective study of 17 cases. J Vet Int Med 6:235–244, 1992.

63. Morse EV, Duncan MA. Salmonellosis—an environmental problem affecting animals and man. Proc 78th Ann Meeting US Anim Health Assoc 288–299, 1974.

64. Morse EV, Duncan MA. Canine Salmonellosis: Prevalence, epizootiology, signs, and public health significance. J Am Vet Med Assoc 16:817–820, 1975.

65. Morse EV, Duncan MA, Estep DA, et al. Canine Salmonellosis—a review and report of dog to child transmission of *Salmonella* enteritis. Am J Pub Health 66:82–84, 1976.

66. Uhaa IJ, Hird DW, Hirsh DC et al. Case-control study of risk factors associated with nosocomial *Salmonella krefeld* infection in dogs. Am J Vet Res 49:1501–1505, 1988.

67. Shimi A, Barin A. *Salmonella* in cats. J Comp Pathol 87:315–318, 1977.

68. Calvert CA, Leifer CE. Salmonellosis in dogs with lymphosarcoma. J Am Vet Med Assoc 180:56–58, 1982.

69. Scott FW. *Salmonella* implicated as a cause of song bird fever. Feline Health Topics 3:5–6, 1988.

70. Dow SW, Jones RL, Henik RA, et al. Clinical features of salmonellosis in cats: Six cases (1981–1986). J Am Vet Med Assoc 194:1464–1466, 1989.

71. Timoney JF, Neibert HC, Scott FW. Feline salmonellosis. Cornell Vet 68:211–219, 1978.

72. Cookson SL, Edelman R. Treatment of gastrointestinal infections. Curr Opin Gastroenterol 10:105–111, 1994.

73. Varela G, Perez-Rebelo R, Olarte J. *Salmonella* and *Shigella* organisms in the intestinal tract of dogs in Mexico City. J Am Vet Med Assoc 119:385–386, 1951.

74. Keusch GT, Jacewicz M, Levine MM, et al. Pathogenesis of *Shigella* diarrhea. J Clin Invest 57:194–202, 1976.

75. Lee A, Hazell SL, O'Rourke J, et al. Isolation of a spiral-shaped bacterium from the cat stomach. Infect Immun 56:2843–2850, 1988.

76. Paster BJ, Lee A, Fox JG, et al. Phylogeny of *Helicobacter felis* sp. nov., *Helicobacter mustelae*, and related bacteria. Int J Syst Bacteriol 41:31–38, 1991.

77. Weber AF, Hasa O, Sautter JH. Some observations concerning the presence of spirillia in the fundic glands of dogs and cats. Am J Vet Res 19:677–680, 1958.

78. Feinstein RE, Olsson E. Chronic gastroenterocolitis in nine cats. J Vet Diagn Invest 4:293–298, 1992.

79. Kapral FA, O'Brien AD, Ruff PD, et al. Inhibition of water absorption in the intestine by *Staphylococcus aureus* delta-toxin. Infect Immun 13:140–145, 1976.

80. Carpenter JL, Myers AM, Conner MW, et al. Tuberculosis in five Basset hounds. J Am Vet Med Assoc 192:1563–1568, 1988.

81. Qureshi SR, Carlton WW, Olander HJ. Tyzzer's disease in a dog. J Am Vet Med Assoc 168:602–604, 1976.

82. Jones BR, Johnstone AC, Hancock WS. Tyzzer's disease in kittens with familial hyperlipoproteinemia. J Sm Anim Pract 26:411–419, 1985.

83. Ramirez-Romero R, Gonzalez-Spencer DJ, Robinson RM, et al. Tyzzer's disease associated with distemper: A case report. Veterinaria Mexico 20:61–64, 1989.

84. Yong CW, Nutting G, Hupkabutz D. Tyzzer's disease in a dog. Can Vet J 33:827, 1992.

85. Schneck G. Tyzzer's disease in an adult cat. VM/SAC 70:155–156, 1975.

86. Wilkie JS, Barker IK. Colitis due to *Bacillus piliformis* in two kittens. Vet Pathol 22:649–652, 1985.

87. Pai CH, Mors V. Production of enterotoxin by *Yersinia enterocolitica*. Infect Immun 19:908–911, 1978.
88. Hariharan H, Bryenton J. Prince Edward Island. Isolation of *Yersinia* spp. from cases of diarrhea. Can Vet J 31:799, 1990.
89. Fenwick SG, Madie P, Wilks CR. Duration of carriage and transmission of *Yersinia enterocolitica* biotype 4, serotype 0:3 in dogs. Epidemiol Infect (in press).
90. Adesiyun AA, Mdirmbita MT, Abdullahi SU, et al. Experimental infection of dogs with *Yersinia enterocolitica* using three routes. Trop Vet 8:39–46, 1990.
91. Papageorges M, Higgins R, Gosselin Y. *Yersinia enterocolitica* enteritis in two dogs. J Am Vet Med Assoc 182:618–619, 1983.
92. Vantrappen G, Agg HO, Ponette E, et al. *Yersinia* enteritis and enterocolitis: Gastroenterological aspects. Gastroenterology 72:220–227, 1977.
93. Wilson HD, McCormick JB, Feeley JC. *Yersinia enterocolitica* infection in a 4 month old infant associated with infection in household dogs. J Pediatr 89:767–769, 1976.
94. Carlson JH, Scott FW, Duncan JR. Feline panleukopenia. I. Pathogenesis in germ-free and specific pathogen-free cats. Vet Path 14:79–88, 1977.
95. England JJ, Fry CS, Enright EA. Negative contrast electron microscopic diagnosis of viruses of neonatal calf diarrhea. Cornell Vet 66:172–182, 1976.
96. Hammond MM, Timoney RJ. An electron microscope study of viruses associated with canine gastroenteritis. Cornell Vet 73:82–97, 1983.
97. Hoffmann R, von Pock U. Zur epidemiologie und symptomatolgie der parvovirusinfektion des hundes. Praktische Tierarzt 62:16–23, 1981.
98. Roseto A, Lema F, Cavalieri F, et al. Electron microscopy detection and characterization of viral particles in dog stools. Arch Virol 66:89–93, 1980.
99. Williams FP. Astrovirus-like, coronavirus-like, and parvovirus-like particles detected in the diarrheal stools of beagle pups. Arch Virol 66:215–226, 1980.
100. Marshall JA, Healey DS, Studdert MJ, et al. Virus and virus-like particles in the faeces of dogs with and without diarrhoea. Aust Vet J 612:33–37, 1984.
101. Vandenberghe J, Ducatelle R, Debauck P, et al. Coronavirus infection in a litter of pups. Vet Q 2:136–141, 1980.
102. Chalifoux A, Elazhary Y, Frechette JL. Canine parvovirus enteritis: Possible role of endoparasites. Méd Vét du Québec 11:66–70, 1981.
103. Tennant BJ, Gaskell RM, Jones RC, et al. Studies on the epizootiology of canine coronavirus. Vet Rec 132:7–11, 1993.
104. Tennant BJ, Gaskell RM, Kelly DF, et al. Canine coronavirus infection in the dog following oronasal inoculation. Res Vet Sci 51:11–18, 1991.
105. Keenan KP, Jervis HR, Marchwicki RH, et al. Intestinal infection of neonatal dogs with canine coronavirus 1–71: Studies by virologic, histologic, histochemical, and immunofluorescent techniques. Am J Vet Res 37:247–256, 1976.
106. News: Infectious canine enteritis caused by a coronaviral type virus. J Am Vet Med Assoc 173:247–248, 1978.
107. Takeuchi A, Binn LN, Jervis HR, et al. Electron microscope study of experimental enteric infection in neonatal dogs with a canine coronavirus. Lab Invest 34:539–549, 1976.
108. Grahn BH. The feline coronavirus infections: Feline infectious peritonitis and feline coronavirus enteritis. Vet Med, 376–393, April 1991.
109. Van kruiningen HJ. The classification of feline colitis. J Comp Path V 93:275–294, 1993.
110. Pollock RVH, Coyne MJ. Canine parvovirus. Vet Clin N Am 23:555–568, 1993.
111. Kariatsumari T, Horiuchi M, Hama E, et al. Construction and nucleotide sequence analysis of an infectious DNA clone of the autonomous parvovirus mink enteritis virus. J Gen Virol 72:867–875, 1991.
112. Glickman LT, Domanski LM, Patronek GJ, et al. Breed-related risk factors for canine parvovirus enteritis. J Am Vet Med Assoc 187:589–594, 1985.
113. Brunner CJ, Swango LJ. Canine parvovirus infection: Effects on the immune system and factors that predispose to severe disease. In: Burrows CF (ed) Gastroenterology in Practice. The Compendium Collection, 289–298, 1993.
114. Turk J, Miller M, Brown T, et al. Coliform septicemia and pulmonary disease associated with canine parvoviral enteritis: 88 cases (1987–1988). J Am Vet Med Assoc 196:771–773, 1990.
115. Isogai E, Isogai H, Onuma M, et al. *Escherichia coli*–associated endotoxemia in dogs with parvovirus infection. Jap J Vet Sci 51:597–606, 1989.
116. Difruscia R, Chalifoux A, Elazhary Y. Enteric parvovirus and coronavirus infections in dogs: Frequency in Quebec. Méd Vét du Québec 21:16–17, 1991.
117. van den Broek AHM. Serum protein electrophoresis in canine parvovirus enteritis. Br Vet J 146:255–259, 1990.
118. Jacobs RM, Weiser MG, Hall RL, et al. Clinicopathologic features of canine parvoviral enteritis. J Am Anim Hosp Assoc 16:809–814, 1980.
119. Pollock RVH. The Parvoviruses. Part II. Comp Cont Ed Pract Vet 6:653–664, 1984.
120. Hebeler V. Systematic study of morphologic changes in dogs during naturally acquired infection with canine parvovirus type 2. Dissertation, Fachbereich Veterinarmedizin, Frei Universitat, Berlin, 1991.
121. Waldvogel AS, Hassam S, Stoerckle N, et al. Specific diagnosis of parvovirus enteritis in dogs and cats by in situ hybridization. J Comp Path 107:141–146, 1992.
122. Dimmitt R. Clinical experience with cross-protective anti-endotoxin antiserum in dogs with parvoviral enteritis. Canine Pract 16(3):23–26, 1991.
123. Hinshaw L. Effect of high-dose glucocorticoid therapy on mortality in patients with clinical signs of systemic sepsis. N Eng J Med 317:659–665, 1987.
124. Foley JB. Concomitant onset of central nervous system and gastrointestinal disease associated with panleukopenia in an adult feral cat. Feline Pract 21:12–16, 1993.
125. McNulty MS, Curran WL, McFerran JB, et al. Viruses and diarrhea in dogs. Vet Rec 106:350–351, 1980.
126. Evermann JF, McKeirnan AJ, Smith AW, et al. Isolation and identification of caliciviruses from dogs with enteric infections. Am J Vet Res 46:218–220, 1985.
127. Mochizuki M, Kawanishi A, Sakamoto H, et al. A calicivirus isolated from a dog with fatal diarrhoea. Vet Rec 132:221–222, 1993.
128. Mochizuki M, Tamazumi T, Kawanishi A, et al. Serotype-2 reoviruses from the feces of cats with and without diarrhea. J Vet Med Sci 54:963–968, 1992.
129. Mebus CA. Infectious enteric viruses of neonatal animals. J Clin Nutr 30:1851–1856, 1977.
130. Schreiber DS, Trier JS, Blacklow NR. Recent advances in viral gastroenteritis. Gastroenterology 73:174–183, 1977.
131. McNultey MS, Allan GM, Thompson DJ, et al. Antibody to rotavirus in dogs and cats. Vet Rec 102:534–535, 1978.
132. Harbour DA, Williams PD, Gruffydd-Jones TJ, et al. Natural and experimental astrovirus infection of cats. Vet Rec 120:555–557, 1987.
133. Rice M, Wilks CR, Jones BR, et al. Detection of astroviruses in the feces of cats with diarrhea. NZ Vet J 41:96–97, 1993.
134. Snodgrass DR, Angus KW, Gray EW. A rotavirus from kittens. Vet Rec 104:222–223, 1979.
135. Snodgrass DR, Angus KW, Gray EW, et al. Pathogenesis of diarrhea caused by astrovirus infections. Arch Virol 60:217–226, 1979.
136. Yamamoto JK, Hansen H, Ho EW, et al. Epidemiologic and clinical aspects of feline immunodeficiency virus infection in cats from the continental United States and Canada and possible mode of transmission. J Am Vet Med Assoc 194:213–220, 1989.
137. Ishida T, Washizu T, Toriyabe K, et al. Feline immunodeficiency virus infection in cats of Japan. J Am Vet Med Assoc 194:221–225, 1989.
138. Hopper CD, Sparkes AH, Gruffydd-Jones TJ, et al. Clinical and laboratory findings in cats infected with feline immunodeficiency virus. Vet Rec 125:341–346, 1989.
139. Reinacher M. Feline leukemia virus–associated enteritis. A condition with features of panleukopenia. Vet Pathol 24:1–4, 1987.
140. Hayes KA, Rojko JL, Tarr MJ, et al. Atypical localised viral expression in a cat with feline leukaemia. Vet Rec 124:344–346, 1989.
141. Johnson CA, Snider TG, Fulton RW, et al. Gross and light microscopic lesions in neonatal gnotobiotic dogs inoculated with a canine rotavirus. Am J Vet Res 44:1687–1693, 1983.
142. Fulton RW, Johnson CA, Person NJ, et al. Isolation of a rotavirus from a newborn dog with diarrhea. Am J Vet Res 42:841–843, 1981.
143. Osterhaus AD, Drost GA, Wirahadiredja RM, et al. Canine viral enteritis: Prevalence of parvo-, corona-, and rotavirus infections in dogs in the Netherlands. Vet 2:181–190, 1980.
144. Oldenburg VU, Danner K, Krass H. Importance of rotavirus infections in the dog. Zentralblatt fur Veterinarmedizin 31:297–302, 1984.
145. Johnson CA, Snider TG, Henk WG, et al. A scanning and transmission electron microscopic study of rotavirus-induced intestinal lesions in neonatal gnotobiotic dogs. Vet Pathol 23:443–453, 1986.
146. Muir P, Harbour DA, Gruffydd-Jones TJ, et al. A clinical and microbiological study of cats with protruding nictitating membranes and diarrhea: Isolation of a novel virus. Vet Rec 127:324–330, 1990.
147. Voderfecht SL, Miskuff RL, Eiden JJ, et al. Enzyme immunoassay inhibition assay for the detection of rat rotavirus-like agent in intestinal and fecal specimens obtained from diarrheic rats and humans. J Clin Micro 726–730, 1985.
148. Evas P, Goldstein M, Sherlock P. *Candida* infection of the gastrointestinal tract. Medicine 51:367–379, 1972.
149. Stone HH, Geheber CE, Kolb LD, et al. Alimentary tract colonization by *Candida albicans*. J Surg Res 14:273–276, 1973.
150. Buttner DW, Matthieesen B. Gelangen lebende Hefezellen beim Gesunden regelmassig aus dem dermlungen in die blutbahn? Mykosen 12:387–390, 1969.
151. Anderson PG, Pidgeon G. Candidiasis in a dog with parvoviral enteritis. J Am Anim Hosp Assoc 23:27–30, 1987.
152. McClausland IP. Systemic mycoses of two cats. NZ Vet J 20:10–12, 1972.
153. Ossent P. Systemic aspergillosis and mucormycosis in 23 cats. Vet Rec 120:330–333, 1987.
154. Kuttin ES, Burtscher H, Weissenbock H. Canine parvovirus-2 infection—a predisposing factor for alimentary tract mycoses. Israel J Vet Med 46:97–101, 1991.

155. Clinkenbeard KD, Cowell RL, Tyler RD. Disseminated histoplasmosis in cats: 12 cases (1981–1986). J Am Vet Med Assoc 190:1445–1448, 1987.

156. Stark DR. Primary gastrointestinal histoplasmosis in a cat. J Am Anim Hosp Assoc 18:154–156, 1982.

157. Sherding RG, Johnson SE. Intestinal histoplasmosis. In: Kirk RW, Bonagura JD (eds) Current Veterinary Therapy XI. WB Saunders, Philadelphia, 609–613, 1992.

158. Ader PL. Phycomycosis in fifteen dogs and two cats. J Am Vet Med Assoc 174:1216–1223, 1979.

159. Stokes K. Intestinal mycosis in a cat. Aust Vet J 49:499–500, 1973.

160. Legendre AM. Itraconazole: A new antifungal drug. Proc 11th ACVIM Forum, Washington, DC, 277–278, 1993.

161. Taboada J, Werner BE, Legendre AM. Successful management of gastrointestinal pythiosis with itraconazole in two dogs. J Vet Int Med 8:176, 1994.

162. Mahmood NA, Carmichael WW, Pfahler D. Anticholinesterase poisonings in dogs from a cyanobacterial (blue-green algae) bloom dominated by Anabaena flos-aquae. Am J Vet Res 49:500–503, 1988.

163. Kelly DF, Pontefract R. Hepatorenal toxicity in a dog following immersion in Rutland water. Vet Rec 127:453–454, 1990.

164. Migaki G, Font RL, Sauer RM, et al. Canine prototothecosis: Review of the literature and report of an additional case. J Am Vet Med Assoc 181:794–797, 1982.

165. Thomas JB, Preston N. Generalized prototothecosis in a collie dog. Aust Vet J 67:25–27, 1990.

166. Dillberger JE, Homer B, Daubert D, et al. Prototothecosis in two cats. J Am Vet Med Assoc 192:1557–1559, 1988.

167. Roudebush P. An updated guide to the chemotherapy of small animal intestinal parasites. Canine Pract 12:7–20, 1985.

168. Brightman AH, Slonka GF. A review of five clinical cases of giardiasis in cats. J Am Anim Hosp Assoc 12:492–497, 1976.

169. Erlandsen SL. Scanning electron microscopy of intestinal giardiasis: Lesions of the microvillous border of villus epithelial cells produced by trophozoites of giardia. In: Johari O (ed) Scaning Electron Microscopy. IIT Research Institute, Chicago, 775–782, 1973.

170. Levine HD. Protozoan Parasites of Domestic Animals and of Man, 2nd ed. Minneapolis, Burgess, 1973.

171. Petersen H. Giardiasis (lambliasis). Scand J Gastroenterol 7 (suppl) 14:1–44, 1972.

172. Roberts-Thomson IC, Stevens DP, Mahmoud AAF, et al. Giardiasis in the mouse: An animal model. Gastroenterology 71:57–61, 1976.

173. Oakley GA. Anthelmintics for cats and dogs. Anpar, Berkhamsted, UK, 1991.

174. Zajac AM. Developments in the treatment of gastrointestinal parasites of small animals. Vet Clin N Am 23:671–681, 1993.

175. Lloyd S, de Wijesundera S, Soulsby EJL. Intestinal changes in puppies infected with Toxocara canis. J Comp Path 105:93–104, 1991.

176. Harvey JB, Roberts JM, Schantz PM. Survey of veterinarians' recommendations for treatment and control of intestinal parasites in dogs: Public health implications. J Am Vet Med Assoc 199:702–707, 1991.

177. Prociv P, Croese J. Human eosinophilic enteritis caused by dog hookworm Ancylostoma caninum. Lancet 335:1299–1302, 1990.

178. Mansfield LS, Schad GA. Ivermectin treatment of naturally acquired and experimentally induced Strongyloides stercoralis infections in dogs. J Am Vet Med Assoc 201:726–730, 1992.

179. Greiner EC, Brenner DG, Cox DD, et al. Comparison of febantel tablets and Vercom paste against gastrointestinal nematodes of dogs. Vet Parasitol 41:151–156, 1992.

180. Bowman DD, Johnson RC, Helper DI. Effects of milbemycin oxime on adult hookworms in dogs with naturally acquired infections. Am J Vet Res 51:487–490, 1990.

181. Akao N, Konishi Y, Kondo K. Anthelmintic effects of milbemycin oxime on the intestinal parasites of dogs and cats. J Vet Med Japan 44:653–657, 1991.

182. Dubey JP. Intestinal protozoa infections. Vet Clin N Am 23:37–55, 1993.

183. Dacasto M, Farca AM, Re G, et al. Chlortetracycline treatment of coccidiosis in dogs and cats. Veterinaria-Cremona 6:95–98, 1992.

184. Bennett M, Baxby D, Blundell N, et al. Cryptosporidiosis in the domestic cat. Vet Rec 116:73–74, 1985.

185. Goodwin MA, Barsanti JA. Intractable diarrhea associated with intestinal cryptosporidiosis in a domestic cat also infected with feline leukemia virus. J Am Anim Hosp Assoc 26:365–368, 1990.

186. Turnwald GH, Barta O, Taylor HW, et al. Cryptosporidiosis associated with immunosuppression attributable to distemper in a pup. J Am Vet Med Assoc 192:79–81, 1981.

187. Wilson RB, Holsscher MA, Lyles SJ. Cryptosporidiosis in a pup. J Am Vet Med Assoc 183:1005–1006, 1983.

188. Green CE, Jacobs GJ, Prickett D. Intestinal malabsorption and cryptosporidiosis in an adult dog. J Am Vet Med Assoc 197:365–367, 1990.

189. Lappin MR. Cryptosporidiosis in dog and cat. Proc 11th ACVIM Forum, Washington, DC, 265–268, 1993.

190. Tzipori S, Campbell I. Prevalence of Cryptosporidium antibodies in 10 animal species. J Clin Microbiol 14:455–456, 1981.

191. Mtambo MMA, Nash AS, Blewett DA, et al. Cryptosporidium infection in cats: Prevalence of infection in domestic and feral cats in the Glasgow area. Vet Rec 129:502–504, 1991.

192. Uga S, Matsumura T, Ishibashi K, et al. Cryptosporidiosis in dogs and cats in Hyogo prefecture, Japan. Jap J Parasitol 38:139–143, 1989.

193. Mtambo MMA, Nash AS, Blewett DA, et al. Comparison of staining and concentration techniques for detection of cryptosporidium oocysts in cat faecal specimens. Vet Parasitol 45:49–57, 1992.

194. Barr SC, Guilford WG, Jamrosz GF, et al. Paromomycin for the treatment of cryptosporidium in dogs and cats (abstract). J Vet Int Med 8:177, 1994.

195. Dubey JP, Cosenza SF, Lipscomb TP, et al. Acute sarcocystosis-like disease in a dog. J am Vet Med Assoc 198:439–443, 1991.

196. Lappin MR, Gasper PW, Rose BJ, et al. Effect of primary phase feline immunodeficiency virus infection on cats with chronic toxoplasmosis. Vet Immunol Immunopathol 35:121–131, 1992.

197. O'Neill SA, Lappin MR, Reif JS, et al. Clinical and epidemiological aspects of feline immunodeficiency virus and Toxoplasma gondii coinfections in cats. J Am Anim Hosp Assoc 27:211–220, 1991.

198. Peterson JL, Willard MD, Lees GE, et al. Toxoplasmosis in two cats with inflammatory intestinal disease. J Am Vet Med Assoc 199:473–476, 1991.

199. Green CE, Lappin MR, Marks A. Effect of clindamycin on clinical, hematological and biochemical parameters in clinically healthy cats. J Am Anim Hosp Assoc 28:323–326, 1992.

200. Wittnich C. Entamoeba histolytica infection in a German shepherd dog. Can Vet J 17:259–262, 1976.

201. Kirkpatrick CE. Feline giardiasis: A review. J Sm Anim Pract 27:69–80, 1986.

202. Zajac AM. Giardiasis. In: Burrows CF. (ed) Gastroenterology in Practice. The Compendium Collection, 307–312, 1993.

203. Douglas H, Reiner DS, Gault MJ et al. Advances in Giardia trophozoites in the small intestine of naturally infected dogs in San Diego. In: Wallis PM, Hammond BR (eds) Advances in Giardia Research. Proc Calgary Giardia Conference, 65–69, 1988.

204. Baker DG, Strombeck DR, Gershwin LJ. Laboratory diagnosis of Giardia duodenalis infection in dogs. J Am Vet Med Assoc 190:53–56, 1987.

205. Hahn NE, Glaser CA, Hird DW, et al. Prevalence of Giardia in the feces of pups. J Am Vet Med Assoc 192:1428–1429, 1988.

206. Tonks MC, Brown TJ, Ionas G. Giardia infection of cats and dogs in New Zealand. NZ Vet J 39:33–34, 1991.

207. Swan JM, Thompson RCA. The prevalence of Giardia in dogs and cats in Perth, Western Australia. Aust Vet J 63:110–112, 1986.

208. Katelaris PH, Farthing MJG. Diarrhoea and malabsorption in giardiasis: A multifactorial process? Gut 33:295–297, 1992.

209. Belosevic M, Faubert GM, Maclean JD. Disaccharidase activity in the small intestine of gerbils (Meriones unguiculatus) during primary and challenge infections with Giardia lamblia. Gut 30:1213–1219, 1989.

210. Abaza H, El-Mallah S, et al. Symptomatic giardiasis and intestinal bacterial overgrowth. J Trop Med 1:19–22, 1991.

211. Leib MS, Zajac AM, Hahn N, et al. Comparisons of diagnostic tests in dogs experimentally infected with Giardia (abstract). J Vet Int Med 6:129, 1992.

212. Zimmer JF, Burrington DB. Comparison of four techniques of fecal examination for detecting canine giardiasis. J Am Anim Hosp Assoc 22:161–167, 1986.

213. Zajac AM, Leib MS, Burkholder WJ. Giardia infection in a group of experimental dogs. J Sm Anim Pract 33:257–260, 1992.

214. Zimmer JF. Treatment of feline giardiasis with metronidazole. Cornell Vet 77:383–388, 1987.

215. Zimmer JF, Burrington DB. Comparison of four protocols for the treatment of canine giardiasis. J Am Anim Hosp Assoc 22:168–172, 1986.

216. Barr SC, Bowman DD, Heller RL, et al. Efficacy of albendazole against giardiasis in dogs. Am J Vet Res 54:926–928, 1993.

217. Barr SC, Bowman DD, Heller RL. Efficacy of fenbendazole against giardiasis in dogs (abstract). J Vet Int Med 8:175, 1994.

218. Kirkpatrick CE, Farrell JP. Feline giardiasis: Observations on natural and experimental transmission. Am J Vet Res 45:2182–2188, 1984.

219. Ferrer L, Juanola B, Ramos JA, et al. Chronic colitis due to Leishmania infection in two dogs. Vet Path 28:342–343, 1991.

220. Gonzalez JL, Fermin ML, Garcia P, et al. Erosive colitis in experimental canine Leishmaniasis. J Vet Med (B) 37:377–382, 1990.

221. Bailey EM. Emergency and general treatment of poisonings. In: Kirk RW (ed) Current Veterinary Therapy X. WB Saunders, Philadelphia, 116–125, 1989.

222. Clark ML. Poisoning. In: Chandler EA, Sutton JB, Thompson DJ (eds) Canine Medicine and Therapeutics. Blackwell Scientific, Oxford, 482–498, 1984.

22

Acute Hemorrhagic Enteropathy (Hemorrhagic Gastroenteritis: HGE)

W. GRANT GUILFORD AND DONALD R. STROMBECK

Clinical Synopsis

Diagnostic Features

- Peracute onset of vomiting and bloody diarrhea
- Often aged between 2 and 4 years
- Toy and miniature breeds predisposed
- History does not support parvovirus or toxicosis
- Usually do not appear dehydrated
- Markedly elevated PCV (> 60 in most dogs)

Standard Treatment

- NPO 2 to 3 days
- Lactated Ringer's solution: 45 to 90 mL/kg in first hour followed by sufficient fluid to meet maintenance needs and ongoing losses
- Broad-spectrum parenteral antibiotics

INTRODUCTION

Bloody diarrhea (dysentery) has a number of known causes in dogs including parvovirus, salmonella, and heavy metal poisoning (Table 22–1). Over the years, an idiopathic hemorrhagic diarrhea syndrome, clearly differentiable from other forms of dysentery, has emerged.[1,2] The syndrome is characterized by acute onset and marked hemoconcentration without clinically obvious dehydration. Unlike other causes of dysentery, fluid therapy usually results in rapid recovery.[1] The stomach is rarely involved in the syndrome, and necrosis and inflammation are not prominent features of the histopathology.[1] The most commonly used name for the disorder, "hemorrhagic gastroenteritis," or "HGE," is not an accurate description of the syndrome because it incorrectly implies that gastric and intestinal inflammation are usually present. More preferable terms for this disorder are "acute intestinal hemorrhage syndrome"[1,2] or, more simply, acute hemorrhagic enteropathy (AHE), which is the term we use in this chapter.

Acute hemorrhagic enteropathy usually affects dogs 2 to 4 years of age.[2] The prevalence of the disease is particularly high in miniature schnauzers but other small or toy breeds

such as dachshunds, toy poodles, King Charles spaniels, shelties, and Pekingese are frequently affected.[1,2,4]

Dogs developing AHE are usually well cared for and in good health. Vaccinations are usually up to date. Contact with other animals is not necessary for development of the disease. The problem can suddenly occur in spite of no obvious change in daily routine, environment, or diet.[1,2]

ETIOPATHOGENESIS

The cause(s) of AHE is not known. It is probable that an acute, massive increase in small intestinal vascular and mucosal permeability plays an important role in the pathophysiology of the disease. Highly permeable vasculature allows leakage of fluid, plasma proteins, and eventually red blood cells into the mucosa and bowel lumen (see Chapter 18). Splenic contraction and loss of protein-rich fluid from the permeable vasculature explains why the PCV in AHE is markedly elevated but the serum total protein level remains low or normal.[3]

One likely cause of an acute increase in bowel permeability is intestinal anaphylaxis.[1] As discussed in Chapter 23, type I hypersensitivities of the bowel result in significant increases in bowel permeability and plasma protein leakage without marked accumulation of inflammatory cells. Potential triggers of intestinal anaphylaxis include food allergens, storage mites, bacterial secretions, or intestinal parasites. It is difficult to explain the sporadic nature of the attacks of AHE with this hypothesis, when it is considered that no changes in the the daily routine of affected dogs usually precede the attack.[2] However, sometimes a combination of events is required to trigger anaphylaxis (see Chapter 23). For instance, in many animal models of immune-mediated intestinal inflammation, bowel permeability must be mildly increased (e.g., by a virus or toxin) before sufficient concentrations of antigen can leave the bowel lumen and interact with antibody in the lamina propria.

There is no evidence that a transmissible infectious agent is involved in AHE. The problem appears sporadically in dogs that live in relative isolation, and usually does not occur in outbreaks. Known pathogens such as Salmonella, Shigella, *E. coli*, and *Clostridium perfringens* can cause dysentery but, unlike AHE,

Table 22–1

CAUSES OF HEMORRHAGIC DIARRHEA
(DYSENTERY)

Infectious Agents
  Canine viral hepatitis
  Clostridium perfringens
  Leptospirosis
  Neorickettsia helminthoeca
  Parvovirus
  Prototheca
  Salmonella
Toxicities
  Amanita mushrooms
  Arsenic
  Thallium
  Miscellaneous household products (e.g., phenol)
Metabolic Disorders
  Addison disease
  Uremia
Ischemia
  Intestinal volvulus
  Intussusception
  Shock
Miscellaneous
  "Idiopathic hemorrhagic gastroenteritis" (HGE)
  Neoplasia
  Warfarrin toxicity

*See also Table 5–25.

inflammation is a prominent feature of the histopathology caused by these organisms. Cultures of diseased tissues have not revealed any specific enteropathogens, but cultures of intestinal contents usually yield large numbers of *Clostridium perfringens*. This has led to suggestions that overgrowth of the bowel with *C. perfringens* is responsible for the disease. It is more likely, however, that the clostridial overgrowth complicates rather than causes AHE. The dysentery associated with *C. perfringens* is usually not associated with the marked rise in PCV characteristic of AHE and, as already described, inflammation and necrosis are prominent features of the histopathology, unlike AHE.[5] Similarly, clostridial overgrowth frequently complicates parvoviral infection[6] but in spite of being present in massive numbers the bacteria do not induce the profound hemoconcentration that is the hallmark of AHE. It is important to note, however, that the clinical spectrum of clostridial diarrhea is broad,[5] and a primary role for the organism in AHE cannot be ruled out.

Other possible causes of AHE are endotoxic shock, autoimmune reactions, and hypovolemic shock. As yet there is little direct evidence to implicate any of these processes in naturally occurring AHE. However, several experimental models of acute enteropathy are similar to the naturally occurring disease.

Intravenous administration of bacterial endotoxins cause severe mucosal congestion and hemorrhage within 24 hours.[1,7] Elevated plasma endotoxin concentrations have been detected in dogs with hemorrhagic enteritis irrespective of cause.[8] Endotoxin elevations are to be expected whenever the bowel mucosal barrier becomes compromised. As yet no evidence suggests that the absorption of endotoxin precedes the disease.

The clinical signs and lesions in AHE resemble some experimentally induced models of immune-mediated colitis in dogs.[9–12] Injection of anticolon antibodies into normal dogs causes diarrhea, severe mucosal hemorrhage, and varying degrees of inflammation and necrosis. It is uncertain, however, how dogs with AHE could become naturally sensi-

tized and how they could develop such an acute autoimmune response.

Hypovolemic shock complicates recovery from untreated AHE but is unlikely to cause the disease. In naturally occurring AHE, bloody diarrhea is evident before signs of shock, not vice versa. Shock (and other causes of bowel ischemia that involve venous stasis) can produce marked gastrointestinal congestion and hemorrhage, but necrosis is also usually a prominent feature (unlike AHE).

CLINICAL FINDINGS

The clinical signs of acute hemorrhagic enteropathy include bloody diarrhea, vomiting, anorexia, and depression.[1,2] The diarrhea may rapidly progress from liquid stools to dysentery, or the animal may be presented with peracute onset of dysentery without the preceding period of blood-free diarrhea.[2] The bloody stools have been likened to dark raspberry jam. The history usually does not reveal any changes in diet, environment, animal contact, or daily routine.

Physical examination typically reveals a well cared for dog in good body condition. Fever is uncommon.[1] Mucous membrane abnormalities that can be seen include hyperemia, pallor, slow capillary refill time, and/or petechia. Signs of shock may be apparent, but skin turgor and other indicators of dehydration are usually not abnormal in the early stages of the disease. Palpation often reveals the abdomen and/or colon to be sensitive and the colon to be enlarged and doughy.[1,12] Rectal examination identifies the characteristic dark bloody feces. Abdominal radiographs commonly suggest ileus.[2]

Affected dogs can rapidly develop shock if fluid therapy is not prompt. In contrast, even without treatment, less severely affected dogs can spontaneously go into remission within 24 hours. More often, bloody diarrhea persists and becomes more severe.

LABORATORY FINDINGS

A complete blood count is indicated to help differentiate AHE from parvovirus. The white blood cell count is usually normal or indicative of a stress leukogram, but sometimes a degenerative left shift with toxic leukocytes is seen. The profound leukopenia characteristic of parvovirus infection is usually not present. The PCV is usually significantly elevated above the normal range but plasma proteins are most often normal or low, in contrast to simple dehydration.[3] To be comfortable with the diagnosis of AHE, most clinicians prefer to see a markedly elevated PCV (60–85). It is probable, however, that mild forms of the disease do not necessarily have such markedly elevated PCV.

Measurement of serum electrolytes and blood gas analysis sometimes reveals hypokalemia and acidosis. Results of serum chemistry panels occasionally reveal increased ALT and BUN. The elevated ALT is probably due to hepatocellular damage from absorbed toxins, and from hypoxia developing from shock-induced hepatic ischemia. Increased BUN reflects prerenal uremia, and measurement of urine production often reveals oliguria. Evaluation of coagulation profiles may reveal evidence of disseminated intravascular coagulation.

MANAGEMENT

Successful treatment of acute hemorrhagic enteropathy depends on managing fluid and electrolyte abnormalities and minimizing bacterial invasion of the body. Dietary management is important during recovery.

Fluid Therapy

Management of fluid and electrolyte derangements is the most important facet of treatment. Lactated Ringer's solution is the fluid of choice. Volume replacement should be rapid (up to 90 mL/kg IV over the first hour). Once mucous membrane color, capillary refill time, heart rate, and pulse pressure return to normal and PCV decreases to the reference range, the fluid rate is decreased to match maintenance fluid requirements and ongoing losses (see Chapter 39). Potassium chloride should be added to the maintenance fluids. The amount of potassium added is guided by the serum potassium level (see Table 39–3) but at least 15 to 20 mEq/L is required. Sodium bicarbonate treatment is recommended if blood gases or clinical signs suggest marked acidemia (see Chapter 39).

Antimicrobial Therapy

Antibiotics are indicated in AHE because there is a high risk of bacterial translocation from the bowel as a result of shock and deranged mucosal permeability. Four-quadrant protection (aerobes, anaerobes, gram positives, and gram negatives) is required in dogs showing evidence of shock. A suitable combination is gentamicin (2.2 mg/kg SC q 8 hours) and intravenous ampicillin (20 mg/kg IV q 8 hours). Gentamicin should not be used until after volume replacement has been largely completed. Amikacin can be substituted for gentamicin. In less severely affected dogs clavulanic acid-amoxicillin, trimethoprim-sulfa, fluoroquinilones, or cephalosporins may be used successfully.

Miscellaneous Medical Therapy

Dogs with evidence of shock may benefit from an intravenous injection of corticosteroids. Motility modifiers and antiemetics are rarely necessary. Intestinal protectives appear to be of little value.[3] Treatment for disseminated intravascular coagulation may be required.

Dietary Management

Dogs with AHE are usually kept off food for 24 to 48 hours. Once vomiting has ceased, food can be reintroduced. The type of food offered must be carefully chosen, however, because it is theoretically possible that acquired food allergies (resulting from the compromised mucosal permeability barrier) can delay recovery from the disease (see Chapters 23 and 38 for the mechanism of acquired food allergy). This theoretical concern is supported by the observation that, after a bout of AHE, dogs can often no longer tolerate many foods they were previously able to eat.[12] Therefore, it is sensible to base the diet for dogs with AHE on protein sources that are not contained in the usual diet of the affected dog. These might include chicken, cottage cheese, lamb, or tofu,

for example. As described in Chapter 38, these protein sources can be mixed with boiled white rice (see Table 38–9). One to 2 weeks after resolution of the diarrhea, the dog can be cautiously weaned back onto its old diet.

PROGNOSIS

Most dogs recover completely and rapidly from AHE if they are promptly and adequately treated with fluids. Those dogs that take longer than a few days to recover should be double-checked for causes of dysentery other than AHE (Table 22–1). A small number of dogs (< 10%) die from AHE in spite of adequate fluid therapy, and approximately 10% to 15% develop repeated recurrences of the disease.[24] The mortality is high in untreated dogs, and the prognosis is guarded in dogs with very high PCVs (> 70%).

NECROPSY FINDINGS

Necropsy reveals dark reddish-black congested loops of bowel. The entire intestinal tract or just isolated segments of small or large bowel can be affected[1,2] Blood is found in the bowel lumen. Detailed description of the histologic appearance of the disease has not been reported because the low mortality of the syndrome, and rapid autolysis of affected bowel, has precluded extensive study.[2] However, it appears that inflammation and necrosis are rarely seen in spite of marked congestion and hemorrhage in the mucosa of the small and large bowel.[1] Necrosis is most often observed in the more severely affected dogs, and might be due to shock or clostridial overgrowth rather than the primary disease process.

REFERENCES

1. Hill FWG. Acute intestinal haemorrhage syndrome in dogs. In: Grunsell GSG, Hill FWG (eds) Vet Annual. John Wright, Bristol, 98–101, 1972.
2. Burrows CF. Canine hemorrhagic gastroenteritis. J Am Anim Hosp Assoc 13:451–458, 1977.
3. Bernstein M. Hemorrhagic gastroenteritis. In: Kirk RW (ed) Current Veterinary Therapy VI. WB Saunders, Philadelphia, 951–952, 1977.
4. Simpson JW, Else RW. Diseases of the intestine. In: Digestive Disease in the Dog and Cat. Blackwell Scientific, Oxford, 101–139, 1991.
5. Kruth SA, Prescott JF, Welch K, et al. Nosocomial diarrhea associated with enterotoxigenic Clostridium perfringens infection in dogs. J Am Vet Med Assoc 195:331–334, 1989.
6. Turk J, Fales W, Miller M, et al. Enteric Clostridium perfringens infection associated with parvoviral enteritis in dogs: 74 cases (1987–1990). J Am Vet Med Assoc 200:991–994, 1992.
7. Weipers WL, Hagy L, Pirie HM, et al. A comparison of the toxic effects of intestinal obstruction fluid with those of certain endotoxins. J Path 110:295–304, 1973.
8. Wessels BC, Gaffin SL, Wells MT. Circulating plasma endotoxin (lipopolysaccharide) concentrations in healthy and hemorrhagic enteritis dogs: Antiendotoxic immunotherapy in hemorrhagic enteric endotoxemia. J Am Anim Hosp Assoc 23:291–295, 1986.
9. Bicks RO, Walker RH. Immunologic "colitis" in dogs. Am J Dig Dis 7:574–584, 1962.
10. LeVeen HH, Falk G, Schatman B. Experimental ulcerative colitis produced by anticolon sera. Ann Surg 154:275–280, 1961.
11. Shean FC, Barker WF, Fonkalsrud EW. Studies on active and passive antibody induced colitis in the dog. Amer J Surg 107:337–339, 1964.
12. Strombeck DR. Acute hemorrhagic enterocolitis and gastroenteritis. In: Strombeck DR, Guilford WG (eds) Small Animal Gastroenterology, 2nd ed. Stonegate, Davis, CA, 338–343, 1990.

23 Adverse Reactions to Food

W. GRANT GUILFORD

INTRODUCTION

Adverse reactions to food are frequently observed in dogs and cats. They are comprised of a variety of subclassifications including food allergies, food anaphylaxis, food intolerances, food poisoning, food idiosyncrasy, anaphylactoid reactions to food, pharmacologic reactions to food, metabolic adverse reactions to food, and dietary indiscretions. In general, the pathogenic mechanisms that lead to an adverse reaction include interaction of the food with a biologic amplification system that leads to inflammation and the generation of clinical signs (Figure 23–1).[1] The amplification system varies considerably with the inciting agent but may include the immune system, the arachidonic acid cascade, the complement cascade, chemotaxis of phagocytes, and generation of kinins. At times, sufficient toxic material may be present in the food to produce clinical signs without need for amplification.

TERMINOLOGY

The terminology applied in the past to the various subclassifications of adverse reactions to food has been misleading. To rectify this situation, the terms and definitions listed in Table 23–1 and Figure 23–2 were recommended by the American Academy of Allergy and Immunology.[2] These terms are also preferred for description of adverse reactions to foods in animals.[3] The term *food allergy* has been greatly misused in the veterinary literature. Although there seems little reason to doubt that food allergies occur in dogs and cats, adequate documentation of an allergic response to food has rarely been provided in spite of a wealth of literature on the subject.

Clinical Signs and Differential Diagnosis

Adverse reactions to food are usually suspected when a client or veterinarian establishes an historical association between the ingestion of a certain foodstuff and the appearance of clinical signs. The signs are usually dermatologic or gastrointestinal.[4–10]

The diet has a vast array of influences on the gastrointestinal tract (see Chapter 38). As a result, the clinician must be careful not to diagnose food sensitivity solely on the basis of improvement in a patient's condition following a change of diet. Several abdominal disorders other than food sensitivity can be associated with acute signs following food ingestion. Examples include chronic gastritis, pancreatitis, biliary neoplasia, portosystemic shunts, and diaphragmatic hernias. These diseases can be differentiated from food sensitivity because the initiating food is usually nonspecific.

DIAGNOSIS OF ADVERSE REACTIONS TO FOOD

The diagnosis of food sensitivity is confirmed by elimination-challenge trials. In food allergic patients, resolution of clinical signs occurs after elimination of the responsible food from the diet followed by recrudescence of the signs when the patient is rechallenged with the food. Subsequent resumption of the elimination diet should again alleviate the signs. To rule out coincidental improvement in patients with chronic relapsing conditions (e.g., inflammatory bowel disease), reproducible clinical signs must be produced in more than one elimination-challenge cycle to diagnose food sensitivity definitively.[11]

Elimination-Challenge Trial Design

Correct design of elimination-challenge trials is imperative for reliable diagnosis.[11] The initial elimination period chosen is usually 2 to 4 weeks in duration. This period is sufficient for partial improvement or remission of clinical signs of most food-sensitive humans and animals.[6,7,9,12–15] Recently, an elimination period of at least 10 weeks has been recommended for the diagnosis of pruritus due to food allergy in dogs.[16] It is unknown if such long elimination periods are necessary for diagnosis of gastrointestinal allergy. In chronic relapsing conditions, the elimination period chosen must be greater than the usual symptom-free period of the patient to allow reliable assessment of the contribution of food sensitivity to the patient's signs.[13]

The degree of improvement of the clinical abnormality during the elimination trial will only be 100% if food sensitivity is the sole cause of the clinical signs. This is often not the

436

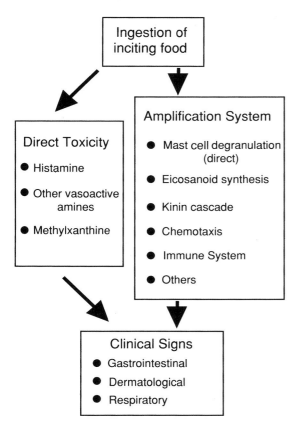

FIGURE 23-1. Pathogenic mechanisms involved in the generation of an adverse reaction to food.

case. For instance, resolution of allergies acquired as a result of gastrointestinal disease (see later) will not eliminate the clinical signs due to the primary gastrointestinal disease process.

Once the clinical signs have resolved (or partially resolved), the patient is rechallenged with its old diet. If signs recur, and then resolve for a second time once the patient is again fed the elimination diet, a diagnosis of food sensitivity is made. Further cycles of elimination-challenge trials may then be undertaken in an attempt to identify the responsible allergens or additives (Figure 23-3). Reintroduction of the offending allergen usually causes recurrence of clinical signs within a few hours to 3 days but may take as long as 7 days particularly if the responsible allergen has been removed from the diet for longer than 1 month.[4,7]

Practical constraints have limited the application of single and double-blind placebo trials in veterinary medicine. This is unfortunate, because the placebo effect has been shown to be of great importance in humans participating in food trials,[17–19] and is also likely to play a role in the reporting by the client or veterinarian of clinical signs expressed by a small animal patient. Nevertheless, open challenges, in which both owner and clinician are aware of the test food, are considered adequate for routine clinical work in veterinary medicine by most investigators.[6,7,9]

Constituents of the Elimination Diet

The constituents of a suitable elimination diet are primarily determined by diet history. As a general rule, the protein

and carbohydrate source chosen should not have formed a significant part of the patient's diet in the previous 6 months. Formulation of elimination diets is discussed in more detail in Chapter 38.

Constituents of the Challenge Diets

Challenge testing should be performed with every suspected diet or foodstuff. Diets, additives, and food proteins likely to be responsible for food sensitivity are usually identified by diet history. The results of radioallergosorbent test (RAST), enzyme-linked immunoabsorbent assay (ELISA), and/or skin test may also assist selection of food proteins for inclusion in the challenge diets.[13] The animal should be fed approximately the same quantity of the challenge diet it normally consumes. This is particularly important in the diagnosis of food intolerance, a disorder in which clinical signs are often dose dependent. An appropriate challenge dose of protein for diagnosis of suspected allergic gastroenteropathy is 0.6 g/kg body weight.[20]

Drawbacks of Elimination-Challenge Trials

Less than strict adherence to the dietary trial may result in misleading results. False negatives may occur if the food used in the test is not in the same form as that usually ingested (e.g., cooked versus raw), or if exacerbating factors have not been identified.[8,13] Lastly, and perhaps most importantly, subclinical disease is difficult to detect by elimination-challenge test.

Summary of Elimination-Challenge Trials

To reiterate, such dietary trials confirm or rule out adverse reactions to food but do not indicate the underlying mecha-

Table 23-1

ADVERSE REACTIONS TO FOODS:
PREFERRED TERMINOLOGY

"Adverse reaction to food" (food sensitivity): General term for a clinically abnormal response attributed to an ingested food or food additive.

"Food allergy" (hypersensitivity): Adverse reaction to a food or food additive with a proven immunologic basis.

"Food anaphylaxis": Acute food allergy with systemic consequences resulting from an IgE-mediated release of chemical mediators.

"Food intolerance": Abnormal response to an ingested food or food additive that does not have an immunologic basis. It includes idiosyncratic, metabolic, pharmacologic, or toxic responses to foods.

"Food poisoning": Direct nonimmunologic action on the host of a toxin contained within the food or released by organisms contaminating the food.

"Food idiosyncrasy": Quantitatively abnormal response to a food substance or additive that resembles a hypersensitivity response but does not involve immune mechanisms.

"Pharmacologic reactions to food": Adverse reactions as a result of a drug-like or pharmacologic effect in the host.

"Metabolic reactions to food": Adverse reactions as a result of an effect of the substance on the metabolism of the host or as a result of defective metabolism of the nutrient by the host.

"Dietary indiscretion": Adverse reactions resulting from such behaviors as gluttony, pica, or ingestion of indigestible materials.

Immunologic

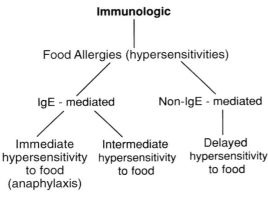

Non-immunologic

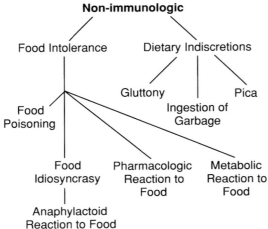

FIGURE 23-2. Classification of adverse reaction to foods.

nism.[13] To make a diagnosis of food allergy, the clinician must go on to establish that the adverse reaction has an immunologic basis.[3,13,21] The latter step is often omitted from the diagnostics because the management of most patients will not be altered whether the clinical signs result from food allergy or from food intolerance.

FOOD ALLERGY

Clinical Synopsis

Diagnostic Features

- Historical association between a particular diet and gastrointestinal, dermatologic, or multisystemic signs compatible with an adverse reaction to food
- Elimination trial identifies suspect food antigen
- Recrudescence of clinical signs on reexposure
- Documentation of an immunologic pathomechanism

Treatment

- Avoidance of the food antigen to which the animal has confirmed hypersensitivity
- Avoidance of related food antigens
- Benadryl (2.0–4.0 mg/kg PO q 8 hours; 0.5–1.0 mg/kg IV once) for mild to moderate acute to subacute clinical signs

- Epinephrine (0.1–0.5 mL SC, IM, IV of 1:1000 aqueous solution q 15–20 minutes as required) for food anaphylaxis

FOOD ALLERGENS

Chemistry

Food allergens are almost exclusively proteins, and in particular glycoproteins with a molecular weight in the range of 10,000 to 70,000 daltons.[1,2,22–24] Although all food proteins are antigenic, often only a small component of the total protein content of a food is allergenic.[25] The reasons for the propensity of some antigens to produce a hypersensitivity response (particularly type I) is incompletely understood. Most food allergens are partially resistant to heat and digestion, two properties that help ensure the maintenance of antigenic-

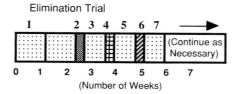

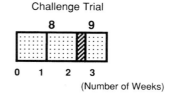

FIGURE 23-3. Suggested protocol for elimination-challenge trials to determine the foodstuff responsible for adverse reactions to food.

Elimination Trial: (1) Place the patient on a controlled diet of a single protein source and a single carbohydrate source until signs resolve: e.g., lamb and boiled white rice, or cottage cheese and rice, or tofu and rice. (2) After 2 symptom-free weeks, add a small quantity (100 g) of a protein source to which the patient has been previously exposed, and which may be the cause of the clinical signs, to the controlled diet and feed for 3–4 days (or less if clinical signs are observed). (3) Observe for clinical signs during the feeding period and 3–4 days thereafter. (4–7) If no evidence of clinical abnormality, repeat the procedure using another protein or foodstuff every week until a dietary component is identified that appears to cause clinical signs. If a prolonged trial becomes necessary supplement the diet with appropriate quantities of vitamins and minerals.

Challenge Trial: (8) After a suspect allergen has been identified, remove the protein from the diet, and observe for evidence of resolution of signs. (9) Wait a minimum of 1–2 weeks from the last ingestion of the suspected allergen and until the patient is symptom free and then, under close observation, challenge the patient again with the suspected allergen to ensure that similar signs are manifest on the second exposure.

ity.[1,22,23] The more frequently a protein is found in a diet, the more likely the animal eating the diet will become allergic to that protein.[4,25,26] Furthermore, there are apparently other as yet undefined physicochemical properties that result in the higher allergic potential of some proteins such as shellfish and nuts.[27,31]

Food carbohydrates, fats, and vegetable oils do not appear to be important food allergens[28] although allergic reactions to peanut oil have occasionally been observed in humans.[29] These reactions may be due to residual peanut proteins contaminating the oil.[29]

Influence of Processing

Food processing influences the allergenicity of foods. Denaturing of proteins by heat (or their partial digestion) may destroy old epitopes and expose new ones, thus increasing or decreasing allergenicity. The overall importance of this phenomenon in food allergy is under debate but it appears that the allergenicity of most foods is either unchanged or reduced by cooking or partial digestion.[1,2,9,12,13,22,23,25,30] Formation of Maillard reactant products will reduce the allergenicity of some foods and increase the allergenicity of others.[2,25,31] Maillard reaction products are formed when proteins are cooked with carbohydrate. This phenomenon may explain the apparent increase in allergenicity of proteins in canned pet foods (as compared to fresh proteins).

Common Allergens

Foods responsible for allergy in dogs include milk, soybeans, wheat, oats, beef, eggs, horse meat, chicken, cornmeal, pork, yeast, and a variety of commercial foods of varying protein base.[5,6,8,9,14,15,32] In the cat, the foods most often incriminated are fish and dairy products.[4,7] These suggestions need to be confirmed by well-designed elimination-challenge trials. It is worthy of note that psyllium is a documented cause of IgE-mediated anaphylaxis in humans. Most food sensitivities affecting the skin are due to single foods.[4] In contrast, multiple allergies to foods are quite common in animals suffering from gastrointestinal diseases.

Information is accumulating about the allergenic makeup of many common foods. For instance, of the nearly 30 identified proteins in cow's milk, the most allergenic are thought to be casein, alpha-lactalbumin, bovine gamma globulin, bovine serum albumin, and particularly beta-lactoglobulin. Casein may also have direct proinflammatory properties in the gastrointestinal mucosa.[33] Soy proteins consist of a globulin and whey fraction. The globulin fraction comprises 85% of the total protein and consists of four subgroups with different sedimentation constants. The 2S globulin subfraction has been found to be the most allergenic.[23,34] The 2S subfraction is the most heat stable of the soy globulin fractions.[23] Another allergenic soy protein is soybean trypsin inhibitor found in the whey fraction. This protein is resistant to acid pH and proteolytic digestion.[2] Allergy to soybean in dogs has been reported occasionally.[9] Soybeans are likely to be an important cause of food allergy in dogs because of the widespread use of soy in dog foods and the documented allergenicity of soy proteins in humans and farm animals.[35,36] Unfortunately, the allergen composition of the meats and animal by-products commonly included in pet foods is poorly understood.

Table 23–2

FOODS GROUPED ACCORDING TO BIOLOGIC RELATIONSHIP AND POTENTIAL IMMUNOLOGIC CROSS-REACTIVITY

Birds	Eggs	Milk Products
Chicken	Ovomucoid	Milks
Turkey	Ovovitellin	Milk replacers
Others	White	Creams
Bovidae	Yolk	Cheeses
Beef	**Fish**	Cottage cheese
Goat	Salmonidae	Yogurt
Sheep meats	Tuna	Ice cream
Gelatin	Others	Casein and other milk products
Sweetbread	**Legumes**	**Suidae**
Cereals	Peas	Bacon
Barley	Beans	Pork
Corn	Lentils	Ham
Oat	Licorice	Sausage
Rice	Peanut	
Rye	Soybean	
Sorghum	Others	
Wheat*		
Others		

*Bran, germ, gliadin, globulin, glutenin, leucosin, proteose.

Allergen Cross-Reactivity

In some food groups, allergy to one member of the group may result in a variable degree of allergy to other members of the same group.[25,37] This cross-reactivity is particularly common among seafoods and legumes, and has also been demonstrated with the grains.[2,37] Cross-antigenicity is less apparent in other foods even when derived from the same species.[2] For example, dogs allergic to cow's milk can often tolerate beef.[4,9] Some foods with an increased likelihood of cross-reactivity are listed in Table 23–2.

ETIOPATHOGENESIS OF FOOD HYPERSENSITIVITY

The defense against hypersensitivity to dietary antigens is a well-developed, multitier system dependent on an effective mucosal barrier in association with oral tolerance generated by the cellular immune system of the gut-associated lymphoid tissue (GALT). The mucosal barrier and oral tolerance are discussed in more detail in Chapters 3, 18, and 24.

The Mucosal Barrier

The first component of the defense against food allergy is an effective mucosal barrier that prevents overwhelming uptake of food antigens.[38–41] The mucosal barrier is composed of a number of interrelated immunologic and nonimmunologic components that include effective digestion (renders proteins nonantigenic); the epithelial cell and its mucus (mucus glycoproteins act as receptors for the attachment of bacteria and other antigens); IgA; and the mononuclear-phagocyte system of the liver.[38–43] Efficient functioning of the mucosal barrier excludes the majority of antigen, thus minimizing the exposure of GALT and the systemic immune system to reaginic antigens. Defective barrier function is the most likely cause of acquired food allergies secondary to gastrointestinal disease.

Absorption of Proteins Across the Mucosal Barrier

It is known that the mucosal barrier is not impervious to macromolecules.[26,41,44,45] Dietary proteins cross the intact mucosa into the portal venous system and mesenteric lymphatics of normal animals in small but immunologically significant amounts.[44,46] This phenomenon was demonstrated in dogs as early as 1913 by Van Alstyne.[47] The rate of entry in the jejunum of normal animals is 2 to 4 μg/hour/cm² of intestine.[45] This is approximately 100th the rate of glucose absorption in the jejunum. Protein absorption also occurs across the stomach and colonic mucosa but at approximately one-tenth of the jejunal rate.[45] These rates of protein absorption are sufficient to produce cutaneous weal-and-flare reactions within 15 to 60 minutes of eating fish in normal people sensitized with dermal injections of serum from fish-allergic patients.[26] Approximately 0.02% of daily dietary protein intake is absorbed intact, although claims that up to 2% of fed protein may be absorbed in this manner have been made.[42,44,48,49] In normal humans, for example, systemic absorption of ingested milk proteins results in a serum level of 2 to 4 ng/mL of milk antigens.[50]

In the normal animal, almost all of the absorbed protein enters the enterocyte by endocytosis and is released to the lamina propria by exocytosis.[44,45] Paracellular absorption is prevented by the tight junctions.[45] After internalization by the enterocyte, 90% of the absorbed protein is partially degraded within lysozymes to yield new antigenic determinants with a molecular weight of 2000 to 4000.[45] The remaining 10% of the internalized protein passes intact across the enterocyte. In the M cell of the Peyer's patch the degradative pathway is not as active as that of other enterocytes. In some species, proteins are transported to a greater extent across Peyer's patches than the adjacent epithelium.[45]

The rate of protein absorption is influenced by the degree of maturation of the enterocyte, nutritional state, composition of the meal, effectiveness of digestion, and the presence of inflammation.[26,38,40,41,44,45] The maturation of the enterocyte depends on the age of the animal and the stage of development along the crypt-villus axis.[45] Neonatal permeability to food macromolecules can be high for various periods, depending on the species.[40,51] Immature crypt cells have twice the endocytotic capacity of mature villus cells. Malnutrition and maldigestion increase intestinal permeability to macromolecules.[40,41,45,52] Consuming a protein along with other proteins decreases individual absorption rates of the proteins.[26] In contrast, ingesting a protein along with glucose increases the absorption of the protein.[44] Gastrointestinal inflammatory diseases including viral enteritis, bacterial infections, parasitism, wheat-sensitive enteropathy, milk-sensitive enteropathy, and type 1 food sensitivity reactions increase gut permeability in humans and animals.[36,40,41,44,45,53–56] Enteric bacterial infections result in increased protein absorption through transcellular and/or paracellular pathways.[45] Nonsteroidal anti-inflammatory drugs induce increased food antigen absorption in humans.[57] IgA deficiency also increases food antigen absorption.[42]

Consequences of Increased Mucosal Permeability

In normal animals and people, only very small amounts of gut antigens reach the systemic immune system. In normal people, the levels of circulating antibodies and immune complexes to food antigens are correspondingly low.[1,42,58,59] They increase, however, when any of the processes that contribute to exclusion of gut antigens from the systemic circulation are compromised. For instance, increased serum antibodies and, in some cases, increased food antigen-antibody immune complexes have been clearly demonstrated in human patients with IgA deficiency, portosystemic shunts, and gastrointestinal inflammation.[1,27,40,41] The consequences of increased mucosal permeability and increased circulating immune complexes to foods are unpredictable, depending on such factors as species, age, type and quantity of antigen absorbed, location of the absorption, the pathophysiologic state, and the genetic makeup.[41,45] In some instances oral tolerance to the absorbed antigen is maintained.[55] In other situations the suppressor response of the GALT is bypassed, local inflammation results, and hypersensitivity rather than tolerance to the absorbed proteins develops.[40,45,60] Thus, it should not be surprising that patients with defective barrier function due to acute gastroenteritis frequently do not recover normal intestinal function rapidly and completely. Many must be managed with controlled diets, because transient food allergies are often in evidence for some time after the initial insult.[36,61]

Oral Tolerance

Protein absorbed by the M cell (and perhaps intestinal epithelial cells) is presented to GALT in such a manner that a potent gut-associated, cell-mediated suppressor response to that antigen develops.[49,40,58] It is this suppressor response that is the basis of oral tolerance[49,58,62,63] and may be the primary site of the defect in food allergic animals.[26,64] In addition to the suppressor response, the gut-associated humoral immune system generates IgA antibody, which acts to reinforce the mucosal barrier against that antigen and to eliminate antigen in the lamina propria by forming immune complexes that do not fix complement but can be taken up by the liver and excreted in the bile.[38,40,42,58,65]

Etiopathogenesis Summary

A food protein, therefore, has the potential to incite an allergic response if it is incompletely digested in the bowel, absorbed across the mucosa intact (or partially intact), and then escapes to the systemic lymphoid tissue in excessive quantities. Alternatively, the allergic response may result if small amounts of antigen encounter a defective suppressor arm of GALT. In either case, the result is the stimulation of the synthesis of immunoglobulins such as IgE and IgG and the sensitization of peripheral lymphocytes, both of which can go on to generate immunosensitivity to the food antigen rather than tolerance. Thus, the feeding of poorly digestible proteins, incomplete digestion, increased mucosal permeability, decreased IgA secretion, deranged cell-mediated responses of GALT, and portosystemic shunts all predispose patients to food allergies.[2,22,36,40]

PATHOPHYSIOLOGY AND CLASSIFICATION OF FOOD ALLERGY

Immediate Hypersensitivities to Food

Immediate hypersensitivities to food occur within a few minutes to several hours of ingestion of the offending antigen.[1,14,43,47] Immediate hypersensitivity responses are mediated by IgE.[43,66] This is probably true even for cats, a species in which IgE has not as yet been identified. In susceptible individuals an IgE immune response develops in response to certain food antigens instead of an IgA response. The basic defect that results in the preferential production of IgE in these individuals is unknown. Genetic factors and age appear to influence the propensity to produce a specific IgE response.[43] In rats, the IgE response appears to be maximal in the young as a result of reduced suppressor activity. Predisposing factors such as a defective mucosal barrier were discussed earlier. As mentioned in Chapter 3, the source of the IgE in the lamina propria is uncertain but is probably primarily the mesenteric lymph nodes. The IgE binds to gastrointestinal and, on occasion, peripheral mast cells, priming them for a response to the inciting antigen if it is represented. The exposure of the sensitized mast cells to the inciting antigen leads to mast cell degranulation and the release of a variety of mediators, including histamine, kinins, prostaglandins, leukotrienes, and proteases (see Chapter 4).

Gastrointestinal type 1 hypersensitivity reactions have been well characterized.[43,66] The mediators released by mast cell degranulation cause loss of fluid, plasma proteins, and even blood from the capillaries into the lumen of the gut. They stimulate mucosal mucus and chloride secretion, and cause disaccharidase and motility derangements.[1,36,43,66–73] These changes culminate in vomiting, diarrhea, and if chronic, weight loss. Repeated mast cell degranulation may eventually lead to eosinophil accumulation in the bowel and may be the cause of some cases of eosinophilic gastroenteritis.[74,75] Another consequence of gastrointestinal type 1 hypersensitivity is increased macromolecule absorption, potentially exacerbating the allergic reaction or leading to multiple sensitivities by increased absorption of bystander proteins.[1,53,66,73,76–79]

If the sensitized mast cells are restricted to the gastrointestinal tract, the ingestion of antigen will cause a local intestinal type 1 hypersensitivity. More generalized reactions occur when antigen escapes from the intestine to reach sensitized basophils or IgE-bearing mast cells in the skin.[26] Release of gastrointestinal mast cell mediators into the systemic circulation may also contribute to nongastrointestinal manifestations of IgE-mediated food allergy.[43]

Intermediate Hypersensitivities to Food

Intermediate hypersensitivities to food appear to be frequent in dogs and cats judging by the reported timing of occurrence of adverse reactions after food challenges.[4,7,9] Intermediate reactions occur several hours after antigen ingestion. They are a poorly defined intergrade between immediate and delayed reactions. Intermediate hypersensitivity responses are probably the result of a late-phase response to IgE-mediated mast cell degranulation and/or a type 3 hypersensitivity response to immune complexes.[26] Qualitative and quantitative differences in food immune complexes have been demonstrated in normal versus food-allergic human patients.[59] In food-allergic people, IgE and IgG complexes are thought to accumulate in the gastrointestinal mucosa[1,22,43,80–82] and other organs[1] leading to an inflammatory response by the fixation of complement and the attraction of phagocytes. IgG and IgE immune complexes are another stimulus for mast cell degranulation and eosinophil migration (as well as other phagocytes) and may contribute to the eosinophilic infiltration seen in some cases of food allergy.[43,75] This contrasts to normal individuals in which IgA complexes predominate in the lamina propria. IgA complexes are noninflammatory and are rapidly cleared by the liver.

Delayed Hypersensitivities to Food

Delayed hypersensitivity responses to food are considered by some the most prevalent classification of food allergy in humans.[83] In spite of their probable importance, delayed hypersensitivities remain poorly documented with the exception of those in children suffering from milk-sensitive enteropathy and those in laboratory animals with experimentally induced delayed hypersensitivity.[1,36,43,84] Delayed hypersensitivity reactions appear several hours to 2 to 3 days after ingestion of the allergen[43,85] and produce nonspecific diverse symptoms such as recurrent abdominal pain, fatigue, arthropathies, oral ulcers, and gastrointestinal upsets.[43,89]

Little is known about the pathophysiology of delayed hypersensitivities to food but limited evidence suggests they are mediated by type 3 and 4 reactions.[1,27,36,43,86]

The prevalence of delayed hypersensitivity responses to food in the canine and feline population is unknown, but clinical experience indicates they do occur[4,7,9,47] and that, as in humans, they may be a relatively prominent classification of food allergy.

CLINICAL FEATURES OF FOOD ALLERGY

Food allergy is usually nonseasonal and often occurs suddenly after months or years of consuming the diet containing the inciting foodstuff.[4,5,7,10,14,47] A wide age range of patients can be affected including dogs and cats as young as 2 to 6 months.[4,5,7,9] No breed or sex predilections have been established.[4,5–9,47]

The clinical signs vary from gastrointestinal reactions such as vomiting and diarrhea to dermatologic reactions such as pruritus, papules, and erythema.[3,5–9,14] Head and neck pruritus is reputed to be a particularly common manifestation of food allergy in cats. Dermatologic signs need not be present to attribute a gastrointestinal abnormality to food allergy.[4,5,14] The adverse reactions are usually uniform in manifestation and occur consistently on subsequent rechallenges. On rare occasions a suspected food may fail to lead consistently to the expected clinical signs. Reasons for such inconsistency in patients with food allergy include variations in dose of the allergen ingested, the presence of simultaneously ingested foods that interfere with the reaction, and altered methods of preparation of the food.

Every level of the gastrointestinal tract (including the oral cavity) can be affected by food allergies. On most occasions, the clinical signs relate to gastric and small bowel dysfunction but colitis can also occur.[83,87] The diarrhea can be profuse and watery, mucoid, or hemorrhagic.[8,14,87] At least five subacute to chronic gastrointestinal conditions that are thought to involve food allergy are recognized in humans. These are food protein-induced enterocolitis, food-induced proctitis syndrome, food-induced malabsorption (enteropathy) syndrome, gluten-sensitive enteropathy, and allergic eosinophilic gastroenteritis.[20,27,39] All of these conditions can occur in dogs and cats. The severity and nature of the immune response depends on the type of ingested antigen to which the animal is sensitive, the sensitivity of the patient (in part determined by the number of mast cells that bear IgE antibody), and the amount of allergen ingested.

Involvement of organ systems other than the skin and gastrointestinal tract has been reported in humans[88] but is poorly documented in the cat and dog. Clinical experience suggests, however, that food sensitivity (and perhaps food allergy) may on occasion be responsible for such diverse signs as anorexia, rhinitis, conjunctivitis, bronchoconstriction, seizures, malaise, feline lower urinary tract disease, urinary incontinence, and glomerulonephritis in dogs and cats.[3,4,6,7,14] These clinical impressions need more objective confirmation. Such diverse symptomology is within the realms of scientific possibility because undigested food antigens and food immune complexes can be readily detected in blood, urine, and tissues of humans where they have the potential to cause inflammation.[50,55] The clinical signs associated with food allergies in humans are listed in Table 23–3. Some or all of these signs may occur in animals.

DIAGNOSIS OF FOOD ALLERGY

The diagnosis of food allergy requires that an adverse reaction to a food is proven to have an immune-mediated basis.[13,89] This is not a simple matter. The enormous number of possible dietary allergens is one stumbling block.[1,25] Furthermore, whether or not an animal manifests clinical signs following the ingestion of an antigen to which it is sensitive may depend on a number of different factors including synergism with sensitivities to other allergens, and emotional and various environmental factors that may influence the allergy threshold. Another problem is the high incidence of asymptomatic sensitization whereby patients demonstrate positive immunologic tests to food antigens but do not show signs on subsequent challenge with the incriminated food.[26] It is important to realize that a positive reaction to an allergy test is an immunologic phenomenon that must not be the only basis for diagnosis. Both positive and negative results provide only a part of the accumulated evidence in the clinician's final judgment.[25]

Some dogs and cats with food allergy have a persistent eosinophilia. Unfortunately, eosinophilia is not consistently present in all affected animals and it is not specific for food allergy. Tests that have been employed to confirm food allergy in animals and humans include skin testing, measurement of serum antibodies to foods, tests of cell-mediated immune reactions, assay of the products of mast cell degranulation, and endoscopic challenge tests. The diagnostic value of many of these tests is limited.[9,10,12,90]

Skin Tests

Skin tests are performed by inoculation of a small quantity of the suspected antigen into the skin along with a positive control (histamine) and a negative control (saline). A positive reaction appears as an area of swelling and induration sometimes with erythema. Skin tests are a sensitive technique for the detection of antigen-specific IgE in the skin. Unfortunately, the presence or absence of IgE in the skin need not bear any relation to the presence or absence of IgE in the lamina propria of the bowel. Thus, allergies with signs restricted to the gastrointestinal tract may not necessarily be confirmed by skin tests[47] or, for that matter, measurement of serum IgE levels. Furthermore, nonreaginic (non-IgE) food allergies, such as delayed hypersensitivity reactions, will not be diagnosed by this technique.[36,43] It should not be surprising, therefore, that skin testing has poor accuracy for the prediction of adverse reactions to foods in most veterinary studies.[9,30] One study in humans demonstrated that only 10% of people allergic to milk proteins had positive skin tests.[91]

Skin tests should not be considered a test for adverse reactions to foods but more properly a test to assist determination of which adverse reactions have an IgE-mediated pathogenesis. Even for this purpose, the reliability of skin tests is ham-

Table 23–3

PROVEN OR SUSPECTED SYMPTOMS OR DISORDERS ASSOCIATED WITH FOOD ALLERGIES IN HUMANS

Dermatologic
  Angioedema
  Dermatitis herpetiformis
  Pruritus
  Urticaria
Gastrointestinal
  Abdominal pain
  Anal pruritus
  Constipation
  Diarrhea
  Eosinophilic gastroenteritis
  Gastrointestinal bleeding
  Gastrointestinal protein loss
  Gluten-sensitive enteropathy
  Hemorrhagic proctocolitis
  Irritable bowel syndrome
  Milk-sensitive enteropathy
  Oral and pharyngeal pruritus
  Oropharyngeal ulcers and fissuring
  Pancreatitis
  Vomiting
Respiratory
  Allergic (eosinophilic) rhinitis
  Asthma
  Bronchitis
  Pulmonary infiltrates
Miscellaneous
  Allergic (eosinophilic) conjunctivitis
  Anaphylaxis
  Arthropathies
  Headache
  Hyperactivity
  Lassitude
  Urinary incontinence
  Vasculitis

pered by poor standardization of food extracts used for testing and the high incidence of false positive reactions. Furthermore, the optimal concentration of allergen for skin testing in dogs and cats has not been established.[10]

Measurement of Antibodies to Foods

Antibodies (IgG and IgA) specific to food antigens have been demonstrated in the serum of human patients with suspected food allergies but also in the serum of normal individuals and in patients with inflammatory bowel disease but no evidence of food allergy.[2,92] The significance of the majority of these antibodies is unknown. A small percentage may have a pathogenic role but many appear to be epiphenomena.

Fecal antibodies (IgG) against food proteins have also been demonstrated, and again do not have a confirmed pathologic role.[93] Increased levels of IgE have been observed in the intestinal juice of humans with food allergies and may provide a means of screening for food allergies.[94]

Total serum IgE levels tend to be elevated in humans with food allergy but there is considerable overlap with the normal range.[43] The concentration of antigen-specific IgE in the serum can be measured by a radioallergosorbent test (RAST) or ELISA. The diagnostic value of in vitro tests for food-specific IgE antibodies varies widely in reported studies.[90] The consensus view emerging from human studies is that the primary diagnostic benefit of measuring food-specific IgE is the good negative predictive value of the test. That is, food proteins with low circulating IgE levels are highly unlikely to be responsible for acute allergic reactions.[90] Furthermore, a positive challenge test along with an elevated IgE level to a food protein strongly implies food allergy (rather than intolerance) to that protein.[90] Because of the high incidence of asymptomatic sensitization, a positive RAST or ELISA test without an associated positive oral challenge does not permit a diagnosis of food allergy to a particular protein.[90] The significance of such asymptomatic sensitization in dogs and cats is uncertain but in children it can be a warning that clinically significant allergy will develop to the sensitizing food protein in the future.[92] Not surprisingly, RAST and ELISA are less sensitive when the food allergic signs are primarily gastrointestinal or delayed in onset.[9,36,83] Canine and feline ELISA tests are available (Bio-Medical Services; Austin, TX; Iatric Corp; Tempe, AZ). Objective evaluation of the tests in the diagnosis of canine and feline food allergy has begun. As with skin tests, RAST and ELISA are committed to the diagnosis of only one form of food sensitivity (immediate hypersensitivity mediated by IgE released in sufficient quantities to enter the systemic circulation in measurable amounts).

Gastroscopic Food Sensitivity Testing

Gastroscopic food sensitivity testing (GFST) has been used to diagnose food allergies in humans and dogs.[95,96] As described in Chapter 7, antigen solutions are dripped on to an area of gastric mucosa and the mucosal response observed. In hypersensitive patients, erythema or blanching, edema, and petechiation can appear within minutes of application of the food extract.[95,96] To establish an immune-mediated basis to the inflammation, the tissues can be sampled and histamine or other mediators measured, or the degree of mast cell degranulation assessed.[95] The pathophysiologic basis of these gastric reactions appears to involve rapid penetration of the gastric mucosa by antigen, a phenomenon that has been confirmed experimentally in a number of species including the dog.[8,45,97]

GFST has application in the diagnosis of gastrointestinal food sensitivity mediated by mast cell degranulation. The diagnostic accuracy of the method in clinical cases is unknown, but in dogs experimentally sensitized to cod the technique was able to identify correctly 75% of dogs that subsequently vomited on oral challenge with cod.[87] GFST may find a niche in screening for acute gastrointestinal food sensitivities in patients already undergoing endoscopy for other diagnostic purposes.

Gastrointestinal Biopsy

An isolated gastrointestinal biopsy specimen rarely confirms food allergy because many of the acute changes are not detectable by light microscopy or are transient, such as edema.[43] Furthermore, in diseases such as celiac sprue and milk-sensitive enteropathy that produce morphologic changes easily recognizable by light microscopy, there are no pathognomonic histologic features that differentiate food hypersensitivity from the other causes of chronic intestinal inflammation.[12,36] Eosinophilic infiltration is suggestive of food allergy but not pathognomonic.[39,43,75] Eosinophilic infiltration need not be a prominent feature of intestinal biopsy specimens from food-allergic animals.[98]

Few biopsy findings have been reported in dogs and cats with documented food allergy. The small intestine and colon of a cat allergic to milk showed congestion, edema, villous degeneration, hemorrhage, and an increase in the number of plasma cells after 4 days of milk challenge.[98]

In food-sensitive humans and laboratory animals, histologic abnormalities can be observed in stomach, small bowel, and/or colon.[36,39,43] Histology can be normal or can show mucosal edema, separation of the epithelium from the lamina propria, fat accumulation in the epithelium, sloughing of villus tip epithelium, increased mucus secretion, increased intraepithelial lymphocytes, infiltration of the lamina propria with round cells, IgA, IgM, and IgG plasma cells and/or IgE bearing cells, villus atrophy, and widespread ultrastructural disruption of the basement membrane and collagenous matrix of the lamina propria.[22,27,36,39,43,68,70,99,100] The histologic changes resulting from food protein–induced enteropathies are usually patchy and the villus atrophy partial rather than complete.[43] Decreased villous and epithelial height and increased intraepithelial lymphocyte numbers are considered hallmarks of delayed hypersensitivity reactions by some,[58] but these changes, along with increased numbers of plasma and mast cells in the lamina propria, have also been observed 6 hours after milk challenge in milk-sensitive children.[36]

IgE containing plasma cells increase in the lamina propria of humans with type 1 hypersensitivity reactions to food.[68,83,101] This may help differentiate some food allergies from idiopathic inflammatory bowel disease on a single biopsy specimen. Caution in interpretation is required, however, because it has also been observed that IgE plasma cells will increase in number as a secondary complication of a variety of chronic gastrointestinal inflammatory disorders.[102]

Repeated gastrointestinal biopsy specimens acquired during elimination-challenge trials are of considerably more diagnostic value than single biopsy specimens.[39] For instance, comparing the initial tissue sample to a second sample, taken after several weeks of an elimination diet and a third sample acquired several days after reexposure to the incriminated food is a tedious but reasonably effective way to diagnose some diet-induced enteropathies such as those due to milk and gluten.[36,39,103]

Assay of Products of Mast Cell Degranulation

Marked increases in the serum concentrations of histamine have been observed following challenge in children with suspected food allergies.[90,104,105] Assay difficulties and the rapid metabolism of histamine have prevented routine application of this test.[43] Histamine is also known to increase in concentration in the intestinal fluid following challenge of food-sensitive rats.[106] In rats sensitized to egg albumin, oral challenge is associated with the local and systemic release of a protease (rat mast cell protease II) that is a specific product of mucosal mast cells. The systemic release of such a product may prove a useful serum test for food allergies associated with intestinal mast cell degranulation.[43] Assays of human mast cell tryptase have been recently developed and are under investigation for food allergy diagnosis.[90]

Measurements of Cell-Mediated Responses

Techniques to measure cell-mediated responses to food antigens are at present in their infancy. Skin tests with food antigen have not produced characteristic delayed hypersensitivity reactions.[107] Lymphocyte blastogenesis and measurement of migration inhibition factor production in response to food antigens can detect immunologically mediated delayed responses to foods.[108] They are sometimes abnormal in food-allergic patients but are not sufficiently specific to be reliable.[36,90,109-112] Normal patients and patients with nonallergic gastrointestinal disease frequently show cell-mediated reactivity to foods without evidence of clinically significant food sensitivity.[27,112]

Miscellaneous Techniques

The basophil or leukocyte histamine release assay is a specific and reproducible diagnostic technique based on measurement of the release of histamine from peripheral blood leukocytes exposed to food antigen.[3,90] The phenomenon depends on basophil-fixed IgE.[113] Technical difficulties have limited this assay to the research setting. Measurement of food-specific IgE immune complexes shows promise in the diagnosis of human food allergy but remains unproven.[59,90]

Measurement of changes in intestinal permeability to mannitol and lactulose following oral challenge with food allergens may be a useful way to objectively confirm gastrointestinal food sensitivity.[76] Injection of a food extract into the rectal mucosa has also been used to detect gastrointestinal allergy[114] as has fluoroscopy to detect spastic changes on food challenge.[25]

A test to evaluate dogs or cats for food allergies that is based on the appearance of cytotoxic changes in neutrophils (and on platelet agglutination) when blood from allergic animals is reacted with food antigens has been described.[115] The test has not been validated. The cytotoxic test has been used in humans, but the American Academy of Allergy has stated that the technique is inaccurate and does not recommend its use.[59]

TREATMENT OF FOOD ALLERGY

Treatment depends on identification of the responsible food proteins by elimination-challenge diets. These antigens should then be omitted from the diet for a minimum of 6 months. Care should be taken to ensure that the therapeutic diet remains balanced, palatable, and practical. Ninety percent of homemade elimination diets are not nutritionally adequate.[116] Acquisition of food allergy to the protein source in the therapeutic diet can occur and may be responsible for a recurrence of signs.[47] To avoid acquisition of additional sensitivities, patients with food allergy in association with gastrointestinal inflammatory disorders are ideally fed diets based on protein hydrolysates. Such hydrolysates have proved successful in the treatment of gastrointestinal sensitivity to cow's milk and soy protein in humans.[36]

Antihistamines (H₁ blockers) administered prior to meals may decrease some of the systemic symptoms of food hypersensitivity but usually do not prevent gastrointestinal symptoms.[3] Corticosteroids are not very effective at blocking immediate hypersensitivity reactions and their efficacy in inhibiting mucosal mast cell mediator release has not been reported.[117] Corticosteroids are, however, very valuable in reducing late phase inflammatory reactions. Corticosteroids are reserved for the induction of a more rapid remission in severe conditions such as allergic chronic gastroenteropathies, and for those patients in which avoidance of the offending antigen is impossible. Animals with food allergy do not respond as consistently as those with atopy to anti-inflammatory doses of corticosteroids but will usually partially improve.[3,14] Disodium cromoglycate has no proven benefit in gastrointestinal allergic conditions. Theophylline appears to have broad-spectrum

antiallergic properties and may prove to be of value in gastrointestinal allergic conditions.[117] Hyposensitization therapy, either through oral or parenteral routes, has no proven benefit in food hypersensitivity.

FOOD INTOLERANCES

Clinical Synopsis

Diagnostic Features

- Historical association between a particular diet and gastrointestinal, dermatologic, or multisystemic signs compatible with an adverse reaction to food
- May occur on first exposure to offending food or additive
- Elimination trial identifies suspected inciting food or food additive
- Recrudescence of clinical signs on reexposure
- *No* documentation of an immunologic pathomechanism

Treatment

- Avoidance of the suspected food or food additive

FOOD IDIOSYNCRASY

A wide variety of food additives have been noted to produce adverse reactions to food in susceptible people.[118] These reactions can closely mimic food allergies. One distinguishing feature is that they usually do not require prior sensitization and thus may occur on the first exposure to the inciting agent. By far the majority of reactions to food additives are due to idiosyncratic food intolerances and not immunologic mechanisms. The reactions may be dermatologic, respiratory, gastrointestinal, or behavioral.[14,17,119,120]

The prevalence of adverse reactions to food additives has been estimated to range from 0.3% to 0.15% of the whole human population.[17] The same reactions are likely to occur in animals[8] but remain to be documented. Diagnosis of food idiosyncrasy most often requires the use of elimination-challenge diets. No in vitro tests are available. It is difficult to rule out an immunologic basis to a food idiosyncrasy. RASTs for food additives are not available, and skin testing using chemicals, many of which are known contact irritants, has received little evaluation. A partial list of potentially adverse additives commonly added to pet foods and pet treats is shown in Table 23–4. In addition, penicillin-contaminated food has been reported to cause adverse reactions in a cat.[4]

The mechanisms by which these chemical additives produce such clinical symptoms without involvement of the immune system is a matter of continuing investigation. Suggested possibilities include triggering of eicosanoid pathways, alteration of cell membrane permeability, inhibition of enzymes, direct release of histamine, changes in neurotransmitter levels, and independent activation of the complement and kinin cascades.[17,121,122]

ANAPHYLACTOID REACTIONS TO FOOD

Anaphylactoid reactions mimic anaphylactic reactions yet laboratory tests fail to establish an immune basis. Anaphylactoid reac-

Table 23–4

FOOD ADDITIVES WITH THE POTENTIAL TO CAUSE FOOD SENSITIVITY

Metabisulfite
Sulphur dioxide
Monosodium glutamate
Sodium nitrate
Sorbic acid
Butylhydroxytoluene (BHT)
Butylhydroxyanisole (BHA)

tions can occur after ingestion of spoiled tuna, mackerel, or mahi-mahi, which contain large amounts of histamine.[2] The contamination of the fish with *Proteus morganii* or *Klebsiella pneumoniae* results in microbial decarboxylation of histidine to yield histamine.

PHARMACOLOGIC REACTIONS TO FOOD

A number of foods contain vasoactive amines and other pharmacologically active substances capable of inducing a wide variety of signs that particularly affect the gastrointestinal tract and nervous system.[123] The vasoactive amines include tyramine, tryptamine, phenylethylamine, dopamine, norepinephrine, serotonin, and histamine.[123] They are usually produced by bacterial decarboxylation of amino acids. Tyramine is common in cheese, histamine in spoiled tuna, and phenylethylamine in chocolate.[2,123]

Psychoactive agents and stimulants are contained in some foods. The most important example in dogs is chocolate toxicosis resulting from methylxanthines. Another example is myristin in nutmeg.[123]

METABOLIC ADVERSE REACTIONS TO FOOD

Metabolic adverse reactions to food usually occur only in a susceptible subpopulation.[123] Reasons for susceptibility to a particular food include disease states, malnutrition, and inborn errors of metabolism.[123] The diarrhea, bloating, and abdominal discomfort that occur following ingestion of milk by animals with lactose intolerance is a metabolic adverse reaction that is relatively common in dogs and cats.[124] Inborn errors of metabolism collectively are important causes of metabolic adverse reactions to food in humans and also occur in animals (for example, urea cycle enzyme deficiencies). The site of the defect in the metabolic pathway determines the specificity of the resultant clinical signs for a particular nutrient. For example, inherited defects in the metabolism of most of the amino acids occur in humans. Many of these defects cause vomiting, diarrhea, or skin rashes, and many can be controlled by modifications in the type or quantity of amino acids or protein provided in the diet. Defective enzymatic handling of fermented colonic food residues has also been proposed as an important cause of food intolerance.[125] Occasionally an excessive intake of a food will produce a metabolic derangement. For instance, avidin ingestion in raw egg white can induce biotin deficiency.

FOOD POISONING

Food poisoning is a frequent cause of gastrointestinal disease in dogs and cats. Food poisoning is thought to be increasing in prevalence in people, a change that has been attributed to decreased use of preservatives.[123] The increasing sales of preservative-free pet foods may precipitate a similar trend in small animals.

The diagnosis of food poisoning is usually made when a pet is suspected to have eaten inadequately prepared, spoiled, or contaminated food. Clinical signs will occur within a few hours of ingestion when the poisoning is due to a toxin inherent to the food or a secreted toxin derived from a microorganism. More delayed symptoms result if the food poisoning is due to a microorganism that must colonize the bowel for pathogenicity.[126] Examples of microorganism-induced food poisoning include aflatoxins, which cause hepatotoxicity and liver cancer; ergot, which results in ischemic necrosis of extremities; a wide variety of other mycotoxins that cause vomiting and diarrhea; and bacterial exotoxins such as that produced by *Clostridium botulinum*, *Clostridium perfringens*, and *Staphylococcus aureus*.[123]

Ingestion of a variety of toxic plants mistaken as food can cause poisoning. An important example is *Amanita* mushrooms. Ingestion of commonly used foods after inadequate preparation or in excessive quantities can result in food poisoning. For example, green potatoes have high levels of glycoalkaloids; excessive quantities of onions cause Heinz body anemia probably due to N-propyl disulfide; large quantities of inadequately cooked lima beans, sorghum sprouts, maize, or chick peas can lead to cyanide toxicity; excessive quantities of spinach or preserved meats contain nitrates and nitrites that can lead to methemoglobinemia; high levels of oxalates and anthraquinone glycosides contained in rhubarb, spinach, and beet can lead to a corrosive gastroenteritis; and large quantities of spices such as peppers can cause abdominal discomfort.[123,126]

DIETARY INDISCRETIONS

Gluttony by dogs can result in gastric dilatation with or without subsequent volvulus. "Garbage can enteritis" is a frequent problem in unrestrained dogs. The history usually provides the diagnosis. Clinical signs vary with the toxic principals concerned but usually include an acute onset of vomiting and diarrhea sometimes with blood. The condition is usually self-limiting but dogs often require symptomatic therapy to maintain fluid, electrolyte, and acid-base homeostasis. The pathophysiology of the disorder involves a multitude of potential injurious products found in decomposing garbage. They include bacterial and fungal toxins, vasoactive amines such as histamine, and indigestible materials such as bone and tin foil that can physically abrade the mucosa.

GLUTEN-SENSITIVE ENTEROPATHY

Clinical Synopsis

Diagnostic Features

- Historical association between gluten-containing diets and malabsorption
- Elimination of gluten-containing grains results in resolution of signs
- Recrudescence of clinical signs on reexposure to one or, preferably, more than one gluten-containing grain
- Intestinal biopsy usually showing some degree of villus atrophy and cellular infiltration

Standard Treatment

- Elimination of wheat, barley, rye, buckwheat, and oats from the diet

Introduction

Gluten-induced enteropathy (celiac disease) is an important chronic inflammatory disease of the small intestine of humans. In some populations the prevalence of the disease may reach as high as 1 in 300 people.[127] The prevalence of gluten intolerance in dogs and cats is unknown. Recent work has conclusively demonstrated that an analogous disorder affects the Irish setter dog,[56,128–131] and clinical experience suggests that other breeds may also be affected. It is possible that some dogs with gluten intolerance are incorrectly diagnosed as having idiopathic lymphocytic- plasmacytic enteritis. On many occasions lymphocytic-plasmacytic enteritis is associated with villus atrophy and the other histologic features found in gluten-induced enteropathy. These diseases are difficult to separate without properly conducted elimination-challenge trials.

Cereal Grain Proteins

Flour from cereal grains contains various proteins including the water-soluble albumins, the saline-soluble globulins, the ethanol-soluble prolamins, and the acid- or alkali-soluble glutelins.[24] There is marked sequence homology between the prolamins of wheat, rye, and barley but not between the prolamins of rice and corn, which do not exacerbate the disorder.[132] The prolamin protein of wheat is gliadin, and the glutelin protein of wheat is glutenin. Gliadin is a glutamine and proline-rich polypeptide with a molecular weight of 15,000 daltons. Gliadin is comprised of four major electrophoretic fractions, the most toxic of which in humans appears to be alpha-gliadin.[133] "Gluten" is a crude mixture of gliadin and glutenin. These peptides are normally digested by pancreatic enzymes in the intestinal lumen, and the process is completed by brush border and intracellular enzymes of the mucosa. Completely hydrolyzed gliadin is nontoxic. It is worthy of note that there at least 18 allergenic proteins in wheat,[24] suggesting that adverse reactions to wheat in dogs should not be automatically attributed to gluten.

Etiopathogenesis

The cause of gluten sensitivity is unknown. Affected humans have an increased incidence of certain histocompatibility antigens, suggesting a genetic role. Recently, immunologic cross-reactivity between alpha-gliadin and a human adenovirus protein has been observed.[134,135] This raises the possibility that viral infection may be the initiating event in the development of sensitivity to gliadin. Intestinal permeability is significantly higher in human patients with celiac disease and their healthy relatives when compared to healthy controls and patients with nonspecific gastrointestinal symptoms.[136] Whether the increased permeability in the relatives is a secondary phenomenon due to undetected low-grade inflammation to gluten or results from primary mucosal barrier dysfunction that is involved in the genesis of the disease remains to be determined. Intestinal permeability improves rapidly in gluten-sensitive humans placed on a gluten-free diet, but some degree of abnormal permeability persists.[137] Similarly, studies of gluten intolerant Irish setters have demonstrated that increased mucosal permeability predates the development of the disease.[56] This finding supports the possibility that increased mucosal permeability may be the basis for an acquired sensitivity to gluten.

The pathogenesis of gluten-sensitive enteropathy has been debated for many years.[127,132,138–140] An early theory suggesting that the disease was caused by defective mucosal digestion of gluten, resulting in accumulation of a toxic fraction that directly damaged the mucosa, has been largely discredited in humans.[132] Brush border enzyme defects have been demonstrated in gluten-induced enteropathy of Irish setters.[129] These brush border defects include a decrease in the activity of alkaline phosphatase and aminopeptidase N, the most abundant brush border peptidase.[131] As with humans, the activity of these enzymes is normal in gluten-sensitive dogs reared on a wheat-free diet,[131] suggesting the changes in enzyme activity are a result and not a cause of the disease. It is possible, however, that the reduced aminopeptidase activity contributes to the perpetuation of the disease by causing reduced degradation of gliadin.[131]

It is now considered probable that gluten sensitivity in humans is mediated by the immune system. Knowledge of the complete sequence of immunologic events is far from complete, but it appears the immune damage is not mediated by IgE. Instead, evidence suggests that delayed hypersensitivity to gluten is responsible.[132] It is thought that gliadin-activated macrophages recruit lamina propria lymphocytes, resulting in a delayed hypersensitivity response and various inflammatory changes such as infiltration of inflammatory cells, mast cell degranulation, production of eicosanoids, increased microvascular permeability, and complement activation.[132,141] In gluten-sensitive dogs the mucosal intraepithelial lymphocyte density is increased and serum total IgA levels are elevated.[142] In comparison to humans, anti-gliadin antibody (IgG) levels are lower in affected dogs than age-matched controls and serum immune complex levels are not elevated.[142] These findings do not support a role for a systemic immune response in the pathogenesis of canine gluten-sensitive enteropathy but do not rule out a mucosal delayed hypersensitivity response.

Histopathology

The lesions of gluten-induced enteropathy are more prominent in the cranial part of the small intestine, where the exposure to gluten is the greatest. In severe cases, the entire length of the small intestine is affected.

Marsh describes three distinctive but interrelated patterns of mucosal change in gluten-sensitive enteropathy of humans.[132] These three patterns have been called infiltrative, hyperplastic, and destructive (flat). The infiltrative lesion comprises normal mucosal architecture in which the villous epithelium is markedly infiltrated by a gluten-dependent population of intraepithelial lymphocytes. The hyperplastic lesion is similar to the infiltrative lesion but with enlarged crypts whose epithelium is also infiltrated by lymphocytes. The destructive lesion is the flat mucosa (villus atrophy) considered classical for gluten-sensitive enteropathy. Thus, villus atrophy is now considered the end of a spectrum of change induced by gluten. The absence of villus atrophy does not eliminate a diagnosis of gluten sensitivity.[132] When villus atrophy is present, the number of intraepithelial lymphocytes increases per unit length of epithelium, but the total number of intraepithelial cells is not increased because the absorptive surface area is markedly decreased.[127,143] Granulomas can be seen.[144] As with any chronic inflammatory process, a persistent contact with glutens will cause more permanent changes to develop, such as fibrosis. Otherwise, the lesions are largely reversible

The histopathologic changes in dogs with gluten-induced enteropathy are similar, although less severe, to those of humans with the disorder. Morphologically, gluten-sensitive enteropathy in dogs is characterized by partial villus atrophy of the jejunum, accompanied by an increase in the relative numbers of intraepithelial lymphocytes.[130]

It is important to note that villus atrophy and infiltration of the lamina propria are nonspecific changes that accompany many other pathologic processes in the intestinal tract including the idiopathic inflammatory bowel diseases, marked bacterial overgrowth, parasitism, and neoplasia. Villus atrophy is not pathognomonic of gluten-induced enteropathy.

Pathophysiology

The initial clinical signs associated with gluten-induced enteropathy are related to the changes in the small intestinal mucosa. Villus atrophy and crypt hyperplasia result in a reduced absorptive capacity and increased secretion by the crypt epithelium. Lymphedema and protein loss into the bowel may occur.[145] Mucosal mast cell degranulation occurs on gluten challenge[146] and may partly explain these permeability changes. Many mucosal enzymes that contribute to the digestive absorption process are decreased. The pathology is most striking in the cranial part of the small intestine, however, and because there is a large reserve capacity for absorption, the pathologic changes must be advanced and extensive to cause malabsorption. Another important cause of the gluten-induced malassimilation, at least in humans, is maldigestion due to reduced cholecystokinin and secretin release as a result of the pathologic changes in the duodenal mucosa.[127] Enterogastric reflexes may also be impaired. The result of these changes is inadequate secretion of bile and pancreatic enzymes, and perhaps deranged gastric emptying, all of which contribute to maldigestion. Chronic malassimilation in humans has resulted in deficiencies of the fat soluble vitamins, iron, folate, cobalamin, and various electrolytes including calcium, potassium, sodium, chloride, magnesium, and zinc.

Clinical Findings and Diagnosis

The clinical-laboratory findings are those of malassimilation (Chapter 19). In Irish setters with the disease, the onset of clinical signs occurs between 4 to 7 months of age. The dogs present with poor weight gain or weight loss, in many cases accompanied by chronic intermittent diarrhea.[130,131,147] Serum folate concentrations are low in a few dogs whereas cobalamin concentrations are unaltered. Xylose absorption is subnormal in a small number of affected animals. A promising screening test for the disease in humans is the assay of serum levels of IgA-antigliadin antibody.[145,148]

The diagnosis is made by an elimination-challenge trial.[49] The usual test diet contains a single source of carbohydrates and a single source of proteins. They are selected so they are gluten free. The most common nutrients used are rice, to meet carbohydrate needs, and cottage cheese, eggs, or meat, to supply protein. With chronic mucosal changes, several weeks are required for morphology and function to begin to return to normal. The controlled diet should be fed for 2 weeks before evaluations or changes are made. A presumptive diagnosis is

made if the patient responds to the gluten-free diet and signs recur when gluten-containing grains are reintroduced. A more definitive diagnosis of gluten sensitivity is provided by the observation that the clinical signs may be induced by the use of purified gluten, or by challenge by more than one gluten-containing grain. These precautions rule out or reduce the likelihood (respectively) that the diarrhea arises from an allergy to a grain antigen other than gluten.

A significant number of humans with gluten-induced enteropathy do not respond to a gluten-free diet. They are usually longstanding cases, with mucosal changes that are irreversible. Thus, the possibility of gluten-induced enteropathy should not be excluded if a dog with advanced mucosal changes does not respond well to a gluten-free diet.

Biopsy of the small intestine supports but does not confirm the diagnosis because the histologic changes seen in gluten enteropathy are nonspecific. Histologic quantitation of rectal mucosal intraepithelial lymphocytes before and after rectal gluten challenge is an accurate way to diagnose gluten-sensitive enteropathy in humans.[150]

Management and Prognosis

The treatment for gluten-induced enteropathy is to exclude grains such as wheat, barley, rye, buckwheat, and oats from the diet. These grains can all exacerbate the disease, presumably because of similar prolamin structure.[132] Homemade diets can be safely formulated from rice and animal proteins. Many foods prepared for human consumption contain cereal by-products, and so must be excluded from the diet. Low-fat diets may be advantageous if villus atrophy and malabsorption are marked. Many commercial pet foods contain glutens. Prescription Diets d/d and i/d (Hills Pet Products) contain no wheat glutens. Eukanuba (Iams Co.) and Science Diet (Hills Pet Products) dry diets are also free of wheat.

Corticosteroids cause a remission of clinical signs, and mucosal morphology returns to normal. Both in vivo and in vitro studies in humans show that when corticosteroids are given and glutens are not removed from the diet, the mucosa regains normal morphology.[151] Corticosteroids must be used indefinitely because the pathologic changes return when the drug is discontinued. The amount of steroids to use has not been precisely defined but initial doses of 1 to 2 mg/kg body weight per day may be required. Corticosteroids are best reserved for patients that have marked histologic changes and do not respond well to the gluten-free diet. They should be used as adjunct therapy to a gluten-free diet, not as a substitute for gluten exclusion.

Two weeks is the earliest to expect improvement from severe mucosal changes complicated by hypoproteinemia, anemia, and mineral imbalances. Clinical improvement often occurs despite little improvement in mucosal morphology. Any improvement in mucosal pathology is noted first in the caudal small intestine, where the mucosa has been exposed to fewer glutens than in the cranial part.

The prognosis is generally good as long as the enteropathy is not advanced.

Prevention

Humans are less likely to develop gluten-induced enteropathy when feeding of gluten-containing cereals to young children is delayed.[152] A similar phenomenon has been observed in dogs.[130]

CONCLUSION

There is now a wealth of good scientific literature on the causes, pathophysiology, diagnosis, and clinical manifestations of adverse reactions to foods. The confusion and controversy that surround this topic are no longer necessary[21] and will be further dispelled in coming years by carefully designed studies that systematically examine both immunologically mediated and non-immunologically mediated food sensitivity.

REFERENCES

1. Kniker WT. Immunologically mediated reactions to food: State of the art. Ann Allergy 56:60–69, 1987.
2. Anderson JA, Sogu DD (eds). Adverse reactions to foods. National Institute for Health Publication, no. 84-2442, July 1984.
3. Halliwell REW. Management of dietary hypersensitivity in the dog. J Sm Anim Pract 33:156–160, 1992.
4. Walton GS. Skin responses in the dog and cat to ingested allergens: Observations on one hundred confirmed cases. Vet Rec 81:709–713, 1967.
5. White SD. Food hypersensitivity in 30 dogs. J Am Vet Med Assoc 188:695–698, 1986.
6. White SD. Food hypersensitivity. Vet Clin N Am 18:1043–1048, 1988.
7. White SD. Sequoia D. Food hypersensitivity in cats: 14 cases (1982–1987). J Am Vet Med Assoc 194:692–695, 1989.
8. Baker E. Food allergy. In: Small Animal Allergy: A Practical Guide. Lea & Febiger, Philadelphia, 94–118, 1990.
9. Jeffers JG, Shanley KJ, Meyer EK. Diagnostic testing of dogs for food allergy in dogs. J Am Vet Med Assoc 198:245–250, 1991.
10. Kunkle G, Horner S. Validity of skin testing for diagnosis of food allergy in dogs. J Am Vet Med Assoc 200:677–680, 1992.
11. Metcalfe DD, Sampson HA (eds). Workshop on experimental methodology for clinical studies of adverse reactions to foods and to food additives. J Allergy Clin Immunol 86:421–442, 1990.
12. Bahna SL. Diagnostic tests for food allergy. Clin Rev Allergy 6:259–284, 1988.
13. Bahna SL. Practical considerations in food challenge testing. Immunol Allergy Clin N Am 11:843–850, 1991.
14. August JR. Dietary hypersensitivity in dogs: Cutaneous manifestations, diagnosis, and management. Comp Contin Ed Pract Vet 7:469–477, 1985.
15. Harvey RG. Food allergy and dietary intolerance in dogs: A report of 25 cases. J Sm Anim Pract 34:175–179, 1993.
16. Rosser EJ. Diagnosis of food allergy in dogs. J Am Vet Med Assoc 203:259–262, 1993.
17. Hannuksela M, Haahtela T. Hypersensitivity reactions to food additives. Allergy 42:561–575, 1987.
18. Farah DA, Calder I, Benson L, et al. Specific food intolerance: Its place as a cause of gastrointestinal symptoms. Gut 26:164–168, 1985.
19. Sampson HA. Immunologically mediated food allergy: The importance of food challenge procedures. Ann Allegy 60:262–269, 1988.
20. Lake AM. Food protein-induced gastroenteropathy in infants and children. In: Metcalfe DD, Sampson HA, Simon RA (eds) Food Allergy, Adverse Reactions to Foods and Food Additives. Blackwell Scientific, Oxford, 174–185, 1991.
21. May CD. Are confusion and controversy about food hypersensitivity really necessary? J Allergy Clin Immunol 75:329–333, 1985.
22. Sampson HA, Buckley RH, Metcalfe DD. Food allergy. JAMA 258:2886–2890, 1987.
23. Lemanske RF, Taylor SL. Standardized extracts, foods. Clin Rev Allergy 5:23–26, 1987.
24. Yunginger JW. Food antigens. In: Metcalfe DD, Sampson HA, Simon RA (eds) Food Allergy, Adverse Reactions to Foods and Food Additives, Blackwell Scientific, Oxford, 36–51, 1991.
25. Perlman F. Food Allergens. In: Castimpoolas N (ed) Immunological Aspects of Foods. AVI, Westport, CT, 279–316, 1977.
26. Sampson HA. IgE-mediated food intolerance. J Allergy Clin Immunol 81:495–504, 1988.
27. Sampson HA. Immunologic mechanisms in adverse reactions to foods. Immunol Allergy Clin N Am 11:701–716, 1991.
28. Bush RK, Taylor SL, Nordlee JA, et al. Soybean oil is not allergenic to soybean-sensitive individuals. J Allergy Clin Immunol 76:242–245, 1985.
29. Moneret-Vautrin DA, Hatahet R, Kanny G, et al. Allergenic peanut oil in milk formulas (letter). Lancet 338:1149, 1991.
30. Schwartz RH. IgE-mediated allergic reactions to cow's milk. Immunol Allergy Clin N Am 11:717–741, 1991.
31. Lietze A. Laboratory research in food allergy I. Food allergens. J Asthma Res 7:25–40, 1969.
32. Stogdale L, Bomzon L, Bland van den Berg P. Food allergy in cats. J Am Anim Hosp Assoc 18:188–194, 1982.
33. Miller MJS, Zhang XJ, Gu X, et al. Acute intestinal injury induced by acetic acid and casein: Prevention by intraluminal misoprostol. Gastroenterology 101:22–30, 1991.
34. Shibasaki M, Suzuki S, et al. Allergenicity of major component of soybean. Int Arch Allergy Appl Immun 61:441–448, 1980.
35. Barratt MEJ, Strachan PJ, Porter P. Antibody mechanisms implicated in digestive disturbances following ingestion of soya protein in calves and piglets. Clin Exp Immunol 31:305–312, 1978.
36. Gryboski JD. Gastrointestinal aspects of cow's milk protein intolerance and allergy. Immunol Allergy Clin N Am 11:733–797, 1991.
37. Block G, Tse KS, Kijek K, et al. Baker's asthma. Clin Allergy 14:177–185, 1984.
38. Walker WA. Pathophysiology of intestinal uptake and absorption of antigens in food allergy. Ann Allergy 59:7–20, 1987.
39. Proujansky R, Winter HS, Walker WA. Gastrointestinal syndromes associated with food sensitivity. Adv Pediatr 35:219–238, 1988.
40. Schreiber RA, Walker WA. Food allergy: Fact and fiction. Mayo Clinic Proc 64:1381–1391, 1989.
41. Sanderson IR, Walker WA. Uptake and transport of macromolecules by the intestine: Possible role in clinical disorders (an update). Gastroenterology 104:622–639, 1993.
42. Levinsky RJ. Factors influencing intestinal uptake of food antigens. Proc Nutrition Soc 44:81–86, 1985.
43. Patrick MK, Gall DG. Protein intolerance and immunocyte and enterocyte interaction. Pediatr Clin N Am 35:17–34, 1988.
44. Gardner MLG. Gastrointestinal absorption of intact proteins. Ann Rev Nutr 8:329–350, 1988.
45. Heyman M, Desjeux JF. Significance of intestinal food protein transport. J Pediatr Gastroenterol Nutr 15:48–57, 1992.
46. Gallagher PJ, Goulding NJ, Gibney MJ, et al. Acute and chronic immunological response to dietary antigen. Gut 24:831–835, 1983.
47. Baker E. Food allergy. Vet Clin N Am 4:79–89, 1974.
48. Warshaw AL, Walker WA, Isselbacher KJ. Protein uptake by the intestine: Evidence for absorption of intact macromolecules. Gastroenterology 66:987–992, 1974.
49. Mowat AM. The regulation of immune responses to dietary protein antigens. Immunology Today 8:93–98, 1987.
50. Lovegrove JA, Osman DL, Morgan JB, et al. Transfer of cow's milk B-lactoglobulin to human serum after a milk load: A pilot study. Gut 34:203–207, 1993.
51. Hamburger RN, Heller S, Mellon MH, et al. Current status of the clinical and immunologic consequences of a prototype allergic disease prevention program. Ann Allergy 51:281–290, 1983.
52. Worthington BS, Boatman ES, Kenny GE. Intestinal absorption of intact proteins in normal and protein-deficient rats. Am J Clin Nutr 27:276–286, 1974.
53. Ramage JK, Stanisz A, Scicchitano R, et al. Effect of immunologic reactions on rat intestinal epithelium. Gastroenterology 94:1368–1375, 1988.
54. Heyman M. Antigen absorption by the jejunal epithelium of children with cow's milk allergy. Pediatr Res 24:197–202, 1988.
55. Powell GK, McDonald PJ, Van Suckle GJ, et al. Absorption of food protein antigen in infants with food protein-induced enterocolitis. Dig Dis Sci 34:781–788, 1989.
56. Hall EJ, Batt RM. Enhanced permeability to ^{51}Cr-EDTA in canine small intestinal disease. J Am Vet Med Assoc 196:91–95, 1990.
57. Fagiolo V, Paganelli R, Ossi E, et al. Intestinal permeability and antigen absorption in rheumatoid arthritis. Effects of acetylsalicylic acid and sodium chromoglycate. Int Arch Allergy Appl Immunol 89:98–102, 1989.
58. Ferguson A. Immunological response to food. Proc Nutrition Soc 40:73–80, 1985.
59. Goldberg BJ, Kaplan MS. Controversial concepts and techniques in the diagnosis and management of food allergies. Immunol Allergy Clin N Am 11:863–884, 1991.
60. Nicklin S, Miller K. Local and systemic immune responses to intestinally presented antigen. Int Archs Allergy Appl Immun 72:87–90, 1983.
61. Iyngkaran N, Robinson MJ, Sumithran E, et al. Cow's milk protein sensitive enteropathy: An important factor prolonging diarrhea of acute infectious enteritis in early infancy. Arch Dis Child 53:1503–1512, 1978.
62. Richman LK, Chiller JM, Brown WR, et al. Enterically induced immunologic tolerance. I. Induction of suppressor T lymphocytes by intragastric administration of soluble proteins. J Immunol 121:2429–2434, 1978.
63. Miller SD, Hanson DG. Inhibition of specific immune responses by feeding protein antigen. IV. Evidence for tolerance and specific active suppression of cell-mediated immune response to ovalbumin. J Immunol 123:2344–2350, 1979.
64. Mowat AM, Strobel S, Drummond HE, et al. Immunological responses to

fed protein antigens in mice. I. Reversal of oral tolerance to ovalbumin by cyclophosphamide. Immunology 45:105–113, 1982.

65. Dobbins WO. Gut immunophysiology: A gastroenterologist's view with emphasis on pathophysiology. Am J Physiol 242:G1–G8, 1982.

66. Crowe SA, Perdue MH. Gastrointestinal food hypersensitivity. Basic mechanisms of pathophysiology. Gastroenterology 103:1075–1095, 1992.

67. Sissons JW. Effects of soy-bean products on digestive processes in the gastrointestinal tract of preruminant calves. Proc Nutr Soc 41:53–61, 1982.

68. Patrick MK, Dunn IJ, Buret A, et al. Mast cell protease release and mucosal ultrastructure during intestinal anaphylaxis in the rat. Gastroenterology 94:1–9, 1988.

69. Catto-Smith AG, Patrick MK, Hardin JA, et al. Intestinal anaphylaxis in the rat: Mediators responsible for the ion transport abnormalities. Agents Actions 28:185–191, 1989.

70. Curtis GH, Patrick MK, Catto-Smith AG, et al. Intestinal anaphylaxis in the rat. Effect of chronic antigen exposure. Gastroenterology 98:1558–1566, 1990.

71. Scott RB, Gall DG, Mario M. Mediation of food protein-induced jejunal smooth muscle contraction in sensitized rats. Am J Physiol 259:G6–G14, 1990.

72. Scott RB, Maric M. Mediation of anaphylaxis-induced jejunal circular smooth muscle contraction in rats. Dig Dis Sci 38:396–402, 1993.

73. Hatz RA, Bloch KJ, Harmatz PR, et al. Divalent hapten-induced intestinal anaphylaxis in the mouse enhances macromolecular uptake from the stomach. Gastroenterology 98:894–900, 1990.

74. Metcalfe DD. Diseases of food hypersensitivity. N Engl J Med 321:255–257, 1989.

75. Min K, Metcalfe DD. Eosinophilic gastroenteritis. Immunol Allergy Clin N Am 11:815–829, 1991.

76. Andre C, Andre F, Colin L, et al. Measurement of intestinal permeability to mannitol and lactulose as a means of diagnosing food allergy and evaluating therapeutic effectiveness of disodium cromoglycate. Ann Allergy 59:127–130, 1987.

77. Kleinman RE, Harmatz PR, Hatz RA, et al. Divalent hapten-induced intestinal anaphylaxis in the mouse: Uptake and characterization of bystander proteins. Immunology 68:464–468, 1989.

78. Turner MW, Barnett GE, Strobel S. Mucosal mast cell activation patterns in the rat following repeated feeding of antigen. Clin Exper Allergy 20:421–427, 1990.

79. Suomalainen H, Isolauri E, Kaila M, et al. Cow's milk provocation induces an immune response to unrelated dietary antigens. Gut 33:1179–1183, 1992.

80. Matthews TS, Soothill JF. Complement activation after milk feeding in children with cow's milk allergy. Lancet 2:893–895, 1970.

81. Shiner M, Ballard J, Smith ME. The small intestinal mucosa in cow's milk allergy. Lancet 1:136–140, 1975.

82. Bock SA, Remigio LK, Gordon B. Immunochemical localization of proteins in the intestinal mucosa of children with diarrhea. J Allergy Clin Immunol 72:262–268, 1983.

83. Heyman MB. Food sensitivity and eosinophilic gastroenteropathies. In: Sleisinger MH, Fordtran JS (eds) Gastrointestinal Disease, 4th ed. WB Saunders, Philadelphia, 1113–1134, 1989.

84. Mowat AM, Ferguson A. Hypersensitivity in the small intestinal mucosa V. Induction of cell-mediated immunity to dietary antigen. Clin Exp Immunol 43;574–582, 1981.

85. Atkins FM, Metcalfe DD. The diagnosis and treatment of food allergy. Ann Rev Nutr 4:233–255, 1984.

86. Saalman R, Carlsson B, Fallstrom SP, et al. Antibody-dependent cell-mediated cytotoxicity to beta-lactoglobulin-coated cells with sera from children with intolerance of cow's milk protein. Clin Exp Immunol 85:446–452, 1991.

87. Guilford WG. Development of a model of food allergy in the dog. J Vet Int Med 6:128, 1992.

88. Panush RS, Bahna SL. Connective tissue reactions to foods. In: Metcalfe DD, Sampson HA, Simon RA (eds) Food Allergy, Adverse Reactions to Foods and Food Additives. Blackwell Scientific, Oxford, 382–391, 1991.

89. Lessof MH. Clinical reactions to food. Br J Hosp Med, 138–142, February 1988.

90. Ownby DR. In vitro assays for the evaluation of immunologic reactions to foods. Immunol Allergy Clin N Am 11:851–862, 1991.

91. Bock SA. The natural history of food sensitivity. J Allergy Clin Immunol 69:173–177, 1982.

92. Bjorksten B. In vitro diagnostic methods in the evaluation of food hypersensitivity. In: Metcalfe DD, Sampson HA, Simon RA (eds) Food Allergy, Adverse Reactions to Foods and Food Additives. Blackwell Scientific, Oxford, 67–80, 1991.

93. Davis SD, Bierman CW, et al. Clinical nonspecificity of milk coproantibodies in diarrhea stools. N J Med 282:612–613, 1970.

94. Belut D, Moneret-Vautrin DA, Nicolas JP, et al. IgE levels in intestinal juice. Dig Dis Sci 25:323–332, 1980.

95. Reimann HJ, Ring J, Ultsch B, et al. Intragastral provocation under endoscopic control (IPEC) in food allergy: Mast cell and histamine changes in gastric mucosa. Clin Allergy 15:195–202, 1985.

96. Guilford WG, Olsen J, Riel D, et al. Gastroscopic food sensitivity testing in the dog. J Vet Int Med 5:132, 1991.

97. Catto-Smith AG, Patrick MK, Scott RB, et al. Gastric response to mucosal IgE-mediated reactions. Am J Physiol 257:G704–G798, 1989.

98. Walton GS, Parish WE, Coombs RRA. Spontaneous allergic dermatitis and enteritis in a cat. Vet Rec 83:35–41, 1968.

99. Perkkio M, Savilahti E, Kuitunen P. Morphometric and immunohistochemical study of jejunal biopsies from children with intestinal soy allergy. Eur J Pediatr 137:63–69, 1981.

100. Stern M, Dietrich R, Muller J. Small intestinal mucosa in coeliac disease and cow's milk protein intolerance: Morphometric and immunofluorescent studies. Eur J Pediatr 139:101–105, 1982.

101. Rosekrans PCM, Meijer CJ, Van Der Wal AM, et al. Allergic proctitis, a clinical and immunopathological entity. Gut 21:1017–1023, 1980.

102. Van Spreeuwel JP, Lindeman J, et al. Increased numbers of IgE containing cells in gastric and duodenal biopsies. An expression of food allergy secondary to chronic inflammation? J Clin Pathol 37:601–606, 1984.

103. Iyngkaran N, Yadav M, Boey CG. Rectal mucosa in cow's milk allergy. Arch Dis Child 64:1256–1260, 1989.

104. Sampson HA, Jolie PA. Increased plasma histamine concentrations after food challenges in children with atopic dermatitis. N Engl J Med 311:372–375, 1984.

105. Ohtsuka T. Changes in plasma histamine concentration following food challenges in children with food allergy. Jap J Allergology 41:394–401, 1992.

106. Lake AM, Kagey-Sobotka A, Jakubowicz T, et al. Model for the study of immediate hypersensitivity mechanisms in the intestine. J Immunol 133:1529–1534, 1984.

107. May CD, Alberto R. In vitro responses of leukocytes to food proteins in allergic and normal children: Lymphocyte stimulation and histamine release. Clin Allergy 2:335–344, 1972.

108. Kondo N, Agata H, Fukutomi O, et al. Lymphocyte responses to food antigens in patients with atopic dermatitis who are sensitive to foods. J Allergy Clin Immunol 86:253–259, 1990.

109. Minor JD, Tolber Sg, Frick OL. Leukocyte inhibition factor in delayed-onset food allergy. J Allergy Clin Immunol 66:314–321, 1980.

110. Valverde E, Vich JM, et al. In vitro stimulation of lymphocytes in patients with chronic urticaria induced by additives and food. Clin Allergy 10:691–698, 1980.

111. Van Sickle GJ, Powell GK, McDonald PJ, et al. Milk- and soy protein-induced enterocolitis: Evidence for lymphocyte sensitization to specific food proteins. Gastroenterology 88:19151921, 1985.

112. Baudon JJ, Mougenot JF, Didry JR. Lymphoblastic stimulation test with food proteins in digestive intolerance to cow's milk and infant diarrheas. J Pediatr Gastroenterol Nutr 6:244–251, 1987.

113. Lichtenstein LM, Ishizaka K, et al. IgE antibody measurements in ragweed hayfever: Relationship to clinical severity and the results of immunotherapy. J Clin Invest 52:472–482, 1973.

114. Rider JA, Moeller HC. Food hypersensitivity in ulcerative colitis. Further experience with an intramucosal test. Am J Gastroenterol 37:497–507, 1962.

115. Cheung G, Plechner AJ. Diagnosis of canine and feline food sensitivities. A new method. New Methods, 20–25, October 1982.

116. Roudebush P, Cowell CS. Results of a hypoallergenic diet survey of veterinarians in North America with a nutritional evaluation of homemade diet prescriptions. Vet Dermatol 3:23–28, 1992.

117. Barrett KE. Mast cells, basophils and immunoglobulin E. In: Metcalfe DD, Sampson HA, Simon RA (eds) Food Allergy, Adverse Reactions to Foods and Food Additives. Blackwell Scientific, Oxford, 13–35, 1991.

118. Metcalfe DD, Sampson HA, Simon RA (eds). Food Allergy, Adverse Reactions to Foods and Food Additives. Blackwell Scientific, Oxford, 1991.

119. Gross PA, Lance K, Whitlock RJ, et al. Additive allergy: Allergic gastroenteritis due to yellow dye #6. Ann Intern Med 111:87–88, 1989.

120. Wilson N, Scott A. A double-blind assessment of additive intolerance in children using a 12 day challenge period at home. Clin Exp Allergy 19:267–272, 1989.

121. Collins-Williams C. Intolerance to additives. Ann Allergy 51:315–316, 1983.

122. Dipalma JR. Tartrazine sensitivity. AFP 42:1347–1350, 1990.

123. Furukawa CT. Nonimmunologic food reactions that can be confused with allergy. Immunol Allergy Clin N Am 11:815–829, 1991.

124. Hill FWG, Kelly DF. Naturally occurring intestinal malabsorption in the dog. Am J Dig Dis 19:649–665, 1974.

125. Hunter JO. Food allergy—or enterometabolic disorder? Lancet 338:495–496, 1991.

126. Anderson JA. Non-immunologically-mediated food sensitivity. Nutr Rev 42:109–116, 1984.

127. Trier JS. Celiac sprue. In: Sleisinger MH, Fordtran JS (eds) Gastrointestinal Disease, 4th ed. WB Saunders, Philadelphia, 1134–1152, 1989.

128. Batt RM, Carter MW, McLean L. Morphological and biochemical studies

of a naturally occurring enteropathy in the Irish setter dog: A comparison with coeliac disease in man. Res Vet Sci 37:339–346, 1984.

129. Batt RM, Carter MW, McLean L. Wheat-sensitive enteropathy in Irish setter dogs: Possible age-related brush border abnormalities. Res Vet Sci 39:80–83, 1985.

130. Hall EJ, Batt RM, Development of wheat-sensitive enteropathy in Irish setters: Morphologic changes. Am J Vet Res 51:978–982 1990.

131. Hall EJ, Batt RM. Development of wheat-sensitive enteropathy in Irish setters: Biochemical changes. Am J Vet Res 51:983–989, 1990.

132. Marsh MN. Gluten, major histocompatibility complex, and the small intestine. Gastroenterology 102:330–354, 1992.

133. Kasadra DD, Bernardin JE, Nimmo CC. Wheat proteins. In: Pomeranz Y (ed). Advances in Cereal Science and Technology, Vol. 1. American Association of Cereal Chemists, St. Paul, 158–236, 1976.

134. Kagnoff M, Austin RK, Hubert JJ, et al. Possible role for a human adenovirus in the pathogenesis of celiac disease. J Exp Med 160:1544–1549,1984.

135. Mantzaris GJ, Karagiannis JA, et al. Cellular hypersensitivity to a synthetic dodecapeptide derived from human adenovirus 12 which resembles a sequence of A-gliadin in patients with celiac disease. Gut 31:668–673, 1990.

136. Van Elburg RM, Uil JJ, Mulder CJJ, et al. Intestinal permeability in patients with coeliac disease and relatives of patients with coeliac disease. Gut 34:354–357, 1993.

137. Cummins AG, Penttila IA, LaBrooy JT, et al. Recovery of the small intestine in coeliac disease on a gluten-free diet: Changes in intestinal permeability, small bowel morphology and T-cell activity. J Gastroenterol Hepatol 6:53–57, 1991.

138. Peters TJ, Bjarnason I. Coeliac syndrome: Biochemical mechanisms and the missing peptidase hypothesis revisited. Gut 25:913–918,1984.

139. Davidson AGF, Bridges MA. Coeliac disease: A critical review of aetiology and pathogenesis. Clinica Chimica Acta 163:1–40, 1987.

140. Mercer J, Eagles MF, Talbot TC. Brush border enzymes in celiac disease: A histo-chemical evaluation. J Clin Pathol 43:307–312, 1990.

141. Loft DE, Marsh MN, Sandle GI, et al. Studies of intestinal lymphoid tissue. XII. Epithelial lymphocyte and mucosal responses to rectal gluten challenge in celiac sprue. Gastroenterology 907:29–1989.

142. Hall EJ, Carter SD, Barnes A, et al. Immune responses to dietary antigens in gluten sensitive enteropathy of Irish setters. Res Vet Sci 53:293–299, 1992.

143. Lancaster-Smith M, Packer C, Kumar PJ, et al. Cellular infiltrate of the jejunum after re-introduction of dietary gluten in children with treated coeliac disease. J Clin Path 29:587–591, 1976.

144. Bjorneklett A, Fausa O, Refsum SB, et al. Jejunal villous atrophy and granulomatous inflammation responding to a gluten-free diet. Gut 18:814–815,1977.

145. Kumar PJ. Clinical pathology of celiac disease. Cur Opin Gastroenterol 7:232–235,1991.

146. Horvath K, Nagy, L, Horn G, et al. Intestinal mast cells and neutrophil chemotactic activity of serum following a single challenge with gluten in celiac children on a gluten-free diet. J Pediatr Gastroenterol Nutr 9:276–280, 1989.

147. Batt RM, Hall EJ, Chronic enteropathies in the dog. J Sm Anim Pract 30:3–12, 1989.

148. Kelly J, O'Farrelly C, Rees JPR, et al. Humoral response to alpha gliadin as serological test for coeliac disease. Arch Dis Child 62:469–473,1987.

149. Chua YY, Bremner K, Lakdawalla N, et al. In vivo correlates of food allergy. J Allergy Clin Immunol 58:299–307, 1976.

150. Loft DE, Marsh MN, Crowe PT. Rectal gluten challenge and a diagnosis of coeliac disease. Lancet 335:1293–1295, 1990.

151. Katz AJ, Falchuck ZM, Strober W, et al. Gluten-sensitive enteropathy. Inhibition by cortisol of the effect of gluten protein in vitro. Engl J Med 295:131–135, 1976.

152. Logan RFA, Rifkind EA, Busuttil A, et al. Prevalence and "incidence" of celiac disease in Edinburgh and the Lothian region of Scotland. Gastroenterology 90:334–342, 1986.

24 Idiopathic Inflammatory Bowel Diseases

W. GRANT GUILFORD

Introduction

The idiopathic inflammatory bowel diseases (IBD) are a group of disorders characterized by persistent clinical signs of gastrointestinal disease associated with histologic evidence of inflammation of undetermined cause in the lamina propia of the small or large intestine. The inflammatory bowel diseases are currently considered the most common causes of *chronic* vomiting and diarrhea in both cats and dogs. The diagnosis of these disorders carries stringent diagnostic obligations, not the least of which is establishing their idiopathic nature. By definition, this means ruling out known causes of gastrointestinal inflammation, of which there are many (Tables 24–1 to 24–4). If clinicians diagnose IBD without eliminating known causes of gastrointestinal inflammation, the diagnosis of IBD becomes a meaningless garbage can diagnosis into which the majority of gastrointestinal diseases can be tossed. IBD may strike the small intestine, the large intestine, or both. In cats the disease complex most commonly affects the small intestine, whereas with dogs it is common in both the large and small intestine.

Table 24–1

CAUSES OF EOSINOPHILIC INTESTINAL INFLAMMATION

Parasites
  Trichuris
  Visceral larval migrans
  Miscellaneous nematode parasites
Immune-Mediated Disorders
  Food allergy
  Type 1 hypersensitivities
  Complement-mediated diseases
  Delayed cell-mediated hypersensitivity
Mast Cell Neoplasia
Miscellaneous Causes of Mast Cell Degranulation
  Neurogenic?
Idiopathic
  Eosinophilic gastroenteritis
  Eosinophilic enteritis
  Eosinophilic enterocolitis
  Eosinophilic colitis
  Hypereosinophilic syndrome
  Granulomatous enteritis

CLASSIFICATION OF IDIOPATHIC INFLAMMATORY BOWEL DISEASES

The idiopathic inflammatory bowel diseases are usually classified according to the type of inflammation present and the area of the gastrointestinal tract in which the inflammation predominates. It is important to realize that this classification is an arbitrary system forced onto disease processes that have overlapping clinical-pathologic features. Thus, it is not surprising to find inflammatory bowel diseases that do not fit easily into the standard classifications. For the purposes of this discussion, canine and feline idiopathic inflammatory bowel diseases are classified into lymphocytic-plasmacytic enteritis, chronic (lymphocytic-plasmacytic) colitis, eosinophilic gastroenteritis, eosinophilic colitis, eosinophilic granulomas, the hypereosinophilic syndrome, histiocytic coli-

Table 24–2

CAUSES OF GRANULOMATOUS INTESTINAL INFLAMMATION

Food Starch
Foreign Bodies
Nonsteroidal Anti-inflammatory Drugs
Tissue Trauma
  Collagen breakdown
Chronic Infections
  Salmonella
  Campylobacter
  Cryptococcosis
  FIP
  Histoplasmosis
  Leishmania
  Mycobacteria
  Phycomycosis
  Prototheosis
  Toxoplasmosis
Parasitic Granulomas
Whipworms
Hookworms
Immune Mediated
  Miscellaneous delayed hypersensitivity reactions
  Miscellaneous complement-mediated disease
Idiopathic
  Histiocytic colitis of boxers
  Granulomatous enterocolitis

Table 24–3

CAUSES OF LYMPHOCYTIC/PLASMACYTIC INTESTINAL INFLAMMATION

Bacterial Infection
  Campylobacter
  Spiral-shaped organisms?
Bacterial Overgrowth (sometimes)
Parasitic Disorders
  Giardiasis (sometimes)
  Cryptosporidiosis
Wheat-Sensitive Enteropathy
Neoplasia
  Lymphosarcoma
  Adenocarcinomas
Immune-Mediated Disease
  Food sensitivity
  Miscellaneous chronic antigenic stimulation

tis, granulomatous colitis, transmural granulomatous entero-colitis, suppurative colitis, and the diarrheal syndromes of the basenji and Ludenhund.

Canine chronic colitis has similarities to ulcerative colitis of humans. Canine granulomatous enteritis resembles Crohn's disease of humans. Current evidence in humans suggests that ulcerative colitis and Crohn's disease are the two ends of a spectrum of idiopathic inflammatory bowel diseases.[1] These two diseases are commonly grouped together under the term *inflammatory bowel disease*. The justification for such a communal grouping is that in 5% to 10% of cases they share overlapping clinical-pathologic features, a patient with one disease not infrequently has a relative with the other disease, the diseases share certain immunologic abnormalities, and finally they are both idiopathic.[2] Although the etiopathogenesis of the idiopathic inflammatory bowel diseases of dogs and cats has been inadequately examined, there is no doubt the pathophysiology of these diseases has an immune-mediated component, they have overlapping clinical-pathologic features, some breeds are predisposed to more than one type of idiopathic inflammatory bowel disease (boxers, German shepherds), and the disorders are idiopathic. Therefore, for purposes of this discussion the diverse group of canine and feline idiopathic inflammatory bowel diseases are placed in one clinical-pathologic category and given the general term *inflammatory bowel disease* (IBD). The pathomechanisms that

Table 24–4

CAUSES OF SUPPURATIVE INTESTINAL INFLAMMATION

Bacterial Infection
  Yersinia
  Toxigenic *E. coli*
  Salmonella
Absorption of Bacterial Products
  FMLP
Ischemic Injury
  Shock
Trauma
  Bone particles
  Indigestible food debris
  Fur?
Neoplasia
  Necrotizing masses
Immune-Mediated Disease
  Miscellaneous complement mediated
  Miscellaneous immune complex mediated

result in these different morphologic expressions of inflammatory bowel disease are as yet poorly defined.

ETIOLOGY

Introduction

The cause or causes of IBD in animals and humans remain unknown, in spite of intensive research into the etiopathogenesis of human ulcerative colitis and Crohn's disease. Proposed causes include defective immunoregulation of the gut-associated lymphoid tissue; genetic,[2] ischemic,[3] biochemical,[4,5] and psychosomatic[6] disorders; infectious[7] and parasitic agents; permeability defects;[8] dietary allergies;[9–11] and adverse drug reactions.[9–10]

Whatever the cause of IBD, there is a general consensus that the pathogenesis of the syndrome involves hypersensitivity responses to antigens in the bowel lumen or mucosa. In the dog, such a conclusion is supported by several experimental studies which have demonstrated that sensitizing dogs to fecal or colonic antigens can produce chronic colitis.[12,13] Although there is agreement that hypersensitivity reactions are important in the pathogenesis of IBD, there is as yet no widespread agreement about the cause of the hypersensitivity responses. Whether the hypersensitivity results from a primary immune disorder or whether the numerous immunologic events associated with the disease are simply secondary to mucosal damage from an undefined primary cause remains to be settled. The nature of the inciting antigens and the reason for the unrestrained immune response against these putative antigens remains unresolved. In addition, which of the immunologic events associated with the disease are pathologic and which are epiphenomena has yet to be determined.

The Immunopathology of IBD

MUCOSAL IMMUNOPATHOLOGY. The immunopathology of IBD has been extensively investigated in humans.[1,14] Discrepancies exist in the data, partially as a result of variations in the methodology and stage and class of IBD studied. Most investigators are in agreement with the following observations (in humans). IBD lesions contain a twofold to fourfold increase in inflammatory cells, with B lymphocytes somewhat more prominent than T lymphocytes. The B lymphocytes are composed of an increased proportion of IgG-secreting lines. IgA secretion at the mucosal level may be depressed in spite of raised serum levels, and there is evidence that a higher percentage of monomeric IgA is secreted than in normal patients.[15] The T lymphocyte population, however, contains a more or less normal proportion of subpopulations as defined by various monoclonal antibodies. In addition to the increased numbers of lymphocytes, there are increased numbers of macrophages, neutrophils, mast cells, eosinophils, plasma cells, and intraepithelial lymphocytes, the proportion of which varies with the particular class of IBD. Opinion as to the relative numbers of NK cells in the tissues of IBD patients is divided. Their numbers probably change little, but their activity seems to decline.

The mucosal immunopathology of canine and feline IBD is currently under investigation in dogs and cats. A recent study in dogs with lymphocytic-plasmacytic enteritis has demonstrated an increase in the number of IgA-, IgG-, and IgM-containing plasma cells in the lamina propria of the small intestine and cecum.[16] As described for humans, the greatest increase was in the number of IgG-containing cells.

CIRCULATING IMMUNOLOGIC ELEMENTS IN IBD.[1,14,17]

Humans with IBD generally manifest normal or mildly increased immunoglobulin levels, particularly of the IgA class. In addition, they demonstrate elevated titers to various bacterial antigens, such as bacterial cell wall constituents of Enterobacteriaceae (the common antigen of Kunin) and food antigens such as bovine serum albumin. Antibodies to various colonic epithelial antigens and mucus glycoproteins are also increased in many patients.

In contrast to the increased serum antibody levels, the percentage and number of circulating B lymphocytes are decreased during active IBD, either as a consequence of sequestration at sites of inflammation or exudation into the bowel lumen. Circulating T lymphocytes are generally normal to decreased. The activity of B lymphocytes, especially those that secrete IgA, as judged by lymphocyte blastogenesis tests is often increased. The reactivity of T lymphocytes to mucosal antigens, such as subcellular fractions of colonic epithelial cells and the common antigen of Kunin, is also often increased, although peripheral blood T cell responsiveness to nonmucosal antigens is often slightly depressed. The increased immunoreactivity of mucosal lymphocytes to mucosal antigens may result from increased exposure of the immune system to these antigens as a result of increased permeability. Alternatively, it may be due to a fundamental mucosal immunoregulatory defect.

DEFECTIVE IMMUNOREGULATION IN IBD.

Unlike most other lymphoid tissues, GALT cannot rely on elimination of antigen to terminate an immune response. Instead, GALT has evolved a complex system to suppress the interminable immune response to familiar, nonreplicating, enteric antigens.[18] The details of this oral tolerance are discussed in Chapter 3. Essential components of tolerance are an effective permeability barrier to macromolecules; maintenance of the nonphlogistic, predominantly IgA antibody response of GALT; and effective T suppressor cell activity. Effective T suppressor cell function requires constant surveillance and active suppression by the suppressor limb of the gut-associated lymphoid tissue.

A breakdown in the suppressor function of GALT is currently thought to be an important cause of the hypersensitivity response characteristic of IBD[1,8,9,19] (Figure 24–1). It is hypothesized that a defect in this system results in the escape of a reactive clone of lymphocytes that goes on to incite an immune response against a gut antigen, whether that antigen be a bacterial product, a food antigen, or a self-antigen (autoimmunity). The ensuing immune response would induce gastrointestinal inflammation, which in turn would increase bowel permeability, flooding the lamina propria with additional antigen of a variety of types. Eventually, the suppressor function of GALT to a variety of antigens is thought to be overwhelmed, resulting in a vicious cycle of further inflammation, further permeability increase, and eventually overt tissue damage.[1]

In support of this hypothesis, defects in the activity of both circulating and mucosal T suppressor cells have been detected in humans with IBD. However, these defects have not been demonstrated in all patients or in all in vitro assay systems, and their importance remains to be established.[1,17,20] An important role for intestinal epithelial cells in the gut suppressor response has recently been discovered.[21] Intestinal epithelial cells act as antigen-presenting cells that selectively activate suppressor cells. Any derangement of the epithelium might therefore compromise the immunosuppressive activities of GALT. Defective immunoregulation by gut epithelium has

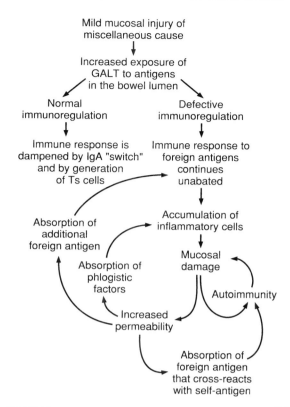

FIGURE 24–1. A defect in the suppressor function of the gut-associated lymphoid tissue has been proposed as the cause of inflammatory bowel disease.

recently been demonstrated in humans with IBD, and has been hypothesized to be the primary defect in the development of the disease.[21]

AUTOIMMUNITY IN IBD.

Autoimmune disease of the bowel could result from a number of mechanisms. As already discussed, a T suppressor cell failure may result in the escape of an autoreactive lymphocyte clone. Alternatively, an immune response against a foreign gut antigen that shares antigenic determinants with self-tissue could result in an inappropriate attack against self-tissue in addition to the inciting agent. The latter suggestion has received some prominence because of the demonstration that antibodies to the common enterobacterial antigen of Kunin will cross-react with antigenic determinants on colonic epithelial cells.[22] Similarly, cross-reactivity between *Klebsiella nitrogenase* and human leukocyte antigen B27 has been observed.[23] The gut is a huge reservoir of microbial antigens, and it is probable that other examples of molecular mimicry will be discovered. Furthermore, it is possible that absorption of "superantigens" (such a Staphylococcal enterotoxins) would predispose to autoimmunity.

To establish an autoimmune basis for the disease, researchers must first prove that IBD is associated with disease-specific and tissue-specific autoantibodies or self-reactive lymphocytes, that these antibodies or lymphocytes precede the intestinal damage, and finally that they are capable of causing tissue damage. It has been clearly demonstrated that autoantibodies and cytotoxic cells with specificity for intestinal epithelial cells are present in the sera of humans with IBD and that they can precede overt clinical disease.[1,17] What remains to be convincingly shown is that these autoreactive immune components have an important damaging role and are not simply epiphenomena.[23]

GALT = gut assoc. lymphoid tissue

As many as 60% to 70% of humans with ulcerative colitis have circulating antibodies to colonic tissue, whereas only 10% to 15% of normal people are antibody positive.[1] The importance of these antibodies has been questioned because the titer often bears no correlation to the severity of the disease and because the tissue specificity of the initial autoantibody preparations is poor. More recently, however, the existence of antibodies specific for gastrointestinal tract mucin-associated glycoproteins[24] and basolateral membranes of colon epithelial cells[25] has been confirmed. Furthermore, these antibodies were shown to be present in nondiseased relatives of patients with IBD.[26] Moreover, it has been established that some of these antibodies can prime mucosal leukocytes to cause cytotoxicity of colonic epithelial cells via antibody-dependent cellular cytotoxicity.[27] These observations go against the supposition that all the anti-intestinal antibodies are merely secondary to mucosal injury. In spite of these advances, it remains to be shown how important autoantibodies are to the tissue injury of IBD. Antibody-mediated, complement-dependent cytotoxicity of colon cells does not appear to be important in the pathogenesis of IBD.[28] It is probable that many of the antibodies produced are not pathogenic, but occur as a consequence of the tissue injury.

Autoreactive T cell clones are also present in the intestinal tissues of humans with IBD and are capable of cytotoxicity.[29] As with autoantibodies, however, it remains to be established how important this MHC-restricted T lymphocyte cytotoxicity is in comparison to nonspecific tissue destruction resulting from the multitude of cytotoxic mediators released in inflammatory processes.

The importance of autoimmunity in canine and feline IBD requires further investigation. An acute onset of a hemorrhagic diarrhea can be induced in dogs by the injection of antisera prepared against canine colonic mucosa.[30,31] The colonic tissues show edema, neutrophil infiltration, and multifocal hemorrhagic necrosis. A mild, persistent colitis has been induced in two dogs by the repeated injection of a homogenate of the dogs' own colonic mucosa, derived by colectomy.[12] Unfortunately, inadequate attempts to ensure sterility of the antigenic material were made in these studies. Nevertheless, they suggest that immune-mediated mechanisms and perhaps autoimmunity may be involved in the pathogenesis of canine enterocolitis.

Genetic Influences

There is a well-recognized familial tendency toward IBD in humans. Multiple occurrences of IBD in the same family are identified in 20% to 40% of IBD cases.[17] To date, however, a consistent genetic marker of disease predisposition has not been identified. A genetic influence is also well recognized in dogs. The boxer and the French bulldog are the only two dog breeds in which histiocytic colitis has been reported. Furthermore, the basenji and the Ludenhund have well-recognized protein-losing enteropathies with a familial component. It is probable that the genetic makeup of the patient establishes susceptibility to IBD, but the actual disease is precipitated by other factors.

Environmental Influences

Striking differences in the prevalence of IBD occur in human populations throughout the world. Westernization of populations leads to a higher incidence of the disease. The reasons for these environmental variations are unknown.[11]

Drug Therapy

The prostaglandin synthetase inhibitors, cinchophen and indomethacin, can induce colitis with a resemblance to early Crohn disease when used in dogs.[32] Lesions develop as early as one day after the initiation of therapy and are centered over the Peyer's patches. Similarly, a strong association occurs between the use of nonsteroidal anti-inflammatory drugs (NSAIDs), small intestinal inflammation, and IBD in humans.[33–35]

The reason for the proinflammatory effect of NSAIDs on the intestine is unknown, but proposed causes have included removal of the protective effect of prostaglandins,[34] interference with mucus secretion, increase in bowel permeability,[36] and interference with T suppressor activity resulting in an unrestrained interaction of lymphoid tissue and intestinal antigen.[32]

Chronic hypermotility of the bowel induced by the repeated administration of cholinergic agents can cause an ulcerative colitis in dogs.[37]

Dietary Influences

It is well established that the clinical signs of some dogs and cats with chronic colitis and, to a lesser extent, eosinophilic gastroenteritis will resolve if the patient is placed on a controlled diet.[38,39] Similarly, in humans, convincing data suggests that bowel rest by parenteral nutrition or use of elemental diets can reduce the symptoms of Crohn's disease.[11] These observations are useful from the therapeutic point of view, and suggest dietary factors influence the pathophysiology of IBD, but they do not establish a role for diet in the *etiology* of the disease.

The apparent response of some patients to dietary management may have a number of explanations (Table 24–5). The diet may contain additives that irritate the mucosa or antigens to which the patient is allergic. The diet directly influences intestinal morphology and physiologic functions such as the rapidity of cell renewal, mucus secretion, fluid and electrolyte absorption, and motility patterns.[40] The type and amount of fiber influences mucus synthesis and secretion, colonic morphology, and fluid and electrolyte absorption. Experimental dietary deficiencies of vitamin A, folic acid, and pantothenic acid can cause colitis. Deficiency of essential fatty acids delays bowel healing. The composition of the diet has a profound influence on the composition of the intestinal microbial flora.[41–43] Alteration of the bacterial flora in turn has wide-ranging effects on bowel morphologic, physiologic, and immunologic function. Furthermore, many patients with IBD are malnourished for a variety of reasons (Table 24–6), and their clinical improvement may simply result from improved nutritional status.

It is difficult to determine which of these influences of diet is the most important in the responsiveness of IBD to dietary manipulation. The wide variety of diets that have met with apparent success (high protein, low protein, high fiber, low fiber, hypoallergenic, easily digestible, enteral, and parenteral) suggests that the beneficial response may operate through more than one mechanism. Of the diverse influences of diet on gastrointestinal function, dietary additives and antigenic dietary proteins have received the most attention as possible causes of IBD.

FOOD ADDITIVES. Carrageenans are a group of sulfated polygalactones that are frequently used as gelling agents in canned pet foods. Lignosulfonate is often used as a binding

Table 24–5

POSSIBLE INFLUENCES OF DIET ON THE ETIOPATHOGENESIS OF IBD

Mucosal disease resulting from dietary deficiencies
Provision of toxic food additives
Provision of antigenic dietary proteins
Provision of protein substrate for ammonia generation
Alteration of cell renewal rate
Alteration of bowel morphology
Alteration of bowel motility
Alteration of absorption
Alteration of mucus secretion
Alteration of the number of bowel microflora
Alteration of the composition of bowel microflora
Reconstitution of depressed immunity resulting from malnutrition

agent in pelleted animal feeds. Exposure to carrageenan and several closely related sulfated polysaccharides, such as ligno-sulfonates, sulfated amylopectin, and dextran sulfate sodium, is a well-recognized method of producing experimental colitis in laboratory animals.[49,50] The precise mechanism of the colitis is unknown, but mucosal macrophages swollen with polysaccharides are common to these models, and there is evidence that carrageenan can influence cytokine secretion by lamina propria macrophages.[50,51] The bacterial flora also appears to play a role in the development of carrageenan-induced colitis because pretreatment with metronidazole[49] or trimethoprim-sulfamethoxazole[52] will protect guinea pigs against ulcerative colitis induced by the administration of carrageenan.

It is not known whether the incidence of colitis has changed since the feeding of prepared foods became popular. As yet, no binding agents, food colorings, or preservatives have been shown to be responsible for human, canine or feline IBD, although the vast array of these products precludes discounting this possibility.

DIETARY ANTIGENS. An influence of dietary antigens on the etiopathogenesis of IBD seems likely, but the relative importance of that influence is as yet undetermined. The absorption of intact antigenic macromolecules into the lamina propria of patients with IBD increases because of increased mucosal permeability. Human patients with IBD have an enhanced immunoresponsiveness to food antigens, but also to other antigens in the gut, particularly bacteria and bacterial products.[11] Antibodies against a variety of dietary antigens are found in the plasma of both normal humans and humans with IBD.[53] There is disagreement about the correlation between their titers, the severity of the disease process, and the responsiveness of the patient to an elimination diet.[54,53] It is most likely that these antibodies are a consequence of the disease rather than a cause. That is, dietary antigens aggravate but do not cause IBD.[55]

An investigation of one dog for the presence of fecal and serum antibodies against a variety of food and parasitic antigens was unrewarding.[56] Currently 10% of dogs with IBD diagnosed at Massey University have positive gastroscopic food sensitivity tests (GFST) to food antigens. Positive GFST results to foods used in the treatment of the disease are often detected during follow-up endoscopic studies. This strongly implies that food allergy is involved in the perpetuation of IBD, but it may not be the primary cause. That is, inflammation of the mucosa predisposes to the development of acquired food allergies. Therefore, a change in dietary antigens may temporarily reduce the immune-mediated mucosal

inflammatory response. The longevity of this amelioration is questionable, however, since the so-called hypoallergenic diets in common use in veterinary medicine contain intact proteins that are hypoallergenic primarily by virtue of their novelty to the host's immune system. The duration of their novelty to GALT is likely to be very limited if the antigen is fed to an animal with a highly porous mucosal barrier.

The results of elimination diets in humans have been inconsistent. Earlier reports of widespread hypersensitivity to cow milk proteins among patients with IBD have not been confirmed,[17] with the exception of patients with eosinophilic gastroenteritis, in which evidence of hypersensitivity to milk is common.[57] Dogs with eosinophilic gastrointestinal inflammation occasionally show a complete clinical response to controlled diets, but no information has been accumulated as to which specific nutrients, if any, the dogs are hypersensitive.

In summary, the apparent success of dietary therapy in the treatment of IBD most likely relates to direct effects of diet on bowel physiologic functions such as digestion and absorption, motility and secretion, and to indirect effects such as altered bowel microflora. The elimination of toxic food additives or allergenic proteins may also play an important role. The most likely disorder in which hypersensitivity to dietary antigens plays a causal role is eosinophilic IBD.

Pathogenic Microorganisms in IBD

A role for pathogenic microorganisms in IBD has been long suspected but, in spite of intensive efforts in humans over the last 50 years, no pathogenic microorganisms have been conclusively identified as a cause of IBD. Most investigators have been unable to incite intestinal inflammation following the administration to various species of materials obtained from human intestinal tissues affected by IBD. An exception to this statement is the work of Van Kruiningen and associates, who were able to isolate an as yet unclassified Mycobacterium from the tissues of humans with Crohn's disease, which when administered to goats incited a granulomatous enteritis similar in nature to human Crohn's disease.[7] Other investigators have also been able to culture Mycobacteria from tissues of patients with Crohn's disease.[44] The possibility that the Mycobacteria isolated are simply commensals of ulcerated mucosal membranes has been raised.[1] Another group has suggested that cell wall–defective variants of

Table 24–6

CAUSES OF MALNUTRITION IN INFLAMMATORY BOWEL DISEASE

Inadequate Intake
  Anorexia
Maldigestion
  "Functional" exocrine pancreatic insufficiency
Malabsorption
  Bacterial overgrowth
  Brush border enzyme derangements
  Villus atrophy
  Diffusion barriers
Excessive Losses
  Protein-losing enteropathy
  Gastrointestinal bleeding
  Increased cellular desquamation
Increased Requirements
  Inflammation
  Fever

pseudomonas-like bacteria can be consistently isolated from humans with Crohn's disease.[45] Viruses have inconsistently been isolated from the tissues of humans with IBD.[46]

Evidence of a role for pathogenic microorganisms in canine and feline IBD is similarly scanty. Coccoid bodies resembling Chlamydia particles have been observed in the macrophages of boxers with histiocytic colitis,[47] but no evidence could be found for an infectious cause in a comparable study.[48] Feline infectious peritonitis virus can cause a granulomatous colitis in cats, and FeLV and FIV viral infections have been associated with a chronic enteropathy that resembles IBD.

The inability to isolate a pathogen consistently, the lack of epidemiologic data supportive of contagion, and the responsiveness of the condition to immunosuppressive therapy strongly rule against an infectious cause in most cases of human and animal IBD.[1] The apparent response of IBD to antibacterial agents such as tylosin, metronidazole, and sulfasalazine has been taken by some to indicate a role for a pathogenic bacteria. This need not be the case, however, because both metronidazole and sulfasalazine have well-established immunoregulatory and anti-inflammatory effects, respectively. The possibility that tylosin and metronidazole exert their beneficial effects through alteration of the composition of normal flora must also be considered.

Normal Flora in IBD

Although it is unlikely that pathogenic microorganisms are an important cause of IBD, strong evidence suggests normal bacterial flora are involved in the pathogenesis of the disease. Bacterial flora influence numerous anatomic, physiologic, and immunologic parameters of the host. Bacterial flora stimulate peristalsis; induce a heavier, thicker intestinal wall; accelerate the transit time of epithelial cells moving from the crypts to the villous tips; accelerate the process of epithelial renewal; influence the activity of brush border enzymes; increase the number of intraepithelial lymphocytes, plasma cells, and Peyer's patches; and modify bile acids by deconjugation and dehydroxylation.[58] Which enteric bacterial species are of most importance in the pathogenesis of IBD has yet to be established. Studies of the bowel microflora in ulcerative colitis in humans are as yet indecisive.[17]

Small intestinal bacterial overgrowth can induce lymphocytic-plasmacytic infiltrates in the small intestine of dogs.[59] Experimental sensitization of laboratory animals to bacterial flora (such as *E. coli*) will exacerbate the severity and prolong the duration of transient mild bowel inflammation.[60,47] Similar results were seen following sensitization of dogs with a bacterial-rich fecal extract.[13] Chronic granulomatous inflammation can be induced in the bowel of rats by injecting cell wall fragments of group A Streptococcus.[61] Antibodies reacting with anaerobic but not aerobic fecal bacteria can be demonstrated in the mucosa of patients with ulcerative colitis.[17]

Additional evidence for a role for bacterial flora in IBD is provided by the observation that pretreatment with antibiotics will protect guinea pigs against ulcerative colitis induced by the administration of carrageenan (see earlier). Furthermore, immunization against urease-producing bacteria will reduce the severity of experimental ulcerative colitis resulting from uremia and irradiation.[30]

Recently, evidence has emerged that certain bowel bacteria secrete small phlogistic peptides, the most well characterized of which is N-formly-methionyl-leucyl-phenylalanine (FMLP). These peptides attract leukocytes, in particular neutrophils,

and cause them to degranulate. It appears that these peptides can cross intact bowel mucosa, raising the possibility that the secretory products of bacterial flora may be directly involved in the initiation of IBD. Infusion of N-formylated peptides into the colon of laboratory animals can induce experimental colitis.[62,63] Neutrophils from human patients with ulcerative colitis have increased responsiveness to FMLP. Furthermore, any factor that increases bowel permeability or increases the number of proportion of enteric bacteria that secrete these agents is likely to predispose to IBD.

Parasites

Parasitism frequently causes local inflammatory reactions in the intestine, and occasionally results in more generalized inflammation. For instance, *Trichuris vulpis* infection is sometimes associated with an extensive colonic inflammatory infiltrate, which may have lymphocytic, plasmacytic, granulomatous, and eosinophilic components. Similarly, giardiasis is occasionally associated with generalized small intestinal lymphocytic-plasmacytic inflammation, and hookworm infection can cause generalized infiltrates of lymphocytes, neutrophils, and eosinophils. Thus, trichuris, giardia, and hookworm infections are important differential diagnoses for IBD but little evidence suggests that occult parasitism is responsible for the generalized (idiopathic) lymphocytic-plasmacytic inflammation seen in many cases of IBD. In contrast, it has been suggested that eosinophilic gastroenteritis may be due to visceral larval migrans.[64] The association between ascarid infections and eosinophilic IBD is particularly common in young animals. In young German shepherds the association may indeed be a causal one. However, ascarids or their migrating larvae are rarely identified in older animals with eosinophilic gastroenteritis, suggesting the existence of causes other than occult parasitism.

Permeability Alteration

Inflammation of many causes is known to increase intestinal permeability in humans and animals.[65,66] The increase is thought to relate to epithelial denudation or, in less severe cases, to the development of a less differentiated epithelium as a result of increased cell turnover.[67] In addition, gamma interferon will increase epithelial tight junction permeability.[68] It is highly likely that increased mucosal permeability from transient viral infections may be the initiating cause of some cases of IBD. For example, small intestinal biopsy specimens from puppies developing chronic diarrhea following parvoviral enteritis have similar features to those from dogs with severe IBD. It is likely that the increased mucosal permeability floods the lamina propria with bacterial and food antigens, compromising the development of oral tolerance and causing inflammation that perpetuates the mucosal barrier dysfunction.

Not surprisingly, humans with inflammatory bowel disease have increased bowel permeability. However, it has been demonstrated (in some but not all studies) that relatives of people with IBD also have increased bowel permeability. This raises the likelihood that disordered permeability is the primary lesion in human IBD and that the intestinal inflammation is a result of chronic excessive antigenic exposure (Figure 24–2). As yet no cause of the increased permeability in the relatives has been defined, although altered IgA secretion may play a role in some people.[15] In a similar fashion, it is likely

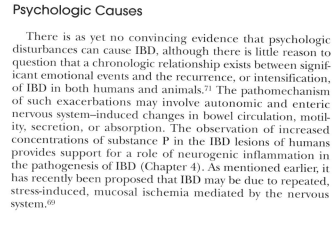

FIGURE 24–2. A defect in the mucosal permeability barrier has been proposed as the cause of inflammatory bowel disease.

that some cases of intractable IBD in dogs and cats are due to primary dysfunction of the mucosal permeability barrier.

Ischemia

It has been proposed that intermittent ischemia-reperfusion injury of the colonic mucosa due to intermittent excessive sympathetic activity could result in IBD in humans.[69] Vascular lesions have been identified in histiocytic ulcerative colitis in dogs but appear to be a result and not a cause of the ulceration.[70] Suppurative inflammation and necrosis are common histologic findings following ischemia but are uncommon in cats and dogs with IBD. Thus, ischemia would seem to be an unlikely cause of IBD in dogs or cats.

Biochemical Causes

Diminished incorporation of ^{14}C-labeled amino acids into colonic mucosal proteins of humans with colitis has been reported, suggesting a defective mucosal regenerative capacity.[17] Rectal biopsies of humans with ulcerative colitis have decreased concentrations of various enzymes, but these are thought to be a consequence rather than a cause of the disease. The metabolism of affected colonic epithelial cells allegedly differs from normal in that butyrate oxidation is impaired and glutamine and glucose oxidation is increased.[17] The significance of these observations is unknown. Alterations in colonic mucin profiles have been reported in human ulcerative colitis.[4,5] The significance of this observation is also unknown, but it is of interest to note that mucin is thought to be a potent scavenger of oxygen-free radicals; furthermore, it affords mucosal protection by way of its lubricant properties and a cooperative role with IgA.

Psychologic Causes

There is as yet no convincing evidence that psychologic disturbances can cause IBD, although there is little reason to question that a chronologic relationship exists between significant emotional events and the recurrence, or intensification, of IBD in both humans and animals.[71] The pathomechanism of such exacerbations may involve autonomic and enteric nervous system–induced changes in bowel circulation, motility, secretion, or absorption. The observation of increased concentrations of substance P in the IBD lesions of humans provides support for a role of neurogenic inflammation in the pathogenesis of IBD (Chapter 4). As mentioned earlier, it has recently been proposed that IBD may be due to repeated, stress-induced, mucosal ischemia mediated by the nervous system.[69]

PATHOPHYSIOLOGY

Hypersensitivity Responses in IBD

Hypersensitivity responses are exuberant inflammatory reactions of immunologic origin. It appears that much of the tissue damage of IBD results from hypersensitivity to enteric antigens. As already discussed, it is not clear whether the hypersensitivities result from a primary defect in immunoregulation or whether they are a result of overwhelmed suppressor activity pursuant to a defective mucosal permeability barrier. More than one type of hypersensitivity response is involved in IBD.

TYPE 1, IMMEDIATE-TYPE HYPERSENSITIVITY. Eosinophilic gastroenteritis and eosinophilic colitis are probably mediated (at least in part) by an immediate (type 1) hypersensitivity response. Type 1 hypersensitivities are inflammatory reactions mediated by IgE bound to mast cells. Antigens binding to the IgE induce mast cell degranulation. Mast cells release a number of inflammatory mediators, some of which attract eosinophils (Chapter 4). Eosinophils temper some aspects of the inflammatory response but also release toxic products such as major basic protein (see Chapter 4).[72] Type 1 hypersensitivity responses also result in acute damage to the enterocytes.[73] The mechanism for this damage is unknown, but the secretory products of mast cells or eosinophils (e.g., major basic protein) are probably involved.

The antigens that induce IgE have no discernable unique features separating them from the antigens that induce IgG responses.[74] Potent stimulators of this response include pollens, helminth antigens, and some bacteria. In animals and humans, there are recognizable genetic predispositions to type 1 hypersensitivities. Evidence that food antigens, such as milk proteins, can induce eosinophilic responses has been presented.[57] Dietary alteration will resolve some cases of canine eosinophilic gastroenteritis or colitis, suggesting, but by no means proving, that dietary antigens may be involved in the pathogenesis of the inflammation. If eosinophilic gastroenteritis is due to a dietary antigen that incites a type 1 hypersensitivity response, it is likely the inciting antigen would have to be a regular component of the diet to maintain chronic excitation of what is usually an acute and self-limiting hypersensitivity.

TYPE 2, CYTOTOXIC-TYPE HYPERSENSITIVITY. Type 2 hypersensitivity refers to antibody-mediated destruction of cells, either by the activation of complement or through the activities of cytotoxic cells that bind to the antibody-coated cell and induce lysis (antibody-dependent cellular cytotoxicity). This subject is discussed more fully under the section of autoimmunity in IBD. It is possible that antibody-mediated cytotoxicity is important in canine and feline lymphocytic-plasmacytic IBD.

TYPE 3, ANTIGEN-ANTIBODY COMPLEXES. Immune complexes deposited in tissues can fix complement and incite an inflammatory process. Experimental models of colitis induced by immune complexes have been reported.[75] The majority of human patients with IBD have circulating immune complexes,[1] and in some patients immune complexes can be detected in IBD lesions.[17] However, the pathologic role of immune complexes in human IBD is thought to be minor. There is no evidence that immune complex deposition is essential for the development of IBD lesions, and systemic consequences of circulating immune complexes such as vasculitis and glomerulonephritis are not common.[1] The prominent presence of antibody-secreting plasma cells in the IBD lesions of dogs and cats suggests that type 3 hypersensitivity may be more important in the inflammatory bowel diseases of dogs and cats than it is in humans.

TYPE 4, CELL-MEDIATED HYPERSENSITIVITY. Cell-mediated or delayed-type hypersensitivity depends on sensitized T lymphocytes. The primed T lymphocyte releases chemotactic substances that result in inflammation, phagocyte infiltration, and cell death. Expression of this reaction requires several days. Cell-mediated hypersensitivity plays a role in IBD in humans.[29] Because of methodologic problems in the in vitro study of these more delayed processes, there is little definitive information on the importance of T cell–mediated cytotoxicity. Some authors have hypothesized that it is a key mechanism of injury.[1] Certainly, T cell–mediated colitis can be readily induced in laboratory animals by the administration of the contactant dinitrochlorobenzene (DNCB).[76,77] Furthermore, the central role of the cellular immune system has been underscored by a report of the rapid and persistent remission of Crohn's disease in a patient with AIDS.[20]

In canine and feline IBD, T cell–dependent hypersensitivity is likely to be of prime importance in the few cases of granulomatous enteritis that have been reported. Lymphokines released by activated T cells may also play a role in the induction of the villous atrophy that accompanies many of the inflammatory gastrointestinal disorders.

Gastrointestinal Inflammation in IBD

Gastrointestinal inflammation is the final common pathway resulting in the tissue damage of IBD. The classification, mediators, consequences, and regulation of gastrointestinal inflammation are discussed in Chapter 4. As mentioned earlier, it is probable that immune-initiated inflammation (hypersensitivity) is an important cause of the persistent inflammation that characterizes IBD, but other factors such as absorbed bacterial peptides and neurotransmitters are also involved. If inflammation is persistent, fibrosis will result.

Leukotriene B_4 and HETEs are found in high concentrations in rectal mucosal samples taken from humans with ulcerative colitis. The severity of the inflammation positively correlates with the concentration of leukotriene B_4. Inhibitors of leukotriene synthesis have resulted in significant decreases in inflammation in various experimental colitis models. It is likely that these eicosanoids are important proinflammatory mediators in inflammatory bowel disease. Other mediators that may be of importance are interleukin-1, lymphokines, tumor necrosis factor, oxygen-derived free radicals, phagocyte proteases, substance P, platelet derivatives, growth factors, nitric oxide, and prostaglandins.[20,78–82]

Pathogenesis of Vomiting in IBD

Vomiting is a frequent sign of IBD in dogs and cats, whether the disease process is centered in the stomach, small bowel, or large bowel. The vomiting probably results from stimulation of the vomiting center by way of visceral afferent fibers, or the chemoreceptor center by absorbed toxins. Disrupted gastrointestinal motility and in particular delayed gastric emptying and/or ileus may exacerbate the vomiting in some animals.

Pathogenesis of Diarrhea in IBD

IBD frequently results in diarrhea in dogs and cats. The diarrhea has more that one pathogenesis. Inflammatory processes centered in the small bowel result in increased leakage of fluid and electrolytes and, if severe, protein and blood into the bowel lumen. The accumulated inflammatory cells result in a diffusion barrier and release mediators that result in brush border enzyme damage, villous atrophy, and motility changes (Chapter 4). These changes result in malabsorption of nutrients and osmotic diarrhea. Malabsorbed fat and bile acids lead to secretory diarrhea. Bacterial overgrowth resulting from intestinal hypomotility, malabsorption, or partial obstruction may contribute to the diarrhea. Concomitant maldigestion as a result of functional pancreatic insufficiency can also occur.

The diarrhea associated with colitis results primarily from disordered colonic motility, reduced water and electrolyte absorption, and/or increased water and electrolyte secretion.[83,84] The inflammation increases bowel permeability and interferes with the absorption of fluid and electrolytes.

Motility abnormalities have been readily demonstrated in experimental models of feline and canine colitis. In experimental feline colitis, a significant overall reduction in both basal- and urecholine-stimulated colonic motility was observed coincident with the worst colonic ulceration and diarrhea.[85] In experimental canine colitis, the total duration of contractile activity of the colon is also reduced, but the incidence of giant migrating contractions in the middle and distal colon increases significantly.[83] These giant contractions result in defecation or the expulsion of gas or mucus. Thus, the reservoir (urge) fecal incontinence and classical large-bowel-type diarrhea of colitis are probably due to the large number of giant migrating contractions induced by colonic inflammation.[83] It is possible that the inflammatory mediators released in colitis result in initiation of the defecation reflex at lower thresholds of chemical and physical stimulation.[83]

Colitis will occasionally result in watery diarrhea rather than the small pasty stools of classical large-bowel-type diarrhea. It is probable that this watery diarrhea is due to secretory diarrhea and/or a reduction in the reverse peristalsis that characterizes the motility of the ascending and transverse colon in cats and, to a lesser extent, dogs. Disturbed motility in this segment would result in more rapid transit of colonic content through the cranial colon, less absorption of water, and a watery diarrhea.

The pathogenesis of the motility disturbances in colitis are not clear but probably result either from a direct effect of the mediators, such as PGE_2 or leukotrienes, on smooth muscle function or from an indirect effect of these mediators on the enteric nervous system (Chapter 4).

The fresh blood that tinges the feces of dogs and cats with colitis results from vascular engorgement, ulceration, and the development of friable mucosa and granulation tissue.

Pathogenesis of Abdominal Pain in IBD

Occasionally, animals with inflammatory bowel disease will show evidence of abdominal pain. The cause of the abdominal pain is probably multifactorial. Gastrointestinal inflammation releases mediators that can directly stimulate visceral pain receptors. The same mediators also reduce the threshold at which muscular stretch is perceived as painful. Thus, bowel contractions of normal strength can induce a pain response. In addition, gastrointestinal inflammation is occasionally associated with painful muscular spasms. Furthermore, hypomotility or carbohydrate malabsorption can result in the accumulation or generation of intestinal gas, which causes abdominal pain by overdistension of the intestinal tract. Lastly, an association between gastroduodenal ulceration and abdominal pain has been observed in dogs.[86]

Pathogenesis of Extraintestinal Signs of IBD

A large variety of extraintestinal signs accompany IBD in humans and animals (Table 24–7).[87] Similarly, immunization with intestinal antigens produces striking inflammatory changes in the extraintestinal tissues of laboratory animals.[88] The pathogenesis of these changes remains uncertain. Antibodies to bile ductal cells, liver, kidney, and pancreatic extracts have been observed in the sera of human patients with IBD. The presence of immune complexes does not correlate with the presence of many of the extraintestinal manifestations of IBD,[1] although a correlation has been noted in sclerosing cholangitis. It is possible that the same immunoregulatory defect hypothesized as a cause for IBD result in hypersensitivities in other organs. The increased absorption of bowel toxins into the portal system may also be involved.

Summary of Etiology and Pathophysiology

In summary, the high prevalence of IBD, the diversity of the age, breed, and sex of animals affected, and the variations in

Table 24–7

EXTRAINTESTINAL MANIFESTATIONS OF IBD

Weight loss
Growth retardation
Polyarthritis
Ankylosing spondylitis
Nephrolithiasis (oxalate)
Coagulopathies (pulmonary embolism)
Hepatobiliary disease
Skin disease (Pyoderma gangrenosum, erythema nodosum, cutaneous vasculitis)
Autoimmune hemolytic anemia
Hypercoagulability
Uveitis
Pericholangitis and sclerosing cholangitis
Fatty infiltration of the liver
Chronic active hepatitis
Amyloidosis
Chronic obstructive pulmonary disease

the site and pathologic appearance of the inflammation suggest there is more than one cause of IBD in dogs and cats (Figure 24–3). The most likely causes are an as yet undefined abnormality in the immune response of the suppressor arm of the GALT or a defect in the mucosal permeability barrier. In some breeds, these defects may have a genetic basis. Either of these abnormalities are capable of inducing a hypersensitivity response to gut antigens, the most important of which are probably normal bacterial flora, but which in some animals may be self-antigens or food antigens. The relative importance of the different hypersensitivity responses in the pathogenesis of IBD has not been determined in the cat or dog, but it is probable that type 1 hypersensitivity predominates in eosinophilic IBD, and that antibody-mediated hypersensitivities (type 2 and 3) predominate in lymphocytic-plasmacytic IBD. It is likely that inflammation resulting from the absorption of phlogistic factors, as well as neurogenic inflammation, can exacerbate the inflammation resulting from hypersensitivity responses. Neutrophilic infiltrates would be expected to characterize the absorption of phlogistic factors such as FMLP and so might be relatively more important in suppurative IBD. The inflammatory mediators of most importance in IBD appear to be lymphokines, leukotrienes, oxygen-derived free radicals, and leukocyte proteases. The primary clinical signs of IBD directly pertain to gastrointestinal inflammation and its effects on gastrointestinal permeability and motility, nutrient absorption, and the vomiting center. The pathogenesis of the extraintestinal clinical signs remains to be elucidated.

DIAGNOSIS OF INFLAMMATORY BOWEL DISEASE

To make a definitive diagnosis of IBD, the clinician must fulfill certain diagnostic obligations. First, the clinician or owner must observe primary or secondary clinical signs of gastrointestinal disease. Secondly, the clinical signs must be determined to be persistent. In general, the duration of such signs should be in terms of weeks rather than days to help differentiate IBD from the inflammatory changes of acute enteritis. Thirdly, the clinician must go on to demonstrate that the observed clinical signs are associated with chronic inflammation in the lamina propria of the small or large intestine. This is best achieved by endoscopic examination and biopsy of the small and/or large bowel, followed by careful pathologic assessment. Finally, the clinician and pathologist must establish that the gastrointestinal inflammation has no demonstrable cause. This latter step in the diagnostics is commonly overlooked by clinicians, yet it is essential for the diagnosis of IBD.

Clinical Findings

The primary clinical signs compatible with IBD include vomiting, diarrhea, anorexia or increased appetite, lethargy, weight loss, flatulence, borborygmus, abdominal pain, hematochezia, tenesmus, or mucoid stools. In general, the clinical signs in a particular patient reflect the area of the bowel affected rather than the type of infiltrate. That is, few, if any, clinical findings differentiate the various forms of colitis and enteritis from one another. Signalment provides some help, in that boxers and French bulldogs are the breeds most likely to be affected by histiocytic colitis, whereas basenjis and Ludenhunds have their own specific diarrheal syndromes.

Secondary (extraintestinal) signs of IBD seen in humans

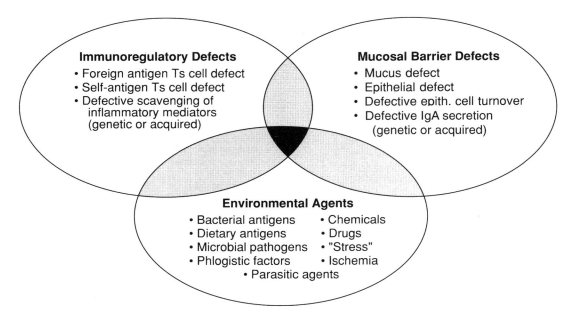

Immunoregulatory Defects
- Foreign antigen Ts cell defect
- Self-antigen Ts cell defect
- Defective scavenging of inflammatory mediators (genetic or acquired)

Mucosal Barrier Defects
- Mucus defect
- Epithelial defect
- Defective epith. cell turnover
- Defective IgA secretion (genetic or acquired)

Environmental Agents
- Bacterial antigens
- Dietary antigens
- Microbial pathogens
- Phlogistic factors
- Chemicals
- Drugs
- "Stress"
- Ischemia
- Parasitic agents

FIGURE 24–3. The interaction of immunoregulatory defects, increased mucosal permeability, and environmental pathogens in the genesis of inflammatory bowel disease.

are listed in Table 24–7. The most frequent clinically overt complication is joint disease (26% of patients), closely followed by skin disease (19%).[89] In humans, colitic arthritis is migratory, pauciarticular, and preferentially affects larger joints.[89] In those patients that are affected by joint disease, the severity of the joint disease tends to parallel the severity of the colitis. Common subclinical abnormalities reported in humans with IBD include pericholangitis, fatty liver, and a variety of other hepatic disorders.[90]

In dogs and cats with IBD, extraintestinal clinical signs are rarely noticed. In a retrospective review of the dogs with chronic colitis presented to the University of California VMTH, the most common concurrent problems were pruritic skin diseases and otitis externa, but these conditions did not have a greater prevalence in dogs with colitis than in the general hospital population. A nonerosive polyarthritis has been recognized in the occasional dog with colitis.[91] Polyarthritis has not been recognized as a complication of IBD in cats, although the sedentary nature of this species may have obscured this clinical sign. Fatty livers are not uncommon in canine and feline IBD,[92] and many animals have mild elevations of liver enzymes.[86,93,94] The cause of the liver abnormalities is unknown but might include anorexia (lipidosis), absorption of bacteria and bacterial products, or concomitant specific immune-mediated reactions against hepatobiliary tissue (see Chapter 37).

Diagnostic Tests and Differential Diagnosis

Inflammatory bowel disease is a diagnosis of exclusion. The known causes of intestinal inflammation resembling IBD are many (Table 24–1 to 24–4). As a result, the diagnostic testing required to eliminate all known causes of intestinal inflammation is quite laborious and will, by necessity, become more so as our knowledge of the causes of intestinal inflammatory disease increases. Important diagnostic procedures are listed in Table 24–8.

As in most diagnostic workups, the investigation should begin with a database consisting of a CBC, serum chemistry profile, urinalysis, and fecal flotation. Fecal flotations are necessary to rule out parasites such as trichuris. In areas in which giardiasis is prevalent, three serial $ZnSO_4$ flotations are recommended to rule out giardia. Alternatively, a treatment trial with albendazole can be instituted. Direct smears of warm feces diluted in saline can be useful for detecting a variety of protozoal diseases. Acid-fast staining of fecal smears assists recognition of cryptosporidia. Rectal scrapes are useful for the diagnosis of histoplasmosis. Furthermore, the presence of significant numbers of eosinophils, neutrophils, or clostridial spores in the scrapes are suggestive of eosinophilic colitis, enteropathogens, and *Clostridium perfringens*–associated diarrhea, respectively. Fecal cultures are valuable to rule out zoonotic enteropathogens but are only occasionally positive.

Table 24–8

PROCEDURES COMMONLY REQUIRED TO RULE OUT KNOWN CAUSES OF INTESTINAL INFLAMMATION

TEST	RULE OUT
Controlled diet	Food allergy, wheat-sensitive enteropathy
Fecal flotation	Trichuris, hookworms, Giardia
Fecal smear/rectal scrape	Giardia, Entamoeba, Cryptosporidia, Clostridia, Histoplasmosis
Fecal enterotoxin assay	*Clostridial perfringens*
Quantitative intestinal bacterial count	Bacterial overgrowth
Breath hydrogen	Bacterial overgrowth
Serum cobalamin/folate	Bacterial overgrowth
Fecal culture	Campylobacter, Salmonella?
Serum T4	Feline hyperthyroidism
FIP titer?	FIP
FeLV and FIV titer	FeLV or FIV
Endoscopy and intestinal biopsy	Neoplasia, cryptosporidia, fungi, algae
Celiotomy and intestinal biopsy	Neoplasia, cryptosporidia, fungi, algae

Measurement of fecal enterotoxin levels can help diagnose *Clostridial perfringens*–associated diarrhea.

Useful serum tests include measurement of trypsin-like immunoreactivity (TLI), thyroxine (T4), FIP, FeLV, and FIV titers. Assay of serum TLI is useful in dogs with small-bowel diarrhea, to rule out exocrine pancreatic insufficiency. Because the clinical signs of hyperthyroidism and IBD are similar, it is prudent to run a serum T4 in middle-aged or older cats. A relationship between feline hyperthyroidism and lymphocytic-plasmacytic infiltrates has been observed[95,96] but remains to be confirmed. FIP can produce a granulomatous colitis in cats. An FIP titer may help rule out this condition, but interpretation of the titer is difficult. Serum tests for FeLV and FIV are helpful because both of these viral infections can be associated with inflammatory conditions of the bowel.

Once systemic diseases and parasitism have been eliminated as causes of the clinical signs, a dietary trail with a controlled (hypoallergenic) diet to detect food sensitivity (food intolerance or food allergy) is indicated. Dietary trials are of particular importance in the differential diagnosis of IBD, but careful interpretation of the results is required. If there is no response to the controlled diet, food allergy and food intolerance can be tentatively ruled out, whereas IBD remains a possibility. Resolution of clinical signs on the controlled diet and recrudescence when the previous diet is again fed establishes that the patient is food sensitive, and obviates the need for further workup if the clinical signs can be controlled satisfactorily by dietary management. It is important to note, however, that patients with IBD often acquire food sensitivity secondary to the gastrointestinal inflammation. Unfortunately, the improvement resulting from a diet change in animals with IBD is often transient and incomplete. In contrast, long-lasting and complete clinical response to controlled diets is usually seen with primary food sensitivity. In other words, the clinical conunundrum of which came first—IBD-induced food sensitivity or food-sensitivity-induced gastrointestinal inflammation—can be partially resolved by dietary history. That is, IBD is more likely than primary food sensitivity if the patient has chronic relapsing gastrointestinal complaints in spite of strict adherence to previously successful controlled diets.

Tests for small intestinal bacterial overgrowth (SIBO) are a valuable part of the diagnostic workup of patients with suspected IBD because SIBO can result in lymphocytic-plasmacytic enteritis. Conversely, malabsorption from any form of IBD can cause bacterial overgrowth, complicating the disease. The ideal test for SIBO remains to be determined, but choices include quantitative duodenal culture, serum B_{12} and folate levels, and breath hydrogen analysis.

Survey and contrast radiography with barium suspensions are usually unremarkable but occasionally will detect obstructive processes such as intussusceptions. Transit studies with barium-impregnated polyethylene spheres (BIPS) are useful to detect concurrent gastric emptying disorders and rule out subtle partial obstructions of the bowel that can produce similar clinical signs to IBD.

Intestinal biopsy is required to rule out other known causes of intestinal inflammation such as lymphoma, mastocytosis, phycomycosis, prototheca infection, and cryptosporidiosis. A search should also be made for spiral-shaped organisms that have been associated with lymphocytic-plasmacytic infiltrates in the gastrointestinal tract of cats.[97] The significance of these spirochetes remains to be determined. Intestinal biopsy provides a more reliable assessment than clinical signs do of whether both small and large bowel are involved in the disease process.

BIOPSY INTERPRETATION. As befits a loose collection of diseases, the syndrome of IBD lacks pathognomonic histopathologic features. It is important to reiterate that IBD cannot be diagnosed on the basis of a biopsy sample alone because many chronic diseases can result in intestinal inflammation with the same histopathologic appearance as IBD. Furthermore, highly discriminant histopathologic criteria for the differentiation of IBD from acute inflammatory conditions, or even from normal intestine in the dog and cat, have not been published.[98] Evaluation of endoscopic intestinal biopsy specimens, in particular, is predominantly subjective and varies greatly from pathologist to pathologist.[98] In an attempt to reduce the subjective nature of these interpretations, histopathologic grading systems for endoscopic biopsy specimens from dogs and cats with IBD have been developed.[86,94,99,100,101] Unfortunately, because of the constraints of endoscopic biopsy, many of these grading systems still must rely on subjective assessments of the severity of cellular infiltration, rather than on more objective morphologic parameters such as villus and crypt architecture.[102] It is important to remember that the normal intestine has a complement of mucosal leukocytes which varies considerably in number between individual animals and between different bowel locations. For instance, the complement of mucosal leukocytes in the duodenum is usually greater than that of the jejunum.[103] The important message for the clinician is to use consistency in his or her diagnostic technique. Take tissue specimens from the same regions of the stomach and intestinal tract by use of a consistent biopsy technique. Do not allow the tissues to dry, and preserve them in a uniform manner. Where possible, send the biopsy specimens to the same pathologist so you become familiar with his or her interpretations. Lastly, demand a detailed report that mentions some or all of the parameters in Table 24–9 so you can assess the abnormalities on which the diagnosis was made.

Greater confidence should be placed in the diagnosis of IBD if the pathologist reports moderate or severe infiltration of immunocytes rather than mild infiltration. Similarly, it is reassuring if at least some architectural abnormalities (such as thinning of the epithelium, villus blunting, or crypt hyperplasia or irregularity; see Table 24–9) are observed. Beware of the diagnosis of mild inflammatory bowel disease based only on a subjective assessment of mildly increased lymphocytes or plasma cells. This tissue may be interpreted as normal by another pathologist. In addition, underlying causes for mild infiltration of lymphocytes and plasma cells are more commonly found than for moderate or severe infiltrations of these cells (i.e., mild infiltration is less specific for IBD). Furthermore, beware the diagnosis of IBD if the pathologist reports extensive submucosal infiltration of lymphocytes. Incipient lymphosarcoma is highly likely if large numbers of lymphocytes are observed infiltrating the submucosa as well as the lamina propria.[101]

DISCORDANCE OF CLINICAL SIGNS AND TEST RESULTS. Discordant results between clinical signs, endoscopic examination, and biopsy results are sometimes observed. For the clinician, it is disappointing to receive a normal biopsy report when the clinical signs or endoscopic findings are suggestive of significant intestinal disease. In my experience the most common discordance is that of essentially normal colon biopsies in spite of concomitant evidence of moderate to severe signs of large-bowel function, including tenesmus and hematochezia. It is less common for biopsies of the small intestine to be normal when there is concurrent evidence of moderately severe small-bowel disease, but these situations certainly do occur. The reasons for discordance have not been examined systematically. Variation in the severity of the lesions

Table 24–9

HISTOPATHOLOGIC ABNORMALITIES OF THE SMALL AND LARGE INTESTINE*,+

Small-Bowel Biopsy Specimens
  Atrophy or hyperplasia of the mucosa (normal dog duodenum ≈ 1800 μm)
  Villus atrophy or fusion (villus:crypt ratio dog duodenum ≈ 1.0)
  Excessive separation of crypt bases from muscularis mucosae
  Separation of crypts by edema, cellular infiltrates, or fibrosis
  Increased numbers of lymphocytes, plasma cells, or eosinophils
  Increased numbers of IgG-containing immunocytes
  Presence of neutrophils anywhere in the mucosa
  Presence of granulomas
  Focal loss of epithelium
  Flattening of epithelium to a cuboidal or squamous form
  Loss of brush border
  Epithelial hyperplasia (hyperchromatism, increased mitoses)
  Increased intraepithelial lymphocytes (> 15 per 100 enterocytes)
  Dilated lacteals
  Mucosal edema, fibrosis, or necrosis
  Vascular changes: congestion, vasculitis, hemorrhage, thrombosis
  Presence of microorganisms in or adherent to the mucosa

Colonic Biopsy Specimens
  Atrophy or hyperplasia of the mucosa (normal in dogs ≈ 400 μm)
  Irregularly distributed, tortuous crypts
  Separation of crypt bases from muscularis mucosae by > 20 μm
  Separation of crypts by edema, cellular infiltrates, or fibrosis
  Increased numbers of lymphocytes, plasma cells, or eosinophils
  Increased numbers of IgG-containing immunocytes
  Presence of eosinophils in superficial half of the lamina propria
  Presence of neutrophils anywhere in the mucosa
  Presence of granulomas
  Excessive basophilia in the basal third of crypts
  Mitotic figures in superficial third of crypts
  Cryptitis or abscesses
  Accumulation or depletion of mucus from goblet cells
  Focal loss of epithelium
  Flattening of epithelium to a cuboidal or squamous form
  Epithelial hyperplasia (hyperchromatism, increased mitoses)
  Increased intraepithelial lymphocytes (> 1–2 per 100 enterocytes)
  Mucosal edema, fibrosis, or necrosis
  Vascular changes: congestion, vasculitis, hemorrhage, thrombosis
  Presence of microorganisms in or adherent to the mucosa

*Not all of these criteria can be reliably assessed in endoscopic biopsy specimens.
+After Wilcox B. Endoscopic biopsy interpretation in canine or feline enterocolitis. Sem Vet Med Surg 7:162–171, 1992.

between areas is quite common in IBD,[101] and may explain some cases of discordance. Some other suggested causes of discordance are provided in Table 24–10.

POSTTREATMENT BIOPSIES. Some veterinarians recommend follow-up biopsies of the intestinal mucosa of all patients with moderate to severe IBD after several months of therapy.[95] The author has found follow-up biopsies to be helpful in those patients whose clinical signs are not responsive to therapy, because they provide an objective assessment of the response of the intestinal inflammation to the therapeutic regimen. Clinically nonresponsive patients whose follow-up intestinal biopsies show a reduction in inflammation are maintained on the same therapy, and the client is instructed to allow more time for the disease to resolve. Clinically nonresponsive patients whose biopsies show no improvement are changed to a different therapeutic protocol, usually involving another controlled diet and more aggressive immunosuppression.

The question of whether it is justified to rebiopsy patients in clinical remission cannot as yet be answered. There is no doubt that many patients with IBD have evidence of persistent intestinal inflammation in spite of clinical remission. Furthermore, it is not uncommon for patients with such subclinical gastrointestinal inflammation to have a rapid recurrence of their clinical signs after the conclusion of the medical therapy. Moreover, it is possible that in the long term this residual inflammation will lead to intestinal fibrosis and eventually a recurrence of untreatable clinical signs. Whether these theoretical concerns justify the expense of repeated intestinal biopsy can only be determined by carefully controlled prospective studies.

MANAGEMENT OF INFLAMMATORY BOWEL DISEASE

Introduction

The management of IBD varies widely and includes the use of controlled diets, immunosuppressive agents, antimicrobials, and motility modifiers. No controlled studies have been done to evaluate any of these therapies in cats or dogs. Evaluation of therapeutic response in IBD is difficult because of the often cyclical nature of the signs.

It is important to understand that the therapy of IBD must be tailored according to each patient's response. The rapidity with which the clinical signs resolve and the severity and nature of drug side effects vary tremendously among patients. The details of the treatment regimens for each of the different types of IBD are described in the sections pertaining to each disease. The following discussion consists of general comments on the management of IBD.

Client Education

Good client education is of paramount importance in achieving successful management of IBD. The client is informed that the problem is chronic, and in many cases control, rather than cure, is all that can be achieved. Regardless of

Table 24–10

REASONS FOR DISCORDANCE OF BIOPSY RESULTS WITH CLINICAL AND ENDOSCOPIC FINDINGS

Incorrect Localization of Disease Process by Clinician
  Failure to separate large- and small-bowel diarrheas
Incorrect Endoscopic Assessment of Gastrointestinal Mucosa
  Inexperience
  Inadequate insufflation misread as mucosal thickening, mucosal granularity, or obscured submucosal blood vessels
  Scope-induced trauma misread as spontaneous disease
Incorrect Biopsy Evaluation by Pathologist
  Inexperience
  The unknown significance of mild inflammation
  Sample handling error
Nonrepresentative Biopsies
  Poor biopsy technique
  Biopsied incorrect aspect of a lesion (e.g., necrotic center)
  Patchy mucosal lesions
Presence of Functional Rather Than Morphologic Disease
  Brush border defects
  Motility abnormalities (e.g., irritable bowel syndrome)
  Secretory diarrheas
  Permeability defects

the therapeutic program, relapses are to be expected in many animals. Time must be committed to discussing the importance of the controlled diet so the client does not alter the diet or give the patient unsanctioned treats. Moreover, it must be explained that there is no foolproof recipe for the therapy of IBD, and the treatment of each patient has to be individualized. Once warned of the constraints and difficulties of IBD treatment, and provided with appropriate expectations of the outcome, the client will be less likely to lose confidence in the veterinarian during the management of difficult cases.

Fluid and Electrolyte Therapy

An important component of the symptomatic therapy of IBD is providing adequate fluid and electrolyte replacement. In general, fluid and electrolyte derangements are not as frequent in chronic gastrointestinal diseases as in acute gastroenteritis.

Dietary Management of IBD

The dietary management of IBD has two basic tenets. First, the patient's nutritional requirements must be provided and, second, highly digestible nutrients must be fed. The IBD patient is often malnourished (Table 24–6), probably has increased energy and protein requirements, and at times must receive intensive nutritional support. The provision of adequate quantities of easily assimilated nutrients improves the nutritional status of the patient, provides bowel rest, and reduces the quantity of unabsorbed nutrients that can result in osmotic diarrhea, bacterial overgrowth, and antigenic stimulation of the mucosa. A third consideration of probable importance in the nutritional management of IBD is the use of hypoallergenic diets. Hypoallergenic diets may be beneficial because acquired allergies to food proteins are likely to perpetuate IBD. Dietary management is a very important component of the treatment of all IBD patients. In the author's experience, the types of IBD most responsive to dietary manipulation are chronic colitis, "mild" lymphocytic-plasmacytic enteritis, and, to a lesser extent, eosinophilic IBD.

PARENTERAL NUTRITION. Complete bowel rest can be achieved through parenteral nutrition. Results of the treatment of humans with IBD by parenteral nutrition have been mixed.[104–106] There is little doubt that such aggressive nutritional support improves the patient's nutritional status. The severity of the diarrhea is also reduced but the degree of mucosal inflammation is not necessarily modified. The greatest success of parenteral nutrition in assisting disease control occurs in patients with newly diagnosed Crohn's disease or in patients with the clinical signs of abdominal pain, anorexia, and weight loss.[107] Ulcerative colitis appears to be more refractory to nutritional therapy that Crohn's disease.[108] The disappointing response to parenteral nutrition in many patients should not come as a surprise, in view of the probable role of bacterial flora in the pathogenesis of the condition. Dietary changes by no means eliminate bowel flora, and so the bowel mucosa is still inundated with potentially highly antigenic products.

Experience with parenteral nutrition in the therapy of canine and feline IBD has been limited. The primary indication for this type of nutritional supplementation is the support of the anorexic and debilitated patient, particularly if that patient vomits persistently and has small-bowel disease which may limit absorption of nutrients. Maintaining nutri-

tional parity is particularly important in those animals destined for full-thickness bowel biopsy.

If carefully performed, parenteral nutrition is practical in dogs and cats for periods of up to a week. The benefits to the animal's attitude and strength are at times remarkable. The severity of the diarrhea also decreases dramatically. It is not known, however, if these short periods of complete bowel rest speed the resolution of the gastrointestinal inflammation.

ENTERAL DIETS. Enteral diets share a number of potentially beneficial features in the treatment of IBD. These include low antigenicity, high digestibility, and ease of administration in anorexic patients. Furthermore, many enteral diets are deficient in purines and pyrimidines. Nucleotide deficient diets are immunosuppressive (in an analogous way to azathioprine, discussed later).[53] Both elemental and polymeric enteral diets have proved useful in the induction of disease remission in Crohn disease but not ulcerative colitis of humans.[53,109–111] In spite of the lower antigenicity of elemental diets than polymeric diets (see Chapter 38), few studies have been able to demonstrate that elemental diets are more effective than polymeric diets in inducing remission of IBD.[53,110,111]

In addition to positive effects on disease activity in some forms of human IBD, enteral diets have been shown to improve consistently the nutritional status and well-being of humans with IBD.[107] Similarly, tube feeding with enteral diets is also a valuable method of meeting the nutritional requirements of anorexic dogs and cats with IBD. Furthermore, the vomiting frequency of some severely affected animals with IBD can be significantly reduced by changing to an enteral diet. The decreased vomiting might relate to the relative hypoallergenicity of the enteral diet or to the greater ease with which liquid diets leave the stomach in comparison to solid foods. Products available for enteral nutrition of dogs and cats are discussed in Chapter 38.

CONTROLLED DIETS. Controlled diets are the most common dietary manipulation used in veterinary medicine for the therapy of IBD. Controlled diets may be defined as diets in which the clinician has control over all or the majority of the dietary ingredients. The weak link in this scheme is the client, and in general the effectiveness of the dietary control is directly related to the effectiveness of the client education. The client must be informed that the controlled diet may be less palatable than the animal's standard diet, and persistence may be required to encourage acceptance of the diet. Furthermore, it should be explained that no unsanctioned treats can be fed. If the provision of treats is an important part of the owner-animal bond, rice cakes can be substituted for the more detrimental meat or cereal-containing treats.

The ideal controlled diet for IBD is based on highly digestible protein and carbohydrate sources, is gluten free, low in lactose and fat, hypoallergenic, isotonic, and contains generous overages of potassium and water soluble and fat soluble vitamins. Good palatability, nutritional balance, and convenience are also required. The diet should incorporate the fewest ingredients possible, so that the influence of each ingredient on the patient's bowel function can be assessed. Strict adherence to the controlled diet is essential and depends on the effectiveness of client education. Suitable homemade recipes are provided in Chapter 38.

Digestibility. Nutrients of high digestibility are more completely absorbed in the cranial small intestine, permitting the remainder of the bowel to rest. Highly digestible diets reduce the likelihood of gaseousness and osmotic diarrhea due to malabsorption. Highly digestible protein is less antigenic because little dietary protein is absorbed intact into the mucosa. Furthermore, less protein will enter the colon, preventing excessive colonic ammonia generation. Diets needing minimal digestion stimulate gastric, pancreatic, biliary, and intestinal secretion less than regular diets. The rate of bacterial growth is directly related to nutrient availability. Total intestinal bacterial counts decline with the feeding of highly digestible diets such as elemental diets. These diets are virtually completely absorbed in the proximal small intestine. Thus, the bacterial flora is "starved," and its total population is reduced. By reducing the total number of bacteria, the number of potential invaders, the amount of enterotoxin produced, and the total antigenic load in the intestinal tract is limited.

Protein Sources. Protein used in the treatment of IBD should be derived from one food source and, as described earlier, should be highly digestible to limit antigenicity. A protein source not commonly included in the animal's usual diet is advantageous because it reduces the likelihood of feeding a protein to which the animal is allergic. Furthermore, acquired allergy to an infrequently fed protein is less problematical than acquired allergy to a dietary staple.

Suitable protein sources for dogs include cottage cheese, tofu, eggs, chicken, venison, lamb (except Australasia), and rabbit, but any other highly digestible meat not commonly included in the animal's diet is also likely to be well tolerated. Cottage cheese is advantageous because it contains less lipid than eggs and meat, and less lactose than yogurt. Furthermore, it is noteworthy that cottage cheese is low in nucleotides in comparison to meat-based diets. As already mentioned, this is of potential importance in the treatment of IBD because purine deficient diets are immunosuppressive.[53] Cottage cheese is less palatable to cats than dogs, but chicken, turkey, fish, and liver (provided liver is not fed continuously) are readily accepted alternatives.

The amount of protein fed should comfortably meet the animal's protein requirements. Excess protein should be avoided to minimize dietary antigenicity and to limit the amount of protein in the ileal effluent. Malabsorbed protein results in the generation of ammonia, which can contribute to colonic injury.[112]

Sacrificial Protein Sources. As discussed above, oral tolerance is difficult to maintain in the inflammatory milieu, and so animals with IBD are at risk of becoming rapidly sensitive to undigested food proteins entering the lamina propria. That is, novel protein sources fed to an animal with an inflamed gut may result in only transient benefit because the intact protein will soon find its way into the mucosa where it can contribute to the inflammatory response. This theoretical concern has led to the concept of feeding a sacrificial protein source. The first novel protein fed to the patient in the early phase of therapy is referred to as a sacrificial protein because it is being offered when the bowel is inflamed and the mucosal barrier porous. Therefore, there is a distinct possibility that the patient may acquire an allergy to this protein, perpetuating the IBD. To avoid this potential problem, the dietary protein source is changed after approximately the first 6 weeks of therapy. In animals receiving concurrent prednisone therapy, this diet change is made just prior to the lowering of the prednisone dose from the immunosuppressive to the anti-inflammatory range, by which time it is hoped the mucosal inflammation is largely under control and the mucosal barrier has substantially recovered. As a result, the second dietary protein source is less likely to result in acquired food allergy and delayed recovery from IBD. The benefit of this recommendation is currently under investigation. This type of nutritional management is likely to be of most value in those animals in which IBD has resulted from a transient injury to the gut-associated lymphoid tissue or the

mucosal barrier (e.g., from a viral infection) rather than those in which IBD is due to an inherent (permanent) defect in these structures.

Carbohydrate Sources. Rice is the preferred carbohydrate source for IBD because it is more completely assimilated than other carbohydrates.[113] Furthermore, rice does not induce gluten enteropathy and there are few reported allergies to rice proteins in dogs or cats. Boiled white rice is suitable for dogs and baby rice cereals for cats. Other carbohydrates that can be used include corn, potatoes, or tapioca. These are all gluten free. Potato and tapioca starches are less digestible than rice starch, however. Corn starch is very well digested but, because corn is widely used in pet foods the prevalence of allergies to corn proteins is likely to be higher than that of rice. Pasta is another alternative but is not gluten free. As discussed in Chapter 38, the advisability of including carbohydrate in the diet of cats with diarrhea has been questioned because of concern about the palatability and digestibility of carbohydrate in cats. Certainly, for the first few weeks of treatment, there is no compelling reason to include carbohydrate in the diet of cats with diarrhea. However, in the author's experience, boiled chicken diced into rice baby cereal that has been reconstituted with chicken soup or chicken broth is reasonably palatable to cats and is well tolerated by cats with IBD (see Chapter 38).

Lactose and Gluten Content. Diets for the treatment of IBD are preferably gluten free in case the diarrhea is due to gluten enteropathy. Diets for use in IBD should also be low in lactose to avoid lactose intolerance.

Fat Content and Type of Fat. Restriction of fat is usually necessary because fat malassimilation commonly complicates IBD. Unabsorbed fatty acids and bile acids can promote colonic secretion and increase colonic permeability.[114] It has been suggested that cats with diarrhea tolerate high-fat diets better than high-carbohydrate diets. This suggestion needs further investigation before widespread application. Low-fat foods include vegetables, cereals, low-fat milk products, most fish, and lean meats such as boiled poultry (without skin).

Medium chain triglycerides can be used to increase the fat content and caloric density of the diet fed to IBD patients but unfortunately have negative effects on palatability (see Chapter 38). The fatty acids contained in fish oils have anti-inflammatory effects in the gastrointestinal tract (see Chapter 38). Addition of fish oil to the diets of humans with IBD has shown beneficial effects,[53,115,116] and is likely to prove useful in dogs and cats with IBD.

Vitamin and Mineral Content. For reasons discussed in Chapter 38, diets used for the treatment of diarrhea should be adequately supplemented with vitamins and minerals. This is particularly important in cats, a species in which thiamin and potassium depletion are not infrequently seen. Oral vitamin and mineral supplements should be avoided in the first few weeks of the controlled diet. They can be carefully reinstituted once remission is attained. In the interim period, parenteral supplementation of B vitamins should be considered in cats. In general, no home made controlled diet should be used for longer than 2 to 3 weeks without adequate vitamin and mineral supplementation. In animals with IBD it is advisable to use fractionated doses from a multivitamin and mineral capsule to avoid accidental inclusion in the diet of the potentially allergenic proteins contained in so-called palatable or chewable veterinary vitamin and mineral supplements. In addition to the multivitamin and mineral capsule, it is usually necessary to provide supplementary calcium, phosphorus, potassium, and essential fatty acids (see Chapter 38).

Fiber Content. Low-fiber diets have been recommended

for the treatment of IBD on the assumption that fiber results in adverse mechanical trauma to the mucosa and interferes with dietary digestibility. This practice is in need of reevaluation, however, because the gelling and binding properties of fiber are potentially of benefit in the treatment of small-bowel diarrhea, and fiber has a variety of well-documented beneficial influences on the large bowel (see Chapter 38).

Osmolality. High dietary osmolality in undesirable in IBD because of the likelihood of osmotic diarrhea. Furthermore, high osmolality is one stimulus for gastrointestinal inflammation and can also disrupt tight junction structure.

Palatability. Controlled diets for the treatment of IBD should be reasonably palatable to ensure adequate caloric intake. If a malnourished animal with IBD persistently refuses to eat controlled diets, but will eat more palatable commercial diets, the clinician must not be overly zealous in his or her insistence on the feeding of a controlled diet. Sufficient caloric intake (no matter what the diet) is more beneficial to the malnourished patient than the insufficient intake of a theoretically suitable diet.

COMMERCIAL SELECTED PROTEIN DIETS. The last few years has seen a proliferation of high-quality commercial selected protein diets. Most can be used with confidence as controlled diets. The hallmarks of these products include fixed formulation, single protein and carbohydrate sources, high digestibility, and minimal use of unnecessary additives. They have the advantage of convenience and guaranteed dietary balance. Either homemade or commercial selected protein diets can be used in the early phases of IBD treatment, but in my opinion commercial selected protein diets are advisable whenever long-term use in anticipated (e.g., in the maintenance of remission) because of their nutritional completeness. Useful products include (but are not limited to) those from Hills Pet Products, The Iams Company, Innovative Veterinary Diets, and Ralston Purina.

WEANING OFF THE CONTROLLED DIET. Homemade controlled diets can be impractical for long-term use because of expense, inconvenience, or lack of dietary balance. Many commercial controlled diets are more expensive than regular grocery store brands. Therefore, it is common practice to attempt to wean animals with IBD back to less expensive mixed-protein source commercial diets once the disease is in remission. If dietary expense is not of concern to the owner, my advice is not to attempt this change of diet for at least 6 months and preferably 1 year. If dietary expense is an issue, or if the clinical signs have been in remission for 6 months, a change of diet can be carefully tried. Where practical, the choice of the grocery store brand to recommend should be based on oral challenge testing. That is, modify the selected protein diet by introducing one new dietary ingredient every 1 to 2 weeks. The animals is closely observed for adverse effects due to the new ingredient. If there is any evidence of flatulence (an early sigh of malabsorption) or diarrhea the new ingredient is eliminated from the diet. With time, a number of dietary ingredients are identified that are well tolerated, and others may be recognized that provoke clinical signs. Eventually an inexpensive commercial food that is free of the poorly tolerated ingredients can usually be chosen.

Pharmacologic Therapy of IBD

In my opinion, medical therapy is indicated as an adjunctive therapy to controlled diets in all moderate to severe cases of IBD. Although clinical remission can be obtained in some cases of moderate or severe cases of IBD without medical therapy, it is my experience that remission will be more rapid,

complete, and prolonged if the patient is placed on a short course of anti-inflammatory drugs. The rationale for this recommendation is that the more rapidly intestinal inflammation can be controlled, the more rapidly the intestinal permeability barrier will be restored and the less exposure the patient will have to luminal antigens, including the antigens in the controlled diet. A large variety of medications have been used on an empirical basis for the treatment of IBD in cats and dogs.

ORAL CORTICOSTEROIDS. Clinical experience suggests that corticosteroids are the drugs of choice for the treatment of all inflammatory bowel diseases except chronic (lymphocytic-plasmacytic) colitis. Controlled studies in humans have show that corticosteroids are effective in treating an initial attack or an acute relapse of ulcerative colitis. With prolonged use, however, their effectiveness decreases and the incidence of side effects increases. Similarly, many dogs with acute exacerbations of chronic colitis will respond quickly and completely to corticosteroid therapy but, if at all possible, sulfasalazine and not corticosteroids should be used to maintain remission of colitis.

The effectiveness of corticosteroids primarily relates to the potent anti-inflammatory and immunosuppressive properties of these drugs.[20,79] Additional beneficial effects are appetite stimulation, increased small and large intestinal sodium and water absorption,[117] and enhanced uptake of glutamine by the small intestinal mucosa.[118] The effect of glucocorticoids on colonic water absorption, at least in the rat, appears to be mediated via specific colonic glucocorticoid receptors that increase sodium conductance through the apical enterocyte membrane. These effects have been seen with pharmacologic doses of methylprednisolone and dexamethasone.[117]

The side effects of corticosteroid therapy are legion. Prolonged usage is associated with predictable iatrogenic hyperadrenocorticism. The onset of this disease is delayed, but not necessarily prevented, by adopting an alternate-day treatment regimen. Systemic side effects of glucocorticoids that are commonly seen include polyuria, polydipsia, steroid hepatopathy, urinary tract infection, and hyperventilation. Behavioral abnormalities are occasionally noted. Rare side effects of great concern are acute pancreatitis, gastric ulceration, and colonic perforation. These adverse drug reactions are most commonly associated with high doses and are rarely apparent during alternate-day therapy. The advent of new oral corticosteroids with low systemic bioavailability, such as fluticasone propionate, is likely to reduce the frequency of these systemic side effects.[119,120]

The adverse effects of pharmacologic doses of corticosteroids on the gastrointestinal tract include the stimulation of increased gastric acid and pepsin secretion and gastrin cell mass, decreased gastric mucus secretion, and decreased gastric and duodenal epithelial mitotic rate leading to moderate (betamethasone) to mild (prednisolone) epithelial hypoplasia. The latter effect is offset by glucocorticoid-induced increased activity of certain brush border enzymes.[121]

In general, cats show fewer adverse clinical signs due to corticosteroids than dogs, but both species demonstrate marked hypothalamo-pituitary axis depression at the doses utilized for the therapy of IBD. Thus, a tapered withdrawal from the steroid medication is essential. The veterinarian must discuss the potential complications of corticosteroid therapy with the client.

The corticosteroid most frequently used for the therapy of canine and feline IBD is prednisone. Prednisone is suitable because of its availability in a wide range of tablet sizes, its lack of expense, and its short duration of action. Dexamethasone is less desirable because it has a longer duration of action than prednisone and therefore is not suitable for alternate-day therapy. The prednisone dosages employed in the treatment of canine and feline have been chosen empirically. The initial dose is chosen according to the severity and type of inflammation. Thereafter, it is modified according to clinical response. Consistent beneficial responses are obtained by the short-term use of immunosuppressive doses (1–2 mg/kg q 12 hours PO) in association with controlled diets. Higher doses (2–3 mg/kg q 12 hours PO) are required in the cat for the treatment of eosinophilic enteritis, which is considerably less responsive than eosinophilic IBD in dogs.[122] The details of suggested dosage regimens are provided in the discussion of the particular types of IBD.

The eventual aim of IBD therapy is to maintain remission by use of a controlled diet rather than chronic glucocorticoid use. Relapses may require repeated courses of prednisone. If prednisone must be used for maintenance therapy of refractory cases, then it is best combined with another drug or drugs such as sulfasalazine, metronidazole, or azathioprine to reduce the required prednisone dosage and to facilitate alternate-day prednisone therapy.

PARENTERAL CORTICOSTEROIDS. Parenteral corticosteroid therapy should be considered in nonresponsive patients with severe disease. There is evidence that high-dose parenteral therapy will provide a more rapid and predictable remission than oral therapy in humans and dogs with some immune-mediated diseases. Furthermore, in a patient that is vomiting and has diffuse intestinal disease the absorption of oral preparations is likely to be compromised.

Injections of depot preparations of glucocorticoids should be avoided because they produce rapid and profound depression of the hypothalamo-pituitary axis. The only indication for these preparations is in the treatment of intractable cats that cannot be medicated orally. Methylprednisolone acetate (Depo-Medrol; UpJohn) is the most commonly employed product. It is usually used at a dose of 20 mg SQ and repeated at 2 to 3 week intervals for three injections. Thereafter, injections are administered on an as needed basis to control the signs. Consistent control of IBD is more difficult to obtain with this drug than with oral corticosteroids.[122]

CORTICOSTEROID ENEMAS. Patients in the active phase of severe chronic colitis are sometimes treated locally with corticosteroid enemas. In humans these steroids are very effective because very little is absorbed and a high drug concentration is maintained. The value of corticosteroid enemas in the dog and cat remains to be established. Poor retention of the enema is likely to reduce the effectiveness of this therapy in animals.

SULFASALAZINE. Sulfasalazine (Azulfidine; Pharmacia Laboratories) is a combination of 5-aminosalicylic acid and sulfapyridine, joined through an azo bond.[123] Well-controlled studies have verified that sulfasalazine is an effective drug for the treatment of human ulcerative colitis of mild to moderate severity. No comparable controlled studies have been conducted in small animals, but the drug is in wide usage and has demonstrated convincing clinical benefit in the treatment of chronic colitis in dogs and cats. In one study of canine chronic colitis, in which sulfasalazine was used alone or in combination with other drugs, over 80% of the patients improved.[124] Results were poorer with other forms of therapy. Sulfasalazine remains the drug of choice for the pharmacological therapy of chronic colitis in the dog and perhaps the cat. It must be realized that the drug is not a panacea, however, and a significant number of animals do not respond to it, or initially respond but later relapse.

After administration of sulfasalazine, a small amount of the intact drug is absorbed in the small intestine (20%–30% in humans), but the majority of the sulfasalazine passes unabsorbed to the colon. The small amount of sulfasalazine absorbed in the small intestine is excreted unchanged in the urine and bile. About 75% of the sulfasalazine reaches the colon, where bacteria break the azo bond and release the component parts of the drug. In humans most of the cleaved sulfapyridine and about 30% of the 5-aminosalicylate is absorbed from the colon. The remainder of the 5-aminosalicylate remains in the colon and is eventually excreted in the feces. After absorption, sulfapyridine is largely metabolized in the liver via acetylation, hydroxylation, and glucuronide formation. The small amount of 5-aminosalicylic acid that is absorbed is metabolized by the liver and excreted in the urine. Because sulfasalazine needs bacterial metabolism to release its active moiety, the drug is effective only against large-bowel inflammation. One reason for treatment failure with sulfasalazine is failure by the clinician to recognize that the patient has concomitant small-bowel signs.

The majority, but by no means all, of the activity of sulfasalazine resides with the 5-aminosalicylate moiety, not sulfapyridine as previously assumed.[20,79] The 5-aminosalicylate has an anti-inflammatory action. It inhibits both cyclooxygenase and lipoxygenase activities, depressing prostaglandin and leukotriene synthesis. In addition, 5-aminosalicylate is thought to have an oxygen-free radical scavenging action, to interfere with phagocyte chemotaxis and function, and to inhibit cytokine and immunoglobulin production.[119,125] It is worthy of note that nonsteroidal anti-inflammatory drugs such as aspirin and indomethacin, which inhibit prostaglandin but not leukotriene formation, are ineffective in treating colonic inflammation and may actually worsen IBD.

The most common side effects of sulfasalazine in dogs are anorexia and vomiting. Depression, vomiting, and anemia have been observed in cats. Keratoconjunctivitis can occur as a result of sulfasalazine therapy.[126] The keratoconjunctivitis is reversible or partially reversible in only 30% of dogs.[126] The keratoconjunctivitis has been attributed to the sulfapyridine moiety, but this view has been challenged by the observation that beagles developed keratoconjunctivitis sicca (KCS) in toxicity trials of 5-aminosalicylate.[127] Dogs maintained on long-term sulfasalazine therapy should have periodic Schirmer's tear testing to identify KCS early. The relatively high incidence of side effects with sulfasalazine has led to the development of analogues of sulfasalazine that contain 5-aminosalicylate but not sulfapyridine (see later).

Sulfasalazine (Azulfidine) is supplied as 500 mg tablets or as a 50 mg/mL liquid formulation, which is particularly useful for the therapy of cats and small dogs. Various dose regimens have been successfully used. The regimen most commonly employed in dogs by the author is 12.5 mg/kg q 6 hours for 2 weeks, followed by 12.5 mg/kg q 12 hours for a further 4 weeks. Others have had success with 20 to 30 mg/kg q 8 hours administered for 3 to 6 weeks. The anti-inflammatory effects of sulfasalazine are dose dependent, and some dogs with intractable colitis have been reported to require doses as high as 50 mg/kg q 8 hours.[38] Similarly, in cats a variety of dosages have been reported. The author has found 10 to 20 mg/kg q 24 hours safe and effective, although others have used higher doses without apparent ill effect from salicylate toxicity.

5-AMINOSALICYLATE (MESALAZINE, MESALAMINE). Preparations of 5-aminosalicylate are now in use in human medicine for the treatment of ulcerative colitis.[128,129] In most studies, 5-aminosalicylate appears to preserve the effectiveness of sulfasalazine but reduce the incidence of side effects by dispensing with the sulfonamide moiety.[125] The drug is administered as a suppository, enema, or enteric-coated tablet to ensure the majority of the drug reaches the colon without absorption in the small intestine.[119,125] The mesalazine preparations currently available for humans have questionable value for dogs and cats because of potential compliance problems and differences in transit times between the species.

OLSALAZINE. Olsalazine is a drug composed of two molecules of 5-aminosalicylic acid linked by an azo bond, thus serving as their own carriers.[119,130] The drug is effective against human ulcerative colitis.[119] However, not all trials in humans have demonstrated that olsalazine is of equivalent effectiveness to sulfasalazine or that the incident of side effects is significantly reduced.[131] Furthermore, olsalazine can induce a secretory diarrhea in some people.[125] I have used olsalazine (25 mg/kg divided q 8 hours) with mixed success in a small number of dogs with colitis that were intolerant of sulfasalazine. That value of this product (and other azo-bond preparations such as Balsalazine) in the treatment of chronic colitis in the dog and cat remains to be established.

AZATHIOPRINE. Azathioprine (Imuran; Coopers Animal Health) is a synthetic purine that interferes with DNA and RNA formation, resulting is inhibition of antigen-induced lymphocyte transformation.[20] It has value in maintaining remission of IBD in humans.[119,125] The drug is very useful in cats and dogs as adjunctive therapy in severe or refractory IBD. Azathioprine can also be used if the dosage of prednisone requird to maintain remission is unacceptably high. The addition of azathioprine to the treatment regimen usually allows the prednisone dose to be at least halved and sometimes eliminated. The azathioprine dose most often used in dogs is 50 mg/m² or 1 to 1.5 mg/kg once daily for 2 weeks, followed by alternate-day therapy as required. A lower dose has been recommended in cats (0.3–0.5 mg/kg q 48 hours).[96,122] A lag effect of several weeks should be expected before the beneficial effects of azathioprine become apparent.

The most important side effect is bone marrow suppression. Mild suppression is common with this drug and of little concern. Severe depression is rare, is most often seen early in the treatment protocol, is more common in cats than in dogs, and is usually reversible on discontinuation of therapy. A complete blood count should be performed every 10 to 14 days for the first 2 to 3 months of therapy and should be repeated at monthly to bimonthly intervals thereafter. Treatment with azathioprine should stop if marked neutropenia or thrombocytopenia develop. Other side effects of azathioprine include anorexia and, rarely, pancreatitis and hepatic damage. The drug is supplied in 50 mg tablets. For use in cats, the tablets should be crushed and suspended in a carrier by a pharmacist.

CYCLOPHOSPHAMIDE AND CYCLOSPORIN. Cyclophosphamide (Cytoxan, Cycloblastin) is a potent immunosuppressive agent that is occasionally of value in the therapy of refractory IBD in dogs and cats. Cyclophosphamide is easier to administer to cats than azathioprine because it requires less frequent dosage and is supplied in a more suitable tablet size (25 mg). The dose is 50 mg/m² given four times per week. In most cats this equates to one-quarter to one-half of a 25 mg tablet at each administration. Side effects include bone marrow suppression and, particularly in dogs, hemorrhagic cystitis. Regular complete blood counts must be performed when using this agent. Cyclosporin is showing promise in humans for the therapy of refractory IBD.[20,119]

5-LIPOXYGENASE INHIBITORS. Inhibition of 5-lipoxygenase, with drugs such as zileuton, has shown promise in the treatment of human IBD.[125] The role of these drugs in IBD of dogs and cats is unknown.

METRONIDAZOLE. Metronidazole (Flagyl) has beneficial effects in the therapy of human,[20] canine, and feline IBD. Metronidazole has a number of different actions. It is an antiprotozoal agent, inhibits cell-mediated immunity,[132,133] has a broad spectrum of activity against anaerobic bacteria, and has positive effects on brush border enzyme levels and the uptake of nutrients like glucose and amino acids by the intestine.[134] It is unknown which of the immunosuppressive, antibacterial, or metabolic actions of this drug best explain its apparent efficacy in the treatment of IBD. The antibacterial action of metronidazole is likely to be more important in the small bowel than the large bowel, particularly if bacterial overgrowth is present. Experimental and clinical studies have shown that it is not possible to suppress the colonic microflora with antibiotics for more than a few days.[135] Metronidazole reduces the number of Bacteroides species in the feces of humans with IBD but has little influence on the fecal flora of healthy individuals.

Metronidazole can be used successfully as a single pharmaceutical agent in the treatment of mild IBD.[136] However, the drug is rarely effective as a single agent in the treatment of moderate to severe IBD. Metronidazole is most often used in combination therapeutic protocols to facilitate control of refractory cases or allow reduction in prednisone dosage. The dosage of metronidazole used in cats and dogs is usually 10 to 20 mg/kg q 8 to 12 hours. Metronidazole is supplied as 250 and 500 mg tablets or as a 5 mg/mL oral solution. Side effects are rare, but nausea, vomiting, and neurotoxicity (disorientation, ataxia, seizures) are occasionally seen in dogs and cats.[96,137] Salivation following administration is not uncommon in cats.[96] The drug is carcinogenic and mutagenic in laboratory animals, and so prolonged high-dose therapy and therapy during pregnancy should be avoided.

TYLOSIN. Tylosin has been reported to be effective in a variety of IBD-like disorders.[138] The mechanism of action is unknown. Anecdotal reports exist for a response to tylosin in some cases of IBD that have been unresponsive to more conventional therapy. Tylosin is supplied as a powder for use in pigs. The reported dose range used in small animals is broad: 11 to 200 mg/kg q 12 hour[138] and 20 to 40 mg/kg q 12 hours.[139] Side effects have yet to be reported.

MISCELLANEOUS ANTIBIOTICS. Parenteral antibiotic therapy is required in those animals showing clinical or laboratory signs of sepsis. Sepsis is not a frequent complication of IBD, but is occasionally observed in those animals with severe mucosal ulceration. Because of the wide variety of possible pathogens, the choice of antibiotic therapy is best based on blood cultures. If expedient therapy is required, trimethoprim-sulfa drugs may be utilized prior to the receipt of blood culture results. These antibiotics combine the advantages of reasonably broad spectrum activity, minimal disturbance of enteric microbial flora, and low toxicity. If life-threatening acute sepsis is suspected, combinations of parenteral aminoglycosides and ampicillin may be utilized.

Oral antibiotics such as tetracycline may be useful in cases in which the IBD is associated with bacterial overgrowth of the small intestine. There is no place for the use of unabsorbable oral antibiotics in the treatment of any form of bowel disease.

MOTILITY MODIFIERS. Short courses of opiates such as loperamide (Imodium 0.1 mg/kg q 8 hours PO) and diphenoxylate (Lomotil 0.1–0.2 mg/kg q 8 hours PO) are occasionally useful to reduce the severity of watery diarrhea associated with small intestinal and upper colonic IBD. These agents promote segmental contraction of bowel, thus slowing transit time of luminal content and prolonging the period available for water and electrolyte absorption. They should not be used in severe cases of hemorrhagic diarrhea because the retention of necrotizing material and pathogenic microbes may facilitate toxemia and sepsis.

Metoclopramide (Reglan, Maxalon) is an antiemetic and prokinetic. It hastens gastric emptying of solids and liquids and improves upper intestinal motility. It is useful in IBD patients with delayed gastric emptying. The drug has a short duration of action and is best administered by IV infusion, or given at least four times per day or just prior to meals. A suitable dose is 0.2 to 0.5 mg/kg PO. Cisapride (Jansen Pharm) is another prokinetic. It appears to be a more reliable agent for the acceleration of gastric emptying of solids in the dog.[140] The effective dose is 0.3 to 0.5 mg/kg q 8 hours PO administered prior to eating.

Anticholinergics have little value in the treatment of IBD. They may exacerbate the delayed gastric emptying seen in some animals with IBD. They are thought to have only minimal influence on colonic motility,[141] and so their benefit in treating the colonic motility abnormalities associated with colitis is in doubt. Anticholinergics are most often used for the treatment of intermittent acute abdominal pain demonstrated by some dogs with colitis, on the assumption the pain results from colonic spasm. Their effectiveness in the treatment of this problem has not been proven. If the pain results from accumulation of gas in the hypomotile colon rather than from colonic spasm, anticholinergics are likely to exacerbate the pain rather than relieve it.

IBD: PROGNOSIS AND TREATMENT FAILURES

The prognosis for most patients with IBD is good. Exceptions include those patients with severe mucosal damage and fibrosis, cats with the hypereosinophilic syndrome, and cats or dogs with granulomatous or histiocytic IBD. Treatment failures are usually due to (1) inadequate client education; (2) noncompliance of owners with management program; (3) reliance on drug therapy alone for managing the problem; (4) use of inappropriate nutritional therapy (especially choice of wrong protein source); (5) lack of aggression, persistence, and patience in the tailoring of therapy for individual patients; (6) failure to address the common complications of gastrointestinal inflammation such as delayed gastric emptying, disordered intestinal motility, or bacterial overgrowth; and (7) misdiagnosis. The most common misdiagnoses are lymphoma and partial obstructions of the bowel (such as intussusceptions or annular adenocarcinoma of the distal small intestine). Occasionally, immunosuppressive therapy is associated with the activation of previously quiescent diseases, such as toxoplasmosis,[142] giardiasis, cryptosporidiosis, or histoplasmosis, that may be responsible for apparent resistance to treatment for IBD.

LYMPHOCYTIC-PLASMACYTIC ENTERITIS

Clinical Synopsis

Diagnostic Features

- Vomiting or small-bowel diarrhea of greater than several weeks duration
- Biopsy evidence of small intestinal inflammation in which the predominant cells are lymphocytes and plasma cells
- No cause found after a thorough workup

Standard Treatment

- Selected protein, highly digestible controlled diet(s)
- Prednisone: 1 to 2 mg/kg q 12 hours PO for 1 to 2 weeks; followed by 1.0 mg/kg q 24 hours PO for 4 weeks; followed by 0.5 to 1.0 mg/kg qod PO for 4 weeks; followed by a tapered withdrawal over 2 weeks

Follow-up

- Withdraw the pharmacologic therapy and attempt to maintain on a selected protein diet for 6 to 12 months
- Thereafter, consider oral challenge trials to help determine suitability of standard (mixed- protein source) pet foods
- Repeat pharmacologic therapy if recurrence occurs

Lymphocytic-plasmacytic enteritis (LPE) is a chronic, idiopathic, inflammatory disease of the small bowel characterized by a mixed inflammatory infiltrate in the lamina propria in which lymphocytes and plasma cells predominate.

Prevalence and Signalment

The prevalence of the disease is unknown, but reviews[86,93,95,96,101,136,143–146] suggest that small intestinal LPE is one of the most frequent causes of chronic vomiting and diarrhea in cats and dogs. LPE is the most prevalent IBD variant affecting the small bowel of the dog and cat. No sex predisposition has been recognized. In both cats and dogs the disease is most common in middle age and older animals. However, PLE has been observed in cats as young as 4 months and dogs as young as 8 months.[95,96,143,144] German shepherds[101] and sharpeis, two breeds that have a high incidence of IgA deficiency, may be predisposed. The basenji and the Ludenhund have their own particular variant of LPE. No breed predisposition has been observed in cats.

Etiopathogenesis

The cause of LPE is unknown.[147] In many animals, the disease resembles food protein-induced enteropathy of humans.[148] In others,[149] it has similarities to immunoproliferative enteropathy (Mediterranean lymphoma) of humans in which a monoclonal expansion of benign-appearing plasma cells diffusely infiltrates the gastrointestinal tract. As with LPE in dogs and cats, immunoproliferative enteropathy can progress to lymphosarcoma if untreated.[150]

The presence of increased numbers of lymphocytes and plasma cells in canine and feline LPE suggests chronic antigenic challenge of the gut-associated lymphoid tissues. It remains to be established whether this chronic challenge results from a damaged or defective mucosal permeability barrier, or a failure of tolerance to self-, dietary, or bacterial antigens. Moreover, the extent of the role of genetic makeup, psychologic factors, enteric pathogens, and mucosal biochemical defects remains to be defined. In all probability there is more than one cause of LPE.

Clinical Findings

Chronic small-bowel type diarrhea is the most common clinical sign in the dog, whereas chronic intermittent vomiting is the most common sign in the cat. The diarrhea can be semiformed and/or watery. Cats and, less commonly, dogs may manifest vomiting as their only clinical sign. In cats, a presumptive diagnosis of hair balls often figures prominently in the history. The clinical signs have a cyclical course, but as the disorder worsens episodes become progressively more frequent and severe. Unless concomitant delayed gastric emptying has developed, patients with LPE will usually vomit small amounts of food or scant volumes of bile-stained or clear fluid. The history helps differentiate IBD from gastrointestinal neoplasia. Neoplasia has a relentlessly progressive rather than cyclical course, and if gastrointestinal obstruction occurs the volume of the vomitus tends to be copious. Hematemesis and melena are uncommon in LPE and suggest concurrent gastroduodenal ulceration.[86] Occasionally diarrhea is precipitated by a stressful episode. Additional clinical signs that are often present include weight loss, lethargy, dehydration, and borborygmus. Rarely, abdominal pain, ascites, pica, polydipsia, polyuria, and pyrexia may be apparent. An association between abdominal pain and gastrointestinal ulceration has been observed in some but not all dogs with LPE.[86] Appetite is usually decreased, but in milder cases, polyphagia may be apparent. Weight loss is the most consistent observation during the physical examination. Palpation of the abdomen may reveal abdominal discomfort and thickened loops of intestine.

Laboratory Findings

Hematologic findings are nonspecific.[86,101] Leukocytosis as a result of stress or chronic inflammation may be observed. In severely affected animals leukocyte counts can reach 40,000 to 50,000/mm.[3,95,143,101] Left-shifted leukograms are rarely observed but can occur, particularly if mucosal erosion and ulceration or neutrophilic infiltration of the mucosa has occurred.[86,101] Monocytosis, lymphopenia, and eosinopenia are not uncommon, presumably as a result of stress. Occasionally, eosinophilia is observed, and may or may not be associated with an eosinophilic component to the mucosal infiltrate.[86,101] Mildly elevated PCV may be seen, presumably due to dehydration. Mild normocytic-normochromic-nonregenerative anemia, assumedly due to chronic inflammation, is sometimes present. Occasionally, regenerative anemias are detected, and should encourage the clinician to consider gastrointestinal hemorrhage from mucosal ulceration. In cats, mild hyperglycemia and mild hypokalemia are often observed.[86,93] These changes are also seen in dogs but less frequently.[86,101] Liver enzymes are frequently mildly elevated. For instance, 26% of dogs and 12% to 33% of cats with lymphocytic/plasmacytic enteritis have been reported to have elevated serum ALT.[86,93] Hyperamylasemia is also relatively frequent in affected dogs.[86] Hypoalbuminemia and hypoglobulinemia as a result of malnutrition and protein-losing enteropathy are common in dogs with moderate to severe disease. In contrast, panhypoproteinemia is uncommon in cats with LPE unless the disease is particularly severe.[95,96] When panhypoproteinemia is detected in cats, intestinal lymphosarcoma is an important differential diagnosis.[96] Hypoalbuminemia (without hypoglobulinemia) is seen in approximately 15% to 25% of cats, and mild hyperglobulinemia is periodically noted. With the exception of basenjis, hyperglobulinemia as a result of LPE is infrequent in dogs. When present, hyperglobulinemia is usually polyclonal, but a monoclonal IgG gammopathy has been reported in a dog with chronic plasmacytic enterocolitis.[149] Tests of exocrine pancreatic function are usually normal but laboratory evidence of malabsorption is often noted. Thus, excessive fatty acid

droplets in the stool and abnormal absorption tests may occur.[101] Moderate steatorrhea (5–13 g/day) and excessive fecal nitrogen loss (8.4–11.7 g/day) have been reported in affected dogs.[56] Results of xylose, cobalamin, folate, and vitamin A absorption tests are inconsistent. Breath hydrogen tests are usually abnormal. Coagulopathies in association with suspected vitamin K malabsorption due to LPE have been reported in cats.[151] but appear to be rare. Tests for parasites are usually negative. Fecal cultures do not reveal enteric pathogens, but test for small intestinal bacterial overgrowth are occasionally positive. In cats, hyperthyroidism can have a similar presentation and so it is important to evaluate a serum T_4. FeLV and FIV titers are usually negative. A partial response to an elimination diet may be observed but, with the exception of mildly affected animals, it is uncommon to get complete resolution of signs except on a transient basis.[122]

Radiographic Findings

Survey and contrast radiographs with liquid barium reveal nonspecific abnormalities. Gas-and/or fluid-distended loops of small bowel are frequently observed in cats and dogs with LPE.[86] Flocculation and segmentation of barium sulfate suspension is observed in some dogs.[56] Mucosal irregularity and narrowed dye columns can be seen in severely affected cats and dogs. Transit studies with barium-impregnated polyethylene spheres (BIPs) have revealed delayed gastric emptying of food in some affected dogs and cats. Delayed transit of barium sulfate liquid has also been observed in some cats with the disorder.

Ultrasound Findings

Ultrasonography will occasionally reveal a diffusely thickened bowel wall or mild mesenteric lymphadenopathy. Marked mesenteric lymphadenopathy is unusual in LPE and should raise suspicion for lymphosarcoma and to a lesser extent hypereosinophilic syndrome. Aspiration of the lymph nodes may provide a diagnosis.

Endoscopy Findings

The endoscopic appearance of the duodenum may be normal in as many as 50% of animals with LPE.[86] In many cases, however, the duodenal mucosa will appear more granular and friable than normal (Figure 24–4). Erosions and ulcers may be seen.[152] Likewise, during celiotomy the bowel may appear normal, which should not discourage biopsy.

Biopsy Findings

Multiple gastric and small intestinal biopsies should be obtained from different sites of the stomach and small bowel because the severity of the infiltrate can vary between areas of the gastrointestinal tract in individual dogs.[101] If concurrent large bowel signs are observed, colon biopsies should also be obtained. It is not unusual for the lymphocytic-plasmacytic infiltrates to involve stomach or colon in addition to the small bowel.[86,101] Biopsy not only helps confirm the diagnosis of LPE but also provides information pertinent to prognosis and assists determination of how aggressive the pharmacologic therapy needs to be.

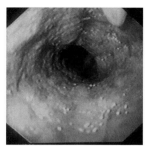

FIGURE 24-4. Endoscopic view of the duodenum of a dog with severe lymphocytic-plasmacytic enteritis. Note the irregular mucosal granularity.

The cardinal finding in the intestinal biopsy is an increase in the number of lymphocytes and plasma cells in the lamina propria. The distribution of these cells may widen to extend in heavier numbers into the villi, a position where plasma cells are not commonly found in the normal intestine.[101,153] The distribution may be patchy, with areas of markedly increased cellular infiltrate interdispersed with areas of slightly increased infiltrate.[101] A layer of lymphocytes, plasma cells, eosinophils, and histiocytes may be present above the muscularis mucosae. Scattered neutrophils and increased numbers of intraepithelial lymphocytes may be seen. Neutrophils are often associated with foci of mucosal erosion or ulceration.[86] The surface epithelium may appear normal or low columnar to cuboidal with an indistinct brush border.[153] In more severe cases there may be villus clubbing, atrophy, and fusion.[101,146] Multifocal coalescing erosions or increased basophilia and flattening of the surface epithelium, suggestive of recent erosion, may be seen.[98,101] The crypt architecture may be distorted or hypertrophic. Some crypts may obstruct and dilate with mucus. Occasionally, evidence of rupture of obstructed crypts will be seen, such as mucus in the lamina propria in association with reactive histiocytes and the occasional giant cell.[153] There may be edema of the lamina propria and mildly dilated lacteals[98,101] presumably secondary to increased vascular permeability and lymph formation. The lymphatic dilation must not be overinterpreted as diagnostic of idiopathic lymphangiectasia, a disease in which the lymphatic dilation is usually massive and in which other mucosal changes are usually absent.[98] The submucosa is normally not involved in LPE.

Differential Diagnosis

As discussed previously, the clinician and the pathologist must take great care to differentiate LPE from a variety of known causes of intestinal lymphocytic-plasmacytic infiltrates and from normal intestine that routinely has a small complement of mucosal leukocytes. A general discussion of the differential diagnosis of IBD was provided earlier, and important differential diagnoses are provided in Table 24–3. Lymphosarcoma, in particular, can be difficult to differentiate from LPE, and the occasional patient initially diagnosed as having LPE will later manifest lymphosarcoma.[96,101] Whether this represents a progression of the disease from LPE to lymphosarcoma or an initial misdiagnosis is as yet uncertain. A similar condition to LPE has been reported in dogs in Britain, and is referred to as "tropical sprue-like enteropathy."[154] The information published to date on this enteropathy has not allowed clear differentiation of this disorder from LPE.

Treatment

Important details concerning the controlled diets and pharmacologic treatment regimens useful in LPE may be found in the previous section discussing therapy of inflammatory bowel disease. The treatment protocol described in the clinical synopsis is suitable for the therapy of moderate to severe LPE. The higher end of the prednisone dosage range (provided in the synopsis) is recommended for the more severe cases. If the inflammatory infiltrates or clinical signs are milder, smaller doses of prednisone may be sufficient to obtain remission. In general, controlled diets used alone are not satisfactory for the induction of long-lasting remission in patients with LPE unless the infiltration is classified as mild.[95,143,144] In moderate or severe LPE, controlled diets often ameliorate the signs, but they rarely induce complete long-lasting remission.

Most patients show signs of improvement within a week of beginning prednisone and nutritional therapy. If the clinical signs of affected patients are nonresponsive after 2 weeks, consider the adjunctive use of metronidazole or more aggressive immunosuppressive therapy with azathioprine. If the response is still poor, consider the common reasons for treatment failure discussed earlier.

Combination therapy with prednisone and azathioprine is also useful if remission can only be achieved at doses of prednisone that cause an unacceptably high frequency of side effects. Furthermore, if the clinical signs and histopathology results reveal a severely affected animal, it is often sensible to use combination prednisone/azathioprine from the start of therapy.

Some patients require continued medical therapy throughout their lives, but many can be weaned from medication after 3 months and maintained in remission on controlled diets. Some patients can eventually be returned to commercial mixed-protein diets. If recurrence of signs occurs, the pharmacologic treatment regimen should be reinstituted for the same duration. If recurrence of signs occurs at the end of the second episode of drug therapy, it is probable that indefinite drug administration will be required.

Prognosis

The prognosis for most patients with LPE is good. The concomitant presence of protein-losing enteropathy, melena, or severe histopathologic changes, however, merits a guarded to poor outlook.[144] In one study, 30% of the dogs were nonresponsive to therapy.[155] Forty percent of cats with histologically severe disease are nonresponsive.[156]

CHRONIC IDIOPATHIC (LYMPHOCYTIC-PLASMACYTIC) COLITIS

Clinical Synopsis

Diagnostic Features

- Large-bowel signs of greater than several weeks duration
- Frequent passage of small quantities of mucoid diarrhea
- Hematochezia and tenesmus are common
- Significant weight loss is unusual
- Biopsy evidence of colonic inflammation in which the predominant cells are lymphocytes and plasma cells
- No cause apparent after a thorough workup

Standard Treatment

- Selected protein, highly digestible controlled diets(s) containing fermentable fiber
- Add Metamucil (1–6 teaspoons per meal) if controlled diet low in fiber
- Sulfasalazine: Dogs, 12.5 mg/kg q 6 hour PO for 14 days followed by 12.5 mg/kg q 12 hour for 28 days; cats, 10 to 20 mg/kg q 24 hour PO for 14 days.

Follow-up

- Withdraw the drug therapy and attempt to maintain on selected-protein/fermentable fiber diet for 6 to 12 months
- Thereafter, consider oral challenge trials to help determine suitability of standard pet foods
- Repeat drug therapy if recurrence occurs

Chronic idiopathic colitis is characterized by persistent large-bowel-type diarrhea and a mixed inflammatory infiltrate in the lamina propria of the large bowel in which lymphocytes and plasma cells predominate. The disease must be carefully differentiated from other types of colitis of known and unknown cause (see this chapter and Chapters 21 and 22).

Prevalence and Signalment

Chronic idiopathic colitis is the most prevalent large-bowel disease in dogs,[33,157,158] and is one of the most common causes of chronic diarrhea in this species. At the UCD VMTH, approximately 130 cases of the disease are presented each year, accounting for 5 cases per 1000 canine submissions. A study of clinically normal dogs in a beagle colony revealed that the prevalence of subclinical colonic inflammation is higher, reaching 40 out of every 1000 dogs.[159]

Although chronic idiopathic (lymphocytic-plasmacytic) colitis is also the most common form of colitis recognized in cats, the prevalence of the disease appears to be lower in cats than dogs. Idiopathic colitis accounts for 3.2 cases per 1000 feline submissions at the UCD VMTH, and 1.7 cases per 1000 feline submissions at Michigan State University Veterinary Hospital.[94] However, the prevalence of feline colitis may be higher than these numbers would suggest because the signs of large-bowel dysfunction are often less overt in cats than in dogs.

Predisposed dog breeds include boxers[160] and perhaps German shepherds. Purebred cats may also be predisposed.[94] At the UCD VMTH, most dogs first present for chronic colitis before 6 years of age but as many as 30% of dogs are first presented before 1 year of age. Similarly, young to middle-aged cats are most commonly affected.[94] No sex predisposition to chronic colitis has been recognized in cats or dogs.

Etiopathogenesis

The etiopathogenesis of chronic colitis is unknown. The disease has similarities to ulcerative colitis, microscopic colitis, and food protein–induced proctitis of humans. It is likely that some or all of the factors described earlier in the general discussion of the etiopathogenesis of IBD are important. In addition, recent experimental observations in dogs and clinical findings in humans have raised the possibility that insufficient fiber, or the inclusion of the wrong type of dietary fiber, may play a role in the etiopathogenesis of some forms of colitis. Dogs fed a poorly fermentable fiber (cellulose) have atrophied colons in comparison to dogs fed fermentable fibers.[161] Furthermore, there is some suggestion that the accumulation of inflammatory cells and/or necrotic crypt enterocytes (cryptitis) is higher in dogs fed a cellulose-based diet compared to dogs fed a diet containing beet pulp, a moderately fermentable fiber.[161] Moreover, butyrate enemas are effective therapy for diversion colitis and distal ulcerative colitis in humans.[162] As discussed in Chapter 38, the beneficial effect of fermentable fibers is thought to relate to their provision of volatile fatty acids, which are the principal energy sources of colonocytes.[163]

Clinical Findings

The history usually reveals a prolonged history of intermittent large-bowel disease, characterized by some or all of the following signs: tenesmus, defecation urgency, reservoir fecal incontinence, and the frequent passage of diarrhea with fresh blood and mucus. Hematochezia is the most common sign in cats with chronic colitis, and hematochezia without diarrhea is occasionally seen in this species.[94] Mucoid diarrhea is usually the earliest sign seen in dogs. In both cats and dogs, tenesmus is usually not observed until the disease worsens. Vomiting occurs in as many as 30% of dogs with colitis, and is occasionally seen in affected cats. The presence of this sign should not mislead the clinician into ruling out a large-bowel problem. Anal pruritus is occasionally seen in dogs. Infrequently, the only sign is marked dyschezia. Borborygmus and excessive flatus are rare, and if present suggest concomitant small-bowel disease. As the severity of the disease increases, other signs develop, including anorexia, weight loss, fever, and abdominal pain. In multipet households only one animal is affected and there should be no evidence of contagion to people. Concurrent lymphocytic-plasmacytic infiltrates in the small intestine is not uncommon (enterocolitis). This can lead to animals presented for a mixture of small- and large-bowel signs.

The physical examination is usually unremarkable with the exception of the digital examination of the rectum. The rectal examination often reveals stool with fresh blood or mucus, and occasionally detects a cobblestone mucosal surface. On some occasions rectal spasms or a rectal stricture will be felt.

Laboratory Findings

Laboratory abnormalities are usually mild and are nonspecific. Stress leukograms may be seen in cats and dogs. Liver enzymes are mildly elevated in about 20% of dogs with colitis. Mild elevations in ALT, and hypokalemia occurs in approximately half of affected cats.[94] A small number of cats with colitis develop hypoproteinemia.[94] Fecal flotations for parasites such as whipworm are negative. Rectal scrapes are usually unremarkable in dogs with chronic idiopathic colitis, but neutrophils may be seen in the smears from animals with marked colonic erosion or ulceration. The presence of many eosinophils in a rectal scrape is strongly suggestive of eosinophilic colitis rather than chronic idiopathic colitis. If large numbers of clostridial spores are observed in fecal smears, consideration should be given to measurement of the fecal level of *Clostridium perfringens* enterotoxin to rule out *Clostridium perfringens*–associated colitis. Fecal cultures for enteropathogens such as Campylobacter should be negative. In cats, a positive FeLV titer or a markedly elevated FIP titer raise the possibility that the colitis is FeLV or FIP associated.

Radiographic Findings

Survey radiographs rarely provide useful information for the diagnosis of chronic colitis. Similarly, barium enemas have poor sensitivity for the diagnosis of this disease and are rarely performed. The few indications for barium enemas are discussed in Chapter 5 and 6 and primarily pertain to the examination of the upper colon if flexible colonoscopy cannot be performed. Changes compatible with chronic colitis that can be recognized by a barium enema include poor colonic distensibility, generalized mucosal thickening and irregularity, and mucosal ulcerations or strictures. The colon can be markedly shortened in severe chronic cases (Figure 24–5). Endoscopic examination and or blind biopsy is necessary following barium enemas to determine the cause of any suspected radiographic abnormality.

Endoscopic Findings

Endoscopy greatly assists the diagnosis of chronic colitis and its differentiation from the other common causes of large-bowel diarrhea. Most cases of chronic idiopathic colitis in the dog and cat are associated with mucosal abnormalities that can be recognized with an endoscope. The characteristic findings are generalized hyperemia and friability, with patchy or complete loss of the submucosal vascular pattern due to the overlying inflammatory infiltrate and edema in the lamina propria (Figures 24–6A and B). Additional observations are excessive accumulations of mucus, mucosal granularity, and areas of erosion or spontaneous hemorrhage. The colon is often more difficult to insufflate than the colon of normal dogs, perhaps due to edema, increased muscular tone, or mucosal infiltration by cells. Occasionally circumferential mucosal folds are present that will not yield to the proctoscope (Figure 24–7). Well-circumscribed deep ulcers or strictures may be seen but are relatively rare in chronic idiopathic colitis (see histiocytic colitis). It is important to emphasize that these features are not specific for chronic idiopathic colitis, but can be seen in any inflammatory large-bowel disease. Furthermore, the colon can appear grossly normal in spite of significant histologic abnormalities. Therefore, biopsy samples should be acquired even from bowel that appears normal.

Biopsy Findings

Colonic biopsy is a very useful procedure in the diagnosis of chronic colitis. Biopsy findings help eliminate some impor-

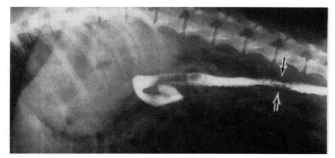

FIGURE 24–5. Radiograph of 1-year-old miniature dachshund with signs of severe bloody diarrhea. Barium enema reveals the colon to be shortened. The transverse colon is at the level of the first lumbar vertebrae instead of its usual position at the level of the twelfth thoracic vertebrae. The cecum cannot be identified. Stricture of the colon is most evident at the arrows.

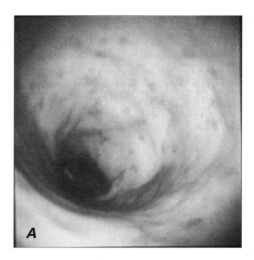

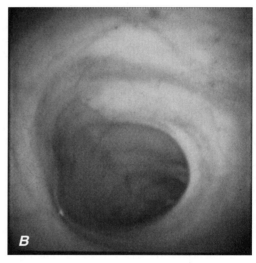

FIGURE 24–6. Endoscopic view of the colon of a dog before (A) and after (B) treatment for chronic (idiopathic) colitis. Note the mucosal erosions and the lack of submucosal vessels prior to treatment.

tant differential diagnoses (e.g., neoplasia), determine the histopathologic classification of the colitis (i.e. idiopathic vs. eosinophilic, etc.), and occasionally determine the cause of the colitis (e.g., histoplasmosis). Moreover, the severity of the histopathologic changes assists choice of therapy and facilitates provision of an accurate prognosis. Histologic grading systems to assess the severity of chronic colitis in dogs and cats have been published.[94,100]

The earliest histopathologic change in chronic idiopathic colitis is hyperplasia of crypt cells, reflective of a more rapid epithelial turnover. Additional mild changes include infiltration of the lamina propria with plasma cells, lymphocytes, and, to a lesser extent eosinophils and neutrophils. In contrast to histiocytic colitis, there is an absence of periodic acid–Schiff (PAS) positive histiocytes. The inflammatory process is confined to the mucosa with the exception of hyperplasia of submucosal lymphoid aggregates. A photomicrograph showing the typical changes of mild chronic idiopathic colitis is shown in Figure 24–8.

In severe cases of chronic colitis, infiltration by leukocytes is more extensive. The crypt cells in the glands appear markedly hyperplastic and show increased numbers of mitotic figures. Dilation of the colonic glands and mucus clearance are also

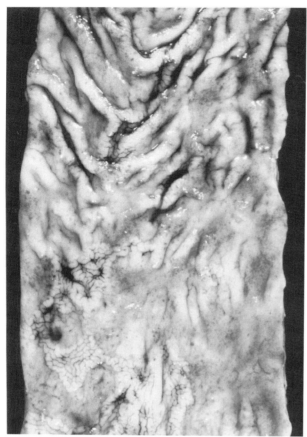

FIGURE 24-7. Chronic colitis. Inflammation has caused mucosal folds that remain with distension of the colon during endoscopy or barium enema.

observed. With increased severity the goblet cells may virtually disappear from the glandular epithelium. Degeneration of the surface epithelial cells becomes apparent. In the early stages, the degenerating surface mucosal cells are characterized by basophilia, reductions in height so they become cuboidal or flattened, and the appearance of cytoplasmic vacuoles (Figure 24–9). This condition can progress to epithelial desquamation, erosion, and ulceration. Epithelial erosion is followed by the appearance of acute inflammatory changes characterized by neutrophil accumulation in the lamina propria directly beneath the epithelial surface. The erosions are usually focal but almost complete loss of the surface epithelium can occur (Figure 24–10).

Fibrosis in the lamina propria becomes apparent as the colitis becomes more persistent. Widespread fibrosis at this site eventually results in mucosal distortion, the loss of colonic glands, and failure of the colon's absorptive functions. Rarely, stricture can result if the inflammation extends into the submucosa. Additional advanced lesions include microabscesses in the lamina propria and submucosa. Occasionally, focal chronic inflammatory changes can result in the formation of granulomas (Figure 24–10), an unusual feature of colitis. Granulomas contribute to stricture formation.

Differential Diagnosis

It is important to remember that the clinical signs, endoscopic changes, and histopathologic findings discussed ear-lier are not specific for chronic idiopathic colitis and can be caused by various infectious and irritative conditions of the large bowel (see Chapters 21 and 26 and Table 26–1). A discussion of the differential diagnosis of IBD is provided in the general section on IBD, and important differential diagnoses of lymphoplasmacytic infiltration are provided in Table 24–3. A very important rule-out for chronic idiopathic colitis in dogs is whipworm infection. Occasionally, it is difficult, clinically and histopathologically, to differentiate chronic colitis from intestinal lymphosarcoma. If the pathologist has difficulty differentiating between lymphoma and colitis, clients should be warned that their dogs will most likely go on to develop overt lymphosarcoma at a later date.[160] It is worthy of note that a recent report has described bloody diarrhea in a group of Persian cats with lymphocytic-plasmacytic gastroenterocolitis associated with a spiral-shaped organism.[97]

Another important differential diagnosis in dogs is the functional bowel disorder termed irritable bowel syndrome (IBS). Some veterinary gastroenterologists diagnose IBS in dogs with large-bowel-type diarrhea that have mild or no histologic abnormalities in the colon. It is important to note, however, that these findings bear a close resemblance to those of the so-named microscopic colitis of humans. In microscopic colitis minimal inflammatory infiltrates and mild reactive changes in the epithelium are associated with markedly abnormal colonic absorption of water and electrolytes and clinical signs that include persistent diarrhea with urgency, mild abdominal cramping, but no hematochezia.[164,165] The diagnostic approach to large-bowel-type diarrhea is covered in more detail in Chapter 5.

Treatment

Nutritional management is the cornerstone of treatment. Many patient with mild to moderate chronic idiopathic colitis will respond to dietary management without the need for drug therapy. Unfortunately, controversy surrounds the best diet for use in the treatment of colitis. Several studies have shown good results with the use of selected-protein highly digestible diets.[38,39,166] For example, retrospective evaluation of the records of the UCD VMTH showed that approximately 50% of dogs with chronic idiopathic colitis placed exclusively on cottage cheese and rice had a complete resolution of clinical signs. Approximately 20% showed no improvement, and the remainder of the dogs showed partial remission. In another study, 85% of dogs with chronic colitis showed resolution of their clinical signs within 2 weeks of the initiation of a cottage cheese and rice diet, and 100% of the dogs were in remission within 6 weeks.[39] The majority of these dogs initially treated with cottage cheese and rice could subsequently be fed a lamb-based selected-protein diet (Prescription diet d/d, Hills Pet Products) without adverse reactions.[39] Other authors have recommended the use of high-fiber diets in the treatment of chronic colitis, with some finding success using soluble fibers such as psyllium (hemicellulose) and others preferring insoluble fibers such as bran. As discussed in Chapter 38, the use of soluble (fermentable) fiber in preference to insoluble (nonfermentable) fiber in the treatment of colitis has theoretical support because most soluble fibers generate volatile fatty acids that nurture the large bowel and discourage growth of bacterial pathogens. Nevertheless, Prescription Diet r/d, a diet high in insoluble fiber, has been used successfully in cats with colitis.[94]

In the author's experience, the nutritional management of colitis that gives the best short-term and long-term results is a highly digestible diet containing moderate amounts of a

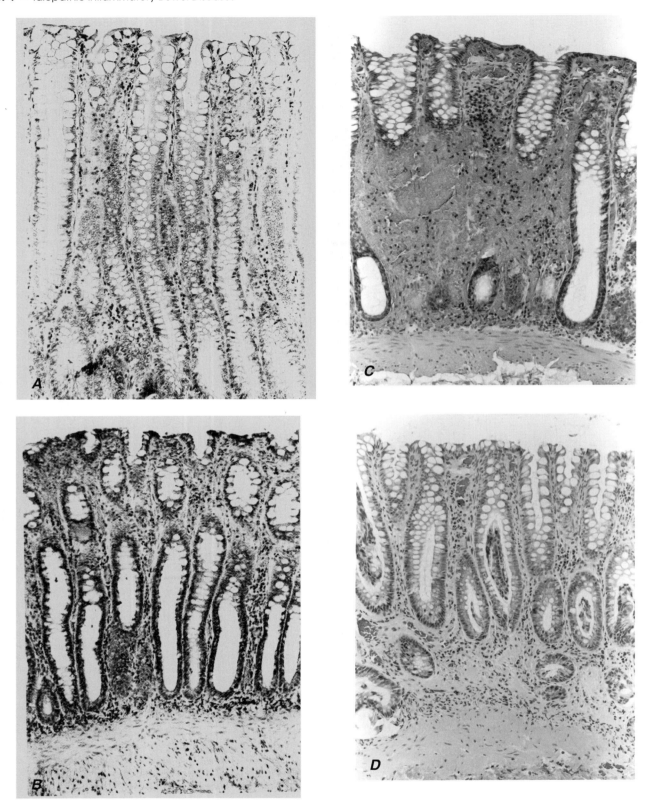

FIGURE 24–8. *(A)* Biopsy of normal canine colon. *(B)* Colitis. Changes include moderate crypt dilation, accelerated regeneration of crypt epithelium (identified by low cuboidal epithelial cells with dark staining nuclei and absence of differentiation to goblet cells) in deepest part of crypt, increased number of inflammatory cells, and degeneration and erosion of surface epithelium. *(C)* Colitis. Normal mucosal thickness. Surface epithelium is low cuboidal to squamous. Crypts are moderately dilated; lower crypt epithelium is cuboidal with dark nuclei and few goblet cells. Widespread hemorrhage in lamina propria. *(D)* Colitis. Mucosal atrophy caused by inflammatory changes in lower mucosa. Changes characterized by infiltration of inflammatory cells and fibrosis. Surface epithelium is normal.

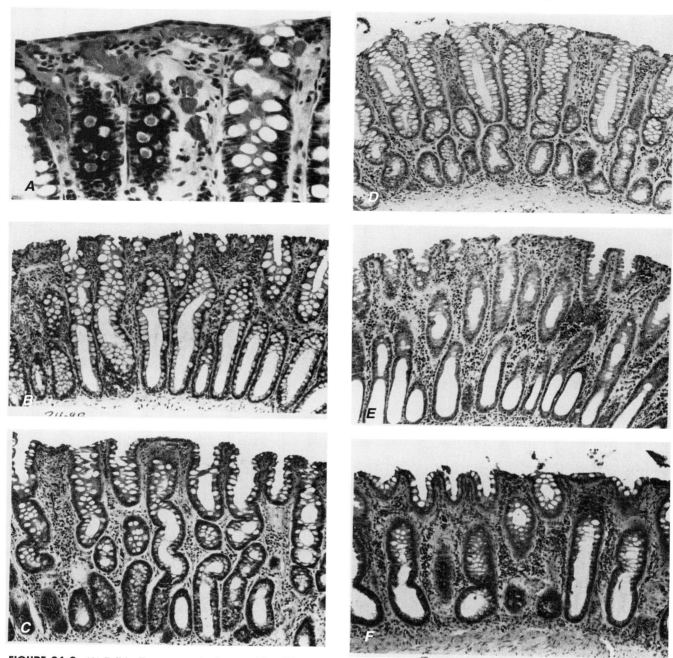

FIGURE 24-9. *(A)* Colitis. Frequent early change with colitis is appearance of squamous or low cuboidal epithelium on absorptive surface. Section also exhibits hemorrhage in lamina propria. High power magnification. *(B)* Colitis with atrophy. Reduced mucosal thickness is associated with moderate crypt dilation. Crypt epithelium is normal except in bottom of crypts where many cells are low cuboidal with dark nuclei, suggesting augmented regeneration. Differentiation to goblet cells is normal throughout crypts. Increased inflammatory cells in lamina propria contribute to mild splaying (irregular spacing) of crypts. *(C)* Colitis. Changes are similar to *(B)* except that atrophy is not as severe but mucosal surface epithelium is eroded in places. *(D)* Colitis. Reduced mucosal thickness. Increased number of inflammatory cells in lamina propria. Number of goblet cells on mucosal surface is reduced. *(E)* Colitis. Reduced mucosal thickness. Moderate dilation of crypts with epithelium in lower crypts being cuboidal with few goblet cells. Mild to moderate infiltration of inflammatory cells in lamina propria with few areas of hermorrhage. *(F)* Colitis. Mucosal thickness is 50% to 60% of normal. Moderate crypt dilation and splaying. Epithelial cells in deeper half of crypts are cuboidal with dark nuclei, suggesting increased regeneration. Few goblet cells in crypt depths. Increased number of inflammatory cells in lamina propria. Surface epithelium exhibits thinning and erosions.

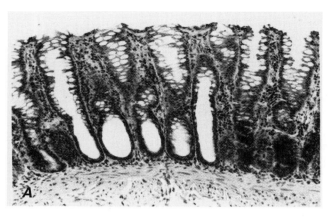

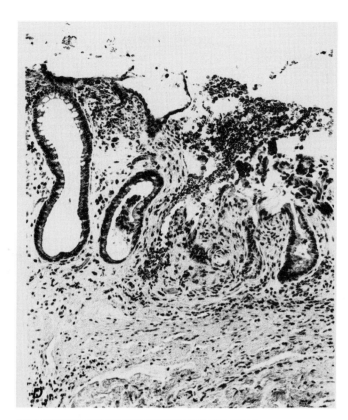

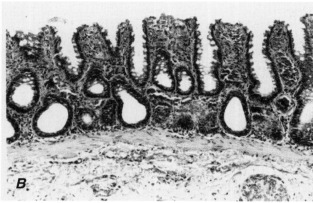

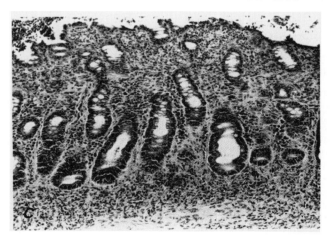

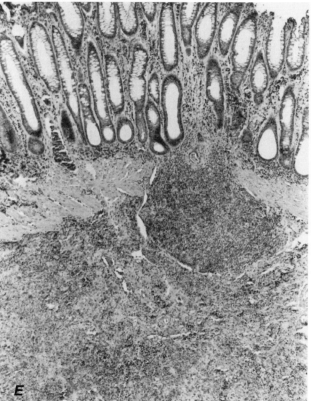

FIGURE 24-10. (A) Colitis with mucosal atrophy. Mucosal thickness is about 50% of normal. Moderate crypt dilation with cuboidal epithelium possessing dark nuclei in lower half. Epithelial surface is eroded. Number of inflammatory cells is increased in lamina propria. (B) Colitis with atrophy. Changes are similar to (A) but are more severe and with hemorrhage. (C) Colitis. Changes include erosion of surface epithelium and ulceration into lamina propria with hemorrhage. Marked infiltration by inflammatory cells. Fibrous tissue is increased. Crypt changes are similar to those with milder forms of colitis. (D) Ulcerative colitis with mucosal atrophy. Changes include ulceration of surface, dilation of crypts, cuboidal crypt epithelium, inflammatory cell infiltration and fibrosis of lamina propria, and hemorrhage. (E) Colitis with severe involvement of submucosa. Marked infiltration by inflammatory cells with granuloma formation. Normal lymphoid follicle is seen in right half at junction of mucosa with submucosa. (F) Colitis in cat with feline infectious peritonitis. Biopsy specimen showing changes that include marked crypt dilation. FIP titer was 1 to 1600.

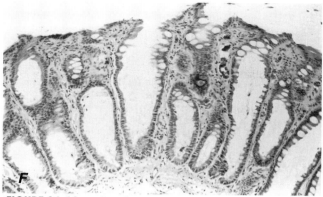

(FIGURE 24-10 *continued*)

selected protein, in association with the addition of a fermentable fiber such as psyllium, soy fiber, or oat bran. To minimize the chance of food protein–induced allergic colitis, the protein source chosen should not have been included in the animal's staple diet in recent months. The amount of fiber added is empirical. For instance, Metamucil is usually added to the diet at a rate of 1 to 6 teaspoons per meal, depending on the body weight of the patient.

In moderate to severe chronic idiopathic colitis the treatment protocol described in the clinical synopsis is suitable. Nutritional management remains an integral part of the treatment plan but therapy with sulfasalzine is also usually necessary to induce a more rapid and long-lasting remission. If sulfasalazine at the doses recommended in the clinical synopsis fails to induce remission, higher doses can be used (see the recommendations made in the section on sulfasalazine in this chapter). Alternatively, prednisone can be used instead of, or in addition to, sulfasalazine Prednisone is also indicated if side effects from sulfasalazine develop (see earlier). Disagreement exists over the relative merit of prednisone and sulfasalazine in the treatment of chronic colitis.[122,143,167,168] In my experience and that of others, both drugs are efficacious in the control of acute flareups of the disease, but sulfasalazine is the preferred drug for maintaining remission. The prednisone dosage schedule described for the treatment of lymphocytic-plasmacytic enteritis (see earlier) is also a suitable regimen for the management of chronic idiopathic colitis. Olsalazine is an alternative to prednisone if side effects from sulfasalazine develop. As already mentioned, however, the value of olsalazine in chronic colitis in dogs and cats remains to be established.

Azathioprine and, to a lesser extent, metronidazole, can be useful in the treatment of colitis if prednisone (or prednisone and sulfasalazine) fails to induce remission. These drugs are also valuable if unacceptable side effects from high doses of prednisone develop. The doses and precautions required when using these drugs are described in the earlier section on therapy.

Surgical resection of the diseased colon is a last resort in managing patients with irreversible changes that cannot be treated medically.

Prognosis

The prognosis is good. Few cases of chronic idiopathic colitis fail to respond to medical management. Stricture formation and extensive fibrosis of the lamina propria is associated with a poorer prognosis. Another common reason for lack of treatment success is reliance on sulfasalazine therapy when

there is unrecognized, but clinically significant, small intestinal involvement in addition to the colitis. Other reasons for treatment failures were discussed above in the earlier section on prognosis and treatment failures.

EOSINOPHILIC GASTROENTERITIS, ENTERITIS, AND ENTEROCOLITIS

Clinical Synopsis

Diagnostic Features

- Vomiting, small-bowel diarrhea, or mixed small- and large-bowel diarrhea of greater than several weeks duration
- Peripheral eosinophilia often present
- Biopsy evidence of gastric and/or intestinal inflammation in which the predominant feature is eosinophil infiltration
- No cause found after a thorough workup

Standard Treatment

- Selected protein, highly digestible controlled diet(s)
- Dogs: Prednisone 1 to 2 mg/kg q 12 hours PO for 1 to 2 weeks; followed by 1.0 mg/kg q 24 hours PO for 4 weeks; followed by 0.5 to 1.0 mg/kg qod PO for 4 weeks; followed by a tapered withdrawal over 2 weeks
- Cats: Prednisone 2 to 3 mg/kg q 12 hours PO for 2 to 4 weeks; followed by 1 to 1.5 mg/kg q 12 hours for 2 to 4 weeks; followed by 0.5 to 1.0 mg q 24 hours for 2 to 4 weeks; followed by alternate-day therapy for another 4 months

Follow-up

- Withdraw the pharmacologic therapy and attempt to maintain on a selected-protein diet for 6 to 12 mouths
- Thereafter, consider oral challenge trials to help determine suitability of standard pet foods
- Repeat pharmacologic therapy if recurrence occurs

Eosinophilic gastroenteritis is a chronic, idiopathic inflammatory disease of the stomach and small intestine that is characterized by a mixed inflammatory infiltrate in which the predominate feature is eosinophil infiltration. If the process involves the small intestine but not the stomach the disease is called eosinophilic enteritis; if it involves both the small and large intestine, it is called eosinophilic enterocolitis. In dogs, eosinophilic gastroenteritis is the most common variant of this disease. In cats, concomitant involvement of the colon rather than the stomach is more frequently seen.[122,169] In cats, eosinophilic involvement of other tissue in addition to the bowel is also common (hypereosinophilic syndrome).[170,171] Because the cause of eosinophilic IBD has not been proven, it is best classified as a variant of the inflammatory bowel diseases rather than a consequence of food allergy as is commonly done in the literature on humans.

Prevalence and Signalment

Eosinophilic IBD is less common than LPE.[146] No sex predispositions are apparent. German shepherds[172] and Rottweilers appear to be predisposed. At the UCD VMTH the disease is less common in cats than in dogs. In dogs, the disorder is most common in animals 5 years of age or younger.[172] In cats, most common in animals 5 years of age or younger.[172] In cats, a median age of 8 years has been reported with a range of 1.5 to 11 years.[122,169]

Etiopathogenesis

The etiopathogenesis of eosinophilic gastroenteritis is unknown. The disease has been reported in a specific-pathogen-free cat[173] establishing that parasitic and infectious agents are not necessarily involved in the pathogenesis. A recent report described a high prevalence of superficial eosinophilic gastritis in beagles fed a particular commercial diet.[174] The relevance of these observations to other clinical cases of eosinophilic IBD is unknown, however, because the diet appeared to induce chronic irritation of the gastric mucosa and, unlike classic descriptions of eosinophilic gastroenteritis, macrophages containing foreign material were a prominent histologic finding. Hypersensitivity (especially type 1) to dietary antigens absorbed from the intestine is a likely cause of eosinophilic gastroenteritis. However, dietary elimination trials have established that in many affected animals food sensitivity is not cause, suggesting the disease may also result from an immune response to other antigens such a enteric bacteria and migrating parasites (see Table 24–1). Further discussion of the etiopathogenesis of eosinophilic IBD may be found elsewhere in this chapter (see sections on type 1 hypersensitivity and the relationship of food and parasitic antigens to IBD).

Clinical Findings

Clinical findings in dogs and cats with eosinophilic IDB are similar to those for other types of chronic gastroenteritis. No pathognomonic signs are seen. Chronic vomiting, small-bowel type diarrhea, weight loss, and anorexia are the most common clinical signs observed. If the process extends to the colon, signs of large-bowel dysfunction may be observed. Occasionally, evidence of chronic blood loss is manifested by anemia and melena. In one report, 50% of affected cats had evidence of hematochezia and melena.[169] Similarly, hematemesis, hematochezia, or melena are thought to be more common in dogs with eosinophilic IDB than in other forms of IBD.[171] In cats, physical examination often reveals a markedly thickened, rigid intestine, and may detect peripheral lymphadenopathy, hepatomegaly, or splenomegaly if eosinophilic infiltration of other organs has occurred (hypereosinophilic syndrome).[122] On rare occasions, clinical signs of intestinal obstruction or perforation may develop.[171]

Diagnostic Findings

LABORATORY FINDINGS. A peripheral eosinophilia is present in most cats with eosinophilic IBD, but is an inconsistent finding in dogs. Basophilia is also sometimes seen. Ninety percent of cats with eosinophilic enteritis have eosinophilic infiltration of their bone marrow.[169] In severe cases, the laboratory work may reveal a panhypoproteinemia suggestive of protein-losing enteropathy. Hyperglobulinemia is sometimes seen.[171] Enteric blood loss may be associated with a regenerative anemia.

ENDOSCOPIC, RADIOGRAPHIC, AND ULTRASONOGRAPHIC FINDINGS. The endoscopic and radiographic findings are similar to those described for LPE. In severe eosinophilic enteritis

the bowel can appear rigid, and insufflation is difficult. In dogs, there may be increased friability of the gastric mucosa, and erosions or ulcers may be apparent. Rugal folds may appear thickened and edematous. Just as with LPE, the mucosa can look normal to endoscopic examination in spite of the presence of significant disease. Radiography or ultrasonography may reveal organomegaly or mesenteric lymphadenopathy, particularly in cats.

BIOPSY FINDINGS. A prominent, diffuse infiltration of the lamina propria with eosinophils is consistently present in biopsy samples (Figure 24–11). Globule leukocytes have been conspicuous in the mucosal samples from some affected dogs at Massey University, and have also been observed by others.[171] Mucosal atrophy with villus atrophy is seen in advanced disease.[146] Concomitant granulomatous infiltration is occasionally seen.[171] Miscellaneous other histopathologic findings seen in some animals include mucosal ulceration, perivascular accumulations of eosinophils, fibrosis, and muscular hypertrophy.[171]

It is important to note that eosinophils are conspicuous normal inhabitants of the small intestinal mucosa and the basilar portion of the colonic mucosa.[98] Therefore, for a diagnosis of eosinophilic gastroenteritis to be made the pathologist must be sure the complement of eosinophils observed is in excess of that seen in healthy animals. Furthermore, the eosinophil must constitute the "dominant" cell in the inflammatory infiltrate. Unfortunately, pathologists use different criteria to define cellular dominance. Because the longevity of leukocytes in tissues differs, the cell type present in greatest number among the newly infiltrating cells is not necessarily the cell type that accumulates in the most numbers in a chronic lesion.[98] Thus, most chronic lesions come to be dominated in number by long-lived lymphocytes and plasma cells, in spite of differing initiating causes. As a result, patients with a mixed infiltrate of lymphocytes, plasma cells, and eosinophils will be diagnosed by some pathologists as having

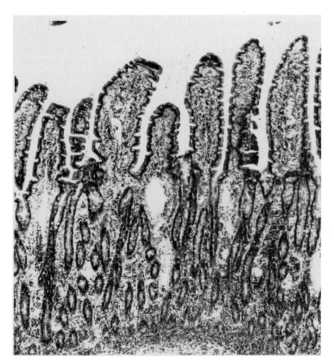

FIGURE 24–11. Eosinophilic enteritis. Diffuse infiltration of villi and crypts by eosinophils. Dilation of some lymphatics. Changes caused in villus height and crypt depth are minor.

lymphocytic-plasmacytic IBD and by others as having eosinophilic IBD.

In dogs with eosinophilic IBD, the eosinophilic infiltration is largely confined to the lamina propria but will spill into the submucosa and rarely into the muscularis.[98,175] In cats, the infiltration is often transmural.[170] In dogs, gastric involvement is usually evident; less commonly the eosinophilic infiltrate will also affect the colon. Figure 24–11 is an example of a biopsy sample confirming eosinophilic enteritis. Multiple intestinal biopsies should be obtained because the morphologic changes of eosinophilic enteritis can be discontinuous.

Differential Diagnosis

Gastrointestinal parasites, heartworms, hypoadrenocorticism, eosinophilic pulmonary diseases, flea-allergic dermatitis, and food allergy must be ruled out before an eosinophilia can be attributed to eosinophilic gastroenteritis. Eosinophilia may also occur with mast cell neoplasia and transmural granulomatous enteritis, both of which can mimic many of the clinical signs of eosinophilic gastroenteritis. Negative fecal flotations are of particular importance in ruling out gastrointestinal parasitism. Some authors recommend treatment trials with broad-spectrum anthelmentics, such as fenbendazole (50 mg/kg q 24 hours for 3 days) to ensure occult parasitism is not missed.[171] Resolution of peripheral eosinophilia and gastrointestinal signs after placement of a patient on a controlled diet supports the diagnosis of food sensitivity–induced eosinophilic gastroenteritis. Other causes of eosinophilic inflammation of the gastrointestinal tract are listed in Table 24–1.

Treatment

Important details concerning the controlled diets and drugs used in the treatment of eosinophilic IBD can be found in the general section on therapy of inflammatory bowel disease. In some, but not many, cases of canine eosinophilic gastroenteritis, remission of clinical signs will occur in response to a selected protein controlled diet.[168] In those dogs that do not respond to controlled diets alone, prednisone therapy should be begun. In cats, concurrent dietary and prednisone therapy is routinely used. The dosage of prednisone listed in the clinical synopsis controls the disease in most dogs. In cats, the refractory nature of the disease demands high prednisone dosages for prolonged periods.[122] Lower prednisone doses in cats (1–2 mg/kg q 24 hours) are associated with temporary remissions but rapid and refractory recurrence of the disease.[169] Additional immunosuppressive drugs such as azathioprine may be useful in some cases. In those animals manifesting a peripheral eosinophilia, the eosinophil count may be used as a guide to the adequacy of therapy. Once the clinical signs have been in remission for greater than 6 months, attempts can be made to return the patients back to mixed-protein source commercial foods if so desired. Prior to relaxation of the dietary restrictions, it is advisable to consider a series of oral-challenge trials with the aim of identifying foods that are tolerated and those that are not.

Prognosis

Treatment of eosinophilic gastroenteritis is usually successful in dogs, although controlled diets and glucocorticoids may have to be continued indefinitely in some dogs. In cats, the disease has been traditionally associated with a poor prognosis but recent publications have suggested that very aggressive immunosuppressive therapy can result in resolution.[122] Given these observations, a guarded rather than poor prognosis would seem warranted in cats.

HYPEREOSINOPHILIC SYNDROME

The hypereosinophilic syndrome is a common variant of eosinophilic enteritis in the cat, in which the eosinophilic infiltration affects not just the bowel but also other parenchymal organs such as the liver, spleen, mesenteric lymph nodes, kidney, adrenal glands, and heart.[169,170] The skin, lungs, and peripheral lymph nodes can also be affected.[176] Dogs do not appear to suffer from a similar disorder. Involvement of the mesenteric lymph nodes has been reported in dogs,[175] but more extensive extraintestinal infiltration is rare.

The etiopathogenesis of the syndrome is presumably similar to that of eosinophilic enteritis. The reason why some cats (and humans) develop a multisystemic eosinophilic response is poorly understood. Proposed causes are the absorption and widespread dissemination of the inciting antigen or the involvement of the bowel in a multisystemic eosinophilic infiltration due to some defect in eosinophil regulation. The disease is thought to be distinct from eosinophilic leukemia, although the two disorders can be difficult to distinguish.[170] Only morphologically normal eosinophils have been seen in feline hypereosinophilic syndrome.[176]

No sex predisposition has been established. The syndrome is most common in cats 7 years and older, although cats as young as 4 years of age have been affected.[170] Clinical findings are similar to the other IBD disorders, with the exception that intestinal thickening is more marked, hepatosplenomegaly may be detected, and bloody diarrhea is frequent. Furthermore, cough, peripheral lymphadenopathy, and erythematous alopecia have been reported.[176]

Peripheral eosinophilia is invariably present and sometimes reaches dramatically high proportions. The diagnosis is usually made by biopsy of the intestinal tract and a variety of abdominal organs at exploratory celiotomy. The characteristic finding is multiorgan invasion of eosinophils. The treatment most commonly used is aggressive high-dose prednisone therapy (3 mg/kg q 12 hours).[122] Most cats have to be maintained on high doses of prednisone to prevent relapse. An alternative or adjunctive therapy that holds some promise is hydroxyurea (Hydrea; Squibb) used at a dose of 7.5 mg/kg PO q 12 hours for 3 to 14 day courses as required to maintain remission.[176] Prognosis is guarded to poor.

EOSINOPHILIC COLITIS

Eosinophilic colitis is a chronic, idiopathic inflammatory disease of the large bowel characterized by a mixed inflammatory infiltrate in which eosinophils are the dominant cell type. The clinical signs are indistinguishable from chronic (lymphocytic-plasmacytic) colitis.

The etiopathogenesis of eosinophilic colitis is unknown. Similar pathomechanisms to those of eosinophilic gastroenteritis are presumably involved, and it is not uncommon to find eosinophilic infiltration affecting both the large and small intestine concurrently.

Eosinophilic colitis is an uncommon disorder in comparison to chronic idiopathic (lymphocytic-plasmacytic) colitis.[157]

The condition is most frequent in dogs but is occasionally seen in cats. In cats, the eosinophilic infiltration is most often a component of eosinophilic enterocolitis or the hypereosinophilic syndrome. It is most common in middle-aged patients. No sex predisposition has been reported.

A peripheral eosinophilia may be present, but otherwise the laboratory work is unremarkable. Particular care must taken to be rule out large-bowel parasitism by whipworms. Rectal scrapes may reveal large numbers of eosinophils. Endoscopic findings are identical to those with chronic colitis. The dominance of eosinophils in the biopsy distinguishes the disorder from chronic idiopathic colitis. In dogs, the eosinophilic infiltrate is most commonly confined to lamina propria, but on occasion it can affect all bowel layers and mesenteric lymph nodes.[175]

The response of patients with eosinophilic colitis to dietary therapy alone is inconsistent. In dogs and cats, the treatment most often used is a selected protein controlled diet with the concomitant administration of prednisone at the doses listed in the clinical synopsis for eosinophilic gastroenteritis. Sulfasalazine has not found as much favor as prednisone in the treatment of eosinophilic colitis but it can be successfully used in some animals. As discussed in the section on chronic idiopathic colitis, the addition of certain fibers (such as Metamucil) to the controlled diet is useful. If pharmacologic therapy was used to assist remission, it should be withdrawn after 8 to 12 weeks and the patient maintained on a controlled diet for a further few months before relaxing the dietary restrictions. Oral challenge trials should be considered to help determine which diets will be tolerated. Recurrences can occur, but in general the prognosis is favorable.

GASTROINTESTINAL EOSINOPHILIC GRANULOMA

Gastrointestinal eosinophilic granulomas are chronic, idiopathic inflammatory masses of the esophagus, stomach, small intestine, or large intestine in which the dominant cell is the eosinophil. The major importance of this rare disorder is its mimicry of gastrointestinal neoplasia, a resemblance that may result in inappropriate euthanasia. A similarly named disorder has been reported to occur in the mouth of Siberian huskies and the mouth and lips of cats. The following comments apply only to eosinophilic granulomas of the stomach and intestine.

Gastrointestinal eosinophilic granulomas are an uncommon cause of vomiting or diarrhea in the dog.[171] They are most common in middle-aged dogs but can occur as early as 1 year of age. Rottweillers may be predisposed. The most consistent sign of eosinophilic granuloma is vomiting, reflective of either gastric involvement in the granulomatous process or intestinal obstruction. Peripheral eosinophilia may be present. Ultrasonographic evidence of a gastric or intestinal mass may be noted. Endoscopy may reveal focal thickenings of the mucosa.

Eosinophilic granulomas often involve the entire thickness of the bowel wall, as shown in Figure 24–12. Concurrent mesenteric eosinophilic lymphadenopathy may occur. Important differential diagnoses include neoplasia, visceral larval migrans, and other cause of granulomatous inflammation such as phycomycosis and regional enteritis (Table 24–2).[171] A similar process has been described in association with actinobacillosis-like club colonies in the ileocolic region of a dog.[177]

Eosinophilic granulomas can be successfully removed surgically, but limited experience has shown that they recur if controlled diets and glucocorticoid therapy are not continued postsurgically.

HISTIOCYTIC COLITIS

Clinical Synopsis

Diagnostic Features

- Intractable large-bowel diarrhea of greater than several weeks duration
- Boxers are commonly affected
- Endoscopy usually reveals colonic ulceration
- Histopathology shows colonic inflammation in which PAS-positive histiocytes are conspicuous

Standard Treatment

- Selected protein, highly digestible controlled diet(s) containing fermentable fiber
- Add Metamucil (1–6 teaspoons/meal) if controlled diet low in fiber
- Sulfasalazine (12.5 mg/kg q 6 hours PO for 14 days followed by 12.5 mg/kg 12 hours for 28 days) in combination with prednisone
- Prednisone: 1 to 2 mg/kg q 12 hours PO for 1 to 2 weeks; followed by 1.0 mg/kg q 24 hours PO for 4 weeks; followed by 0.5 to 1.0 mg/kg qod PO for 4 weeks; followed by a tapered withdrawal over 2 weeks

Follow-up

- Withdraw the drug therapy and attempt to maintain on selected-protein/fermentable fiber diet for 6 to 12 months
- Thereafter, consider oral challenge trials to help determine suitability of standard (mixed-protein source) pet foods
- Repeat drug therapy if recurrence

Histiocytic colitis is a chronic, idiopathic inflammatory disease of the large bowel characterized by a mixed inflammatory infiltrate in which PAS-positive histiocytes (engorged macrophages) are a prominent feature. The disease tends to have a more ulcerative nature than chronic idiopathic (lymphocytic-plasmacytic) colitis and is more refractory to treatment.

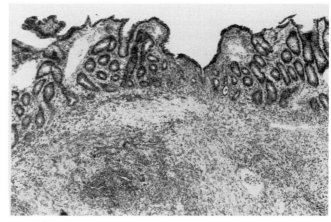

FIGURE 24–12. Eosinophilic granuloma in intestine. Granuloma in submucosa produced signs of intestinal obstruction. Diffuse infiltration of mucosa by eosinophils. Total villus atrophy at site of granuloma and partial loss of crypt epithelium.

Prevalence and Signalment

Boxer dogs are predisposed to histiocytic colitis,[178,179] but the disease has also been reported in the French bulldog[180] and the cat.[181] The disease has a relatively high prevalence in boxers as does chronic idiopathic colitis. It affects primarily young dogs.

Etiopathogenesis

The etiopathogenesis of histiocytic colitis is unknown. In early lesions, normal-appearing macrophages can often be seen near the luminal surface of the lamina propria, whereas the basilar regions of the mucosa contain distended periodic acid–Schiff (PAS) positive histiocytes. This observation has been taken to suggest that the histiocytes are transporting engulfed foreign material from the mucosa which they are unable to digest. Therefore, the pathogenesis of the disease may have similarities to the ulcerative colitis induced by carrageenan and related sulfated polysaccharides (see earlier). An infectious etiology has also been suggested. An ultrastructural study of the histiocytes suggested they contain a Chlamydia-like agent.[47] However, a second study failed to confirm these findings[48] and no studies to date have shown that histiocytic colitis is a transmissible disease. Similarly, the disease does not appear to be due to a vascular abnormality. Vascular dilation and hypervascularity can be seen late in the course of the disease. Ulceration results in complete disruption of the normal mucosal microvascular bed, which is replaced with an unorganized tangle of ectatic vessels. However, microangiography has demonstrated that vascular changes do not appear in the early stages of the disease.[70]

Ulceration of the mucosa in histiocytic colitis is thought to result from a failure of crypt cell proliferation to keep pace with the degenerating and desquamating surface epithelial cells. The engorgement of the lamina propria with histiocytes does not cause mechanical rupture.

Clinical and Diagnostic Findings

In general the clinical signs are those of large-bowel-type diarrhea. The clinical signs are similar to chronic idiopathic colitis but are usually more severe. About one-third of the animals with histiocytic colitis show tenesmus, and nearly all pass blood in the feces. Laboratory findings are usually unremarkable. The endoscopy findings are similar to chronic colitis, with the exception of a greater prevalence of well-circumscribed ulcers.

BIOPSY FINDINGS. Morphologic changes characteristic of chronic histiocytic colitis have been well described.[48,178,182,183] The earliest morphologic change discernible is epithelial cell degeneration and focal, acute inflammation at the luminal surface of the colon. Electron microscopy indicates that epithelial cell injury is the initial morphologic lesion, followed by acute inflammation and then necrosis and ulceration. The inflamed lamina propria contains neutrophils and a heavy infiltration of eosinophilic foamy macrophages (histiocytes).[98] Neutrophils appear in response to the ulceration and do not participate in producing the initial lesion. Histiocytes are normally only present in small numbers in the colonic lamina propria. In histiocytic colitis their numbers increase markedly once the colonic epithelium is disrupted, and they become engorged with PAS-positive polysaccharides (Figure 24–13). Some report that granulomas are a consistent feature of chronic histiocytic ulcerative colitis, whereas others claim this

is not the case. The disagreement may be due to differences in chronicity and severity. Epithelioid and giant cell granulomas, found with advanced disease, can become transmural.

Treatment

The treatment of histiocytic colitis must be more aggressive than that of chronic colitis. A combination of controlled diet, sulfasalazine, and prednisone, as described in the clinical synopsis, is a useful starting point. Some dogs will respond to this treatment regimen. Other dogs will require more potent immunosuppression, whereupon combination prednisone and azathioprine therapy can be utilized. Important details concerning the controlled diets and drugs used in the treatment of histiocytic colitis can be found in the general section on therapy of inflammatory bowel disease.

Prognosis

The prognosis is guarded to poor unless treatment is begun very early in the disease course.

GRANULOMATOUS INFLAMMATORY BOWEL DISEASE

Granulomatous Enteritis, Colitis, and Enterocolitis

Granulomatous enteritis, colitis, and enterocolitis are rare idiopathic inflammatory diseases of the small or large bowel characterized by the presence of aggregates of histiocytes in the lamina propria.[153] PAS-positive histiocytes are not a feature. In contrast to transmural granulomatous enterocolitis, this process is more diffuse in distribution. These diseases are seen in both the cat and the dog. Clinical signs and diagnostic procedures are similar to the other inflammatory bowel diseases. Treatment is also similar. Great care must be taken to rule out the infectious causes of granulomatous enteritis such as FIP, histoplasmosis, phycomycosis, and tuberculosis (Table 24–2) before a patient is placed on immunosuppressive therapy. The prognosis is guarded.

Transmural Granulomatous Enterocolitis (Regional Enteritis)

Transmural granulomatous enterocolitis is seen rarely in dogs and cats.[98,138] The majority of affected dogs have been males of less than 4 years.[184] The disease is usually segmental and discontinuous in distribution and most often affects the lower ileum, cecum, colon, and draining lymph nodes.[153] Clinical signs are similar to chronic colitis with the exception that weight loss is prominent and that violent vomiting, hematemesis, and constipation can occur due to obstruction of the ileum, colon, or rectum by the granulomatous process. Abdominal palpation may reveal an abdominal mass in the ileocecal area. Rectal palpation occasionally will detect strictures or mucosal thickenings. Perianal location of the granulomatous inflammation can lead to perianal fistulation. Mild to moderate peripheral eosinophilia is common, and

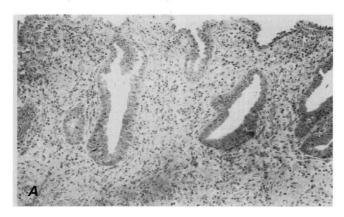

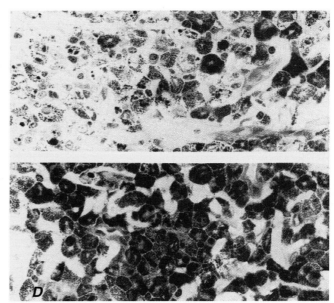

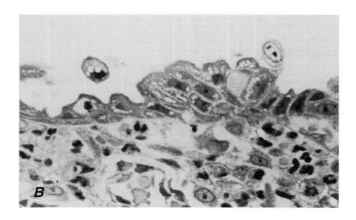

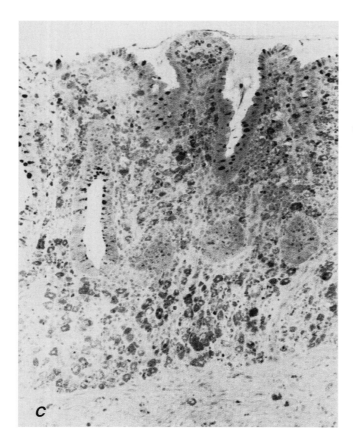

FIGURE 24–13. (A) Biopsy of colon from boxer with chronic histiocytic ulcerative colitis. Marked infiltration of lamina propria with histiocytes. Other forms of inflammatory cells are numerous. Few goblet cells are evident. Cell infiltrate has caused marked splaying of glands. Pathologic changes extended throughout submucosa (not shown). (B) Epithelial changes involve all cells lining mucosal surface. (C) PAS-stained section shows granules in histiocytes with varying amounts of PAS staining material. Goblet cells also stain dark with PAS stain. Relative numbers of goblet cells is low. (D) Higher magnification of PAS-staining granules in histiocytes showing different degrees of severity.

eosinophils form a significant component of the inflammatory infiltrate.[184,185] Colonoscopy reveals single or multiple discontinuous areas of mucosal proliferation associated with mucosal rigidity, ulceration, and luminal narrowing. Important differential diagnoses are listed in Table 24–2 and include parasitic granulomas from whipworms or hookworms,[186] scirrhous intestinal carcinoma,[98] and Campylobacter-associated proliferative enteritis.[187] Treatments attempted to date have included surgical resection of affected areas, tylosin, and prednisone therapy. Temporary improvement has been seen following surgery or prednisone therapy, but relapses are common. The prognosis is poor.

CHRONIC SUPPURATIVE COLITIS

Neutrophils are a minor component of the inflammatory infiltrate of many chronic gastrointestinal inflammatory disorders and a major component of the cellular response in acute gastrointestinal inflammation. The ubiquitous presence of neutrophils is not surprising given the variety of products that causes their chemotaxis (Chapter 4) and the diverse range of pathologic processes that incite the release of these mediators. On rare occasions, the neutrophil is a prominent or even dominant cell in chronic idiopathic inflammation. This condition is referred to as chronic suppurative colitis. In the author's experience, and that of others,[188] this entity is most common in cats. The cause of the chronic suppurative inflammation is unknown. The most important differential diagnoses are bacterial enteropathogens such as Salmonella and Clostridia. Chronic colonic abrasion from ingested hair has also been suggested as a possible cause. Suggested treatments have included sulfasalazine or antibiotics such as calvulinic acid-amoxicillin. For cats suspected of hair-induced colitis, the administration of laxatives and more frequent brushing of the cat's coat may be useful.

IMMUNOPROLIFERATIVE ENTEROPATHY OF BASENJIS

Immunoproliferative enteropathy of basenji dogs is characterized by chronic diarrhea, and a spectrum of gastrointestinal pathology including hypertrophic-gastropathy and lymphocytic plasmacytic inflammation of the small intestine.[189-193] It is distinguished from LPE by its high prevalence in basenjis; by its more severe, progressive, and refractory nature; by concomitant hypergammaglobulinemia and elevated serum IgA concentrations; and by the high incidence of a concurrent hypertrophic gastropathy. The prevalence in the basenji breed may approach 3%.[191]

The etiopathogenesis of the disease is unknown, although both genetic and environmental factors appear to be involved. Altered gastric acid secretory capacity may play a role, particularly in the dogs with diarrhea.[194] The disease is thought to bear similarities to immunoproliferative enteropathy of humans.

There is no sex predisposition. Most affected basenjis develop diarrhea by the time they are 3 years of age. The clinical signs include anorexia, progressive weight loss, and intractable diarrhea. Vomiting is occasionally noted. The gastrointestinal signs are frequently precipitated by stressful events. Ulcerative dermatitis of the pinnae is occasionally seen. Neurologic signs, including incoordination, paresis, circling, and seizures, were seen in some affected basenjis after vaccination. Progression of the disease to abdominal lymphoma can occur.

Hypoproteinemia, hypoalbuminemia, hypergammaglobulinemia, mature leukocytosis, and mild nonregenerative anemia are present in many basenji dogs.[192] Malabsorption is often present, and concurrent maldigestion is suspected. The maldigestion has been attributed to functional pancreatic insufficiency because the pancreas is histologically normal.[189]

The pathologic findings vary considerably. Gastric rugal hypertrophy, lymphocytic gastritis, and gastric mucosal atrophy occur in 50% of affected basenjis.[189] All affected dogs have moderate or severe intestinal lesions dominated by villus clubbing and fusion, increased tortuosity of intestinal crypts, and diffuse infiltration of mononuclear inflammatory cells of which lymphocytes and plasma cells predominate.[189] The colon is usually not affected by the disease but a mild glomerulonephritis is often present. Examination of the gastrointestinal tracts of asymptomatic basenjis reveals lesions that are similar to but milder than those of affected dogs.

Immunosuppressive doses of corticosteroids and therapy with tylosin, metronidazole, or trimethoprim sulfa can ameliorate the signs, but the beneficial effect is usually temporary. Affected basenjis tolerated Iam's diets well. The prognosis is guarded to poor. Most dogs die within 2 years of diagnosis, although survival for as long as 5 years has been reported.

DIARRHEAL SYNDROME IN LUDENHUNDS

A diarrheal syndrome in Ludenhunds characterized by chronic, idiopathic lymphocytic-plasmacytic inflammation of the small intestine has been described.[195] A mixed infiltrate is present in which lymphocytes and plasma cells predominate. Intestinal protein loss is common. The disease is distinguished from LPE by its progressive nature and breed predisposition. The prognosis is poor.

REFERENCES

1. Strober W, James SP. The immunological basis of inflammatory bowel disease. J Clin Immunol 6:415–432, 1986.
2. Geller AJ, Das KM. Etiology of inflammatory bowel disease. Cur Opin Gastroenterol 6:561–564, 1990.
3. Matthews JGW. Experimental ischemic colitis in the dog. In: Pfeiffer CJ (ed) Animal Models of Colitis. CRC Press, Boca Raton, FL, 161–180, 1985.
4. Podolsky DK, Isselbacher KJ. Composition of human colonic mucin: Selective alteration in inflammatory bowel disease. J Clin Invest 72:142–153, 1983.
5. Podolsky DK, Isselbacher KJ. Glycoprotein composition of colonic mucosa. Gastroenterology 87:991–998, 1984.
6. Mayer EA, Raybould H, Koelbel C. Neuropeptides, inflammation, and motility. Dig Dis Sci 33:71S–77S, 1988.
7. Chiodini RJ, Van Kruiningen HJ, Thayer WR, et al. Possible role of mycobacteria in inflammatory bowel disease. I. An unclassified Mycobacterium species isolated from patients with Crohn's disease. Dig Dis Sci 29:1073–1079, 1984.
8. Jewell DP, Patel C. Immunology of inflammatory bowel disease. Scan J Gastroenterol (suppl) 114, 20:120–126, 1985.
9. Strober SP, Quinn TC, Danovitch SH. Crohn's disease. New concepts of pathogenesis and current approaches to treatment. Dig Dis Sci 32:1297–1310, 1987.
10. Strober W, James SP. The immunopathogenesis of gastrointestinal and hepatobiliary diseases. J Am Med Assoc 258:2962–2969, 1987.
11. Hodgson HJF. Inflammatory bowel disease and food intolerance. J Royal College Physicians, London 20:45–48, 1986.
12. Shean FC, Barker WF, Fonkalsrud EW. Studies on active and passive antibody induced colitis in the dog. Am J Surg 107:337–339, 1964.
13. Guilford WG, Olander H, Strombeck DR. Experimental canine colitis. Unpublished observations, 1988.
14. Strickland RG, Jewell DP. Immunoregulatory mechanisms in nonspecific inflammatory bowel disease. Ann Rev Med 34:195–204, 1983.
15. MacDermott RP, Nash GS, Bertovich MJ, et al. Altered patterns of secretion of monomeric IgA and IgA subclass 1 by intestinal mononuclear cells in inflammatory bowel disease. Gastroenterology 91:379–385, 1986.
16. Peterson JL, Willard MD, Lees GE, et al. Toxoplasmosis in two cats with inflammatory intestinal disease. J Am Vet Med Assoc 199:473–476, 1991.
17. Kirsner JB. Chronic inflammatory bowel disease: Overview of etiology and pathogenesis. In: Berk JE, Haubrich WS, Kalser MH, et al. (eds) Bockus Gastroenterology, 4th ed. WB Saunders, Philadelphia, 2093–2126, 1985.
18. Wold AE, Dahlgren UIH, Hanson LA, et al. Difference between bacterial and food antigens in mucosal immunogenicity. Infect Immun 57:2666–2673, 1989.
19. Targan SR, Kagnoff MF, Brogan MD, et al. Immunologic mechanisms in intestinal diseases. UCLA Conference. Ann Int Med 106:853–870, 1987.
20. Markowitz J, Daum F, Cohen, SA, et al. Immunology of inflammatory bowel disease: Summary of the subcommittee on immunosuppressive use in IBD. J Pediatr Gastroenterol Nutr 12:411–423, 1991.
21. Mayer L, Eisenhardt D. Lack of induction of suppressor T-cells by gut epithelial cells from patients with inflammatory bowel disease: The primary defect? Gastroenterology 92:1524, 1987.
22. Lagercrantz R, Hammarstrom S, Perlmann P, et al. Immunological studies in ulcerative colitis. IV. Origin of autoantibodies. J Exp Med 128:1339–1352, 1968.
23. Snook J. Are the inflammatory bowel diseases autoimmune disorders? Gut 31:961–963, 1990.
24. Roche JK, Fiocchi C, Youngman K. Sensitization to epithelial antigens in chronic mucosal inflammatory disease. I. Purification, characterization, and immune reactivity of murine epithelial cell-associated components. J Immunol 131:2796–2804, 1983.
25. Vecchi M, Sakamaki S, Diamond B, et al. A human colon specific antigen reactive with ulcerative colitis colon tissue–bound IgG. Gastroenterology 90:1679A, 1986.
26. Fiocchi C, Roch JK, Sapatnekar W. Familial immune reactivity to intestinal epithelial cell-associated components in inflammatory bowel disease. Gastroenterology 90:1415, 1986.
27. Shorter RG, Huizenga KA, ReMine SG, et al. Effects of preliminary incu-

bation of lymphocytes with serum on their cytotoxicity for colonic epithelial cells. Gastroenterology 58:843–850, 1970.

28. Broberger O, Perlmann P. In vitro studies of ulcerative colitis. I. Reactions of patient's serum with human fetal colon cells in tissue cultures. J Exp Med 117:705–716, 1963.
29. Roche JK, Fiocchi C, Youngman K. Sensitization to epithelial antigens in chronic mucosal inflammatory disease. J Clin Invest 75:522–530, 1985.
30. LeVeen HH, Falk G, Schatman B. Experimental ulcerative colitis produced by anticolon sera. Ann Surg 154:275–280, 1961.
31. Bicks RO, Walker RH. Immunologic colitis in dogs. Am J Dig Dis 7:574–584, 1962.
32. Stewart THM, Hetenyi C, et al. Ulcerative enterocolitis in dogs induced by drugs. J Pathol 131:363–378, 1980.
33. Bjarnason I, Giuseppe Z, Smith T, et al. Nonsteroidal antiinflammatory drug-induced intestinal inflammation in humans. Gastroenterology 93:480–489, 1987.
34. Kaufmann HJ, Taubin HL. Non-steroidal antiinflammatory drugs activate quiescent inflammatory bowel disease. Ann Int Med 107:513–516, 1987.
35. Bjarnason I, Peters TJ. Intestinal permeability, non-steroidal anti-inflammatory drug enteropathy and inflammatory bowel disease: An overview. Gut Festschrift, 22–28, 1989.
36. Bjarnason I, Williams P, Smethurst P, et al. Effect of non-steroidal anti-inflammatory drugs and prostaglandins on the permeability of the human small intestine. Gut 27:1292–1297, 1986.
37. Moeller HC, Kirsner JB. The effect of drug-induced hypermotility on the gastrointestinal tract of dogs. Gastroenterology 26:303–310, 1954.
38. Leib MS, Hiler LA, Roth L, et al. Plasmacytic-lymphocytic colitis in the dog. Sem Vet Med Surg 4:241–246, 1989.
39. Nelson RW, Stookey LJ, Kazacos E. Nutritional management of idiopathic chronic colitis in the dog. J Vet Int Med 2:133–137, 1988.
40. Dobesh GD, Clemens T. Effect of dietary protein on porcine colonic microstructure and function. Am J Vet Res 48:862–865, 1987.
41. Finegold SM, Attebry HR, Sutter VL. Effect of diet on human fecal flora: Comparison of Japanese and American diets. Am J Clin Nutr 27:1456–1469, 1974.
42. Bruns P, Hood LF, Seeley HW. Effect of modified starch on the microflora of the small intestine and caecum of rats. Nutr Rep Intl 15:131–138, 1977.
43. Smith HW. Observations on the flora of the alimentary tract of animals and factors affecting its composition. J Path Bact 89:95–122, 1965.
44. Graham DY, Markesich DC, Yoshimura HH. Mycobacteria and inflammatory bowel disease. Results of culture. Gastroenterology 92:436, 1987.
45. Parent K, Mitchell P. Cell wall-defective variants of pseudomonas-like (Group Va) bacteria in Crohn's disease. Gastroenterology 75:368–372, 1978.
46. Gitnick GL, Rosen VJ, Arthur MH, et al. Evidence for the isolation of a new virus from ulcerative colitis patients. Dig Dis Sci 24:609–619, 1979.
47. Van Kruiningen HJ. The ultrastructure of macrophages in granulomatous colitis of boxer dogs. Vet Path 12:446–459, 1975.
48. Gomez JA, Russell SW, Trowbridge JW, et al. Canine histiocytic ulcerative colitis: An ultrastructural study of the early mucosal lesion. Am J Dig Dis 22:485–496, 1977.
49. Onderdonk AB, Hermos JA, et al. Protective effect of metronidazole in experimental ulcerative colitis. Gastroenterology 74:521–526, 1978.
50. Okayasu I, Hatakeyama S, Yamada M, et al. A novel method in the induction of reliable experimental acute and chronic ulcerative colitis in mice. Gastroenterology 98:694–702, 1990.
51. Nicklin S, Miller K. Intestinal uptake and immunological effects of carrageenan—current concepts. Foods Additives Contaminants 6:425–436, 1989.
52. van der Waaij D, Cohen BJ, Anver MR. Mitigation of experimental inflammatory bowel disease in guinea pigs by selective elimination of the aerobic gram-negative intestinal microflora. Gastroenterology 67:460–472, 1974.
53. Seidman E, LeLeiko N, Ament M, et al. Nutritional issues in pediatric inflammatory bowel disease. J Pediatr Gastroenterol Nutr 12:424–438, 1991.
54. Kraft SC, Kirsner JB. Immunological apparatus of the gut and inflammatory bowel disease. Gastroenterology 60:922–951, 1971.
55. Harris ML, Bayless TM. Dietary antigens as aggravating factors in Crohn's disease. Dig Dis Sci 34:1613–1614, 1989.
56. Hayden DW, Van Kruiningen HJ. Lymphocytic-plasmacytic enteritis in German shepherd dogs. J Am Anim Hosp Assoc 18:89–96,1982.
57. Heyman MB. Food sensitivity and eosinophilic gastroenteropathies. In: Sleisinger MH, Fordtran JS (eds) Gastrointestinal Disease: Pathophysiology, Diagnosis, Management, 4th ed. WB Saunders, Philadelphia, 1113–1134, 1989.
58. Rolfe RD. Interactions among microorganisms of the indigenous intestinal flora and their influence on the host. Rev Infect Dis 6:S73–S79, 1984.
59. Leib MS. Stagnant loop syndrome. Sem Vet Med Surg 2:257–265, 1987.
60. Halpern B, Zweibaum R, et al. Experimental immune ulcerative colitis. In: Immunopathology International Symposium, Schwarbe, Basel-Stuttgart, 161–178, 1967.

61. Sartor RB, Schwab JH, et al. Granulomatous enterocolitis induced by bacterial cell wall fragments. Gastroenterology (abstract) 80:1271, 1981.
62. Chester JF, Ross JS, Malt RA, et al. Acute colitis produced by chemotactic peptides in rats and mice. Am J Pathol 121:284–290, 1985.
63. LeDuc LE, Nast CC. Chemotactic peptide-induced acute colitis in rabbits. Gastroenterology 98:929–935, 1990.
64. Hayden DW, van Kruiningen HJ. Eosinophilic gastroenteritis in German shepherd dogs and its relationship to visceral larva migrans. J Am Vet Med Assoc 162:379–384, 1973.
65. Hall EJ, Batt RM. Enhanced intestinal permeability to 51Cr-labeled EDTA in dogs with small intestinal disease. J Am Vet Med Assoc 196:91–95, 1990.
66. Strober W. Animal models of inflammatory bowel disease—an overview. Dig Dis Sci 30:3s–11s, 1985.
67. Ramage JK, Hunt RH, Perdue MH. Changes in intestinal permeability and epithelial differentiation during inflammation in the rat. Gut 29:57–61, 1988.
68. Madara JL. Gamma-interferon (Gamma-IFN) enhances intestinal epithelial permeability by altering tight junctions. Gastroenterology 94:A276, 1988.
69. Grisham MB, Granger DN. Neutrophil-mediated mucosal injury. Dig Dis Sci 33:6S–15S, 1988.
70. Lawson TL, Gomez JA, Margulis AR. Vascular alterations in canine histiocytic ulcerative colitis. Invest Radiol 10:212–224, 1975.
71. Whorwell PJ, Wright R. Immunological aspects of inflammatory bowel disease. Clin Gastroenterol 5:303–321, 1976.
72. Talley NJ, Kephart GM, McGovern TW, et al. Deposition of eosinophilic granule major basic protein in eosinophilic gastroenteritis and celiac disease. Gastroenterology 103:137–145, 1992.
73. Perdue MH, Forstner JF, Roomi NW, et al. Epithelial response to intestinal anaphylaxis in rats: Goblet cell secretion and enterocyte damage. Am J Physiol 247:G632–G637, 1984.
74. Tizard I. Veterinary Immunology. WB Saunders, Philadelphia, 1987.
75. Ferguson A. Models of intestinal hypersensitivity. Clin Gastroenterol 5:271–288, 1976.
76. Rabin BS, Rogers SJ. A cell-mediated immune model of inflammatory bowel disease in the rabbit. Gastroenterology 75:29–33, 1978.
77. Glick ME, Falchuk ZM. Dinitrochlorobenzene-induced colitis in guinea pigs. Gut 22:120–125, 1981.
78. Simmonds NJ, Allen RE, Stevens TRJ, et al. Chemiluminescence assay of mucosal reactive metabolites in inflammatory bowel disease. Gastroenterology 103:186–196, 1992.
79. Brynskov J, Nielsen OH, Ahnfelt-Ronne I, et al. Cytokines in inflammatory bowel disease. Scand J Gastroenterol 27:897–906, 1992.
80. Lichtman SN, Sartor RB. Examining the role of inflammatory cytokines in chronic inflammatory bowel disease. J Pediatr Gastroenterol Nutr 16:239–240, 1993.
81. Tran DD, Visser JJ, Pool MO, et al. Enhanced systemic nitric oxide production in inflammatory bowel disease (letter). Lancet 341:1150, 1993.
82. Cominelli F, Kam L. Inflammatory mediators of inflammatory bowel disease. Cur Opin G 9:534–543, 1993.
83. Sethi AK, Sarna SK. Colonic motor activity in acute colitis in conscious dogs. Gastroenterology 100:954–963, 1991.
84. Travis SPL, Jewel DP. Mechanisms of diarrhea in ulcerative colitis (correspondence). Gastroenterology 105:643, 1993.
85. MacPherson BR, Shearin NL, Pfeiffer CJ. Experimental diffuse colitis in cats: Observations on motor changes. J Surg Res 25:42–49, 1978.
86. Jergens AE, Moore FM, Haynes JS, et al. Idiopathic inflammatory bowel disease in dogs and cats: 84 cases (1987–1990). J Am Vet Med Assoc 201:1603–1608, 1992.
87. Danzi JT. Extraintestinal manifestations of idiopathic inflammatory bowel disease. Arch Int Med 148:297–302, 1988.
88. Rabin BS, Rogers SJ. Pathologic changes in the liver and kidney produced by immunization with intestinal antigens. Am J Pathol 84:201–210, 1976.
89. Cello JP, Schneiderman DJ. Ulcerative colitis. In: Sleisenger MH, Fordtran JS (eds) Gastrointestinal Disease: Pathophysiology, Diagnosis, Management, 4th ed. WB Saunders, Philadelphia, 1435–1475, 1989.
90. Desmet VJ, Geboes K. Liver lesions in inflammatory bowel disorders. J Pathol 151:247–255, 1987.
91. Pedersen NC, Weisner K, Castles JJ, et al. Noninfectious canine arthritis: The inflammatory non-erosive arthritides. J Am Vet Med Assoc 169:304–310, 1976.
92. Center SA, Crawford MA, Guida L, et al. A retrospective study of 77 cats with severe hepatic lipidosis: 1975–1990. J Vet Int Med 7:349–359, 1993.
93. Leib MS. Feline inflammatory bowel disease—a critical review. Proc Am Col Int Med, Washington DC, 114–117, May 1993.
94. Dennis JS, Kruger JM, Mullaney TP. Lymphocytic/plasmacytic colitis in cats: 14 cases (1985–1990). J Am Vet Med Assoc 202:313–318, 1993.
95. Tams TR. Chronic feline inflammatory bowel disorders. I. Idiopathic inflammatory bowel disease. Comp Contin Ed Pract Vet 8:371–376, 1986.
96. Tams TR. Feline inflammatory bowel disease. Vet Clin N Am 23:569–586, 1993.

97. Feinstein RE, Olsson E. Chronic gastroenterocolitis in nine cats. J Vet Diag Invest 4:293–298, 1992.

98. Wilcox B. Endoscopic biopsy interpretation in canine or feline enterocolitis. Sem Vet Med Surg 7:162–171, 1992.

99. Leib MS. Gastrointestinal endoscopy: Endoscopic and histologic correlation. Proc 7th ACVIM Forum, 784–786, 1989.

100. Roth L, Walton AM, Leib MS, et al. A grading system for lymphocytic plasmacytic colitis in dogs. J Vet Diag Invest 2:257–262, 1990.

101. Jacobs G, Collins-Kelly L, Lappin M, et al. Lymphocytic-plasmacytic enteritis in 24 dogs. J Vet Int Med 4:45–53, 1990.

102. Surawicz CM, Belic L. Rectal biopsy helps to distinguish acute self-limited colitis from idiopathic inflammatory bowel disease. Gastroenterology 86:104–113, 1984.

103. Hart IR. The distribution of immunoglobulin-containing cells in canine small intestine. Res Vet Sci 27:269–274, 1979.

104. Payne-James JJ, Silk DBA. Total parenteral nutrition as primary treatment in Crohn's disease—RIP? Gut 29:1304–1308, 1988.

105. Jones VA. Comparison of total parenteral nutrition and elemental diet in induction of remission of Crohn's disease. Dig Dis Sci 32:100S–107S, 1987.

106. Whittaker JS. Nutritional therapy of hospitalized patients with inflammatory bowel disease. Dig Dis Sci 32:89S–94S, 1987.

107. Fuchs GJ, Grand RJ Motil KJ. Malnutrition and nutritional support in inflammatory bowel disease. Nutritional Support Services 5:28–33, 1985.

108. Rhodes J, Rose J. Does food affect acute inflammatory bowel disease? The role of parenteral nutrition, elemental and exclusion diets. Gut 27:471–474, 1986.

109. Teahon K, Bjarnason I, Pearson M, et al. Ten years' experience with an elemental diet in the management of Crohn's disease. Gut 31:1133–1137, 1990.

110. Rigaud D, Cosnes J, Le Quintrec Y, et al. Controlled trial comparing two types of enteral nutrition in treatment of active Crohn's disease. Elemental vs polymeric diet. Gut 32:1492–1497, 1991.

111. Raouf AH, Hildrey V, Daniel J, el al. Enteral feeding as sole treatment for Crohn's disease: Controlled trial of whole protein v amino acid based feed and a case study of dietary challenge. Gut 32:702–707, 1991.

112. LeVeen EG, Falk G, Ip M, et al. Urease as a contributing factor in ulcerative lesions of the colon. Am J Surg 135:53–56, 1978.

113. Washabau RJ, Strombeck DR, Buffington CA, et al. Evaluation of intestinal carbohydrate malabsorption in the dog by pulmonary gas excretion. Am J Vet Res 47:1402–1406, 1986.

114. Cummings JH, Wiggins HS, Jenkins DJA, et al. Influence of diets high and low in animal fat on bowel habit, gastrointestinal transit time, fecal microflora, bile acid, and fat excretion. J Clin Invest 61:953–963, 1978.

115. Lorenz R, Weber PC, Szimnau P, et al. Supplementation with n-3 fatty acids from fish oil in chronic inflammatory bowel disease—a randomized placebo-controlled double-blind cross-over trial. J Internal Med 225:(suppl) 225–232, 1989.

116. Stenson WF, Cort D, Rodgers J, et al. Dietary supplementation with fish oil in ulcerative colitis. Ann Internal Med 116:609–614, 1992.

117. Binder HJ, Sandle GI. Electrolyte absorption and secretion in the mammalian colon. In: Johnson LR (ed) Physiology of the Gastrointestinal Tract, 2nd ed. Raven Press, New York, 1389–1418, 1987.

118. Souba WW, Herskowitz K, Salloum RM, et al. Gut glutamine metabolism. J Parenteral Enteral Nutr 14:45S–50S, 1990.

119. Selby W. Current management of inflammatory bowel disease. J Gastroenterol Hepatol 8:70–83, 1983.

120. Hawthorne AB, Record CO, Holdsworth CD, et al. Double blind trial of oral fluicasone propionate v prednisolone in the treatment of active ulcerative colitis. Gut 34:125–128, 1993.

121. Johnson LR. Regulation of gastrointestinal growth. In: Johnson LR (ed) Physiology of the Gastrointestinal Tract, 2nd ed. Raven Press, New York, 301–333, 1987.

122. Tams TR. Chronic feline inflammatory bowel disorders. II. Feline eosinophilic enteritis and lymphosarcoma. Comp Contin Ed Pract Vet 8:464–471, 1986.

123. Schroder H, Lewkonia RM, Price Evans DA. Metabolism of salicylazosulfapyridine in healthy subjects and in patients with ulcerative colitis. Clin Pharm Ther 14:802–809, 1973.

124. Ewing GO, Gomez JA. Canine ulcerative colitis. J Am Anim Hosp Assoc 9:395–406, 1973.

125. Hanauer SB. Medical therapy of ulcerative colitis. Lancet 342:412–417, 1993.

126. Morgan RV, Bachrach A. Keratoconjunctivitis sicca associated with sulfonamide therapy in dogs. J Am Vet Med Assoc 180:432–434, 1982.

127. Barnett KC. Keratoconjunctivitis sicca and the treatment of canine colitis. Vet Rec 119:363, 1986.

128. Schroeder KW, Tremaine WJ, Ilstrup DM. Coated oral 5-aminosalicylic acid therapy for mildly to moderately active ulcerative colitis. N Eng J Med 317:1625–1629, 1987.

129. McPhee MS, Swan JT, Biddle WL, et al. Proctocolitis unresponsive to conventional therapy. Response to 5-aminosalicylic acid enemas. Dig Dis Sci 32:76S–81S, 1987.

130. Hawkey CJ, Hawthorne AB. Medical treatment of ulcerative colitis: Scoring the advances. Gut 29:1298–1303, 1988.

131. Ferry GD, Kirschner BS, Grand RJ, et al. Olsalazine versus sulfasalazine in mild to moderate childhood ulcerative colitis. J Pediatr Gastroenterol Nutr 17:32–38, 1993.

132. Grove DI, et al. Suppression of cell-mediated immunity by metronidazole. Int Arch Allergy Appl Immunol 54:422, 1977.

133. Miller JJ. The imidazoles as immunosuppressive agents. Transplant Proc 12:300–303, 1980.

134. Sanyal SN, Jamba L, Channan M. Effect of the antiprotozoal agent metronidazole (Flagyl) on absorptive and digestive functions of the rat intestine. Ann Nutr Metab 36:235–243, 1992.

135. Kikuchi T, Oikawa T, Inoue K, et al. The effect of antibiotics against the intestinal bacterial flora. In: Heneghan JB (ed) Germ-Free Research. Academic Press, New York, 355–359, 1973.

136. Jergens AE. Feline idiopathic inflammatory bowel disease. Comp Contin Ed Pract Vet 14:509–520, 1992.

137. Chiapella A. Diagnosis and management of chronic colitis in the dog and cat. In: Kirk RW (ed) Current Veterinary Therapy IX. WB Saunders, Philadelphia, 896–903, 1986.

138. Van Kruiningen HJ. Clinical efficacy of Tylosin in canine inflammatory bowel disease. J Am Anim Hosp Assoc 12:498–501, 1976.

139. De Novo RC. Therapeutics of gastrointestinal diseases. In: Kirk RW (ed) Current Veterinary Therapy. WB Saunders, Philadelphia, 862–872, 1986.

140. Gue M, Fioramonti J, Bueno L. A simple double radiolabeled technique to evaluate gastric emptying of canned food meal from dogs. Gastroenterol Clin Biol 12:425–430, 1988.

141. Christensen J. Motility of the colon. In: Johnson LR (ed) Physiology of the Gastrointestinal Tract, 2nd ed. Raven Press, New York, 665–693, 1987.

142. Vibe-Petersen G. Canine lymphocytic plasmacytic enteritis: An immunopathological investigation of intestinal plasma cells. Acta Vet Scand 32:221–232, 1991.

143. Tams TR. Canine lymphocytic plasmacytic enteritis. Comp Cont Ed Pract Vet 9:1184–1192, 1987.

144. Magne ML. Canine lymphocytic-plasmacytic enteritis. In: Kirk RW (ed) Current Veterinary Therapy X. WB Saunders, Philadelphia, 922–926, 1989.

145. Dennis JS, Kruger JM, Mullaney TP. Lymphocytic/plasmacytic gastroenteritis in cats: 14 cases (1985–1990). J Am Vet Med Assoc 200:1712–1718, 1992.

146. van der Gaag I, Happe RP. The histologic appearance of peroral small intestinal biopsies in clinically healthy dogs and dogs with chronic diarrhea. J Vet Med (A) 37:401–416, 1990.

147. Magne ML. Lymphocytic-plasmacytic enteritis. Pathogenesis. Proc ACVIM, 521–523, 1988.

148. Lake AM. Food protein-induced gastroenteropathy in infants and children. In: Metcalfe DD, Sampson HA, Simon RA (ed) Food Allergy, Adverse Reactions to Foods and Food Additives. Blackwell Scientific, Oxford, 174–185, 1991.

149. Diehl KJ, Lappin MR, Jones RL, et al. Monoclonal gammopathy in a dog with plasmacytic gastroenterocolitis. J Am Vet Med Assoc 201:1233–1236, 1992.

150. Salem PA, Nassar VH, Shadid MJ, et al. Mediterranean abdominal lymphoma or immunoproliferative small intestinal disease. Cancer 40:2941–2947, 1977.

151. Edwards DF, Russell RG. Probable vitamin K-deficient bleeding in two cats with malabsorption syndrome secondary to lymphocytic-plasmacytic enteritis. J Vet Int Med 1:97–101, 1987.

152. Jergens AE, Moore FM, March P, et al. Idiopathic inflammatory bowel disease associated with gastroduodenal ulceration-erosion: A report of 9 cases in the dog and cat. J Am Anim Hosp Assoc 28:21–26, 1992.

153. Barker IK, Van Dreumel AA. The alimentary system. In: Jubb KVF, Kennedy PC, Palmer N (eds) Pathology of Domestic Animals. Academic Press, Orlando, 1–202, 1985.

154. Batt RM, Bush BM, Peters TJ. Subcellular biochemical studies of a naturally occurring enteropathy in the dog resembling chronic tropical sprue in human beings. Am J Vet Res 44:1492–1496, 1983.

155. Jacobs G, Lappin M, Collins L. Lymphocytic-plasmacytic enteritis in 17 dogs. Proc ACVIM, 745, 1988.

156. Magne ML. Unpublished observations.

157. Houston DM. An intergrated study of colonic disease in the dog. Dissertation Abstracts International (B, Sciences and Engineering). 50:1278–1279, 1989.

158. Henroteaux M. Results of an endoscopic study of colitis in dogs; predominance of idiopathic colitis. Ann Med Vet 134:389–392, 1990.

159. Hottendorf GH, Hirth PS. Lesions of spontaneous sub-clinical disease in beagle dogs. Vet Path 11:240–258, 1974.

160. van der Gaag I, Happe RP. Follow-up studies by large intestinal biopsies and necropsy in dogs with clinical signs of large bowel disease. Can J Vet Res 53:473–476, 1989.

161. Reinhart GA, Moxley RA, Clemens ET. Dietary fiber source and its effects on colonic microstructure and histopathology of beagle dogs. Proc

Waltham Symposium on the Nutrition of Companion Animals, Adelaide (abstract) 79, 1993.

162. Scheppach W, Sommer H, Kirchner T, et al. Effect of butyrate enemas on the colonic mucosa in distal ulcerative colitis. Gastroenterology 103:51–56, 1992.

163. Penn D, Lebenthal E. Intestinal mucosal energy metabolism—a new approach to therapy of gastrointestinal disease. J Pediatr Gastroenterol Nutr 10:1–4, 1990.

164. Bo-Linn GW, Vendrell DD, Lee E, et al. An evaluation of the significance of microscopic colitis in patients with chronic diarrhea. J Clin Invest 75:1559–1569, 1985.

165. Kingham JGC. Microscopic colitis. Gut 32:234–235, 1991.

166. Yam PS, Simpson JW, Maskell IE, et al. Dietary management of chronic canine colitis (abstract). Proc Brit Sm Anim Vet Assoc Congress 206, 1994.

167. Bush BM. Colitis in the dog. Vet Ann 25:337–347, 1985.

168. Pidgeon GL. Chronic disorders of the exocrine pancreas, small bowel and large bowel. Vet Clin N Am 13:541–550, 1983.

169. Moore RP. Feline eosinophilic enteritis. In: Kirk RW (ed) Current Veterinary Therapy VIII. WB Saunders, Philadelphia, 791–793, 1983.

170. Hendricks M. A spectrum of hypereosinophilic syndromes exemplified by six cats with eosinophilic enteritis. Vet Pathol 18:188–200, 1981.

171. Johnson SE. Canine eosinophilic gastroenterocolitis. Sem Vet Med Surg 7:145–152, 1992.

172. Van der Gaag I, Happe RP, Wolvekamp WTC. Eosinophilic gastroenteritis complicated by partial ruptures and a perforation of the small intestine in a dog. J Sm Anim Pract 24:575–581, 1983.

173. Griffin HE, Meunier LD. Eosinophilic enteritis in a specific-pathogen-free cat. J Am Vet Med Assoc 197:619–620, 1990.

174. Narama I, Kuroda J, Nagatani M, et al. Superficial eosinophilic gastritis in laboratory beagle dogs attributable probably to diet. Jpn J Vet Sci 52:581–589, 1990.

175. Quigley PJ, Henry K. Eosinophilic enteritis in the dog: A case report with a brief review of the literature. J Comp Pathol 91:387–392, 1981.

176. Muir P, Gruffydd-Jones TJ, Brown PJ. Hypereosinophilic syndrome in a cat. Vet Rec 132:358–359, 1993.

177. van der Gaag I, van der Linde-Sipman JS, van Sluys FJ, et al. Regional eosinophilic coloproctitis, typhlitis and ileitis in a dog. Vet Q 12:1–6, 1990.

178. Van Kruiningen HJ. Granulomatous colitis of boxer dogs: Comparative aspects. Gastroenterology 53:114–122, 1967.

179. Hall EJ, Tennant BJ, Payne-Johnson CE, et al. Boxer colitis. Vet Rec 130:148, 1991.

180. Van der Gaag. I. Histiocytic ulcerative colitis in a French bull dog. J Sm Anim Pract 19:283–290, 1978.

181. Van Kruiningen HJ, Dobbins WO. Feline histiocytic colitis. A case report with electron microscopy. Vet Pathol 16:215–222, 1979.

182. Russell SW, Gomez JA, Trowbridge JO. Canine histiocytic ulcerative colitis. The early lesion and its progression to ulceration. Lab Invest 25:509–515, 1971.

183. Kennedy PC, Cello RM. Colitis of boxer dogs. Gastroenterology 51:926–931, 1966.

184. DiBartola SP, Rogers WA, Boyce JT, et al. Regional enteritis in two dogs. J Am Vet Med Assoc 181:904–908, 1982.

185. Van der Gaag I, van der Linde-Sipman JS. Eosinophilic granulomatous colitis with ulceration in a dog. J Comp Path 97:179–185, 1987.

186. Fletcher WD. Advanced granulomatous colitis in a Siberian husky. VM/SAC 73:1409, 1978.

187. Collins JE, Libal MC, Brost D. Proliferative enteritis in two pups. J Am Vet Med Assoc 183:886–889, 1983.

188. Leib MS, Sponenberg DP, Wilcke JR, et al. Suppurative colitis in a cat. J Am Vet Med Assoc 188:739–741, 1986.

189. MacLachlan NJ, Breitschwerdt EB, Chambers JM, et al. Gastroenteritis of basenji dogs. Vet Path 25:36–41, 1988.

190. Breitschwerdt EB, Halliwell WH, Foley CW, et al. A hereditary diarrhetic syndrome in the basenji characterized by malabsorption, protein losing enteropathy and hypergammaglobulinemia. J Am Anim Hosp Assoc 16:551–560, 1980.

191. Breitschwerdt EB, Waltman C, Hagstad HV, et al. Clinical and epidemiologic characterization of a diarrheal syndrome in basenji dogs. J Am Vet Med Assoc 180:914–920, 1982.

192. Breitschwerdt EB, Barta O, Waltman C, et al. Serum proteins in healthy basenjis and basenjis with chronic diarrhea. Am J Vet Res 44:326–328, 1983.

193. Breitschwerdt EB. Immunoproliferative enteropathy of basenjis. Sem Vet Med Surg 7:153–161, 1992.

194. Breitschwerdt EB, MacLachlan J, Argenzio RA, et al. Gastric acid secretion in basenji dogs with immunoproliferative enteropathy. J Vet Int Med 5:34–39, 1991.

195. Flesja K, Yri T. Protein-losing enteropathy in the Lundenhund. J Sm Anim Pract 18:11–23, 1977.

25 Intestinal Obstruction, Pseudo-Obstruction, and Foreign Bodies

W. GRANT GUILFORD AND DONALD R. STROMBECK

INTRODUCTION

Intestinal obstruction is a familiar presentation to most practitioners. Obstruction can occur in any part of the intestinal tract but most often develops in the small intestine as a result of its narrower caliber. Obstructions are usually classified as "simple" or "strangulated." In strangulated obstructions the enteric blood supply is compromised and in simple obstructions it is not. Obstruction can be partial of complete and in some cases partial obstructions progress to become complete. Partial intestinal obstruction can be very difficult to diagnose.

CAUSES OF INTESTINAL OBSTRUCTION

Intestinal obstruction (ileus) can result from a large number of causes (Table 25–1). Anatomic intestinal obstruction (mechanical ileus) can be caused by intraluminal foreign objects, intramural masses such as leiomyomas and hematomas, or extramural compression by such abnormalities as abdominal adhesions or entrapment.[1,2] Functional intestinal obstruction can result from transient hypomotility (paralytic or adynamic ileus) or from chronic intestinal neuromuscular derangements that cause persistent hypomotility (pseudo-obstruction) or spasticity (spastic or hyperdynamic ileus).

PATHOPHYSIOLOGY OF INTESTINAL OBSTRUCTION

Intestinal obstruction results in life-threatening complications such as dehydration, hypovolemia, electrolyte imbalances, and toxemia (Figure 25–1).

Fluid and Electrolyte Homeostasis

Fluid and electrolyte imbalances from gastrointestinal obstructions are caused primarily by vomiting but some fluid is lost by sequestration into the intestinal tract. After approximately 24 hours, the intestinal mucosa immediately cranial to the obstruction secretes instead of absorbs fluid. The stimulus for the secretion is unknown. It has been suggested that the fluid accumulating in obstructed loops may generate sufficient hydrostatic pressure to cause vascular stasis, ischemia-induced mucosal damage, and resultant fluid secretion. However, this seems unlikely because fluid accumulated orad of intestinal obstructions does not generate pressures greater than 5 to 10 mm Hg, and the mucosal changes above the obstruction are limited to blunted villi and shortened crypts rather than the necrosis more typical of ischemia (below the obstruction, villus atrophy is seen). Moreover, it has been demonstrated that the intestinal mucosa above an obstruction maintains its ability to absorb electrolytes, glucose, and amino acids at normal rates.[3] The only change is an increase in the flux of ions and water from the extracellular fluid into the intestine, suggesting the presence of a secretagogue. It now seems likely that enterotoxins, secreted by the large numbers of bacteria that accumulate in the obstructed loop, activate cyclic AMP–driven intestinal secretion. This suggestion is supported by recent findings, which show that intestinal obstruction in germ-free dogs does not result in secretion of fluid.[4]

The fluid lost contains potassium at three to four times higher concentrations than those in the extracellular fluid.[2] Hence, hypokalemia is likely, and depletion of total body potassium is a consistent feature of intestinal obstruction. Potassium losses contribute to general muscle weakness and to a loss of normal intestinal motility.

If the intestine is strangulated, blood loss can become a significant problem. Blood is lost into the lumen of the intestine, the wall of the bowel, and eventually the peritoneal cavity.[5] The quantity of blood lost will depend on the length of the intestinal segment incarcerated, and whether there is arterial and/or venous obstruction. Blood loss is greater when only venous drainage is obstructed.[5]

Bacterial Flora and Toxins

The numbers of intraluminal bacteria increase in obstructed intestinal segments as a result of mechanical obstruction to flow and/or loss of the migratory myoelectric

Table 25–1

CAUSES OF INTESTINAL OBSTRUCTION

Anatomic Obstruction
  Intraluminal obstruction
    Linear foreign bodies
    Nonlinear foreign bodies
  Intramural masses
    Neoplasia (adenocarcinoma, leiomyoma, leiomyosarcoma)
    Inflammatory bowel disease (eosinophilic granuloma, transmural
      granulomatous enteritis)
    Phycomycosis
    Strictures
    Hematoma
  Congenital lesions
    Atresia
  Extramural compression
    Adhesions
    Hernias
    Strangulation
    Intussusception
    Volvulus

Functional Obstruction
  Adynamic ileus
    Surgical operations
    Peritonitis
    Unrelieved mechanical obstruction
    Intestinal ischemia
    Gram negative sepsis
    Electrolyte imbalance (hypokalemia)
    Uremia
    Dysautonomia
    Spinal cord injury
    Anticholinergics
    Lead poisoning
  Spastic ileus
    Hirschsprung disease
  Pseudo-obstruction
    Lymphosarcoma
    Idiopathic sclerosing enteropathy
    SLE
    Amanita mushroom poisoning
    Phenothiazines
    Diabetes mellitus
    Others

complex. The migratory myoelectric complex functions to sweep small intestinal contents in the aboral direction, maintaining bacteria at low numbers.[6,7] The number of bacteria in the obstructed loops may approach that usually seen in the large bowel. The composition of the microflora changes toward that found in the feces or mouth.[8,9]

Overgrowth of bacteria and subsequent endotoxic shock is the most important cause of mortality with intestinal obstruction.[10] In conventionally reared animals, strangulation of the intestine usually results in death within 24 hours. In contrast, germ-free animals usually survive at least 23 weeks after intestinal strangulation. The survival of germ-free animals is due entirely to the absence of bacteria in the gastrointestinal tract. Instillation of broad-spectrum antibiotics into loops of strangulated intestine in conventionally reared animals converts a fatal problem to a nonfatal one, provided fluid and electrolyte balance is maintained.

Clostridia are the most important bacteria contributing to the death of obstructed animals. In particular, *Clostridium perfringens* is a very toxic organism in strangulated loops of intestine.[11] It is numerically one of the most important microorganisms in the microflora of the dog, and its numbers

increases further with bacterial overgrowth. *C. septicum* and *C. histolyticum* are also quite deadly, whereas most other species are nonpathogenic. Clostridial species produce toxins that are capable of killing the animal if absorbed into the circulation. Some of the lethal factors can cross a histologically normal mucosa but breaks in the mucosal barrier allow even more rapid absorption. The sites of many foreign body obstructions are ischemic and become necrotic and ulcerated, conditions that allow bacterial toxins to be readily absorbed. Abdominal surgery also compromises the mucosal barrier to toxins.[12] The toxic products pass from the intestine into the peritoneal cavity from whence absorption into the systemic circulation is very rapid.[5] Fluid collected from an obstructed intestine is rapidly lethal when injected into normal animals. Peritoneal fluid collected during strangulation obstruction of the intestine is also lethal when injected into normal animals.

CLINICAL SIGNS OF INTESTINAL OBSTRUCTION

The clinical signs of intestinal obstruction vary with the site of the lesion (Table 25–2), the degree of luminal obstruction, and the severity of the cardiovascular compromise. In general, the higher the obstruction and the more complete the luminal narrowing, the more acute and severe the clinical signs and the more rapid the progression to life-threatening physiologic derangements. The history will reveal the likelihood of the ingestion of a foreign body. Young animals, animals living in an unknown environment, and those with a persistently ravenous appetite are most likely to swallow foreign bodies. A history of recent ovariohysterectomy may be relevant because this procedure can be complicated by colonic stricture.[13,14] One consistent feature of the history is that the clinical signs persist despite medical treatment.

Vomiting

Vomiting is a consistent sign in all but the early phases of intestinal obstruction. In an experimental study in which the intestine of dogs was completely obstructed at a cranial site and the dogs then allowed to drink water ad libitum, only 10% of dogs vomited over a period of four days, and the amounts of vomitus were small.[15,16] During the first few days after experimental obstruction, fluid does not accumulate in

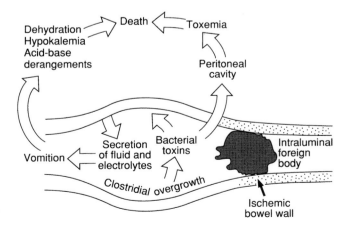

FIGURE 25–1. The pathophysiology of intestinal obstruction. Bacterial toxins induce intestinal secretion of fluid and electrolytes that is ultimately lost through vomition. Bacterial toxins absorbed through ischemic bowel wall produce toxemia.

Table 25–2

CLINICAL SIGNS OF INTESTINAL OBSTRUCTION AT DIFFERENT SITES
IN THE GASTROINTESTINAL TRACT

HIGH SMALL BOWEL	LOW SMALL BOWEL/ HIGH LARGE BOWEL	LOW LARGE BOWEL
Acute onset	Subacute onset	Subacute; chronic
Frequent vomiting	Vomiting less frequent	Vomiting infrequent
Fulminant progression	Insidious	Insidious
Large-volume vomitus	Smaller volume of vomitus	May be scant volume
May be feculent odor	Often feculent odor	Rarely feculent
Minimal abdominal distension	Often abdominal distension	Often abdominal distension
No constipation	No constipation	Often constipation
No tenesmus	No tenesmus	Tenesmus
Diarrhea	Diarrhea	Diarrhea

the intestine proximal to the site of obstruction. Vomiting at this stage is thought to be reflexive. As a result it is intermittent, and the volume of the vomitus may be scant. Thereafter, vomiting became more frequent, as fluid is eventually secreted at a rate sufficient to cause it to accumulate.

Following obstruction of the duodenum and proximal jejunum, vomiting is very frequent and voluminous whereas with obstruction of the ileum vomiting is less frequent and often of smaller volume. Proximal intestinal obstruction results in the vomiting of the large volumes of fluid that enter the intestine from the upper gastrointestinal tract. Distal obstructions, in contrast, result in the loss of lesser volumes of fluid because of the greater intestinal area available for absorption of secreted fluid. Complete intestinal obstruction usually produces persistent vomiting of copious volumes of fluid even in anorectic animals. In contrast, animals with partial obstructions may eat readily and vomit infrequently. The vomitus from animals with intestinal obstruction may have a fecal odor due to overgrowth of fecal-type bacteria.

The vomiting pattern that should raise the most suspicion of intestinal obstruction is the vomiting of copious amounts of feculent fluid by a depressed and anorectic animal. It is important to reemphasize, however, that intestinal obstruction can result in a wide variety of vomiting patterns, none of which are pathognomonic for the disease. In fact, some animals continue to eat and pass normal bowel movements with almost no vomiting at a time when a slowly progressive mass has nearly completely obstructed the intestine.

Diarrhea

Diarrhea is common in animals with partial obstruction of the small bowel. The diarrhea usually results from bacterial overgrowth. Bloody diarrhea is frequently seen in dogs with intussusceptions and is due to venous obstruction and ischemic necrosis of the entrapped intestinal segment. Complete obstructions do not usually cause diarrhea. On the contrary, they are often associated with a dry and tacky rectal mucosa, presumably as a result of hypovolemia and incipient shock.

Miscellaneous Clinical Signs

Additional clinical signs demonstrated by animals with intestinal obstruction are partial to complete anorexia, weakness, and depression. These signs often persist even when the fluid and electrolyte abnormalities have been corrected, probably because of continued absorption of toxins from the

obstructed intestinal loops. Abdominal pain may be apparent. In humans, abdominal pain from an intestinal obstruction is said to be initially episodic and to result from distension of the bowel and peristaltic efforts at moving the foreign body.[5] Early acute obstruction results in increased intestinal motility cranial to the obstruction and reduced motility caudal to the obstruction. The changes are due to stimulation of cholinergic nerves and the toxic effects of luminal contents.[17,18] Thereafter, the pain becomes more continuous and dull, a reflection of the onset of adynamic ileus or peritonitis.

PHYSICAL EXAMINATION FINDINGS IN INTESTINAL OBSTRUCTION

The diagnosis of intestinal obstruction is usually made by physical examination. Dehydration is a consistent finding, with the degree paralleling the frequency of vomiting. The oral cavity must be carefully examined for linear foreign bodies. Thorough palpation of the abdomen is essential. The abdominal palpation of deep-chested dogs is assisted by placing the front paws of the dog on a chair. This displaces movable abdominal contents caudally where they are more accessible to palpation. In intractable patients tranquilization may be necessary for an adequate examination. If the animal requires anesthesia during the course of diagnostic workup, it can be profitable to repeat the abdominal palpation because the anesthesia-induced muscle relaxation facilitates deep abdominal palpation. Great care must be taken to differentiate obstructive masses or foreign bodies from normal abdominal structures. Particular care must be taken not to confuse kidneys, fecal material, or the ileocecal area with an obstructive lesion. Palpation of an obstruction usually causes the animal more discomfort than the palpation of normal structures. Furthermore, accumulations of excessive intestinal gas and fluid orad to the obstruction are often palpable. Intestinal intussusceptions palpate as firm, tubular structures. Rectal examination may reveal rectal impactions or strictures. As mentioned earlier, complete obstructions are sometimes associated with a dry and tacky rectal mucosa.

Auscultation of the abdomen can contribute information on intestinal motility. Excessive noise is sometimes heard early in the obstructive process, possibly as a result of peristaltic rushes. Peristaltic rushes are thought to represent an attempt by the intestine to force content past the point of obstruction. The noise results from frequent peristaltic movements that propel fluid and gas rapidly through flaccid loops of intestine. These types of movement require the disappearance of segmentation motility. A silent abdomen identifies the loss of motility (adynamic ileus) and is suggestive of protracted obstruction or peritonitis.

Frequent reevaluation of patients suspected of intestinal obstruction is mandatory. Subsequent physical examination may reveal an obstruction initially overlooked or one that has developed after the initial examination. For instance, a foreign body may move from the stomach into the intestine where it can be palpated. Furthermore, young dogs with diseases such as acute gastroenteritis can develop secondary intussusception.

LABORATORY FINDINGS IN INTESTINAL OBSTRUCTION

Hemograms in animals with intestinal obstruction usually show nonspecific changes such as a stress response. A degenerative left shift is occasionally seen in severely affected animals, particularly following intestinal perforation.

Serum chemistry, electrolyte, and blood gas estimations are a valuable aid in selecting the appropriate fluid therapy for the patient. The laboratory findings with intestinal obstruction are variable and primarily reflect the severity of fluid and electrolyte imbalances. Hypokalemia. acidosis or alkalosis, and hyponatremia or hypernatremia may be seen. Pyloroduodenal obstructions often result in alkalosis and at times paradoxical aciduria. The PCV and total protein concentration may be elevated. The serum chemistry panel helps rule out renal, hepatic, and metabolic diseases as a cause of the clinical signs. Measurement of plasma electrolytes aids in identifying adrenocortical insufficiency. A normal serum lipase helps rule out acute pancreatitis, a disease with clinical signs that resemble those of intestinal obstruction. Provided it is carefully interpreted, the urinalysis provides valuable information on renal and liver function as well as hydration status.

RADIOGRAPHIC FINDINGS IN INTESTINAL OBSTRUCTION

If the patient's history, physical examination findings, and laboratory result are nondiagnostic but the clinician remains suspicious of intestinal obstruction, abdominal radiography should be performed. Radiography is an important aid in identifying intestinal obstruction but it is not a substitute for a well-conducted physical examination of the patient's abdomen.[19,20]

Survey Radiographs

Initial radiographic evaluation involves the use of survey radiographs. Obstructed loops of small intestines usually accumulate fluid or gas and consequently appear distended (Figure 25–2). In the obstructed intestine, the volume of gas formed usually exceeds the amount that can dissolve in the accumulated fluid and the excess appears as free gas. However, some obstructing lesions do not cause gas retention in the small bowel (Figure 25–3). The absence of accumulated gas makes the diagnosis of obstruction by survey radiography more difficult, but careful examination of the film may reveal fluid-distended loops or "hairpin bends." The latter refers to sharp bends in the small intestine caused by the weight of accumulated fluid in distended loops.

Although the detection of distended small-bowel loops suggests intestinal obstruction, it does not necessarily differ-

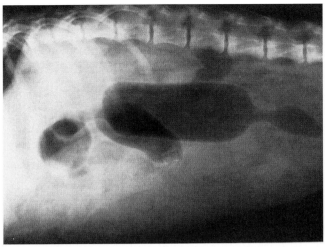

FIGURE 25-2. Lateral radiograph of abdomen of dog presented with clinical signs of intestinal obstruction. The loops of bowel are distended with fluid and gas. Diagnosis was made of intestinal obstruction, which ultimately was shown to be due to an intussusception in the caudal small intestine. Homogenous pattern of abdomen is due to accumulation of abdominal fluid.

entiate between physical and functional causes of obstruction. It is important that this differentiation is made because adynamic ileus is managed medically whereas mechanical obstruction requires surgical intervention. In many cases, discriminating between adynamic ileus and physical obstructions requires considerable clinical acumen. The factors that help clinicians differentiate between functional and anatomic ileus are listed in Table 25–3.

Radiopaque foreign bodies are readily demonstrated by survey radiography. Consideration should be given as to whether the foreign body is a "red herring" or whether it is causing an obstruction. Distended bowel loops associated with the foreign body are highly suggestive of obstruction (Figure 25–3).

Partial obstructions of the intestine often do not produce markedly dilated bowel loops but occasionally will be revealed by the "graveling sign." The graveling sign refers to the accumulation of indigestible material orad to the partial obstruction (Figure 25–4).

HORIZONTAL BEAM RADIOGRAPHS. Horizontal beam radiographs are helpful in confirming the presence of an obstruction but are usually performed to assist the differentiation of adynamic ileus and physical obstructions. Radiographs taken with a horizontal beam show separation of the fluid and gas in the stagnant bowl loops (Figure 25–5). Multiple gas-capped fluid lines scattered about different horizontal planes are characteristic of the early phases of anatomic intestinal obstruction. The fluid at different levels indicates that sufficient gastrointestinal motility is present to move fluid through the intestine (Figure 25–6). The level of the obstruction determines the number of gas-capped loops of intestine. A greater number indicates obstruction in a more caudal part. With adynamic ileus, loss of motility is complete and horizontal beam radiographs reveal gas-capped fluid levels in the same horizontal plane throughout the obstructed intestine. The fluid accumulates at the same level because there is no resistance by the intestine to gravitational pull.

AIR ENEMAS. If difficulty is experienced in determining whether a large-diameter loop of bowel is abnormally dilated small intestine or large intestine of normal caliber, an air

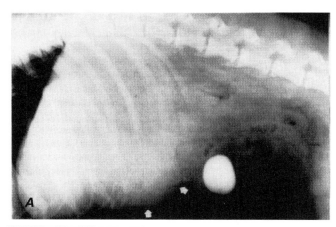

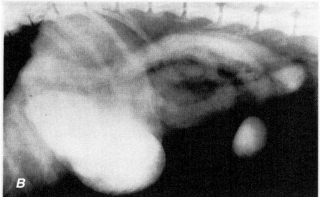

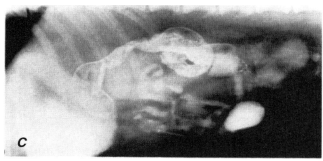

FIGURE 25–3. Lateral films of a dog with clinical signs suggestive of intestinal obstruction. *(A)* Plain film reveals a large radiopaque foreign body that produces no typical signs of intestinal obstruction. Distended stomach (arrows) reflects accumulation of gastric and refluxed intestinal secretions of fluid. *(B)* Lateral film taken 2 hours after administration of positive contrast medium shows dilated loops of jejunum and duodenum proximal to site of obstruction; very little contrast medium has passed this point. *(C)* Lateral film taken at 24 hours shows that obstruction was not complete. The dog had been eating a small amount of food and passing bowel movements. Obstruction was caused by a stone, which was surgically removed.

enema is a convenient method of outlining the large bowel. The procedure is simple to perform. Air (approximately 10–20 mL/kg) is introduced via a Foley catheter and the abdominal radiographs are repeated.

BARIUM-IMPREGNATED POLYETHYLENE SPHERES (BIPS). (Ken Bowman Associates, Diamond Bar, CA; Arnolds, Shrewsbury, UK) are radiopaque plastic spheres that have recently been introduced for the diagnosis of gastrointestinal obstructions and motility problems in dogs and cats.[21] Each set of BIPS

consists of 1 large large capsule or 4 small capsules containing ten 5 mm diameter and thirty 1.5 mm diameter spheres (Figure 25–7). The primary function of the large BIPs is to detect gastrointestinal tract obstructions and that of the small BIPs is to assess quantitatively the gastrointestinal transit time of food. BIPs are convenient to use because they are administered in capsules. Additionally, the large diameter of the 5 mm BIPS improves the likelihood of detecting a partial obstruction. Other advantages and disadvantages of BIPS in comparison to barium sulfate suspensions are listed in Table 25–4. BIPS should not be used to detect obstructions in animals showing evidence of shock because the markers may take 8 hours or more to reach the site of the obstruction.

BIPS have been successfully used at the Massey University Small Animal Clinic to detect physical obstructions (including partial obstructions), functional obstructions (ileus), and delayed gastric emptying (see Chapter 15). When used to detect obstructions BIPS are usually given on an empty stomach. Improved sensitivity for the detection of partial obstructions is achieved by feeding the BIPS in a high-fiber diet.

BIPS ON AN EMPTY STOMACH. BIPS capsules are administered per os and symptomatic management (fluids, etc.) is initiated (or continued). Survey abdominal radiographs are taken at a convenient time 6 to 24 hours later. If delayed gastrointestinal transit of markers or bunching of markers in the small intestine is observed, one or two more radiographs at 1 to 2 hourly intervals are taken to confirm that the radiographic findings are persistent. The gastric emptying time and orocolic transit time of the patient is then compared to the normal gastric emptying and orocolic transit curves provided in the packaging leaflets. If transit time is normal, gastrointestinal obstruction is highly unlikely. If transit time is delayed, the cause might be physical obstructions (e.g., foreign bodies, intussusceptions, tumors), functional obstructions (adynamic ileus), or both (Figure 25–8). The decision as to whether an obstruction is functional or physical is made by a combination of history, clinical signs, laboratory findings, survey radiographic findings, the BIPS radiographic pattern, and response to treatment (see Table 25–3). Persistent bunching of the BIPS in the small intestine (the "stagnant loop" sign) is highly suggestive of physical obstruction of the small bowel (Figure 25–9). It is important to note, however, that in cats and some small dogs there will be a brief bunching of the markers just cranial to the ileocolic junction. Delayed transit associated with a wide scattering of the BIPs throughout the small bowel is usually due to ileus (Figure 25–10). Failure of the markers to leave the stomach can be due to either physical obstruction of the stomach or small bowel with a secondary adynamic ileus, or can be due to ileus resulting from other causes (such as pancreatitis) (Figure 25–11).

BIPS FED WITH PRESCRIPTION DIET R/D. Administration of BIPS in a high-fiber diet is more sensitive than administration of BIPS on an empty stomach for the diagnosis of partial obstructions of the intestinal tract with a luminal diameter of 5 mm or more. The fiber accumulates oral to the partial obstruction, arresting the passage of the markers. This results in delayed transit and persistent bunching of the markers in the abnormal intestinal segment. Careful examination of the area of bowel containing the static markers may reveal an intestinal segment dilated by ingesta Figure 25–12). High-fiber BIPS studies are indicated in animals with intermittent vomiting and/or chronic diarrhea that are suspected of a partial obstruction of the small intestine.

To perform the study, the patient is fasted for 24 hours and then fed the BIPS dispersed in Prescription diet r/d (Hills Pet Products) at a dose of approximately 50 g of r/d per kg

Table 25–3

FACTORS ASSISTING DIFFERENTIATION OF ADYNAMIC ILEUS AND PHYSICAL OBSTRUCTIONS*

FACTOR	ADYNAMIC ILEUS	PHYSICAL OBSTRUCTION
Clinical findings		
History	Supportive of gastroenteritis, systemic diseases, etc.	Exposure to foreign bodies
Abdominal palpation	Usually normal	Often abnormal
Abdominal auscultation	Few or absent sounds	Increased, decreased, or absent sounds
Laboratory findings		
Evidence of systemic disease	Often present	Usually not present
Radiographic findings		
Dilated loops:number	Multiple	Often singular
Dilated loops:diameter	Mildly to moderately increased	Mildly to markedly increased
Graveling sign	No	Yes, especially partial obstructions
Horizontal beam	Gas/fluid lines in one horizontal plane	Gas/fluid lines in multiple horizontal planes
BIPS	Delayed passage; scattered	Delayed passage; bunched
Barium liquid	Delayed passage; no physical lesion outlined	Delayed passage; ± physical lesion outlined
Response to treatment		
Fluids and potassium	Often respond	Vomiting continues
Prokinetics	Often respond	Vomiting continues

*Not infrequently physical obstructions and adynamic ileus occur concurrently, confusing the clinical picture.

body weight. Lateral and D-V radiographs are taken at three or four convenient times between 6 to 24 hours after the meal of r/d. If delayed transit or bunching of markers is observed, one or two more radiographs should be taken at 1 to 2 hourly intervals to confirm the radiographic findings.

Contrast Studies with Barium Sulfate Suspension

Radiographic contrast studies of the upper gastrointestinal tract using barium sulfate suspension are frequently used to detect intestinal obstruction. Barium sulfate suspension is less convenient to use than BIPS and does not provide quantitative information on transit times but has the advantages of more rapid transit through the gastrointestinal tract and the ability to outline the mucosal surface (Table 25–3). The latter is advantageous because it can allow experienced radiologists to detect nonobstructing diseases of the mucosa, such as ulcers and polyps, for which BIPS are not an appropriate diagnostic modality.

Marked obstruction of the small intestine delays gastric emptying and the transit of liquid contrast media through the small intestine. Unfortunately, because of the subjective

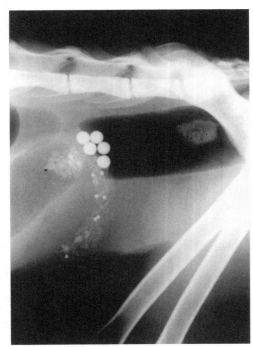

FIGURE 25–4. Lateral abdominal radiograph of a cat with an intestinal stricture following a subtotal colectomy. BIPS have lodged at the stricture and indigestible material can be seen in the stagnant loop (the "graveling sign").

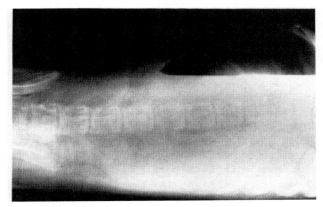

FIGURE 25–5. Lateral radiograph of the same dog as in Figure 25–2. Radiograph was taken with a horizontal beam and shows gas-capped fluid level. Gas accumulation at only one horizontal plane is evidence of bowel stasis.

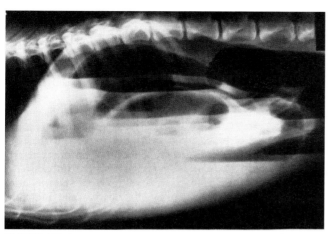

FIGURE 25–6. Lateral radiograph of a 1-year-old German shepherd with clinical signs of intestinal obstruction. Radiograph was taken with a horizontal beam. Multiple gas-capped fluid levels are seen in different horizontal planes. This suggests that motility is present in the intestine and is able to move the gas and fluid from one segment to another. The homogenous appearance of the abdomen suggests that either peritonitis or peritoneal fluid is present.

(rather than quantitative) information on orocolic transit provided by liquid barium, it can be difficult to determine if gastrointestinal passage is significantly delayed. The more complete the intestinal obstruction the greater the delay and the easier it is to interpret the barium study (Figure 25–13). In an obstructed animal, radiographs may show dilution of the contrast agent as it enters the fluid-filled stagnant loop. Occasionally, radiolucent foreign bodies are outlined by contrast medium. Annular lesions, produced by neoplastic or inflammatory disease, often cause the column of contrast medium to taper into a relatively thin line (Figure 25–14).[22] When intestinal obstruction is complete, regardless of the cause, the leading edge of the contrast column may never reach the point of obstruction, presumably because of concurrent ileus. Thus, it is not always possible to define the site of the lesion with barium liquid (or for that matter BIPS).

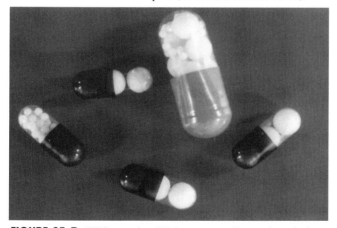

FIGURE 25–7. BIPS capsules. BIPS are a new diagnostic technique of value for the diagnosis of gastrointestinal obstructions and motility abnormalities. Each set of BIPS consists of 1 large capsule or 4 small capsules containing ten 5 mm diameter and thirty 1.5 mm diameter radiopaque spheres. The small capsules are administered per os primarily to cats. The large capsule is administered per os to dogs or can be opened and the BIPS mixed with food prior to administration.

Table 25–4

ADVANTAGES AND DISADVANTAGES OF BIPS

Advantages of BIPs over Barium Suspensions
More convenient
  Administered by capsule or in food
  No mess
  Radiographs do not need to be taken at set intervals
Provide quantitative information on emptying and transit times
Mimic the transit of food not liquid
Better safety
  Less risk of aspiration into the lungs
  Less risk of peritonitis if bowel is perforated
May have improved sensitivity for the detection of partial obstructions
Do not obscure abdominal detail
  By administering BIPs a few hours prior to taking the survey films,
    both anatomic and functional information is gained from one
    set of radiographs

Advantages of Barium Sulfate Suspensions over BIPS
Provides greater information on mucosal detail
  May have greater sensitivity for nonobstructing gastrointestinal diseases such as ulcers and polyps
Outlines luminal margins
  May have improved sensitivity for congenital anomalies such as
    short colon
More rapid transit through the gastrointestinal tract

Enteroclysis

As discussed in Chapter 6, enteroclysis is a sensitive contrast radiographic technique for the diagnosis of intestinal obstructions. Unfortunately, the procedure is technically difficult to perform and requires the use of a fluoroscope.

Ultrasonography

Ultrasonography is a valuable tool for the detection of intestinal obstructions.[23,24] Both radiopaque and radiolucent foreign bodies may be revealed.[24] Intussusception has a characteristic ultrasonographic appearance, in which the multiple layers of overlapping intestinal wall are readily apparent.

MANAGEMENT OF INTESTINAL OBSTRUCTION

Preoperative Management

FLUIDS AND ELECTROLYTES. Intestinal obstruction should be expediently corrected by surgery, but celiotomy must be preceded by effective management of fluid and electrolyte derangements and toxemia.

The volume of fluid to be administered and the rapidity of administration are based on clinical assessment of the severity of dehydration and the presence or absence of shock. The type of fluid administered is determined by the particular fluid, electrolyte, and acid-base derangements present in each individual patient. The wide variation in these derangements makes laboratory assessment of these parameters very helpful for developing an accurate fluid therapy plan. If laboratory assessments of electrolyte and acid-base abnormalities are unavailable, the most appropriate replacement fluid is a balanced electrolyte solution such as lactated Ringer's solution, supplemented with potassium chloride to approximately 20 mEq/L of fluid. If the obstruction is known to be pyloric or upper duodenal, 0.9% sodium chloride supplemented

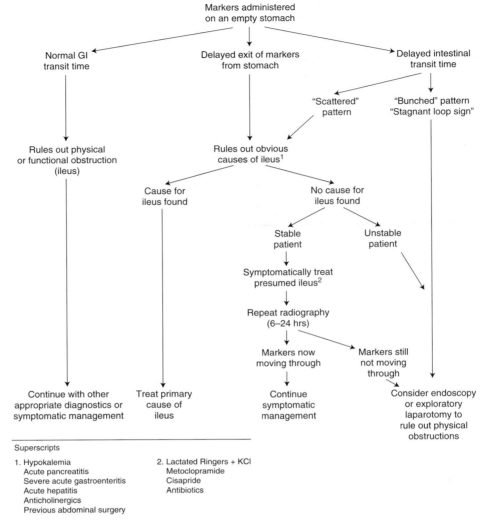

Markers administered
on an empty stomach

Normal GI
transit time

Delayed exit of markers
from stomach

Delayed intestinal
transit time

"Scattered"
pattern

"Bunched" pattern
"Stagnant loop sign"

Rules out physical
or functional obstruction
(ileus)

Rules out obvious
causes of ileus[1]

Cause for
ileus found

No cause for
ileus found

Stable
patient

Unstable
patient

Symptomatically treat
presumed ileus[2]

Repeat radiography
(6–24 hrs)

Markers now
moving through

Markers still
not moving
through

Continue with other
appropriate diagnostics or
symptomatic management

Treat primary
cause of
ileus

Continue
symptomatic
management

Consider endoscopy
or exploratory
laparotomy to
rule out physical
obstructions

Superscripts

1. Hypokalemia
   Acute pancreatitis
   Severe acute gastroenteritis
   Acute hepatitis
   Anticholinergics
   Previous abdominal surgery

2. Lactated Ringers + KCl
   Metoclopramide
   Cisapride
   Antibiotics

FIGURE 25–8. Algorithm demonstrating use of BIPS on an empty stomach for diagnosis of obstructions.

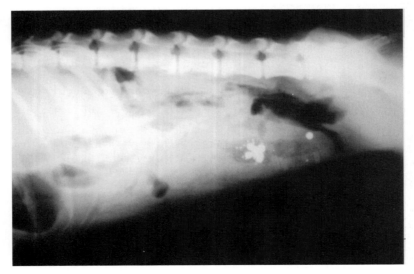

FIGURE 25–9. Lateral abdominal radiograph of a dog with a partial obstruction (luminal diameter approximately 5 mm) of the small bowel. The BIPS have bunched tightly in mid-abdomen, strongly suggesting an anatomic obstruction of the small bowel.

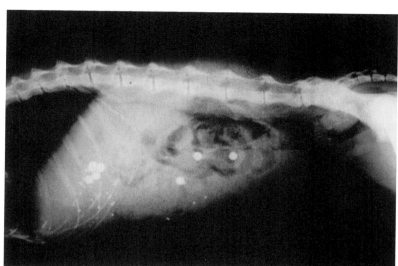

FIGURE 25–10. Lateral abdominal radiograph of an aged cat with renal failure and vomiting. Twenty-four hours after administration, the BIPS are still widely distributed throughout the stomach and small intestine. This delayed transit associated with a scattered distribution of the BIPS is strongly suggestive of adynamic ileus.

FIGURE 25–11. Lateral abdominal radiograph of a dog with a rock obstructing the small intestine. BIPS or barium sulfate "follow-through" studies usually identify small intestinal obstructions but, if a concomitant ileus is present, neither of these contrast agents may reach the level of the obstruction because of lack of peristalsis. In this dog, the BIPS have failed to leave the stomach after 6 hours, suggesting profound adynamic ileus induced by the foreign body.

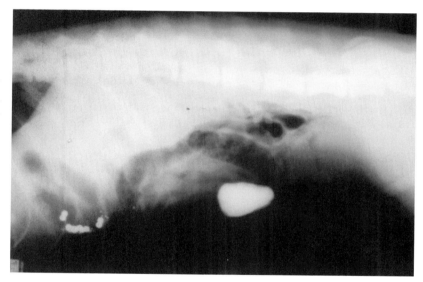

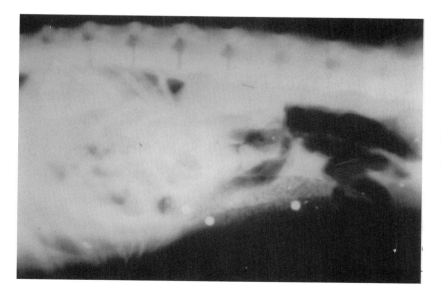

FIGURE 25–12. Lateral abdominal radiograph of a dog with a partial obstruction of approximately 7 mm luminal diameter. The dog was clinically normal until fed a high-fiber diet, following which abdominal discomfort and occasional vomiting became apparent. The radiograph shows a small-bowel loop markedly distended with poorly digestible ingesta. BIPS can be seen scattered through the stagnant loop.

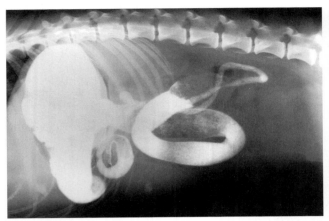

FIGURE 25-13. Lateral radiograph of a 10-year-old beagle with signs of acute intestinal obstruction. Positive contrast medium was administered. The film shows retention of contrast medium in the stomach, a distended loop of small intestine, and an abrupt end to the movement of the contrast through the small intestine. This film suggests the presence of a complete obstruction because the contrast medium is not seen caudal to this point. The obstruction was caused by a corn cob.

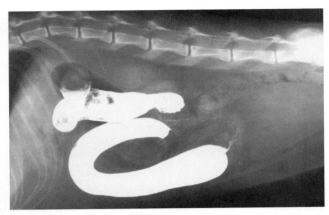

FIGURE 25-14. Lateral radiograph of an 8-year-old cat with clinical signs of anorexia and intermittent vomiting. Positive contrast medium was administered and the 3 hour film shows an obstruction that is partial because there is considerable contrast in the colon at this time. An adenocarcinoma of the small intestine caused the annular constriction.

with potassium is the most suitable fluid because of likely alkalosis (see Chapter 39). Potassium-free solutions are contraindicated in treating obstruction. Administration of glucose or bicarbonate promotes potassium movement into cells and may aggravate hypokalemia. In animals with ischemic loops of bowel, sufficient plasma and blood can be lost into the bowel to require plasma or whole blood administration.

Experimental evidence suggests that colloidal fluids, such as plasma or dextran, have considerably different effects than crystalloid fluids during the resuscitation of dogs with intestinal obstruction.[25] Both colloids and crystalloids increase systemic arterial pressure and intestinal blood flow, but crystalloid fluids result in a marked decrease in plasma oncotic pressure and enhanced transmucosal movement of fluid into the bowel. In comparison to crystalloid fluids, colloidal fluids maintain plasma oncotic pressure and result in net fluid movement from the gastrointestinal lumen to the blood. Thus, colloids provide better cardiovascular volume support but, in view of the toxic nature of intestinal fluid in obstructed bowel loops, it remains to be seen whether colloidal fluid administration will increase or decrease survival rate in obstructed animals.

ANTIBIOTICS. The adverse effects of the bacterial flora in the intestine of the obstructed patient are more difficult to manage than the fluid and electrolyte derangements. Antibiotics are indicated in obstructed animals to reduce the number of bacteria in the intestine and to prevent bacterial translocation through the mucosal barrier. Broad-spectrum antibiotics must be used to cover both aerobic and anaerobic spectra. In life-threatening situations, suitable choices include combinations of ampicillin (20 mg/kg IV q 8 hours) and gentamicin (2 mg/kg IV, SC q 8 hours) for a maximum of 5 days. Cephalosporins such as sodium cephalothin (15 mg/kg IV q 6 hours) or penicillin G (20,000 units/kg q 6 hours) may be used instead of the ampicillin. Amikacin (5 mg/kg IV, SC q 8 hours) is a suitable replacement for the gentamicin. The aminoglycosides should not be administered until fluid therapy has successfully rehydrated the patient. Small intestinal bacterial overgrowth due to partial obstructions can be treated with tetracyclines (20 mg/kg PO q 12 hours) or metronidazole (20 mg/kg PO q 12 hours). The effectiveness of antibiotics against aerobes is quite variable because some, such as coliforms, can develop resistance to antibiotics within 24 hours.

NASOGASTRIC TUBES. During the stabilization period, gastrointestinal fluid can be aspirated by a nasogastric tube. The removal of the accumulated fluid minimizes the absorption of bacterial toxins and lessens the chance of leakage of fluid into the abdomen before and during surgery. In humans it has been demonstrated that nasogastric drainage provides decompression comparable to drainage provided by longer intestinal tubes.[26] Data on survival of obstructed germ-free animals indicate that any reduction of intestinal bacterial numbers will benefit the patient.

Celiotomy

Once the animal is adequately stabilized, celiotomy is performed to relieve the obstruction. The surgical management of the obstructed intestine may require enterotomy only or, in cases of intestinal ischemia, may demand bowel resection and end-to-end anastomosis. The surgical management of intussusceptions can also include some form of prophylactic enteropexy or enteroplication (see later).[27]

Complications of surgery to relieve intestinal obstruction include wound dehiscence and peritonitis. Wound dehiscence is particularly common in debilitated patients. These patients benefit greatly from adequate preoperative and postoperative parenteral nutrition. In anorectic or debilitated patients, consideration should be given at the time of surgery as to whether to place an enteral or gastrostomy feeding tube. The patient should be allowed to drink within 12 to 24 hours of the surgery and should be offered small amounts of soft food within 24 to 48 hours. Intravenous fluid therapy should be continued until the animal is maintaining its own fluid and electrolyte homeostasis.

Adynamic ileus is a common complication of mechanical intestinal obstruction. Intestinal myoelectric activity is depressed in affected animals and the longer the obstruction is present the longer the abnormal activity persists.[28] Abnormal motility persists for at least 48 hours after correction of the obstruction. Restoring intracellular potassium is essential for recovery of normal motility. Postsurgical administration of metoclopramide and other prokinetics, such as cisapride, may also be beneficial in correcting the deranged motility.

SPECIFIC CAUSES OF INTESTINAL OBSTRUCTIONS

Linear Foreign Bodies[29–31]

Most linear foreign bodies, such as pieces of string, cord, or fabrics, pass through the gastrointestinal tract with few clinical signs. However, if one end of the foreign body lodges at some point it will eventually result in intestinal obstruction and perforation. The two most frequent points at which linear foreign bodies lodge are the oral cavity and the pylorus. In the oral cavity, the string most commonly loops around the base of the tongue as it is swallowed. The free end is then propelled through the esophagus and stomach and into the small intestine. Linear foreign bodies become snagged at the pylorus if one end of the object bunches up in the stomach. Eventually the free end of the material moves through the pylorus and unfurls in the small intestine. Peristaltic activity then causes the intestine to become pleated or clumped around the object. The pleating occurs because peristalsis causes the gut and luminal contents to move in opposite directions. The linear foreign body is fixed in position and cannot move aborally. As a result, the intestine must slide in an orad direction over the string until it eventually forms a clump. The taut linear object abrades the wall of the pleated intestinal loops until eventually multiple intestinal perforations develop and peritonitis occurs.

CLINICAL FINDINGS. Linear foreign bodies are more common in cats than in dogs. The clinical signs include anorexia, vomiting, diarrhea, and abdominal pain. The signs are usually of acute onset, but partial obstruction due to the foreign body may persist for weeks before diagnosis. Careful examination of the oral cavity may reveal a string or similar foreign body looped around the base of the tongue. On palpation of the abdomen, pleated loops of intestine bunched into a small area of the abdomen can usually be felt. Radiography of the abdomen is often diagnostic (see later). Evidence of peritonitis may be apparent on the radiograph and can usually be confirmed by a peritoneal tap. Chronic intestinal damage from linear foreign bodies may lead to peritoneal adhesions.

RADIOGRAPHIC APPEARANCE OF LINEAR FOREIGN BODIES. Linear foreign bodies produce characteristic but at times subtle changes that are frequently overlooked.[31] On survey radiographs, affected loops of small intestine appear gathered or convoluted and may be clumped at one site (Figure 25–15). Multiple gas bubbles can appear throughout the affected loops. Contrast studies reveal eccentric pleating, convolution, and foreshortening of the duodenum and jejunum. The duodenum's position often appears fixed in successive films. The radiographic appearance of linear foreign bodies must be differentiated from the changes resulting from an increased amount of segmentation activity in the small intestine. Hypersegmentation can produce a pleating appearance to the gut, but the constrictions in the small intestine are symmetrical with centrally located air bubbles, whereas linear foreign bodies create asymmetric convolutions and eccentrically located gas bubbles. The radiographic findings resulting from a linear foreign body can also resemble those from intestinal adhesions and occasionally from ascarids. A linear foreign body is difficult to distinguish radiographically from peritoneal adhesions but, fortunately, surgical intervention is necessary for the treatment of both conditions.

TREATMENT OF LINEAR BODIES. Conservative management of linear foreign bodies that loop about the tongue of cats is successful in many cases.[30] The string is cut free from around the tongue and allowed to pass through the intestinal tract. During the transit of the foreign body the cat is supported with parenteral fluid therapy if required and encouraged to eat. In many cats the string passes in the feces within 1 to 3 days. Conservative management is contraindicated if the cat shows evidence of depression, cardiovascular compromise, or peritonitis, and should not be contemplated if careful observation of the cat is not guaranteed.

Celiotomy is indicated if intestinal perforation has occurred, if the foreign body is fixed in a position where it cannot be freed, or if it is considered unlikely that the foreign body will pass through the gastrointestinal tract after being released. An enterotomy is performed at one or more sites and the foreign body removed. Perforated areas of bowel are repaired and the abdomen thoroughly lavaged with saline. If bowel perforation had occurred, broad-spectrum antibiotic coverage is indicated. A combination of amoxicillin, metronidazole, and gentamicin is a suitably aggressive regimen (see Chapter 26).

Nonlinear Foreign Bodies

A wide variety of foreign bodies can be ingested by dogs and, to a lesser extent, cats. Foreign bodies that commonly lodge in the intestine include bones, corn cobs, stones, fruit stones, tampons, fabrics, food wrappings, chew toys, children's toys, bottle caps, plant material, hair, fishhooks, and sewing needles.[32] Foreign bodies can lodge at any point

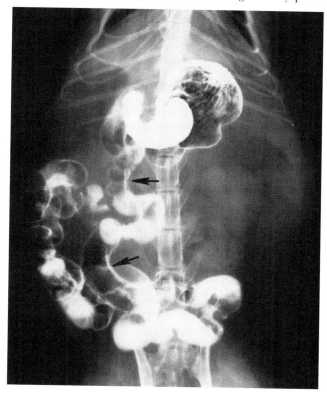

FIGURE 25–15. Dorsoventral radiograph of a 10-year-old cat with clinical signs of vomiting and anorexia. Positive contrast medium was administered. The small intestine is distended and pleated, and the position of the duodenum is altered. A linear foreign body, in this case string, absorbed the contrast medium and can be seen (arrows). The contrast medium in the string and air in the intestine provides double contrast, which assists in evaluation of the abnormality. The string had lodged by forming a clumped mass in the stomach, which retained barium and became radiographically visible. Examination of the film should include reading carefully for localized peritonitis.

throughout the gastrointestinal tract, but common sites are the esophagus, the pylorus, and the ileocolic junction. The consequences of foreign body ingestion depend on the size of the object, its chemical composition, and whether it has sharp points (Table 25–5). Small foreign bodies with smooth surfaces such as stones will often be passed without difficulty. In a recent study, stones as large as $38 \times 32 \times 24$ mm were found to pass uneventfully through the gastrointestinal tract of dogs over a 2 to 24 day period after ingestion.[33] Larger foreign bodies or those with sharp edges may wedge in the bowel lumen, where they mechanically obstruct the gastrointestinal tract and eventually lead to pressure necrosis of the intestinal wall. Many sharp foreign bodies will pass uneventfully, possibly as a result of the mural withdrawal reflex, which consists of local intestinal dilation in response to mucosal contact with a sharp object.[34] Not uncommonly, however, sharp foreign bodies may penetrate the intestinal tract, where they can lead to peritonitis and a functional intestinal obstruction through adynamic ileus. Toothpicks are seemingly innocuous foreign bodies that are an important cause of intestinal perforation in humans (Figure 25–16).

The chemical composition of the foreign body determines its digestibility and the likelihood of the release of toxic products. Lead objects in the gastrointestinal tract rapidly solubilize under the influence of gastric acid. Absorption of lead is fast, particularly in young animals. The ensuing clinical signs include abdominal pain, vomiting, bizarre behavior, and seizures. The clinical signs of lead toxicity are often accompanied by characteristic hematologic changes, including a neutrophilic leukocytosis, moderate anemia, and large numbers of nucleated and basophilic stippled red blood cells.

MANAGEMENT OF NONLINEAR FOREIGN BODIES. Foreign bodies may be managed by endoscopic, surgical, or conservative means. Factors that influence this decision include the type of foreign object and its anatomic location, the clinical appearance of the animal, and the attentiveness with which the owner observes the pet.

Foreign bodies suspected of containing lead, zinc, or caustic materials (batteries) must be removed from the gastrointestinal tract immediately. Intervention to remove lead foreign bodies must be accompanied by suitable medical therapy such as calcium EDTA (20 mg/kg IV or SQ q 8 hours for 4–5 days). Zinc objects in the intestinal tract can result in

Table 25–5

CONSEQUENCES OF GASTROINTESTINAL FOREIGN BODIES

Passage Without Complication
Small-diameter, smooth foreign bodies
Mechanical Obstruction
Linear foreign bodies
Nonlinear foreign bodies
Functional Obstruction Through Peritonitis
Penetrating foreign bodies
Peritonitis
Penetrating foreign bodies
Mural Necrosis
Impacted foreign bodies
Laceration of Adjacent Organs
Penetrating foreign bodies
Esophageal Stricture
Impacted foreign bodies
Caustic foreign bodies
Toxicity
Lead foreign bodies
Zinc foreign bodies

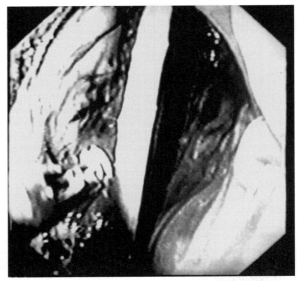

FIGURE 25-16. Endoscopic picture of a shish kebab stick spanning the cardia of a dog. The dog had stolen the shish kebab during a barbecue but had not had the decorum to remove the stick before eating. Like toothpicks, shish kebab sticks are highly dangerous foreign bodies and often penetrate the gastrointestinal tract. This stick had penetrated the stomach and was embedded in the liver. Surgical removal was required.

vomiting, diarrhea, and life-threatening hemolytic crises.[35] The most common sources of zinc are newly minted pennies and hardware such as nuts from zinc cages.

All esophageal foreign bodies should be rapidly removed because of the accompanying pain and dysphagia and the possibility of esophageal stricture. Endoscopic removal is particularly desirable in view of the possible complications of esophageal surgery and thoracotomy. Timely endoscopic removal of all nondigestible sharp objects from the stomach is recommended because of the risk of perforation of the stomach or, should the object leave the stomach, perforation of the intestine. To avoid gastrointestinal obstruction, the early endoscopic or surgical removal of foreign bodies judged too large to pass through the gastrointestinal tract is suggested. Most small-bowel foreign bodies are out of reach of the endoscope. Considerable expertise and discretion is required to safely remove foreign bodies via endoscopy (see Chapter 7).

Surgical removal of a foreign body is indicated if signs of gastrointestinal perforation are observed or if an intestinal foreign body remains stationary for several days. If a hazardous foreign body is out of reach of the endoscope (for example, in the periesophageal tissues or intestinal tract), or if a foreign body can be reached but not removed by the endoscope, surgical removal is necessary. If endoscopy reveals significant laceration or pressure necrosis of a viscus, surgical exploration to determine its mural extent is prudent.

Conservative management, consisting of close observation, high-fiber diets, and radiographic observation of the aboral progress of the foreign object are usually recommended for nontraumatic, small-sized foreign bodies (e.g., pebbles) detected in the stomach or small intestine. Small gastric foreign objects may be given 3 to 4 weeks to pass before endoscopic removal, if the owner is capable of appropriately close observation and the animal remains asymptomatic. Notwithstanding this recommendation, it is questionable whether a high-fiber diet is of any value in hastening the transit of a foreign body because foreign objects usually do not pass through the pylorus in the fed state. Phasic contractions of the pylorus are maximum during the digestive period.[36] As a result gastric foreign bodies with a diameter greater than 7 mm pass through the pylorus in the unfed state during phase III contractions of the migrating motility complex ("housekeeper contractions"). Phasic pyloric contractions are minimal during the interdigestive periods, allowing large-diameter particulate material to leave the stomach.

Emetic drugs, such as apomorphine (given to effect subconjunctivally), low-dose xylazine (cats: 0.2–0.4 mg/kg IV, SC), or sodium carbonate crystals (dogs and cats: 40 mg/kg PO) can be considered if the foreign body does not have sharp edges that could damage the esophagus or result in the object lodging in the esophagus during vomition. Prior to administering the emetic the veterinarian should feed the patient, and he or she must be confident that it is in a sufficiently fit state to protect its airway adequately from the vomitus. Prokinetic drugs, such as metoclopramide, are not recommended to promote the movement of gastric foreign bodies through the pylorus because the exaggerated antral contractions induced by these drugs are likely to exacerbate mechanical damage to the gastric mucosa by the foreign body.

Intussusception

Intussusception is a unique type of obstructive lesion that is produced by the invagination and telescoping of one segment of the intestine into an adjacent loop.[27,37] Intussusceptions usually occur in the direction of normal peristalsis but will occasionally be retrograde (Figure 25–17).[27] Single intussusceptions are most common, but occasionally multiple intussusceptions or compounded intussusceptions occur (Figure 25–17). The latter results when an entire intussusception undergoes a second invagination. Gastroesophageal, gastrogastric, pylorogastric, duodenogastric, enteroenteric, enterocolic, colocolic, and colorectal intussusceptions have been reported in small animals (by convention the invaginating segment is listed first and the recipient segment second).[27,38-40] Intussusceptions most commonly occur at the ileocolic junction.[37,41,42]

Eighty percent or more of intussusceptions arise in animals younger than 1 year of age.[37,42] They occur as a sequelae to a number of conditions, including intestinal parasitism, linear foreign bodies, parvovirus, intestinal neoplasms or granulomas, ingestion of bones, and prior abdominal surgery.[27,42,43] However, most intussusceptions in young animals are idiopathic. An association between idiopathic intussusception and recent dietary change has been observed.[41,44]

PATHOPHYSIOLOGY. The pathophysiologic events that result in intussusception remain to be elucidated, but an important feature appears to be the failure of coordinated motor activity in the affected segments. This can result from diseases that produce discontinuous segmental intestinal flaccidity or induration.[27] Another proposed cause is mechanical linkage of nonadjacent segments that result in a kink in the bowel. Such mechanical linkage can occur with linear foreign bodies or fibrous adhesions.[27] Peristaltic activity continues to invaginate the bowel once the intussusception has begun. The length of the intussusception is limited by tension on the mesentery of the invaginated loop. The consequences of intussusception are intestinal obstruction and ischemia. The lymphatic and venous drainages are obstructed early in the process, resulting in vascular engorgement, intramural edema and hemorrhage, and loss of plasma and blood into the lumen of the gastrointestinal tract. Exudation of fibrin can, within a short time, render the intussusception irreducible. Mural necrosis may eventually result, but perforation is rare because the ensheathing intestinal segments usually retain their viability.[27] Self-cures

can result if the intussuscipiens adheres to the normal bowel at the neck of the intussusception and the intussusceptum necrotizes and sloughs.

CLINICAL SIGNS. Intussusception usually results in partial rather than complete obstruction of the bowel. As a result, the clinical signs are often subacute or chronic and are usually relatively low grade. Some animals with chronic intussusception will continue to eat and pass regular bowel movements. Intermittent vomiting and chronic diarrhea are common, particularly in dogs. In cats, the most consistent signs are anorexia, weight loss, and a palpable abdominal mass.[42] In some affected animals (particularly dogs) the diarrhea is bloody as a result of venous obstruction and ischemic necrosis of the entrapped intestinal segment.

DIAGNOSIS. Most intussusception can be diagnosed by abdominal palpation. The intussusception feels like a firm tubular structure with well-demarcated ends. They are usually located cranially and/or ventrally in the abdomen. Intussusceptions must be differentiated from feces. In contrast to intussusceptions, formed feces usually lie dorsally in the abdomen. Furthermore, sustained digital pressure through the abdominal and rectal walls will usually indent the surface of feces. In contrast, digital pressure applied to an intussusception does not cause any indentation and often results in abdominal discomfort. In the event of uncertainty, the diagnosis can usually be confirmed by radiography.

RADIOGRAPHIC APPEARANCE OF INTUSSUSCEPTION. Intussusceptions usually have a radiographic appearance suggestive of partial obstruction.[37] Gas and fluid accumulation occur cranial to the lesion, and horizontal beam radiography can often detect a gas-fluid interface. Accumulations of gas are frequently noted in segments of intestine on the side of the abdomen opposite to the intussusception. Most intussusceptions are ileocolic, in which case the radiographs show an increase in tissue density caudal to the stomach, with displacement of the small-bowel segments to the right side and caudally. Contrast studies better identify such obstructive lesions (Figure 25–18). BIPS or barium sulfate "follow-through" studies usually identify small intestinal intussusceptions but, if a concomitant ileus is present, neither of these contrast agents may reach the level of the obstruction because of lack of peristalsis.[27,45] Barium enemas can be used to outline ileocolic or cecocolic intussusceptions into the colon. The radiographic findings include distenstion of the segment of colon into which the cecum or ileum is telescoped. The space occupied by the inverted segment of bowel contains no contrast and appears radiolucent. It is outlined only by the small amount of contrast medium that surrounds it. In addition, in comparison to normal animals, the cecum of dogs with cecal inversion will not fill with contrast agent nor be observed in its normal anatomic position (Figure 25–19).

MANAGEMENT. Intussusceptions are managed surgically. Acute intussusceptions can usually be readily reduced by gentle traction. Chronic intussusceptions often require surgical resection of the affected bowel and end-to-end anastomosis. Pneumatic reduction by way of a gas enema has been used successfully in children with ileocolic intussusceptions[46] and has been employed effectively by one of us (WGG) to reduce a gastroesophageal intussusception in a dog. However, pneumatic reduction is unlikely to be valuable in most dogs and cats because most are affected by chronic intussusceptions that are not readily reducible.

The recurrence rate of intussusceptions (either at the same or a different site) can be high if the primary cause is not identified and attended to. Recurrence usually occurs within 3 days of surgery but can occur as late as 20 days post-surgery.[27] In one study of intussusception, the recurrence rate was 20%.[27] However, in our experience, and that of others, the recurrence rate is lessened by resection of the intussus-

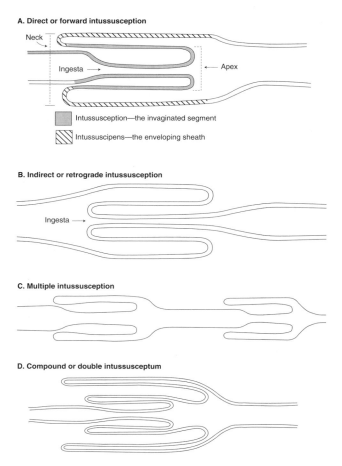

FIGURE 25-17. Terminology commonly applied to describe intussusceptions. *(A)* Direct or forward intussusception. *(B)* Indirect or retrograde intussusception. *(C)* Multiple intussusception. *(D)* Compound or double intussusception.

ception rather than just manual reduction.[47] In order to further reduce the likelihood of recurrence, some surgeons perform prophylactic enteropexy or enteroplication.[27] A recent retrospective study has suggested that enteroplication does, indeed, reduce the frequency of recurrence.[27] Other clinicians use anticholinergics to help prevent recurrence of intussusception. In spite of some experimental support,[48] the use of anticholinergics for this purpose does not seem sensible because these agents produce gastrointestinal hypomotility, a phenomenon that is also a feature of many of the conditions that predispose to intussusception (e.g., parvoviral diarrhea). Furthermore, in a recent report in cats, all recurrent intussusceptions were seen in animals with a concurrent adynamic ileus.[42] Thus, it would seem likely that anticholinergics may even predispose the animal to a recurrence. With this rationale in mind, the authors have successfully used prokinetics (such as cisapride) in several pups with recurrent intussusception resulting from acute gastroenteritis. The aim of the prokinetics is to normalize gastrointestinal motility in the affected pups. Prokinetics are probably not indicated if the intussusception has been resected because the resection itself is likely to reduce the rate of recurrence and because the increased intestinal motility induced by the prokinetic may compromise the healing of the intestinal anastomosis. Prospective trials are required to determine if prokinetics are

indeed valuable in the prevention of intussusception as our limited experience suggests.

Adynamic Ileus

Adynamic ileus is defined as intestinal obstruction resulting from inhibition of bowel motility. The lack of peristaltic activity results in a functional obstruction because intestinal content pools in the dependent areas of the gastrointestinal tract instead of being propelled in an aboral direction. More detailed description of ileus is found in Chapter 28.

Intestinal Hypertrophy Syndrome

On rare occasions, cats and dogs develop mechanical obstruction of the bowel secondary to idiopathic hypertrophy of the intestine. A similar condition affecting the antrum and pylorus (antral pylorus hypertrophy syndrome) of dogs has been well described (see Chapter 15) but little is known about the analogous intestinal syndrome. The disorder seems most prevalent in elderly cats. The intestinal hypertrophy is usually located in the ileum and is most often due to hypertrophy of the external muscle layers with little involvement of the mucosa. However, mucosal proliferation at this site can also occur, and in dogs has been seen in association with Campylobacter-like organisms. An analogous muscular hypertrophy syndrome occurs in horses and pigs. The cause and pathogenesis of the syndrome in any of these species is unknown. In mildly affected cats, the condition can be an incidental observation made at necropsy. Surgical resection of affected areas is recommended when the muscle hypertrophy is marked.

Pseudo-Obstruction Syndrome

Pseudo-obstruction is a poorly defined term used to describe patients that develop clinical and radiographic evidence of mechanical intestinal obstruction but have no evidence of mechanical blockage at subsequent exploratory surgery.[26] The terms *pseudo-obstruction* and *adynamic ileus* overlap somewhat, but pseudo-obstruction has a more chronic duration and often a more segmental appearance than does adynamic ileus. Adynamic ileus, not pseudo-obstruction syndrome, is the most common reason for negative exploratory celiotomy results in dogs and cats with suspected intestinal obstructions.

The primary pathophysiologic process in pseudo-obstruction is distension of a loop or loops of bowel because the smooth muscle of the intestinal muscularis is incapable of normal contraction and maintaining tone.[26] The intestinal hypomotility can be caused by intrinsic disease of the smooth muscle, infiltration of the muscle by some abnormal material (amyloid, fibrous tissue), visceral neuropathy, or by impaired neurohormonal regulation of intestinal muscle motility (neuropathic, idiopathic).[49,50] The sites of intestinal motility dysfunction may be single or multiple, and it can occur in the small or large bowel. Pseudo-obstruction in humans can develop secondary to a variety of systemic diseases such as uremia, SLE, diabetes mellitus, hypoparathyroidism, pheochromocytoma, *Amanita* mushroom poisoning, and phenothiazine administration.[49] However, most reported cases are due to idiopathic familial or degenerative visceral myopathies or neuropathies.[50] Most of the myopathies and neuropathies can be recognized by light microscopy of full

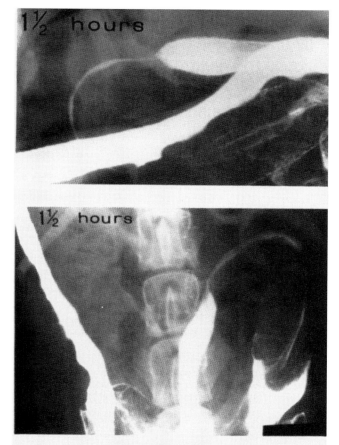

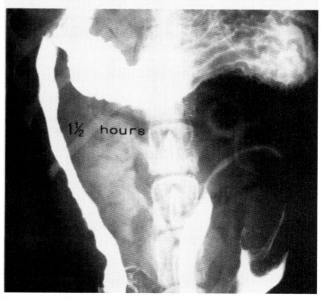

FIGURE 25–18. Lateral and dorsoventral radiographs of a 1-year-old golden retriever with signs of intestinal obstruction. Positive contrast medium was administered and radiographs taken 1.5 hours later show intussusception of a loop of jejunum into the adjacent distal part. The size of the lumen is reduced in the intussuscepted part and some contrast outlines the apex of the intussusceptum.

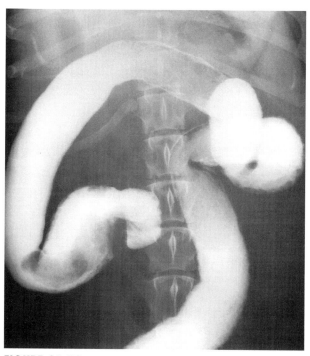

FIGURE 25–19. Dorsoventral radiograph of a 1-year-old basset hound that was presented with clinical signs of an enterocolitis. Barium enema shows a filling defect in the cranial end of colon, which is distended. The cecum is not filled with positive contrast medium. The diagnosis was cecal inversion.

thickness intestinal biopsy specimens, but the recognition of some neuropathies requires specialized histologic techniques such as en face visualization of the myenteric plexus.[50] In addition, noninvasive manometric diagnosis is now possible. In visceral myopathies, the phasic pressure waves of the migrating motor complex (MMC) are weak or absent. In contrast, in visceral neuropathies, the pressure waves are present but incoordinated, interfering with propagation of the MMC or resulting in sustained bursts of contraction.[50]

Intestinal "pseudo-obstruction" is rarely recognized in the dog or cat.[51–53] Idiopathic sclerosing enteropathy is the most commonly reported cause.[52,53] At the UCD VMTH, we have observed the occasional dog with pseudo-obstruction syndrome in which no abnormality could be demonstrated by routine histology at the site of the intestinal obstruction. We have also recognized the syndrome in a cat with intestinal lymphoma. The lymphoma was diffuse and not grossly visible at surgery, but it was presumably associated with disordered intestinal motility. Treatment of pseudo-obstruction is, where possible, directed at the primary cause. Additional potentially beneficial therapy includes prokinetic agents such as metoclopramide, cisapride, and erythromycin, but in advanced visceral myopathies or neuropathies these drugs are of little value and patients must be maintained with enteral and/or parenteral nutrition.[50,54]

REFERENCES

1. Moore R, Carpenter J. Intramural hematoma causing obstruction in three dogs. J Am Vet Med Assoc 184:186–188, 1984.
2. Lantz GC. The pathophysiology of acute mechanical small bowel obstruction. In: Burrows CF (ed) Gastroenterology in Practice. The Compendium Collection. Veterinary Learning Systems, Trenton, 157–164, 1993.

3. Mirkovitch V, Cobo F, Robinson JWL, et al. Morphology and function of the dog ileum after mechanical occlusion. Clin Sci Mol Med 50:123–130, 1976.

4. Heneghan JB, Robinson JWL, Menge H, et al. Intestinal obstruction in germ-free dogs. Eur J Clin Invest 11:285–290, 1981.

5. Cohn I. Intestinal obstruction. In: Berk JE (ed) Gastroenterology, 4th ed. WB Saunders, Philadelphia, 2056–2080, 1985.

6. Donaldson RM. Small bowel bacterial overgrowth. Adv Intern Med 16:191–212, 1970.

7. Summers RW, Helm J, Christensen J. Intestinal propulsion in the dog. Its relation to food intake and the migratory myoelectric complex. Gastroenterology 70:753–758, 1976.

8. Bishop RF, Allcock EA. Bacterial flora of the small bowel in acute intestinal obstruction. Brit Med J 1:776–770, 1960.

9. Sykes PA, Boulter KH, Scofield PF. Alterations in small bowel microflora in acute intestinal obstruction. J Med Micro Biol 9:13–22, 1976.

10. Yale CE, Balish E. The importance of six common bacteria in intestinal strangulation. Arch Surg 104:438–442, 1972.

11. Yale CE, Balish E. The importance of Clostridia in experimental intestinal strangulation. Gastroenterology 71:793–796, 1976.

12. Rhodes RS, Karnovsky MJ. Loss of macromolecular barrier function associated with surgical trauma to the intestine. Lab Invest 25:220–229, 1971.

13. Remedios AM, Fowler JD. Colonic stricture after ovariohysterectomy in two cats. Can Vet J 33:334–336, 1992.

14. Muir P, Goldsmid SE, Bellenger CR. Megacolon in a cat following ovariohysterectomy. Vet Rec 129:512–513, 1991.

15. Mishra NK, Appert HE, Howard JM. The effects of distension and obstruction on the accumulation of fluid in the lumen of small bowel of dogs. Ann Surg 180:791–795, 1974.

16. Shields R. The absorption and secretion of fluid and electrolytes by the obstructed bowel. Brit J Surg 52:774–779, 1965.

17. Summers RW, Yanda R, Prihoda M, et al. Acute intestinal obstruction: An electromyographic study in dogs. Gastroenterology 85:1301–1306, 1983.

18. Prihoda M, Flatt A, Summers RW. Mechanisms of motility changes during acute intestinal obstruction in the dog. Am J Physiol 247:G37–G42, 1984.

19. Gomez JA. The gastrointestinal contrast study. Methods and interpretation. Vet Clin N Am 4:805–842, 1974.

20. O'Brien TR. Radiographic Diagnosis of Abdominal Disorders in the Dog and Cat. WB Saunders, Philadelphia, 1978.

21. Allan FJ, Guilford WG. Radiopaque markers: Preliminary clinical observations (abstract). J Vet Int Med 8:151, 1994.

22. Feeney DA, Klausner JS, Johnston GR. Chronic bowel obstruction caused by primary intestinal neoplasia: A report of five cases. J Am Anim Hosp Assoc 18:67–77, 1982.

23. Penninck DG, Nyland TG, Kerr LY, et al. Ultrasonographic evaluation of gastrointestinal diseases in small animals. Vet Radiol 31:134–141, 1990.

24. Tidwell AS, Penninck DG. Ultrasonography of gastrointestinal foreign bodies. Vet Radiol Ultrasound 33:160–169, 1992.

25. Allen D, Kvietys PR, Granger N. Crystalloids versus colloids: Implications in fluid therapy of dogs with intestinal obstruction. Am J Vet Res 47:1751–1755, 1986.

26. Bynum TE. Intestinal obstruction and peritonitis. In: Stein JH (ed) Internal Medicine, 2nd ed. Little, Brown, Boston, 152–156, 1987.

27. Lewis DD, Ellison GW. Intussusception in dogs and cats. In: Burrows CF (ed) Gastroenterology in Practice. The Compendium Collection. Veterinary Learning Systems, Trenton, 171–181, 1994.

28. Brolin RE, Reddell MT. Gastrointestinal myoelectric activity in mechanical intestinal obstruction. J Surg Res 38:515–523, 1985.

29. Felts JF, Fox PR, Burk RL. Thread and sewing needles as gastrointestinal foreign bodies in the cat: A review of 64 cases. J Am Vet Med Assoc 184:56–59, 1984.

30. Basher AWP, Fowler JD. Conservative versus surgical management of gastrointestinal linear foreign bodies in the cat. Vet Surg 16:135–138, 1987.

31. Root CR, Lord PF. Linear radiolucent gastrointestinal foreign bodies in cats and dogs: Their radiographic appearance. J Am Vet Radiol Soc 12:45–53, 1971.

32. Mantri MB, Asha M, Vishwasrao SV, et al. Incidence of foreign body syndrome in dogs. Indian Vet J 69:346–348, 1992.

33. Capak D, Butkovic V. On the etiology of foreign body induced ileus in dogs. Veterinarski Arhiv 61:297–306, 1991.

34. Carp L. Foreign bodies in the intestine. Ann Surg 85:575, 1927.

35. Torrance AG, Fulton RB. Zinc-induced hemolytic anemia in a dog. J Am Vet Med Assoc 191:443–444, 1987.

36. Keinke O, Ehrlein HJ. Effect of oleic acid on canine gastroduodenal motility, pyloric diameter, and gastric emptying. J Exp Physiol 68:675–686, 1983.

37. Wilson GP, Burt JK. Intussusception in the dog and cat: A review of 45 cases. J Am Vet Med Assoc 164:515–518, 1974.

38. Bowersox TS, Caywood DD, Hayden DW. Idiopathic, duodenogastric intussusception in an adult dog. J Am Vet Med Assoc 199:1608–1609, 1991.

39. Huml RA, Konde LJ, Sellon RK, et al. Gastrogastric intussusception in a dog. Vet Radiol Ultrasound 33:150–153, 1992.

40. Lansdown ABG, Fox EA. Colorectal intussusception in a young cat. Vet Rec 129:429–430, 1991.

41. Weaver AD. Canine intestinal intussusception. Vet Rec 100:524–527, 1977.

42. Bellenger CR, Beck JA. Intussusception in 12 cats. J Sm Anim Pract 35:295–298, 1994.

43. Okewole PA, Odeyemi PS, Cole T, et al. Double intussusception fatally complicated by Clostridial infection in a dog. Br Vet J 145:291–292, 1989.

44. Cunnane SC, Bloom SR. Intussusception in Syrian hamsters. Br J Nutr 63:231–237, 1990.

45. Guilford WG. Unpublished observations, 1994.

46. Katz M, Phelan E, Carlin JB, et al. Gas enema for the reduction of intussusception—relationship between clinical signs and symptoms and outcome. Am J Roentgenology 160:363–366, 1993.

47. Wolfe DA. Recurrent intestinal intussusception in the dog. J Am Vet Med Assoc 171:553–556, 1977.

48. Olsen PR, Boserup F, Mikkelsen AM, et al. Intussusception following renal transplant in dogs. Nord Vet Med 29:36–40, 1977.

49. Jones RS, Schirmer BD. Intestinal obstruction, pseudo-obstruction and ileus. In: Sleisenger MH, Fordtran JS (eds) Gastrointestinal Disease. WB Saunders, Philadelphia, 369–381, 1989.

50. Schuffler MD. Chronic intestinal pseudo-obstruction: Progress and problems. J Pediatr Gastroenterol Nutr 10:157–163, 1990.

51. Arrick RH, Kleine LJ. Intestinal pseudoobstruction in a dog. J Am Vet Med Assoc 172:1201–1205, 1978.

52. Moore R, Carpenter J. Intestinal sclerosis with pseudoobstruction in three dogs. J Am Vet Med Assoc 184:830–833, 1984.

53. Swayne DE, Tyler DE, Farrell RL, et al. Sclerosing enteropathy in a dog. Vet Pathol 23:641–643, 1986.

54. Weber FH, Richards RD, McCallum RW. Erythromycin: A motilin agonist and gastrointestinal prokinetic agent. Am J Gastroenterol 88:485–490, 1993.

26 Miscellaneous Disorders of the Bowel, Abdomen, and Anorectum

W. GRANT GUILFORD AND DONALD R. STROMBECK

VOLVULUS, TORSION, AND STRANGULATION OF THE BOWEL

Introduction

Volvulus, torsion, or strangulation of the bowel rapidly results in ischemic damage. Prolonged ischemia causes irreversible damage to tissues as a result of adenosine triple phosphate (ATP) depletion, intracellular acidosis, failure of ion pumps, calcium influx, and proteolytic destruction of metabolic machinery and cytoskeleton. In contrast, the majority of damage to *transiently* ischemic tissues occurs not during the period of ischemia per se but rather when the ischemia is relieved and the tissues reperfused.[1,2] The pathogenesis of this so-called reperfusion injury includes the release of oxgen-free radicals (see Chapter 16). Ischemia-reperfusion injury has been shown to affect most tissues of the body but is particularly well studied in the intestinal tract.[1,3,4]

INTESTINAL RECOVERY FROM ISCHEMIA. The length of time for recovery of normal intestinal function has been studied in dogs following complete experimental ischemia of the colon and small intestine for 1 to 2 hours.[5–7] Immediate changes are severe, including necrosis and desquamation of villus tips, edema, vascular stasis, and hemorrhage in the lamina propria. Within 24 hours the mucosa has regained almost completely normal histologic appearance and circulation. The ileum is more sensitive than the colon to the effects of ischemia, but its mucosa returns to a normal appearance more rapidly. Mucosal functions return quite rapidly. Net absorption of fluid and nutrients is apparent in 24 hours, and within 1 week the regenerated mucosa has fully regained normal function.

Small Intestinal Volvulus

Small intestinal volvulus is a rare and often fatal disorder resulting from a rotation of the intestine about its mesenteric axis.[8–10] The duodenum is usually not involved in the volvulus because of its relatively fixed position in the abdominal cavity. Small intestinal volvulus is most common in German shepherds, and exocrine pancreatic insufficiency may predispose to the disease.[9] Vigorous activity, dietary indiscretion, or trauma may precede the volvulus.[10] The degree of rotation, the severity of the ensuing gaseous distension of the intestine, and the duration of volvulus determine the seriousness of the ischemic insult. The clinical signs are those of intestinal obstruction. Anorexia, vomiting, abdominal distension, abdominal pain, distress, and defecation of small amounts of bloody mucoid feces are common, and death is rapid.[9]

The diagnosis of small intestinal volvulus is usually made by survey radiography or emergency exploratory celiotomy. Radiography reveals marked gaseous distension of the small intestine, and celiotomy confirms the volvulus. Hypoproteinemia, hypoalbuminemia, hypokalemia, and serosanguinous abdominal fluid are commonly seen in affected dogs.[10]

Unfortunately, the mortality rate due to mesenteric volvulus is very high.[9] In the future, this high mortality may be reduced by measures aimed at minimizing reperfusion injury, such as gradual reperfusion of the ischemic tissues and premedication of the patient with oxyradical scavengers before surgical derotation.

The prognosis depends on the clinical condition of the patient at presentation and the extent of the bowel requiring resection. Dogs presented in shock rarely survive the surgery. If very extensive small-bowel resection is required, malassimilation is a likely sequela (the short bowel syndrome).[11] The management of short bowel syndrome is discussed later.

Cecal-Colic Volvulus

Cecal-colic volvulus is a rare disorder of dogs in which the cecum and colon undergo volvulus about their mesenteric root. The clinical signs are those of an "acute abdomen" (see Chapter 5) and are not specific for large-bowel volvulus.[12,13] Affected dogs may demonstrate a peracute to acute onset of vomiting, abdominal pain, mild abdominal distension, and

503

tenesmus.[12] Radiographs usually reveal marked dilation of the affected bowel loops. The disease is often fatal.

Small Intestinal Strangulation

Strangulation of the small intestine by entrapment in mesenteric openings, tears, hernias, or adhesions results in similar signs to small intestinal volvulus. The amount of bowel involved is usually less extensive, but the prognosis is still guarded because of potential complications such as peritonitis, toxemia, and septicemia.[14]

Colon Torsion

Colon torsion is a rare disorder that results from a twist of the colon around its long axis. The cause is unknown. The condition has been reported in dogs.[15,16] The clinical signs include acute onset of abdominal pain and distension in association with the rapid onset of shock. Physical examination may reveal a gas-distended abdomen or a painful mass in the caudal abdomen. Radiography shows gas or fluid distension of the colon that ends abruptly at the pelvic inlet. Ischemic necrosis of the colon is rapid, and death usually occurs within 24 hours. Surgical resection of the involved ischemic colon can be attempted. If the period of ischemia is less than 2 hours, the colon may retain its viability and resection may not be necessary. In these cases, reduction of the torsion and colopexy are advised.

Short Bowel Syndrome

Short bowel syndrome is an aptly named disorder resulting from resection of long lengths of small intestine. Many diseases can lead to extensive bowel resection but the most common in dogs and cats are ischemic diseases, such as small intestinal volvulus, strangulation, or intussusception.[17] Insufficient length of small intestine results in malabsorption, maldigestion, weight loss, and chronic diarrhea. Gastric hyperacidity and small intestinal bacterial overgrowth may complicate the disorder.[17,18] Hyperplastic changes occurring in the remaining bowel may compensate for the loss of absorptive area, but if greater than 85% of the small intestine has been resected the chances of recovery are poor.[17] However, as little as 30 to 40 cm of small intestine in a dog and 18 to 20 cm in a cat have been reported to be sufficient to maintain nutritional homeostasis.[17,19] The compensatory adaptive changes by the remaining intestine are stimulated by a variety of intraluminal nutrients including protein, protein hydrolysates, glutamine, and fats.[18,20] Mucosal hyperplasia begins within 1 to 2 days and within 2 weeks can lead to as much as a fourfold increase in mucosal surface area.[18] In humans, full adaptation may not be completed for several years.

Treatment of short bowel syndrome requires aggressive nutritional support. Initially, total parenteral nutrition coupled with small quantities of glutamine-containing oral sustenance is required. As compensatory changes in the small bowel occur, greater reliance can be placed on oral feeding. Highly digestible, low-fat diets should be used. The inclusion of small quantities of a gel-forming fiber such as Metamucil may be useful to delay gastric emptying. Cholestyramine powder may help bind malabsorbed bile acids, particularly if the ileum has been resected. Cholestyramine must be used with discretion in cats because it accelerates taurine excretion.

Broad-spectrum antibiotics can be useful because small intestinal bacterial overgrowth is a frequent complication of short bowel syndrome. Occasionally, gastric hyperacidity due to hypergastrinemia complicates the syndrome and can be managed with H_2 blockers such as cimetidine. Loperamide (Imodium; 0.8 mg/kg q 8 hours) may reduce the severity of the diarrhea. Surgical options for the treatment of short bowel syndrome have been utilized in human medicine.[21] These include creation of intestinal valves, reversed intestinal segments, and tapering enteroplasty.[21]

The prognosis is guarded. In an appropriately managed patient, diarrhea that persists for longer than 2 months after bowel resection is unlikely to resolve.

CONGENITAL DISORDERS OF THE BOWEL

Intestinal Atresia

Atresia (agenesis) of the intestine of dogs and cats has been infrequently reported. The small bowel is more commonly affected in dogs and the large bowel in cats.[22] Van der Gaag (1980) distinguishes three types of intestinal atresia: membrane atresia, a thin membranous intraluminal obstruction; cord atresia, two blind ends linked by a small fibrous or muscular cord; and blind-end atresia, two blind ends without any connection (Figure 26–1). One proposed cause of intestinal atresia is an in utero vascular accident.[23] Certainly, the disorder can be created experimentally by occluding fetal intestinal blood supply.[22] Inherited forms of the disease have been recognized rarely in humans and farm animals, but the sporadic incidence suggests that most cases are not inherited.[22,23] Intestinal stenosis also occurs infrequently. It is similar to intestinal atresia but the intestinal obstruction is incomplete (Figure 26–1).

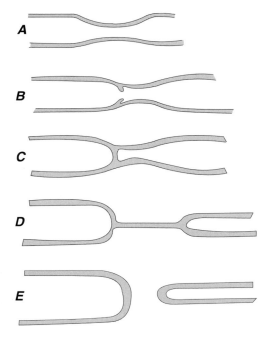

FIGURE 26–1. Classification of intestinal atresia and stenosis (after van der Gaag and Tibboel, 1980).[22] *(A)* Stenosis of the bowel. *(B)* Stenosis of the bowel with a perforate diaphragm. *(C)* Membrane atresia. *(D)* Cord atresia. *(E)* Blind-end atresia.

Intestinal Diverticular Malformations

Intestinal diverticular malformations are rare congenital malformations of the small intestine. They have been reported in both dogs and cats, and occur most frequently in the jejunum.[24] Diverticula are often subclinical, but gastrointestinal signs such as vomiting, diarrhea, a palpable abdominal mass, or abdominal pain may develop.[24] The clinical signs are usually precipitated by diverticulitis, diverticular perforation, or gastrointestinal obstruction at the site of the diverticulum. The obstructions occur secondary to intussusceptions, diverticular impactions, or invagination of the diverticulum into the lumen of the intestine.[24] Diagnosis usually requires exploratory surgery. Surgical resection is curative.

Imperforate Anus

Imperforate anus is a congenital disorder with a number of different causes that include persistence of the anal membrane, atresia ani, and rectal agenesis. Imperforate anus results from abnormal embryologic development. Atresia ani results from failure of the rectum and embryologic cloaca to fuse. The deformity may be noticed within days of birth, or the owner may not realize there is a problem until the pup or kitten is several weeks old by which time constipation is marked, abdominal distension is apparent, and the neonate has lost its vigor. Radiography helps differentiate these three conditions by delineating where the rectal gas shadow stops. The view of choice is a horizontal beam radiograph of the neonate suspended by its hind limbs. Treatment of a persistent anal membrane simply consists of perforating the anal membrane with an instrument such as a thermometer followed by trimming of the remaining tissue tags. Treatment of the other conditions involves more extensive surgery. The prognosis is favorable for imperforate anus and atresia ani, but is guarded for rectal agenesis.

Other anorectal deformities can be associated with imperforate anus. These include anovaginal fistula, rectovaginal fistula, and rectourethral fistula.[25–28] Diagnosis of these disorders is usually made by physical examination and contrast radiography. Surgical repair can be attempted, but the prognosis is guarded.

Miscellaneous Congenital Disorders

Additional congenital abnormalities of the bowel of dogs and cats include colonic and enteric duplication,[29,30] enterocyst formation,[32] and agenesis of the cecum and ascending and transverse colon.[31] Cats and dogs with a congenitally short small intestine or colon have been reported.[19,33] Short colon may be an incidental observation or may result in chronic passage of soft feces.[33] As mentioned in Chapter 28, aganglionosis (Hirschsprung disease) is a hypothesized cause of congenital megacolon in neonatal dogs and cats. A congenital hypoganglionosis of the distal colon has been described in a pup.[34] The affected area was narrowed and convoluted, resulting in constipation. Congenital heterotopic gastric mucosa of the small intestine has been reported in 4% of laboratory beagles.[35] Grossly, the lesions appear as an ulcerous focus but they do not produce clinically apparent problems. Lastly, intractable rectal hemorrhage in a young dog associated with vascular ectasia in the bowel and anus has been reported.[36] The lesion may have been congenital. Surgical intervention resulted in only temporary remission of the bleeding.

DISEASES OF THE CECUM

The cecum can be involved in a number of disease processes including ileocolic intussusception, typhlitis, and cecal abscessation,[37] perforation,[38] dilatation, neoplasia, and inversion. Typhlitis is most commonly due to whipworm infection or occurs along with generalized inflammatory diseases of the large bowel. Ileocolic intussusception is a common cause of intussusception that often involves the cecum. Intussusception is discussed in Chapter 25. Cecal dilatation usually occurs as a component of ileus and of itself has unknown significance. Cecal neoplasia is discussed in Chapter 27. With the exception of typhlitis and cecal dilatation due to ileus, most diseases of the cecum are treated by typhlotomy or typhlectomy.

Cecal Inversion

Cecal inversion is a rare disorder in which the cecum invaginates into the colon. The cause is unknown, but presumably prolapse of the cecum into the colon requires laxity in the ileocecal colic ligament. Whipworm infection is thought to predispose to the condition.[39] The most consistent clinical sign is chronic intermittent diarrhea with hematochezia. Tenesmus is often absent, as would be expected in a lesion that does not involve the distal colon and rectum. The inverted segment will occasionally produce intestinal obstruction resulting in vomiting and rapid deterioration of the patient's condition. Careful abdominal palpation may detect a mid-abdominal mass. Diagnosis is made by barium enemas, air enemas, or colonoscopy. Treatment is surgical resection.

MISCELLANEOUS CAUSES OF COLITIS

There are over 25 known causes of colitis in the dog and cat (Table 26–1). The most common cause is idiopathic chronic (lymphocytic-plasmacytic) colitis. This disease, along with eosinophilic, suppurative, granulomatous, and histiocytic colitis, is classified as an idiopathic inflammatory bowel disease and is discussed in Chapter 24. Colitis can also be caused by a wide variety of infectious agents. These disorders are discussed in Chapter 21. There are a number of other causes of colitis that are less common than the infectious and idiopathic inflammatory conditions.

Acute Nonspecific Colitis

Acute onset of large-bowel diarrhea is a reasonably frequent clinical presentation in dogs and cats. The signs are probably a manifestation of a group of poorly defined diseases, and the specific cause is rarely determined. Fecal cultures are indicated to rule out known enteric pathogens. Proposed etiologies have included toxin ingestion (particularly as a component of so-called garbage can enteritis), abrasion of the colonic mucosa by indigestible material such as bone fragments, enterotoxigenic *E. coli* and *C. perfringens*, and allergic proctocolitis. Coagulation necrosis of the colonic mucosa is a feature of mercury, bismuth, and arsenic poisoning.[40] An important differential diagnosis is ileocolic intussusception.

The clinical signs are an acute onset of explosive watery diarrhea, often with blood and tenesmus. Vomiting and depression are frequent in affected animals. Treatment is usu-

Table 26–1

CAUSES OF COLITIS IN THE DOG AND CAT

Idiopathic Inflammatory Disorders
    Acute nonspecific colitis
    Chronic (lymphocytic-plasmacytic) colitis
    Eosinophilic colitis
    Granulomatous colitis
    Histiocytic colitis
    Suppurative colitis
Bacterial
    Bacillus piliformis
    Campylobacter
    Clostridium perfringens
    Clostridium difficile?
    Enterotoxigenic *E. coli?*
    Salmonella
    Yersinia enterocolitica?
    Spiral-shaped organisms?
Viruses
    FeLV
    FIP
    FIV
Protozoa
    Giardia*
    Balantidium coli
    Entamoeba histolytica
    Leishmania
Fungi or Algae
    Aspergillosis
    Histoplasmosis
    Mucormycosis
    Prototisosis
Parasites
    Hookworms*
    Whipworms
Miscellaneous
    Antibiotic-associated colitis?
    Hemorrhagic gastroenteritis (HGE)
    Pancreatitis
    Traumatic colitis
    Uremic colitis

*Usually small-bowel infections.

ally symptomatic and can include fluids, bismuth subsalicylate, anthelmentics (those effective against whipworms), and antibiotics (e.g., fluoroquinilones, trimethoprim-sulfa, or amoxicillin/clavulinic acid). Food is withheld for 24 to 48 hours after which an easily digestible, hypoallergenic diet such as cottage cheese and rice is fed for 5 to 7 days. The addition of Metamucil (1–6 teaspoons per meal) may hasten recovery of normal colonic function. The prognosis is good. If the diarrhea becomes intractable, a diagnostic workup can be instituted. The diagnostic approach to large-bowel diarrhea is described in Chapter 5.

Antibiotic-Associated Pseudomembranous Colitis

Antibiotic-associated pseudomembranous colitis has been reported in dogs in association with the administration of clindamycin.[41] The clinical signs include severe mucoid diarrhea beginning 10 days after commencement of the antibiotic. At colonoscopy, the mucosa appeared erythematous and friable and was covered by 1 to 5 mm raised yellowish white plaques. The dog recovered when the medication was withdrawn. Fecal culture results were not reported. In humans, the disorder is

due to *Clostridium difficile* infection. Antibiotics most often incriminated in the disorder are clindamycin and lincomycin.

Colitis Associated with Pancreatitis

Acute, severe, necrotizing pancreatitis can be associated with a segmental colitis. The presumed pathogenesis is involvement of the transverse colon (against which the pancreas is anatomically apposed) in the peripancreatic inflammation. The disorder should be suspected in dogs showing concomitant signs of colitis and clinical or laboratory evidence of pancreatitis, or in patients in which colonoscopy determines that colonic inflammation is confined to the transverse colon. The treatment is directed at the pancreatitis (see Chapter 20).

Traumatic Colitis

Trauma to the colon can result from abdominal trauma or the ingestion of indigestible material such as stones, bones, sticks, aluminum foil, plastic, and wire. Most often such objects are passed with few clinical signs except the occasional fresh blood streak on the stool. If the mucosal damage is sufficiently widespread, however, acute colitis may result, presumably from secondary bacterial invasion. Occasionally, a foreign body may lodge in the colon or rectum and result in tenesmus and dyschezia. Traumatic colitis is usually self-limiting and only supportive therapy is required. Occasionally a short course (7–10 days) of sulfasalazine is necessary to quiet the inflammation. Lodged foreign bodies may require endoscopic removal.

Uremic Colitis

Colitis can be a complication of advanced renal insufficiency. It is usually but one of a constellation of gastrointestinal signs that are associated with uremia. Other common gastrointestinal signs of uremia in dogs and cats include anorexia, nausea, halitosis, oral ulceration, ischemic necrosis of the distal tip of the tongue, vomiting, gastritis, and gastroduodenal ulceration (see Chapter 14). In humans, additional gastrointestinal disorders have been ascribed to uremia. These include xerostomia, parotitis, esophagitis, duodenitis, bacterial overgrowth, adynamic ileus, mucosal edema, intestinal perforation, constipation, colonic intussusception, and acute pancreatitis.[42,43]

The pathogenesis of uremic gastrointestinal lesions is probably multifactorial. Factors that are involved include hypergastrinemia, secondary hyperparathyroidism, uremic vasculitis, and altered bile salt metabolism.[42] The treatment is directed at the renal insufficiency.

Ischemic Colitis

Colitis associated with submucosal necrotic vasculitis has been described in cats, and similar lesions occur infrequently in dogs.[44] The overlying mucosa develops varying degrees of infarction and necrosis. The cause has not been identified. The vasculitis due to FIP or uremia will occasionally cause ischemic enterocolitis, but the lesions due to these disorders tend to be transmural rather than just submucosal.[44] Patchy ischemic colitis can also occur in dogs without any evidence of associated vasculitis. The cause of the lesion is unknown, but ischemia-reperfusion injury secondary to stress-induced or hypovolemia-induced vasoconstriction seem likely. Colonic perforation is a catastrophic complication of ischemic colitis. As discussed later, it is likely that the colonic perforation occasionally seen in dogs following concurrent neurosurgery and dexamethasone therapy[45] has an ischemic basis. The treatment of ischemic colitis is directed at the underlying cause if identifiable.

PNEUMATOSIS COLI

Pneumatosis coli refers to the presence of gas in the submucosa or subserosa of the large bowel. The condition has been reported in dogs.[46,47] Rectal examination of affected dogs may reveal crepitus of the rectal or anal wall. The disorder is most often identified radiographically, appearing as linear radiolucency in the wall of the large bowel. The cause is usually not identified but pneumatosis coli has been associated with enema procedures and heavy growth of *Clostridium perfringens* in the feces. The condition is typically incidental, although complications such as bowel rupture and peritonitis are possible.[46] The gas accumulation usually resolves spontaneously, but if infection with gas-forming organisms, such as *C. perfringens,* is suspected, antibiotic therapy is indicated.

IDIOPATHIC (NONINFLAMMATORY) LARGE-BOWEL DIARRHEA

As many as 15% to 20% of dogs presenting for signs of large-bowel diarrhea have no evidence of "significant" colonic inflammation on proctoscopy or biopsy.[41] In other studies of large-bowel diarrhea the percentage without significant morphologic disease is even higher.[48] The clinical appearance of these patients is similar to that of dogs with inflammatory colitis. The appearance of the diarrhea can range from small volumes of soft feces with occasional blood to watery diarrhea. The cause of the condition is unknown. Analogies have been drawn to the irritable bowel syndrome in humans based on the favorable response of many affected dogs to supplemental dietary fiber.[49] Some dogs with the syndrome may indeed be suffering from a disorder analogous to irritable bowel syndrome, but in our experience few affected dogs show any of the other clinical signs consistently demonstrated by human patients with the disorder, such as abdominal distension or abdominal pain (see Chapter 28). Furthermore, responsiveness to fiber can occur in a number of secretory large-bowel diarrheas including those induced by malabsorbed bile and fatty acids. If a comparison must be made to a human disease, a closer analogy might be microscopic colitis. In this syndrome minimal inflammatory infiltrates and mild reactive changes in the epithelium are associated with markedly abnormal colonic absorption of water and electrolytes and clinical signs that include persistent diarrhea with urgency, mild abdominal cramping, but no hematochezia.[50] The responsiveness of the diarrhea in this condition to fiber supplementation has not been established, but one publication, linking microscopic colitis and bile salt malabsorption, described a clinicopathologic response to cholestyramine.[51]

The treatment of noninflammatory large-bowel diarrhea is based on fiber administration to which 50% of dogs reportedly respond.[49] The best type of fiber and the optimal dose has yet to be determined but Metamucil (1–6 teaspoons per meal), oat bran (0.5–2 tablespoons), wheat bran (0.5–2 tablespoons), and beet pulp (in Eukanuba; Iams Co.) are worth trying. A trial with cholestyramine may be of value and opioids may be effective in some cases. If irritable bowel syndrome is suspected, a variety of motility modifiers can be tried and attempts to identify and eliminate stressors are usually undertaken (see Chapter 28).

ANORECTUM: NORMAL STRUCTURE AND FUNCTION[52]

The rectum serves as a reservoir, collecting and holding fecal material. The rectum has a similar morphology to the colon, but the rectal mucosa contains glands with more mucous cells than the colon. At the rectal-anal junction the mucosal surface changes to stratified squamous epithelium and the rectal muscle layers thicken to form the internal anal sphincter. Surrounding the internal anal sphincter are layers of well-defined striated muscle bundles that form the external anal sphincter (Figure 26–2).

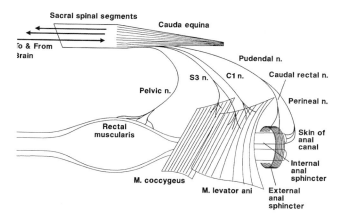

FIGURE 26–2. Neural control of defecation. Sensory information from wall of rectum and anal canal relayed to sacral synaptic centers. Response carried by parasympathetic fibers is to stimulate contraction of rectal muscles and inhibit motor activity in the internal sphincter. Response carried by somatic efferents is to inhibit the external anal sphincter muscle. These events mediate defecation, which is reinforced by local reflexes within the rectal wall to stimulate contraction and by voluntary reinforcement of external anal sphincter relaxation and contraction of abdominal perineal muscles. Sympathetic innervation (not shown) is inhibitory to rectal wall and facilitory to internal anal sphincter.

The rectum contains receptors that are sensitive to changes in intraluminal pressure but not to touch or pain. In contrast, the anal canal possesses receptors that respond to pressure, temperature, touch, and pain. The afferent nerve pathway for the rectal receptors is in pelvic nerves; that for the anal receptors is in the pudendal nerve (Figure 26–2). Afferent fibers synapse in the sacral spinal cord, and efferent motor fibers are contained in the pudendal, hypogastric, and pelvic nerves. Parasympathetic fibers in the pelvic nerves provide the motor input to the rectum but are inhibitory to the internal anal sphincter. In contrast, sympathetic fibers, carried in the hypogastric nerves, are inhibitory to the rectum and excitatory to the internal anal sphincter. The external anal sphincter is innervated by somatic nerve fibers in the pudendal nerve.

The accommodation to, storage, and defecation of feces is controlled by reflex events in the rectum that can be modified by voluntary control of the external anal sphincter. Initially, as fecal material enters the rectum, receptive relaxation occurs, keeping rectal pressure low. Eventually, the rectum is distended sufficiently to stimulate rectal receptors that initiate the defecation reflex. The reflex consists of sensory reception in the rectum (and perhaps pelvic girdle), afferents in the pelvic nerves, synapses in the sacral cord, and efferents in the pelvic nerves to the rectal muscles to cause contraction. Another component of the reflex inhibits tone in the internal anal sphincter, so that as the rectum contracts the internal anal sphincter relaxes. Fecal contents distending the more sensitive anal mucosa stimulate receptors which inform the central nervous system, via the spinal cord and pudendal nerves, that defecation is imminent. At this point, conscious control can be evoked to facilitate or inhibit defecation. To inhibit defecation the external sphincter is voluntarily constricted, closing the anal canal. Facilitation of defecation is mediated by relaxation of external anal sphincter muscles and an increase in intra-abdominal pressure caused by contraction of the diaphragm and abdominal muscles in association with closure of the glottis.

FECAL INCONTINENCE

Definition and Prevalence

Fecal incontinence is the inability to retain feces until defecation is appropriate. Failure of fecal continence is a disastrous occurrence for the household pet. Fifty percent of dogs and cats with fecal incontinence are euthanized within several days of presentation. The recorded prevalence of fecal incontinence is 43 out of 260,000 admissions to the University of Missouri and University of California Veterinary Medical Teaching Hospitals. This is probably an underestimation of the true incidence of the disease. There is no sex predilection, but the majority of affected animals are 11 years of age or older. Two major subcategories of fecal incontinence are recognized: "reservoir incontinence" and "sphincter incontinence."[54] The putative anatomic structures involved in the maintenance of fecal continence are depicted in Figure 26–2.

RESERVOIR INCONTINENCE. A reservoir mechanism is essential for continence because the maximum period of sustained voluntary contraction of the striated anal sphincter muscles is brief.[55,56] Reservoir incontinence results from a failure of the large bowel to accommodate to, and contain within its length, the colorectal content. Animals with reservoir incontinence are usually aware of feces in the rectum and are able to sense the imminence of defecation. Reservoir incontinence is most often characterized by frequent, con-

scious defecation and not by inadvertent anal dribbling. The adequacy of large-bowel reservoir function is affected by colorectal irritability, capacity, compliance, and motility, and by the volume of feces.

SPHINCTER INCONTINENCE. Sphincter incontinence is due to a failure of the sphincteric mechanisms to resist the propulsive forces of the rectum.[55,56] It is characterized by the involuntary passage of feces. Sphincter continence depends on adequate resting tone in the internal anal sphincter and the "continence reaction," a reflexive or conscious contraction of the muscles of the external anal sphincter and the pelvic girdle after sensation of the fecal mass.[57,58]

Physiology of Fecal Continence

NERVOUS PATHWAYS OF THE CONTINENCE REACTION. Three afferent nervous pathways, each with different sensory triggers, may be involved in the continence reaction (Figure 26–3). Which of these nervous pathways are the more important is somewhat controversial. The majority of evidence in humans favors the afferent nervous pathways triggered by stimulation of the anal epithelium, or stretching of the muscles of the pelvic girdle.[57,59,60] The issue has not been adequately addressed in the dog or cat. The hypogastric nerves transmit pain resulting from excessive dilatation of the bowel,[61] and probably do not have an important role in the maintenance of fecal continence. The information derived from the three major afferent pathways is integrated in the sacral spinal cord. The reflex arc is completed by efferent nerve fibers to the muscles of the pelvic girdle (via S1, S2, S3, C1, and the pudendal nerve) and to the external anal sphinc-

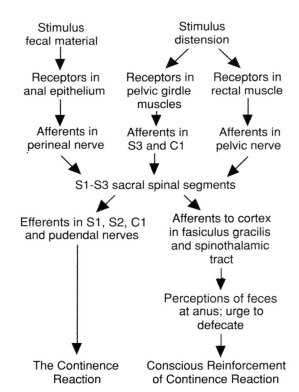

FIGURE 26–3. Hypothetical reflexes involved in the continence reaction. This figure has been compiled from often conflicting papers and texts that deal with the problem of human and, to a lesser extent, canine incontinence.

ter (via the caudal rectal nerve, a distal branch of the pudendal nerve).[62-64] Very little specific information exists on the areas of the brain involved in the control of continence and the perception of the urge to defecate, but similar brain stem centers to those which control micturition are thought to be important.[65]

MUSCLES OF THE CONTINENCE REACTION. In humans, the muscle that is most important in the resistance of the anal canal to propulsive waves appears to be the puborectalis.[57] Contraction of the external anal sphincter can further raise pressure in the anal canal. It appears that the external anal sphincter and puborectalis muscles are closely related and synergistic in action, acting as consecutive sphincteric muscular loops.[66]

In dogs, it is likely that the external anal sphincter plays an important role in the maintenance of continence. The levator ani muscle may also play a role. The levator ani is the most likely canine equivalent of the human puborectalis muscle.[67]

MISCELLANEOUS FACTORS CONTRIBUTING TO SPHINCTER CONTINENCE. Factors other than the continence reaction may also play a contributory role in maintaining sphincter continence.[68] Their relative importance is controversial in humans[68] and poorly addressed in dogs and cats.[67] The internal anal sphincter appears to be important in maintaining the resting pressure of the anal canal, but in response to a propulsive wave, and even slight distension of the rectum of humans or dogs, this muscle relaxes (rectosphincteric reflex).[57,69-71] Therefore, contraction of the internal sphincter is unlikely to be important in maintaining continence when pressure in the rectum becomes high, but may help guard against incontinence of small amounts of liquid stool.[72] Certainly, humans with fecal incontinence frequently have abnormalities in internal anal sphincter function.[58] These abnormalities include more frequent and more profound episodes of spontaneous sphincter relaxation than continent people, resulting in transient decreases in anal pressure.[58] In addition, lower than normal rectal volumes are required in some patients to induce sphincter relaxation, suggesting that the control of sphincter function may be abnormal in some incontinent people.

If low intrarectal pressures are maintained by effective reservoir function, passive factors are able to preserve some semblance of continence, even in those animals in which the neuromuscular components of the sphincter mechanisms are damaged. These passive mechanisms include a proposed flutter-valve-like action of the anorectum in response to increase in intra-abdominal pressure,[68,73] the inherent resistance to expansion exhibited by any tissue in a collapsed state,[67,73] and the horizontal stance of the dog and cat.

Causes of Fecal Incontinence

The causes of fecal incontinence are varied (Table 26–2). Important causes include anal diseases that interfere with sensory information from the anal epithelium and may disrupt the integrity of the anal canal; colonorectal diseases, such as colitis and neoplasia that compromise the reservoir function of the large bowel; constipation ("overflow" fecal incontinence); diarrhea; damage to the muscles and nerves of the continence reaction, in particular due to cauda equina syndrome; CNS injury; and aging. Aging is a common cause of fecal incontinence in humans[74] and dogs. The exact site of the defect or defects is unknown. It is likely that multiple factors are involved. Suggested contributory causes include senility, neuropathies, weakness and atrophy of the muscles of fecal continence, diminished rectal compliance,

Table 26–2

POSSIBLE CAUSES OF FECAL INCONTINENCE

Anorectal Disease
  Lacerations
  Neoplasia
  Anal sac removal
  Perianal fistulas and fistula repair
  Perineal hernia repair
  Rectovaginal fistula
Colonorectal Disease
  Proctitis
  Colitis
  Neoplasia
  Constipation
Myopathies or Neuromuscular Junction Disorders
  Trauma
  Myopathies?
  Myasthenia?
Peripheral Neuropathies
  Trauma
  Drug-induced (e.g., vincristine)
  Polyneuropathies
  Dysautonomia
  Chronic tenesmus?
  Obstetric trauma?
  Diabetes mellitus?
  Pelvic radiation?
Cauda Equina
  Congenital vertebral malformations
  Compressive vertebral malformations
  Traumatic vertebral damage (e.g., sacrococcygeal subluxation)
  Lumbosacral instability
  Anomalous lumbosacral vertebral nerve roots
  Infection
  Neoplasia
  Vascular compromise
CNS Disease
  Congenital (e.g., spina bifida)
  Traumatic
  Infectious (e.g., distemper)
  Degenerative myelopathy
  Vascular compromise
  Neoplasia
  Confusional states
Miscellaneous
  Aging
  Constipation
  Loose fecal consistency
  Increased fecal volume
  Anury

?: Causes of fecal incontinence documented in the human literature only.

and a higher incidence of diarrhea in the older patient.[74-76] Loss of house training in elderly animals can also be associated with problems such as degenerative joint disease.[77]

Diagnosis of Fecal Incontinence

It is important to determine the site and the cause of fecal incontinence because the treatments and prognoses of the different conditions vary considerably. As is evident from the earlier discussion, in order to determine the cause, the clinician must first obtain a meticulous history, perform a thorough physical examination, and, if necessary, complete a number of diagnostic tests. Diagnostic procedures of value in the investigation of fecal incontinence are listed in Table 26–3.

Table 26-3

DIAGNOSTICS USEFUL FOR THE DIFFERENTIAL
DIAGNOSIS OF FECAL INCONTINENCE

History
Physical Examination
Neurologic Examination
  Perception of perineal and anorectal sensation
  Perineal reflex
  Pudendal-anal reflex
  Rectal-inflation reflex
  Manual stimulation of erection
Database
  CBC
  Serum chemistry profile
  Urinalysis
  Fecal
Radiography
  Lumbosacral survey radiographs
  Radiographs of stressed lumbosacrum
  Myelogram
  Epidurogram
  Discogram
  Intraosseous vertebral venogram
  Intrarectal ultrasound
  CT scan
Electrodiagnostics
  Conventional EMG
  Single-fiber EMG
  Anal mapping
  Pudendal-anal reflex
  Pudendal and perineal nerve motor latencies
  Spinal motor latencies
  Hind limb NCV and evoked potentials
CSF Tap
  Fluid analysis
  Distemper titer
Colonoscopy
Anorectal/Colorectal Pressure Profiles
Surgical Exploration

HISTORY. The history may help determine if systemic diseases are involved, may suggest cause (e.g., poor diet, trauma, difficult whelping, drug or toxin exposure, chronic constipation, etc.), and is invaluable in the differentiation of reservoir and sphincter incontinence.

The history should include inquiry as to whether the animal consciously defecates (i.e., adopts a posture appropriate to defecation) and, if it does posture to defecate, whether the time and place chosen is appropriate. Failure to make any attempt at conscious defecation suggests a severe anorectal sensory derangement. These animals usually have a history of unconscious anal dribbling, often occurring at times of increased abdominal or rectal pressures such as while coughing or during exertion. In a previously house-trained animal, conscious defecation at inappropriate times or places, without the associated distress and urgency of reservoir incontinence, is more suggestive of a behavioral problem or a confusional state. In a young animal, inappropriate defecation may be simply due to a failure of house training.

Inquiry should also be made as to whether the animal has the ability to urinate normally and, in intact males, if the dog can attain an erection and subsequently achieve normal detumescence. Both micturition and erection rely on similar nervous pathways to those of fecal continence,[78] and, therefore, concurrent abnormalities in these functions suggest that the fecal incontinence is of neurogenic origin.

PHYSICAL EXAMINATION. Careful inspection of the anal area must be accompanied by digital examination of the anorectum to facilitate the detection of anorectal lesions. At this time anal tone may be assessed, but anal tone is poorly correlated with more objective measures of anal sphincter function.[75] This may relate to the fact that a denervated external anal sphincter does not readily atrophy.[54] Abdominal palpation assesses colonorectal content and bladder tone. Bladder tone may be altered by neurologic lesions. The skin of the hind limbs should be carefully examined for areas of self-trauma, which may be suggestive of paresthesias, and the dorsal lumbosacral skin and musculature should be palpated for evidence of hyperesthesia. Such hindlimb paresthesia and hyperesthesia are both suggestive of cauda equina syndrome.

NEUROLOGIC EXAMINATION. A thorough neurologic examination including observation of gait, cranial nerves, myotatic reflexes and postural reactions is an integral part of the workup. Depressed hindlimb myotatic reflexes may occur with lumbosacral spinal lesion, cauda equina syndrome, polyneuropathies, neuromuscular junction diseases, or myopathies. Special attention should be paid to the presence or absence of the anal reflex, the rectal-inflation reflex, the pudendal-anal (bulbocavernosus) reflex, and the central recognition of perineal and anorectal sensation. The anal reflex is evaluated by pricking or pinching the perianal skin and looking for contraction of the anal sphincter. The rectal-inflation reflex is induced by inflating with 15 to 30 mL of air a Foley catheter that has been placed in the caudal extremity of the rectum. This induces anal contraction in both dogs and humans. The pudendal-anal reflex is evaluated by applying digital pressure to the penis while observing for anal contraction. All three reflexes assess sacral spinal segments, motor neurons in the pudendal nerves, and the external anal sphincter. The anal and pudendal-anal reflexes test perineal nerve afferents, whereas it is likely that the "rectal-inflation reflex" tests pelvic or S3 and C1 nerve afferents (Figure 26-3). These reflexes are usually preserved in patients with suprasacral spinal transverse myelopathies, whereas the conscious perception of perineal and anorectal sensation (induced by the inflated Foley catheter) is not.

DIAGNOSTIC EVALUATIONS. Proctoscopy with biopsy is indicated if reservoir incontinence is suspected. Radiography may reveal diseases of the vertebral column responsible for the incontinence. Myelography, epidurograms, discography,[79] and CT scans are valuable for the diagnosis of deforming lesions affecting the spinal cord and cauda equina. Electrodiagnostic evaluation of the fecal incontinent animal greatly facilitates diagnosis. Electromyographic examination of the continence muscles may reveal denervation or myopathy.[80] The clinical assessment of the pudendal-anal reflex can be made more objective by the electrophysiologic evaluation of the reflex.[81] The CSF examination may include a CSF distemper titer to assist diagnosis of canine distemper.

Treatment of Fecal Incontinence

Before treatment of fecal incontinence is instituted, the veterinarian should discuss with the owner the public health risks of canine and feline feces. Therapy of fecal incontinence is more likely to be successful following identification and treatment, where possible, of the primary cause. For instance, resolution of the incontinence may follow successful treatment of diarrhea.[68,82] Symptomatic surgical therapy by way of implantation of a perianal silastic sling is of demonstrated value for the therapy of fecal incontinence in dogs.[83] Symptomatic medical management aims at reducing fecal water content, decreasing fecal bulk, slowing colonic transit time, and increasing anal sphincter tone. The use of low-residue diets such as cottage cheese and rice reduces fecal volume by up to 85%. They also reduce the frequency of defecation. Bowel transit time may be slowed by the use of opioids such as diphenoxylate or loperamide. These drugs also increase the tone of the anal sphincter in humans.[84] They may be given for prolonged periods with little development of tolerance to their effects.[84] A suggested dosage is diphenoxylate or loperamide (0.1–0.2 mg/kg PO) given every 8 hours initially and to effect thereafter. In addition, limited success has been reported with alpha agonists such as phenylpropanolamine (1.5–2.0 mg/kg PO q 8–12 hours).[85] Presumably, alpha agonists improve resting tone in the internal anal sphincter in an analogous way to opioids.

It is possible to manage the occasional patient with a dedicated and competent owner by the use of daily warm water enemas administered in a place where defecation is appropriate. Alternatively, many animals may be induced to defecate by the inflation of a Foley catheter in their rectums. This technique will not produce conscious defecation in animals with anorectal anesthesia but it will often produce involuntary rectal evacuation, a phenomenon also described in humans suffering from traumatic spinal lesions.[70] In animals with chronic posterior paralysis due to spinal cord damage, a minor stimulus to the hindlimbs or perineum, such as a light toe pinch or warm washcloth, may stimulate appropriate elimination (the mass reflex).

CONSTIPATION[86,87]

Constipation is defined as infrequent or absent defecation associated with fecal retention in the colon and rectum. The term *obstipation* refers to intractable constipation in which fecal retention is so marked that defecation cannot occur without medical intervention. Both disorders should be differentiated from megacolon, which is defined as marked colonic dilatation (see Chapter 28 for a discussion of megacolon). Not all constipated animals have megacolon whereas those with megacolon are almost always constipated.[86]

Constipation is a common presenting complaint, but the reason a client believes his or her pet is constipated should be sought. Many owners confuse constipation with tenesmus. It is important to differentiate these complaints (by questions about fecal frequency and form) because tenesmus can be caused by many disorders other than constipation (e.g., colitis and urogenital abnormalities.) The prevalent causes of constipation are listed in Table 26–4 and the diagnostic approach to tenesmus is described in Chapter 5. In addition to tenesmus, constipated animals may vomit or be depressed, anorexic, or show signs of mild abdominal discomfort. Paradoxically, passage of small quantities of liquid feces and fecal incontinence may be seen. The liquid feces are thought to result from irritation of the rectal mucosa by the impacted fecal mass, and the fecal incontinence to develop because the large fecal mass interferes with anal sphincter function.

The evaluation of patients with constipation should include a detailed history, particularly regarding diet. The ingestion of highly refined diets or large quantities of bone, hair, grass, or other indigestible material, such as cat litter, can lead to constipation. Inactivity predisposes animals to constipation. A history of recent ovariohysterectomy may be relevant because rectal strictures have been reported secondary to adhesion of the remaining uterine tissue with the colon and mesocolon.[88]

A careful visual and digital examination of the anorectum is important. Painful anorectal lesions, such as perianal fistula, can cause a reluctance to defecate and can be easily missed during a cursory examination. Rectal examination

Table 26–4

CAUSES OF CONSTIPATION[86]

Ingestion of Indigestible Material
  Bones, wool, cloth, hair, plant material, gravel, cat litter
Lack of Exercise
  Hospitalization
  Obesity
Painful Defecation
  Anorectal lesions (perianal fistula, tumors, anal sac abscess)
  Pelvic trauma
  Painful hindlimb musculoskeletal diseases
Mechanical Obstruction
  Colorectal mass
  Congenital anorectal lesions (imperforate anus, intestinal atresia)
  Healed pelvic fracture
  Intrapelvic mass
  Perineal hernia
  Prostatomegaly
  Pseudocoprostasis
  Rectal diverticulum
  Strictures (fibrous, neoplastic, postovariohysterectomy)
Neurologic Disease
  Dysautonomia
  Idiopathic megacolon
  Meningoencephalomyelitis
  Paraplegia
  Sacral spinal cord deformity (Manx cats)
Miscellaneous
  Debility
  Dehydration
  Drugs (anticholinergics, opioids, cholestyramine, sucralfate)
  Endocrinopathies (hypothyroidism, hyperparathyroidism)
  Hypokalemia
  Soiled litter tray

may reveal prostatomegaly, pelvic masses, abnormal pelvic bone structure (e.g., from old fractures), rectal stricture, masses in the rectum or anus, rectal diverticula, or perineal hernia.

If the cause of the constipation cannot be identified by the clinical examination, additional diagnostic procedures are indicated. Blood work may identify evidence of hypothyroidism or electrolyte abnormalities that can lead to constipation. Survey radiographs of the pelvis should be taken to rule out obvious obstructive lesions. Endoscopy or barium enema is of value if rectal strictures or masses are suspected. Ultrasonographic examination of the prostate and other pelvic structures can be helpful. If the etiology of the constipation is still elusive, full thickness rectal biopsy, radiopaque marker studies, manometric procedures, or electrodiagnostic testing may be required to detect certain rectal neuromuscular disorders, to differentiate anal from rectal dysfunction, to determine if colorectal failure is focal or generalized, and to identify lumbosacral spinal cord lesions.[89]

The first considerations in the treatment of constipation are correction of any fluid and electrolyte derangements and attention to the primary cause if one can be identified. For instance, pelvic osteotomy is an effective treatment for obstipation secondary to acquired stenosis of the pelvic canal provided it is not delayed for greater than 6 months from the onset of clinical signs of rectal obstruction.[90] After this period, the surgery is less successful, presumably due to colorectal damage from the chronic dilation.

The treatment of obstipated patients should include anesthesia, the administration of a lubricating warm water enema, and manual fragmentation and removal of the hardened stool. Precautions include adequate preparation of the patient for anesthesia and the use of endotracheal intubation to prevent aspiration of regurgitated gastrointestinal content (which can be induced by the enema procedure). The enema is performed and the fecal mass is carefully but firmly kneaded through the abdominal wall until it softens and can be fragmented into small pieces. These pieces can be subsequently removed by a gloved finger or with the use of whelping forceps. A suitable enema solution is warm water mixed with generous quantities of methylcellulose lubricant. Enema fluid is best run into the rectum under the force of gravity only. In inexperienced hands, pumping the fluid in under pressure can lead to through-and-through rectal to oral lavages. A standard volume used is 5 to 10 mL/kg. High concentrations of soap should not be used in enema fluids because they can damage the colonic mucosa. Phosphate (Fleet) enemas are contraindicated because of the likelihood of intoxication.[91]

Animals with less severe constipation do not require anesthesia and manual breakdown of the stool. They can be treated by twice daily warm water, lubricating enemas in association with softening agents (emollient laxatives) such as dioctyl sodium sulfosuccinate (Colace; Surfak; Coloxyl; 50 mg (cats), 50–200 mg (dogs) q 12–24 hours PO), and bulk-forming laxatives such as psyllium (Metamucil; 1–6 teaspoons mixed with each meal) or bran (1–2 tablespoons per 400 g canned food).

Prevention of subsequent constipation is best achieved by educating the client about suitable diet and exercise for his or her pet, and the use of bulk-forming laxatives or lubricant laxatives (white petrolatum: Katalax, Laxatone). Lactulose syrup (Chronulac or Duphalac) at a dose of 0.25 to 1 mL/kg q 12 hours PO is a useful osmotic laxative, particularly in cats because of relative ease of administration. Mineral oil, a lubricant laxative, should be avoided because of the risk of aspiration. Similarly, chronic use of irritant laxatives such as bisacodyl or castor oil is discouraged because of potential damage to the large bowel. More detailed discussion of laxatives can be found in several reviews.[87,92]

PROCTITIS

Inflammation of the rectum (proctitis) usually occurs in association with acute or chronic colitis. Occasionally, proctitis occurs in isolation from more generalized large-bowel disease. On most occasions the cause of such regional proctitis is not identified, although rectal prolapse and incarceration of the rectum in the sac of a perineal hernia can lead to localized inflammation. The clinical signs of proctitis are similar to those of colitis, but tenesmus and dyschezia predominate over diarrhea. The diagnostic evaluation of animals with suspected proctitis is the same as that for those with tenesmus or large-bowel diarrhea (see Chapter 5). Biopsy usually reveals lymphocytic-plasmacytic inflammation, although eosinophilic proctitis can occur. In addition, focal areas of suppuration are not uncommon. Treatment of idiopathic proctitis is similar to that of idiopathic colitis (see Chapter 24) and utilizes selected protein (hypoallergenic) diets with added fermentable fiber in combination with anti-inflammatory therapy (sulfasalazine or prednisone). In intractable cases, several intrarectal products containing corticosteroids with or without local anesthetics have been found useful (e.g., Proctofoam-HC; Reed & Carnrick).[85]

PERINEAL HERNIA

Perineal hernia is a relatively common problem in older dogs and is also seen in cats.[93,94] In both species, males are more commonly affected than females. The disorder is characterized by failure of the pelvic diaphragm and herniation of the rectum and, at times, other pelvic organs such as the bladder, into the ischiorectal fossa.[93] The result is tenesmus, dyschezia, and constipation. Incarceration of the bladder in the hernial sac causes more severe clinical signs as a result of urinary obstruction.

In most dogs the herniation is idiopathic, but in up to 50% of affected cats, associated conditions causing chronic tenesmus can be identified (e.g., megacolon, perineal masses, feline urologic syndrome, perineal urethrostomy).[94] Idiopathic perineal herniation appears to result from age-related changes in the muscles of the pelvic girdle, particularly the levator ani muscle, which undergoes significant atrophy in affected dogs.[64] Recent electromyographic and histologic examinations of the levator ani and other muscles of the pelvic girdle have suggested that the probable cause of the atrophy is damage to the sacral plexus or to the muscular branches of the pudendal nerves.[64]

The diagnosis is usually made by physical examination of the perineal area. In most dogs and some cats a fluctuant swelling lateral to the anus will be observed. Rectal palpation reveals atrophy of the muscles of the pelvic girdle and/or dilatation or lateral deviation of the rectum. The process is usually unilateral, but bilateral hernias can occur in both dogs and cats. The deviation of the rectum into the hernial sac can lead to the development of a rectal diverticulum or rectal sacculation. In a rectal diverticulum the mucosa and submucosa of the rectum is forced through a defect in the muscular wall of the rectum. In rectal sacculation, the distal rectum dilates to fill the space formed by the atrophied pelvic girdle muscles. Feces are often retained in the sacculated area.

Definitive treatment of perineal hernia requires perineal herniorrhaphy.[94,95] Fecal softeners may palliate the condition in some animals. In cats, attention to the primary cause is particularly important.[94]

RECTAL PROLAPSE

Rectal prolapse is occasionally seen in dogs and cats. It is particularly common in young animals and usually occurs secondary to other diseases causing persistent diarrhea and tenesmus (see Chapter 5). It is occasionally observed as a complication of the megacolon syndrome in cats. On most occasions, just the rectal mucosa prolapses, but sometimes the prolapsed segment involves the entire rectal wall. Prolapsed mucosa usually appears as a small rosette-like area of red and swollen mucosa in the anal canal. When the entire rectal wall is prolapsed, a tubular mass will be observed. The major differential diagnosis in the latter case is intussusception of a more proximal section of bowel through the anus. The two conditions are differentiated by use of a rectal probe. In the case of a proximal intussusception no rectal "cul-de-sac" will be encountered by a probe placed between the anal skin and the rectal prolapse.

Small prolapses can usually be replaced manually. Lubrication and use of topical dessicants such as powdered dextrose may facilitate replacement. Once the prolapse is reduced it is usually held in place with a temporary purse string suture, and medical treatment is directed at any identifiable cause of tenesmus. Intrarectal administration of topical anesthetic/steroid ointments or enemas can be useful in the immediate postoperative period.[96] More extensive prolapse, particularly if the tissue appears to have questionable viability, requires surgical excision of the mucosa or rectum. A colopexy procedure is indicated if the rectum repeatedly prolapses.

ANORECTAL STRICTURES

Anorectal strictures are unusual in the dog and cat. They most commonly result from neoplasia and occasionally from severe inflammatory diseases of the large bowel or anus. They are a recognized complication of perianal fistula. The clinical signs usually pertain initially to the primary disease process, and then are superseded by progressively greater tenesmus, dyschezia, and thinning of the diameter of the stool. Diagnosis may be made by digital palpation in many cases or by contrast radiography or proctoscopy (Figure 26–4). Treatment is surgical resection. The prognosis is guarded because stricturing may reoccur at the surgical site.

ANAL PRURITUS AND ANAL SAC DISEASES

In dogs, anal pruritus is usually manifested by scooting of the perineal region on the ground or frequent licking of the anal area. The most common cause in dogs is anal gland disorders. At times, badly inflamed anal glands will lead to dyschezia and hematochezia, mimicking colitis. Occasionally, an impacted anal gland will abscess and lead to a skin lesion reminiscent of a perianal fistula. Apocrine adenocarcinomas of the anal sacs are occasionally seen. These tumors are discussed in Chapter 27. Cats are rarely presented for anal gland impaction. On the rare occasion cats are affected by anal gland diseases, they lick their perianal area rather than scoot. The cause of impacted or inflamed anal sacs is usually not apparent. Occasionally the disorder is precipitated by a period of diarrhea during which incomplete evacuation of the sac results. It may also be a component of a generalized seborrheic disease.

Other postulated causes of perianal pruritus include tapeworm segments, irritant substances passed in the stool, and frequent perianal soiling by feces. Occasionally, perineal diseases such as perianal fistula, perianal dermatitis, fold pyodermas, vaginitis, and flea bite allergies may be apparent. When no specific cause can be determined, treatment considered should be regular baths or frequent gentle perianal washes (to minimize fecal soiling), a change of diet, and the discontinuation of any nonessential medications. Impacted anal sacs are usually evacuated by digital pressure. Concurrent anal saculitis may be treated by instillation of antibacterial corticosteroid ointments into the anal sac. If repeated evacuations prove necessary, chemical cautery with 1 to 2 mL of tincture of iodine or a variety of other chemical agents may be performed.[97] Alternatively, surgical resection may be undertaken.

PERIANAL FISTULA

Perianal fistulas are chronic inflammatory lesions of perianal tissues (Figure 26–5). The disease is most frequently seen in the middle-aged to older German shepherd dog and, to a lesser extent, in Irish setters and Labradors, but a wide variety of dog breeds and occasionally cats[98] can be affected. Perianal fistulas cause sufficient pain that affected dogs often cannot be examined without sedation. Similarly, the owner is seldom able to examine the area under the tail and may be unaware of the extent of the lesions. Clinical signs include licking of the anal area and scooting to relieve the irritation, which may leave a discharge of pus or blood on the floor. More advanced cases show signs of dyschezia and tenesmus.

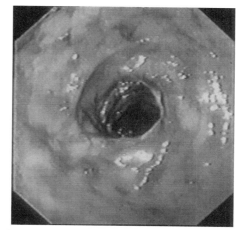

FIGURE 26–4. Endoscopic appearance of a rectal stricture in a dog. The cause of the stricture was never determined.

The cause of perianal fistulas is unknown. One proposed pathomechanism is fecolith impaction in the anal sinuses, which is thought to lead eventually to pressure necrosis and fistulation. Another proposed cause is contamination of the hair follicles or anal, tubular, or sebaceous glands with a film of feces that eventually leads to infection and fistulation.[99] Detailed histopathologic studies of the early lesions (see later) support this latter proposal as do some peculiarities of the German shepherd breed. It is entirely possible that both pathomechanisms are operative.

The German shepherd has a broad tail base and a low tail carriage, which predisposes it to the maintenance of a moist perianal fecal film in which bacteria can proliferate. In a detailed histologic analysis of the perianal area of dogs, German shepherds were noted to have an increase in density of apocrine sweat glands in the zona cutanea and increased evidence of chronic inflammation in the perianal glands (modified tubuloalveolar sweat glands that ring the anal canal).[100] German shepherds are predisposed to deep pyodermas in other parts of the body, and as a breed they are known to have low serum IgA levels, perhaps implying a deficient defense of cutaneous follicular structures. Of 5 consecutive German shepherds presented to the UCD VMTH with perianal fistula, 3 were observed to have moderately low IgA levels (0.20–0.26 mg/dl).[53] In a more extensive evaluation of immune function

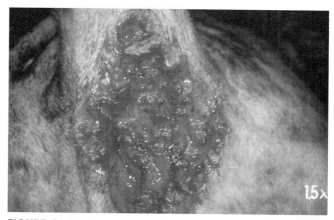

FIGURE 26–5. Severe perianal fistulation in a German shepherd dog.

in German shepherds, however, only 2 of 15 dogs had a low serum IgA.[101] Lymphocytic blastogenesis tests were persistently abnormal in 5 of 33 dogs.[101] There is also a high incidence of concomitant diarrhea in affected dogs. This diarrhea often persists after surgical correction of the perianal disease. Thus, tenesmus caused by the anal problem is not the sole cause of the diarrhea. Colonic biopsy often identifies chronic colitis. The chronic diarrhea may contribute to the condition by encouraging more frequent perianal soiling.

Perianal fistula lesions appear initially as small ulcerations in the perianal area, and when they are probed it is discovered that considerable adjacent subepithelial tissue is involved. In addition to the involvement of the subepithelial space, chronically infected tracts often extend into the tissue between the anal sphincters and the wall of the pelvis. Occasionally they can penetrate to depths cranial to both sphincters. The tracts do not usually penetrate the rectal mucosa, submucosa, or the anal sacs. In one study, histopathology of the anal area demonstrated five distinct lesions.[102] Four of these were relatively common and included hidradentitis of the cutaneous zone of the anal canal that was responsible for superficial cutaneous sinuses; fistulas of the anal sinuses which extended either directly to the skin or into large perianal subcutaneous abscesses that in turn opened to the skin; rupture of the anal sac; and submucosal sinuses of the terminal third of the rectum. A less frequently observed lesion was rectal fistulation. In another study, early lesions were classified as inflammation associated with epidermal appendages; intermediate lesions were considered inflammation of the epidermal appendages in association with cutaneous ulceration and nonarborizing sinus tracts; and late lesions were described as arborizing epithelial-lined sinus tracts extending through the perirectal stroma.[103] Aerobic cultures of deep perianal tissues revealed bacterial growth in 85% of dogs with *E. coli* being the predominant isolate.

Antibiotic therapy of perianal fistulas at best only ameliorates the disease temporarily. The disease is managed surgically, although the most effective surgical technique remains mired in controversy. The most frequent complication of the surgery is fecal incontinence. In dogs with concomitant diarrhea, a colon biopsy should be obtained at the time of the surgical correction of the fistulas. If concurrent chronic colitis is present it should be managed by standard measures. Recurrence is common. The prognosis is guarded.

BOWEL PERFORATION AND PERITONITIS

Etiology

Perforation of the bowel is an infrequent but extremely serious condition. Perforation may accompany a variety of conditions including ingestion of foreign bodies, neoplasia, hyperadrenocorticism, anti-inflammatory drug administration, intestinal torsion or incarceration, penetrating abdominal wounds, perforating peptic ulcers, pelvic fractures, and dehiscence of intestinal anastomoses or enterotomy sites. The gastrointestinal tract is the source of peritoneal contamination in approximately 60% of the cases of peritonitis in dogs, and surgical dehiscence of the bowel is the most frequent cause of this contamination.[104,105] The dehiscence rate for dogs undergoing small intestinal surgery is as high as 15.7% with an associated mortality rate of approximately 70%.[105]

Colonic ulcerations and perforations are most frequently observed in patients treated surgically for neurologic disease and concurrently medicated with dexamethasone.[45] In addi-

tion, combination corticosteroid and nonsteroidal anti-inflammatory drug (NSAID) therapy has been associated with colonic perforation in dogs undergoing non-neurologic surgical procedures. The colonic perforations in these situations are most commonly found on the antimesenteric border of the proximal portion of the descending colon but can appear anywhere in the large bowel including the cecum.

Glucocorticoids or NSAIDs can cause upper as well as lower gastrointestinal ulceration and perforation (see Chapter 14).[106] When NSAIDs and corticosteroids are combined, the development of the lesions is particularly rapid.[107]

Pathogenesis

The pathogenesis of most intestinal perforations is self-explanatory although that of drug-associated and neurosurgery-associated perforation has not been completely resolved. Proposed precipitating factors of colonic perforation in neurosurgical cases include the administration of glucocorticoids, surgical stress, neurologic damage, and fecal retention.[45] Localized colonic ischemia as a result of pain-induced increased sympathetic tone is a likely contributor, especially in view of the location of the lesions at the antimesenteric border. Inadequate postsurgical fluid therapy with resultant hypovolemia and release of angiotensin II is likely to compound the intestinal vasoconstriction. Angiotensin II is a potent vasoconstrictor and, in dogs, the vasculature of the canine colonic muscularis is particularly sensitive to angiotensin-induced vasoconstriction.[108] The release of angiotensin is also stimulated by opiates, agents that are frequently used during anesthesia or for pain relief of animals undergoing neurosurgery.[109] Once mucosal injury occurs, ischemia may be perpetuated because of the absorption of bacterial endotoxins that are known to increase sympathetic tone and, albeit transiently, portal pressure.

Possible mechanisms by which corticosteroids could predispose the colon to perforation include the inhibition of the immune response and collagen synthesis and damage to the mucosal barrier. The pathogenesis of bowel injury resulting from NSAIDs is also thought to be multifactorial and includes inhibition of cytoprotective prostaglandins, compromised bowel permeability, and depressed gut-associated lymphoid tissue suppressor activity (see Chapter 14).

Once the bowel is perforated, a complex series of events is initiated.[110] Intraperitoneal fluid circulation can result in rapid dispersion of the contaminants about the abdomen. Bacteria are readily absorbed into the lymphatics of the diaphragm and can be found in thoracic lymph within as short a time as 6 minutes.[110] Peritoneal injury leads to the peritoneal inflammation, leukocyte chemotaxis, exudation of plasma, release of thromboplastin, and eventually the formation of fibrin.[110] The plasma and phagocytes have antibacterial activities. Fibrinous adhesions of abdominal organs may occur, particularly in the presence of foreign material.[110] Fibrinous adhesions help prevent continual leakage of bowel content and may reduce the extent of their spread but, in excess, adhesions are detrimental to normal gastrointestinal tract function. A dynamic ileus develops rapidly, minimizing further contamination of the abdomen but complicating recovery by preventing alimentation once the perforation has been repaired. In animals succumbing to peritonitis, death results from a combination of hypovolemic, endotoxic, and septic shock, and DIC.

Diagnosis

The clinical signs of bowel perforation and peritonitis include depression, anorexia, vomiting, abdominal pain, and evidence of sepsis. In some animals, melena may be apparent. An important differential diagnosis is acute pancreatitis. The clinical signs of pancreatitis and intestinal perforation are similar and furthermore, at least in humans, serum amylase can be high in both conditions. Animals with intestinal perforation frequently have a left-shifted leukogram.[105] The diagnosis of perforation is usually made by observation of free fluid or gas on abdominal radiographs, and a septic exudate containing a mixed bacterial flora and particulate debris on paracentesis. If an animal has recently undergone an abdominal surgery, be careful in interpreting the presence of free abdominal gas as indicative of a perforation because air entering the abdomen during the surgery can remain there for as long as 3 to 4 weeks before resorption is complete.[111] Culture of the abdominal fluid may be necessary to differentiate septic from nonseptic peritonitis in some patients. Amylase concentration may be high in the abdominal fluid as a result of leakage from the bowel. On occasion, particularly following neurosurgery-associated colonic perforation, the diagnosis can be elusive because of the anti-inflammatory nature of concomitantly administered corticosteroids, peracute onset of clinical signs, and rapid death (within 24 hours) of the patient.[45] Perforations that result in a localized area of peritonitis may require diagnostic peritoneal lavage to detect. Ultrasonography or exploratory surgery may be necessary to locate walled-off abscesses resulting from previous perforation.

Treatment

The treatment for perforation and peritonitis is surgical. The patient is first rapidly stabilized with intravenous fluids in association with intravenous ampicillin (20 mg/kg IV). As soon as any hypovolemia has been corrected, gentamicin therapy (2.2 mg/kg IV) is begun. During surgery the cause of the perforation is determined and corrected, adhesions are broken down, and the abdominal cavity is flushed with copious quantities of warm sterile saline.[112] No antimicrobials need be added to the flush solution. At the conclusion of the surgery, the abdomen is closed if the perforation was very recent and the peritonitis incipient. However, if the peritonitis is well established, the abdominal incision is only partly closed (with a loosely applied simple continuous suture pattern) and the abdomen is carefully bound with a sterile absorptive wrap that is replaced two to four times daily. This open abdominal drainage technique is the preferred technique for the drainage of heavily contaminated abdomens.[113-115] It is the only means by which effective drainage can be facilitated, and it provides an unfavorable environment for anaerobic bacteria and allows the abdomen to be repeatedly flushed with sterile saline.[112-115] In the authors' experience, and that of others, dogs and cats tolerate open abdominal drainage well and demonstrate minimal signs of discomfort.[112] Hypoproteinemia is a common complication of the procedure.[113-115]

Antimicrobial therapy is continued during the postoperative period. A combination protocol is essential to prevent abscess formation by the intestinal anaerobic bacteria, and sepsis from the intestinal (and perhaps nosocomial) gram negative bacteria. A suitable antimicrobial combination is ampicillin (20 mg/kg q 6–8 hours IV, PO) to cover the aerobic gram positive spectrum, gentamicin (2.2 mg/kg q 8 hours IV, SC) to cover the gram negative aerobic spectrum, and metronidazole (10–15 mg/kg q 12 hours PO, SC) to broaden the anaerobic coverage to include Bacteroides species. Another suitable combination is clindamycin and gentamicin. The use of gentamicin combined with first-generation cephalosporins has been recommended but is not likely to cover the anaerobic spectrum adequately. The duration of antibiotic therapy is dictated by the animal's response to therapy, but a minimum of 7 to 10 days is usual. It is advisable to restrict the gentamicin course to 5 days or less to reduce the probability of clinically significant renal toxicity. When the gentamicin is stopped, the gram negative spectrum should be covered by the addition of a fluorquinilone antibiotic, such as norfloxacin (3–7 mg/kg q 12 hours PO) or enrofloxacin (5 mg/kg q 12 hours PO), to the treatment regimen.

In animals undergoing open abdominal drainage, the peritoneal discharge usually abates 3 to 5 days after the surgery. At this point a sample of the abdominal fluid is cultured (aerobically and anaerobically), the abdominal lavage is repeated, and the abdomen closed. Subsequent antibacterial therapy is based on these culture results.

Prognosis and Prevention

In spite of properly applied open drainage techniques, the mortality attributable to generalized peritonitis in dogs and cat ranges from 20% to 48%.[113,115] The mortality associated with anti-inflammatory drug-associated or neurosurgery-associated colonic perforation is close to 100%, presumably because of late detection.

The postoperative patient (particularly following neurosurgery) should be considered at high risk for gastrointestinal perforation.[45] Preventative measures are important to avoid this complication. Maintain adequate hydration status and plasma protein concentration by the use of parenteral fluids or plasma administration to prevent hypovolemia and angiotensin II release. Do not use glucocorticoids in the postoperative peroid if at all possible but, if they are essential, restrict the use of high doses to as short a period as feasible (e.g., 2–3 days postsurgery). Avoid the use of NSAIDs and, in particular, do not administer these drugs in association with glucocorticoids. In our experience, this adverse interaction can still occur even if the administration of the glucocorticoids precedes the NSAIDs by as long as 3 days. If NSAIDs must be used, consider the concurrent usage of misoprostol (Cytotec, Searle; 1–4 µg/kg q 8 hours) to minimize mucosal damage. Misoprostol may also prove superior to drugs such as sucralfate and H_2 blockers in the prevention of glucocorticoid-induced mucosal injury (see Chapter 14). In addition, correct fecal retention before surgery and prevent constipation by using bulk-promoting agents and laxatives.

SCLEROSING ENCAPSULATING PERITONITIS; MESENTERIC SCLEROSIS

Sclerotic thickening of the peritoneum, serosa, and/or mesentery with encapsulation and clumping of the bowel are relatively uncommon disorders in dogs and cats (Figure 26–6). They are usually idiopathic, but similar disorders have been reported in association with multiple bowel perforations due to linear foreign bodies and to abdominal carcinomatosis and sclerosing mesotheliomas.[117-120] In the latter situation, the pri-

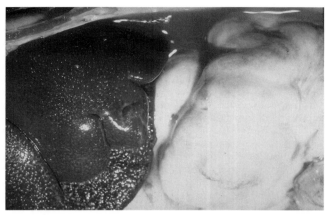

FIGURE 26–6. Abdominal sclerosis secondary to mesothelioma in a dog. Note the bunching of the small intestine into a sclerotic sac. (Courtesy of Dr. Keith Thompson)

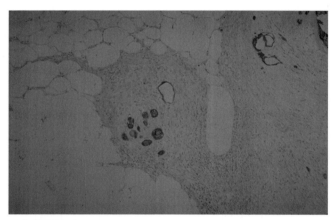

FIGURE 26–7. Photomicrograph of a marked sclerotic reaction surrounding a small focus of neoplastic cells in the peritoneum of a dog with abdominal carcinomatosis.

mary tumors can be located in the stomach, bowel, or pancreas, and histologically small islands of neoplastic cells are found surrounded by abundant proliferating connective tissue (Figure 26–7).[117] The clinical signs associated with the abdominal sclerosis include anorexia, vomiting, borborygmus, abdominal distension, and abdominal effusion. The prognosis is poor but one dog with sclerosing encapsulating peritonitis that occurred postovariohysterectomy responded to surgical drainage and abdominal lavage.[119]

REFERENCES

1. Granger DN, Rutili G, McCord JM. Superoxide radicals in feline intestinal ischemia. Gastroenterology 81:22–29, 1981.
2. McCord JM, Wong K. The pathophysiology of superoxide: Roles in inflammation and ischemia. Can J Physiol Pharmacol 60:1346–1352, 1982.
3. Parks DA, Buckley GB, Granger DN, et al. Ischemic injury in the cat small intestine: Role of superoxide radicals. Gastroenterology 82:9–15, 1982.
4. Kubes P, Hunter J, Granger N. Ischemia/reperfusion-induced feline intestinal dysfunction: Importance of granulocyte recruitment. Gastroenterology 103:807–812, 1992.
5. Robinson JWL, Haroud M, Winistorfer B, et al. Recovery of function and structure of dog ileum and colon following two hours acute ischaemia. Eur J Clin Invest 4:443–452, 1974.
6. Robinson JWL, Menge H, Sepulveda FV, et al. The functional response of the dog ileum to one hour's ischaemia. Clin Sci Mol Med 50:115–122, 1976.
7. Robinson JWL, Mirkovitch V. The recovery of function and microcirculation in small intestinal loops following ischaemia. Gut 13:784–789, 1972.
8. Harvey HJ, Rendano VT. Small bowel volvulus in dogs. Vet Surg 13:91–94, 1984.
9. Westermarck E, Rimailia-Parnanen E. Mesenteric torsion in dogs with exocrine pancreatic insufficiency: 21 cases (1978–1987). J Am Vet Med Assoc 195:1404–1406, 1989.
10. Shealy PM, Henderson RA. Canine intestinal volvulus: A report of nine new cases. Vet Surg 21:15–19, 1992.
11. Williams DA, Burrows CF. Short-bowel syndrome—a case report in a dog and discussion of the pathophysiology of bowel resection. J Sm Anim Pract 22:263–275, 1981.
12. Carberry CA, Flanders JA. Cecal-colic volvulus in 2 dogs. Vet Surg 22:225–228, 1993.
13. Camble PJ, Page CA. Mesenteric torsion in a toy dog. Vet Rec 130:166–167, 1992.
14. Hosgood G, Bunge M, Dorfman M. Jejunal incarceration by an omental tear in a dog. J Am Vet Med Assoc 200:947–950, 1992.
15. Marks A. Torsion of the colon in a rough collie. Vet Rec 118:400, 1986.
16. Endres WA, Remondini DJ, Graver ER. A case report of torsion of the descending colon in a six-month-old female collie. VM/SAC, 954–960, October 1968.
17. Yanoff SR, Willard MD. Short bowel syndrome in dogs and cats. Sem Vet Med Surg 4:226–231, 1989.
18. Vanderhoof JA, Langnas AN, Pinch LW, et al. Short bowel syndrome. J Pediatr Gastroenterol Nutr 14:359–370, 1992.
19. Zenger E, Evering WN, Willard MD. Chronic diarrhea associated with intestinal anomalies in a 6 year old dog. J Am Vet Med Assoc 201:1737–1740,1992.
20. Gouttebel MC, Astre C, Briand D, et al. Influence of N-acetylglutamine or glutamine infusion on plasma amino acid concentrations during the early phrase of small-bowel adaptation in the dog. J Parenter Enteral Nutr 16:117–120, 1992.
21. Warner BW, Chaet MS. Nontransplant surgical options for management of the short bowel syndrome. J Pediatr Gastroenterol Nutr 17:1–12, 1993.
22. Van der Gaag I, Tibboel D. Intestinal atresia and stenosis in animals: A report of 34 cases. Vet Pathol 17:565–574, 1980.
23. Johnson R. Intestinal atresia and stenosis: A review comparing its etiopathogenesis. Vet Res Commun 10:95–105, 1986.
24. Ablin LW, Moore FM, Shields Henney LH, et al. Intestinal diverticular malformations in dogs and cats. Comp Contin Ed Pract Vet 13:426–430, 1991.
25. Amand WB. Nonneurogenic disorders of the anus and rectum. Vet Clin N Am 4:535–551, 1974.
26. Osborne CA, Engen MH, Yano BL. Congenital urethrorectal fistula in two dogs. J Am Vet Med Assoc 166:999–1002, 1975.
27. Rawlings CA, Capps WS. Rectovaginal fistula and imperforate anus in a dog. J Am Vet Med Assoc 159:320–326, 1971.
28. Suess RP, Martin RA, Moon ML, et al. Rectovaginal fistula with atresia ani in three kittens. Cornell Vet 82:141–153, 1992.
29. Jakowski RM. Duplication of colon in a Labrador retriever with abnormal spinal column. Vet Pathol 14:256–260, 1977.
30. Spaulding KA, Cohn LA, Miller RT, et al. Enteric duplication in two dogs. Vet Radiol 31:83–88, 1990.
31. Schlesinger DP, Philibert D, Breur GJ. Agenesis of the cecum and the ascending and transverse colon in a twelve year old cat. Can Vet J 33:544–546, 1992.
32. Runyon CL, Merkley DF, Hagemoser WA. Intussusception associated with a paracolonic enterocyst in a dog. J Am Vet Med Assoc 185:443, 1984.
33. Fluke MH, Hawkins EC, Elliot GS, et al. Short colon in two cats and a dog. J Am Vet Med Assoc 195:87–90, 1989.
34. Forbes DC, Dalla-Tina K, Lester S. Plasmacytic enterocolitis with hypogangliosis in a puppy. Can Vet J 32:624–625, 1991.
35. Iwata H, Arai C, Koike Y, et al. Heterotopic gastric mucosa of the small intestine in laboratory beagle dogs. Toxicol Pathol 18:373–379, 1990.
36. Rogers KS, Butler LM, Edwards JF, et al. Rectal hemorrhage associated with vascular ectasia in a young dog. J Am Vet Med Assoc 200:1349–1351, 1992.
37. Levine SH. Ruptured cecum due to abscessation in a dog. A case report. J Am Anim Hosp Assoc 18:337–340, 1982.
38. Moore MP, Robinette JD. Cecal perforation and adrenocortical adenoma in a dog. J Am Vet Med Assoc 191:87–88, 1987.
39. Miller WW, Hathcock JT, Dillon AR. Cecal inversion in eight dogs. J Am Anim Hosp Assoc 20:1009–1013, 1983.
40. Bush BM. Colitis in the dog. Vet Ann 25:337–347, 1985.
41. Burrows CF. Diseases of the colon rectum and anus in the dog and cat. In: Anderson NV (ed) Veterinary Gastroenterology. Lea & Febiger, Philadelphia, 553–592, 1980.

42. Sack TL, Sleisenger MH. Effects of systemic and extraintestinal diseases on the gut. In: Sleisenger MH, Fordtran JS (eds) Gastrointestinal Disease. Pathophysiology, Diagnosis, Management, 4th ed. WB Saunders, Philadelphia, 488–528, 1989.
43. Kang JY. The gastrointestinal tract in uremia. Dig Dis Sci 38:257–268, 1993.
44. Wilcox B. Endoscopic biopsy interpretation in canine or feline enterocolitis. Sem Vet Med Surg 7:162–171, 1992.
45. Toombs JP, Collins LG, Graves GM, et al. Colonic perforation in corticosteroid-treated dogs. J Am Vet Med Assoc 188:145–150, 1986.
46. Morris EL. Pneumatosis coli in a dog. Vet Radiol Ultrasound 33:154–157, 1992.
47. Degner DA. Pneumatosis coli in a dog. Can Vet J 33:609–611, 1992.
48. Spinato MT, Barker IK, Houston DM. A morphometric study of the canine colon: Comparison of control dogs and cases of colonic disease. Can J Vet 54:477–486, 1990.
49. Leib MS. Dietary fiber and large bowel diarrhea. Proc 7th ACVIM Forum, 359–360, 1989.
50. Bo-Linn GW, Vendrell DD, Lee E, et al. An evaluation of the significance of microscopic colitis in patients with chronic diarrhea. J Clin Invest 75:1559–1569, 1985.
51. Rampton DS, Baithun SI. Is microscopic colitis due to bile-salt malabsorption? Dis Colon Rectum 30:950–952, 1987.
52. Schuster MM. Motor action of rectum and anal sphincters incontinence and defecation. In: Code CF (ed) Handbook of Physiology. Sec. 6, Alimentary Canal, Vol. 4. American Physiological Society, Washington DC, 2121–2146, 1968.
53. Guilford WG. Unpublished observations, 1987.
54. Gaston EA. The physiology of fecal continence. Surg Gynecol Obstet 87:280–290, 1948.
55. Gaston EA. Physiological basis for the preservation of fecal continence after resection of rectum. J Am Med Assoc 146:1486–1489, 1951.
56. Karlan M, McPherson RC, Watman RN. An experimental evaluation of fecal continence- sphincter- and reservoir- in the dog. Surg Gynecol Obstet 108:469–475, 1959.
57. Scharli AF, Kiesewetter WB. Defecation and continence: Some new concepts. Dis Colon Rectum 13:81–107, 1970.
58. Speakman CTM, Kamm MA. The internal anal sphincter—new insights into faecal incontinence. Gut 32:345–346, 1991.
59. Parks A. Anorectal incontinence. Proc Royal Soc Med 68:681–690, 1975.
60. Duthie HL, Bennett RC. The relationship of sensation in the anal canal to the functional anal sphincter: A possible factor in anal continence. Gut 4:179–182, 1963.
61. De Lahunta A. Veterinary Neuroanatomy and Clinical Neurology. WB Saunders, Philadelphia 288–295, 1977.
62. Martin WD, Fletcher TF, Bradley WE. Innervation of feline perineal musculature. Anat Rec 180:15–30, 1974.
63. Evans HE, Christensen GC. Miller's Anatomy of the Dog, 2nd ed. Philadelphia, WB Saunders, 331–337, 1979.
64. Sjollema BE, Venker-van Haagen AJ, van Sluijs FJ, et al. Electromyography of the pelvic diaphragm and anal sphincter in dogs with perineal hernia. Am J Vet Res 54:185–190, 1993.
65. De Lahunta A. Veterinary Neuroanatomy and Clinical Neurology. WB Saunders, Philadelphia, 110–124, 1977.
66. Shafik A. A new concept of the anatomy of the anal sphincter mechanism and the physiology of defecation. Invest Urology 12:412–419, 1975.
67. Ashdown RR. Symposium on canine recto-anal disorders. 1. Clinical anatomy. J Sm Anim Pract 9:315–322, 1968.
68. Duthie HL. Anal continence. Gut 12:844–852, 1971.
69. Wunderlich M, Parks AG. Physiology and pathophysiology of the anal sphincters. Int Surg 67:291–298, 1982.
70. Frenckner B. Function of the anal sphincters in man. Gut 16:638–644, 1975.
71. Strombeck DR, Harrold D. Anal sphincter pressure and the rectosphincteric reflex in the dog. Am J Vet Res 49:191–192, 1988.
72. Schuster MM. Tests related to the colon, rectum, and anus. In: Berk JE (ed) Gastroenterology, 4th ed. WB Saunders, Philadelphia, 388–401, 1985.
73. Phillips SF, Edwards DAW. Some aspects of anal continence and defaecation. Gut 6:396–406, 1965.
74. Goldberg SM. Anal incontinence. In: Goldberg SM, Gordon PH, Nivatongs S (eds) Essentials of Anorectal Surgery. JB Lippincott, Philadelphia, 282–290, 1980.
75. Read NW, Harford WV, Schmulen CA, et al. A clinical study of patients with fecal incontinence and diarrhea. Gastroenterology 76: 747–756, 1979.
76. Schoetz DJ. Operative therapy for anal incontinence. Surg Clin N Am 65:35–46, 1985.
77. Chapman BL, Voith VL. Behavioral problems in old dogs: 26 cases (1984–1987). J Am Vet Med Assoc 196:944–946, 1990.
78. De Groat WC, Booth AM. Autonomic systems to the urinary bladder and sexual organs. In: Dyck PJ (ed) Peripheral Neuropathy, 2nd ed. WB Saunders, Philadelphia, 285–299, 1984.
79. Morgan JP. Vertebral column. In: Radiology in Veterinary Orthopedics. Lea & Febiger, Philadelphia, 219–300, 1972.
80. Swash M. Anorectal incontinence: Electrophysiological tests. Br J Surg (suppl) 72:14–15, 1985.
81. O'Brien DP, Dean PW. Pudendo-anal (bulbocavernosus) reflex electrophysiology in the dog. Abstract ACVIM Proc, 1988.
82. Pemberton JH, Kelly KA. Achieving enteric continence: Principles and applications. Mayo Clin Proc 61:586–599, 1986.
83. Dean PW, O'Brien DP, Turk AM, et al. Silicone elastomer sling for fecal incontinence in dogs. Vet Surg 17:304–310, 1988.
84. Jaffe JH, Martin WR. Opioid analgesics and antagonists. In: Goodman-Gilman A, Goodman LS, et al. (eds) The Pharmacological Basis of Therapeutics, 7th ed. Macmillan, New York, 503, 1985.
85. Richter KP. Diseases of the rectum and anus. In: Kirk RW, Bonagura JD (eds) Current Veterinary Therapy XI. WB Saunders, Philadelphia, 613–618, 1992.
86. Burrows CF. Constipation. In: Kirk RW (ed) Current Veterinary Therapy IX. WB Saunders, Philadelphia, 905–908, 1986.
87. Dimski DS. Constipation: Pathophysiology, diagnostic approach, and treatment. Sem Vet Med Surg 4:247–254, 1989.
88. Muir P, Goldsmid SE, Bellenger CR. Megacolon in a cat following ovariohysterectomy. Vet Rec 129:512–513, 1991.
89. Shafik A. Constipation, pathogenesis and management. Drugs 45:528–540, 1993.
90. Schrader SC. Pelvic osteotomy as a treatment for obstipation in cats with acquired stenosis of the pelvic canal: Six cases (1978–1989). J Am Vet Med Assoc 200:208–213, 1992.
91. Atkins CE. Hypertonic sodium phosphate enema intoxication. In: Kirk RW (ed) Current Veterinary Therapy IX. WB Saunders, Philadelphia, 213–216, 1986.
92. DeNovo RC, Bright RM. Chonic feline constipation/obstipation. In: Kirk RW, Bonagura JD (eds) Current Veterinary Therapy XI. WB Saunders, Philadelphia, 619–625, 1992.
93. Hayes HM, Wilson GP, Tarone RE. The epidemiologic features of perineal hernia in 771 dogs. J Am Anim Hosp Assoc 14:703–707, 1978.
94. Welches CD, Scavelli TD, Aronsohn MG, et al. Perineal hernia in the cat: A retrospective study of 40 cases. J Am Anim Hosp Assoc 28:431–438, 1992.
95. Orsher RJ, Johnston DE. The surgical treatment of perianal hernia in dogs by transportation of the obturator muscle. Comp Contin Educ Pract Vet 7:233–239, 1985.
96. Seim HB. Diseases of the anus and rectum. In: Kirk RW (ed) Current Veterinary Therapy IX. WB Saunders, Philadelphia, 916–921, 1986.
97. Halnan CRE. Therapy of anal sacculitis in the dog. J Sm Anim Pract 17:685–691, 1976.
98. Johnson ME. Perianal fistula-like disease in a cat. Comp Anim Pract 1:16–19, 1987.
99. Harvey CE. Perianal fistula in the dog. Vet Rec 91:25–32, 1972.
100. Budsberg SC, Spurgeon TL, Liggitt HD. Anatomic predisposition to perianal fistulae formation in the German shepherd dog. Am J Vet Res 46:1468–1472, 1985.
101. Killingsworth CR, Walshaw R, Reimann KA, et al. Thyroid and immunologic status of dogs with perianal fistula. Am J Vet Res 49:1742–1746, 1988.
102. Johnston DE. Rectum and anus: Surgical diseases. In: Slatter DH (ed) Textbook of Small Animal Surgery. WB Saunders, Philadelphia, 770–794, 1985.
103. Killingsworth CR, Walshaw R, Dunstan RW, et al. Bacterial population and histologic changes in dogs with perianal fistula. Am J Vet Res 49:1736–1741, 1988.
104. Hosgood G, Salisbury K. Generalized peritonitis in dogs: 50 cases (1975–1986). J Am Vet Assoc 193:1448–1450, 1988.
105. Allen DA, Smeak DD, Schertel ER. Prevalence of small intestinal dehiscence and associated clinical factors: A retrospective study of 121 dogs. J Am Anim Hosp Assoc 28:70–76, 1992.
106. Sorjonen DC, Dillon AR, Powers RD, et al. Effects of dexamethasone and surgical hypotension on the stomach of dogs: Clinical, endoscopic, and pathologic evaluations. Am J Vet Res 44:1233–1237, 1983.
107. Dow SW, Rosychuk AW, McChesney AE, et al. Effects of flunixin and flunixin plus prednisone on the gastrointestinal tract of dogs. Am J Vet Res 51:1131–1138, 1990.
108. MacDonald PH, Dinda PK, Beck IT. The role of angiotensin in the intestinal vascular response to hypotension in a canine model. Gastroenterology 103:57–64, 1992.
109. Livingston EH, Passaro EP. Postoperative ileus. Dig Dis Sci 35:121–132, 1990.
110. Hosgood GL, Salisbury SK. Pathophysiology and pathogenesis of generalized peritonitis. Prob Vet Med 1:159–167, 1989.
111. Probst CW, Stickle RL, Bartlett PC. Duration of pneumoperitoneum in the dog. Am J Vet Res 47:176–178, 1986.

112. Salisbury SK, Hosgood GL. Management of the patient with generalized peritonitis. Prob Vet Med 1:168–182, 1989.
113. Greenfield CL, Walshaw R. Open peritoneal drainage for treatment of contaminated peritoneal cavity and septic peritonitis in dogs and cats: 24 cases (1980–1986). J Am Vet Med Assoc 191:100–105, 1987.
114. Orsher RJ, Rosin E. Open peritoneal drainage in experimental peritonitis in dogs. Vet Surg 222–226, 1984.
115. Woolfson JM, Dulisch ML. Open abdominal drainage in the treatment of generalized peritonitis in 25 dogs and cats. Vet Surg 15:27–32, 1986.
116. Green CE. Gastrointestinal, intra-abdominal, and hepatobiliary infections. In: Green CE (ed) Clinical Microbiology and Infectious Diseases. WB Saunders, Philadelphia, 247–268, 1984.
117. Roth L, King JM. Mesenteric and omental sclerosis associated with metastases from gastrointestinal neoplasia in the dog. J Sm Anim Pract 31:27–30, 1990.
118. Boothe HW, Lay JC, Moreland KJ. Sclerosing encapsulating peritonitis in three dogs. J Am Vet Med Assoc 198:267–270, 1991.
119. Bellenger CR, Rothwell TLW. Sclerosing encapsulating peritonitis in a dog. Aust Vet Pract 21:131–132, 1991.
120. Rothwell TLW. Retractile mesenteritis in a cat. Vet Rec 130:492, 1992.

27

Neoplasms of the Gastrointestinal Tract, APUD Tumors, Endocrinopathies and the Gastrointestinal Tract

W. GRANT GUILFORD AND DONALD R. STROMBECK

NEOPLASMS OF THE GASTROINTESTINAL TRACT[1-6]

Prevalence of Gastrointestinal Tumors

Neoplasms of the gastrointestinal tract of dogs and cats occur infrequently in comparison to neoplasms of other body systems. In a recent study of 400 dogs with cancer, 5.5% of the tumors were located in the digestive tract and 70% of these gastrointestinal cancers originated in the oral cavity.[7] Tumors of the canine and feline esophagus are very rare, accounting for less than 1% of all neoplasms and less than 5% of gastrointestinal tract neoplasms.[4] Similarly, gastric cancer is uncommon in dogs and cats, accounting for less than 1% of all canine neoplasms.[4] In dogs, neoplasms of the small intestine are less frequently recognized than those of the stomach or colonorectum, but in cats intestinal neoplasms occur most frequently in the small intestine.[1] In the intestine of dogs, the most common sites for cancer are the rectum, colon, and duodenum. Excluding the oral cavity, tumors of the large intestine represent 36% to 60% of all canine gastrointestinal tract neoplasms and 10% to 15% of all feline gastrointestinal neoplasms. At the VMTH at Davis the prevalence of all intestinal and rectal tumors is 9.9 cases per 10,000 in the dog and 8.8 cases per 10,000 in the cat.

Over two-thirds of gastrointestinal neoplasms in dogs and cats are malignant.[8] In general, older animals are affected and male dogs appear predisposed (at least to adenocarcinoma and lymphosarcoma).

The cause of gastrointestinal neoplasia is rarely evident with the exception of *Spirocerca lupi*–induced esophageal sarcoma. Other postulated causes are listed in Table 27–1 and discussed later in the section on gastric cancer.[9]

Clinical Findings and Diagnosis of Gastrointestinal Neoplasia

A variety of clinical signs can accompany gastrointestinal neoplasia. At times, the signs result from the local "mass effect" of the tumor, where the clinical manifestation primarily depends on the site of the tumor in the gastrointestinal tract. Thus, the most prominent manifestation of esophageal neoplasia is regurgitation, that of gastric neoplasia is vomiting, that of small intestinal neoplasia is small-bowel–type diarrhea with or without vomiting, and that of large-bowel neoplasia is large-bowel–type diarrhea. Alternatively, the clinical signs may result from metastatic lesions. Examples include the compression of adjacent organs by expansile lymph nodes, or infiltration of distant organs such as the liver, spleen, and central nervous system producing dysfunction of these organs and signs such as jaundice, abdominal hemorrhage, and seizures. Moreover, the clinical signs of gastrointestinal neoplasia can result from paraneoplastic syndromes. For example, apocrine adenocarcinoma is often associated with hypercalcemia, which in turn results in bowel stasis, renal disease, and polyuria/polydipsia.

Diagnosis of gastrointestinal neoplasia follows the principles outlined in Chapter 5. It is important to remember that not all nodular or ulceroproliferative lesions of the gastrointestinal tract are neoplastic. Important differential diagnoses include granulomas from inflammatory bowel disease, fungal infections, or foreign body penetration.

Table 27–1

POSTULATED PREDISPOSING CAUSES OF GASTROINTESTINAL NEOPLASIA

Esophageal Sarcoma
  Chronic esophagitis
  Spirocerca lupi
  Thermal injury
Gastric Carcinoma
  Achlorhydria
  Chronic gastritis
  Dietary carcinogens (mycotoxins, nitrosamines)
  Reflux gastritis
  Gastric polyps
  Helicobacter spp.
Alimentary Lymphosarcoma
  FeLV
  Lymphocytic-plasmacytic enteritis
Colonorectal Adenocarcinoma
  Bile salt malabsorption
  Chronic colitis
  Low-fiber diets
  High-fat diets
  Nitrosamines
  Polyposis

Treatment of Gastrointestinal Neoplasia

The treatment of gastrointestinal neoplasia still largely depends on surgical excision. If complete excision of the primary tumor is impossible or metastasis has occurred, adjuvant chemotherapy can be attempted. Unfortunately, with the principal exception of lymphosarcoma, chemotherapy has very limited value in the treatment of gastrointestinal neoplasia. Veterinarians interested in administering chemotherapeutic agents should do so only after consulting with a veterinary oncologist or reading recent in-depth reviews on the subject of cancer therapy because of the complexities of chemotherapeutic usage and the inherent danger to patient, owner, and veterinary staff.[1,4,6,10]

Gastrointestinal Toxicoses Resulting from Cancer Therapy

Damage to the bone marrow and gastrointestinal tract have long been the foremost toxicoses limiting the dose of many current chemotherapy drugs. In recent years, gastrointestinal toxicosis has assumed a relatively greater importance than bone marrow suppression because of the advent of products such as granulocyte-stimulating factor, which are capable of minimizing bone marrow toxicosis from chemotherapy.

Most drugs commonly used for cancer treatment in veterinary practice have adverse effects on the gastrointestinal system. For example, doxorubicin therapy in dogs not infrequently results in vomiting, diarrhea, colitis, and anorexia.[11] Vomiting is a frequent complication of high-dose cisplatin therapy and occasionally results from use of methotrexate, cyclophosphamide, and dacarbazine.[12,13] Methotrexate will occasionally produce a gastroenterocolitis.[13] Vomiting and diarrhea with or without blood are common signs resulting from 5-fluorouracil toxicosis in dogs.[14] Severe gastroenteritis occurred in 27% of dogs treated with a combination of vincristine, cyclophosphamide, and doxorubicin in one study.[15]

The gastroenterocolitis induced by chemotherapy drugs usually develops 3 to 7 days after administration and is characterized by hemorrhagic large-bowel–type diarrhea.[13] The condition usually resolves within 3 to 5 days, but severe hemorrhagic gastroenterocolitis is sometimes fatal (Figure 27–1). Anecdotal evidence suggests that treatment with Pepto-Bismol and antiemetics such as metoclopramide and/or prochloperazine is usually helpful.[13] Sucralfate appears to be valuable in reducing chemotherapy-induced nausea and vomiting in humans.[16]

The gastrointestinal tract is also vulnerable to ionizing radiation used for cancer therapy. Both acute (within 2 weeks of treatment) and delayed (months to years after treatment) gastrointestinal complications occur. Damage to the rapidly dividing gastrointestinal epithelium causes the acute gastrointestinal radiation syndrome (anorexia, vomiting, diarrhea) but is not responsible for the chronic syndrome (diarrhea, abdominal pain, and weight loss).[17] Microscopic changes in chronic radiation enteropathy in dogs include villus blunting, large bizarre fibroblasts, vascular sclerosis, thickening of the muscle layer, and submucosal and serosal fibrosis.[17] The clinical signs of the delayed syndrome are thought to be most often due to impaired motility and gastrointestinal transit (pseudo-obstruction), but aggressive radiation therapy in humans can produce other severe prob-

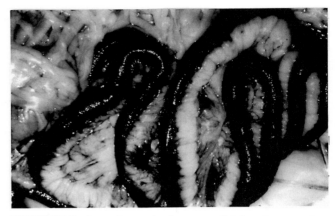

FIGURE 27–1. Severe hemorrhagic enterocolitis in a dog secondary to chemotherapy. (Courtesy of Dr. Keith Thompson)

lems including intestinal bleeding, stenosis, fistulation, and peritonitis.[17] Not only the dosage of irradiation administered but also the timing and fractionation of the dose are important in determining the degree of damage.[17] In dogs, 938 cGy on four separate occasions, 2 weeks apart, is sufficient to produce chronic diarrhea associated with mild histologic abnormalities and marked jejunal myoelectrical abnormalities including irregular slow wave rhythm with frequent uncoupling.[17] The cytotoxic effects of the radiation appear to be largely mediated by oxygen-derived free radicals and can be reduced in rats by the administration of vitamin E.[18] Sucralfate has also been found to be beneficial in reducing the symptoms of both acute and chronic radiation enteropathy in humans.[19]

Oropharyngeal Neoplasia

The oropharynx is the most frequent site of neoplasia in the gastrointestinal tract and accounts for approximately 4% to 7% of all canine neoplasia.[7,8] In dogs, the most frequent oropharyngeal neoplasms are melanoma and squamous cell carcinoma, followed in prevalence by fibrosarcoma and the epulides. In the feline oropharynx, the neoplasm with the highest prevalence is squamous cell carcinoma. About 50% of all feline oral neoplasms occur in the tongue. Oropharyngeal tumors are discussed more fully in Chapter 9.

Esophageal Neoplasia

Secondary esophageal cancers (e.g., thyroid carcinoma, tonsillar squamous cell carcinoma) are diagnosed more frequently than primary esophageal tumors but are still uncommon. In cats and dogs the most frequent primary esophageal cancers are squamous cell carcinomas and fibrosarcomas. In endemic areas, the esophageal sarcomas in dogs are usually associated with the parasite *Spirocerca lupi*. Other reported primary tumors include leiomyosarcoma, osteosarcoma, and undifferentiated carcinomas. Benign tumors are uncommon in the esophagus with the exception of leiomyomas, which have a high prevalence in older dogs and are usually found at the gastroesophageal junction. The occurrence of esophageal neoplasms is age related with the prevalence reaching 80% in 17- to 18-year-old beagles. Esophageal neoplasia is discussed more fully in Chapter 11.

Gastric Neoplasia

The prevalence of gastric cancer in dogs and cats is low, accounting for less than 1% of all canine tumors. At the UCD VMTH, the prevalence is 3 cases per 10,000 submissions. Similarly, most other institutions report only a scattering of cases over a prolonged period.[20] Primary gastric neoplasms occur predominantly in older dogs. The mean age of dogs affected by gastric cancer is 8 to 10 years, with by far the majority of affected dogs being older than 6 years.[20–26] The mean age of affected cats is lower than that of dogs because of the higher prevalence of lymphosarcoma, a neoplastic disease which frequenty affects young adult animals. Male dogs are more commonly affected with gastric cancer than females.[6,20] A higher risk has been noted for rough collies and Staffordshire bull terriers in one study.[26] In addition, Belgian shepherds appear to be predisposed to gastric carcinoma.[20,27]

The most prevalent gastric neoplasms in dogs are malignant epithelial tumors referred to as gastric carcinomas or adenocarcinomas. A variety of histologic subclassifications including signet ring cell carcinoma, undifferentiated carcinoma, mucinous adenocarcinoma, tubular adenocarcinoma, and scirrhous adenocarcinomas have been reported[27] but to date appear to have similar clinical behavior (Figure 27–2). In contrast, in cats, lymphosarcoma is the most common gastric neoplasm and adenocarcinoma is very rare (Figure 27–3). In dogs, the next most prevalent gastric neoplasm is leiomyoma, a benign tumor of smooth muscle. Other gastric tumors occasionally reported in dogs are adenomatous polyps, lymphosarcoma, leiomyosarcoma, fibroma, fibrosarcoma, squamous cell carcinoma, and plasmacytoma.

Most gastric cancers are malignant. One survey of gastric cancer recorded benign tumors in 31% (8% epithelial and 23% mesenchymal in origin) and malignant tumors in 68% of animals (53% epithelial and 15% mesenchymal in origin).[25] Malignant tumors spread early to regional lymph nodes and then to the liver and lungs.

Primary gastric neoplasms can occur anywhere in the stomach, but carcinomas often originate on the incisura angularis of the lesser curvature or elsewhere in the pyloric antrum. Leiomyomas are frequently found at the gastroesophageal junction (Figure 27–4).[21,22,24,27]

ETIOLOGY AND PATHOGENESIS. Little is known about the pathogenesis of gastric neoplasms in any species of animals. The incidence of gastric neoplasms in humans has long been thought to be influenced by diet, but it has been difficult to identify specific foods or food additives that result in increased risk.[28] Gastric atrophy and reduced acid secretion predispose to gastric cancer in people. The secondary increase in gastric bacterial numbers that accompanies atrophic gastritis may contribute to the pathogenesis by encouraging the conversion of chemicals such as nitrates into carcinogens. Recently, a strong link between *Helicobacter* spp. and gastric cancer has been discovered in humans[29] and may eventually prove to be of importance in dogs and cats. Chronic gastroduodenal reflux is also a risk factor for gastric cancer.[30]

The influence of growth factors and their receptors on the biologic behavior of gastric cancers is receiving close attention.[29,31] Human gastric cancer cells secrete and respond to such factors (by growth and proliferation) in an autocrine fashion. In an analogous manner, escape from growth inhibition by transforming growth factor beta may contribute to tumor cell proliferation.[29] Recent studies have indicated that transforming growth factor beta can induce apoptotic cell death. This observation is important because apoptosis appears to be a natural mechanism of counteracting cellular proliferation.[29]

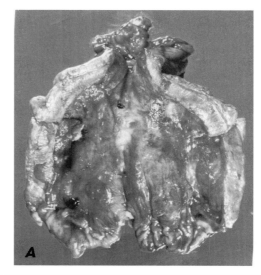

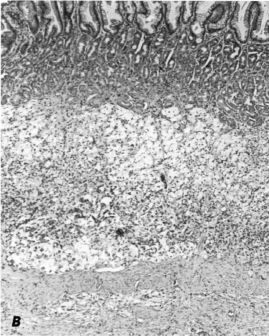

FIGURE 27–2. *(A)* Photograph of the stomach of a dog with schirrous carcinoma. Note the markedly thickened walls. *(B)* Photomicrograph of the stomach in *(A)*. The entire submucosa and part of the mucosa is infiltrated by adenocarcinoma cells. In other sections the muscularis and entire mucosa were involved.

CLINICAL FINDINGS. The clinical signs of gastric neoplasia usually have an insidious onset and a relentlessly progressive course. Consistent findings are vomiting, anorexia, and progressive weight loss. Hematemesis, diarrhea, and/or melena are often seen and abdominal pain is occasionally detected. Anemia can result when blood loss is chronic or marked.[32] Occasionally, advanced gastric neoplasia will be palpable as a cranial abdomen mass.

RADIOGRAPHIC AND ENDOSCOPIC FINDINGS. Positive contrast radiographic studies will detect some cases of stomach cancer but, even in animals with advanced neoplasms, these radiographic studies are often normal. In affected animals, positive contrast studies may identify gastric ulceration, a lack

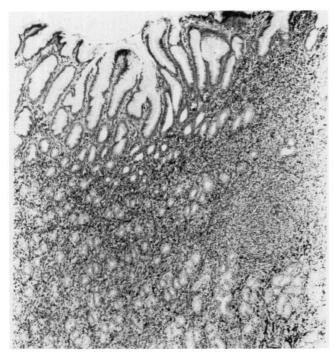

FIGURE 27-3. Photomicrograph of a gastric biopsy from a cat showing diffuse infiltration of lymphocytes, diagnostic for lymphosarcoma. No evidence of lymphosarcoma was found in any other tissue at necropsy.

of distensibility, thickening or roughening of the gastric wall, and delayed gastric emptying.[20] Most gastric ulcerations identified radiographically are caused by gastric carcinomas. Endoscopy is more sensitive than radiography for identifying gastric cancers that involve the mucosa. However, neoplasms located in the submucosa or muscularis are difficult to detect endoscopically unless they are sufficiently extensive to limit gastric distensibility whereupon the stomach wall feels stiff and unyielding against the tip of the endoscope. The endoscopic appearance of gastric carcinoma is quite variable. In some animals, gastric carcinomas will appear as single large ulcers raised from the surrounding mucosa with a thickened margin.[20] In other cases, carcinoma will be diffusely infiltrative causing mucosal discoloration, irregularity, necrosis, ulceration, and hemorrhage (Figure 27–5).[20] On occasion, carcinoma will infiltrate widely, distorting the lumen and rugal folds but without producing ulceration (Figure 27–6).[20]

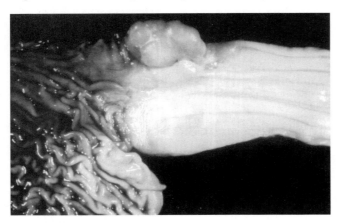

FIGURE 27-4. Photograph of a leiomyoma at the gastroesophageal junction of a dog. (Courtesy of Dr. Keith Thompson)

DIAGNOSIS. Although radiographic, endoscopic, or surgical findings may be highly suggestive of gastric neoplasia, definitive diagnosis can be made only by cytology or biopsy. It is important not to diagnose gastric cancer just on the gross appearance of the lesion because a variety of potentially treatable granulomatous diseases can grossly resemble gastric neoplasia. Chest radiographs should be taken because advanced gastric adenocarcinoma frequently metastasizes to the lungs.

MANAGEMENT. Gastric neoplasms are primarily treated by surgical resection. A successful adjuvant chemotherapy protocol for gastric carcinoma is yet to devised for dogs and cats. Promising avenues in human medicine include intraperitoneal 5-fluorouracil and cisplatin along with intravenous 5-fluorouracil, or the combination of cisplatin, etoposide, and doxorubicin, but survival rates remain very poor.[29,33] Gastric lymphosarcoma can be successfully treated with chemotherapeutic drugs (see later). An ulcerating gastric extamedullary plasmacytoma in a dog has been successfully treated with doxorubicin.[34] It is noteworthy that improved survival of humans with gastric cancer after treatment with cimetidine has been reported.[33] Furthermore, the growth of several human gastric tumor cell lines is enhanced by histamine and can be inhibited by cimetidine.[33] These observations suggest that histamine acting locally in the stomach may enhance the proliferation of gastric tumors and support the use of H_2 blockers as adjuvants in the treatment of gastric carcinoma.

Small Intestinal Neoplasia

The most common small intestinal neoplasms of dogs are adenocarcinoma, lymphosarcoma, and smooth muscle tumors (see later for additional discussion of these tumors). In the small intestine of cats, lymphosarcoma is the most common neoplasm, followed by adenocarcinoma (particularly of the ileum). Siamese cats are predisposed to intestinal adenocarcinoma.[3] The duodenum of both species is more likely to be invaded by carcinomas from other organs such as the pancreas and liver than to develop primary neoplasia. The majority of intestinal neoplasms are malignant (e.g., lymphosarcoma, adenocarcinomas, leiomyosarcomas, mast cell tumors, and hemangiosarcomas). The most common benign tumors are leiomyomas, adenomas, fibromas, and adenomatous polyps.[35] Less frequent intestinal tumors include plasmacytomas,[36] fibrosarcomas,[2] extraskeletal osteosarcoma,[37] ganglioneuromas,[38,39] and neurilemmomas.[40]

CLINICAL SIGNS. Prominent clinical signs of small intestinal neoplasia are anorexia, chronic diarrhea, vomiting, and weight loss. The pathogenesis of the diarrhea is probably multifactorial, but may include malassimilation as a result of widespread mucosal infiltration, deranged intestinal motility, and bacterial overgrowth secondary to partial obstruction. Not infrequently, anemia and/or melena may be observed,[32] and abdominal masses or thickened intestines palpated. Rarely, the initial presentation is acute abdomen as a result of intestinal perforation. An important differential diagnosis is inflammatory bowel disease (IBD). In contrast to IBD, however, the clinical signs resulting from neoplasia tend to be steadily progressive rather than waxing and waning. Furthermore, if the vomitus becomes odiferous and of large volume, an obstructive neoplasm such as annular adenocarcinoma should be suspected more so than IBD.

DIAGNOSIS. Laboratory evidence of inflammation, blood loss, protein-losing enteropathy, bacterial overgrowth, or malassimilation may be apparent. Survey radiography may reveal an abdominal mass or an obstructive intestinal pattern.[3] Contrast radiographic studies may reveal mucosal

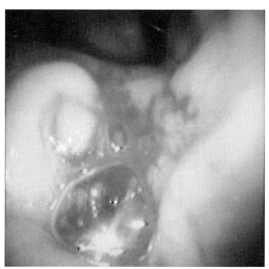

FIGURE 27-5. Endoscopic photograph of an ulcerating gastric carcinoma.

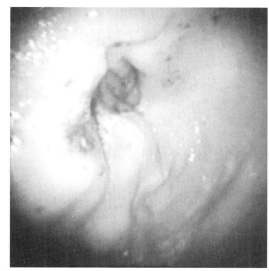

FIGURE 27-6. Endoscopic photograph of an infiltrative gastric

filling defects or obstructive lesions. Barium impregnated polyethylene spheres (BIPS, Ken Bowman Associates, Diamond Bar, CA; Arnolds, Shrewsbury, UK) will bunch at the site of any neoplastic stricture with a diameter of 5 mm or less (Figure 27-7). If the neoplasm has not narrowed the bowel to this degree, BIPS may not bunch, but their transit through the small intestine will usually be delayed, particularly if they are fed with a high-fiber diet (see Chapter 25). Ultrasonography is a major advance in the diagnosis of gastrointestinal neoplasia. The ultrasonographic appearance of gastrointestinal neoplasms in the dog has been described.[41] Ultrasonography may reveal bowel thickenings, localized ileus, or enlarged mesenteric nodes. Enlarged mesenteric nodes are highly suggestive of neoplasia but can also occur with other conditions (Table 27-2).

Ultimately, diagnosis requires a biopsy of the neoplastic tissue. Tissue samples can be obtained by ultrasound-guided aspiration or biopsy. Alternatively, intestinal biopsy via celiotomy is effective. Endoscopy is of limited value in the diagnosis of small-bowel neoplasia because the tumor often lies out of reach of the endoscope. If surgical biopsy specimens are taken from the intestine of a debilitated patient, placement of a gastrostomy tube to allow nutritional support should be considered at the time of the celiotomy. This is important because intestinal biopsy sites in animals with small intestinal neoplasia undergo dehiscence reasonably frequently[5] and it is probable that good postoperative nutrition will reduce the risk of this complication.

TREATMENT AND PROGNOSIS. If the process is localized to one segment of the bowel, surgical resection is indicated. If metastasis has occurred, adjuvant chemotherapy can be attempted but offers little benefit.[5] Unfortunately, the prognosis for all nonresectable gastrointestinal neoplasia is guarded to poor.

Large-Bowel Neoplasia[4,36,42]

After the oral cavity, the large bowel is the next most common site of gastrointestinal neoplasia. The prevalence of tumors of the colon and rectum in dogs presented to the VMTH are 2.8 and 4.1 per 10,000, respectively. These

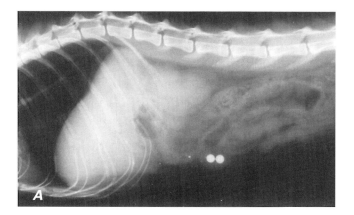

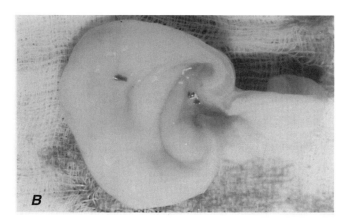

FIGURE 27-7. (A) Barium-impregnated polyethylene sphere (BIPS) study in a cat with chronic vomiting. The majority of BIPS failed to leave the stomach and were eventually vomited after 8 hours, indicating delayed gastric emptying. However, two large BIPS entered the small intestine and bunched at one point in the small intestine, failing to move further aborally. (B) Exploratory celiotomy in the cat in (A) revealed an annular small intestinal adenocarcinoma (pictured) that was successfully removed.

Table 27–2

CAUSES OF MESENTERIC LYMPHADENOPATHY

Reactive Lymph Node
Lymphocytic-plasmacytic enteritis (mild lymphadenopathy)
Eosinophilic enteritis
Toxoplasmosis
Idiopathic
Lymphadenitis
Campylobacter spp.
Ehrlichia
FIP
Histoplasmosis
Leishmania
Mycobacteria
Parvovirus
Prototophecosis
Salmon poisoning
Salmonella spp.
Staphylococcus intermedius
Yersinia pseudotuberculosis
Zygomycosis
Other enteric pathogens
Neoplasia
Lymphosarcoma
Mast cell neoplasia
Metastatic adenocarcinoma
Metastatic leiomyosarcoma
Other neoplasia

data are similar to findings elsewhere.[21,43,44] In the large bowel of dogs, the most frequent neoplasm is adenocarcinoma followed by lymphosarcoma and smooth muscle tumors. In cats, lymphosarcoma is the most common neoplasm of the large bowel, followed in frequency by adenocarcinoma. Extramedullary plasmacytomas have been reported in the large bowel of dogs.[45–47] Most large-bowel neoplasms are located in the rectum or distal one-third of the colon.[6]

CLINICAL SIGNS. The clinical signs associated with colonic and rectal neoplasia are essentially the same as colitis or large-bowel obstruction. The signs are caused by neoplastic invasion of the bowel wall that causes inflammation, stricture formation, and obstruction (Figure 27–8). Neoplasms cause the mucosa to become friable and bleed easily. Adenocarcinomas spreading from the colon into adjacent blood vessels and lymphatics sometimes obstruct regional circulation, resulting in marked edema of the inguinal area and the rear legs. Occasionally, the edema will develop before signs of intestinal disease appear. Rectal prolapse is frequent in dogs with rectal plasmacytomas.[45]

DIAGNOSIS. Few abnormalities are observed in blood tests from affected animals. Rarely, rectal or cecal plasmacytomas are associated with a monoclonal gammopathy.[46,47] Many large-bowel neoplasms are detectable by digital examination and most are within view of a proctoscope.[42] In the absence of an endoscope, ultrasonography, survey radiography, and barium, air, or double-contrast enemas are sometimes useful in gaining more information on colonic lesions (Figure 27–8). Survey radiographs and, in particular, ultrasonography are also helpful in detecting metastatic spread to sublumbar nodes. The diagnostic workup of large-bowel diarrhea is described in more detail in Chapter 5.

TREATMENT AND PROGNOSIS. The treatment of colorectal neoplasia is usually surgical (adenocarcinoma) or medical (lymphoma). Occasionally, radiation therapy is utilized for rectal carcinoma (see later). The prognosis for malignant

lesions is guarded. Mean survival time for malignant tumors of the rectal wall irrespective of tumor type was 6.9 months in one study.[42]

Alimentary Lymphosarcoma[10,48–51]

Lymphosarcoma is the most common gastrointestinal neoplasm in cats and is also relatively common in dogs. Lymphopoietic neoplasms are classified as alimentary lymphosarcoma if the organs involved are restricted to the mesenteric nodes, gastrointestinal tract, liver, kidney, and spleen. Alimentary lymphosarcoma constitutes 36% of feline lymphosarcoma and 7% of canine lymphosarcoma. The intestinal tract can also be affected by multicentric lymphosarcoma, which comprises 18% of feline lymphosarcoma and 84% of canine lymphosarcoma. Alimentary lymphosarcoma is usually of B cell origin but in cats not infrequently involves the large granular lymphocyte lineage.[51] Similarly, globular leukocyte tumors have been reported in the lower small intestine of cats.[52] Globular leukocyte tumors are characterized by small round cells containing numerous intracytoplasmic eosinophilic granules.[52] They can be metastatic but appear to be slow growing.[52]

Clinical signs of lymphoma usually include anorexia, vomiting, diarrhea, weight loss, and pyrexia.[5,51] Thickened bowel loops, enlarged mesenteric nodes, and organomegaly may also be palpated. Lymphosarcoma can occur at any site along the length of the gastrointestinal tract. The neoplasm may appear as a solitary mass, a generalized diffuse thickening of the wall, and perhaps as "skip" lesions (Figure 27–9). In cats, alimentary lymphosarcoma is particularly common at the ileocolic junction. Concomitant involvement of other organs resulting in hepatosplenomegaly is frequent, and a variety of paraneoplastic findings and extraintestinal manifestations may be apparent.

Hematologic and serum biochemical abnormalities are usually nonspecific, but hypoproteinemia and hyperbilirubinemia occur with greater frequency in lymphoma than in inflammatory bowel disease, an important differential diagnosis. Occasionally lymphoblasts will be seen in peripheral blood, especially if a buffy coat examination is performed. Affected cats usually test negative for feline leukemia. Diagnosis is made by gastrointestinal tract biopsy. Histologic differentiation of lymphosarcoma and lymphocytic-plasmacytic enteritis can be difficult, particularly on the basis of endoscopic biopsy samples.[5,48] Lymphomatous foci are often surrounded by an extensive lymphocytic- plasmacytic inflammatory infiltrate.[48] Furthermore, it appears likely that some cases of lymphocytic-plasmacytic enteritis eventually mutate into lymphosarcoma.[5]

Treatment of the localized form of alimentary lymphosarcoma is usually by surgical resection followed by adjuvant chemotherapy. Large lymphomatous masses involving the bowel wall should not be treated by chemotherapy alone because necrosis of the tumor mass can result in perforation of the intestine.[6] Surgical resection of large masses prior to chemotherapy minimizes the likelihood of this complication. The generalized form of the disease is treated by combination chemotherapy only. A popular regimen is cyclophosphamide, vincristine, and prednisone, but because alimentary lymphosarcoma is more refractory to treatment than multicentric lymphosarcoma, it is often advisable to incorporate doxorubicin into the chemotherapy protocol.[5,10,42,48]

Alimentary lymphoma has a guarded prognosis. Response rates of 30% to 60% can be expected with median remissions

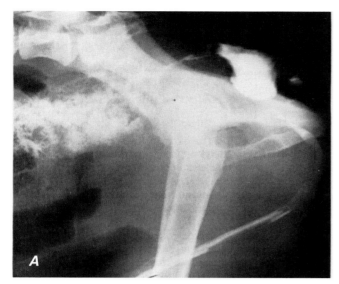

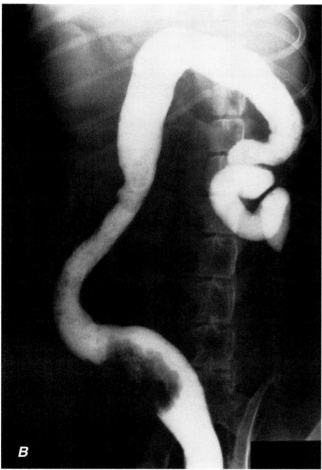

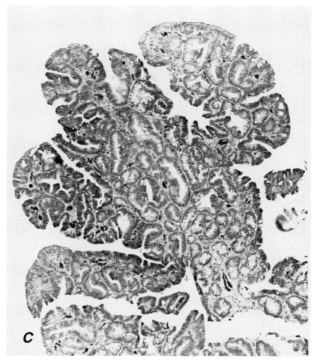

FIGURE 27-8. *(A)* Lateral radiograph of a 9-year-old German shepherd that presented with signs of tenesmus and chronic diarrhea. Rectal examination revealed a stricture, the length of which could not be determined. Positive contrast medium was introduced into the rectum with a bulb syringe. The mural lesion produced a "ring-like" constriction of the rectum. A urethrogram done at this time revealed that the suspected tumor did not involve the urethra. Biopsy identified the cause of the stricture to be an adenocarcinoma. *(B)* Dorsoventral radiograph of an 8-year-old Airedale terrier with chronic signs of passing blood in the feces. Proctoscopy was done but with its use the dimensions of the lesion and its involvement could not be ascertained. A barium enema revealed a mural lesion that invades the lumen. The lesion is pedunculated and creates an intra-luminal mass. The filling defects proximal to the lesion are due to an inability to completely clean the bowel. The mass was an adenoma that was surgically resected. *(C)* Adenoma of colon. Epithelium is tall columnar, cells are hyperchromatic with large nuclei and several with mitotic figures. There was no evidence for invasion through the basement membrane.

Gastrointestinal Mast Cell Neoplasia[1,53,54]

Visceral mastocytosis is uncommon in the dog but is seen with reasonable frequency in cats. Occasionally, the viscera become involved in systemic mastocytosis. The clinical signs of mast cell neoplasia include vomiting, diarrhea, and weight loss. The diagnosis is usually made by detection of large numbers of mast cells in a blood smear, buffy coat, or aspirates of bone marrow, spleen, liver, or an abdominal mass. Mast cell tumors can appear anywhere throughout the small intestine. They usually result in segmental thickening of the bowel wall. Occasionally, mast cell tumors will occur in the colon. They commonly infiltrate the liver and spleen. Prolonged survival times have been reported following splenectomy to remove part of the tumor burden, prednisone therapy (as a chemotherapeutic), and H_2 receptor blockers to limit histamine-induced gastric acid secretion. The prognosis remains poor.

of 4 to 8 months reported.[4,5,50] The prognosis appears to be better for localized rather than generalized alimentary lymphosarcoma.[5] It is particularly good for dogs with localized lesions confined to the large bowel.[5] The response to chemotherapy is poor in visceral lymphoma involving large granular lymphocytes in cats.[51]

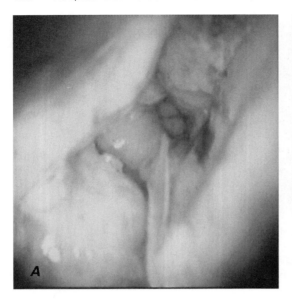

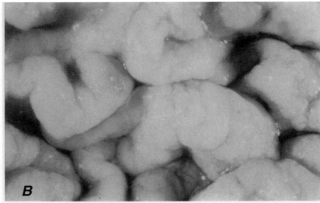

FIGURE 27-9. *(A)* Endoscopic picture of canine colonic lymphosarcoma. Note the fibrin and swollen mucosa. *(B)* Photograph of a dog's stomach with swollen rugal folds resulting from the infiltrative form of lymphosarcoma. (Courtesy of Dr. Keith Thompson)

Intestinal Adenocarcinoma

Adenocarcinoma is the most common large-bowel neoplasm of dogs (Figures 27–10 and 27–11).[2] In dogs, small intestinal adenocarcinomas are less common than their large intestinal counterparts, but in cats, particularly of the Siamese breed, the lower small intestine is the site of predilection.[3,55,56] Adenocarcinomas are most often seen in older animals, but dogs as young as 2 years have been afflicted with large-bowel adenocarcinoma.[57] Adenocarcinoma of the small intestine tends to be annular and produce signs of intestinal obstruction after several weeks of vague inappetence and lethargy (Figure 27–12). Large-bowel adenocarcinoma more often manifests as rectal bleeding with or without tenesmus and dyschezia. The gross appearance of adenocarcinomas is variable. They may appear as expansive, plaque-like, ulcerated masses; they may invade adjacent bowel wall producing an annular or fusiform obstruction; they may cause discrete ulcers or polypoid growths; or may widely infiltrate the submucosa causing diffuse thickening without causing obstruction. Metastasis to mesenteric lymph nodes is common in cats but need not necessarily warrant a poor prognosis.[55] Occasionally, marked mesenteric and omental sclerosis develops in association with metastases from gastrointestinal adenocarcinomas.[58]

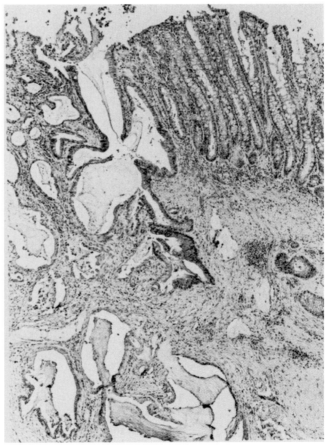

FIGURE 27-11. Adenocarcinoma of the colon. Neoplastic involvement of the wall of the colon has resulted in loss of normal mucosa on the left side of the photomicrograph.

FIGURE 27-10. Adenocarcinoma of the jejunum of a cat. Neoplastic involvement of the greater part of the luminal circumference produces partial obstruction and vomiting and/or diarrhea.

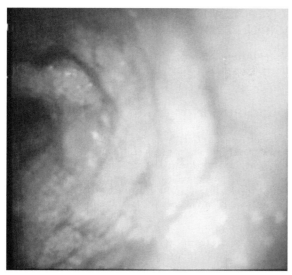

FIGURE 27-12. Endoscopic picture of annular adenocarcinoma of the duodenum of a dog with chronic vomiting.

Reviews of gastrointestinal adenocarcinomas have been published.[55–57] Treatment of localized disease is by surgical excision. Pelvic splitting can usually be avoided during the excision of large-bowel adenocarcinoma by prolapsing the rectum or using appropriate rectal pull-through techniques.[6] Single high-dose radiation therapy has been reported to be effective for the treatment of small rectal carcinomas.[59] If sublumbar or mesenteric metastasis is apparent, adjuvant chemotherapy can be attempted but is rarely helpful.

The prognosis is guarded but long-term survival is common if patients with well-differentiated adenocarcinomas survive the immediate postoperative period.[55] Local recurrence or distant metastasis can occur as late as 1 year after excision.[4] Polypoid forms of adenocarcinoma have a better prognosis than annular lesions.[57]

Gastrointestinal Polyps

Hyperplastic polyps can occur in the stomach, duodenum, and rectum of dogs.[2] The cause of polypoid growths is unknown. Rectal polyps are the most common, but gastric polyps are seen with reasonable frequency during endoscopy.[36,42,60,61] Gastric polyps are most often singular but occasionally numerous polypoid growths will be observed.[62] Gastric polyps are not thought to become malignant and are usually considered an incidental finding. Occasionally they will produce clinical signs by obstructing gastric outflow.

Rectal polyps appear as friable, lobulated, sessile, or pedunculated growths protruding from the mucosa. They can be single or multiple and are most often located in the distal rectum. Occasionally they protrude through the anus during defecation. Most canine rectal polyps are benign although precancerous polyps have been reported.[42,63] Large polyps are particularly likely to be precancerous. Rectal polyps often result in hematochezia. Laboratory work is usually nondiagnostic but a paraneoplastic leukocytosis has been reported in association with a rectal polyp.[64] The treatment is surgical and the prognosis is good, but local recurrence is common.[42] Rectal polyps should be differentiated from rectal plasmacytomas, which appear as red to ulcerated solid nodules on the rectal mucosa of dogs.[45] As with polyps, surgical resection of rectal plasmacytomas is usually curative.[45]

Adenomatous polyps can occur in the stomach, duode-

num, ileum, and colon of cats.[35,65] The most common site appears to be the duodenum.[35] Cats of Asian ancestry are predisposed to duodenal polyps. Cats with duodenal polyps are usually elderly and are often presented for acute or chronic vomiting and hematemesis. Anemia is common and the diagnosis is usually made by positive contrast radiography or gastroduodenoscopy. Examination of the duodenum will usually reveal one polyp but up to three polyps have been reported.[35] Surgical resection of the polyp at its base via an enterotomy incision is usually curative. Malignant transformation of duodenal polyps is unlikely.

Smooth Muscle Tumors[2,4,66–69]

Leiomyomas and leiomyosarcomas can appear at any level of the gastrointestinal tract, but sites of predilection include the gastroesophageal junction (leiomyomas) and jejunum and cecum (leiomyosarcomas) (Figure 27–4). They usually appear as single nodules with or without ulceration. Smooth muscle tumors are often subclinical but may eventually cause anemia, hypoglycemia, obstruction, or perforation.[32,69,70] On most occasions, anemia due to these tumors is classified as hypochromic, most probably due to iron deficiency from chronic blood loss.[32] Colorectal leiomyomas frequently result in tenesmus or narrowed stools because of their compressive nature.[69]

Treatment of smooth muscle tumors is by surgical resection. Prognosis is good with leiomyomas[69] and guarded to good with leiomyosarcomas.[68] Fortunately, leiomyosarcomas are slow to metastasize, and long-term survival after resection is not uncommon.[67,68]

Apocrine Adenocarcinomas

Apocrine adenocarcinomas are malignant tumors of the anal sacs. They are most common in older spayed females. They should be differentiated from benign perianal adenomas, which are almost exclusively seen in older, uncastrated males. Apocrine adenocarcinomas often produce hypercalcemia due to the secretion of a parathyroid hormone-like substance. The presenting signs most often pertain to the hypercalcemia rather than the perianal mass. Signs include weakness, anorexia, constipation, polyuria, and polydipsia. The prognosis is guarded. Local recurrence can occur, and metastasis to the regional lymph nodes occurs in approximately 50% of the dogs.[42]

AMINE PRECURSOR UPTAKE AND DECARBOXYLATION TUMORS[71–75]

Amine precursor uptake and decarboxylation (APUD) cells are a diffuse system of endocrine cells that have in common certain cytochemical, ultrastructural, and metabolic features that allow them to secrete biogenic amines from amino acid precursors. Most APUD cells share a common neuroectodermal source. They often retain the ability to secrete more than one hormone.[76,77] They are found in many organs of the body including the pituitary, intestine, pancreas, adrenal medulla, and thyroid. These features of APUD cells are responsible for the potent secretory function of many APUD tumors and occasionally for the development of concomitant neoplasia at apparently disparate sites (i.e., multiple endocrine neoplasm syndromes).

APUD tumors are rare neoplasms in the dog and cat. Those that have been reported include insulinomas, gastrinomas, pheochromocytomas, thyroid medullary carcinoma, a pancreatic polypeptide secreting tumor, and carcinoid tumors of the small intestine.

Gastrinomas (Zollinger-Ellison Syndrome)

Gastrinomas are rare neoplasms in dogs and cats. Detailed description is provided elsewhere.[71,72,75,78–81] They are most common in older dogs, although a dog as young as 3.5 years has been affected. Gastrin-secreting tumors are usually located in the pancreas. The clinical signs include vomiting, weight loss, anorexia, and diarrhea particularly with steatorrhea. Hematemesis, melena, abdominal pain, and polydipsia may be seen. The most frequent laboratory findings are regenerative anemia and leukocytosis. Hyperglycemia, hypoalbuminemia, hypocalcemia, hypokalemia, and increased serum alkaline phosphatase are seen occasionally. Endoscopy usually reveals gastric and/or duodenal ulceration and gastric mucosal hypertrophy. Reflux esophagitis and ulcers of the esophagus and jejunum may also occur.

Diagnosis is usually made by exploratory celiotomy. The tumor most commonly occurs in the left lobe or body of the pancreas. In two-thirds of affected animals the pancreatic tumor is a solitary nodule. In the remainder of animals multiple masses are seen. Metastasis to the liver is very common. High gastrin levels support but do not confirm a diagnosis. Provocative testing with calcium or secretin, or the assessment of gastric pH, may enhance the discriminatory value of the serum gastrin level (see Chapter 6). A gastrin assay is available for the dog.[82]

Because of early metastasis, treatment is usually only palliative. Therapy includes surgical removal of visible tumor and administration of H_2 receptor blockers to decrease gastric acid secretion. Treatment with a somatostatin analogue was reported to provide successful palliation in a dog. The prognosis is poor. Average survival time is 5 months.

Carcinoid Tumors of the Stomach and Intestine

These tumors have been reported infrequently in the dog and cat.[2,4,83,84] They arise from enterochromaffin cells, which produce a variety of vasoactive amines capable of producing secretory diarrhea. Most carcinoids reported to date in dogs and cats have been clinically silent.[73]

Pancreatic Polypeptide Secreting Pancreatic Tumor

A pancreatic polypeptide secreting adenocarcinoma in a dog has been reported.[85] Associated clinical signs were chronic vomiting, anorexia, and weight loss. The tumor was metastatic and was associated with duodenal ulcers and hypertrophic gastritis. The affected dog did not respond to treatment with H_2 receptor antagonists.

ENDOCRINOPATHIES AND THE GASTROINTESTINAL TRACT

Many other endocrinopathies in addition to the APUD tumors can adversely affect the gastrointestinal tract.

Hypoadrenocorticism

Hypoadrenocorticism results in depression, weakness, vomiting, and diarrhea. The vomitus and diarrhea may contain blood, and abdominal pain may be present. In dogs, severe gastrointestinal hemorrhage occasionally complicates hypoadrenocorticism.[86] Regurgitation can accompany the vomiting as a result of a concomitant megaesophagus. The megaesophagus is reversible, and is thought to result from the generalized muscle weakness that affects these patients.[87] The cause of the vomiting and diarrhea remain uncertain, but it is thought that corticosteroids in physiologic amounts have a trophic action on the gastrointestinal mucosa. Adrenalectomized cats undergo gastric and intestinal atrophy[88] and gastritis accompanies hypoadrenocorticism in some dogs.[87] Gastric blood flow is reduced in adrenalectomized rats[89] and gastric motility is depressed in affected dogs. The hypomotility may be a result of the electrolyte imbalances that accompany the disease or perhaps the inhibitory influence of elevated corticotropin-releasing factor on gastric contractions.[90]

Electrolyte changes compatible with hypoadrenocorticism include a low serum sodium and a high serum potassium concentration. Gastrointestinal fluid loss from primary gastrointestinal diseases can also produce these electrolyte changes, however, and they should not be considered pathognomonic for hypoadrenocorticism.[91] Additional laboratory findings include the presence of an azotemia that responds rapidly to fluids, hypercalcemia, low urine specific gravity, eosinophilia, and lymphocytosis. Diagnosis may be confirmed rapidly by a modified Thorn's test and more definitively with an ACTH test. Therapy is described elsewhere.[71,72,92]

Hyperadrenocorticism

Aside from the characteristic hepatic vacuolization and cholestasis associated with elevated serum concentrations of glucocorticoids, Cushing syndrome is generally thought to have minimal effect on the bowel. However, two cases of bowel perforation have been associated with hyperadrenocorticism.

Hypoparathyroidism

Hypoparathyroidism leads to hypocalcemia, which depresses gut motility. Constipation and even pseudo-obstruction can occur in hypoparathyroid humans. Vomiting and diarrhea are also seen in some patients. Similar signs can occur in dogs, but they are usually overshadowed by other signs of hypocalcemia such as seizures.

Hyperparathyroidism

Constipation, vomiting, anorexia, and peptic ulcers are common in humans with hyperparathyroidism. Pancreatitis is a rare complication.[93] In hyperparathyroid dogs, constipation and vomiting have been observed.[71] The signs appear to be due to the hypercalcemia, but the exact pathogenesis is unknown. High calcium concentrations dampen neuronal transmission and may be responsible for gastric atony. Acute elevations in serum calcium cause increased gastric acid secretion via gastrin release, but this is not a feature of chronic hypercalcemia.[94] The relationship between hypercalcemia and pancreatitis is also obscure. One explanation is that high calcium concentration in pancreatic fluid can activate trypsinogen.[93,95]

Hyperthyroidism

Hyperthyroid cats show a number of gastrointestinal signs. Diarrhea occurs in 45% of cases and vomiting in one-third.[71] Additional signs include increased fecal volume, foul-smelling stools, increased frequency of defecation, and steatorrhea.[71,72] The causes of these signs in hyperthyroid cats are unknown, but more rapid orocolic transit time has been detected in affected cats.[96] Rapid small intestinal transit has also been observed in hyperthyroid people and correlates well with the presence of diarrhea. In experimental hyperthyroidism in dogs, the frequency of intestinal contractions and, in particular, giant migrating contractions is increased.[97] This deranged intestinal motility is thought to be of prime importance in the pathogenesis of the diarrhea due to thyrotoxicosis.[97,98] Additionally, increased thyroid hormone is able to produce a secretory diarrhea via elevating cyclic AMP in the enterocyte. Furthermore, a relative deficiency of pancreatic trypsin secretion and some brush border enzyme levels is likely to occur.[99,100] The resultant malassimilation is likely to be compounded by mucosal edema and round cell infiltration, which have been observed in the small bowel of humans and cats with hyperthyroidism.[50,101,102] In addition, the polyphagia of hyperthyroid cats would increase the total amount of nutrient presented to the bowel for digestion and absorption.

Similarly, the pathogenesis of the vomiting in hyperthyroid cats is unknown. In humans, hyperthyroidism is associated with a myopathy that can interfere with the striated musculature of the pharynx and upper esophagus, resulting in dysphagia. In addition, gastric hypoacidity, hypergastrinemia, and superficial gastritis occur in some people.[93] Gastric emptying time is usually normal. In addition to the possibility that the vomiting exhibited by hyperthyroid cats is due to gastritis or esophageal dysfunction, a direct effect of thyroid hormone on the chemoreceptor trigger zone has been proposed.[71,103]

Hyperthyroid cats commonly have elevated plasma activities of SAP and ALT liver enzymes. In some cats, a periportal mixed inflammatory reaction and focal areas of fatty degeneration may be seen in the liver. The cause of these lesions is unknown.

Medullary Carcinoma of the Thyroid

Diarrhea has been described in association with medullary carcinoma of the thyroid in dogs.[104] The diarrhea is proposed to result from the secretion of serotonin and/or prostaglandins by the tumor.[71,72]

Hypothyroidism

Hypothyroidism in humans can be associated with reflux esophagitis, gastric hypomotility, constipation, rectal prolapse, and rarely megacolon or diarrhea.[93] The cause of these signs is depressed gastrointestinal motility resulting from myxedema and decreased electrical control activity. Similarly, hypothyroid dogs have been shown to have depressed gastrointestinal motility.[105] In dogs with marked hypothyroidism, both diarrhea and, alternatively, constipation have been reported.[71,72,87] The cause of the diarrhea is unknown, but experiments have demonstrated that hypothyroid rats have reduced mucosal thickness and villus height in comparison to hyperthyroid rats.[100] Furthermore, hypothyroid humans have depressed exocrine pancreatic function.[106]

Diabetes Mellitus

Diabetes mellitus has been associated with chronic vomiting due to delayed gastric emptying and gastric hypomotility in dogs.[71] The vomiting responded to metoclopramide therapy. Diabetic gastroparesis is a common complication of human diabetics. The cause appears to be a diabetes-induced degeneration of the parasympathetic innervation of the gastrointestinal tract, but hyperglycemia per se also inhibits gastric emptying.[107] Idiopathic chronic diarrhea has also been seen in a diabetic dog, and may have been analogous to idiopathic diabetic diarrhea of humans. The pathogenesis of diabetic diarrhea is multifactorial.[108] In affected humans, bacterial overgrowth, exocrine pancreatic insufficiency, deranged intestinal motility, bile acid catharsis, and secretory diarrheas have been documented. Fecal incontinence in conjunction with anorectal dysfunction has also been reported in humans.[108]

Management of diabetic diarrhea is usually by trial and error. Suggested therapies have included antibiotics for bacterial overgrowth, pancreatic enzyme replacements, opioids, psyllium, cholestyramine, somatostatin, or clonidine.[93,108] The latter agent has shown considerable promise.

Diabetes mellitus in humans has a wide range of additional deleterious effects on the gastrointestinal system including esophageal dysfunction, chronic gastritis, idiopathic abdominal pain, constipation, and fatty liver.[93] The cause of these conditions is not completely clear, but suggestions have included autonomic degeneration, microcirculatory disease, electrolyte imbalances, and metabolic derangements.

Diabetic ketoacidosis is a well-recognized cause of acute vomiting and diarrhea in dogs and cats. Abdominal pain and abdominal distension may also be apparent. Proposed causes for these acute gastrointestinal signs are impaired gastrointestinal motility with resultant gaseous abdominal distension or a direct effect of the acidosis on the vomiting center.

AGE-RELATED CHANGES IN THE GASTROINTESTINAL TRACT[109]

A variety of age-related changes have been reported in the gastrointestinal tract of humans and laboratory animals.[109] Parenchymal atrophy and sclerotic changes in the stroma are often observed. Constipation is common in the elderly and is associated with a marked decline in contractile strength of the rectal wall. Digestion and absorption are somewhat reduced by aging, but these changes have little clinical significance because of the large functional reserves of the gastrointestinal system. The function of the gastrointestinal immune system is slightly impaired in aging mice. Young mice produce more dimeric IgA to bacterial antigens in the intestine than older mice. It is likely that many of the aging changes just described also occur in cats and dogs.

REFERENCES

1. Theilen GH, Madewell BR. Tumors of the digestive tract. In: Veterinary Cancer Medicine. 499–534, 1987.
2. Head KW, Else RW. Neoplasia and allied conditions of the canine and feline intestine. Vet Ann 21:190–208, 1981.
3. Birchard SJ, Couto CG, Johnson S. Nonlymphoid intestinal neoplasia in 32 dogs and 14 cats. J Am Anim Hosp Assoc 22:533–537, 1986.
4. Crow SE. Tumors of the alimentary tract. Vet Clin N Am 15:577–596, 1985.
5. Couto CG. Gastrointestinal neoplasia in dogs and cats. In: Kirk RW (ed) Current Veterinary Therapy XI. WB Saunders, Philadelphia, 595–601, 1993.
6. White RAS. The alimentary system. In: White RAS (ed) Manual of Small Animal Oncology. British Small Animal Veterinary Association, Cheltenham, 237–263, 1991.
7. Adamu D. Pathomorphological assessment and classification of spontaneous neoplasms in the dog. Medycyna-Weterynaryjna 48:200–201, 1992.
8. Priester WA, McKay FA. The occurrence of tumors in domestic animals. National Cancer Institute Monograph 54. U.S. Department of Health and Human Services, Bethesda, 1980.
9. Haubrich WS, Berk JE. Malignant tumors of the colon and rectum. In: Bockus HL (ed) Gastroenterology, 3rd ed. WB Saunders, Philadelphia, 1009–1044, 1976.
10. Cotter SM. Treatment of lymphoma and leukemia with cyclophosphamide, vincristine, and prednisone. II. Treatment of cats. J Am Anim Hosp Assoc 19:166–172, 1983.
11. Ogilvie GK, Richardson RC, Curtis CR, et al. Acute and short-term toxicoses associated with the administration of doxorubicin to dogs with malignant tumors. J Am Vet Med Assoc 195:1584–1587, 1989.
12. Ogilvie GK, Moore AS, Curtis CR. Evaluation of cisplatin-induced emesis in dogs with malignant neoplasia: 115 cases (1984–1987). J Am Vet Med Assoc 195:1399–1403, 1989.
13. Couto CG. Management of complications of cancer chemotherapy. Vet Clin N Am 20:1037–1053, 1990.
14. Dorman DC, Coddington KA, Richardson RC. 5-fluorouracil toxicosis in the dog. J Vet Int Med 4:254–257, 1990.
15. Hammer AS, Couto CG, Filppi J, et al. Efficacy and toxicity of VAC chemotherapy (vincristine, doxorubicin, and cyclophosphamide) in dogs with hemangiosarcoma. J Vet Int Med 5:160–166, 1991.
16. Kotzmann H, Gisslinger H. Treatment and prophylaxis of chemotherapy-induced gastrointestinal complaints. Scand J Gastroenterol 27 (suppl) 191:12–15, 1992.
17. Summers RW, Glenn CE, Flatt AJ, et al. Does irradiation produce irreversible changes in canine jejunal myoelectric activity? Dig Dis Sci 37:716–722, 1992.
18. Empey LR, Papp JD, Jewell LD, et al. Mucosal protective effects of vitamin E and misoprostol during acute radiation-induced enteritis in rats. Dig Dis Sci 37:205–214, 1992.
19. Henriksson R, Franzen L, Littbrand B. Prevention and therapy of radiation-induced bowel discomfort. Scan J Gastroenterol 27 (suppl) 191:7–11, 1992.
20. Fonda D, Gualtieri M, Scanziani E. Gastric carcinoma in the dog: A clinicopathological study of 11 cases. J Sm Anim Pract 30:353–360, 1989.
21. Brodey RS, Cohen D. An epizootiologic and clinicopathologic study of 95 cases of gastrointestinal neoplasms in the dog. Proc 101st annual meeting AVMA, Chicago, 167–179, 1964.
22. Murray M, Robinson PB, McKeating FJ, et al. Primary gastric neoplasia in the dog: A clinicopathological study. Vet Rec 91:474–479, 1972.
23. Patnaik AK, Hurvitz AI, Johnson GV. Canine gastrointestinal neoplasms. Vet Pathol 14:547–555, 1977.
24. Sautter JH, Hanlon GF. Gastric neoplasms in the dog: A report of 20 cases. J Am Vet Med Assoc 166:691–696, 1975.
25. Landes C, Sandersleben JV. Primare Neoplasien und schleimhauthyperplasien in magen des hundes. Tierarztl Prax Suppl 1:139–158, 1985.
26. Sullivan M, Lee R, Fisher EW, et al. A study of 31 cases of gastric carcinoma in dogs. Vet Rec 120:79–83, 1987.
27. Scanziani E, Giusti AM, Gualtieri M, et al. Gastric carcinoma in the Belgian shepherd dog. J Sm Anim Pract 32:465–469, 1991.
28. Shils ME. Nutrition and diet in cancer. In: Shils ME, Young VR (eds) Modern Nutrition in Health and Disease, 7th ed. Lea & Febiger, Philadelphia, 1380–1422, 1988.
29. Sinicrope FA, Levin B. Gastric cancer. Curr Opin G 9:930–937, 1993.
30. Taylor PR, Mason RC, Filipe MI, et al. Gastric carcinogenesis in the rat induced by duodenogastric reflux without carcinogens: Morphology, mucin, histochemistry, polyamine metabolism, and labelling index. Gut 32:1447–1454, 1991.
31. Lemoine NR, Leung HY, Gullick WJ. Growth factors in the gastrointestinal tract. Gut 33:1297–1300, 1992.
32. Comer KM. Anemia as a feature of primary gastrointestinal neoplasia. Comp Contin Ed Pract Vet 12:13–19, 1990.
33. Watson SA, Wilkinson LJ, Robertson JFR, et al. Effect of histamine on the growth of human gastrointestinal tumours: Reversal by cimetidine. Gut 34:1091–1096, 1993.
34. Brunnert SR, Dee LA, Heron AJ, et al. Gastric extramedullary plasmacytoma in a dog. J Am Vet Med Assoc 200:1501–1502, 1992.
35. MacDonald JM, Mullen HS, Moroff SD. Adenomatous polyps of the duodenum in cats: 18 cases (1985–1990). J Am Vet Med Assoc 202:647–651, 1993.
36. Holt PE, Lucke VM. Rectal neoplasia in the dog. A clinicopathological review of 31 cases. Vet Rec 116:400–401, 1985.
37. Patnaik AK. Canine extraskeletal osteosarcoma and chondrosarcoma: A clinicopathologic study of 14 cases. Vet Path 27:46–55, 1990.
38. Patnaik AK, Hurvitz AI, Johnson GF. Canine intestinal adenocarcinoma and carcinoid. Vet Pathol 17:149–163, 1980.
39. Ribas JL, Kwapien RP, Pope ER. Immunohistochemistry and ultrastructure of intestinal ganglioneuroma in a dog. Vet Pathol 27:376–379, 1990.
40. Patnaik AK, Hurvitz AI. Neoplasms of the digestive tract in the dog. In: Kirk RW (ed) Current Veterinary Therapy VI. WB Saunders, Philadelphia, 393–394, 1977.
41. Penninck DG, Nyland TG, Kerr LY, et al. Ultrasonographic evaluation of gastrointestinal diseases in small animals. Vet Radiol 31:134–141, 1990.
42. White RAS, Gorman NT. The clinical diagnosis and management of rectal and pararectal tumors in the dog. J Sm Anim Pract 28:87–107, 1987.
43. Cotchin E. Some tumors in dogs and cats of comparative veterinary and human interest. Vet Rec 71:1040–1054, 1959.
44. Hayden DW, Nielsen SW. Canine alimentary neoplasia. Zen Tralbl Veterinaer Med 20:1–22, 1973.
45. Rakich PM, Latimer KS, Weiss R, et al. Mucocutaneous plasmacytomas in dogs: 75 cases (1980–1987). J Am Vet Med Assoc 194:803–810, 1989.
46. Trevor PB, Saunders GK, Waldron DR, et al. Metastatic extramedullary plasmacytoma of the colon and rectum in a dog. J Am Vet Med Assoc 203:406–409, 1993.
47. Jackson MW, Helfand SC, Smedes SL, et al. Primary IgG secreting plasma cell tumor in the gastrointestinal tract of a dog. J Am Vet Med Assoc 204:404–406, 1994.
48. Couto CG, Rutgers HC, Sherding RG, et al. Gastrointestinal lymphoma in 20 dogs. J Vet Int Med 3:73–78, 1989.
49. Couto CG. Canine extranodal lymphomas. In: Kirk RW (ed) Current Veterinary Therapy IX. WB Saunders, Philadelphia. 473–477, 1986.
50. Tams TR. Chronic feline inflammatory bowel disorders. II. Feline eosinophilic enteritis and lymphosarcoma. Comp Contin Ed Pract Vet 8:464–471, 1986.
51. Wellman ML, Hammer AS, DiBartola SP, et al. Lymphoma involving large granular lymphocytes in cats: 11 cases (1982–1991). J Am Vet Med Assoc 201:1265–1269, 1992.
52. McPherron MA, Chavkin MJ, Powers BE, et al. Globule leukocyte tumor involving the small intestine in a cat. J Am Vet Med Assoc 204:241–245, 1994.
53. Allroy J, Leav I, De Ellis RA, et al. Mast cell tumors. Lab Invest 33:159–167, 1975.
54. O'Keefe DA, Couto CG, Burke-Schwartz C, et al. Systemic mastocytosis in 16 dogs. J Vet Int Med 1:75–80, 1987.
55. Kosovsky JE, Matthiesen DT, Patnaik AK. Small intestinal adenocarcinoma in cats: 32 cases (1978–1985). J Am Vet Med Assoc 192:233–235, 1988.
56. Cribb AE. Feline gastrointestinal adenocarcinoma: A review and retrospective study. Can Vet J 29:709–712, 1988.
57. Church EM, Mehlhaff CJ, Patnaik AK. Colorectal adenocarcinoma in dogs: 78 cases (1973–1984). J Am Vet Med Assoc 191:727–730, 1987.
58. Roth L, King JM. Mesenteric and omental sclerosis associated with metastases from gastrointestinal neoplasia in the dog. J Sm Anim Pract 31:27–30, 1990.
59. Turrel JM, Theon AP. Single high-dose irradiation for selected canine rectal carcinomas. Vet Radiol 27:141–145, 1986.
60. Seiler RJ. Colorectal polyps of the dog: A clinicopathologic study of 17 cases. J Am Vet Med Assoc 174:72–75, 1979.
61. Seim HB. Diseases of the anus and rectum. In: Kirk RW (ed) Current Veterinary Therapy IX. WB Saunders, Philadelphia, 916–921, 1986.
62. Happe RP, Van der Gaag I, Wolvekamp WTC, et al. Multiple polyps of the gastric mucosa in two dogs. J Sm Anim Pract 18:179–189, 1977.
63. Silverberg SG. Carcinomas arising in adenomatous polyps of the rectum of a dog. Dis Colon Rectum 14:191–194, 1971.
64. Thompson JP, Christiopher MM, Ellison GW, et al. Paraneoplastic leukocytosis associated with a rectal adenomatous polyp in a dog. J Am Vet Med Assoc 201:737–738, 1992.
65. van Niel MHF, van der Gaag I, van der Ingh TS, et al. Polyposis of the small intestine in a young cat. A comparison with polyposis in man and dogs. J Vet Med A 36:161–165, 1989.
66. Culbertson R, Branam JE, Rosenblatt LS. Esophageal/gastric leiomyoma in the laboratory beagle. J Am Vet Med Assoc 183:1168–1171, 1983.
67. Brueckner KA, Withrow SJ. Intestinal leiomyosarcomas in six dogs. J Am Anim Hosp Assoc 24:281–284, 1988.
68. Kapatkin AS, Mullen HS, Matthiesen DT, et al. Leiomyosarcoma in dogs: 44 cases (1983–1988). J Am Vet Med Assoc 201:1077–1079, 1992.
69. Mcpherron MA, Withrow SJ, Seim HB, et al. Colorectal leiomyomas in seven dogs. J Am Anim Hosp Assoc 28:43–46, 1992.
70. Bagley RS, Levy JK, Malarkey DE. Hypoglycemia associated with intra-abdominal smooth muscle tumors in 6 dogs (abstract). J Vet Int Med 8:148, 1994.

71. Feldman EC, Nelson RW. Canine and Feline Endocrinology and Reproduction. WB Saunders, Philadelphia, 1987.
72. Chastain CB, Ganjam VK. Clinical Endocrinology of Companion Animals. Lea & Febiger, Philadelphia, 1986.
73. Morrison WB. The clinical relevance of APUD cells. Comp Contin Ed Pract Vet 6:884–890, 1984.
74. Willard MD, Schall WD. APUDomas. In: Kirk RW (ed) Current Veterinary Therapy VIII. WB Saunders, Philadelphia, 771–773, 1983.
75. Johnson SE. Pancreatic APUDomas. Sem Vet Med Surg 4:202–211, 1989.
76. O'Brien TD, Hayden DW, O'Leary TP. Canine pancreatic endocrine tumors: Immunohistochemical analysis of hormone content and amyloid. Vet Pathol 24:308–314, 1987.
77. Boosinger TR, Zerbe CA, Grabau JH, et al. Multihormonal pancreatic endocrine tumor in a dog with duodenal ulcers and hypertrophic gastropathy. Vet Pathol 25:237–239, 1988.
78. Middleton DJ, Watson ADJ. Duodenal ulceration associated with gastrin-secreting pancreatic tumor in a cat. J Am Vet Med Assoc 183:461–462, 1983.
79. Shaw DH. Gastrinoma (Zollinger-Ellison syndrome) in the dog and cat. Can Vet J 29:488–452, 1988.
80. Wolfe MM, Jensen RT. Zollinger-Ellison syndrome. Current concepts in diagnosis and management. N Eng J Med 317:1200–1209, 1987.
81. Zerbe CA. Gastrinoma. Proc 11th ACVIM Forum, Washington, DC, 378–381, 1993.
82. Gabbert NH, Nachreiner RF, Holmes-Wood P, et al. Serum immunoreactive gastrin concentrations in the dog: Basal and postprandial values measured by radioimmunoassay. Am J Vet Res 45:2351–2353, 1984.
83. Brodey RS. Alimentary tract neoplasms in the cat. A clinicopathologic survey of 46 cases. Am J Vet Res 27:74–80, 1966.
84. Giles RC, Hildebrandt PK, Montogomery CA. Carcinoid tumor in the small intestine of a dog. Vet Pathol 11:340–349, 1974.
85. Zerbe CA, Boosinger TR, Grabau JH, et al. Pancreatic polypeptide and insulin-secreting tumor in a dog with duodenal ulcers and hypertrophic gastritis. J Vet Int Med 3:178–182, 1989.
86. Medinger TL, Williams DA, Bruyette DS. Severe gastrointestinal tract hemorrhage in 3 dogs with hypoadrenocorticism. J Am Vet Med Assoc 202:1869–1872, 1993.
87. Burrows CF. Reversible mega-oesophagus in a dog with hypoadrenocorticism. J Sm Anim Pract 28:1073–1078, 1987.
88. Johnson LR. Regulation of gastrointestinal growth. In: Johnson LR (ed) Physiology of the Gastrointestinal Tract. Raven Press, New York, 301–333, 1987.
89. Takeuchi K, Nishiwaki H, Okada M, et al. Bilateral adrenalectomy worsens gastric mucosal lesions induced by indomethacin in the rat. Gastroenterology 97:284–293, 1989.
90. Hall JA, Twedt DC, Burrows CF. Gastric motility in dogs. II. Disorders of gastric motility. Comp Contin Ed Pract Vet 12:1373–1390, 1990.
91. Di Bartola SP, Johnson SE, Davenport DJ, et al. Clinicopathologic findings resembling hypoadrenocorticism in dogs with primary gastrointestinal disease. J Am Vet Med Assoc 187:60–63, 1985.
92. Lynn RC, Feldman EC, Nelson RW, et al. Efficacy of microcrystalline desoxycorticosterone pivalate for treatment of hypoadrenocorticism in dogs. J Am Vet Med Assoc 202:392–396, 1993.
93. Sack TL, Sleisenger MH. Effects of systemic and extraintestinal disease on the gut. In: Sleisenger MH, Fordtran JS (eds) Gastrointestinal Disease. Pathophysiology, Diagnosis, Management. WB Saunders, Philadelphia, 488–528, 1989.
94. Wilson SD, Singh RB, Kalkhoff RK, et al. Does hyperparathyroidism cause hypergastrinemia? Surgery 80:231–237, 1976.
95. Geokas MC, Baltaxe HA, Banks PA, et al. Acute pancreatitis. Ann Intern Med 103:86–100, 1985.
96. Papasouliotis K, Muir P, Gruffydd-Jones TJ, et al. Decreased orocecal transit time as measured by the exhalation of breath hydrogen in hyperthyroid cats. Res Vet Sci 55:115–118, 1993.
97. Karaus M, Wienbeck M, Grussendorf M, et al. Intestinal motor activity in experimental hyperthyroidism in conscious dogs. Gastroenterology 97:911–919, 1989.
98. Thomas FB, Caldwell JH, Greenberger NJ. Steatorrhea in thyrotoxicosis. Relation to hypermotility and excessive dietary fat. Ann Int Med 78:669–675, 1973.
99. Wiley ZD, Lavigne ME, Liu KA, et al. The effect of hyperthyroidism on gastric emptying in pancreatic exocrine biliary secretion in man. Am J Dig Dis 23:1003–1008, 1978.
100. Hodin RA, Chamberlain SM, Upton MP. Thyroid hormone differentially regulates rat intestinal brush border enzyme gene expression. Gastroenterology 103:1529–1536, 1992.
101. Hellesen C, Friis T, Larsen E, et al. Small intestinal histology, radiology, and absorption in hyperthyroidism. Scan J Gastroenterol 4:169–175, 1969.
102. Tams TR. Feline inflammatory bowel disease. Vet Clin N Am 23:569–586, 1993.
103. Rosenthal FD, Jones C, Lewis SI. Thyrotoxic vomiting. Br Med J 2:209–211, 1976.
104. Rijnberk A, Leav I. Thyroid tumors. In: Kirk RW (ed) Current Veterinary Therapy VI. WB Saunders, Philadelphia, 1020–1024, 1977.
105. Kowalewski K, Kolodej A. Myoelectrical and mechanical activity of stomach and intestine in hypothyroid dogs. Am J Dig Dis 22:235–240, 1977.
106. Gullo L, Pezzilli R, Bellanova B, et al. Influence of the thyroid on exocrine pancreatic function. Gastroenterology 100:1392–1396, 1991.
107. Fraser R, Horowitz M, Dent J. Hyperglycaemia stimulates pyloric motility in normal subjects. Gut 32:475–478, 1991.
108. Valdovinos MA, Camilleri M, Zimmerman BR. Chronic diarrhea in diabetes mellitus: Mechanisms and an approach to diagnosis and treatment. Mayo Clin Proc 68:691–702, 1993.
109. Hosoda S, Bamba T, Nakago S, et al. Age-related changes in the gastrointestinal tract. Nutr Rev 50:374–377, 1992

28 Motility Disorders of the Bowel

W. GRANT GUILFORD

IRRITABLE BOWEL SYNDROME

Clinical Synopsis

Diagnostic Features

- Chronic, intermittent, gastrointestinal dysfunction of variable character
- Signs often exacerbated or initiated by stress
- Large-bowel diarrhea common
- Little or no deterioration in physical condition despite chronic course
- Clinical signs should preferably include at least two of the following: abdominal gaseousness, abdominal pain, more frequent and/or more fluid bowel movements during periods of abdominal discomfort
- Diagnostic evaluations including intestinal biopsy reveal no evidence of organic disease

Standard Treatment

- Identify and remove stressors
- Controlled diet plus supplementary dietary fiber (wheat bran 0.5–2 tablespoons per meal)
- Various motility modifiers (see text)

Introduction

Irritable bowel syndrome is a gastrointestinal motility disorder of humans that is characterized by irregular bowel habits, abdominal pain, and the absence of detectable organic disease.[2] Irritable bowel syndrome has been variously referred to as nervous colon, nervous colitis, unstable colon, spastic colon, spastic colitis, and mucus colitis. The term *irritable bowel syndrome* (IBS) is at present favored because the disorder is thought to be a conglomerate of diseases of different causes, because inflammation is not a feature (thus *colitis* is inappropriate), and because areas of the bowel other than the colon are thought to be involved.[2] The syndrome is considered a functional bowel disorder. The term *functional* is used in this context to denote a disease syndrome with a definable group of symptoms but no organic lesion or at least no lesion that can be consistently demonstrated at our present level of expertise.[3,4] As time has passed, the syndrome of irritable bowel disease has become more defined. In humans it is now not just a diagnosis of exclusion, but can be confirmed by the presence of certain clinical and motility findings.[2,4]

It seems likely that a disorder analogous to IBS occasionally afflicts dogs, but not all stress-associated gastrointestinal complaints should be classifed as IBS. For instance, stressful situations can precipitate acute diarrhea in dogs and to a lesser extent in cats. Many of these instances, however, are acute responses to extremely stressful situattions (such as the waiting room of a veterinary clinic) occurring in animals with no history of preexisting gastrointestinal dysfunction. The acute so-called nervous diarrheas are presumably mediated by the autonomic and enteric nervous systems and are not analogous to IBS, which has a chronic course. Other causes of stress-induced diarrhea are due to recognizable organic diseases of the large bowel that reduce its reservoir and absorptive capacity predisposing the animal to diarrhea from any precipitating cause. In these patients stress no longer results in diarrhea once the underlying disease (usually chronic colitis) is successfully treated. However, there is a subgroup of animals with stress-related diarrhea (particularly dogs) that have chronic gastrointestinal signs compatible with irritable bowel disease, in which we and others[5–8] have been unable to demonstrate any organic lesion and that have responded to fiber, motility modifiers, or avoidance of stressful situations. This latter group of patients have been tentatively designated as suffering from IBS.

Prevalence

Irritable bowel syndrome is one of the most commonly encountered human gastrointestinal disorders. Veterinarians are perhaps fortunate that this often vague and frustratingly intractable disease is not a major cause of gastrointestinal disease in animals. The precise prevalence of IBS in dogs is unknown. At the author's Massey University practice, the syndrome is uncommon, accounting for approximately 1 in 3000 submissions and fewer than 1 in 20 patients with large-bowel diarrhea. However, others find the disease more common. For instance, "spastic colon" has been reported to account for as many as 17% of dogs with clinical evidence of colitis.[7] These contrasting opinions probably represent differing definitions as to what constitutes IBS, rather than true differences in prevalence (see later).[5,8,9]

Etiology, Pathogenesis, and Pathophysiology

The cause(s) of IBS is unknown.[10] The pathogenesis appears to involve myoelectric abnormalities in the bowel, disturbances in visceral afferent function, and perhaps, to a lesser extent, generalized autonomic dysfunction.[4,10–12] A variety of pathophysiologic abnormalities have been observed and are listed in Table 28–1.

During the times when humans with IBS have diarrhea, pressures within the colon are low and segmentation motility is reduced.[13] However, when constipation prevails, pressure within the colon is high, reflecting increased motility. In this state resistance provided by the segmentation type of motility is high, retarding the movement of colonic contents, with the result that they are maximally dehydrated. Thus, motility responses in the irritable colon are exaggerated in both directions, suggesting there is a dysfunction in the control mechanisms that normally modulate motility.

The mechanisms by which stress influences IBS remain speculative, but it is known that emotional stress can trigger gastrointestinal hypermotility in normal humans and it appears that the threshold of this effect appears lower in IBS patients. Furthermore, much progress has been made in our understanding of how CNS neuropeptides influence gastrointestinal motility[14] and the type of motility derangements that occur due to stress.[15] In addition, the importance of neurogenic inflammation mediated by neurotransmitters such as substance P is now understood (see Chapter 4).

The stimuli that initiate the abnormal motility in IBS are not limited to psychologic factors. The abnormal responses are also stimulated by food, at times before the meal has had a chance to reach the colon. This suggests that the response is mediated by abnormal events in physiologic reflexes such as the neural reflexes that affect colonic motility when feeding begins. It is possible that gastrointestinal hormones mediate some of the abnormal motor responses in IBS. In particular, gastrin and cholecystokinin have been suggested to play a role in functional bowel disorders. CCK infusion in affected patients produces colonic hypermotility and abdominal pain. In addition, humans with IBS develop abnormal colonic motility responses to bile acids at concentrations one-third of that required to produce abnormal responses in normal

Table 28–1

MYOELECTRIC AND MOTILITY ABNORMALITIES PROMINENT IN HUMANS WITH IRRITABLE BOWEL SYNDROME

High-amplitude pressure waves a prominent feature of basal motility
Clustered contractions in the small bowel
Spastic response to rectal distension
Delayed but prolonged colonic hypermotility in response to ingestion of food (particularly fats)
Pronounced colonic hypermotility to cholinergic agents
Increased colonic motility and abdominal pain in response to CCK
Increased frequency of basal electrical rhythm
Colonic motor activity is increased by low concentrations of bile acids
Small-bowel transit time is faster when diarrhea is predominant
Small-bowel transit time is slower when constipation is predominant
Lowered gastroesophageal sphincter pressure

humans. In healthy dogs, infusion of bile acids has been shown to induce increased motor activity in the small intestine[16] and colon, raising the possibility that a similar phenomenon could occur in dogs. A spastic response of the large bowel to distension is a consistent feature of patients with IBS, although it is also seen in some normal individuals.

In humans, the abdominal pain due to IBS has been attributed to bowel spasms. Alternatively, during periods of intestinal hypomotility the pain may result from gas distension of the paralyzed intestine. Surprisingly, the actual volume of gas generated by most human patients with IBS is not increased and the abdominal pain and gaseous distension reported by affected humans is thought to relate to slower intestinal transit, reduced tone in the intestinal wall, and perhaps increased sensitivity to gaseous distension of the bowel.[4,11,17] The latter suggestion is supported by the observation that human patients with IBS appear to have a lower colonic pain threshold during endoscopy.[18] In an analogous manner to humans, breath hydrogen concentrations were normal in a small number of dogs with abdominal gaseousness associated with IBS that were tested by the author. This suggests that the abdominal gas noted in dogs with IBS is predominantly derived from aerophagia rather than fermentation.

Clinical Findings

Dogs with IBS have clinical signs of gastrointestinal dysfunction that are often (but not always) associated with an identifiable stress, and that are chronic, intermittent, and usually somewhat variable in nature. Affected animals are often timid, behave nervously, or are under performance stress such as police or show animals. The signs most often seen in affected dogs include a combination of diarrhea and abdominal discomfort, alternating with periods of normality or even mild constipation.

Diarrhea due to IBS usually has a large-bowel character, most often consisting of small volumes of loose stools. Sometimes the diarrhea is explosive, consisting of a mixture of gas and fluid. Mucus may be seen but hematochezia is uncommon. Tenesmus may occur and, in humans, is usually attributed to a sensation of incomplete evacuation rather than colonic irritation.

Episodic abdominal pain is an important feature of the disease. In humans the pain is usually poorly localized and of variable character ranging from sharp to dull, and acute to chronic. In dogs the "pain" is difficult to characterize because it is usually reported by the owner but not present during the physical examination. Not infrequently the pain is relieved by eructation or defecation. In some dogs, eating precipitates the discomfort and in others it relieves it. Abdominal gaseousness manifested by borborygmus, mild abdominal distension, and frequent belching and flatulence are common.

Nausea, vomiting, and excessive gastroduodenal and gastroesophageal reflux can also occur in dogs and people with IBS. Other signs such as urinary bladder dysfunction and difficult or painful coitus are not infrequent in affected people and have raised the possibility that the disorder results from a generalized autonomic disturbance.

Diagnosis

If the term *irritable bowel syndrome* is to retain meaning, the onus is on the veterinary profession not to apply it without discretion to any form of diarrhea that defies definition by current methods. Unknown disease entities are better described as *idiopathic* because that term honestly describes a problem as having an unknown cause. Suggested criteria to be fulfilled before a diagnosis of IBS is made are provided in the clinical synopsis. If analogy is to be drawn to the human disease, the signs in animals with IBS should preferably include two or more of the following signs in addition to the other clinical features listed in the clinical synopsis: abdominal gaseousness; abdominal pain; more frequent and/or more fluid bowel movements during periods of abdominal discomfort.[2,17] The abdominal gaseousness may manifest as frequent eructation, borborygmus or flatulence, and/or mild abdominal distension. Often the signs are temporarily relieved by eructation or defecation. A dog presented with idiopathic chronic diarrhea (large or small bowel) without evidence of abdominal discomfort or gaseousness is unlikely to be suffering from a disorder analogous to human IBS.

Before diagnosing IBS, an extensive workup must be performed to ensure that serious organic disease is not overlooked. Important differential diagnoses are chronic pancreatitis, food sensitivity, lymphocytic-plasmacytic enteritis, eosinophilic gastroenteritis, idiopathic colitis, *Clostridium perfringens*–associated colitis, and chronic idiopathic large-bowel diarrhea (see Chapters 24 and 26). Appropriate diagnostic evaluations are dictated by the particular spectrum of clinical signs shown by the patient but, as a minimum, should include CBC, serum chemistry profile, fecal flotations, dietary trials, diagnostic imaging of the abdomen, and endoscopic examination with mucosal (particularly colon) biopsy.

Tentative diagnosis of IBS is thus largely made by exclusion of organic disease in a patient with history and clinical signs compatible with a functional motility disorder. The observation of pronounced large-bowel segmental contractions (either by barium enema or endoscopy) is suggestive, but not diagnostic, of the disorder. Increased colonic mucus is sometimes observed during endoscopy. In a small number of affected dogs examined by the author, fluoroscopy and barium-impregnated polyethylene sphere studies have been normal with the exception of one dog that showed a subjective increase in the frequency of intestinal contractions. In human medicine, application of electrodiagnostic and manometric techniques to the diagnosis of gastrointestinal disease has revealed a spectrum of motility abnormalities that allow positive confirmation of the disorder (Table 28–1). Unfortunately, these diagnostic evaluations have not yet been applied to the confirmation of IBS in dogs.

Long-term successful remission of signs following the addition of fiber to the diet and stress reduction helps confirm the disease. However, fiber responsiveness in and of itself should not be considered diagnostic of IBS. Fiber has a variety of favorable effects on the bowel in addition to its influences on colonic motility (see Chapter 38), and many diseases of diverse cause will respond or partially respond to supplementation of the diet with fiber. For instance, in people (and perhaps animals) bile salt malabsorption produces signs of large-bowel diarrhea (in spite of a morphologically normal colon mucosa) that will respond to fiber supplementation.

Management

Well-designed clinical trials have yet to be conducted in humans or dogs with the syndrome.[20] The principal aspects of treatment are identification and elimination of stressors, dietary modification, and, during flare-ups of the disease, symptomatic drug therapy. Both nutritional and pharmacologic management must be painstakingly individualized according to the predominant manifestation of IBS in the particular dog under

treatment. For instance, if diarrhea is the predominant clinical sign shown, opioids are indicated, but this class of drugs is usually unhelpful in dogs in which the predominant sign is abdominal pain and may even exacerbate the pain.

IDENTIFYING STRESSORS. A large number of different stressful situations can precipitate the disorder. In my experience, the most common stressors are a tense owner, work or show stress, separation anxiety, territorial challenges, and new additions (both human and animal) to the family. Many owners of dogs with IBS are of anxious dispositions themselves and some even suffer from similar disorders. In this situation, there is often a very strong bond between the affected dog and its owner. Owner anxiety, of course, can result from many causes, but one of the more important can be worry about the dog's clinical signs, creating a vicious cycle. Once careful diagnostic procedures rule out serious organic diseases and the syndrome of IBS is carefully explained to the owner, this vicious cycle can be broken. Other endeavors that are at times helpful are behavioral modification, reducing the work hours to which the dog is subjected, and even moving house. Tranquilizers are to be avoided because they are poorly effective and impractical for long-term use.

DIETARY MODIFICATION. High-fiber diets have been the cornerstone of the nutritional management of IBS in humans and dogs, but in both species doubts have been expressed about their therapeutic value.[8,17] In humans, the best results with fiber are achieved in IBS patients in which constipation is the predominant sign.[17] In my experience, and that of others,[8] the clinical signs of dogs with IBS are often dampened by the addition of fiber to the diet, but complete remission is only occasionally seen. The best type of fiber for the treatment of IBS has not been determined. Considerable individual variation occurs, with some dogs doing better on a fermentable fiber (e.g., Metamucil, 1–6 teaspoons per meal; or oat bran 0.5–2 teaspoons per meal) and others doing best on a nonfermentable fiber (e.g., wheat bran 0.5–2 teaspoons per meal). Paradoxically, the clinical signs of some human patients and dogs with IBS are aggravated by fiber. The reasons why fiber sometimes exacerbates the condition are unknown but might include allergic reactions to the protein components of the fiber or, more likely, excessive use of fermentable fiber resulting in increased abdominal gaseousness. Changing the type of fiber will often relieve the aggravation.

In addition to adding fiber to the diet, the author feeds dogs with IBS a controlled diet for the first month of treatment. If the controlled diet meets with success it is continued; otherwise, dietary restrictions are relaxed. Desirable features of the controlled diet include hypoallergenicity (achieved by use of selected protein sources), low fermentability (achieved by using highly digestible diets), and a low fat content. Controlled diets are used because food allergy or intolerance has been reported to be an important trigger of irritable bowel–like symptoms in humans.[21] Gas-producing foods, such as milk and legumes, and situations that promote aerophagia, should be avoided. Low dietary fat is valuable in some dogs with IBS. The reason for the beneficial effect of low-fat diets in these individuals is uncertain but may relate to a reduction in the severity of gastroesophageal reflux that often accompanies the disease or a reduction in irritant bile acids reaching the colon.

MOTILITY MODIFIERS. Short courses of opioids, such as diphenoxylate (Lomotil; Searle: 0.1 mg/kg PO q 8 hours) or loperamide (Imodium; Janssen: 0.08 mg/kg PO q 8 hours) are sometimes helpful during periods of diarrhea due to IBS. Anticholinergics may be useful for temporary relief of intestinal spasms, but they are poorly effective at controlling the other clinical signs of the disease and at times may exacerbate abdominal pain associated with ileus and intestinal gas distension. Librax (Roche), a combination of an anticholinergic (clidinium bromide) and a sedative/smooth muscle relaxant (chlordiazepoxide), at a dose of 0.1 to 0.25 mg/kg PO q 8–12 hours (based on the clidinium fraction) is useful for the control of abdominal discomfort associated with IBS.[8] Mebeverine hydrochloride (Colofac; Jansen-Cilag) is available in many countries for the treatment of IBS in people. The drug is an antispasmodic that acts as a direct smooth muscle relaxant but also has local anesthetic properties and mild anticholinergic effects. The author has used this drug with mixed success in dogs with IBS at a dose of approximately 2 mg/kg PO q 8 hours. Cisapride and metoclopramide are useful in dogs with reflux esophagitis associated with IBS (see Chapter 11) and may also be helpful if depressed gastrointestinal motility is the predominant abnormality in an affected dog.

MISCELLANEOUS MEASURES. In the author's experience, eliminating potent organophosphate flea treatment products (such as fenthion) is valuable, particularly in dogs in which the predominant manifestation of IBS is abdominal pain. Simethicone is occasionally helpful in dogs with abdominal gaseousness associated with IBS. The drug is inert and nonabsorbed. It acts as a defoaming agent that coalesces gas bubbles in the gastrointestinal tract, thereby assisting their eructation or passage as flatus. The dose is empirical but usually ranges from 2 to 10 mg/kg PO q 6 to 8 hours. Cholestyramine (a bile acid binding resin) is useful in some humans with IBS and a short trial with cholestyramine is worthwhile in affected dogs. Similarly, verapamil has met with limited success in some people with IBS. The drug relaxes gastroenteric smooth muscle, delays colonic transit time, and has a favorable effect on intestinal absorption and secretion.[17]

ADYNAMIC ILEUS

Introduction

Adynamic ileus is defined as a transient and reversible intestinal obstruction resulting from inhibition of bowel motility. It affects the stomach, small bowel, and large bowel. The lack of peristaltic activity results in a functional obstruction because intestinal content pools in the dependent areas of the gastrointestinal tract, instead of being propelled in an aboral direction.

Intestinal obstruction (ileus) can result from a large number of causes in addition to adynamic ileus (Table 25–1) including persistent intestinal neuromusclar derangements that cause hypomotility (pseudo-obstruction). The terms pseudo-obstruction and adynamic ileus overlap somewhat, but pseudo-obstruction has a more chronic duration and often a more segmental appearance than adynamic ileus. The etiopathogenesis, pathophysiology, and management of intestinal obstruction are described in Chapter 25. What follows is a brief additional discussion of adynamic ileus with particular reference to its etiopathogenesis.

Cause

Adynamic ileus is a relatively common problem with a variety of causes (Table 25–1). It is seen most frequently as a complication of abdominal surgery, electrolyte imbalance, or acute inflammatory lesions of the bowel, peritoneal cavity, or other abdominal organs. It is a particularly common complication of canine parvoviral gastroenteritis and acute pancreatitis. Intestinal ischemia transiently increases but then inhibits intestinal motility. Neuropathies affecting the autonomic nervous system can produce intestinal stasis. Anti-

cholinergic drugs inhibit gastrointestinal motility. When disease has reduced normal motility, anticholinergics will compound the situation, leading to ileus[22] and potentially bacterial overgrowth. Intestinal distension, if pronounced, results in inhibition of motility via the intestinointestinal reflex. Frequently, potassium deficits must be corrected before normal motor function returns. Diarrhea causes an accelerated loss of potassium from the body. The potassium depletion is often compounded by inadequate intake.

Pathogenesis

Several neural, humoral, and metabolic factors appear to interact to cause ileus.[23–25] In most models of adynamic ileus, electrical slow waves still occur in the longitudinal muscle of affected bowel but do not initiate action potentials and associated contractile activity within the circular muscle layers. This electromechanical dissociation appears to result from a tonic discharge of inhibitory neurons and an absence of spike waves.[25] Increased adrenergic tone may be partly responsible for the tonic inhibitory discharge. The sympathetic nervous system interacts presynaptically with excitatory synaptic connections in the enteric nervous system. Release of norepinephrine appears to inhibit release of excitatory neurotransmitters such as acetylcholine, thus allowing tonic discharge of inhibitory neurons to dominate. The result is a decrease in intestinal motor activity, blood flow, and other gastrointestinal functions.

It is thought that other factors in addition to increased sympathetic discharge are necessary for the development of ileus because in most species, including cats and dogs, nonselective alpha and beta blockade or splanchnicectomy improves but does not prevent ileus.[25,26] Interestingly, selective alpha$_2$ blockade with yohimbine or atipamezole lessens endotoxin-induced ileus in horses[27] and surgical-induced ileus in rats,[28] respectively.

Humoral factors are known to contribute to the pathogenesis of ileus because the motility of transplanted (denervated) intestinal loops is inhibited during experimental peritonitis in dogs.[23] Proposed humoral inhibitory factors have included circulating catecholamines but this is unlikely because adrenalectomy does not prevent the disorder.[25] However, vasopressin levels increase during laparotomy and are likely to have an inhibitory effect on small-bowel motility.[25] Release of endogenous opiates has also been proposed as a cause of postoperative ileus.[25] Although naloxone does not relieve postoperative ileus, fedotozine, a k-opioid agonist, restores intestinal motility in rats.[25,29] It is noteworthy that fedotozine has been shown to stimulate gastrointestinal motility in dogs.[30] Impaired release of prokinetic hormones such as neurotensin or motilin may also play a role in ileus.

Hypokalemia interferes with the normal ionic movements on which smooth muscle contraction depends. Potassium deficits may contribute more to the loss of motility than does stimulation of the sympathetic nervous system.[31] In addition, following surgery anesthetic agents may exacerbate the loss of motility.[25]

Clinical Signs and Diagnosis

The clinical signs of ileus include anorexia, vomiting, and depression. Occasionally, mild abdominal distension or abdominal pain may occur, probably as a result of accumulation of gas in the hypomotile bowel. Adynamic ileus should be suspected in any animal with these clinical signs, particularly if it is affected by one of the predisposing diseases listed in Table

25–1. Auscultation of the abdomen in affected patients reveals the absence of gut sounds. Abdominal radiographs usually show loops of bowel distended wtih gas and fluid. Adynamic ileus can be confirmed by a BIPS study that will show delayed gastrointestinal transit along with retention of BIPS in the stomach or a scattering of BIPS throughout the entire upper gastrointestinal tract (Figures 25–10 and 25–11).

Management

Treatment of adynamic ileus is important because affected patients are uncomfortable and the disorder prevents the use of the gastrointestinal tract for feeding. Furthermore, animals with ileus are predisposed to the development of small intestinal bacterial overgrowth, magnifying the potential for bacterial translocation and sepsis. Adynamic ileus is initially managed by treatment of any identifiable primary cause and by the correction of electrolyte abnormalities. Gastrointestinal decompression can be maintained by use of a nasogastric tube but is rarely necessary. The administration of prokinetic agents such as metoclopramide (0.4 mg/kg IV q 6 hours) or cisapride (0.25–0.5 mg/kg PO q 8 hours) is likely to be helpful.[25,32,33] It is worthy of note that in one study of humans with adynamic ileus, erythromycin failed to have a prokinetic effect.[34]

DYSAUTONOMIA

Dysfunction of the autonomic nervous system is referred to as dysautonomia and has been reported in humans, horses,[35] cats,[36-38] and dogs[39-41] both in Europe and the United States. Characteristic clinical signs of dysautonomia include dilated pupils, dry mucous membranes, regurgitation, vomiting, constipation, a fixed or bradycardic heart rate, and dysuria (Figure 28–1). Generalized megaesophagus is common in cats with dysautonomia and is occasionally seen in affected dogs. Delayed gastric emptying is usually present. In humans, dysautonomia has been related to a number of different causes including diabetes mellitus, paraneoplastic syndromes, genetic defects, CNS lesions, chronic renal failure, drug reactions, and heavy metal toxicoses.[42] In animals, the causes of dysautonomia remain obscure.[35]

The clinical signs result from a widespread degeneration of the autonomic ganglia. Both parasympathetic and sympathetic systems are affected. The gastrointestinal signs primarily pertain to failure of parasympathectic regulation of esophageal, gastric, and colonic motility. Diagnosis is usually made by the characteristic clinical appearance. If the diagnosis is in doubt various diagnostic procedures can be instituted including the 0.1% pilocarpine and 0.25% physostigmine ocular response tests.[38] Plasma and urinary catecholamines can be assayed. In affected cats, catecholamine levels are low or absent.[38]

Treatment relies on prolonged nutritional support in association with the use of 0.25% pilocarpine eye drops q 6 to 8 hours, metoclopramide (0.2–0.4 mg/kg PO, SC q 8 hours) or bethanechol (2.5–5.0 mg (cats) or 5–25 mg (dogs) PO q 8 hours). The prognosis is guarded particularly if megaesophagus is present.

MEGACOLON SYNDROME

Megacolon is simply defined as colonic dilatation. In humans, the syndrome of megacolon encompasses a variety

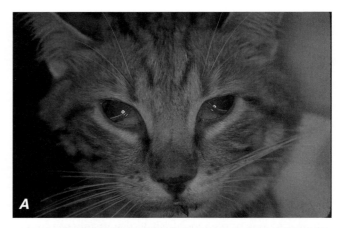
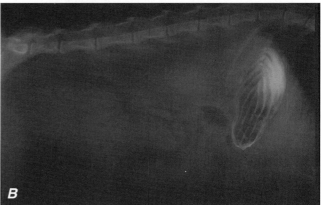

FIGURE 28–1. *(A)* Domestic shorthaired cat affected by dysautonomia. Note the dilated pupils and prolapsed third eyelids. *(B)* Lateral abdominal radiograph of the cat in *(A)*. Note the distended bladder and barium retained in the stomach, 36 hours after administration.

of diseases that result in colonic dilatation. The syndrome is usually classified into two categories, congenital megacolon (Hirschsprung disease) and acquired megacolon. Acquired megacolon in turn is subdivided according to the suspected cause of the disorder or is labeled as idiopathic if no cause is apparent. Megacolon has been reported in both dogs and cats.[6] It is uncommon, occurring in about 1 case per 10,000 in both dogs and cats at the VMTH at Davis, and many of those are referrals. Both congenital and acquired forms are recognized, but it is unclear if the congenital form is analogous to Hirschsprung disease.[43] The syndrome is most common in the cat, and on most occasions it is idiopathic.

Pathogenesis

CONGENITAL MEGACOLON.[44-46] Congenital megacolon has been studied in humans and in experimental animals. In most affected individuals, the pathologic lesion that causes fecal retention is a congenital absence of myenteric and submucosal intramural plexi (aganglionosis) in the caudal part of the colon. The aganglionosis is thought to occur due to a defect in the caudal migration of cells from the neural crest.[47] The absence of the ganglionic cells releases the gastrointestinal smooth muscle from phasic inhibition by the enteric nervous system, which in turn results in tonic smooth muscle contraction and intestinal obstruction. The colon cranial to the contracted segment dilates because of retained fecal material.

There is considerable heterogeneity in congenital mega-colon. In most humans with the disorder, only the rectum and sigmoid colon are affected, but in others almost the entire extent of the colon is involved. The variability in the length of the large bowel involved results from fetal events. Plexuses containing the ganglia are formed by neuroblasts that lay them down in order from cranial to caudal. Thus, the terminal colon is the last to be innervated. Aganglionosis results from arrested development, and when the arrest occurs early in gestation most of the colon is involved. When the arrest is late, only the caudal rectum and internal anal sphincter or, in unusual cases, just the anal sphincter are affected. Further confusion has arisen because there is a vari-ety of clinical presentations for what appears to be a similar lesion. Some patients require immediate surgical relief of obstruction in the neonatal period whereas other patients present much later in life with only constipation. Moreover, there is variability in the histopathologic lesion. Patchy or zonal loss of ganglia and abnormal or dysplastic neurons have been reported. Immunohistochemical staining of affected segments has yielded a variety of results ranging from deficits of adrenergic (relaxant) innervation, increased cholinergic (excitatory) innervation, and a deficit or absence of nerves containing enkephalin, gastrin-releasing peptide, VIP, and substance P.[48,49] Another suggestion is that there is a deficit of inhibitory interneurons of the enteric nervous system.[24] It is this heterogeneity of lesion in the complex neurologic con-trol of the colon that presumably explains the variability in the clinical picture.

Diagnosis of Hirschsprung disease in humans is usually made by manometry. Normally the internal anal sphincter relaxes when the rectum is distended. It remains contracted in patients with Hirschsprung disease.[50] As mentioned earlier, it is unclear if true Hirschsprung disease exists in the dog and cat. Differential diagnoses of importance include intestinal atresia and imperforate anus. Most cases of congenital mega-colon seen in dogs and cats would be more appropriately termed idiopathic congenital megacolon.

ACQUIRED MEGACOLON. There are a number of known causes for acquired megacolon in animals (Table 28–2). The most frequent are pelvic trauma and chronic constipation. Megacolon can also be associated with active colonic inflam-mation. Severe colitis is a prerequisite, and the loss of normal motor function is exacerbated by complicating factors such as potassium depletion. Megacolon is a frequent complaint in older Manx cats. The pathogenesis of the disorder in these cats is not understood but likely relates to interference with the defecation reflex by the sacral spinal cord deformities that plague this breed. Hypothyroidism is an established cause of megacolon in humans, and thyroid replacement can be dramatically effective. Constipation has also been noted in hypothyroid dogs.

Megacolon is idiopathic in many cats. Idiopathic mega-colon can strike cats of a variety of ages. In one report, affected cats ranged from 1 to 15 years with a mean of 4.9 years.[51] Kittens of weaning age have also been seen with the problem. It is unclear whether idiopathic megacolon in these kittens, and for that matter in many adults, is truly an acquired lesion or whether the origin is congenital. The hall-marks of the disorder are a dilated colon with no evidence of physical or functional obstruction, and normal or near nor-mal numbers of ganglion cells observed histologically in affected segments. A similar condition is seen in humans.[46] In humans as in cats, the "sluggish" colonic activity has no defined cause. Proposed etiologies include an ultrashort area of aganglionosis or a functional defect in the intrinsic inner-vation of the colon. In humans, rectosphincteric manometry

is considered the most definitive diagnostic technique for the differentiation of idiopathic megacolon from Hirschsprung disease. In cats, the primary differential diagnoses are spinal cord injury, pelvic fractures, neoplasia, and fur-associated constipation.

Clinical Findings

Megacolon causes constipation as the principal sign. With neglect, complications can appear, including signs of obstruc-tion such as anorexia and vomiting. The pathogenesis of these systemic signs is uncertain but most likely results from a breakdown of the mucosal barrier and absorption of toxic luminal products such as those produced by Clostridia, thought to multiply in the static colonic content. Chronically affected animals take on an unthrifty appearance. Paradoxi-cally, colonic impaction and megacolon can also cause diar-rhea. Fecal incontinence is also often associated with the con-dition. Abdominal palpation and rectal examination are usually sufficient to identify an impacted colon and to rule out prostatomegaly, intestinal atresia, and imperforate anus.

Radiographic, Proctoscopic, and Biopsy Findings

Survey radiographs confirm megacolon and allow assess-ment of pelvic bones. After evacuation a barium, or air enema will help establish if a narrowed rectal or colonic segment is present. Proctoscopic evaluation followed by surgical resec-tion of the affected segment differentiates fibrous strictures, neoplastic proliferations, and aganglionosis. Full thickness (usually excisional) biopsy is required to detect aganglionosis.

Management and Prognosis

Acquired megacolon can occasionally be successfully man-aged medically, but ultimately most patients undergo colec-

Table 28–2

CAUSES OF MEGACOLON IN DOGS AND CATS

Extraluminal Constriction
Pelvic deformity (trauma, congenital, nutritional osteodystrophia fibrosa)
Prostatomegaly
Pelvic masses
Strictures
Intraluminal Constriction
Constipation*
Foreign bodies
Neoplasia
Non-neoplastic strictures
Metabolic
Hypokalemia
Hypothyroidism
Neuromuscular Abnormalities
Sacral spinal cord deformities (Manx cats)
Pseudo-obstruction*
Ileus*
Dysautonomia
Idiopathic
Aganglionosis?

*These disorders in turn have a variety of rule-outs (see text and Chapter 26).

tomy or are euthanized. Even when the cause of the colonic obstruction that resulted in the acquired megacolon is identified and readily corrected, the changes in the dilated colon are often irreversible.

Palliative medical therapies most often utilized are enemas, bulk-promoting agents such as psyllium derivatives, and various other laxatives. Animals showing systemic signs such as depression or anorexia related to their obstipation should be immediately treated with fluids and antibiotics such as trimethoprim-sulfonamide combinations or ampicillin. Unexpected deaths from obstipation are not uncommon in patients showing such systemic signs. Once the animal's clinical condition has improved, enemas may be administered. Suitable enema procedures are discussed in Chapter 26. Once the retained feces are removed, laxatives can be utilized with the aim of preventing recurrence. Bulk-promoting agents reduce rectal retention time and limit water absorption from the stool. The stool can also be made softer by laxatives such as dioctyl sodium sulfosuccinate, which, in addition to softening the feces, causes colonic secretion of fluid and alterations in the colonic mucosa.[52] Another useful agent, better tolerated by cats than many other laxatives, is lactulose (Chronulac). An appropriate starting dose is 1 mL/5 kg PO q 8 hours, after which the dosage is individualized depending on response. Mineral oil is not advised for long-term use because of the danger of aspiration during administration. Cisapride, a new prokinetic agent, has been used with variable success in humans recovering from acquired megacolon and may be valuable in cats with idiopathic megacolon.[53]

The treatment of choice for idiopathic megacolon is subtotal colectomy.[51,54–59] In cats, this results in minimal adverse clinical or laboratory abnormalities.[60] In dogs, reservoir fecal incontinence is a common complication. Removal of the proximal two-thirds of the canine colon results in frequent passage of liquid or, at best, semiformed feces.[61]

INTESTINAL GASEOUSNESS[62,63]

Gaseous abdominal distension is a common complication of ileus and may also be partly responsible for the clinical signs of irritable bowel syndrome. The two most common sources of intestinal gas in dogs and cats are thought to be swallowed air and bacterial fermentation of nutrients. Additional sources are the chemical release of carbon dioxide from bicarbonates and diffusion of gas from the blood.

Intestinal gas consists of nitrogen, carbon dioxide, hydrogen, and small amounts of methane and oxygen. Nitrogen makes up 20% to 90% of intestinal gas. The nitrogen is derived primarily from swallowed air and by diffusion from blood. As other gases are produced in the gut, nitrogen diffuses into the lumen, so its partial pressure remains the same in the lumen as in the blood. Up to 50% of intestinal gas can be hydrogen, which is produced by colonic bacteria metabolizing unabsorbed nutrients. Malabsorption of carbohydrates provides substrates to the colon for hydrogen production. Thus, pancreatic insufficiency, intramural mucosal disease, and disaccharidase deficiency all cause excessive hydrogen production and abdominal gaseousness. Certain foodstuffs contain nutrients that are fermented in the colon, contributing to intestinal gas. Carbon dioxide is the third most abundant gas in the intestine. Carbon dioxide is formed as acid contents leaving the stomach are neutralized by the bicarbonate secretions of the pancreas. Most of the gas in the duodenum is carbon dioxide, but most has been absorbed by the level of the caudal intestine, and the amount in the flatus is less than 20%. As much as 1 to 2L of carbon dioxide can be produced by the hydrochloric acid-bicarbonate reaction in a 25 kg animal. Carbon dioxide is also produced by colonic bacteria and by secreted colonic bicarbonate reacting with short chain acids produced by fermentation. An increase in the amount of unabsorbed fermentable substrates entering the colon causes an increase in the amount of carbon dioxide produced. Small amounts of methane are produced by colonic bacteria. In humans, it is recognized that only certain individuals have the ability to produce methane. The factors that determine its production are not dietary, but may reflect the population of the normal resident microflora.

Gas normally passes rapidly from one region to another because there is little resistance to its flow, and little peristaltic activity is needed to propel it. When the intestine has lost its normal motility, gas accumulates and distends the bowel. Gaseous distention of the intestines apperars as bloat and causes discomfort. The quantity of gas normally present in the gastrointestinal tract is small and, in humans, only minor quantities of additional gas are necessary to produce signs of bloat that are disproportionate to the amount introduced. The amount of gas accumulated is difficult to assess radiographically.

Excessive gas production in association with normal motility most often manifests as flatulence (Chapter 5). In contrast, motility problems that do not allow the normal evacuation of intestinal gas lead to bloating and abdominal discomfort. It is possible that a vicious circle can eventually develop because disordered motility results in bacterial overgrowth, which in turn results in increased intestinal gas production. Moreover, accumulation of intesinal gas leads to intestinal distension, which in turn can exacerbate ileus through the intestinointestinal inhibitory reflex.

REFERENCES

1. Schuster MM, Whitebread WE. Physiologic insights into irritable bowel syndrome. Clin Gastroenterol 15:839–853, 1986.
2. Schuster MM. Irritable bowel syndrome. In: Sleisenger MH, Fordtran JS (eds) Gastrointestinal Disease. Pathophysiology, Diagnosis, and Management. WB Saunders, Philadelphia, 1402–1418, 1989.
3. Haubrich WS. Recognition of functional disorders. In: Berk JE (ed) Bockus Gastroenterology. WB Saunders, Philadelphia, 236–246, 1985.
4. Zighelboim J, Talley NJ. What are functional bowel disorders? Gastroenterology 104:1196–1201, 1993.
5. Leib MS. Dietary fiber and large bowel diarrhea. Proc 7th ACVIM Forum, 359–360, 1989.
6. Lorenz MD. Diseases of the large bowel. In: Ettinger SJ (ed) Textbook of Veterinary Internal Medicine. WB Saunders, Philadelphia, 1346–1372, 1983.
7. Henroteaux M. Results of an endoscopic study of colitis in dogs; predominance of idopathic colitis. Ann Med Vet 134:389–392, 1990.
8. Tams TR. Irritable bowel syndrome. In: Kirk RW, Bonagura JD (eds) Current Veterinary Therapy XI. WB Saunders, Philadelphia, 604–608, 1992.
9. Leib MS. Fiber-responsive large bowel diarrhea. Proc 8th ACVIM Forum, Washington, DC, 817–819, 1990.
10. Christensen J. Pathophysiology of the irritable bowel syndrome. Lancet 340:1444–1447, 1992.
11. Mayer EA, Raybould HE. Role of visceral afferent mechanisms in functional bowel disorders. Gastroenterology 99:1688–1704, 1990.
12. Camilleri M, Fealey RD. Idiopathic autonomic denervation in eight patients presenting with functional gastrointestinal disease. A causal association? Dig Dis Sci 35:609–616, 1990.
13. Christensen J. Myoelectric control of the colon. Gastroenterology 68:601–609, 1975.
14. Tache Y, Garrick T, Raybould H. Central nervous system action of peptides to influence gastrointestinal motor function. Gastroenterology 98:517–528, 1990.
15. Wittmann T, Crenner F, Angel F, et al. Long-duration stress. Immediate and late effects on small and large bowel motility in rats. Dig Dis Sci 35:495–500, 1990.
16. Romanski K. Bile acids and the electrical activity of canine stomach and small bowel during the interdigestive period. Polskie Archiwum Weterynaryjne 29:125–137, 1989.

17. Weber FH, McCallum RW. Clinical approach to irritable bowel syndrome. Lancet 340:1447–1452, 1992.
18. Cullingford GL, Coffey JF, Carr-Locke DL. Irritable bowel syndrome: Can the patient's response to colonoscopy help with diagnosis? Digestion 52:209–213, 1992.
19. Haderstorfer B, Whitehead WE, Schuster MM. Intestinal gas production from bacterial fermentation of undigested carbohydrate in irritable bowel syndrome. Am J Gastroenterol 84:375–378, 1989.
20. Klein KB. Controlled treatment trials in the irritable bowel syndrome; a critique. Gastroenterology 95:232–241, 1988.
21. Nanda R, James R, Smith H, et al. Food intolerance and the irritable bowel syndrome. Gut 30:1099–1104, 1989.
22. Murtaza A, Khan SR, Butt KS, et al. Paralytic ileus, a serious complication in acute diarrheal disease among infants in developing countries. Acta Paediatrica Scandinavica 78:701–705, 1989.
23. Jones RS, Schirmer BD. Intestinal obstruction, pseudo-obstruction, and ileus. In: Sleisenger MH, Fordtran JS (eds) Gastrointestinal Disease. Pathophysiology, Diagnosis, and Management. WB Saunders, Philadelphia, 369–381, 1989.
24. Wood JD. Physiology of the enteric nervous system. In: Johnson LR (ed) Physiology of the Gastrointestinal Tract. Raven Press, New York, 67–109, 1987.
25. Livingston EH, Passaro EP. Postoperative ileus. Dig Dis Sci 35:121–132, 1990.
26. Smith J, Kelly KA, Weinshiboum M. Pathophysiology of postoperative ileus. Arch Surg 112:203–209, 1977.
27. Eades SC, Moore JN. Blockade of endotoxin-induced cecal hypoperfusion and ileus with an alpha$_2$ antagonist in horses. Am J Vet Res 54:586–590, 1993.
28. Tanila H, Kauppila T, Taira T. Inhibition of intestinal motility and reversal of postlaparotomy ileus by selective alpha$_2$-adrenergic drugs in the rat. Gastroenterology 104:819–824, 1993.
29. Riviere PJM, Pascaud X, Chevalier E, et al. Fedotozine reverses ileus induced by surgery or peritonitis: Action at peripheral k-opioid receptors. Gastroenterology 104:724–731, 1993.
30. Pascaud X, Honde C, Le Gallou B, et al. Effects of fedotozine on gastrointestinal motility in dogs: Mechanism of action and related pharmacokinetics. J Pharm Pharmacol 42:546–552, 1990.
31. Mishra NK, Appert HE, Howard JM. Studies of paralytic ileus. Effects of intraperitoneal injury on motility of the canine small intestine. Am J Surg 129:559–563, 1975.
32. Graves GM, Becht JL, Rawlings CA. Metoclopramide reversal of decreased gastrointestinal myoelectric and contractile activity in a model of canine postoperative ileus. Vet Surg 18:27–33, 1989.
33. Gerring EL, King JN. Cisapride in the prophylaxis of equine postoperative ileus. Equine Vet J (suppl 7), Proc 3rd Equine Colic Research Sympos, 52–55, 1989.
34. Bonacini M, Quiason S, Reynolds M, et al. Effect of intravenous erythromycin on postoperative ileus. Am J Gastroenterol 88:208–211, 1993.
35. Pollin MM, Griffiths IR. A review of the primary dysautonomias of domestic animals. J Comp Path 106:99–199, 1992.
36. Rochilitz I. Feline dysautonomia (the Key-Gaskell or dilated pupil syndrome): A preliminary review. J Sm Anim Pract 25:587–598, 1984.
37. Sharp NJH, Nash AS, Griffiths IR. Feline dysautonomia (the Key-Gaskell syndrome): A clinical and pathological study of forty cases. J Sm Anim Pract 25:599–615, 1984.
38. Guilford WG, O'Brien DP, Allert A, et al. Diagnosis of dysautonomia in a cat by autonomic nervous system function testing. J Am Vet Med Assoc 193:823–828, 1988.
39. Rochilitz I, Bennet AM. Key-Gaskell syndrome in a bitch. Vet Rec 112:614–615, 1983.
40. Wise LA, Lappin MR. A syndrome resembling feline dysautonomia (Key-Gaskell syndrome) in a dog. J Am Vet Med Assoc 198:2103–2106, 1991.
41. Schrauwen E, van Ham L, Maenhout T, et al. Canine dysautonomia: A case report. Vet Rec 128:524–525, 1991.
42. Bannister R. Autonomic failure: A textbook of clinical disorders of the autonomic nervous system. Oxford University Press, Oxford, 1983.
43. Burrows CF. Constipation. In: Kirk RW (ed) Current Veterinary Therapy IX. WB Saunders, Philadelphia, 904–908, 1986.
44. Wood JD. Physiological studies on the large intestine of mice with hereditary megacolon and absence of enteric ganglion cells. In: Proceedings of the Fourth International Symposium on Gastrointestinal Motility. Mitchell Press, Vancouver, 177–187, 1974.
45. Christensen J. Motility of the colon. In: Johnson LR (ed) Physiology of the Gastrointestinal Tract. Raven Press, New York, 665–693, 1987.
46. Phillips SF. Megacolon: Congenital and acquired. In: Sleisenger MH, Fordtran JS (eds) Gastrointestinal Disease. Pathophysiology, Diagnosis, and Management. WB Saunders, Philadelphia, 1389–1402, 1989.
47. Okamoto E, Veda T. Embryogenesis of intramural ganglia of the gut and its relation to Hirschsprung's disease. J Pediatr Surg 2:437–443, 1967.
48. Larsson LT, Malmfors G, Sundler F. Peptidergic innervation in Hirschprung's disease. Z Kinderchir 38:301–304, 1983.
49. Tsuto T, Okamura H, Fuukui K, et al. An immunohistochemical investigation of vasoactive intestinal polypeptide in the colon of patients with Hirschsprung's disease. Neurosci Lett 34:57–62, 1982.
50. Howard ER, Nixon HH. Internal anal sphincter. Arch Dis Child 43:569–578, 1968.
51. Rosin E, Walshaw R, Mehlhaff C, et al. Subtotal colectomy for treatment of chronic constipation associated with idiopathic megacolon in cats: 38 cases (1979–1985). J Am Vet Med Assoc 193:850–853, 1988.
52. Saunders DR, Sillery J, Rachmilewitz D. Effect of dioctyl sodium sulfosuccinate on structure and function of rodent and human intestine. Gastroenterology 69:380–386, 1975.
53. Washabau RJ, Zhukovskaya N. Effect of smooth muscle pro-kinetic agents on feline colonic smooth muscle function (abstract). J Vet Int Med 8:149, 1994.
54. Horney FD, Archibald J. Colon, rectum and anus. In: Archibald J (ed) Canine Surgery, 2nd ed. American Veterinary Publications, Santa Barbara, 602–628, 1974.
55. Swenson O. The pull-through operation for congenital megacolon. Rev Surg 24:229–232, 1967.
56. Yoder JJ, Dragsted LR, Starch CJ. Partial colectomy for correction of megacolon in a cat. Vet Med/Sm Anim Clin 63:1049–1052, 1968.
57. Webb SM. Surgical management of acquired megacolon in the cat. J Sm Anim Pract 26:399–405, 1985.
58. Bright RM, Burrows CF, Goring R, et al. Subtotal colectomy for treatment of acquired megacolon in the dog and cat. J Am Vet Med Assoc 188:1412–1416, 1986.
59. Holt D. Idiopathic megacolon in cats. Comp Contin Ed Pract Vet 13:1411–1417, 1991.
60. Gregory CR, Guilford WG, Berry CR, et al. Enteric function in cats after subtotal colectomy for treatment of megacolon. Vet Surg 19:216–220, 1990.
61. Peck DA, Hallenbeck GA. Fecal continence in the dog after replacement of rectal mucosa with ileal mucosa. Surg Gynecol Obstet 119:1312–1320, 1964.
62. Lasser RB, Levitt MD, Bond JH. Studies of intestinal gas after ingestion of a standard meal. Gastroenterology 70:906, 1976.
63. Levitt MD. Intestinal gas. Postgrad Med 57:77–80, 1975.

29 Liver: Normal Structure and Function

SHARON A. CENTER AND DONALD R. STROMBECK

LIVER: NORMAL STRUCTURE

The liver is the largest solid organ in the body and is strategically positioned between the digestive tract and the systemic circulation. Its highly vascular structure receives venous blood draining from the abdominal viscera and arterial blood circulated from the aorta. It has central importance in intermediary metabolism. It provides important synthetic, detoxification, biotransformation, storage, and host defense activities and also intercedes in other homeostatic mechanisms such as regulation of fluid and electrolyte balance, temperature, and circulation.

LIVER: GROSS STRUCTURE

Anatomic Relationships

The liver comprises approximately 3.4% of body weight in the adult and a greater percentage in the young animal.[1-4] Its convex surface is beneath and attached to the diaphragm. Its concave visceral surface is in contact with the stomach, duodenum, pancreas, and right kidney, each of these organs producing surface impressions in adjacent liver lobes. The normal liver is positioned cranial to the last rib. On deep cranial abdominal palpation, a sharp liver margin may be felt in some healthy dogs and in most cats. The division of the liver into lobes allows it to adapt to changes in position as the lobes slide over one another.

The liver consists of four major lobes that are distinct at the periphery of the liver but which merge near the hilus. These include right, left, quadrate, and caudate lobes (Figure 29–1). The left lobe is the largest, comprising 30% to 50% of the hepatic mass; this lobe is also the most mobile and usually has an irregular margin. The right and left lobes can be divided into lateral and medial regions. The quadrate lobe is situated between the right and left medial lobes; the gallbladder is positioned in a fossa between the right medial and the quadrate lobes. The caudate lobe, divided into a papillary process and a caudate process, lies almost entirely on the visceral surface of the liver. The papillary process lies in the gastric impression of the left lobe and the caudate process comprises the most caudal portion of the liver. The caudate process is commonly palpated when a liver becomes diffusely enlarged. The duodenal impression crosses the caudate process and the renal fossa lies in its most caudal aspect. The relationship of the liver to other abdominal organs is shown in Figure 29–2.

The peritoneum almost completely covers the liver and

contributes to six ligaments that anchor the organ to the body wall and adjacent visceral structures: (1) coronary, (2) right triangular, (3) left triangular, (4) falciform, (5) hepatorenal, and (6) hepatogastric and hepatoduodenal. A strong attachment exists between the caudal vena cava as it courses through the liver. The coronary ligament attaches the liver to the diaphragm at the foramen venae cavae. The triangular ligaments attach the central portions of the right and left lobes to the diaphragm. The falciform ligament may be incomplete in its union with the liver but typically houses the cushion of fat that provides radiographic contrast against which the caudal-ventral margins of the liver may be identified. The hepatorenal ligament courses from the cranial pole of the right kidney to the renal fossa of the caudate process. The hepatogastric and hepatoduodenal ligaments are associated with the lesser omentum; these ensheath the bile duct, hepatic artery, portal vein, lymphatics, and nerves entering the porta hepatis, that area where vessels enter and ducts leave the liver. The nerves and arteries enter the porta dorsally, the biliary duct leaves ventrally, and the portal vein enters in between.

Vasculature: Blood Vessels and Lymphatics

The liver has a unique circulatory system in that it has a dual blood supply derived from the hepatic artery and the portal vein. In health and at rest, approximately 25% to 33% of car-

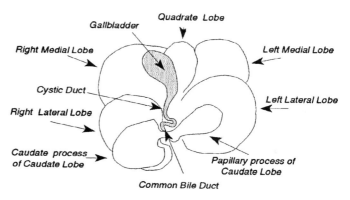

FIGURE 29-1. Gross appearance of the liver structure from a ventral visceral aspect. Adapted from reference 1.

540

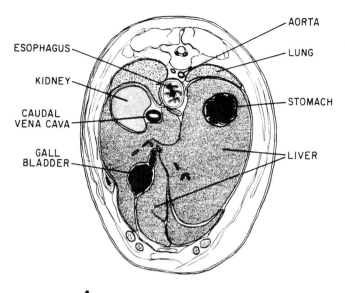

A

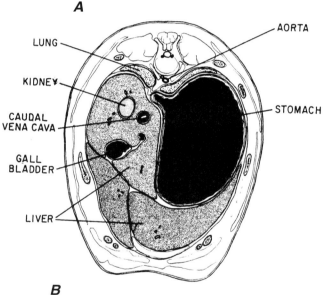

B

FIGURE 29–2. Drawings of transverse sections of dog showing relationship of liver to adjacent structures. Drawing *(A)* is at the level of the thoracic vertebrae 12, and *(B)* at the level of thoracic vertebrae 13.

diac output perfuses the liver.[4] Total flow to the liver averages 30 to 45 mL/minute/kg and can be estimated using ultrasonography.[5] More than 40% of the hepatic blood is contained in the capacitance vessels (hepatic arteries, portal veins, hepatic veins) with the remainder in the hepatic sinusoids. Approximately 15% of hepatic volume is comprised of vascular or sinusoidal spaces. These can be rapidly expanded or contracted as the need arises, accommodating up to 20% of rapidly infused fluid volumes and compensating for 25% of a lost blood volume. The ability of the liver to serve as a blood reservoir can markedly affect hepatic size.[6] Animals with chronic passive congestion can develop remarkable hepatomegaly attributable to blood storage of up to 60 mL blood per 100 g of liver.[7]

The hepatic artery and portal vein enter the liver at the porta hepatis. The hepatic artery is a branch from the celiac trunk which eventually arborizes into three proper hepatic

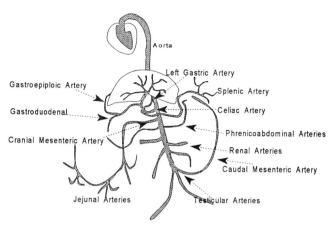

FIGURE 29–3. Diagrammatic representation of abdominal arteries derived from the aorta, including the hepatic artery, a branch of the celiac artery.

arteries before continuing as the gastroduodenal artery (Figures 29–3 and 29–4). The hepatic arteries supply well-oxygenated blood to the liver, the source of between 25% to 30% of the total afferent blood flow and approximately 50% of the oxygen used by the liver. Evidence suggests that a large component of the blood derived from the hepatic artery is delivered to a peribiliary plexus, a microcirculatory bed surrounding bile ducts as they pass through the portal canals. This arrangement results in the passage of arterial blood into this plexus before reaching the sinusoidal circulation.[4] This blood mingles with blood in the portal vein at the level of the portal triad.

The portal vein carries blood derived from the visceral alimentary capillary beds including those from the stomach, pancreas, spleen, and intestines (Figures 29–5 and 29–6). This blood is rich in nutrients as well as noxious substances from the alimentary canal, but is comparatively poor in oxygen. The portal vein provides approximately 70% to 75% of the total afferent blood flow.[4,8] Portal blood is delivered directly to the sinusoids and provides a rich source of nutrients, metabolic substrates, and trophic influences. In health, the portal venous circulation is a low-pressure system; the capacitance of this system is great. Because the portal vein does not contain valves, obstructive flow

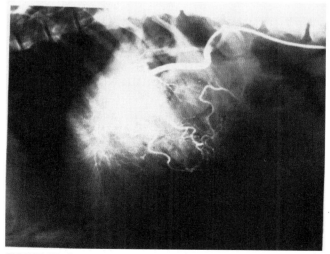

FIGURE 29–4. Arteriogram of hepatic artery in a normal dog. Number of branches is variable, two in this case. (By permission, Sibylle Schmidt)

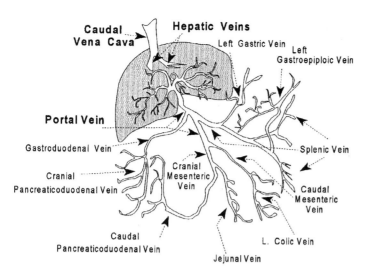

FIGURE 29–5. Diagrammatic representation of the portal vein tributaries and its distribution in the liver.

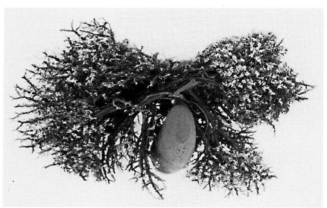

FIGURE 29-7. Corrosion cast of hepatic circulatory and biliary systems after injection of the portal, arterial, and biliary system with different color plastex. The smaller vessels have been removed from parts of the periphery to show distribution of larger vessels. The gallbladder appears in the center of the model.

or hypertension developing in one segment will be reflected in the entire circulatory bed proximal to the abnormality. Throughout the liver, arborization of the portal vessels accompanies that of the hepatic arteries and distribution of the biliary tree (Figure 29–7).[9] The lumen of portal vessels greatly exceed those of accompanying branches of the hepatic artery. The portal vein enters the liver from the root of the mesentery as it traverses along the short ventral boundary of the epiploic foramen. Here the portal vein is susceptible to occlusion or twisting as a result of abnormalities of adjacent viscera, as occurs for example in gastric dilatation-volvulus.[10] The portal vein dispatches seven major tributaries that perfuse the liver.[1,11] Their anatomic pattern is remarkably consistent (see Figure 29–5).

The hepatic venules drain blood collected from the hepatic arterioles and portal venules that has percolated through the sinusoidal beds (see Figure 29–8). Hepatic venules arborize into vessels with increasing diameters until they become hepatic veins that join the inferior vena cava. None of the branches of the hepatic vein has any substantial

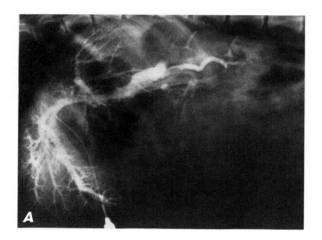

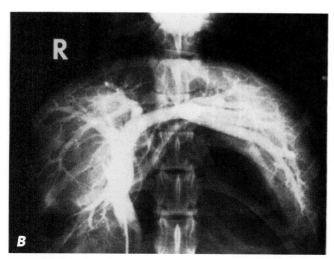

FIGURE 29–6. Venograms of portal vein of a normal dog shown in lateral *(A)* and ventrodorsal *(B)* views. (By permission, Sibylle Schmidt)

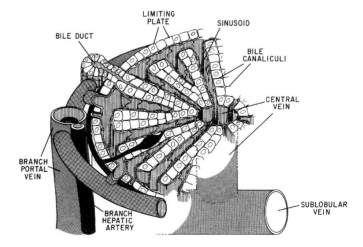

FIGURE 29-8. Drawing of hepatic lobule showing circulation entering the liver by the branches of the portal vein and hepatic artery. After circulation through hepatic capillaries (sinusoids), blood leaves the lobule by central sublobular veins.

extrahepatic variation; these vessels are short and broad and enter the vena cava as it courses through the dorsal portion of the liver. Obstruction of flow in the hepatic veins from any cause (cardiac failure, pericardial tamponade, vena caval stricture) leads to intrahepatic passive venous congestion, hepatomegaly, and often the development of ascites.[12]

The hepatic lymphatics carry ultrafiltrate transported from the space of Disse. Lymphatic vessels are not present between parenchymal cells. The perisinusoidal space, the space of Disse, is the major site of hepatic lymph formation. Lymph flows from the perisinusoidal space to the periportal space delimited by portal connective tissue and the limiting plate of hepatocytes.[13] From this site, lymph is collected into lymphatic capillaries within the portal canal. It is estimated that 80% of the hepatic lymph is transported through lymphatic vessels which progressively enlarge as they approach the liver hilus. The deep lymphatic vessels accompany small branches of the portal vein, hepatic artery, and bile ducts throughout the parenchyma. An intimate association between bile ducts and lymphatics permits biliary constituents to enter lymph vessels in some circumstances. Lymphatic vessels repeatedly divide and anastomose and form a network around the portal triad. The connective tissue encircling the central (hepatic) vein also contains lymphatics of varying sizes. Superficial lymphatic channels have also been identified on the surface of the liver and these may sometimes appear distended when passive congestion is severe. Ultimately, lymphatic drainage from the liver is delivered to hepatic lymph nodes (located adjacent to the portal vein near the liver hilus), to the splenic nodes (adjacent to the splenic artery), and to the gastric nodes (located in the lesser omentum near the pylorus).[1] However, it is not widely believed that lymph nodes are necessarily involved in lymphatic drainage. In humans, hepatic lymph flows into larger lymph channels and then into the cisternae chylii and thoracic duct. The remainder leaves the liver either through small networks of lymphatics around the hepatic veins and inferior vena cava or through the diaphragm to enter the retrosternal lymphatics that ascend to the neck.[4] It is probable that similar flow occurs in animals.

Innervation

Nerves enter the liver at the hilus and are derived from the autonomic nervous system. Generally, these are unmyelinated fibers and are occasionally discovered during histopathologic examination of larger portal tracts, gallbladder, and liver capsule. Afferent and efferent parasympathetic innervation of the liver and biliary system is derived via branches that leave the vagal trunk at the level of the gastroesophageal cardia and celiac plexus. Sympathetic innervation is derived from the splanchnic nerves, celiac ganglia, and celiac plexus. These follow the hepatic arteries within the liver and the smooth muscle of the gallbladder. The biliary system may also receive afferent fibers from the phrenic nerves.[14] The sphincter of Oddi in the duodenal papilla receives rich cholinergic innervation.[15,16]

Hepatic Capsule and Reticulin Framework

The liver is almost completely encapsulated by flat peritoneal mesothelium. This serous layer is fused to an underlying fibrous connective tissue capsule that adheres to the surfaces of the liver and extends interlobular trabeculae into the parenchyma. The fibrous capsule is more substantial at the

porta hepatis where it ensheaths vessels, biliary structures, and nerves as they distribute within the hepatic tissue. This connective tissue layer provides an internal supporting framework for the hepatic parenchyma, surrounds most of the vessels and nerves, and subdivides the parenchyma into lobules. A fine reticular framework interdigitates between the sinusoidal endothelium and the hepatic parenchymal cells (Figure 29–9). These fibers presumably support the parenchyma and assist in keeping sinusoids open. The reticular framework provides a scaffold on which a rapid and organized hepatic regeneration occurs following injury. If it is destroyed, regenerative nodules and sinusoidal disorganization ensue.

STRUCTURE OF THE BILIARY TREE AND GALLBLADDER

The biliary system is comprised of gallbladder, cystic duct, common bile duct, hepatic ducts, segmental, septal, and interlobular bile ducts, bile ductules, and hepatic canaliculi, as illustrated in Figure 29–10. Bile ductules are a synonym for cholangioles, the smallest branches of the biliary system lined by bile duct epithelium and having a basement membrane. These lack an individual capillary supply and conduct bile received from canaliculi. They terminate at the (interlobular) bile ducts. The interlobular bile ducts are the smallest branches of the intrahepatic biliary tree, accompanied by branches of the hepatic artery and portal vein. These are lined by cuboidal epithelium. Septal bile ducts are the small

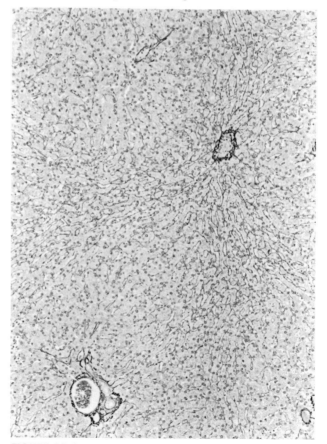

FIGURE 29–9. Photomicrograph of recticulin fibers in the hepatic parenchyma of a healthy dog. (Reticulin stain: 87× magnification)

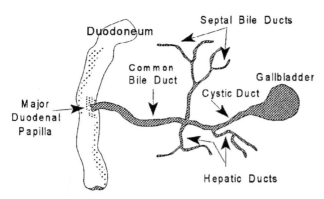

FIGURE 29-10. Diagrammatic representation of the normal anatomic divisions of the biliary tree.

branches of the intrahepatic biliary system that begin with the union of two or more interlobular bile ducts. These eventually fuse into segmental bile ducts, the medium sized branches of the intrahepatic biliary system located at the main drainage areas of the liver lobes. These are distinguished on the basis of their anatomic location as they carry bile to the hepatic bile ducts. In the dog, hepatic ducts enter the cystic duct and common bile duct separately. The cystic duct extends from the neck of the gallbladder to its junction with the first hepatic duct. Distal to this, it continues to the duodenum still receiving hepatic ducts as it becomes the common bile duct.

Bile is initially formed in canaliculi, the smallest component of the biliary tree. These are formed from contiguous portions of adjacent hepatocyte membranes that have become specially adapted (Figure 29–11). These membranes have elongated fingerlike microvilli that extend into the canalicular lumen. Canaliculi remain separated from the hepatocyte and perihepatic space by junctional complexes of desmosomes (macula adherens) and tight junctions (zonula occludens).[17] The desmosomes provide adhesion between the cell surfaces. The tight junction provides a high-resistance barrier to leakage of water and solutes into and from the bile canaliculus. This permits the bile canaliculus to contain fluid that is markedly different from that of the other pericellular fluids. Tight junctions become injured with certain toxins (CCl_4) and cholestasis.[18] When damaged, they permit a paracellular flow of micromolecular solutes, including enzymes, bile acids, and bilirubin. It is this pathway that is thought to be an origin of substances "regurgitated" into the plasma compartment. Gap junctions (macula communicans) are cellular organelles comprised of gated channels that are adjacent to but distinctly separate from canaliculi, and that permit communication between adjacent hepatocytes.[18] These consist of channels that bridge the membrane of adjacent cells to permit a low-resistance intercellular pathway. These channels permit the passage of ions and uncharged molecules with molecular weight below 1000 daltons including current-carrying ions, second messenger molecules, and tissue metabolites that function in intercellular signal exchange.

Bile formation begins near the hepatic veins (zone 3) and flows toward the portal triad (zone 1). The canaliculi keep bile compartmentalized and separated from blood by a barrier at least half a cell thick. This barrier is secure in health permitting little bile to regurgitate into the circulation. Bile canaliculi merge with larger ducts called cholangioles (canals of Hering), which are formed by four or five modified liver cells organized in a circular or acinar arrangement. These cells demonstrate ultrastructural features of both hepatocytes

and bile duct cells. Compared to hepatocytes, they possess fewer organelles and more intracellular fibrils. Cholangioles are supported by interstitial tissue between hepatic lobules; these deliver bile to lobar bile ducts in the portal triad. Bile ducts are lined with cuboidal or columnar epithelial cells with some mucin-secreting cells that stain positive with PAS. As ducts merge and enlarge, they sequentially become the hepatic, cystic, and common bile ducts. The large extrahepatic bile ducts are lined by columnar epithelium, their walls resembling those of the intestines: a mucosa, submucosa, muscularis, and adventitia are recognized.

The hepatic ducts are characterized as that segment of the biliary tract which emerges from the surface of the liver. These are highly variable both in number and in their pattern of fusion into the common bile duct. In dogs two to seven ducts have been reported, five branches being most common.[19–21] The segment of the extrahepatic bile duct from the neck of the gallbladder to the point where the first hepatic duct enters is called the cystic duct, and the remainder of the main duct transporting bile to the duodenum is the common bile duct. The cystic duct is short and straight in the dog and longer and more tortuous in the cat.[19,21]

Communication of the common bile duct with the duodenum is anatomically unique in the dog and cat. In a medium-sized dog, the common bile duct is approximately 5 cm long and 2.5 mm in diameter.[1] It empties into the duodenum 1.5 to 6.0 cm distal to the pylorus at the major duodenal papilla after coursing intramurally for 2 cm.[1] In the dog, the common bile duct opens near the pancreatic duct, the smaller of two pancreatic ducts. The larger duct is the accessory pancreatic duct; this opens into the duodenum a few centimeters caudal to the common bile duct on the minor duodenal papilla. In the cat, the common bile duct and the pancreatic duct are usually fused prior to entrance in the duodenal papilla, located 3 cm distal to the pylorus. In some cats, the major pancreatic duct opens separately but immediately adjacent to the common bile duct. Approximately 2 cm caudal to the major duodenal papilla, the accessory pancreatic duct enters the duodenum at the minor duodenal papilla. This duct is sometimes absent in the cat. Although the pancreas in dogs and cats is almost always drained by two ducts, a great deal of variation occurs. Pancreatic and biliary diseases (extrahepatic and intrahepatic) are commonly associated in the cat, seemingly as a result of the anatomic fusion of the pancreatic and common bile ducts. Despite the separation of these systems in the dog, acute and chronic pancreatitis also is commonly associated with extrahepatic biliary obstruction (partial or complete) as a result of regional inflammation and duodenitis. The intramural course of the common bile duct within the muscularis of the duodenum functions as a sphincter. The sphincter of Oddi is located at the papilla and is comprised of muscle fibers that are subject to great variation; their anatomic features are complex, inconsistent, and a topic of conflicting reports.[22,23] One muscle layer of the sphincter of Oddi is derived from the duodenal wall. Release of bile into the intestines is controlled by neurohumoral factors that stimulate gallbladder contraction and relaxation at the sphincter of Oddi.

The gallbladder is positioned in a fossa between the quadrate and right medial lobes of the liver on its visceral surface. It may not be readily apparent on gross inspection unless distended, because it normally lies deep within the liver. The most dependent portion of the gallbladder may juxtapose the diaphragm[28] (Figure 29–12). The gallbladder provides four distinct functions: reservoir, absorptive, secretory, and motor. It functions as a bile reservoir and is under neuroendocrine influence that coordinates its contraction with digestive interval. The gallbladder modifies bile through reabsorption of iso-

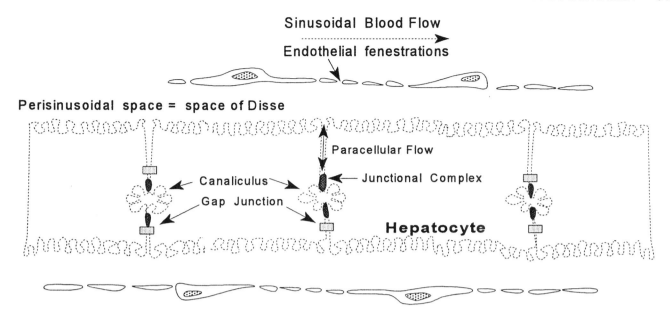

FIGURE 29-11. Diagrammatic representation of the normal canaliculus and adjacent functional domains of the hepatocellular membranes. Modified from reference 17.

tonic fluid (water absorption is coupled to active transport of sodium and chloride across the gallbladder mucosa) and secretion of glycoproteins and H^+ ions. In dogs, bile has a pH of less than 6.0. Acidification is accomplished as a result of H^+ secretion rather than HCO_3^- reabsorption.[24,25] More than 90% of the biliary solids are comprised of bile acids. In concentrated bile, total bile salt concentration may exceed 300 mM/L. Bile salts are kept in solution by incorporation into micelles that maintain an isosmotic balance with plasma. The gallbladder resorbs more than 50% of the calcium in bile. In health this is believed to maintain free calcium at a relatively low concentration and protects against cholelith precipitation. Lipid solubility is the major determinant of absorption of organic compounds in the gallbladder. Conjugation of bilirubin, steroid hormones, biliary contrast media, and bile acids increases their water solubility and is believed to inhibit their

reabsorption by the gallbladder epithelium.[26] Concentrated gallbladder bile thus contains large amounts of conjugated bile acids and bilirubin and lesser quantities of lipid soluble cholesterol. Increased absorption of conjugated bile acids and cholecystographic contrast agents can occur in the presence of gallbladder inflammation or sepsis owing to deconjugation reactions. This results in greater cholesterol saturation of bile and hence greater bile lithogenicity. This also contributes to the inability to visualize the inflamed and infected gallbladder during cholecystography.

Regionally, the gallbladder can be divided into a fundus, body, and neck that is continuous with the cystic duct. Although the capacity of the gallbladder has been suggested to be about 1 cc per kg of body weight, a recent study showed that body weight is not significantly associated with gallbladder volume. In that study gallbladder volume was reliably determined by ultrasonography and application of a regression formula to the determined lumen diameter.[27] The wall of the gallbladder, from inside to outside, consists of (1) epithelial cells on a lamina propria, (2) a smooth muscle muscular layer, (3) a perimuscular layer of connective tissue, and (4) a peritoneal covering. The internal surface of the gallbladder is lined by columnar epithelial cells containing microvilli on their luminal surface (Figure 29-13). The muscular layer consists of poorly defined groups of longitudinal, transverse, and oblique fibers.

The circulation to the gallbladder and common bile ducts is derived from the left branch of the proper hepatic artery.[1] This circulation must be preserved when decompressive biliary surgery is performed.

A double gallbladder has been described as a congenital malformation in clinically healthy cats.[28]

THE HEPATIC PARENCHYMA

Microscopic Structure

The liver is comprised of hepatocytes, bile ducts, blood vessels, sinusoidal cells (Kupffer cells, endothelial cells), perisinusoidal cells (fat-storing, or Ito cells), and pit cells. Hepato-

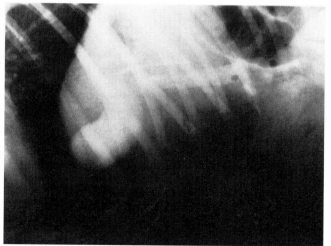

FIGURE 29-12. Lateral radiograph of a healthy dog 60 minutes after administration of iodipamide. The normal position of the gallbladder is demonstrated adjacent to the diaphragm and deep within the liver.

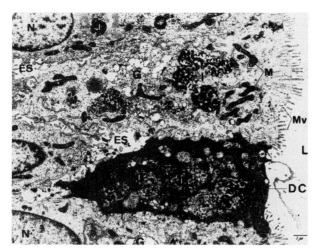

FIGURE 29-13. Ultrastructural anatomy of an epithelial cell from the gallbladder. L = lumen of gallbladder, MV = microvillus, M = mitochondrion, I = Inclusion, G = Golgi apparatus, ES = extracellular space, N = nucleus, DC = degenerating cell.

cytes represent about 60% of cells in the liver and approximately 80% of the parenchymal volume.

Structural and Functional Concept of Liver Lobulation and Its Circulation

The classic structural concept of liver lobulation is defined as single cords of hepatocytes radiating around a central (hepatic) vein and delimited by portal triads (Figure 29-14). This interpretation of microscopic anatomy lent simplicity for the purpose of structural identification. It is not, however, representative of functional anatomy. The functional concept of liver lobulation is described using the hepatic acini. The simple liver acinus is a three-dimensional mass of liver cells in which all hepatocytes are perfused by the same vascular axis: a terminal portal venule and a terminal hepatic arteriole.[29,30] This vascular axis is the core of the acinar unit and is associated with bile ductules, lymphatics, and nerves to comprise the *portal triads*. The central (hepatic) veins lie at the periphery of this functional unit. The acinus as the functional unit

of the liver provides a foundation on which a better pathophysiologic understanding of hepatobiliary disease is accomplished.

Merging of the high-pressure hepatic arterial and low-pressure circulations occurs within the sinusoidal microcirculation. Perfusion of hepatocytes is unidirectional and therefore sequential. Consequently, hepatocytes within different circulatory "zones" are perfused with blood that contains varied concentrations of oxygen, nutrients, hormones, and noxious materials (Figure 29-15). Hepatocytes immediately surrounding the vascular axis receive blood with the highest concentration of incoming solutes and oxygen: this is zone 1. Periacinar hepatocytes surrounding central (hepatic) venules are perfused with blood that has already been processed by preceding hepatocytes: this is zone 3. Between these two zones, there is a mass of hepatocytes denoted as zone 2.[4,29-31]

Portal triads appear as diamond-shaped islands of vessels and bile ducts accompanied by fibrous supporting tissue. Branches of vessels from triads radiate to meet branches from other local triads, creating a three-dimensional interconnecting circulatory system. Portal triads are associated with more connective tissue than other portions of the hepatic lobule; this difference underlines the slight hyperechoic ultrasonographic image of the triad areas. Branches of the hepatic artery enter the acinus via the portal triads and terminate in arterioles to sinusoids. Sphincters at the end of arterioles influence the rate of blood flow and sinusoidal pressure. Arterioles terminate at all levels of the acinus, near the central (hepatic) vein as well as near the portal triads. Most arterial blood, however, is supplied by short vessels that terminate close to the central vascular axis of the acinus.[8,31,32]

Sinusoidal blood flow is subject to many levels of regulation.[8,31,32] Consequently, a red blood cell entering the portal vein is not committed to flow the shortest route to the central (hepatic) vein. An inherent contractibility of sinusoids enables them to promote uniform perfusion to all hepatocytes. Distribution of blood is also influenced by sphincters in distributing branches of the portal veins and in portal venules. Sphincters at the level of the central (hepatic) veins also influence the rate of blood flow through a particular area. There also are sphincters that adjust blood flow where central (hepatic) veins merge to form sublobular veins. A subendothelial mast cell population and an adventitial lymphatic plexus are associated with the sublobular hepatic veins in dogs.[33] Collectively, a variety of mechanisms continuously adjust sinusoidal circulation,

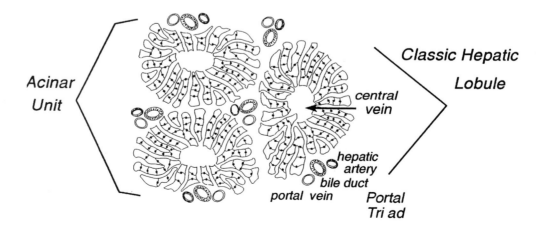

FIGURE 29-14. Diagrammatic representation of the acinar/lobular units of the liver. The classical anatomic description is that of the lobular unit with the hepatic vein coinciding with the terminology as the "central vein." The modern functional concept is of the acinar unit because it better describes the functional relationships between hepatic perfusion, bile flow, and patterns of tissue injury.

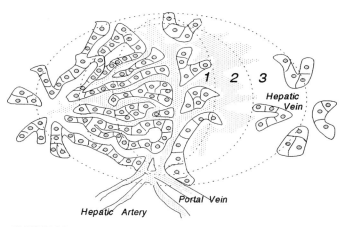

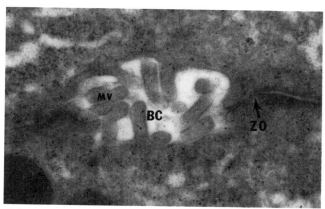

FIGURE 29-16. Ultrastructural photomicrograph of canine liver showing a bile canaliculus (BC), MV = microvilli, ZO = zonula occludens (tight junction).

FIGURE 29-15. Diagrammatic representation of the zonal distribution of blood flow in the liver. Modified from Gumucio JJ, Chianale J. Liver cell heterogeneity and liver function. In: Arias IM, Jakoby WB, Popper H, et al. (eds) *The Liver: Biology and Pathobiology,* 2nd ed. Raven Press, New York, 1988, 931–948.

although most evidence supports a major dependency on the local accumulation of adenosine realized by the hepatic arterioles. At any one time each sinusoid has differential flow.[34] This phenomenon helps explain why multifocal pathologic lesions develop in some hepatobiliary disorders. This seems reasonable, particularly if the insult depends on delivery of noxious or infectious material during a short interval.

Autoregulation of hepatic blood inflow is important in relation to health and disease. Autoregulation denotes the tendency for local blood flow to be maintained in the circumstance of reduced inflow from its afferent source. The arterial side of hepatic perfusion has major autoregulatory abilities; the portal circuit does not. Autoregulation in the arterial bed occurs mainly though nervous stimulation, hormones, metabolites, and bile salts. A reciprocal compensatory response between arterial and portal flow has been shown in most species, although the precise mechanisms remain ill defined.

Hepatocytes

Hepatocytes are large, metabolically active, and occasionally binucleate polyhedral cells with eight or more sides. Their cell membranes possess receptors for many hormones, plasma proteins, and glycoproteins. A unique surface membrane antigen, liver-specific membrane lipoprotein, has been associated with autoimmune injury in chronic liver diseases in humans.[35] Each hepatocyte has three major structural surfaces: (1) a basolateral surface endowed with numerous microvilli, (2) a straight or continuous segment, and (3) a bile canalicular surface[36-38] (Figure 29–11). The basolateral surface abuts the sinusoids and is designed for exchange of fluid and substances with plasma ultrafiltrate in the space of Disse. The microvilli greatly magnify this surface area that comprises 70% of the hepatocyte cell membrane. The straight domain forms the boundary between adjacent hepatocytes. These membranes form a relatively impermeable barrier to the movement of fluid and ions between adjacent cells. However, this also is the site of the gap junction that provides gated channels for communication between cells. This intercellular communication system permits adjacent hepatocytes to respond to stimuli as a "mass" of cells rather than as independent entities. The bile canalicular surface comprises approximately 15% of the hepatocyte surface area. In health, canaliculi contain numerous microvilli (Figure

29–16). On either side of a bile canaliculus, appositional surfaces of hepatocytes are joined by tight junctions, previously described. This area permits the canaliculus to maintain an isolated lumenal system separated from the space of Disse and hepatocellular cytosol. On the cytoplasmic side of the canalicular wall, a zone of condensed cytoplasm provides reinforcement. Actin filaments are located in this area and extend into the microvilli. These are believed to impart contractile ability and play a role in intracellular transport, bile flow, and tone of the canalicular wall.

Hepatocytes are arranged in one-cell-thick radiating cords or plates; these are perfused with plasma ultrafiltrate on two sides (Figures 29–8, 29–17). This anatomic arrangement optimizes cell perfusion, the ability of hepatocytes to remove substances derived from the intestinal tract, and the exchange of substances with the vascular compartment. The vascular channels on each side of the hepatic cords are called *sinusoids*. These are valveless conduits and interconnect in a three-dimensional honeycomb pattern.

Each hepatocyte is in direct contact with adjacent parenchymal cells, the biliary space, and the space of Disse. The cytoskeleton of the hepatocyte provides its structural sup-

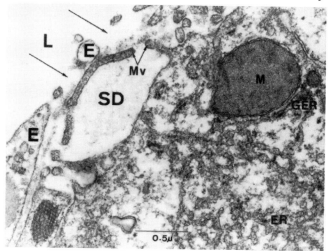

FIGURE 29-17. Electron photomicrograph of canine liver showing relationship of hepatocyte, space of Disse, and sinusoid. ×26,930. L = lumen of sinusoid, E = part of endothelial cell, SD = space of Disse, Mv = microvilli of hepatocyte, M = mitochondria, GER = granular (rough) endoplasmic reticulum, ER = agranular (smooth) endoplasmic reticulum. Arrows from sinusoidal lumen = pores in endothelial lining.

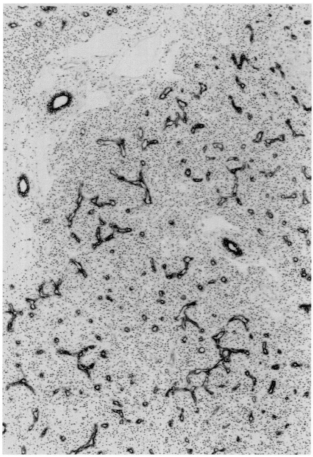

FIGURE 29-18. Photomicrograph of the liver of a healthy cat that has been stained with an immunoperoxidase stain specific for biliary cytokeratins. This stain specifically marks the location of biliary epithelial cells. (Courtesy Dr. P. Rowland, Department of Pathology, College of Veterinary Medicine, Cornell University)

port. This is composed of microfilaments, intermediate filaments, and microtubules comprised of actin, tubulin, and protein subunits assembled into helical fibers.[39] The intermediate filaments are considered to be "mechanical integrators of cellular space" and are classified as cytokeratins.[39] Cytokeratins are constituents of adhesion plaques between adjacent cells. Specific cytokeratins are found in differentiated epithelia and can be used for immunohistochemical characterization. A photomicrograph showing immunohistochemically stained biliary cytokeratin is shown in Figure 29–18. Microfilaments are involved with the contractile system of hepatocytes and, as previously discussed, are associated with bile transport into canaliculi.

Hepatocytes are richly endowed with organelles and membrane systems (Figure 29–19) that comprise about one-half of the cell volume.[36,37,40] The membranous system divides the cytoplasm into two compartments: cytoplasmic and intracisternal. Specialized metabolic functions are carried out in organelles defined by membranous boundaries. Hepatocytes contain a plethora of endoplasmic reticulum (ER). The relative proportion of the rough and smooth endoplasmic reticulum varies according to the species and the metabolic demands of the individual. In healthy dogs, the rough ER represents approximately 40% of the total.[40] Rough ER is usually arranged in flattened cisternae around the nucleus and mitochondria and at the margin of the sinusoidal border adjacent

to smooth ER. Protein synthesis occurs in the rough ER. The smooth ER is involved with synthesis of triglycerides from free fatty acids; synthesis and metabolism of cholesterol and bile acids; metabolism of glycogen; and metabolism and detoxification drugs, steroids, and bilirubin. It is the smooth ER that undergoes hypertrophy after exposure to phenobarbital. This can cause diffuse organ enlargement. The Golgi apparatus is a specialized area of the smooth ER that assumes the appearance of a group of flat saccules, vacuoles, and small vesicles. The Golgi apparatus is commonly located adjacent to canaliculi and often associated with lysosomes. This is the site for assembly and packaging of substances destined for export from the cell and the source of residual bodies in the cell (lysosomal storage granules). Many substances are prepared for further use by the Golgi apparatus; notable examples include lipoproteins and glycoproteins destined for export or incorporation into intracellular components. Mitochondria are abundant in hepatocytes where they have been estimated to comprise 24% of the cytoplasmic volume in dogs.[40] Hepatocytes in zone 3 generally contain more mitochondria than hepatocytes in zone 1. Mitochondria demonstrate morphologic heterogeneity owing to their ability and tendency to constantly alter their shape. Megamitochondria (giant mitochondria) have been described in association with many different hepatobiliary disorders in human beings and animal models of disease. Mitochondria are bounded by a double membrane, the inner membrane convoluted into folds defined as cristae. A multitude of biochemical reactions occur on mitochondrial membranes and within the organelle matrix. Examples include the tricarboxylic acid cycle; fatty acid elongation, activation, and oxidation; steroid metabolism; respiration (oxidative phosphorylation); nucleic acid and protein synthesis; urea cycle ammonia detoxification; and heme biosynthesis.[36,41] Lysosomes are heterogenous spherical organelles that develop into secondary lysosomes or residual bodies. These are limited by a single membrane and contain a variety of inclusions. Secondary lysosomes are a storage form, either temporary or committed, of degradation products of normal cell metabolism and auto- or heterophagocytosis. In hepatocytes, most residual bodies are located around the bile canaliculi and include autophagic vacuoles, multivesicular bodies, ferritin (iron) and lipofucin-containing granules, and excessive stores of copper. Peroxisomes (microbodies) are present in all tissues, but are most plentiful in the liver. These are limited by a single membrane and are ordinarily arranged in clusters in close proximity to areas rich in smooth ER and glycogen. Hepatic peroxisomes may be derived from dilations of smooth ER or be self-replicating; this remains controversial. Peroxisomes of dogs and cats contain a crystalline inclusion or core believed to be comprised of urate oxidase, and many have a marginal plate (Figure 29–20). Peroxisomes are involved in respiration, oxidation of very long chain fatty acids, purine catabolism, alcohol metabolism, gluconeogenesis, and bile acid synthesis and conjugation.[42] Peroxisomal respiration is responsible for 20% of the oxygen consumed by the liver; this respiration differs from mitochondrial respiration in that derived energy dissipates as heat rather than in ATP production. Hydrogen peroxide is produced from molecular oxygen, and is decomposed by peroxisomal catalase; this enzyme can be used as a marker for histochemical staining of the organelle (Figure 29–21).

Hepatocytes store substances with metabolic value, such as glycogen, triglycerides, and lipid soluble vitamins. They also store substances with little to no value or that are noxious. Examples include lipofuscin, copper, and iron. Excessive glycogen and triglyceride is initially suspected on routine light microscopy on hematoxylin and eosin (H and E) stained specimens; each creates the impression of a lacy or

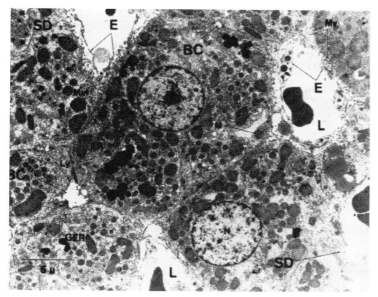

FIGURE 29-19. Electron micrograph of normal canine liver. N = nucleus of hepatocyte, BC = bile canaliculus, L = lumen of sinusoid, E = part of endothelial cell, SD = space of Disse, Mv = microvilli of hepatocyte membrane, M = mitochondrion, Ly = lysome, Lf = lipofuscin, GER = granular endoplasmic reticulum, ER = agranular endoplasmic reticulum.

vacuolated cytoplasm. Glycogen is periodic acid–Schiff (PAS) positive and diastase resistant. Triglycerides stain with oil red O or Sudan stains. The best staining for glycogen and triglyceride is done on tissue that has not been routinely processed, tissue sectioned without embedment in paraffin. Lipofuscin is a normal wear and tear pigment, comprised of peroxidated lipid. It assumes a golden granular slightly refractile appearance on routine light microscopy and accumulates in lysosomes, forming residual bodies. A similar appearing substance is ceroid pigment. Copper assumes a pale red-orange hue and appears as fine granules on routine H and E staining. Iron-containing granules appear as dark brown-blue granules with routine staining and are somewhat refractile. Specific staining with copper stains (Rubeanic acid, Rhodanine, Timms) or iron stain (Perls' Prussian Blue) confirms the constituency of these inclusions.

Considerable evidence indicates that hepatocytes in the portal triad area differ both structurally and functionally from cells in the central (hepatic) vein area.[43] Ultrastructurally, hepatocyte heterogeneity is reflected in a differing balance of organelle proportions. Hepatocyte heterogeneity

is believed to reflect functional requirements dependent on variations in oxgyen availability, hepatocyte maturity, and concentration gradients. These variables are associated with blood flow patterns that are believed to impart important heterogenous influences. Zonal localization of major parenchymal cell functions are summarized in Table 29–1.[43,44] The surface to volume ratio of sinusoids in zone 1 is greater than that of zone 3; this suggests a greater access to circulating components in zone 1. These hepatocytes tend to accumulate solutes taken up by simple diffusion. The presence of specific binding proteins/surface receptors on hepatocellular sur-

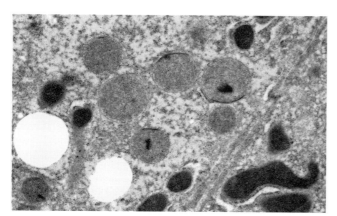

FIGURE 29-20. Electron micrograph of a normal feline hepatocyte showing peroxisomes as they appear without special staining. Notice the dense nucleoid present in the center of the organelle and the marginal plate (thin black line at margin of organelle).

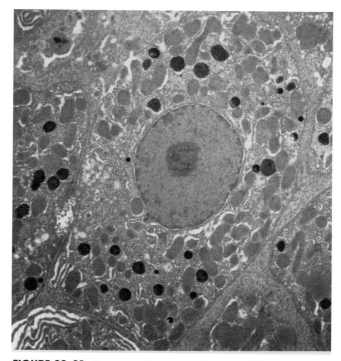

FIGURE 29-21. Electron micrograph of a normal feline hepatocyte showing peroxisomes histochemically stained with diaminobenzidine. Peroxisomes appear as dark oval organelles, mitochondria as light gray organelles.

Table 29-1

ZONAL LOCALIZATION OF MAJOR METABOLIC FUNCTIONS[4]

PERIPORTAL	CENTRILOBULAR

Solute Uptake Influenced By:
Concentration of incoming solute
Protein binding
Specificity of receptor uptake mechanisms
Zonal concentration of intracellular binding proteins for that solute

Solutes Taken Up By Simple Diffusion
Initial high uptake Zone 1 > Zone 2

PERIPORTAL	CENTRILOBULAR
↑ **Glucose Release** Glycogenolysis Gluconeogenesis	↑ **Glucose Uptake** Glycogen synthesis Glycolysis
Oxidative Energy Metabolism Oxidation of fatty acids Citric acid cycle Respiratory chain	**Liponeogenesis** **Biotransformation** Phase 1 and 2 activity ↑ concentration cytochrome p450 ↑ sulfation and glucuronidation reactions (varies with circulatory saturation) steroid hormone, bil acid 3α-hydroxylation
Oxidative Protection Increased glutathione availability	
Amino Acid Utilization/Ammonia **Detoxification** Amino acid degradation/gluconeogenesis Urea cycle: Amino acid nitrogen	**Ammonia Detoxification** Glutamine synthesis
Organic Anion Uptake Nonprotein-bound moieties	**Organic Anion Uptake** Protein-bound moieties
Bile Acid Uptake and Excretion Depends upon uptake mechanisms: variability among bile acid moieties	**Bile Acid Uptake and Excretion** Increases with higher concentrations
Canalicular Bile Excretion of bile salt dependent fraction of canalicular bile	**Canalicular Bile** Excretion of bile salt independent fraction of canalicular bile
Bilirubin Excretion	
Cytogenesis	

---

faces influences the zonal uptake of substances. The unique metabolic activities of hepatocytes in certain zones makes them preferentially susceptible to some toxins and infectious agents. Nevertheless, it is important to remember that the specific functional designations of a particular hepatocyte remain flexible. They can divert their activities and accommodate novel metabolic activities when hepatocellular reserves are impaired by injury or disease. This ability underlies the tremendous regenerative capability and functional reserve in the liver and allows recovery following substantial injury or 70% hepatectomy.

Sinusoidal Lining Cells: Kupffer Cells, Endothelial Cells, Ito Cells, Pit Cells

The sinusoidal wall consists of endothelial cells, Kupffer cells, fat-storing cells or lipocytes (Ito cells), and pit cells. Kupffer cells, pit cells, and endothelial cells are in direct contact with blood in the sinusoidal lumen; lipocytes, located in the space of Disse (perisinusoidal space), are in contact only with a plasma ultrafiltrate (Figure 29—22). Collectively, the cells of the sinusoid and perisinusoidal space function as a cooperative system with hepatic parenchymal cells; this allows for initiation and integration of many important biologic processes and organ response to disease or injury.

The sinusoidal capillaries differ from typical capillaries in that they are large and more variable in size and their walls are lined by two distinct cell types: endothelial cells and Kupffer cells. Hepatic endothelial cells are unique compared to others in the body. These cells are devoid of an underlying basement membrane and have well-developed endocytic capabilities. Sinusoidal endothelial cells have pores or fenestrae in slender cytoplasmic processes that cluster in small patches called sieve plates. These fenestrae may change in size depending on a variety of factors; this dynamic nature permits compensatory adaptations in certain pathologic conditions. A major function of a sinusoidal endothelial cell is to maintain a selective or semipermeable barrier between blood and the liver parenchyma. In health, the fenestrae exclude passage of particles larger than 10 nm; for example, newly formed chylomicra cannot enter the space of Disse until circulatory preprocessing has reduced their size.[8] Sinusoidal endothelial cells are able to engulf a large variety of exogenous and endogenous particles and molecules, including but

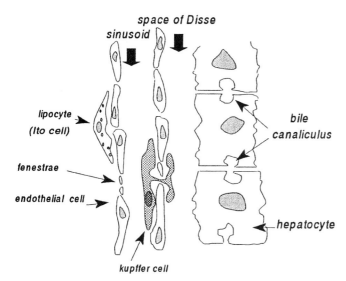

FIGURE 29-22. Diagram showing the anatomic localization of Kupffer cells, lipocytes (Ito cells), and endothelial cells in the hepatic sinusoids. Notice the marked fenestration of the endothelial cells. This characteristic is lost in chronic fibrosing liver disease, creating a poorly permeable barrier resulting in the intrahepatic shunting of blood by the hepatocytes. The Kupffer cell is extending into the space of Disse and the Ito cell shows lipid vacuoles filled with vitamin A stores.

not limited to inert particles, denatured albumin, glycoproteins, and some lipoproteins. In addition, these cells may also be capable of antigen processing and presentation, and function as effector cells in hepatic fibrosis.

Fat-storing cells are also known as Ito cells, perisinusoidal cells, lipocytes, or stellate cells. Their most prominent feature is cytoplasmic lipid droplets or vacuoles. The Ito cell is the major physiologic site of vitamin A storage in the mammalian body. The presence of lipid droplets in these cells is entirely for the purpose of vitamin A storage. Ito cells contain high concentrations of binding proteins for retinol and retinoic acid and enzymes reactive with vitamin A. It is currently believed that the Ito cells play an important role in the production of collagen in the normal and fibrotic liver; they are capable of forming types I, II, and IV collagen. They are also believed to be the cell from which the (myo)fibroblastic cells originate.[45–49]

The hepatic macrophages or Kupffer cells are star shaped or stellate in gross appearance. These are believed to be derived from circulating monocytes, although they also can self-replicate. Kupffer cells comprise 80% to 90% of the fixed macrophages of the reticuloendothelial system in the body,[37] and about 10% of all cells in the liver.[48,49] Kupffer cells are anchored to endothelial cells by long cytoplasmic processes. Occasionally, they extend thin cytoplasmic processes through the fenestrae of sinusoidal endothelium reaching into the perisinusoidal space (Figure 29–22). The largest proportion of Kupffer cells are distributed around the periportal areas in zone 1, purportedly for the purpose of policing blood entering the sinusoids for foreign and noxious material. In conjunction with other sinusoidal cells, Kupffer cells play a critical role in maintaining normal liver function. They clear and degrade effete endogenous or exogenous particulate matter by pinocytosis or phagocytosis, detoxify endotoxin, influence hepatic microcirculation, process antigens, mediate a variety of immune reactions, and are involved in the uptake and

catabolism of lipids and glycoproteins including many enzymes.[50] Examples of materials engulfed by Kupffer cells include virus particles; test substances such as latex particles, Thorotrast, colloidal gold, and denatured or aggregated albumin; enzymes leaked from cells or the gastrointestinal tract; fibrin derivatives and complexes; altered platelets; damaged or senescent erythoctyes; aggregated immunoglobulin and immune complexes; complement; tumor cells; bacteria and their toxins; ferritin and hemosiderin; lysosomal hydrolases; mitochondrial enzymes, membranes, and subcellular organelles released from dying cells; thrombin; heparin; carcinoembryonic antigen; collagen chains; and a variety of hormones including growth hormone, parathyroid hormone, insulin, and glucagon.[48–50] The phagocytic capacity of Kupffer cells is influenced by their functional status, humoral factors, and hepatic blood flow. Portal venous rather than arterial flow appears to facilitate phagocytosis presumably because slow flow allows more time for phagocytic removal; the velocity of sinusoidal flow and phagocytosis by Kupffer cells is reciprocally related.[51] Phagocytosis by Kupffer cells can be invoked by nonimmunospecific opsonin-mediated mechanisms best characterized by fibronectin coating; immunospecific opsonin-mediated phagocytosis involving Fc receptor binding to antigen or particles bound by IgG, IgM, or C3; and by mechanisms that do not require opsonization.[44,48] The limiting factor in Fc and C3 receptor-mediated phagocytosis is the volume of Kupffer cells rather than the number of cell surface receptors. Kupffer cells also synthesize factors that can stimulate or block hepatocellular protein synthesis; they are known to stimulate acute-phase protein synthesis through liberation of interleukin-1. They also are known to secrete erythropoietin and colony-stimulating factor that regulates granulocyte growth and to participate in lipoprotein metabolism. They also participate as a site of albumin degradation, and are believed to be important in immune surveillance for the elimination of mutated or neoplastic cells.

Endotoxin or bacterial lipopolysaccharide (LPS) is derived from the enteric flora and is a normal constituent of portal venous plasma.[49,50] In health, LPS is efficiently and selectively pinocytosed by Kupffer cells. In human patients with seriously compromised liver function, particularly those with portosystemic shunting, systemic concentrations of endotoxin increase. This has not been documented in clinical disease in dogs or cats.[51] The ability of Kupffer cells to phagocytose bacteria is crucial in control of many infections. They also provide important defense against parasitic infections.[47]

In addition to the other functional capabilities of Kupffer cells just described, they are now believed to play a pivotal role in the generation of fibrous connective tissue in response to hepatic injury and to participate in the perpetuation of hepatic inflammation. Kupffer cells produce soluble factors (including transforming growth factor β) that promote fibroblast and Ito cell proliferation, an effect associated with the development of hepatic fibrosis.[46] Activated Kupffer cells consume an increased quantity of oxygen and glucose and release oxygen-derived free radicals in response to particulate or soluble stimuli. Although release of oxygen-derived free radicals and lysosomal enzymes is advantageous for microbicidal effect, growing evidence indicates that this contributes to hepatocyte damage in endotoxin-mediated acute liver injury and other forms of disease.[52]

Pit cells have been described in the sinusoids of some species. These cells are in contact with both the hepatocytes and the lumenal portion of the sinusoids. These cells are believed to represent large granular lymphocytes and function as natural killer cells that have tumoricidal capabilities. Pit cells located in the hepatic sinusoids are thus considered important components of host defense given their strategic location.

REFERENCES

1. Evans HE. Miller's Anatomy of the Dog, 3rd ed. WB Saunders, Philadelphia, 1993.
2. Nickel R, Schummer A, Seiferele E, et al. The viscera of the domestic animals. Springer-Verlag, New York, 1973.
3. Popesko P. Atlas of topographical anatomy of the domestic animals. WB Saunders, Philadelphia, 1977.
4. Jones AL. Anatomy of the normal liver. In: Zakim D, Boyer TD (eds) Hepatology: A Textbook of Liver Disease. WB Saunders, Philadelphia, 3–29, 1990.
5. Kantrowitz BM, Nyland TG, Fisher P. Estimation of portal blood flow using duplex realtime and pulsed doppler ultrasound imaging in the dog. Vet Radiol 30:222–226, 1989.
6. Greenway CV, Lister GE. Capacitance effects and blood reservoir function in the splanchnic vascular bed during non-hypotensive haemorrhage and blood volume expansion in anesthetized cats. J Physiol 237:279–294, 1974.
7. Hanson KM. Liver. In: Johnson PC (ed) Peripheral Circulation. John Wiley, New York, 285–314, 1978.
8. Campra JL, Reynolds RB. The hepatic circulation. In Arias IM, Jakoby WB, Popper H, et al. (eds) The Liver: Biology and Pathobiology. Raven Press, New York, 911–932, 1988.
9. Ohtani O. Corrosion casts in liver and stomach microcirculation. In: Cells and Tissues: A Three-Dimensional Approach by Modern Techniques in Microscopy. Proceedings of the VIIIth International Symposium on Morphological Science, Rome, Italy. New York, Alan R. Liss, 317–326, 1989.
10. Wingfield WE, Betts CW, Rawlings CA. Pathophysiology associated with gastric dilation-volvulus in the dog. J Am Anim Hosp Assoc 12:136–142, 1976.
11. Sleight DR, Thomford NR. Gross anatomy of the blood supply and biliary drainage of the canine liver. Anat Rec 166:153–160, 1970.
12. Kershner D, Hooton TC, Shearer EM. Production of experimental portal hypertension in the dog: anatomy of the hepatic veins in the dog. Arch Surg 53:425–434, 1946.
13. Mall FP. A study of the structural unit of the liver. Am J Anat 5:227–232, 1906.
14. Alexander WF. The innervation of the biliary system. J Comp Neurol 72:357–370, 1940.
15. Chiu SL. The superficial hepatic branches of the vagi and their distribution to the extrahepatic biliary tract in certain mammals. Anat Rec 86:149–155, 1943.
16. Kyosola AK, Rechardt L. The anatomy and innervation of the sphincter of Oddi in the dog and cat. Am J Anat 140:497–512, 1974.
17. Introduction: Organizational principles. In: Arias IM, Jakoby WB, Popper H, et al. (eds) The Liver: Biology and Pathobiology, 2nd ed. Raven Press, New York, 3–6, 1988.
18. Spray DC, Saez JC, Hertzberg EL. Gap junctions between hepatocytes: Structural and regulatory features. In: Arias IM, Jakoby WB, Popper H, et al. (eds) The Liver: Biology and Pathobiology, 2nd ed. Raven Press, New York, 851–866, 1988.
19. Bragulla H, Vollmerhaus B. Korrosions anatomischer Beitrag zum Gallengangsystem in der Katzenleber. Berl Munch Tieraztl Wochenschr 100:78–82, 1987.
20. Florentin P, et al. Topographie des voies biliaires du chien. Bull l'Assoc Anatomists 48th Reunion, Toulouse, 605–608, 1962.
21. Bourdelle E, Bressou C. Anatomie régionale des animaux domestiques. 4. Carnivores: Chien et chat. J-B Baillière, Paris, 1953.
22. Casas AP. Contribution à l'étude du sphincter d'Oddi chex Canis familiaris. Acta Anat 34:130–153, 1958.
23. Eichhorn EP, Boyden EA. The choledochoduodenal junction in the dog—a restudy of Oddi's sphincter. Am J Anat 97:431–451, 1955.
24. Hueman DM, Moore EW, Vlahcevic ZR. Pathogenesis and dissolution of gallstones. In: Zakim D, Boyer TD (eds) Hepatology: A Textbook of Liver Disease. WB Saunders, Philadelphia, 1480–1516, 1990.
25. Rege RV, Moore EW. Evidence for H$^+$ secretion by the canine gallbladder. Gastroenterology 92:281–289, 1987.
26. Scharschmidt BF. Bile formation and cholestasis. In: Zakim D, Boyer TD (eds) Hepatology: A Textbook of Liver Disease. WB Saunders, Philadelphia, 303–340, 1990.
27. Finn-Bodner ST, Park RD, Tyler JW, et al. Ultrasonographic determination, in vitro and in vivo, of canine gallbladder volume, using four volumetric formulas and stepwise-regression models. Am J Vet Res 54:832–835, 1993.
28. Carlisle CH. Radiographic anatomy of the cat gallbladder. J Am Vet Radiol Soc 18:170–176, 1977.
29. Rappaport AM. Anatomic considerations. In Schiff L, Schiff ER (eds) Diseases of the Liver. JB Lippincott, Philadelphia, 1–46, 1987.
30. Jones AL, Schmucker DL. Current concept of liver structure as related to function. Gastroenterology 73:833–851, 1977.
31. Rappaport AM. The acinus-microvascular unit of the liver. In: Lautt WW (ed) Hepatic circulation in health and disease. Raven Press, New York, 1981, 175–192.
32. Withrington PG, Richardson PDI. Liver blood flow. In: Zakim D, Boyer TD (eds) Hepatology: A Textbook of Liver Disease. WB Saunders, Philadelphia, 30–48, 1990.
33. Takahashi-Iwanaga H, Fujita T, Takeda M. Canine hepatic vein branches associated with subendothelial mast cells and an adventitial lymphatic plexus. Arch Histol Cytol 53:189–197, 1990.
34. Lautt WW, Greenway CV. Conceptual review of the hepatic vascular bed. Hepatology 7:952–963, 1987.
35. Meyer Zum Buschenfelde KM, Manns M, et al. Immunological aspects of chronic hepatitis. J Gastroenterol and Hepatol 3:177–185, 1988.
36. Millward-Sadler GH, Jezequel AM. Normal histology and ultrastructure. In: Wright R, Millward-Sadler GH, Alberti KGMM, et al. (eds) Liver and Biliary Disease: Pathophysiology, Diagnosis, Management, 2nd ed. WB Saunders, Philadelphia, 13–44, 1985.
37. Orlandi F, Koch M. The fine structure of liver cells. In: Taylor W (ed) The Hepatobiliary System. Plenum Press, New York, 145–177, 1976.
38. Blouin A, Bolender RP, Weibel ER. Distribution of organelles and membranes between hepatocytes and non-hepatocytes in the rat liver parenchyma. J Cell Biol 72:441–455, 1977.
39. Lazarides E. Intermediate filaments as mechanical integrators of cellular space. Nature 283:249–256, 1980.
40. Hess FA, Weibel ER, Preisig R. Morphometry of dog liver. Normal baseline data. Virch Archiv Abteilung B 12:303–307, 1973.
41. Hinkle PC. Mitochondria. In: Arias IM, Jakoby WB, Popper H, et al. (eds) The Liver: Biology and Pathobiology. Raven Press, New York, 269–278, 1988.
42. Goldfisher S, Reddy JK. Peroxisomes (microbodies) in cell pathology. Int Rev Exp Pathol 26:45–84, 1984.
43. Gumucia JJ, Chianale J. Liver cell heterogeneity and liver function. In: Arias IM, Jakoby WB, Popper H, et al. (eds) The Liver: Biology and Pathobiology. Raven Press, New York, 931–947, 1988.
44. Jones EA, Summerfield JA. Functional aspects of hepatic sinusoidal cells. Sem Liver Dis 5:157–174, 1985.
45. Mak KM, Leo MA, Liever CS. Alcoholic liver injury in baboons: Transformation of lipocytes to transitional cells. Gastroenterology 87:188–200, 1984.
46. Matsuoka M, Tsukamoto H. Stimulation of hepatic lipocyte collagen production by Kupffer cell-derived transforming growth factor β: Implication for a pathogenetic role in alcoholic liver fibrogenesis. Hepatology 11:599–605, 1990.
47. Gressner AM, Bachem MG. Cellular sources of noncollagenous matrix proteins: Role of fat storing cells in fibrogenesis. Sem Liver Dis 10:30–46, 1990.
48. Jones EA, Summerfield JA. Kupffer cells. In: Arias IM, Jakoby WB, Popper H, et al. (eds) The Liver: Biology and Pathobiology. Raven Press, New York, 683–705, 1988.
49. Biozzi G, Stiffel C. The physiopathology of the reticuloendothelial cells of the liver and spleen. Prog Liver Dis 2:166–191, 1965.
50. Nolan JP. Endotoxin, reticuloendothelial function and liver injury. Hepatology 1:458–465, 1981.
51. Peterson SL, Koblik PD, Whiting PG, et al. Endotoxin concentrations measured by a chromogenic assay in portal and peripheral venous blood in ten dogs with portosystemic shunts. J Vet Intern Med 5:71–74, 1991.
52. Saba RM. Physiology and pathophysiology of the reticuloendothelial system. Arch Intern Med 126:1031–1052, 1970.

30

Pathophysiology of Liver Disease: Normal and Abnormal Function

SHARON A. CENTER

INTRODUCTION

The liver occupies a central role in many different biologic processes essential to life. It provides regulatory, synthetic, storage, detoxification, hematopoietic, and excretory functions that are necessary for normal homeostasis. Many of these functions are not duplicated elsewhere in the body. Consequently, disorders of the hepatobiliary system can have diverse effects on a variety of different physiologic functions and organ systems. Table 30–1 summarizes the major functions of the hepatobiliary system. This chapter discusses the basic physiology of the hepatobiliary system and the pathophysiologic mechanisms of disease and their consequences.

THE ROLE OF THE LIVER IN ENERGY PRODUCTION

The normal liver provides energy substrates for itself and other organs. It occupies a central position in interchange of energy substrates between tissues and is critical for integrating the metabolic adaptations during the transition from the fed to the fasted condition. The adequacy of liver function is not critical in the fed state because absorbed substrates are directly circulated to other tissues. However, it becomes critical in the fasted state because hepatic production of glucose provides energy for erythrocytes and the central nervous system (CNS). In the event of a prolonged fast (> 48 hours), normal liver also produces ketone bodies for oxidation. This spares by approximately 50% the normal glucose requirements for energy production in the brain. The liver is the primary source of fatty acids used for energy in the chronic fasted condition. An overview of the metabolic distribution and regulation of energy substrates and the central role of the liver in permitting these metabolic adaptations is provided in Figure 30–1.[1]

CARBOHYDRATE METABOLISM

The liver has central importance in carbohydrate metabolism due to its role in maintaining euglycemia. Complete hepatectomy results in hypoglycemic shock and death within a few hours unless continuous infusions of glucose are pro-

vided. Hepatic carbohydrate metabolism includes the storage and release of glucose from glycogen, gluconeogenesis, and the metabolic conversion of nonglucose hexoses to glucose.

In the fed state, glucose absorbed from the gut is circulated to all tissues where it is either oxidized, producing energy, or is stored. In the fed condition, glucose taken into a healthy liver is converted to glycogen to a maximum storage capacity of 65 g glycogen per kg liver tissue.[1] This equates to approximately 1 g of carbohydrate per kilogram of total body weight. When hepatic stores of glycogen are saturated, excess glucose can be utilized in several different ways including fatty acid synthesis.

Glucose uptake by the liver occurs via facilitated, non-insulin-dependent diffusion. Uptake is rapid so that glucose concentrations in hepatocytes remain equivalent to the glucose concentration in the hepatic sinusoids.[2] Less than 50% of ingested glucose is removed by the normal liver; the remainder is distributed to extrahepatic tissues.[3,4]

Glucose is stored as glycogen after entering hepatocytes. Glycogen synthesis is highest after a meal when portal venous glucose and insulin concentrations are increased. Low blood glucose stimulates glucose-6-phosphatase activity, which initiates glycogenolysis, a process stimulated during hypoglycemia by catecholamines, glucagon, glucocorticoids, and growth hormone. Starvation for only 24 hours depletes hepatic glycogen stores. It is during this adaptive interval that liver function is essential for provision of CNS energy. Because the brain's daily requirement of glucose exceeds the amount of glucose stored in the liver as glycogen, gluconeogenesis is necessary to prevent neuroglycopenia. After a 12 hour fast, glucose produced from lactate, pyruvate, and glycerol exceeds that derived from hepatic glycogenolysis. Gluconeogenesis from amino acids is the most important source of glucose when carbohydrate intake is minimal and glycogen stores are depleted. Alanine, glutamine, and serine are the principal amino acids used for gluconeogenesis.

The enzymes of glycogen synthesis, glycolysis, and gluconeogenesis are not distributed uniformly in the liver lobule.[5,6] Cells in the perivenous zone are more active in glycogenolysis. Periportal hepatocytes are more active in gluconeogenesis and glycogen synthesis. Although distribution of glycogen appears uniform throughout the hepatic acinus in the well-fed condition, glycogen in periportal areas is used more rapidly and replenished sooner than glycogen in perivenous cells.

Table 30-1

SUMMARY OF MAJOR HEPATOBILIARY FUNCTIONS

Carbohydrate Metabolism
  Glucose homeostasis
    gluconeogenesis
    glycogenolysis
  Insulin metabolism
  Glucagon metabolism

Glycogen	metabolism and storage
Insulin	degradation
Glucagon	degradation
Growth hormone	regulation

Lipid Metabolism

Cholesterol	synthesis, esterification, excretion
Bile acid	synthesis and regulation
Ketogenesis	
Fatty acid	oxidation and mobilization
Triglyceride	metabolism and storage
Lipoprotein	synthesis and release
Phospholipid	metabolism

Protein Metabolism

Albumin	synthesis
	turnover

  Globulins
    acute-phase proteins
    transport proteins
    certain immunoglobulins (bile)

Apoproteins	synthesis (some)

  Coagulation proteins

procoagulants	synthesis
activators	procoagulants and inhibitors
inhibitors	procoagulants and inhibitors
Amino acid	regulation
Ammonia	synthesis and detoxification
Urea	synthesis

Vitamin Metabolism

Water soluble	activation, synthesis, storage (B_1, B_6 (pyridoxine), B_{12} (cyanocobalamin), folic acid, nicotinic acid, and riboflavin)
Fat soluble	activation, synthesis, storage (vitamins E, D, A, and K)

Immunologic Functions

Kupffer cell	population, function
	phagocytic protection
	gut bacteria, toxins, particulate debris

  Complement metabolism, interleukin production
  Immunomodulation (metabolic products)
  IgA production for biliary excretion

Endocrine Hormone Metabolism

Polypeptide hormones	target organ influence
	degradation
Steroid hormones	conjugation
	degradation/excretion

Storage Functions

Water soluble vitamins	Fat soluble vitamins
Triglycerides	Glycogen
Copper, iron, zinc	Blood

Hematologic Functions

In utero	hematopoiesis
Extramedullary hematopoiesis	severe anemia
Coagulation system	factor synthesis, activation
	inhibitor synthesis, activation
	overall homeostasis
Reticuloendothelial	senescent RBC breakdown
Transferrin synthesis	
Bilirubin	uptake, conjugation, excretion, enterohepatic circulation
Hematopoietic factor storage/activation	B_{12}, folate, iron
Iron homeostasis	

Digestive Functions

Bile acids	synthesis, regulation, enterohepatic circulation
Bile	component synthesis-excretion, digestive release
Gallbladder	bile storage, bile digestive interval release

Detoxication and Excretory Functions

Bilirubin	conjugation, uptake, biliary excretion
Ammonia	urea cycle
Steroid hormones	cortisol, androgens, estrogens, aldosterone

Xenobiotics examples	barbiturates	propoxyphene
	chloramphenicol	pentozocine
	clindamycin	diazepan
	metronidazole	meperidine
	propranolol	lidocaine
	theophylline	aminophylline
Copper	biliary excretion, lysosomal storage	
Cholesterol	biliary excretion	

The liver has great metabolic reserve for maintaining euglycemia. It has been estimated that less than 30% of normal functioning hepatic mass is necessary to maintain a normal blood glucose concentration because a 70% hepatectomy does not produce hypoglycemia. When hepatic insufficiency causes hypoglycemia, pathogenic mechanisms may include any of the following: (1) inadequate gluconeogenic enzymic activity for converting amino acids to glucose, (2) reduced hepatic mass for sufficient gluconeogenesis, (3) insufficient storage of glycogen to sustain euglycemia during interdigestive intervals, and (4) abnormal response to glucagon. Patients with severe hepatic insufficiency may develop increased insulin concentrations during pathologic hypoglycemia suggestive of a functional insulin-secreting neoplasm. Generally, the insulin to glucose ratio in these patients is lower than that associated with a pancreatic tumor. Hypoglycemia is rare in cats with severe liver disease. This is related to their greater propensity for hyperglycemia

as a result of glucocorticoid or catecholamine stimulation. With severe diffuse hepatic necrosis, such as occurs with toxic or infectious disorders (e.g., infectious canine hepatitis virus infection), hypoglycemia may develop along with its attendant clinical signs of lethargy, weakness, ataxia, seizures and coma. Hypoglycemia may occur before other signs of hepatic failure. Similarly, following complete hepatectomy, maintenance of blood glucose concentration is one of the earliest hepatic functions to be lost. Portosystemic vascular anomalies in dogs are often associated with mild hypoglycemia. Only small breeds of dogs seem to display obvious clinical signs relating to this hypoglycemia. Any animal with a portosystemic vascular anomaly is at increased risk of hypoglycemia during a prolonged fast, general anesthesia, and surgery. Any animal with clinically significant liver disease should be frequently monitored for development of hypoglycemia during diagnostic or surgical interventions or a prolonged fast. Patients with small body stature, limited mus-

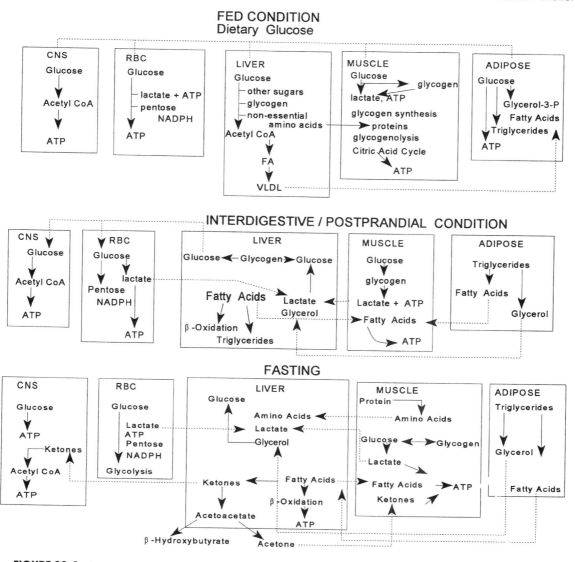

FIGURE 30-1. An overview of the metabolic distribution and regulation of energy substrates and the central role of the liver in providing metabolic adaptation.[1] (Adapted, with permission)

cle mass, and young patients with high brain metabolic needs relative to hepatic mass are at greatest risk. Hypoglycemia associated with hypoinsulinemia may develop in dogs with large hepatic tumors.[7] A variety of non-beta cell tumors have been associated with hypoglycemia in the dog.[8] The differential causes of fasting hypoglycemia are presented in Table 30–2.

Rare congenital enzyme deficiencies causing glycogen storage disease can also cause hypoglycemia. Abnormal glycogen retention can result from a deficiency of one of several different enzymes; the enzymes involved in hepatic glycogen and glucose metabolism are shown in Figure 30–2. A deficiency of glucose-6-phosphatase impairs the hydrolysis of glucose-6-phosphate to free glucose; a deficiency of amylo-1,6-glucosidase, the debrancher enzyme, reduces the liver's ability to convert glycogen to glucose-6-phosphate; a deficiency of lysosomal acid alpha-glucosidase also results in the accumulation of glycogen. These disorders cause hypoglycemia and hepatomegaly due to abnormal hepatic glycogen accumulation.[9] Enzyme deficiencies are initially suspected on the basis

of an animal's early age of presentation, persistent or recurrent hypoglycemia, and absence of other organ system abnormalities. Definitive diagnosis requires glucagon response testing, hepatic biopsy, and specific enzyme assays.

In some small animal patients, hyperglycemia rather than hypoglycemia is associated with hepatic insufficiency. This has been shown in dogs with experimentally created cirrhosis and chronic bile duct occlusion.[10] In human beings, 80% of cirrhotic patients demonstrate glucose intolerance, which is believed to reflect peripheral insulin resistance. The normal liver metabolizes about 50% of insulin secreted into the portal vein.[11] Defective metabolism of insulin by the cirrhotic liver results in the delivery of an abnormally large proportion of insulin to the peripheral circulation. Increased plasma concentrations of catecholamines, glucocorticoids, and glucagon appear to overcompensate for increased concentrations of insulin. The result is hyperglycemia during the fasting or interdigestive interval. Development of glucose intolerance and difficult to control diabetes mellitus has been documented in dogs with cirrhosis having peculiar cutaneous

Table 30-2

DIFFERENTIAL DIAGNOSES FOR FASTING HYPOGLYCEMIA

↑ **Glucose Utilization**
Polycythemia vera
Leukemia
Neoplasia (solid tumors)
  hepatic neoplasia
    hepatocellular carcinoma, hepatoma, heman-
    giosarcoma, leiomyosarcoma
  others
    hemangiosarcoma, oral melanoma, plasma
    cell tumors, salivary adenocarcinoma
Severe endoparasitism (neonate)
Protracted grand mal seizure activity
Exercise (severe in unconditioned animal)
Hunting dog hypoglycemia (?)
Endotoxemia
Sepsis

↑ **Insulin or Insulin-like Activity**
Beta-cell pancreatic neoplasia
  adenoma, adenocarcinoma
Iatrogenic insulin overdosage
Sulfonylurea administration
Reactive insulin receptor antibodies

↑ **Glucose Excretion**
Renal tubular glucosuria

Spurious Hypoglycemia
Laboratory error
In vitro glucose consumption
  Leukemia cell
  RBC

↓ **Gluconeogenesis** ↓ **Glycogenolysis**
Neonate (toy dog breeds especially)
Congenital portosystemic vascular anomaly
  (PSVA)
Hepatic cirrhosis
Massive hepatic necrosis
Starvation/cachexia (severe)
Maldigestion/malabsorption
Severe endoparasitism
Hypoadrenocorticism
Hypopituitarism
Pregnancy toxemia
Endotoxemia

Insufficient Glycogen Mobilization
Glycogen storage disorders (rare)
PSVA
Hepatic cirrhosis
Starvation/cachexia
Hunting dog hypoglycemia (?)
Sepsis

lesions denoted as hepatocutaneous disease or necrolytic migratory erythema.[12-14] This disorder is discussed comprehensively in Chapter 33.

Excessive hepatocellular storage of glycogen is a peculiar metabolic response in dogs with a variety of disorders. Dogs fed a protein deficient but calorically adequate diet develop glycogen-laden (15- to 25-fold greater than normal) swollen hepatocytes referred to by some pathologists as hydropic degeneration.[15] Puppies receiving excessive calories by parenteral nutrition develop glycogen-engorged hepatocytes.[16] Accumulated glycogen pushes organelles to the peripheral and perinuclear portions of the cell. Glycogen-laden cells have slightly reduced glucose-6-phosphatase activity that would correspond with a reduced rate of glycogenolysis. This lesion may develop in dogs treated with glucocorticoids and dogs that are chronically ill due to any cause that, presumably, are producing increased amounts of endogenous glucocorticoids. It is associated with increased liver enzyme activity, especially alkaline phosphatase, and when severe with moderately increased serum bile acid concentrations typical of intrahepatic cholestasis.

Lactate Metabolism

The metabolism of lactic acid in the liver can become compromised in severe liver disease leading to lactic acidosis. This, however, rarely occurs in clinical patients. In health, the liver utilizes lactate in glucose production during fasting. Otherwise, the liver normally metabolizes only very small amounts of lactate, even during vigorous exercise.[17] The only circumstances where compromised liver function leads to increased plasma lactate concentrations is in humans with cirrhosis following ethanol ingestion and in patients with glucose-6-phosphatase deficiency.[1]

LIPID METABOLISM

The liver plays a central role in many aspects of lipid metabolism. In liponeogenesis, the liver converts excess carbohydrates and proteins to fatty acids that may be esterified into triglycerides and exported as very low density lipoproteins (VLDLs). The liver also mediates the metabolic fate of lipids absorbed from the alimentary canal and released from adipose tissue, determining whether hepatic triglyceride storage, or synthesis and export of lipoproteins, or energy production by beta-oxidation, acetyl CoA oxidation, and ketone body production is appropriate for the current metabolic conditions. An overview of hepatic lipid metabolism is provided in Figure 30-3.

Lipoproteins

Three major lipid components exist in plasma: cholesterol, triglycerides, and phospholipids. The natural water insolubility of these compounds is modified by their incorporation in large macromolecular complexes, the lipoproteins. Lipoproteins are dynamic particles in a constant state of flux between synthesis, degradation, exchange of structural moieties, and removal from the circulation. Several classes of lipoproteins are recognized, characterized by laboratory procedures that detail particular physicochemical characteristics including hydrated density using ultracentrifugation, size using gel filtration, net surface charge using electrophoresis, or other surface properties using precipitation techniques[18,19] (Table 30-3[20,21]). Chylomicrons are very large particles that float. These can be separated from plasma by overnight refrigeration and routine centrifugation. These remain at the origin when electrophoresis is used to characterize plasma lipids. Other categories of lipoproteins include the very low density lipoproteins (VLDLs), low density

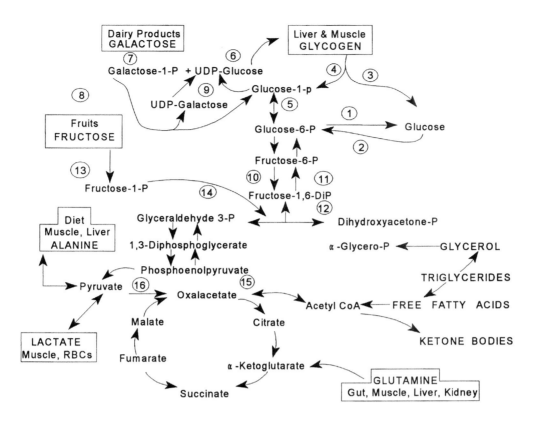

FIGURE 30-2. Enzymes and substrates involved in hepatic glucose and glycogen metabolism. Metabolic pathways involved in glycogen synthesis and degradation and gluconeogenesis. Enzymes designated by number are (1) glucose-6-phosphatase, (2) glucokinase, (3) amylo-1,6-glucosidase, (4) phosphorylase, (5) phosphoglucomutase, (6) glycogen synthetase, (7) galactokinase, (8) galactose-1-phosphate uridyl transferase, (9) uridine diphosphogalactose-4-epimerase, (10) phosphofructokinase, (11) fructose-1,6-diphosphatase, (12) fructose-1,6-diphosphate aldolase, (13) fructokinase, (14) fructose-1-phosphate aldolase, (15) phosphoenolpyruvate carboxykinase, (16) pyruvate carboxylase.

lipoproteins (LDL), and high density lipoproteins (HDL). Subclasses of these categories have been identified. Each class of lipoproteins contains particles that are heterogenous with respect to chemical composition and metabolism. The composition of a lipoprotein determines its physical properties. Generally, the greater the triglyceride content, the larger and more buoyant it becomes.[18]

Only the intestine and liver appear to synthesize and secrete plasma lipoproteins. Chylomicrons are initially produced in enterocytes during dietary fat absorption. Their precise size and composition depend on dietary constituents. Free fatty acids , derived from dietary fat, are taken into enterocytes where they are reesterified with monoglycerides, combined with small amounts of free and esterified cholesterol, phospholipids, and protein, to form chylomicrons. These particles are secreted into mesenteric lymphatics from which they reach the systemic circulation. Chylomicrons are enriched with apoprotein B_{48} before entering lymphatics and with apolipoprotein C_{II} and E within the circulation. Chylomicrons normally have a short residence in the circulation, usually less than 30 minutes.[18] They bind to endothelial cells in a variety of tissues where they are substrates for the enzyme lipoprotein lipase (LPL). LPL hydrolyzes most of the chylomicron triglyceride, freeing fatty acids for diffusion into

nearby cells. Within cells, fatty acids are either metabolized for energy or converted to triglycerides for storage. The residual component of the chylomicron particle is called a chylomicron remnant. This particle has a very short half-life because of rapid and selective hepatic clearance. These particles are taken into the liver through action of apoprotein E.

VLDL are produced in the liver and intestine. VLDL is the primary form of triglyceride transported from the liver. The metabolism of VLDL is quite similar to that of chylomicrons except after LPL binding, they generate an intermediate density lipoprotein (IDL). These IDL may be removed by the liver or undergo further lipolysis under the action of hepatic lipase (HL) to yield an LDL. Species differences in the fate of VLDL remnants have been shown and may explain particular susceptibilities to atherosclerosis. Their metabolism involves receptor-mediated cell internalization (primarily in the liver) of the lipoprotein moiety and subsequent degradation in lysosomes. Cholesterol esters are hydrolyzed to free cholesterol and the apoproteins degraded to small peptides and amino acids. Any abnormality in the pathway leads to hypercholesterolemia.

HDL are synthesized by the gut and liver and from redundant cholesterol and phospholipid released from the surface of chylomicrons and VLDL during triglyceride hydrolysis.

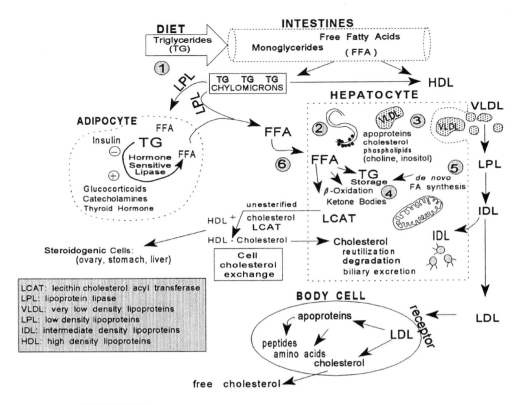

FIGURE 30-3. A simplified overview of hepatic and systemic lipid metabolism.

The metabolism of HDLs is not clear. The free cholesterol of HDL can exchange with plasma membranes and other lipoproteins and their associated apoproteins transfer between HDLs and VLDLs. Even their cholesterol esters can be exchanged with other lipoproteins. The half-life of an HDL particle is difficult to estimate because none of its constituents are fixed. The HDL provides a reservoir for cholesterol as it accepts unesterified cholesterol from peripheral cells. It transports this cholesterol to the liver for biliary excretion, degradation, or reutilization.

Thus, lipoprotein metabolism is complex. It centrally involves three enzymes: lipoprotein lipase (LPL), hepatic lipase (HL), and lecithin-cholesterol acyltransferase (LCAT). Transfer of constituent lipids and lipoproteins between the various lipoprotein classes, either by specific transfer proteins or by equilibration, is known to occur. The LPLs are synthesized in cells but the active form is extracellular, loosely bound to the surface of capillary endothelium. Injection of heparin can release LPL from its endothelial binding. This maneuver is sometimes used to clear chylomicronemic blood because LPL catalyzes the hydrolysis of triglyceride in chylomicrons and VLDL. Certain apoproteins are required as cofactors for optimal activity of LPL. As triglyceride lipolysis proceeds, the lipoprotein particles become smaller, more dense, and poorer substrates for LPL. These are lipoprotein remnants. HL is synthesized by hepatocytes and is a membrane-bound enzyme. It is also is released into plasma following heparin injection. After hepatocyte formation and excretion, HL binds to endothelium in the liver, adrenal gland, and ovary. Like LPL, HL hydrolyzes triglycerides in LDL and HDL$_2$ to free fatty acids and glycerol. LCAT is synthesized and secreted by the liver. This enzyme esterifies and sequesters cholesterol in HDL.[18,20,22] This reaction is responsible for interconversion among the HDL subclasses and is thought to retard athero-

sclerosis. Once cholesterol is esterified, it is transferred to other lipoprotein classes. This reaction may be important in atherogenesis associated with diabetes mellitus and uremia in human beings. Once the HDL has made a "new" space for cholesterol, it can pick up a new molecule of free cholesterol from the plasma membrane of any cell ready to unload it. This is believed to be the mechanism for "unloading" cholesterol from tissues and for transporting cholesterol to tissues that need it for structural or metabolic functions. Patients with liver disease can have varying degrees of LCAT and HL deficiency. Galactosamine, a toxin used to model liver failure in animals experimentally, causes LCAT deficiency.

Apoprotein

The protein components of lipoproteins are called apoproteins, which are classified into several groups alphabetically. A single lipoprotein class may contain several different apoproteins, and certain apoproteins occur in more than one lipoprotein class. Apoproteins provide three major functions: (1) binding core lipids into the soluble lipoprotein particle, (2) binding to cell surface receptors, facilitating lipoprotein cellular uptake, and (3) activating enzymes that modify or mobilize lipoprotein particles. The major functions of lipoproteins are summarized in Table 30-3.[20,21]

HEPATIC SYNTHESIS AND EXPORTATION OF VLDL. Apoprotein B$_{100}$ is synthesized on ribosomes and is joined to lipoprotein in the smooth endoplasmic reticulum adjacent to the enzymes responsible for lipogenesis. Once synthesized, VLDL are transferred to the Golgi apparatus, where carbohydrate is attached. Here they accumulate in secretory vesicles that migrate to and fuse with the lateral plasma membrane of the hepatocyte from which they discharge their contents into the

Table 30–3

CHARACTERISTICS OF LIPOPROTEINS IN THE DOG AND CAT
AND THE ASSOCIATED APOPROTEINS[20,21]

Particle	Species (d = dog) (c = cat)	Size Diameter (nm)	Electrophoretic band	Density	TG	Chol	Phospholipids	Protein	Apoproteins
					\% Composition				
Chylomicron	d, c	75–1200	Origin	< 0.960	90	3	5	2	A, B_{48}, C, E
VLDL	d, c	26–80	Pre-beta	0.930–1.006	62	12	14	12	B_{100}, C, E
LDL	d, c	16–25	beta	1.019–1.087 (d) 1.030–1.043 (c)	8	42	23	27	B_{100}
HDL_1	d	10–35	$alpha_2$	1.025–1.100	1	36	40	23	A, C, E
HDL_2	c	9–12	$alpha_1$	1.063–1.100	2	30	35	33	A, C, E
HDL_3	d, c	5–9	$alpha_1$	1.100–1.210	1	21	35	35	A, C

Adapted from reference 20, with permission.

Pertinent Apoproteins and Their Functions

A_1 Structural to HDL, activates LCAT.

B_{48} Structural to lipoproteins.

B_{100} Structural to VLDL and LDL, bind to LDL receptor.

C_{11} Activates LPL.

E Binds to remnant receptor, facilitates hepatic uptake of VLDL and HDL remnants.
Binds to LDL receptor

space of Disse.[28] Movement of the secretory vesicles is thought to involve microtubules. Protein synthesis is necessary for lipoprotein formation. Inhibitors of protein synthesis, such as tetracycline, orotic acid, cycloheximide, and puromycin, inhibit secretion of hepatic VLDL. Because these substances do not impair triglyceride synthesis, triglycerides accumulate in the liver causing hepatic lipidosis. Many other variables influence hepatic lipid metabolism, for example, estrogens that cause a marked increase in secretion of VLDL, a high carbohydrate diet that increases VLDL production, and insulin that inhibits VLDL secretion.

Cholesterol

Cholesterol is the precursor sterol nucleus for the synthesis of bile acids, steroid hormones, and vitamin D. It is present as a structural component in all mammalian cell membranes, and although all mammalian tissues are capable of cholesterol synthesis, up to 50% occurs in the liver.[19] Serum cholesterol concentrations are adjusted by feedback mechanisms according to the balance among ingestion, synthesis, degradation, and excretion. Alimentary sources of cholesterol are derived from the diet, enteric epithelial exfoliation, and bile. The rate of hepatic cholesterol synthesis depends on the functional condition of the liver, the animal species studied, and its metabolic condition. Cholesterol biosynthesis involves three distinct groups of reactions: (1) metabolic conversion of acetyl coenzyme A (CoA) to beta-hydroxy-beta-methylglutaryl (HMG) CoA; this reaction is catalyzed by HMG-CoA reductase, (2) conversion of mevalonate to squalene, a long chain hydrocarbon, and (3) conversion of squalene to cholesterol; these reactions are catalyzed by membrane-bound enzymes and are the targets for several drugs used to control hypercholesterolemia. Cholesterol exists in an esterified form and in a free form. Esterified cholesterol is much less soluble than the free form and is believed to provide an inactive stor-

age pool. In the normal dog, 60% to 80% of the circulating cholesterol is esterified.[18] Cholesterol esterification is catalyzed by acyl coenzyme A:cholesterol-acyltransferase (ACAT) and lecithin-cholesterol acyl transferase (LCAT), which act on cholesterol incorporated in lipoproteins.[18,19,22]

Cholesterol undergoes an enterohepatic circulation, excretion largely occurring via fecal elimination of biliary and dietary cholesterol, and metabolites of unabsorbed cholesterol. Minor losses are incurred through the shedding of cellular cholesterol from skin and intestinal epithelia. Synthesis of bile salts is the major catabolic pathway.

Intestinal absorption of cholesterol occurs by passive diffusion into enterocytes where it is esterified and packaged with triglycerides, apoproteins, and newly synthesized cholesterol into chylomicrons. In some patients that develop portal hypertension due to hepatic fibrosis, the enteric absorption of cholesterol, other lipids, and protein is impaired and a malabsorption syndrome develops.

Diet appears to be an important determinant of the serum total cholesterol content in normal dogs. Despite increases in serum cholesterol induced by dietary cholesterol, dogs do not develop atherosclerotic lesions unless they have some other metabolic derangement such as hypothyroidism.[24-26]

FATTY ACIDS

The fate of a fatty acid presented to the liver is determined by a number of factors. Metabolic designation can include (1) reesterification for formation of triglyceride for hepatic storage, (2) reesterification for formation of triglycerides used in synthesis of VLDL slated for export from the liver, or (3) utilization for energy production by beta-oxidation and production of ketone bodies. In the circumstance of chronic consumption of excessive calories, de novo hepatic synthesis of fatty acids may add to the hepatic lipid burden. In health, there are limits to the rate of fatty acid oxidation, but not esterification, and there is relatively limited triglyceride secretion as VLDL.[18,19]

During fasting, adipose fat is released as free fatty acids for energy production in liver, skeletal, and cardiac muscle. Hormone sensitive lipase (HSL) mediates this process. Adipose lipolysis is promoted by several hormones including catecholamines, glucocorticoids, growth hormone, glucagon, and thyroxine, and is inhibited by insulin and hyperglycemia. The release of fatty acids from adipose tissue in not well controlled and may exceed the quantity of fat that can be effectively used for energy production. Most circulating fatty acids are rapidly taken up by the liver and esterified to triglycerides, a process that maintains the circulating fatty acids within nontoxic concentrations. If hepatic uptake is increased, excessive stores of triglyceride may accumulate, particularly if VLDL dispersal is also compromised. In almost all metabolic circumstances, the uptake of fatty acids by the liver exceeds its capabilities for rapid fatty acid utilization in lipid oxidation and ketogenesis. Even during starvation, only 10% of the fatty acids taken up are rapidly used. The amount of ketones generated varies between 10% to 60% of the fatty acids taken up, depending on the metabolic circumstances and the animal's condition.

Utilization of fatty acids for energy involves metabolism to a two-carbon metabolite, acetyl coenzyme A (Acetyl CoA). This occurs in mitochondria and peroxisomes. Peroxisomes or microbodies are important for the preprocessing of fatty acids with carbon lengths exceeding C_{12}.[27] Once chain lengths are reduced by peroxisomal oxidation, fatty acids diffuse into mitochondria. Passage of fatty acids from peroxisomes and entry into mitochondria is facilitated by carnitine. The liver has a limited capacity for oxidizing fatty acids to carbon dioxide and water. It can, however, metabolize large amounts of fatty acid to acetyl CoA. Acetyl CoA serves as a substrate for either direct energy production or ketogenesis. Utilization for energy involves condensation with oxaloacetate to form citrate, a metabolite oxidized in the citric acid cycle. Oxaloacetate must be continuously replenished by glucose metabolism to sustain entry of acetyl CoA into the citric acid cycle. When oxaloacetate becomes deficient, as occurs in diabetes mellitus, excess Acetyl CoA condenses to form acetoacetate, a ketone body.

Hepatic esterification of fatty acids to triglycerides designated for hepatocellular storage occurs whenever there is a bottleneck in other utilization pathways. Esterification and storage increase when beta-oxidation or ketogenesis is blocked, when hepatic apoprotein synthesis is impaired, when VLDL exportation is disabled, or when excessive calories are continuously fed or administered via intravenous glucose administration. An interplay of lipogenic and lipotropic factors regulate hepatic deposition and mobilization of lipid and control fatty acid synthesis and degradation. The balance between anabolism and catabolism is upset when caloric delivery to the liver is inadequate, excessive, or imbalanced. Such derangements can develop by consumption of high-fat or protein deficient diets, overnutrition, starvation, and endocrine abnormalities. The ability of the liver to regulate fatty acid metabolism may also be impaired by exposure or ingestion of certain toxins.

Disorders of Hepatic Lipid Metabolism

Alterations in the composition of plasma lipids and lipoproteins occur in patients with liver disease. These abnormalities are associated with changes in lipoprotein and cholesterol synthesis, LCAT deficiency, defective lipolysis, abnor-

mal recognition and uptake of lipoproteins by the liver, and regurgitation of biliary lipids into plasma.

CHOLESTEROL. Many different factors have been shown to influence hepatic cholesterol synthesis. As previously discussed, experimentally, hypercholesterolemia can be induced in dogs by feeding high cholesterol, high saturated fat diets, along with induction of hypothyroidism.[24–26]

Obstructive jaundice may lead to hypercholesterolemia and hypertriglyceridemia.[28–36] The increased serum cholesterol concentration is attributed to increased hepatic cholesterol synthesis, presumably in response to reflux of lecithin from the obstructed biliary system or deranged feedback inhibition normally provided by chylomicron remnants. Lecithin is a potent stimulus for cholesterol synthesis. An additional factor is regurgitation of biliary phospholipid into the systemic circulation because this also contributes a component of cholesterol to the circulating pool.

Although cholesterol esterification is usually reduced in cholestasis, studies of obstructive jaundice in the dog have shown either no change in cholesterol esterification or a transient (2 to 6 days postobstruction) decrease followed by a gradual rise to normal.[35,37] The reduced concentration of esterified cholesterol is believed to be related, at least in part, to reduced LCAT function or activity possibly related to bile salt inhibition of LCAT or accumulation of lipoprotein X, which is a poor substrate for LCAT cholesterol esterification.[38–40]

Reduced cholesterol esterification also develops due to hepatic synthetic failure, such as that occurring with diffuse hepatic necrosis. This is attributed to a decline in LCAT activity. Although acute necrosis induced by CCl_4 in the dog has no effect on the total serum cholesterol concentration, within 5 to 6 days, a 35% reduction in cholesterol esters develops.[35] The net result is an increase in the unesterified or free cholesterol to esterified cholesterol ratio, similar to that which occurs in extrahepatic bile duct obstruction.

In normal dogs, the ratio of esterified to nonesterified cholesterol ranges from 0.64 to 0.88.[37] A retrospective study of dogs with histologically verified hepatic disease demonstrated that 90% had a reduced esterified to unesterified cholesterol ratio (< 0.52 in most dogs.) Approximately 20% of these dogs had ratios of 0.4. Dogs with acute hepatitis had the highest incidence of abnormal ratios. In most circumstances, the abnormal cholesterol ester ratio was associated with hyperbilirubinemia. The degree of alteration in the ratio was not significantly associated with the estimated severity of hepatic disease.

Hypocholesterolemia has received more attention than other lipid aberrations in patients with hepatic disease. Low serum total cholesterol concentrations have been recognized in animals with surgically created portosystemic shunts, congenital portosystemic vascular anomalies, and acquired hepatic insufficiency.[41–50] The mechanism of hypocholesterolemia in the patient with portosystemic shunting remains undetermined but is conjectured to involve decreased synthesis of cholesterol, triglyceride, or lipoproteins, or a shift in the localization of cholesterol away from the routinely measured pool. Acute hepatic failure can also be associated with hypocholesterolemia. This only occurs when loss of hepatic mass is severe or portosystemic shunting coexists.[51] Both esterified and nonesterified cholesterol fractions decline.

The hypocholesterolemia noted in animals with portosystemic vascular anomalies or acquired hepatic insufficiency is associated with markedly increased concentrations of serum bile acids. Bile salts may have a direct inhibitory effect on some of the key enzymes essential for cholesterol synthesis.[18]

Hypocholesterolemia may be a response to certain drugs. Examples in the dog include methyltestosterone when given at high doses and administration of high doses of primidone.[50,52,53]

TRIGLYCERIDE. Low serum triglyceride concentrations have been shown in dogs with experimentally created portosystemic shunts.[41,49] This has been verified in clinical patients. The mechanism involved is not understood. Experimentally induced hepatic necrosis in dogs with CCl_4 results in reduced serum triglyceride concentrations for at least 2 days.[51]

LIPOPROTEINS. A distinct lipoprotein has been shown to accumulate in the serum of human patients and dogs with cholestatic liver disease.[54–59] This moiety is called lipoprotein X and is an abnormal VLDL characterized by reduced cholesterol ester and triglyceride components. It is composed primarily of free cholesterol and phospholipid, contains little apoprotein C, and has albumin as its major protein.[18] It is believed to be formed in bile canaliculi from which it is transported through the hepatic cytosol to the space of Disse. Explanations for the occurrence of lipoprotein X include regurgitation of biliary lipids, substrate accumulation secondary to LCAT deficiency, or because it is a poor substrate for LCAT. The latter consideration is most widely accepted. In retrospective study of human patients, more than 90% of those with major bile duct occlusion have detectable lipoprotein X. It has thus been shown to be a sensitive indicator of this disorder. Unfortunately, measurement of lipoprotein X does not differentiate intrahepatic from extrahepatic cholestatic disorders. Lipoprotein X has been measured in normal dogs after experimentally created complete bile duct occlusion.[59]

Lipid and lipoprotein abnormalities characterized in human beings with different forms of hepatobiliary disease are shown in Table 30–4. Relatively little is known about the lipoprotein moieties in dogs or cats with liver disease.

An inherited hyperlipoproteinemia of miniature schnauzers has been described.[60,61] Some dogs may develop an accompanying hepatopathy; see Chapter 34 for a discussion of this condition. A hyperlipidemic syndrome has also been recognized in Shetland sheepdogs and beagles. Hyperlipidemia in these dogs and in schnauzers is associated with signs consistent with recurrent pancreatitis and liver disease (profound

Table 30–4

LIPID AND LIPOPROTEIN CHANGES IN LIVER DISEASE

Parenchymal Disease	
Acute	↑ Triglycerides
	↓ Triglycerides*
	↓ Cholesterol esters
	↓ VLDL, ↓HDL
	↓ LCAT, ↓HL, ±↓ LPL
Chronic	↑ free: ester cholesterols*
	↓ VLDL, ↓HDL, ↓ LCAT, ↓ HL
Major Bile Duct Occlusion	↑ Cholesterol (free and total)*
	↓ Cholesterol esters*
	↓ LCAT, ↑ Lipoprotein X*
Portosystemic Shunting	↓ Cholesterol (total)*
	↓ Triglycerides*

*   Humans and dogs
VLDL: Very low density lipoproteins
HDL: High density lipoproteins
LCAT: Lecithin cholesterol acyl transferase
HL: Hepatic lipase
LPL: Lipoprotein lipase

increases in ALP activity, moderate to marked increases in serum bile acids).

An inherited hyperchylomicronemia has been characterized in cats with reduced activity of LPL.[62–66] Affected animals have profound lipemia and develop xanthomas and pathologic tissue stores, which cause hepatomegaly.

Although the ramifications of abnormal lipoprotein metabolism are multisystemic, we remain naive about many of these effects. Immunosuppression secondary to abnormal HDLs that develop in certain forms of liver disease has been suggested.[67] The best recognized systemic effects of aberrant lipoprotein metabolism are those resulting from cell membrane adsorption of abnormal lipids. Membrane effects include deleterious changes in membrane permeability, surface receptors, transport proteins, enzymes, and reduced concentrations of prostaglandin and thromboxane precursors.[67] Abnormal platelet function and conformational changes in the shape of circulating erythrocytes have been attributed to these effects.

Hepatic Lipidosis

Abnormalities in the transport of VLDL from the liver or any imbalance resulting in a greater accumulation than dispersal of triglycerides can result in hepatic lipidosis. These mechanisms are conceptualized in Figure 30–4. This syndrome can lead to hepatic failure and death in the cat (see Chapter 34).

Hepatic lipidosis has been reported in human beings, cows, horses, dogs, and cats as a spontaneous hepatobiliary disorder.[68–92] Development of lipid vacuoles in hepatocytes is not directly noxious to the cell but is a common response to a variety of metabolic aberrations or underlying liver disorders. Physiologically, lipid accumulation is benign and potentially reversible. If severe in humans, it can lead to cirrhosis. When severe in cats, it leads to death rather than cirrhosis. Compared to the dog, the cat seems to have a propensity for the formation of fatty vacuoles in hepatocytes, and similar to the human, may develop lipid vacuolation in association with other clinically significant liver diseases.

Lipid metabolism becomes abnormal in many different endocrine conditions, nutritional and metabolic derangements, and in some forms of hepatic disease. The lipid content of the liver is normally only 5% of the organ weight. When increasing amounts of triglyceride accumulate, the liver enlarges so that it may become easily palpable. In severe hepatic lipidosis the liver weight may double or triple due to retained triglyceride. Abnormal hepatic fat accumulation may occur as a result of (1) increased de novo hepatic synthesis of fatty acids and triglycerides, (2) increased mobilization of fatty acids from adipose tissue, (3) decreased hepatic oxidation of fatty acids, or (4) impaired dispersal of lipids as VLDLs from the liver (Figure 30–4). Specific causes include (1) obesity, (2) excessive or insufficient caloric intake, (3) imbalanced nutrition, (4) hepatotoxins, and (5) miscellaneous derangements such as diabetes mellitus, inflammatory bowel disease, hypoxia, congestive heart failure, or severe anemia. Many of the metabolic conditions and toxins associated with hepatic lipidosis and their pathogenetic mechanisms are provided in Table 30–5. The relationship of obesity related causes of hepatic lipidosis are discussed in Chapter 34.

HEPATOTOXINS. A number of toxins have been associated with hepatic lipidosis in human beings and experimental animals. Chronic alcohol ingestion is the best known lipidosis-producing intoxicant. In general, toxins causing hepatic lipid accumulation impair lipoprotein exportation or membrane-associated enzymes essential for fat oxidation.

A classic toxin causing hepatic lipid accumulation is carbon

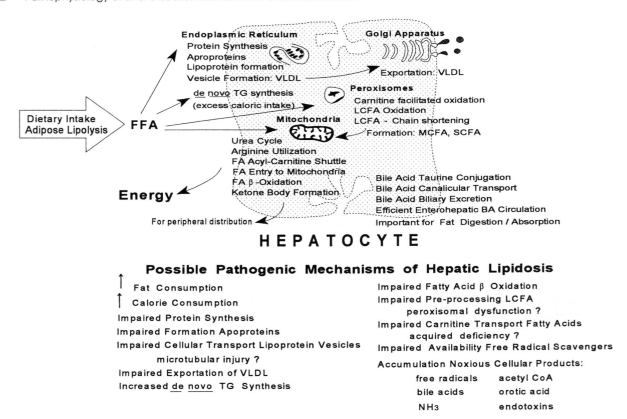

FIGURE 30–4. Hepatic functions important in lipid metabolism that can lead to hepatic triglyceride accumulation if dysfunctional.

tetrachloride (CCl$_4$). Hepatotoxicity due to CCl$_4$ results from metabolites produced in the P-450 microsomes. This toxin, and many others similarly metabolized, yield free radicals that initiate lipid peroxidation, causing organelle and cell membrane injury and inhibition of protein synthesis. Injury to microsomes impairs the ability of the hepatocyte to synthesize and export lipoproteins. Small nonlethal doses of CCl$_4$ depress microsomal enzyme function by causing organelle injury, such that the compound cannot be biotransformed into its injurious metabolites. Subsequent exposures to CCl$_4$ have a muted effect. Naturally occurring antioxidants can provide some protection against toxin-induced lipid peroxidation. Vitamin E and glutathione can provide protection if available in very high concentrations immediately before toxin exposure. They are not effective if administered after exposure. CCl$_4$ also causes a substantial reduction in available ATP or its precursor in the liver, which may lead to impaired fatty acid mobilization.

Ethionine, phosphorus, and puromycin are similar to CCl$_4$ in impairing hepatic protein synthesis. Each impairs apolipoprotein synthesis, whereupon triglycerides cannot be dispersed from the hepatocyte. Specifically, these compounds disrupt protein synthesis by damaging ribosomes and endoplasmic reticulum. Hepatic lipidosis does not develop with these toxins unless there is an ongoing fatty acid influx into the liver. Increased mobilization of free fatty acids has been shown with each of these toxins and can be prevented by glucose infusions or by feeding.[93,94] Ethionine has also been shown to impair the availability of hepatic ATP by competing with methionine, making the liver more susceptible to membrane injury and other toxins. Provision of ATP can reverse the influence of ethionine.

Hypoglycin, a toxin in the fruit and seed of the Akee tree,

causes a disorder known as Jamaican vomiting sickness in human beings. A metabolite of this toxin impairs fatty acid oxidation and cellular metabolism by conversion to nonmetabolizable derivatives of coenzyme A and carnitine.[91]

Aflatoxins, mycotoxins produced by strains of *Aspergillus flavus* and *A. parasiticus,* occur worldwide but are most common in crops grown in tropical and subtropical areas. Aflatoxins are potent inhibitors of RNA synthesis. The metabolic effects include inhibited synthesis of protein, enzymes, clotting factors, and fatty acids; suppressed glucose metabolism; and loss of feedback control on cholesterol synthesis.[95] Liver changes in aflatoxicosis include fatty infiltration, biliary proliferation, acute toxic necrosis, and portal fibrosis. It has been shown that a high protein intake protects against aflatoxin injury and that a protein-deficient diet increases susceptibility. In experimental animals exposed to aflatoxin, vitamin A deficiency is associated with high mortality. Toxicity can be favorably modified by additions of selenium, methionine, choline, and fat as dietary constituents.

Orotic acid has been shown to induce hepatic lipidosis in rats.[96] Some consider that it may be involved in the genesis of the feline hepatic lipidosis syndrome (see Chapter 34).[82,86,97]

Toxic substances produced by intestinal bacteria have been suggested to induce hepatic lipid vacuolation. Endotoxin has received the most attention. Mild hepatic lipidosis associated with moderate choline deficiency can become severe when endotoxin is given intraperitoneally. Bacterial overgrowth in the bowel, as occurs with the stagnant loop syndrome, can also induce hepatocellular vacuolation. The etiopathogenesis may include formation of toxic bile salts or be related to dietary inadequacies. Hepatic lipidosis has been diagnosed in human beings with chronic inflammatory bowel disease, coli-

Table 30–5

CONDITIONS OR AGENTS ASSOCIATED WITH PRODUCTION OF HEPATIC LIPIDOSIS

CONDITION	MECHANISMS
Overnutrition	
Chronic ↑↑ calorie ingestion→ obesity	↑ mobilization fatty acids
Abnormal Calorie Intake	
Undernutrition/starvation	↑ mobilization FA and amino acids
	↓ lipoprotein synthesis
Imbalanced Nutrition	
lipotrope deficiency	↓ apoprotein synthesis
(choline, B_{12}, folate	↓ lipoprotein dispersal
methionine, inositol)	
protein deficiency	↓ apoprotein synthesis, ↓ lipoprotein dispersal
	↑ protein catabolism, ↑ FA mobilization
	↑ susceptibility to free radical injury
carbohydrate excess	↑ hepatic triglyceride synthesis
carbohydrates *but* inadequate calories in anorexia	incomplete adaptation to FA and ketone metabolism
	↓ beta-oxidation, ↓ ketone bodies
Hepatotoxins	
ethanol	↑ lipolysis, ↓ oxidation FA, ↑ FA esterification, ↑ synthesis FA
carbon tetrachloride	↓ protein synthesis, ↓ apoprotein, ↓ VLDL dispersal
ethionine	↓ VLDL formation and dispersal
phosphorus	↓ VLDL formation and dispersal
puromycin	↓ VLDL formation and dispersal
Ackee fruit (Jamaican vomiting sickness)	↓ FA oxidation, ↓ Acetyl CoA, ↓ carnitine
bacterial endotoxin	↓ FA oxidation, ↓ apoprotein synthesis,
	toxic bile acids → membrane injury
orotic acid	↓ assembly VLDL, ↓ dispersal VLDL
aflatoxins	↓ protein synthesis, ↓ assembly VLDL, ↓ dispersal VLDL
salicylates	mitochondrial injury (children) ↓ FA oxidation
tetracycline	impaired protein metabolism, apoprotein synthesis,
	↓ VLDL dispersal, ↑ hepatic FA uptake
valproic acid	↓ FA oxidation, ↓ Acetyl CoA, ↓ carnitine
coconut oil in cats (?)	mechanism unknown
Metabolic Disorders	
diabetes mellitus	↑ FA mobilization
inborn errors FA oxidation	↓ FA oxidation
cellular hypoxia (severe anemia, posthepatic portal hypertension)	↓ apoprotein synthesis, ↓ VLDL dispersal
parenteral hyperalimentation	protein deficiency, FA overload
Fatty liver of pregnancy	mitochondrial defect, ↓ FA oxidation
Reye's syndrome (children)	mitochondrial defect, ↓ FA oxidation
glucocorticoid excess	↑ FA mobilization, ↑ gluconeogenesis, ↑ appetite → obesity
jejunoileal bypass	protein calorie imbalance, catabolism
inflammatory bowel disease	malabsorption, malnutrition, catabolism, ↑ glucocorticoids (Rx),
	bacterial endotoxins, toxic bile acids, ↓ VLDL dispersal

---

tis, or jejunoileal bypass performed for control of obesity.[70,72–74] Bacterial toxins, toxic bile acids (such as lithocholate), and catabolism associated with starvation, malnutrition, exogenous or endogenous glucocorticoids may independently or collectively promote lipidosis in these conditions. Fat accumulates in large droplets and is usually diffusely distributed. Certain bacterial toxins can impair fatty acid oxidation and decrease apoprotein synthesis. In some human beings, an overgrowth of intestinal anaerobes is believed to generate lipidosis-inducing toxins. In these cases, hepatic fat deposition was reversed by eliminating anaerobic overgrowth with metronidazole.[73]

DRUGS. Many drugs, chemicals, and plant toxins may produce lipidosis if chronic exposure to small quantities occurs. Acute severe intoxications are usually associated with hepatic necrosis or inflammation rather than lipidosis. Because lipid vacuolation is one of the few morphologic responses the hepatocyte can make to metabolic injury, different toxins producing diverse biochemical defects may provoke this lesion. Few toxins have been specifically identified that can induce clinical hepatic lipidosis in dogs or cats. In one study a diet composed of safflower seed oil (5%), chicken fat (5%), and hydrogenated coconut oil (15%) produced a moderate degree of lipidosis in the cat.[98] The medium chain triglycerides in the coconut oil were suggested to be the underlying noxious agent.

Tetracyclines accumulate in the liver and undergo enterohepatic circulation. Administration of tetracycline produces microvesicular hepatic lipid vacuolation in human beings.[99] Hepatic fatty vacuolation develops in humans within 3 to 12 days of tetracycline administration. Suspected hepatic toxicity associated with tetracycline administration in a cat has been reported.[100] The major clinical finding was a markedly increased serum ALT activity. Hepatic biopsy revealed a mild degree of hepatic lipidosis. Based on experimental work of tetracycline-induced lipidosis, the most plausible toxic mechanisms involve impaired protein metabolism most likely associated with inhibition of apoprotein production or impaired VLDL exportation.[101-105] The histologic lesion in rats, mice, and humans is a microvesicular vacuolation with localization in zone 3 and zone 2 (perivenular and midzonal areas). The most notable serum biochemical abnormality is a markedly increased serum ALT activity.[101,105]

Valproic acid, an anticonvulsant, is a branched medium chain fatty acid that can lead to hepatotoxicity. The etiology of liver injury is unknown but has been proposed to involve impaired fatty acid oxidation and decreased availability of coenzyme A and carnitine, similar to hypoglycin.[106-108]

Methotrexate, an antimetabolite used as a chemotherapeutic agent in cancer therapy and treatment of immune-mediated disorders, can cause hepatic lipidosis, fibrosis, and cirrhosis.[91] Toxic effects seem dose related and can be avoided if the dosage is minimized to a low level and given as weekly pulse therapy. The mechanism of toxicity remains undetermined. Because this drug is a folate inhibitor, a deleterious influence on lipotropic agents is suspected. This would curtail hepatic dispersal of VLDL and impair other folate-dependent metabolic processes.

Glucocorticoids increase adipocyte lipolysis and fatty acid mobilization to the liver. These effects may promote hepatic lipidosis if an underlying abnormality of hepatic fat dispersal or beta-oxidation exists. Hepatic lipid vacuolation can develop in cats receiving high doses of glucocorticoids and that are partially anorectic. Hepatic lesions observed in dogs with a glucocorticoid hepatopathy are primarily associated with hepatocellular swelling with glycogen. Dogs generally do not develop large numbers of lipid-containing vacuoles in hepatocytes unless they have diabetes mellitus or a hyperlipoproteinemia.

FATTY LIVER OF PREGNANCY. Acute fatty liver is a potentially fatal complication of the third trimester of pregnancy in humans.[109-111] Ultrastructural mitochondrial changes suggest an association with impaired fatty acid oxidation. The exact etiopathogenesis of this disorder remains undetermined. It can lead to disseminated intravascular coagulation and death of mother and baby. Pregnancy-associated fatty liver in the dog and cat has also been observed but has not been well studied. Affected animals demonstrate signs of systemic illness.

CARNITINE DEFICIENCY. Carnitine is essential for enzyme-mediated uptake of fatty acids into mitochondria. Congenital (primary) and acquired (secondary) carnitine deficiency in human beings is associated with severe lipid accumulation in liver and other tissues and can be associated with hepatic dysfunction.[112] Acquired carnitine deficiency may be related to the development of feline hepatic lipidosis syndrome (see Chapter 34).

MISCELLANEOUS IMBALANCES. Fatty liver is associated with diabetes mellitus; about 50% of human patients with diabetes have a fatty liver.[91] An absolute or relative insulin deficiency promotes fasting hyperglycemia, glucose intolerance, and increased adipocyte lipolysis. These effects encourage hepatic lipid accumulation.

Hepatic lipidosis has been reported as a syndrome in puppies of toy breeds between the ages of 4 to 16 weeks.[113] Anorexia was strongly associated as an etiopathogenic event. Hepatic fat content of affected puppies was comprised largely of triglycerides and contributed up to 54% of the liver dry weight.

Hypernatremia has been shown to induce hyperlipemia and fatty liver in rats. It was postulated that the hyperosmolal state in the liver leads to enhanced triglyceride formation and impaired conversion of fatty acids to ketone bodies.[114]

Cellular hypoxia, due to abnormal hepatic circulation or impaired oxygen transport, can lead to mild forms of hepatic lipidosis. Vacuolation in zone 3 (perivenular) is most common. Congestive heart failure, pericardial tamponade, and other causes of posthepatic portal hypertension can cause this lesion. Hypotension, such as that caused by endotoxic, hemorrhagic, or hypovolemic shock, anesthetic agents, and drugs or toxins with vasoactive properties, can also induce this effect. It is postulated that lipid vacuolation develops as a result of the diverted effort of the hepatocyte to maintain euglycemia. Consequently, there are reduced available resources for fatty acid oxidation as an alternative source of energy. With chronicity, hypoxia may lead to more severe hepatic lipid deposition and necrosis. It can lead to cirrhosis in human beings.

LIVER REGENERATION. Hepatic lipid vacuole formation develops in the liver remnant almost immediately following a two-thirds hepatectomy.[115] Lipid vacuole formation is believed to be associated with reduced synthesis and/or release of VLDL, purportedly because protein synthesis is deviated to reparative and regenerative processes.

PROTEIN METABOLISM

The liver is of central importance to normal protein homeostasis; hepatic synthesis of constituent and export proteins provides about 20% of the total body protein turnover.[116] It is the exclusive or primary site for synthesis of a majority of the plasma proteins and is the site of degradation, activation, or regulation for many others. The liver synthesizes albumin, most of the procoagulant and many anticoagulant proteins, as well as the activators and inhibitors important in maintaining homeostasis of the coagulation pathways. In addition, most of the alpha-globulins, half of the beta-globulins, some of the gamma-globulins, most of the transport globulins, and many serum enzymes are derived from the liver. A list of important proteins synthesized by the liver is provided in Table 30–6. The total serum protein concentration is influenced by liver disease in a number of diverse ways. Inflammation can induce production of acute-phase proteins that may substantially increase the total protein concentration. Reduced Kupffer cell function results in an increased systemic challenge with foreign or noxious substances such as endotoxin, bacteria, and particulate material derived from the portal circulation. This stimulates increased systemic production of immunoglobulins. Hepatic synthetic failure can be marked by development of severe hypoalbuminemia and inadequacy of many of the proteins involved in coagulation.

Protein Synthesis and Regulation

One of the most important secretory functions of the hepatocyte is production of the circulating plasma proteins. The most abundant and best characterized is albumin, which comprises 60% of the total plasma proteins in most mammals.[117] The remainder of the plasma proteins are an heterogenous group of glycosylated proteins (glycoproteins). Many of these have specialized functions essential for life.

Numerous factors influence hepatic protein production. One of the most important factors permitting synthesis of export proteins (albumin) is amino acid availability. Reduced intake of amino acids or protein rapidly leads to reduced albumin synthesis. Following long-term amino acid and protein deprivation, albumin synthesis is not restored until hepatic organelles necessary for protein synthesis and secre-

Table 30–6

PLASMA PROTEINS SECRETED BY THE LIVER

PROTEIN MOIETY	ACUTE PHASE	FUNCTION
Albumin	No	Binding/carrier protein: hormones, amino acids, steroids, bilirubin, bile acids, BSP, ICG, vitamins, copper, calcium, fatty acids; regulates osmotic pressure
Alpha$_1$-Acid glycoprotein	Yes	Modulates coagulation, binds drugs, interaction in inflammation
Alpha$_1$-Antitrypsin	Yes	Trypsin and general protease inhibitor: proteases in serum and tissues
Alpha$_1$-Fetoprotein	No	Synthesized by fetal liver, hepatic tumors, regenerating hepatocytes
Alpha$_2$-Macroglobulin	Yes	Endoprotease inhibitor
Antithrombin III	Yes	Serine protease inhibitor, anticoagulant, requires heparin
Ceruloplasmin	Yes	Copper transport protein, oxidase activity
C-reactive protein	Yes	Regulation of inflammation and microbial defense: activates complement, enhances phagocytosis of bacteria, RBCs
Fibrinogen	Yes	Fibrin precursor necessary for hemostasis
Haptoglobin	Yes	Free hemoglobin binding and transport
Hemopexin	Yes	Oxidized heme/porphyrin binding, essential for heme recycling
Transferrin	No	Iron transport: may decrease in inflammation due to vascular leakage
Immunoglobulins IgG, IgM	±	Immunoprotection
Steroid hormone	No	
Binding globulins		Circulatory transport of hormones
thyroid-binding protein		thyroxine
sex hormone–binding globulin		estrogen, testosterone
vitamin D–binding globulin		vitamin D
transcortin		cortisone

tion are revitalized.[118] Insulin and physiologic concentrations of thyroxine and glucocorticoids exert an anabolic effect on protein metabolism. Excessive concentrations of glucocorticoids simultaneously increase both albumin synthesis and degradation. Low concentrations of thyroxine and glucocorticoids reduce hepatic protein synthesis.

Although hepatic protein synthesis generally has a high metabolic priority, it remains secondary to gluconeogenesis. During fasting, liver structural proteins are used as the first source of substrates for gluconeogenesis, before branched chain amino acids are solicited from muscle. Hepatic autophagy, driven by fasting and by increased glucagon or catecholamine concentrations, is mediated by lysosomal proteases. Increased concentrations of ammonia and certain amino acids (alanine, glutamate, and glutamine) can blunt hepatic proteolysis and may participate in the etiopathogenesis of hypoglycemia in some patients with hepatic insufficiency. Regulation of the synthesis and degradation of proteins dependent on hepatic metabolism is reflected in their plasma half-lives. The estimated half-life of albumin is less than 10 days, of coagulation proteins ranges between 5 hours and 5 days, of certain alpha-globulins is 8 to 10 days, and for gamma-globulins is 20 to 35 days.

Albumin

Albumin is the major secretory protein of the liver. Its relatively small size (molecular weight of 66,000 daltons) allows it to be lost through injured vasculature, gut, or glomeruli.[117] Albumin represents 25% of all protein synthesized by the liver.[118] The serum albumin concentration is the net result of three active physiologic processes: (1) synthesis and secretion from the hepatocyte, (2) distribution, and (3) degradation. An overview of the details of the following discussion is provided in Figure 30–5.

ALBUMIN SYNTHESIS. The liver manufactures albumin at a massive rate. The normal adult human liver produces 200 mg of albumin per kg body weight per day.[119] A large synthetic reserve capacity is available for albumin. When necessary, the basal synthetic rate can be more than doubled. Initiation of synthesis and release of albumin from hepatocytes is a rapid process. It only takes an average of 20 to 30 minutes for the appearance of an albumin molecule in the plasma from the onset of its synthesis.[119] Albumin is not considered to be a high-priority protein; its synthesis fluctuates depending on other physiologic requirements. The most important factors regulating albumin synthesis are nutrition and the intravascular colloidal osmotic pressure. Synthesis of albumin is maintained during periods of adequate nutrition but is curtailed when nutrition is deficient.[120–126] Albumin synthesis also is reduced following exposure to certain hepatotoxins or if the hepatocyte senses an increased colloidal osmotic pressure at its surface. Clinically, when animals are deprived of food or fed a protein-deficient diet, albumin synthesis declines by 50% within 24 hours. Following an abrupt decline in albumin synthesis, the concentration of albumin in plasma requires a lag time of days or weeks to reflect the change. This occurs because it takes time to establish a new homeostatic balance between the exchangeable pools. Upon refeeding a starved animal, albumin synthetic activity returns within minutes. Dietary depletion of branched chain amino acids substantially reduces albumin synthesis.[119,124] Feeding of excessive calories in a low-protein diet augments the development of hypoalbuminemia due to reduced albumin synthesis more than feeding a similar diet containing inadequate calories.[127]

Albumin synthesis is also influenced by a number of hormones including glucocorticoids, growth hormone, sex hormones, thyroxine, and insulin. Glucocorticoids act directly by stimulating hepatic RNA synthesis and indirectly by increasing the hepatic pool of amino acids. Thyroxine also stimulates hepatic RNA synthesis. Glucagon suppresses hepatic protein synthesis.

ALBUMIN DISTRIBUTION. Between 50% to 70% of the total albumin mass is located extravascularly in the normal animal.[127] The greatest amount is found in the interstitial spaces of skin and muscle. Because of the large volume of distribution and physiologic mechanisms that influence albumin distribution, the plasma albumin concentrations do not necessarily reflect the size or adequacy of the total body albumin pool.

Following secretion of albumin from the hepatocyte it passes into the space of Disse and from there into the hepatic sinusoids where it joins the systemic circulation. From the systemic circulation, albumin may enter the interstitial spaces from which it returns to the intravascular compartment via the lymphatics and thoracic duct. It is believed that regulation of albumin synthesis occurs via minute amounts of albumin distributed in the hepatic interstitial matrix. It is theorized that it is from this region that the surface of the hepatocyte senses and regulates the colloid osmotic pressure.[128-131] Hypoalbuminemia due to reduced albumin synthesis may occur as a result of hyperglobulinemia as well as intravascular treatment with dextrans; these circumstances stimulate osmotic "sensors" that suspend further production of albumin.[119,132,133]

ALBUMIN CATABOLISM. The rate of albumin catabolism is highly variable; in humans (healthy individuals and patients with protein-losing disease), the daily albumin breakdown ranges from 2% to 57% of the plasma pool per day.[134] Degradation regulates the size of the albumin pool by maintaining a fractional rate of catabolism directly proportional to the plasma albumin concentration and pool size. When the pool size increases, degradation of albumin increases to maintain the status quo. With reductions in pool size, albumin degradation decreases.

The half-life of plasma albumin has been estimated in dogs to range between 6.7 and 9.4 days.[135-136] The site of albumin catabolism has not been precisely clarified although it is believed to be the vascular endothelium.[128,137] The plasma concentration of albumin directly influences the rate of albumin catabolism. In nearly all conditions producing hypoalbuminemia, the fractional as well as the absolute rate of albumin catabolism declines.[128] The overall rate of catabolism is augmented by adding albumin to plasma, perhaps by increasing flow through catabolic sites.

In patients with chronic inflammatory disorders, infections, or neoplasia, plasma albumin may undergo structural changes that promote its catabolism.[138] This may be coupled with reduced albumin synthesis due to production of cytokines, which are inhibitory. Stress associated with trauma, surgery, or hospitalization can increase albumin degradation to such an extent that the albumin pool decreases by 20% to 75%.[128]

ALBUMIN FUNCTIONS. Serum albumin has two major functions: (1) maintenance of colloid osmotic pressure (albumin provides 80%), and (2) plasma transport of a variety of substances. Plasma albumin represents greater than 50% of the plasma protein mass. In comparison to the other plasma proteins, albumin is a relatively small molecule and thus it is the most important mediator of the plasma colloid osmotic pressure. Severe hypoalbuminemia (serum albumin ≤ 1.5 g/dl) promotes development of interstitial edema and body cavity effusions. Formation of ascites in patients with hepatic insufficiency usually develops concurrent with portal hypertension when the serum albumin concentration falls below 1.5 g/dl. Mild hyperglobulinemia commonly observed in patients with liver disease probably does not contribute to the colloid osmotic pressure.

A multitude of substances are transported bound to albumin including endogenous substances such as bilirubin, fatty acids, hormones, and bile acids, metals such as copper and zinc, and ions such as calcium. Albumin also serves as a transport protein for a large number of exogenous substances including drugs and toxins. A list of drugs that have been recognized as having a high degree of binding to albumin is provided in Table 30-7.[139,140] In the circumstance of hypoalbuminemia, the clinician must recognize which drugs have a high degree of protein binding in order to anticipate adverse drug effects or interactions. This is clinically relevant because it is the unbound drug component that distributes and interacts with receptors and diffuses into normally inaccessible body spaces (e.g., CNS), causing unexpected or amplified effects.

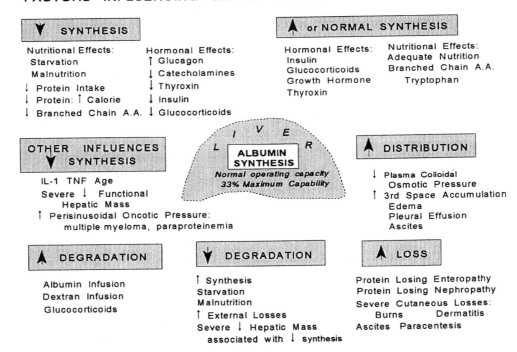

FIGURE 30-5. Variables influencing the serum albumin concentration.

CLINICAL CONSIDERATIONS OF ALTERED ALBUMIN CONCENTRATION. Because albumin synthesis occurs exclusively in the liver, lowered production would be expected in hepatobiliary disorders associated with synthetic failure. However, subnormal serum concentrations of albumin develop in many but not all patients with hepatic insufficiency. This reflects the multitude of interacting factors that influence the serum albumin concentration.

In most cases, a reduced albumin concentration observed in a nonascitic cirrhotic patient is believed to be due to decreased albumin synthesis.[141-145] When ascites develops, expansion of the exchangeable albumin pool has a dilutional influence as protein is sequestered in a "third space." In the presence of ascites, high rates of albumin synthesis commonly develop. In part, this is due to the fact that a major fraction of the newly synthesized albumin is released directly into the ascitic fluid, bypassing the plasma pool.[146,147] This third-spaced albumin may require weeks to achieve equilibrium with the plasma pool where it can impart an influence on the hepatic osmotic regulators. These physiologic interactions are discussed more fully in the section of this chapter dealing with ascites formation.

The rate of albumin synthesis is actively suppressed by inflammation and varies inversely with the rates of synthesis of acute-phase reactants such as fibrinogen, haptoglobin, alpha$_2$-macroglobulin, and alpha$_1$-acid glycoprotein.[148-152] This is mediated through tumor necrosis factor (TNF) and interleukin-1 (IL-1).[152,153] This phenomenon further complicates the diagnostic significance of hypoalbuminemia in the patient with inflammatory hepatic or systemic disease.

A further complicating variable in the liver patient is the influence of anorexia. Any cause of nutritional deficiency results in hepatocyte atrophy and a reduction in albumin-synthesizing organelles. If branched chain amino acids become restricted, reduced synthesis leads to a gradual decline in plasma and total body albumin concentrations. The decline is gradual because of the concurrent conservation of albumin due to a readjustment of its catabolism. With reduced protein consumption, there is also a fall in the level of the urea cycle enzymes.[154,155] Arginine and other amino acids such as ornithine, involved in the urea cycle, stimulate albumin synthesis after they are converted to polyamines: putrescine, spermidine, and spermine.[156,157] These amines play many varied and important roles in DNA and RNA metabolism, cell regeneration, and protein synthesis.[158] Polyamines are also derived from methionine metabolism, which can become impaired in the patient with hepatic insufficiency. An absence of polyamines has been shown to block amino acid stimulation of albumin synthesis. The role of polyamines is not fully understood, and it is postulated that as their role is more fully defined, the urea cycle will be found to be important in protein synthesis in addition to its traditionally recognized role in nitrogen detoxification.[156]

In formulating diets for animals with hepatic insufficiency, it is important to consider that both adequate calorie and protein intake are essential for normal albumin production. Diets adequate in caloric content but restricted in protein are more deleterious on albumin synthesis and albumin body stores than diets containing the same amount of protein but deficient in total calories.[128] Unfortunately, there have not been any studies of the protein requirements of dogs or cats with spontaneous hepatobiliary disorders. One study of dogs with experimentally created portosystemic shunts showed that they required maintenance level of dietary protein.[159] Most clinicians are too ready to use protein-restricted diets when liver disease is suspected. It is possible that in some of these animals, protein restriction is detrimental to the patient's albumin status and particularly recovery from acute necrotizing insults.

Considerable increases in the rate of albumin catabolism occur after albumin infusions.[123] Consequently, most patients with pathologic conditions associated with hypoalbuminemia do not derive long-term benefit from intravenous albumin administration. Albumin transfusions are generally reserved for support of colloid osmotic pressure during critical situations. Administration of frozen plasma as a source of albumin is problematic for the patient with hepatic insufficiency because substantial amounts of ammonia may generate during plasma storage. A patient demonstrating hypoalbuminemia as a sign of synthetic failure most likely also has a problem with ammonia detoxification.

Most hypoalbuminemias in animals are due to an increased rate of albumin degradation, an expanded volume of distribution, or albumin loss rather than albumin synthetic failure. Even in patients with spontaneous or experimentally created cirrhosis, synthetic failure is only a partial cause. Interestingly, some dogs with portosystemic shunts are unable to maintain normal plasma albumin concentrations despite being clinically normal and consuming adequate proteins and calories to maintain albumin synthesis.[49] An algorithm for the differential diagnoses of hypoproteinemia is provided in Figure 30–6.

Alpha-, Beta-, and Gamma-Globulins

The serum globulin concentration represents a myriad of different proteins; (Table 30–7). Most of the nonimmunoglobulin serum globulins are synthesized and stored in the liver.[160] This includes 75% to 90% of the alpha-globulins and 50% of the beta-globulins. Many of the nonimmunoglobulin moieties are considered to be "acute-phase proteins." These include a variety of functionally diverse plasma proteins normally present in only very small amounts.[161-163] The synthesis of acute-phase proteins is rapidly and markedly increased in response to tissue injury or inflammation.[163-172] This response is stimulated by cytokines, including IL-1, IL-6, and TNF-alpha that are released within the injured liver or transported to the liver from other sites of tissue damage.[170-172]

Cellulose acetate electrophoretic separation of serum globulins has been studied in detail in human patients with liver disease. The alpha$_1$-globulin fraction contains high density and very high density lipoproteins, ceruloplasmin, and alpha$_1$-glycoprotein. The alpha$_2$-globulin fraction includes haptoglobin, alpha$_2$-macroglobulin, plasminogen, prothrombin, and alpha$_2$-glycoprotein. The beta-globulin fraction consists of low density and very low density lipoproteins and transferrin. The gamma-globulin fraction largely consists of immunoglobulins although dimers of IgA can migrate in the beta-globulin fraction. The cellulose acetate electrophoretogram has limited utility in the diagnosis of liver disease because of the diverse overlap between protein moieties. Some generalities have been reported for patients with different disorders. The alpha$_2$-globulins may increase with extrahepatic bile duct obstruction, malignancy, and bacterial or viral infections. The beta-globulins are more consistently increased in parenchymal hepatobiliary disorders; examples include acute and chronic hepatitis, cirrhosis, and extrahepatic bile duct obstruction.

The control of synthesis of most globulins is more specific than that for albumin. Proteins that are catabolized as they complete their functions require steady state production. An example of such a globulin is haptoglobin,

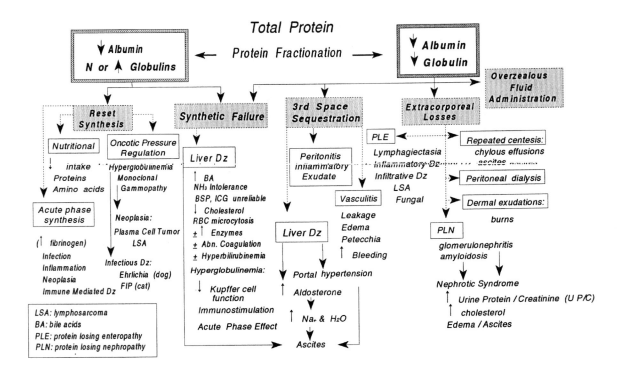

FIGURE 30–6. Diagnostic algorithm for the differentiation of causes of hypoproteinemia.

which binds and transports hemoglobin in the circulation. Once taken into an RE cell, haptoglobin delivers hemoglobin for catabolism and is degraded into subunit amino acids. Globulins having procoagulant and anticoagulant functions also are similarly degraded once they have been utilized. Some globulins are conserved and recycled after completion of their specific function. An example is transferrin, which binds and transports iron in the circulation. Upon delivery of iron to the RE cell, transferrin undergoes endocytosis, the iron is removed, and the apotransferrin globulin (transferrin devoid of iron) is recycled for further use. As already discussed, the synthesis of acutephase globulins is under the influence of several different cytokines. Globulins dependent on hepatic production can become depleted in the patient with protein synthetic failure. This is difficult to document unless specific globulin moieties are quantitatively measured. Those which can be specifically determined are discussed individually in the following section.

Hyperglobulinemia is common in animals with acquired hepatobiliary disorders. Increased globulin concentrations develop as a result of an immunologic response elicited by reduced Kupffer cell function, disturbed B and T cell function, development of autoantibodies, and induction of acute-phase hepatic proteins.[173–175] As a result of hepatic injury, Kupffer cell function may be reduced because of quantitative cell loss, redesignation of cell function, abnormal sinusoidal blood flow, or portosystemic shunting causing Kupffer cell bypass. Humans with serious chronic liver disease may develop antinuclear antibodies, anti-DNA antibody, antismooth muscle antibody, antimitochondrial antibody, bile canalicular antibody, and liver membrane–directed antibodies. Some of these antibodies may participate in continued hepatic inflammation. Their role in chronic liver disorders in dogs and cats has not been defined.

Fibrinogen

Fibrinogen is synthesized only in the liver. It is an essential component of the coagulation system and also is an acutephase protein. In steady state, fibrinogen disappearance follows first-order kinetics. The fractional rate of degradation remains constant, so that the amount catabolized is directly proportional to its level in plasma. Hyperfibrinogenemia represents increased synthesis and release by the hepatocyte. Hypofibrinogenemia can reflect reduced fibrinogen synthesis or increased consumption. Synthetic failure only occurs in severe end-stage hepatic disease or acute massive necrosis. Differentiation of synthetic failure from increased consumption as the cause of hypofibrinogenemia can be difficult because dysregulation of the coagulation system may manifest as DIC in severe liver disorders.

Antithrombin III

Antithrombin III (AT III) is synthesized in the liver and is recognized as one of the most important naturally occurring anticoagulants in the body. It is discussed in detail in the coagulation section that follows.

Alpha-Fetoprotein

Alpha-fetoprotein is the major plasma protein synthesized by the yolk sac and liver during fetal life. Synthesis declines during the perinatal period. In humans, increased serum alpha-fetoprotein concentrations develop in patients with hepatocellular carcinoma, hepatomas, malignant disease of yolk-sac cell origin (gonadal carcinomas), and a variety of liver diseases including viral hepatitis, chronic active hepatitis, and cirrhosis.[176–178] In dogs, alpha-fetoprotein has been shown to reflect hepatic regeneration more consistently than conventional serum enzyme activities and total bilirubin concentration following 70% hepatectomy.[179,180] Increased alpha-fetoprotein values have been reported to serve as a paraneoplastic marker in dogs with a variety of hepatic tumors including hepatocellular carcinoma, cholangiocarcinomas, and hepatic lymphosarcoma.[181–183]

AMINO ACID METABOLISM

The liver plays a key role in amino acid metabolism; an overview of amino acid metabolism is presented in Figure 30–7. The total body amino acid pool is derived from degradation of body protein and proteins absorbed from the alimentary tract. The liver is efficient in adjusting the amino acid balance in the portal circulation; it preferentially retains aromatic amino acids (AAA, phenylalanine, tyrosine, and tryptophan) but passes on the branched chain amino acids (BCAA, valine, isoleucine, and leucine) to the systemic circulation. When alimentary intake of protein results in a positive nitrogen balance, only 20% to 25% of the portal venous nitrogen is passed to the peripheral circulation. Circulating plasma amino acid concentrations are similar during the postabsorptive interval following protein-rich and protein-restricted meals and during a fast.

The liver synthesizes amino acids from intermediates of carbohydrate and lipid metabolism by amination and transamination reactions. An amine group can be transferred from one amino acid to many alpha-keto acids to synthesize nonessential amino acids in particular demand. Branched

chain amino acids are the major carriers of amino nitrogen from the liver to the peripheral tissues for synthesis of nonessential amino acids. The keto derivatives of BCAA are an essential source of pyruvate, which is oxidized for energy or undergoes transamination to alanine and glutamine.

There are at least eight different amino acid transport systems in the liver; some are Na+ dependent and responsive to nutritional status, amino acid availability, or hormones important in regulating amino acid and glucose metabolism.[184] The influence of variables on amino acid metabolism are exemplified by consideration of alanine, a major gluconeogenic branched chain amino acid. The so-called glucose-alanine cycle is illustrated in Figure 30–7. The anabolic-catabolic balance of the alanine-glucose cycle is under the influence of insulin and glucagon. Insulin is highest after feeding, at which time it limits hepatic uptake of alanine and thus restricts its utilization for gluconeogenesis. Glucagon, which increases during fasting, promotes muscle protein and BCAA degradation, stimulates alanine synthesis and uptake by liver, and promotes gluconeogenesis and ureagenesis. A variety of enzymes in liver and muscle adjust intermediary amino acid metabolism and are subject to feedback autoregulatory influences. Most of the essential amino acids are catabolized primarily in the liver. Hepatic catabolism prevails when amino acid levels exceed those necessary to sustain protein synthesis for export or hepatic utilization. Amino acid degradation provides carbon for gluconeogenesis, ketogenesis, or fatty acid synthesis.

Glutamine is the most abundant plasma amino acid; it is present in concentrations that are twice that of the next most prevalent amino acid, alanine. Glutamine increases dramatically with hyperammonemia while it provides a temporary protective mechanism against ammonia toxicity; see Figure

Table 30–7

DRUGS WITH STRONG BINDING TO PLASMA PROTEINS[139,140]

CATEGORY	APPROXIMATE % PROTEIN BINDING	CATEGORY	APPROXIMATE % PROTEIN BINDING
CNS Active		**Anti-infectives**	
Acepromazine	99	Cephalothin	79
Benzodiazepines	95	Clindamycin	93
Chlordiazepoxide	95	Cloxacillin	95
Chlorpromazine	95	Dicloxacillin	98
Imipramine	96	Oxacillin	94
Phenytoin	78	Doxycycline	86
Thiopental	87	Rifampin	90
Valproic acid	80	Sufadimethoxine	90
		Sulfamethoxypyridazine	90
Anti-inflammatory		Sulfisoxazole	84
Fenoprofen	99	Trimethoprim/sulfa	70
Indomethacin	97		
Oxyphenbutazone	95	**Miscellaneous**	
Phenylbutazone	99	Butorphanol	80
Salicylic acid	84	Coumadin	97
		Chlorpropamide	96
Cardiovascular		Clofibrate	90
Digitoxin	90	Methotrexate	50
Hydralazine	85	Tolbutamide	99
Prazosin	97	Tolazamide	94
Propranolol	90		
Quinidine	90		
Verapamil	90		
Renal			
Chlorothiazide	95		
Ethacrynic acid	90		
Furosemide	95		
Probenicid	99		
Spironolactone	98		

30–7. After resolution of hyperammonemia, glutamine levels normalize within hours.

The primary amino acid substrates for gluconeogenesis are alanine, serine, and threonine. Branched chain amino acids, with central importance in both hepatic and muscle protein metabolism, may function in the following capacities: (1) undergo degradation providing a source of energy for muscle, (2) provide carbon skeletons for pyruvate formation, (3) provide nitrogen for transamination of pyruvate to alanine and glutamine, or (4) be used for protein synthesis. After an overnight fast, both alanine and glutamine are released from muscle protein stores. Alanine is destined for hepatic use in gluconeogenesis, liponeogenesis, and nitrogen donation for transamination reactions or for ureagenesis. Transamination permits formation of other amino acids. Glutamine is destined for use by the gut, where it is a primary source of energy, or to be used by the kidney for ammoniagenesis necessary for renal acid-base regulation.[185] Glutamine metabolism in the gut also supplies precursors and nitrogen for hepatic gluconeogenesis, urea synthesis, and synthesis of intraluminal ammonia that may be involved in sodium and water transport.[185] Glutamine-derived nitrogen is essential for protein and nucleic acid synthesis in enterocytes required for their rapid replication.

In health, the AAAs are efficiently extracted from the portal circulation and metabolized by the liver. Thus, reduced liver function is associated with impaired hepatic metabolism of AAAs and their increased passage into the systemic circulation. Hepatic insufficiency is also associated with increased plasma levels of insulin, glucagon, and catecholamines because these hormones are not adequately removed by the injured liver[186–188] and because hyperammonemia directly or indirectly stimulates their release.[189] Normally, 40% to 50% of insulin in the portal circulation is extracted during first pass through the liver.[190] In hepatic insufficiency both insulin and glucagon increase in the systemic circulation; the effect on

glucagon supersedes that on insulin. The resulting decreased insulin to glucagon molar ratio stimulates gluconeogenesis at the expense of body proteins. Continued mobilization of amino acids for gluconeogenesis results in a sustained increase in blood levels of amino acids metabolized only by the liver (AAAs). Catecholamine release is believed to be a major determinant of amino acid metabolism in hepatic insufficiency. The plasma concentrations of BCAA and most other amino acids metabolized in peripheral tissues are reduced when catecholamines increase. This influence has been studied in adrenalectomized and intact dogs.[189,191] A long-term study of plasma amino acid changes in dogs with chronic hepatic insufficiency has shown an absence of a significant correlation between amino acid changes and the insulin and glucagon plasma concentrations. It is assumed that the catecholamine influence is therefore more important.[192]

The diseased liver maintains it ability to metabolize alanine. As compared to the aromatic amino acids the liver has a 10-fold greater innate capacity to handle alanine.[193] In health, the molar ratio between the BCAAs and the AAAs (BCAA:AAA) usually ranges between 3.0 and 3.5. In patients with severe hepatic insufficiency, this is usually reduced to less than 1.0. The BCAA to AAA ratios for normal dogs and dogs with various hepatic disorders are provided in Table 30–8.[189,194–196] The plasma amino acid profiles reported for dogs with various forms of experimental hepatic injury are shown in Figure 30–8.[192,194–197] The plasma concentrations of most amino acids increase in dogs with massive hepatic necrosis.[194] The exceptions are arginine, which becomes undetectable, and citrulline, cystathionine, hydroxyproline, and isoleucine, which do not change.[194,195] Increased amino acid concentrations develop due to their reduced hepatic utilization and release from damaged hepatocytes.[198] High levels of catecholamines, insulin, and glucagon associated with diffuse hepatic necrosis promote catabolism of extra-

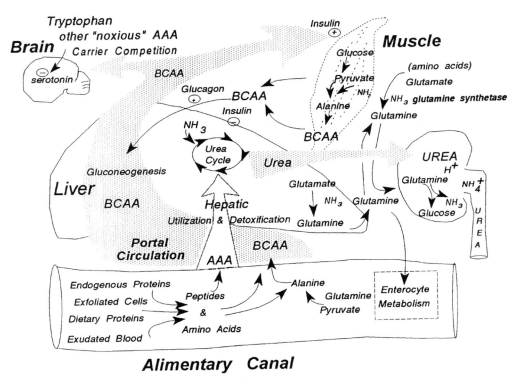

FIGURE 30–7. A simplified overview of amino acid metabolism important in the patient with hepatic disease.

Table 30–8

BRANCHED CHAIN AMINO ACID TO AROMATIC
AMINO ACID RATIO REPORTED IN CLINICALLY
HEALTHY DOGS AND DOGS WITH DIFFERENT
HEPATIC DISORDERS[191,192,197]

HEPATOBILIARY CONDITION	DOGS (N)	BCAA:AAA (MEAN VALUE ± SEM)
Clinically healthy dogs	13	4.14 ± 0.2
	18	3.50 ± 0.2
Congenital portosystemic vascular anomalies	8	0.94 ± 0.1
Spontaneous chronic active hepatitis	8	1.31 ± 0.1
Experimental bile duct occlusion	5	2.95 ± 0.3
Chronic nitrosamine exposure	3	0.75
	4	1.17 ± 0.1

hepatic proteins and increased release of amino acids that cannot be metabolized by the injured liver. The reduced concentration of plasma arginine develops as a result of increased plasma arginase activity due to enzyme release from the cytosol of injured hepatocytes. Arginase rapidly converts plasma arginine to urea and ornithine. Two dogs with hepatocellular carcinoma developed marked increases in alpha-amino-N-butyric acid, and moderate increases in the BCAAs and 3-methylhistidine; the significance of these changes remains undetermined.[194]

Inborn errors of metabolism can cause derangements in plasma amino acid levels. In humans, deficiencies in either the transport mechanisms or the enzymes involved in the metabolism of an amino acid cause the imbalances.[199,200] Hyperammonemia is frequently an associated abnormality.

When the AAAs increase relative to the BCAA, important neurologic consequences can develop. Because BCAAs share membrane transporters with AAAs, some of the more noxious AAAs like tryptophan have increased passage across the blood-brain barrier. High levels of AAAs can result in neurotoxicity. Tryptophan, for instance, can result in overproduction of brain serotonin, an inhibitory neurotransmitter believed to contribute to hepatic encephalopathy. These

changes are discussed more fully in the section on hepatic encephalopathy.

Blood Ammonia

An overview of ammonia metabolism is provided in Figure 30–9. Ammonia is an important product of amino acid metabolism. In health, it is produced in several organs including the brain, small intestines, colon, and kidney. The liver is the only organ able to convert large amounts of ammonia efficiently to an excretable product. The gastrointestinal tract is the largest source of ammonia. Most (75%) of the alimentary ammonia is produced in the colon, through the action of microbial ureases on endogenous urea and degraded dietary amines. The intestinal mucosa does not produce ureases that reduce urea to ammonia because germ-free animals produce little ammonia from urea in the gut.[201] Anaerobic microorganisms and coliforms are the major source of colonic ureases.[202] The most potent gram negative aerobic producers include *E. coli, Klebsiella, Proteus,* and *Pseudomonas* species; the most potent anaerobic producers include *Bacteroides, Bifidobacteria,* and *Clostridium* species. A substantial amount of intestinal ammonia is derived from urea that diffuses into the gut from the peripheral circulation; this occurs largely in the small intestines. Approximately 25% of the endogenous urea diffuses into the alimentary canal where it is transformed into ammonia. This accounts for 40% of the colonic ammonia production. Acidification of the alimentary lumen reduces the hydrolysis of urea by urease, the prevalence of urease-producing organisms, and the intestinal absorption of ammonia. The nonionized form of ammonia (NH_3) is relatively lipid soluble and readily crosses cell membranes. The ammonium ion (NH_4^+) favored by a low pH is poorly absorbed across the bowel wall. Variables favoring the alimentary generation of ammonia may be modified by dietary manipulations and administration of certain nondigestible disaccharides. Effective dietary changes include restriction of meat-derived protein, reduction in protein-derived calories, and increased ingestion of vegetable fiber and poorly digested disaccharides. Therapeutic manipulations targeted at altering the enteric substrates and biochemi-

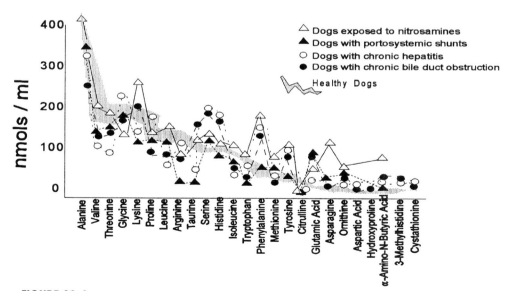

△ Dogs exposed to nitrosamines
▲ Dogs with portosystemic shunts
○ Dogs with chronic hepatitis
● Dogs wtih chronic bile duct obstruction
〜 Healthy Dogs

FIGURE 30–8. Plasma amino acid profiles in dogs with different forms of experimental liver injury. (Adapted from references 192, 194–197)

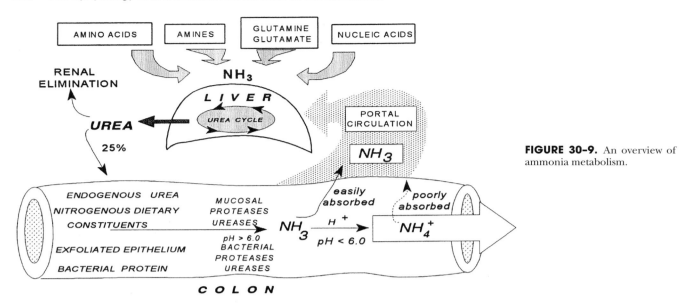

FIGURE 30-9. An overview of ammonia metabolism.

cal reactions permitting ammonia production and absorption are discussed in Chapters 33 and 35.

Following absorption into the portal vein, ammonia is delivered to the liver where most is extracted during the first pass. The concentration of ammonia in portal venous blood has been reported as 350 μg/dl in fasting dogs and 700 μg/dl in fasting cats. This is reduced to 50 μg/dl in the hepatic vein, reflecting the great hepatic capacity for ammonia removal.[203] The difference in the portal venous ammonia concentrations between dogs and cats is related to the greater dietary protein requirement for cats and demonstrates the cat's enormous hepatic capacity to metabolize ammonia.[204] In normal animals, an increased ammonia load absorbed into the portal circulation is not reflected in hepatic venous or peripheral circulating blood since ammonia entering the normal liver is removed at a constant percentage of 85% to 90% and there is considerable reserve capacity for this function.[203] Consequently, hyperammonemia does not develop unless liver damage is extensive and severe or portal blood flow bypasses the liver.

The liver converts most of the circulating ammonia and glutamine to urea in the Krebs-Hensleit urea cycle, a cyclical chain of reactions controlled by five major enzymes. The urea cycle is illustrated in Figure 30–10. In health, the urea cycle operates at only 60% of its maximal capacity. The activity and quantity of urea cycle enzymes self-adjust according to demands for dietary protein detoxification.[154,155] Up to two- or threefold increases in urea cycle enzymes and urea formation occur with high protein intake or with starvation whereas a two- to fivefold decrease occurs with protein-free diets. Arginosuccinate synthetase and carbamyl phosphate synthetase are lower in activity than the other enzymes of the urea cycle and thus represent the rate-limiting steps in cycle function. The intermediate products of the cycle must be continuously supplied to maintain its activity. In dogs, a large ammonia infusion depletes one intermediate, arginine, so that its concentration falls.[189] In cats, the availability of dietary arginine is critical for urea cycle function; an elemental arginine deficient but high-protein diet fed to cats following a 24 hour fast results in hyperammonemia and neurologic sequelae within a few hours of eating.[204]

Regulation of the urea cycle is not well understood. Ammonia detoxification to urea increases when a high-protein diet is fed, during fasting, and under the influence of increased glucocorticoids or glucagon. Each of these variables increases activities of the urea cycle enzymes. Glucocorticoids and glucagon increase ammonia formation by stimulating gluconeogenesis from amino acids. Certain amino acids must be available for incorporation in urea cycle substrates or enzymes for the cycle to function properly. An example is aspartate, which is required for conversion of citrulline to arginosuccinate (Figure 30–10). Ammonia is essential for carbamylphosphate formation (Figure 30–10). The activity of carbamylphosphate synthetase is augmented by N-acetylglutamate and by bicarbonate and is normally low. Reduced bicarbonate concentrations associated with acidosis or administration of carbonic anhydrase inhibitors (certain diuretics) can reduce urea cycle activity and urea formation by interference at this step. There are other important interrelations between hepatic ammonia metabolism and metabolic substances. Mercaptans produced in the intestine and liver from methionine interfere with the conversion of ammonia to urea. Small amounts of mercaptans have been shown to increase blood ammonia concentrations proportedly through this mechanism.[206] Fatty acids have a similar effect via inhibition of carbamyl phosphate synthetase and arginosuccinate synthetase; octanoic acid is more suppressive than oleic acid.[207] Zinc also influences plasma ammonia metabolism.[208,209] In humans with cirrhosis, zinc deficiency is associated with hyperammonemia and reduced urea production. Supplementation with zinc may ameliorate clinical signs of hepatic encephalopathy (HE) in some of these patients.[210] Zinc is an important component of many metalloenzymes and thus may improve intermediary metabolism in a number of ways.[211] The section on metals in this chapter discusses zinc in patients with hepatic disease.

In addition to the urea cycle, the liver can also detoxify ammonia by its use in aminating ketoacids and in the formation of glutamine. Ammonia detoxification by production of glutamine occurs in the liver, skeletal muscle, brain, and kidney and is considered a temporary storage form rather than a means of permanent ammonia detoxification. Glutamine formation proceeds at rates comparable to urea synthesis providing that the necessary substrates, (alpha-ketoglutarate and ATP) are available. In the kidneys, glutamine serves as a carrier for ammonia elimination across renal tubules. Overall,

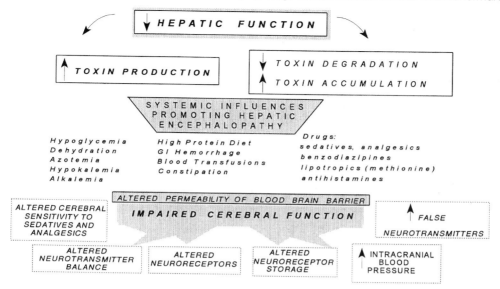

FIGURE 30-10. Diagrammatic representation of the urea cycle and its important enzymes.

renal excretion of ammonia provides quantitatively little elimination of excess nitrogen from the body. This, however, may increase in importance in the patient with hepatic insufficiency.

Ammonia is also taken up and released from peripheral tissues. The most important peripheral tissue participating in ammonia detoxification is skeletal muscle, where ammonia is condensed with glutamate to form glutamine under the influence of glutamine synthetase (Figure 30–7).[212] In general, there is a small uptake during rest but there may be considerable release upon exercise. In animals with HE, signs may improve with cage rest and this is speculated to be related to a reduced output of ammonia from muscle. Muscle detoxification of ammonia is why arterial concentrations of ammonia exceed venous concentrations at rest.[213,214] The loss of muscle mass in patients with serious liver disease reduces this systemic capacity for ammonia detoxification and augments development of hyperammonemia. Other peripheral influences affect the plasma ammonia concentration. Hypokalemia is associated with a shift of potassium from intracellular stores to extracellular location. Exchange of cellular potassium for sodium and hydrogen ions results in reduced intracellular and increased extracellular pH. This pH gradient favors the movement and containment of ammonia inside cells. Greater toxic effects may be realized due to CNS involvement in this effect. This phenomenon may explain why some patients with falling or low blood ammonia concentrations have worsening signs of HE. An augmentation of renal ammonia production and increased efflux to the peripheral circulation is also believed to occur in hypokalemia.[215–217]

HEPATIC ENCEPHALOPATHY

Hepatic encephalopathy (HE) is a neurophysiologic disorder of the central nervous system that develops as a result of hepatic insufficiency.[218–221] Disorders causing loss of critical functional hepatic mass (65%–70%) and those associated with portosystemic shunting (hepatofugal blood flow) result

in HE. Hepatic encephalopathy is best considered a clinical syndrome that has a multifactorial etiology. Onset of clinical signs can be acute, chronic, progressive, or episodic. Early or mild signs of HE are underdiagnosed because they may consist of subclinical effects such as drowsiness, anorexia, or lethargy. The spectrum of clinical signs associated with HE in dogs and cats is presented in Table 8–2. It is unknown whether acute and chronic HE share common pathogenetic mechanisms because the events leading to episodes differ. Acute HE may be accompanied by cerebral edema, increased intracranial pressure, and brain herniation. Chronic HE develops in relationship to severe long-standing metabolic derangements in which neuronal responsivity and brain energy requirements may become markedly altered, leading to subtle neurologic consequences.

Pathogenesis

The pathogenesis of HE is controversial despite its intense study by a multitude of investigators and methods over 40 years. The healthy liver acts as an important protective barrier against potentially neurotoxic substances imported from the alimentary canal. When liver function is compromised and/or portosystemic shunting exists, the liver cannot perform its essential metabolic, regulatory, and guardian functions. Subsequently, a number of toxic substances gain entry to the peripheral and cerebral circulation. Numerous toxins have been implicated in the pathogenesis of HE; these and their mechanisms are summarized in Table 30–9. These substances may alter CNS function through a variety of mechanisms, including (1) depression of neuronal electrical activity via modulation of neurotransmitters or their receptors, (2) inhibition of electrogenic pumps or ion channels, or (3) interruption of neuronal oxidative metabolism.

An overview of the mechanisms responsible for the clinical manifestations of HE and the conditions leading to it are provided in Figure 30–11. The clinical signs of HE are variable among patients and in a single patient at different times. Most signs are consistent with neuroinhibitory effects

Table 30–9

PUTATIVE TOXINS IMPLICATED IN THE PATHOPHYSIOLOGY OF HEPATIC ENCEPHALOPATHY

TOXINS	MECHANISMS DESCRIBED BY EXPERIMENTAL EVIDENCE
Ammonia	↓ Microsomal Na, K-dependent ATPase in brain ↓ ATP availability (ATP consumed in glutamine production) ↑ Excitability (if mild ↑ NH_3) Disturbed malate-aspartate shuttle ↑ Glycolysis Brain edema (acute liver failure) ↓ Glutamate, altered glutamate receptors ↑ BBB transport: glutamate, tryptophan, octopamine
↓ Alpha-ketoglutaramate	Diversion from Krebs cycle for NH_3 detoxification ↓ ATP availability
Glutamine	Alters BBB amino acid transport
Aromatic amino acids	↓ Neurotransmitter synthesis: ↓ DOPA Altered neuroreceptors ↑ Production false neurotransmitters
Short chain fatty acids	↓ Microsomal Na, K ATPase in brain Uncouple oxidative phosphorylation Impairs oxygen utilization Displaces tryptophan from albumin → ↑ free tryptophan

False neurotransmitters
  Tyrosine → Octopamine
  Phenylalanine →
    Phenylethylamine
  Methionine → Mercaptans
  (methanethiol and dimethydisulfide)
	
	Impairs norepinephrine action
	Impairs norepinephrine action
	
	Synergistic with other toxins: NH_3, SCFA
	↓ NH_3 detoxification in brain urea cycle
	Are gut derived → fetor hepaticus (distinct breath odor in HE)
	↓ Microsomal Na, K ATPase

Tryptophan	Directly neurotoxic ↑ Serotonin: neuroinhibition
Phenol (derived from phenylalanine/tyrosine)	Synergistic with other toxins ↓ A multitude of cellular enzymes Neurotoxic and hepatotoxic
Bile acids	Membranocytolytic effects alter cell/membrane permeability Blood-brain barrier more permeable to other HE toxins Impaired cellular metabolism due to cytotoxicity
GABA	Neural inhibition: hyperpolarize neuronal membrane ↑ BBB permeability to GABA in HE
Endogenous benzodiazepines	Neural inhibition: hyperpolarize neuronal membrane

although excitatory phenomenon such as seizures, aggression, and hyperexcitability may also develop. In an individual patient, the role of one toxin cannot easily be discerned from that of a combination of toxins. Assessment of causal factors has been complicated by the presence of the numerous metabolic derangements that develop in the circumstance of hepatic insufficiency. It is believed that synergistic and complex metabolic derangements underlie the variations in expression of HE and the contradictory results of investigative efforts of individual causal factors. Electroencephalographic evidence of altered brain function in humans has been used to detect subclinical HE. As veterinarians, we remain unaware of subclinical HE in dogs and cats because of lack of sensitive measures.

Theoretically, the characteristics of important hepatoencephalopathic toxins should fulfill the following criteria based on experimental and clinical studies: (1) they should be nitrogenous, (2) they should be derived from the alimentary canal, (3) they should be either synthesized by gastrointestinal flora or be consumed in the diet, (4) they should be easily detectable in the portal circulation, (5) they should be

metabolized or detoxified in the normal liver, and (6) they should be able to cross the blood-brain barrier and affect the CNS.[219,221] Considering these criteria, a number of hypotheses have been put forward regarding the etiopathogenesis of HE. It is important to remember that although the individual hepatoencephalopathic agents discussed here may play individual roles in HE, their potency may be markedly increased when more than one of them coexist.

Ammonia

The strongest arguments for an encephalopathic agent have been made for ammonia, which is undisputedly neurotoxic.[221,222] If ammonia is infused into animals, it causes profound cerebral signs, including convulsions, somnolence, coma, and death.[223] Hyperammonemia caused by nonhepatic disorders can also result in encephalopathic signs.[199,200,224–229] Ammonia toxicity can develop in the patient with compromised liver function after ingestion of ammonia-generating substances. Therapeutic measures that decrease intestinal

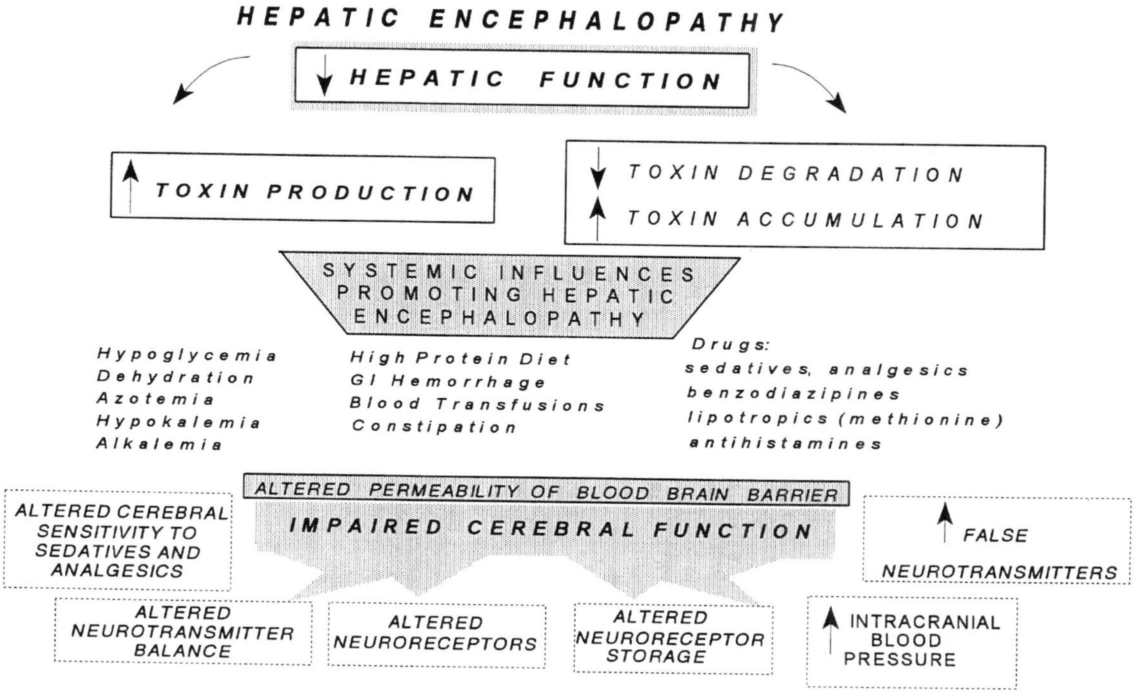

HEPATIC ENCEPHALOPATHY

FIGURE 30-11. Diagrammatic overview of the mechanisms involved with the genesis of hepatic encephalopathy and the conditions leading to it.

production and absorption of ammonia improve clinical status in both human and companion animal patients with hepatic insufficiency.

In HE, ammonia is not adequately detoxified and enters the systemic circulation. Increased alimentary production of ammonia can thus have important clinical consequences. Production of ammonia in the intestines increases following the ingestion of meat, fish, or other high-protein foods, gastrointestinal hemorrhage, constipation, and the ingestion of ammonium salts. Patients showing encephalopathic tendencies that become azotemic are in danger of continued hyperammonemia as a result of alimentary ammonia production from endogenous urea that diffuses into the small bowel. Constipation is detrimental because of the increased risk of ammonia and other alimentary toxin production and absorption from retained colonic residue.

Evidence indicates that a heightened sensitivity to ammonia or an increased blood-brain transfer of ammonia occurs in patients prone to HE. These patients may have high brain ammonia concentrations despite nearly normal systemic blood ammonia concentration.[230,231] This may explain the lack of correlation between circulating plasma ammonia concentrations and HE that has been observed in clinical patients.[231-237] A variety of factors may contribute to these contradictive results including an increased rate of ammonia generation from muscle contraction, variation in individual ammonia tolerance, altered ammonia distribution associated with pH and electrolyte imbalances, and technical difficulties in sample collection and ammonia determinations.

Ammonia has multiple known toxic effects. In modestly increased concentrations, ammonia appears to suppress postsynaptic neuroinhibition resulting in transient excitation. Higher levels of ammonia are inhibitory and are associated with glutamate depletion and altered glutamate receptors.[238,239] Neuroinhibition occurs because glutamate is one of the important excitatory neurotransmitters. Glutamate is considered a major underlying mechanism of HE by some inves-

tigators. Other adverse effects attributed to ammonia include inhibition of Na,K-dependent ATPase, blockade of the GABA receptor complex, altered amino acid membrane transport and impaired cerebral energy metabolism.[240,241] Ammonia is detoxified in the brain by conversion to glutamine.[242] Glutamine synthetase is mainly located in astrocytes where it catalyzes the formation of glutamine from ammonia and glutamate. The CSF levels of ammonia metabolites (glutamine and alpha-ketoglutaramate) correlate with the clinical severity of HE in human patients in some studies but not in others.[237,243-247] Alkalosis facilitates brain uptake of ammonia and precipitates HE in patients with hepatic insufficiency.[248,249] Severe hypokalemia may also precipitate HE by causing metabolic alkalosis or by facilitating ammonia entry into nervous tissue.

GABAergic Hypothesis

The neuronal CNS network functions by continuously balancing inhibitory and excitatory signals. Depending on whether they depolarize or hyperpolarize receptive neurons, transmitters are classified as excitatory or inhibitory.[219] The major excitatory neurotransmitter in the mammalian brain is glutamate; major inhibitory neurotransmitters are glycine and gamma-aminobutyric acid (GABA).[250,251] Neurotransmitters alter the transmembrane potential of neurons bearing specific receptors for them on their surface; hyperpolarization is associated with a neuroinhibitory influence.

The most popular theory regarding the mediation of HE is related to the GABA receptor complex, a member of a family of ion channels that includes the nicotinic acetylcholine receptor and the glycine receptor.[219] There is much experimental evidence that altered GABAergic and glutamatergic neural transmission is associated with HE. An intimate relationship between GABA, glutamine, glutamate, and ammonia

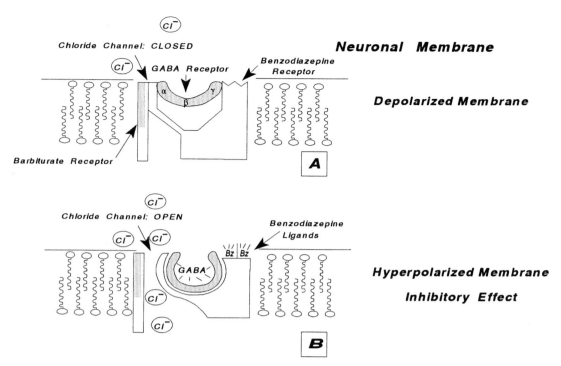

FIGURE 30–12. Diagrammatic representation of the traditional concept of the GABA$_{alpha}$ receptor. *(A)* resting potential, *(B)* hyperpolarized and neuroinhibitory state. (Adapted from Jones EA, Gammal SH. Hepatic Encephalopathy. *In* Arias IM, Jakoby WB, Pepper H, et al. (eds.) The Liver: Biology and Pathology, 2nd ed. New York: Raven Press, 1988, pp. 985–1005.)

that makes scrutiny of individual variables difficult. More than one-third of the central nervous system synapses are GABAergic.[219] Virtually all neurons in the CNS respond to GABA because each bears thousands of synaptic connections. Several types of GABA receptor complexes have been characterized. The GABA$_{alpha}$ complex, as it is traditionally represented, is shown in Figure 30–12.[219] This complex is the receptor for many sedative-hypnotic drugs and other substances such as purines, nicotinamide, proteins, and peptides. The pharmacology of the GABA receptor is complex; it is subdivided into a GABA$_{alpha}$ receptor, a benzodiazepine receptor, and a chloride ionophore (channel through which Cl⁻ passes into the cell), which is thought to contain receptors for barbiturates and other substances (e.g., ethanol and certain gaseous anesthetics). These regions are physically and pharmacologically joined to form a "supramolecular complex."[219] A change in the GABAergic tone can markedly influence cortical and subcortical functions, thus influencing consciousness and motor control.[219]

Thousands of compounds interact at the benzodiazepine site. These may alter the GABA receptor in at least three different ways: (1) *agonists:* act with GABA to promote chloride movement; (2) *benzodiazepine antagonists:* compete with agonists at the binding site but do not promote chloride movement, for example, flumazenil; or (3) *inverse agonists:* compete with other agonists and decrease the ability of GABA to promote chloride movement (these are proconvulsant and can cause anxiety). It is known for certain that agonist drugs which interact with the GABA receptor complex have the ability to worsen hepatic coma; these include benzodiazepines and barbiturates. The overall importance of the GABA-ergic neurotransmitter system in HE is not yet clarified. Some studies have shown increased plasma, CSF, and brain extract concentrations of GABA or GABA-like activity in humans and animals with HE; others have not.[252–262] An increase in brain GABA receptors has been shown in rats and

rabbits with experimentally induced fulminant hepatic failure[263–266] but not in subsequent studies using other models and in humans with HE.[253–256,267–275] It is possible that an as of yet unidentified substance could displace GABA from its receptor and have the same inhibitory influence. One suggested possibility is taurine, which has been isolated from rats with acute and chronic HE.[276] Currently, increased GABA is thought to be associated with HE but its importance in the etiopathogenesis is questionable. GABA is produced in the gut by bacterial action on protein and is normally detoxified in the liver.[277] Thus, increased GABA concentrations are not unexpected in the circumstance of hepatic insufficiency.

Plasma concentrations of benzodiazepine-like activity have been shown to correlate with the degree of HE in humans with hepatic cirrhosis.[219,278] Because benzodiazepines augment GABAergic tone, they may be important contributors to the neuroinhibition that typifies HE.[219] Treatment with flumazenil (a benzodiazepine antagonist) has provided short-term improvement in the mental capacity of some humans with hepatic cirrhosis and in some animal models of HE.[219,279–287] The evidence linking GABA, benzodiazepines, and HE still remains controversial. The administration of benzodiazepine antagonists are not universally effective in reversing the behavioral effects of HE in cirrhotic humans or in animal models of fulminant hepatic failure.[219, 288–290] When they do produce an improved clinical status, the effects are often transient.

The origin of the apparent elevated benzodiazepine concentrations in HE remains unclarified. There is indirect evidence for de novo synthesis of benzodiazepines in mammalian cells. In addition, both diazepam and N-desmethyldiazepam may be produced by gut microorganisms and may also be derived from the diet.[219] Foods such as wheat, potatoes, soybeans, rice, and mushrooms contain a family of 1,4 benzodiazepines, including diazepam and n-desmethyldiazepam. Benzodiazepine agonists, regardless of their source, should be extracted and metabolized by a normal liver. Hepatic disease could permit an increase in free benzodiazepine in peripheral blood as a result of reduced detoxification, decreased concentration of plasma albumin that binds them in the circulation, or portal systemic shunting.

Studies of brain GABA and glutamate concentrations have been complicated by the fact that their metabolism is highly compartmentalized and because ammonia plays a crucial role in regulating their interrelationships.[291] Only a small portion of total GABA and glutamate function as neurotransmitters. As a result, whole tissue amino acid concentrations do not reflect availability or activity of these amino acids in the neurotransmitter pool. Variant results have been generated by different studies of the importance of GABA and glutamate in HE because of this compartmentalization and differences between tissue extraction methods. Glutamate functions as a neurotransmitter by interacting with the excitatory amino acid receptor system as well as interfering with GABA binding. Only minimal information is available regarding the role of glutamine and glutamate as hepatoencephalopathic toxins. Recent determination of cellular uptake and release of L-glutamate have suggested that it is increased immediately adjacent to the neuroreceptor in animals with HE.[292,293]

Amino Acid Balance

Profound abnormalities in plasma amino acid concentrations have been related to HE in human patients and in animal models with HE.[194,294–300] Dogs with portosystemic shunts develop abnormal plasma amino acid concentrations, as previously discussed.[194,301] The role of plasma amino acids in the genesis of HE remains controversial. Changes in the serum BCAA to AAA ratio parallel the severity of liver injury rather than the presence or degree of encephalopathy.[219,302] Alteration in the CSF concentration of amino acids has been shown to correlate with the grade of HE in humans with cirrhosis.[303]

An increased plasma concentration of AAAs relative to BCAAs favors transport of AAAs across the blood-brain barrier. This occurs not only as a result of the increased relative concentration of the AAAs but also because of their competition with BCAA for membrane transport (Figure 30–13). Ammonia-induced increases in brain glutamine may also facilitate brain AAA uptake because they share the same antiporter system.[219] There are several proposed mechanisms by which AAA to BCAA imbalance should generate HE.

These include (1) altered synthesis of brain neurotransmitters derived from amino acids; (2) genesis of false neurotransmitters; and (3) a direct inhibitor influence of tryptophan on brain function. The AAAs may be directly neurotoxic or may exhibit indirect neurotoxicity by suppressing catecholamine neurotransmitter synthesis or by serving as synthetic precursors of false neurotransmitters. Transport of greater amounts of AAA into the brain, particularly tryptophan, could augment neuroinhibition by increasing the cerebral synthesis of serotonin. This could promote deficiency of true neurotransmitters such as noradrenaline and dopamine, which have been associated with HE in some studies.[304,305] Evidence for this is conflicting. Brain concentrations of serotonin and a metabolite of serotonin, 5-hydroxyindole acetic acid (5-HIAA), have been increased in some humans and animal models with HE and in the CSF of humans with fulminant hepatic failure.[306–312] This is contradicted by the finding that brain serotonin concentrations decrease in rats with portocaval anastomoses[313] and that interventional therapy with serotonin does not alter HE.[314]

A reduced synthesis of brain catecholamines may develop due to phenylalanine inhibition of tyrosine hydroxylation to dopamine, the first step in catecholamine synthesis.[315] Depletion of brain noradrenaline and reduced affinity of brain dopamine receptors have also been reported in animal models of HE. The significance of these findings are contradicted by the observation that depletion of brain dopamine and noradrenaline does not induce coma in normal rats.[316]

Tryptophan has received individual attention as a pathogenetic mechanism of HE because profound alterations in its metabolism have been shown in the brain of rats with portacaval anastomosis.[317] Increased plasma free tryptophan levels in HE may result from its displacement from albumin by nonesterifed fatty acids and hypoalbuminemia.[219] Tryptophan concentrations in CSF were shown to differentiate between human patients in HE coma and those with cirrhosis but not in coma. Tryptophan is highly toxic and can produce neurologic signs including sleepiness, attitude changes, and gait disturbances in normal humans[318] and drowsiness, headaches, vomiting, and dizziness in humans with hepatic insufficiency.[319] Coma can be induced in normal dogs by combination tryptophan/phenylalanine infusion; tryptophan alone only causes drowsiness. A mechanism different from HE has been suggested.[320]

Modification of the plasma amino acid balance by infusion of solutions rich in BCAA has been proposed by a number of investigators as an effective therapy in HE. The bene-

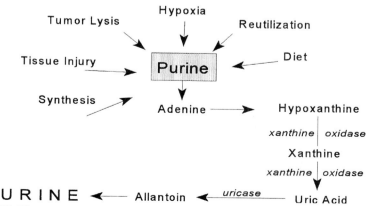

FIGURE 30–13. Diagrammatic representation of the interactions between branched chain amino acids and aromatic amino acids in the etiopathogenesis of hepatic encephalopathy. Consult text for explanation.

fit of such therapy remains controversial.[321-324] Early results of infusion of BCAAs on HE showed benefit; subsequent controlled trials and meta-analysis of previously published clinical trials have not.[325-327] The relevancy of plasma amino acid concentrations to HE remains controversial because plasma amino acid imbalances in humans with chronic HE and dogs with congenital portosystemic shunts also occur in humans with cirrhosis[328] and dogs with chronic active hepatitis[194] lacking clinical signs of HE. These observations argue against plasma amino acid balance having a central role in HE. The many conflicting results regarding the role of altered amino acid balance in HE have led to a unifying theory that relates ammonia and amino acid hypotheses.[329] An example is the ammonia-augmented passage of glutamine, tryptophan, and octopamine (discussed later) across the blood-brain barrier.[330]

Abnormal or False Neurotransmitters

Production of abnormal or "false" neurotransmitters probably contributes to the genesis of HE. Decreased concentrations of the normal excitatory neurotransmitters norepinephrine and dopamine and increased concentrations of the normal inhibitory neurotransmitter serotonin have been shown. Of particular concern are neuroinhibitory metabolites derived from tyrosine and phenylalanine (Figure 30–13). Impaired catecholamine synthesis associated with tyrosine accumulation may result in increased production of octopamine, a weak "false" neurotransmitter that can be stored and released at nerve endings. High intracellular concentrations of phenylalanine compete with tyrosine for binding to the enzyme tyrosine-3 hydroxylase. This impedes formation of dopamine necessary for norepinephrine synthesis. Phenylalanine can be metabolized to phenylethylamine, another "false" neurotransmitter.[331,332] Both octopamine and phenylethylamine can displace norepinephrine and dopamine from synaptic vesicles; once released, the normal neurotransmitters are degraded, leading to their depletion. When a "false" neurotransmitter acts, it replaces a normal neurotransmitter and results in neuroinhibition. "False" neurotransmitters also suppress synthesis of normal neurotransmitters by competitive enzyme inhibition and can act as low-potency catecholamine receptor agonists. Study of the association between the "false" neurotransmitters and HE has produced inconsistent and contradictory evidence. Both increased octopamine and phenylethylamine concentrations in brain and CSF have been demonstrated in animals with HE.[333-335] A positive correlation between the degree of HE and the plasma concentrations of octopamine was shown in humans and dogs. However, in other studies, neither reduced brain catecholamine concentrations nor increased octopamine concentrations were found at autopsy in humans with HE, and infusions of large amounts of octopamine into the cerebroventricular system of rats did not produce HE. In consideration of the concentrations that false neurotransmitters attain in liver disease and their behavioral and electrophysiologic effects, it is unlikely that they play a key role in HE.[219]

Mercaptans/Methionine

The toxicity of methionine administered to dogs and humans with hepatic insufficiency has implicated its importance in the genesis of HE where it is believed to act synergis-

tically with ammonia and short chain fatty acids (discussed later).[206,336,337] Methionine can be metabolized to mercaptans such as methanethiol and dimethyl disulfide by intestinal organisms. The liver may also directly contribute to the formation of methanethiol.[338] High concentrations of mercaptans can reversibly induce coma in animals and suppress brain Na/K ATPase activity. However, the concentration of mercaptans in patients with liver failure are not sufficient to induce overt HE. Furthermore, studies of the association of mercaptans and methionine to HE have yielded contradictory results, complicated by invalid biochemical determinations. The latest work has not shown a primary role for mercaptans in the pathogenesis of HE.[219,338-341]

Short Chain Fatty Acids

Short chain fatty acids (SCFAs) are considered to be minor HE toxins that act synergistically with ammonia and methionine, and possibly other factors.[206,207,337] Infusion of fatty acids has been shown to displace tryptophan from albumin binding, thus increasing neurotoxic free tryptophan. Infusion of fatty acids has also been shown to inhibit the Na/K ATPase in neurons. The blood concentration of SCFAs necessary to induce coma in experimental animals is greater than that found in humans with HE. In addition, the circulating blood concentration of SCFA in cirrhotic humans correlates better with the severity of the hepatic disease than with the expression of HE.[342-343]

Impaired hepatic oxidation of long chain fatty acids has been shown to generate SCFA. Most SCFAs are generated during intestinal bacterial metabolism of carbohydrates, principally fiber components metabolized by anaerobic bacteria in the colon. Acetic, propionic, and butyric acid represent the major SCFAs produced in the colon where they are rapidly absorbed. The administration of medium chain triglycerides can lead to the accumulation of SCFAs in humans with cirrhosis where they have been incriminated as inducing HE.[267] Most experience however suggests that direct administration of SCFAs is not deleterious in patients susceptible to HE.[219,315,344]

Phenols

Phenols are lipophilic substances, derived from the aromatic amino acids phenylalanine and tyrosine, that are neurotoxic and hepatotoxic. Plasma-free phenol concentrations have been shown to be increased in fulminant hepatic failure.[345] Little is known about their importance as an initiating factor for HE. Concentrations of phenols in patients with hepatic coma are at least four times lower than those that induce coma in normal animals.[219]

Bile Acids

Bile acids increase in the peripheral circulation in patients with hepatic insufficiency or portosystemic shunting. An accumulation of membranocytolytic bile acids (bile acids that undesirably alter membrane permeability) has been shown in peripheral circulation, in bile, and in liver tissue in many forms of serious liver disease. Bile acid concentrations also increase in the CSF and brain tissue of patients with hepatic failure. A direct association between HE and the concentration of bile acids in plasma or tissues has not been demonstrated. Bile acid concentrations in blood do not correlate with the severity of HE, and many patients with high bile acid concentrations are not encephalopathic. Bile acids may play an adjunctive role with other factors in the production of HE through their ability to modify cell membrane permeability allowing greater distribution of other toxins. In addition, they may impair cell energy production or metabolism in other ways. Increased permeability of the blood-brain barrier is one possible mechanism whereby bile acids may facilitate development of HE.

Blood-Brain Barrier

The blood-brain barrier (BBB) is the anatomic structure composed of tight junctions between adjacent endothelial cells in cerebral capillaries. It provides a less permeable barrier than typical systemic capillaries and thus restricts passage of a wide range of substances into the brain. In liver failure, there may be increased permeability of the BBB, allowing brain access to normally excluded neuroreactive agents.[346-348] Studies of the BBB permeability in animal models of HE have produced conflicting results. Although increased permeability has been persuasively shown in acute hepatic failure, these changes have been argued to reflect agonal microvascular changes.[349,350] It is uncertain that a major change in BBB permeability develops in chronic hepatic failure because the nature and extent of the lesions remain controversial.[351-354] It is unknown whether abnormal permeability of the BBB contributes to HE or indicates the presence of other metabolic derangements. An increase in the blood-brain transfer of ammonia has been suggested by results of some studies.[230,355] It is argued that increased plasma concentrations of substances such as ammonia, octanoate, mercaptans, phenol, or bile acids may increase permeability of the BBB by acting on capillary enzymes involved in the regulation of cerebral blood flow, altering the function of membrane transporters and/or increasing vessel membrane fluidity or vessel patency.[219,356,357]

Neurologic Lesions

The development of gross pathologic changes in the CNS depends on whether HE is acute or chronic. Histologic changes are usually mild and nonspecific.[358-360] In most patients with portosystemic encephalopathy, no significant changes in neuron structure are observed.[361-362] Neuronal necrosis is rare unless the cause of HE is an hepatic toxin that has widespread cellular toxicity. Cerebral atrophy has been reported in CT scans of cirrhotic humans that have had recurrent HE. The causal mechanism(s) remains unknown, although it has been shown that the brains of these patients use less oxygen and have reduced blood flow. Ammonium salt infusion into experimental animals results in signs consistent with HE and polymicrocavitation and Alzheimer type II astrocyte proliferation in the brain.[363] Similar histologic lesions have been described in humans and animals dying after a protracted course of HE.[343,360,363-365] High intracranial pressure, cerebral edema, and brain herniation may be complications of acute HE. Vasogenic edema may also develop and is believed to be associated with increased BBB permeability, failure of cell osmotic regulation, and expansion of the extracellular space.[366,367]

Uric Acid Metabolism

Serum uric acid concentrations are increased in animals with surgically created portosystemic shunts and in some clinical patients with hepatic insufficiency.[49,368] Uric acid is an organic acid that is a by-product of purine nucleotide catabolism.[369] Purines are synthesized from nonpurine compounds such as simple carbon or nitrogen compounds or are derived from reutilization of other protein subunits. The scheme of uric acid synthesis is illustrated in Figure 30–14. Uric acid is produced from oxidation of hypoxanthine and xanthine by xanthine oxidase.[369] In most dogs, uric acid is further oxidized to allantoin, a water soluble product eliminated in urine. Most uric acid is transformed into allantoin via the action of uricase, an enzyme present in high concentration within hepatic peroxisomes. In the dog, other tissues also contain high amounts of xanthine oxidase including the lungs, intestines, and blood.[369] Uric acid that is not converted to allantoin is distributed throughout the body as monosodium urate. Some dogs, particularly Dalmatians, have an inborn error of uric acid metabolism whereby they cannot transform uric acid to allantoin. The exact nature of the metabolic defect is controversial.[370-375] It is believed this breed has subnormal transport of uric acid across the hepatocyte cell membrane and a lower ability to oxidize uric acid to allantoin. Dalmatians develop hyperuricosuria, relative hyperuricemia (compared with other dogs), hypoallantoinemia, and hypoallantoinuria.[375-377] Serum urate concentration in Dalmatians ranges from 0.3 to 4.0 mg/dl,[374-376,378] roughly two to four times as much as other dog breeds.[377,379,380] In animals with normal uric acid metabolism but insufficient hepatic function or portosystemic shunting, serum uric acid concentration may increase due to impaired availability or function of hepatic uricase. Hyperuricemia also develops in patients with diffuse tissue destruction or inflammation causing increased catabolism of purine nucleotides.[381,382] Examples of such conditions include pyometritis, diffuse tissue trauma, hypoxia, hemorrhagic shock, multicentric lymphosarcoma (before chemotherapy), and tumor lysis syndrome.[381-383] Study of uric acid as a clinical test for liver disease in the dog showed it was relatively insensitive.[384]

Ammonium urate crystalluria may develop during hyperammonemia. When urine pH is more than 6.0, ammonium ion can combine with uric acid to form insoluble ammonium acid urate.[385,386] Ammonium ions enhance precipitation of urates. When increased uric acid concentrations develop in a patient with hepatic insufficiency, the stage is set for ammonium biurate precipitation. Ammonium biurate crystalluria and/or calculi, especially in young animals, indicates the need for a thorough investigation for a congenital portosystemic shunt. See Chapters 8 and 35 for further discussion of biurate crystalluria and illustration of their morphology.

Coagulation Proteins

The liver plays a central role in coagulation homeostasis. In humans, it is estimated that hemostatic problems develop in approximately 70% to 85% of patients with confirmed serious liver disease. However, only a small number of these demonstrate pathologic bleeding.[387-389] It is unknown what percentage of dogs or cats with liver disease demonstrate bleeding tendencies because no large population of such patients has been studied.

The liver is the single site of origin of all the coagulation proteins except Factor VIII, von Willebrand's factor

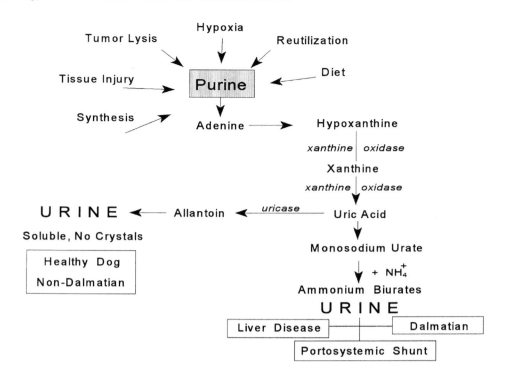

FIGURE 30-14. Diagrammatic representation of the metabolism of uric acid in health and in the patient with hepatic disease.

(FVIII:RA), calcium, and locally released tissue thromboplastin; a summary of these is provided in Table 30–10. It also synthesizes and/or regulates anticoagulant and fibrinolytic proteins, including the activity of plasminogen, the physiologic inhibitor of plasmin, antithrombin III (AT III), alpha$_2$-antiplasmin, and alpha$_2$-macroglobulin, and the plasmin activators.[388-391] The normal coagulation, anticoagulation, and fibrinolytic systems as they are conventionally drawn are shown in Figures 30–15 and 30–16. Tests evaluating the coagulation system are discussed in Chapter 8.

The prothrombin complex factors, Factors II, VII, IX, and X, and protein C (a coagulation inhibitor), depend on vitamin K for normal activity. The active forms of these factors contain carboxylated glutamic acid residues that require vitamin K for formation. The carboxyglutamate residues bind calcium essential for adherence of the coagulation proteins to phospholipid-rich surfaces (platelets, collagen). Lack of vitamin K impairs normal carboxylation, resulting in nonfunctional precursor proteins. These nonfunctional factors are present in plasma and may be measured as evidence of insufficient vitamin K activation; they are referred to as "proteins induced by vitamin K absence or antagonism" (PIVKAs).[392-399] Prothrombin formed in the absence of vitamin K is not converted to thrombin; this disables both sides of the coagulation cascade in the common pathway.

In health, vitamin K deficiency is rare. The adequacy of vitamin K depends on an individual's diet, intestinal bacterial flora, and adequacy of intestinal absorption. Phylloquinone (K$_1$), the major source in most mammals, is derived in the diet from green leafy vegetables. This form of vitamin K is actively absorbed in the proximal small intestine and is lipid soluble.[399] Menaquinone (K$_2$) is produced by intestinal bacteria in the ileum and colon; E. coli and Bacteroides organisms have been shown to be largely responsi-

ble.[400] Vitamin K is rapidly concentrated in the liver following absorption, but without continued repletion a deficiency develops within weeks. An overview of vitamin K interaction with the coagulation system, the epoxidase cycle, and differences in the sources of this vitamin is presented in Figure 30–17.

Deficiency of vitamin K may develop in a number of different clinical circumstances including dietary restriction of foodstuffs containing K$_1$; gut sterilization; fat malabsorption; or ingestion of vitamin K antagonists. Inadequate ingestion of preformed vitamin K in food only leads to deficiency if intestinal microbial synthesis is concurrently compromised.

Table 30-10

ORIGINS AND BIOLOGIC HALF-LIVES OF COAGULATION PROTEINS

PROTEIN	SITE OF SYNTHESIS	HALF-LIFE
Factor XIII	Liver	3–4 days
Prekallikrein	Liver	3–4 days
Factor XII	Liver	3–4 days
Factor XI	Liver	4–5 days
Factor X	Liver	3–4 days
Factor IX	Liver	20–24 hours
Factor VIII:C	Liver/Endothelial cells	5–12 hours
Factor VIII:Ag	Liver/Endothelial cells	8–24 hours
Factor VIII:vWF	Endothelial cells	24–40 hours
Factor VII	Liver	2–6 hours
Factor V	Liver	12–36 hours
Prothrombin	Liver	2–3 days
Fibrinogen	Liver	2–4 days
Plasminogen	Liver	2 days
Antithrombin III	Liver	12 hours
Protein C	Liver	?

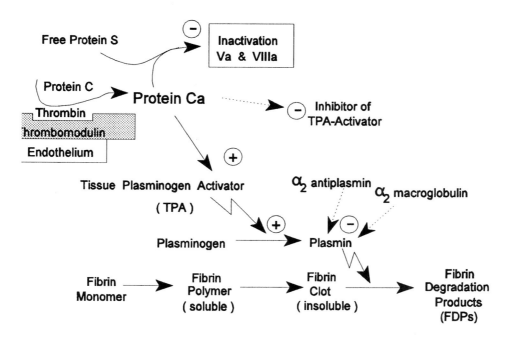

FIGURE 30-15. Diagrammatic representation of the classical coagulation pathways including the sites of action of antithrombin III and protein C.

In this scenario, vitamin K deficiency develops within 14 to 30 days.[387,401–403] Certain antibiotics have been shown to directly induce vitamin K deficiency in humans and animals. The most common problems have been reported with the beta-lactam antibiotic second-generation cephalosporins such as moxalactam and cefoperazone[404–407] and with certain sulfa drugs (sulfaquinoxaline).[408–411] Beta-lactam antibiotics inhibit vitamin K carboxylase.[419] Sulfaquinoxaline induces hypoprothrombinemia due to a synergistic inhibitory effect from the component drug moieties on vitamin K epoxide reductase,

impairing reuse of a single vitamin K molecule in procoagulant activation.[413]

Protein C, a vitamin K–dependent serine protease zymogen synthesized in the liver, is activated by exposure to thrombin in the presence of endothelial cofactor (thrombomodulin).[391] In vitro, protein C neutralizes an inactivator of plasminogen activator, thereby activating plasminogen. It also inhibits activated Factors VIII and V; see Figure 30–16. It is thus recognized as a natural inhibitor of blood coagulation, which also participates in fibrinolysis. Low levels of protein C

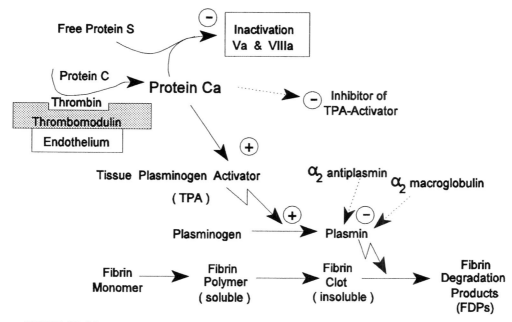

FIGURE 30-16. Simplified representation of the fibrinolytic cascade and anticoagulant effects of proteins C and S.

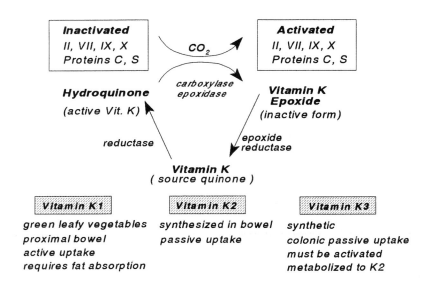

FIGURE 30–17. Vitamin K epoxidase cycle and the different forms and origins of vitamin K.

activity and antigen have been detected in humans with hepatocellular disease. It is unknown to what extent vitamin K deficiency disables the normal modulation of clotting by its influence on protein C in the clinical patient.

Fibrinogen is exclusively synthesized in hepatocytes. The liver has a huge capacity for fibrinogen synthesis and it is only with acute hepatic failure or decompensated chronic hepatic disease that synthetic failure occurs. Normally, about 75% of the total fibrinogen is located in the intravascular compartment where it is readily available for coagulation purposes.[414] Excessive catabolism of fibrinogen may occur when liver disease is associated with disseminated intravascular coagulation (DIC). Once fibrinogen is transformed to fibrin, proteolysis by plasmin releases fibrin monomers and other degradation products that are cleared by the reticuloendothelial cells in the liver and spleen. Increases in fibrin degradation products (FDPs) occur as a result of accelerated fibrinolysis or because of impaired clearance of fibrin monomers by the liver.

Antithrombin III (AT III) is an alpha$_2$-globulin synthesized primarily by the liver.[415–417] It is the principal plasma protein responsible for the progressive inactivation of thrombin. In the absence of heparin, AT III slowly inactivates the serine proteases by irreversibly binding with their activated forms. Factors II, VII, IX, X, XI, and XII, plasmin, and kallikrein are inactivated by AT III; see Figure 30–15. The binding of AT III to coagulation proteins is markedly increased in the presence of heparin. Heparin assumes a catalytic role in this inactivation and dissociates when the irreversible AT III-serine protease complex forms. Heparin is then available to catalyze multiple rounds of protease inactivation. Patients with low AT III concentrations are predisposed to thrombosis because they lack the ability to abolish coagulation factor activation. Unrestricted coagulation becomes a risk in this circumstance. The thromboembolic potential of a patient with AT III between 50% and 75% of normal is moderate, and becomes marked when less than 50% of control plasma. AT III concentrations have been proposed as a reliable index of the severity of cirrhosis.[418–422] Low AT III levels develop as a result of synthetic failure, increased catabolism, altered transcapillary flux, or as a result of a consumptive coagulopathy. Low AT III levels are a principal marker of DIC. In the patient with serious liver disease, the presence of low concentrations of coagulation factors and platelet dysfunction overshadows the thrombotic tendency induced by low AT III concentrations. These patients have a greater potential for bleeding problems than for thromboembolism.

In dogs with chronic liver disease induced by dimethylnitrosamine administration, the decline in AT III concentration paralleled that of albumin, implying synthetic failure or third space protein distribution; some of these animals developed ascites.[423] Considering that the size of the AT III molecule is very similar to albumin (65,000 daltons), it is possible that AT III extravasated into ascitic effusion. In the author's hospital, measurements of AT III in dogs with liver disease have shown that values decline as hepatic function worsens; values equal to or less than 50% normal plasma activity are associated with severe dysfunction and can develop in dogs with either acute or chronic liver injury. The AT III concentration was the most discriminant of the routinely evaluated coagulation parameters in differentiating parenchymal and cholestatic disorders in humans with serious liver disorders. Patients with parenchymal disease had low AT III concentrations that indicated synthetic failure or DIC.[421] Other studies have confirmed that AT III concentrations are usually low in human patients with histologically confirmed cirrhosis.[419–428]

The fibrinolytic system normally assists in the overall homeostatic balance of coagulation.[414,429,430] This system depends on the production of the serine protease plasmin, which is derived from plasminogen, a protein synthesized in hepatocytes and endothelium. Plasmin is responsible for maintaining vascular patency by digestion of fibrin.[429] About 60% of plasminogen is present in the intravascular compartment where its activity is controlled by specific antiproteases (alpha$_2$-antiplasmin, alpha$_2$-macroglobulin) which also are synthesized by hepatocytes (Figure 30–16). Liver disease may disrupt the coagulation inhibitor and fibrinolytic systems in a number of ways. There may be increases in plasminogen activators due to impaired hepatic clearance, reduced levels of plasminogen and alpha$_2$-antiplasmin due to impaired hepatic synthesis, reduced protein C due to vitamin K deficiency, or accelerated consumption secondary to DIC.[388,390,414]

Coagulation Disorders in Liver Disease

Coagulation abnormalities that develop in patients with liver disease are complex because they are multifactorial and depend on the balance between various components of the coagulation, anticoagulation, and fibrinolytic reactants. Hemorrhagic complications in patients with liver disease are usually associated with provocative local factors such as gastritis, gastrointestinal ulcers, invasive procedures, or other medical problems. Spontaneous hemorrhage is rare.[431-433] Numerous pathophysiologic mechanisms can be involved as detailed in general in Table 30–11. Specific abnormalities characterized in human beings and dogs with spontaneous or experimentally induced liver disease are listed in Table 30–12.

Deficiency of clotting factors develops in spontaneous and experimentally induced hepatic disease. Coagulation factor deficiency may develop in patients with liver disease as a result of synthetic failure, acquired qualitative factor defects, excessive factor consumption, excessive proteolysis, or inadequate clearance of activated factors by the hepatic Kupffer cells; these are detailed in Table 30–11. The severity of coagulation abnormalities seems to depend on the degree and type of hepatocellular injury; these are discussed in detail later.[414,434,435] Specific factor deficiencies have been described in dogs with various types of liver disease.[434,435] In dogs undergoing experimental CCl_4 hepatic injury, dramatic reductions in Factors II, VII, and IX developed within 48 hours and resolved within 5 days. Hepatectomized dogs given intravenous glucose survive for 20 hours and then succumb to hemorrhagic diathesis owing to coagulation factor deficiencies.[436-438] Blood transfusions can prolong survival. During synthetic failure, the onset of factor deficiency is influenced by factor utilization, factor activation, and factor half-life. The factor half-lives vary from hours to days and are shown in Table 30–10. Although one would expect that factor half-life would largely determine the expression of factor deficiency in acute severe hepatic failure, experimental study of hepatectomized dogs has shown that factor disappearance is more rapid than is predicted on the basis of factor half-life (Table 30–13). Comparison of the PT and APTT in dogs (n = 32) with naturally occurring hepatic disease showed that abnormal clotting times (prolongation or shortening) may develop, but that neither test is consistently superior.[439] Prolongation was more common than shortening of the coagula-

Table 30–11

CAUSES OF COAGULOPATHIES ASSOCIATED WITH HEPATOBILIARY DISORDERS

↓ Factor Availability	↓ synthesis:	procoagulants activator proteins inhibitor proteins
	↑ utilization:	DIC
↓ Activation procoagulants anticoagulants plasminogen		
↑ Fibrinolysis	↑ plasminogen activators ↓ plasminogen inhibitors	
↑ Tissue Thromboplastin Release	↑ activation coagulation cascade massive hepatic necrosis	
↑ Activity Anticoagulants	Acute-phase protein response ↓ synthesis inhibitors ↓ hepatic clearance (FDPs) ↑ rate of production	
↓ Activity Anticoagulants	synthetic failure vitamin K inadequacy (proteins C and S)	
Synthesis Abnormal Coagulants	secondary to hepatic disease (e.g., dysfibrinogenemia)	
↓ Platelet Function	acquired thrombasthenia expression of latent von Willebrand's diagnosis	
↓ Platelet Numbers	splenic sequestration due to portal hypertension immune-mediated thrombocytopenia impaired bone marrow production	

Table 30–12

HEMOSTATIC DEFECTS IDENTIFIED IN HUMAN AND CANINE* PATIENTS WITH VARIOUS HEPATOBILIARY DISORDERS

COAGULATIVE FACTOR	SPECIFIC ABNORMALITIES	ASSOCIATED CONDITIONS
Platelets		
Thrombocytopenia	↓ platelets	Cirrhosis* Neoplasia* Congestive splenomegaly DIC* Hepatectomy
Thrombocytosis	↑ platelets	Hepatoma Hepatoblastoma
Thrombocytopathia Defects	↓ platelet aggregation	Cirrhosis Viral hepatitis
Vitamin K–Dependent Factors (II, VII, IX, X)	↓ factor activation ↓ synthesis	Extrahepatic cholestasis* Hepatic failure Hepatectomy* Hepatic failure* Hepatic necrosis* Cirrhosis*
Factor V	↓ synthesis	Hepatic failure*
Factor VIII	↑ or normal synthesis	Acute or chronic disease* Extrahepatic cholestasis* Biliary cirrhosis Hepatoma Neoplasia* Viral hepatitis
Fibrinogen	↑ synthesis	Acute or chronic disease* Extrahepatic cholestasis Biliary cirrhosis Hepatoma Metastatic neoplasia Hepatic necrosis*
	↓ synthesis	Hepatic failure* Cirrhosis*
	↑ consumption	DIC* Hemorrhage* Loss into ascites
	dysfibrinogenemia	Viral hepatitis Cirrhosis Severe necrosis Hepatoma
Protein C	↓ synthesis	Hepatic failure
Factor XI, XII, XIII	↓ synthesis	Cirrhosis* Severe hepatitis Hepatoma Degeneration*
Prekallikrein	↓ synthesis	Cirrhosis Viral hepatitis
Plasminogen Activator	↓ clearance	Cirrhosis
Plasminogen	↓ synthesis or ↑ consumption	Hepatic failure Hepatic lipidosis Hepatic necrosis
Antithrombin III	↓ synthesis or ↑ consumption	Viral hepatitis Cirrhosis* Hepatoma DIC* Hepatic necrosis*
	↑ or normal synthesis abnormal protein	Extrahepatic cholestasis Primary biliary cirrhosis Diffuse liver disease Cirrhosis
Fibrin Degradation Products (FDPs)	↓ clearance	Diffuse liver injury

*Characterized also in dogs and cats.

tion times, but abnormalities were not frequent enough to warrant use of either test for screening or diagnostic purposes in the detection of liver disease. The sensitivity of the PT and APTT for recognizing borderline "bench test" coagu-

Table 30–13

EFFECT OF HEPATECTOMY ON CLOTTING FACTORS, PROTHROMBIN TIME (PT),
PARTIAL THROMBOPLASTIN TIME (APTT), THROMBIN TIME (TT),
AND FDPS IN THE DOG

CLOTTING FACTOR	PRE	0.5 HR	3 HR	6 HR	8 HR
			% of Presurgical Factor Level		
Factor V	100	90	38	18	5
Factor VII	100	81	35	14	5
Factor VIII	100	73	38	25	10
Factor VIII:RA	100	236	298	374	266
Factor X	100	91	40	17	10
Fibrinogen	100	93	38	16	5
Antithrombin	100	63	62	38	14
PT, APTT, TT			each test $>\uparrow$ 10 X		
			FDP expressed as μg/dl		
FDPs	< 10	< 10	< 10	< 10	< 10

Unpublished observations of BF Feldman, DR Strombeck.

lopathies was improved by using a dilution of the patient's citrated platelet-poor plasma. Only 15% of dogs with hepatic disease showed abnormal PT and APTT when routinely measured, but with testing done on diluted plasma this increased to 66%. In dinitrosamine-induced hepatic injury in the dog, a model for chronic hepatopathy, a prolongation of the APTT developed before prolongation of the PT.[423]

Hepatitis caused by infectious canine hepatitis adenovirus results in a precipitous decline in Factor VII activity within 2 days and a comparatively modest decline in fibrinogen.[440] In dogs with 70% hepatectomy, Factor VII activity decreases to almost zero within 1 to 2 days; Factor V reduces by 50%.[437]

Vitamin K deficiency can occur in the hepatobiliary patient that has completely obstructed bile flow. In the absence of bile, steatorrhea and vitamin K malabsorption occurs. Vitamin K deficiency may also occur as a result of inadequate rejuvenation of the vitamin in the epoxidase cycle (see Figure 30–17) in patients with severe hepatic parenchymal disease. In the author's experience, a substantial number of animals with severe parenchymal and intrahepatic cholestatic liver disease develop increased PIVKAs in the presence of a normal PT; these normalize following implementation of vitamin K therapy. When this response is documented, chronic weekly or biweekly treatment with vitamin K$_l$ is used in management of chronic liver disease.

Disseminated intravascular coagulation may be a sequela to a variety of hepatic disorders as well as viral diseases that can lead to hepatic disease.[387,414,440–444] Pathogenetic mechanisms include release of thromboplastic substances from damaged hepatocytes, decreased hepatic clearance of gut origin endotoxins that trigger coagulation, impaired hepatic clearance of activated coagulation factors, reduced concentration or activity of AT III and stagnation of blood flow in mesenteric collaterals.[414]

Clotting factors are depleted by DIC. As clotting factors are consumed, the patient with hepatic insufficiency is incapable of regenerating adequate quantities of new factors to restore the escalating coagulant needs. At first, only a few factors are consumed, such as Factor VIII, which is one of the first to be depleted. A cascade of events soon follows including development of hypofibrinogenemia, production of nonfunctional fibrinogen (dysfibrinogenemia), and depletion of clotting factors, platelets, plasminogen, and protease inhibitors. The severity of DIC worsens when the liver loses the ability to "clear" activated factors and plasminogen activators from the circulation. A considerable increase in the production of FDPs develops as DIC worsens. Plasmin activators stimulate digestion of fibrinogen and fibrin. When the ability of the liver to remove FDPs is overwhelmed, they accumulate in the circulation and interfere with fibrin polymerization and platelet function and thus encourage pathologic bleeding. The liver is the recipient of the most devastating consequences of DIC. Preexisting hepatobiliary disorders can worsen under the influence of these circumstances. The development of microthrombi occlude sinusoidal flow and can cause local damage to hepatic parenchyma.

If synthetic failure is associated with chronic liver disease, there is little chance of recovery from DIC. However, if hepatic functional insufficiency is reversible, aggressive support may be successful and should consist of fresh blood transfusions supplying coagulation factors, functional platelets, the activators and inhibitors of plasminogen and plasma AT III, combined with minidose heparin (50 to 75 μ/kg SQ TID) and mini-dose aspirin (0.5 mg/kg PO or rectal BID). It is essential to remember that AT III is required for heparin to provide an anticoagulant effect. For this reason, whole fresh blood or plasma transfusions are necessary when using heparin to treat the liver patient that has DIC. Heparin therapy for treating coagulapathies associated with severe hepatic disease remains controversial. High-dose heparin can cause massive bleeding in coagulopathies due to deficiency of clotting factors, high levels of circulating anticoagulants, or abnormal clotting factors. Mini-dose heparin is much safer and clinically appears to be efficacious in the veterinary patient with hepatic insufficiency and DIC in the author's experience. Care is warranted if low-dose aspirin is used in a cirrhotic patient with ascites because even low levels of salicylates may impair renal prostaglandin synthesis. Aspirin is a highly protein-bound drug and increased quantities of free drug will occur in the hypoalbuminemic patient. If aspirin is used in this circumstance, concurrent treatment with furosemide may protect renal prostaglandin production.

Thrombocytopenia associated with liver disease can result

from increased clearance of platelets by the spleen associated with portal hypertension or immune-mediated events, from increased consumption as in DIC, and occasionally from secondary reduction of thrombocyte production in the bone marrow. Abnormal platelet function is probably more common than considered or documented in these patients. This likely underlies some of the bleeding tendencies observed in patients that are subsequently shown to have normal coagulation profiles. The high prevalence of von Willebrand's disease in dogs must also be considered as a cause of platelet dysfunction. Thrombocytopathy may be identified by evaluation of a mucosal bleeding time or platelet aggregation studies using an aggregometer or, more simply, by observation of clot retraction.

As previously mentioned, serious hemorrhage seldom spontaneously develops in hepatic disease even when the liver is severely damaged.[445] Bleeding tendencies after venipuncture or upon biopsy are recognized most often. Spontaneous bleeding associated with hepatic disease is usually in the gastrointestinal tract. In humans, liver disease is associated with a gastric microvasculopathy that leads to gastrointestinal hemorrhage. A tendency to develop gastroduodenal ulcerations has been noted in veterinary patients with hepatic disease, particularly patients with cirrhosis and chronic bile duct occlusion.[446]

The patient with serious liver disease should remain a suspect for hemorrhagic complications no matter what the results of a clotting profile. The tenuous balance of the coagulation/anticoagulation systems can be upset by a procedure that initiates only small amounts of bleeding. An upset in this hemostatic balance can turn into critical bleeding, hypotensive shock, DIC, and death. The clinician therefore should always anticipate this eventuality and have on hand a ready source of fresh blood or plasma for crisis intervention.

Bilirubin Metabolism

BILIRUBIN FORMATION. Bilirubin, the major pigment in bile, is a product of hemoprotein catabolism. Hemoprotein sources include hemoglobin from senescent erythrocytes and ineffective erythropoiesis, myoglobin from muscle, and a number of hemoproteins having short half-lives (cytochromes, catalase, and peroxidases).[448] Hemoglobin constitutes greater than 90% of all heme in the body. Considering that it is largely derived from senescent erythrocytes, it has a slow turnover: 120 days in dogs and 90 days in cats. The turnover of myoglobin is very low and contributes only a small fraction of heme for bilirubin synthesis. Collectively, the many short-lived hemoproteins contribute 25% to 35% of the total heme pigment. In normal dogs, it is estimated that 67% of total bilirubin produced is derived from erythrocytes, 28% from hepatic hemoproteins, and 5% from ineffective erythropoiesis. An overview of heme degradation and bilirubin synthesis is provided in Figure 30–18.

Senescent erythrocytes are engulfed by phagocytic cells of the RE system where they are hemolyzed. Macrophages located in the bone marrow, spleen, liver, and lymph nodes can participate in this process. Hemoglobin released in circulation combines with haptoglobin, an alpha$_2$-globulin, and is transported to the RE system. The carrier protein is degraded along with hemoglobin during heme catabolism. Heme is dissociated from globin and transferred to heme oxygenase in the endoplasmic reticulum of the RE cell; this also may occur in hepatocytes.[449] Heme oxygenase is one of the rate-limiting factors in bilirubin formation; it is inhibited by large concentrations of other protoporphyrin complexes. The globin moiety of hemoglobin is eventually degraded to amino acids for reutilization.

A reduction of ferric (Fe^{+3}) heme to ferrous (Fe^{+2}) heme occurs through the action of microsomal NADPH-cytochrome c reductase. This complex is further modified to a ferric iron-biliverdin complex and carbon monoxide, which is eliminated through the lungs. Released iron binds to iron-carrying proteins, transferrin, and ferritin for storage or reutilization. Biliverdin is subsequently converted to unconjugated bilirubin via biliverdin reductase, an enzyme abundant in most mammalian tissues but having highest concentration in the liver, spleen, and kidney. The average daily production of bilirubin from hemoprotein in normal adult mammals is approximately 3 to 5 mg/kg.[450]

HEPATOCELLULAR UPTAKE. Approximately 75% of unconjugated or indirect reacting bilirubin is released into the circulation. At physiologic pH, unconjugated bilirubin is relatively insoluble in aqueous solutions and must bind with plasma proteins for circulatory transport. Albumin is the

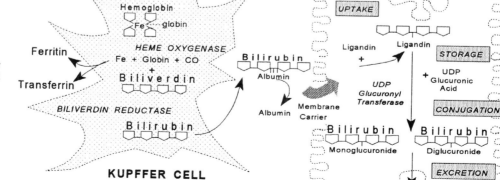

FIGURE 30–18. An overview of heme degradation and bilirubin synthesis.

major transport protein. Albumin-bound bilirubin in the vascular compartment equilibrates with protein-bound bilirubin in the extravascular pool and pigment bound to intracellular organelles. Albumin has a great capacity and high binding affinity for unconjugated bilirubin, which limits its glomerular filtration. Only a very small amount of unconjugated bilirubin remains unbound. Because it is readily miscible with phospholipids it is readily distributed to the intracellular compartment where it can remain for long intervals.[451] At high concentrations (exceeding 35 mg/dl), which are relatively uncommon, unconjugated bilirubin can bind to sites on albumin that have a low binding affinity. These "loosely" bound molecules can be easily displaced by other compounds that compete for protein binding; this increases tissue deposition of unconjugated bilirubin. Some of these agents and circumstances that promote displacement are shown in Table 30–14.

Albumin-bound unconjugated bilirubin is transferred to hepatocytes for conversion to the water soluble form: conjugated or direct-reacting bilirubin. This form can be excreted either through the biliary system or by renal filtration. The large fenestrae in the hepatic sinusoids permit albumin-bound unconjugated bilirubin direct access to the hepatocyte. Uptake at the hepatocellular surface is rapid and efficient. Like any substance avidly bound to a carrier protein, the rate of uptake is determined by the efficiency of the extraction mechanism rather than hepatic blood flow. Uptake competes with many other organic anions including BSP and ICG but *not* bile acids.[448] Uptake is not influenced by high intracellular concentrations of bilirubin. Jaundice due to unconjugated hyperbilirubinemia occurs transiently in hemolytic disease when the concentration of newly released pigment exceeds the hepatic capacity for extraction. Other circumstances causing unconjugated hyperbilirubinemia include impaired pigment uptake as occurs with hepatobiliary disease or certain inherited transport or conjugation abnormalities, or when large amounts of unconjugated bilirubin reflux into plasma before conjugation can occur. Kinetic studies of the hepatocellular uptake of bilirubin indicate a bidirectional transfer across the cell membrane; one-third of unconjugated bilirubin entering the liver can reflux unaltered back into plasma.[448]

HEPATOCELLULAR BILIRUBIN STORAGE AND CONJUGATION. In the hepatocyte, bilirubin binds to specific intracellular storage proteins. The most important of these are ligandin and Y protein. Ligandin is a member of the glutathione-S-transferase enzyme system that catalyzes conjugation of many different substances with glutathione. It has a nonspecific affinity for many organic anions. Z protein (fatty acid binding protein) has a lower affinity for unconjugated bilirubin than ligandin and is thought to be of primary importance in uptake and metabolism of fatty acids. It is hypothesized that the storage proteins provide important and related cytoprotective functions. Binding to ligandin or Y protein prevents the precipitation of insoluble materials within the hepatocyte. Binding also reduces potentially toxic effects, such as the uncoupling of oxidative phosphorylation, that occurs upon exposure to large amounts of bilirubin. Function of ligandin in the capacity of glutathione-S-transferase also provides intracellular detoxification and transport for a variety of non-bilirubin organic anions.[448] Binding of the storage proteins to large amounts of bilirubin impairs the processing of other organic anions (BSP and ICG) that are sometimes used diagnostically to appraise liver function and perfusion.

Each of the cytosolic storage proteins has a delayed appearance in humans and some animals until 5 to 10 days after birth. During this neonatal interval, the paucity of stor-

Table 30–14

Agents or Conditions That Displace "Loosely" Protein-Bound Unconjugated Bilirubin

Acidemia	Organic anions: BSP, ICG
Digitoxin	bile acids
Diazepam	cholecystographic agents
Free fatty acids	Oxacillin
Furosemide	Phenylbutazone
Hydrocortisone	Salicylates
Hypoalbuminemia	Thyroxine
Mercuhydrin	

Agents That Compete with Bilirubin for Net Hepatic Uptake

Probenecid	Rifamycin SV
Rifampin	Iodinated radiographic contrast

Agents That Compete with Bilirubin for Binding to Hepatocellular Storage Proteins: Ligandin and Z Protein

Indicator dyes	Antimicrobials
BSP	nitrofurantoin
ICG	penicillins
Rose bengal	sulfonamides
Ethacrynic acid	tetracycline
Fatty acids	Cholecystographic agents
Heme	Certain carcinogens
Steroids: glucocorticoids	
hormones	

Agents Competing with Bilirubin for Conjugation: for Glucoronic Acid or Glucuronyl Transferase

Chloramphenicol	Morphine
Estradiol	Testosterone

age proteins causes a marked delay in circulatory clearance of organic anions, including bilirubin. The synthesis of the storage proteins can be induced by certain drugs, most notably phenobarbital. Treatment with phenobarbital has been used in some hyperbilirubinemic conditions in humans to facilitate resolution of jaundice.

Conjugation of bilirubin occurs in the smooth endoplasmic reticulum of the hepatocyte, where a particular UDP-glucuronosyl transferase (bilirubin UDP-glucuronyl transferase) catalyzes conjugation with glucuronic acid.[452] Small amounts of bilirubin are also conjugated to xylose and glucose in the dog and cat.[453–454] Conjugation with glucuronide (mono- or diglucuronidation) occurs by transfer of glucuronic acid from uridine diphosphate glucuronic acid (UDPGA). Conjugation changes lipid soluble bilirubin to a water soluble form by the addition of the polar glucuronic acid group(s). The rate of conjugation is determined by the activity of glucuronyl transferase and the availability of glucuronic acid. Approximately 70% of the bilirubin in the liver is in the unconjugated form; this emphasizes the importance of enzymic activity and glucuronic acid as rate-limiting variables influencing bilirubin conjugation. Reduced activity of glucuronyl transferase, a deficiency of glucuronic acid, or competition for either enzyme or substrate can delay bilirubin conjugation and lead to jaundice. Certain drugs and hormones conjugated with glucuronic acid or that require glucuronyl transferase for metabolism compete with bilirubin for conjugation; some of these are shown in Table 30–14. Administration of phenobarbital or clofibrate has been used to stimulate bilirubin-glucuronyl transferase activity in humans when it is suspected that enzyme activity has become a rate-limiting factor. This scenario applies to infants with neonatal jaundice (unconjugated jaundice) and for some types of inborn errors of bilirubin metabolism (Crigler-Najjar Type II).[452]

BILIRUBIN EXCRETION. In most mammals, virtually all bilirubin excreted in bile is conjugated; less than 3% loss is in the unconjugated form. Transport of conjugated bilirubin into canaliculi occurs by a poorly understood process. Movement against a concentration gradient is believed to involve a saturable, presumably carrier-mediated and energy dependent process. This can be modulated by a variety of factors, including anoxia, infection, age, certain medications, and hypothermia. Carrier mechanisms for canalicular excretion are shared by certain other organic anions (BSP, ICG) but *not* by bile acids.[448] In humans, maximal bilirubin excretion is about 55 mg/kg/day but this can be increased by bile salt dependent and independent choleresis (infusion of bile salts or treatment with phenobarbital).[455] In rats, the canalicular transport rather than conjugation of bilirubin is the rate-limiting process of bilirubin excretion.[456] It is believed by some that canalicular excretion occurs as bilirubin simply diffuses across membranes in a nonmicellar phase. After reaching bile canaliculi, it then becomes incorporated into bile micelles. This theory maintains that a low relative concentration of bilirubin develops on the canalicular side of the membrane as bilirubin conjugates become concentrated in bile salt mixed micelles. This results in canalicular excretion of bilirubin along a downhill gradient into a so-called micellar sink created by the presence of bile acids.[456]

The liver has a large reserve capacity for bilirubin excretion as it can accommodate a 30- to 60-fold increase above normal. The maximum rate of bilirubin excretion in dogs is reported to range between 52 and 126 µg/kg/minute.[457] In health, only a small amount of conjugated bilirubin is refluxed into the circulation. This immediately binds to albumin, but with less affinity than unconjugated bilirubin. At any given time less than 2% of the plasma conjugated bilirubin is in the unbound or free form. As a result, less than 2% is filtered through the glomerulus. The dog's renal threshold for bilirubin is low because the renal tubules are capable of active bilirubin excretion. Consequently, bilirubinuria is routinely detected. The cat, unlike the dog, does not demonstrate bilirubinuria without associated hyperbilirubinemia. Consequently, bilirubinuria in the cat always warrants evaluation for hemolytic or hepatobiliary disease.[458] Renal excretion of bilirubin is not efficient compared with biliary excretion.

However, in the circumstance of profound hyperbilirubinemia, renal excretion can become important.[459,460] In most circumstances, unconjugated bilirubin does not appear in urine because of its avid protein binding. The exception is in the dog with hemoglobinemia in which renal tubules produce bilirubin that is secreted into tubular urine.[461–464] This only occurs with large amounts of circulating hemoglobin; experimentally it occurs when free plasma hemoglobin exceeds 50 mg/dl. Male dogs have a greater ability for this than females.

BILIRUBIN METABOLISM IN THE GASTROINTESTINAL TRACT. Following expulsion of bile into the alimentary canal, conjugated bilirubin is deconjugated and hydrogenated by colonic bacteria (Figure 30–19). This produces a colorless pigment, mesobilirubinogen,[466] which is oxidized to a group of colorless tetrapyrolles collectively called urobilinogens. These may be oxidized to urobilin (yellow-orange) or stercobilin (brown fecal pigment). Intestinal bacterial flora determine the final products formed. Small amounts of urobilinogen are absorbed from the intestine and are either re-extracted by the liver (95%) and eliminated in bile or are excreted through the kidneys (5%). Conjugation of bilirubin minimizes its enterohepatic circulation as conjugation impedes absorption in the small bowel. Increased deconjugation occurs during bacterial overgrowth of the small bowel with colonic anaerobes. This leads to an increased enterohepatic turnover of bilirubin pigments. Some animal species are able to absorb small amounts of bilirubin from the gallbladder.[456]

Normal fecal color requires both the presence of bilirubin and bacterial activity that produces different colored pigments. Feces lacking pigmentation are referred to as being "acholic." Lack of the normal brown fecal pigmentation can reflect a deficiency of either bile flow or intestinal bacterial activity. Since only small amounts of bile pigments are necessary to impart normal color, complete biliary obstruction is required for stools to become acholic. An absence of fecal pigmentation develops 7 to 10 days after complete bile duct occlusion by which time jaundice is obvious. To avoid confusion, the clinician should remember that fecal color can change with antibiotics, diarrhea, the ingestion of bismuth (black), iron (black), and with different diets. The consump-

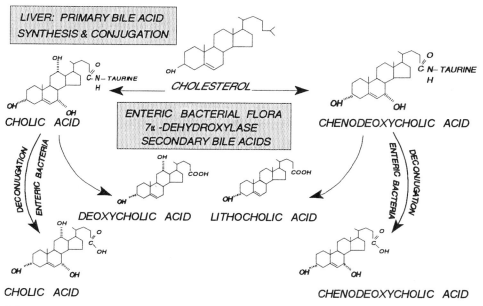

FIGURE 30–19. Enteric metabolism of bilirubin diglucuronide into fecal pigments.

tion of foods rich in hemoglobin/myoglobin, such as raw meat or liver, can cause the spurious appearance of very dark feces similar to melena. Animals with large amounts of bilirubin entering the bowel may produce orange or dark green stool.

UROBILINOGEN METABOLISM. Considerable amounts of bilirubin are reduced to urobilinogen, in the alimentary canal and subsequently lost in feces. Approximately 10% to 20% of urobilinogen is absorbed from the ileum and colon. After absorption, the liver removes most of this urobilinogen from the portal circulation and secretes it into bile without conjugation. The liver has a large reserve capacity for this function. Plasma urobilinogen that is not extracted by the liver and not bound to proteins is excreted in urine by glomerular filtration. Small amounts of urobilinogen can also be secreted by the proximal tubules. Some urobilinogen is passively resorbed in the distal nephron; this is enhanced in acid urine. Distal nephron absorption is augmented by acid urine because the pigment is largely unionized and thus more lipid soluble. Semiquantitation of urinary urobilinogen has been suggested as a useful test for differential diagnoses of hepatobiliary disease. Unfortunately, the presence or absence of urine urobilinogen is an inconsistent and unreliable marker for the differential diagnosis of jaundice. Test interpretation is confused by many variables, discussed in detail in Table 8–8.

ALTERNATE PATHWAYS FOR BILIRUBIN ELIMINATION. Alternate pathways for bilirubin elimination have been characterized.[453] As previously mentioned, only very small amounts of unconjugated bilirubin are excreted in bile. Unconjugated bilirubin may also reach the alimentary lumen by passage across the intestinal wall or by desquamation of enterocytes. In the circumstance of gastrointestinal hemorrhage, plasma bilirubin spills into the alimentary lumen. This can provide a considerable source of bilirubin in the jaundiced patient and thus serves as a mechanism for alimentary production of urobilinogen and normal fecal pigments in a patient with complete bile duct obstruction. The propensity for patients with serious hepatobiliary disease, portal hypertension, or major bile duct occlusion to develop gastrointestinal ulceration and coagulopathies makes this a common clinical occurrence.

Another variable that can complicate clinical interpretation of bilirubin values is that hepatic bilirubin catabolism is enhanced by induction of mixed function oxidases. This may result in production of colorless metabolites not detected by routine tests.

In total biliary obstruction or after hepatectomy, urinary excretion of bilirubin becomes a major route of elimination.[467] When unconjugated hyperbilirubinemia is severe in human neonates, a photochemical reaction resulting from exposure to fluorescent lamps (peak emissions between 457 and 525 nm) is used to transform bilirubin into nontoxic photoisomers. One such isomer is known as lumirubin. The photoisomers are subsequently excreted in bile or urine.[468]

JAUNDICE. Jaundice or icterus develops when the serum bilirubin concentration is equal to or exceeds 2.0 mg/dl. Inspection of nonpigmented body surfaces in "natural" lighting facilitates its early recognition. Examination of the sclera of the eye, oral mucosa (gingiva, sublingual tissues, soft palate), pinna of the ear, periumbilical area, and the mucosal surface of the penis or vagina allows easy recognition. When bilirubin concentration attains 4 to 5 mg/dl, jaundice is obvious. Hyperbilirubinemia does not occur in all hepatobiliary disorders but is the hallmark of major bile duct occlusion, severe intrahepatic cholestasis, and severe diffuse parenchymal failure.

The differential diagnoses of jaundice is facilitated by consideration of (1) prehepatic or hemolytic, (2) hepatic, and (3) posthepatic or obstructive categories. Differential pathophysiologic mechanisms for each category are presented in Table 30–15. Specific differential diagnoses included in these categories are discussed in Chapter 8 and summarized in Table 8–3.

Hepatic causes of jaundice involve several pathophysiologic mechanisms. With inflammatory disorders, occlusion of the intrahepatic biliary tree including canaliculi, bile ductules, and small bile ducts develops due to cellular swelling and inflammation that impedes bile flow. An increase in membrane permeability facilitates regurgitation of bilirubin into the sinusoidal space or back diffusion into the hepatocyte. In addition, the ultrastructural mechanisms involved with canalicular excretion of bilirubin may become compromised. Chronic inflammation in the portal area and involving bile ducts, bile duct hyperplasia, and biliary cirrhosis results in mechanical occlusion of the small- and intermediate-sized biliary pathways. These circumstances cause *cholestasis*, a general term used to indicate impairment of the flow of bile. The zonal localization of a pathologic condition can determine whether or not jaundice develops early in the disease course. For example, moderate inflammatory changes in periportal areas (zone 1) can cause marked hyperbilirubinemia whereas severe parenchymal injury localized away from periportal areas (zone 3) can be free of hyperbilirubinemia until relatively late in the disease process. Loss of normal hepatic architecture due to formation of regenerative nodules can impair normal bile flow when severe, resulting in persistent jaundice. Hepatic atrophy, as seen in animals with congenital portosystemic vascular anomalies, is not usually associated with hyperbilirubinemia. The capacity of the liver to metabolize bilirubin and maintain normal plasma levels is greater than for many of the liver's other functions. Normal concentrations of bilirubin are maintained by a liver less than half its normal size, one that is unable to maintain normal plasma albumin, glucose, and urea concentrations.

Extrahepatic or obstructive jaundice is caused by intraluminal or extraluminal problems that mechanically occlude the biliary tree. The most common causes are neoplasia in and around the gallbladder, cystic duct and common bile duct, and pancreatitis. Less frequent causes are primary disorders involving the walls of the biliary system that obstruct the flow of bile. Extraheptic jaundice can also develop when the biliary tree is ruptured and bile spills into the peritoneal cavity.

The magnitude of hyperbilirubinemia realized in different forms of hepatic and extrahepatic jaundice are discussed in Chapter 8. The concentrations of unconjugated and conjugated bilirubin in hemolytic, hepatic, and extrahepatic jaundice are shown in Table 30–16.[469,470] Scrutiny of these values explains why the van den Bergh test for serum bilirubin fractionation is not useful in the differential diagnosis of jaundice.

Inherited metabolic impairments of bilirubin metabolism have been described in human beings, nonhuman primates, sheep, and rodents. These are summarized in Table 30–17.

Bilirubin Toxicity and Encephalopathy

That bilirubin is toxic to cells has been well established. In vitro studies have detailed that bilirubin depresses cellular respiration, impairs protein synthesis, increases glycolysis, and uncouples mitochondrial oxidative phosphorylation.[471-474] Concern regarding toxicity is warranted when the total serum bilirubin approaches 30 mg/dl in the adult. Unconjugated bilirubin is more toxic than conjugated bilirubin owing to its greater affinity for lipids. Fortunately, the

Table 30-15

DIFFERENTIAL MECHANISMS FOR HYPERBILIRUBINEMIA

↑ **Bilirubin Production**	↑ Destruction RBCs: Hemolysis Abnormal erythropoiesis → Ineffective erythropoiesis ↑ Turnover nonhemoglobin heme: liver, other tissues Phagocytic breakdown extravasated RBCs: hematoma, hemothorax, hemoperitoneum
↓ **Hepatic Uptake**	Competition: cholecystographic agents, BSP, ICG, drugs ↓ Functional hepatic mass Severe ↓ hepatic perfusion Inherited defect (not documented in dogs or cats) Hypoproteinemia: ↓ albumin-bilirubin presentation necessary for bilirubin hepatocyte uptake
↓ **Hepatic Storage**	Competition: drugs and other organic anions ↓ Functional hepatic mass
↑ **Regurgitation Bilirubin**	Severe unconjugated hyperbilirubinemia: hemolysis ↓ Functional hepatic mass Cholestasis → impaired membrane permeability
↓ **Hepatic Conjugation**	Competition: drugs and other organic anions ↓ Functional hepatic mass Inherited defect (not documented in dogs or cats)
↓ **Canalicular Excretion**	↓ Functional hepatic mass Cholestatic disorders: functional with or without morphologic lesions
↓ **Biliary Excretion**	Obstructed bile flow: Extraluminal: stricture, scar strangulation, mass compression, pancreatitis Intraluminal: mass, disease of intrahepatic small pathways, wall inflammation, swelling, hematoma

high avidity of unconjugated bilirubin for binding with albumin reduces its availability for widespread tissue distribution. In the presence of normal albumin concentrations, bilirubin levels up to 20 to 25 mg/dl are normally bound to albumin. Unconjugated bilirubin becomes "toxic" when protein binding is reduced as occurs in hypoalbuminemia or as a result of displacement by competing drugs.[451] Free unconjugated bilirubin easily penetrates the blood-brain barrier, producing neurotoxicity. Experimental work in the adult dog has demonstrated that rapid intravascular infusions of unconjugated bilirubin to achieve concentrations of 60 to 70 mg/dl is associated with hypotensive shock and death.[475] Severe hyperbilirubinemia in adult dogs and cats may also be associated with renal injury, both glomerular and tubular.[476–478] This has been observed as a clinical problem in some animals treated by the author and may be marked by the appearance of granular casts in urine.

Perinatal human and nonhuman primates are at great risk

Table 30-16

SERUM BILIRUBIN FRACTIONATION IN DOGS WITH DIFFERENT FORMS OF JAUNDICE

Histologic and Clinical Diagnoses	Dogs (n)	UNCONJUGATED BILIRUBIN		CONJUGATED BILIRUBIN	
		mg/dl (range)	% Total (range)	mg/dl (range)	% Total (range)
Prehepatic-Hemolytic Jaundice					
Hemolytic disease	11	2.0 (0.5–10)	33 (8–95)	4.2 (0.5–17)	68 (5–92)
Hepatic Jaundice					
Chronic active hepatitis	8	1.6 (0.3–30)	20 (4–30)	6.0 (2–28)	83 (70–96)
Cirrhosis	6	0.3 (0.1–0.9)	29 (11–51)	1.6 (0.6–2.2)	71 (49–89)
Acute hepatitis	9	2.0 (0.1–9.1)	18 (2–86)	5.2 (0.3–18)	83 (14–98)
Hepatic lymphosarcoma	7	0.5 (0.2–1.5)	23 (10–60)	2.1 (0.4–15)	76 (40–90)
Glucocorticoid hepatopathy	2	0.3 (0.2–0.3)	18 (12–24)	1.7 (1–2.5)	82 (76–88)
Posthepatic-Extrahepatic Jaundice					
Extrahepatic bile duct obstruction	10	2.1 (0.2–10.5)	16 (6–31)	9.0 (0.6–34)	84 (71–92)

Data derived and compiled from references 469, 470, and College of Veterinary Medicine, Cornell University, 1993.

Table 30–17

INHERITED METABOLIC IMPAIRMENTS OF BILIRUBIN METABOLISM IN HUMAN BEINGS AND ANIMALS

	MECHANISM/SIGNS
Abnormal Bilirubin Conjugation	
Crigler-Najjar disease	Deficiency of UDP glucuronyl transferase activity
Type I	Unconjugated hyperbilirubinemia: no response to phenobarbital
Type II	Less severe unconjugated hyperbilirubinemia: responds to phenobarbital
Gunn rat Hyperbilirubinemia	Similar to Type I Crigler-Najjar disease
Gilbert's syndrome	Reduced UDP-glucuronyl transferase activity
	Worsens with illnesses of many types
Mutant Southdown sheep	Similar to Gilbert's syndrome
Bolivian Squirrel monkey	Similar to Gilbert's syndrome
Conjugated Hyperbilirubinemia	
Dubin-Johnson syndrome	↓ Hepatic bilirubin storage and canalicular transport
	Normal BSP storage capacity, abnormal BSP conjugation
	Normal ICG and rose bengal elimination (no conjugation needed)
Mutant Corriedale sheep	Similar to Dubin-Johnson syndrome
Mutant rat model	Similar to Dubin-Johnson syndrome
Rotor's syndrome	Chronic intermittent fluctuating jaundice
	Abnormal BSP, ICG, and rose bengal excretion

for bilirubin toxicity. Major factors include defective hepatocellular uptake of bilirubin, deficient bilirubin conjugation, increased enteric reabsorption of bilirubin, and increased bilirubin synthesis.[479–482] Comparatively, the perinatal dog is more resistant to bilirubin toxicity.[482] In the puppy, the hepatic glycosyl transferase activities develop to three-quarters of adult activity prior to birth. Susceptibility of the perinatal cat has not been studied. One report of kernicterus (bilirubin encephalopathy) in a neonatal kitten did not convincingly describe a syndrome solely attributable to bilirubin toxicity.[481] Kernicterus is characterized by hyperbilirubinemia, hyperpyrexia, seizures, paresis, yellow staining of nuclear brain centers, and damaged neurons in basal ganglia, hippocampus, cerebellum, and nuclei adjacent to the fourth ventricle.[482]

SERUM BILE ACIDS

Bile is a digestive secretion that provides a route for cholesterol and bilirubin elimination. Its major lipid components are cholesterol, bile acids, and phospholipids. All three components can be synthesized de novo by the hepatocyte and also can be imported into the liver from the circulation. Bile acids are the predominant component of bile, composing approximately 85% of the biliary solids. Their continuous transhepatocellular secretion from blood into bile serves an important role in the generation of canalicular bile flow (bile acid–dependent flow). Bile acids act as ionic detergents and in that way provide a pivotal role in the intestinal absorption, transport, and secretion of lipids. They have many biologic functions and pathologic effects; these are summarized in Table 30–18.

Bile acids are organic acids derived from cholesterol. Synthesis occurs exclusively in the liver in a series of sequential steps involving numerous intermediates and several different hepatocellular organelles.[483,484] Conversion of the C_{27} neutral sterol cholesterol to the primary bile acids occurs in nine steps, each reaction being catalyzed by distinct enzymes. Conversion of cholesterol to bile acids involves addition of either one or two hydroxyl groups, epimerization of the 3beta

hydroxyl group to a 3alpha hydroxyl group, and degradation of the C_{27} side chain of cholesterol forming a C_{24} structure. The term *bile acid* refers to the molecular configuration in which the carboxylic acid side chain is nonionized; the term *bile salt* refers to the ionized form. At a physiologic pH of 7.4, the bile salt form predominates.[483]

The biologic properties of bile salts depend on the number and position of their hydroxyl groups and the type of conjugation at the carboxyl group. In humans, dogs, and cats, the major bile acids synthesized in the liver are cholic acid (CA) and chenodeoxycholic acid (CDCA). These are the primary bile acids. Dehydroxylation of these moieties by anaerobic intestinal microorganisms produces the more hydrophobic secondary bile acids; CA is converted to deoxycholic acid (DCA) and CDCA acid to lithocholic acid (LCA). A metabolic scheme showing intestinal decarboxylation and dehydroxylation is provided in Figure 30–20. In most mammals, bile acid biosynthesis is regulated primarily by the amount of bile acids returning to the liver. This is determined by the size of the bile acid pool and the number of enterohepatic circulations of this pool each day.[485–495] In humans, approximately 6 to 8 cycles occur per day, 2 at each meal interval. Although healthy humans synthesize approximately twofold more CA than CDCA, more of the CDCA is preserved by efficient hepatic extraction and enterohepatic circulation. A relatively small amount of secondary bile acids are contained within the bile acid pool; only about one-third to one-half of DCA and one-fifth of LCA formed in the intestines is absorbed.

The rate-limiting step in bile acid synthesis is cholesterol 7alpha-hydroxylase, which catalyzes the conversion of cholesterol to 7alpha-hydroxycholesterol.[489] Bile acid wasting syndromes, such as occurs with ileal disease, biliary fistula, certain types of biliary tract diversions, or the administration of a bile acid binding resin (cholestyramine), increases hepatic 7alpha-hydroxylase activity and bile acid synthesis.[490] A number of variables influence the rate of bile acid synthesis via this enzyme (summarized in Table 30–19). Biosynthesis is regulated primarily by the amount of bile acids returning to the liver, which reflects the size of the bile acid pool and the number of enterohepatic circulations of this pool each day.[491–495]

Table 30-18

BIOLOGIC FUNCTIONS AND PATHOLOGIC EFFECTS OF BILE ACIDS

Bile flow: Bile salts generate a portion of the biliary secretions (bile salt–dependent bile flow). Important route for solubilization and excretion of organic compounds, endogenous metabolites, variety of drug and mineral metabolites.

Solubilization of biliary lipids: Combined with lecithin, bile salts solubilize biliary cholesterol, forming mixed micelles and vesicles. This is beneficial in avoiding cholesterol choleliths.

Cholesterol elimination: (1) Bile acids *synthesis* from cholesterol is a principal pathway for cholesterol elimination. (2) Secretion of bile salts into bile is coupled with the *secretion and elimination* of phosphatidylcholine (lecithin) and cholesterol.

Regulation of cholesterol synthesis: Bile salts have regulatory effects on cholesterol synthesis, either by acting directly on the hydroxymethylglutaryl-coenzyme Q (HMG-CoA) reductase, or indirectly by modulating intestinal cholesterol absorption.

Control of bile acid synthesis: Enterohepatic circulation of bile salts regulates bile acid synthesis through feedback on the rate-limiting enzyme (7alpha-hyroxylase).

Regulation of hepatic lipoprotein receptors: Bile acids may modulate the rate of uptake of lipoprotein cholesterol by the liver.

Alimentary fat digestion and absorption: Bile salts form mixed micelles in the intestines and participate in the intraluminal solubilization, transport, and absorption of cholesterol, fat soluble vitamins, and other lipids. Bile salts also optimize certain lipases.

Alimentary transport of calcium and iron: Bile salts may be involved in the transport of calcium and iron from the intestinal lumen to the brush border.

Perpetuation of hepatobiliary membrane injury: Retention of hepatotoxic (hydrophobic, membranocytolytic) bile acids in serum, bile, and liver tissue in patients with serious hepatobiliary disease is thought to promote the self-perpetuation of a chronic inflammatory process. The membranocytolytic effects of certain bile acids have been well established. They alter the ability of hepatocytes and bile duct epithelium to participate in the inflammatory process by altering histocompatibility complex expression.

Modification of blood-brain barrier in hepatic encephalopathy: High concentrations of circulating bile acids may promote increased permeability of the blood-brain barrier, thereby providing CNS access for noxious hepatoencephalopathic substances.

Generation of gastroesophageal and duodenal ulcers: Because of their membrane-damaging capabilities, reflux of bile into duodenum, stomach, and/or esophagus may contribute to the formation and perpetuation of ulcerative lesions in patients with hepatic gastric vasculopathy.

Diarrhea in bile acid malabsorption: Passage of unconjugated bile acids into the distal bowel can result in morphologic injury to enterocytes and colonic villi and development of diarrhea.

Immunosuppression: Certain bile salts inhibit lymphocyte response to mitogens in patients with cholestatic liver disease.

Abnormal platelet function: Bile salts have been shown to reduce normal platelet aggregation when they are exposed to ADP.

After synthesis, bile acids are conjugated in the liver. The normal liver conjugates almost all bile acids before secretion into bile.[495] Conjugation results in the attachment of a second organic substituent, most often glycine or taurine, to the side chain carboxyl group or to one of the ring hydroxyl groups. The relative proportions of glycine and taurine conjugates vary markedly among species.[483,496,497] Humans conjugate with glycine and taurine, depending on the availability of taurine.[498] Dogs and cats conjugate primarily to taurine. The dog has the ability to convert to glycine conjugation, but the cat undergoes obligate conjugation with taurine.[483,499–502]

In illness, alternative conjugation reactions may occur involving glucuronate or sulfate, but in health these reactions are minor.[503–505] Sulfation and glucuronidation occur at the hydroxyl groups of the bile salt and these polar groups increase water solubility allowing increased renal clearance. It is believed that most of these alternative conjugation reactions occur in the liver although some sulfation also occurs in the kidney.[491] Sulfation of bile salts may serve a protective role in cholestasis by stimulating bile flow and/or reducing biliary phospholipid and cholesterol secretion. Increased bile flow may augment bile salt excretion and protect cellular membranes against their detergent effects.[504] Renal clearance of sulfated bile salts is 20 to 200 times greater than clearance of nonsulfated forms.[503] Of the common bile salts, only the most hydrophobic (LCA) normally is found as a sulfate in liver tissue and bile. LCA is highly hepatotoxic and accumulates in the presence of cholestasis. The sulfated form is poorly resorbed from the intestine and is rapidly lost from the enterohepatic circulation.

Conjugation of bile acids impedes their passive intestinal absorption and thus enables participation in intestinal digestion of dietary fats. Conjugation with glycine or taurine decreases the pKa of bile acids without altering their amphipathic properties. Free bile acids have a significantly higher pKa and thus precipitate or are passively absorbed in the proximal intestines. These do not facilitate lipid digestion and absorption. At physiologic intestinal pH, most conjugated forms are ionized and water soluble. These are actively absorbed in the distal ileum via high-affinity receptors. Approximately 95% of bile acids are absorbed here and return to the liver through the portal circulation.

Deconjugation of bile acids occurs in the intestinal lumen through action of bacterial enzymes. This is the first step in their degradation. Increased fecal concentrations of deconjugated bile acids reflects intestinal bacterial activity; this is not a clinically applicable test at the present time. Rapid nonionic passive absorption of unconjugated bile acids, particularly the dihydroxy forms, occurs at all levels of the small intestine. These moieties are efficiently reconjugated in the liver. Many different fecal bile acid metabolites formed by microbial enzymes have been identified. Rehydroxylation of these moieties is minimal in humans and has not been fully investigated in the dog or cat.[488]

Enterohepatic Circulation of Bile Acids

The enterohepatic circulation of bile acids is illustrated in Figure 30–21. After hepatic synthesis and conjugation, primary bile acids are excreted through the biliary tract and are stored and concentrated in the gallbladder. Emptying of the gallbladder is usually, but not exclusively, initiated after meals following release of cholecystokinin. Cholecystokinesis can also occur in the middle of the night in the dog and at random times during a prolonged fast.[506–513] This variation causes some animals to have higher fasting than postprandial bile acid values. This phenomenon seems more common in the dog than in the cat as a variable affecting clinical test results.

After bile enters the alimentary canal, bile salts facilitate intraluminal solubilization and absorption of ingested lipids. They are absorbed throughout the entire intestines, although most prominently in the distal ileum. They are transported exclusively in the portal venous circulation. This cycling between the liver-intestines-portal circulation is referred to as the bile acid enterohepatic circulation. This cycle is highly efficient, recycling more than 95% of bile salts secreted in

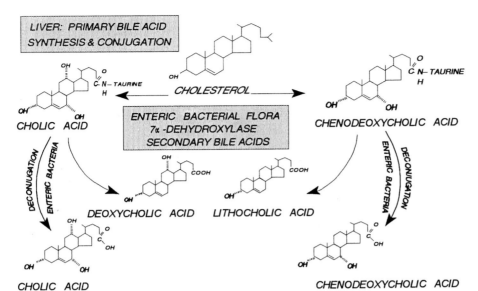

FIGURE 30-20. Mechanism of enteric production of secondary bile acids and bile acid deconjugation.

bile. The very small amounts lost in feces each day are replenished by hepatic synthesis. In health, the rate of intestinal absorption is the major factor determining serum bile acid concentrations in both fasting and postprandial intervals.[514,515] Bile salts returning to the liver are bound to albumin and to a lesser extent, plasma lipoproteins. Uptake into the liver occurs mainly in the periportal areas (zone 1). The load of bile acid returning to the liver during the postprandial interval exceeds the clearing capacity. This allows a small increase in the total bile acid concentration in systemic blood in most healthy animals. It is this endogenous challenge that provides the clinical utility of the postprandial serum bile acid test. Hepatic extraction of bile acids approximates 90%; the trihydroxy forms are more efficiently cleared than are the dihydroxy forms. First-pass extraction for taurocholic, glycocholic, deoxycholic, and chenodeoxycholic acids is 80%, 65%, 55%, and 40%, respectively.[484]

Within the hepatocytes, bile acids may exist as single unbound molecules or bound to carrier proteins. Most evidence supports carrier-mediated hepatic transport against concentration and electrical gradients. Both sodium-independent and sodium-dependent systems have been characterized.[516–519] Movement to canaliculi is facilitated by cytosolic binding proteins and may involve microtubules associated with Golgi. Secretion into canaliculi may occur by simple exocytosis or may be facilitated by a carrier.[519] The path of bile acid secretion from the hepatocyte becomes altered in cholestasis. Transport may be deviated from canaliculi to the basolateral regions of the hepatocyte, resulting in direct excretion of bile across the sinusoidal membrane. This may be the mechanism for the so-called regurgitation of bile acids into plasma.

An overview of the enterohepatic bile acid circulation details four discrete circuits that contribute to the bile acid pool returning to the liver (Figure 30–21). A *cholehepatic circuit* is defined between biliary radicles (canaliculi, bile ductules) and the liver. Regurgitation of bile acids here contributes to the high bile acid levels associated with cholestasis. A *jejunohepatic circuit* is defined for bile acids passively absorbed in the proximal small intestines. This circuit contributes to the increased load of unconjugated bile acids that may develop in the circumstance of bacterial overgrowth of the bowel, a condition that increases bile acid deconjugation.

Approximately 30% of the CDCA is absorbed by nonionic diffusion in this circuit. The *ileal-hepatic circuit* is the major component of the enterohepatic circulation in health. A *colohepatic circuit* allows for the passive uptake of bile acids that escape absorption by the small bowel or that are deconjugated in the distal portion of the alimentary canal. This circuit can become important when bile acid malabsorption occurs as a result of ileal disease or resection. Bile acid absorption in the colon is greatly influenced by the rate of bacterial dehydroxylation. Secondary bile acids tend to precipitate and bind to bacteria in the colon and consequently have low absorption.

Maintenance of an adequate concentration of bile acids in the alimentary canal and of the enterohepatic circulation

Table 30–19

VARIABLES INFLUENCING THE RATE OF BILE ACID SYNTHESIS

VARIABLES	EFFECT ON CHOLESTEROL 7ALPHA-HYDROXYLASE (RATE-LIMITING ENZYME)
Bile fistula	↑
Bile acid malabsorption	↑
Cholestyramine Rx	↑
Lymphatic drainage (bile acid wasting)	↑
Portocaval anastomosis	↑
Glucocorticoids	↑
Adrenalectomy	↓
Thyroxin	↑
Thyroidectomy	↓
Glucose after starvation	↑
Fasting	↓
Oral administration bile acids (hydrophobic bile acids)	↓
Bile duct ligation/obstruction	↑
Diurnal rhythm (feeding time)	↑
Hepatic failure	↓
	↓ (12alpha-hydroxylase activity)

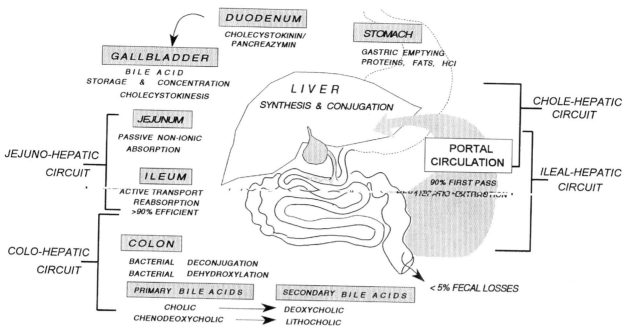

FIGURE 30–21. Enterohepatic circulation of bile acids showing the component circuits involved in absorption and recirculation.

depends on efficient intestinal uptake. Under normal conditions this system is efficient and hepatic bile acid synthesis is maintained at a relatively constant low level sufficient to replace a 5% daily fecal loss.

Variables Influencing Bile Acid Enterohepatic Circulation

Many factors influence the enterohepatic circulation of bile acids. These include (1) the rate of bile acid synthesis, (2) meal synchronization and completeness of gallbladder emptying, (3) gastric emptying and intestinal transit rate, (4) intestinal absorption and (5) the enterohepatic cycling frequency. Variables that influence use of an endogenous bile acid test for evaluation of hepatobiliary function are discussed in Chapter 8, and summarized in Tables 8–13 and 8–14. The dynamics of the enterohepatic circulation influences the maximal bile acid concentration attained in the systemic circulation and the sensitivity of bile acid quantification as a test of hepatobiliary function. Deranged enterohepatic circulation, reduced intestinal absorption, incomplete gallbladder contraction, and an altered intestinal transit rate can each influence the optimal interval for postprandial sample collection. Although bile acid synthesis can be markedly reduced in patients with serious liver disease, a less efficient enterohepatic cycling, the presence of portosystemic shunting, reduced hepatic extraction, and regurgitation due to cholestasis result in elevated systemic bile acid concentrations.

The health and function of the gallbladder can have a major influence on the enterohepatic circulation of bile acids. The physiologic functions of the gallbladder include bile storage, concentration, acidification, and release of bile into the intestines. The gallbladder mucosa has a unique ability to withstand the detergent properties of bile acids. During storage, hepatic bile is concentrated to approximately 10% to 20% of its original volume. As the concentration of bile increases, bile salts form micelles, which eliminates osmolal stresses that would develop in a conventional aqueous solution. Contraction of the gallbladder does not occur only after feeding. Cholecystokinesis during the interdigestive interval has been clearly demonstrated.[506,508–513] The gallbladder undergoes intermittent partial emptying during phase 2 of the migrating myoelectric complex. Interdigestive contraction is also triggered by a variety of gastrointestinal peptides and neuropeptides including gastrin, motilin, vasoactive intestinal peptide, secretin, glucagon, and pancreatic polypeptide.[520] In humans, altered gallbladder kinesis is believed to be involved in gallstone development. Impaired emptying has been shown in humans receiving total parenteral nutrition, and these individuals are particularly prone to formation of biliary sludge and choleliths.[521,522] It is important to remember that the storage and concentration of bile in the gallbladder is not necessary for normal fat digestion. Surgical removal of the gallbladder or cholecystoenterostomy does not lead to fat maldigestion, bile acid malabsorption, or inability to use the serum bile acid test.

Bile Salts and Dietary Lipid Assimilation

Initial digestion of triglycerides and formation of a lipid emulsion occurs in the stomach. As chyme passes into the intestines, fatty acids, amino acids, and a lowered pH stimulate secretion of cholecystokinin, which invokes gallbladder contraction. Bile salts initially prepare dietary fats for lipolysis by production of a stable lipid emulsion. Eventually they enhance absorption of digested fat by formation of mixed micelles. The function of several lipases is optimized by the presence of bile salts so they also contribute to lipid digestion. Digestion of long chain phospholipids and cholesterol esters also requires bile salts.

The major influence of bile acids in the small intestine is dietary lipid solubilization through formation of micelles. As lipids diffuse through the unstirred water layer adjacent to the intestinal mucosa, they are transformed by association with bile acids into mixed micelles. Micelles assist the diffusion of fats to the enterocyte for further digestion and absorption. Complete diversion of bile from the intestines results in steatorrhea, impaired absorption of cholesterol, and malabsorption of fat soluble vitamins. In the absence of bile, a bleeding diathesis due to vitamin K deficiency develops within 21 days. The absorption of triglycerides is not fully dependent on the presence of bile salts because approximately 60% to 70% of triglycerides can be absorbed in their absence. However, only 50% of dietary and biliary free cholesterol can be absorbed in their absence.[523] Bile salts are also thought to enhance the intestinal absorption of iron and calcium.

Influence of Nonhepatic and Hepatic Disorders on Serum Bile Acid Concentrations

A summary of the effects of various disorders on the serum bile acid concentrations is provided in Table 8–13 and discussed below.

Intestinal Disease

Chronic diarrhea can alter intestinal and colonic epithelium as a result of perturbed bile acid metabolism.[524] Small intestinal bacterial overgrowth can result in increased bile acid deconjugation, rapid absorption of free bile acids in the proximal jejunum, and subsequent fat maldigestion and steatorrhea.[525] In this circumstance, steatorrhea may be alleviated following readjustment of the bowel flora. Loss of a critical volume of the terminal ileum as a result of inflammation or resection can cause increased delivery of bile acids to the colon, resulting in diarrhea and/or steatorrhea. If the extent of ileal loss or dysfunction is not severe, patients may develop diarrhea that resolves with administration of cholestyramine (a bile acid–binding agent). Diarrhea develops when increased amounts of deoxycholic and chenodeoxycholic acid are delivered to the colon. Bile salts, particularly the dihydroxy bile salts, inhibit water, sodium chloride, and bicarbonate absorption, promote potassium secretion, and accelerate colonic motility.[526–531]

Cholecystectomy

Cholecystectomy does not abolish diurnal variations of serum CA and CDCA concentrations. However, it does increase the fractional turnover rate and the rate of intestinal degradation of certain bile acids. Cholecystectomy increases the enterohepatic cycling of bile acids in the fasting state. The cholecystectomized patient has slightly high fasting serum bile acid concentrations and slightly low, early, and a less obvious postprandial serum bile acid increase. These patients develop increased quantities of

secondary bile acids due to increased exposure to dehydroxylating intestinal anaerobes, in the distal ileum. Demonstration of higher than normal proportion of DCA relative to CA substantiates increased production of the secondary bile acid. Newly formed DCA is efficiently absorbed from the intestines and CA synthesis is curtailed as a result of feedback inhibition derived from an increased transhepatic flux of bile acids. This leads to a reduced proportion of CA in the bile acid pool.

Bile Acids in Liver Disease

The diagnostic efficacy of fasting and 2 hour postprandial total serum bile acid values in the dog and cat have established that they are useful in the diagnosis of hepatobiliary disorders associated with histologic lesions or portosystemic shunting.[532–543] Bile acid values improve the diagnostic performance of routine tests when used adjunctively. The application of the serum bile acid test to the diagnosis of hepatobiliary disease in the dog and cat is fully discussed in Chapter 8.

Individual bile acid moieties in serum and bile have been thoroughly characterized in human beings with various types of liver injury.[495,544–552] Some of these changes are characterized in Table 8–14. There has only been limited work in this area in the dog and cat.[553–558] Serum bile acid profiles in normal dogs, dogs with portosystemic shunts, a dog with cholestatic neoplasia, normal cats, cats with hepatic lipidosis and cats with major bile duct occlusion have been characterized. For further discussion of the alterations in serum bile acid profiles in patients with hepatic disease, see Chapter 8 and other sources.[495,544–558]

Hepatic Toxicity of Bile Acids

Certain bile acids administered in large doses induce acute hepatocellular injury accompanied by cholestasis. One of the most noxious bile acids is lithocholic acid, which can intercalate into cell membranes, altering both structure and function. Most notably affected are bile canaliculi, which results in cholestasis. CDCA has a greater effect on cell membranes, leading to more immediate cytotoxicity. In addition to cytotoxic membrane damage, bile acids alter cell surface receptors and membrane-signaling systems.[559–563] They also impair cell-mediated immune and macrophage activity, and both LCA and CDCA have been shown to enhance expression of histocompatibility foci on hepatocytes and biliary epithelium, which augments their destruction. It is now well accepted that endogenous bile acids contribute to perpetuation and progression of chronic liver injury. Infusions of taurochenodoxycholate and taurocholate in the rat cause severe biochemical abnormalities. In bile, these include a 30-fold increase in biliary leakage of proteins such as alkaline phosphatase, lactate dehydrogenase, IgG, and albumin.[560,561] Enzyme induction is thought to contribute to the increased enzyme activities; taurocholic acid has been shown to be a potent inducer of alkaline phosphatase. Hepatocytes in zone 1 are most severely affected by bile acid toxicity. Injured hepatocytes exhibit swollen mitochondria and endoplasmic reticulum and loss of surface membrane integrity with extrusion of cytoplasm and organelles. Altered lipid composition of membranes is thought to be involved, as is abnormal transport and signaling.[561–563] Bile acid cytotoxicity is inversely proportional to the degree of hydroxylation: the dihydroxy bile acids (CDCA, DCA) are most injurious. Increased lipid solubility also increases cytotoxicity. Conjugation does not result in significant differences in bile acid toxicity, with the exception of deoxycholate conjugates, which induce enzyme leakage more rapidly.

Bile Acids as Therapeutic Agents

DEHYDROCHOLIC ACID. Dehydrocholic acid (DHCA) is a synthetic bile acid derived by oxidation of cholic acid; it has a keto group in the 3-position rather than an hydroxyl group. It is not detected in serum using the conventional enzymatic assay for bile acids. This bile acid has been used as a potent choleretic in physiologic studies of the biliary system. It is a potent choleretic because its osmotic activity in bile is not diminished by micelle formation.[564] It increases the total volume of bile by stimulating a watery secretion without increasing biliary solids. It does not increase the elimination of bilirubin pigments, but rather has been shown to decrease bilirubin excretion.[565] DHCA does not increase the elimination of other bile acids, cholesterol, or phospholipids. During passage through the liver, 50% of DHCA is believed to become 3alpha-hydroxylated, forming CA.[564] One study has shown that extensive metabolism to other bile acids also occurs.[565] For short-term use, DHCA appears to be minimally hepatotoxic. Studies of patients subjected to chronic DHCA administration have not been completed. Therapeutic use of DHCA is recommended when a "thinning" of biliary secretions is desired. It has been used in dogs and cats with biliary sludge or precipitation confirmed during laparotomy. It should always be used in this context with antibiotics and fluid therapy. Sludged bile or biliary concretions can be associated with biliary tract infection in a causal or secondary role. Fluid therapy is important because these patients must remain well hydrated if hydrocholeresis is to be induced. Observation of biliary sludge on ultrasonographic evaluation is not an indication for use of dehydrocholate. Sludged biliary material is commonly observed in anorectic animals. Currently, ursodeoxycholic acid (UDCA; see following section) is being used in most animals that require hydrocholeresis.

URSODEOXYCHOLIC ACID (UDCA). UDCA has been recommended as a treatment for liver disease for the past 40 years in Asia. It is a powerful choleretic and can be used to treat sludged bile and cholelithiasis. It has limited effect in the gastrointestinal tract as an aid to lipid digestion. UDCA received global attention for use in the treatment of chronic liver disease after it was recognized that it improved the condition of patients with serious liver disease being treated for cholelithiasis. Patients with serious liver disease, unrelated to their cholelithiasis, underwent remarkable improvement in serum biochemical tests (enzymes, total bilirubin, increased albumin) and some had resolution of jaundice and ascites.[566] UDCA has been shown to benefit humans with chronic active hepatitis, primary biliary cirrhosis, sclerosing cholangitis, chronic persistent hepatitis, cirrhosis, biliary atresia in infants, and the hepatic lesions associated with cystic fibrosis. Although its precise mechanism of action remains controversial, it is now believed to alter expression of histocompatibility foci on hepatocytes and biliary epithelium involved in the perpetuation of inflammatory injury. This is believed to suppress the targeting of cytotoxic T cells, block the destruction of bile ducts, and prevent periportal or lobular necrosis, thereby slowing the progression of liver injury. It is clear that UDCA modifies the cytotoxic effects of the most noxious bile acids. Simulta-

neous infusion of the taurine conjugate of UDCA prevents injury caused by other bile acids. Studies on liposomes, erythrocytes, esophageal and gastric mucosa, and in vitro incubation with hepatocytes have shown that UDCA has minimal adverse effects on biologic membranes.

Extensive toxicity studies were conducted in dogs when this product was evaluated for use in humans. It is not toxic to the dog when given in doses much higher than those used therapeutically. A pilot study in healthy cats indicates that it is not toxic to this species; the dose administered was the same as that anticipated for therapeutic use.[567] Although use of any choleretic agent is contraindicated in an animal with major bile duct occlusion, experimental studies of UDCA in rats with major bile duct obstruction demonstrated it could slow the morphologic lesions that typically develop. UDCA is hepatotoxic in rabbits and rhesus monkeys owing to unique differences in metabolism in these species. This drug should not be used without consideration of its potential toxicity.

TRACE METALS: ZINC, COPPER, IRON

The liver plays an influential role in the balance of many trace metals. It is the first organ perfused with blood-carrying alimentary-derived metals. Upon extraction from the portal circulation, some metals are held in an hepatic storage reservoir until needed elsewhere. In the circulation, many metals are bound to transport proteins synthesized in the liver. Examples of such transport proteins include ceruloplasmin, albumin, and transferrin. The concentration of these proteins determines the bioavailability, volume of distribution, and toxicity of metals they transport. Some metals undergo extensive enterohepatic circulation (iron); others rely on the hepatobiliary system for excretion (copper).

Zinc

Zinc is an essential trace metal required for over 200 metalloenzymes involved in intermediary metabolism and collagen homeostasis. It is essential for normal protein metabolism, cell and organelle membrane integrity (membrane stabilization, protection against lipid peroxidation), immune functions, neurosensory functions, wound healing, DNA and RNA replication, gene regulation, and for normal reproduction.[211,568] It has also been shown to increase the concentration of hepatocellular glutathione and in this way functions as an antioxidant.[569]

Zinc is absorbed mainly in the small intestines.[568,570] Only about 25% of ingested zinc is absorbed. Zinc acetate is absorbed more efficiently than the gluconate or sulfate forms. Zinc uptake is significantly regulated by metallothioneins, small sulfhydryl-rich metal-binding proteins located in enterocytes and hepatocytes. During periods of zinc deficiency, the concentration of intestinal metallothionein is reduced and more zinc is absorbed. During periods of high zinc intake, metallothionein increases and intestinal zinc uptake is blocked. Metallothionein has a greater binding affinity for copper than for zinc. As metallothionein concentration increases, copper is bound preventing its absorption. When the intracellular concentration of metallothionein is high, zinc absorption is also reduced, which protects against iatrogenic zinc toxicity when zinc is used as a therapeutic agent. As a result of this physiologic response of metallothionein zinc therapy has become an important means of managing copper storage hepatopathies.[571-573] Pretreatment with zinc and

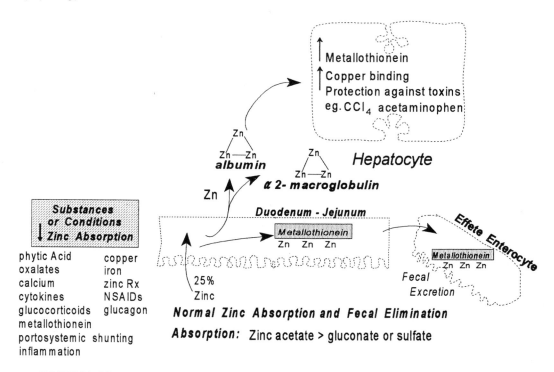

FIGURE 30–22. Diagrammatic representation of zinc uptake.

induction of metallothionein has also been shown to mitigate the hepatotoxic effects of bromobenzene, acetaminophen, carbon tetrachloride, and pyrrolizidine alkaloids in rats.[569,574–577] Metallothionein is considered an important detoxification mechanism. Induction occurs primarily in the liver and intestines and is followed by increased accumulation and/or redistribution of copper and zinc in each tissue. In rats, this protein has a rapid turnover; its concentration falls to negligible levels within 20 hours after discontinuing oral zinc administration.[578,579] An overview of zinc metabolism is provided in Figure 30–22.

Low serum and liver tissue zinc concentrations have been documented in many types of liver disease in humans.[580–585] One study has shown that lowest concentrations develop in humans with cirrhosis associated with acquired portosystemic shunting.[586] The genesis of altered zinc metabolism in patients with hepatobiliary disease is multifactorial (see Table 30–20). These patients tend to have reduced zinc intake because of anorexia, appetite change, and consumption of a restricted protein diet. The main source of dietary zinc is meat and fish. A diet adequate in calories but low in meat-derived protein may contain less than half the "normal" amount of ingested zinc.[568] Patients with liver disease also seem to have reduced intestinal uptake of zinc. This is speculated to be related to metallothionein induction by cytokines, stress hormones such as glucocorticoids and glucagon, and reduced intestinal zinc absorption (especially in the presence of portal hypertension).[586,587] Patients with liver disease also undergo increased urinary zinc excretion.[585,588,589] Hypozincemia is a well-established biologic effect of IL-1, IL-6, and tumor necrosis factor, each known to be increased in humans with liver disease.

Zinc deficiency can have far-reaching consequences, particularly in the patient with liver disease. One important consideration is that low concentrations of zinc promote hyperammonemia as a result of compromised urea cycle enzyme activity.[208–210,590] Oral zinc therapy can improve the clinical

status of humans suffering from HE purportedly thorough this mechanism.[210] Another important consequence of zinc deficiency is that it appears to permit tissue accumulation of potentially hepatotoxic metals such as iron and copper. Zinc-deficient rats develop significant increases in hepatic and total body accumulation of iron and copper. Given zinc's essential association with DNA and RNA polymerases, zinc deficiency would impair hepatocellular regeneration following an ischemic or necrotizing insult. Reduced activity of hepatic microsomal P-450 oxidases has also been associated with zinc deficiency.[591] This adversely influences the metabolism of barbiturates. Insufficient zinc may also increase susceptibility to oxidative injury.[592] Zinc deficiency in patients with hepatic disease may increase their sensitivity to drugs and their susceptibility to toxins. Because zinc deficiency can produce disorders of taste and smell that impair normal appetite, this could influence the nutritional status of patients with liver disease.

Zinc toxicity can cause acute hepatic necrosis. Midzonal mineralization and vacuolation around the hepatic vein in zone 3, mineralization of portal vasculature, and biliary hyperplasia have been described in calves.[593]

Iron

Iron is the most abundant trace metal in the body. The liver is central to iron metabolism because it contains the largest depot of stored iron and is the principal site of synthesis of iron transport proteins. Kupffer cells assist in iron reutilization. After phagocytosis of senescent RBCs and heme extraction, most iron is returned to the circulation. The liver is particularly vulnerable to iron overload; hepatic failure is a central cause of death in acute or chronic iron overload.[594]

In health, most body iron is incorporated in heme.

Table 30–20

ESSENTIAL FUNCTIONS OF ZINC OF SPECIAL CONCERN IN HEPATIC DISEASE

DNA and RNA polymerases: promotes hepatocellular repair

Microsomal enzymes: drug metabolism

Antioxidant effect: stabilizes membranes; inhibits membrane peroxidation

Urea cycle enzymes: improves NH_3 tolerance

Metallothionein induction: protection against hepatic toxicity, copper, acetaminophen, bromobenzene, carbon tetrachloride, pyrrolizadine alkaloids

Repression of certain toxin-metabolizing enzyme systems

MECHANISMS OF ZINC DEFICIENCY IN HEPATIC DISEASE

Dietary insufficiency

Anorexia

Reduced intestinal absorption:
  metallothionein induction: cytokines IL-1, IL-6, tumor necrosis factor, glucocorticoids, glucagon
  portal hypertension

Redistribution of zinc
  cytokine effect
  metallothionein induction

Increased urinary excretion

Remaining iron is stored in tissues including the hepatocytes, reticuloendothelial cells of the bone marrow and spleen, and skeletal muscles.[594] Iron is stored in the form of ferritin, hemosiderin, and hematin. Only a very small amount of iron is in the extracellular compartment bound to transferrin, the most important of the iron transport proteins. Estimation of the adequacy of systemic iron stores is best accomplished by determining the serum ferritin concentration; low values indicate iron depletion. Serum iron is an unreliable indicator of total body iron adequacy because it is affected by many factors unrelated to the iron status. Examples include inflammation, which decreases the circulating iron concentration, and corticosteroids, which increase the serum iron concentration.[595] The reliability of the serum total iron binding capacity (a reflection of transferrin) for estimation of iron adequacy varies among species. During iron deficiency it is unreliable in dogs.[596,597]

Iron uptake by reticuloendothelial cells primarily involves phagocytosis and hemolysis of senescent red blood cells. Heme released from hemoglobin is degraded by heme oxygenase in microsomes. Kupffer cells and other macrophages also phagocytize damaged erythrocytes; it is estimated that individual macrophages have the capacity to take up more than 10 erythrocytes should the need arise.[598] In the circumstance of unrestricted erythrophagocytosis instigated by immunosensitized erythrocytes, Kupffer cells can ingest a tremendous load of iron. This is particularly noxious in the circumstance of hypoxia, which often accompanies a critical hemolytic process. In most cases, iron derived from phagocytized RBCs is either released for binding to transferrin or is incorporated into ferritin.[599] Some Kupffer cell ferritin may be passed to hepatocytes. Lactoferrin released from degranulating neutrophils sequesters iron in the vicinity of inflammation. Sequestration of iron in this way is believed to inhibit growth of foreign cells and microorganisms and to minimize damage initiated by iron catalyzed free radical formation. Much of the released lactoferrin is scavenged by macrophages. That which escapes into plasma may be taken up by hepatic endothelium and Kupffer

cells and subsequently deposited as ferritin. Ferritin released at sites of inflammation may also be taken up by hepatocytes. Hepatic deposition of iron in these ways can lead to an apparent hepatic iron "overload" in inflammatory disorders. This may explain the accumulation of iron in hepatocytes and Kupffer cells in some hepatic diseases. Chronic hepatitis observed in Doberman pinschers, for example, is associated with increased accumulations of iron in areas of inflammation. Small lipid granulomas containing iron are commonly observed in liver tissue from both dogs and cats with chronic inflammatory hepatopathies. Even animals with portosystemic vascular anomalies can develop these small lipogranulomas that stain positively for iron.

Hepatic distribution and concentration of iron is important in the development of liver disease in chronic iron overload. Humans with hereditary hemochromatosis (a disorder of excessive hepatic iron storage) have a predominant hepatocellular iron deposition. These patients develop hepatic disease when liver iron concentrations attain 5,000 to 6,000 μg iron/g wet liver weight. Occasionally, liver injury occurs at concentrations of iron as low as 3,000 μg/g wet liver weight.[594] In humans with iron overload resulting from repeated blood transfusions, excess iron is deposited in both hepatocytes and Kupffer cells and liver disease is not seen until the hepatic iron concentration exceeds 9,000 to 10,000 μg/g wet tissue weight.[600,601] Oral rather than parenteral iron loading (with carbonyl ion) causes a gradual increase in hepatic parenchymal iron stores. Iron deposits in zone 1 (periportal distribution), a pattern analogous to that seen in human hereditary hemochromatosis. Parenteral administration of iron chelates (iron-dextran, iron-sorbitol, or FeNTA) results in a diffuse lobular deposition of iron in RE cells and hepatocytes. Hepatic iron loading is an important pathophysiologic concern not only because iron is a potent free radical, but also because hepatocellular iron overload can culminate in hepatic fibrosis, cirrhosis, and hepatocellular carcinoma. Each of these conditions are sequelae to the syndrome of hemochromatosis in human beings.

Iron-associated hepatic injury is believed to evolve from iron-induced lipid peroxidation of membranes, including those of the mitochondria, lysosomes, and peroxisomes. Organelle injury leads to cellular dysfunction.[600–603] It is the low molecular weight iron rather than the storage forms that are responsible for production of free radicals and subsequent lipid peroxidation. In health, the hepatocyte is able to maintain iron in a nontoxic protein-bound ferric state. When overload occurs, excessive amounts of iron generate hydroxyl radicals (OH·) by reacting with H_2O_2. Free ferrous iron Fe^{+2} can independently initiate membrane peroxidation by formation of perferryl ion (FeO^{2+}) or by formation of a free radical complex involving polyunsaturated fatty acids, ferrous iron, and oxygen. In rats with chronic dietary iron loading, hepatic lipid peroxidation depends on the extent of iron loading. The proposed mechanisms of iron toxicity are summarized in Figure 30–23. Hepatic iron overload can impair activity of certain microsomal enzymes, the cytochrome P-450 enzymes being most susceptible.[602–604] Several studies have shown impaired drug metabolizing systems.[610–613]

Copper

Copper is an essential element that is an important component of numerous metalloenzymes critical for a broad repertoire of metabolic functions including mitochondrial energy

Proposed Mechanisms of Copper & Iron Hepatoxicity

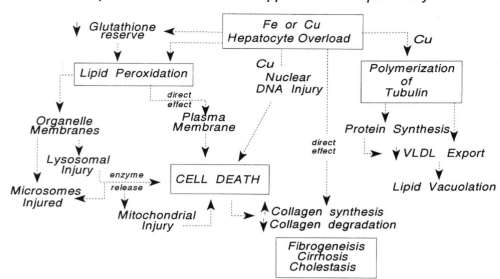

FIGURE 30–23. Diagrammatic representation of the proposed mechanisms of iron- and copper-related injury to the hepatocyte.

production, cross-linkage of elastin and collagen fibrils, scavenging of oxygen radicals, and production of melanin.

Approximately 30% to 60% of ingested copper is absorbed. Most absorption occurs in the upper portion of the small intestines. Enterocyte copper absorption is highly regulated by metallothionein. High levels of metallothionein bind copper within the enterocyte; complex formation prohibits systemic copper absorption. The copper-metallothionein complex is retained within the enterocyte and is lost from the body when the enterocyte is sloughed into the alimentary canal. The highest tissue concentration of copper is found in the liver, where 50% is located in the cytosol associated with metallothionein, superoxide dismutase, and ceruloplasmin. The remainder is located in the nuclear fraction (20%), in the large granule fraction (20%, lysosomes and mitochondria as cytochrome c oxidase and monoamine oxidase), and in microsomes (10%).[605] A schematic representation of hepatic copper metabolism is provided in Figure 30–24.

The major determinant in copper homeostasis is biliary excretion. Glucocorticoids are known to promote biliary copper secretion. Cholestatic liver disorders are believed to increase liver copper concentrations as a result of impaired biliary copper elimination.[606] The concentration of copper is usually less than 400 µg/g dry liver in healthy dogs and cats.[607–612] Hepatotoxicity associated with excess copper deposition varies with the species studied.[613] Some animals can sequester large amounts of copper within lysosomes and thus protect their liver from toxicity; the dog seems to be moderate in its tolerance. A disorder associated with excess copper storage has been well defined in the Bedlington terrier and is suspected in a few other pure breeds; these are discussed in Chapter 33.[607–612,614] The cat seems to be relatively tolerant of copper in comparison to the dog.

There are several proposed mechanisms of copper-associated hepatic toxicity. These include (1) stimulation of mitochondrial lipid peroxidation leading to abnormal cell respiration; (2) impaired protein sulfhydryl groups that promotes polymerization of cytosolic proteins such as tubulin in microtubules; (3) impaired cell protein synthesis decreasing cell survival and growth; (4) lysosomal dysfunction associated with increased fragility and release of enzymes into the cytosol; and (5) impaired formation and exportation of constituent proteins and lipoproteins. These effects may result in altered plasma and organelle membrane permeability, disfigured and dysfunctional cytosolic proteins, destabilized nuclear DNA, depleted glutathione reserves, stimulation of fibrogenesis, and cell death. Mechanisms of hepatoxicity of copper are summarized in Figure 30–23.

The morphologic pattern of copper deposition in dogs with excessive hepatic copper stores varies among breeds and the suspected underlying factors. Acute copper toxicity due to ingestion of toxic quantities causes perivenular, submassive, or massive necrosis. This is relatively uncommon but can occur in the late stages of copper storage hepatopathy in the Bedlington terrier when sudden massive release of copper from the liver can result in a hemolytic crisis and hepatic necrosis. In Bedlingtons and West Highland white terriers, early deposition of copper is in perivenular hepatocytes (adjacent to the hepatic vein). In the Bedlington, as the consumption of copper continues, the lesions progress from focal hepatitis to a diffuse distribution. High concentrations of hepatic copper can accumulate in any type of cholestatic liver disease including chronic bile duct occlusion, biliary cirrhosis, and chronic cholestatic hepatitis. Periportal copper deposition seems common in the early stages of cholestatic disease. This type of copper retention is observed in the hepatopathy described in the Doberman pinscher.[610,615] When hepatic fibrosis and nodular regeneration are well established in chronic liver disease, the concentration of tissue copper declines as a result of cell regeneration. New cells are comparatively free of copper storage and displacement of hepatocytes by connective tissue reduces the quantity of cells that can store copper.

THERAPEUTIC BENEFITS OF TRACE METAL REGULATION. Theoretically, zinc supplementation is beneficial in the patient with liver disease associated with increased hepatocellular accumulation of copper, and possibly in those associated with excess iron stores. Zinc induction of enterocyte metallothionein, results in effective blockade against enteric copper absorption. Zinc also induces hepatic metallothionein which sequesters excessive copper into an innocuous form. Zinc has also been shown to be hepatoprotective against experimentally induced toxin-associated hepatic injury.[569,571–577] These hepatoprotective effects include zinc repression of certain

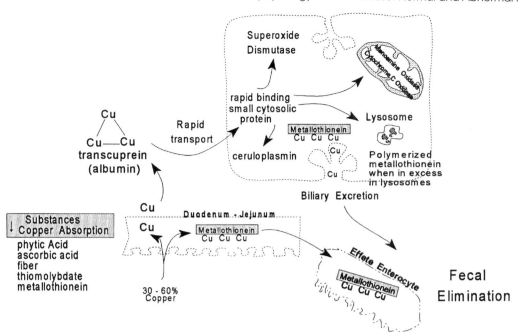

FIGURE 30-24. Diagrammatic representation of copper uptake, transport, and hepatic storage.

cytochrome P-450 microsomal enzymes essential for generation of toxic metabolites; the induction of metallothionein rich in SH groups used in detoxication; stabilization of membranes; and inhibition of membrane peroxidation. [569,571-577] Similar benefits may be realized in the patient with iron-associated liver injury, but confirmatory work has not been completed. In addition to the cytoprotective benefits of zinc, an improvement in the mental capacity of humans with cirrhosis and HE has been shown, possibly due to improved ammonia detoxification.[210] Treatment with D-penicillamine to chelate excessive copper was the mainstay of therapy for copper-associated hepatopathies for many years. Side effects of drug therapy have focused increasing attention on alternative treatments with zinc or other copper chelators (tetramine). These are discussed in Chapter 33.

Treatment of seemingly pathologic hepatic iron stores (iron in hepatocytes) in dogs or cats with liver disease has not been adequately discussed in the veterinary literature because such lesions are comparatively rare.

DRUG AND TOXIN METABOLISM

The liver occupies a central position in the metabolism of drugs and toxins. Of particular importance is its location in the portal circulatory pathway, which permits immediate access to substances absorbed from the intestines. The liver can profoundly influence the bioavailability of a drug or toxin acquired through the gastrointestinal tract. After a substance has entered the hepatocyte, it may be excreted with or without biotransformation, initially into the biliary system and then into the gastrointestinal tract where it may be resorbed in an enterohepatic circulation. Such enterohepatic cycling may prolong its systemic availability. If a substance is completely removed from the portal circulation on a single circulatory pass through the liver, its bioavailability after an oral dose will be low and first-pass extraction will be high. The presence of hepatoportal circulatory derangements and

hepatic architectural injury may profoundly change drug or toxin absorption and disposition. Especially influenced are substances that undergo first-pass extraction. Oral bioavailability increases for these when portosystemic shunting develops or when a substantive loss of hepatocellular mass occurs. When shunting is the primary derangement, the bioavailability of highly extracted drugs parallels the fraction of blood shunted around the liver.

Hepatic metabolism of drugs and toxins converts lipid soluble substances into a water soluble form. This permits biliary or urinary excretion. A number of chemical pathways in the liver are capable of increasing the polarity of xenobiotics (substances foreign to the body). Some systems are specialized and used exclusively for this purpose; others catalyze normal endogenous reactions. Many of the enzymes involved with drug and toxin metabolism are associated with the endoplasmic reticulum.

Hepatic metabolism of xenobiotics is catalyzed by three classes of enzymes: oxidoreductases, hydrolases, and transferases. Oxidation-reduction and hydrolytic reactions usually insert reactive groups in a drug molecule.[616] These are referred to as *phase I* reactions. Examples include addition of carboxyl, epoxide, or hydroxyl groups on a parent compound. Addition of these groups tends to increase polarity and water solubility and thereby enhance the potential for urinary or biliary excretion. They also provide a site for further chemical modification in phase II reactions. Phase I reactions usually detoxify a parent compound; however, in some cases they generate toxic metabolites.

Synthetic reactions catalyzed by transferase enzymes modify phase I reaction products. These are referred to as *phase II* reactions. Acetate, amino acids, sulfate, glucuronic acid, and glutathione are transferred to phase I products, and generally enhance their water solubility and potential for biliary or urinary excretion.[616] These products are less toxic or less biologically active compared to the parent compound. Although the combination of phase I and phase II reactions provides a powerful mechanism for detoxification, many substances are metabolized by phase II reactions directly. Phase II reactions are involved in the metabolism of endogenous steroids, hormones, bile acids, and bilirubin.

The most important phase I drug-metabolizing enzymes are those comprising the P-450 microsomal enzyme system. The *P* refers to pigment, and the *450* refers to the absorption spectrum of the enzymes.[616] This system is an electron transport chain comprised of several distinct forms of cytochrome P-450 associated with membranes of the endoplasmic reticulum and nucleus. At least nine different forms have been characterized in humans. The P-450 microsomal enzyme system is more prominent in the liver compared to other tissues and it is here that more than 50% of drugs are metabolized. It also activates many potential toxins. Although a number of different chemical reactions are catalyzed by this system, their general function is to catalyze substrate mono-oxygenation.[616] The P-450 enzymes are thus referred to as mono-oxygenases or mixed function oxidases. Some xenobiotics are metabolized at more than one site by this system. The predominant reactions catalyzed include aliphatic hydroxylations, aromatic hydroxylation, O-, N-, and S-dealkylations, dehalogenations, N-hydroxylation, and N-oxide formation. The demethylation of aminopyrine and the dehydroxylation and demethylation of antipyrine have been used as in vivo measurements of the activity of this enzyme system. In a clinical patient this can reflect their capacity for drug metabolism. Application of these tests is complicated by the fact that metabolism is accomplished by some rather than all of the P-450 enzymes, and because there are intrinsic differences in clearance rates among individuals. There have been limited studies of the clinical utility of these agents in companion animals.[617]

There are other microsomal pathways for drug oxidation that are not associated with the cytochrome P-450 system. Most notable are those involved with metabolism of nitrogen or sulfur; examples include flavoprotein (FAD)-containing amine oxidases, now called microsomal FAD-containing mono-oxyganase or mixed function oxidase, and monoamine oxidase. These enzymes are located in the cytosol and outer mitochondrial membranes.

Phase II reactions are familiarly called *conjugation reactions*. The most common conjugate is glucuronic acid. In these reactions, uridine diphosphate glucuronic acid (UDPGA) is conjugated to a substance under the influence of UDP-glucuronyltransferase, a membrane-bound enzyme of the endoplasmic reticulum. Bilirubin is conjugated using this system (see Figure 30–18). There are several forms of this enzyme. Each form is susceptible to induction by different types of compounds. The glucuronidating capacity of the liver is dependent on the rate of UDPGA generation from UDP-glucose; in some animals this has been shown to correlate with their hepatic glycogen stores and nutritional condition.[618,619] Variables or conditions that impair formation of UDP-glucose can impair the glucuronication capacity and lead to adverse drug effects; examples include hypoxia, ingestion of galactosamine (a potent hepatotoxin), and alcohol ingestion. Agents that impair glucuronyltransferase activity also can impair glucuronidation and cause adverse drug effects.

A large number of xenobiotics and endogenous substances are sulfated in the liver. There are several different sulfating enzymes; at least eight are involved with xenobiotic metabolism. Examples of endogenous substances metabolized by sulfation include bile acids, estrone, and 3 beta-hydroxysteroids. In general, sulfate conjugation leads to inactive or less active compounds that are more water soluble and more readily excreted in urine or bile. However, a few compounds become more toxic by this process.[620]

A family of similar enzymes, glutathione S-transferases, catalyze glutathione conjugation. Active electophilic toxins can react spontaneously with glutathione, which functions as a free radical scavenger. The presence of cytosolic glutathione S-transferase ensures their reaction with glutathione. Unfortunately, rapid conjugation of toxins with glutathione can lead to its cellular depletion. This occurs, for example, following exposure to acetaminophen. Administration of cysteine or N-acetylcysteine enhances the rate of glutathione synthesis and is effective in protecting against acetaminophen hepatotoxicity if given before or early (within 10 hours) following intoxication. One form of glutathione S-transferase serves as a cellular transport protein for organic anions. This form, referred to as ligandin, is operational in the metabolism of sulfobromophthalein and bilirubin. In general, conjugation with glutathione prepares a compound for biliary excretion.

Certain phase II reactions render a parent molecule less water soluble. These include certain methylation and acetylation reactions. Nevertheless, these still seem to inactivate or detoxify the parent compound. Acetylation is an important pathway for inactivation of amine-containing drugs. These enzymes are found in white blood cells and in many other tissues besides the liver, where they can be measured. Acetylation is important in detoxification of sulfonamides, procainamide, serotonin, p-aminobenzoate, aspirin, and hydralazine. Considerable polymorphism has been shown for acetylation capacity in humans and in the dog. Certain Doberman pinschers have been shown to be slow acetylators.[621–623] Such differences can profoundly affect drug pharmacokinetics.

A final phase II mechanism of xenobiotic modification is conjugation of carboxyl groups with amino acids. This differs from other conjugation reactions in that it occurs in mitochondria or peroxisomes via several different enzyme catalyzed steps. Amino acid conjugation with glycine or taurine is the final step in formation of bile acids. Virtually all bile acids undergo such conjugation prior to biliary elimination.

Factors Affecting Drug-Metabolizing Enzymes

More than 200 compounds have been identified that can stimulate or inhibit some type of microsomal enzyme activity. These include drugs, insecticides, organic solvents, carcinogens, and environmental pollutants. Adverse drug interactions result when one drug influences the metabolism of another. Activity of the P-450 system can be either decreased or increased. Decreased activity can develop from reduced cellular content of P-450 enzymes or from enzyme inhibition. Decreased enzyme production can result from impaired heme availability because heme is an essential component of the cytochrome structure. Heme availability can be restricted following induction of heme oxygenase activity by cobalt or organotin compounds and by chloramphenicol.[624] A number of xenobiotics are metabolically activated by cytochrome P-450 to reactive intermediates that cause so-called suicidal destruction of system enzymes. This can lead to a 20% to 80% decrease in enzyme activity and complete loss of certain hydroxylating activities.

Increased activity of xenobiotic-metabolism may be related to increased enzyme synthesis, decreased enzyme turnover, or enhanced cellular concentration of substrates. A biphasic effect is seen with some enzyme inducers. Initially, they inhibit P-450 catalyzed reactions by competing for system enzyme(s). Later they promote appearance of new enzyme, which increases the net drug-metabolizing activity. Two different general categories of inducer effects have been recognized. One is typified by phenobarbital with features that include increase in overall liver size and weight, proliferation of endoplasmic reticulum, increased microsomal protein and hemoprotein content, activities of a variety of enzymes, and UDPGT conjugation activity. The other type is typified by a more limited effect on a small group of enzymes. Many forms of P-450 are inducible; barbiturates and phenytoin induce the metabolism of many drugs via this mechanism.

Some drugs stimulate their own metabolism as well as that of others. This leads to drug tolerance and may require clinical dosing adjustments. This occurs with barbiturates, the most notable example being phenobarbital. Spironolactone, a diuretic commonly used in the treatment of ascites in the dog, induces the metabolism of a variety of steroids including prednisone. In addition to interfering with drug metabolism, some enzyme inducers enhance the metabolism of xenobiotics to toxic intermediates. Phenobarbital augments the toxic effects of acetaminophen, carbon tetrachloride, and nitrosamines through increased formation of toxic adducts. Examples of substances that modify the activity or availability of microsomal enzymes are listed in Table 30–21. There are species differences in effects on microsomal enzymes; these have not been distinctly defined for the dog and cat. The influence of phenobarbital enzyme induction on metabolism of a limited number of drugs and toxins has been studied in the dog.[625–633]

Age also influences drug metabolism. Neonatal dogs achieve maximal activity of drug-metabolizing enzymes by the fifth to eighth week after birth.[634] With old age, the rates of drug metabolism, volume of distribution, and impaired hepatic blood flow can all contribute to altered drug pharmacokinetics. In healthy geriatric dogs up to 10 years old, normal activity of most drug-metabolizing enzymes are maintained.[634]

Nutritional condition can influence xenobiotic metabolism. Mild to moderate malnutrition usually does not have much of an influence. However, fasting or an exclusive mono-carbohydrate diet in rats has been shown to impair the availability of glutathione and consequently to enhance toxicity of certain drugs and toxins.[635] Dietary protein intake also appears to modify metabolism of some drugs. Examples include enhanced metabolism of antipyrine and theophylline on a high-protein diet.

The influence of liver disease on the elimination and metabolism of drugs is highly variable and often unpredictable. The clinician should learn to anticipate the unexpected and to consult pharmacologic references frequently when choosing medications for a patient with compromised hepatic function. Studies have shown that altered drug metabolism may be related to decreased activity of drug-metabolizing enzymes, cholestasis, altered (increased or decreased) hepatic blood flow, reduced liver cell volume, and decreased availability of NADPH due to altered cell energy metabolism. The activity of some of the P-450 microsomes

Table 30–21

AGENTS THAT MODIFY MICROSOMAL ENZYME ACTIVITY

↓ Microsomal Enzyme Activity

↓ P-450 availability
cobalt
organotin compounds
chloramphenicol

↑ P-450 destruction
chloramphenicol
phencyclidine
secobarbital
17-alpha ethinylestradiol
certain insecticide synergists
quinidine

↑ Formation Inactive P-450
propoxyphen (Darvon)
troleandomycin
piperonyl butoxide

↓ P-450 Activity by Competitive Binding
carbon monoxide
metyrapone
quinine
imidazole antimycotics:
   ketoconazole, clotrimazole, miconazole
   cimetidine
   ranitidine

Inherited deficiencies
humans: 5% to 10% of population has a defect

Nonspecific inhibitors microsomal enzymes

allopurinol	monoamine oxidase inhibitors
quinidine	organophosphates
methylphenidate	oxyphenbutazone
metronidazole	sulfonamides
morphine	valporic acid

↑ Microsomal Enzyme Activity
↑ P-450 Activity

alcohol	phenylbutazone*
chlorinated hydrocarbons: DDT, others	phenytoin*
chlorphenoxy herbicides	polycyclic aromatic hydrocarbon
dexamethasone*	pregnenolone
imidazoles	primidone*
isoniazid	pyrazole
pentobarbital	rifampin
phenobarbital*	triacetyloleandomycin

↑ Drug-Metabolizing Enzymes (nonspecified)

carbamazepine, chlorpromazine, diphenhydramine, glutethimide, griseofulvin, imipramine, lithium,* mebrobamate, methoxyflurane, nikethamide, spironolactone

*May be associated with "marked" enzyme induction in the dog.

can be reduced from 30% to 50% in humans with severe liver disease (cirrhosis and intrahepatic cholestasis).[636-641] It is important to recognize that there is a high degree of variation among patients with similar histologic lesions. Most notable is the discrepancy reported among patients with extrahepatic cholestasis. Another confusing finding is that in severe liver disease, the influence of enzyme inducers is inconsistent.

METABOLICALLY INDUCED LIVER DISEASE. As a result of the major detoxification role of the liver, it is not surprising that it can be the primary site of injury when a toxic product is made. Adverse drug reactions are a leading cause of hepatotoxicity in humans and have received enormous attention in the medical literature. A list of the histopathologic reactions of the liver to hepatotoxic drugs in humans, dogs, and cats is provided in Table 30–22.[641-643] Most of the recorded adverse reactions have been documented in humans. Drug-induced liver injury is classified as either predictable (usually dose related) or unpredictable ("idiosyncratic," usually unrelated to dose).[641] The mechanisms by which drugs and their metabolites injure hepatocytes or alter their function are unknown for most agents. Known mechanisms include (1) alteration of the physicochemical properties of membranes; (2) inhibition of membrane enzymes; (3) impairment of hepatic uptake processes; (4) altered cytoskeletal function; (5) precipitation of insoluble complexes in bile; (6) alterations in cell calcium homeostasis; and (7) metabolic conversion to reactive intermediates. Metabolically generated toxins are most often derived from reactions catalyzed by the cytochrome P-450 system. These toxins are potentiated by microsomal enzyme induction and are impaired by exposure to enzyme blockers such as cimetidine.

The biochemical basis for hepatotoxicity among different toxins is variable. Generally they are classified either as free radicals or as containing strong electrophilic centers. Carbon tetrachloride is the best studied of the free-radical-type hepatotoxins. Although the basic underlying toxic mechanism remains to be demonstrated, it leads to peroxidation of membrane phospholipids. Carbon tetrachloride must be metabolized in order to inflict cellular injury. It is not toxic to species that do not metabolize it, such as the chicken. A diagram of the specific proposed mechanisms of carbon tetrachloride hepatotoxicity is provided in Figure 30–25. Perivenular (zone 3) hepatocyte necrosis is the dominant lesion and this is accentuated by pretreatment of experimental animals with phenobarbital. A free-radical-based mechanism of toxicity is also suggested for halothane, diethylstilbestrol, morphine, phenothiazines, doxorubicin, and daunorubicin.[640]

Electrophilic toxins are molecules that can form covalent bonds with tissue macromolecules (proteins). These toxins deactivate enzymes or modify normal regulatory or structural proteins, causing abnormalities in metabolism that lead to cell necrosis. Electrophilic toxins can also lead to oncogenic mutations. Metabolically generated electrophiles are usually detoxified with glutathione before they can react with cell constituents. Unfortunately, the cellular pool of glutathione is limited and in some circumstances is rapidly depleted. The electrophile then becomes injurious. Acetaminophen is an example of an electrophilic toxin, although it also generates free radical injury. Acetaminophen toxicity leads to massive perivenular (zone 3) hepatic necrosis. Its metabolism and mechanism of toxicity are illustrated in Figure 30–26. Toxicity from acetaminophen can be reduced by early treatment (less than 10 hours after ingestion) with oral or intravenous cysteine or N-acetylcysteine. These drugs restore glutathione levels by enhancing its synthesis. Glutathione is not beneficial when administered directly because hepatocytes are unable to transport it into the cytosol.[644] Protein depletion, fasting, or concurrent ingestion of other electrophiles that reduce hepatocellular glutathione enhance acetaminophen toxicity.[635] Treatment either with large doses of ranitidine (120 mg/kg) or cimetidine before administration of toxic amounts of acetaminophen is hepatoprotective because these drugs block production of the electrophile metabolites via an inhibition of P-450 enzymes.[632]

Dimethylnitrosamine, formed in the intestine from nitrates, is also derived from processed foods, agricultural chemicals, and polluted air.[616] This is an important hepatotoxin used to model chronic liver disease in animals.[192,423,645,646] Demethylation of dimethylnitrosamine by cytochrome P-450 microsomal enzymes is believed to generate diazomethane, a potent electrophile. This toxin reacts with cell proteins, leading to hepatotoxicity and carcinogenicity.

Halothane toxicity has been studied extensively. Approximately 20% of halothane is metabolized and toxic effects are related to its metabolic product(s). Animals pretreated with microsomal enzyme inducers and subjected to halothane in a relatively oxygen-deficient environment regularly develop perivenular (zone 3) necrosis. In an oxygen-limited environment, halothane metabolism is diverted to an alternate metabolic pathway generating electrophile intermediates and free radicals. These react with sulfhydryl groups of cell proteins and membranes. In humans, individual susceptibility to halothane toxicity is related to a number of variables including intraoperative hypoxemia, microcirculatory insult, inherent biotransformation activity, adequacy of cellular protective mechanisms, dose, genetic factors, and immunologic responses.

Aflatoxicosis has been well described in dogs.[647-652] Toxicity is associated with an active metabolite that impairs nucleic acid synthesis. Toxic effects can develop within 15 minutes of exposure to the active metabolite. Early lesions are characterized by severe (zone 3) perivenular fatty degeneration extending to the periportal areas. Perivenular canaliculi are distended with bile and a mild round cell inflammatory response is notable in the perivenular and periportal areas. In subacute toxicity, scattered single cell necrosis, bile ductule proliferation, and a mild to severe degree of bridging fibrosis develop. With chronicity, extensive fibrosis is the most striking feature. Most hepatocytes within the fibrous network show fatty degeneration or necrosis. Hepatocytes outside the fibrous matrix may appear normal. Chronically affected dogs develop portal hypertension, hepatic synthetic failure, and ascites. Disseminated intrahepatic coagulation also may complicate the clinical condition.[653]

Other important hepatotoxins are listed in Table 30–23. Some of these have been examined in dogs and cats.[654-676] A summary of the effects of oxidation injury to the liver is shown in Figure 30–27.

Drug Toxicity

Histopathologic changes implicating drug toxicity can range from cholestasis indicated only by canalicular plugging to profound hepatocellular injury associated with zonal or massive cell degeneration, inflammation, or necrosis. Pure cholestasis due to drug therapy, such as occurs with androgens, is characterized by bile retention in canaliculi and hepatocytes.[677] With other drugs there may be distinct zonal involvement accompanied by infiltration with eosinophils or granulomatous inflammation.[678] In some cases, drug toxicity can lead to permanent histologic changes and perpetuating inflammation categorized pathologically as chronic hepatitis. This can proceed to cirrhosis and is believed to occur in some dogs exposed to oxibendazole, mebendazole, methoxyflu-

Table 30–22

HISTOLOGIC INJURIES ASSOCIATED WITH DRUG TOXICITY IN HUMANS, DOGS, AND CATS

Necrosis Perivenous/Mid-zonal Lesions	Necrosis Periportal	Cholestatic	Granulomatous Inflammation	Veno-Occlusive Disease
acetaminophen[d,c]	acetaminophen	acetaminophen	acetaminophen[d, c]	azathioprine
allopurinol	aminosalicylic acid	allopurinol	allopurinol	combination
chlorotetracycline	aspirin	aminosalicylic acid	aspirin	chemotherapy
danorubicin	chlorothiazide	amitryptyline	carbamazepine	contraceptives
diazepam	chlorpropamide	androgens	cephalexin	estrogens
enflurane	cyproheptadine	azathioprine	chlorpropamide	dacarbazine
halothane[d]	dantrolene	captopril	contraceptives	daunorubicin
imipramine	docusate calcium	carbamazepine	diazepam	6-thioguanine
indomethacin	erythromycin	cephalopsporins	halothane	
iodipamide	halothane	chlorambucil	hydralazine	**Cholestasis, No Lesion**
meglumine	isoniazid	chlorothiazide	isoniazid	contraceptives
isoniazid	methyldopa	chlorpropamide	methyldopa	androgens
mercaptopurine	nicotinic acid	chlortetracycline	nitrofurantoin	methyltestosterone[d]
methoxyflurane	nitrofurantoin	cimetidine	oxacillin	gold sodium thiomalate
methyldopa	oxacillin	cisplatin	oxyphenbutazone	phenothiazines
mithramycin	oxibendazole[d]	clorazepate	penicillin	
quinidine	oxyphenbutazone	dacarbazine	phenylbutazone	**Cirrhosis**
rifampin	penicillin	danazol	phenytoin	acetaminophen
sulfasalazine	phenothiazines	dantrolene	procainamide	acetoheximide
tolzamide	propylthiouracil	diazepam	procarbazine	chlorothiazide
	sulfonamide(s)	erythromycin	quinidine	ferrous: fumarate,
Necrosis Submassive/Massive Lesions	trimethoprim/sulfa[d]	flurazepam	sulfonamide(s)	gluconate, sulfate
	tolazamide	griseofulvin	sulfasalazine	halothane
allopurinol		haloperidol		mercaptopurine
amitriptyline	**Inflammation, Necrosis, Lobular**	halothane	**Destructive Nonsuppurative Cholangitis**	methotrexate[d]
carbamazepine		imipramine		methyldopa
carparsolate	aminosalicylic acid	indomethacin	acetaminophen	methyltestosterone
chlordiazepoxide	amitryptyline	iodipamid	chlorpropamide	oxibendazole[d]
cimetidine	aspirin	meglumine	cromolyn sodium	phenobarbital[d]
dacarbazine	carbenicillin	mercaptopurine	haloperidol	phenothiazines
dantrolene	dantrolene	methyldopa	imipramine	phenylbutazone
diazepam[c]	enflurane	oxacillin	methyltestosterone	phenytoin[d]
ethacrynic acid	halothane	oxibendazole[d]	phenylbutazone	primidone[d]
halothane[d]	hydrazine	nicotinic acid	probenecid	valproic acid
hydralazine	h. chlorothiazide	penicillamine	tolbutamide	
indomethacin	isoniazid	penicillin	phenothiazines	**Nodular/Regenerative Hyperplasia**
ketoconazole	ketoconazole	phenothiazines		
mebendazole	mercaptopurine	phenobarbital	**Lipid Vacuolation**	azathioprine
methimazole[c]	methimazole	phenylbutazone		clofibrate
mephobarbital	methoxyflurane	phenytoin	acetaminophen	contraceptives
methoxyflurane	methyldopa	rifampin	asparaginase	oxymethalone
methyldopa	nicotinic acid	sulfonamide(s)	bleomycin	
mitomycin	nitrofurantoin	sulfasalazine	chlortetracycline	**Neoplasia**
nitrofurantoin	penicillin	thiabendazole	cantrolene	contraceptives
phenobarbital	phenazopyridine	trimethobenzamide	flurasepam	methotrexate
phnylbutazone	phenylbutazone	trimethoprim	halothane	methyltestosterone
phenytoin	phenytoin	valproic acid	indomethacin	oxymethalone
probenecid	sulfasalazine		isoniazid	stanozolol
prochlorperazine	sulfonamide(s)		methimazole	thioguanine
propylthiouracil			methyldopa	
sulfadizine			nitrofurantoin	
sulfamethoxazole			oxacillin	
sulfasalizine			rifampin	
valproic acid			spironolactone	
			sulfonamide(s)	
			tetracycline[d,c]	
			valproic acid	

c: cats; d: dogs
Adapted from references 641–643, 655–669, 677–684.

rane, phenobarbital, primidone, and phenytoin. Immunologic mechanisms may promote drug- or toxin-initiated tissue injury, although this is rarely proven. A drug or toxin interacting with hepatocellular proteins or membranes may function as an antigen. The location of drug fixation determines the initial morphologic lesion. After inflammation is established, a self-perpetuating and expanding lesion is speculated to evolve.

The mechanisms discussed previously for generation of hepatotoxins also pertains to hepatic injury caused by some drugs. Toxic metabolites are now implicated as mediators of hepatic injury from a variety of medications. These metabolites appear to be highly reactive and, if not cleared from the liver, fix to cellular organelles and produce hepatic damage and necrosis.[677] Conjugation reactions are of particular impor-

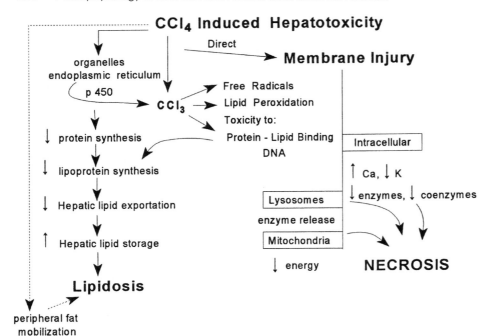

FIGURE 30–25. Diagrammatic representation of the proposed mechanism of carbon tetrachloride–induced hepatic injury.

tance for rapid elimination of toxic drug metabolites. Depletion of glutathione, glucuronide, or sulfates by other toxins can set the stage for drug-induced injury. Nutrition, enzyme induction, and genetically determined rates of drug metabolism can make some patients more susceptible to toxicity. A compilation of the types of hepatotoxic lesions recognized in human beings treated with commonly used medications, relevant to companion animals, and those reported in dogs and cats, is provided in Table 30–22.[655–669,677–684] In most circumstances, drug-associated hepatotoxicity is uncommon. Most reports have been made in human patients and reflect only a few involved individuals.

Hepatic Function and Pharmacokinetics

The influence of liver disease on pharmacokinetics cannot be as clearly estimated as that of renal disease. This occurs due to numerous biochemical intricacies influencing drug metabolism and the influence of liver function on whole animal health. A number of important variables are summarized in Table 30–24. Drug therapy must always be individually tailored with the clinician remaining vigilant for adverse drug responses and drug interactions. Determining the appropri-

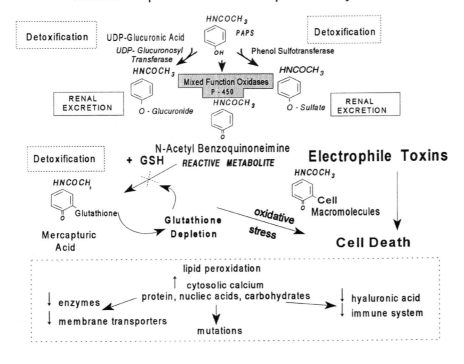

FIGURE 30–26. Diagrammatic representation of the proposed mechanism of acetaminophen-induced hepatic injury.

Table 30–23

RECOGNIZED HEPATOTOXIC CHEMICALS[654]

TOXIN	SOURCE
Aflatoxin	grain contamination
Amanita phalloides	death cap mushroom
Arsenic	insecticides, well water, "home remedies"
Blue-green algae	stagnant water
Beryllium	
Benzyl chloride	manufacture of dyes, perfumes, and pharmaceuticals
Carbon tetrachloride	carpet cleaner, solvent, fire extinguisher, grain fumigant
Chlorphenoxy	herbicide (2, 4, 5-trichlorophenoxy acetic acid)
Chlordecone (Kepone)	factory pollutant
Dinitrobenzene	industrial solvent
Dinitrophenol	old vermifuge
Dioxane	solvent, degreaser, cement component, used in production of adhesives, deodorants, detergents, glue, lacquer, oil, paint, polish, varnish remover
Hexachlorobenzene	fungicide
Metals	antimony, cadmium, copper, iron, lead
Methyl bromide	fumigant, insecticide
Nitroparaffins	nitromethane, nitroethane, 1-nitro-propane, 2-nitro-propane, solvents, protective coatings, adhesives, printing inks
Organochlorine pesticides	DDT, methoxychlor, chlordane, heptachlor, aldrin, dieldrin, lindane, chlordecone
Paraquat	herbicide
Phosphorus	
Phthalate esters	plasticizers dioctyl phthalate (DOP) di-(2-ethylhexyl) phthalate (DEHP)
Picric acid	(2, 4, 6 trinitrophenol) used as copper etcher, laboratory chemical, in a variety of products (batteries, colored glass, disinfectants, drugs, dyes, explosives, matches, photography chemicals, tanneries)
Polychlorinated biphenyls (PCBs)	manufacture of plastics
Pyrrolizidines	Senecio toxin, bush tea
2, 3, 7, 8 Tetrachloro-dibenzo-p-dioxin	commercial contaminant
Tetrachloroethane	solvent
Tetrachloroethylene	solvent, degreaser, fumigant, used in production of gums, soap, rubber, vacuum tubes, wax, wool
Thallium	diagnostic agent, old rodenticide
Toluene	solvent in glue, paint
Trichloroethane	industrial degreasing agent
Trichloroethylene	dry cleaning solvent
2, 4, 5 Trinitrotoluene	munitions plant pollutant (TNT)
Selenium	semiconductor technology, electrical engineering, glass, rubber, steel, lubricants, fungicides, medications, by-product of petroleum, coal energy generation
Vinyl chloride	solvent, production of polyvinyl chloride and resins

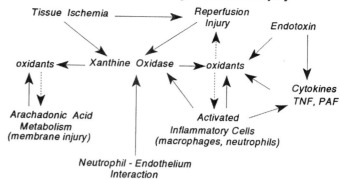

FIGURE 30–27. Diagrammatic representation of proposed mechanisms of oxidant injury to the liver.

elimination. Drugs that are efficiently extracted by the liver are also heavily influenced by impaired intrinsic hepatic clearance. Several studies of humans have shown that clearance of efficiently extracted drugs is more consistently influenced by liver disease than clearance of poorly extracted drugs. In general, it is usually expected that clearance of efficiently extracted drugs is reduced by approximately 50% in patients with hepatic cirrhosis. Clearance of poorly extracted drugs is difficult to predict because it may be unaltered, reduced, or increased. Clinical dose recommendations should be made on the basis of knowledge of the clearance of a particular drug in patients with hepatic insufficiency, whenever that information is available. Unfortunately, that is the exception rather than the rule.

Protein binding of a drug is an important determinant of its hepatic disposition, especially for drugs poorly extracted by the liver. In the presence of hypoalbuminemia, poorly extracted but normally highly protein bound drugs achieve greater distribution to intrahepatic sites of biotransformation or elimination. This results in increased hepatic clearance and a minimized pharmacologic effect. The overall influence on drug pharmacokinetics becomes complicated when one considers that some drugs are not highly protein bound. For these drugs, a change in plasma albumin concentration will have minimal if any influence on hepatic clearance. The primary influence will be an increased volume of distribution, which will require a greater initial loading dose to attain steady state conditions. For drugs that are highly protein bound, hypoalbuminemia results in increased amounts of unbound or free drugs permitting greater interaction with receptors. This precipitates increased or aberrant pharmacologic responses. For drugs efficiently extracted by the liver, decreased protein binding will minimally influence hepatic clearance. Hypoalbuminemia is the major factor effecting a change in plasma drug-protein binding. Other variables that influence drug-protein binding include reduced concentrations of alpha$_1$-acid glycoprotein (a common transport protein), and displacement of drugs from their transport binding sites by endogenous substances accumulating as a result of impaired hepatic function. In patients with inflammatory disorders associated with acute-phase proteins, there may be increased transport of highly protein bound drugs in combination with newly synthesized proteins.

Some drugs are eliminated in the liver by biliary excretion into the gastrointestinal tract. Once within the gastrointestinal tract, the fate of the drug depends on its polarity and its metabolism by enteric organisms. Biliary elimination of

ate body weight on which to calculate drug dosages is important in the patient with ascites or edema. In this circumstance, an estimated reduction of body weight is necessary for drugs not distributed into the third space fluid compartment.

Classically, the pharmacokinetics of drugs that are efficiently extracted by the liver are primarily influenced by alterations in hepatic perfusion. In liver disease, sinusoidal blood may shunt past hepatocytes, impairing hepatic uptake and

Table 30-24

INFLUENCE OF HEPATIC DISEASE ON PHARMACOKINETICS	
↓ Gastrointestinal drug absorption	Portal hypertension Gastroduodenal ulceration
Deviated portal circulation	Congenital portosystemic shunting Acquired portosystemic shunting
↑ Volume of distribution	Altered drug transport: ↓ Albumin concentration ↓ Alpha₁-acid glycoprotein Altered lipoprotein
↓ Hepatic uptake	↓ Hepatic blood flow Impaired sinusoidal perfusion (sinusoidal collagenization, capillarization) ↓ Functional hepatic mass ↓ Albumin-receptor interactions
↓ Hepatic biotransformation	↓ Functional hepatic mass Impaired enzyme synthesis
↓ Canalicular excretion	↓ Functional hepatic mass Impaired bile flow
↓ Biliary excretion	↓ Functional hepatic mass Intrahepatic cholestasis Extrahepatic cholestasis

unchanged drug and its subsequent reabsorption results in an enterohepatic circulation. This contributes only as a distributional process rather than an excretory process if the enterohepatic resorption is efficient. For drugs excreted in bile but not reabsorbed, obstructed bile flow has a major pharmacokinetic impact . Drugs that are relatively polar, ionized, and those with relatively high molecular weights (> 500 kd) are often excreted in bile. Drugs that are nonpolar and unionized at physiologic pH may be secreted into bile but are reabsorbed, and undergo enterohepatic circulation.

Dosage reductions for certain drugs are necessary in patients with severely compromised hepatic function. In some cases, when a drug has a high therapeutic index (wide margin of dosage safety), drug dosage may be maintained as is conventionally recommended despite marked changes in its pharmacokinetics. For other drugs, although no alteration in pharmacokinetics are predicted, their use is contraindicated on the basis of adverse interaction with neuroreceptors that contribute to the signs of HE. Such is the circumstance for many sedative agents, an example being the benzodiazepines. Many of the known pharmacokinetic changes for drugs in human patients with severe hepatic insufficiency, having relevancy to companion animal medicine, are provided in Table 30–25.[641,642,685] When clearance of a drug is reduced, the maintenance dose of the drug may be proportionally reduced or the dosing interval may be proportionally increased. When the volume of distribution of a drug is increased the necessity of a loading dose should be considered. When the half-life of a drug is increased the dosage interval should be proportionally increased. Unfortunately, few studies have been done in animals with liver disorders, and caution is required when making adjustments for dogs or cats based on the figures in Table 30–25. An example of species differences is that dogs metabolize digoxin in the liver to a greater extent than humans.[686,687]

HORMONE METABOLISM

The hepatobiliary system and endocrine hormones interface in numerous ways (see summary in Table 30–26). The liver can function in the following respects with the endocrine

system: (1) as a major target organ for hormone effect, (2) to activate prohormones, (3) to provide second-messenger hormones, (4) in the production of transport proteins for hormone dispersal, (5) in the maintenance and health of tissue hormone receptors, and (6) in the biotransformation, degradation, or excretion of hormones or their metabolites. Certain hormones undergo efficient enterohepatic circulation. The breadth of interaction between these systems results in disrupted endocrine physiology when hepatobiliary function is substantially impaired. Due to the complexities of the interactions that occur, prediction of clinicopathologic consequences is often impossible. Many of the specific aberrations that may develop are shown in Table 30–27.

ADRENAL STEROIDS. Natural and synthetic steroid hormones are largely metabolized in the liver. Adrenocortical hormones are lipid soluble and must be converted to water soluble derivatives before excretion by the kidneys. The transformation to nonbiologically active substances is followed by conjugation with glucuronide or sulfate, which renders them water soluble. Some therapeutic forms of glucocorticoids must be biotransformed in the liver before they are biologically active; prednisone is activated to prednisolone in this manner. Studies of the pharmacokinetics of prednisone in humans with cirrhosis have shown that despite delayed activation to prednisolone, alterations in protein binding and excretion maintain adequate therapeutic plasma concentrations with conventional dose recommendations.[637-640]

Glucocorticoids are avidly protein bound to albumin and to transcortin, a corticosteroid-binding globulin synthesized in the liver. Any pathologic process that reduces the plasma protein binding of glucocorticoids results in an increased availability of free or reactive hormone. This can lead to relative overdosing when drug therapy is continued with conventional regimens. Increased availability of free or unbound drug will create a condition of glucocorticoid excess. Synthetic glucocorticoids, such as dexamethasone, do not bind to corticosteroid-binding globulin.[688] Animals that are chronically ill have increased release of endogenous glucocorticoids. These patients are at increased risk for the detrimental effects of high circulating glucocorticoids if protein binding is insufficient. This may contribute to the Cushingoid appearance of some dogs with end-stage liver disease.

Table 30–25

INFLUENCE OF HEPATIC DISEASE ON DRUG DISPOSITION AS DETERMINED IN HUMANS WITH SEVERE HEPATIC DISEASE/INSUFFICIENCY[641,642,685]

DRUG	PLASMA CLEARANCE	VOLUME OF DISTRIBUTION	HALF-LIFE
Antibiotics			
Amikacin	—	↑ 200%	No change
Ampicillin	No change	↑ 46–200%	↑ 30–45%
Carbenicillin	—	—	↑ 90%
Cefoperazone	↓ 0–40%	↑ 150%	↑ 200%
Cefotaxime	↓ 30–40%	—	Increased
Chloramphenicol	↓ 65–70%	↓ 20%	↑ 130–150%
Clindamycin	↓ 25–60%	↓ 40%	↑ 15–40%
Erythromycin	↓ 30%	↑ 50%	↑ 60–65%
Gentamicin		No change	↑ 85%
Metronidazole	No change	No change	↑ 40–150%
Mezlocillin	↓ 50%	—	↑ 170%
Norfloxacin	No change	—	No change
Pefloxacin	↓ 70%	↓ 20%	↑ 255%
Vancomycin	↓ 70%	No change	↑ 1300%
Isoniazid	—	—	↑ 110%
Rifampin	—	—	↑ 90%
Sedatives			
Chlordiazepoxide	↓ 50–65%	↑ 45%	↑ 160–250%
Diazepam	↓ 50%	↑ 55–130%	↑ 130–410%
Oxazepam	No change	No change	No change
Pentobarbital	—	—	—
Phenobarbital			↑ 50%
Narcotics			
D-propxyphene	↓ 50%	—	—
Fentanyl	No change	No change	No change
Meperidine	↓ 40–50%	No change	↑ 70–120%
Morphine	No change	No change	No change
Pentazocine	↓ 50%	No change	↑ 70–110%
Diuretics			
Furosemide	↓ 0–35%	↑ 0–40%	↑ 0–75%
Spironolactone	—	—	↑ 40–65%
Cardiac Drugs			
Atenolol	No change	No change	No change
Digoxin	—	—	↓ (?)
Digitoxin	No change	No change	No change
Propranolol	↓ 25–90%	↑ 30%	↑ 180–400%
Lidocaine	↓ 45–50%	↑ 30–60%	↑ 220%
Mexiletine	↓ 70%	No change	↑ 190%
Quinidine	↓ 60%	↑ 50–170%	↑ 50–560%
Tocainide	No change	—	↑ 50%
Verapamil	↓ 50%	↑ 50%	↑ 280%
Miscellaneous			
Metoclopramide	↓ 25%	—	—
Cimetidine	↓ 35–55%	↓ 30–50%	↑ 35–50%
Ranitidine	↓ 10–35%	No change	↑ 35–55%
Tolbutamide	45%	No change	↑ 110%
Atracurium	No change	↑ 30%	No change
Pancuronium	↓ 20%	↑ 50%	↑ 55%
Cytoxan	↓ 30%	—	↑ 65%
Methotrexate	No change	—	No change
Diphenhydramine	No change	No change	↑ 60%
Aspirin	No change	—	No change
Phenylbutazone	0–240%	No change	↓ 0–40%
Prednisolone	No change	No change	No change
Prednisone	No change	No change	No change
Theophylline	↓ 30–80%	↑ 0–45%	↑ 250–750%

Aldosterone, a natural mineralocorticoid, is also inactivated and rendered water soluble in the liver. Normal metabolism of aldosterone is impaired in patients with hepatic insufficiency, which can lead to a condition of aldosterone excess. A major stimulus of aldosterone release is angiotensin II, which is under the influence of renin. Hyperreninemia

Table 30–26

MECHANISMS OF ENDOCRINE ABNORMALITIES ASSOCIATED WITH REDUCED HEPATIC FUNCTION

↓ or ↑ hepatic hormone production
↓ or ↑ hepatic hormone activation
↓ hepatic hormone degradation
↓ hepatic hormone excretion
↓ or ↑ hormone receptors in target tissues
↓ or ↑ hepatic synthesis of hormone-binding proteins
↓ or ↑ hormone production and secretion by endocrine organs
↑ hepatic production of variant/inappropriate hormones
↓ hypothalamic-pituitary hormone production/elaboration
Impaired feedback mechanisms regulating hormone production
Inappropriate local hepatic response to hormones
Interference in endocrine balance due to therapeutic interventions
Interference in endocrine balance due to nutritional deficiencies

develops in patients with liver disease as a result of diverse pathophysiologic mechanisms involving body sodium and water stores, renal perfusion, and reduced plasma oncotic pressure. This is described more fully in the section on ascites and in Figure 30–28. Because renin also is metabolized and excreted via the hepatobiliary system, a continued stimulus for aldosterone secretion is maintained. This reinforces a tendency toward hyperaldosteronism.

SEX STEROIDS. Androgens are metabolized by the liver to a variety of 17 ketosteroids.[689,690] Initial conversion to inactive metabolites is followed by conjugation with glucuronic acid and sulfate, which permits urinary excretion. Testosterone enters the blood as a result of secretion from the adrenal cortex, the ovaries, and the testes. Binding to sex hormone-binding globulin is believed to determine the concentration of free or active testosterone in the circulation. Increased estrogen levels and reduced free plasma testosterone concentrations may develop in some men with cirrhosis.[689] Estrogen increases due to its peripheral derivation from circulating androgens.[689,690] In addition to reduced testicular secretion of testosterone in men with cirrhosis, an abundance of the sex hormone–binding globulin limits the availability of testosterone for interaction with tissue receptors.

Estrogens are metabolized in the liver by different enzymes that catalyze hydroxylation, oxidation, reduction, and methylation reactions, producing a number of different metabolites.[690–691] Metabolites (estrone, estriol, and other estradiols) are excreted as glucuronide and sulfate conjugates in urine. Biliary excretion of some estrogens permits them to undergo an efficient enterohepatic circulation. After undergoing intestinal resorption, these are eliminated in urine. Increased concentrations of biologically active estrogen metabolites have been detected in humans with hepatic insufficiency. This may be due, in part, to the efficient enterohepatic circulation of some estrogen metabolites, especially in the circumstance of portosystemic shunting. An additional factor is the increased conversion of androstenedione to estrone in peripheral tissues. Exposure to drugs such as spironolactone can augment the tendency to develop high circulating estrogen levels. These drugs can displace steroids from sex hormone–binding globulin, and they displace estrogen more easily than androgens. The cumulative influence on sex hormone metabolism results in the expression of estrogenic effects such as gynecomastia in human beings with cirrhosis.[691] The changes in sex hormones reported in humans with liver disease have not been verified in dogs or cats.

Table 30–27

SPECIFIC HEPATOBILIARY-HORMONE INTERACTIONS

Estrogens	Biliary excretion and hepatic catabolism: ↓ clearance in cirrhosis Undergoes enterohepatic circulation Influences bile formation and flow ↑ production in hepatic insufficiency ↑ conversion testosterone → estrogens
Androgens: (testosterone)	Binding globulin: ↑ in hepatic insufficiency ↓ free hormone ↓ testicular production
Progesterone	Hepatic catabolism: ↓ in cirrhosis
Glucocorticoids	Induce hepatic protein synthesis: albumin, fibrinogen, enzymes Hepatic clearance/catabolism ↓ binding globulin → ↑ free cortisol
Aldosterone	Hepatic biotransformation → renal elimination ↑ production: stimulation renin: angiotensin axis low oncotic pressure and ↓ renal blood flow
T_4, T_3	Hepatic storage, metabolism, elimination A site of deiodination: $T_4 \rightarrow T_3$ Undergoes enterohepatic circulation Influences bile formation and flow
Growth hormone	Hepatic catabolism: ↓ clearance in cirrhosis ↑ production in cirrhosis: impaired hypothalamic/pituitary control
Somatomedin	Hepatic synthesis: ↓ synthesis with cirrhosis
Vitamin D	Hepatic activation: $D_3 \rightarrow 25\text{-OH}(D_3)$ ↓ with cirrhosis Undergoes enterohepatic circulation
Parathormone	Hepatic catabolism
Glucagon	Hypersecretion in cirrhosis Hepatic and renal catabolism
Insulin	↓ hepatic delivery: portosystemic shunting Hepatic and renal catabolism: 50% first-pass hepatic degradation

Other hormones catabolized (at least partially) by the liver: ACTH, ADH, angiotensin II, bradykinin, calcitonin, LH, oxytocin, TRH, TSH

Progesterone is metabolized mainly in the liver and serves as the precursor for estrogens, androgens, and adrenal steroid hormones. Since progesterone has salt-retaining properties, increased concentrations could contribute to the water-sodium retention that occurs in patients with hepatic insufficiency, portal hypertension, and ascites.

VITAMIN METABOLISM

Vitamins are organic compounds necessary for production of essential cofactors used in intermediary metabolism. Liver function is important in the metabolism, utilization, storage, and degradation of many of the vitamins.[692-696] Decreased dietary intake due to anorexia or feeding of an imbalanced diet, malabsorption due to altered intestinal perfusion (portal hypertension and lymph stasis), malabsorption of fat soluble vitamins due to abnormal bile salt concentrations, and adverse reactions with drugs being concurrently administered, may each lead to vitamin malnutrition. Reduced hepatic storage may occur due to fibrosis, severe lipidosis, hepatocellular degeneration, or necrosis. Increased urinary excretion of vitamins may occur as a result of impaired vitamin-protein binding. Relative vitamin malnutrition occurs when increased demand develops during tissue regeneration or when there is an inability to utilize or transport a nutrient supplied in normally adequate amounts. Function of the hepatobiliary system can be impaired by excess or deficiency of certain vitamins. Examples include the hepatopathy associated with vitamin A toxicity and the inability of the liver to activate certain coagulation factors in the absence of vitamin K.

Most of the water soluble vitamins are essential in coenzymes of intermediary metabolism.[692] Many of these are activated in the liver. Water soluble vitamins are absorbed mainly into the portal vein and circulate directly to the liver where some are retained. Liver stores of riboflavin, nicotinic acid, B_{12}, folic acid, and pantothenic acid are greater than a 1 day supply, whereas stores of B_1, B_6, and biotin are adequate to supply metabolic needs for only 1 day.[696] Hepatocellular necrosis, functional insufficiency, biliary obstruction, and the nutritional and hormonal dysregulations that develop in liver disease contribute to vitamin insufficiency. Therapeutic support of the patient with serious liver disease therefore should include administration of metabolically active forms of these vitamins. Water soluble vitamins include vitamin C and the vitamin B complex.

The liver plays a major role in vitamin A metabolism.[693,697-699] Naturally occurring and synthetic analogues of vitamin A are termed retinoids. Retinal esters are the principal storage form of retinol within lipid droplets in Ito cells (lipocytes) in the liver. Over 90% of total body reserves of vitamin A are located in these cells. Hydrolysis of free retinol from the liver determines the availability of vitamin A to the body, which is dispersed bound to retinal-binding protein (RBP). Parenchymal liver disease, zinc deficiency, and pro-

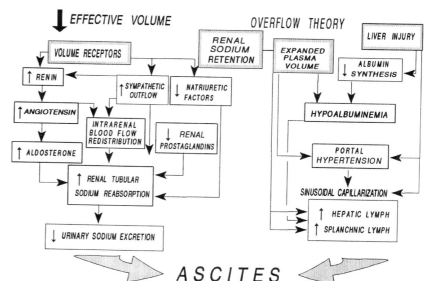

FIGURE 30-28. Pathophysiologic mechanisms responsible for ascites formation.

tein malnutrition can influence the availability of plasma vitamin A. Reduced RBP synthesis, in the absence of true vitamin deficiency, can lead to subnormal plasma vitamin A concentrations when vitamin deficiency itself is not present. Vitamin A toxicity has been described in cats fed an exclusive diet of beef liver. Clinical signs include hepatosplenomegaly and vertebral hyperostosis.[700,701] Similar signs have been described in humans.[702] Histologic changes in the liver include increased fat storage, fibrosis, and central vein sclerosis. Veno-occlusive disease involving the hepatic veins (central veins) of captive cheetahs was attributed to vitamin A toxicity derived from a high meat diet rich in liver.[703]

Vitamin D_3 can be synthesized in the skin from 7-dehydrocholesterol upon exposure to ultraviolet light. The liver converts this to the principal circulating form: 25 OH D_3. The 25 OH D_3 product is further metabolized by the kidney to 24,25-(OH)$_2$ D_3 and the most active form, 1,25- (OH)$_2$ D_3. After oral ingestion, vitamin D_3 is absorbed in the small intestine in the presence of bile salts. The presence of fat in the intestinal lumen decreases vitamin D absorption. In circulation, vitamin D is transported bound to an alpha$_1$-globulin known as vitamin D binding globulin, which is synthesized in the liver. It also can circulate bound to albumin. Parenchymal liver disease can lead to low circulating 25 OH D and 1,25(OH)$_2$D$_3$ due to low vitamin D binding protein. There may also be a reduced intestinal absorption of vitamin D and an impaired ability of the liver to convert vitamin D to the 25-OH D_3 form. Signs referable to vitamin D insufficiency in veterinary patients with liver disease have not been reported. Empirical supplementation with vitamin D is contraindicated.

In the liver, vitamin K is necessary for the activation and regulation of several important coagulation proteins including Factors II, VII, IX, X and the antithrombotic proteins C and S. In severe liver disease, synthetic failure may impair the synthesis of vitamin K–dependent proteins and lead to a coagulopathy. Some hepatic disorders are associated with defective or incomplete vitamin K carboxylation of coagulation factors resulting in the formation of a des-gamma-carboxyglutamate form of prothrombin. This occurs in humans with cirrhosis, acute severe hepatitis, and hepatocellular carcinoma, but it does not contribute to abnormal bleeding.[392,393,704] This does not respond to treatment with vitamin K. Extrahepatic bile duct occlusion and severe intrahepatic cholestasis may lead to vitamin K responsive coagulopathies. Concurrent dietary deficiency, antibiotic suppression of vita-

min K synthesizing gastrointestinal flora, and biliary tract obstruction can produce vitamin K deficiency within 3 weeks.

Vitamin E is a natural antioxidant that inhibits oxidation of unsaturated fatty acids and other susceptible compounds.[705] Tocopherol is taken up slowly from the circulation into tissues and is principally stored in adipose, skeletal muscle, and the liver.

Vitamin E deficiency may develop in patients with severe cholestasis.[706,707] Red blood cell membrane instability and shortened red cell survival is one sequela. Generally, signs of insufficiency are not clinically recognized. Vitamin E and selenium have been shown to modify the noxious effects of hepatotoxins known to produce injury through lipid peroxidation.[708–712]

CIRCULATORY FUNCTION

Under resting conditions, total hepatic blood flow approximates 25% of cardiac output; this varies with exercise, alimentation, and posture.[713] Exercise causes a reduction in hepatic blood flow as a result of splanchnic vasoconstriction. This is why cage rest is advocated for the patient with acute hepatic injury. The liver has a unique circulation, receiving afferent flow from the hepatic artery and portal vein. The hepatic artery provides 80% of the hepatic oxygen supply. The portal venous circulation transports blood from the stomach, spleen, pancreas, intestines, and colon to the liver. Consequently, the portal circulation provides exposure of hepatocytes and Kupffer cells to nutrients, metabolites, toxins, particulate debris, microorganisms, and hormones derived from the abdominal viscera.

Regulation of Hepatic Blood Flow

Portal venous and hepatic arterial blood undergo intrahepatic mixing in zone 1.[713] Regulation of hepatic blood flow occurs largely through the arterial portion of the hepatic circulation. Perfusion through the hepatic arterial system is similar to arterial perfusion in other organs. Pressure is high in the hepatic artery, and the pressure of arterial blood flowing into the hepatic sinusoids is regulated by resistance mechanisms in the network's arterioles. Arteriole resistance vessels are sensitive to vasoactive agents and are capable of autoregulation. Making appropriate responses to changes in arterial pressure, they maintain adequate sinusoidal pressure and flow. Increased portal venous pressure results in constriction of the hepatic arterioles. Hepatic arterial flow increases in response to reduced portal venous flow; a reciprocal compensatory response in the portal system does not occur, although both systems participate in compensatory local sinusoidal flow adjustments.

The portal venous system is a low pressure system. Its vessels lack valves and are relatively insensitive to vasoactive substances. Consequently, the portal system behaves as a passive conduit responding to changes in perfusion pressure. Vasoactive drugs reducing splanchnic blood flow through mesenteric arteriolar vasoconstriction reduce hepatic blood flow due to reduced intestinal venous perfusion. Portal pressure normally exceeds hepatic venous and caudal vena caval pressures, maintaining a flow gradient through the liver.

Both afferent and efferent hepatic vessels have rich innervation (adrenergic fibers) and contractile elements. Sphincters have been demonstrated in hepatic arterioles, portal venules, and terminal hepatic veins. Sinusoids are also believed to have contractile capabilities. A constant vacillation adjusts acinar perfusion and is believed to contribute to the multifocal distribution of some hepatic lesions.

The most important local physiologic vasoregulator of the hepatic circulation is adenosine, which influences hepatic arteriole resistance. Its presence results in arteriolar vasodilation. When portal blood flow is reduced, as in the interdigestive interval, adenosine accumulates and dilates the arteriolar side of the hepatic circulatory bed. When portal blood flow is brisk, adenosine is "washed" away, and arteriolar dilation subsides. This maintains a relatively stable flow of blood through the hepatic sinusoids at any given time. During the postprandial interval, the arterial blood flow is maintained despite an increased portal flow. A variety of factors mediate this vasodilator effect, including bile salts, gastrin, secretin, glucagon, and hypertonicity.

With arterial blood pressure in the normal range (80 to 120 mm Hg), total hepatic blood flow remains constant. When arterial blood pressure is at the high end of this range, the arteriolar contribution to total hepatic blood flow is reduced as more blood is deviated to the mesenteric circulation. This leads to a greater hepatic return of portal venous blood. In this circumstance, the hepatic artery directly contributes only 30% to total hepatic blood flow. When arterial blood pressure is at the low end of the normal range, a smaller proportion of blood is circulated to the mesenteric circulation. The portal circulation is effectively reduced, and the hepatic artery directly contributes up to 70% of the total hepatic blood flow. Reduced pressure in the hepatic artery is accompanied by a substantial reduction in hepatic artery resistance. Increased portal venous flow is accompanied by decreased portal resistance until capacitance vessels expand to their maximum.

Complete diversion of portal circulation to systemic veins, as in the creation of an Eck fistula, results in a 50% to 100% increase in hepatic arterial flow.[714] This compensates for the lost venous perfusion. Following selective reduction of pressure in the hepatic artery, total hepatic circulation is maintained as a result of autoregulatory mechanisms. In some circumstances, loss of the hepatic arterial supply is compensated by development of a collateral arterial supply from mesenteric vessels or from the pericholedochal arterial bed. Impaired hepatic artery inflow or hepatic venous outflow results in ischemic lesions in zone 3 (perivenular), the last acinar area perfused.

Sinusoidal blood volume is maintained by constriction of hepatic venous sphincters, which regulate outflow of blood from the liver. This ensures a uniform distribution of blood. In health, hepatic venous sphincters are responsible for virtually all of the resistance to portal blood flow in the liver as there is essentially no resistance to flow through the presinusoidal portal or sinusoidal vessels. Presinusoidal resistance is realized during infusion of norepinephrine, angiotensin (dogs and cats), and histamine (dogs). Hepatic venous sphincters are located in the third-order branches of the hepatic vein in cats and in the terminal 1 to 2 cm of the lobar veins in dogs. These sphincters constrict to adjust intrahepatic volume expansion and blood pressure, offering some protection against pathologically increased central venous pressure (CVP), as occurs with congestive heart failure and pericardial tamponade. However, large increases in CVP can fatigue these sphincters. These venous sphincters normally respond to norepinephrine, angiotensin, hepatic nerve stimulation, and to histamine in dogs.

Hepatic Oxygen Extraction

Although a majority of the hepatic oxygen is supplied by the hepatic artery, the portal circulation can supply up to 50% of the oxygen requirements. The liver is more efficient in its ability to extract oxygen than most other tissues. It can compensate for reductions in oxygen supply up to 50% of normal. Oxygen uptake is maintained by increasing the efficiency of extraction; consequently, reductions in either afferent blood supply do not impair its oxygen availability as long as systemic blood remains normally oxygenated. This ability supports the contention that all acinar units have mixed arterial and portal blood supplies. Oxygen deprivation, as occurs with hepatic artery ligation, reduces Kupffer cell function, resulting in inadequate removal of bacteria and toxins from the portal circulation.[715] Septicemia has been reported as a frequent sequela to this type of ischemic injury. Survival occurs when experimental animals are pretreated with drugs such as neomycin in doses that "sterilize" the gut.[715–717]

Hepatic Lymphatics

The hepatic lymphatic system transports extracellular fluid and large molecules, such as plasma proteins, tissue debris, and foreign substances, from the liver. The protein content of hepatic lymph is similar to that of plasma because of the large sinusoidal fenestrae that permit passage of large molecules. The rate of lymph flow is directly related to hepatic blood flow and intrahepatic sinusoidal pressure. Approximately 80% of the hepatic lymph passes through the hilar lymphatics and cisterna chyli into the thoracic duct. Hilar lymph flow is greatly increased in cirrhosis, veno-occlusive disorders of the hepatic vein, and glycogen storage diseases.

Blood Storage

The liver is an important blood reservoir. It can accommodate up to 60 mL blood per 100 g tissue in the circumstance of chronic passive congestion.[718–722] It can thus become markedly enlarged as a result of its blood storage capability. More than 40% of hepatic blood is in capacitance vessels (hepatic arteries, portal veins, and hepatic veins) with the remainder being contained within hepatic sinusoids.[721] The liver is dynamic in its ability to store blood and to mobilize it when necessary. In a normal individual, the liver contains 25 to 30 mL blood per 100 g tissue.[718–721] This is estimated as 10% to 15% of total blood volume. The liver can accommodate up to 20% of the volume associated with rapid intravascular fluid expansion in healthy cats.[721,722] During moderate hemorrhage, it can expel enough blood to compensate for a 25% reduction in total blood volume, equivalent to immediate release of approximately 50% of the total hepatic blood volume.[723] This volume can be expelled under the influence of sympathetic stimulation.

Portal Hypertension and Ascites

Portal hypertension results when normal flow from abdominal splanchnic vessels through the portal vein, liver and caudal vena cava, to the right side of the heart, is impeded. The diagnosis of portal hypertension is commonly inferential. The assessment of an affected patient requires careful consideration of the causes and complications of portal hypertension. In human beings, complications include ascites, hepatic encephalopathy, hypersplenism, and esophageal varicoceles. Animals differ in that they do not develop clinical evidence of hypersplenism or esophageal varicoceles.

In health, the portal circulation is a low-resistance low-pressure system. Healthy anesthetized dogs have portal pressures ranging between 6 to 13 cm of water.[724,725] Portal pressure normally exceeds hepatic venous and caudal vena caval pressures, thus providing a flow gradient across the hepatic sinusoids. A number of variables influence portal pressure. Causes of a transiently decreased pressure include inspiration, fasting, exercise, and certain anesthetic agents.[722,723] Portal pressure can be transiently increased during expiration, postprandially, and when intra-abdominal pressure increases, such as when a tight abdominal bandage is applied. Sustained pressure above 40 cm H_2O will decrease portal flow by 90%. Portal venous pressure is a function of both the rate of portal blood flow and the resistance to it. Differential acinar perfusion and autoregulation of sphincters maintains homeostasis among intrahepatic portal blood flow, vascular resistance, and pressure. If any variable increases beyond a certain critical threshold, portal hypertension can develop. The thresholds among these variables are diverse. For example, healthy dogs can tolerate a threefold increase in splanchnic arterial blood flow (and subsequently in hepatic portal blood flow) in the absence of flow restriction, without developing portal hypertension.[725] Any factor that increases vascular resistance in this circumstance will precipitate portal hypertension. A similar degree of vascular resistance without increased afferent flow may not cause portal hypertension. Increased portal vascular resistance can result from changes at the level of the right heart or from obstructed flow in the hepatic vein, its tributaries, the hepatic sinusoids, or portal vein. Classification of portal hypertension into *prehepatic*, *hepatic*, and *posthepatic* causes assists consideration of differential diagnosis. This approach is presented in Tables 30–28 to 30–30.

Posthepatic portal hypertension indicates obstruction of flow at

Table 30–28

PATHOPHYSIOLOGIC MECHANISMS OF PORTAL HYPERTENSION		
POSTSINUSOIDAL/POSTHEPATIC	**HEPATIC/SINUSOIDAL** **IMPAIRED SINUSOIDAL/PORTAL FLOW**	**PRESINUSOIDAL/PREHEPATIC**

Right-Sided Cardiac Disturbance
cardiomyopathy
tricuspid insufficiency
dirofilariasis
pulmonary thromboembolism
intracardiac neoplasia
    atrial, valvular, mural, infiltrative
cor triatrium dexter
	Cirrhosis
	regenerative nodules
	collagenization of sinusoids
	parenchymal collapse
	chronic diffuse hepatitis
	chronic cholangiohepatitis
	postnecrotic
	breed-specific hepatopathies
	drug-related hepatopathies
		Prehepatic Portal Vein Occlusion
		portal vein thrombosis
		portal vein stenosis:
		    trauma
		    congenital
		portal vein neoplasia
		congenital portal atresia
		extraluminal portal vein occlusion:
		    neoplasia
		    lymph nodes
		    abscess
		    granuloma
		    peritonitis

Pericardial Disease
pericardial tamponade
    atrial hemangiosarcoma
    coagulopathy
    trauma
    benign pericardial effusion
    infectious
restrictive pericarditis
constrictive pericarditis
	Biliary Cirrhosis
	severe peribiliary fibrosis
	    bridging fibrosis
	chronic cholangitis/cholangiohepatitis
	chronic major bile duct obstruction	

Obstructed C. Vena Caval/Hepatic Vein congenital "kinked" vena cava posttraumatic vena caval stenosis vena caval syndrome (Dirofilariasis) vena caval/hepatic vein thrombosis diaphragmatic hernia vascular entrapment	**Miscellaneous Causes** congenital portal atresia portal/sinusoidal disseminated neoplasia portal/sinusoidal thromboembolism diaphragmatic hernia: liver entrapment hepatic amyloidosis	

	Portal Blood Flow (Arteriolization of Portal Vasculature)
	hepatic artery/portal vein fistula:
	    congenital
	    traumatic
	    neoplastic
	    splanchnic
	    microanastomosis (cirrhosis) (intrahepatic
	      sinusoidal shunting)	

Table 30-29

PATHOPHYSIOLOGIC MECHANISMS OF HEPATIC
CAUSES OF PORTAL HYPERTENSION

↑ **Hepatic Resistance to Flow**
  Sinusoidal collagenization:
      narrowed vascular lumen
      obliterated space of Disse
  ↓ Hepatic vein flow:
      terminal hepatic vein sclerosis/occlusion (chronic passive
          congestion, Budd-Chiari, venocclusive disease)
  ↑ Hepatocyte size:
      swelling, inflammation
      storage: lipid, glycogen
  ↑ Sinusoidal lining cells (Kupffer cells, Ito cells)
  Obliteration of normal sinusoidal distribution
      regenerative nodules
      regenerative hyperplasia
  ↓ Portal vein flow
      occlusion of small portal venous radicals (thrombus, metasta-
          sis, atresia, inflammation)
      periportal fibrosis
↑ **Hepatic Arterial Flow (arterialization)**
  cirrhosis (microanastomoses)
  congenital hepatic AV anastomosis (haemartoma)
  traumatic hepatic AV anastomosis
  neoplasia hepatic AV anastomosis
  splanchnic AV anastomosis

the level of the hepatic vein tributaries up to and including cardiac, pericardial, or pulmonary outflow lesions. *Hepatic portal hypertension* indicates etiologic conditions within the hepatic parenchyma causing a diminution of sinusoidal flow such as collagenization of the sinusoids (as occurs in cirrhosis), sinusoidal collapse (as occurs in postnecrotic cirrhosis), or restricted portal vein and hepatic artery acinar perfusion due to periportal inflammation/fibrosis. A rare cause of sinusoidal hypertension is increased blood flow such as occurs in congenital or acquired hepatic arteriovenous (AV) fistula. Hepatic causes of portal hypertension can be subdivided into *presinusoidal, sinusoidal, postsinusoidal,* and mixed causes (any combination), depending on pathophysiologic mechanisms and the acinar location of the inciting histologic lesion. *Prehepatic portal hypertension* indicates the presence of restricted blood flow into or through the portal vein; this is a rare cause of portal hypertension in the dog and cat. The most common causes of portal hypertension are disorders in the hepatic sinusoidal or postsinusoidal categories. A summary of the differential diagnoses and diagnostic characteristics associated with each of the general categories is provided in Table 30-30.

When portal hypertension reduces sinusoidal blood flow, increased formation of hepatic lymph occurs. Hepatic lymph normally drains from the perisinusoidal space (space of Disse) into lymphatics in the portal triad area. From there it flows to hepatic lymph nodes in the hilus, the cisternal chyli, and thoracic duct.[726] When hepatic lymph formation exceeds the capacity for drainage through conventional pathways, excess lymph "weeps" from the capsule of the liver into the abdominal cavity. Depending on the etiologic factors responsible for portal hypertension and the capacity for hepatic protein synthesis, the physicochemical characteristics of the abdominal effusion will vary. Evaluation of the difference between the serum albumin concentration and that in the abdominal effusion is used in humans to predict the involvement of mechanisms other than portal hypertension. This has shown better predictive value than categorizing the different forms of effusion based on cell content and total protein quantification. A large difference (> 1.1 g/dl) is associated with conditions causing prehepatic or hepatic portal hypertension and a small difference (< 1.1 g/dl) suggests involvement of other mechanisms.[727] It is unknown at present how this applies to animals.

The pathophysiologic mechanisms leading to portal hypertension are usually associated with overt changes in health parameters that allow deduction of the underlying cause. Experimentally, measurement of wedged hepatic vein pressure (a pressure determination made with a catheter wedged within a small tributary of the hepatic vein) and free hepatic venous pressure (catheter floating within the hepatic vein) can be used to deduce the localization of portal hypertension. Direct pressure determinations are rarely necessary in clinical patients with portal hypertension. Determination of central venous pressure, estimation of hepatic size, evaluation of cardiac function, estimation of caudal vena caval and hepatic vein distension by radiography and ultrasonography, evaluation of liver function using routine screening tests and serum bile acid determinations, and the physicochemical characteristics of an abdominal effusion will permit classification into the prehepatic, hepatic, or posthepatic categories. Abdominal ultrasonography and colonic scintigraphy studies may additionally be used to detail the presence of functional portosystemic collateral circulation. Definitive diagnosis of the cause of hepatic portal hypertension requires liver biopsy.

Posthepatic Portal Hypertension

Posthepatic portal hypertension develops from a variety of disorders that increase resistance to blood flow in the major hepatic veins, the caudal vena cava, or the heart. These are listed in Table 30-28 and typical diagnostic features clarified in Table 30-30. The Budd-Chiari syndrome denotes a unique condition in which hepatic venous outflow becomes obstructed and impairs flow to the right atrium. The characteristic histologic lesion includes severe perivenular (zone 3) and sinusoidal congestion. In human beings, hepatic venous thrombosis is the most common cause.[728] A similar pathologic lesion has rarely been recognized in dogs and cats.[729,730] Other causes include hepatic vein fibrosis, extension of neoplasia (from the liver or kidney), hepatic vein occlusion by adjacent hepatic cyst(s) or abscess, or congenital membranous obstruction (web) of the vena cava. Chronic passive congestion due to cardiac-related abnormalities causes similar histologic changes. A unique lesion classified as veno-occlusive disease is also associated with posthepatic portal hypertension. This lesion is uncommon and is typified by intimal occlusion of small- and medium-sized hepatic veins and perivenular hepatic necrosis. Causes of posthepatic portal hypertension are discussed in detail in Chapter 35.

Hepatic Portal Hypertension

In dogs with cirrhosis and portal hypertension, portal pressures have been reported to range between 18 to 39 cm of water, equivalent to three- to sixfold normal.[731] In health, the quantity of blood perfusing the liver is equivalent to the amount reaching hepatocytes. In cirrhosis, regenerative nodules and collagen deposition distorts the sinusoidal circulatory bed and increases vascular resistance so that blood perfusing the liver does not necessarily reach the hepatocytes. In dogs with portal fibrosis and portal hypertension, total hepatic blood flow can increase up to 60% over normal, yet

Table 30–30

CLINICOPATHOLOGIC FEATURES USED TO DIFFERENTIATE CAUSES OF PORTAL HYPERTENSION

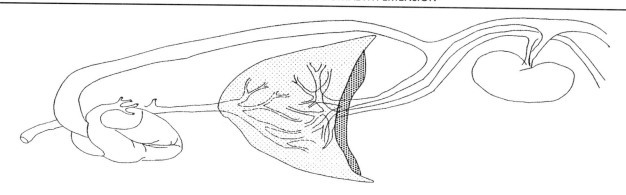

	POSTHEPATIC		HEPATIC		PREHEPATIC
	Cardiac/Pericardial (filling/pump failure)	CVC Occlusion	Numerous Causes	Intrahepatic AV Fistula	Numerous Causes
Central venous pressure	↑	normal	normal	normal	normal
ECG	abnormal	normal	normal	normal	normal
Radiography:					
Cardiac silhouette	↑/normal	normal	normal	normal	normal
Caudal vena caval distension	↑	↓/normal/mass lesion	normal	normal	normal
Liver size	↑	↑	variable/↓	↑/individual lobe	normal
Ultrasonography:					
Liver pattern	hypoechoic	hypoechoic	variable lesions	anechoic foci	normal
Size:					
Hepatic vein	distended	distended	normal	normal	normal
Portal vein	prominent	prominent	variable	segmentally larger	normal
CBC:					
PCV	↑/normal	↑/normal	variable	↓/normalvariable	
MCV	normal	normal	↓	↓	normal
Poikilocytes	rare	rare	common	common	rare
Schistocytes, acanthocytes	↑ if vascular lesions	↑ if vascular lesions	rare	rare	rare
Chemistry profile:					
Albumin	normal	normal	↓/normal	↓/normal	↓/normal
Liver enzymes	↑ ALP, ↑ ALT, ↑ AST	↑ ALP, ↑ ALT, ↑ AST	variable	variable	variable
Glucose	normal	normal	normal/↓		
normal	normal/↓				
Serum bile acids	normal	normal	↑↑ postprandial	↑↑ postprandial (especially)	↑
Ascites:	common	common	chronic disease	common	rare
Pure transudate	uncommon	uncommon	common	common	common
Modified transudate	common	common	rare	possible	possible

this blood does not effectively reach its target cells.[732] In cirrhosis, there are a number of reasons that sinusoidal flow does not functionally perfuse viable hepatocytes and encounters increased sinusoidal resistance. These obliterative and constrictive effects are summarized in Table 30–29.[728] Increased flow from the hepatic artery may aggravate portal hypertension in cirrhosis. As the portal circulation becomes diminished, the hepatic arterial mass relatively increases as it becomes the major source of blood for regenerative nodules. Abnormal communications develop between small hepatic arterioles and portal veins that lead to retrograde flow through the portal venous system. This aggravates preexisting portal hypertension. As a result of intrahepatic portal hypertension, the portal venous circulation may functionally bypass viable hepatocytes or follow hepatofugal flow through portosystemic collateral vessels.[731–735]

An increase in portal blood flow can result from the presence of a large intrahepatic AV communication between an hepatic artery and a portal vein. These congenital malformations, intrahepatic arteriovenous fistulas or hamartomas, have been described as a cause of portal hypertension in dogs and one cat.[736–740] In one dog with an hepatic AV fistula, the portal pressure was measured as 38 mm Hg.[740] Such AV fistulas lead to arterialization of the hepatoportal circulatory system, development of portal hypertension, ascites, and multiple functional portosystemic collaterals (see Chapter 35).

Prehepatic Portal Hypertension

Prehepatic causes of portal hypertension include disorders that constrict or impair the lumen of the portal vein and, consequently, the afferent portal venous flow. With acute portal vein obstruction, portal hypertension may lead to death resulting from impaired visceral perfusion, endotoxemia, and thromboembolism. When portal vein obstruction has a more gradual or insidious development, the ensuing portal hypertension can be tolerated as a result of recruitment of portosystemic collateral circulatory pathways.[741,742] Prehepatic causes of portal hypertension are infrequent in dogs and rare in cats.[743–748]

Rarely, a communication between splanchnic arterial and portal vein tributaries can lead to increased portal flow and portal hypertension. The surgical creation of an aortic-splenic shunt in healthy dogs results in a marked increase in hepatic blood flow and moderate portal hypertension.[749] In humans, an increase in splenic perfusion associated with hematologic disturbances such as leukemia, Hodgkin's disease, polycythemia rubra vera, and other myeloproliferative diseases can be associated with portal hypertension.[728] Obstruction of portal flow associated with cellular infiltrates in hepatic vasculature is also thought to contribute to portal hypertension in these circumstances. These disorders have not been identified in dogs or cats with prehepatic portal hypertension.

Systemic Consequences of Portal Hypertension

After experimental creation of portal hypertension by partial attenuation of the portal vein, compensatory portosystemic shunting through collateral circulation develops within 1 to 2 months.[741,742] Portosystemic collaterals develop in two groups: portoprecaval and portopostcaval. Portoprecaval vessels extend to the cranial vena cava via the azygous vein; these are uncommon in the dog and cat. Portopostcaval vessels connect with the caudal vena cava; these are common. The portopostcaval shunts are often located in the renal and splenic regions where they may be visualized on abdominal ultrasonography or by radiographic portography. In dogs, the portopostcaval vessels usually are comprised of the velar-omental anastomoses; these vessels arise from a branch of the splenic vein and anastomose with radicles of the left gonadal (testicular or ovarian) vein.[741] These empty into the left renal vein. In cats, the anastomoses most likely to develop extend from the left gastric vein to the phrenicoabdominal veins and from the left colic vein to the left gonadal vein.[742] In humans, the most common collateral vasculature develops in the portoprecaval group. This leads to the development of a prominent system of esophageal varices, which are an important cause of patient morbidity and mortality.

In a patient with portal hypertension, the determining factors in the development of portosystemic collateral circulation include (1) the rate of development of the portal hypertension, (2) the magnitude of the hypertension, and (3) the anatomic site of the causal factors. Portosystemic shunting consistently develops in healthy cats and dogs that have undergone surgical attenuation of the portal vein. In addition to the conventional pathways, accessory portal vein radicles may also develop the capacity for substantial blood flow. These vessels allow hepatopedal blood flow (flow to the liver) by shunting blood around the portal vein obstruction. In the veterinary patient with cirrhosis, the development of portosystemic shunting is believed to be more common than is substantiated. The opening of portosystemic collaterals delays or ameliorates ascites formation but increases a patient's susceptibility to hepatic encephalopathy by increasing the systemic concentrations of ammonia, endotoxins, and other alimentary derived substances normally detoxified or removed by the liver. Dogs with chronic hepatobiliary disorders seem to develop portal hypertension and portosystemic shunting more commonly than cats. This is likely due to the very different nature of the chronic hepatobiliary disorders that affect these species.

Posthepatic portal hypertension due to cardiac-related disorders usually does not cause portosystemic shunting. This is because a gradient does not develop between the portal and systemic venous beds that favors collateral vasculature as a pathway of least resistance.[750] Posthepatic portal hypertension due to caudal vena caval occlusion may be associated with portosystemic shunting through portoprecaval anastomoses whereby portal flow is diverted through radicles associated with the azygous, internal thoracic, esophageal, or subcutaneous veins.[751,752] Blood from the systemic venous system may also drain into the cranial vena cava through this collateral vasculature.

The development of portocaval shunts reduces portal pressure by transferring portal circulation into an hepatofugal flow pattern. In most circumstances, pressure in the portal vasculature never completely normalizes, the flow gradient being maintained by the underlying etiologic disorder(s).

Hepatic blood flow can dramatically increase with acute liver inflammation. The increased flow is derived from the hepatic artery. Streaming of blood in the sinusoids permits intrahepatic arteriovenous shunting and reduced availability of oxygen or toxin extraction and nutrient exchange. Blood flow returns to normal when the inflammation subsides. Hepatic blood flow also increases and persists with portal inflammation and fibrosis such as occurs with extrahepatic bile duct occlusion. This is derived primarily from increased splanchnic circulation. Vasodilation produced by bacterial activity in the intestines is thought to be responsible for increased portal flow because oral antibiotics that reduce intestinal microflora can ameliorate the hyperdynamic condition.[753] This increased flow accompanies portal hypertension and occurs weeks before development of collateral circulatory pathways. Dogs with chronic major bile duct occlusion develop hyperdynamic systemic circulation including elevated heart rate, cardiac index, low blood pressure, and decreased systemic vascular resistance, similar to the changes realized in patients with cirrhosis.[754,755] This is accompanied by development of portosystemic collateral circulation. Experimental induction of extrahepatic bile duct obstruction is a well-established method of modeling portal hypertension, portosystemic shunting, and a hyperdynamic splanchnic circulation within 4 to 6 weeks.

Increased Hepatic Lymph Formation

According to Starling's law, which governs transcapillary fluid distribution, an independent increase in capillary hydrostatic pressure results in increased production of interstitial fluid and lymph. As long as lymphatic channels can accommodate the increased lymph production, fluid does not accumulate in interstitial or "potential third spaces." When portal hypertension causes increased hepatic lymph formation, the amount of lymph carried in the thoracic duct increases. When the capacity of the intrahepatic lymphatic system is exceeded, high-protein lymph escapes from the space of Disse and leaks through the hepatic capsule into the peritoneal cavity. This results in formation of ascites that is relatively high in protein. This typifies the abdominal fluid that forms in association with congestive heart failure, pericardial tamponade, restrictive or constrictive pericarditis, and vena caval obstruction.

Intrahepatic portal hypertension associated with cirrhosis leads to the production of a large volume of a relatively low-protein-containing hepatic lymph. Increased formation of hepatic lymph, 20-fold greater in a cirrhotic liver compared to the healthy liver, can easily exceed the capacity of lymphatics to transport it.[756] This occurs because of a reduced capacity for albumin synthesis, which reduces the plasma oncotic pressure, and because of capillarization of hepatic sinusoids.[757,758] Capillarization develops in sinusoids exposed to increased perfusion pressures and represents an increase in their restrictive properties (they become less permeable to proteins). In this process, sinusoids are transformed into passages with fewer permissive endothelial fenestrae. The net effect is formation of a large amount of hepatic lymph (because of increased hydrostatic pressure) that has a relatively low protein concentration. In humans with cirrhosis, hepatic lymph contains approximately 60% of the protein in plasma whereas normal hepatic lymph contains approximately 90%.[756] The protein content of splanchnic lymph averaged 18% of the plasma protein concentration compared to a normal of 60%.[756] The increased flow and pressure in the sinusoids and the capillarization effects result in lymph formation that exceeds the capacity of the hepatic lymphatic system. Excess fluid spills across the capsule of the liver into the peritoneal cavity. In early cirrhosis, a higher protein-containing fluid accumulates compared to that which forms in late cirrhosis, which is typically a pure transudate (very low protein) (Table 30–30). The evaluation of the albumin in the abdominal effusion compared to plasma usually reveals a large difference.[736]

Increase in intestinal lymph formation occurs with prehepatic portal hypertension (portal vein occlusion), and to a lesser extent with intrahepatic portal hypertension. With prehepatic hypertension (portal vein ligation, portal vein thromboembolism) ascites is transient because intestinal lymph production usually does not exceed the capacity for lymphatic absorption and flow and because recanalization of thrombi or establishment of portosystemic collaterals alleviates the portal hypertension. A marked reduction in hepatic lymph formation develops due to the impaired hepatic portal perfusion. Sustained prehepatic portal hypertension is associated with a progressive decline in the concentration of protein in intestinal lymph, regardless of the status of liver function. Initially, a large oncotic gradient develops between splanchnic capillaries and the interstitial space that favors the reabsorption of intestinal lymph. However, with chronicity, the transcapillary fluid balance results in the formation and accumulation of a low-protein ascites derived exclusively from intestinal lymphatics.[759–761]

Ascites

The pathophysiologic mechanisms underlying ascites formation are complex; these are summarized in Figure 30–28. Thus, no clinical characteristics clearly differentiate patients who will develop ascites from those who will not.[762] Ascites associated with portal hypertension is aggravated by alterations in renal sodium handling and systemic conservation of water. There are two alternative theories that have been proposed as major sequences preceding ascites formation.[762,763]

The *traditional concept* of ascites formation focuses on the role of diminished effective circulating volume. Initial derangements occur with imbalance of transcapillary fluid fluxes in the hepatic sinusoids and lymphatics, as previously discussed. This results in excessive lymph formation that exceeds the capacity of the lymphatics and thoracic duct. Excess fluid (lymph) accumulates in the peritoneal cavity and subsequently causes a contraction of the circulating plasma volume. As ascites accumulates, there is a gradual redistribution of plasma resulting in a reduction of the effective circulating plasma volume. Despite the reduction in the plasma volume realized by the kidneys and volume receptors, the total plasma volume may increase by third space fluid entrap-

ment. A reduction in effective intravascular volume invokes renal conservation of sodium (antinatiuresis) and water (ADH), which further promote ascites formation.

The *overflow theory* of ascites formation designates renal sodium retention as the primary pathologic event. This leads to plasma volume expansion, which in the setting of abnormal Starling forces (portal hypertension, reduced plasma oncotic pressure), in the sinusoidal and splanchnic circulations, promotes ascites formation. The abnormal tendency to retain sodium in cirrhosis is caused by a complex constellation of influences. The interplay of forces is suspected to be highly variable among different patients and within a given patient at different stages of their disease.

Fluid in the abdominal cavity may be absorbed by lymphatics of the peritoneal membrane; most absorption occurs through diaphragmatic lymphatics.[764] The accumulation of ascites reflects a balance between the rates of fluid production and peritoneal absorption. The rate of ascites production is determined by the portal pressure, sinusoidal permeability, quantity of lymph exuded from the liver or splanchnic vessels, and the capacity of the lymphatics. The rate of peritoneal fluid absorption is determined by the nature of the peritoneal surface and the pressure in the abdominal cavity (intraperitoneal pressure). When the intraperitoneal pressure increases, equaling or exceeding the sinusoidal and vascular hydrostatic pressure, ascites formation is curtailed and absorption occurs.[765,766] Large-volume paracentesis results in dynamic adjustments in the rate of ascites formation and absorption: An increased rate of ascites formation occurs concurrent with a reduced rate of fluid absorption.[767] These adjustments continue until a new steady state is established. These phenomenon suggest that large-volume therapeutic paracentesis in the cirrhotic patient be delayed as long as possible.

Occasionally, in the dog with liver disease that has ascites, pleural effusion will also develop. Hepatic hydrothorax occurs in 5% to 10% of humans with cirrhosis accompanied by ascites. It is defined as the presence of pleural effusion in a cirrhotic patient lacking primary pulmonary or cardiac disease. The effusion can develop quickly and be unilateral or bilateral. Its physicochemical characteristics usually reflect those of the patient's ascites. Pathogenic mechanisms include (1) flow through defects in the tendinous portion of the diaphragm, (2) azygos vein hypertension, and (3) trans-diaphragmatic lymphatic flow. Flow through the diaphragm is the favored theory. Fluid moves into the pleural cavity as a result of an intrathoracic-peritoneal pressure gradient.

Gastrointestinal Flora: Endogenous Bacterial Population

Gram positive cocci, gram negative bacilli, and clostridial organisms have been cultured from the liver of normal dogs.[768,769] Older experimental work indicated that clostridial organisms become established as resident hepatic flora in dogs after 6 months of age.[769] Other work has shown that adult dogs develop lethal hepatic necrosis following acute interruption of the hepatic artery associated with unabated growth of gut-derived microorganisms, particularly anaerobes. However, it remains controversial whether or not microorganisms inhabit normal canine liver tissue. Older experiments were fraught with problems, a major one being contamination of cultured specimens. Later studies questioned results of prior work, in identification of bacterial species and in number of positive cultures.[768] The clinical impression is that clostridial organisms rarely create a problem in ischemic liver following trauma, surgery, or toxin exposure. This correlates with the observation that intrahepatic abscesses are rare complications of liver disease or biopsy collection.

A complication of ascites is the development of spontaneous bacterial peritonitis. This has been well described in humans with cirrhosis but is uncommon in the dog. Affected patients are variably symptomatic and the disorder is diagnosed on the basis of finding increased numbers of neutrophils in ascitic effusion (> 250/µL) or a positive bacterial culture. Infection is derived from transmural movement of enteric organisms into the abdominal effusion or escape of alimentary microorganisms from poorly perfused Kupffer cells. These patients are predisposed to infection owing to reduced opsonization capabilities in blood and ascitic effusion. The portal route of infection has been shown to be important as a source of bacteria in biliary tract sepsis.[770] It is clear that the intestinal tract is the major source of organisms.[770–776] Intestinal macrophages are suspected to facilitate the passage of organisms into extraintestinal sites.[777,778] The presence of biliary obstruction facilitates penetration of organisms into the biliary tree.[771–776] Although the biliary tract does not harbor bacteria at most times, in the circumstance of impaired bile flow, positive cultures have been reported in between 30% and 80% of humans. Patients undergoing reoperation for biliary tract problems are at highest risk. *Bacteroides fragilis* has been commonly implicated as an important pathogen, although this is inconsistent.[768] Prophylactic antibiotic treatment of any patient undergoing biliary tract surgery is predicated on findings in retrospective studies. There have been no published studies in large numbers of veterinary patients.

Kupffer Cell Function

Particulate debris, bacterial organisms and their toxins, and many other substances (detailed later) have been shown to be removed by the hepatic RE system principally comprised of Kupffer cells. The Kupffer cell mass represents the largest accumulation of fixed macrophages in the body.[778,779] This network is capable of trapping and phagocytosing more antigen than any other component of the mononuclear-phagocytic system.[779] Normally, phagocytosis and antigen degradation proceeds independent of antibody processing and results in rapid elimination without antibody production.

Kupffer cells are tissue macrophages originally derived from monocytic bone marrow precursors.[780] They have a long life and a slow turnover rate but can replicate if stimulated. Like all macrophages, they have numerous important immunologic functions related to antigen presentation, T and B cell interaction, and repair of tissue damage. They also may produce tissue injury as a result of interactions with lymphocytes, expression of cytotoxicity, release of hydrolytic enzymes, and harboring of infectious agents (viruses, intracellular bacteria). Kupffer cells function as accessory cells, processing antigens and presenting them to immunocompetent cells.[779–781] Liver injury may disrupt the hepatic microenvironment facilitating close contact between Kupffer cells and transient inflammatory lymphocytes.[778,780,781] This is thought to be one factor that may promote chronic inflammation.

Kupffer cells have multiple influences over hepatocytes including stimulation of fibrinogen synthesis, inhibition of cytochrome P-450 activity, and inhibition of albumin synthesis. They also are involved in induction of fibroblast proliferation and Ito cell transformation that lead to fibrosis. Clearance of endotoxin derived from the enteric bacterial flora is a normal function of Kupffer cells. In health, the level of endo-

toxin in the systemic circulation is undetectable because Kupffer cells efficiently extract and degrade it.[782] In severe liver disease or in the presence of portosystemic shunting, the ability of the Kupffer cell to extract endotoxin is reduced and it appears in the systemic circulation.[782–797]

Reduced Kupffer cell phagocytosis occurs during systemic infections with certain bacteria and viruses, certain autoimmune disorders, radiation injury, immunologic suppression, starvation, and portosystemic shunting. Kupffer cell function is influenced by hepatic blood flow, oxygen, and glucose availability. Kupffer cells clear large particles faster than smaller particles. Too many particles can saturate the system and lead to system hypofunction or blockade.[798] This can occur when colloids, such as dextrans, are administered.

When liver injury is severe and Kupffer cell function compromised by loss of cell mass, impaired circulation, or altered function, the immunoprotective role they provide becomes compromised. The consequence is illustrated in Figure 30–29. This can result in production of antibodies against material usually restricted from the peripheral circulation and stimulation of acute-phase globulin and interleukin production and systemic hyperglobulinemia.

Endotoxemia in the Patient with Impaired Liver Function

Endotoxemia, in the absence of gram negative bacteremia, is believed to occur in patients with hepatic insufficiency.[782–795] In health, there is a daily entry of endotoxin into the portal circulation from the alimentary canal. Endotoxin can also be transported in intestinal lymphatics and may directly enter the peritoneal cavity by transmural leakage from the gut. Absorption of endotoxin is enhanced by gut inflammation, hypoperfusion, or anoxia. In health, clearance of alimentary-derived endotoxin is accomplished by the hepatic Kupffer cells. In patients with compromised hepatic function, Kupffer cell clearance is reduced and systemic endotoxemia may develop and lead to a variety of abnormalities, listed in Table 30–31. Endotoxemia has been associated with increased incidence of coagulopathy, renal failure, HE, and a high mortality rate in humans with hepatic insufficiency. In experimentally created portosystemic shunts, increased peripheral blood endotoxin concentrations have been shown.[756] However, dogs with congenital portosystemic shunts in one study did not have peripheral endotoxemia.[764]

Endotoxins may directly damage hepatocytes through (1) binding to cell membranes, (2) impairing cell communication, (3) reducing activity of cytochrome P-450s, and (4) impairing mitochondrial function. Endotoxin uptake by tissue macrophages results in their activation and release of products with potential to mediate hepatocellular injury (superoxide and other toxic oxygen radicals, lysosomal enzymes, factors inhibitory to protein synthesis, procoagulants, leukotrienes, interleukins, tumor necrosis factor, and platelet activating factor).

Hepatobiliary Immunoglobulin Production

The liver is an active participant in host defense through macrophage and local IgA activity.

IgA, the major immunoglobulin of the mucosal immune system,[799] is the major protein in bile where it is accompanied by a glycoprotein secretory component (SC), which functions

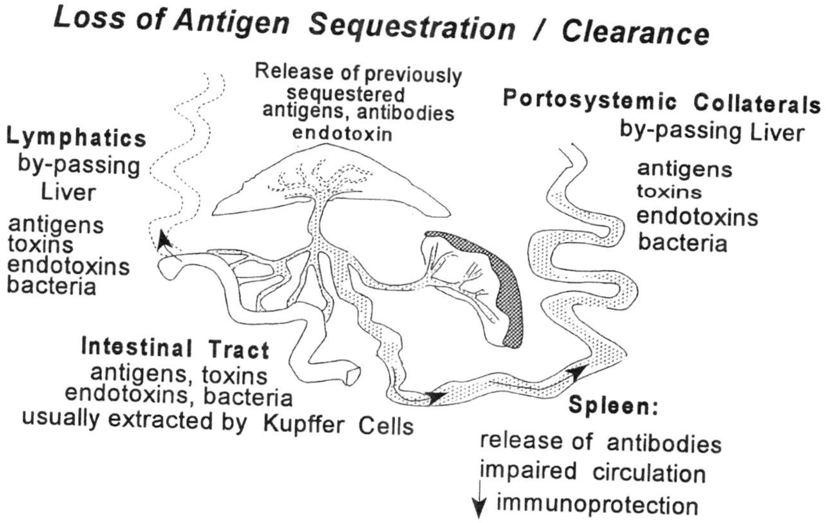

Loss of Antigen Sequestration / Clearance

FIGURE 30-29. Consequences of reduced Kupffer cell function and portosystemic shunting of blood that develop in chronic liver disease.

as the IgA cellular receptor. The IgA transported into bile is either synthesized locally by plasma cells and transported through bile duct epithelium or is cleared from plasma.[799,800] In many species, the hepatocyte extracts and transports most of the IgA released into bile; dogs and humans do not transport IgA as efficiently as rats. Species that are "poor" transporters express SC on intrahepatic and extrahepatic biliary epithelium rather than hepatocytes. The gallbladder may also contribute a substantial amount of biliary IgA.

The delivery of biliary IgA is suppressed by bile duct occlusion. The biologic benefit of biliary IgA includes immunologic protection of the biliary and upper gastrointestinal tract and clearance of harmful antigens. IgA specific against intestinal microbes, certain viruses, and enterotoxins have been shown and these are presumed to prevent attachment or penetration of mucous membranes. IgA can modulate the "violence" of local immunologic responses by preventing complement activation and excessive tissue injury due to cytotoxic reactions induced by other immune interactions.

Table 30-31

ADVERSE EFFECTS OF ENDOTOXINS

KUPFFER CELLS	HEPATOCYTES
Initially activated → suppressed	Lysosomal damage
Enlarge and become vacuolated	↓ microsomal enzymes
↑ response to chemoattractants	impaired mitochondrial function
↑ interaction with lymphocytes	impaired organic anion processing
↑ release collagenase	fatty metamorphosis
↑ release arachadonic acid	hepatocyte necrosis
↑ release prostaglandins	
↑ release soluble factors:	
Ito cells → fibrocytes	
modulates hepatocyte function:	
↑ hepatocyte protein synthesis	
↑ release lysosomal enzymes	
↑ release procoagulants	
↑ release pyrogens	
↑ colony stimulating factors	
↑ release interferon	
↑ tumoricidal factor	

Gastrointestinal Inflammation and Hemorrhage

Gastroduodenal inflammation and ulceration is a well-recognized clinical complication in cirrhotic patients that may lead to HE. Gastrointestinal bleeding may be occult or obvious and life endangering. In humans with cirrhosis and in animal models of cirrhosis, gastric lesions are associated with a hyperdynamic portal circulation.[801–807] The pathogenesis of gastrointestinal ulceration is not well defined but involves mechanisms shown in Figure 30–30.

In humans, two different gastric syndromes are recognized: (1) portal hypertensive gastropathy associated with edema in the lamina propria and submucosa, increased intraluminal gastric pH, hypergastrinemia, and increased back diffusion of H+ into gastric mucosa, and (2) angiodysplasia or vascular ecstasia associated with dilated mucosal vessels representing microvarices.[801–804] Even though total gastric blood flow may increase in the presence of a hyperdynamic portal circulation, effective blood flow to the surface mucosa is reduced. Causal mechanisms include microvascular shunting and extensive mucosal edema.[801–804] Animals with experimental portal hypertension have increased susceptibility to mucosal damage induced by noxious substances; an example is exposure to bile acids.[801,803] Increased susceptibility to injury is related to mucosal ischemia induced by the microvasculopathy. Chronic microvascular lesions are characterized by thinning of vessel walls and expanded lumen diameter leading to the formation of microvarices.[805] These changes develop in rats within 15 days after induction of portal hypertension by portal vein ligation.[805] Hypergastrinemia has been well documented in humans with cirrhosis, portal hypertension, and gastric ulceration.[801,808] High gastrin concentrations are not due to reduced hepatic function because the liver does not appear to play a major role in gastrin clearance[809] but rather is related to the high intraluminal gastric pH.[806] This suggests that use of H_2 blockers are not always indicated in the patient with liver disease that has evidence of gastric ulceration. High gastrin levels may provide a gastric vasodilator effect in this condition. However, contradictory evidence has shown an increase in gastric acid secretion and back diffusion of hydrogen ions develops after surgical creation of portacaval anastomoses.[805,808,810]

The development of gastrointestinal bleeding is devastating in the patient prone to develop HE. Blood is a potent source of HE toxins and is considered to be the most noxious of almost any substance that can precipitate HE. Gastroin-

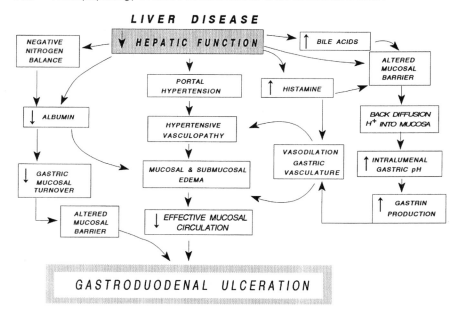

FIGURE 30-30. Etiopathogenic mechanisms associated with gastroduodenal ulceration in patients with hepatic insufficiency.

testinal bleeding may be aggravated by the presence of an acquired coagulopathy due to hepatic synthetic failure or vitamin K deficiency.

Hepatorenal Syndrome

An hepatorenal syndrome (HRS) is recognized in humans with decompensated hepatic insufficiency, either chronic or acute.[811,812] All affected patients have tense ascites. The syndrome is characterized by unexplained oliguric renal failure in a patient with severe liver disease. It is probable that a similar entity occurs in dogs, particularly Doberman pinschers that present in decompensated hepatic failure. Humans with HRS produce urine that contains subnormal quantities of sodium and yet retain the ability to concentrate urine. Although potentially reversible, there is marked clinical variation in expression and in the course of the disorder. Interventional procedures such as therapeutic paracentesis of ascites

or vigorous diuresis and gastrointestinal bleeding seem to precipitate the syndrome.

The HRS is best considered a functional condition of the kidneys. Demonstrable pathologic lesions are minimal and inconsistent.[811] Kidneys transplanted from an affected patient can become functionally normal in a recipient without liver disease. Although the cause of this syndrome is not known, it is believed to be multifactorial, involving activation of the sympathetic system, renin-angiotensin system, endotoxemia, endothelin, nitric oxide, and altered eicosanoid production (Figure 30–31).[811–814] Renal vasomotor instability is the most obvious physiologic abnormality. Patients develop reduced renal cortical perfusion resulting in ischemic injury. Other factors that influence regulation of the glomerular surface area available for ultrafiltration also are believed to be involved. These dynamically regulate the surface of the glomerulus available for ultrafiltration.

When the HRS develops, marked systemic hemodynamic disturbances are also usually found. These include a hyperdynamic circulation, tachycardia, increased cardiac output, and

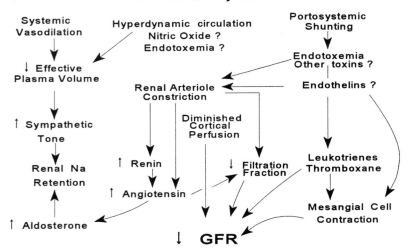

FIGURE 30-31. Simplified algorithm showing the mechanisms involved with the hepatorenal syndrome.

decreased blood pressure and systemic vascular resistance.[811] These findings suggest the likelihood of a vasodilator influence, such as nitric oxide or endotoxin, in the etiopathogenesis of the disorder.

Despite the considerable amount of study of the HRS in humans, intensive supportive care, avoidance or treatment of infection and endotoxemia, and maintenance of systemic perfusion pressures are the mainstay of therapy. Interventional treatments aimed at conjectured disease mechanisms remain investigational. Monitoring and support of the patient undergoing therapeutic paracentesis is advised because of the association of HRS with this procedure. Suspected hepatorenal syndrome in dogs with hepatic insufficiency has been associated with a dismal prognosis.

REFERENCES

1. Zakim D. Metabolism of glucose and fatty acids by the liver. In: Zakim D, Boyer TD (eds) Hepatology: A Textbook of Liver Disease, 2nd ed. WB Saunders, Philadelphia, 65–96, 1982.
2. Cahill GF, Jr, Ashmore J, Earle AS, et al. Glucose penetration into liver. Am J Physiol 192:491–496, 1958.
3. Katz LD, Glickman MG, Rappaport S, et al. Splanchnic and peripheral disposal of oral glucose in man. Diabetes 32:675–679, 1983.
4. Maehlum S, Jervell J, Pruett EDT. Arterial-hepatic vein glucose differences in normal and diabetic man during glucose infusion at rest and after exercise. Scand J Clin Lab Invest 36:415–422, 1976.
5. Matsumura T, Thurman RG. Predominance of glycolysis in pericentral regions of the liver lobule. Eur J Biochem 140:229–234, 1984.
6. Matsumura T, Kashiwagi R, Meren H, et al. Gluconeogenesis predominates in periportal regions of the liver lobule. Eur J Biochem 144:409–415, 1984.
7. Strombeck DR, Krum S, Meyer D, et al. Hypoglycemia and hypoinsulinemia associated with hepatoma in a dog. J Am Vet Med Assoc 169:811–812, 1976.
8. Leifer CE, Peterson ME, Matus RE, et al. Hypoglycemia associated with nonislet cell tumor in 13 dogs. J Am Vet Med Assoc 186:53–55, 1985.
9. Walvoort HC. Glycogen storage disease type II in the Lapland dog. Vet Q 7:187–190, 1985.
10. Yoshiya K, Kishimoto T, Ishikawa Y, et al. Insulin response following intravenous glucose administration in dogs with obstructive jaundice. J Surg Res 43:271–277, 1987.
11. Rojdmark S, Bloom G, Chou MCY, et al. Hepatic extraction of exogenous insulin and glucagon in the dog. Endocrinology 102:806–000, 1978.
12. Walton DK, Center SA, Scott DW, et al. Ulcerative dermatosis associated with diabetes mellitus in the dog: A report of four cases. J Am Anim Hosp Assoc 22:79–88, 1986.
13. Gross TL, Song MD, Havel PJ, et al. Superficial necrolytic dermatitis (necrolytic migratory erythema) in dogs. Vet Pathol 30:75–81, 1993.
14. Miller WH, Scott DW, Buerger RG, et al. Necrolytic migratory erythema in dogs: A hepatocutaneous syndrome. J Am Anim Hosp Assoc 26:573–581, 1990.
15. Ericsson JLE, Orrenius S, Holm I. Alterations in canine liver cells induced by protein deficiency. Ultrastructural and biochemical observation. Exp Mol Path 5:329–349, 1966.
16. Mashima Y. Effect of calorie overload on puppy livers during parenteral nutrition. J Parenteral Ent Nutr 3:139–145, 1979.
17. Hermansen L, Stensvold I. Production and removal of lactate during exercise in man. Acta Med Scand 86:191–201, 1972.
18. Cooper AD. Hepatic lipoprotein and cholesterol metabolism. In: Zakim D, Boyer TD (eds) Hepatology: A Textbook of Liver Disease, 2nd ed. WB Saunders, Philadelphia, 96–123, 1990.
19. Turley SD, Dietschy JM. The metabolism and excretion of cholesterol by the liver. In: Arias IM, Jakoby WB, et al. (eds) The Liver: Biology and Pathobiology. Raven Press, New York, 617–662, 1988.
20. Watson TDG, Barrie J. Lipoprotein metabolism and hyperlipidaemia in the dog and cat: a review. J Small Anim Pract 34:479–487, 1993.
21. Chapman MJ. Animal lipoproteins: chemistry, structure and comparative aspects. J Lipid Res 21:789–853, 1980.
22. Erickson SK, Shrewsbury MA, Brooks C, et al. Rat liver acyl coenzyme A:cholesterol acyltransferase. Its regulation *in vivo* and some of its properties *in vitro*. J Lipid Res 21:930–941, 1980.
23. Glickman RM, Sabesin SM. Lipoprotein metabolism. In: Arias IM, Jakoby WB, Popper H, et al. (eds) The Liver: Biology and Pathobiology, 2nd ed. Raven Press, New York, 331–362, 1988.
24. Mahley RW. Alterations in plasma lipoproteins induced by cholesterol feeding in animals including man. In: Dietshy JM, Gotto AM, Ontko JA

(eds) Disturbances in Lipid and Lipoprotein Metabolism. American Physiological Society, Washington DC, 181–197, 1978.
25. Cho BHS, Erdman JW, Corbin JE. Effects of feeding raw eggs on levels of plasma and lipoprotein cholesterol in dogs. Nutr Reports Inter 30:163–171, 1984.
26. Steiner A, Kendall FE. Atherosclerosis and arteriosclerosis in dogs following ingestion of cholesterol and thiouracil. Arch Path 42:433–444, 1946.
27. Lazarow PB, Moser HW. Disorders of peroxisome biogenesis. In: Scriver CR, Beaudet AL, Sly WS, et al. (eds) The Metabolic Basis of Inherited Disease, 6th ed., Vol. II. McGraw-Hill Information Services, New York, 1479–1509, 1989.
28. Quarfordt SH, Oelschlaeger H, Krigbaum WR, et al. Effect of biliary obstruction on canine plasma biliary lipids. Lipids 8:522–530, 1973.
29. Quarfordt SH, Oelschlaeger H, Krigbawm WR. Liquid crystalline lipid in the plasma of humans with biliary obstruction. J Clin Invest 51:1979–1987, 1972.
30. McIntyre N, Harry DS, Pearson AJG. Progress report: The hypercholesterolemia of obstructive jaundice. Gut 16:379–391, 1975.
31. Cooper AD, Ockner RK. Studies of hepatic cholesterol synthesis in experimental acute biliary obstruction. Gastroenterology 66:586–595, 1974.
32. Fredrickson DS, Loud AV, Hinkelman BT, et al. The effect of ligation of the common bile duct on cholesterol synthesis in the rat. J Exp Med 99:43–53, 1954.
33. McIntyre N, Calandra S, Pearson AJG. Lipid and lipoprotein abnormalities in liver disease: The possible role of lecithin:cholesterol acyl transferase deficiency. Scan J Clin Invest 33 (suppl 137):115–120, 1974.
34. Agorastos J, Fox C, Harry DS, et al. Lecithin-cholesterol acyltransferase and the lipoprotein abnormalities of obstructive jaundice. Clin Sci Mole Med 54:369–379, 1978.
35. Van Vleet JF, Alberts JO. Evaluation of liver function tests and liver biopsy in experimental carbon tetrachloride intoxication and extrahepatic bile duct obstruction in the dog. Am J Vet Res 29:2119–2131, 1968.
36. Center SA, Baldwin BE, Tennant B, et al. Hematologic and biochemical abnormalities associated with induced extrahepatic bile duct obstruction in the cat. Am J Vet Res 44:1822–1829, 1983.
37. Opitz M, Lettow E. Der cholesterinesterquotient im serujm leberkranker hunde. Berl Munch, Tierarztl Wschr 89:28–32, 1976.
38. Simon JB, Scheig R. Serum cholesterol esterification in liver disease: Importance of lecithin-cholesterol acyltransferase. N Engl J Med 283:841–846, 1970.
39. Kepkay DL, Poon R, Simon JB. Lecithin-cholesterol acyltransferase and serum cholesterol esterification in obstructive jaundice. J Lab Clin Med 81:172–181, 1973.
40. Wengeler H, Greten J, Seidel D. Serum cholesterol esterification in liver disease. Combined determinations of lecithin:cholesterol acyltransferase and lipoprotein X. Eur J Clin Invest 2:372–378, 1970.
41. Coyle JJ, Schwartz MZ, Marubbio AT, et al. The effect of portacaval shunt on plasma lipids and tissue cholesterol synthesis in the dog. Surgery 80:54–60, 1976.
42. Francavilla A, Jones AF, Benichou J, et al. The effect of portacaval shunt upon hepatic cholesterol synthesis and cyclic AMP in dogs and baboons. J Surg Res 28:1–7, 1980.
43. Guzman IJ, Schneider PD, Coyle JJ. Combined hypolipidemia of portacaval transposition and ileal resection in the dog. Surg Gyn Obstet 150:475–480, 1980.
44. Coyle JJ, Guzman IJ, Varco RL. Cholesterol pool sizes and turnover following portacaval shunt in the dog. Surg Gyn Obstet 148:723–737, 1979.
45. Guzman IJ, Coyle JJ, Schneider PD, et al. The effect of selective visceral caval shunt on plasma lipids and cholesterol dynamics. Surgery 82:42–50, 1977.
46. Castellanos J, Toledo-Pereyra LH, Mittal VK, et al. Prolonged hypocholesterolemic effects of portacaval transposition in dogs: An experimental study. Eur Surg Res 13:438–443, 1981.
47. Beher WT, Toledo-Pereyra LH. Effect of caval shunts on lipid metabolism. Prog Lipid Res 18:165–177, 1980.
48. Ponz de Leon M, Loria P, Iori R, et al. Cholesterol absorption in cirrhosis: The role of total and individual bile acid pool size. Gastroenterology 80:1428–1437, 1981.
49. Schaeffer MC, Rogers QR, Buffington CA, et al. Long-term biochemical and physiologic effects of surgically placed portacaval shunts in dogs. Am J Vet Res 47:346–355, 1986.
50. Bunch SE. Hypocholesterolemia in dogs. Proc ACVIM 13/7–13/20, 1986.
51. Bass VD, Hoffmann WE, Dorner JL. Normal canine lipid profiles and effects of experimentally induced pancreatitis and hepatic necrosis on lipids. Am J Vet Res 37:1355–1358, 1976.
52. Bunch SE, Castleman WL, Baldwin BH, et al. Effects of long-term primidone and phenytoin administration on canine hepatic function and morphology. Am J Vet Res 46:105–115, 1985.
53. Abell LL, Mosbach EH, Kendall FE. Hypocholesterolemic effect of 17alpha-methyltestosterone in dogs. Circ Res 10:846–850, 1962.
54. Milewski B, Palynyczko Z. Evaluation of the usefulness of serum lipoprotein-X (LP-X) detection test for the diagnosis of cholestasis in chronic liver diseases. Pol Arch Med Wewn, 53:445–452, 1975.

55. Magnani HN, Alaupovic P. Utilization of the quantitative assay of lipoprotein X in the differential diagnosis of extrahepatic obstructive jaundice and intrahepatic disease. Gastroenterology 71:87–93, 1976.
56. Ritland S. Quantitative determination of the abnormal lipoprotein of cholestasis, LP-X, in liver disease. Scand J Gastroenterol 10:5–15, 1975.
57. Seidel D, Buff HU, Bleyl U. On the metabolism of lipoprotein-X (LP-X). Clin Chim Acta 66:195–207, 1976.
58. Danielsson B, Ekman R, Johansson BG, et al. Abnormal low density plasma lipoproteins occurring in dogs with obstructive jaundice (letter). FEBS 63:33–36, 1976.
59. Bauer JE, Meyer DJ, Goring RL, et al. Cholestasis induced changes in canine serum lipids and lipoproteins. Proc ACVIM, (abstract), 14–45, 1986.
60. Rogers WA, Donovan EF, Kociba GJ. Idiopathic hyperlipoproteinemia in dogs. J Am Vet Med Assoc 166:1087–1091, 1975.
61. Whitney MS, Boon GD, Rebar AH, et al. Ultracentrifugal and electrophoretic characteristics of the plasma lipoproteins of miniature schnauzer dogs with idiopathic hyperlipoproteinemia. J Vet Int Med 7:253–260, 1993.
62. Jones BR, Wallace A, Harding DRK, et al. Occurrence of idiopathic familial hyperchylomicronemia in a cat. Vet Rec 112:543–547, 1983.
63. Bauer JE, Verlander JW. Congenital lipoprotein lipase deficiency in hyperlipemic kitten siblings. Vet Clin Path 13:7–11, 1984.
64. Thompson JC, Johnstone AC, Jones BR, et al. The ultrastructural pathology of five lipoportein lipase-deficient cats. J Comp Path 101:251–262, 1989.
65. Jones BR, Johnstone AC, Hancock WS. Inherited hyperchylomicronaemia in the cat. Vet Ann 26:330–340, 1986.
66. Jones BR, Johnstone AC, Cahill JI, et al. Peripheral neuropathy in cats with inherited primary hyperchylomicronaemia. Vet Rec 119:268–272, 1986.
67. Harry DS, Owen JS, McIntyre N. Plasma lipoproteins and the liver. In: Wright R, Millward-Sadler GH, Alberti KGMM (eds) Liver and Biliary Disease, 2nd ed. WB Saunders, Philadelphia, 65–86, 1985.
68. Hoyumpa AM, Greene HL, Dunn GD, et al. Fatty liver: Biochemical and clinical considerations. Digest Dis 20:1142–1170, 1975.
69. Cello JP, Grendell JH. The liver in systemic conditions. In: Zakim D, Boyer TD (eds) Hepatology, a Textbook of Liver Disease. WB Saunders, Philadelphia, 1411–1437, 1990.
70. Holdstock G, Millward-Sadler GH, Wright R. Hepatic changes in systemic disease. In: Wright R, et al. (eds) Liver and Biliary Disease, 2nd ed. WB Saunders, Philadelphia, 1033–1076, 1985.
71. Smuckler EA. Patterns of reaction of the liver to injury. In: Zakim D, Boyer TD (eds) Hepatology, a Textbook of Liver Disease. WB Saunders, Philadelphia, 681–692, 1982.
72. Vierling JM. Hepatobiliary complications of ulcerative colitis and Crohn's disease. In: Zakim D, Boyer TD (eds) Hepatology, a Textbook of Liver Disease. WB Saunders, Philadelphia, 797–824, 1982.
73. Drenick EJ, Fisler J, Johnson D. Hepatic steatosis after intestinal bypass: Prevention and reversal by metronidazole, irrespective of protein calorie malnutrition. Gastroenterology 82:535–548, 1982.
74. Quigley EMM, Zetterman RK. Hepatobiliary complications of malabsorption and malnutrition. Sem Liver Dis 8:218–228, 1988.
75. Klein S, Nealon WH. Hepatobiliary abnormalities associated with total parenteral nutrition. Sem Liver Dis 8:237–246, 1988.
76. Gerloff BJ, Herdt TH. Hepatic lipidosis from dietary restriction in nonlactating cows. J Am Vet Med Assoc 185:223–224, 1984.
77. Herdt TH, Gerloff BJ. Hepatic lipidosis and liver function in 49 cows with displaced abomasums. Proc XIIth World Congress on Diseases of Cattle, the Netherlands, Vol. I, 522–526, 1982.
78. Gerloff BJ, Herdt TH, Emery RS, et al. Inositol as a lipotropic agent in dairy cattle diets. J Anim Sci 59:806–812, 1984.
79. Murray M. Hepatic lipidosis in a post parturient mare. Equine Vet J 17:68–69, 1985.
80. Herdt TH, Goeders L, Liesman JS, et al. Test for estimation of bovine hepatic lipid content. J Am Vet Med Assoc 182:953–955, 1983.
81. Barsanti JA, Jones BD, Spano JS, et al. Prolonged anorexia associated with hepatic lipidosis in three cats. Fel Pract, 52–57, May 1977.
82. Burrows CF, Chiapella AM, Jezyk P. Idiopathic feline hepatic lipidosis: The syndrome and speculations on its pathogenesis. Florida Vet J, 18–20, Winter 1981.
83. Thornburg LP, Simpson S, Digilio K. Fatty liver syndrome in cats. J Am Anim Hosp Assoc 18:397–400, 1982.
84. Percy DH, Jortner BS. Feline lipidosis: light and electron microscopic studies. Arch Path 92:136–144, 1971.
85. Pritchard DH, Jolly RD, Howell LJ, et al. Ceroid-lipidosis: An acquired storage-type disease of liver and hepatic lymph node. Vet Pathol 20:242–244, 1983.
86. Zawie D, Garvey MS. Feline hepatic disease. Vet Clin N Am 14:1201–1230, 1984.
87. Center SA, Thompson M, Wood PA, et al. Hepatic ultrastructural and metabolic derangements in cats with severe hepatic lipidosis. Proc 9th ACVIM Forum 193–196, 1991.
88. Hubbard BS, Vulgamott JC. Feline hepatic lipidosis. Comp Contin Ed 14:459–463, 1992.
89. Akol KG, Washabau RJ, Saunders HM, et al. Acute pancreatitis in cats with hepatic lipidosis. J Vet Int Med 7:205–209, 1993.
90. Center SA, Crawford MA, Guida L, et al. Clinicopathologic features of spontaneous severe hepatic lipidosis in the cat: 77 cases (1977–1990). J Vet Int Med 7:349–359, 1994.
91. Alpers DH, Sabesin SM. Fatty liver: Biochemical and clinical aspects. In: Schiff L, Schiff ER (eds) Diseases of the Liver, 6th ed. JG Lippincott, Philadelphia, 949–978, 1987.
92. Flatt FP. Role of the increased adipose tissue mass in the apparent insulin insensitivity of obesity. Am J Clin Nutr 25:1189–1192, 1972.
93. Campagnari-Visconti L, et al. Inhibition by glucose of the ethionine-induced fatty liver. Proc Soc Exp Biol Med 111:479–482, 1962.
94. Miyai K, Raick AN, Ritchie AC. Effects of glucose on the subcellular structure of the rat liver cells in acute ethionine intoxication. Lab Invest 23:268–277, 1970.
95. Hendricksie RG. The influence of aflatoxins on child health in the tropics with particular reference to kwashiorkor. Royal Soc Trop Med Hyg 78:427–435, 1984.
96. Windmueller HG, Levy RI. Total inhibition of hepatic beta-lipoprotein production in the rat by orotic acid. J Biol Chem 242:2246–2254, 1967.
97. Bauer JE. Feline lipid metabolism and hepatic lipidosis. Feline Medicine. Proc 12th Kal Kan Symp, 75–78, 1988.
98. MacDonald ML, Anderson BC, Rogers QR, et al. Essential fatty acid requirements of cats: Pathology of essential fatty acid deficiency. Am J Vet Res 45:1310–1317, 1984.
99. Read AE. The liver and drugs. In: Wright R, et al. (eds) Liver and Biliary Disease, 2nd ed. WB Saunders, Philadelphia, 1003–1032, 1985.
100. Kaufman AC, Greene CE. Increased alanine transaminase activity associated with tetracycline administration in a cat. J Am Vet Med Assoc 202:628–6630, 1993.
101. Freneaux E, Gilles L, Letteron P, et al. Inhibition of the mitochondrial oxidation of fatty acids by tetracycline in mice and man: Possible role in microvesicular steatosis induced by this antibiotic. Hepatology 8:1056–1062, 1988.
102. Breen KJ, Schenker S, Heimberg M. Effect of tetracyline on the metabolism of (1-¹⁴C) oleate by the liver. Biochem Pharmacol 28:197–200, 1979.
103. Gwee MCE. Can tetracycline-induced fatty liver in pregnancy be attributed to choline deficiency? Med Hypotheses 9:157–162, 1982.
104. Hansen CH, Pearson LH, Schenker S, et al. Impaired secretion of triglycerides by the liver: A cause of tetracycline-induced fatty liver. Proc Soc Exp Biol Med 128:143–146, 1968.
105. Romert P, Matthiessen ME. Tetracycline-induced changes in hepatocytes of mini-pigs and mini-pig foetuses as revealed by electron microscopy. Acta Pathol Microbiol Immunol Scand 94:125–131, 1986.
106. Jezequel AM, Bonazzi P, Novelli G, et al. Early structural and functional changes in liver of rats treated with a single dose of valproic acid. Hepatology 4:1159–1166, 1984.
107. Kesterson JW, Granneman GR, Machinist JM. The hepatotoxicity of valproic acid and its metabolites in rats. I. Toxicologic, biochemical and histopathologic studies. Hepatology 4:1143–1152, 1984.
108. Granneman GR, Wang S-I, Kesterson JW, et al. The hepatotoxicity of valproic acid and its metabolites in rats. II. Intermediary and valproic acid metabolism. Hepatology 4:1153–1158, 1984.
109. Kaplan MM. Acute fatty liver of pregnancy. N Engl J Med 313:367–370, 1985.
110. Scully RE, Galdabini JJ, McNeely BU. Weekly clinicopathological exercises. 304:216–224, 1981.
111. Ockner SA, Brunt EM, Cohn SM, et al. Fulminant hepatic failure caused by acute fatty liver of pregnancy treated by orthotopic liver transplantation. Hepatology 11:59–64, 1989.
112. Rebouche CJ, Engel AG. Carnitine metabolism and deficiency syndromes. Mayo Clin Proc 58:533–540, 1983.
113. van der Linde-Sipman JS, van den Ingh TS, van Toor AJ. Fatty liver syndrome in puppies. J Am Anim Hosp Assoc 26:9–12, 1990.
114. Hayek A, Bryant PD, Woodside WF. Hypernatremia induces hyperlipemia and a fatty liver. Metabolism 32:1–3, 1983.
115. Bengmark S. Liver steatosis and liver resection. Digestion 2:304, 1969.
116. Rothschild MA, Oratz M, Schreiber SS. Albumin synthesis. N Engl J Med 286:748–757, 1972.
117. Putnam FW. Alpha, beta, gamma, omega—the roster of plasma proteins. In: Putnam FW (ed) The Plasma Proteins. Structure, Function and Genetic Control, 2nd ed., Vol. 1. Academic Press, New York, 63, 1975.
118. Morgan EH, Peters T: The biosynthesis of rat serum albumin: V. Effect of protein depletion and refeeding on albumin and transferrin synthesis. J Bio Chem 246:3500–3507, 1971.
119. Rothschild MA, Oratz M, Schreiber SS. Serum albumin. Hepatology 8:385–401, 1988.
120. Kirsch R, Frith L, Black E, et al. Regulation of albumin synthesis and catabolism by alteration of dietary protein. Nature 217:578–579, 1968.
121. Waterlow JC, Stephen JML. The effect of low protein diets on the

turnover rates of serum, liver and muscle proteins in the rat measured by continuous infusion of L-(U[14]C)lysine. Clin Sci 35:287–305, 1968.

122. Rothschild MA, Oratz M, Schreiber SS. Albumin synthesis [first of two parts]. N Engl J Med 286:748–757, 1972.

123. Rothschild MA, Oratz M, Mongelli J, et al. Amino acid regulation of albumin synthesis. J Nutr 98:395–403, 1969.

124. Kirsch RE, Saunders SJ, Frith L, et al. Plasma amino acid concentration and the regulation of albumin synthesis. Am J Clin Nutr 22:1559–1562, 1969.

125. Coward WA, Sawyer MB. Whole-body albumin mass and distribution in rats fed on low-protein diets. Br J Nutr 37:127–134, 1977.

126. Yap SH, Hafkenscheid JCM. Effect of starvation on the synthesis rate of albumin in vivo and its relation to the concentrations of amino acids in the peripheral blood, the portal circulation and in the liver cytosolic fraction. Ann Nutr Metab 25:158–164, 1981.

127. Lunn PG, Austin S. Excess energy intake promotes the development of hypoalbuminemia in rats fed on low-protein diets. Br J Nutr 49:9–16, 1983.

128. Kaysen GA. Albumin metabolism in the nephrotic syndrome: The effect of dietary protein intake. Am J Kid Dis 12:461–480, 1988.

129. Rothschild MA, Oratz M, Mongelli J, et al. Effect of albumin concentration on albumin synthesis in the perfused liver. Am J Physiology 216:1127–1130, 1969.

130. Rothschild MA, Oratz M, Evans CD, et al. Role of hepatic interstitial albumin in regulating albumin synthesis. Am J Physiol 210:57–62, 1966.

131. Dich J, Hansen SE, Thieden HID. Effect of albumin concentration and colloid osmotic pressure on albumin synthesis in the perfused rat liver. Acta Physiol Scand 89:352–358, 1973.

132. Rothschild MA, Oratz M, Franklin ED, et al. The effect of hypergammaglobulinemia on albumin metabolism in hyperimmuned rabbits studied with albumin-I[131]. J Clin Invest 41:1564–1571, 1962.

133. Rothschild MA, Oratz M, Mongelli J, et al. Albumin metabolism in rabbits during gamma globulin infusions. J Lab Clin Med 66:733–740, 1965.

134. Hoffenberg R. Control of albumin degradation in vivo and in the perfused liver. In: Rothschild MA, Waldmann T (eds) Plasma Protein Metabolism: Regulation of Synthesis, Distribution and Degradation. Academic Press, New York, 239–255, 1970.

135. Fink RM, Enns R, Kimball CP, et al. Plasma protein metabolism: Observations using heavy nitrogen in lysine. J Exp Med 80:455–475, 1944.

136. Dixon FJ, Maurer PH, Deichmiller MP. Half-lives of homologous serum albumins in several species. Soc Exp Bio Med 83:287–288, 1953.

137. Yedgar S, Carew RE, Pittman RC, et al. Tissue sites of catabolism of albumin in rabbits. Am J Physiol 244:E101-E107, 1983.

138. Morris MA, Preddy L. Glycosylation accelerates albumin degradation in normal and diabetic dogs. Biochem Med Metabolic Bio 35:267–270, 1986.

139. Plumb DC. Veterinary Drug Handbook. Pharmavet Publishing, White Bear Lake, MN, 1991.

140. McEvoy GE (ed). American Hospital Formulary Service Drug Information 95. American Society of Hospital Pharmacists Inc. Bethesda, MD, 1995.

141. Hasch E, Jarnum S, Tygstrup N, et al. Albumin synthesis rate as a measure of liver function in patients with cirrhosis. Acta Med Scand 182:83–91, 1967.

142. Berson SA, Yalow RS. The distribution of I[131]-labeled human serum albumin introduced into ascitic fluid: Analysis of the kinetics of a three compartment quaternary transfer system in man and speculation on possible sites of degradation. J Clin Invest 33:377–387, 1954.

143. Dykes PW. The rates of distribution and catabolism of albumin in normal subjects and in patients with cirrhosis of the liver. Clin Sci 34:161–183, 1968.

144. Sterling K. Serum albumin turnover in Laennec's cirrhosis as measured by I[131]-tagged albumin. J Clin Invest 30:1238–1242, 1951.

145. Wilkinson P, Mendenhall CL. Serum albumin turnover in normal subjects and patients with cirrhosis measured by I[131]-labelled human albumin. Clin Sci 25:281–282, 1963.

146. Rothschild MA, Oratz M, Zimmon D, et al. Albumin synthesis in cirrhotic subjects with ascites studied with carbonate[14]. J Clin Invest 48:344–350, 1969.

147. Zimmon DS, Oratz M, Kessler R, et al. Albumin to ascites: Demonstration of a direct pathway bypassing the systemic circulation. J Clin Invest 48:2074–2078, 1969.

148. Castell JV, Gomez-Lechon MJ, David M, et al. Acute-phase response of human hepatocytes: regulation of acute-phase protein synthesis by interleukin-6. Hepatology 12:1179–1186, 1990.

149. Cornell RP. Acute-phase responses after acute liver injury by partial hepatectomy in rats as indicators of cytokine release. Hepatology 11:923–931, 1990.

150. Jamieson JC, Kaplan HA, Woloski BM, et al. Glycoprotein biosynthesis during the acute-phase response to inflammation. Can J Biochem Cell Biol 61:1041–1048, 1983.

151. Koj A, Gauldie J, Regoeczi E, et al. The acute-phase response of cultured rat hepatocytes. Biochem J 224:505–514, 1984.

152. Moshage HJ, Janssen JAM, Franssen JH, et al. Study of the molecular mechanism of decreased liver synthesis of albumin in inflammation. J Clin Invest 79:1635–1641, 1987.

153. Perimutter DH, Dinarello CA, Punsal PI, et al. Cachectin/tumor necrosis factor regulates hepatic acute-phase gene expression. J Clin Invest 78:1349–1354, 1986.

154. Schimke RT. Differential effects of fasting and protein-free diets on levels of urea cycle enzymes in rat liver. J Bio Chem 237:1921–1924, 1962.

155. Schimke RT. Adaptive characteristics of urea cycle enzymes in the rat. J Bio Chem 237:459–468, 1962.

156. Tabor CW, Tabor H. Polyamines. Annu Rev Biochem 53:749–790, 1984.

157. Luk GD. Essential role of polyamine metabolism in hepatic regeneration: Inhibition of deoxyribonucleic acid and protein synthesis and tissue regeneration by difluoromethylornithine in the rat. Gastroenterology 90:1261–1267, 1986.

158. Diehl AM, Abdo S, Brown N. Supplemental putrescine reverses ethanol-associated inhibition of liver regeneration. Hepatology 12:633–637, 1990.

159. Laflamme D, Allen SW, Huber TL. Apparent dietary protein requirement of dogs with portosystemic shunt. Am J Vet Res 54:719–723, 1993.

160. Kukral JC, Sporn J, Louch J, et al. Synthesis of alpha- and beta- globulins in normal and liverless dog. Am J Physiol 204:262–264, 1963.

161. Koj A. Metabolic studies of acute-phase proteins. In: Mariani G (ed) Pathophysiology of Plasma Protein Metabolism. Plenum Press, New York, London, 221–248, 1984.

162. Koj A. Liver reponse to inflammation and synthesis of acute phase plasma proteins. In: Gordon AH, Koj A (eds) The Acute Phase Response to Injury and Infection. Elsevier, New York, 139–246, 1985.

163. Conner JG, Eckersall PD. Acute phase response in the dog following surgical trauma. Res Vet Sci 45:107–110, 1988.

164. Harvey JW, West CL. Prednisone-induced increases in serum alpha-2-globulin and haptoglobin concentrations in dogs. Vet Pathol 24:90–92, 1987.

165. Ganrot K. Plasma protein response in experimental inflammation in the dog. Res Exp Med (Berlin) 161:251–261, 1973.

166. Harvey JW. Quantitative determinations of normal horse, cat and dog haptoglobins. Theriogenology 2–3:133–137, 1976.

167. Harvey JW. Comparison between serum haptoglobin and alpha-2-globulin concentrations in dogs. Vet Clin Path 15:4–5, 1986.

168. Caspi D, Snel FWJ, Batt RM, et al. C-reactive protein in dogs. Am J Vet Res 48:919–921, 1987.

169. Jain NC. Acute phase proteins. In: Kirk RW (ed) Current Veterinary Therapy X. WB Saunders, Philadelphia, 468–471, 1989.

170. Castell JV, Gomez-Lechon MJ, David M, et al. Acute-phase response of human hepatocytes: Regulation of acute-phase protein synthesis by interleukin-6. Hepatology 12:1179–1186, 1990.

171. Cornell RP. Acute phase responses after acute liver injury by partial hepatectomy in rats as indicators of cytokine release. Hepatology 11:923–931, 1990.

172. Jamieson JC, Kaplan HA, Woloski RNJ, et al. Glycoprotein biosynthesis during the acute-phase response to inflammation. Can J Biochem Cell Biol 61:1041–1048, 1983.

173. Triger DR, Wright R. Immunological aspects of liver disease. In: Wright R, et al. (eds) Liver and Biliary Disease, 2nd ed. WB Saunders, Philadelphia 215–232, 1985.

174. Canalese J, Gove CD, Gimson AES, et al. Reticuloendothelial system and hepatocyte function in fulminant hepatic failure. Gut 23:265–269, 1982.

175. Rimola A, Soto R, Bory F, et al. Reticuloendothelial system phagocytic activity in cirrhosis and its relation to bacterial infections and prognosis. Hepatology 4:53–58, 1984.

176. Ruoslahti E, Salaspuro M, Pihko H, et al. Serum alpha-fetoprotein diagnostic significance in liver disease. Brit Med J 2:527–529, 1974.

177. Nayak SS, Kamath SS, Kundaje GN, et al. Diagnostic significance of estimation of serum apolipoprotein A along with alpha-fetoprotein in alcoholic cirrhosis and hepatocellular carcinoma patients. Clin Chim Acta 173:157–164, 1988.

178. Liaw Y-F, Chen T-J, Chu C-M, et al. Alpha-fetoprotein changes in the course of chronic hepatitis: Relation to bridging hepatic necrosis and hepatocellular carcinoma. Liver 6:133–137, 1986.

179. Madsen AC, Rikkers LF, Moody RR, et al. Alpha-fetoprotein as a marker for hepatic regeneration in the dog. J Surg Res 28:71–76, 1980.

180. Madsen AC, Rikkers LF. Alpha-fetoprotein secretion by injured and regenerating hepatocytes in the dog. J Surg Res 37:402–408, 1984.

181. Hirao K, Matsumura K, Imagawa A, et al. Primary neoplasms in dog liver induced by diethylnitrosamine. Cancer Res 34:1870–1882, 1974.

182. Shinomiya Y, Hirao K, Matsumura K, et al. Alpha-fetoprotein during hepatocarcinogenesis in dogs treated with chemical carcinogens. In: Hirai H, Miyaji T (eds) GANN Monograph on Cancer Research: Alpha-Fetoprotein and Hepatoma. University Park Press, Tokyo, 301–313, 1973.

183. Lowseth LA, Gillett NA, Chang I-Y, et al. Detection of serum alpha-fetoprotein in dogs with hepatic tumors. J Am Vet Med Assoc 199:735–741, 1991.

184. Tavill AS. Protein metabolism and the liver. In: Wright R, Mullward-Sadler GH, Alberti KGMM, et al. (eds) Liver and Biliary Disease. WB Saunders, Philadelphia, 87–117, 1985.

185. Cersosimo E, Williams P, Geer R, et al. Importance of ammonium ions in regulating hepatic glutamine synthesis during fasting. Am J Physiol 257:E514–E519, 1989.

186. Holdsworth CD, Nye L, Kin E: The effect of portacaval anastomosis on oral carbohydrate tolerance and on plasma insulin levels. Gut 13:58–63, 1972.

187. Lickley HLA, Chisholm DJ, Rabinovitch A, et al. Effects of portacaval anastomosis on glucose tolerance in the dog: Evidence of an interaction between the gut and the liver in oral glucose disposal. Metabolism 24:1157–1168, 1975.

188. Waddell WR, Sussman KE. Plasma insulin after diversion of portal and pancreatic venous blood to vena cava. J Appl Physiol 22:808–812, 1967.

189. Strombeck DR, Rogers QR, Stern JS. Effects of ammonia infusion on plasma glucagon, insulin, and amino acids in intact, pancreatectomized, and adrenalectomized dogs. Am J Vet Res 42:810–818, 1981.

190. Kaden M, Harding P, Field JB. Effect of intraduodenal glucose administration on hepatic extraction of insulin in the anesthetized dog. J Clin Invest 52:2016–2028, 1973.

191. Strombeck DR, Harrold D, Rogers QR. Effects of catecholamines and ammonia on plasma and brain amino acids in dogs. Am J Physiol 247:E276–283, 1984.

192. Strombeck DR, Harrold D, Roberts Q, et al. Plasma amino acid, glucagon and insulin concentrations in dogs with nitrosamine-induced hepatic disease. Am J Vet Res 44:2028–2036, 1983.

193. Felig P. Amino acid metabolism in man. Annu Rev Biochem 44:933–955, 1975.

194. Strombeck DR, Rogers Q. Plasma amino acid concentrations in dogs with hepatic disease. J Am Vet Med Assoc 173:93–96, 1978.

195. Aguirre A, Yoshimura N, Westman T, et al. Plasma amino acids in dogs with two experimental forms of liver damage. J Surg Res 16:339–345, 1974.

196. McMenamy RH, Vang J, Drapanas T. Amino acid and alpha-keto acid concentrations in plasma and blood of the liverless dog. Am J Physiol 209:1046–1052, 1965.

197. Rutgers C, Stradley RP, Rogers WA. Plasma amino acid analysis in dogs with experimentally induced hepatocellular and obstructive jaundice. Am J Vet Res 48:696–702, 1987.

198. Rosen HM, Yoshimura N, Hodgman JM, et al. Plasma amino acid patterns in hepatic encephalopathy of differing etiology. Gastroenterology 72:483–487, 1977.

199. Hsia YE. Inherited hyperammonemic syndromes. Gastroenterology 67:347–374, 1974.

200. Flannery DB, Hsia E, Wolf B. Current status of hyperammonemic syndromes. Hepatology 2:495–506, 1982.

201. Nance FC, Kaufman HJ, Kline DG. Role of urea in the hyperammonemia of germ-free Eck fistula dogs. Gastroenterology 66:108–112, 1974.

202. Vince A, Dawson AM, Park N, et al. Ammonia production by intestinal bacteria. Gut 14:171–180, 1973.

203. Aldrete JS. Quantification of the capacity of the liver to remove ammonia from the circulation of dogs with portacaval transposition. Surg Gyncecol Obstet 141:399–404, 1975.

204. Morris JG, Rogers QR. Ammonia intoxication in the near-adult cat as a result of dietary deficiency of arginine. Science 199:431–432, 1978.

205. Windmueller HG, Spaeth A. Uptake and metabolism of plasma glutamine by the small intestines. J Biol Chem 5070–5079, 1974.

206. Zieve L, Doizaki WM, Zieve FJ. Synergism between mercaptans and ammonia or fatty acids in the production of coma: A possible role for mercaptans in the pathogenesis of hepatic coma. J Lab Clin Med 81:16–28, 1974.

207. Derr RF, Zieve L. Effects of fatty acids on the disposition of ammonia. J Pharmacol Exper Ther 197:675–680, 1976.

208. Rabbani P, Prasad AS. Plasma ammonia and liver ornithine transcarbamylase activity in zinc-deficient rats. Am J Physiol 235:E203–E206, 1978.

209. Burch RE, Williams RV, Hahn HKJ, et al. Serum and tissue enzyme activity and trace-element content in response to zinc deficiency in the pig. Clin Chem 21:568–577, 1975.

210. Reding P, Duchateau J, Bataille C. Oral zinc supplementation improves hepatic encephalopathy. Results of a randomized controlled trial. Lancet 2:493–495, 1984.

211. Vallee BL, Falchuk KH. The biochemical basis of zinc physiology. Physiological Rev 73:79–118, 1993.

212. Lockwood AH, McDonald JM, Reiman RE. The dynamics of ammonia metabolism in man. Effects of liver disease and hyperammonemia. J Clin Invest 63:449–460, 1979.

213. Bessman SP, Bradley JE. Uptake of ammonia by muscle. Its implications in ammoniagenic coma. N Engl J Med 253:1143–1147, 1955.

214. Stahl J. Studies of the blood ammonia in liver disease. Its diagnostic, prognostic, and therapeutic significance. Ann Int Med 58:1–24, 1963.

215. Gabuzda GJ, Hall PW. Relation of potassium depletion to renal ammonium metabolism and hepatic coma. Medicine 45:481–490, 1966.

216. Shear L, Gabuzda GJ. Potassium deficiency and endogenous ammonium overload from the kidney. Am J Clin Nutr 23:614–618, 1970.

217. Warren KS, Iber FL, Dolle W, et al. Effect of alterations in blood pH on distribution of ammonia from blood to cerebrospinal fluid in patients in hepatic coma. J Lab Clin Med 56:687–694, 1960.

218. Fraser CL, Arieff AI. Hepatic encephalopathy. N Engl J Med 313:865–873, 1985.

219. Basile AS, Jones EA, Skolnick P. The pathogenesis and treatment of hepatic encephalopathy: Evidence for the involvement of benzodiazepine receptor ligands. Pharm Rev 43:27–71, 1991.

220. Schafer DF, Jones EA. Hepatic encephalopathy. In: Zakim D, Boyer TD (eds) Hepatology, a Textbook of Liver Disease. WB Saunders, Philadelphia, 447–460, 1990.

221. Maddison JE. Hepatic encephalopathy: Current concepts of the pathogenesis. J Vet Int Med 6:341–353, 1992.

222. Butterworth RF, Giguere J-F, Michaud J, et al. Ammonia: The key factor in the pathogenesis of hepatic encephalopathy. Neurochem Pathol 6:1–12, 1987.

223. Schafer DF. Hepatic coma: Studies on the target organ. Gastroenterology 93:1131–1134, 1987.

224. Canzanello VJ, Rasmussen RT, McGoldrick MD. Hyperammonemic encephalopathy during hemodialysis. Ann Intern Med 99:190–191, 1983.

225. Drayna CJ, Titcomb CP, Varma RR, et al. Hyperammonemic encephalopathy caused by infection in a neurogenic bladder. N Engl J Med 304:766–768, 1981.

226. Watson AJ, Chambers T, Karp JE, et al. Transient idiopathic hyperammonemia in adults. Lancet 2:1271–1274, 1985.

227. Sinha B, Gonzalez R. Hyperammonemia in a boy with obstructive ureterocele and *Proteus* infection. J Urol 131:330–331, 1984.

228. Samtoy B, DeBeaukelaer MM. Ammonia encephalopathy secondary to urinary tract infection with *Proteus mirabilis*. Pediatrics 65:294–297, 1980.

229. Hall JA, Allen TA, Fettman MJ. Hyperammonemia associated with urethral obstruction in a dog. J Am Vet Med Assoc 191:1116–1118, 1987.

230. Ehrlich M, Plum F, Duffy TE. Blood and brain ammonia concentration after portacaval anastomosis. Effects of acute ammonia loading. J Neurochem 34:1538–1542, 1980.

231. Sullivan JF, Linder H, Holdener P, et al. Blood ammonia levels in liver disease and hepatic coma. Am J Med 30:893–898, 1961.

232. Phear EA, Sherlock S, Summerskill WHJ. Blood ammonium levels in liver disease and hepatic coma. Lancet 1:836–840, 1955.

233. Phillips GB, Schwartz R, Gabuzda GJ, et al. The syndrome of impending hepatic coma in patients with cirrhosis of the liver given certain nitrogenous substances. N Engl J Med 247:239–246, 1952.

234. Black M. Hepatic detoxification of endogenously produced toxins and their importance for the pathogenesis of hepatic encephalopathy. In: Zakim D, Boyer TD (eds) Hepatology, a Textbook of Liver Disease. WB Saunders, Philadelphia, 397–414, 1982.

235. Fischer JE. On the occurrence of false neurochemical transmitters. In: Williams R, Murray-Lyons IM (eds) Artificial Liver Support. Pitman Medical, Tunbridge Wells, 31–48, 1975.

236. Warren KS, Schenker S. Drugs related to the exacerbation or amelioration of hepatic coma and their effects on ammonia toxicity. Clin Sci 25:11–15, 1963.

237. Schafer K, Ukida M, Steffen C, et al. Effect of ammonia on plasma and cerebrospinal fluid amino acids in dogs with and without portacaval anastomoses. Res Exp Med 185:35–44, 1985.

238. Hamberger A, Jacobsson I, Molin SO, et al. Regulation of glutamate biosynthesis and release by pathophysiological levels of ammonium ions. In: DiChiara G, Gessa G (eds) Glutamate as a Neurotransmitter. Raven Press, New York, 115–126, 1981.

239. Ferenci P, Pappas SC, Munson PJ, et al. Changes in glutamate receptors on synaptic membranes associated with hepatic encephalopathy or hyperammonemia in the rabbit. Hepatology 4:25–29, 1984.

240. Schenker S, Henderson GI, Hoyumpa AM, et al. Hepatic and Wernicke's encephalopathies: Current concepts of pathogenesis. Am J Clin Nutr 33:2719–2726, 1980.

241. Grippon P, Le Poncin-Laffitte M, Faure G, et al. Role of ammonia in the intercerebral transfer and metabolism of tryptophan. In: Kleinberger G, Ferenci P, Riederer P, et al. (eds) Advances in Hepatic Encephalopathy. S. Karger, Basel, 293–300, 1984.

242. Berl S, Takagaki G, Clarke DD, et al. Metabolic compartments in vivo: ammonia and glutamic acid metabolism in brain and liver. J Biol Chem 237:2563–2569, 1962.

243. Rossle M, Luft M, Herz R, et al. Amino acid, ammonia and neurotransmitter concentrations in hepatic encephalopathy: Serial analysis in plasma and cerebrospinal fluid during treatment with an adapted amino acid solution. Klin Wochenschr 62:867–875, 1984.

244. Oei LT, Kuys J, Lombarts AJ, et al. Cerebrospinal fluid glutamine levels and EEG findings in patients with hepatic encephalopathy. Clin Neurol Neurosurg 81:59–63, 1979.

245. Hourani BT, Hamlin EM, Reynolds TB. Cerebrospinal fluid glutamine as

a measure of hepatic encephalopathy. Arch Intern Med 127:1033–1036, 1971.

246. Vergara J, Plum F, Duffy TE. alpha-Ketoglutaramate: Increased concentrations in the cerebrospinal fluid of patients with hepatic coma. Science 183:81–83, 1974.

247. Watanabe A, Takei N, Higashi T, et al. Glutamic acid and glutamine levels in serum and cerebrospinal fluid in hepatic encephalopathy. Biochem Med 32:225–231, 1984.

248. Zieve L. The mechanism of hepatic coma. Hepatology 1:360–365, 1981.

249. Duffy TE, Plum F. Hepatic encephalopathy. In: Arias I, Popper H, Schachter D, et al. (eds) The Liver: Biology and Pathobiology. Raven Press, New York, 693–715, 1982.

250. Johnson GAR, Allan RD, Skerritt JH. GABA receptors. In: Lajtha A (ed) Handbook of Neurochemistry, Vol. 6. Plenum, New York, 213–237, 1984.

251. Collingridge GL, Lester RAJ. Excitatory amino acid receptors in the vertebrate central nervous system. Pharmacol Rev 40:143–209, 1989.

252. Schafer DF, Waggoner JC, Jones EA. Sera from rabbits in acute hepatic coma inhibit the binding of [³H] GABA in neural membranes. Gastroenterology 78:1320, 1980.

253. Thompson JS, Schafer DF, Schafer GJ, et al. gamma- aminobutyric acid plasma levels and brain GABA binding in Eck fistula dogs. J Surg Res 38:143–148, 1985.

254. Maddison JE, Dodd PR, Johnston GAR, et al. Brain gamma-amino butyric acid receptor binding is normal in rats with thioacetamide-induced hepatic encephalopathy despite elevated plasma gamma-aminobutyric acid like activity. Gastroenterology 93:1062–1068, 1987.

255. Maddison JE, Dodd PR, Morrison M, et al. Plasma GABA, GABA-like activity and the brain GABA-benzodiazepine complex in rats with chronic hepatic encephalopathy. Hepatology 7:621–628, 1987.

256. Maddison JE, Dodd PR, Morrison M, et al. Plasma GABA concentrations and cerebro-cortical GABA receptor binding and function in dogs with congenital portosystemic encephalopathy. In: Soeters PB, Wilson JHP, Meijer AJ, et al. (eds) Advances in Ammonia Metabolism and Hepatic Encephalopathy. Excerpta Medica, Amsterdam, 265–274, 1988.

257. Maddison JE, Yau D, Stewart P, et al. Cerebrospinal fluid gamma-aminobutyric acid levels in dogs with chronic portosystemic encephalopathy. Clin Sci 71:749–753, 1986.

258. Borg J, Warter JM, Schlienger JL, et al. Neurotransmitter modifications in human cerebrospinal fluid and serum during hepatic encephalopathy. J Neurol Sci 57:343–356, 1982.

259. Ferenci P, Schafer DF, Kleinberger G, et al. Serum levels of GABA-like activity in acute and chronic hepatocellular disease. Lancet ii:811–814, 1983.

260. Minuk GU, Winder A, Burgess ED, et al. Serum GABA levels in patients with hepatic encephalopathy. Hepatogastroenterology 32:171–174, 1985.

261. Levy LJ, Losowsky MS. Plasma GABA concentrations provide evidence of different mechanisms in the pathogenesis of hepatic encephalopathy in acute and chronic liver disease. Hepatogastroenterology 36:494–498, 1989.

262. Losher W, Kretz F-J, Tung C, et al. Reduction of highly elevated plasma levels of gamma-aminobutyric acid does not reverse hepatic coma. Hepatogastroenterology 36:504–505, 1989.

263. Baraldi M, Zeneroli ML. Experimental hepatic encephalopathy: Changes in the binding of gamma-aminobutyric acid. Science 216:427–429, 1982.

264. Schafer DF, Fowler JM, Munson PJ, et al. gamma-aminobutyric acid and benzodiazepine receptors in an animal model of fulminant hepatic failure. J Lab Clin Med 102:870–880, 1983.

265. Basile AS, Gammal SH, Jones EA, et al. GABAalpha receptor complex in an experimental model of hepatic encephalopathy: Evidence for elevated levels of an endogenous benzodiazepine receptor ligand. J Neurochem 53:1057–1063, 1989.

266. Basile AS, Ostrowski NL, Gammal SH, et al. The GABAalpha receptor complex in hepatic encephalopathy: Autoradiographic evidence for the presence of elevated levels of a benzodiazepine receptor ligand. Neuropsychopharmacology 3:61–71, 1990.

267. Roy S, Pomier-Layrargues G, Butterworth RF, et al. Hepatic encephalopathy in cirrhotic and portacaval shunted dogs: Lack of changes in brain GABA uptake, brain GABA levels, brain glutamic acid decarboxylase activity and brain postsynaptic GABA receptors. Hepatology 4:845–849, 1988.

268. Watanabe A, Fujiwara M, Shiota R, et al. Amino acid neurotransmitters and their receptors in the brain synaptosomes of acute hepatic failure rats. Biochem Med Metab Biol 40:247–252, 1988.

269. Zanchin G, Maggioni F, Salassa D, et al. GABA and dopamine receptors after chronic porta-caval shunt in the rat. In: Kleinberger G, Ferenci P, Riederer P, et al. (eds) Advances in Hepatic Encephalopathy and Urea Cycle Disorders. Karger, Basel, 360–367, 1984.

270. Ferenci P, Zieve L, Ebner J, et al. Postsynaptic gamma-aminobutyric acid receptors in hepatic coma following portacaval shunt and hepatic artery ligation in the rat. Metab Brain Dis 2:195–200, 1987.

271. Lal S, Quirion R, Lafaille F, et al. Muscarinic benzodiazepine, GABA, chloride channel and other binding sites in frontal cortex in hepatic coma in man. Prog Neuro-Psychopharmacol Biol Psychiatr 11:243–250, 1987.

272. Butterworth RF, Lavoie J, Giguere J-F, et al. Affinities and densities of high affinity [³H]muscimol (GABA-A) binding sites and of central benzodiazepine receptors are unchanged in autopsied brain tissue from cirrhotic patients with hepatic encephalopathy. Hepatology 8:1084–1088, 1988.

273. Rossle M, Deckert J, Jones EA. Autoradiographic analysis of GABA benzodiazepine receptors in an animal model of acute hepatic encephalopathy. Hepatology 10:143–147, 1989.

274. Zimmermann C, Ferenci P, Pifl C, et al. Hepatic encephalopathy in thioacetamide-induced acute liver failure in rats: Characterization of an improved model and study of amino-acidergic neurotransmission. Hepatology 9:594–601, 1989.

275. Rossle M, Deckert J, Mullen KD, et al. Autoradiography determination of the GABA(A) receptor density in the brain of rats with portacaval shunt. Z Gastroenterol 28:142–146, 1990.

276. Maddison JE, Leong DK, Dodd PR, et al. Plasma GABA-like activity in rats with hepatic encephalopathy is due to GABA and taurine. Hepatology 11:105–110, 1990.

277. Schafer DF, Fowler JM, Jones FA. Colonic bacteria: A source of gamma-amino-butyric acid in blood. Proc Soc Exp Biol Med 167:301–302, 1981.

278. Mullen KD, Szauter KM, Kaminsky-Russ K. "Endogenous" benzodiazepine activity in body fluids of patients with hepatic encephalopathy. Lancet 336:81–83, 1990.

279. Butterworth RF, Pomier Layrargues G. Benzodiazepine receptors and hepatic encephalopathy. Hepatology 11:499–501, 1990.

280. Baraldi M, Zeneroli M, Ventura E, et al. Supersensitivity of benzodiazepine receptors in hepatic encephalopathy due to fulminant hepatic failure in the rat: Reversal by a benzodiazepine antagonist. Clin Sci 67:167–175, 1984.

281. Bansky G, Meier PJ, Ziegler WH, et al. Reversal of hepatic coma by benzodiazepine antagonist (Ro 15–1788). Lancet 2:1325, 1985.

282. Scollo-Lavizzari G, Steinmann E. Reversal of hepatic coma by benzodiazepine antagonist (R0 15 1788). Lancet 2:1324–2325, 1985.

283. Bassett ML, Mullen KD, Skolnick P, et al. Amelioration of hepatic encephalopathy by pharmacologic antagonism of the GABAalpha benzodiazepine receptor complex in a rabbit model of fulminant hepatic failure. Gastroenterology 93:1069–1077, 1987.

284. Grimm G, Ferenci P, Katzenschlager R, et al. Improvement of hepatic encephalopathy treated with flumazenil. Lancet 2:1392–1394, 1988.

285. Bansky G, Meier P, Riederer E, et al. Effects of the benzodiazepine receptor antagonist flumazenil in hepatic encephalopathy in humans. Gastroenterology 97:744–750, 1989.

286. Ferenci P, Grimm G, Meryn S, et al. Successful long-term treatment of portal-systemic encephalopathy by the benzodiazepine antagonist flumazenil. Gastroenterology 96:240–243, 1989.

287. Gammal SH, Basile AS, Geller D, et al. Reversal of the behavioral and electrophysiological abnormalities of an animal model of hepatic encephalopathy by benzodiazepine receptor ligands. Hepatalogy 11:371–378, 1990.

288. Zieve L, Ferenci P, Rzepcznski D, et al. A benzodiazepine antagonist does not alter the course of hepatic encephalopathy or neural GABA binding. Metab Brain Dis 2:201–205, 1987.

289. Sutherland LR, Minuk RY. RO 15 1788 and hepatic failure. Ann Intern Med 108:158, 1988.

290. Van der Rijt CCD, Schaln SW, Meulstee J, et al. Flumazenil therapy for hepatic encephalopathy: A double blind cross-over study. Hepatology 10:590, 1989.

291. Balazs R, Machiyama Y, Patel AJ. Compartmentation and the metabolism of gamma-aminobutyrate. In: Balazs R, Cremer JE (eds) Metabolic Compartmentation in the Brain. Macmillan, London, 57–70, 1973.

292. Hamberger A, Nystrom B. Extra- and intra-cellular amino acids in the hippocampus during the development of hepatic encephalopathy. Neurochem Res 9–11:1181–1192, 1984.

293. Moroni F, Lombardi G, Moneti G, et al. The release and synthesis of glutamic acid are increased in experimental models of hepatic encephalopathy. J Neurochem 40:850–854, 1983.

294. Butterworth RF, Lavoie J, Peterson C, et al. Excitatory amino acids and hepatic encephalopathy. In: Butterworth RF, Pomier Layrargues G (eds) Hepatic Encephalopathy: Pathophysiology and Treatment. Humana Press, Clifton, NJ, 417–433, 1989.

295. Wu C, Bollman JL, Butt HR. Changes in free amino acids in the plasma during hepatic coma. J Clin Invest 34:845–849, 1955.

296. Cascino A, Cangiano C, Calcaterra V, et al. Plasma amino acids imbalance in patients with liver disease. Digest Dis 23:591–598, 1978.

297. Fischer JE, Rosen HM, Ebeid AM, et al. The effect of normalization of plasma amino acids on hepatic encephalopathy in man. Surgery 10:463–476, 1974.

298. Fischer JE, Funovics JM, Aquirre A, et al. The role of plasma amino acids in hepatic encephalopathy. Surgery 78:276–290, 1975.

299. Iob V, Mattson WJ, Sloan M, et al. Alterations in plasma-free amino acids in dogs with hepatic insufficiency. Surg Gyn Obstet 794–799, 1970.

300. Rosen HM, Yoshimura N, Hodman JM, et al. Plasma amino patterns in hepatic encephalopathy of differing etiology. Gastroenterology 72:483–487, 1977.

301. Maddison JE. Canine congenital portosystemic encephalopathy. Aust Vet J 65:245–249, 1988.

302. Fischer JE. Amino acids in hepatic coma. Dig Dis Sci 27:97–102, 1982.

303. Cascino A, Cangiano C, Fiaccadori F, et al. Plasma and cerebrospinal fluid amino acid patterns in hepatic encephalopathy. Dig Dis Sci 27:828–832, 1982.

304. James JH, Escourrou J, Fischer JE. Blood-brain neutral amino acid transport activity is increased after portacaval anastomosis. Science 200:1395–1397, 1978.

305. Zieve I, Olsen RI. Can hepatic coma be caused by a reduction of brain noradrenaline or dopamine. Gut 18:688–691, 1977.

306. Simert G, Nobin A, Rosengren E, et al. Neurotransmitter changes in the rat brain after portacaval anastomosis. Eur Surg Res 10:73–85, 1978.

307. Curzon G, Kantamanesi BD, Fernando JC, et al. Effects of chronic portacaval anastomosis on brain tryptophan, tyrosine and 5-hydroxytryptamine. J Neurochem 24:1065–1070, 1975.

308. Cummings MG, Soeters PB, James JH, et al. Regional brain indoleamine metabolism following chronic portacaval anstomosis in the rat. J Neurochem 27:501–509, 1976.

309. Bergeron M, Swain M, Reader TA, et al. Effect of ammonia on brain serotonin metabolism in relation to function in the portacaval shunted rat. J Neurochem 55:222–229, 1990.

310. Bengtsson F, Bugge M, Hohansen KH, et al. Brain tryptophan hydroxylation in the portacaval shunted rat: A hypothesis for the regulation of serotonin turnover *in vivo*. J Neurochem 56:1069–1074, 1991.

311. Bergeron M, Reader T, Pomier Layrargues, et al. Monoamines and metabolites in autopsied brain tissue from cirrhotic patients with hepatic encephalopathy. Neurochem Res 14:853–859, 1989.

312. Knell AJ, Davidson AR, Williams R, et al. Dopamine and serotonin metabolism in hepatic encephalopathy. Br Med J 1:549–551, 1974.

313. Kamata S, Okada A, Watanabe T, et al. Effects of dietary amino acids on brain amino acids and transmitter amines in rats with portacaval shunt. J Neurochem 35:1190–1196, 1980.

314. Rzepcznyski D, Zieve L, Lindblad S. Inhibitory neuromodulators do not alter the course of experimental hepatic encephalopathy. Metab Brain Dis 3:211–216, 1988.

315. Fischer JE, Baldessarini RJ. Pathogenesis and therapy of hepatic coma. In: Popper H, Shaffner F (eds) Progress in Liver Disease. Grune & Stratton, New York, 363–397, 1975.

316. Zieve L, Olsen RL. Can hepatic coma be caused by a reduction of brain noradrenaline or dopamine? Gut 18:688–691, 1977.

317. Moroni F, Lombardi G, Carla V, et al. Content of quinolinic acid and of other tryptophan metabolites increases in brain regions of rats used as experimental models of hepatic encephalopathy. J Neurochem 46:869–874, 1986.

318. Hirayama C. Tryptophan metabolism in liver disease. Clin Chim Acta 32:191–197, 1971.

319. Smith B, Prockop DJ. Central-nervous-system effects of ingestion of l-tryptophan by normal subjects. N Engl J Med 267:1338–1341, 1962.

320. Rossi-Fanelli F, Freund H, Krause R, et al. Induction of coma in normal dogs by the infusion of aromatic amino acids and its prevention by the addition of branched chain amino acids. Gastroenterology 83:664–671, 1982.

321. Rigotti P, Jonung T, James JH, et al. Infusion of branched-chain amino acids and ammonium salts in rats with portacaval shunts. Arch Surg 120:1290–1295, 1985.

322. Bombardieri G, Gigli GL, Bernadi L, et al. Visual evoked potential recordings in hepatic encephalopathy and their variations during branched chain amino acid treatment. Hepatogastroenterology 32:3–7, 1985.

323. Horst D, Grace ND, Conn HO, et al. Comparison of dietary protein with an oral branched-chain-enriched amino acid supplement in chronic portal-systemic encephalopathy: A randomized controlled trial. Hepatology 4:279–287, 1984.

324. Michel H, Bories P, Aubin JP, et al. Treatment of acute hepatic encephalopathy in cirrhotics with a branched-chain amino acids enriched versus a conventional amino acids mixture. Liver 5:282–289, 1985.

325. Warren J, Denis J, Desurmont P, et al. Is intravenous administration of branched chain amino acids effective in the treatment of hepatic encephalopathy: A multicenter study. Hepatology 314:475–480, 1983.

326. Naylor CD, O'Rourke K, Detsky AS, et al. Parenteral nutrition with branched-chain amino acids in hepatic encephalopathy: A meta-analysis. Gastroenterology 97:1033–1042, 1989.

327. Eriksson LS, Conn HO. Branched-chain amino acids in the management of hepatic encephalopathy: An analysis of variants. Hepatology 10:228–246, 1989.

328. Morgan MY, Milson JP, Sherlock S. Plasma ratio of valine, leucine, and isoleucine to phenylalanine and tyrosine in liver disease. Gut 19:1068–1073, 1978.

329. James JH, Ziparo V, Jepson B, et al. Hyperammonemia, plasma amino acid imbalance and blood-brain amino acid transport: A unified theory of portal-systemic encephalopathy. Lancet 2:772–775, 1979.

330. Mans AM, Biebuyck JF, Hawkins RA. Ammonia selectively stimulates neutral amino acid transport across blood-brain barrier. Am J Physiol 245:c74-c77, 1983.

331. Fisher JE. On the occurrence of false neurochemical transmitters. In: Williams R, Murray-Lyons IM (eds) Artificial Liver Support. Pitman Medical, Tunbridge Wells, 31–48, 1975.

332. Fischer JE, Baldessarini RJ. False neurotransmitters and hepatic failure. Lancet 2:75–79, 1971.

333. Smith AR, Rossi-Fanelli F, Ziparo V, et al. Alterations in plasma and CSF amino acids, amines and metabolites in hepatic coma. Ann Surg 187:343–350, 1978.

334. Meredith CG, Wade DN. A model of portal systemic shunting in the rat. Clin Exp Pharmacol Physiol 8:651, 1981.

335. Hilgier W, Zitting A, Albrecht J. The brain octopamine and phenylethanolamine content in rats in thioacetamide-induced hepatogenic encephalopathy. Acta Neurol Scand 71:195–198, 1985.

336. Phear EA, Ruebner B, Sherlock S, et al. Methionine toxicity in liver disease and its prevention by chlortetracycline. Clin Sci 15:93–117, 1956.

337. Zieve L, Lyffogt C, Draves K. Toxicity of a fatty acid and ammonia: Interactions with hypoglycemia and Krebs cycle inhibition. J Lab Clin Med 101:930–939, 1983.

338. Blom HJ, Chamuleau RA, Rothuizen J, et al. Methanethiol metabolism and its role in the pathogenesis of hepatic encephalopathy in rats and dogs. Hepatology 11:682–689, 1990.

339. Al Mardini H, Bartlett K, Record CO. Blood and brain concentrations of mercaptans in hepatic and methanethiol induced coma. Gut 25:284–290, 1984.

340. Al Mardini H, Leonard J, Bartlett K, et al. Effect of methionine loading and endogenous hypermethionianemia on blood mercaptans in man. Clin Chim Acta 176:83–90, 1988.

341. McClain CJ, Zieve L, Doizaki WM, et al. Blood methanethiol in alcoholic liver disease with and without hepatic encephalopathy. Gut 21:318–323, 1980.

342. Lai JC, Silk DBA, Williams R. Plasma short chain fatty acids in fulminant hepatic failure. Clin Chim Acta 78:305–310, 1977.

343. Misra P. Hepatic encephalopathy. Med Clin N Am 65:209–226, 1981.

344. Black M. Hepatic detoxification of endogenously produced toxins and their importance for the pathogenesis of hepatic encephalopathy. In: Zakim D, Boyer TD (eds) Hepatology, a Textbook of Liver Disease. WB Saunders, Philadelphia, 397–414, 1982.

345. Crossley IR, Wardle EN, Williams R. Biochemical mechanisms of hepatic encephalopathy. Clin Sci 64:247–252, 1983.

346. Hoyumpa AM, Schenker S. Perspectives in hepatic encephalopathy. J Lab Clin Med 100:477–487, 1982.

347. Goldstein GW. The role of brain capillaries in the pathogenesis of hepatic encephalopathy. Hepatology 4:565–567, 1984.

348. Livingstone AS, Potvin M, Goresky CA, et al. Changes in the blood brain barrier in hepatic coma after hepatectomy in the rat. Gastroenterology 73:697–704, 1977.

349. Potvin M, Finlayson MH, Hinchey EJ, et al. Cerebral abnormalities in hepatectomized rats with acute hepatic coma. Lab Invest 50:560–564, 1984.

350. Laursen H, Westergaard E. Enhanced permeability to horse-radish peroxidase across cerebral vessels in the rat after portocaval anastomosis. Neuropathol Appl Neurobiol 3:29–43, 1977.

351. Zaki AEO, Silk DBA, Williams R. Increases in blood brain permeability after portacaval anastomosis. Gut 21:A900, 1980.

352. Zaki AEO, Ede RJ, Davis M, et al. Experimental studies of blood brain barrier permeability in acute hepatic failure. Hepatology 4:359–363, 1984.

353. Traber PG, Dal Canto M, Ganger DR, et al. Electron microscopic evaluation of brain edema in rabbits with galactosamine-induced fulminant hepatic failure: Ultrastructure and integrity of the blood-brain-barrier. Hepatology 7:1272–1277, 1987.

354. Butterworth RF, Girard G, Giguere J-F. Regional differences in the capacity for ammonia removal by brain following portocaval anastomosis. J Neurochem 51:486–490, 1988.

355. Horowitz ME, Schafer DF, Molnar P, et al. Increased blood-brain transfer in a rabbit model of acute liver failure. Gastroenterology 84:1003–1011, 1983.

356. Spigelman MK, Zappulla RA: Pathogenesis of hepatic encephalopathy. Gastroenterology 86:778–783, 1984.

357. Spigelman MK, Zappulla RA, Malis LI, et al. Intracarotid dehydrocholate infusion: a new method for prolonged reversible blood-brain barrier disruption. Neurosurgery 12:606–612, 1983.

358. Norenberg MD, Lapham LW. The astrocyte response in experimental portal-systemic encephalopathy: An electron microscopic study. J Neuropath Exp Neurol 33:422, 1974.

359. Norenberg MD. Astrocytes in hepatic encphalopathy. Adv Exp Med Biol 272:81–97, 1990.

360. Rothuizen J, Van den Ingh TS, Voorhout G, et al. Congenital porto-sys-

temic shunts in sixteen dogs and three cats. J Sm Anim Pract 23:67–81, 1982.

361. Conn HO. Cirrhosis: In: Schiff L, Schiff ER (eds) Diseases of the Liver. JB Lippincott, Philadelphia, 725–864, 1987.

362. Jones EA, Gammal SH. Hepatic encephalopathy. In: Arias IM, Jakoby WB, Popper H, et al. (eds) The Liver: Biology and Pathobiology, 2nd ed. Raven Press, New York, 985–1005, 1988.

363. Hooper PT. Spongy degeneration in the central nervous system. III: Occurrence and pathogenesis—hepatocerebral disease caused by hyperammonaemia. Acta Neuropathol 31:343–351, 1975.

364. Cavanagh JB, Lewis PD, Blakemore WR, et al. Changes in the cerebellar cortex in rats after portacaval anastomosis. J Neurosci 15:13–26, 1972.

365. Bradbury M. The concept of the blood-brain barrier. John Wiley, New York, 1979.

366. Ede RJ, Williams R. Hepatic encephalopathy and cerebral edema. Sem Liver Dis 6:107–118, 1986.

367. Condon RE. Effect of dietary protein on symptoms and survival in dogs with an Eck fistula. Am J Surg 121:107–114, 1971.

368. Dauterberg B, Sautter V, Herz R, et al. The defect of uric acid metabolism in Eck fistula rats. J Lab Clin Med 90:91–100, 1977.

369. Sorenson JL, Ling GV. Metabolic and genetic aspects of urate urolithiasis in Dalmations. J Am Vet Med Assoc 203:857–862, 1993.

370. Giesecke D, Tiemeyer W. Defect of uric acid uptake in Dalmatian dog liver. Experientia 40:1415–1416, 1984.

371. Vinay P, Gattereau A, Moulin B, et al. Normal urate tranport into erythrocytes in familial renal hyperuricemia and in the Dalmatian dog. Can Med Assoc J 128:545–549, 1983.

372. Kuster G, Shorter RG, Dawson B, et al. Uric acid metabolism in Dalmatians and other dogs. Arch Intern Med 129:492–496, 1972.

373. Duncan H, Wakim KG, Ward LE. The effects of intravenous administration of uric acid on its concentration in plasma and urine of Dalmatian and non-Dalmatian dogs. J Lab Clin Med 58:876–883, 1961.

374. Briggs OM, Harley EH. The fate of administered purines in the Dalmatian coach hound. J Comp Pathol 96:267–276, 1986.

375. Friedman M, Byers SO. Observations concerning the causes of the excess excretion of uric acid in the Dalmatian dog. J Biol Chem 175:727–735, 1948.

376. Briggs OM, Harley EH. Serum urate concetrations in the Dalmatian coach hound. J Comp Pathol 95:301–304, 1985.

377. Byers SO, Friedman M. Rate of entrance of urate and allantoin into the cerebrospinal fluid of the Dalmatian and non-Dalmatian dog. Am J Physiol 157:394–400, 1949.

378. Duncan H, Curtiss AS. Observations on uric acid transport in man, the Dalmatian and non-Dalmatian dog. Henry Ford Hosp Med J 19:105–115, 1971.

379. Folin O, Berglund H, Derick C. The uric acid problem. J Biol Chem 60:361–471, 1924.

380. Wooliscroft JO, Colfer H, Fox IH. Hyperuricemia in acute illness: A poor prognostic sign. Am J Med 72:58–62, 1982.

381. Fox IH, Palella TD, Kelley WN. Hyperuricemia: A marker for cell energy crises. N Engl J Med 317:111–112, 1987.

382. Page RL, Leifer CE, Matus RE. Uric acid and phosphorus excretion in dogs with lymphosarcoma. Am J Vet Res 47:910–912, 1986.

383. Laing EJ, Carter RF. Acute tumor lysis syndrome following treatment of canine lymphoma. J Am Anim Hosp Assoc 24:691–696, 1988.

384. Hoe CM, Harvey DG. An investigation into liver function tests in dogs. II. Tests other than transaminase estimation. J Sm Anim Pract 21:109–127, 1961.

385. Morgan HC. A comparison of uric acid determinations and sulfobromphthalein retention tests as an index to canine liver dysfunction. Am J Vet Res 20:372–377, 1959.

386. Sorenson JL, Ling GV. Diagnosis, prevention, and treatment of urate urolithiasis in Dalmatians. J Am Vet Med Assoc 203:863–869, 1993.

387. Deutsh E. Blood coagulation changes in liver diseases. In: Popper H, Schaffner F (eds) Progress in Liver Diseases, Vol. II. Grune & Stratton, New York, 69–83, 1965.

388. Roberts HR, Cederbaum AI. The liver and blood coagulation: Physiology and pathology. Gastroenterology 63:297–320, 1972.

389. Walls WD, Losowsky MS. The hemostatic defect of liver disease. Gastroenterology 60:108–119, 1971.

390. Steinberg SE, Hillman RS. The liver and hematopoiesis. In: Zakim D, Boyer TD (eds) Hepatology, a Textbook of Liver Disease. WB Saunders, Philadelphia, 537–545, 1982.

391. Kelly DA, Summerfield JA. Hemostasis in liver disease. Sem Liver Dis 7:182–191, 1987.

392. Friedman PA. Vitamin K-dependent proteins. N Engl J Med 310:1458–1460, 1984.

393. Blanchard RA, Furie BC, Jorgensen M, et al. Acquired vitamin K-dependent carboxylation deficiency in liver disease. N Engl J Med 305:242–248, 1981.

394. Hemker HC, Muller AD. Kinetic aspects of the interaction of blood clotting enzymes. VI. Localization of the site of blood-coagulation inhibition by the protein induced by vitamin K absence (PIVKA). Throm Diath Haemorrh 20:78–87, 1968.

395. Gaudernack G, Prydz H. Studies on PIVKA-X. Thromb Diath Haemorrh 34:455–464, 1975.

396. Mount ME. Proteins induced by Vitamin K absence or antagonists (PIVKA). In: Kirk RW (ed) Current Veterinary Therapy IX. WB Saunders, Philadelphia, 513–515, 1986.

397. Koller F. Die blutgerinnung und ihre klinische bedeutung- Deutsch Med Wochnschr 80:516–534, 1956.

398. Koller F. Theory and experience behind use of coagulation tests in diagnosis and prognosis of liver disease. Scand J Gastroenterol 8(suppl 19):51–61, 1973.

399. Hollander D, Rim E, Muralidhara KS. Vitamin K_1 intestinal absorption in vivo: Influence of luminal contents on transport. Am J Physiol 232:E69-E74, 1977.

400. Ramotar K, Conly JM, Chubb H, et al. Production of menaquinones by intestinal anaerobes. J Infect Dis 150:213–218, 1984.

401. Gustafson BE, Daft FS, McDaniel EG, et al. Effects of vitamin K-active compounds and intestinal microorganisms in vitamin K-deficient germ-free rats. J Nutr 78:461–468, 1962.

402. Conly JM, Ramotar K, Chubb H, et al. Hypoprothrombinemia in febrile, neutropenic patients with cancer: Association with antimicrobial suppression of intestinal microflora. J Infect Dis 150:202–212, 1984.

403. Pineo GF, Gallus AS, Hirsh J. Unexpected vitamin K deficiency in hospitalized patients. Can Med Assoc J 109:880–883, 1973.

404. Sattler FR, Weitekamp MR, Ballard JO. Potential for bleeding with the new beta-lactam antibiotics. Ann Intern Med 105:924–931, 1986.

405. Barza M, Furie B, Brown AE, et al. Defects in vitamin K-dependent carboxylation associated with moxalactam treatment. J Infect Dis 153:1166–1169, 1986.

406. Baxter JG, Margle DA, Whitfield LR, et al. Clinical risk factors for prolonged PT/PTT in abdominal sepsis patients treated with moxalactam or tobramycin plus clindamycin. Ann Surg 210:96–102, 1985.

407. Fainstein V, Bodey GP, McCredie KB, et al. Coagulation abnormalities induced by beta-lactam antibiotics in cancer patients. J Infect Dis 148:745–750, 1983.

408. Neer TM, Savant RL. Hypoprothrombinemia secondary to administration of sulfaquinoxaline to dogs in a kennel setting. J Am Vet Med Assoc 200:1344–1345, 1992.

409. Patterson JM, Grenn HH. Hemorrhage and death in dogs following the administration of sulfaquinoxaline. Can Vet J 16:265–268, 1975.

410. Osweiler GD, Green RA. Canine hypoprothrombinemia resulting from sulfaquinoxaline administration. Vet Hem Toxicol 20:190–192, 1978.

411. Preusch PC, Hazelett SE, Lemasters KK. Sulfaquinoxaline inhibition of vitamin K epoxide and quinone reductase. Arch Biochem Biophys 269:18–24, 1989.

412. Suttie JW. Recent advances in hepatic vitamin K metabolism and function. Hepatology 7:367–376, 1987.

413. Seeler AI, Muskett CW, Graessle O, et al. Pharmacological studies on sulfaquinoxaline. J Pharmacol Exp Ther 82:357–363, 1944.

414. Fiore L, Levine J, Deykin D. Alterations of hemostasis in patients with liver disease. In: Zakim D, Boyer TD (eds) Hepatology, a Textbook of Liver Disease. WB Saunders, Philadelphia, 546–571, 1990.

415. High KA. Antithrombin III, protein C, and protein S. Arch Pathol Lab Med 112:28–36, 1988.

416. Green RA. Pathophysiology of antithrombin III deficiency. Vet Clin N Am 18:95–104, 1988.

417. Williams WJ. Control of coagulation reactions. In: Williams WJ, Beutler E, Ersley AJ, et al. (eds) Hematology, 3rd ed. McGraw-Hill, New York, 1247–1257, 1983.

418. Rodzynek JJ, Urbain D, Leautaud P, et al. Antithrombin III, plasminogen and $alpha_2$ antiplasmin in jaundice. Clinical usefulness and prognostic significance. Gut 25:1050–1056, 1984.

419. Knot E, Cate JW, Drijfhout HR, et al. Antithrombin III metabolism in patients with liver disease. J Clin Pathol 37:523–530, 1984.

420. Boneu B, Sie P, Caranoge C, et al. Progressive antithrombin activity and the concentration of three inhibitors in liver cirrhosis. Thromb Haem 47:78, 1982.

421. Rodzynek JJR, Preux C, Leautaud P, et al. Diagnostic value of antithrombin III and aminopyrine breath test in liver disease. Arch Intern Med 146:677–680, 1986.

422. Leone G, De Stefano V, Garufi C, et al. Antithrombin III in patients with hepatocellular carcinoma. Throm Haem 58:1093, 1987.

423. Boothe DM, Jenkins WL, Green RA, et al. Dimethylnitrosamine-induced hepatotoxicosis in dogs as a model of progressive canine hepatic disease. Am J Vet Res 53:411–420, 1992.

424. Biggs R, Denson KW, Akwan N, et al. Antithrombin III, antifactor Xalpha and heparin. Brit J Haematol 19:283–305, 1970.

425. Feldman BF, Madewell BR, ONeill S. Disseminated intravascular coagulation: Antithrombin, plasminogen, and coagulation abnormalities in 41 dogs. J Am Vet Med Assoc 179:151–154, 1981.

426. Raymond SL, Dodds WJ. Plasma antithrombin activity: A comparative study in normal and diseased animals. Proc Soc Exp Biol Med 161:464–467, 1979.

427. Mannucci L, Dioguardi N, Del Ninno E, et al. Value of Normotest and antithrombin III in the assessment of liver function. Scand J Gastroenterol 8(suppl 19):103–107, 1973.

428. Duckert F. Behaviour of antithrombin III in liver disease. Scand J Gastroenterol 8(suppl 19):109–112, 1973.

429. Violi F, Ferro D, Basili S, et al. Hyperfibrinolysis increases the risk of gastrointestinal hemorrhage in patients with advanced cirrhosis. Hepatology 15:672–676, 1992.

430. Lowe GDO, Prentice CRM. The laboratory investigation of fibrinolysis. In: Thomson JM (ed) Blood Coagulation and Haemostasis. A Practical Guide. Churchill Livingstone, New York, 222–278, 1980.

431. Ewe K. Bleeding after liver biopsy does not correlate with indices of peripheral coagulation. Dig Dis Sci 26:388–393, 1981.

432. Picinino F, Sagnelli E, Pasquale G, et al. Complications following percutaneous liver biopsy. A multicentre retrospective study on 68,276 biopsies. J Hepatol 2:165–173, 1986.

433. Spector I, Corn M. Laboratory tests of hemostasis: The relation to hemorrhage in liver disease. Arch Intern Med 119:577–582, 1967.

434. Osbaldiston GW, Hoffman MW. Coagulation defects in experimental hepatic injury in the dog. Can J Comp Med 35:129–135, 1971.

435. Badylak SF, Dodds WJ, Van Vleet JF. Plasma coagulation factor abnormalities in dogs with naturally occurring hepatic disease. Am J Vet Res 44:2336–2340, 1983.

436. Schenk WG, Fopeano J, Cosgriff JH, et al. The coagulation defect after hepatectomy. Surgery 42:822–826, 1957.

437. Strombeck DR, Feldman E. Unpublished information, 19??.

438. Furnival CM, Mackenzie RJ, MacDonald GA, et al. The mechanism of impaired coagulation after partial hepatectomy in the dog. Surg Gynecol Obstet 81–86, 1976.

439. Badylak SF, Van Vleet JF. Alterations of prothrombin time and activated partial thromboplastin time in dogs with hepatic disease. Am J Vet Res 42:2053–2056, 1981.

440. Wigton DH, Hoover EA. Infectious canine hepatitis: Animal model of viral-induced disseminated intravascular coagulation. Blood 47:287–296, 1976.

441. Green RA. Clinical implications of antithrombin III deficiency in animal diseases. Comp Cont Ed 5:537–545, 1984.

442. Weiss RC, Dodds WJ, Scott FW. Disseminated intravascular coagulation in experimentally induced feline infectious peritonitis. Am J Vet Res 41:663–671, 1980.

443. Carr JM. Disseminated intravascular coagulation in cirrhosis. Hepatology 10:103–110, 1989.

444. Rake MO, Flute PT, Pannell G, et al. Intravascular coagulation in acute hepatic necrosis. Lancet 1:533–537, 1970.

445. Aledort LM. Blood clotting abnormalities in liver disease. In: Popper H, Schaffner F (eds) Progress in Liver Diseases, Vol. II. Grune & Stratton, New York, 350–362, 1976.

446. Murray M, Robinson PB, McKeating FJ, et al. Peptic ulceration in the dog: A clinico-pathological study. Vet Rec 91:441–447, 1972.

447. Blake JC, Sprengers D, Grech P, et al. Bleeding time in patients with hepatic cirrhosis. Brit Med J 301:12–15, 1990.

448. Berk PD, Javitt NB. Hyperbilirubinemia and cholestasis. Am J Med 64:311–326, 1978.

449. Tenhunen R, Marver HS, Schmid R. The enzymatic conversion of heme to bilirubin by microsomal heme oxygenase. Proc Nat Acad Sci 61:748–755, 1968.

450. Gollan J, Schmid R. Bilirubin update: Formation, transport and metabolism. In: Popper H, Schaffner F (eds) Progress in Liver Diseases, Vol. VII. Grune & Stratton, New York, 261–284, 1982.

451. Broderson R. Bilirubin encephalopathy—the preventive role of bilirubin binding to albumin. Critical Rev Clin Lab Sci 11:307–399, 1980.

452. Jansen PLM, Mulder GJ, Burchell B, et al. New developments in glucuronidation research: Report of a workshop on "glucuronidation, its role in health and disease." Hepatology 15:532–541, 1992.

453. Royer M, Noir BA, Sfarcich D, et al. Extrahepatic biliurbin formation and conjugation in the dog. Digestion 10:423–434, 1974.

454. Fevery J, van de Vijver, Michiels R, et al. Comparison in different species of biliary bilirubin-IXalpha conjugates with activities of hepatic and renal bilirubin-IXalpha-uridine diphosphate glycosyltransferases. Biochem J 164:737–746, 1977.

455. Blanckaert N, Fevery J. Physiology and pathophysiology of bilirubin metabolism. In: Zakim D, Boyer TD (eds) Hepatology, a Textbook of Liver Disease. WB Saunders, Philadelphia, 254–302, 1990.

456. Chowdury JR, Wolkoff AW, Arias IM. Heme and bile pigment metabolism. In: Arias IM, Jakoby WB, Popper H, et al. (eds) The Liver: Biology and Pathobiology, 2nd ed. Raven Press, New York, 419–449, 1988.

457. Raymond GD, Galambos JT. Hepatic storage and excretion of bilirubin in the dog. Am J Gastroenterology 55:119–134, 1971.

458. Lees GE, Hardy RM, Stevens JB, et al. Clinical implications of feline bilirubinuria. J Am Anim Hosp Assoc 20:765–771, 1984.

459. Cameron JL, Stafford ES, Schnaufer L, et al. Bilirubin excretion in the dog. J Surg Res 111:39–42, 1963.

460. France D, Preaux AM, Bismuth H, et al. Extrahepatic formation of bilirubin glucuronides in the rat. Biochim Biophys Acta 286:55–61, 1972.

461. De Schepper J. Degradation of haemoglobin to bilirubin in the kidney of the dog. Tijdschr Diergeneesk 99:699–707, 1974.

462. De Schepper J, van der Stock. Increased urinary bilirubin excretion after elevated free plasma haemoglobin levels. Arch Intern Physiol Biochim 80:279–291, 1972.

463. De Schepper J, van der Stock. Increased urinary bilirubin excretion after elevated free plasma haemoglobin levels. II. Variations in the calculated renal clearances of bilirubin in isolated normothermic perfused dog's kidneys. Arch Intern Physiol Biochim 80:339–348, 1972.

464. De Schepper J, van der Stock. Influence of sex on the urinary bilirubin excretion on increased free plasma haemoglobin levels in whole dogs and in isolated normothermic perfused dog kidneys. Experientia 27:1264–1264, 1971.

465. Pimstone NR, Engel P, Tenhunen R, et al. Inducible heme oxygenase in the kidney: A model for the homeostatic control of hemoglobin catabolism. J Clin Invest 50:2042–2050, 1971.

466. Watson CJ. Composition of the urobilin group in urine, bile and feces and the significance of variations in health and disease. J Lab Clin Med 54:1–25, 1959.

467. Fulop M, Brazeau P. The renal excretion of bilirubin in dogs with obstructive jaundice. J Clin Invest 43:1192–1202, 1964.

468. McDonagh AF, Lightner DA. Phototherapy and the photobiology of bilirubin. Sem Liver Dis 8:272–283, 1988.

469. Rothuizen J, Van den Brom WE. Bilirubin metabolism in canine hepatobiliary and hemolytic disease. Vet Q 9:235–240, 1987.

470. Rothuizen J, van den Ingh T. Covalently protein-bound bilirubin conjugates in cholestatic disease of dogs. Am J Vet Res 49:702–704, 1988.

471. Cowger ML. Mechanisms of bilirubin toxicity on tissue culture cells: Factors that affect toxicity, reversibility by albumin and comparison with other respiratory poisons and surfactants. Biochem Med 5:1–16, 1971.

472. Cowger ML, Igo RP, Labbe RF. The mechanism of bilirubin toxicity studied with purified respiratory enzyme and tissue culture systems. Biochem 4:1763–2770, 1965.

473. Karp WB. Biochemical alterations in neonatal hyperbilirubinemia and bilirubin encephalopathy: A review. Pediatrics 64:361–368, 1979.

474. Mustafa MG, Gowger ML, King TE. Effects of bilirubin on mitochondrial reactions. J Bio Chem 244:6403–6414, 1969.

475. Rozdilsky B. Toxicity of bilirubin in adult animals. Arch Path 72:22–30, 1961.

476. Arhelger RB, Davis JT, Evers CG, et al. Experimental cholemia in dogs. Arch Path 89:353–363, 1970.

477. Ayer GD. Renal lesions associated with deep jaundice. Arch Path 30:26–41, 1940.

478. Fajers C. Experimental studies in so-called hepato-renal syndrome. Acta Path Microbiol Scand 44:5–20, 1958.

479. Cornelius CE. In: Bilirubin metabolism in fetus and neonate. Brans YW, Kuehl TJ (eds) Nonhuman Primates in Perinatal Research. John Wiley, New York, 393–410, 1988.

480. Bernstein RB, Novy MJ, Plasecki GJ, et al. Bilirubin metabolism in the fetus. J Clin Invest 48:1678–1688, 1969.

481. Tryphonas L, Rozdilsky B. Nuclear jaundice (kernicterus) in a newborn kitten. J Am Vet Med Assoc 157:1084–1087, 1970.

482. Claireaux AE. In: Sass-Kortsak (ed) Kernicterus. University of Toronto Press, Toronto, 140–149, 1961.

483. Haslewood GAD. The biological significance of chemical differences in bile salts. Biol Rev 39:537–574, 1964.

484. Vlahcevic ZR, Heuman DM, Hylemon PB. Physiology and pathophysiology of enterohepatic circulation of bile acids. In: Zakim D, Boyer T (eds) Hepatology, a Textbook of Liver Disease, 2nd ed. WB Saunders, Philadelphia, 341–377, 1989.

485. Elliott WH, Hyde PM. Metabolic pathways of bile acid synthesis. Am J Med 51:568–579, 1971.

486. Boyd GS, Percy-Robb IW. Enzymatic regulation of bile acid synthesis. Am J Med 51:580–587, 1971.

487. Danielsson H. Mechanisms of bile acid biosynthesis. In: Nair PP, Kritchevsky D, (eds) The Bile Acids: Chemistry, Physiology and Metabolism, Vol. II. Plenum Press, New York, 1–31, 305–306, 1973.

488. Bjorkhem I, Danielsson H. Hydroxylations in biosynthesis and metabolism of bile acids. Mol Cell Biochem 4:79–95, 1974.

489. Kwekkeboom J, Princen HMG, Van Voorthuizen EM, et al. Bile acids exert negative feedback control on bile acid synthesis in cultured pig hepatocytes by suppression of cholesterol 7alpha-hydroxylase activity. Hepatology 12:1209–1215, 1990.

490. Goldman MA, Schwartz CC, Swell L, et al. Bile acid metabolism in health and disease. In: Popper H, Schaffner F (eds) Progress in Liver Disease, Vol. VI. Grune & Stratton, New York, 225–241, 1979.

491. Bjorkhem I, Danielsson H. Biosynthesis and metabolism of bile acids in man. In: Popper H, Schaffner F (eds) Progress in Liver Disease. Grune & Stratton, New York, 215–131, 1976.

492. Boyd GS, Percy-Robb IW. Enzymatic regulation of bile acid synthesis. Am J Med 51:580–587, 1971.

493. Danielsson H. Mechanisms of bile acid biosynthesis. In: Nair PP, Kritchevsky D (eds) The Bile Acids: Chemistry, Physiology and Metabolism, Vol. II. Plenum Press, New York, 1–31, 305–306, 1973.

494. Elliott WH, Hyde PM. Metabolic pathways of bile acid synthesis. Am J Med 51:568–579, 1971.

495. Sjovall J. Bile acids in man under normal and pathological conditions. Clin Chim Acta 5:33–41, 1960.

496. Coleman R, Iqbal S, Godfrey PP, et al. Membranes and bile formation. Composition of several mammalian biles and their membrane-damaging properties. Biochem J 178:201–208, 1979.

497. Alvaro D, Cantafora A, Attili AF, et al. Relationships between bile salts hydrophilicity and phospholipid composition in bile of various animal species. Comp Biochem Physiol (B) 83:551–554, 1986.

498. Hardison WGM, Grundy SM. Effect of bile acid conjugation pattern on bile acid metabolism in normal humans. Gastroenterology 84:617–620, 1983.

499. Rabin B, Nicolosi RJ, Hayes KC. Dietary influence on bile acid conjugation in the cat. J Nutr 106:1241–1246, 1976.

500. Hickman MA, Rogers QR, Morris JG. Taurocholic acid turnover in taurine-depleted and normal cats. J Nutr 121:S185, 1991.

501. Rentschler LA, Hirschberger LL, Stipanuk MH. Response of the kitten to dietary taurine depletion: Effects on renal reabsorption, bile acid conjugation and activities of enzymes involved in taurine synthesis. Comp Biochem Physiol 84B:319–325, 1986.

502. Smallwood RA, Hoffman NE. Bile acid structure and biliary secretion of cholesterol and phospholipid in the cat. Gastroenterology 71:1064–1066, 1976.

503. Stiehl A, Earnest DL, Admirand WH. Sulfation and renal excretion of bile salts in patients with cirrhosis of the liver. Gastroenterology 68:534–544, 1975.

504. Yousef I, Mignault D, Tuchweber B. Effect of complete sulfation of bile acids on bile formation: Role of conjugation and number of sulfate groups. Hepatology 15:438–445, 1992.

505. Frohling W, Stiehl A. Bile salt glucuronides: Identification and quantitative analysis in the urine of patients with cholestasis. Eur J Clin Invest 6:67–74, 1976.

506. Mok HYL, von Bergmann K, Grundy SM. Kinetics of enterohepatic circulation during fasting: Biliary lipid secretion and gallbladder storage. Gastroenterology 78:1023–1033, 1980.

507. Nally CV, McMullin LJ, Clanachan, et al. Periodic gallbladder contraction maintains bile acid circulation during the fasting period: A canine study. Br J Surg 74:1134–1138, 1987.

508. Itoh Z, Takahashi I. Periodic contractions of the canine gallbladder during the interdigestive state. Am J Physiol 240:G183–G189, 1981.

509. DiMagno EP, Hendricks JC, Go VLW, et al. Relationships among canine fasting, pancreatic and biliary secretions, pancreatic duct pressure, and duodenal phase III motor activity—Boldyreff revisited. Dig Dis Sci 24:689–693, 1979.

510. Keane FB, DiMagno EP, Dozois RR, et al. Relationships among canine interdigestive exocrine pancreatic and biliary flow, duodenal motor activity, plasma pancreatic polypeptide, and motilin. Gastroenterology 78:310–316, 1980.

511. Traynor OJ, Dozois RR, DiMagno EP. Canine interdigestive and postprandial gallbladder motility and emptying. Am J Physiol 246:G426–G432, 1984.

512. Scott RB, Strasberg SM, El-Sharkawy TY, et al. Regulation of the fasting enterohepatic circulation of bile acids by the migrating myoelectric complex in dogs. J Clin Invest 71:644–654, 1983.

513. Scott RB, Eidt PB, Shaffer EA. Regulation of fasting canine duodenal bile acid delivery by sphincter of Oddi and gallbladder. Am J Physiol 249:G622–G633, 1985.

514. LaRusso NF, Korman MG, Hoffman NE, et al. Dynamics of the enterohepatic circulation of bile acids. N Engl J Med 291:689–692, 1974.

515. Barbara L, Roda A, Roda E, et al. Diurnal variations of serum primary bile acids in healthy subjects and hepatobiliary disease patients. Rendiconti di Gastroenterologia 8:194–198, 1976.

516. Kramer W, Bickel U, Buscher HP, et al. Bile-salt-binding polypeptides in plasma membrane of hepatocytes revealed by photoaffinity labelling. Eur J Biochem 129:13–24, 1982.

517. Von Dippe P, Levy D. Synthesis and transport characteristics of photoaffinity probes for the hepatocyte bile acid transport system. J Biol Chem 258:8890–8895, 1983.

518. Ziegler K, Frimmer M, Mulner S, et al. 3-Isothiocyanatobenzamido [³H] cholate, a new affinity label for hepatocellular membrane proteins responsible for the uptake of both bile acids and phalloidin. Biochim Biophys Acta 733:11–22, 1984.

519. Erlinger S, Lamri Y, Roda A, et al. Transport of bile acids by the liver cell: Direct evidence for a vesicular mechanism involving the Golgi apparatus. In: Trends in Bile Acid Research, 52nd Falk Symposium, Freiburg, Germany. Kluwer Academic Publishers, Lancaster UK, 115–122, 1988.

520. Yau WM, Makhlouf GM, Edwards LE, et al. Mode of action of cholecystokinin and related peptides on gallbladder muscle. Gastroenterology 65:451–456, 1973.

521. Roslyn JJ, Pitt HA, Mann LL, et al. Gallbladder disease in patients on long-term parenteral nutrition. Gastroenterology 84:148–154, 1983.

522. Messing B, Borries C, Kunstlinger F, et al. Does total parenteral nutrition induce gallbladder sludge formation and lithiasis? Gastroenterology 84:1012–1019, 1983.

523. Pertsemlidis D, Kirchman EH, Ahrens EH. Regulation of cholesterol metabolism in the dog. I. Effects of complete bile diversion and of cholesterol feeding on absorption, synthesis, accumulation and excretion rates measured during life. J Clin Invest 52:2353–2367, 1973.

524. Gracey M, Papadimitriou J, Burke V, et al. Effects on small-intestinal function and structure induced by feeding a deconjugated bile salt. Gut 14:519–528, 1973.

525. Setchell KDR, Harrison DL, Gilbert JM, et al. Serum unconjugated bile acids: Qualitative and quantitative profiles in ileal resection and bacterial overgrowth. Clin Chim Acta 152:297–306, 1985.

526. Mekhjian HS, Phillips SF, Hofmann AF. Colonic secretion of water and electrolytes induced by bile acids; perfusion studies in man. J Clin Invest 50:1569–1577, 1971.

527. Binder HJ, Rowlins CL. Effect of conjugated dihydroxy bile salts on electrolyte transport in rat colon. J Clin Invest 52:1460–1466, 1973.

528. Teem MV, Phillips S. Perfusion of the hamster jejunum with conjugated and unconjugated bile acids: Inhibition of water absorption and effects on morphology. Gastroenterology 62:261–267, 1972.

529. Galapeaux EA, Templeton RD, Borkon EL. The influence of bile on the motility of the dog's colon. Am J Physiol 21:130–136, 1938.

530. Mekhjian HS, Phillips SF, Hofmann AF. Conjugated bile salts block water and electrolyte transport by the human colon (abstract). Gastroenterology 54:1256, 1968.

531. Hofmann AF, Poley JR, Mekhjian HS, et al. Hydroxy fatty acids: An apparent cause of diarrhea in patients with ileal resection and steatorrhea (abstract). J Clin Invest 49:44a, 1970.

532. Hauge JG, Abdelkader SV. Serum bile acids as an indicator of liver disease in dogs. Acta Vet Scand 25:495–503, 1984.

533. Center SA, Baldwin BH, deLahunta A, et al. Evaluation of serum bile acid concentrations for the diagnosis of portosystemic venous anomalies in the dog and cat. J Am Vet Med Assoc 186:1090–1094, 1985.

534. Center SA, Baldwin BH, Erb HN, et al. Bile acid concentrations in the diagnosis of hepatobiliary disease in the dog. J Am Vet Med Assoc 187:935–940, 1985.

535. Center SA, Leveille CR, Baldwin BH, et al. Direct spectometric determination of serum bile acids in the dog and cat. Am J Vet Res 45:2043–2050, 1984.

536. Meyer DJ. Liver function tests in dogs with portosystemic shunts: Measurement of serum bile acid concentrations. J Am Vet Med Assoc 188:168–169, 1986.

537. Center SA, Baldwin BH, Erb H, et al. Bile acid concentrations in the diagnosis of hepatobiliary disease in the cat. J Am Vet Med Assoc 189:891–896, 1986.

538. Center SA, ManWarren R, Slater MR, et al. Evaluation of twelve-hour preprandial and two-hour postprandial serum bile acids concentrations for diagnosis of hepatobiliary disease in dogs. J Am Vet Med Assoc 199:217–226, 1991.

539. Jensen AL. Evaluation of fasting and postprandial total serum bile acid concentration in dogs with hepatobiliary disorders. J Vet Med A 38:247–254, 1991.

540. Aquilera-Tejero E, Mayer-Valor R, Gomez-Cardenas G. Plasma bile acids, lactate dehydrogenase and sulphobromophthalein retention test in canine carbon tetrachloride intoxication. J Sm Anim Pract 29:711–717, 1988.

541. Center SA, Joseph S, Erb HN. The diagnostic efficacy of fasting and 2-hour postprandial serum bile acids in cats (n = 108) hepatobiliary disease. J Am Vet Med Assoc 207:1048–1054, 1995.

542. Johnson SE, Rogers WA, Bonagura JD, et al. Determination of serum bile acids in fasting dogs with hepatobiliary disease. Am J Vet Res 46:2048–2053, 1985.

543. Rutgers HC, Stradley RP, Johnson SE. Serum bile acid analysis in dogs with experimentally induced cholestatic jaundice. Am J Vet Res 49:317–320, 1988.

544. Roda E, Aldini R, Mazzella G, et al. Enterohepatic circulation of bile acids after cholecystectomy. Gut 19:640–649, 1978.

545. Struthers JE, Mehta SJ, Kaye MD, et al. Relative concentrations of individual nonsulfated bile acids in the serum and bile of patients with cirrhosis. Dig Dis 22:861–865, 1977.

546. Patteson TE, Vlahcevic ZR, Schwartz CC, et al. Bile acid metabolism in cirrhosis. VI. Sites of blockage in the bile acid pathways to primary bile acids. Gastroenterology 79:620–628, 1980.

547. Poupon RY, Poupon RE, Lebrec D, et al. Mechanisms for reduced hepatic clearance and elevated plasma levels of bile acids in cirrhosis. Gastroenterology 80:1438–1444, 1981.

548. Akashi Y, Mizazaki H, Yanagisawa J, et al. Bile acid metabolism in cirrhotic liver tissue-altered synthesis and impaired hepatic secretion. Clin Chim Acta 168:199–206, 1987.

549. Vlahcevic ZR, Juttijudata P, Bell CC, et al. Bile acid metabolism in patients with cirrhosis. II. Cholic and chenodeoxycholic acid metabolism. Gastroenterology 62:1174–1181, 1972.

550. Yoshida T, McCormick WC, Swell L, et al. Bile acid metabolism. IV. Characterization of the abnormality in deoxycholic acid metabolism. Gastroenterology 68:335–341, 1975.

551. Bremmelgaard A, Sjovall J. Bile acid profiles in urine of patients with liver diseases. Eur J Clin Invest 79:620–628, 1980.

552. Vlahcevic ZR, Goldman M, Schwartz CC, et al. Bile acid metabolism in cirrhosis. VII. Evidence for defective feedback control of bile acid synthesis. Hepatology 1:146–150, 1981.

553. Thompson MB, Chappell JD, Kunze DJ, et al. Bile acid profile in a dog with cholangiocarcinoma. Vet Pathol 26:75–78, 1989.

554. Thompson MB, Meyer DJ, Laflamme DP, et al. Serum bile acid concentrations and profiles in dogs with surgically created portocaval shunts (abstract). Vet Clin Path 21:34, 1992.

555. Center SA, Thompson MB, Guida L. Serum and urine bile acid profiles in healthy cats, cats with hepatic lipidosis, and cats with extrahepatic bile duct obstruction. Am J Vet Res 54:681–688, 1993.

556. Washizu T, Ikenage H, Washizu M, et al. Bile acid composition of dog and cat gallbladder bile. Jpn J Vet Sci 52:423–425, 1990.

557. Washizu R, Tomoda I, Kaneko JJ. Serum bile acid composition of the dog, cow, horse and human. J Vet Med Sci 53:81–86, 1991.

558. Washizu T, Koizumi I, Kaneko JJ. Postprandial changes in serum bile acids concentration and fractionation of individual bile acids by high performance liquid chromatography in normal dogs. Jpn J Vet Sci 49:593–600, 1987.

559. Schmucker DL, Ohta M, Kanai S, et al. Hepatic injury induced by bile salts: Correlation between biochemical and morphological events. Hepatology 12:1216–1221, 1990.

560. Tanikawa K, Kawahara T, Kumashiro R, et al. Effects of bile acids on the cultured hepatocyte and kupffer cell (abstract). Hepatology 6:779, 1986.

561. Kakis G, Yousef IM. Mechanism of cholic acid protection in lithocholate-induced intrahepatic cholestasis in rats. Gastroenterology 78:1402–1411, 1980.

562. Yousef IM, Tuchweber B, Vonk RJ, et al. Lithocholate cholestasis-sulfated glycolithocholate induced intrahepatic cholestasis in rats. Gastroenterology 80:233–241, 1981.

563. Yousef IM, Fisher MM. In vitro effect of free bile acids on the bile canalicular membrane phospholipids in the rat. Can J Biochem 54:1040–1046, 1976.

564. Hardison WG. Metabolism of sodium dehydrocholate by the rat liver: Its effect on micelle formation in bile. J Lab Clin Med 77:811–820, 1971.

565. Desjeux JF, Erlinger S, Dumont M. Metabolism and influence on bile secretion in the dog of dehydrocholate. Biol Gastroenterol (Paris) 6:9–18, 1973.

566. Podda M, Ghezzi IC, Battezzati PM, et al. Ursodeoxycholic acid for chronic liver diseases. J Clin Gastroenterol 10(suppl 2):S25-S31, 1988.

567. Nicholson B, Center SA, Randolph JF, et al. Clinicopathologic and hepatic light microscopic and ultrastructural effects of chronic ursodeoxycholic acid in healthy cats (abstract). Proc ACVIM 949, 1993.

568. Spencer H, Osis D, Kramer L, et al. Intake, excretion and retention of zinc in man. In: Trace Elements in Human Health and Disease. Academic Press, New York, 345–361, 1976.

569. Szymanska JA, Swietlicka EA, Piotrowski JK. Protective effect of zinc in the hepatotoxicity of bromobenzene and acetaminophen. Toxicology 66:81–91, 1991.

570. McClain CJ. Zinc in malabsorption syndromes. J Am Coll Nutr 4:49–64, 1985.

571. Schilsky ML, Blank RR, Czaja MJ, et al. Hepatocellular copper toxicity and its attenuation by zinc. J Clin Invest 84:1562–1568, 1989.

572. Lee D-Y, Brewer GJ, Wang Y. Treatment of Wilson's disease with zinc. VII. Protection of the liver from copper toxicity by zinc-induced metallothionein in a rat model. J Lab Clin Med 114:639–646, 1989.

573. Brewer GJ, Dick RD, Schall W, et al. Use of zinc acetate to treat copper toxicosis in dogs. J Am Vet Med Assoc 201:566–568, 1992.

574. Clarke IS, Lui EMK. Interaction of metallothionein and carbon tetrachloride on the protective effect of zinc on hepatotoxicity. Can J Physiol Pharmacol 64:1104–1110, 1986.

575. McMillan DA, Schnell RC. Amelioration of bromobenzene hepatotoxicity in the male rat by zinc. Fund Appl Toxicol 5:297–304, 1985.

576. Miranda CL, Henderson MC, Reed RL, et al. Protective action of zinc against pyrrolizidine alkaloid induced hepatotoxicity in rats. J Toxicol Environ Health 9:359–366, 1982.

577. Cagen SZ, Klaassen CD. Protection of carbon tetrachloride induced hepatotoxicity by zinc: Role of metallothionein. Toxicol Appl Pharmacol 51:107–116, 1979.

578. Richards MP, Cousins RJ. Zinc-binding protein, relationship to short-term changes in zinc metabolism. Proc Soc Exp Biol Med 153:52–56, 1976.

579. Chen RW, Vasey EJ, Whanger PD. Accumulation and depletion of zinc in rat liver and kidney metallothionein. J Nutr 107:805–813, 1977.

580. Keeling PWN, Jones RB, Holton PJ, et al. Reduced leukocyte zinc in liver disease. Gut 21:561–564, 1980.

581. Trentini GPP, Dalla Pria AF, Ferrari de Gaetani C, et al. Cirosi epatica e modificazioni del contenuto testicolare di zinco. Possible reuolo della ipozincoemia nella patogenesi del'ipogandismo del cirrotico. Arch Vecchi Anat Patol 52:658–669, 1968.

582. Boyett JD, Sullivan JF. Zinc and collagen content of cirrhotic liver. Dig Dis Sci 15:797–802, 1970.

583. Fredricks RE, Ranaka KR, Valentine WN, et al. Zinc in human blood cells: Normal values and abnormalities associated with liver disease. J Clin Invest 39:1651–1656, 1960.

584. Bode JC, Hanisch P, Henning H, et al. Hepatic zinc content in patients with various stages of alcoholic liver disease and in patients with chronic active and chronic persistent hepatitis. Hepatology 8:1605–1609, 1988.

585. Kahn AM, Helwig HL, Redeker AG, et al. Urine and serum zinc abnormalities in disease of the liver. Am J Clin Pathol 44:426–435, 1965.

586. Scholmerich J, Becher M-S, Kottgen E, et al. The influence of portosystemic shunting on zinc and vitamin A metabolism in liver cirrhosis. Hepatogastroenterology 30:143–147, 1983.

587. Anonymous. Interleukin-1 regulates zinc metabolism and metallothionein gene expression. Nutr Rev 47:285–287, 1989.

588. Cousins RJ, Leinart AS. Tissue-specific regulation of zinc metabolism and metallothionein genes by interleukin 1. FASEB J 2:2884–2890, 1988.

589. Antonow DR, McClain CJ. Nutrition and alcoholism. In: Tarter RE, Thiel DH (eds) Alcohol and the Brain. Plenum, New York, 81–120, 1985.

590. Cossack ZT, Prasad AS. Hyperammonemia in zinc deficiency: Activities of urea cycle related enzymes. Nutr Res 7:1161–1167, 1987.

591. Becking GC, Morrison BA. Hepatic drug metabolism in zinc-deficient rats. Biochem Pharmacol 19:895–902, 1970.

592. Bray TM, Bettger WJ. The physiological role of zinc as an antioxidant. Free Radic Biol Med 8:281–291, 1990.

593. Graham TW, Holmberg CA, Keen CL, et al. A pathologic and toxicologic evaluation of veal calves fed large amounts of zinc. Vet Pathol 25:484–491, 1988.

594. Tavill AS, Bacon BR. Hemochromatosis: Iron metabolism and the iron overload syndromes. In: Zakim D, Boyer TD (eds) Hepatology, a Textbook of Liver Disease. WB Saunders, Philadelphia, 1273–1299, 1990.

595. Weeks BR, Smith JE, Stadler CK. Effect of dietary iron content on hematologic and other measures of iron adequacy in dogs. J Am Vet Med Assoc 196:749–753, 1990.

596. Harvey J, French T, Meyer D. Chronic iron deficiency anemia in dogs. J Am Anim Hosp Assoc 18:946–990, 1982.

597. Weiser G, O'Grady M. Erythrocyte volume distribution analysis and hematologic changes in dogs with iron deficiency anemia. Vet Pathol 20:230–241, 1983.

598. Kondo H, Saito K, Grasso JP, et al. Iron metabolism in the erythrophagocytosing Kupffer cell. Hepatology 8:32–38, 1988.

599. Sibille J-C, Kondo H, Aisen P. Interactions between isolated hepatocytes and Kupffer cells in iron metabolism: A possible role for ferritin as an iron carrier protein. Hepatology 8:296–301, 1988.

600. Bacon BR Park CH, Brittenham GM, et al. Hepatic mitochondrial oxidative metabolism in rats with chronic dietary iron overload. Hepatology 5:789–797, 1985.

601. Bacon BR, Healey JF, Brittenham GM, et al. Hepatic microsomal function in rats with chronic dietary iron overload. Gastroenterology 90:1844–1853, 1986.

602. Bonkowsky HL, Carpenter SJ, Healey JF. Iron and the liver: Subcellular distribution of iron and decreased microsomal cytochrome P-450 in livers of iron-loaded rats. Arch Pathol Lab Med 103:21–29, 1979.

603. Britton RS, O'Neill R, Bacon BR. Hepatic mitochondrial malondialdehyde metabolism in rats with chronic iron overload. Hepatology 11:93–97, 1990.

604. Bonkowsky HL, Healey JF, Sinclair PR, et al. Iron and the liver: Acute and long-term effects of iron loading on hepatic haem metabolism. Biochem J 196:57–68, 1981.

605. Vierling JM. Copper metabolism. In: Current Hepatology: An Update in Science and Practice. AASLD postgraduate course. Chicago, 132–143, 1988.

606. Center SA, Baldwin BH, King JM, et al. Hematologic and biochemical abnormalities associated with induced extrahepatic bile duct obstruction in the cat. Am J Vet Res 44:1822–1829, 1983.

607. Twedt DC, Sternlieb I, Gilbertson SR. Clinical, morphologic, and chemical studies on copper toxicosis of Bedlington terriers. J Am Vet Med Assoc 175:269–275, 1979.

608. Ludwig J, Owen CA, Jr, Barham SS, et al. The liver in the inherited copper disease of Bedlington terriers. Lab Invest 43:82–88, 1980.

609. Keen CL, Lonnerdal B, Fisher GL. Age-related variations in hepatic iron, copper, zinc, and selenium concentrations in beagles. Am J Vet Res 42:1884–1887, 1981.

610. Johnson GF, Zawie DA, Gilbertson SR, et al. Chronic active hepatitis in Doberman pinschers. J Am Vet Med Assoc 1438–1442, 1982.

611. Thornburg LP, Shaw D, Dolan M, et al. Hereditary copper toxicosis in West Highland white terriers. Vet Pathol 23:148–154, 1986.

612. Haywood S, Rutgers HC, Christian MK. Hepatitis and copper accumulation in Skye terriers. Vet Pathol 25:408–414, 1988.

613. Sternlieb I, Goldfischer S. Heavy metals and lysosomes. In: Dingle JT, Dean RT (eds) Lysososmes in Biology and Pathology, Vol. 5. Elsevier, New York, 185–200, 1976.

614. Johnson GF, Morell AG, Stockert RJ, et al. Hepatic lysosomal copper protein in dogs with an inherited copper toxicosis. Hepatology 2:243–248, 1981.

615. Crawford MA, Schall WD, Jensen RK, et al. Chronic active hepatitis in 26 Doberman pinschers. J Am Vet Med Assoc 187:1343–1350, 1985.

616. Vessey DA. Metabolism of drugs and toxins by human liver. In: Zakim D,

Boyer TD (eds) Hepatology, a Textbook of Liver Disease. WB Saunders, Philadelphia, 196–234, 1990.

617. Boothe DM. Drug disposition as diagnostic and prognostic indicators of liver disease. Proc 8th ACVIM Forum 745–752, 1990.

618. Thurman RG, Kauffman FC. Factors regulating drug metabolism in intact hepatocytes. Pharmacol Rev 31:229-251, 1980.

619. Aw TY, Jones DP. Control of glucuronidation during hypoxia. Limitation by UDP-glucose pyrophosphorylase. Biochem J 219:707–712, 1984.

620. Debaun JR, Miller EC, Miller JA. N-hydroxy-2-acetylaminofluorene sulfotransferase: Its probable role in carcinogenesis and in protein-(methion-5-yl) binding in liver. Cancer Res 30:577–595, 1970.

621. Crib AE, Spielberg SP. An in vitro investigation of predisposition to sulfphonamide idiosyncratic toxicity in dogs. Vet Res Comm 14:241–252, 1990.

622. Crib AE. Idiosyncratic reactions to sulfonamides in dogs. J Am Vet Med Assoc 195:1612–1614, 1989.

623. Giger U, Werner LL, Millichamp NJ, et al. Sulfadiazine-induced allergy in six Doberman pinschers. J Am Vet Med Assoc 186:479–484, 1985.

624. Kappas A, Drummond GS. Control of heme and cytochrome P450 metabolism by inorganic metals, organometals and synthetic metalloporphyrins. Environ Health Perspect 57:301–306, 1984.

625. Ali B, Spencer HW, Auyong TK, et al. Selective induction of hepatic drug metabolizing enzymes by lithium treatment in dogs. J Pharm Pharmac 27:131–132, 1975.

626. Vu VT, Bai SA, Abramson FP. Interactions of phenobarbital with propranolol in the dog. 2. Bioavailability, metabolism and pharmacokinetics. J Pharmacol Exp Ther 224:55–61, 1983.

627. Bai SA, Abramson FP. Interaction of phenobarbital with propranolol in the dog. 3. beta blockade. J Pharmacol Exp Ther 224:62–67, 1983.

628. Gascon-Barre M, Valliers S, Huet PM. Influence of phenobarbital on the hepatic handling of [3H] vitamin D in the dog. Am J Physiol 251:G627–G635, 1986.

629. Ravis WR, Pedersoli WM, Turco JD. Pharmacokinetics and interactions of digoxin with phenobarbital in dogs. Am J Vet Res 48:1244–1249, 1987.

630. Breznock EM. Effects of phenobarbital on digitoxin and digoxin elimination in the dog. Am J Vet Res 36:371–373, 1975.

631. Pedersoli WM, Ganjam VK, Nachreiner RF. Serum digoxin concentrations in dogs before, during, and after concomitant treatment with phenobarbital. Am J Vet Res 41:1639–1642, 1980.

632. Francavilla A, Makowka L, Polimeno L, et al. A dog model for acetaminophen-induced fulminant hepatic failure. Gastroenterology 96:470–478, 1989.

633. Berkersky I, Maggio AC, Mattaliano, V, Jr et al. Influence of phenobarbital on the disposition of clonazepam and antipyrine in the dog. J Pharm Biopharm 5:507–512, 1977.

634. Kawalek JC, El Said KR. Maturational development of drug-metabolizing enzymes in dogs. Am J Vet Res 51:1742–1745, 1990.

635. Pessaye D, Dolder A, Artigou J-Y, et al. Effect of fasting on metabolite mediated hepatotoxicity in the rat. Gastroenterology 77:264–271, 1979.

636. Adithan D, Shashindran CH, Gandhi IS, et al. Pharmacokinetics of phenylbutazone in chronic liver disease. Indian J Med Res 71:316–321, 1980.

637. Uribe M, Go VLW. Corticosteroid pharmacokinetics in liver disease. Clin Pharmacokinet 4:233, 1979.

638. Uribe M, Go VLM, Kluge D. Prednisone for chronic active hepatitis: Pharmacokinetics and serum binding in patients with chronic active hepatitis and steroid major side effects. J Clin Gastroenterol 6:331, 1984.

639. Powell LW, Axelsen E. Corticosteroids in liver disease: Studies on the biological conversion of prednisone to prenisolone and plasma protein binding. Gut 13:690–696, 1972.

640. Bergrem H, Ritland S, Opedal I, et al. Prednisolone pharmacokinetics and protein-binding in patients with portosystemic shunt. Scand J Gastroenterol 18:273–276, 1983.

641. Bass NM, Williams RL. Hepatic function and pharmacokinetics. In: Zakim D, Boyer TD (eds) Hepatology, a Textbook of Liver Disease. WB Saunders, Philadelphia, 235–254, 1990.

642. Ludwig J, Axelsen R. Drug effects on the liver: An updated tabular compilation of drugs and drug-related hepatic diseases. Dig Dis Sci 28:651–666, 1983.

643. Bass NM, Ockner RK. Drug-induced liver disease. In: Zakim D, Boyer TD (eds) Hepatology, a Textbook of Liver Disease. WB Saunders, Philadelphia, 754–791, 1990.

644. Hahn R, Oberrauch W. Unidirectional transport of reduced glutathione in rat liver and its metabolization in the extracellular spaces. In: Wendel A, Sies H (eds) Functions of Glutathione in Liver and Kidney. Springer Verlag, New York, 32, 1978.

645. Madden JW, Gertman PM, Peacock EE. Dimethylnitrosamine-induced hepatic cirrhosis: A new canine model of an ancient human disease. Surgery 68:260–268, 1970.

646. Testas P, Benichou J, Perrin N, et al. Comparative models for experimental cirrhosis in the dog. Eur Surg Res 10:146–152, 1978.

647. Liggett AD, Colvin BM. Canine aflatoxicosis: A continuing problem. Vet Hum Toxicol 28:428–430, 1989.

648. Bastianello SS, Nesbit JW, Williams MC, et al. Pathological findings in a natural outbreak of aflatoxicosis in dogs. Onderstepoort J Vet Res 54:635–640, 1987.

649. Armbrecht BH, Geleta JN, Shalkop WT, et al. A subacute exposure of beagle dogs to aflatoxin. Tox App Pharm 18:579–585, 1971.

650. Chaffee VW, Edds GT, Himes JA, et al. Aflatoxicosis in dogs. Am J Vet Res 30:1737–1749, 1969.

651. Newberne PM, Russo R, et al. Acute toxicity of aflatoxin B₁ in the dog. Pathol Vet 3:331–340, 1966.

652. Newberne PM. Chronic aflatoxicosis. J Am Vet Med Assoc 163:1262–1267, 1973.

653. Green CE, Barsanti JA, et al. Disseminated intravascular coagulation complicating aflatoxicosis in dogs. Cornell Vet 67:29–49, 1977.

654. Gitlin N. Clinical aspects of liver diseases caused by industrial and environmental toxins. In: Zakim D, Boyer TD (eds) Hepatology, a Textbook of Liver Disease. WB Saunders, Philadelphia, 791–821, 1990.

655. Kelly DF, Pontefract ??. Hepatorenal toxicity in a dog following immersion in Rutland water. Vet Rec 127:453–454, 1990.

656. Bunch SE, Baldwin BH, Hornbuckle WE, et al. Compromised hepatic function in dogs treated with anticonvulsant drugs. J Am Vet Med Assoc 184:444–448, 1984.

657. Bunch SE, Castleman WL, Hornbuckle WE, et al. Hepatic cirrhosis associated with long-term anticonvulsant drug therapy in dogs. J Am Vet Med Assoc 181:357–362, 1982.

658. Bunch SE, Conway MB, Center SA, et al. Toxic hepatopathy and intrahepatic cholestasis associated with phenytoin administration in combination with other anticonvulsant drugs in three dogs. J Am Vet Med Assoc 190:194–198, 1987.

659. Poffenbarger EM, Hardy RM. Hepatic cirrhosis associated with long-term primidone therapy in a dog. J Am Vet Med Assoc 978–980, 1985.

660. Heywood R, Chesterman H, Ball SA, et al. Toxicity of methyl testosterone in the beagle dog. Toxicology 7:357–365, 1977.

661. Gaunt PS, Meuten DJ, Pecquret-Goad ME. Hepatic necrosis associated with use of halothane in a dog. J Am Vet Med Assoc 184:478–480, 1984.

662. Dayrell-Hart B, Steinberg SA, VanWinkle TJ, et al. Hepatotoxicity of phenobarbital in dogs: 18 cases (1985–1989). J Am Vet Med Assoc 199:1060–1066, 1991.

663. Thornburg LP, Rottinghaus GB, Glassberg R. Drug-induced hepatic necrosis in a dog. J Am Vet Med Assoc 183:327–328, 1983.

664. Nash AS, Thompson H, Bogan JA. Phenytoin toxicity: A fatal case in a dog with hepatitis and jaundice. Vet Rec 100:280–281, 1977.

665. Polzin DJ, Stowe CM, O"Leary TP, et al. Acute hepatic necrosis associated with the administration of mebendazole to dogs. J Am Vet Med Assoc 179:1013–1016, 1981.

666. Swanson JF, Breider MA. Hepatic failure following mebendazole administration to a dog. J Am Vet Med Assoc 181:72–73, 1982.

667. Ndiritu CG, Weigel J. Hepatorenal injury in a dog associated with methoxyflurane. VMSAC 72:545–550, 1977.

668. Hardy RM, Polzen DJ, O'Brien RD. Letter to the editor: Report of drug-associated hepatitis in dogs. J Am Vet Med Assoc 189:850–851, 1986.

669. Pedersoli WM. Serum fluoride concentrations, renal and hepatic function tests results in dogs with methoxyflurane anesthesia. Am J Vet Res 38:949–953, 1977.

670. Setchell KDR, Gosselin SJ, Welsh MB, et al. Dietary estrogens—a probable cause of infertility and liver disease in captive cheetahs. Gastroenterology 93:225–233, 1987.

671. Liggett AD, Weis R. Liver necrosis caused by mushroom poisoning in dogs. J Vet Diag Invest 1:267–269, 1989.

672. Hjelle JJ, Grauer GF. Acetaminophen-induced toxicosis in dogs and cat. J Am Vet Med Assoc 188:742–746, 1986.

673. Eder H. Chronic toxicity studies on phenacetin, N-acetyl-p-aminophenol (NAPA) and acetylsalicylic acid on cats. Acta Pharmacol Toxicol (Copenhagen) 21:197–204, 1964.

674. Gaunt SD, Baker DC, Green RA. Clinicopathologic evaluation of N-acetylcesteine therapy in acetaminophen toxicosis in the cat. Am J Vet Res 42:1982–1984, 1981.

675. Finco DR, Duncan JR, Schall WD, et al. Acetaminophen toxicosis in the cat. J Am Vet Med Assoc 166:469–472, 1975.

676. Ortega L, Landa Garcia JI, Garcia AT, et al. Acetaminophen-induced fulminant hepatic failure in dogs. Hepatology 5:673–676, 1985.

677. Koch-Weser J, Williams RL. Drug therapy: Drug administration in hepatic disease. N Engl J Med 309:1616–1622, 1983.

678. McMaster KR, Hennigar GR. Drug-induced granulomatous hepatitis. Lab Invest 44:61–73, 1981.

679. Center SA, Elston TH, Rowland PH, et al. Idiosyncratic fulminant hepatic failure associated with oral administration of diazepam to cats. J Am Vet Med Assoc, in press.

680. Werner LL, Bright JM. Drug-induced immune hypersensitivity disorders in two dogs treated with trimethoprim sulfadiazine: Case reports and drug challenge studies. J Am Anim Hosp Assoc 19:783–790, 1983.

681. Anderson WI, Campbell KL, Wilson RC, et al. Hepatitis in a dog given sulfadiazine-trimethoprim and cyclophosphamides. Mod Vet Pract 65:115, 1984.

682. Toth DM, Derwelis SK. Drug-induced hepatitis in a dog. VM SAC 75:421–422, 1980.

683. Rowland PH, Center SA, Dougherty SA. Presumptive trimethoprim-sulfa-diazine-related hepatotoxicosis in a dog. J Am Vet Med Assoc 200:348–350, 1992.

684. Crib AE, Miller M, Tesoro A, et al. Peroxidase-dependent oxidation of sul-fonamides by monocytes and neutrophils from humans and dogs. Mol Pharm 38:744–751, 1990.

685. Sanford JP. Guide to Antimicrobial Therapy. Antimicrobial Therapy, Inc., Dallas, 105, 1993.

686. Miyazawa Y, Sato T, Kobayashi K, et al. Influence of induced cholestasis on pharmacokinetics of digoxin and digitoxin in dogs. Am J Vet Res 51:605–610, 1990.

687. Abel RM, Luchi RJ, Peskin GW, et al. Metabolism of digoxin: Role of the liver in tritiated digoxin degradation. J Pharmacol Exp Ther 150:463–468, 1965.

688. Westphal U. Steroid Protein Interactions. Springer, Berlin, 1971.

689. Van Thiel DH. Disorders of the hypothalamic-pituitary-gonadal and thy-roidal axes in patients with liver disease. In: Zakim D, Boyer TD (eds) Hepatology, a Textbook of Liver Disease. Philadelphia, WB Saunders, 791–821, 1990.

690. Braunstein GD. Gynecomastia. N Engl J Med 328:490–495, 1993.

691. Gordon GG, Olivo J, Rafii F, et al. Conversions of androgens to estrogens in cirrhosis of the liver. J Clin Endocrinol Metab 40:1018–1026, 1975.

692. Danford DE, Munro HN. Liver in relation to B vitamins. In: Arias IM, Jakoby WB, Popper H, et al. (eds) The Liver: Biology and Pathobiology. Raven Press, New York, 495–503, 1988; pp 495–503.

693. Goodman DS. Vitamin A metabolism in the liver. In: Arias IM, Jakoby WB, Popper H, et al. (eds) The Liver: Biology and Pathobiology. Raven Press, New York, 467–474, 1988.

694. Bikle DD; Metabolism and functions of vitamins A, D, and K. In: Zakim D, Boyer TD (eds) Hepatology, a Textbook of Liver Disease, 2nd ed. WB Saunders, Philadelphia, 182–196, 1990.

695. Russel RM. Vitamin and mineral supplements in the management of liver disease. Med Clin N Am 63:537–544, 1979.

696. Frank O, Baker H, Leevy CM. Vitamin-binding capacity of experimentally injured liver. Nature 203:302–303, 1964.

697. Underwood BA. Vitamin A in animal and human nutrition. In: Sporn MB, Robert AB, Goodman DS (eds) The Retinoids, Vol. 1. Academic Press, New York, 281–392, 1984.

698. Goodman DS, Blaner WS. Biosynthesis, absorption, and hepatic metabo-lism of retinol. In: Sporn MB, Robert AB, Goodman DS (eds) The Retinoids, Vol. 1. Academic Press, New York, 1–39, 1984.

699. Goodman DS. Vitamin A and retinoids in health and disease. N Engl J Med 310:1023–1031, 1984.

700. Seawright AA, English PB, Gartner RJW. Hypervitaminosis A and hyperos-tosis of the cat. Nature 206:1171–1172, 1965.

701. English PB, Seawright AA. Deforming cervical spondylosis of the cat. Aust Vet J 40:376–381, 1964.

702. Pittsley RA, Yoder FW. Retinoid hyperostosis: Skeletal toxicity associated with long-term administration of 13-Cis-retinoic acid for refractory ichthyosis. N Engl J Med 308;1012–1014, 1983.

703. Gosselin SJ, Loudy DL, Tarr MJ, et al. Veno-occlusive disease of the liver in captive cheetah. Vet Pathol 25:48–57, 1988.

704. Jorgensen MJ, Furie BC, Furie B. Vitamin K dependent coagulation pro-teins. In: Arias IM, Jakoby WB, Popper H, et al. (eds) The Liver: Biol-ogy and Pathobiology. Raven Press, New York, 467–474, 1988.

705. Putnam ME, Comben N. Vitamin E. Vet Rec 121:541–545, 1987.

706. Elias E, Muller DPR, Scott J. Association of spinocerebellar disorders with cystic fibrosis or chronic childhood cholestasis and a very low serum vit-amin E. Lancet ii:1319–1321, 1981.

707. Rosenblum JL, Keating JP, Prensky AL, et al. A progressive neurological syndrome in children with chronic liver disease. N Engl J Med 304:503–508, 1981.

708. Hafeman DG, Hoekstra WG. Protection against carbon tetrachloride-induced lipid peroxidation in the rat by dietary vitamin E, selenium and methionine as measured by ethane evolution. J Nutr 107:656–665, 1977.

709. Tollerz G. Vitamin E, selnium (and some related compounds) and toler-ance towards iron in piglets. Acta Agr Scand(suppl) 19:184–187, 1973.

710. Dougherty JJ, Croft WA, Hoekstra WG. Effects of ferrous chloride and iron-dextran on lipid peroxidation in vivo in vitamin E and selenium adequate and deficient rats. J Nutr 111:1784–1796, 1981.

711. Galagher CH. The effect of antioxidants on poisoning by carbon tetra-chloride. Aust J Exp Biol Med Sci 40:170–181, 1962.

712. Dougherty JJ, Hoekstra WG. Effects of vitamin E and selenium on copper-induced lipid peroxidation in vivo and on acute copper toxicity. Proc Soc Exp Bio Med 169:201–208, 1982.

713. Rappaport AM. Physioanatomic considerations. In: Schiff L, Schiff ER, eds (eds) Diseases of the Liver, 6th ed. JB Lippincott, Philadelphia, 1–46, 1987.

714. Loisance DY, Peronneau PA, Pellet MM, et al. Hepatic circulation after side-to side portacaval shunt in dogs: Velocity pattern and flow rate changes studied by an ultrasonic velocimeter. Surgery 73:43–52, 1973.

715. Schatten WE. The role of intestinal bacteria in liver necrosis following experimental excision of the hepatic arterial supply. Surgery 36:256–269, 1954.

716. Cobb LM, McKay KA. A bacteriological study of the liver of the normal dog. J Comp Pathol 72:92–96, 1962.

717. Gunn C, Gourley IM, Koblik PD. Hepatic dearterialization in the dog. Am J Vet Res 47:170–175, 1986.

718. Lautt WW. Hepatic vasculature: A conceptual review. Gastroenterology 73:1163–1169, 1977.

719. Lautt WW, Greenway CV. Conceptual review of the hepatic vascular bed. Hepatology 7:952–963, 1987.

720. Greenway CV, Stark RD. Hepatic vascular bed. Physiol Rev 51:23–65, 1971.

721. Greenway CV, Lister GE. Capacitance effects and blood reservoir function in the splanchnic vascular bed during non-hypotensive haemorrhage and blood volume expansion in anesthetized cats. J Physiol 237:279–294, 1974.

722. Lautt WW, Greenway CV. Hepatic venous compliance and role of liver as a blood reservoir. Am J Physiol 231:292–295, 1976.

723. Hanson KM. Liver. In: Johnson PC (ed) Peripheral Circulation. John Wiley, New York, 285, 1987.

724. Witte CL, Tobin GR, Clark DS, et al. Relationship of splanchnic blood flow and portal venous resistance to elevated portal pressure in the dog. Gut 17:122–126, 1976.

725. Schmidt S, Suter PF. Indirect and direct determination of the portal vein pressure in normal and abnormal dogs and normal cats. Vet Rad 21:246–259, 1980.

726. Johnson SE. Portal hypertension. I. Pathophysiology and clinical conse-quences. Comp Cont Ed 9:741–750, 1987.

727. Runyon BA, Montano AA, Akriviadis EA, et al. The serum-ascites albumin gradient is superior to the exudate-transudate concept in the differen-tial diagnosis of ascites. Ann Intern Med 117:215–220, 1992.

728. Crossley IR, Westaby D, Williams R. Portal hypertension. In: Wright R, Millward-Sadler GH, Alberti KGMM, et al. (eds) Liver and Biliary Dis-ease, 2nd ed. WB Saunders, Philadelphia, 1283–1317, 1985.

729. Cohn LA, Spaulding KA, Cullen JM, et al. Intrahepatic postsinusoidal venous obstruction in a dog. J Vet Int Med 5:317–321, 1991.

730. Macintire DK, Henderson RH, Banfield C, et al. Budd Chiari syndrome in a kitten, caused by membranous obstruction of the caudal vena cava. J Am Anim Hosp Assoc 31:484–491, 1995.

731. Twedt DC. Cirrhosis: A consequence of chronic liver disease. Vet Clin N Am 15:151–176, 1985.

732. Sugita S, Ohnishi K, Saito M, et al. Splanchnic hemodynamics in portal hypertensive dogs with portal fibrosis. Am J Physiol 252:G748-G754, 1987.

733. Popper H, Elias H, Petty DE. Vascular pattern of the cirrhotic liver. Am J Clin Pathol 22:717–729, 1952.

734. Hales M, Allan J, Hall E. Injection-corrosion studies of normal and cir-rhotic livers. Am J Pathol 35:909–941, 1959.

735. Nakamura T, Nakamura S, Suzuki T. Studies on cirrhosis of the liver. IX. Structure of shunted blood vessels in the autopsied cirrhotic liver. Tohoku J Exp Med 75:1–9, 1961.

736. Strombeck DR, Weiser MG, Kaneko JJ. Hyperammonemia and hepatic encephalopathy in the dog. J Am Vet Med Assoc 166:1105–1108, 1975.

737. Easley JC, Carpenter JL. Hepatic arteriovenous fistula in two Saint Bernard pups. J Am Vet Med Assoc 166:167–171, 1975.

738. Legendre AM, Krahwindel DJ, Carrig CV, et al. Ascites associated with intrahepatic arteriovenous fistula in a cat. J Am Vet Med Assoc 168:589–591, 1976.

739. McGavin MD, Henry J. Canine hepatic vascular hamartoma associated with ascites. J Am Vet Med Assoc 160:864–866, 1972.

740. Rogers WA, Suter PF, Breznock EM, et al. Intrahepatic arteriovenous fistu-lae in a dog resulting in portal hypertension, portacaval shunts, and reversal of portal blood flow. J Am Anim Hosp Assoc 13:470–475, 1977.

741. Vitums A. Portosystemic communications in the dog. Acta Anat (Basel) 39:271–299, 1959.

742. Khan IR, Vitums A. Portosystemic communications in the cat. Res Vet Sci 12:215–218, 1971.

743. Ewing GO, Suter PF, Bailey CS. Hepatic insufficiency associated with con-genital anomalies of the portal vein in dogs. J Am Anim Hosp Assoc 10:463–476, 1974.

744. Hoskins JD, Ochoa R, Hawkins BJ. Portal vein thrombosis in a dog: A case report. J Am Anim Hosp Assoc 15:497–500, 1979.

745. Willard MD, Bailey MQ, Hauptman J, et al. Obstructed portal venous flow and portal vein thrombus in a dog. J Am Vet Med Assoc 194:1449–1451, 1989.

746. Own LN, Hall LW. Ascites due to a metastasis from an adenocarcinoma of the ovary. Vet Rec 74:220–223, 1962.

747. Thornburg LP. Diseases of the liver in the dog and cat. Comp Cont Ed Pract Vet 4:538–547, 1982.

748. Suter PF. Portal vein anomalies in the dog: Their angiographic diagnosis. J Am Vet Radiol Soc 16:84–97, 1975.

749. Siderys H, Judd D, Herendeen TL, et al. The experimental production of elevated portal pressure by increasing portal flow. Surg Gynecol Obstet 120:514–516, 1965.

750. Sugar I, Jakab F, Szabo G. The effect of increased inferior vena cava pressure on hepatic circulation in the dog. Res Exp Med 171:263–270, 1977.

751. Kolata RJ, Cornelius LM, Bjorling DE, et al. Correction of an obstructive lesion of the caudal vena cava in a dog using a temporary intraluminal shunt. Vet Surg 11:100–104, 1982.

752. Cornelius L, Mahaffey M. Kinking of the intrathoracic caudal vena cava in five dogs. J Sm Anim Pract 26:67–80, 1985.

753. Blei AT, Gottsten J, Ganger D. Oral neomycin normalizes hyperdynamic features of awake portal hypertensive rats (abstract). Hepatology 8:1253, 1988.

754. Willems B, Villeneuve J-P, Huet P-M; Effect of propranolol on hepatic and systemic hemodynamics in dogs with chronic bile duct ligation. Hepatology 6:92–97, 1986.

755. Bosch J, Enriquez R, Groszmann RJ, et al. Chronic bile duct ligation in the dog: Hemodynamic characterization of a portal hypertensive model. Hepatology 3:1002–1007, 1983.

756. Witte MH, Witte CL, Dumont AE. Estimated net transcapillary water and protein flux in the liver and intestines of patients with portal hypertension from hepatic cirrhosis. Gastroenterology 80:265–272, 1980.

757. Popper H, Schaffner F. Capillarization of hepatic sinusoids in man. Gastroenterology 44:239–252, 1963.

758. Huet P-M, Goresky CA, Villeneuve J-P, et al. Assessment of liver microcirculation in human cirrhosis. J Clin Invest 70:1234–1244, 1982.

759. Witte CL, Witte MH, Dumont AE. Lymph imbalance in the genesis and perpetuation of the ascites syndrome in hepatic cirrhosis. Gastroenterology 78:1059–1068, 1980.

760. Witte CL, Chung YC, Witte M, et al. Observations on the orgin of ascites from experimental extrahepatic portal congestion. Ann Surg 170:1002–1015, 1969.

761. Shear L, Ching S, Gabuzda GJ. Compartmentalization of ascites and edema in patients with hepatic cirrhosis. N Engl J Med 282:1391–1396, 1970.

762. Witte C, Witte M, Dumont A. Dual origin of ascites in hepatic cirrhosis. Surg Gynecol Obstet 129:1027, 1969.

763. Epstein M. Functional renal abnormalities in cirrhosis: Pathophysiology and management. In: Zakim D, Boyer TD (eds) Hepatology, a Textbook of Liver Disease. WB Saunders, Philadelphia, 493–512, 1990.

764. Lill SR, Parsons RH, Buhac I. Permeability of the diaphragm and fluid reabsorption from the peritoneal cavity in the rat. Gastroenterology 76:997–1001, 1979.

765. Zink J, Greenway CV. Control of ascites absorption in anesthetized cats: Effects of intraperitoneal pressure, protein, and furosemide diuresis. Gastroenterology 73:1119–1124, 1977.

766. Zink J, Greenway CV. Intraperitoneal pressure in formation and reabsorption of ascites in cats. Am J Physiol 233:H185–H190, 1977.

767. Buhac I, Flesh L, Kishore R. Intraabdominal pressure and resorption of ascites in decompensated liver cirrhosis. J Lab Clin Med 104:264–270, 1984.

768. Lykkegaard Nielsen M, Justesen T, Asnaes S. Anaerobic bacteriological study of the human liver—with a critical review of the literature. Scand J Gastroenterol 9:671–677, 1974.

769. Schatten WE, Desprez JD, Holden WD. A bacteriologic study of portal-vein blood in man. AMA Arch Surg 404–408, 1955.

770. Dineen P. The importance of the route of infection in experimental biliary tract obstruction. Surg Gyn Obstet 1001–1008, 1964.

771. Sung JY, Shaffer EA, Olson ME. Bacterial invasion of the biliary system by way of the portal-venous system. Hepatology 14:313–317, 1991.

772. Jackaman FR, Hilson GRF, Smith L. Bile bacteria in patients with benign bile duct stricture. Br J Surg 67:329–332, 1980.

773. Bourgault AM, England DM, Rosenblatt JE, et al. Clinical characteristics of anaerobic bactibilia. Arch Intern Med 139:1346–1349, 1979.

774. Hancke E, Marklein G, Helpap B. Keimbesiedlung der gallenwege: Experimentelle hinweise auf einen entero-heptico-biliaren Bakterienkreislauf. Langenbecks Arch Chir 353:121–127, 1980.

775. Eade MN, Brooke BN. Portal bacteraemia in cases of ulcerative colitis submitted to colectomy. Lancet 1:1008–1009, 1969.

776. Hambraeus A, Laurell G, Nybacka O, et al. Biliary tract surgery: A bacteriologic and epidemiologic study. Acta Chir Scand 156:155–160, 1990.

777. Wells CL, Maddaus MA, Simmons RL. Role of the macrophage in the translocation of intestinal bacteria. Arch Surg 122:48–53, 1987.

778. Hume DA, Doe WF. The role of macrophages in cellular defense. In: Heyworth MF, Jones AL (eds) Immunology of the Gastrointestinal Tract and Liver. Raven Press, New York, 23, 1988.

779. Jones EA, Summerfield JA. Kupffer cells. In: Arias IM, Jakoby WB, Popper H, et al. (eds) The Liver: Biology and Pathobiology. Raven Press, New York, 683–708, 1988.

780. Bradfield JW. Liver sinusoidal cells. J Pathol 142:5–6, 1984.

781. Rogoff TM, Lipsky PE. Role of the Kupffer cells in local and systemic immune responses. Gastroenterology 80:854–860, 1981.

782. Maitra SK, Rachmilewitz D, Eberle D, et al. The hepatocellular uptake and biliary excretion of endotoxin in the rat. Hepatology 1:401–407, 1981.

783. Nolan JP. Intestinal endotoxins as mediators of hepatic injury—an idea whose time has come again. Hepatology 10:887–891, 1989.

784. Bigatello LM, Broitman SA, Fattori L, et al. Endotoxins, encephalopathy and mortality in cirrhotic patients. Am J Gastroenterol 82:11–15, 1987.

785. Lumnsden AB, Henderson JM, Kutner MH. Endotoxin levels measured by a chromogenic assay in portal, hepatic and peripheral venous blood in patients with cirrhosis. Hepatology 8:232–236, 1988.

786. Liehr H, Grun M. Clinical aspects of Kupffer cell failure in liver diseases. In: Wisse E, Knook DL (eds) Kupffer Cells and Other Liver Sinusoidal Cells. Elsevier/North Holland, Amsterdam, 427–436, 1977.

787. Ruiter KJ, van der Meulen J, Wisse E. Some cell biological and pathological aspects of endotoxin uptake by the liver. In: Liehr H, Grun M (eds) The Reticuloendothelial System and the Pathogenesis of Liver Disease. Elsevier/North Holland, Amsterdam, 267–277, 1980.

788. Liehr H, Grun M, Thiel H, et al. Endotoxin-induced liver necrosis and intravascular coagulation in rats enhanced by portacaval collateral circulation. Gut 16:429–436, 1975.

789. Gaeta GB, Perna P, Adinolfi LE, et al. Endotoxemia in a series of 104 patients with chronic liver disease: Prevalence and significance. Digestion 23:239–244, 1982.

790. Prytz J, Holst-Christensen J, Korner B, et al. Portal venous and systemic endotoxemia in patients without liver disease and systemic endotoxemia in patients with cirrhosis. Scand J Gastroenterol 11:857–863, 1976.

791. Bigatello LM, Broitman SA, Fattori L, et al. Endotoxemia, encephalopathy, and mortality in cirrhotic patients. Am J Gastroenterol 82:11–15, 1987.

792. Tarao K, So K, Moroi T, et al. Detection of endotoxin in plasma and ascites of patients with cirrhosis; its clinical significance. Gastroenterology 73:539–542, 1976.

793. Leihr H, Grun M, Brunswig. Endotoxaemia in acute hepatic failure. Acta Hepato-Gastroenterol 23:235–240, 1976.

794. Nolan JP. Endotoxin, reticulendothelial function, and liver injury. Hepatology 5:458–465, 1981.

795. Lumsden AB, Henderson JM, Kutner MH. Endotoxin levels measured by a chromogenic assay in portal, hepatic, and peripheral venous blood in patients with cirrhosis. Hepatology 8:232–236, 1988.

796. Guarner F, Wallace JL, MacNaughton WK, et al. Endotoxin induced ascites formation in the rat: Partial mediation by platelet activating factor. Hepatology 10:788–794, 1989.

797. Peterson SL, Koblik PD, Whiting PG, et al. Endotoxin concentrations measured by a chromogenic assay in portal and peripheral venous blood in ten dogs with portosystemic shunts. J Vet Int Med 5:71–74, 1991.

798. Bradfield JWB. Reticuloendothelial blockade: A reassessment. In: Wisse E, Knook DL (eds) Kupffer Cells and Other Liver Sinusoidal Cells. Amsterdam, Elsevier, 365–372, 1977.

799. Brown WR, Kloppel TM. The liver and IgA: Immunological, cell biological and clinical implications. Hepatology 9:763–784, 1989.

800. Kleinman RE, Harmatz PR, Walker WA. The liver: An integral part of the enteric mucosal immune system. Hepatology 2:379–384, 1982.

801. Sarfeh IJ, Tarnawski A. Gastric mucosal vasculopathy in portal hypertension. Gastroenterology 93:1129–1131, 1987.

802. Lingenfelser T, Krige JE. The stomach in cirrhosis. J Clin Gastroenterol 17:92–96, 1993.

803. Vigneri S, Termini R, Piraino A, et al. The stomach in liver cirrhosis: Endoscopic, morphological, and clinical correlations. Gastroenterology 101:472–478, 1991.

804. Viggiano TR, Gostout CJ. Portal hypertensive intestinal vasculopathy: A review of the clinical, endoscopic, and histopathologic features. Am J Gastroenterol 87:944–954, 1992.

805. Sarfeh IM, Tarnawski A, Malki A, et al. Portal hypertension and gastric mucosal injury in rats. Gastroenterology 84:987–993, 1983.

806. Quintero E, Pique JM, Bombi JA, et al. Gastric mucosal vascular ectasias causing bleeding in cirrhosis: A distinct entity associated with hypergastrinemia and low serum levels of pepsinogen I. Gastroenterology 93:1054–1061, 1987.

807. Albillos A, Colombato LA, Enriquez R, et al. Sequence of morphological and hemodynamic changes of gastric microvessels in portal hypertension. Gastroenterology 102:2066–2070, 1992.

808. Lam SK. Hypergastrinaemia in cirrhosis of liver. Gut 17:700–708, 1976.

809. Strunz UT, Thompson MR, Elashoff J, et al. Hepatic inactivation of gastrins of various chain lengths in dogs. Gastroenterology 74:550–553, 1978.

810. Hein MF, Silen W, Skillman JJ, et al. The effect of portacaval shunting on gastric secretion in cirrhotic dogs. Gastroenterology 44:637–641, 1963.

811. Epstein M. Hepatorenal syndrome. In: Epstein M (ed) The Kidney in Liver Disease, 3rd ed. Williams & Wilkins, Baltimore, 89–118, 1988.

812. Wilkinson SP, Moore KP, Arroyo V. Pathogenesis of ascites and hepatorenal syndrome. Gut (suppl) S12-S17, 1991.
813. Arroyo V, Planas R, Gaya J, et al. Sympathetic nervous activity, renin-angiotensin system and renal excretion and prostaglandin E_2 in cirrhosis. Relationship to functional renal failure and sodium and water excretion. Eur J Clin Invest 13:271–278, 1983.
814. Moore K, Wendon J, Frazer M, et al. Plasma endothelin immunoreactivity in liver disease and the hepatorenal syndrome. N Engl J Med 327:1774–1778, 1992.

31

Hepatic Pathology

DENNY J. MEYER

INTRODUCTION

This chapter is principally written for the veterinarian who performs liver biopsies and interprets the report and the veterinary student who is applying histopathologic concepts to the morphologic basis of liver disease. It offers suggestions to consider when obtaining and submitting the biopsy and is intended to be a practical aid for interpreting the biopsy report. The more common terms and histopathologic findings are defined and illustrated. Woven throughout the chapter is an emphasis on the dynamic response of the liver to injury, the pathophysiologic consequences, and the impact of both primary hepatic disease and extrahepatic events.

MICROSCOPIC STRUCTURE-FUNCTION RELATIONSHIP

The liver is composed of two things: glandular acini and various branches of vessels. Hence if some common work is to result from them, there must be some commerce between the glands and the vessels.

Marcello Malpighi, 1666.

The parenchyma of the liver is histologically composed of lobules or units. The two more commonly accepted models are the classic lobule and the acinar unit defined by histologic and functional criteria, respectively. The development of the classic lobule was predicated on histologic observations made on the pig liver because of the notably dense connective tissue delineation of lobular structures.[1] The raccoon, camel, and polar bear show similar well-defined histology. Dense connective tissue septa define the boundaries of a polygonal area 1 to 2 mm in diameter. Portal triads are located at the corners of the polygon. A portal triad is comprised of a branch of the portal vein, a branch of the hepatic artery, and a bile ductule surrounded by connective tissue. The central vein is located in the center of the lobule, giving rise to the additional nomenclature of central vein unit. Cords of parenchymal cells, supported by a delicate network of reticular tissue and separated by endothelial cell–lined channels of the sinusoids, radiate from the central vein toward the portal tracts located at the periphery of the lob-

ule. Unfortunately, the paucity of connective tissue in the dog and cat make identification of the polygonal structure virtually impossible to visualize without pathology (Figures 31–1 to 31–5).

Later, based on studies of the hepatic microcirculation, the liver acinus concept was developed.[2,3] The acinus is a variably sized clump of hepatocytes oriented around the terminal portal and arterial (afferent) vessels and bile ductules. In humans, the acinus is approximately 2 mm in diameter and comprised of approximately 100,000 parenchymal cells.[4] The afferent vessels form the axis of the acinus from which blood flows through the sinusoids to the terminal hepatic venule (the central vein of the classic lobule). The terminal hepatic venule receives blood from several adjacent acini. The liver acinus is not microscopically visible in formalin-fixed tissue and is discernible only with special dye injection techniques. The characterization of the liver unit based on a functional concept facilitates the subsequent finding of functional hepatocyte heterogeneity.[5,6] Based on the functional heterogeneity within the lobule, three concentric zones around the vascular axis have been suggested. The periportal population of hepatocytes (zone 1) surround the axis of the acinus, and the perivenous (centrilobular, pericentral, periacinar) population of hepatocytes (zone 3) are located most distant from

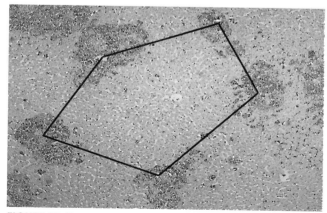

FIGURE 31–1. The pentagonal shape of the classic lobule is approximated by a predominantly portal (zone 1) infiltrate of neoplastic lymphocytes (dark blue). This is a frequent microanatomic location of hepatic lymphoma. Neoplastic foci are scattered throughout the parenchyma. The central vein is located in the center. H&E ×20.

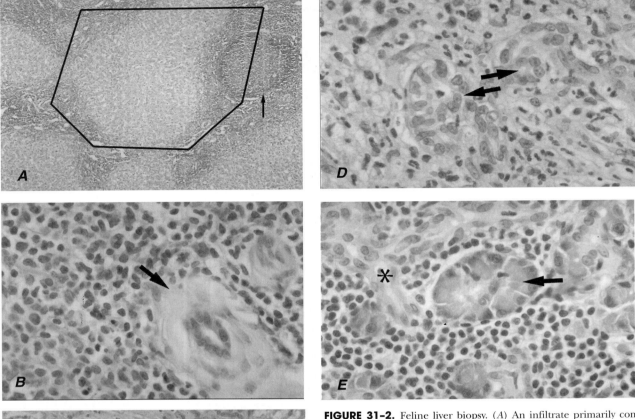

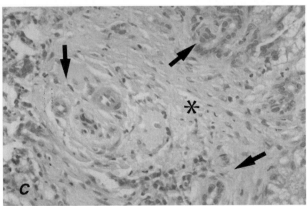

FIGURE 31-2. Feline liver biopsy. (*A*) An infiltrate primarily comprised of lymphocytes and lesser numbers of plasma cells are aggregated in the portal areas. Extension of the infiltrate along zone 1 to adjacent portal tracts provides an outline of the classical lobule. This form of chronic hepatitis is referred to as the chronic lymphocytic "cholangitis/cholangiohepatitis" syndrome and has histopathologic similarities to primary biliary cirrhosis and hepatitis C in humans.[79–80,102–107] A prominent lymphoid follicle is noted to the far right of the central vein (arrow). (*B*) In this high power field, a dense population of primarily small lymphocytes surrounds a thick bile duct (arrow). (*C*) This portal tract is expanded by dense connective tissue (asterisk); hyperplastic bile ducts (arrows) and scattered lymphocytes are located at the periphery of the fibrosis. (*D*) Occasionally, portal tracts (arrows indicate hyperplastic bile ducts) are infiltrated by a mixed inflammatory infiltrate comprised of neutrophils, lymphocytes, and rare eosinophil. This inflammatory variability emphasizes the importance of adequate sampling for an accurate histologic assessment and interpretation. (*E*) Numerous lymphocytes surround pancreatic acinar tissue (arrow) and ducts (asterisk). Lymphocytic infiltrates in the liver and pancreas of the same animal have been noted.[60,102]

the vasculature axis, that is, closest to the terminal hepatic vein. The intermediate (mid-zonal) area of hepatocytes (zone 2) is empirically sandwiched between zones 1 and 3. Zone 1 hepatocytes are the first to be exposed to blood rich in oxygen and nutrients and, among their many functions, they are primarily responsible for the efficient removal of bile acids from the portal blood.[7] In contrast, zone 3 hepatocytes remove canine intestinal alkaline phosphatase by adsorptive endocytosis and are bathed in blood with lowest oxygen content because it has percolated through zones 1 and 2[8] (Figure 31-6). Hepatocytes in zone 1 are the first to be insulted by direct-acting hepatotoxins. However, the enzymatic heterogeneity of hepatocytes, especially the high activity of the cytochrome P-450 monooxygenases in zone 3, gives these hepatocytes a greater capacity for the formation of toxic metabolites from xenobiotics (substances foreign to hepatic metabolism) and increases their risk of damage.[9] In summary, the lobule is comprised of hepatocytes that appear

morphologically uniform, but biochemically and functionally represent a heterogeneous population. The classic hepatic lobule represents a disparity between the structural unit and the functional unit. By convention, pathologic changes often are reported in terms relative to the classic lobule. Investigations into the hepatic pathology, especially those related to vascular disturbances, should utilize the liver acinus concept.[4,10–13]

Hepatocytes account for approximately 60% of the total cell number comprising the liver. In the human liver, there are approximately 200,000 hepatocytes per milligram tissue with an approximate life span of 200 days.[14–16] Nonparenchymal cells constitute the remaining cell population and, because they line the liver sinusoid, are sometimes referred to as sinusoidal cells. Specific phenotypic and functional

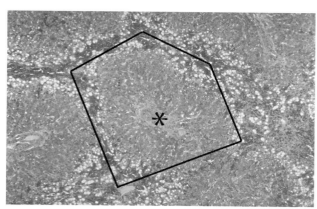

FIGURE 31-3. Marked congestion of zone 3 (centrilobular, periacinar) in a dog with acute congestive heart failure with secondary hydropic degeneration of the hepatocytes is illustrative of that zonal pattern in the liver. A normal portal tract (asterisk) is located in the center and is highlighted with the use of a trichrome stain, ×20.

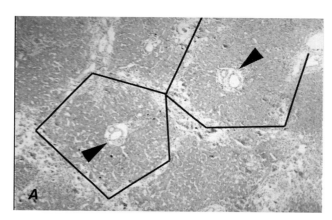

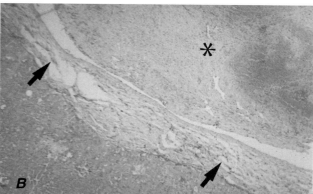

FIGURE 31-4. (*A*) The classic lobule is delineated by zone 3 hepatocellular degeneration and necrosis subsequent to hepatic vein thrombosis (Budd-Chiari-like syndrome)[108,109] of undetermined etiology in a 9-month-old great dane. Two portal tracts are located to the lower left and upper right of center (arrowheads). (*B*) Thrombosed hepatic vein; thrombus is observed to upper right (asterisk), hepatic parenchyma to the lower left, and a thickened vessel wall is diagonally located top left to bottom right (arrow). H&E ×20.

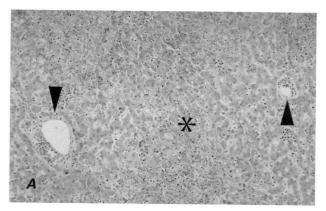

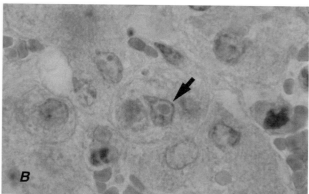

FIGURE 31-5. (*A*) Zone 3 necrosis (asterisk) in a dog with infectious canine hepatitis; unaffected periportal areas (zone 1), to the lower left and upper right of center, are noted by the clear lumen of the bile ducts (arrowheads). H&E ×40. It is not known why the virus has a predilection for zone 3. (*B*) A rare intranuclear inclusion body (arrow) is present. H&E ×1000.

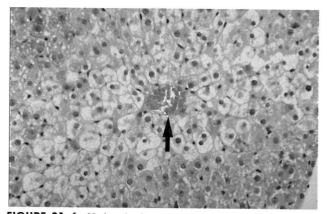

FIGURE 31-6. Hydropic degeneration is prominent in zone 3 hepatocytes secondary to hypoxia in a dog with immune-mediated hemolytic anemia (PCV = 10%). Hepatocellular degeneration probably contributes to the increase in serum aminotransferase activity frequently noted in these patients. A blood-filled central vein is located in the center (arrow). H&E ×200.

characteristics permit the identification of four cell types: endothelial cells, Kupffer cells, lipocytes, and pit cells.[17] Endothelial cells form the sinusoids and have a wide variety of functions including filtration, lipoprotein uptake, endocytosis, and secretion of bioactive factors. Kupffer cells represent the largest population of macrophages in the body. They are involved in the clearance of a variety of substances, antigen processing, and secretion of bioactive factors and cell-mediated cytotoxicity. The term *littoral cells* has been used to collectively define Kupffer cells and endothelial cells. Lipocytes (Ito cells, stellate cells, fat-storing cells, vitamin A–storing cells) are located in the space of Disse and have received considerable attention recently for their role in hepatic fibrosis[18] (Figure 31–7). The cells express transforming growth factor beta and, as the name implies, store and metabolize retinoids. Pit cells morphologically resemble large granular lymphocytes/NK cells. The term *pit* was first used to describe the electron-dense cytoplasmic granules.

In summary, the hepatic lobule is comprised of parenchymal and nonparenchymal cells that demonstrate remarkable biochemical and functional diversity. The cellular heterogeneity, rich blood supply, and sentinel location between the outside of the body (gastrointestinal tract) and the internal milieu permit development of hepatic pathology that is primary in origin as well as a consequence of extrahepatic diseases.

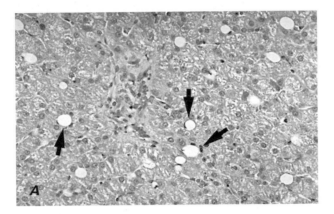

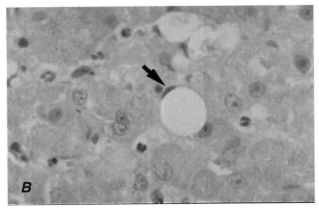

FIGURE 31-7. (*A*) Multiple lipocytes are easily recognized in cats and dogs by the clear punctuated areas left after the fixative has removed the lipid from their cytoplasm (arrows). (*B*) Although they appear to be located in, and in this case, occlude the sinusoid, the cell resides in the space of Disse, which is not microscopically discernable. The nucleus is displaced to the periphery of the cell (arrow) giving it a signet ring appearance. It is not known if their prominence is a physiologic or pathologic phenomenon. The finding is not equivalent to hepatic lipidosis. H&E ×200.

THE BIOPSY SPECIMEN

The establishment of an accurate diagnosis is dependent on sampling an adequate amount of tissue and, more importantly, on a histologic interpretation by someone well versed in liver histopathology.[19]

Types

The liver biopsy provides only a small window for viewing histopathologic changes. Biopsy specimens of the liver are usually obtained with needles, alligator-type cutting instruments, and by surgical excision. Suction/aspiration-type needles (Menghini, Jamshidi) or cutting type (Tru-cut, Vim-Silverman with Franklin modification) provide a core of tissue that represents approximately 1/50,000 of the whole organ. The type of needle used impacts on the volume (amount) of tissue available for sectioning. Differences in tissue volume will vary with the square of the radius of the core for specimens of equal length. For example, a 1 cm specimen obtained with a Menghini needle will have a volume approximately 1.5 times more than one obtained with a Vim-Silverman needle. The cutting-type needle is useful in obtaining successful specimens from cirrhotic livers.[20] Early or subtle changes in liver architecture associated with cirrhosis or nodular regeneration are likely to be missed with a needle biopsy specimen.[21]

The length and management of the specimen are important factors to ensure an adequate number of lobules for evaluation (Figure 31–8). One study noted that a 5 mm length permitted the diagnosis of acute viral hepatitis but was insufficient for the reliable diagnosis of chronic hepatitis; a 15 mm length was reliable.[22,23] The observation of bridging hepatic necrosis and bridging fibrosis are prognostically important to communicate.[24,25] An intact needle biopsy at least 2 cm in length is suggested as minimally adequate for the identification of at least two "bridges"[26,27] (Figure 31–9).

The wedge biopsy provides ample tissue and contains larger portal tracts than those deeper in the hepatic parenchyma. Because of its superficial location relative to blood supply, the margin of the liver is predisposed to fibrosis that may mimic changes of cirrhosis[28] (Figure 31–10). In this location, fibrous septa join portal tracts to the subcapsular connective tissue or to each other, and vessels are sometimes unusually close. This would be particularly problematic if the specimen was obtained with a clam shell–type biopsy forceps used at laparoscopy that may only cut 2 to 4 mm deep. The subcapsular zone of the liver may show more extensive necrosis than deeper parenchyma in chronic hepatitis, resulting in an overly pessimistic interpretation.[29]

Lack of uniformity in selecting the biopsy site for repeat biopsies could affect the evaluation for disease progression and therapeutic efficacy. Varying degrees of crush artifact at the periphery of the biopsy specimen further reduces the area available for adequate evaluation.

A biopsy taken a period of time after the beginning of a surgical procedure can contain neutrophils that accumulate under the capsule and focally in liver cell plates[30] (Figure 31–11). Along with isolated liver cell necrosis, the artifactual process would morphologically resemble focal suppurative hepatitis. Heavy sedation appears to have the potential for producing similar artifact.[31] Changes are thought to be secondary to anoxia. A few inflammatory cells may also be seen in portal tracts; the lesion would be described as mild cholangitis.

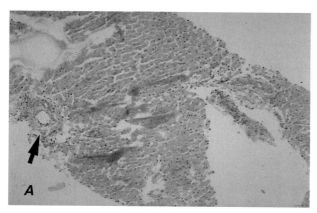

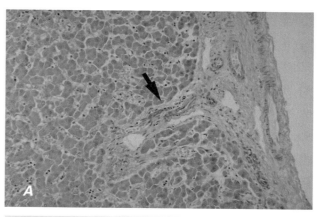

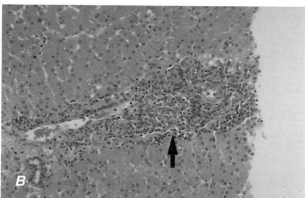

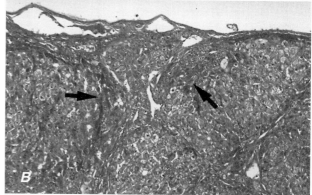

FIGURE 31-8. (*A*) This fragmented specimen obtained during ultrasound examination had only one portal tract located on the edge (arrow) and should be considered an inadequate sample. (*B*) A second specimen obtained with a laparoscopy-guided Tru-cut needle contained multiple portal tracts; an inflammatory infiltrate is readily apparent in one (arrow). H&E ×20; H&E ×40.

Fixatives and Stains

Liver specimens are routinely fixed in 10% buffered formalin. Needle biopsies should be placed on supportive material (e.g., a piece of cardboard, Teflon pad, or absorbable gel-type sponge) prior to being placed into the formalin to protect against fragmentation. Gauze pads should be avoided

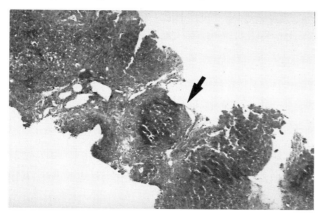

FIGURE 31-9 (see **Plate I**). This needle biopsy, 2 cm long from a 4-year-old German shepherd with ascites (transudate), demonstrates the importance of an adequate specimen for assessing fibrosis. Both bridging fibrosis and micronodule formation (arrow) can be appreciated with a trichrome stain. A Tru-cut needle was used in combination with laparoscopy. Trichrome stain ×12.

FIGURE 31-10. (*A*) The capsule is thick and the portal tract is prominent in this wedge section obtained at necropsy from an aged dog without clinical or biochemical findings of liver disease. Fibrous septa join portal tracts to subcapsular connective tissue (arrow) and, when cut longitudinally, can appear similar to increased portal fibrosis.[28] (*B*) (see **Plate I**) A trichrome stain accentuates two septa (arrow). There are a small number of cells present, predominantly lymphocytes as well, not an uncommon finding in older dogs. Inadvertent needle biopsy of this site or an inadequate tissue specimen could give histologic findings compatible with chronic hepatitis and hepatic fibrosis. H&E ×40; trichrome ×100.

because of the potential for the fibers to compress segments of the specimen, resulting in crush artifact. Fixation in absolute alcohol has been suggested for the reliable demonstration of glycogen.[32] In that study, glycogen-rich liver tissue fixed in 10% buffered formalin or Bouin's solution did not generally stain with periodic acid–Schiff reaction (PAS). An unexpected PAS-negative finding when attempting to define a morphologic change in a formalin-fixed specimen may be a consequence of the type of fixative (Figure 31–12). Fixation for transmission electron microscopy requires 1 mm cubes of tissue be placed in 2.5% glutaraldehyde in 0.1 m phosphate buffer for at least 3 hours and subsequent processing steps by someone knowledgeable with the process. If mucopolysaccharidoses is suspected, tissue is placed in Lindsay's dioxane picrate solution. This storage disease has been described in both cats and dogs,[33] and can present with hepatomegaly and hepatocellular changes that are suggestive of hepatic lipidosis.

Stains required beyond the routine hematoxylin and eosin vary and are often limited by economical considerations. Most diagnostic pathologists suggest a reticulin stain and a collagen stain to complement the evaluation of hepatic architecture and inflammatory liver diseases (Figure 31–13). The former assesses structural changes associated with necrosis by

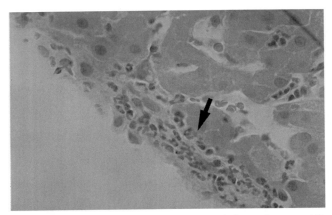

FIGURE 31-11. Focal, subcapsular accumulations of neutrophils (arrow) are present in this wedge biopsy taken to evaluate areas of hepatic discoloration at the completion of a lengthy exploratory laparotomy. Superficial sinusoidal migration of the neutrophils is also observed, but necroinflammatory findings were not observed in the rest of the specimen. It is possible that the neutrophil infiltrate is associated with the anesthesia or surgical procedure.[30,31] H&E ×400.

outlining areas of focal necrosis and parenchymal collapse secondary to extensive necrosis. The latter stain highlights the presence and magnitude of collagen deposition in the process of hepatic fibrosis and is important for the early definition of cirrhosis (Figures 31–14 to 31–16).

Frozen sections of formalin-fixed tissue can be stained with oil red-O for the demonstration of neutral lipid in hepatocytes and the identification of lipocytes. Lipid can be preserved in paraffin sections by postfixation in osmium tetroxide. The Schultz modification of the Liebermann-Burchardt reaction can be used to stain for cholesterol in frozen sec-

tions if cholesterol ester storage disease is suspected. Phospholipid can be identified in frozen sections in Niemann-Pick disease. The disease has been diagnosed in young cats; notable findings include neurologic signs, hepatomegaly, abnormal liver tests, and microscopic findings suggestive of hepatic lipidosis[34,35] (Figure 31–17).

Measurement of Copper and Iron

The increasing routine use of stains for iron and copper in the differentiation of hepatic pigment has identified their presence in a variety of liver diseases (Figure 31–18). In addition to identifying iron with Mallory's stain, it has the advantage of highlighting the green of bile pigment and amplifying the golden color of lipofuscin in the further differentiation of yellow granules. The stain for copper-containing pigment is mandatory in breeds known to be predisposed to the toxic effects of copper accumulation (Figure 31–19). Histochemical identification of copper-containing granules can be correlated to its quantitative analysis for certain stains.[36] Prolonged staining (72 hours) with rubeanic acid has been shown to be the method of choice for the detection of copper in the canine liver. The presence of copper-containing granules is consistently observed with that stain when the copper concentration is above 400 ppm. Orcein does not consistently demonstrate granules when the copper concentration is increased.[36] This study indicates that the identification of copper in formalin-fixed wedge biopsies is a valid procedure. After 7 months of formalin fixation, the reactions for rubeanic acid and rhodanine are lost. The reaction is maintained if the tissue is embedded in paraffin blocks. Consequently, control tissue for histochemical reactions should be stored in paraffin blocks.[36]

Copper can be quantitated from fresh and formalin-fixed

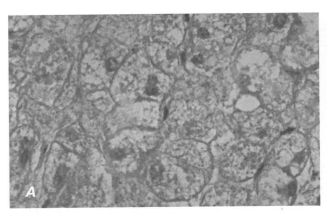

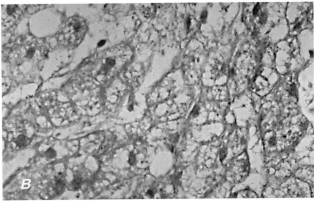

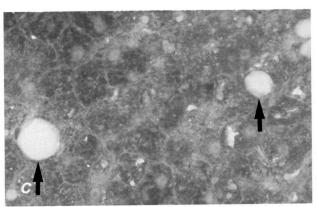

FIGURE 31-12. (A) Diffuse hydropic degeneration was observed in this liver biopsy from a dog with an increased serum alkaline phosphatase activity. (B) The formalin-fixed specimen stained with periodic acid–Schiff reaction (PAS) identifies minimal glycogen in contrast to the specimen fixed in absolute alcohol (C) that demonstrates abundant glycogen; two Ito cells (arrows) are accentuated by the PAS-positive glycogen. (A) H&E ×400; (B) formalin fixed; and (C) fixation in absolute alcohol followed by PAS staining before amylase activity (diastase) ×400.

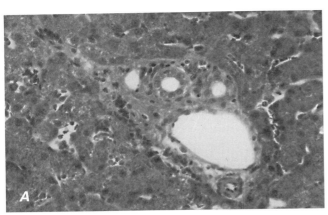

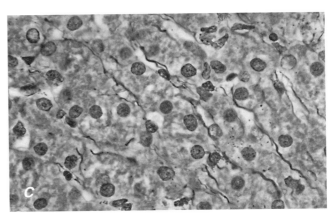

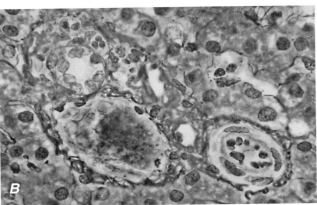

FIGURE 31-13. (*A*) (see **Plate I**) A trichrome stain demonstrates collagen associated with a normal portal tract; note that the surrounding parenchyma does not appreciably stain for collagen. (*B*) A reticulin stain demonstrates the reticular network in and around a normal portal tract, and (*C*) its delicate distribution throughout the parenchyma. Trichrome ×400; Reticulin stain ×400.

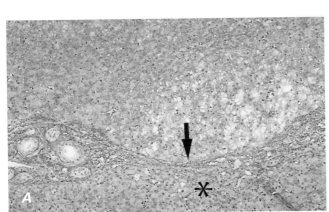

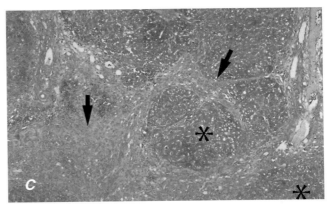

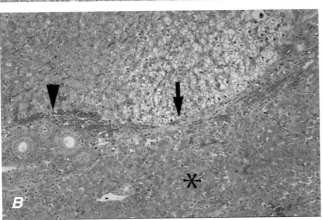

FIGURE 31-14. This wedge biopsy is from a 12-year-old dog with a small liver and numerous variably sized hepatic nodules. (*A*) The reticulin stain demonstrates compression of hepatic tissue (asterisk) by nodular formation (arrow); most of the hepatocytes show varying degrees of hydropic degeneration. (*B*) (see **Plate I**) A trichrome stain demonstrates no excessive connective tissue. A portal tract is located to the far left (arrowhead). (*C*) (see **Plate I**) In contrast, this trichrome-stained specimen from a grossly similar appearing liver demonstrates diffuse, dense connective tissue (arrows) in association with architecturally abnormal regenerative nodules (asterisks) compatible with cirrhosis. Reticulin stain ×40; trichrome stain ×40;

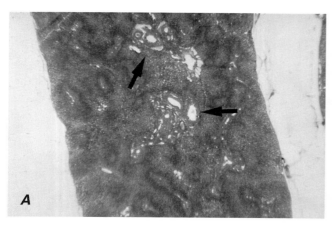

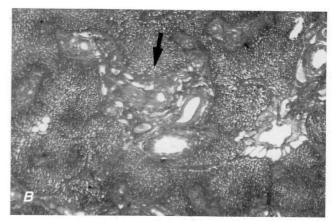

FIGURE 31-15. (*A* and *B*) A trichrome stain demonstrates moderate to marked portal fibrosis involving all portal tracts (arrows) in this 4-month-old boxer with ascites (transudate) and markedly increased serum total bile acid concentration. There is no necrosis or inflammation associated with the fibrosis, suggesting a congenital event. Multiple, presumably acquired, portosystemic shunts were present. This case and others[110,111] highlight the importance of the histologic evaluation of the liver in young dogs with portosystemic shunts. Trichrome stain ×20; ×100.

specimens or, if already embedded for sectioning, deparaffinized tissue used.[36] Although the initial accumulation of copper is generally located in zone 3[37-40] (Figure 31-20), the development of altered architecture can result in pseudolobules that do not contain copper.[36] When the liver appears to be grossly abnormal, it may be prudent to submit more than one specimen for copper measurement.

Iron can be accurately measured in deparaffinized specimens.[41] However, placing fresh liver tissue in saline for as little as 1 hour can result in up to a 50% iron loss.[41]

Cytology

Although histologic examination remains the cornerstone for the evaluation of hepatic pathology, cytologic specimens obtained by the fine needle aspiration technique can provide valuable information and preclude the need for a biopsy. Needle aspiration is a suction-type procedure and relatively safer than a cutting technique. The arrangement of the plump hepatocytes in cords and the limited amount of connective tissue facilitate their exfoliation. Because the speci-

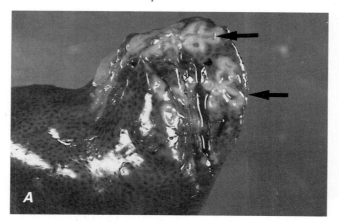

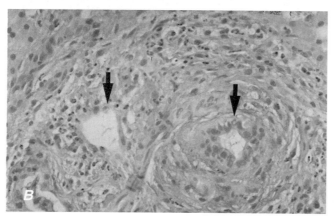

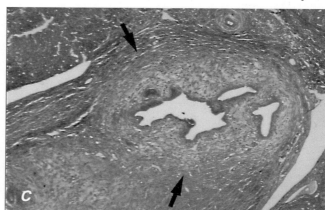

FIGURE 31-16. (*A*) Grossly thickened bile ducts (arrows) are visible in a cat infected with liver flukes. (*B*) Marked periductal fibrosis with edema and a mixed inflammatory cell infiltrate (neutrophils, eosinophils, and lymphocytes) are present. Bile ducts are indicated by arrows. (*C*) The trichrome stain dramatically illustrates the extent of the fibrotic process (arrows). The common bile duct, not shown, is similarly affected. The magnitude of fibrosis indicates why some do not respond to medical management. H&E ×400; trichrome ×40.

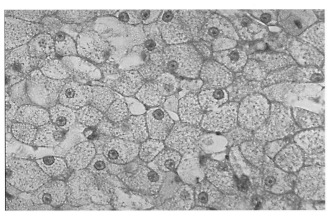

FIGURE 31-17 (see **Plate I**). Diffuse, microvesicular, lipid accumulation in a kitten affected with Niemann-Pick type C disease. H&E ×400. (Courtesy of Dr. Diane E. Brown, Department of Pathology, Colorado State University)

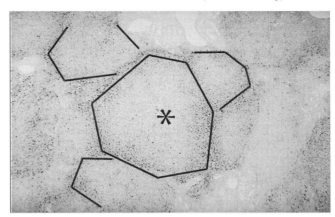

FIGURE 31-20. A rhodanine stain demonstrates the predominantly zone 3 accumulation of copper in this wedge biopsy from a Bedlington terrier and outlines the shape of a classic lobule. A portal tract is centrally located (asterisk). Rhodanine stain ×20.

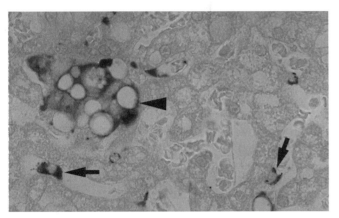

FIGURE 31-18 (see **Plate II**). A Prussian blue stain demonstrates the accumulation of iron in Kupffer cells and a foci (arrowhead) of pigment and lipid-filled cells morphologically compatible with macrophages (lipogranulomata). Arrows indicate Kupffer cells with iron. Prussian blue iron stain ×400.

men represents a smaller part of the hepatic parenchyma than the biopsy and does not permit the assessment of architecture, selection of the appropriate candidate is important for successful application.

In general, the presence of hepatomegaly suggests a change that diffusely involves the hepatic parenchyma. Hepatomegaly facilitates identification of the organ and percutaneous aspiration. Examples of diseases that can be cytologically recognized with relative consistency include lymphoma, mast cell neoplasia, corticosteroid-induced hepatocellular change, lipidosis, amyloidosis, and hepatocellular carcinoma.[42] The cytologic examination of an aspirate or scraping obtained from a focal lesion(s) discovered intraoperatively provides a quick means of evaluation. If inadequate information is obtained, a biopsy can be subsequently taken (Figures 31–21 to 31–27).

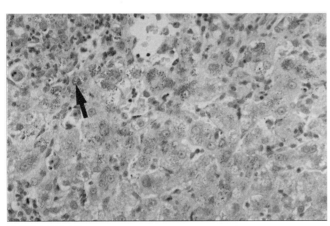

FIGURE 31-19. A rhodanine stain highlights the copper accumulated in the cytoplasm of hepatocytes. A suppurative necroinflammatory process is noted at the upper left in this biopsy from a Bedlington terrier; lesser number of lymphocytes and macrophages are present, ×400.

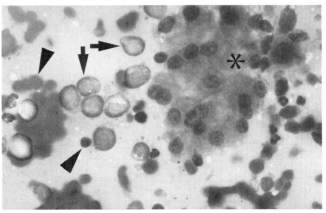

FIGURE 31-21. An aspirate from an icteric 2-year-old dog with hepatomegaly. A clump of hepatocytes (asterisk) with abundant basophilic cytoplasm is associated with a uniform population of large lymphocytes with scant cytoplasm (arrows). The large size of the lymphocytes can be better appreciated by comparing them to the diameter of the pale yellow to yellow-green erythrocytes, often clumped, scattered throughout the field (arrowheads). These findings are consistent with hepatic lymphoma. Diff-Quik stain ×400.

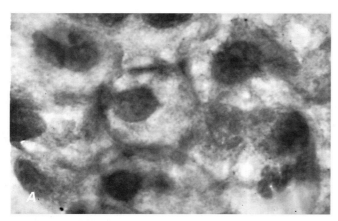

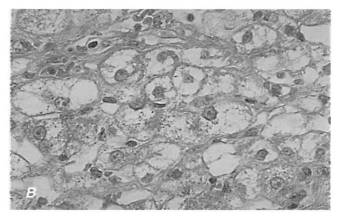

FIGURE 31-22. (*A*) An aspirate from a dog with hepatomegaly, moderately increased serum alkaline phosphatase activity, and serum total bilirubin concentration within reference range. Most hepatocytes have lacy to wispy indistinct cytoplasm consistent with glycogen accumulation. (*B*) Similar changes are histologically observed from a needle biopsy. The dog had been given a long-acting corticosteroid parenterally 2 weeks earlier. Diff-Quik stain ×1000; H&E ×400.

THE ROLE OF THE PATHOLOGIST

Upon examining the liver biopsy the pathologist performs two functions. The first is to describe the histopathologic changes, assess their severity, and define their location in the lobule or unit. The second responsibility is to attempt to relate these findings with the clinicopathologic information. It is intuitive that to execute the second responsibility, the appropriate information needs to be part of the submission process.

When submitting the specimen, it may be useful to ask specific questions on the form so the pathologist can address them during the microscopic examination. The questions often will reflect the indication for the biopsy. Why is hepatomegaly present? Why is the patient jaundiced? Why are multiple serum liver enzyme tests increased (and provide the values)? Why is only the serum alkaline phosphatase activity increased? Why are the serum bile acid concentrations markedly increased in association with a normal serum bilirubin concentration? Are there findings that help define the cause of an abdominal effusion? Providing the pathologist with a classification of the ascites (transudate or modified transudate)[43] can assist in the assessment of the microscopic findings.

In many cases, the examination of the liver biopsy is an art honed by experience. The most meaningful interpretation of the findings is predicated by a dialogue between clinician and pathologist.

RESPONSE TO INJURY AND DISEASE

Regeneration

Although most tissues demonstrate a similar repertoire of responses to injury, the liver demonstrates several unique features. One of the most fascinating characteristics is the capacity to regenerate rapidly following injury.

HEPATIC STEM CELL. A probable candidate for a stem or progenitor cell identified in the rat liver is the oval cell. They are small, bland-appearing epithelial-like cells located in zone 1, near the portal tract, and appear to be associated with the bile ductule cells or a distinct population of periductual cells.[44,45] These cells are involved in the embryogenesis of liver and can proliferate and migrate into zones 2 and 3.[46,47] The cell compartment can be induced to differentiate into hepatocytelike cells, biliary-type cells, and neoplastic cells of hepatobiliary derivation.

HEPATOCELLULAR PROLIFERATION. A widely accepted the-

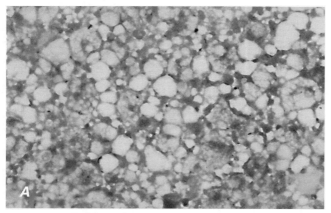

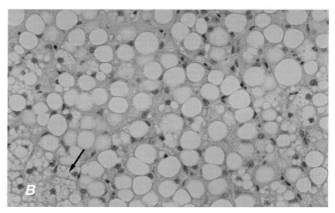

FIGURE 31-23. (*A*) An aspirate from an icteric cat with moderately increased serum alkaline phosphatase activity. Most hepatocytes contain a large clear vacuole that displaces the nucleus to the periphery of the cell. Other hepatocytes have multiple small clear vacuoles. These findings are consistent with hepatic lipidosis. (*B*) Similar morphologic changes are histologically observed; microvesiculated hepatocytes are located to the lower left (arrow). Diff-Quik stain ×200; H&E ×200.

Plate I

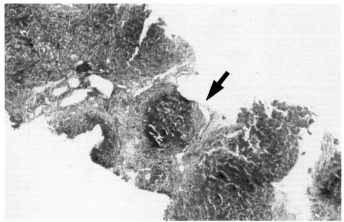

FIGURE 31-9. This needle biopsy, 2 cm long from a 4-year-old German shepherd with ascites (transudate), demonstrates the importance of an adequate specimen for assessing fibrosis. Both bridging fibrosis and micronodule formation (arrow) can be appreciated with a trichrome stain. A Tru-cut needle was used in combination with laparoscopy. Trichrome stain ×12.

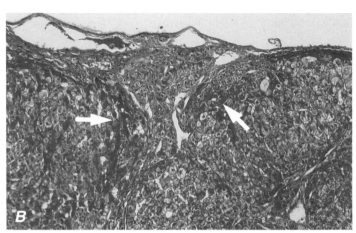

FIGURE 31-10. (*B*) A trichrome stain accentuates two septa (arrow). There are a small number of cells present, predominantly lymphocytes as well, not an uncommon finding in older dogs. Inadvertent needle biopsy of this site or an inadequate tissue specimen could give histologic findings compatible with chronic hepatitis and hepatic fibrosis. H&E ×40; trichrome ×100.

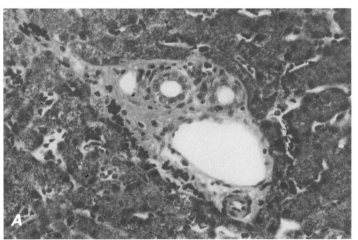

FIGURE 31-13. (*A*) A trichrome stain demonstrates collagen associated with a normal portal tract; note that the surrounding parenchyma does not appreciably stain for collagen.

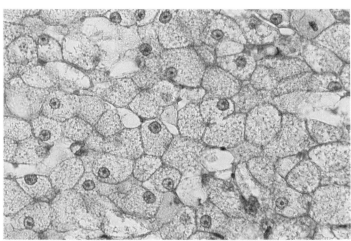

FIGURE 31-17. Diffuse, microvesicular, lipid accumulation in a kitten affected with Niemann-Pick type C disease. H&E ×400. (Courtesy of Dr. Diane E. Brown, Department of Pathology, Colorado State University)

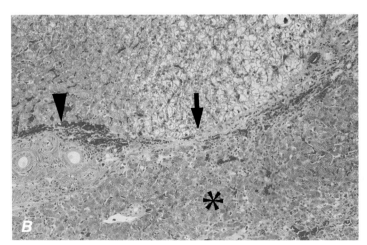

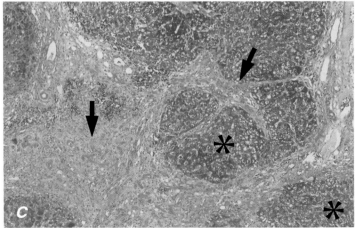

FIGURE 31-14. This wedge biopsy is from a 12-year-old dog with a small liver and numerous variably sized hepatic nodules. (*B*) A trichrome stain demonstrates no excessive connective tissue. A portal tract is located to the far left (arrowhead). (*C*) In contrast, this trichrome-stained specimen from a grossly similar appearing liver demonstrates diffuse, dense connective tissue (arrows) in association with architecturally abnormal regenerative nodules (asterisks) compatible with cirrhosis. Reticulin stain ×40; trichrome stain ×40; trichrome ×40.

Plate II

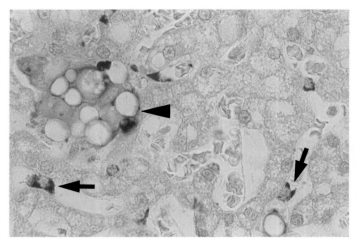

FIGURE 31-18. A Prussian blue stain demonstrates the accumulation of iron in Kupffer cells and a foci (arrowhead) of pigment and lipid-filled cells morphologically compatible with macrophages (lipogranulomata). Arrows indicate Kupffer cells with iron. Prussian blue iron stain ×400.

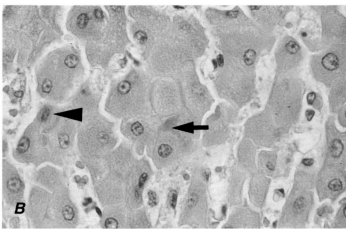

FIGURE 31-29. This liver specimen is from a 2-year-old dog that rapidly developed icterus (total serum bilirubin = 11.0 mg/dl and minimal to no increase in the serum hepatic enzymes) in association with a severe bacterial cellulitis secondary to a bite (B) Bile stasis, canilicular plug (arrow), and bile "casts" of the longitudinally cut canaliculi on the surface of hepatocytes (arrowhead) is the predominant histopathologic finding.[57]

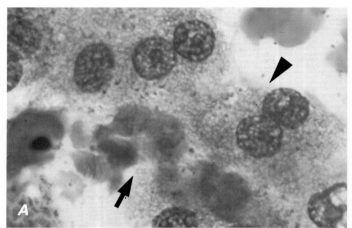

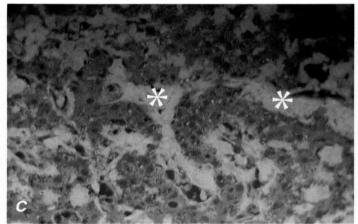

FIGURE 31-24. (A) Homogeneous eosinophilic ribbons of material (arrow) are laced among clumps of hepatocytes (arrowhead) in this aspirate from a dog with chronic osteomyelitis (2 years duration) that developed hepatomegaly. (C) There is positive staining (asterisk) of the material (green birefringence on polarization) with Congo red. Congo red positive following treatment with trypsin digestion and oxidation with potassium permanganaté indicates that the amyloid is composed of immunoglobulin light chain moieties; loss of Congo red affinity subsequent to treatment indicates a nonimmunoglobulin (AA) type amyloid. The recent reports of hepatic amyloidosis in cats and its presentation without renal involvement in Chinese shar pei dogs increase our awareness for this disorder as a cause of hepatomegaly and liver dysfunction.[112,113] Diff-Quik stain ×500; H&E ×400; Congo red stain with polarization ×400.

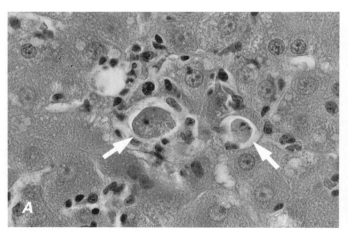

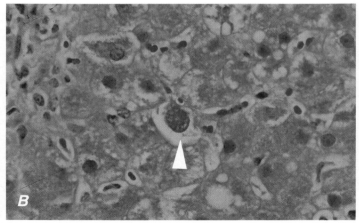

FIGURE 31-34. (A) An acidophilic body (arrow) with hypereosinophilic cytoplasm and pyknotic nuclear remnant is observed from specimen depicted in Figure 31–5. A less conspicuous one is located to the right of center. (B) Apoptosis is reflected by this small, densely eosinophilic anuclear mass (arrowhead) in this Doberman pinscher with chronic hepatitis. Note the absence of inflammatory cells. H&E ×500; ×400.

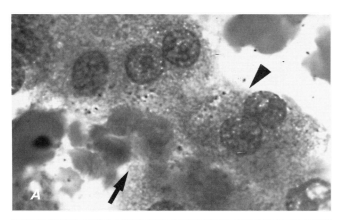

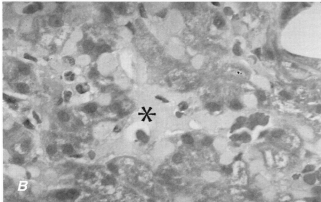

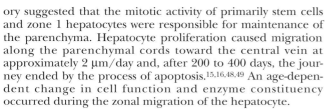

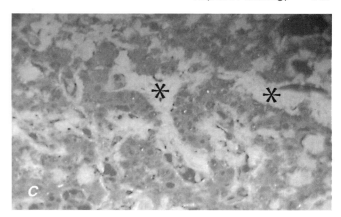

FIGURE 31–24. (*A*) (see **Plate II**) Homogeneous eosinophilic ribbons of material (arrow) are laced among clumps of hepatocytes (arrowhead) in this aspirate from a dog with chronic osteomyelitis (2 years duration) that developed hepatomegaly. (*B*) Hepatic amyloidosis was histologically confirmed; note the lightly stained eosinophilic material (asterisk) separating and compressing the cords of hepatocytes. (*C*) (see **Plate II**) There is positive staining (asterisk) of the material (green birefringence on polarization) with Congo red. Congo red positive following treatment with trypsin digestion and oxidation with potassium permanganaté indicates that the amyloid is composed of immunoglobulin light chain moieties; loss of Congo red affinity subsequent to treatment indicates a nonimmunoglobulin (AA) type amyloid. The recent reports of hepatic amyloidosis in cats and its presentation without renal involvement in Chinese shar pei dogs increase our awareness for this disorder as a cause of hepatomegaly and liver dysfunction.[112,113] Diff-Quik stain ×500; H&E ×400; Congo red stain with polarization ×400.

ory suggested that the mitotic activity of primarily stem cells and zone 1 hepatocytes were responsible for maintenance of the parenchyma. Hepatocyte proliferation caused migration along the parenchymal cords toward the central vein at approximately 2 μm/day and, after 200 to 400 days, the journey ended by the process of apoptosis.[15,16,48,49] An age-dependent change in cell function and enzyme constituency occurred during the zonal migration of the hepatocyte.

This concept has recently been refuted by a study employing a novel retroviral gene transfer method to tag replicating hepatocytes and their progeny.[50] The findings indicate that hepatocytes locally proliferate, forming clusters. A mature hepatocyte can repetitively cycle approximately five or six

times to produce 30 progeny and the life span is compatible with previously established values. Thus, stem cells are not involved in the formation of new hepatocytes during postnatal growth, although they can be stimulated to form hepatocytes under certain pathologic conditions.[51]

Compensatory liver growth is a complex and poorly understood process comprised of hyperplasia and hypertrophy.[52] Following partial hepatectomy, regeneration is complete in approximately 10 days and 8 months in the rat and human being, respectively. Regeneration of the canine liver appears to be closer to the proliferative response of the rat.[53–55] The process is more rapid following injury than surgical amputation as long as the reticular framework is not injured. This

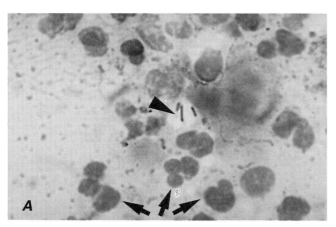

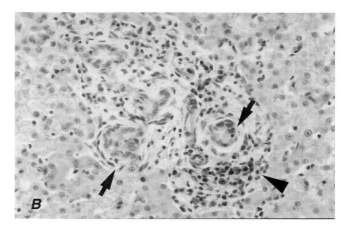

FIGURE 31–25. (*A*) Cytology of bile obtained during a laparotomy of an icteric cat with recurrent fever, leukocytosis, and abdominal discomfort for 3 weeks. Abundant "mushy" neutrophils (arrows) and rod-shaped bacteria (arrowhead) are present; an *E. coli* was later cultured. Histologic examination of the gallbladder following its removal was consistent with suppurative cholecystitis. (*B*) Mild bile duct proliferation (arrows), portal edema, and an infiltrate of predominately lymphocytes confined to the portal tract (arrowhead) were observed in the liver biopsy. Diff-Quik stain ×1000; H&E ×200.

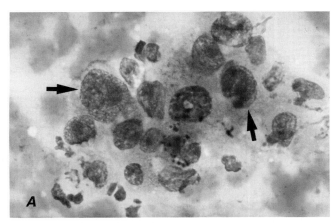
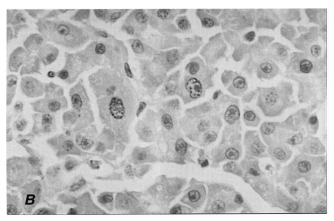

FIGURE 31-26. (*A*) An aspirate from a cat with an asymmetrically enlarged liver. Small clumps of cells with marked anisokaryosis (arrows), prominent variably sized nucleoli, and granular to lacy chromatin pattern are indicative of a neoplasm. The basophilic cytoplasm is suggestive of a hepatocyte origin. (*B*) Similar morphologic features are noted histologically, the findings compatible with a hepatocellular carcinoma. Notable in this limited field of view is the architectural disorganization, anisokaryosis, and prominent variably sized nucleoli. Diff-Quik ×400; H&E ×400.

scant connective tissue stroma acts as a scaffolding for the parenchymal cells, and regeneration of a large lesion may be complete with 10 to 20 days in the dog.

BILIARY PROLIFERATION. Following complete bile duct ligation, biliary epithelial cell proliferation predominates, but hepatocellular proliferation also occurs.[56] Proliferation of preexisting biliary epithelial cells is responsible for the elongation of the newly formed tortuous ductular network.[56] Following prolonged biliary obstruction, ductular metaplasia of hepatocytes appears to contribute to the formation of biliary ductular structures. However, cholestasis is not a prerequisite for cholangiolar proliferation; it is associated with a variety of intra- and extrahepatic insults (Figure 31–28).

Functional Cholestasis

Functional cholestasis develops when the physiologic mechanisms responsible for bile flow, bile acid excretion, and canalicular membrane activity are impaired without overt tissue damage. A relatively common clinical cause for this type of bile stasis is extrahepatic bacterial infections.[57] Despite moderate to marked increases in the serum bilirubin concentration, there usually are minimal histopathologic changes other than cellular and canalicular bile retention (Figure 31–29). The cholestasis spontaneously resolves with successful management of the bacterial infection. The icterus that occasionally develops in cats with hyperthyroidism may be another example of functional cholestasis which is metabolic in origin.[58,59]

Extramedullary Hematopoiesis

Hematopoiesis, a normal function of the fetal liver, ceases within a couple of weeks of birth. Chronic anemia, chronic extrahepatic inflammation, and chronic hepatic disease can stimulate the liver to produce one or more hematopoietic elements, referred to as extramedullary hematopoiesis or myeloid metaplasia. In the dog, small to large foci of

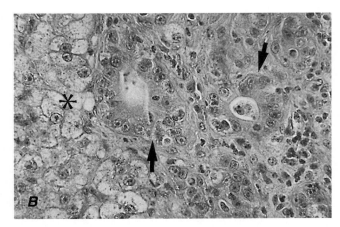

FIGURE 31-27. (*A*) An ultrasound-guided aspirate from a cat with multiple lesions. Dense clumps of large cohesive cells with minimal cytoplasm are observed; their morphology is best evaluated by examining the periphery (arrowhead). Notable is the relatively large nuclear size and increased nuclear to cytoplasm ratio of the neoplastic cells. Two hepatocytes (arrow) just to the left of center can be used to guess at cell and nuclear size. These findings are compatible with a cholangiocellular carcinoma. (*B*) The architecture of the neoplasm can be appreciated with histologic examination. A dense mass of variably sized atypical ductular structures (arrows) is compressing hepatocytes with hydropic degeneration (asterisk). Diff-Quik ×400; H&E ×400.

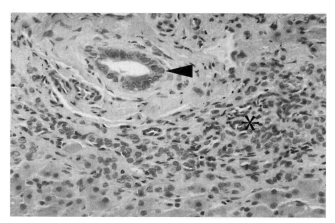

FIGURE 31-28. Moderate bile ductular proliferation (asterisk) and mild to moderate portal inflammation (predominantly lymphocytes) in a dog with increased serum liver enzymes activities and lymphocytic, plasmacytic enteritis. A large bile duct is noted by an arrowhead. Similar histopathologic changes develop in experimental models of small intestinal bacterial overgrowth.[114] This lesion will resolve within a few weeks once the inciting cause is eliminated. Contrast the uniformity of this proliferative process with the preceding neoplastic growth.

hematopoietic cells appear to frequently accompany chronic inflammatory liver disease and nodular hyperplasia. Focal accumulations of the granulocytic series in the portal and periportal areas are notable. When the majority of the cellular elements formed are mature neutrophils, the benign process can be misinterpreted as suppurative inflammation (Figure 31–30).

Hepatocellular Degeneration

Hepatocellular degeneration is a common response to a variety of inflammatory, toxic, metabolic, and ischemic insults. Light microscopy often cannot discern between reversible and irreversible change. Hydropic degeneration is an early cytoplasmic change (Figure 31–31). Other terms used to describe this morphologic change include cloudy swelling and feathery degeneration. Subcellular studies indicate that altered function of mitochondria and the cytoplas-

mic cytocavitary system are responsible for cloudy swelling and that feathery degeneration is a bile (acid)-induced change subsequent to cholestatic disease.[60,61] Hydrophobic bile acids have been shown to be cytotoxic and increased concentrations injurious to subcellular organelles.[62–64] Perhaps the adverse subcellular effects of accumulated bile acids are a cause of the degenerative change (Figure 31–32). It is interesting to note that one study did not find this change to be a reliable morphologic feature of cholestasis in the dog.[65]

As the name implies, hydropic degeneration represents the presence of cytoplasmic fluid. This may occur subsequent to the metabolism of glycogen or the consequence of cell injury allowing the cell membrane or organelles to take up water. Hydropic degeneration is often considered a reversible change but can be the earliest microscopic indication of hepatocellular necrosis. The accumulation of glycogen can have a similar light microscopic appearance as hydropic degeneration in formalin-fixed tissue stained with H&E. A periodic acid–Schiff (PAS) stain is required to differentiate glycogen from fluid. Even early fatty change can be mistaken for hydropic degeneration without the use of special stains.

Accumulation of Lipid

HEPATIC LIPIDOSIS. Hepatic lipidosis (fatty liver, fatty degeneration, steatosis) refers to an increase in hepatocellular lipid. It may be associated with conditions such as starvation and dietary excess and pathologic conditions such as diabetes mellitus, hypoxia, and a syndrome in cats. Because of the intimate role of the hepatocyte in the energy-dependent, multiple-step process associated with the synthesis and transport of lipoproteins, any disturbance in (apo)protein and phospholipid synthesis or impairment in generation of adenosine triphosphate (ATP) can result in lipid accumulation.

The term *vacuole* denotes a cavity in the cytoplasm that is bounded by a distinct membrane. Because the accumulation of lipid is within an organelle and surrounded by its membrane, the term is an appropriate descriptor. However, the membrane may be difficult to observe with certainty using light microscopy. Consequently, it is sometimes used, probably inappropriately, to describe any cytoplasmic change in which open or clear areas are observed. This connotative usage of the term *vacuole* leads to nonspecificity in interpreta-

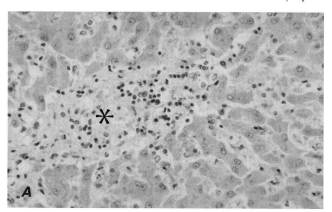
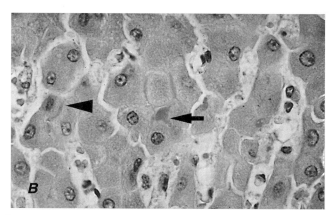

FIGURE 31-29 (see **Plate II**). This liver specimen is from a 2-year-old dog that rapidly developed icterus (total serum bilirubin = 11.0 mg/dl and minimal to no increase in the serum hepatic enzymes) in association with a severe bacterial cellulitis secondary to a bite. (*A*) The portal tract (asterisk) contains a small number of lymphocytes and the surrounding parenchyma shows no necroinflammatory changes. (*B*) Bile stasis, canilicular plug (arrow), and bile "casts" of the longitudinally cut canaliculi on the surface of hepatocytes (arrowhead) is the predominant histopathologic finding.[57]

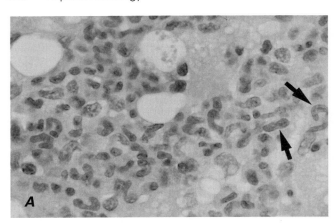
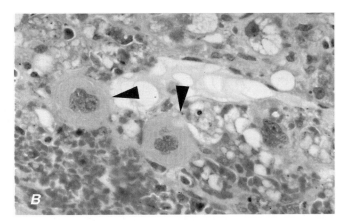

FIGURE 31-30. (*A*) A dense accumulation of granulocytes is present near the compressed portal tract in a liver biopsy from a dog with abnormal hepatic enzyme activities and irregular hepatic surface. The prominence of band neutrophils and lesser numbers of metamyelocytes (arrows) indicates this is a focus of extramedullary hematopoiesis. The differentiation between a suppurative inflammatory process and extramedullary hematopoiesis becomes more subjective when the segmented neutrophil predominates. (*B*) Megakaryocytes (arrowheads) are prominent in other areas of this biopsy from a dog with severe nodular regeneration.

tive meaning. Clarification of the use of the term in a report may be required to determine if the described change is most compatible with lipid, glycogen, or water accumulation (hydropic degeneration).

Hepatic lipidosis is a common finding in a variety of metabolic disturbances and toxic injuries because of these complex, interdependent pathways for lipid metabolism located within the hepatocyte. The formation of small vacuoles is usually associated with acute cell injury (Figure 31–33). The more commonly observed large cytoplasmic vacuole or globule that displaces the nucleus to the periphery of the cell probably forms from fusion of the small vacuoles over time (Figure 31–22). Consequently, the finding of predominantly large vacuoles is more commonly associated with nutritional and metabolic disorders.

LYSOSOMAL STORAGE DISEASE. Lysosomal storage diseases also cause fatty change in hepatocytes and Kupffer cells (Figure 31–17). Because the accumulation is often more severe in the central nervous system, neurologic signs predominate. In

a young (< 1 year of age) animal with hepatic lipidosis and prominent central nervous system dysfunction, a storage disease should be suspected.

LIPOCYTE PROMINENCE. The lipocyte (Ito cell) becomes readily apparent when filled with lipid. The diffuse accumulation of lipid in lipocytes gives the liver a "Swiss cheese" appearance in both dogs and cats (Figure 31–7). The term *fatty liver* has been used to describe this finding, but the etiopathogenesis is probably quite different.

PATTERNS OF INJURY AND INFLAMMATION

Necrosis and Apoptosis

The recognition of cell death (necrobiosis) is more common in the liver than most other organs due to the routine measurement of the hepatocellular specific enzyme activity in the serum, alanine aminotransferase (ALT), and ease of

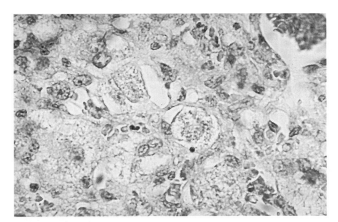

FIGURE 31-31. Diffuse hydropic degeneration, bile retention (not visible in this field), and distorted architecture with minimal inflammation in a 4-month-old dog that became icteric 5 days following a second treatment with mebendazole (ALT = 2670 IU/L, AST = 1243 IU/L, ALP = 320 IU/L, total bilirubin = 4.8 mg/dl). These histologic findings are typically referred to as toxic hepatitis or toxic hepatopathy. Reversibility or cause of the lesion cannot be determined histologically. H&E ×400.

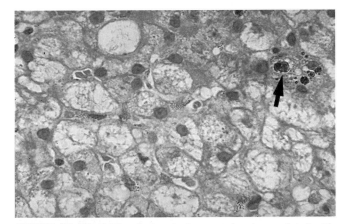

FIGURE 31-32. Diffuse hydropic degeneration is associated with bile accumulation (arrow) secondary to partial obstruction of the common bile duct by a pancreatic carcinoma. The bile (acid)-associated morphologic change is referred to as feathery degeneration and appears histologically similar to glycogen accumulation. (Compare to Figure 31–22*B*.) H&E ×400.

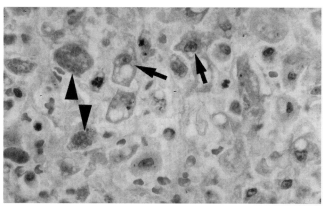

FIGURE 31–33. There is a diffuse loss of hepatocytes throughout the liver in this dog that died from massive necrosis associated with the administration of trimethoprim-sulfadiazine. The few remaining hepatocytes (arrows) show small variably sized vacuoles in the cytoplasm compatible with lipid. Pigmented-filled macrophages (arrowheads) are noted to the left of center. The histopathological findings are generically associated with a variety of insults that cause a "toxic" liver injury. H&E ×400.

biopsy. A variety of infectious, toxic, metabolic, and nutritional disturbances can initiate the sequence of hepatocellular degenerative events that may culminate in cell death.

APOPTOSIS. Apoptosis refers to programmed cell death by cellular fragmentation. The deeply eosinophilic membrane-bound anuclear fragments are not commonly observed in the nondiseased liver as a consequence of normal cell turnover. They are phagocytized and digested; the golden pigment observed in hepatocytes and Kupffer cells referred to as lipofuscin results from this degradative process. Thus, this form of cell death does not usually provoke an inflammatory reaction because the intracellular contents are not released. Apoptosis in the liver may be increased by cytokines and amplified by interferon-gamma associated with inflammation, a mechanism that may be responsible for their formation in chronic hepatitis.[66,67]

COAGULATIVE AND LYTIC NECROSIS. Coagulative necrosis indicates a group or zone of dead hepatocytes that uniformly stain intensely with eosin. There is minimal or no inflammation. The lesion suggests an acute hepatocellular insult. Single cell coagulative necrosis (extrusion of water and organelle condensation) results in a shrunken hepatocyte referred to as an acidophil body (Councilman body) (Figure 31–34). Their formation may be prominent in acute viral and drug-mediated injury, but sporadic occurrence is observed in cryptogenic chronic hepatitis. Acidophil body formation is a prominent feature of acute and chronic hepatitis in dogs with findings suggestive of a viral etiology.[68,69] Acidophil bodies also develop during the process of apoptosis; microscopically both appear similar.[70,71]

Another form of rapid hepatocellular death in which they disintegrate often in groups is lytic necrosis (Figure 31–35). When the lytic process is associated with a moderate to dense infiltration of neutrophil, it is probable that the release of their lysosomal (hydrolytic) enzymes is, in part, responsible for the hepatocellular dissolution.

ZONAL AND MASSIVE NECROSIS. Two properties predispose zone 3 hepatocytes to injury: a high activity of cytochrome P-450 mixed function oxidases and perfusion by sinusoidal blood with the lowest oxygen content. Consequently, in anemia and shock these cells are most susceptible to hypoxia (Figure 31–6). Any posthepatic process (e.g., right-sided

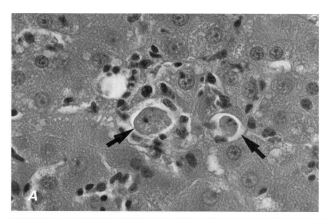

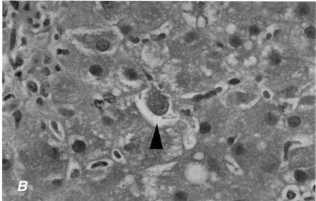

FIGURE 31–34 (see **Plate II**). (*A*) An acidophilic body (arrow) with hypereosinophilic cytoplasm and pyknotic nuclear remnant is observed from specimen depicted in Figure 31–5. A less conspicuous one is located to the right of center. (*B*) Apoptosis is reflected by this small, densely eosinophilic anuclear mass (arrowhead) in this Doberman pinscher with chronic hepatitis. Note the absence of inflammatory cells. H&E ×500; ×400.

heart failure) that impairs the drainage of sinusoidal blood from the liver also results in an hypoxic injury to these hepatocytes (Figure 31–3). Xenobiotics that undergo metabolism by the mixed function oxidase system (e.g., acetaminophen) can result in toxic metabolites that injure zone 3 hepatocytes. The term *zonal necrosis* is also used to describe this type of pathologic event that primarily involves a specific microanatomic region of the lobule or acinus.

Massive necrosis refers to necrobiosis of hepatocytes comprising one or more acini (Figure 31–33). Because no hepatocytes remain to divide and the stem cells are dead, no regeneration can occur. The reticulin framework collapses, trapping macrophages filled with pigmented debris. Along with a variable degree of fibroplasia, the lesion has been referred to as postnecrotic scarring. It is probable that nodules of hepatocellular regeneration develop in lesser affected acini. The left lobe of the liver appears to be predisposed to massive necrosis. One suggestion to explain this phenomenon is "streamlined" portal blood flow, that is, preferential flow of portal blood from segments of the gastrointestinal tract to specific lobes of the liver. This blood flow pattern has been demonstrated to occur in dogs and rats. In the latter, portal blood from the spleen and colon tend to go to the left lobe while the right lobe receives relatively nutrient-rich blood from the small intestine. It is probable that hepatic insults of gut origin may have varying severity and magnitude in different lobes of the liver as well. Consequently, when

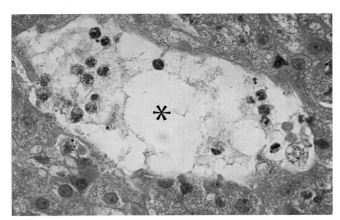

FIGURE 31-35. Random areas of hepatocellular lysis (asterisk), sometimes associated with small numbers of neutrophils, were observed in this ultrasound-guided needle biopsy obtained from an icteric dog with acute pancreatitis. The remarkable hepatocellular dissolution prompts the suggestion that the pancreatic proteases released from the inflamed organ are causative. A variety of histopathologic changes develop in the canine liver in association with acute pancreatitis, the severity of which parallel the intensity of the pancreatic necrosis.[116,117] Hydropic degeneration with focal accumulations of bile pigment were prominent throughout the specimen (refer to Figure 31-32).

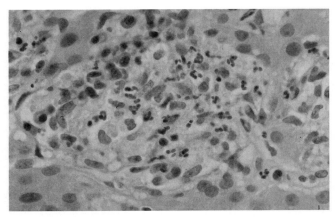

FIGURE 31-36. Scattered focal areas of macrophages, neutrophils, and hepatocellular necrosis are present in this hepatic wedge biopsy from a dog with increased serum liver enzyme activities associated with severe inflammatory bowel disease. Translocation of bacteria and bacterial "toxins" are probably involved in the pathogenesis of the inflammatory foci. H&E ×400.

investigating abnormal liver tests, it would appear prudent to biopsy both the left and right lobes of the liver whenever possible.

FOCAL AND PIECEMEAL NECROSIS. Focal necrosis, often with a random distribution, is caused by a variety of viral and bacterial infections, parasitic migration, and extrahepatic inflammatory disease. Septicemia and inflammation of the gastrointestinal tract that permits increased translocation of gut microbes can cause this lesion (Figure 31-36). It is probable that cytokines released from the Kupffer cell consequent to phagocytosis often cause cytolysis of the hepatocyte in the immediate area.[72,73] Either the cytokines or cellular degeneration per se attract neutrophils, resulting in a focal suppurative lesion. These lesions heal with little or no residual scar tissue.

Piecemeal necrosis refers to portal and periportal inflammation with hepatocellular necrosis. The inflammatory cells, primarily lymphocytes and plasma cells, violate the limiting plate (Figure 31-37) and extend into the hepatic parenchyma. The inflammatory process may isolate small islands of hepatocytes, insulating them from adequate perfusion (Figure 31-38).

The Inflammatory Response

When the insult to the liver is less intense than that observed with coagulative and lytic necrosis, a gradation of degenerative changes develop in concert with the formation of an inflammatory infiltrate. In general, the initial inflammatory cell often is the neutrophil and the release of their enzymes can cause additional injury to cell membranes. The presence of neutrophils in tissue is often used as an indication of "acute" or "active" in the inflammatory "time line." As the process continues (days), other inflammatory cell types, usually lymphocytes and macrophages, become apparent. Their presence is usually equated with "chronicity" in the inflammatory time line. An increase in fibrous tissue and magnitude of deposition is another, perhaps better indication

of chronicity. Thus, an inflammatory liver lesion with neutrophils, lymphocytes, and macrophages is morphologically designated as hepatitis, active, chronic. The rearrangement of these terms to "chronic active hepatitis" may stimulate an erroneous cognitive association with a specific disease process.

CHRONIC LIVER DISEASE. The classification of most liver diseases is historically based on morphologic observations. In humans, the emphasis on the histologic characterization of chronic active hepatitis and chronic persistent hepatitis evolved into a primarily histomorphologic meaning for the terminology.[74] The clinical contribution to the original definition of chronic, that is, the presence of symptoms and abnormal liver tests for at least 6 months, being minimized. Consequently, chronic active hepatitis and chronic persistent hepatitis have become a histologically driven clinical diagnosis.[74]

Many causes of chronic liver disease can appear histologically similar. For example, in human beings, autoimmune hepatitis and chronic hepatitis B cannot be reliably differentiated histologically. Prednisolone can be effective treatment in the former but lacks efficacy in the relatively more common latter disease, despite studies that support immune-mediated cell injury in both diseases.[75] In the medical profession, the discovery of the Australian antigen and the detection of hepatitis A virus and hepatitis C viruses have paved the way for remarkable progress in the classification of inflammatory liver disease with serologic markers.[76–78] It is now known that hepatitis C (formerly non-A, non-B hepatitis) is also difficult to differentiate histologically from autoimmune hepatitis and is not responsive to prednisolone.[79] Interestingly, by studying the inflammatory pattern in serologically defined cases of chronic hepatitis caused by hepatitis C virus, characteristic histomorphologic features were identified.[80]

In dogs and cats, clinical, serologic, immunologic, and histopathologic correlates have not been studied sufficiently to permit a meaningful classification of chronic liver disease. One notable exception is the association of copper accumulation in the Bedlington terrier. Consequently, the pathogenesis of chronic hepatitis in animals based on histomorphology is often shrouded in opinion not predicative of therapeutic modalities. A morphologic description identifying the pre-

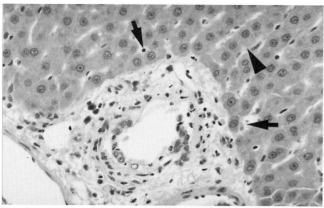

FIGURE 31-37. This partial view of a large portal tract demonstrates the innermost row of hepatocytes referred to as the "limiting plate" (arrows). It is not readily apparent in most specimens. Also note that some cords of hepatocytes, one cell thick, appear to "radiate" from the portal tract (arrowhead); others appear to intersect each other. The conceptual depiction of single cords of hepatocytes branching in straight lines between portal tracts and terminal hepatic veins is inconsistent with the structural complexity of the lobule. Adjacent hepatic cords frequently branch and intersect.[51] H&E ×100.

dominant lobular location of the necroinflammatory process with gradation of the severity is prudent. Similarly, the medical profession supports the discontinuation of the terms *chronic active hepatitis* and *chronic persistent hepatitis* in favor of assessing (grading) severity by the degree of inflammation and necrosis and using the magnitude of fibrosis to stage the disease.[74,81,82] It is suggested that prognosis be related to etiologic (serologic) terminology supplemented by the grade and stage of the disease process.

BRIDGING NECROSIS AND FIBROSIS. Realizing its interpretive limitations, the light microscopic examination of the liver tissue can provide diagnostic and prognostic information and guide patient management.[24,37–40] Bridging hepatic necrosis indicates an extensive form of necrosis and inflammation that links ("bridges") portal tracts or a portal tract to a terminal hepatic (central) vein. Collapse of the hepatic parenchyma in these regions can be best demonstrated with the use of a reti-

culin stain. In humans, the development of this lesion, especially when associated with signs or symptoms greater than 3 to 6 months in duration, is considered an adverse prognostic finding.[83,84] Bridging hepatic fibrosis indicates the presence of connective tissue that links portal triads or a portal triad to a terminal hepatic vein (Figure 31–14). It is implicit that alteration of the hepatic architecture by fibrosis will violate the intimate relationship between the sinusoidal blood and hepatocyte causing a deterioration of a variety of liver functions and, ultimately, the patient. This is supported by the finding that the degree of bridging fibrosis correlates with survival time; the more fibrosis, the shorter the survival time.[24] In that study, the severity of necrosis and fibrosis was greater in dogs dying within 1 week. The presence of piecemeal necrosis was not indicated to have prognostic importance.

Nodular Hyperplasia

The dog shows a propensity for the development of nodular hyperplasia of the liver. It is not known if the proliferative change is a response to previous hepatic injury or metabolic disorders. In human patients, nodule formation, which appears to differ histomorphologically from that described in dogs, has been associated with altered hepatic blood flow and the use of azathioprine.[85,86] In the dog, the lesion is common and appears to be age related, suggesting, perhaps, a factor common to many dogs or a similar type of hepatic response to a variety of factors.[87–89] Nodules are present by 6 years of age and, in one study, were present in all dogs older than 14 years.[89] The expansile process compresses existing parenchyma, resulting in hepatocellular atrophy and approximation of the reticular fibers. Grossly, their appearance mimics macronodular cirrhosis and neoplasia. Microscopically, hepatocytes can develop a variety of cytoplasmic changes including lipidosis, hydropic degeneration, and glycogen accumulation. This may be problematic in needle biopsy specimens because the identification of nodular regeneration is very difficult due to size limitations, and the histomorphologic findings can be suggestive of a metabolic disorder (Figure 31–39).

Nodular hyperplasia is associated with lipocyte prominence and the formation of lipogranulomata.[89] Prussian blue

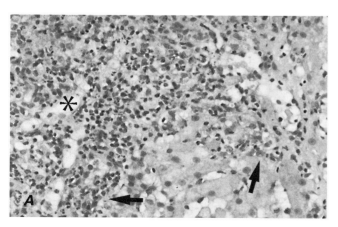

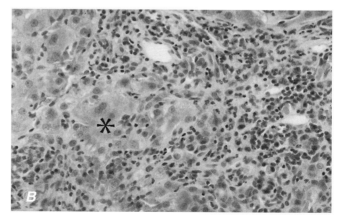

FIGURE 31-38. (*A*) A predominantly mononuclear inflammatory infiltrate is located in the periportal area (asterisk) and extends into the surrounding parenchyma (arrows). *Piecemeal necrosis* is the term given to this histopathological finding. There is moderate bile duct proliferation and acidophil bodies are present (not visible in this field). (*B*) The inflammatory process "dissects" small clumps of hepatocytes away from the parenchyma (asterisk), violating their oxygen and nutrient supply. H&E ×200; H&E ×400.

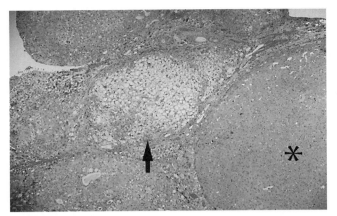

FIGURE 31-39. Wedge biopsy from a 10-year-old mixed breed with hepatic encephalopathy and hyperammonemia. The liver was small and comprised of numerous variably sized nodules. In this microscopic field, a large nodule is located to the lower right (asterisk) and a fatty nodule is located in the center (arrow). Most of the hepatocytes comprising the other nodules show minimal hydropic degeneration. It would be difficult to identify architecturally the nodules with a percutaneous needle biopsy. If the center nodule was biopsied with a needle, the histologic findings could erroneously suggest an underlying metabolic disorder. A pedunculated nodule emanates at the top. Reticulin and trichrome stains were used to help differentiate these changes from a cirrhotic process. H&E ×20.

staining demonstrates an abundance of iron accumulation in these foci of pigmented macrophages. An increase in serum hepatic enzyme activities, especially alkaline phosphatase, has been associated with nodular hyperplasia (D.J. Meyer, David Cameron Twedt, personal observations). The etiopathogenesis may be a reflection of two physioanatomic processes. First, the distorted hepatic architecture impairs bile flow and precludes adequate blood supply to hepatocytes, resulting in cholestatic induction of enzyme synthesis (alkaline phosphatase) and compromised membrane integrity (leakage of aminotransferases). Alternatively, the increase in at least the aminotransferases may be directly related to the hepatocyte proliferative process because an increase in the serum aminotransferase activities has been shown to be related to an increased production of these enzymes following an injury.[90-92] Interesting, an increase in the serum alkaline

phosphatase activity was consistently present in the patients with azathioprine-associated nodular hyperplasia.[85]

A syndrome is described in the dog that may represent an extreme of nodular hyperplasia.[60] The liver is atrophied and is comprised of variably sized nodules. The extensive nodule formation grossly appears similar to cirrhosis but, histologically, fibrosis is not a prominent feature. Consequently, the use of agents to reduce or impair the formation of collagen is not a rational strategy in these patients. There is sufficient disruption of the architecture to cause liver insufficiency (increased serum total bile acid concentration and plasma ammonia concentration), but the author does not believe jaundice frequently develops as it can with cirrhosis. Special stains may be warranted to separate this disorder histologically from cirrhosis because a recent study noted the potential for histopathologic confusion or misinterpretation.[93]

Changes Associated with Congenital Portosystemic Shunts

HEPATIC ATROPHY. Hepatocellular atrophy, a reduction in cell volume, not numbers, is associated with congenital portosystemic shunts. Portal blood carries hepatotrophic factors (e.g., insulin, glucagon, amino acids) to the liver. The reduction in factors necessary for maintaining normal hepatocellular size can result in smaller lobules and, consequently, portal tracts that appear closer to each other. The portal tracts may be devoid of a recognizable portal vein and can have abnormal structures that resemble vessels and bile ducts (Figure 31-40). The relationship between these abnormal intrahepatic structures and the extrahepatic congenital portal vascular anomaly is not known. Multifocal areas of hydropic degeneration may be present.

IRON ACCUMULATION AND LIPOGRANULOMATA. Increased iron content involving hepatocytes, Kupffer cells, or both has been observed in the liver of dogs with congenital portosystemic shunts[94] (Figure 31-18). Microcytosis, hypoferremia, and a decreased hematocrit were frequently present. Similar hematologic changes and iron accumulation in hepatic tissue developed in dogs with a surgically created portocaval anastomosis.[95] The reason for the iron accumulation in the liver is not known. Foci of lipid- and pigment-containing macrophages ("lipogranulomata") that often stain intensely

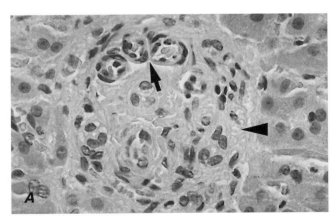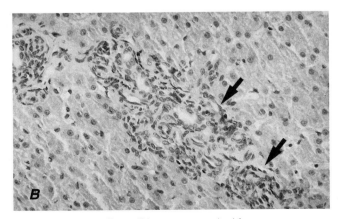

FIGURE 31-40. (A) Inappropriate numbers of arterioles are present (three discernible at top, arrow) without an identifiable portal vein in a dog with a congenital portosystemic shunt. Some of the other structures may be bile ductules (arrowhead). (B) In other cases, a proliferative lesion is observed in which either vascularlike or bile-duct-like structures, or both, are present (arrows). The observation suggests the possibility of hepatic stem cell involvement in their formation. H&E (A) ×400; (B) ×200.

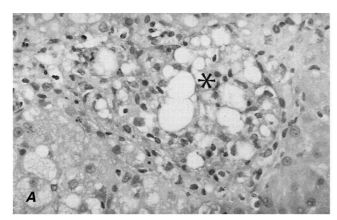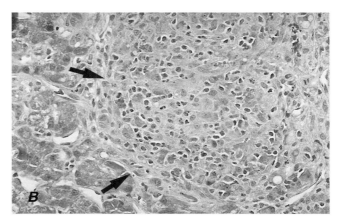

FIGURE 31-41. (*A*) A focus of pigment and lipid-laden cells (asterisk) compatible with macrophages is noted in this wedge biopsy from a 1-year-old pug with a congenital portal systemic shunt. The term *lipogranulomata* is sometimes used to define this structure. It often stains intensely for iron (refer to Figure 31–17). The terminology for this lesion and a similar one common in aged dogs should not be confused with granuloma formation. It is morphologically different, uncommon, and is associated with parasitic and fungal infections and a variety of extrahepatic diseases.[118] (*B*) A foci of uniform histiocytes (arrows) with a small number of lymphocytes sprinkled throughout is noted in this liver biopsy from a dog with fever of unknown origin and increased serum liver enzyme activities. Special stains for infectious agents were negative. Note the morphologic differences between granulomatous hepatitis observed here and the preceding "lipogranulomata." H&E ×400.

for iron are observed in naturally occurring cases (Figure 31–41). Their formation may be a consequence of iron-induced cellular injury resulting from peroxidative decomposition of organelle membrane phospholipids.[96,97] The diversion of portal blood over a long period of time may predispose to oxidative stress.[98] An injurious effect of secondarily accumulated iron is not supported by a recent study in humans following portocaval shunting.[99]

"Lipogranulomata" formation is an unusual finding in relatively young dogs (< 6 years of age) and their presence should stimulate the consideration of a congenital portosystemic shunt, either as a serendipitous discovery or as an explanation of the clinical signs or abnormal serum hepatic enzyme tests.

Similar iron-rich accumulations of macrophages have been reported in copper-associated liver disease and nodular hyperplasia.[40,89] It is apparent that a variety of liver cell types containing lipid can have similar histomorphologic and ultrastructural characteristics.[100] Further investigations into defining the cell type comprising lipogranulomata may be informative in defining their development.

If injurious in selected types of diseases such as congenital portosystemic shunts, iron accumulation could act as an oxidative stress that is amplified by inadequate blood to sufficiently meet nutritional and oxygen needs. This would predispose to hepatocellular injury accompanied by a proliferative reparative response (nodular regeneration). Surgically created portosystemic shunts in rats are associated with nodular regeneration,[101] and altered hepatic blood flow appears related to their formation in humans.[86] It is possible that in some dogs with severe nodular regeneration and apparent "acquired" shunts that the process reflects the end stage of a degenerative/regenerative sequence of events in which a congenital anomaly of the portal circulation is the inciting event.

REFERENCES

1. Kiernan, F. The anatomy and physiology of the liver. Philos Trans R Soc (London), 711–770, 1833.
2. Rappaport AM, Borowy ZJ, Longheed WM. Subdivision of hexagonal liver lobules into a structural and functional unit: Role in hepatic physiology and pathology. Anat Rec 119:11–34, 1954.
3. Rappaport AM. The microcirculatory acinar concept of normal and pathological hepatic structure. Beitr Pathol 157:215–243, 1976.
4. Lautt WW, Greenway CV. Conceptual review of the hepatic vascular bed. Hepatology 7:952–963, 1987.
5. Jungermann K, Katz N. Functional specialization of different hepatocyte populations. Physiol Rev 69:708–764, 1989.
6. Sokal EM, Trivedi P, Cheeseman P, et al. The application of quantitative cytochemistry to study the acinar distribution of enzymatic activities in human liver biopsy sections. J Hepatol 9:42–48, 1989.
7. Gumucio J, Chianale J. Liver cell heterogeneity and liver function. In: Arias IW, Jakoby W, Popper H (eds) The Liver: Biology and Pathobiology, 2nd ed. Raven Press, New York, 931–947, 1988.
8. Scholtens HB, Meijer DKF, Hardonk MJ. A histochemical study on the distribution of injected canine intestinal alkaline phosphatase in rat liver. Liver 2:14–21, 1982.
9. Plaa G. Toxicology of the liver. In: Casarett L, Doull J (eds) Toxicology: The Basic Science of Poisons. Macmillan, New York, 170–189, 1975.
10. Mitra SK. The terminal distribution of the hepatic artery with special reference to arterio-portal anastomosis. J Anat 100:651–663, 1966.
11. Gumucio JJ. Functional and anatomic heterogeneity in the liver acinus: Impact on transport. Am J Physiol 244:G578–G582, 1983.
12. Molino G. The functioning liver mass. Res Clin Lab 21:9–40, 1991.
13. Dioguardi N. Liver system. IV. Res Clin Lab 21:41–68, 1991.
14. Gates GA, Henley KS, Pollard HM, et al. The cell population of human liver. J Lab Clin Med 57:182–184, 1961.
15. Zajicek G, Oren R, Weinreb M. The streaming liver. Liver 5:293–300, 1985.
16. Zajicek G, Ariel I, Arber N. The streaming liver. III. Littoral cells accompany the streaming hepatocytes. Liver 8:213–218, 1988.
17. Bouwens L, De Bleser P, Vanderkerken K, et al. Liver cell heterogeneity: Functions of non-parenchymal cells. Enzyme 46:155–168, 1992.
18. Freedman S. The cellular basis of hepatic fibrosis: Mechanisms and treatment strategies. N Engl J Med 328:1828–1835, 1993.
19. Ishak KG, Schiff ER, Schiff L. Needle biopsy of the liver. In: Schiff L, Schiff ER (eds) Diseases of the Liver. J.B. Lippincott, Philadelphia, 399–441, 1987.
20. Colombo M, del Ninno E, de Franchis R, et al. Ultrasound-assisted percutaneous liver biopsy: Superiority of the Tru-Cut over the Menghini needle for diagnosis of cirrhosis. Gastroenterology 95:487–489, 1988.
21. Levison DA, Kingham JG, Dawson AM, et al. Slow cirrhosis or no cirrhosis? A lesion causing benign intrahepatic portal hypertension. J Pathol 137:253–272, 1982.
22. Holund B, Poulsen H, Schlichting P. Reproducibility of liver biopsy diagnosis in relation to the size of the specimen. Scan J Gastroenterol 15:329–335, 1980.
23. Schlichting P, Holund B, Poulsen H. Liver biopsy in chronic aggressive hepatitis: Diagnostic reproducibility in relation to size of specimen. Scan J Gastroenterol 18:27–32, 1983.
24. Strombeck DR, Miller LM, Harrold D. Effects of corticosteroid treatment

on survival in dogs with chronic hepatitis: 151 cases (1977–1985). J Am Vet Med Assoc 193:1109–1113, 1988.

25. Boyer JL, Klatskin G. Pattern of necrosis in acute viral hepatitis—prognostic value of bridging (subacute hepatic necrosis). N Engl J Med 283:1063–1071, 1970.

26. Boyer JL. Chronic hepatitis. A perspective on classification and determinants of prognosis. Gastroenterology 70:1161–1171, 1976.

27. Henley KS, Appelman HD. The fading menace of chronic hepatitis. Ann Int Med 82;840–841, 1975.

28. Petrelli M, Scheur PJ. Variation in subcapsular liver structure and its significance in the interpretation of wedge biopsies. J Clin Pathol 20:743–748, 1967.

29. Scheur PJ. General considerations. In: Liver Biopsy Interpretation, 4th ed. Bailliere Tindall, Philadelphia, 1–9, 1988.

30. Christoffersen P, Poulsen H, Skeie E. Focal liver cell necroses accompanied by infiltration of granulocytes arising during operation. Acta Hepato Splenologica 17:240–245, 1970.

31. McDonald GS, Courtney M. Operation-associated neutrophils in a percutaneous liver biopsy: Effect of prior transjugular procedure. Histopathology 10:217–222, 1986.

32. Fittschen C, Bellamy JE. Prednisone-induced morphologic and chemical changes in the liver of dogs. Vet Pathol 21:399–406, 1984.

33. Haskins ME, Otis EJ, Hayden JE, et al. Hepatic storage of glycosaminoglycans in feline and canine models of mucopolysaccharidoses in I, VI, and VII. Vet Pathol 29:112–119, 1992.

34. Snyder SP, Kingston RS, Wenger DA. Niemann-Pick disease: Sphingomyelinosis of Siamese cats. Am J Pathol 108:252–254, 1982.

35. Lowenthal MC, Cummings JF, Wenger DA, et al. Feline sphingolipidosis resembling Niemann-Pick disease type C. Acta Neuropathol 81:189–197, 1990.

36. Thornburg LP, Beissenherz M, Dolan M, et al. Histochemical demonstration of copper-associated protein in the canine liver. Vet Pathol 22:327–332, 1985.

37. Twedt DC, Sternlieb I, Gilbertson ST. Clinical, morphologic and chemical studies in copper toxicosis of Bedlington terriers. J Am Vet Med Assoc 175:269–275, 1979.

38. Thornburg LP, Shaw D, Dolan M, et al. Hereditary copper toxicosis in West Highland white terriers. Vet Pathol 23:148–154, 1986.

39. Thornburg LP, Rottinghaus G, McGowan M, et al. Hepatic copper concentrations in purebred and mixed-breed dogs. Vet Pathol 27:81–88, 1990.

40. Haywood S, Rutgers HC, Christian MK. Hepatitis and copper accumulation in Skye terriers. Vet Pathol 25:408–414, 1988.

41. Colynyk JK, O'Neill R, Britton RS, et al. Determination of hepatic iron concentration in fresh and paraffin-embedded tissue: Diagnostic implications. Gastroenterology 106:674–677, 1994.

42. Meyer DJ, French TW. The liver. In: Cowell RL, Tyler RD (eds) Diagnostic Cytology of the Dog and Cat. American Veterinary Publications, Goleta, CA, 189–197, 1989.

43. Meyer DJ, Coles EH, Rich L. Evaluation of effusions. In: Veterinary Laboratory Medicine: Interpretation and Diagnosis. WB Saunders, Philadelphia, 125–130, 1992.

44. Fausto N. Oval cells and liver carcinogenesis: An analysis of cell lineages in hepatic tumors using oncogene transfection techniques. Prog Clin Biol Res 331:325–334, 1990.

45. Sigal SH, Brill S, Fiorino AS, et al. The liver as a stem cell and lineage system. Am J Physiol 263:G139–G148, 1992.

46. Fausto N, Lemire JM, Shiojiri N. Cell lineages in hepatic development and the identification of progenitor cells in normal liver. Proc Soc Exp Biol Med 204:237–241, 1993.

47. Thorgeirsson SS, Evarts RP, Bisgaard HL, et al. Hepatic stem cell compartment: Activation and lineage commitment. Proc Soc Exp Biol Med 204:253–260, 1993.

48. Thorgeirsson SS. Hepatic stem cells. Am J Pathol 142:1331–1333, 1993.

49. MacDonald RA: Lifespan of liver cells. Arch Int Med 107:335–343, 1961.

50. Bralet M, Branchereau S, Brechot C, et al. Cell lineage study in the liver using retroviral mediated gene transfer: Evidence against the streaming of hepatocytes in normal liver. Am J Pathol 144:896–905, 1994.

51. Grisham JW. Migration of hepatocytes along hepatic plates and stem cell-fed hepatocyte lineages. Am J Pathol 144:849–854, 1994.

52. Chamuleau RA, Bosman DK. Liver regeneration. Hepatogastroenterology 35:309–312, 1988.

53. Bucher NLR. Experimental aspect of hepatic regeneration. N Engl J Med 277:686–696, 1967.

54. Zoli M, Marchesini H, Melli A. Evaluation of liver volume and liver function following hepatic resections in man. Liver 6:286–291, 1986.

55. Francavilla A, Porter KA, Benichou J, et al. Liver regeneration in the dog: Morphologic and chemical changes. J Surg Res 25:409–419, 1978.

56. Slott PA, Liu MH, Tavolini N. Origin, pattern, and mechanism of bile duct proliferation following biliary obstruction in the rat. Gastroenterology 99:463–477, 1990.

57. Taboada J, Meyer DJ. Cholestasis associated with extrahepatic bacterial infection in five dogs. J Vet Int Med 3:216–221, 1989.

58. Peterson ME, Kintzer PP, Cavanagh PG, et al. Feline hyperthyroidism: Pretreatment clinical and laboratory evaluation of 131 cases. J Am Vet Med Assoc 183:103–110, 1983.

59. Fong TS, McHutchison JG, Reynolds TB. Hyperthyroidism and hepatic dysfunction. J Clin Gastroenterol 14:240–244, 1992.

60. Kelly WR. The liver and biliary system. In: Jubb KVF, Kennedy PC, Palmer N (eds) Pathology of Domestic Animals, 4th ed. Academic Press, San Diego, 319–406, 1993.

61. Greim H, Trulzsch D, Czygan P, et al. Mechanism of cholestasis. 6. Bile acids in human livers with or without biliary obstruction. Gastroenterology 63:846–850, 1972.

62. Scholmerich J, Becher M, Schmidt K, et al. Influence of hydroxylation and conjugation of bile salts on their membrane-damaging properties—studies on isolated hepatocytes and lipid membrane vesicles. Hepatology 4:661–666, 1984.

63. Miyazaki K, Nakayama F, Koga A. Effect of chenodeoxycholic and ursodeoxycholic acids on isolated adult human hepatocytes. Dig Dis Sci 29:1123–1130, 1984.

64. Velardi ALM, Groen AK, Oude Elferink RPJ, et al. Cell type-dependent effect of phospholipid and cholesterol on bile salt cytotoxicity. Gastroenterology 101:457–464, 1991.

65. van den Ingh TSGAM, Rothuizen J, van den Brom WE. Extrahepatic cholestasis in the dog and the differentiation of extrahepatic and intrahepatic cholestasis. Vet Q 8:150–157, 1986.

66. Kerr JFR, Cooksley WGE, Searle J, et al. The nature of piecemeal necrosis in chronic active hepatitis. Lancet 2:827–828, 1979.

67. Shinagawa T, Yoshioka K, Kakumu S, et al. Apoptosis in cultured rat hepatocytes: The effects of tumour necrosis factor-alpha and interferon-gamma. J Pathol 165:247–253, 1991.

68. Jarrett WFH, O'Neill BW. A new transmissible agent causing acute hepatitis, chronic hepatitis and cirrhosis in dogs. Vet Record 116:629–635, 1985.

69. Jarrett WFH, O'Neill BW, Lindholm I. Persistent hepatitis and chronic fibrosis induced by canine acidophil cell virus. Vet Record 120:234–235, 1987.

70. Ledda-Columbano GM, Coni P, Curto M, et al. Induction of two different modes of cell death, apoptosis and necrosis, in rat liver after a single dose of thioacetamide. Am J Pathol 139:1099–1109, 1991.

71. Eastman A. Apoptosis: A product of programmed and unprogrammed cell death. Toxicol Appl Pharmacol 121:160–164, 1991.

72. Mochida S, Ohta Y, Ogata I, et al. Gut-derived substances in activation of hepatic macrophages after partial hepatectomy in rats. J Hepatol 16:266–272, 1992.

73. Nolan JP. Intestinal endotoxins as mediators of hepatic injury: An idea whose time has come. Hepatology 10:887–891, 1989.

74. Ludwig J. The nomenclature of chronic active hepatitis: An obituary. Gastroenterology 105:274–278, 1993.

75. Dienes HP. Viral and Autoimmune Hepatitis: Morphologic and Pathogenetic Aspects of Cell Damage in Hepatitis and Potential Chronicity. Gustav Fischer Verlag, New York, 90–92, 1989.

76. Blumberg B. A serum antigen (Australian antigen) in Down's syndrome, leukemia, and hepatitis. Ann Int Med 66:924–931, 1967.

77. Feinstone S, Kapikian A, Purcell R. Detection by immune electron microscopy of a virus-like antigen associated with acute illness. Science 182:1026.

78. Kuo G, Choo Q, Alter H, et al. An assay for circulation antibodies to a major etiologic virus of human non-A, non-B hepatitis. Science 244:362–364, 1989.

79. Czaja AJ, Carpenter HA. Sensitivity, specificity, and predictability of biopsy interpretations in chronic hepatitis. Gastroenterology 105:1824–1832, 1993.

80. Bach N, Thung S, Schaffner F. The histological features of chronic hepatitis C and autoimmune chronic hepatitis: A comparative analysis. Hepatology 15:572–577, 1992.

81. Czaja AJ. Chronic active hepatitis: The challenge for a new nomenclature. Ann Int Med 119:510–517, 1993.

82. Borhan-Manesh F. Nomenclature of chronic hepatitis: A plea for change. Scand J Gastroenterol 29:193–194, 1994.

83. Boyer JL, Klatskin G. Patterns of necrosis in acute viral hepatitis. Prognostic value of bridging (subacute hepatic necrosis). N Engl J Med 283:1063–1069, 1970.

84. Okuno T, Okanoue T, Takino T, et al. Prognostic significance of bridging necrosis in chronic active hepatitis. Gastroenterol Japan 18:577–584, 1983.

85. Gane E, Portmann B, Saxena R, et al. Nodular regenerative hyperplasia of the liver graft after liver transplantation. Hepatology 20:88–94, 1994.

86. Wanless IR. Micronodular transformation (nodular regenerative hyperplasia) of the liver: A report of 64 cases among 2,500 autopsies and a new classification of benign hepatocellular nodules. Hepatology 11:787–797, 1990.

87. Fabry A, Benjamin SA, Angleton GM. Nodular hyperplasia of the liver in the beagle dog. Vet Pathol 19:109–119, 1982.

88. Prichard DH, Jolly RD, Howell LJ, et al. Ceroid-lipidosis: An acquired storage-type disease of liver and hepatic lymph node. Vet Pathol 20:242–244, 1983.

89. Bergman JR. Nodular hyperplasia in the liver of the dog: An association with changes in the Ito cell population. Vet Pathol 22:427–438, 1985.

90. Pappas NJ, Jr. Increased rat liver homogenate, mitochondrial, and cytosolic aspartate aminotransferase activity in acute carbon tetrachloride poisoning. Clin Chim Acta 106:223–229, 1980.

91. Pappas NJ, Jr, Wisecarver JL, Becker S. Effect of cycloheximide on increased aspartate aminotransferase in carbon tetrachloride hepatotoxicity. Ann Clin Lab 14:40–46, 1984.

92. Pappas NJ, Jr. Source of increased serum aspartate and alanine aminotransferase: Cycloheximide effect on carbon tetrachloride hepatotoxicity. Clin Chim Acta 154:181–190, 1986.

93. Gross TL, Song MD, Havel PJ, et al. Superficial necrolytic dermatitis (necrolytic migratory erythema) in dogs. Vet Pathol 30:75–81, 1993.

94. Meyer DJ, Harvey JW. Hematologic changes associated with serum and hepatic iron alterations in dogs with congenital portosystemic vascular anomalies. J Vet Int Med 8:55–56, 1994.

95. Laflamme DP, Mahaffey EA, Allen SW, et al. Microcytosis and iron status in dogs with surgically induced portosystemic shunts. J Vet Intern Med 8:212–216, 1994.

96. Bacon BR, Britton RS. Hepatic injury in chronic iron overload: Role of lipid peroxidation. Chem Biol Interact 70:183–226, 1989.

97. Bacon BR, Britton RS. The pathology of hepatic iron overload: A free radical-mediated process? Hepatology 11:127–137, 1990.

98. Benoit JN, Grisham MB, Mesh CL, et al. Hepatic oxidant and antioxidant systems in portacaval shunted rats. J Hepatol 14:253–258, 1992.

99. Adams PC, Bradley C, Frei JV. Hepatic iron and zinc concentrations after portocaval shunting for nonalcoholic cirrhosis. Hepatology 19:101–105, 1994.

100. Dixon D, Yoshitomi K, Boorman GA, et al. "Lipomatous" lesions of unknown cellular origin in the liver of B6C3F1 mice. Vet Pathol 31:173–182, 1994.

101. Weinbren K, Washington SLA. Hyperplastic nodules after portacaval shunts in rats. Nature 264:440–442, 1976.

102. Prasse KW, Mahaffey EA, DeNovo R, et al. Chronic lymphocytic cholangitis in three cats. Vet Pathol 19:99–108, 1982.

103. Kanel GC, Korula J. Cholestasis and biliary tract disorders. In: Atlas of Liver Pathology. WB Saunders, Philadelphia, 35–52, 1992.

104. Portmann B, Popper H, Neuberger J, et al. Sequential and diagnostic features in primary biliary cirrhosis based on serial histologic study in 209 patients. Gastroenterology 88:1777–1790, 1985.

105. Ludwig J, Czaja AJ, Dickson ER, et al. Manifestations of nonsuppurative cholangitis in chronic hepatobiliary diseases: Morphologic spectrum, clinical correlations and terminology. Liver 4:105–116, 1984.

106. Gerber MA. Chronic hepatitis C: The beginning of the end of a time-honored nomenclature? Hepatology 15:567–571, 1992.

107. Scheuer PJ, Ashrafzadeh P, Sherlock S, et al. The pathology of hepatitis C. Hepatology 15:567–571, 1992.

108. Miller MW, Bonagura JD, DiBartola SP, et al. Budd-Chiari-like syndrome in two dogs. J Am Anim Hosp Assoc 25:277–283, 1989.

109. Cohn LA, Spaulding KA, Cullen JM, et al. Intrahepatic postsinusoidal venous obstruction in a dog. J Vet Int Med 5:317–321, 1991.

110. van den Ingh TSGAM, Rothuizen J. Hepatoportal fibrosis in three young dogs. Vet Rec 110:575–577, 1982.

111. Rutgers HC, Haywood S, Kelly DF. Idiopathic hepatic fibrosis in 15 dogs. Vet Record 133:115–118, 1993.

112. Loeven KO. Hepatic amyloidosis in two Chinese Shar Pei dogs. J Am Vet Med Assoc 204:1212–1216, 1994.

113. Blunden AS, Smith KC. Generalised amyloidosis and acute liver haemorrhage in four cats. J Sm Anim Prac 33:566–570, 1992.

114. Lichtman SN, Sartor RB, Keku J, et al. Hepatic inflammation in rats with experimental small intestinal bacterial overgrowth. Gastroenterology 98:414–423, 1990.

115. Polzin DJ, Stowe CM, O'Leary TP, et al. Acute hepatic necrosis associated with the administration of mebendazole to dogs. J Am Vet Med Assoc 179:1013–1016, 1981.

116. Andrzejewska A, Dlugosz J, Kurasz S. The ultrastructure of the liver in acute experimental pancreatitis. Exp Pathol 28:167–176, 1985.

117. Weiner S, Gramatica L, Voegle LD, et al. Role of the lymphatic system in the pathogenesis of inflammatory disease in the biliary tract and pancreas. Am J Surg 119:55–61, 1970.

118. Chapman BL, Hendrick MJ, Washabau RJ. Granulomatous hepatitis in dogs: Nine cases (1987–1990). J Am Vet Med Assoc 203:680–684, 1993.

32

Acute Hepatic Injury: Hepatic Necrosis and Fulminant Hepatic Failure

SHARON A. CENTER

Clinical Synopsis

Diagnostic Features

- Subclinical if mild hepatic injury
- Acute onset of depression, vomiting, polydipsia, or jaundice may occur if damage more severe
- ALT, AST, and, to a lesser extent, SAP are increased
- Hyperbilirubinemia may be present (especially cats)
- Hyperbilirubinuria may be present (especially dogs)
- Hepatic function tests abnormal if damage marked
- Biopsy reveals hepatic degeneration and necrosis

Standard Management

- Address primary cause if identified
- NPO for 1 to 3 days followed by cottage cheese and rice
- IV fluid therapy including dextrose and potassium as needed
- Control of hepatic encephalopathy if required (see later)
- Additional therapy sometimes indicated (see text) includes H$_2$ blocker, plasma, heparin, antibiotics, and glucocorticoids

INTRODUCTION

Acute hepatic injury can result from a variety of disorders, summarized in Table 32–1. Mechanisms leading to hepatic degeneration and necrosis are discussed in Chapter 30. The morphologic patterns of hepatic injury are described in Chapter 31 and briefly reviewed here. Although liver injury can be categorized using descriptive morphologic characteristics, it is important to realize that the underlying cause may never be established. The zonal distribution of involved cells suggests possible pathogenesis (Figure 32–1). General patterns associated with some well-known hepatotoxins are summarized in Table 32–2.

Massive hepatic necrosis is associated with canine infectious hepatitis virus infection and drug-induced hepatitis (mebendazole in the dog and diazepam in the cat). Focal necrosis, involving any acinar zone, is a nonspecific form of hepatic injury seen with viral, drug, and hepatotoxin exposure as well as with biliary obstruction. Focal hepatic necrosis

is a frequent finding in liver biopsies obtained during surgery.[1] This is thought to result from hypotension and local hypoxia, caused by the effects of anesthesia and surgery.

Periacinar necrosis (centrilobular necrosis, zone 3 necrosis) commonly occurs as a result of hypoxemia, hypoperfusion, or stagnated hepatic blood flow. It is associated with shock and with clinical and pathologic sequelae of systemic hypotension. Periacinar degeneration and necrosis occur in animals that have a slow, agonal death and the lesions are worsened and become more expansive in the presence of anemia or hypoxemia. Chronic passive congestion due to heart failure or pericardial disease leads to periacinar necrosis. The lesions observed with chronic passive congestion and hypotension are discussed later. Severe periacinar necrosis may be followed by complete repair and restoration of normal structure and hepatic function within a few weeks.[2]

Midzonal hepatic necrosis is uncommon. In cases of shock, midzonal necrosis is always associated with centrilobular necrosis. In experimental animals, midzonal necrosis has been produced after pharmacologic doses of furosemide, and following intoxication with beryllium, ngaione, and paraquat.[3,4]

Periportal or zone 1 necrosis is an uncommon lesion but is seen more commonly than midzonal necrosis. Causes include exposure to certain hepatotoxins and endotoxins. Periportal necrosis can be observed as a chronic ongoing process in animals with inflammatory bowel disease and chronic pancreatitis.

Paracentral necrosis is coagulative necrosis that involves a complete hepatic acinus: This is believed to reflect an ischemic lesion or infarct produced by occlusion of a terminal portal venule and hepatic artery such as could occur with thromboembolism. It also can reflect the synergistic effect of hepatotoxin accumulation or production and reduced or impaired perfusion within an acinar unit. Spotty involvement of acini indicates physiologic differences in acinar blood flow at the moment of the pathogenic event (e.g., toxin distribution or embolic shower).

Simultaneous occurrence of varied combinations of hepatocellular degeneration and necrosis explain the clinical expression of hepatic injury. Hepatocellular degeneration occurs in viable cells with damaged organelles and is reflected by increased concentrations of leakage enzymes (transaminases) and impaired hepatic function if the injury is diffuse and involves a critical number of hepatocytes. In the

Table 32–1

DISORDERS IN DOGS AND CATS ASSOCIATED WITH HEPATIC NECROSIS OR DEGENERATION WITH OR WITHOUT INFLAMMATION

Infectious

Viral
Infectious canine hepatitis*
  (Adenovirus I)
Canine herpesvirus (neonatal)*
Feline herpesvirus (neonatal)
Feline infectious peritonitis

Bacterial
Gram negative septicemia
Gram positive septicemia
Endotoxema*
Francisella tularensis (tularemia)
Salmonella spp.
Clostridia spp.
Leptospira spp.
  icterohemorrhagiae canicola,
  grippotyphosa
Bacillus piliformis (Tyzzer's disease)
Mycobacteria:
  M. fortuitum

Rickettsial
Rickettsia rickettsii
Ehrlichia canis
Haemobartonella felis, canis

Mycotic
Histoplasmosis
Blastomycosis
Coccidioidomycosis
Aspergillosis (disseminated)
Candidiasis
Phaecomycoses

Protozoal
Toxoplasma gondi
Neospora caninum
Coccidiosis
Leishmania donovoni
Cytauxzoon felis

Parasitic
Heterobilharzia americana
Liver fluke migration
  Platynosomum spp.
  Pseudoamphistomum spp.
  Metorchis spp.
  Opisthorchis spp.
  Capillaria hepatica
Visceral larval migrans
Dirofilariasis

Algae
Protothecosis

Miscellaneous
Disseminated Intravascular
  Coagulation
Neoplasia:
  primary or secondary
  pressure necrosis
  thromboembolism
Pancreatitis:
  severe hemorrhagic
  severe necrotizing
Inflammatory bowel disease:
  lymphocytic-plasmacytic
  eosinophilic
  protein-losing enteropathy
  lymphangiectasia
  ulcerative colitis
Gastric dilation / volvulus
Hemolytic anemia:
  type III immune destruction
  intravascular hemolysis
  autoagglutination
Thromboembolic disease:
  hyperadrenocorticism
  protein-losing nephropathy:
    glomerulonephritis
    amyloidosis
  protein-losing enteropathy
  immune-mediated hemolytic
    anemia
  neoplasia

Cardiac Disease
Congestive heart failure
  AV insufficiency
  dilated cardiomyopathy
  congenital malformations
  reduced cardiac output: any
    cause
Severe passive congestion:
  right-sided heart failure
  dirofilariasis
  symptomatic cardiac
    arrhythmias
  pericardial disease:
    tamponade
    restrictive or constrictive
  vena caval occlusion: kink,
    thrombi
  Cor triatum dextor
  Vena caval syndrome:
    dirifilaria

Drugs: Also Consult Chapter 30
  Aspirin: cat
  Acetaminophen: dog, cat*
  Aprindine: dog
  Diazepam: cat*
  Halothane: dog*
  Ketoconazole: dog, cat
  Mebendazole: dog*
  Methotrexate: dog, human
  Phenobarbital: dog
  Phenytoin: dog
  Primidone: dog
  Phenazopyridine: cat
  Tetracycline: cat, dog
  Thiacetarsamide*
  Tolbutamide: dog
  Trimethoprim-sulfadiazine: dog
  Valproic acid: dog

Toxins: Also Consult Chapter 30
Arsenic: thiacetarsimide*
Chlorinated hydrocarbons*
  CCl_4, naphthalenes,
    chloroform
Dimethylnitrosamines*
Endotoxins*
Galactosamine*
Metals: copper, zinc, mercury*
Phosphorus: rat poison*

Biologic Substances
Aflatoxins*
  Aspergillus flavus
  Aspergillus parasitucus
  Penicillium puberulum
Ochratoxin A
  Aspergillus ochraceus
  Penicillium viridicatum
Rubratoxin
  Penicillium rubrum
  Penicillium purpurogenum
Penitrem A
  Penicillium crustosum
Blue-green algae
  Microcystis aeruginosa
  Anabena, Aphanizomenon
Sporidesmin
  Pithomyces chartarcum
Mushroom Poisoning: alpha-
  amanitin
  Amanita phalloides
  Amanita virosa
  Amanita verna

*= Can result in fulminant hepatic failure.

---

dog it seems hepatocellular degeneration is associated with induced production of ALP, which may appear in the systemic circulation in prodigious quantities. The histologic verification of hepatocellular degeneration is inconsistent owing to the inability to document organelle changes other than by variations in size and staining qualities of hepatocytes, which can be confused with processing artifacts. Thus the clinician may discount substantial degenerative injury if the pathologic description discounts cellular changes to collection or processing artifacts. Areas of degeneration are less impressive than areas of necrosis because the latter is accompanied by an inflammatory reaction. Diffuse degenerative lesions can have more impact on overall hepatic function than does focal, spotty, or zonal necrosis. Necrosis must be confluent or massive to damage sufficient numbers of hepatocytes and limit hepatic functions. Massive confluent necrosis can result in fulminant hepatic failure, but is an unusual clinical presen-

tation. Fulminant hepatic failure is described later in this chapter.

MECHANISMS OF HEPATOCELLULAR DEATH

The pathogenesis of hepatocellular degeneration leading to cell necrosis and death is complex and incompletely understood. A number of primary and secondary mechanisms leading to cell necrosis have been clarified through experimental work in animals, (Figure 32–2). These studies have permitted the characterization of causal factors and mechanisms of cell injury. Major categories are discussed in the following section.[5,6]

TISSUE ISCHEMIA AND HYPOXIA. The pathogenesis of ischemic liver injury remains to be clearly elucidated. An overview is illustrated in Figure 32–3. Hepatocytes are espe-

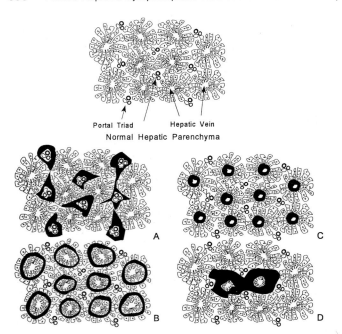

Portal Triad   Hepatic Vein
Normal Hepatic Parenchyma

FIGURE 32-1. Drawing showing the microanatomic distribution of (*A*) periportal or zone 1 lesions, (*B*) midzonal or zone 2 lesions, (*C*) periacinar or centrizonal or centrilobular, zone 3 lesions, and (*D*) paracentral lesion involving an entire acinar unit.

cially susceptible to anoxia. Tissue hypoxia rapidly leads to plasma membrane and cytosolic organelle injury.[1,3–15] Impairment of mitochondrial metabolism and resulting ATP depletion plays a pivotal role in the structural and functional ischemic injury.[16] Other important aspects of the pathogenesis include accumulation of lactic acid, impaired membrane ion pumps, accumulation of cytosolic Ca^{2+}, compromised cellular protein synthesis, and activation of xanthine oxidase. Leakage of lysosomal enzymes is a major terminal event causing irreversible tissue injury and organ failure.[17–19] Destruction of sinusoidal beds, hepatocellular swelling that compresses sinusoidal flow causing microsludging, and vascular spasm promote continued ischemia.[15,18,20] Failure of the reticuloendothelial system in providing host defense complicates injury by permitting endotoxins to enter liver tissue.[21]

Experimentally, alleviation of hepatic ischemia within 60 minutes results in only a partial recovery of the cellular injury.[16] In the dog, after 30 minutes of hepatic ischemia, lysosomal enzymes can be detected in the systemic circulation.[22] Normothermic hepatic ischemia of 40 minutes duration can be tolerated, but ischemia lasting between 50 and 70 minutes has a 60% survival, and ischemia lasting for 80 minutes or longer is fatal.[22] Cytoprotective agents given before ischemia is induced improves tolerance.[23–26] Death after hepatic ischemia occurs during the first 24 hours, usually 8 to 10 hours after hepatic perfusion is reinstated. Serum biochemistry studies show a profound increase in hepatic transaminases immediately following ischemic injury, which decline during the next several days. The serum ALP activity is modestly increased as early as 90 minutes after revascularization and remains high for as long as 4 to 6 weeks in dogs that survive diffuse ischemic injury.

FREE RADICALS AND OXIDATIVE INJURY. Free radicals are atoms, ions, or molecules having odd numbers of electrons.[5,6] Those behaving as hepatotoxins are subdivided into two groups. One group is comprised of metabolic products of organic compounds and is exemplified by CCl_4, nitrofuran-

toin, paraquat, and other aromatic compounds. The other group involves activated toxic oxygen species. If the balance between toxic oxygen species and the cellular antioxidant potential is not maintained, oxidative cell injury occurs.

MEMBRANE LIPID PEROXIDATION AND INTERACTIONS WITH PHOSPHOLIPIDS. Lipid peroxidation always accompanies hepatocellular damage by oxidative injury and results when free radicals attack the unsaturated bonds of fatty acids. A cleavage chain reaction results in membrane breakdown that permits dislocation and dysfunction of membrane proteins and enzymes.[5,6,27] Examples of toxins injurious via lipid peroxidation include CCL_4, halothane, chloroform, ionizing radiation, dimethylnitrosamines, and hepatocellular iron overload.

The degradation of phospholipids is an early effect of many hepatotoxins. In addition to peroxidative damage, another process causing membrane injury involves the Ca^{2+}-dependent activation of phospholipases A and C, as occurs with CCl_4, bromobenzene, and galactosamine toxicities and in ischemic liver injury.[5,6] These lipases normally are essential in the generation of secondary messengers from phosphatidyl inositol, which is an important mechanism of cell signaling.

DEPLETION OF ESSENTIAL INTRACELLULAR COMPOUNDS AND COFACTORS. In a select few forms of hepatic injury, depletion of a specific factor has been shown to be the central causal factor. The best examples are the glutathione depletion that occurs with acetaminophen and bromobenzene intoxication. These toxins produce irreversible cell injury related to lipid peroxidation. Glutathione depletion results in

Table 32-2

KNOWN HEPATOTOXINS AND THEIR MOST COMMON ZONAL DISTRIBUTION OF HEPATOCELLULAR INJURY	
NECROSIS	**NECROSIS AND FATTY DEGENERATION**
Albitocin (PP)	Acetaminophen (M)
Alloxan (PP)	Aflatoxins (PV, PP)
Allyl compounds (PP)	Alpha-Amanitin (PV)
Aniline (M)	Arsenicals (inorganic) (PV, M)
Berylium (MZ)	Bromobenzene (PV)
Chlorinated benzenes (M)	Carbon tetrachloride (PV)
Dioxane (M)	Chlorinated diphenyls (M)
Ferrous sulphate (PP)	Chlorinated naphtalene (M)
Manganese compounds (PP)	Chloroform (PV)
Ngaione (MZ)	Chloroprene (PV)
Paracetamol (PV)	2-Chloropropane (PV)
Paraquat (PV, MZ)	Dichloropropane (PV)
Phalloidin (PV)	Dimethylnitrosamine
P. Vulgaris endotoxin (PP)	Dinitrobenzone (PV, M)
P. multocida (M)	Dinitrophenol (M)
Rubratoxin (PV)	Dinitrotoluene (PV, M)
Selenium (M)	Ethylene dibromide (PV)
Sporidesmin (PP)	Ethylene dichloride (PV)
Thiacetarsimide (PV)	Galactosamine (M)
Urethane (PV)	Iodoform (PV)
	Islandicum (PV)
	Luteoskyrin (PV)
	Methylchloroform
	Naphthalene (PV)
	Pyrrolizidine alkaloids (PV)
	Synthalin (PP)
	Tannic acid (PV)
	Tetrachloroethane (M)

Key: (PP) = Periportal (zone 1), (M) = Massive, (MZ) = Midzonal (zone 2), (PV) = Perivenular (centrilobular, zone 3)

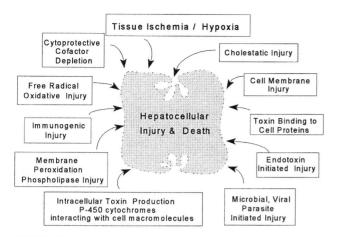

FIGURE 32-2. Drawing showing an overview of the mechanisms of cellular injury and death (corresponds with discussion in the text).

a failure of antioxidant protection from reactive electrophile metabolites.

INTRACELLULAR TOXIN PRODUCTION AND INTERACTION WITH CELL MACROMOLECULES. Most hepatotoxic agents enter the hepatocyte as lipid-soluble compounds. Many undergo biotransformation in the cell yielding metabolites that adversely interact with cell components. The sequential modification

of a nonreactive parent compound into a bioreactive toxin mainly occurs via the cytochrome P-450 system. The tropism of bioreactive toxins is variable and thus different metabolites may induce a different type of injury and regional acinar distribution. The pathogenic effects of a particular toxin depends on the quantity and life span of the toxic metabolite and its regional metabolism within the acinus.

CELLULAR INJURY DERIVED FROM BINDING OF TOXINS TO CELL PROTEINS, RNA, DNA. Idiosyncratic binding to proteins may result in unpredictable hypersensitivity reactions that can be metabolic or immunogenic.[5,6] Altered metabolic pathways as a result of previous exposure to an inducing or inhibiting agent or to genetic factors can explain some of the unpredictable responses to seemingly benign medications. In some cases, known drug interactions can explain hepatocellular toxicity.

Some toxins bind to nucleic acids or to enzymes essential for protein synthesis. Necrogenic mushroom poisoning due to alpha-amanitine inhibits RNA polymerase, which is requisite for messenger RNA formation. Aflatoxin binds DNA and also interferes with RNA polymerase. It is not conclusively known that these effects lead to cell necrosis or that some other toxic product induces cell death. Exposure to OH· has been shown to break the DNA backbone and induce abnormal cell growth in vitro. Certain chemical carcinogens inhibit DNA synthesis in cell cultures of proliferating hepatocytes. Despite these recognized adverse interactions, a close association with hepatic necrosis in vivo is not consistent. The hepatocyte may be

Consequences of Hepatic Ischemia / Hypoxia

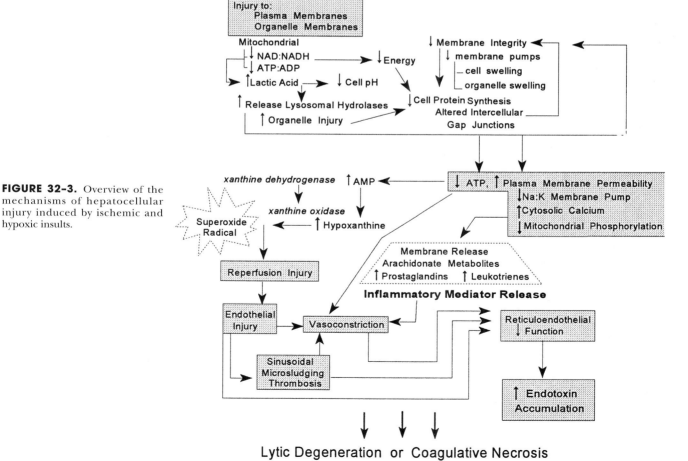

FIGURE 32-3. Overview of the mechanisms of hepatocellular injury induced by ischemic and hypoxic insults.

somewhat tolerant to cytotoxic effects depending on DNA involvement owing to its long life span and limited replication unless provoked. However, if cell injury induces hepatic regeneration, oncogenic transformation of cells may occur. Chronic aflatoxin exposure has been implicated as a promoter of hepatocellular carcinoma in human beings.

CHOLESTATIC INJURY. Any hepatic process that induces cholestasis has the potential to cause hepatocellular injury and necrosis. Retention of bile acids produces organelle injury and destroys portions of the cytochrome P-450 system. The dihydroxy bile acids are more deleterious than the trihydroxy bile acids. In prolonged severe cholestasis, hepatocytes undergo degenerative and lytic necrosis, although the exact mechanisms are not fully understood.

ENDOTOXIN, MICROBIAL, VIRAL, PARASITIC, AND IMMUNOLOGIC MECHANISMS OF INJURY. Hepatocellular degeneration and necrosis caused by bacteria and parasites have been well established. Infectious agents that can be associated with hepatic necrosis are summarized in Table 32–1 and are discussed individually in the latter portions of this chapter. Shock due to septicemia and endotoxemia is responsible for the periacinar distribution in some of these conditions. Hepatic necrosis due to septicemia or bacterial infection in a nonhepatic location usually produces a diffuse multifocal distribution of necrosis twice as often as it is restricted to zone 3.

The role of bacterial products, most notably endotoxins, have been investigated as a cause of hepatic injury.[28-35] Endotoxin is now proposed as a unifying mechanism of hepatocellular necrosis in a diverse number of primary hepatic disorders. The noxious effects of endotoxins are mediated by mononuclear phagocytes, most notably hepatic Kupffer cells, which become stimulated to produce inflammatory mediators including prostaglandins and leukotrienes. Endotoxins also impair the elimination of certain leukotrienes. These interactive effects potentiate the injurious effects of endotoxins and are believed to promote the necroinflammatory reactions commonly observed around the portal triads in patients showing signs of endotoxemia, inflammatory bowel disease, and pancreatitis.

Endotoxins potentiate the effects of other hepatotoxins.[29] In rodents, endotoxin derived from *E. coli* has a vasoconstrictive effect on liver blood flow.[28] Among the systemic effects of endotoxic shock are hypotension and altered microvascular perfusion.[30] Hypoxemia, a complication of endotoxin-induced pulmonary edema and ventilation/perfusion mismatching, may amplify their direct hepatotoxic effects as well as those of inflammatory mediators whose release they promote.

Jaundice in patients with bacteremia may develop due to intrahepatic cholestasis with or without associated multifocal hepatocellular necrosis.[4,36-38] Kupffer cell hyperplasia, mild accumulation of lymphocytes in portal areas, and mild to moderate "fatty" vacuolation has been referred to as nonspecific "reactive hepatitis" seen in a variety of conditions, including bacteremia and endotoxemia. In the patient with suspected bacteremia, hyperbilirubinemia associated with a disproportionate (mild) increase in liver enzymes is unlikely to directly involve hepatic tissue. Rather, the impaired ability to normally process and excrete bilirubin should be suspected.[36,37] Endotoxin and other toxic bacterial components or products, distinct from exotoxins, may also produce this effect. The lipid A moiety of endotoxin may inhibit hepatocyte excretion of bilirubin into bile canaliculi.[39] A bacterial derivative associated with hyperbilirubinemia in staphylococcal bacteremia is teichoic acid, a component of the bacterial wall.[38]

Relatively few viruses have been recognized to have direct cytopathic effects on hepatocytes of companion animals. The infectious canine hepatitis virus (canine adenovirus 1) is one of these (see later). Another virus, more recently identified in dogs, causes an acidophil cell hepatitis.[40] Although this virus is linked with chronic hepatitis, it is likely that episodes of acute necrosis predominate as early events. Some human hepatitis viral agents appear to survive long enough in animals to cause a serologic response. Their pathogenicity, however, has not been studied long term in these alternative host species. Viruses can cause secondary hepatic lesions in the cat, but the induced lesion is usually not hepatic necrosis. Feline infectious peritonitis is associated with pyogranulomatous inflammation in the liver. Recently, a retrospective study of hepatic lesions in cats infected with the feline leukemia virus disclosed the presence of hepatocellular degeneration, often in association with other systemic conditions related to their immunosuppression.[41] Parasitic diseases involving the liver cause either endothelial injury or inflammatory or ischemic insults that secondarily damage the hepatocyte.

Immunologic reactions generating inflammatory mediators, such as complement and perforin, lymphocytotoxins, and reactive radicals, can result in hepatocellular lysis. Acquired directed attack against hepatocellular membrane antigens, such as the liver-specific lipoproteins and the asialoglycoprotein receptor, can serve to perpetuate tissue necrosis as discussed in Chapter 33 for chronic hepatitis.

INJURY TO THE HEPATOCYTE PLASMA MEMBRANE. Injury to the plasma membrane of the hepatocyte is an important factor inducing loss of cell integrity and may occur secondary to chemical or immunologic mechanisms. This leads to leakage of enzymes, coenzymes, and electrolytes from the cell, permits entry of calcium ions and other electrolytes, and may progress to an irreversibly altered intracellular milieu such that recovery is impossible. Injury to the plasma membrane is the best documented initiating event in many forms of hepatic necrosis.

CLINICAL FINDINGS

Focal, mild, or moderate hepatic necrosis or degeneration is rarely associated with clinical signs that draw attention to the liver. Rather, the underlying cause in another organ system usually produces the dominant physical signs.

Acute massive hepatic necrosis produces consistent clinical signs, which are usually severe and reflect the degree of hepatic damage. Signs of acute hepatic failure are nonspecific and often include anorexia, depression, vomiting, polydipsia, and dehydration. Jaundice develops early if hepatic toxicity is focused on the periportal region but develops later when lesions involve other portions of the acinus. Fever occurs with infectious hepatitis, with release of pyrogens from damaged tissue, and when Kupffer cell dysfunction and abnormal parenchymal perfusion reduce clearance of microorganisms and toxins derived from the portal circulation. Surface petechial and ecchymotic hemorrhages are manifested infrequently. When present, clinical signs of hemorrhage usually include hematemesis, melena, and hematochezia. Overt signs of hepatic encephalopathy usually develop after it is clear that hepatic failure is established.

CLINICAL PATHOLOGY

The clinicopathologic features documented in dogs and cats with biopsy-confirmed hepatic necrosis are summarized in Figures 32–4. Comparison of the diagnostic sensitivities for different tests are shown in Figure 32–5.

Hepatic necrosis causes a loss of hepatocyte structure and

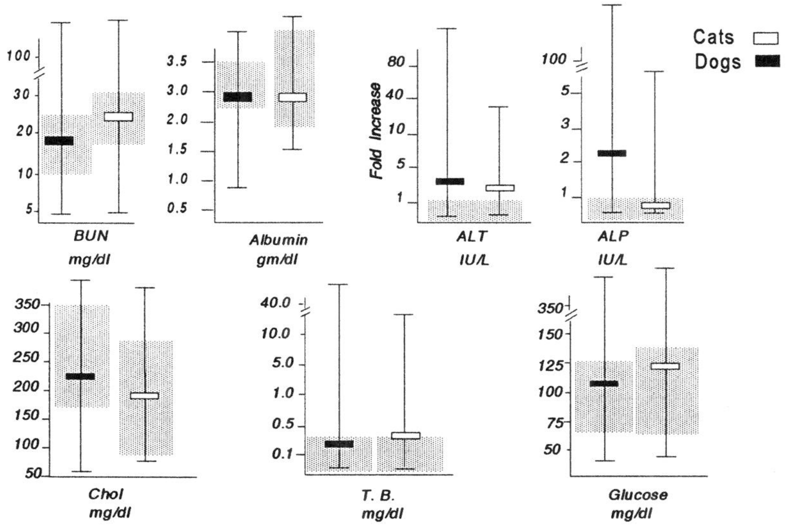

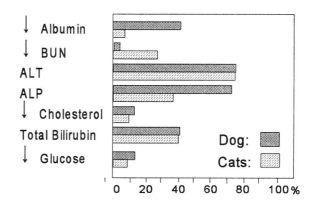

FIGURE 32-4. Clinicopathologic features of dogs and cats with histologically confirmed acute hepatic injury. Data is represented as the mean and range. Hatched area represents the normal values for each parameter. Data derived from the College of Veterinary Medicine, University of California at Davis.

function. Structural injury results in a loss in integrity of constraining cell and organelle membranes such that soluble intracellular components are released into surrounding tissues. The hepatic circulation quickly distributes released soluble moieties to the point they can be detected in the peripheral circulation. The hepatic transaminases, ALT and AST, are freely discharged from the cytosol when cell membrane permeability is reversibly altered, leaky gap junctions develop, or the cell undergoes necrosis. The serum half-lives of the transaminases are relatively short (<5 hours), which permits a chronologic profile of ongoing injury by sequential serum measurements. Detection of increased serum activity of ALT and AST is the first overt clinicopathologic feature of hepatocellular injury and becomes apparent within hours of a significant cellular insult. There is considerable individual variation in the magnitude of serum enzyme activity for a comparatively equivalent histologic lesion. Consequently, the serum activity of the transaminases do not reliably parallel the degree or severity of hepatic injury. In animals given an hepatotoxin, the degree of necrosis correlates well with the immediate increase in serum ALT activity, which may increase by a 50-fold margin compared to normal values in the first 24 hours.[42] Within 3 days after the toxic injury, the histologic appearance of necrosis remains unchanged yet the serum ALT values have resolved or remain only 4- to 5-fold normal values. In spontaneous necrosis, measurement of the serum ALT and AST activities reflects recent necrosis in only 50% of animals if several days have lapsed since the toxic insult occurred. Sequential measurements of serum transaminase activity can be used diagnostically to increase the index of suspicion of necrosis and prognostically to monitor remission or continuation of hepatocellular injury. Because so many factors can alter the plasma membrane and health of the hepatocyte, serum ALT and AST determinations are not specific for hepatic necrosis or degeneration. In human beings, the ratio between ALT and AST has been suggested to reflect the severity of hepatocellular injury. The serum AST activity can be comprised of several different isoenzymes. The hepatocellular mitochondria are particularly rich in a unique AST isoenzyme. Severe hepatocellular injury that damages mitochondria can thus be detected through documentation of a marked increase in the serum AST to ALT ratio.[43] Clarification that the AST is comprised of the mitochondrial isoenzyme improves the diagnostic utility of this enzyme as an estimate of the degree or severity of hepatocellular injury.

Caution is warranted to rule out muscle injury with measurement of the creatine kinase (CK) activity when marked increases in ALT and AST activities are detected. Rich stores of transaminase are present in muscle and these may be released in the circumstance of a myopathy, for example in dogs with muscular dystrophy or rhabdomyolysis.[44]

Serum ALP activity can be comprised of several different isoenzymes. In the dog, primarily the hepatic, glucocorticoid, and bone isoenzymes, and in the cat, primarily the hepatic and bone isoenzymes, are detected in serum. The ALP derived from liver is associated with the hepatocellular canalicular structures and the biliary epithelium. When ALP is detected in abnormal amounts in serum, a previous increase in its rate of production has been initiated. Seemingly, many conditions in the body can initiate increased ALP production, resulting in its lack of diagnostic specificity. In the dog, serum ALP activity behaves similar to an acute-phase protein that is stimulated by inflammation and cytokine messengers. In addition, many primary and secondary hepatic disorders can result in biliary epithelial proliferation that is usually associated with increased serum ALP activity. Examples include intrahepatic cholestasis, cholangitis, extrahepatic biliary obstruction, hepatic regeneration following necrosis, and certain hepatic tumors.[45] Although increased release of hepatic ALP occurs during hepatic necrosis, during the acute phase (first 2 days) the magnitudes of increase are minor in

FIGURE 32-5. Sensitivity of different laboratory tests in the diagnosis of hepatic necrosis in the dog and cat. Data derived from the College of Veterinary Medicine, University of California at Davis.

comparison to changes in hepatic transaminases. Hepatic necrosis caused by infectious canine hepatitis results in increased serum ALP activity, although not until 3.5 days after virus inoculation.[46] Serum activity of ALP increases until death, reflecting an increased synthesis of the enzyme by proliferating biliary epithelia. A continued increase in plasma ALP activity while plasma ALT returns to normal can signify an unresolved biliary stasis, reactive biliary hyperplasia, or hepatic regeneration.

The serum gamma-glutamyltransferase (GGT) activity largely reflects hepatic origin of the enzyme. In the dog, the serum GGT activity used in series with the ALP activity improves the diagnostic performance of the latter enzyme. Nevertheless, the serum GGT activity undergoes changes similar to that observed with ALP.[47] These are exemplified by the enzyme changes that have been quantified in dogs intoxicated with carbon tetrachloride (CCl_4). The use of GGT in the cat assists in the early detection of most conditions causing parenchymal inflammation, necrosis, and cholestasis. In the cat, the serum GGT activity used in parallel with ALP improves the sensitivity of the latter enzyme as a diagnostic indicator.[48] It is interesting but remains unexplained why the disproportionate increase in serum ALP to GGT activity occurs in cats with severe hepatic lipidosis. Nevertheless, this unique difference assists in recognizing necroinflammatory disorders in the cat that may clinically mimic the lipidosis syndrome.

Hyperbilirubinemia can be produced by hepatic necrosis especially when it is centered in zone 1 around the portal triad. Swelling of degenerated cells and disruption of canaliculi by hepatocyte necrosis can obstruct bile flow and produce cholestasis. The serum bile acid concentrations become markedly increased before hyperbilirubinemia becomes overt. This is the major reason that serum bile acid determinations are useful in appraising early cholestatic changes. Hyperbilirubinemia is a relatively late development in animals with necrosis or degeneration in zone 3 and also in those with florid necrosis.[49] Only a small percentage of the total liver capacity is required to catabolize the small quantity of heme pigment recycled each day. With normal periportal hepatocytes and an intact and functioning biliary system, the liver can manage normal daily bilirubin processing.[49] In spontaneous hepatic necrosis in dogs and cats, hyperbilirubinemia is a variable finding. In the dog with widespread necrosis, hyperbilirubinemia may not exceed 2.0 to 3.0 mg/dl. In the cat, bilirubin concentrations tend to increase to a greater magnitude at a faster rate.

Function tests such as total serum bile acids, BSP 30 minute percentage retention, random blood ammonia, and ammonia tolerance testing usually are normal in patients with hepatic necrosis unless the distribution is periportal or there is massive tissue involvement.

Changes in other clinicopathologic parameters reflecting hepatic injury also usually do not develop unless massive necrosis causes fulminant hepatic failure. As shown in Figure 32–4 the most common abnormalities observed in natural cases of hepatic necrosis are increases in the serum enzyme activities. Hepatic necrosis cannot be diagnosed from biochemical tests because moderately to markedly increased plasma ALT activity can not differentiate necrosis from acute or chronic hepatitis, steroid-induced hepatopathy, portosystemic vascular anomalies, hepatocellular carcinoma, or a variety of other hepatic conditions. A diagnosis of hepatic necrosis or degeneration can only be made on the basis of histologic examination of liver tissue. It is important for the clinician to consider that most animals with clinicopathologic evidence of hepatic necrosis have a nonhepatic primary disease process and liver biopsy is less important than diagnostic effort directed at the underlying problem.

TREATMENT OF FOCAL HEPATIC NECROSIS

By virtue of the paucity of clinical signs produced by focal hepatic necrosis, it is seldom identified as a single diagnosis. Focal necrosis is frequently an incidental finding easily dismissed or ignored as unimportant. The pathologic sequela to persistent focal necrosis is unknown but is speculated to include chronic hepatitis and development of hepatic fibrosis and possibly primary hepatic neoplasia. Because chronic hepatic disease remains covert until it reaches an advanced stage, focal hepatic necrosis should not be ignored once discovered.

Whenever focal necrosis is diagnosed, primary treatment is directed to removal of the etiologic agent or condition. As previously discussed, many factors causing focal necrosis are related to the gastrointestinal tract. These include drugs, exogenous toxins, endogenous toxins produced by enteric microorganisms, dietary and bacterial antigens, antigens initiating immune complex formation and cell-mediated immune responses, microorganisms, and pancreatitis. The primary treatment goal is to minimize enteric absorption of noxious substances. The patient should be evaluated for pancreatitis and intestinal disease, and if found, these are managed appropriately. A diet free of food additives and preservatives is advised because some of these chemicals can be hepatotoxic. For example nitrites used as preservatives in meat products are converted in the bowel to hepatotoxic nitrosamines. An effective controlled diet consists of a source of carbohydrate (boiled white rice) and a single protein such as cottage cheese. This diet is also free of many antigens that could be primary initiating factors for an inflammatory bowel response. Because this diet also influences the quantity and types of bacteria in the intestines, it is believed to reduce the amount of absorbable toxins. Unlike diets formulated for patients with hepatic insufficiency, the diet for a patient recovering from hepatic necrosis should contain as much protein as tolerated without precipitating or aggravating signs of HE. Recovery from hepatic necrosis is more rapid on a high-protein than on a low-protein diet. Any drug suspected as a cause of the hepatic injury must be discontinued.

MASSIVE HEPATIC NECROSIS: FULMINANT HEPATIC FAILURE

Clinical Synopsis

Diagnostic Features

- Anorexia, depression, and behavioral abnormalities progressing to obtundation and coma
- Vomiting, diarrhea, and seizures are common
- Hepatomegaly, cranial abdominal pain, and bleeding tendencies may be seen
- ALT markedly increased followed by increased SAP
- Hyperbilirubinemia and/or hyperbilirubinuria are common
- Progressive reduction in blood glucose, urea, and albumin
- Abnormal coagulation tests likely
- Biopsy reveals massive hepatic necrosis or degeneration

Standard Management (see Figures 32–7 and 32–8)

- Address primary cause if identified
- NPO for 1–3 days followed by cottage cheese and rice

- IV fluid therapy with 0.45% saline and 5% dextrose with 20 mEq/L of KCl (minimum)
- Plasma (20 mL/kg) or other colloids often valuable
- Saline enemas to cleanse rectum of feces
- Neomycin retention enema (15–20 mL of a 1% solution)
- Lactulose enema (5–15 mL of a 1 to 3 dilution every 4–6 hours)
- Additional therapy sometimes indicated (see text) includes cimetidine, famotidine, antibiotics, blood, heparin, phosphate, diuretics, corticosteroids, N-acetylcysteine, flumazenil.

Fulminant hepatic failure is used to define the occurrence of acute liver failure in an otherwise healthy individual. It is complicated by hepatic encephalopathy and the sequelae of lost hepatic synthetic, excretory, and regulatory functions. It develops when acute hepatocellular necrosis or degeneration involves a large proportion of the liver. As applied to human beings, the definition of fulminant hepatic failure implies a lack of preexisting hepatocellular disease. Recovery is possible because (1) the underlying pathogenetic factor can be removed or inactivated; (2) the failed hepatic functions can be compensated by therapeutic support; (3) the reticulin framework of the liver remains intact; and (4) the organ retains its ability to regenerate.[50]

The causes of fulminant hepatic failure have been characterized into four categories: (1) infections, (2) toxins, chemicals, and drugs, (3) ischemic and hypoxic injury, and (4) metabolic anomalies. Disorders that can lead to fulminant hepatic failure in the dog and cat are listed in Table 32–1.

There are two distinct morphologic forms of hepatic injury in fulminant hepatic failure. One type is characterized by massive hepatocellular necrosis involving large confluent areas of tissue. A second type of lesion is characterized by a microvesicular hepatocyte appearance with cells appearing swollen and pale. A microvesicular fatty infiltration may be verified by application of a fat-specific stain. Minimal histologic features of hepatocellular necrosis are apparent. Failure of organ function is attributed to organelle dysfunction. In humans this lesion may be invoked by metabolic disorders and certain drugs. This is an uncommon cause of fulminant hepatic failure in the dog and cat with the exception of cats with severe hepatic lipidosis syndrome.

A typical response to massive hepatic necrosis due to toxic chemicals is a marked increase in the serum activities of plasma ALT and AST when the toxin is administered or consumed, and a return to normal values soon after discontinuation of the insulting agent.[51-60] The increased activity of serum ALP follows that of serum ALT and AST and persists for several weeks longer than peak transaminase activities, (Figure 32–6). As with focal necrosis, the serum ALP activity

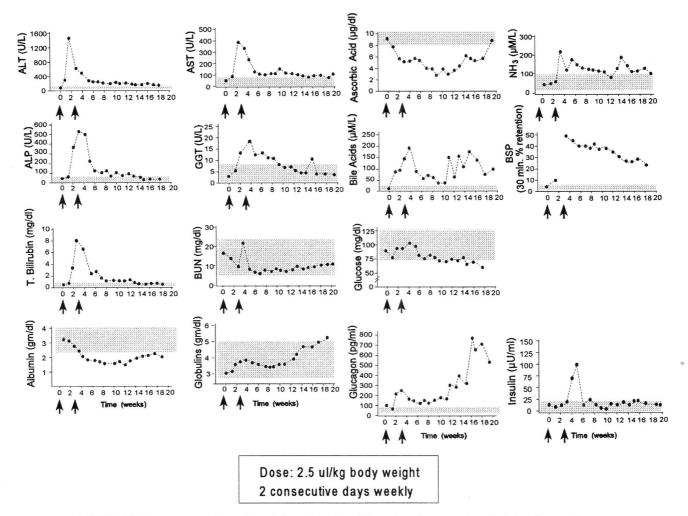

Dose: 2.5 ul/kg body weight
2 consecutive days weekly

FIGURE 32–6. Laboratory data collected from dogs (n = 12) undergoing acute hepatic injury from oral administration of dimethylnitrosamine. The hatched area represents the normal values for each parameter. Arrows represent the interval during which the toxin was administered.[53]

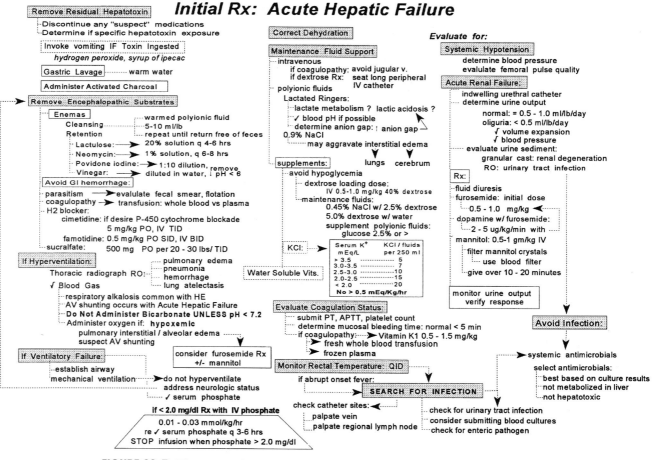

FIGURE 32–7. Therapeutic algorithm (Part 1) for the initial management of animals with acute hepatic failure.

reflects intrahepatic cholestasis and hepatocellular regeneration. The scenario of a progressive decline in serum transaminases with increasing or persisting high activities of serum ALP is viewed as a favorable indication of hepatic regeneration.

Hepatic function is compromised to varying degrees with massive hepatic necrosis. Increased serum bilirubin concentration lags slightly behind the initial massive release of hepatic transaminases. Total serum bile acid determinations are increased during the acute phase of injury and remain elevated for as long as cholestasis and sinusoidal blood flow is impaired by stromal collapse. Baseline resting blood ammonia values usually progressively increase but are not reliable indicators of hepatic injury. Better estimation is made using an ammonia tolerance test. Impaired circulation, hepatic uptake or processing, or biliary excretion of the organic anion indicator dyes (BSP and ICG) can provide the earliest indication of the severity of the hepatic injury. Abnormalities in plasma elimination of BSP or ICG have been shown experimentally before marked increases in the serum enzymes occur.

The liver's major functions in carbohydrate and nitrogen metabolism are impaired at the time of peak enzyme abnormalities, or shortly thereafter. A relative hypoglycemia reflects compromised carbohydrate metabolism, (Figures 32–5 and 32–6). A progressive reduction in the serum concentration of BUN, albumin, and certain globulins reflect impaired nitrogen and protein metabolism.

Coagulopathies including DIC may complicate hepatic necrosis (see Chapter 30).[61–65] The change in routinely used coagulation tests and specific coagulation factors in dogs undergoing chronic exposure to dimethylnitrosamines causing severe hepatic necrosis are summarized in Table 32–3.[66] In these dogs, hepatic injury was severe and resulted in chronic functional insufficiency.

Platelet numbers and function are also compromised by massive hepatic failure. Platelet numbers decrease and their smaller size indicates an older population and the possibility of delayed release of young platelets. Platelets show abnormal ultrastructural morphology and have intrinsic functional defects resulting in abnormal aggregation and adhesion.

Animals developing massive hepatic necrosis have deranged nitrogen detoxification causing hyperammonemia and signs of HE, whereas animals with focal or moderate hepatic necrosis or degeneration do not develop these abnormalities. Following massive hepatic necrosis, the plasma concentrations of almost all amino acids increase markedly (Table 32–4).[53,67] The exceptions are the branched chain amino acids arginine and citrulline (see Chapter 30). Currently, it is thought abnormalities in plasma amino acids are a consequence of hepatic injury and probably contribute little to clinical signs. The exception is the importance given to plasma arginine concentrations and the ability for supplemental arginine to improve function of the urea cycle in patients hyperammonemic due to hepatic failure.

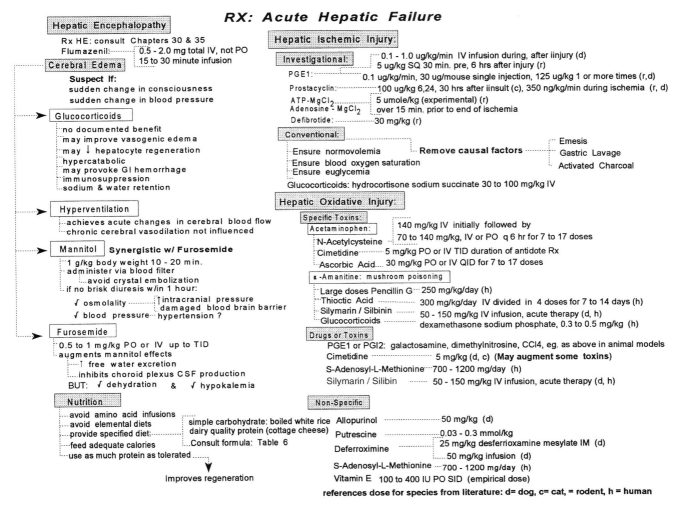

FIGURE 32–8. Therapeutic algorithm (Part 2) for management of animals with acute hepatic failure.

Clinical Consequences of Fulminant Hepatic Failure

Fulminant hepatic failure leads to the full spectrum of biochemical and coagulation abnormalities expected with synthetic, excretory, and regulatory dysfunction.

HEPATIC ENCEPHALOPATHY (HE). Hepatic encephalopathy that accompanies fulminant hepatic failure remains potentially reversible. As for HE in other forms of liver injury, the metabolic disturbances are multifactorial and impair cerebral function through a variety of diverse mechanisms. These are discussed in detail in Chapter 30. Many secondary factors can contribute to HE associated with fulminant hepatic failure. These include hypoglycemia, hypoxia, systemic hypoperfusion as a consequence of impaired cardiac function, impaired cerebral perfusion, gastrointestinal hemorrhage, dehydration, and cerebral edema.

CEREBRAL EDEMA. Increased intracranial pressure is associated with the syndrome of fulminant hepatic failure in humans and some animal models as a neurologic complication distinct from the syndrome of HE and terminal hypoxemia.[50,68–70] Up to 30% of humans with cerebral edema also show evidence of cerebellar herniation, a significant cause of death.[50,68,69] The pathogenetic mechanisms responsible for cerebral edema in patients with fulminant hepatic failure have not been clearly defined, although there are several hypotheses (Figure 32–9). These include (1) development of vasogenic edema in which there is an increased transfer of extracellular fluid across the blood-brain barrier, (2) development of cytotoxic edema due to a failed ability to regulate cellular osmotic balance, and (3) expansion of the intracranial extracellular space either diffusely in the intercellular space or as compartmentalized hydrocephalus. Altered integrity of endothelial tight junctions in cerebral capillaries or an increase in transport processes across these cells may promote development of vasogenic edema.[71–76] This may be augmented by a generalized vasodilation or an increase in cerebral blood flow. Toxins, hypoxia, and impaired mitochondrial function, which impair cell sodium osmoregulation, may induce cytotoxic cerebral edema. Development of microthrombi occluding cerebral microvasculature has also been shown in humans who have died of fulminant hepatic failure.[77] In humans and experimental animal models, fulminant hepatic failure is associated with a reduced systemic blood pressure, decreased cerebral blood flow, and reduced cerebral oxygen consumption. Cerebral ischemia occurs if cerebral-perfusion pressure (systemic blood pressure minus intracranial pressure) is not maintained above 40 to 50 mm Hg.

Table 32–3

ROUTINE COAGULATION TESTS AND COAGULATION FACTORS
IN DOGS AFTER DIMETHYLNITROSAMINE TOXICITY[66]

TESTED VARIABLE	NORMAL VALUES	WEEKS			
		1	2	3	4
Prothrombin time (seconds)	< 8.2	10.7	11.7	10.4	9.2
Partial thromboplastin time (seconds)	< 12.0	17.4	24.2	27.4	16.7
Thrombin time (seconds)	5 to 10	10.7	12.9	12.4	15.2
Fibrinogen (mg/dl)	> 200	76	61	66	73
Factor V (%)	100	32	53	41	54
Factor VII (%)	100	23	19	19	28
Plasminogen (%)	100	50	75	81	89

Dimethylnitrosamines given weeks 1 through 3, two consecutive days each week at a dose of 2.5 µl/kg body weight.

COAGULOPATHY. Severe diffuse hepatic necrosis causing fulminant hepatic failure usually leads to a severe coagulopathy and hemorrhagic diathesis (see Chapter 30). The changes in humans patients have been well characterized; little investigation has been done in veterinary patients. As with other forms of severe liver dysfunction, bench tests appraising the coagulation status may be profoundly abnormal in the absence of overt signs of hemorrhage. Thrombocytopenia and reduced plasma concentrations of liver synthesized or activated coagulation proteins are the major mechanisms involved.

The development of a coagulopathy is usually more clinically important than the expression of DIC. However, the expression of DIC and subsequent organ damage may be exacerbated by infection, endotoxemia, or by infusion of activated clotting factors. The most common site of clinically overt bleeding is the gastrointestinal tract. Evidence of impaired vascular integrity and platelet dysfunction is visible as surface petechiation at areas of catheter insertion or mechanical trauma. In severely affected patients, intracranial bleeding may culminate in death.[50]

HYPOTENSION. Although systemic hypotension may develop in humans with fulminant hepatic failure, approximately 60% of the time, the cause remains undetermined. In the remainder, hypotension is related to reduced circulating volume due to increased capillary permeability, hemorrhage, decreased peripheral vascular resistance acquired secondary to bacteremia, endotoxemia, cardiac or pulmonary abnormalities, use of extracorporeal perfusion devices, or as an indication of impending death. Fulminant hepatic failure is associated with high cardiac output, systemic vasodilation, and reduced peripheral resistance. Association of an inappropriate systemic vasodilation with a relatively bradycardic heart rate suggests central vasomotor dysfunction that may be linked to systemic infection, circulating toxins, or cerebral edema. Although many theories have been suggested including increased serum concentrations of octopamine, abnormal end-organ sensitivity to norepinephrine, and altered serum concentrations of angiotensin II and prostaglandins, the pathogenesis of hypotension in these patients is likely multifactorial.[78–81]

CARDIAC DYSFUNCTION. Massive hepatic necrosis leading to hepatic failure is associated with a severe circulatory problem characterized by a low systemic vascular resistance with a compensatory increase in cardiac output. With generalized hypotension, mesenteric blood flow falls, so that both hepatic arterial and portal flow is reduced. The maintenance of hepatic perfusion is further compromised by hepatocellular swelling, accumulated cellular debris, and the deposition of fibrin that collectively impairs sinusoidal blood flow.

Development of cardiac arrhythmias is common in humans with fulminant hepatic failure. Sinus tachycardia is the most common arrhythmia, but many others including ectopic ventricular contractions, heart block, and sinus bradycardia have been documented. Arrhythmias other than sinus tachycardia are seemingly associated with hypoxemia, acidosis, or hyperkalemia. The most common cardiac findings at necropsy are petechial hemorrhages, small-volume pericardial effusions, and fatty, pale-appearing flabby ventricles.[82] These changes are believed to reflect tissue hypoxia and DIC.

PULMONARY ABNORMALITIES. Approximately one-third of humans with fulminant hepatic failure develop clinical and radiologic evidence of pulmonary edema in the presence of normal left ventricular function and without pulmonary hypertension.[83] Change in osmotic forces due to hypoalbuminemia is not implicated as a major pathogenic factor. However, an association between the development of cerebral edema and pulmonary edema suggests that common factors are responsible for an increased accumulation of extravascular fluid. It is proposed that altered permeability of pulmonary capillaries and intrapulmonary vasodilation results in edema formation. These factors may be augmented by development of endotoxemia, which promotes vascular leakage.[50]

Table 32–4

PLASMA AMINO ACIDS IN DOGS WITH
MASSIVE HEPATIC FAILURE DUE TO
DIMETHYLNITROSAMINE[53]

AMINO ACID	% OF NORMAL
Taurine	436
Aspartic acid	345
Glutamic acid	403
Proline	323
Glycine	301
Alanine	538
Citrulline	72
Valine	172
Isoleucine	123
Leucine	165
Tyrosine	594
Phenylalanine	392
Ornithine	1070
Lysine	301
Arginine	0

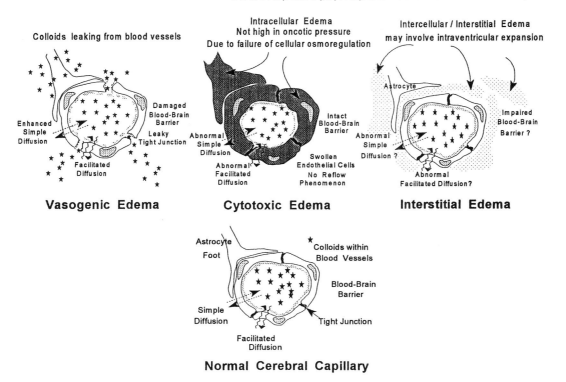

FIGURE 32–9. Diagrammatic representation of the mechanisms causing cerebral edema in the patient with fulminant hepatic failure and hepatic encephalopathy.

Pulmonary edema may be aggravated by injudicious administration of sodium-containing fluids and excessive fluid volumes.

ACID-BASE AND ELECTROLYTE DISTURBANCES. Altered concentrations of serum electrolytes can adversely influence progression of neurologic and cardiac dysfunction in these patients. Hyponatremia is common in humans despite increased renal retention of sodium and increased total body sodium content. Impaired renal excretion of free water is the proposed mechanism. This explains the perceived hemodilution that aggravates hyponatremia. Failure of cell sodium pumps may permit abnormally increased intracellular concentrations of sodium. Changes in the serum sodium concentration are not consistent among patients as some rapidly become hypernatremic in response to intravenous administration of polyionic fluids.

Hypokalemia may develop due to inadequate potassium intake, vomiting, secondary aldosteronism, and use of potassium-wasting diuretics.[50] Hypokalemia is dangerous because it may exacerbate expression of HE. There is no demonstrable association between the severity of liver cell failure and the degree of hypokalemia, owing to the numerous variables that influence the serum potassium concentration. Management of hypokalemia may require administration of prodigious amounts of potassium in some humans.[50] This is believed to occur in response to a central nervous system–induced respiratory alkalosis and renal exchange of potassium for hydrogen ions.

In some patients, hypophosphatemia may become severe. Low serum phosphorus in these patients develops in relation to respiratory alkalosis, which causes phosphate to move into the intracellular space. Hypocapnia results in a shift of intracellular CO_2 into the extracellular fluid. A rise in intracellular pH accelerates the intracellular utilization of phosphate in phosphorylation of glucose. Inorganic phosphate rapidly moves intracellularly resulting in hypophosphatemia. Prolonged, severe hyperventilation may lead to profound hypophosphatemia requiring intravenous phosphate supplementation.[84,85] Hypophosphatemia can have multiple debilitating effects on a patient's clinical status, summarized in Table 32–5.

Severe peripheral shunting of blood has been shown in patients with fulminant hepatic failure. This is believed to be associated with plugging of small vessels by platelets, interstitial edema, and/or abnormal vasomotor tone. Tissue oxygen extraction falls and arterial oxygen saturation is limited by development of arteriovenous pulmonary shunting.[86] Alterations in tissue oxygen extraction resemble those described in the adult respiratory distress syndrome.[71,82,86] Structural changes in pulmonary blood vessels have been shown in humans who have died from fulminant hepatic failure.[49,71,87] The resulting tissue hypoxia leads to anaerobic metabolism and generation of lactic acidosis.[86,88] Because lactic acid depends on hepatic metabolism for conversion to energy, the syndrome of lactic acidosis is fostered. Lactic acid accumulates because of poor circulation or shunting of blood away from the liver or because of the liver's inadequate metabolic function. High lactate concentrations are not sufficient by themselves to cause lactic acidosis unless circulatory failure and shock intervenes. Hypoxemia is detrimental to cerebral function and aggravates brain damage produced by other factors such as cerebral hypotension, hemorrhage, and edema.

The ventilatory response to hypoxia may initially be increased due to an enhanced sensitivity of peripheral chemoreceptors. However, the response to prolonged hypoxia seems impaired by hypoxic depression of the respiratory center.[49] Pulmonary complications of fulminant hepatic failure, including pneumonia, atelectasis, or edema, further

Table 32–5

ADVERSE EFFECTS OF HYPOPHOSPHATEMIA IN FULMINANT HEPATIC FAILURE

Respiratory	**Renal**
Ventilatory failure	↓ bicarbonate regeneration
↓ diaphragmatic contractility	↓ renal acid excretion
Skeletal muscle	**Cardiac**
rhabdomyolysis	impaired myocardial function
generalized weakness	congestive cardiomyopathy
myopathy	
	Hematologic
Neurologic	erythrocytes
metabolic encephalopathy	↑ RBC fragility
ataxia	↓ intracellular ATP
seizures	left shift oxyhemoglobin
coma	dissociation curve
	↓ 2,3 diphosphoglycerate
Gastrointestinal	leukocytes
anorexia	↓ chemotaxis
nausea	↓ phagocytosis
diarrhea	↓ bactericidal activity
	platelets
Endocrine	↓ number
insulin resistance	shortened survival
	↓ adhesion / aggregation

predispose these patients to hypoxemia and depression of ventilatory drive, which worsens their neurologic status. Hypocapnia due to hyperventilation is a typical finding in early fulminant hepatic failure in humans.[50] As the syndrome progresses, impaired responses to inhaled CO_2 (both ventilatory and cerebral blood flow responses) along with hypoxic depression of the central respiratory center lead to hypoventilation.[89–91] Respiratory arrest of central origin or muscle weakness can be a complication that requires institution of ventilatory support.

There is a wide spectrum of acid-base disturbances in patients with fulminant hepatic failure, and complex mixed abnormalities may develop due to a multitude of factors that influence acid-base balance. Massive hepatic necrosis may result in metabolic acidosis associated with lactic acidosis and accumulations of pyruvate, acetoacetate, citrate, succinate, fumarate, and free fatty acids.[50] In the final stages, depression of the respiratory center and complications due to pulmonary edema or infections lead to hypercapnia and respiratory acidosis.[82,92,93]

PANCREATIC INJURY. Morphologic evidence of pancreatic injury is found in some humans with fulminant hepatic failure. Increased serum activities of amylase and lipase may provide antemortem evidence of pancreatic injury. Because other medical complications, such as reduction in glomerular filtration, may augment the observed enzyme elevations, the presence of pancreatic injury is only confirmed by tissue examination or highly suspected on the basis of abdominal ultrasonography. If pancreatitis becomes clinically overt, it contributes to acid-base, fluid, and electrolyte imbalances and promotes the development of systemic hypotension that can further compromise hepatic perfusion and oxygen availability.

RENAL DYSFUNCTION. A serious complication of fulminant hepatic failure is the development of renal failure.[50,71,94] This has been well described in human beings and has been recognized in dogs and cats with fulminant hepatic failure. In addition to prerenal azotemia attributable to dehydration and digestion of blood lost into the gut, a spectrum of renal

insufficiency develops due to renal vasoconstriction.[49,82,94] As described in humans, the renal injury may be primarily a functional failure or be associated with acute tubular necrosis. Some hepatotoxins also are nephrotoxins directly causing renal tubular injury. There is no close correlation between the severity of hepatocellular failure and the severity of the renal failure.[94–96] When fulminant hepatic failure is associated with renal injury, the clinical course of the renal dysfunction is best followed using the serum creatinine concentration and urine volume. Determination of the serum concentration of urea fails to reflect accurately the glomerular filtration rate owing to reduced synthesis of urea in the liver due to reduced hepatic mass or arginine depletion, and because of prerenal nitrogen challenge resulting from blood in the alimentary canal.

HYPOGLYCEMIA. Because the liver is of major importance in the maintenance of euglycemia, abnormalities in glucose metabolism are common in the circumstance of fulminant hepatic failure (see Chapter 30). Severe hypoglycemia may develop in dogs and in some cats undergoing massive hepatic necrosis. Hypoglycemia can develop rapidly and result in overt neurologic signs that can be confused with and augment HE.

INFECTION SUSCEPTIBILITY. Humans with fulminant hepatic failure are at high risk for developing systemic infections. Plasma from affected patients contains a substance(s) that can be removed which inhibits the metabolic activity of granulocytes and compromises their chemotaxis.[49,97–99] Impaired cell Na-K-ATPase, reduced ability to regulate intracellular sodium, and impaired cell adhesion have been shown in neutrophils.[100,101] An acquired defect in opsonization also predisposes these patients to infection. This has been linked to low levels of plasma complement and plasma fibronectin.[102–106] Although hepatic Kupffer cells show reduced phagocytic ability, there no strong evidence that this alone leads to impaired host defense.[49] The requirement for intravenous catheterization and indwelling or intermittent urethal catheterizations permit a potential route for iatrogenic infection. The impaired mental state of the patient reduces normal pharyngeal reflex mechanisms that guard against aspiration of saliva, food, and vomitus. Reduced ventilatory capability and recumbency leads to hypostatic pulmonary congestion and lung atelectasis. All of these factors predispose the patient to pulmonary infections.

PORTAL HYPERTENSION. In some patients with fulminant hepatic failure, massive sinusoidal collapse creates a blockade against intrahepatic circulation and development of ascites. These patients develop portal hypertension and may develop splenomegaly. Portal hypertension in this circumstance is a grave prognostic sign.

CHOLESTASIS. Cholestasis may develop early or late in fulminant hepatic failure. Although it remains undetermined why biliary hyperplasia occurs in response to massive hepatocellular injury, this morphologic response is associated with the large increases in the serum ALP activity. In most cases, hyperbilirubinemia develops several days after the onset of the fulminant necrosis. It is the impression of the author that serum bilirubin concentrations increase at a faster rate in the cat as compared to the dog in the circumstance of florid necrosis.

HEPATIC REGENERATION. The tremendous hepatic reserve for regeneration makes recovery from fulminant hepatic failure possible if the underlying cause of injury is eliminated and intensive supportive care is provided. Unfortunately, despite survival for several days along with biochemical evidence of improved hepatobiliary status, some patients will unexpectedly expire. Failure of hepatocytes to rapidly undergo a regenerative response makes recovery due to some toxic and infectious insults difficult. Although it is known that rapid hepatic regeneration follows partial hepatectomy, regeneration following certain toxins, for example CCl_4, is slower and marred by aberrant mitotic attempts probably as a result of membrane injury and impaired ability for protein synthesis.[107–109] It is speculated that substances circulate in plasma of these patients which inhibit DNA synthesis and cell regeneration.[109–111] Hepatotrophic factors extracted and purified from humans and animals with acute liver failure and from neonatal liver are currently undergoing investigation in hope that a therapeutic product may be developed.[112–114]

Recovery from fulminant hepatic failure is possible following injury from a drug or toxin that destroys more than 50% of the liver. Dogs recovering from nitrosamine toxicity with liver mass judged to be 42% to 48% of normal appear clinically well for at least 18 months, although biochemical evidence of hepatic insufficiency persists.[53]

Prognosis and Sequelae Fulminant Hepatic Failure

Despite effort to predict the outcome of fulminant hepatic failure in human beings, there are no reliable clinical or histologic features.[71] General guidelines indicate that a poor prognosis is warranted when the prothrombin time is greater than 100 seconds, the patient is very young or old, a viral or idiosyncratic drug reaction is the suspected underlying cause, and the serum bilirubin is markedly increased. When a known hepatotoxin is involved, such as in the case of acetaminophen poisoning, use of antidotes and metabolic interruption of toxin production can markedly improve survival. The most important issue in planning the course of critical support is determining whether there is a recognizable underlying cause. Better survival is attained in hospitals where aggressive intensive care is available.

The morphologic sequelae to massive hepatic necrosis is variable. Although the outcome can include fibrosis, regenerative nodules, cirrhosis, and possibly chronic hepatitis, there is good evidence that the liver is not committed to inevitable fibrosis, nodular regeneration, and cirrhosis. Following nitrosamine-induced hepatic necrosis, dogs can develop cirrhosis or chronic hepatitis, or they can completely recover. In some studies, chronic lesions persisted in dogs that had relatively modest hepatic biochemical abnormalities.[51] In another study, dogs recovering from acute necrosis, characterized by severe biochemical abnormalities, had normal liver biopsies a number of months later.[53] The difference between these morphologic outcomes may be due to differences in the clinical management provided. Animals fed commercial dog food developed chronic liver lesions. Dogs fed restricted diets, with casein or soybeans providing the source of protein, recovered with nearly normal hepatic histology.[53] The basic recipe for that diet is shown in Table 32–6. Rather than a direct nutritional benefit, it is possible that the diet alters both the production and absorption of harmful antigens and toxins in the alimentary canal.

FLUID THERAPY. General supportive care should include provision of fluid therapy using intravenous infusions of polyionic fluids with judicious potassium and glucose supplementations. Jugular catheters should only be used after consideration of the patient's coagulation status. Catheter insertion into the jugular vein may induce intractable hemorrhage and should be avoided until bench tests of coagulation, an estimated platelet count, and a mucosal bleeding time have

Table 32–6

BASIC DIETARY FORMULATION FOR THE CANINE PATIENT WITH FULMINANT HEPATIC NECROSIS

INGREDIENT	g/100 g DRY DIET
Casein	9.0
Animal fat	20.0
Sucrose	32.4
Cornstarch	32.4
Vitamin mix*	1.0
Mineral mix*	5.0
Choline chloride	0.3

*Consult Table 35–6 for further information.

been assessed. Remember that the mucosal bleeding time shows a better correlation with the clinical tendency to bleed than do the prothrombin and activated partial thromboplastin times. Infusion of whole fresh blood or frozen plasma may be necessary to provide coagulation factor support. Fresh whole blood is preferred to provide functional platelets and to minimize exposure to ammonia, pyrogens, and contaminating microorganisms that may be generated in stored blood products. Catheter placement and infusion lines and their connectors must be handled with strict asepsis to avoid induction of bacteremia. The blood glucose concentration should be evaluated at least four times daily, or more often, if hypoglycemia is detected. Intravenous dextrose supplementation is necessary when hepatic failure restricts gluconeogenesis and glycogen stores become depleted. If hypertonic dextrose-containing solutions are required to maintain euglycemia, a catheter with access to a central vein is advised to avoid small-vessel thrombophlebitis. Placement of a long indwelling jugular catheter into a peripheral vein so that the catheter extends into a larger segment of the vessel can assist in avoiding rapid development of phlebitis and frequent catheter replacement. Daily palpation of regional lymph nodes and the vessel for pain, heat, or swelling can assist in recognizing early inflammation and/or infection. The rectal temperature should be recorded frequently. If fever suddenly develops, a search for infection should be immediately undertaken considering the immunocompromised condition of the patient and the association between fever and bacteremic showers. Sudden development of fever should initiate reconsideration of current antimicrobial therapy. However, because pyrexia is a nonspecific indicator of many complications associated with hepatic injury (e.g., interleukin release), infection will not always be detected.

An indwelling urinary catheter is advised to monitor urine production so oliguric renal failure will be immediately recognized should it occur. Maintenance of a urethral catheter, however, carries the hazard of urothelial trauma and retrograde urinary tract infection that can lead to bacteremia and sepsis. Urine sediment should be evaluated daily looking for evidence of renal tubular injury (casts), bacteriuria, and pyuria. Bacterial culture of urine is indicated if urinary sediment suggests infection.

In the event of oliguric renal failure, peripheral blood pressure should be evaluated and the adequacy of hydration appraised. If dehydration exists, initial treatment requires shock fluid volume replacement (90 mL/kg) and concern directed toward the patient's intravascular oncotic pressure. Low oncotic pressure should be corrected by either plasma, low molecular weight dextran, or hetastarch. Plasma and low molecular weight dextran have been shown to normalize hepatic blood flow and circulation to other organs in a model of hemorrhagic shock.[115] Use of hetastarch and dextran have not been evaluated in patients with fulminant hepatic failure. If a coagulopathy is recognized, low molecular weight dextran should be avoided as this may worsen DIC. Once vascular volume is reinstated, systemic blood pressure is reassessed. If hypotension persists despite volume replacement and oliguria continues, an electrocardiogram should be evaluated to rule out the presence of a complicating cardiac arrhythmia. Coadministration of furosemide and dopamine are used to induce diuresis if intravascular volume replacement is adequate and a cardiac problem is inapparent.

Management of Acid-Base and Electrolyte Disturbances

Acid-base balance may be disturbed in numerous ways such that empirical treatment of suspected abnormalities is absolutely contraindicated. Acquisition of arterial samples for blood gas analysis is hazardous because of bleeding tendencies. Rather, venous samples from the intravenous catheter are collected. Evaluation of blood pH and an estimation of oxygen extraction can provide helpful information regarding peripheral circulatory adequacy and can assist in guiding fluid therapy. Lactic acidosis can be a serious consequence of fulminant hepatic failure and may be worsened by continued administration of lactated Ringer's solution. Administration of sodium bicarbonate should be restricted unless a blood pH equal to or less than 7.2 is recognized and acidemia does not reflect a respiratory acidosis (hypoventilation primarily). If gas exchange seems impaired by pulmonary edema or arteriovenous shunting, supplemental oxygen may be beneficial. If hypoventilation develops due to neurologic complications, mechanical ventilation becomes necessary. It is important that respiratory alkalosis be avoided as this may precipitate signs of HE. Hypoalbuminemia severe enough to augment development of interstitial edema should be managed with infusion of adequate volumes of fresh frozen plasma to reestablish normal intravascular oncotic pressure. Use of furosemide may be necessary to stimulate excretion of free water.

If hypophosphatemia develops, values less than 2.0 mg/dl require treatment. An initial dose of 0.01 to 0.03 mmol/kg/hour has been recommended for small animals.[85] The serum phosphate concentration should be monitored at 3 to 6 hour intervals once infusions are begun. Phosphate supplementation should be suspended when the serum phosphate concentration exceeds 2.0 mg/dl. The rapid transcellular shifts between the various compartments equilibrating with total body phosphate stores make it impossible to predict exact requirements. Most commercially available parenteral phosphate solutions contain 3 mmol/mL phosphate or 93 mg/mL of elemental phosphorus.[85]

THERAPY OF HEPATIC ENCEPHALOPATHY. Conventional therapy aimed at management of HE is undertaken. Efforts are made to minimize formation of noxious nitrogenous compounds in the gut by first mechanically cleansing the colon and then administering a retention enema that changes the enteric environment. Cleansing enemas comprised of warmed saline are recommended. Neomycin, used as a 1% solution, and given at a maximal dose of 22 mg/kg, or lactulose diluted with water and mixed with the neomycin, are effective retention enemas. Complications rarely encountered with oral or repeated rectal administration of neomycin include ototoxicity, nephrotoxicity, and based on experimental evidence, an increased formation of enteric endotoxin. Treatment with oral lactulose is continued when the patient can tolerate medications per os. A full discussion of HE and appropriate clinical management is provided in Chapters 30, 33, and 35.

MANAGEMENT OF CEREBRAL EDEMA. If cerebral edema is suspected on the basis of sudden deterioration in the level of consciousness, sudden change in systemic blood pressure, or loss of oculovestibular reflexes (in human beings but not documented in companion animals), efforts should be made to intervene.[75,116] Therapy directed at alleviation of cerebral edema is summarized in Figure 32–8. Unfortunately, many of these treatments remain controversial.

Postural tilting of a patient in a head-up position is deleterious as it impairs the cerebral-perfusion pressure.[117] Control of systemic blood pressure may reduce the risk of developing cerebral edema or limit its severity. Barbiturates, which are helpful in some forms of cerebral edema, are hazardous in these patients because they lower systemic blood pressure and may augment the encephalopathic state by interaction with the GABA receptor.

Corticosteroids are proposed to reduce the leakiness of cerebral blood vessels that may contribute to vasogenic edema formation. Studies in animals with cerebral edema suggest that early intervention with corticosteroids is beneficial. However, studies in human beings and animals with cerebral edema established in the context of hepatic failure suggest that glucocorticoids are probably ineffective.[49,75,118] The lack of an established benefit from glucocorticoids and the potential adverse consequences associated with their use should be carefully considered before treatment is initiated. In cases of massive hepatic necrosis, one concerning complication of glucocorticoid therapy is a potential reduction in the mitotic rate of regenerating liver.[118] Glucocorticoids also stimulate catabolism that can lead to release of low molecular weight nitrogenous substances, including amino acids and ammonia, which may worsen HE. Other complications with high-dose short-term glucocorticoid therapy include gastroenteric ulceration, increased susceptibility to infections, and increased water and sodium retention.

Although a short-term course of hyperventilation may reduce intracranial pressure via hypocapnia, long-term hyperventilation is ineffectual in avoiding or reducing the severity of established cerebral edema.[119,120] Long-term benefit is thwarted by the renal compensatory response negating changes in pCO_2.

Theoretically, administration of mannitol would reduce accumulation of cerebral edema due to cytotoxic or interstitial mechanisms. Administration of 1 g/kg body weight as a 20% solution by rapid intravenous infusion through a blood filter has been recommended. Doses as low as 0.3 to 0.4 g/kg body weight have been used successfully in humans. Mannitol appears to reduce intracranial pressure (without normalizing it), and seems to improve survival.[121,122] This may be repeated at least once after several hours.[122] This treatment must be used with caution in patients with renal failure because fluid overload and prolonged hyperosmolarity may increase intracranial pressure and further damage the blood-brain barrier.[106] If a brisk diuresis does not follow within an hour of mannitol infusion, the plasma osmolarity and systemic blood pressure should be measured and furosemide administered. A complication of unfiltered mannitol administration is microvascular infarcts due to embolization with mannitol crystals. This can lead to cerebral as well as other organ injury and thus must be avoided.

A synergistic effect between mannitol and furosemide has been shown in dogs with cerebral edema unrelated to hepatic failure.[123] Furosemide is believed to complement mannitol by virtue of its ability to cause preferential water excretion over solute. Consequently, the effect of mannitol in eliminating excess body water is encouraged. Use of furosemide may also optimize the effect of plasma administration when reestablishment of intravascular oncotic pressure is the therapeutic goal. Furosemide encourages redistribution of water from interstitial spaces into the vascular compartment replacing intravascular fluid lost as free water through renal tubules. The loop diuretics may also be beneficial by virtue of their ability to inhibit choroid plexus secretion of CSF.[75] Administration of furosemide is not without complications as hypovolemia and hypokalemia may develop unless careful attention is given to the patient's fluid and electrolyte balance. Hypokalemia is especially dangerous in that it augments expression of HE.

Management of Seizures

Treatment of seizure activity with sedatives or tranquilizers is contraindicated in these patients. Such drugs can intensify HE and depress vital neurologic centers controlling respiration, blood pressure, and consciousness. Opiates, barbiturates, and benzodiazepines are theoretically contraindicated. There may be increased sensitivity of the central nervous system to drugs interacting GABA receptors such that encephalopathic signs are exacerbated. If seizures are recurrent, intervention is focused on removing or minimizing encephalopathic toxins and ensuring euglycemia. Intractable seizure activity is a grave prognostic sign and warrants consideration of euthanasia. More likely than seizure activity, however, is deep hepatic coma.

ANTIBIOTICS. Prophylactic administration of antimicrobials remains controversial. Many clinicians prefer to await development of infection so that specifically targeted therapy can be administered. Prompt treatment with antibiotics is recommended in the event of fever, leukogram suggestive of infection or endotoxemia, urinary tract infection, or other evidence of bacteremia, sepsis, or localized infection. Care must be taken to avoid selection of antimicrobials that require hepatic biotransformation for activation or elimination or that depend on biliary excretion.

Gastrointestinal Drugs

If gastrointestinal ulceration is suspected, administration of an H_2 blocking agent, such as famotidine or cimetidine, is recommended. Cimetidine is preferentially selected only if inhibition of the P-450 cytochrome system is desired, as is the case with acetaminophen toxicity. Otherwise, famotidine is used in an effort to avoid drug interactions associated with cimetidine. Sucralfate can be used for gastric cytoprotection if orally administered medications are tolerated. If vomiting becomes a persistent problem, metoclopramide given either subcutaneously or as a slow intravenous infusion can be used to ameliorate the patient's discomfort and, to permit oral drug administration and alimentation.

Nutritional Management

Oral administration or enteric administration of amino acid solutions or elemental nutrition is not recommended because of the potential worsening of HE due to nitrogenous toxin production. Supplemental vitamin K_1 and water soluble vitamins are empirically given. As previously discussed, the nature of the diet consumed once the patient is eating is an important determinant of the outcome. Recovery seems to be optimized with a defined diet rather than a commercial diet, as outlined in Table 32–6, and as discussed in Chapter 35. The protein source should be soybeans (tofu) or milk products (cottage cheese or yogurt). Commercially prepared enteral diets having milk and soybeans as the protein source have also been used successfully.

Management of Hemorrhagic Diatheses

Intervention of a hemorrhagic diathesis optimally requires administration of fresh whole blood. A complication

observed in some humans, but not yet recognized in animals, is citrate intoxication and hypocalcemia if large quantities of citrate anticoagulated blood are administered. If DIC is suspected, treatment with fresh whole blood or frozen plasma and continued administration of critical nursing care are necessary. Use of heparin remains controversial in these patients because of the hazards of heparinization in the circumstance of hepatic failure. Study of the benefit of frozen plasma with and without heparin administration in humans with fulminant hepatic failure due to acetaminophen toxicity has not verified that heparin improves patient recovery or coagulation status.[124]

Protection Against Oxidative Injury

S-ADENOSYL-L-METHIONINE. Humans with liver disease have reduced levels of glutathione (GSH) in plasma and liver tissue, unrelated to the cause of their liver disease.[125–136] In the cirrhotic liver, the transsulfuration pathway that converts methionine to cysteine is impaired at the level of S-adenosyl-L-methionine synthetase, the enzyme which catalyzes formation of S-adenosyl-L-methionine (SAMe) (Figure 32–10). This results in subnormal concentrations of GSH and decreased clearance of methionine. Administration of oral SAMe as para-toluene-sulfonate (700 to 1200 mg/day) to humans with cirrhosis of diverse origins causes an improvement in GSH concentration and a reduction in plasma methionine concentration. Both of these are beneficial effects. Concurrent increases in cystine and taurine concentrations also develop. This is expected because of an increase in the transsulfuration of cysteine to GSH and taurine. A decrease in serum aminotransferase and GGT activities, and serum concentrations of total bilirubin and total bile acids, have been observed in humans with intrahepatic cholestasis treated with SAMe.[125,137,138] Cholestasis associated with pregnancy, oral contraceptive use, alcoholic liver disease, and nonalcoholic chronic hepatopathies have also shown improvement. A cytoprotective effect is suggested to result from improved membrane fluidity through restored ability to perform membrane phospholipid methylation (Figure 32–10). S-adenosyl-L-methionine has also been shown to attenuate alcohol-induced mitochondrial injury in baboons.[139] It has been suggested as a beneficial therapy in humans with acute hepatic necrosis acquired from drugs or toxins. The positive response to SAMe shown in human studies seems irrefutable. Because GSH deficiency has been recognized as a risk factor for drug hepatotoxicity and because cells are unable to take up the intact tripeptide, its use in patients with acute hepatic injury also seems appropriate.[140] It has consequently been suggested as a standard addition to the maintenance regimen of patients with chronic liver disease considering it is hepatoprotective against a number of toxins known to deplete hepatic GSH activity, including acetaminophen.[141] It has also been proposed for prophylactic administration to avoid drug toxicities related to reduced transsulfuration pathway activity and oxidant injury and is recommended for humans taking anticonvulsants often associated with idiosyncratic hepatotoxicity. Giving methionine may not achieve the same benefit as use of SAMe because of the possibility of impaired SAMe synthetase activity and the toxic side effects sometimes encountered with orally administered methionine in patients with hepatic insufficiency.

N-ACETYLCYSTEINE. N-acetylcysteine has been shown to improve survival in humans with fulminant hepatic failure due to acetaminophen overdosage even after the effective antidotal window (15 hours postingestion) has passed.[142,143]

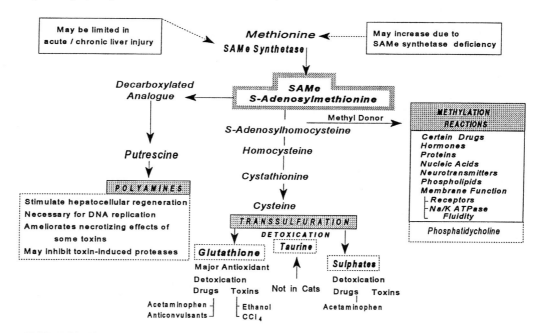

FIGURE 32-10. Diagrammatic representation of the transsulferation pathway, polyamine pathway, and benefit derived from treatment with S-adenosyl-L-methionine in acute hepatic injury.[125]

Patients so treated experienced less cerebral edema, hypotension, and renal failure requiring dialysis. Acetylcysteine appears to enhance oxygen delivery and consumption, a benefit similar to that observed with prostacyclin in critically ill patients.[142,144,145] The mechanisms permitting this effect are not established but have been hypothesized to include a relaxing effect on vascular smooth muscle, inhibition of leukocyte chemotaxis, and inhibition of platelet aggregation and adhesion.[144–148] Acetylcysteine may produce vascular effects through endothelium-derived relaxing factor or nitric oxide. In acetaminophen toxicity, the toxic metabolite leads to a rapid 15-fold increase in neutrophil accumulation, with a consequent plugging of hepatic microvasculature.[149,150] These secondary microcirculatory changes exacerbate the original injury and expand the region of necrosis. This can be subdued by treatment with antioxidants such as allopurinol, discussed next. Unfortunately, marked improvement in patients with fulminant hepatic failure due to causes other than acetominophen have not been documented.

ALLOPURINOL. Allopurinol has been investigated as an antioxidant that protects against ischemic tissue injury.[151–154] It has been evaluated as an early treatment of ischemic liver damage to curb generation of membrane-damaging oxygen radicals. Allopurinol is an effective free radical inhibitor because of its competitive action on xanthine oxidase. It is also suggested that allopurinol may dampen release of arachidonate metabolites from injured membranes. The effect of allopurinol has been studied in experimentally created hepatic ischemia in the dog.[151,153] Results indicate it reduces accumulation of $PGF_{1\alpha}$ when administered intravenously before ischemia but it does not reduce accumulation of thromboxane unless given directly into the hepatic artery or portal vein.

VITAMIN E. Vitamin E is a natural antioxidant that protects the liver from injury by oxygen-free radicals. In the circumstance of vitamin E deficiency, it is more likely that lipid peroxidation will develop following chemical injury. Vitamin E can be used to minimize or help prevent ongoing peroxida-

tive injury and has been shown to protect against lipid peroxidation produced by excess copper in the liver. Vitamin E has also been shown to be hepatoprotective against some known hepatotoxins.[155–159]

DESFERROXAMINE. Another drug imparting antioxidant effects is desferroxamine, a powerful iron chelator and free radical inhibitor.[160] Its use is suggested based on studies conducted in dogs in which desferroxamine protected against clinical and hepatic histopathologic consequences of hemorrhagic shock. In these studies, desferroxamine was shown to hasten recovery and to increase survival.[161] Increased serum iron concentrations develop in animals with hepatic hypoxemia due to hemorrhagic shock. A possible role of iron in tissue injury has been suggested following its release from ferritin during hypoxia. Desferroxamine firmly binds iron, preventing its participation in oxidant formation. It may work best when available during the reperfusion stage of tissue injury.

EXPERIMENTAL THERAPIES. Hepatotrophic substances derived from regenerating livers after hepatectomy and from neonatal liver may be available through molecular biologic engineering in the near future.[108,112] Coadministration of insulin and glucose and insulin and glucagon have been studied as possible hepatotrophic factors in humans with fulminant hepatic failure and in experimental animal models.[162–166] Results are inconsistent in clinical patients that have damaged hepatic tissue. This treatment strategy is currently not advised in the management of patients with fulminant hepatic failure because they have an impaired ability to maintain euglycemia.

Specific interventions to block effects of toxins associated with HE have been intensely studied over the past 30 years (see Chapter 30). The most intriguing recent investigations have been with the benzodiazepine antagonist flumazenil.[167,168] Humans with fulminant hepatic failure seem to respond better than those with chronic portosystemic encephalopathy, but response is inconsistent. For a full discussion of HE and appropriate clinical management see Chapters 30, 33, and 35.

A number of agents have been studied that have the potential to reduce tissue injury resulting from ischemia. Application of findings in experimental work to clinical patients is complicated by the fact that in many models, animals are pretreated before ischemic injury is produced.

Prostaglandin therapy, studied in animal models and humans with fulminant hepatic failure, appears to reduce hepatic damage and improve survival.[169–174] Clinical studies have indicated that prostacyclin (PGI_2) has microcirculatory vasodilatory effects that increase peripheral oxygen uptake.[71,82,86]

A recent study suggests that PGE_1 inhibits the release of cytotoxic factors from macrophages and Kupffer cells stimulated by endotoxins.[175] Prostaglandin E_1 has also been shown to enhance recovery of mitochondrial respiratory function following ischemic injury and to improve in vitro survival of canine liver cells.[193,194]

The administration of ATP-$MgCl_2$ or adenosine-$MgCl_2$ improves survival of animals and enhances hepatic function after induced hepatic ischemia.[24,25,178] It is speculated that this therapy replaces the ATP content of ischemic cells. It is proposed that $MgCl_2$ diminishes ATP breakdown by inhibiting its deamination and dephosphorylation.[178] It is also possible that ATP and adenosine induce vasodilation, which improves blood flow to the ischemic area.[24,25]

Defibrotide, a drug that increases release of PGI_2 and tissue plasminogen activating factor, has been studied in ischemic rat liver as a cytoprotective agent and for its protective influence on endothelial function.[179,180] This drug has been shown to sustain ATP production in ischemic hepatocytes. A beneficial influence on thrombolysis has also been proposed through its action on plasminogen activators; this would assist in recovery from hepatic ischemia associated with microthrombi.[181–183]

Putrescine augments regeneration of remnant liver after partial hepatectomy and is believed to function cooperatively with epidermal growth factor(s).[184] Supplemental putrescine reverses ethanol-associated inhibition of hepatic regeneration.[184,185] Administration of putrescine (0.3 mmol/kg) ameliorates necrosis produced by some hepatotoxins, which suggests it may become important in the management of clinical patients.[184,186]

Artificial Liver Support

This is an area of intense study in human medicine because provision of temporary hepatic support permits a grace period during which hepatic regeneration can occur.[187] In addition, there is a need to improve a patient's metabolic condition prior to hepatic transplantation. Unfortunately, little has been accomplished to make these therapeutic interventions practically applicable to veterinary patients. All of the methods investigated to date are expensive, labor intensive, and associated with severe adverse side effects. Mechanisms of artificial liver support used in human beings and under investigation are summarized in Table 32–7. Controversy regarding the pathogenic importance of specific metabolites and waste products continues to slow development of an optimal device. Retention of drugs and toxins that become hepatotoxic following hepatic metabolism results in a steady source of toxin that continues to damage hepatocytes as they regenerate. A major goal in development of artificial liver support has been optimal removal of toxins from the blood so the cause of hepatic necrosis is eliminated. Some of these mechanisms can also remove endogenous substances that suppress hepatic regeneration which persist in the blood of patients with massive hepatic necrosis for several weeks.[183a]

MISCELLANEOUS DISORDERS ASSOCIATED WITH HEPATIC NECROSIS

A number of diverse disease processes can cause acute liver injury as a result of trauma, reduced hepatic perfusion, accumulation of inflammatory mediators, or the systemic distribution of infectious organisms or their products. In many cases, the cause of the acute hepatic injury is another primary disease or medical problem. In dogs, nonhepatic problems cause nearly 80% of hepatic necrosis; in cats that percentage is even higher at 90% (Table 32–8). In both dogs and cats the most severe hepatic damage is found in association with primary hepatic necrosis and necrosis caused by coagulopathies, thromboembolism, and other conditions causing hepatic hypoxia and ischemia. The most frequent cause of moderate to severe hepatic necrosis is an underlying problem that impairs delivery of oxygen and nutrients to the liver. Such conditions account for 24% of hepatic necrosis in dogs and 34% in cats (Table 32–8).

Mild hepatic necrosis is infrequently reported as a pathologic lesion even though it may be a frequent finding on liver biopsy. This may be because clinicians choose to biopsy only animals with suspected severe diffuse lesions associated with functional insufficiency and otherwise symptomatically treat animals having only mild lesions. Of nonhepatic diseases causing mild hepatic necrosis or degeneration, the steroid-induced hepatopathy in dogs is most frequently reported.

Liver Lobe Rupture

Rupture or tearing of a liver lobe can occur as a result of blunt abdominal trauma to an ostensibly normal liver. Liver rupture may be clinically occult except for the accumulation of fresh blood within the abdominal cavity. Localization of the site of bleeding requires surgical inspection of the surface of the liver or may be identified using ultrasonography with careful inspection given to the locale of fluid accumulation. Initially, blood forms an adherent clot in the area of rupture but then becomes defibrinated and accumulates in the abdomen. Occasionally, spontaneous rupture of a liver lobe occurs in tissue with predisposing pathologic conditions causing friable parenchyma. Examples include tissue infiltrated by amyloidosis, severe passive congestion, fatty degeneration, primary or metastatic hepatic neoplasia, or during the acute swollen stage of diffuse hepatitis.[2]

Table 32–7

MECHANISMS OF PROVIDING TEMPORARY
HEPATIC SUPPORT USED IN HUMAN BEINGS OR
IN EXPERIMENTAL ANIMALS[187]

Exchange blood transfusion
Plasmapheresis
Cross circulation
   using same species
   neurologically stable donor
Hemoperfusion
   isolated cadaveric liver
   isolated liver from a different species
   over microencapsulated charcoal
   over albumin-covered Amberlite XAD-7 resin
Hemodialysis
   conventional as for renal hemodialysis
   special polyacrylonitrile membrane

Table 32–8

PERCENTAGE DISTRIBUTION ACCORDING TO ETIOLOGY OF HEPATOCELLULAR
NECROSIS AND DEGENERATION IN DOGS AND CATS

ETIOLOGY	CANINE (n = 113)		FELINE (n = 49)	
Primary	22	(M,S)	10	(S)
Secondary to other liver disease	16		12	
DIC, thromboembolic disease	14	(S)	8	(M,S)
Hypoxia, ischemia, congestion, anemia	10	(S)	26	(M,S)
Generalized or local infection	11	(M)	8	(M)
Neoplasia: nonhepatic	9	(M,S)	12	(M)
Steroid-hepatopathy lesion	9	(Mild)	0	
Pancreatitis	6	(M)	2	(S)
Drugs	2	(S)	0	
Hyperthyroidism	0		6	(M)
Intestinal disease	2	(S)	4	(M,S)
Renal disease	< 1	(M)	6	
Other	< 1		6	

(M) = moderate, (S) = Severe
Data derived from the College of Veterinary Medicine, University of California at Davis.

Liver Lobe Torsion

Liver lobe torsion is an uncommon cause of hepatic disease. Torsion and entrapment of a liver lobe is most commonly observed in animals with a diaphragmatic hernia. Death from liver lobe torsion is usually a result of endotoxic shock or hemorrhage. If partial rotation of a liver lobe occurs, an effusion is usually produced. If a liver lobe extends through a diaphragmatic rent, fluid usually accumulates within the thoracic cavity. Liver lobe torsion may be a rare iatrogenic consequence of surgical manipulation and resection of hepatic tumors or other abdominal surgeries.[188]

The degree of lobe rotation determines the extent of vascular compromise. Hepatic necrosis develops when perfusion is impaired for longer than 40 minutes. Replication of anaerobic gas-producing bacterial organisms results in formation of gas pockets within affected tissue. This can be visualized radiographically or suspected on the basis of abdominal ultrasonography. Immediately following ischemic insult, the plasma activities of hepatic transaminases increase. Release of tissue degradation products, bacterial products and endotoxins, and bioreactive eicosinoids results in the rapid development of clinical signs and shock. Surgical resection of a torsed liver lobe is the best course of therapy when tissue ischemia is obvious. Venous outflow from an affected liver lobe should be occluded before the lobe is manipulated. This avoids release of noxious and potentially lethal toxins from the ischemic tissue into the systemic circulation. Patients undergoing surgical removal of a torsed or ischemic liver lobe should be treated as if they were endotoxemic with broad-spectrum antimicrobials, adequate volume expansion with polyionic fluids, replacement of lost oncotic pressure with whole plasma, hetastarch, or low molecular weight dextran, and treatment with glucocorticoids. Use of nonsteroidal anti-inflammatory agents such as flunixin meglumine (Banamine; Schering) remains controversial. Blood pressure of the patient should be closely monitored during surgery to avoid hypotension and secondary acute renal failure. Aerobic and anaerobic bacterial culture and sensitivity of material from the interior of the removed tissue is used to guide long-term antimicrobial therapy.

Circulatory Failure

Circulatory failure due to any form of right-sided heart failure, pericardial disease, or vena caval obstruction results in venous hypertension and congestion that is transmitted back through the hepatic vein and into zone 3 of the acinus. Pathogenetic factors include (1) reduced hepatic blood flow resulting in a decreased hepatocellular oxygen supply; (2) increased hepatic venous pressure causing pressure atrophy of zone 3 hepatocytes and edema formation in the perivenous area, which subsequently impairs sinusoidal blood flow; and (3) reduced systemic arterial oxygen saturation due to impaired cardiac output and pulmonary edema leading to zone 3 hypoxia. The critical common denominator is the development of hypoxia in zone 3 hepatocytes.

The major contributing factors to hepatocellular injury in the patient with congestive heart failure is the overall reduction in hepatic blood flow and the increased hepatic venous pressure, rather than hepatic arterial hypoxia.[11] In cardiac failure causing peripheral circulatory failure (left-sided heart failure), only zone 3 necrosis without congestion is observed. Acute circulatory failure or shock, producing zone 3 necrosis, can be caused by a multitude of systemic disorders, including but not limited to severe trauma, hemorrhage, septic shock, surgery, anesthesia, endotoxemia, pulmonary thrombosis or embolism, and heat stroke. Thromboembolic disorders can regionally or focally restrict circulation to the liver, as a result of thrombosis of hepatic sinusoidal and venous pathways.

Impaired acinar outflow causing zone 3 hypoxia can induce biochemical abnormalities consistent with impaired hepatic perfusion (Figure 32–11). Diagnosis usually relies on demonstration of coexisting cardiovascular dysfunction and compatible biopsy findings. The morphologic and temporal sequence of change in the liver with passive congestion has been characterized.[11] Initially, mild hepatic congestion and moderate hepatic venous hypertension causes compression and atrophy of the zone 3 hepatocytes. The adjacent sinusoids appear blood engorged. As congestion worsens, more marked hepatocellular compression and atrophy develop in zone 3 along with a progressive encroachment into zone 2. Cells in varying states of degeneration and necrosis may be

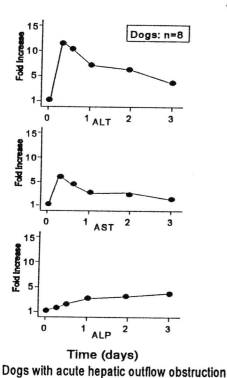

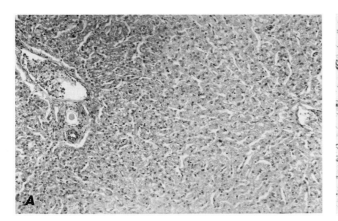

Time (days)
Dogs with acute hepatic outflow obstruction

FIGURE 32-11. Serum enzyme changes after experimental obstruction of hepatic venous outflow in the dog.[12]

observed depending on the extent of acinar hypoxia. Collapse of zone 3 cells around the hepatic vein is associated with condensation of the reticulin stroma, and a thickening of the central vein (Figure 32–12). A proliferation of fibroblasts results in the deposition of collagen. The increase in reticulin and collagen causes sclerosis of the hepatic venule. As more severe hepatic congestion develops or persists, the severity of zone 3 necrosis worsens, fibrosis becomes established, and connective tissue radiates along the acinar margins. As the process continues, a pattern of reverse lobulation may develop in which fibrous tissue connects hepatic venules, sparing relatively normal portal areas. This is rarely seen in dogs and cats. In some cases, liver injury may also involve portal areas resulting in connective tissue encircling portal triads.

The gross morphologic characterization of liver tissue in the patient with congestive heart failure is typically described as "nutmeg" in appearance. This results from the contrast between congested zone 3 areas that appear reddened, and the paler or yellower appearing portal areas. Often the postmortem appearance of the liver is less dramatic than is anticipated from antemortem clinical evaluations. This occurs because of reductions in the hepatic venous pressure occurring at the time of death and loss of blood held within sinusoids. Evaluation of biopsied tissue is believed to be more reliable than that obtained postmortem from patients dying of heart failure. During the agonal stage of death, and within the first 12 hours after death, the hepatocytes and cords of a congested liver shrink, cells undergo rapid autolysis, and glycogen is lost.[11] Cells dissociate from one another and the perisinusoidal spaces enlarge. Consequently, postmortem tissues often show exaggerated histologic changes. Treatment of hepatic injury is largely directed at the primary cause of the poor perfusion.

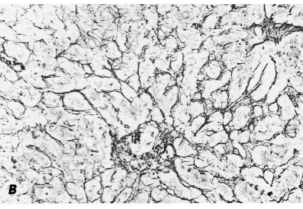

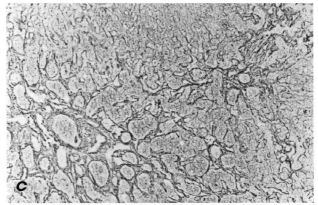

FIGURE 32-12. Photomicrograph of liver biopsies stained with reticulin stain showing collapse of the structural framework of lobules that can accompany hepatic necrosis and degeneration. Comparisons are made between (A) normal tissue, (B) focal necrosis, and (C) centrizonal necrosis due to impaired venous outflow. In (A), the organized normal alignment of hepatic cords is obvious. In (B), collapse of parenchyma is seen in the left portion of the field. In (C), chronically impaired venous outflow due to cardiac failure has resulted in increased fibrous tissue that has distorted the normal appearance of the hepatic lobule. Connective tissue is observed bridging between adjacent hepatic venules.

Disseminated Intravascular Coagulation (DIC)

Conditions that disturb the homeostatic balance of coagulation, anticoagulant, and fibrinolytic pathways can initiate changes that evolve into unrestricted clot formation and coagulation factor consumption (see Chapter 30). Thromboembolic phenomenon can cause acute increases in the serum activities of the hepatic transaminases and GGT, and later on in serum ALP activity. The morphologic injury to hepatocytes develops in response to impaired perfusion, inflammatory mediator release, or directly to the initiating disease condition. Treatment is discussed elsewhere.

Pancreatitis

Among the many injurious substances released from an inflamed pancreas are proteolytic enzymes including trypsin, pancreatic elastase, and phospholipase A, vasoactive polypeptides, and lysolecithin. Injurious pancreatic enzymes are more concentrated in the portal blood than in the systemic circulation and are believed to remain in the liver longer than usual because of reduced hepatic circulation. Consequently, they are able to cause considerable hepatocellular injury. Of particular importance in the cascade of pathogenic events is liberation of elastase, which damages vascular endothelium, and phospholipase A, which damages cell membranes. Together, these enzymes appear to be significant initiators of coagulation necrosis and vascular injury. Disseminated intravascular coagulation is commonly seen in the patient with pancreatitis and may exist as a restricted local process, low-grade coagulopathy, or cause an overt hemorrhagic diathesis. The systemic impact of injurious mediators released from an inflamed pancreas is worsened by development of hypovolemia acquired from dehydration and hemorrhage, hypoperfusion due to cardiac arrhythmias and hypovolemia, portal bacteremia or endotoxemia due to duodenal inflammation and bowel wall devitalization, and thromboembolism. The liver can receive the full impact of each of these effects. In addition, entrapment or occlusion of the common bile duct as a result of pancreatic inflammation or fibrosis, and/or retrograde movement of inflammatory mediators, enzymes, or bacteria into the biliary tree, can directly involve the extrahepatic and intrahepatic biliary structures and induce overt cholestasis. Increased activities of serum enzymes are common in animals with pancreatitis. In most, the fold increase in the serum ALP activity greatly exceeds the fold increases in hepatic transaminases.

Histologic changes described in the liver of animals with pancreatitis have included hepatocellular degeneration, necrosis, and congestion in zone 3; diffuse suppurative cholangitis; thromboembolism of hepatic vasculature and subsequent hepatocellular ballooning degeneration and necrosis; mild to severe hepatocellular fatty change; and mild to marked intracellular and intracanalicular bile stasis. Necrosis of hepatocytes may vary from individual cell necrosis to small areas of coagulative necrosis accompanied by neutrophilic infiltration. In some cases a prominent infiltration by lymphocytes occurs in the portal triad areas. Hepatic atrophy, fibrosis, and cirrhosis have been described in some dogs.[189-191] Treatment of pancreatitis is discussed in Chapter 20.

Gastric Dilatation-Volvulus Complex

The gastric dilatation-volvulus (GDV) complex causes profound impairment of portal and vena caval circulation and can lead to the development of hypovolemic shock, endotoxemia, DIC, cardiac arrhythmias, and pancreatitis.

Increased serum activities of hepatic transaminases are common in response to the altered liver perfusion. Hypoxic changes in zone 3, ballooning degeneration, and lytic necrosis have been observed in dogs that have died from gastric dilatation. In cases that recover, liver enzyme abnormalities usually resolve within 1 to 2 weeks. Treatment of GDV is discussed in Chapter 16.

Immune-Mediated Hemolytic Anemia

Animals with severe anemia due to immune-mediated erythrocyte destruction can develop hepatic injury and increased serum enzyme activities due to hypoxia. Approximately 70% and perhaps more of these patients develop increased serum ALT activities.[192] In some animals, severe intravascular hemolysis liberates large concentrations of hemoglobin and unconjugated bilirubin concentrations that may induce hepatocellular damage. The presence of autoagglutination in patients with immune-mediated hemolytic anemia portends a poor prognosis because of their increased propensity to develop thromboembolism and ischemic injury.[192,193] Endothelial-mediated injury related to circulating immune complexes, complement activation, and the direct effect of hemoglobin on endothelial cells are proposed underlying mechanisms.[194,195] Various organs, including the liver, may be affected by romboembolism, although clinical signs have most often been related to the pulmonary system.[192,193]

Vasculitis

Diseases associated with vascular inflammation include those having a primary infectious cause, those having an immune-mediated basis, those inducing inflammatory mediator release and neutrophil migration, and those involving combinations of these mechanisms. Infectious agents that have primary interaction with vascular endothelium include some of the rickettsial agents, for example *Rickettsia rickettsii*, the cause of Rocky Mountain spotted fever, certain viruses such as canine adenovirus I and the feline infectious peritonitis virus, protozoa such as *Cytauxzoon felis*, and parasites that influence the health and integrity of the vascular endothelium such as *Dirofilaria immitis*. Any of these agents can involve the vasculature of the liver as part of a systemic infection. A number of poorly characterized "collagen" diseases can cause vasculitis as a result of in situ immune-complex formation or immune-complex deposition and subsequent complement fixation. Systemic lupus erythematosis (SLE) represents one form of vasculitis within this category.

Animals manifesting signs of a vasculitis may have increases in the serum activities of the hepatic transaminases and ALP. Histologically there may be localized areas of lymphoid aggregations, focal necrosis, and "reactive" hepatitis (mild to moderate mononuclear cell infiltrates within portal triads and mild fatty change or focal hepatocyte degeneration). Kupffer cells may proliferate, forming a poorly defined granuloma, a nonspecific histologic finding. When vasculitis is a suspected cause of hepatic injury, needle biopsies may miss the vascular lesion that would be apparent upon examination of a larger wedge biopsy.

Inflammatory Bowel Disease

Inflammatory bowel disease (IBD), can be associated with increases in liver enzyme activities and with histologic evidence of liver injury. Inflammation of the gut wall leads to a degradation of its integrity, permitting inflammatory mediators, endotoxins, and enteric microorganisms access to the mesenteric circulation. Transport of these substances to the liver may result in their entrapment within Kupffer cells and cellular injury in the area where portal venous admixture first occurs. The most common histologic lesions observed in patients with IBD is "portal triaditis" (pericholangitis). However, focal periportal or random necrosis, fatty change, periportal fibrosis, chronic hepatitis, and cirrhosis have each been observed in clinical patients.

The increased mucosal permeability that occurs with IBD and other inflammatory intestinal problems permits greater absorption of bacterial, dietary, and epithelial cell antigens. Reaction of these antigens with immunoglobulins forming immune complexes may exceed the capacity of the hepatic Kupffer cells to remove and degrade them. With incomplete removal, immune complexes may deposit in the liver and, by fixing and activating complement, may produce hepatic necrosis.[196,197] Some colonic epithelial cell antigens are similar to those found in epithelial cells of the hepatobiliary system and renal tubules. Some of these antigens are also similar to those found in *E. coli*. Antibodies produced against the common colonic or bacterial antigens may therefore also react with similar antigens within the liver and kidneys. Thus, permeability changes that allow absorption of excess antigen from the intestine may promote production of autoreactive antibodies which can damage both the liver and kidney. This is clinically suspected to occur in animals with chronic bowel disease where the incidence of hepatic and renal lesions seems to be greater than anticipated.

Patients with acute severe enterocolitis all potentially have hepatic lesions. The restoration of normal enzyme activity and the return of normal liver morphology following remission of clinical signs and institution of a diet restricted in antigens is most likely due to reduced enteric absorption of toxins and antigens. The treatment of IBD is discussed in Chapter 24.

Hyperthermia

Hyperpyrexia to the extent of heat stroke can cause moderate to marked increases in the serum activities of hepatic transaminases and, eventually, ALP. Hypoxia and hypovolemia are believed to be important factors contributing to hepatic injury, although DIC also is a frequent complication. Histologically, necrosis in zone 3 associated with marked hydropic degeneration and intracellular cholestasis has been observed.

Neoplasia

Extrahepatic neoplasia can cause acute increases in the serum activities of hepatic enzymes as a result of dissemination of tumor cells to the liver, impaired hepatic perfusion, or production of biologically active or vasoactive substances circulated to the liver. Production of cytokines such as tumor necrosis factor and interleukin-1 activate endothelial cells and increase vascular permeability. Biogenic amines liberated from mast cell tumors or reactive mammary carcinoma can cause a nonspecific reactive hepatitis and DIC. Neoplastic conditions involving the alimentary canal can regionally reduce the integrity of the normal gut barriers that protect against dissemination of endotoxins and enteric organisms through the portal venous circulation.

Intrahepatic neoplasia, either metastatic or primary, can produce hepatocellular injury secondary to mechanical compression of normal tissue, impairment of normal perfusion, or as a result of inflammation induced by tumor cell growth and necrosis.

VIRAL INFECTIONS ASSOCIATED WITH HEPATIC NECROSIS

Infectious Canine Hepatitis

Clinical Synopsis

Diagnostic Features

- Young unvaccinated dogs
- Acute vomiting, diarrhea, abdominal pain, and fever
- Hematemesis, melena, hematochezia, and petechia common
- Tonsilitis, pharyngitis, cough, and anasarca may be seen
- Corneal edema, uveitis, and chronic hepatitis may develop if pups survive acute phase
- Leukopenia and increased ALT common
- Histology reveals hepatic congestion and necrosis often with inclusion bodies

Standard Management

- Intravenous fluid therapy with glucose and potassium supplementation
- Plasma or blood transfusions may be required
- Treatment for hepatic encephalopathy if needed (see elsewhere)

Infectious canine hepatitis (ICH) is an uncommon clinical disease in communities following standard vaccination protocols. This virus causes disease in dogs, foxes, other Canidae, and in Ursidae.[198–201] Viral infection spreads to involve all body tissues and virus can be recovered from secretions during the acute stage of disease. Shedding in urine can persist for 6 to 9 months following infection. Initial exposure usually occurs by the oral or nasal route. Virus disseminates to regional lymph nodes and lymphatics and then to blood. A 4 to 8 day viremia rapidly spreads the virus systemically. A viral tropism for hepatocytes and vascular endothelium has been shown. Acute development of DIC may follow cytotoxic injury to the liver and vascular endothelium.[48] Viral cytoxicity initiates the first injury within liver, kidney, and eye. If a sufficient antibody response neutralizes the virus, clearing it from blood and tissue, the extent of liver injury is restricted. Dogs with a low antibody titer undergo severe and often fatal hepatic necrosis.[202] If a dog survives the peracute phase of necrosis, hepatic regeneration may occur with no evidence of the prior tissue injury. Dogs developing only a partial neutralizing antibody titer by day 4 or 5 may develop a chronic hepatitis that eventually proceeds to cirrhosis.[202] Both the wild virulent adenovirus I and the modified live strains can produce renal injury involving the glomeruli.[203,204] Glomeruli are injured by in situ formation of immune complexes. After an adequate antibody response, virus remains only in the renal tubules and can initiate progressive injury and histologic lesions consistent with chronic interstitial nephritis.

Clinical signs of ICH are usually recognized in young unvaccinated dogs. Some dogs undergo a short interval of acute severe illness and rapidly die. Clinical signs in dogs surviving the acute viremic stage include lethargy, anorexia, vomiting, abdominal pain, and diarrhea.[199] Hematemesis, melena, and hematochezia may also be observed. Physical abnormalities in the initial stages of illness include fever, tachycardia, and tachypnea. Pharyngitis, tonsillar enlargement, coughing, and harsh respiratory sounds may be observed, and some dogs develop pneumonia. Cervical lymphadenopathy and anasarca of the head, neck, and ventrum of the thorax and abdomen may develop. This is thought to be due to vascular and lymphatic involvement. Bleeding tendencies typical of a vasculitis may appear and an abdominal effusion accumulates in some. Central nervous system signs may also develop. Severe signs usually persist for 1 week before improvement is noted. If chronic hepatitis develops, signs of liver disease may temporarily resolve or rapidly worsen. Ocular signs associated with corneal edema and anterior uveitis may develop concurrent with improvement in other clinical signs because antibody-mediated cytotoxicity is associated with these lesions.

Clinicopathologic features of ICH include an initial leukopenia characterized by a neutropenia and lymphopenia attributable to viral infection of lymph nodes and bone marrow. Upon recovery, a neutrophilia and lymphocytosis are usually observed. Gradual increases in the serum activities of ALT and AST are observed during the first 2 weeks of infection (Figure 32–13).[205] Thereafter the enzymes slowly normalize if the dog has cleared the infection and a chronic immune-mediated hepatitis has not been initiated. Serum activity of ALP may increase after the initial week of infection. Most dogs with infectious canine hepatitis do not become hyperbilirubinemic to the point of overt jaundice. If necrosis is severe and hepatic failure induced, the dog dies before bilirubin pigments can accumulate. In dogs that develop chronic hepatitis, the bilirubin value may gradually increase when liver function is substantially compromised. Coagulation abnormalities in dogs with severe acute infection are variable and may include normal or prolonged prothrombin time, normal or prolonged partial thromboplastin time, thrombocytopenia, normal or increased FDPs, abnormal platelet function, and prolonged bleeding times.

Histologic lesions in the liver involve marked congestion and multifocal coagulation necrosis of hepatocytes in zone 3. Hepatocytes and Kupffer cells may contain large basophilic intranuclear inclusion bodies during the first week of infection. These have been shown to contain viral antigen. Edema of the gallbladder is usually obvious. There are many other lesions in different organ systems. See several of the cited references for a more in-depth description.[199,201]

Dogs that develop chronic hepatitis have histologic lesions in the acute phase of viral infection that are mild in comparison to dogs with acute severe disease. Small foci of coagulation necrosis in zone 3 is associated with a neutrophilic inflammatory infiltrate and small numbers of lymphocytes and plasma cells in the acute phase of injury. In dogs that survive for 2 weeks and then succumb to hepatic necrosis, there are round cell infiltrates in zone 3 and in the portal areas. At that time, virus cannot be demonstrated by finding either inclusion bodies or by direct fluorescent antibody tech-

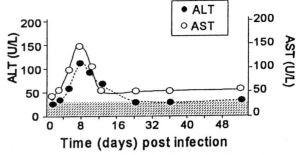

FIGURE 32–13. Serum transaminase activity in dogs following infection with the infectious canine hepatitis virus. Hatched area represents the normal range for each enzyme.[205]

nique.[202] In dogs surviving for 6 months or more, subsequent liver biopsy has shown dense accumulations of lymphoid cells and plasma cells throughout the liver. In some dogs, infiltration is dense in the portal area and is associated with developing portal fibrosis. Virus cannot be demonstrated in liver tissue at this stage, although a recent study of paraffin-fixed liver tissue from dogs with chronic hepatitis suggested the presence of viral antigen in some animals.[206]

Affected dogs should be given intravenous fluids to maintain adequate hydration and to replace ongoing losses due to vomiting and diarrhea. It must be considered that puppies require 130–200 mL/kg of fluid just for maintenance requirements. Glucose supplementation is necessary if hypoglycemia develops. Electrolytes should be monitored and potassium deficits judiciously replaced. If hypoalbuminemia develops during the phase of edema and anasarca formation, plasma transfusions may be necessary. If a coagulopathy is evident, whole blood replacement may be required. Administration of hyperimmune globulin to an exposed unvaccinated neonate would protect them from the most devastating effects of ICH. However, there is danger associated with giving inadequate quantities of antibodies to completely neutralize virus because this promotes more aggressive hepatic injury. Consideration of other treatments discussed in the section dedicated to fulminant hepatic failure and hepatic encephalopathy is advised.

Neonatal Canine and Feline Herpesvirus Infection

Clinical Synopsis

Diagnostic Features

- Neonates usually affected; often die acutely
- Anorexia, diarrhea, abdominal pain common
- Petechia, vesicles, and subcutaneous edema may be seen.
- Histology reveals perivascular necrosis, hemorrhage +/- inclusions.

Standard Care

- Supportive (warmth, fluids, milk replacer)
- Hyperimmune serum (1–2 mL IP) may be useful

Infection of neonates with the canine herpesvirus can result in diffuse necrotizing vasculitis and focal hemorrhagic necrosis of many tissues including the liver.[207–210] Puppies may be infected in utero, during passage through the birth canal, from contacting infected littermates, from excretions from the dam or by other dogs.[211] Neonates infected when less than 1 week of age are particularly susceptible to fatal generalized infections. In older dogs, viral infection is usually limited to the respiratory tract, genital tract, and retropharyngeal and bronchial lymph nodes. Initial infection in the neonate occurs via the nasopharynx. The virus replicates in local epithelial cells and enters the bloodstream through macrophages within 3 to 4 days.[211] Viral localization in the mononuclear phagocytes in lymph nodes and spleen permit local cellular spreading, lymphoid hyperplasia, and necrosis. Hemorrhage is associated with parenchymal tissue necrosis and is augmented by thrombocytopenia.[207] Vascular endothelial damage and tissue necrosis may promote development of a consumptive coagulopathy and subsequent thrombocytopenia.[211]

Unfortunately, clinical signs are vague and puppies between 1 and 3 weeks of age often have acutely fatal disease. Initial signs of illness include listlessness, anorexia, diarrhea, persistent crying, pain upon abdominal palpation, and the conspicuous absence of a febrile response.[211] Petechial hemorrhages may become obvious and an erythematous rash associated with papules or vesicles. Subcutaneous edema of the ventral abdomen and inguinal areas may also develop. Vesicular lesions may be observed on mucous membranes. Neurologic signs may immediately precede death.[211,212] Puppies older than 3 to 5 weeks may develop only mild upper respiratory signs. Although systemic infection is rare, some puppies become anorectic, depressed, vomit, and develop serous ocular discharges and hepatomegaly.[211]

Hepatic histologic findings include diffuse multifocal hemorrhagic lesions associated with perivascular necrosis. Intranuclear inclusions have been observed in parenchymal cells adjacent to foci of necrosis. Viral antigen has been identified within necrotic lesions.[213] The most severe necrotizing lesions are found in the kidneys. A peritoneal effusion is often found in puppies that have died of herpesvirus infection.

Feline herpesvirus infection can also result in systemic infection in the very young kitten. Initial infection occurs by close contact with an infected cat or by fomite transfer. Multifocal necrosis has been observed in the liver of neonates with disseminated infection. In older cats, herpesvirus effects are restricted to the respiratory system.

Supportive symptomatic care is the mainstay of treatment for the neonate with herpesvirus infection. In puppies, intraperitoneal injection of 1 to 2 mL of hyperimmune sera has been suggested for exposed littermates.[211] Only a single treatment is advised owing to the short susceptibility interval. Once a puppy is infected, hyperimmune sera is ineffective. Use of antiviral drugs in affected puppies has not been recommended because viral damage to tissues may persist, most notably in the central nervous system, causing cerebellar dysplasia.[209,212] The use of human alpha-interferon (at a dosage of 10^8 U/kg given parenterally) has been shown to reduce the severity of clinical signs in cats infected with herpesvirus when given early or before infection.[211,214]

Feline Infectious Peritonitis

Infection with the coronavirus causing feline infectious peritonitis (FIP) is believed to result from ingestion or inhalation of virus as a result of close contract with infected cats or by fomite transmission.[215–217] In utero transmission has also been shown. This virus does not survive long external to the host and is easily inactivated by detergents and disinfecting agents (common household bleach).[215,217] Vasculitis is initiated by interactions between monocytes infected with virus, immune complexes, and complement fixation and can lead to accumulation of fluid rich in fibrin in the interstitial space.[215–217] If the exudation of fluid is notable, a condition of "wet or effusive" FIP is characterized as body cavity effusions accumulate. If an effusion does not develop, the "dry" form of FIP is characterized.[218]

Clinical signs in infected cats are variable but usually include weight loss, anorexia, vomiting, depression, and cyclic fever. Clinical signs depend on the severity and localization of the viral-induced vasculitis. Any organ in the body may be affected by FIP including the central nervous system. In cats with hepatic involvement, increased activities of ALT and AST are common. Jaundice may appear when hepatic lesions have progressed. Histologic lesions in the liver are characterized by multifocal hepatic necrosis with associated infiltration by neutrophils and macrophages. Pyogranulomatous lesions may appear on the capsule of the liver. In cats with the "wet" form of the disease, lymphocytic cholongitis is an important differential diagnosis.

There is no definitive therapy for FIP. Once the liver and other parenchymal organs are involved, the disease is always fatal. Supportive care tailored to the patient's status is provided as a palliative measure. Immunosuppressive dosages of glucocorticoids, cytotoxic chemotherapeutic agents (such as cyclophosphamide), broad-spectrum antimicrobials, and nutritional support have been used to extend the life of some cats.

BACTERIAL DISEASES ASSOCIATED WITH HEPATIC NECROSIS

Liver Abscesses

Abscess formation in the liver can develop in association with infections in other portions of the body or, less commonly, may occur as an isolated lesion. Hepatic abscesses can be large and contain caseated or liquified material or be small and disseminated throughout the liver. Abscess formation is most common in the right lobes because of the dynamics of the portal circulation to the liver lobes.

The pathogenesis of hepatic abscess formation is linked to portal bacteremia and extension from biliary tract infections.[219,220] Experimental work suggests that impaired perfusion to liver tissue augments development of infection.[219] Portal thromboembolism related to enteric and mesenteric disease processes or necrosis of tumor tissue are likely causes. Immunodeficient patients and those with diabetes mellitus are at greatest risk.[221] Patients with solitary abscesses may have no discernable underlying predisposing conditions; those with multiple abscesses usually have some other disease in the abdominal cavity or have been bacteremic. In humans, polymicrobial infections are common in large abscesses with gram negative facultative rods, anaerobic gram negative rods, and microaerophilic *Streptococcus* the most common isolates.[221,222]

When an hepatic abscess is an isolated lesion, clinical signs may remain vague and include lethargy, anorexia, and weight loss. Tenderness in the cranial abdominal regions may be detected. In some animals, the diagnosis becomes apparent when signs of septicemia develop or intra-abdominal rupture of the abscess occurs. Most patients are febrile and have unexplained increases in hepatic enzyme activity. Many patients develop a neutrophilic leukocytosis intermittently associated with a left shift, toxic neutrophils, and a monocytosis. Increased serum concentrations of fibrinogen may indicate the presence of an appropriate acute-phase response. Hyperbilirubinemia occurs inconsistently. Ultrasonographic imaging of the liver will disclose the presence of focal lesions greater than 0.5 cm and may reveal patterns consistent with an internal fluid consistency, dystrophic mineralization, or the presence of gas. The latter changes may also be evident on abdominal radiographs. Miliary abscessation cannot be differentiated from other multifocal hepatic parenchymal diseases using ultrasonography.

Treatment of large hepatic abscesses involves drainage or resection of the involved hepatic tissue. Cytologic examination of abscess contents, including gram staining, anaerobic and aerobic cultures of affected as well as normal tissue, and routine histopathologic evaluations, are essential diagnostic evaluations. Anaerobic organisms may be difficult to culture and should be suspected if organisms are seen cytologically but no anaerobes are cultured. Microabscessation of liver tissue has been observed with many different infectious agents in dogs and cats.

Initial antimicrobial therapy should be broad spectrum until culture results are available. Use of an aminoglycoside with an anti-anaerobic drug (clindamycin or metronidazole) with the addition of ampicillin or penicillin has been recommended for human beings.[221] Parenteral therapy is recommended during the first 10 days followed by oral drug administration.

Bacteremia

Seeding of liver tissue with bacteria can occur following bacteremia. Bacteria most commonly isolated from bacteremia in dogs include *Staphylococcus* (coagulase positive and negative), gram negative organisms of the Enterobacteriaceae family, and *Streptococcus* sp.[223–225] Anaerobic bacteria also are considered important bacteremic pathogens.

Confirming the presence of bacteremia can be difficult in companion animals because of the low numbers of bacteria that are usually present in blood. The likelihood of obtaining a positive culture increases with the volume of blood used as inoculum. Furthermore, inadvertent contamination of the collection apparatus or culture media during sample collection or storage can result in spurious positive test results.

Gram negative bacteremia precipitates DIC more readily than gram positive bacteremia.[30] Important clinical complications include hemorrhage, thrombosis, microangiopathic hemolysis, and shock. Damage to the microvascular perfusion of organs, such as the liver, may lead to death. Impaired vascular perfusion to the liver and within the liver causes hypoxia to zone 3 hepatocytes, ballooning degeneration, and thrombotic showers of clots or bacterial organisms that can induce inflammatory lesions in the portal triads. Each of these events leads to increased activity of liver enzymes and clinical signs of an "acute" hepatic disorder.

Anaerobic Bacterial Infections

The normal bacterial flora is predominantly anaerobic with large numbers of obligate anaerobes on mucous membrane surfaces. Three groups of anaerobes predominant in the colon of the dog are *Bacteroides, Clostridium,* and *Fusobacterium.* Disorders associated with altered gut wall permeability, rupture, or mesenteric venous bacteremia can send these organisms to the liver via the portal circulation resulting in either disseminated miliary abscess formation or single large abscesses located in one or a few liver lobes. Recent reviews of anaerobes isolated from domestic animals has shown that *Bacteroides,* and *Fusobacterium,* followed by *Clostridium, Proprionibacterium, Actinomyces, Peptostreptococcus,* and *Peptococcus,* are the most commonly isolated pathogens.[226–229] Spurious contamination with *Clostridium perfringens* seems to be common because this organism is aerotolerant and widespread in the environment and on the surface of the skin.[230]

Recommended antimicrobial treatment of anaerobic bacterial infections is summarized in Table 32–9.[231–233] Penicillins remain the cornerstone of therapy with the exception of some strains of *Bacteroides.* Intravenous therapy for 7 to 10 days is recommended for serious life endangering infections followed by oral drug administration. First-generation cephalosporins cannot be relied upon. If cephalosporins are used, a second-generation drug should be tried. The anaerobic bacteria are uniformly resistant to aminoglycosides and sulfonamides are poor choices.

Tyzzer's Disease: "*Bacillus*" *piliformis*

Tyzzer's disease is caused by a gram negative spore-bearing fusiform bacteria, which can cause spontaneous disease in a wide range of host species, including laboratory animals, dogs, cats, horses, cows, and monkeys. Most affected animals are neonates less than 2 months of age. "*Bacillus*" *piliformis* is an unclassified bacterium, and is not a member of the *Bacillus* genus. It may be found in vegetative or spore stages. Infection is thought to occur through ingestion of spores or contamination of the umbilicus. Neonates are believed to be infected by organisms shed from carrier adults.[235] Wild animals are believed to serve as a reservoir.[234] Dissemination to the liver occurs via the portal or umbilical veins. A number of clinical reports involving dogs and cats without predisposing illnesses have been published.[236–241] However, the disease is more common in immunocompromised animals including neonates and animals treated with glucocorticoids or cytotoxic drugs and those suffering from overcrowding or nutritional deficiencies.[235,242–244] Tyzzer's disease has been diagnosed in animals with other disorders commonly associated with immune incompetence including cryptosporidiosis, canine distemper, feline panleukopenia, feline infectious peritonitis, FeLV, and trypanosomiasis.[245–249] Tyzzer's disease also has been reported in kittens with familial primary hyperlipoproteinemia.[250]

Clinical signs of infection with *B. piliformis* include fever, inappetence, diarrhea, and vomiting. Icterus develops in some animals. Typical histologic lesions include the presence of characteristic bacteria in the lamina propria of the intestinal tract and in hepatocytes at the margins of necrotic foci. Multiple, variably sized foci of coagulative necrosis develop in portal areas. A mild to moderate, variable, mixed inflammatory response is observed at the margins of necrotic areas. Organisms are best visualized within degenerate and intact hepatocytes at the margins of these necrotic areas. The bacteria appear as numerous, long, filamentous bacilli arranged in bundles or crisscross patterns. They are visualized using routine hematoxylin and eosin staining or special staining with Giemsa, PAS, Warthin-Starry, or Gomori's (silver impregnation) methods. Impression smears of liver tissue can be stained with methylene blue or Diff-Quik (American Scientific Products) to demonstrate the filamentous and spore forms of the organism.

The diagnosis of Tyzzer's disease is made on the basis of postmortem findings. Up to now, treatment of affected dogs

Table 32-9

SENSITIVITIES OF IMPORTANT ANAEROBIC PATHOGENS TO ANTIMICROBIALS[231-233]

GRAM STAINING CHARACTERISTICS	GRAM NEGATIVE RODS NONSPORE FORMING		GRAM POSITIVE RODS SPORE FORMING	GRAM NEGATIVE RODS NONSPORE FORMING		GRAM POSITIVE COCCI
Antimicrobial	Bacteroides	Fusobacterium	Clostridium	Propionibacterium	Actinomyces	Peptostreptococcus
Penicillin G	– to +	++	– to ++	+++	+++	+++
Penicillin and beta lactamase inhibitor	+++	+++	+++	+++	+++	+++
Ticarcillin	+++	+++	+++	+++	+++	+++
Cephalosporins						
Cephalothin (1st generation)	–	–	–	–	++	–
Cefoxitin (2nd generation)	++	++ to +++	– to ++	+++	–	+++
Metronidazole	+++	+++	+++	–	+++	++ to +++
Clindamycin	++ to +++	+++	+++	+++	–	+++
Chloramphenicol	+++	+++	+++	+++	+++	+++
Tetracycline	–	–	–	–	–	–
Doxycycline	–	–	–	–	–	–
Fluorinated Quinolones	–	–	–	–	–	–
Aminoglycosides*	–	–	–	–	–	–
Sulfonamides**	–	–	–	–	–	–

*Aminoglycosides require transport enzyme systems to gain entrance to the interior of the bacteria; these are lacking in anaerobes.[227]
**Sulfonamides are usually not effective despite in vitro sensitivity testing results. Tissue necrosis and suppuration commonly associated with anaerobic infections result in competitive inhibition of sulfonamide activity.[231-233]

or cats has not been successful. It is noteworthy, however, that tetracycline administered in drinking water controlled mortality and eradicated the disease in a colony of mice and in a rabbitry.[251,252]

Salmonella

Enteric *Salmonella* infection is the most frequent form of salmonellosis seen in small animals. Following invasion of the intestinal mucosa, *Salmonella* may gain access to the portal circulation, and disseminate to other organ systems, including the liver. Endotoxemia may subsequently develop leading to severe systemic consequences. The clinical signs of salmonellosis in small animals have been subcategorized into (1) gastroenteritis, (2) bacteremia and endotoxemia, (3) organ localization, and a (4) persistent nonsymptomatic carrier state.[253] All animals with hepatic infection with *Salmonella* have concurrently or have recently had enteric signs of infection. Jaundice may develop just before death in puppies with gastroenteritis and endotoxemia due to *Salmonella*.[254]

Histologic lesions in the liver can include congestion and randomly scattered small foci of hepatocellular necrosis infiltrated with macrophages and neutrophils. Lesions may appear hemorrhagic and may be associated with Kupffer cell hyperplasia. Thrombi may occasionally be identified. Mesenteric lymphadenopathy is common and corresponds with recent enteric infection. *Salmonella* can be cultured from liver tissue and bile. *Salmonella* infection can also cause cholecystitis in dogs.[255]

Diagnosis of salmonellosis is made on the basis of clinical signs and isolation of a pathogenic strain of bacteria. It is important to remember that *Salmonella* can be isolated from the feces of healthy dogs. Organisms isolated from blood, tissue, urine, CSF, synovial fluid, or body effusions directly implicate pathogenicity.

Treatment of salmonellosis has been complicated by the emergence of highly resistant organisms attributed to the increased use of antimicrobials in food animals. Initial therapy for confirmed disease should be with chloramphenicol, trimethoprim-sulfonamides, or fluorquinolones until sensitivity results are available. Animals presenting for *Salmonella* gastroenteritis require intensive supportive care aimed at restoration of their hydration status (see Chapter 21). Plasma transfusions may be indicated if hypoalbuminemia develops due to loss of protein into the alimentary canal. Plasma transfusions have reduced mortality from *Salmonella* endotoxin given to dogs experimentally.[256] Antimicrobials are recommended in patients showing systemic signs of endotoxemia, sepsis, or increased serum activities of hepatic transaminases and ALP. Although sensitivity testing usually guides the clinical selection of appropriate antimicrobials, the in vitro sensitivity results for *Salmonella* spp. do not reliably correlate with patient clinical response.

Streptococcal Infections

Group B and group G streptococci are a cause of neonatal sepsis in cats and dogs.[257–259] Group G are the most common streptococcal pathogens in the cat, specifically *S. canis*.[260–265] Neonatal infection in kittens has been acquired from vaginal exposure to organisms. Infection ascends the umbilicus into the peritoneal cavity or via the ductus venosus resulting in bacteremia.[261,266] Several kittens in one litter may be affected. Queens younger than 2 years of age are most often involved, usually with their first litter. Occurrence of multiple infec-

tions in different litters of kittens in a single cattery can result after introduction of the organism into a previously naive environment. Neonatal puppies also can develop septicemia with *S. canis*. Histologic lesions associated with streptococcal hepatitis and septicemia in the neonate include omphalophlebitis, peritonitis, and embolic hepatitis. Local infections with group G streptococci can also develop as a result of wounds, trauma, or viral infections that permit a route of entrance into the body. It is proposed that cervical lymphadenitis can develop in young cats, 3 to 7 months old, after clinically silent pharyngitis or tonsillitis.[262,263] Cervical lymphadenitis can lead to septicemia and dissemination of the bacteria to the liver and other organs.

Recommended treatments for streptococcal infections include penicillin G: 10,000 to 20,000 U/kg IM or SQ BID for 7 days; penicillin V: 8 to 30 mg/kg PO TID for 7 days; cephalexin: 10 to 40 mg/kg PO BID for 7 days; chloramphenicol: 15 to 25 mg/kg for dogs PO, IV, or SQ TID and 10 to 15 mg/kg for cats, PO, IV, or SQ BID for 7 days; or erythromycin: in dogs at 3 to 20 mg/kg PO SID to BID for 7 days.[260] Specific recommendations for neonatal kitten prophylaxis in a cattery with a history of neonatal infections with *S. canis* include ampicillin or amoxicillin at a dose of 25 mg/kg PO or SQ TID for 7 days, or procaine/benzathine penicillin 6250 IU per kitten SQ every 48 to 72 hours for 5 days.[261]

Listeria monocytogenes

Listeria monocytogenes is a gram positive, facultative anaerobe with varying pathogenicity. Systemic infection with *Listeria monocytogenes* has been reported in dogs and cats after ingestion of contaminated food, usually meat or dairy products.[267–269] Following intestinal mucosal penetration, *Listeria* is disseminated in blood causing septic embolization. This results in microabscessation. Persistent tissue infection is enabled by macrophage uptake of organisms. Clinical signs associated with acute infection usually include fever, diarrhea, and vomiting. If the organism forms hepatic microabscesses, clinicopathologic features of hepatic inflammation develop. It is important to realize that *Listeria* can be isolated from feces of healthy animals; thus fecal culture is not a reliable diagnostic test.

Successful treatment of hepatic infections with *Listeria* have not been reported. It is recommended that combination therapy with gentamicin and ampicillin be used.[270]

Mycobacterial Infections

Disseminated infection with mycobacteria is a rare cause of hepatic infection in dogs and cats.[271–285] *Mycobacterium avium*, *M. fortuitum* (atypical or nontuberculous mycobacteria), and *M. tuberculosis* (tuberculous mycobacteria) have each been confirmed as causing systemic infections in companion animals. The atypical forms of mycobacteria are the most common isolates. These have been recovered from soil, natural water supplies, tap water, air, and distilled water. Some have also been discovered as nosocomial pathogens in human health-care facilities. As is the case in humans, animals acquiring systemic mycobacterial infections are believed to be immunodeficient.[274,277–279,286,287] An X-linked recessively inherited, presumed combined immunodeficiency in a kindred of basset hounds is believed to underlie their propensity for mycobacterial infections.[273,274,277,279] Basset hounds with mycobacterial infections have had visceral rather than diffuse pulmonary involvement suggesting an enteric route of infection.[274] Infection with an atypical mycobacteria was reported in association with feline immunodeficiency virus infection in cats.[287]

Hepatic infection usually results in randomly distributed discrete aggregates of macrophages and giant cells that cause compression and necrosis of adjacent hepatocytes. Sinusoidal congestion occurs adjacent to granulomas. Short-chained beaded or rod-shaped intracytoplasmic acid-fast organisms can be visualized within giant cells and macrophages when a Zeil-Neelsen's stain is applied. Routine hematoxylin and eosin staining will not define mycobacterial organisms. Bacteria are most commonly observed in the periphery of necrotic areas. Portal thrombophlebitis and lymphangitis have also been described.[274] In dogs with *M. tuberculosis* infection, dystrophic mineralization has been observed within the liver on examination by abdominal radiography.[281,282] At necropsy, mineralization of liver and bile ducts has been associated with caseous exudates. Histologically, multifocal necrosis with mineralization is evident in larger lesions in lungs, liver, and regional lymph nodes and has been associated with acid-fast organisms. Rarely, mycobacterial septicemia can be recognized by detection of the organisms within circulating neutrophils.[284]

Treatment of mycobacterial infection depends on the species isolated. See a review of commonly used drugs and their side effects.[280] *Mycobacteria fortuitum* is often resistant to standard antimycobacterial and antibacterial treatments and it is advised that accurate susceptibility testing be completed before embarking on long-term therapy.[286,287] If *M. tuberculosis* is isolated, consideration should be given to the significance of the current human health problems associated with emergence of drug-resistant strains in densely populated cities.[288-291]

Leptospirosis

Clinical Synopsis

Diagnostic Features

- Variable signs but concurrent liver and kidney damage is common
- Fever, myalgia, vomiting, tachycardia, jaundice, uveitis, and bleeding tendencies often seen
- Increased BUN, creatinine, and urinary casts common
- Percentage rise in ALP often greater than that of ALT
- Leptospire titers often negative
- Histology may reveal necrosis, cholestasis, or chronic hepatitis

Standard Treatment

- Institute isolation procedures (public health risk)
- Intravenous fluid therapy
- Management of DIC
- Diuresis if oliguric
- Ampicillin (10–20 mg/kg PO, SQ, or IV q 12 hours) during acute phase of illness
- Doxycycline (5 mg/kg PO q 12 hours for 1 day then q 24 hours for 14 days) to eliminate leptospiuria

Infection with *Leptospira interrogans*, serovars icterohaemorrhagiae, canicola, pomona, hardjo, grippotyphosa, and bataviae can lead to either acute or chronic hepatic disease in

dogs.[292-296] Cats have been shown to be relatively resistant to infection with leptospira but can develop hepatic lesions.[297] The leptospires are spirochetes that are transmitted between animals by direct contact, ingestion of infected food or water, contamination of mucous membranes, through bite wounds, or in utero.[292] This is an important disease to diagnose definitively because of its zoonotic potential. Organisms survive well in stagnant or slow-moving water that often serves as the reservoir of infectious agent.[292] Infected dogs may intermittently shed organisms in urine for months after clinical recovery.

Infection usually occurs through mucous membranes whereupon the organism rapidly replicates within microvasculature. Organ tropism of different serovars and the individual host susceptibility (age, immunity) determine the clinical course following acute infection. Recovery corresponds to host antibody production within the first week.

Clinical signs include fever, generalized myalgia, vomiting, anorexia, tachycardia, tachypnea, and jaundice. Severe dehydration and microvascular injury lead to poor peripheral perfusion and microvascular collapse. Vascular injury and coagulopathy manifest as surface bruising, hematemesis, hematochezia, melena, and epistaxis. Acute uveitis and scleral injection are often obvious. Some dogs develop intussusception and some dogs produce acholic feces as a result of extrahepatic and intrahepatic interruption of bile flow.[298]

Hematologic features include a leukopenia during initial leptospiremia. This evolves into a neutrophilic leukocytosis associated with a left shift. Initial tissue injury is related to vascular damage and its consequences. Thrombocytopenia and increased fibrin degradation products have been shown in dogs with experimental infection with *L. icterohaemorrhagiae*.[299] Endothelial damage may result from toxins released from the organisms or from DIC. Hyperfibrinogenemia reflects an acute-phase response in some dogs. Colonization of the kidneys is common because the organisms can evade serum neutralizing antibodies in the renal interstitium and tubular epithelium. Acute renal injury is common due to swelling of the renal interstitium and impaired renal perfusion.[292] Increased BUN and serum creatinine concentrations and an active urine sediment revealing granular or cellular casts reflect the severity of renal injury. Permanent damage to the kidneys may develop in dogs that survive acute infection. Hepatic damage may occur in association with overt necrotizing perivascular lesions or due to subcellular injury attributable to toxins released by the spirochetes. In the dog, icterus reflects hepatic involvement rather than hemolysis as occurs in ruminants. Hepatic injury is indicated by acute increases in the serum activities of ALT, AST, and ALP within the first week of infection with serovars having tropism for the liver.[299] The fold increase in ALP activity may greatly exceed the fold increase in the transaminase activity. Of 36 dogs with confirmed infections with leptospirosis in the author's hospital, over the past 10 years, 12 (33%) developed hepatic involvement. Of the total number of dogs infected, 78% had increased serum ALP activity, 53% had an increased AST activity, 44% an increased ALT activity, and 19% were hyperbilirubinemic.[294] In a recent retrospective report of leptospirosis in 17 dogs from another university hospital, 59% had increased serum ALP activity, 29% had increased AST activity, 35% had increased ALT activity, and 24% were hyperbilirubinemic.[293] In both these hospital populations, serovars pomona and grippotyphosa were most common.

Histologic lesions in the liver of dogs usually include multifocal coagulative necrosis with infiltration of lymphocytes and fewer quantities of neutrophils and macrophages. Organisms may be demonstrable in the sinusoids using a silver stain and visualized on impression smears of liver tissue stained with Giemsa. Histologic lesions in the liver tissue from cats experimentally infected with *L. pomona* included periacinar congestion and marked periportal ballooning degeneration. Fluorescent antibody techniques are used to identify leptospiral serovars in tissues and body fluids, particularly urine. Confirmation of infection using serologic titers (microscopic agglutination test, MAT) can be frustrating because dogs may test negative during the first week of infection and thereafter (2 to 6 weeks) demonstrate only a short phase of antibody production. A more comprehensive discussion on the value of different methods of antibody determination and measurement of specific IgG and IgM responses is available.[292] Isolation of the infectious agent is difficult because of their fastidious growth requirements.[292] Urine is the best substance to submit for culture and must be collected before antimicrobials are administered.

In some dogs with chronic or subclinical infection, chronic hepatitis progressing to hepatic fibrosis and cirrhosis may occur.[295] These animals develop the full gamut of clinical signs and clinicopathologic features typical of a chronic progressive hepatopathy. The grippotyphosa serovar was implicated in one kennel where five dogs were affected.[295] A cell-mediated immune response with or without persistence of organisms in the liver is suspected.

Fluid therapy is essential in severely affected animals and should be given intravenously. If petechia and bleeding tendencies are prominent, treatment for DIC should be instituted. Attention must be given to early recognition of oliguric or anuric renal failure. Use of mannitol or combination of furosemide and dopamine may be used in an attempt to improve urine production once the patient is adequately hydrated. Once low output renal failure develops, a poor prognosis is warranted, although some patients may recover if the leptospiral infection is controlled. Penicillins (penicillin G 25,000–40,000 µ/kg IM or IV BID to TID, ampicillin 10 to 20 mg/kg PO, SQ, IV TID, or amoxicillin 10 mg/kg PO BID) are the antibiotics of choice for eliminating leptospiremia.[292,300] Clearing the organism from the kidney is accomplished with doxycycline (5 mg/kg PO BID day 1, then 5 mg/kg PO SID) given for 14 days.[301–303] Doxycycline therapy is reserved until the patient has recovered from the acute disease and can tolerate oral medications. Fluorinated quinolones, such as enrofloxacin, also are believed to clear the organisms.[304] Previously, dihydrostreptomycin was recommended for renal clearance of the persistent leptospiremia. Its lack of availability and renal toxicity have limited its use.

Tularemia

Infection with *Francisella tularensis* has been diagnosed in both dogs and cats. Wild lagomorphs and rodents serve as reservoirs of the disease that can be transmitted by ticks and flies.[305–310] Infection occurs by ingestion, mucous membrane contamination, inoculation by biting insects, and inhalation. Cats appear to be more susceptible to infection than dogs, and have been shown to serve as a reservoir and transmitter of tularemia to human beings.[307,309] After inoculation, infection spreads via local lymphatics and hematogenously to other regions of the body.

Clinical signs of tularemia include fever, lethargy, weight loss, and jaundice. Physical examination usually reveals profound submandibular lymphadenopathy. Abdominal palpation may reveal splenomegaly and mesenteric lymphadenopathy. Hematologic features usually include panleukopenia, toxic changes in neutrophils, and thrombocytopenia. Serum biochemical abnormalities reflect dehydration and hepatic

inflammation with increased serum activities of ALT, AST, and ALP. Hyperbilirubinemia is common. The infective organisms may be cultured from blood, lymph node aspirates, or bone marrow specimens antemortem, but diagnosis is more conveniently confirmed using direct or indirect fluorescent antibody tests on aspirated or biopsied material.[308]

Liver lesions are characterized as multiple discrete foci of necrosis. Well-circumscribed areas of coagulative necrosis are observed histologically lacking a zonal orientation. Macrophages and fibroblasts are observed at the margins of the lesions. Lymph nodes develop necrotic foci within follicles and extend into parafollicular areas, resulting in large areas of cortical necrosis.

In humans, aminoglycosides are used as first-line therapy. Streptomycin and gentamicin are usually recommended. Alternative choices include tetracycline and chloramphenicol, but these are believed to be less effective in clearing the organisms. Cephalosporins may also be effective. There have not been reports of successful treatment in dogs or cats because diagnosis is usually made postmortem.

RICKETTSIAL DISEASES ASSOCIATED WITH HEPATIC NECROSIS

Ehrlichia canis

Canine ehrlichiosis is caused by an obligate intracellular parasite, *Ehrlichia canis*, transmitted mainly via *Rhipicephalus sanguineus*, the brown dog tick.[311–313] The most common severe organ injury associated with chronic *Ehrlichiosis* is renal failure. However, approximately 15% of infected dogs develop increased serum ALT activity, 8% develop increased ALP activity, and 4% become hyperbilirubinemic. Liver lesions are characterized by lymphoplasmacytic infiltrates around hepatic venules and in the portal triads. The accumulation of lymphocytes in tissue lesions is not surprising because intact T lymphocyte function is important in host defense against rickettsial diseases.[314,315] Sinusoidal congestion and necrosis in zone 3 of the acinus has been observed in dogs in the chronic phase of infection.[316] Expanding foci of macrophages, lymphocytes, and plasma cells may compromise sinusoidal perfusion and cause necrosis of adjacent hepatocytes.[312,313] *Ehrlichia* organisms occasionally are observed in tissue macrophages after routine hematoxylin and eosin staining. A peribiliary infiltration of neutrophils and lymphocytes was observed in one cat with a spontaneous *Ehrlichia canis* infection.[317]

Diagnosis is confirmed using an IFA test for demonstration of antibodies against *E. canis*.[311] Serum IgG titers cannot be detected until 21 days postinfection and so there is a short lag time between development of clinical illness and an ability to confirm infection with routinely used IFA tests.

Successful treatment of *Ehrlichia canis* involves administration of antirickettsial drugs and provision of supportive nursing care. Doxycycline is the drug of choice and is given at a dosage of 5 to 10 mg/kg PO or IV SID to BID for 7 to 10 days. For further information regarding recommended therapies in refractory cases, see another textbook.[311]

Rocky Mountain Spotted Fever: *Rickettsia rickettsii*

Rocky mountain spotted fever (RMSF) is caused by an obligate intracellular rickettsial organism, *Rickettsia rickettsii*. It is pathogenic for people and animals and is primarily distributed through two ticks, *Dermacentor andersoni* (the wood tick) and *D. variabilis* (the brown dog tick).[318]

After a tick bites its host, *R. rickettsii* enters the microcirculation and invades and replicates in endothelial cells of small blood vessels.[314,318–320] Invasion of the endothelium results in a progressive necrotizing vasculitis, which initiates a sequence of events including vascular leakage and activation of platelets and coagulation and fibrinolytic proteins.[321]

Serum biochemical abnormalities include mild hyperglycemia, hypercholesterolemia, and increased activities of ALP, ALT, and AST. The liver enzyme abnormalities are more common in dogs with RMSF than in dogs with *Ehrlichia canis* infection.[322] Azotemia develops due to dehydration and compromised renal vasculature in the terminal stages of infection. Histologic changes in liver usually consist of focal hepatic necrosis. Rickettsiae are difficult to visualize in routinely processed tissues but have been observed in Giemsa-stained sections.[323]

Definitive diagnosis is usually made on the basis of serology. See other resources for a complete discussion of the methods of diagnosis and treatment.[318,324]

PARASITIC INFECTIONS ASSOCIATED WITH HEPATIC NECROSIS

Toxoplasma gondii

Toxoplasma gondii is an obligate intracellular coccidian parasite that can infect all mammalian species. The definitive hosts are Felidae. All nonfeline hosts serve as intermediate hosts. *Toxoplasma* has three infectious stages: sporozoites in oocysts, tachyzoites, and encysted bradyzoites.[325] Oocysts are formed only in feline species and are excreted in feces. Tachyzoites are the tissue invasive, actively replicative stage, and bradyzoites are the encysted slowly, replicative stage. Infection with *Toxoplasma* can occur via consumption of undercooked tissues containing bradyzoites, ingestion of sporulated oocysts contaminating food or water, by inhalation of sporulated oocysts, congenitally from mother to offspring, and rarely, via lactation, blood transfusion, or organ transplantation.[325]

Initial infection through the intestinal epithelium results in invasion of mesenteric lymph nodes. Epithelial and lymphoid tissue necrosis develops due to formation and multiplication of tachyzoites. As host cells die, tachyzoites released into blood or lymph are transported to other tissues. Usually, multiple organs are "seeded" with tachyzoites and the clinical syndrome associated with acute infection is determined by the extent of injury to infected tissues. The liver can be infected early on in the disease process through organism transport in the portal venous circulation. Hepatic necrosis occurs as a result of macrophage and hepatocyte infection, tachyzoite multiplication, and cell lysis. Delayed hypersensitivity reactions and immune complex vasculitis are additional mechanisms of tissue injury.[326] Coagulative necrosis may be observed randomly scattered in the hepatic parenchyma. Degenerate and nondegenerate hepatocytes containing variable numbers of intracytoplasmic tachyzoites are usually seen.[327,328] A neutrophilic or mononuclear cell infiltration may be observed in the area of hepatic necrosis. Cysts containing bradyzoites may also be observed, which are more easily visualized after PAS staining. Cats with fatal neonatal toxoplasmosis have shown extensive periportal and periacinar infiltration with mononuclear cells associated with tachyzoites

and cysts.[329] Animals with hepatic infection usually develop severe clinical signs and do not survive long.

In most immunocompetent animals, the initial phase of infection with *Toxoplasma* resolves after about 3 weeks as tachyzoites disseminate and form bradyzoite tissue cysts. Reactivation of disease may occur at some future time when immunosuppression permits new release of bradyzoites.

Clinicopathologic features in animals infected with *Toxoplasma* developing hepatic necrosis may include leukopenia (in invariably fatal infections) or leukocytosis, and marked increases in the serum ALT and AST activities. In dogs, an increase in the serum activity of ALP is also usually observed. Definitive diagnosis is made by demonstration of organisms in tissue aspirates or biopsy, or by demonstration of significant IgM antibody titers or *Toxoplasma* antigen in host sera. If IgG antibody titers are used, demonstration of a significant increase in convalescent titers is necessary to confirm infection. During the acute phase of infection, the IgG antibody titers may be negative. A number of different serologic methods for detection of toxoplasmosis have been developed. See several excellent discussions of their diagnostic utility.[330–332]

Treatment of the dog or cat with hepatic necrosis attributable to toxoplasmosis should involve supportive fluid, electrolyte, and nutritional care. Clindamycin is the antimicrobial of choice and is used for 2 week intervals either orally or intramuscularly at dosages of 3 to 13 mg/kg TID or 10 to 20 mg/kg BID in the dog and 8 to 17 mg/kg TID or 12.5 to 25 mg/kg BID in the cat.[325,333,334] Oral clindamycin can cause anorexia, vomiting, or diarrhea when given at the higher dosages.[325,334] An alternative, less effective treatment consists of trimethoprim-sulfa combined with pyrimethamine.

Neospora caninum

Neospora is a recently recognized fatal protozoan parasite of dogs, cats, and other mammals.[325,335–339] The protozoa has a worldwide distribution. Until the organism was definitively distinguished from *Toxoplasma gondii* by immunologic and ultrastructural methods, infection with *Neospora* was consistently misdiagnosed.[325,340] The currently understood life cycle of *Neospora* is simpler than that of *Toxoplasma*: tachyzoites and tissue cysts are the only recognized stages. The source of organisms causing natural infection is not known. Both tachyzoites and tissue cysts of *Neospora* are infectious following oral ingestion; it is believed carnivores become infected by ingestion of infected tissue. Transplacental transmission has also been demonstrated.[325,341,342] In infected animals, tachyzoites are found intracellularly and also may be found free within areas of necrosis and in spinal fluid.[325,335] Tissue cysts have only been found in the brain and spinal cord.[335,339,343,344]

Unlike *Toxoplasma*, *Neospora* is believed to be a primary pathogen in dogs. Clinical signs are most common in young dogs and often are neuromuscular and typically involve ascending paralysis with primary involvement of the pelvic limbs. A rigid contraction of muscles of the rear limbs has been repeatedly recognized. Neonatal infections become obvious when pups are 5 weeks old.[339] Disease may be localized or disseminated and it is in the latter group that hepatic necrosis may develop.[339] Prenatally and neonatally infected kittens developed encephalomyelitis, polymyositis, and hepatitis when given methylprednisolone acetate.[336,337,342] Lytic ballooning degeneration rather than coagulative necrosis predominated in liver lesions. Many extracellular tachyzoites were observed in necrotic and adjacent normal tissues. Similar severe infection was diagnosed in an 8 month old basset hound in which over 75% of the hepatocytes were necrotic and contained masses of tachyzoites.[338] Neonates with hepatic involvement develop hepatomegaly and a small quantity of abdominal effusion.

Treatments for *Neospora caninum* infections have been investigated but as of yet, no conclusive recommendations have been given. Use of clindamycin, trimethoprim-sulfa, and trimethoprim combined with pyrimethamine has been clinically evaluated in infected dogs. Little response was observed in dogs treated after overt clinical signs of rear limb paralysis and muscle contracture were demonstrated.[325,343,344,345] Improvement, however, was noted in some dogs showing mild clinical signs. In experimental *Neospora* infections in mice, use of sulfadiazine has reduced the severity of clinical signs.[346]

Intrahepatic Biliary Coccidiosis in Dogs

A single case report of an intrahepatic biliary coccidiosis in a dog has been recently published.[347] Clinical signs included icterus, weight loss, and vomiting. Hepatomegaly and a minor increase in the serum ALT activity were observed. Infection of biliary epithelium with an asexual stage of an unidentified coccidium was identified. The infectious organism was different from other coccidiums known to infect the dog and was not definitively identified. The bile ducts were enlarged and there was inflammation and desquamation of biliary epithelium. Examination of liver tissue revealed a severe chronic suppurative cholangiohepatitis. This dog was a Doberman pinscher and had been exposed to a trimethoprim-sulfa antimicrobial, which may have contributed to the hepatic lesions.

Leishmania donovoni

Leishmania parasitizes and multiplies within macrophages of the reticuloendothelial system.[348–351] There are several different species of *Leishmania* and each has a particular tissue tropism. Syndromes are classified into simple cutaneous, diffuse, mucocutaneous, or visceral. Most reported cases of canine visceral leishmaniasis have been traced to Mediterranean origin, although infection in closed-colony raised dogs in the United States has also been documented.[351–353] Transmission usually occurs through the bite of sand flies of the genera *Phlebotomus* and *Lutzomyia*. Transmission also can occur through blood transfusions and direct contact with infected skin.[351,354]

Clinical signs develop following a prolonged incubation period (3 weeks to 18 months). Visceral forms of infection are characterized by weight loss, vomiting, anorexia, diarrhea, intermittent lameness, fever, and skin lesions. On physical examination, viscerally infected animals may appear cachectic and have peripheral lymphadenopathy, splenomegaly, and cutaneous lesions. Icterus is rare. Cutaneous lesions are characterized by alopecia and desquamation, a diffuse nonsuppurative dermatitis with macrophages containing organisms, or a generalized nodular pattern with nodules containing macrophages, multinucleated giant cells, and lymphocytes along with large numbers of parasites.[355] Hematologic changes commonly include a mild to moderate nonregenerative anemia, leukopenia, and thrombocytopenia. Some dogs develop a leukocytosis with a left shift. Serum biochemical features reflect tissue involvement. With liver infection, increased serum ALT, AST, and ALP activities develop.[348,356] Hyperglobulinemia and hypoalbuminemia are typical and a monoclonal gammopathy was characterized in one dog.[348,356,357] Diagnosis is made by identification of organisms

in macrophages on lymph node aspirates, bone marrow examination, or parenchymal tissue aspirates or biopsy.

Liver lesions are characterized by multifocal to coalescing hepatocellular necrosis, vacuolar degeneration in portal regions, and a marked macrophage infiltration.[352,358,359] Hepatocytes have been observed to develop progressive cellular swelling that terminates in cytolysis, presumably due to noxious materials released from organisms or related to cell-mediated immune responses.[359] Organisms are usually visible in hepatic macrophages. Hemosiderosis and erythrophagocytosis may be marked within and adjacent to areas of inflammation and necrosis. In some dogs, amyloid deposits also are recognized in liver tissue.[360,361]

Serologic diagnosis is possible using a variety of methods; see more in-depth discussions in reference material.[348,362–364]

Pentavalent antimonial compounds are recommended for treatment of visceral leishmaniasis.[348] Unfortunately, these are not approved for use in dogs in the United States. Repeated courses of treatment may be necessary.[357] Recommended drugs and their dosages include meglumine antimonate (100 mg/kg, IV or SQ SID for 3 to 4 weeks) and sodium stibogluconate (30 to 50 mg/kg IV or SQ SID for 3 to 4 weeks).[348] See a more detailed discussion before initiating patient treatment.[348,357]

Cytauxzoon felis

Cytauxzoonosis is a fatal protozoal disease of cats, involving a tissue phase in which large schizonts develop within macrophages and monocytes disseminated within all body systems. The natural host for this parasite appears to be the bobcat (*Felis rufus*). It is believed that *Cytauxzoon* is passed by tick vectors.[365] Most cases have been described in midwestern to southern states. Infected phagocytes locate in the lumen of veins in many organs and enlarge to such an extent that they compromise blood flow causing vascular occlusion and thromboembolism.[366,367]

Clinical signs are initially vague but are rapidly progressive. Anorexia, dyspnea, lethargy, dehydration, anemia, icterus, and high fever are typically observed. The course of the disease often lasts less than 1 week.[368] Blood smears may reveal the parasite within erythrocytes during the late stage of infection.[369] Wright's Giemsa and Diff Quik stains can be used to demonstrate organisms. Occasionally, large mononuclear phagocytes containing merozoites may be seen in peripheral blood smears.[494] Bone marrow aspirates may reveal large mononuclear cells containing schizonts. Serum biochemical abnormalities usually include moderate to markedly increased serum activities of ALT and AST and hyperbilirubinemia.[368,370]

Hepatic lesions are characterized by accumulations of parasitized macrophages. Macrophages containing large numbers of parasites are observed in the lumen of small and medium-sized veins and arteries and in hepatic sinusoids. The vascular lumen appear nearly occluded, imposing hypoxia on surrounding tissues. Multiple partial thromboses of hepatic veins were observed in naturally infected cats. Cytologic touch preparations made from liver and lung tissue reveals macrophages filled with schizonts using routine blood stains. Death usually occurs before diffuse coagulative hepatic necrosis develops from a terminal shock-like state.

No specific therapy can be recommended for successful treatment of feline cytauxzoonosis. Supportive care with polyionic fluids, broad-spectrum antibiotics, and nutritional support has permitted survival in rare cases.[368] Parvaquone (Clexon, Cooper's Animal Health, Hertz, England, or Wellcome Research Labs, Beckenham, Kent, England) has been used beginning 2 to 12 days postinfection.[368] A dose of 10 to 30 mg/kg IM or SQ SID for 2 to 3 weeks has been advised. In a single study, only 2 of 18 cats treated survived. Anecdotally, sodium thiacetarsamide (Caparsolate, Ceva Laboratories, Overland Park, KS) has been used successfully in one cat.[368] Tetracycline has not been effective.

Heterobilharzia americana

Canine schistosomiasis is caused by infection with *Heterobilharzia americana*, a digenetic trematode endemic to the southern Atlantic and Gulf Coast states within North America.[371–374] The major intermediate host is a freshwater snail (*Lymnaea cubensis*). Rapidly motile cercaria are shed by the snail into water and penetrate the intact skin of definitive hosts. Cercaria transform into schistosomula upon entering skin where they remain for a few days prior to migrating through vasculature to the lungs and then to the liver. After maturation in the liver, male and female schistosomes migrate to the mesenteric veins where they undergo sexual reproduction. Eggs are deposited in terminal branches of mesenteric veins. The eggs induce a delayed hypersensitivity reaction resulting in a granulomatous response that prohibits their egress into the bowel and favors dispersal to other tissues. Heavy deposition of eggs in the liver can cause substantial tissue injury. During the acute stage of egg dissemination, increases in serum activity of liver enzymes reflect their delivery to portal triads. With chronicity, massive periportal fibrosis develops and portal venous perfusion becomes impaired. A reciprocal increase in the hepatic arterial blood flow maintains sufficient circulation to the liver. Acquired portosystemic vascular communications may develop in the late stages of granuloma formation after heavy infestation and development of portal hypertension.

Clinical signs of schistosome infection include dermatitis followed by cough and then anorexia, a profuse mucoid diarrhea, and dehydration. When intestinal infestation is severe, anemia, hypoalbuminemia, edema, and weight loss may follow. In rare cases, neurologic signs develop.[372,374]

Histologic lesions in the liver associated with *H. americana* infection include the formation of granulomas around eggs, primarily in the portal triads, and the presence of macrophages distended with coarse granular black pigment. A marked chronic active portal hepatitis, perilobular fibrosis, and hepatocellular necrosis in zone 3 of the acinus have been detailed. Partial thrombosis of portal venules has also been verified. Eggs appear with a thick hyaline or yellow wall and fragments of eggshells, rather than intact eggs, may only be observed.

Diagnosis is confirmed upon discovery of the spineless egg of *H. americana* in feces. The eggs are approximately 88 × 74 μm in diameter.[374]

Recommended treatment of canine schistosomiasis is with praziquantel using a dose approximately 10-fold greater than that conventionally recommended for cestode elimination. This approximates a dosage of 25 mg/kg given TID for two days. Fenbendazole also has been used successfully in experimentally induced *H. americana* infection in the dog and was used as supplemental therapy in a spontaneous clinical case.[375,376]

Visceral Larval Migrants

Prolonged migration of infective nematode larvae through visceral structures can result in eosinophilia, allergic pneumonitis, and hepatic inflammation and necrosis.[377] Infective larva can be found associated with eosinophilic inflammation and granulomas. Cats experimentally infected intragastrically with large numbers of embryonated eggs of *Toxocara canis* developed multifocal, irregular, raised white-gray foci within the liver ranging in size up to 2 mm in diameter. Living larva of *T. canis* were found within these lesions. Microscopic examination of liver tissue from cats between 18 and 39 days postinfection revealed mild to moderate lymphoplasmacytic portal hepatitis and mild periportal fatty vacuolation. Areas directly involved with larval migration contained more eosinophils. Liver tissue examined in the early phase of infection had areas of acute necrosis intermixed with eosinophils and neutrophils. These lesions were scattered throughout liver lobules with no particular zonal distribution. Focally extensive granulomas associated with epithelioid cells, giant cells, and a mantle of intermixed eosinophils, lymphocytes, and plasma cells were also seen in cats in the later stages of infection. How often parasitic migration contributes to spontaneous hepatic inflammation and necrosis is unknown. Tissue injury is believed to result from hypersensitivity response against larval products or structural components.

MYCOTIC INFECTIONS ASSOCIATED WITH HEPATIC NECROSIS

Disseminated Histoplasmosis, Blastomycosis, and Coccidioidomycosis

Disseminated infections with *Histoplasma capsulatum, Coccidioides immitis*, and, rarely, *Blastomyces dermatitidis* have been reported as a cause of hepatic necrosis and pyogranulomatous inflammation in dogs and cats. In these cases, the hepatic involvement contributes to the clinical signs but is not the principal site of infection. Systemic infection is usually obvious by the time the hepatic parenchyma becomes involved.

Animals with disseminated histoplasmosis often have serum biochemical abnormalities reflecting hepatic injury.[378–387] Tissue damage is believed to be the result of excessive or unregulated host inflammation against the organism rather than the direct effect of noxious fungal products. Granulomatous lesions are characterized by accumulations of monocytes, macrophages, lymphocytes, and plasma cells. Formation of granulomas injures adjacent tissues and compromises local microcirculation. Animals with hepatic involvement develop hepatomegaly. Accumulations of macrophages laden with organisms are observed in the hepatic sinusoids, randomly in small granulomas throughout the liver, or predominantly in the periportal areas.[379–384]

Coccidioides immitis can cause local or systemic infections in the dog.[388–391] If the liver is involved, serum enzymes indicate the presence of hepatocellular necrosis and pyogranulomatous inflammation. Liver involvement has never been identified as a solitary site of infection.

Blastomyces dermatitidis also can cause systemic infections in which the liver is one of many organs damaged. Pathologic lesions produced by blastomycosis are characterized as purulent and pyogranulomatous. The large broad-based budding yeast forms are intermixed with neutrophils, macrophages, and multinucleated giant cells. Hepatic injury occurs by displacement of normal parenchyma by granulomatous foci and tissue injury due to inflammatory mediator release.

Consult a detailed discussion on the most current treatments and drug dosages for systemic mycosis in the dog and cat in several references.[391,392,393]

Aspergillosis

Disseminated infection with *Aspergillus* is uncommon in the dog and cat. In the dog, the German shepherd appears predisposed. Hematogenous spread disseminates the fungus to body organs including the liver. Most animals have been terminally ill when presented for health care and have been sick for several months. Fungal hyphae may be evident in urine, blood smears, purulent material draining from chronic wounds, lymph nodes, bone, intervertebral disc material, and aspirates of parenchymal organs. Definitive diagnosis is usually made on the basis of culture of *Aspergillus*. Serologic tests may provide a rapid confirmation of infection, although some dogs with disseminated infection lack detectable *Aspergillus* antibodies.[394]

Liver lesions are usually associated with fungal emboli that impair hepatic perfusion. Hepatocellular necrosis results from hypoxia and possibly from noxious materials emitted from the fungi. A purulent or granulomatous inflammatory reaction may develop in the area where hyphae are observed.

There is no established recommended treatment for disseminated aspergillosis.

Miscellaneous Mycotic Infections

Hyalohyphomycosis is the term used to encompass opportunistic infections caused by nondematiacious fungi with hyaline hyphal elements as the basic tissue form.[395] Included are infections with *Paecilomyces, Pseudallescheria, Geotrichum,* a variety of species causing eumycotic mycetomas (white grains), *Aspergillus,* and *Penicillium.* These organisms, by extension from their primary site of infection, spread into the liver.[395–408]

Eumycotic mycetoma defines granulomatous nodules of the subcutaneous tissues or body cavities that contain tissue grains or granules comprised of dense colonies of fungal organisms and host-derived debris. Usually these involve chronic deforming lesions characterized by swelling and formation of sinus tracts.[403] In the dog and cat, eumycotic mycetomas have been caused by *Curvularia geniculata, Pseudallescheria boydii, Acremonium hyalinum,* and *Bipolaris specifera,* and in the cat by *Madurella grisea.*[401,402,406–408] A diagnosis of mycetoma is made on the basis of cytologic examination and culture of the grains derived from draining material. Dark or black grains may require digestion in 10% KOH prior to microscopic examination.[395] Specific antibody staining of formalin-fixed tissues or agar-gel immunodiffusion may be used to confirm fungal identity.[395] Prognosis for abdominal mycetoma that involves viscera and liver or spleen is guarded because it is difficult to attain therapeutic drug concentrations within fungal grains.

Paecilomyces spp. have been reported to cause multisystemic infection in dogs and cats. The liver is just one of the many organ systems infected.[396–399] Generalized lymphadenopathy and pulmonary signs are common clinical abnormalities. In one cat, dissemination from the intestines was surmised considering the periportal distribution of fungi in the liver. Hepatic lesions are comprised of necrotizing pyogranulomatous foci surrounding fungal hyphae. This fungus is saprophytic, ubiquitous in soil and decaying organic matter, a common airborne contaminant, and resistant to most sterilizing techniques.[400] It may be visualized within pyogranulomatous foci in tissues or be cultured on Sabouraud's dextrose agar.

Pseudallescheria boydii has been shown to cause eumycotic mycetomas (white grains) in the abdomen of the dog. Infections have developed subsequent to dehiscence of laparotomy incisions.[401,402]

Geotrichosis (*Geotrichum candidum*) has been reported in dogs as a disseminated infection.[404,405] It is believed to be an opportunist invader. Dogs with systemic infection have had severe pulmonary signs due to pneumonia characterized by coalescing foci of necrosis and associated pyogranulomatous inflammation. Hepatic signs are attributed to a similar necrotizing and pyogranulomatous reaction. Routine tissue staining can reveal both free and phagocytized fungi.

Candida albicans is an opportunist causing infections in both dogs and cats.[409–417] In one dog, concurrent hepatic cirrhosis was recognized.[416] It was not determined if the hepatic lesions developed before or after onset of the systemic infection. In immunocompromised humans, hepatic candidiasis is an important problem.[417] Immunoincompetence is also a predisposing condition in companion animals.[410–412] The origin of infection is believed to be the gastrointestinal tract. Fungemia of the portal vein results in hepatic dissemination.

Diagnosis of systemic candidiasis is made on the basis of histologic confirmation of the infection. This is necessary because false positive cultures of *Candida* can occur when samples are acquired from or through contaminated surfaces. Body cavity effusions or urine repeatedly showing large quantities of the fungus would be the exception. In humans, false negative cultures have also been a problem despite histologic demonstration of fungal organisms in the cultured specimen.

Treatment of disseminated candidiasis involves amphotericin B if renal function is adequate, or ketaconazole. Recommended ketaconazole treatment for the dog is 5 to 11 mg/kg PO BID for 4 weeks, and for the cat is 50 to 100 mg total dose PO SID to BID for 4 weeks. Alternatively, itraconazole has been recommended at a dosage of 5 to 7 mg/kg PO BID for 4 weeks in the dog or cat.[409] Liposome-encapsulated amphotericin B has been somewhat effective and nontoxic in preliminary work.[417–419]

Zygomycosis describes infection of humans and animals by fungi of the orders Mucorales and Entomophthorales.[395] Mucormycosis is the most common type of phycomycosis reported in humans and animals. Disseminated phycomycosis has been reported in dogs and cats.[420,421] Dogs with intestinal infarction due to fungal invasion may develop embolic showers of organisms into the liver. Hepatic necrosis and inflammation in the area of embolization follows. These fungi are opportunistic invaders that usually gain entrance to the body via the respiratory system or spore implantation in skin or mucous membranes.[421] The disseminated form reflects the systemic dispersal of mycotic emboli. The histologic lesions associated with mucormycosis involve local vessel invasion resulting in acute vasculitis, thrombus formation, and ischemic necrosis.

Miscellaneous Infectious Agents

PROTOTHECA. Disseminated infection with *Prototheca,* a colorless or achlorophyllous alga, can result in a granulomatous necrotizing infection in multiple body systems, including the liver.[422–439] Infected animals are believed to be immunocompromised because this organism is ubiquitous in the environment. *Prototheca* causing polysystemic infection is believed to enter the body through the gastrointestinal tract from which it disseminates by hematogenous and lymphatic routes. Clinical signs commonly include persistent hemorrhagic diarrhea, blindness due to panuveitis, secondary glaucoma, focal retinal hemorrhages and retinal detachment, and neurologic abnormalities.

Histologic lesions in the liver are always associated with disseminated infection. These are comprised of multifocal to coalescent areas of necrosis containing masses of yeast-like organisms. Infiltrates of plasma cells, macrophages, and neutrophils are observed within necrotic foci and at the periphery of these lesions. In tissue, the organism is round to oval in shape and 10 to 30 μm in diameter with a PAS-positive capsule.[438]

Successful treatment in dogs has not been reported for ocular or disseminated prototheciosis but liposome-encapsulated amphotericin B holds promise. The organism is resistant to ketoconazole, clotrimazole, flucytosine, and miconazole.

HEPATOCELLULAR INJURY DUE TO DRUGS, TOXINS, AND CHEMICALS

Hepatic injury can be caused by toxins, drugs, and certain other chemicals. Although few clinical cases of hepatic necrosis are documented as having such causes, there are undoubtedly many cases where these causes are suspected but cannot be proven. Many drugs can cause hepatic injury and when this problem is suspected, the drug is usually withdrawn, the injury resolves, and a tissue biopsy is never collected. Hepatic injury can range from milder forms of degeneration and lipidosis to hepatic necrosis. Some forms of chemical injury manifest themselves as cholestasis caused by either intrahepatic canalicular bile stasis or portal inflammation. Most of the information concerning hepatotoxicity is obtained from the effects of drugs and toxins on humans and experimental animals.[4,440] Many, if not most, cause a repeatable histologic pattern of injury. In Tables 32–2 and 32–10, drugs and toxins a small animal patient is likely to encounter as well as some no longer posing an important risk are cited. See also Chapter 30 where specific morphologic injuries of different drugs and toxins are tabulated.

Anticonvulsants are the most notorious of drugs known to cause hepatotoxicity in veterinary patients.[441] Primidone given at therapeutic doses can cause hepatic necrosis in some dogs. High doses, or use in combination with other anticonvulsants such as phenytoin, may cause lesions that are more severe. Although phenytoin used alone also may cause hepatic degeneration and necrosis, the rapid plasma clearance in the dog limits its use as an effective anticonvulsant and possibly protects against hepatotoxicity. Phenobarbital has also recently been shown to be associated with hepatotoxicity, necrosis, and cirrhosis in the dog.[442] Typically, phenobarbital stimulates proliferation of the smooth endoplasmic reticulum, causing hepatomegaly in the absence of hepatocellular injury. Hyperplastic smooth endoplasmic reticulum permits an increased capacity for metabolizing a wide variety of chemicals acted on by the cytochrome P-450 enzymes. This influence places a treated animal at greater risk for hepatotoxicity when exposed to chemicals metabolized to toxic products by the P-450 cytochrome system. It is possible that the apparent hepatotoxicity of phenobarbital in certain dogs is a result of enhanced toxin formation rather than an idiosyncratic drug reaction.

Some antibiotics metabolized in the liver have been shown to cause hepatic degeneration and necrosis. It is possible that a preexisting hepatic disorder places a patient at an increased risk. Tetracycline, given to healthy dogs, can cause a mild to moderate hepatic lipidosis. The same therapeutic dose given to a dog with a portosystemic shunt can precipitate fatal hepatic and renal failure.[443] The half-life of tetracycline increases almost threefold in dogs with shunts, which may be an important factor promoting organ injury. Increased systemic exposure to enteric-derived toxins normally cleared during first-pass circulation through the liver may also be an important variable in these animals. Several other drugs, including chloramphenicol, erythromycin, and metronida-

zole, and a constant influx of new drugs such as the fluorinated quinolones, are metabolized by the liver and are potential causes of hepatic injury. Sulfonamides are a well-known cause of hepatotoxicity in humans and animals, causing hepatic degeneration, necrosis, and cholestasis in susceptible patients.[444,445] Penicillin products also are known to cause hepatotoxicity in some humans. It is often difficult to determine whether a specific antimicrobial is hepatotoxic because they are used in the circumstance of infection and septicemia, conditions that in themselves produce hepatic injury.

Nonsteroidal anti-inflammatory agents are used to manage a wide spectrum of problems associated with inflammation and pain. These drugs are used more conservatively in veterinary medicine than human medicine because of the great potential for gastroenteric side effects in the dog and overt systemic toxicity in the cat. Nevertheless, acetaminophen toxicity is still encountered in both dogs and cats (see later).

Several chemicals used to treat parasitic infestations can cause hepatic injury. Arsenicals used in the treatment of adult heartworms are an important cause of hepatic necrosis that can sometimes result in fatal intoxication. Mebendazole, an anthelmintic once widely used in veterinary practice, caused severe hepatic toxicity in a small group of dogs.[446] Investigations of mebendazole in healthy dogs, at a dose several times the dose associated with fatal hepatotoxicity, failed to detect

Table 32–10

DRUGS WITH POTENTIAL HEPATOTOXICITY

Anesthetics		Cardiovascular
Chloroform		Captopril
Halothane		Dehydralazine
Methoxyflurane		Enalopril
Enflurane		Furosemide
		Hydralazine
Anticonvulsants	**Tranquilizers**	Methyldopa
Carbamazepine	Diazepam	Procainamide
Phenobarbital	Haloperidol	Quinidine
Phenytoin	Phenothiazines	Thiazides
Primidone		Warfarin
Valproic acid		
Diazepan		**Antineoplastics**
		Busulfan
Antimicrobials		Cyclophosphamide
Amoxicillin	Isoniazid	L-asparaginase
Ampicillin	Ketoconazole	6-Mercaptopurine
Arsenicals	Metronidazole	Methotrexate
Amphotericin	Nitrofurantoin	Mithramycin
Carbenicillin	Oxacillin	Urethrane
Cephalosporins	Penicillin G	
Chloramphenicol	Quinacrine	**Endocrine Agents**
Clindamycin	Sulfonamides	Anabolic steroids
Erythromycin estolate	Tetracyclines	(C$_{17}$ alkylated)
5-Fluorocytosine	Thiabendazole	Danazol
Fluorinated	Trimethoprim-sulfa	Glucocorticois
quinolones		Methimazole
Grieofulvin		Propylthiouracil
Analgesics/NSAIDs		**Other Drugs**
Acetaminophen	Indomethacin	BAL
Allopurinol	Naproxen	Cimetidine
Benoxaprofen	Penicillamine	Danthron
Colchicine	Phenylburazone	Dapsone
Ibuprofen	Salicylates	Iodochlorhydroxyquin
		Iodine
		Stibophen
		Tannic acid
		Vitamin A

Also consult Tables 30–26 and 30–27.

adverse effects. This suggested that hepatotoxicity was likely idiosyncratic.[446]

Tranquilizing agents and inhalation anesthetics can also cause hepatic injury. Halothane hepatotoxicity is precipitated by hypoxic conditions in the liver and possibly by immune-mediated mechanisms. Methoxyflurane can also cause hepatotoxicity that has been more commonly observed in veterinary patients. Newer agents such as enflurane have been associated with hepatotoxic reactions in human beings. Recently, repeated oral administration of diazepam has been associated with lethal fulminant hepatic toxicity in certain cats.[52] This is discussed in detail later.

Anabolic steroids containing a C-17 alkylated structure can cause cholestasis and significant hepatic lesions with long-term use. Propylthiouracil and methimazole, drugs used to manage hyperthyroidism in the cat, can cause clinical illness associated with marked increases in the serum activities of hepatic transaminases and ALP and hyperbilirubinemia. Withdrawal of these drugs usually permits recovery within several weeks.

Just a few of the drugs known to be associated with hepatotoxicity have been specifically mentioned here. The list of drugs and toxins offered in Tables 32–2 and 32–10 were constructed to provide a global perspective on the types of agents you should pay particular attention to if unexplained hepatic injury develops in a patient receiving treatment. This list is not all-inclusive. Several reference texts are available in most pharmacies to further research your suspicions.[42,447] In most cases of suspected drug-associated hepatotoxicity, the serum biochemical profile indicates the existence of hepatic injury through unexpected increases in the serum activities of hepatic transaminases and ALP and in the total bilirubin concentration. The suspected drug(s) should be withdrawn and sequential serum chemistry profiles reevaluated. If the biochemical abnormalities resolve within several weeks, it is likely the injury was drug associated. Although reexposure of the patient to the drug would prove the association, this is usually not an ethical option.

Hymenoptera Toxins

Stings from insects in the order Hymenoptera can cause severe systemic allergic or nonimmunologic toxicity. Multiple stings can cause nonimmunologic intoxication manifesting as hemolysis, rhabdomyolysis, neurotoxicity, coagulopathies, and hepatotoxicity. Hymenopteran venoms have been shown to contain a variety of toxins. The hepatotoxic component of hornet venom has not been identified, although its influence on hepatocytes has been evaluated in vitro.[448–458] Dogs have died as a result of hundreds of stings from hornets.[448,449] Hemolysis, systemic hypotension, acute renal failure, acute hepatic necrosis, and DIC have been recognized causes of death. Hepatocellular necrosis has been documented in human beings stung by hornets.[450,451] Study of the influence of hornet venom on the feline liver showed a 10-fold increase in ALT, 6-fold increase in AST, and a 4.5 fold increase in ALP activities in anesthetized instrumented cats within 3 hours of invenomnation.[452] Dogs receiving multiple hornet stings usually develop hemorrhagic diarrhea and undergo increased vascular permeability resulting in loss of plasma into interstitial tissues. Some dogs develop DIC, seizures, and become comatose. Severe hyperthermia and hypothermia have each been observed.

Animals known to have received hymenopteran stings should be treated for anaphylaxis immediately with 1:10,000 aqueous dilution of epinephrine SQ (1 to 5 mL depending on animal size). Glucocorticoids and antihistamines should also be given. Anaphylaxis may be delayed for several hours in some patients. Animals with multiple stings should be immediately placed on intravenous polyionic fluids. Maintenance potassium should not be added to the fluids because some toxins cause hyperkalemia as a result of tissue injury. Shock levels of fluid (90 mL/kg) may need to be given initially and whole blood transfusion may be needed in the circumstance of hypoproteinemia, edema, and DIC. Broad-spectrum antibiotics should be used prophylactically because of gastrointestinal hemorrhage, potential endotoxemia, and septicemia. Urine production must be monitored to avert oliguric renal failure. If hepatic necrosis is severe, maintenance of euglycemia may require intravenous dextrose supplementation.

Acetaminophen

Clinical Synopsis

Diagnostic Features

- Cats more susceptible than dogs
- Cyanosis, dyspnea, and facial edema often seen
- Methemoglobinemia common, especially cats
- Hemolytic anemia and abnormal RBC morphology
- Elevated ALT, hyperbilirubinemia, and hemoglobinuria common

Standard Management

- Emetics, enemas, charcoal, sodium sulfate useful if ingestion recent
- Fluid therapy, blood transfusions, and oxygen therapy as needed
- N-acetylcysteine (Mucomyst) 140 mg/kg PO or IV once, followed by 70 to 140 mg/kg q 6 hours for 7 to 17 treatments
- Ascorbic acid 30 mg/kg PO, SQ q 6 hours for 7 or more treatments
- Cimetidine 5 mg/kg q 8 to 12 hours for 3 days minimum

Acetaminophen, an analgesic and antipyretic drug, has dose-related hepatotoxicity in dogs, cats, and humans.[84–86,598–609] The popularity of acetaminophen for use in humans has made it a commonly available household medication that may be inappropriately given to dogs and cats. Cats are exceedingly susceptible to acetaminophen toxicosis with signs occurring after as little as one-half of a 320 mg tablet. Dogs are more resistant and toxicity does not occur until the acetaminophen dose reaches 200 mg/kg of body weight.[598–600]

The toxic mechanisms of acetaminophen have been widely researched (see Chapter 30). At therapeutic levels, acetaminophen is detoxified primarily by conjugation with glucuronide and sulfates whereby it is made water soluble and eliminated through the kidneys. This pathway is summarized in Figure 32–14.[459–463] Compared to the dog, the cat is deficient in hepatic acetaminophen-directed UDP glucuronosyltranferase activity.[464] Consequently, cats have a much smaller capacity to glucuronidate the drug. The sulfation pathway is the predominant detoxification mechanism for acetaminophen in the cat but this is capacity limited at dosages as low as 60 and 120 mg/kg. Any remaining acetaminophen that escapes conjugation is biotransformed within the P-450

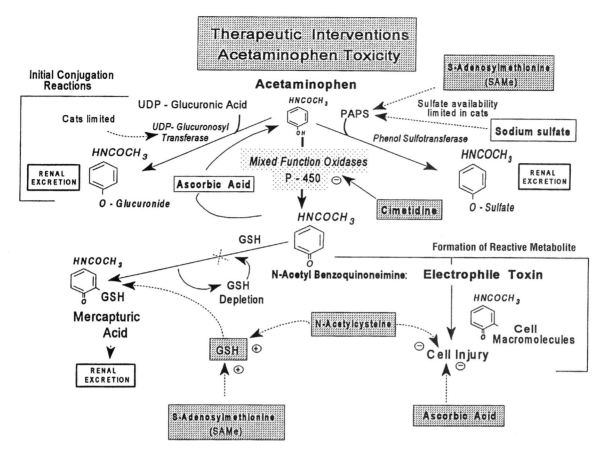

FIGURE 32–14. Diagrammatic representation of the metabolic detoxification of acetaminophen and the sites of antidote intervention.

cytochromes to a toxic adduct, N-acetyl benzoquinoneimine. Because the glucuronidation and sulfation pathways are capacity limited, large doses of acetaminophen result in increased formation of the toxic adduct. This metabolite of acetaminophen is exceedingly toxic, but when produced in small amounts is detoxified by glutathione (GSH) conjugation. The availability of intracellular GSH is of considerable importance in averting toxicity.[56] Formation of GSH is suppressed by high doses of acetaminophen and this further impairs the capacity for adduct detoxication.

As a result of GSH depletion, acetaminophen toxicity leads to marked oxidative stress in cells, including hepatocytes and erythrocytes. High doses result in formation of methemoglobin due to oxidative injury of hemoglobin sulfhydryl groups. The cat is predisposed to hemoglobin oxidation owing to an increased number of vulnerable sulfhydryl groups as compared to other species.[465] Methemoglobinemia results in a critically reduced oxygen-carrying capacity that produces tissue hypoxia and vascular injury.

Hepatic injury acquired from acetaminophen toxicity has been well described. In the cat, acute toxicity may not produce histologic lesions in the liver if the animal succumbs within the first several days to the other systemic effects. In chronic toxicity, with smaller doses of acetaminophen, or following several bouts of acute toxicity, moderate bile duct proliferation, pericholangitis, mononuclear cell infiltrates, biliary stasis, hepatocellular necrosis, degenerative vacuolation, and lipid accumulation have been described.[466,467] In dogs, diffuse severe necrosis of zone 3 (periacinar) of the acinus involves all liver lobules.[55-57] Reticulin collapses around hepatic venules and bridging necrosis may develop between adjacent hepatic lobules. Congestion, hemorrhage, and a small influx of neutrophils are observed in necrotic areas. The few remaining viable periportal hepatocytes appear swollen and microvacuolated. A granulomatous hepatitis was observed in several dogs in one study.[55]

CLINICAL SIGNS. The clinical signs of acetaminophen toxicity in the dog and cat may be recognized within 1 to 4 hours of ingestion. Common signs in 89 cases reported to the Animal Poison Control Center included cyanosis (46%), dyspnea (14.6%), facial edema (14.6%), depression (12.3%), hypothermia (8.9%), and vomiting (7.8%).[468] Less common signs included generalized weakness and coma. Dose relationship between clinical signs and methemoglobinemia have been recognized; dogs require fourfold higher doses than cats to demonstrate similar toxicity. Comparable toxic effects are realized with comparable concentrations of induced methemoglobinemia (Figure 32–15).[466] Methemoglobinemia induces cyanosis, depression, tachycardia, tachypnea, vomiting, and facial and peripheral edema. Endothelial damage has been recognized in humans and likely explains the pulmonary and peripheral edema observed in affected animals.[56] Pulmonary edema and hemorrhagic congestion of the liver and kidneys are observed in dogs and cats dying of acetaminophen toxicity.

LABORATORY FINDINGS. Hematologic evaluations may

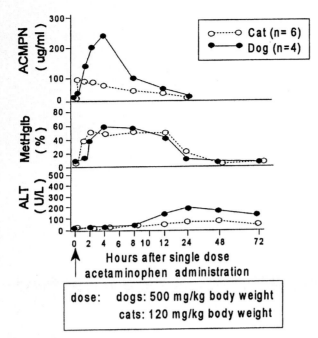

FIGURE 32-15. Relationship between serum acetaminophen (Acmpn) concentration, methemoglobin (MetHglb) percentage, and serum ALT activity in dogs and cats with acetaminophen toxicity. This information highlights the increased susceptibility of the cat to methemoglobin formation.

reveal increased numbers of eccentrocytes (erythrocytes with hemoglobin dense and contracted to one side of the cell).[469a] Heinz bodies faintly staining with new methylene blue become more visible with methyl violet stain.[469] Small numbers of schistocytes and acanthocytes may be observed reflecting endothelial injury and subsequent erythrocyte damage. A regenerative response to anemia may be apparent after 2 to 3 days. Increased numbers of nucleated red cells and a mature neutrophilic leukocytosis are observed after acute toxicity, reflecting a response to hypoxemia and stress.

The serum biochemical abnormalities in the dog and cat with acetaminophen toxicity are summarized in Figure 32–16. In dogs, the serum activities of ALT and AST increase within 24 hours and are profoundly (up to 200-fold or greater) increased within 48 hours. By 60 to 72 hours the transaminase activity may increase 1500-fold normal in dogs destined to succumb to drug toxicity. With untreated severe toxicity, dogs die within 3 days in fulminant hepatic failure. Progressive reductions in the serum concentrations of cholesterol, albumin, and urea, and progressive hyperbilirubinemia reflect severe hepatic dysfunction. In cats, notable increases in hepatic transaminases may develop within 3 to 6 days following drug ingestion. Hyperbilirubinemia causing overt jaundice occurs within 2 days and is associated with erythrocyte hemolysis. Hemoglobinemia and hemoglobinuria are severe during the first 4 to 5 days.

TREATMENT. If acetaminophen overdosage is recognized during the first several hours after dosing, the stomach should be emptied, cleansing enemas administered, and efforts made to reduce gastroenteric absorption. Activated charcoal at a dose of 2 g/kg body weight along with a saline cathartic such as sodium sulfate (0.5 g/kg body weight, given as a 20% mixture) has been advised.[468] Supportive fluid therapy should be provided for dehydration, acid-base, and electrolyte abnormalities. Specific antidotal therapy consists of administration of N-acetylcysteine, ascorbic acid, cimetidine, and possibly blood transfusions and oxygen therapy (Figures

32–8 and 32–14).[465,468,470–472] Blood transfusions may be necessary due to hemolysis that accompanies severe toxicity. Oxygen supplementation will not greatly benefit an intoxicated animal with severe methemoglobinemia unless this is corrected. However, oxygen is beneficial when pulmonary edema is a complicating problem. Corticosteroids are not indicated for treatment of acute toxicity because studies in rats have shown either no protective effect or a dose-dependent increase in mortality.[473]

The use of N-acetylcysteine permits formation of L-cysteine by deacetylases located predominately in the kidney.[465] The derived L-cysteine can act as a precursor for synthesis of GSH or can be oxidized in the liver to inorganic sulfate. Increased availability of sulfate improves the availability of cosubstrates necessary for sulfate conjugation/detoxication of acetaminophen. This would be particularly advantageous in the cat where sulfate availability is thought to limit sulfate conjugation. N-acetylcysteine also is believed to augment hepatocellular synthesis of GSH. Increased availability of GSH can reduce the reactive N-acetyl benzoquinoneimine to the parent drug as well as conjugate the toxic electrophile for elimination.[474] Glutathione cannot be used for direct treatment of acetaminophen toxicity because it is normally synthesized in situ and does not penetrate well into intact cells. Use of GSH precursors, such as N-acetylcysteine, are therefore preferentially used to permit in situ GSH formation. Alternative methods of increasing GSH synthesis in humans include supplementation with methionine and with propylthiouracil.[475] These have not been investigated clinically in veterinary patients. N-acetylcysteine has other beneficial effects that make it a desirable antidote for acetaminophen toxicosis. Collectively, these include reduction in the duration of methemoglobinemia; reduced covalent binding of N-acetyl benzoquinoneimine to hepatic proteins; inhibition of lipid peroxidation; increased intracellular production of GSH; and enhancement of the rate of acetaminophen sulfation and elimination of nontoxic moieties.[461–463,471,474] The treatment regimen for acetaminophen toxicity is outlined in Figure 32–8.[468] This regimen has been extrapolated from experimental work in animals and protocols established for humans. A dose of N-acetylcysteine of 140 mg/kg is initially given orally or intravenously, followed by repeated 70 to 140 mg/kg doses every 6 hours for 7 to 17 treatments. In cats demonstrating clinical signs, and in animals concurrently treated with cimetidine, N-acetylcysteine should be given irrespective of the amount of time that has lapsed since ingestion. Treatment should be continued if following 7 doses and transient discontinuation of N-acetylcysteine, an improved clinical status deteriorates within 6 to 24 hours. N-acetylcysteine is available as Mucomyst (Mead Johnson & Company) as a sterile 10% or 20% solution. This has been used intravenously directly and diluted in 5% dextrose. A problem with oral administration is that treatment is complicated by prior administration of activated charcoal and episodic vomiting. However, orally administered drug is rapidly absorbed from the gastrointestinal tract and is postulated to allow more rapid access to the liver.[471] N-acetylcysteine protects humans with acetaminophen overdosage if treatment is begun within 10 hours of drug ingestion. However, treatment in humans and cats given N-acetylcysteine after a 24 hour delay have also been successful.

An alternative antidote to N-acetylcysteine is administration of sodium sulfate given intravenously. This has been studied in experimentally intoxicated cats. A dose of 50 mg given as a 12.6% solution, at 4.5, 8.5, and 12.5 hours after oral acetaminophen administration, was shown to be as effective as N-acetylcysteine in countering toxic effects. There are two important advantages of N-acetylcysteine over sodium sulfate as an antidote for acetaminophen toxicity. One advan-

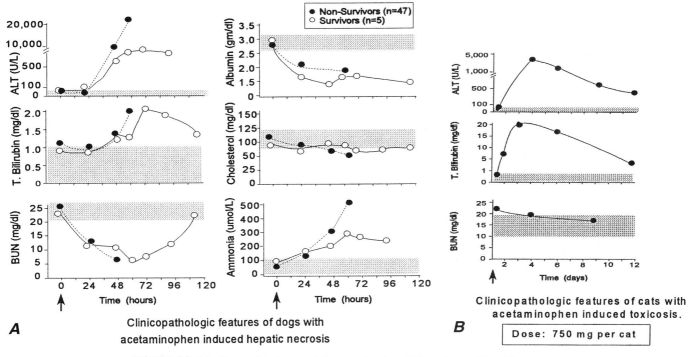

FIGURE 32-16. Serum biochemical features in dogs (*A*) and cats (*B*) with acetaminophen toxicity.

tage is that N-acetylcysteine imparts a beneficial modulatory influence on blood neutrophil and monocyte function that may reduce tissue injury associated with their accumulation.[146-149] Antioxidant effects of N-acetylcysteine are the proposed mechanisms. A second advantage is that N-acetylcysteine improves oxygen delivery and consumption in patients with fulminant hepatic failure due to acetaminophen toxicity, similar to the effects realized with prostacyclin in patients with multisystemic organ failure.[142-145] Patients derive this benefit despite the fact that hepatic toxicity is already established. An effect on microvasculature via endothelium-derived relaxing factor or nitric oxide is proposed.

Ascorbic acid is used in conjunction with N-acetylcysteine to enhance the nonenzymatic reduction of methemoglobin to functional hemoglobin.[472] The reaction is slow and thus ascorbic acid is used as adjunctive therapy. The efficacy of ascorbic acid is controversial. It has been shown to range in efficacy between 2.7 to 5.8 times lower than sulfhydryl compounds such as N-acetylcysteine. However, its effects are noncompetitive, additive, and nontoxic.[472] Although controversial, it is also possible that ascorbate may deter covalent binding of the reactive adduct to cell proteins by converting the toxic moiety back into the parent drug.[472] The dosage of ascorbate given orally or parenterally is 30 mg/kg every 6 hours for seven or more treatments.

Methylene blue has been administered to control methemoglobinemia in dogs during experimental investigation of the acute hepatotoxic effects of acetaminophen. Given at a dose of 10 mg/kg in water at 2 to 5 hour intervals, efficacy was judged on the basis of blood and mucous membrane color. A response was observed within 1 hour. Methylene blue is not recommended for use in clinical patients, especially cats, because it can lead to lethal Heinz body hemolytic anemia.[476,477]

Administration of cimetidine or ranitidine to the patient intoxicated with acetaminophen is suspected to suppress hepatic formation of the toxic adduct produced by the P-450 cytochrome oxidases.[475,478] It is important to administer ade-

quate doses of these drugs; small doses of ranitidine have been shown to potentiate hepatotoxicity of acetaminophen in rats.[475] Normal therapeutic doses of cimetidine cause inhibition of the P-450 oxidases reactive with acetaminophen, and enzyme inhibition persists as long as cimetidine treatments are continued. Recovery of the enzyme system occurs rapidly after cimetidine is discontinued such that recrudescence of clinical signs may occur due to further metabolism of retained acetaminophen. Cimetidine should therefore be continued as adjunctive therapy throughout antidote administration. Experimentally, pretreatment with phenobarbital has been shown to enhance acetaminophen hepatotoxicity through induction of the P-450 oxidases. Phenobarbital or other enzyme inducers should therefore be avoided in animals with acetaminophen toxicity.

Another recently investigated antidotal therapy for acetaminophen is S-adenosylmethionine (SAMe), discussed previously in the section on ischemic injury (Figure 32-10).[141] By virtue of its ability to promote GSH synthesis via the transsulfuration pathway and beneficial effects on transmethylation and polyamine pathways in the hepatocyte, SAMe is believed to provide benefit in humans with acetaminophen hepatotoxicity. A dose of 800 mg/kg body weight per day has been recommended for humans. Use of SAMe has also been shown to attenuate the hepatotoxicity of acetaminophen in animal models.[141]

Aflatoxins

Clinical Synopsis

Diagnostic Features

- Group outbreak of liver disease
- Exposure to spoiled peanuts, corn, rice, or packaged contaminated foods
- Vomiting and diarrhea common

- Bleeding tendencies frequent
- Variable hepatic histopathology
- Elevated aflatoxin concentrations in biologic specimens

Standard Management

- Supportive care
- Vitamin K_1 if coagulopathy
- Oxytetracycline may be protective.

Aflatoxins are coumarin mycotoxins produced by *Aspergillus flavus, Aspergillus parasiticus,* and *Penicillium puberulum.*[479] Not all strains of these fungi produce aflatoxin. Many different food items have been contaminated by aflatoxins.[479] Commonly implicated foods are peanuts, corn, cassava, dried fish, and rice. Aflatoxin can also be ingested through contaminated milk and can be inhaled from contaminated corn and peanut dust.[479] The amount of aflatoxin ingested determines whether or not toxic signs occur. Diagnosis of aflatoxicosis as a cause of hepatic necrosis usually depends on recognition of a group outbreak that initiates measurement of serum or hepatic aflatoxin concentrations. Documentation of aflatoxin concentrations in biologic specimens is necessary to confirm a diagnosis. Unfortunately, the histologic lesions associated with aflatoxicosis are variable among species and among individuals. The lesions vary with the particular toxin ingested, the quantity ingested, and the presence or absence of preexistent hepatic disease or dietary (micronutrient) deficiencies in the host.[479–493] It is currently believed that chronic ingestion of aflatoxins may increase a host's susceptibility to infectious diseases because defects in neutrophil, monocyte, and lymphocyte functions have been shown.[479]

The toxic effects of aflatoxin are mediated through its reactions with DNA, RNA, and proteins that require metabolic activation to a 2,3 epoxide. Aflatoxins also have direct toxic effects on lysosomal and mitochondrial membranes. The metabolic activation of aflatoxin occurs via the P-450 mixed function oxygenases. The effects of toxicity include impaired DNA and RNA synthesis and interference with the glucocorticoid receptor complex.[479] Total cellular protein synthesis is impaired as well as specific protein synthesis by ribosomes and mitochondria. Other effects of aflatoxins do not require metabolic activation. These appear to involve free radical–associated injury of cell membranes and organelles. Membrane-mediated effects may involve protein kinase C and it may be through this interaction that aflatoxins are oncogenic. In humans chronically exposed to aflatoxins, there is an increased occurrence of hepatoma and hepatocellular carcinoma. Because aflatoxins are coumadins, they also are effective anticoagulants, which can complicate the clinical presentation of intoxicated animals.

The typical histologic lesions associated with aflatoxicosis in the dog are described according to their acute, subacute, or chronic status.[480–489] In acute toxicity, periacinar hepatocytes (zone 3 of the acinus) develop severe fatty degeneration. The zone of involvement is wide and may extend to the portal areas. Coagulative or lytic necrosis is observed in some cells adjacent to hepatic venules. Canaliculi in the periacinar areas become distended with bile and Kupffer cells contain fine globular gold-brown pigment granules. Mild congestion is generally observed. A mild round cell infiltrate is seen in portal areas and around hepatic venules. There is minimal bile ductule proliferation.

In subacute toxicity, the hepatic venules may be replaced by dilated sinusoids. Bridging portal fibrosis is common. A vacuolar fatty degeneration is evident throughout the hepatic lobule with rare sparing of hepatocytes adjacent to hepatic venules. Regenerating hepatocytes are seen in zone 1 of the acinus adjacent to portal triads. Many of these cells are bizarre in shape and have prominent nucleoli, anisonucleosis, binucleation, or multinucleation, and mitotic figures may be common. In some areas, cells are apposed as if forming regenerative nodules; in others they form acinar or duct-like structures. In some animals, foci of coagulative or lytic necrosis involving 20 to 50 hepatocytes are surrounded by a mantle of neutrophils. Bile ductule proliferation is marked in all subacute cases. Larger bile ducts within the portal triads disappear and are replaced by proliferating bile ductules. Larger calibre intrahepatic bile ducts persist and show evidence of epithelial injury. Some contain necrotic debris within their lumen and mucin. Occasional ducts have periductal edema and lymphocytic infiltrates.

In chronic cases, extensive fibrosis is the most obvious feature. Hepatic venules are replaced with dilated, tortuous sinusoids surrounded by fibrous connective tissue that dissects through individual lobules. Fibrous tissue is also associated with severe bile ductule proliferation. Remaining hepatocytes are surrounded by connective tissue and show fatty degeneration or lytic necrosis. Regenerative nodules and biliary tract changes are similar to those described in subacute injury. In ruminants, veno-occlusive disease is described as a feature of chronic aflatoxicosis, but this has not been described in dogs or cats. In cats, hepatocellular necrosis in zone 1 of the acinus is most common and acute toxicity results in death within 72 hours.[493]

Acute toxicity with aflatoxins in dogs usually also results in severe gastrointestinal signs and hemorrhage. Impaired activation of vitamin K–dependent coagulation factors results in bleeding tendencies.[494] With chronic exposure, signs of chronic progressive liver disease develop.

Treatment of aflatoxicosis is directed at providing supportive care while the source of toxin is eliminated from the diet. If a coagulopathy is recognized, vitamin K_1 should be administered. If possible, determination of a PIVKA clotting time will assist in determining the need for continued vitamin administration. In rabbits, concurrent treatment with oxytetracycline at the time of aflatoxin administration provides a protective effect, presumably through competition with or inhibition of metabolic processes that produce toxic products.[491,492] In acute aflatoxicosis in goats, cysteine, methionine or methionine, and sodium thiosulfate prolong survival time, presumably because they boost cell availability of glutathione. The use of cysteine, methionine, and sodium thiosulfate do not confer protection from aflatoxicosis in rabbits. Rather, in rabbits, cysteine and methionine are reported to enhance toxicity. It is proposed that differences between species in metabolism of aflatoxin explains these disparate responses. Differences in metabolism also explains the differences in morphologic distribution of primary lesions. In species that metabolize aflatoxin rapidly, the morphologic lesion in acute toxicity is centrilobular (zone 3 of the acinus). In those that metabolize it slowly, zone 1 of the acinus (periportal) lesions predominate.[492] Because a number of metabolites are derived from different aflatoxins and there are inherent species differences in toxin metabolism, no single antidote is recognized. Furthermore, toxicity is usually insidious, developing after ingestion of aflatoxins over several days or longer such that blocking toxin metabolism would confer no benefit. Because aflatoxins can be directly toxic to cell membranes, use of P-450 cytochrome oxidase inhibitors, such as cimetidine or chloramphenicol, has not been recommended. Treatment with prostaglandins (PGE_2) has modulated aflatoxin hepatotoxicity somewhat in the rat.[133]

Penitrem A is a mycotoxin derived from *Penicillium crusto-*

sum, which has been linked to neurotoxicity in a puppy having consumed moldy cream cheese and with hepatic necrosis, hyperthermia, and a coagulopathy in other dogs.[495,496] Experimental work with this toxin has shown that it disrupts lysosomes.

Rubratoxins are hepatotoxic metabolites of *Penicillium rubrum* and *P. purpurogenum,* fungi commonly found in soil and frequently contaminating animal feeds.[497] These toxins have been shown to create hepatic lesions similar to aflatoxin B₁ in dogs. Rubratoxins have been shown to be more toxic in mice than aflatoxins.[498]

Ochratoxin A is an hepatotoxic and renally toxic metabolite derived from *Aspergillus ochraceus* and *Penicillium viridicatum.* This toxin had been found as a contaminant in certain cereal and legume crops used as food for animals and human beings.[499] In ducklings and weanling rats, ochratoxin A induces acute hepatic injury characterized by periportal necrosis and fatty vacuolation. In adult sheep, massive periacinar (zone 3 of the acinus) necrosis and periportal vacuolation was described. It is unknown if this toxin has been the cause of naturally occurring hepatic disease in dogs.

Amanita Mushroom Poisoning

Clinical Synopsis

Diagnostic Features

- Exposure to Amanita mushrooms
- Abdominal pain, vomiting, diarrhea or dysentery
- Coagulopathies, oliguria, hepatic encephalopathy
- Increased ALT activity
- Massive hepatocellular necrosis

Standard Management

- Supportive care
- Vitamin K₁ if coagulopathy
- Silybin 20 to 50 mg/kg per day
- Large doses of penicillin G or glucocorticoids might be helpful

Occasionally, dogs are poisoned by consumption of toxic mushrooms. Poisonous mushrooms are categorized into four groups on the basis of the type of toxin, physical effect on the host, and time of onset of clinical signs.[500] Mushrooms in category A cause hepatic and renal damage after a latent period and are the most common causes of fatalities among human beings. These have also been reported to cause hepatic necrosis in dogs.[501,502] Mushrooms in categories B, C, and D have a precipitous onset of clinical signs and affect the autonomic nervous system, central nervous system, and gastrointestinal tract, respectively.[502] These also have been reported as causing toxicity in dogs.[503,504] Amanita intoxication results from the ingestion of *Amanita phalloides* (the death cap mushroom), *A. virosa, A. verna, A bisporigera,* and *A. ocreata.* The lethal dose for humans of *A. phalloides* is about 50 g, equivalent to three medium-sized mushrooms or about 7 mg of amatoxins.[505,506] This approximates a lethal dose of amatoxins of 0.1 mg/kg body weight. This fungus contains two hepatotoxins: phallodin and alpha-amanitine. The amatoxins are 10- to 20-fold more toxic than the phallotoxins. Phallodin adversely affects cell membranes causing polymerization of actin microfilaments. The amatoxins are cytotoxic and are among the most lethal of all toxins known. These appear to have preferential entry into hepatocytes. The α-amanitine inhibits hepatocellular RNA polymerase, thereby interfering with transcription of DNA, which inhibits cellular protein synthesis.[506–508] These are heat-stable toxins that can persist in cooked meals and desiccated foodstuffs. The amatoxins are secreted in bile and undergo extensive enterohepatic circulation that potentiates their toxic effects. The toxin is also resorbed in the kidney from the glomerular filtrate.

Clinical signs associated with Amanita poisoning have been experimentally studied in dogs. Latent, gastrointestinal, and hepatorenal phases are recognized.[60,509] The latent phase lasts from 5 to 24 hours. The gastrointestinal phase manifests as cramping, abdominal pain, vomiting, and diarrhea that may be bloody. Direct effects of toxin on the intestinal mucosa explains the gastroenteric signs and these may precede the hepatorenal phase by 1 to 5 days. The hepatorenal phase is characterized by hypotension, coagulopathies, oliguria, and signs of HE. Acute hepatic necrosis results in marked increases in the serum ALT and AST activities by 24 hours (Figure 32–17). The serum ALP activity may only become mildly increased or may remain within the normal range. Hypoglycemia, hypokalemia, and hyperbilirubinemia may also develop. There may be no evidence of nephrotoxicity in dogs.

Histologic lesions in dogs have been characterized by massive hepatocellular necrosis.[501] Areas of hemorrhage involving

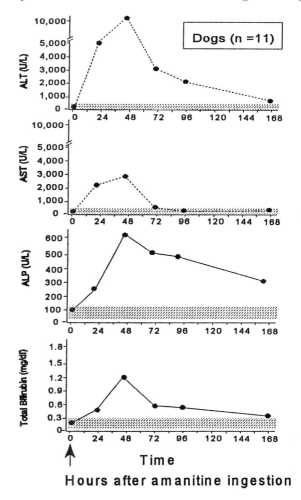

FIGURE 32–17. Serum biochemical features observed in dogs with experimentally induced *Amanita phalloides* hepatotoxicity.[60]

portions of lobules are randomly distributed and confined to necrotic areas. Hepatic cords are disrupted by hepatocellular swelling. Karyorrhexis and karyolysis are pronounced in acinar zones 2 and 3. Periportal hepatocytes develop vesicular nuclei with loss or fragmentation of nucleoli. This latter morphologic change has been suggested to be a useful indicator of Amanita toxicity if clinical evidence is consistent. In massive necrosis, bile ducts remain unaffected and appear as islands surrounded by necrotic parenchyma.

Treatment is focused on providing fluid and electrolyte support and general interventions at ameliorating signs of HE. A chronic active hepatitis persists in approximately 20% of humans intoxicated with Amanita.[507] Death usually occurs within 1 week of mushroom ingestion and results from hepatic and renal failure, hemorrhagic complications, and secondary effects on the cardiovascular and central nervous systems.[507]

There are no specific proven antidotes for the toxins of mushroom poisoning.[60,507,510,511] The patient should be made to vomit if the mushroom has been ingested during the prior 6 hours. Activated charcoal should be given to bind any residual toxin. In children, it is recommended that magnesium sulfate purgation be initiated to hasten removal of residual fungal fragments. This may also be beneficial in dogs. Fluid therapy is necessary because vomiting and diarrhea associated with acute intoxication lead to dehydration and electrolyte aberrations. Institution of a brisk diuresis is recommended to rapidly reduce the total body pool of amatoxins. Although there is concern this procedure may expose the kidneys to greater toxicity, it has not been substantiated. Vitamin K_1 supplementation is empirically given and correction of coagulation deficiencies with frozen plasma or fresh whole blood is recommended. Several anecdotal therapies are recommended for humans intoxicated with Amanita based on perceived, but unproven clinical

benefit. These include administration of large doses of intravenous penicillin G (250 mg/kg/day), thioctic acid, high doses of glucocorticoids, cytochrome c, and silybin (Figure 32–8).[60,511] Silybin (silibinin), an active component of silymarin, a mixture of flavones found in the milk thistle *Silybum marianum*, is given as an antitoxin at a dose of 20 to 50 mg/kg per day in humans. This too has not been substantiated as effective therapy but has been studied in dogs where it was shown to provide benefit.[60] Silibinin has been suggested to protect hepatocytes from injury derived from other hepatotoxic substances, including ethanol, ethionine, and from certain viruses (the murine hepatitis virus).

Carbon Tetrachloride

Carbon tetrachloride (CCl_4) has been studied experimentally as a mechanism of producing acute and chronic hepatic injury.[58,59] Toxicity results following inhalation, topical, intraperitoneal, intravenous, and oral exposure. Acute intoxication with a nonlethal dose leads to hepatocellular necrosis in zone 3, lipid vacuolation, and congestion.[58] Necrotic parenchymal cells undergo lysis within 1 or 2 days. Lobular stroma remains in the areas of necrosis and provides a framework for parenchymal regeneration. Necrotic areas may be recognized up to 12 days after a single exposure to CCl_4.[58] Serum enzyme activities in the dog and cat following a single episode of CCl_4 intoxication are illustrated in Figure 32–18.[58,59] With repeated dosing, a fairly predictable morphologic injury resembling spontaneous hepatic cirrhosis develops. The acute severe toxicity of CCl_4 requires metabolism by microsomal enzyme systems in the liver; a more complete discussion of CCl_4 toxicity is presented in Chapter 30.

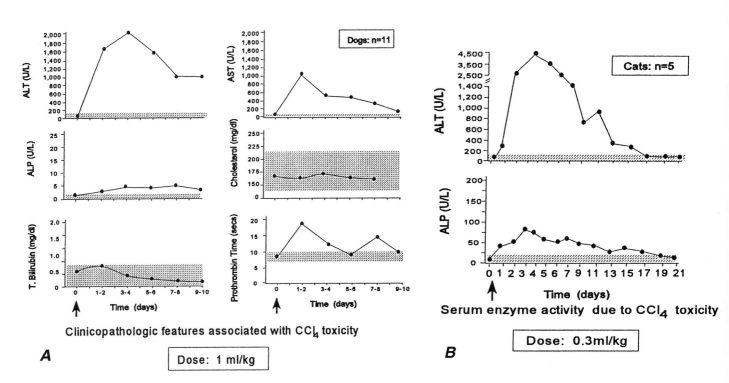

FIGURE 32–18. Serum biochemical features associated with acute carbon tetrachloride hepatotoxicity in the dog (*A*) and cat (*B*).

Dimethylnitrosamine

That dimethylnitrosamine is a potent specific hepatotoxin was recognized after industrial accidents in human beings.[512] As small a dose as 20 mg per kg body weight causes massive liver necrosis and death in all species.[51] Metabolic products of dimethylnitrosamine inhibit protein synthesis and result in lethal hepatocyte injury. Single doses are metabolized in 24 hours, but the enzymatic and morphologic evidence of cell injury continues for several days. The biochemical features associated with administration of dimethylnitrosamine at a dose of 2.5 mg/kg body weight on 2 consecutive days per week for 3 weeks in dogs is shown in Figure 32-6.[53] After a single acute exposure, hepatocellular necrosis associated with a neutrophilic and mononuclear infiltrate develops primarily in zone 3 of the acinus. If only a single intoxication occurs, tissue injury can resolve and the hepatic architecture returns to normal. If exposure is chronic, over several weeks in small doses, irreparable injury permanently alters the hepatic architecture, regenerative nodules form, and hepatic fibrosis bridges between portal triads and hepatic venules. As the liver becomes cirrhotic, the ensuing portal hypertension leads to development of ascites and functional acquired portosystemic shunts. Chronic dosing with dimethylnitrosamine has been used to create hepatic cirrhosis in the dog as an experimental model of chronic liver disease.[51,53,54] Experience with dimethylnitrosamine demonstrates how a small quantity of an hepatotoxin inadvertently mixed in food could induce severe hepatic injury over a period of exposure of as little as several weeks. Signs of mild anorexia and increased serum enzyme activities may be the only clinical signs during early intoxication.

Diazepam-Associated Fulminant Hepatic Failure in Cats

Acute massive hepatic necrosis causing fulminant hepatic failure has been recognized in more than 20 cats in the past 5 years that were treated with oral diazepam for inappropriate urination and behavioral modification.[52] Doses ranging between 1.25 and 2.5 mg PO SID or BID have been involved. Most cats became lethargic, ataxic, and anorectic within 96

hours of initial drug administration. Cats are jaundiced when presented for veterinary care during the first 11 days of illness. A summary of the clinicopathologic features in five affected animals is shown in Figure 32-19. Profound increases in the serum activity of ALT and AST are consistently present. Affected cats also show a tendency to become hypoglycemic and hypocholesterolemic, which may indicate the severity of their hepatic insufficiency. Abnormalities consistent with DIC have been shown in the few cats that have had their coagulation status evaluated. Most cats die from hepatic failure within 15 days of initial drug administration. In those from which a liver biopsy has been obtained, florid hepatocellular necrosis primarily involving zone 3 of the acinus but extending into zones 2 and 1 has been observed. Profound biliary ductule proliferation and hyperplasia and suppurative intraductal inflammation have been consistent features.

Idiosyncratic hepatotoxicity is suspected due to the rarity of this presumed drug reaction. Prior sensitization to diazepam was possible in only one affected cat. No risk factors could be identified that explained the susceptibility of individual cats to drug toxicity. Rare occurrences of idiosyncratic hepatotoxicity from benzodiazepine administration have also been reported in humans.

Benzodiazepines are metabolized mainly by conjugation and oxidation reactions.[513] It is possible that the toxicity of diazepam in cats relates to their inherent deficiency for glucuronide and sulfate conjugation and glutathione detoxification of reactive intermediates.

Based on findings in intoxicated cats, a recommendation is given to evaluate baseline ALT and AST activities in cats prior to initiating daily oral treatment with diazepam and then again within 5 days after treatment has been started. An acquired increase in transaminase activity indicates a need to suspend drug administration and to provide critical supportive care. Cats presented in an obtunded condition have a grave prognosis.

Galactosamine

Intoxication with D-galactosamine has been widely used to model hepatic disease experimentally.[514–517] Intraperitoneal

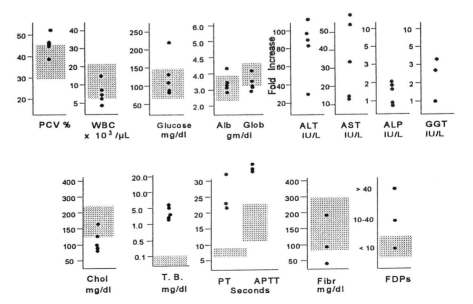

FIGURE 32-19. Serum biochemical features associated with diazepam-induced fulminant hepatic failure in 5 cats.[52] (Alb = albumin, Glob = globulins, Chol = total cholesterol, T.B. = total bilirubin, PT = prothrombin time, APTT = activated partial thromboplastin time, Fibr = fibrinogen, FDPs = fibrin degradation products).

injection of D-galactosamine given to rodents and rabbits depletes hepatocytes of pyrimidine derivatives of uridine.[514-517] This drug is not biotransformed and is not associated with reactive intermediates. Intoxicated rats have deranged lipoprotein metabolism associated with depletion of liver-derived apoproteins. The histologic lesions caused by D-galactosamine are characterized by severe diffuse or multifocal hepatocellular necrosis associated with lipid vacuolation in remaining viable hepatocytes. Prominent periportal and parenchymal inflammation and an increase in the number of Ito cells (fat-storing cells) have been shown. Within the first 24 hours, a granulocytic inflammatory infiltrate predominates. Thereafter, infiltration with T lymphocytes and macrophages predominates. Experimental evidence suggests that endotoxins, cell-mediated immune responses, and cytokine production augment hepatotoxicity of D-galactosamine.[518,519] Prostaglandin E$_2$ treatment has been shown to have a cytoprotective effect on hepatocytes if it is concurrently administered.[134]

Metals Causing Hepatotoxicity

Phosphorus, in the form of yellow phosphorus, is extremely toxic and has been used as rat poison. A dose of 60 mg may be fatal to a human being. The course of illness is peracute with death occurring within 24 hours. When a smaller dose is ingested, clinical signs may be more slowly progressive, with the patient seeking medical care within 4 days. Even with mild illness, the mortality rate in humans approximates 50%. Histologic lesions include a massive fatty degeneration in zone 1 of the acinus (periportal) and hepatic necrosis.[507] Acute renal tubular necrosis and myocardial lesions are also induced. Periportal fibrosis may develop in long-term survivors.

Iron intoxication can result in depression, nausea, vomiting, diarrhea, gastrointestinal hemorrhage, tremors, shock, and death. Ingestion of greater than 60 mg/kg of elemental iron causes signs of toxicity, and doses exceeding 200 mg/kg are potentially lethal.[520,521] Iron toxicity may be acquired by pets ingesting iron-containing tablets used as human mineral supplementations.

The manifestations of acute iron poisoning are divided into three stages. Within the first 6 to 12 hours, the direct effect of gastrointestinal irritation results in nausea, vomiting, diarrhea, and gastrointestinal hemorrhage. Within 6 to 24 hours, a quiescent phase is observed. Thereafter, clinical signs rapidly worsen and include severe lethargy, recurrent gastrointestinal signs, metabolic acidosis, hepatic necrosis, hemorrhagic diathesis, and cardiovascular collapse and shock. Serum transaminase activity increases within the first 24 to 36 hours following severe intoxication and coincides with hepatic necrosis. Hyperbilirubinemia and a prolonged prothrombin time develop by day 3 in human beings. Hepatic histology demonstrates zone 1 acinar necrosis (periportal) and steatosis. There is no remarkable increase in hepatic iron content.[507]

If a patient is seen immediately after ingestion of a toxic source of iron, vomiting should be induced. Gastric lavage should also be considered because activated charcoal does not bind iron.[522,523] Abdominal radiographs may disclose the presence of residual iron containing intoxicant and may indicate a need for endoscopic removal of retained debris. Intravenous fluid therapy is used to maintain the hydration status and replace dehydration deficits. Desferrioxamine may be used by intravenous infusion for iron chelation at a rate of 15 mg/kg per hour.[522,523] Rapid infusions must be avoided because they may aggravate hypotension and initiate cardiac arrhythmias. If intravenous infusion is not possible, desferrioxamine may be administered by intramuscular injection at a dose of 40 mg/kg every 4 to 8 hours. Chelation therapy is continued until serum iron values normalize (<350 μg/dl), which may require 2 to 3 days.[522,523]

Lead intoxication can lead to acute mild hepatic injury associated with a mild hepatitis, fatty vacuolation, and hemosiderosis in zone 3 of the acinus. Liver injury rapidly resolves after removal of the source of lead. Hepatic necrosis is not one of the leading signs of lead intoxication in dogs and cats and is rarely diagnosed.

Copper intoxication can occur in dogs due to ingestion of copper sulfate algacides. In humans, hepatotoxic effects have been associated with absorption of copper ions from the topical use of cupric sulfate as an astringent antiseptic. Acute intoxication leads to nausea, vomiting, gastric pain, and diarrhea. In human beings, increased serum transaminase activity, hyperbilirubinemia, and hepatomegaly develop within 3 days. Erythrocyte hemolysis leads to hemoglobinemia and hemoglobinuria. Signs of acute toxicity are progressive and can culminate in acute renal tubular necrosis, melena, hematuria, shock, and coma. Histologic lesions in the liver include necrosis in zone 3, dilated hepatic venules, cholestasis, and bile thrombi. Death is usually due to acute renal failure.

Treatment is supportive and should include aggressive attempts to remove any residual gastrointestinal copper and to maintain circulating perfusion pressure and renal function. In humans, there is no evidence that chelation with penicillamine is effective or that glucocorticoid therapy alters survival.

REFERENCES

1. McDonald GSH, Courtney MG. Operation-associated neutrophils in a percutaneous liver biopsy: Effect of prior transjugular procedure. Histopathology 10:217–222, 1986.
2. Kelly WR. The liver and biliary system. In: Jubb KVT, Kennedy PC, Palmer N (eds) Pathology of the Domestic Animal, 4th ed. Academic Press, Harcourt Brace Jovanovich, New York, 319–406, 1993.
3. Mitchell JR, Potter WZ, Hinson JA, et al. Toxic drug reactions. In: Gillette JR, Mitchell JR, Randall PS (eds) Concepts in Biochemical Pharmacology, Part 3. Springer-Verlag, New York, 1975.
4. Zimmerman HJ, Ishak KG. Hepatic injury due to drugs and toxins. In: MacSween RN, Anthony PP, Scheuer PJ (eds) Pathology of the Liver. Churchill Livingstone, New York, 335–386, 1979.
5. Popper H. Hepatocellular degeneration and death. In: Arias IM, Jakoby WB, Popper H, et al. (eds) The liver: Biology and Pathobiology, 2nd ed. Raven Press, New York, 1087–1103, 1988.
6. Popper H, Keppler D. Networks of interacting mechanisms of hepatocellular degeneration. Prog Liv Dis 8:209–235, 1986.
7. Shibuya A, Unuma T, Sugimoto M, et al. Diffuse hepatic calcification as a sequela to shock liver. Gastroenterology 89:196–201, 1985.
8. Popper H. Pathological aspects of cirrhosis: A review. Am J Pathol 87:228–264, 1977.
9. Sherlock S. The liver in circulatory failure. In: Schiff L (ed) Diseases of the Liver, 4th ed. Philadelphia, JB Lippincott, 1033–1050, 1975.
10. de la Monte SM, Arcidi JM, Moore GW, et al. Midzonal necrosis as a pattern of hepatocellular injury after shock. Gastroenterology 86:627–631, 1984.
11. Dunn GD, Hayes P, Breen KJ, et al. The liver in congestive heart failure: A review. Am J Med Sci 265:174–189, 1973.
12. Nagasue N, Inokuchi K. Enzymatic and hemodynamic changes after short term hepatic outflow occlusion in the dog. Surg Gynecol Obstet 144:179–184, 1977.
13. Arcidi JM, Moore GW, Hutchins GM. Hepatic morphology in cardiac dysfunction. A clinicopathologic study of 1000 subjects at autopsy. Am J Pathol 104:159–166, 1981.
14. Cook GD. Hepatic changes associated with shock. Int Anesthesiol Clin 7:883–894, 1969.
15. Chaudry IH, Clemen MG, Baue AE. Alteration in cell function with ischemia and shock and their correction. Arch Surg 116:1309–1317, 1981.
16. Gaja G, Ferrero ME, Piccoletti R, et al. Phosphorylation and redox states in ischemic liver. Exp Mol Pathol 19:248–265, 1973.

17. Araki H, Lefer AM. Cytoprotective actions of prostacyclin during hypoxia in the isolated perfused cat liver. Am J Physiol 238:H176–H181, 1980.

18. Glenn TM, Lefer AM, Beardsley AC, et al. Circulatory responses to splanchnic lysosomal hydrolase in the dog. Ann Surg 176:120–127, 1992.

19. Loegering DJ, Kaplan JE, Saba TM. Correlation of plasma lysosomal enzyme levels with hepatic reticuloendothelial function after trauma. Prox Soc Exp Biol Med 152:42–46, 1976.

20. Otto G, Wolff H, David H. Preservation damage in liver transplantation: Electron-microscopic findings. Transplant Proc 16:1247–1248, 1984.

21. DiLuzio NR, Trejo RA, Crafton CC. Influence of endotoxin administration on hepatic function of rats with altered endotoxin sensitivity. J Reticuloendothel Soc 11:637–653, 1972.

22. Farkouh EF, Daniel AM, Beaudon JG, et al. Predictive value of liver biochemistry in acute hepatiac ischemia. Surg Gynecol Obstet 132:832–838, 1971.

23. Kono Y, Ozawa K, Tanaka J, et al. Significance of mitochondrial enhancement in restoring hepatic energy charge after revascularization of isolated ischemic liver. Transplantation 33:150–155, 1982.

24. Clemens MG, McDonagh PF, Chaudry IH, et al. Hepatic microcirculatory failure after ischemia and reperfusion: Improvement with ATP-MgCl$_2$ treatment. Am J Physiol 248:H804–H811, 1985.

25. Fredricks WM, Fronik GM. Quantitative analysis of the effect of ATP-MgCl$_2$ on the extent of necrosis in rat liver after ischemia. J Surg Res 41:518–523, 1986.

26. Hayashi T, Nagasue N, Kohno H, et al. Beneficial effect of cyclosporine pretreatment in canine liver ischemia. Transplantation 52:116–121, 1991.

27. Tribble DL, Aw TY, Jones DP. The pathophysiological significance of lipid peroxidation in oxidative cell injury. Hepatology 7:377–387, 1987.

28. Nolan JP, O'Connel CJ. Vascular response in the isolated rat liver. I. Endotoxin, direct effect. J Exp Med 122:1063–1073, 1965.

29. Nolan JP. Endotoxin, reticuloendothelial function, and liver injury. Hepatology 1:458–465, 1981.

30. Harris RL, Musher DM, Bloom K, et al. Manifestations of sepsis. Arch Intern Med 147:1895–1906, 1987.

31. Boler RK, Bibighaus AJ. Ultrastructural alterations of dog livers during endotoxin shock. Lab Invest 17:537–561, 1967.

32. Kurtz HJ, Quast J. Effects of continous intravenous infusion of *Escherichia coli* endotoxin into swine. Am J Vet Res 43:262–269, 1982.

33. Gans H, Mori K, Lindsey E, Kaster B, et al. Septicemia as a manifestation of acute liver failure. Surg Gynecol Obstet 132:783–790, 1971.

34. Liehr H, Grun M, Thile H, et al. Endotoxin-induced liver necrosis and intravascular coagulation in rats enhanced by portacaval collateral circulation. Gut 16:429–436, 1975.

35. Liehr H, Grun M, Brunswig D. Endotoxemia in acute hepatic failure. Acta Hepato-Gastroenterol 23:235–240, 1976.

36. Zimmerman HJ, Utilli R, Seeff LB, et al. Jaundice due to bacterial infection. Gastroenterology 77:362–374, 1979.

37. Franson TR, Hierholzer WJ, Jr, LaBrecque DR. Frequency and characteristics of hyperbilirubinemia associated with bacteremia. Rev Inf Dis 7:1–9, 1985.

38. Rose HD, Lentino JR, Mavrelis PG, et al. Jaundice associated with nonhepatic *Staphylococcus aureus* infection: Does teichoic acid have a role in pathogenesis? Dig Dis Sci 27:1046–1050, 1982.

39. Oelberg DG, Lester R. Cellular mechanisms of cholestasis. Ann Rev Med 37:297–317, 1986.

40. Jarrett WFH, O'Neil BW. A new transmissible agent causing acute hepatitis, chronic hepatitis, and cirrhosis in dogs. Vet Rec 116:629–635, 1985.

41. Reinacher M. Diseases associated with spontaneous feline leukemia virus (FeLV) infection in cats. Vet Immunol Immunopath 21:85–95, 1989.

42. Olin BR (ed) Facts and Comparisons, Wolters Kluwer Co., Facts and Comparisons, Inc., St. Louis, MO, 1994.

43. Dixon MF, Fulker MJ, Walker BE, et al. Serum transaminase levels after experimental-induced hepatic necrosis. Gut 16:800–807, 1975.

44. Valentine BA, Blue JT, Shelley SM, et al. Increased serum alanine aminotransferase activity associated with muscle necrosis in the dog. J Vet Int Med 4:140–143, 1990.

45. Desmet VJ. Morphologic and histochemical aspects of cholestasis. In: Popper H, Schaffner F (eds) *Progress in Liver Diseases*, Vol. 4. Grune & Stratton, New York, 97–132, 1972.

46. Wigton DH, Kociba GJ, Hoover EA. Infectious canine hepatitis: An animal model for viral-induced disseminated intravascular coagulation. Blood 47:287–296, 1976.

47. Center SA, Slater MR, Manwarren T, et al. Diagnostic efficacy of serum alkaline phosphatase and gamma glutamyltransferase in dogs with histologically confirmed hepatobiliary disease: 270 cases (1980–1990). J Am Vet Med Assoc 201:1258–1264, 1992.

48. Center SA, Baldwin BH, Dillingham S, et al. Diagnostic value of serum gamma glutamyltransferase and alkaline phosphatase activities in hepatobiliary disease in the cat. J Am Vet Med Assoc 188:507–510, 1986.

49. Gopinath C, Ford EJH. Location of liver injury and extent of bilirubinemia in experimental liver lesions. Vet Path 9:99–108, 1972.

50. Jones AE, Schafer DF. Fulminant hepatic failure. In: Zakim D, Boyer ED (eds) *Hepatology: A Textbook of Liver Disease*, 2nd ed. WB Saunders, Philadelphia, 460–492, 1990.

51. Madden JW, Gertman PM, Peacock EE. Dimethylnitrosamine-induced hepatic cirrhosis: A new canine model of an ancient human disease. Surgery 260–268, 1970.

52. Center SA, Elston TH, Rowland PH, et al. Fulminant hepatic failure associated with oral administration of diazepam in 12 cats. In press.

53. Strombeck DR, Harrold D, Rogers Q, et al. Plasma amino acid, glucagon, and insulin concentrations in dogs with nitrosamine-induced hepatic disease. Am J Vet Res 44:2028–2036, 1983.

54. Boothe DM, Jenkins WL, Green RA, et al. Dimethylnitrosamine-induced hepatotoxicosis in dogs as a model of progressive canine hepatic disease. Am J Vet Res 53:411–420, 1992.

55. Ortega L, Landa Garcia JI, Torres Garcia A, et al. Acetaminophen-induced fulminant hepatic failure in dogs. Hepatology 5:673–676, 1985.

56. Kelly JH, Koussayer T, He D, et al. An improved model of acetaminophen-induced fulminant hepatic failure in dogs. Hepatology 15:329–335, 1992.

57. Frankavilla A, Makowka L, Polimeno L, et al. A dog model for acetaminophen induced fulminant hepatic failure. Gastroenterology 96:470–478, 1989.

58. Van Vleet JF, Alberts JO. Evaluation of liver function tests and liver biopsy in experimental carbon tetrachloride intoxication and extrahepatic bile duct obstruction in the dog. Am J Vet Res 2119–2131, 1968.

59. Everett RM, Duncan JR, Prasse KW. Alkaline phosphatase, leucine aminopeptidase, and alanine aminotransferase activities with obstructive and toxic hepatic disease in cats. Am J Vet Res 38:963–966, 1977.

60. Vogel G, Tuchweber B, Trost W, et al. Protection by silibinin against *Amanita phalloides* intoxication in beagles. Toxicol Appl Pharmacol 73:355–362, 1984.

61. Clark R, Rake MO, Flute PT, et al. Coagulation abnormalities in acute liver failure: Pathogenesis and therapeutic implications. Scand J Gastroenterol (suppl) 8:63–70, 1973.

62. Hillenbrand P, Parbhoo SP, Jedrychowski A, et al. Significance of intravascular coagulation and fibrinolysis in acute hepatic failure. Gut 15:83–88, 1974.

63. Roberts H, Cederbaum AI. The liver and blood coagulation: Physiology and pathology. Gastroenterology 62:297–320, 1972.

64. Furnival CM, Mackenzie RJ, MacDonald GA, et al. The mechanism of impaired coagulation after partial hepatectomy in the dog. Surg Gynecol Obstet 143:81–86, 1976.

65. Verstraete M, Vermylen J, Collen D. Intravascular coagulation in liver disease. Ann Rev Med 25:447–455, 1974.

66. Strombeck DR, Feldman BF. Unpublished observations.

67. Aquirre A, Yoshimura N, Westman T, et al. Plasma amino acids in dogs with two experimental forms of liver damage. J Surg Res 16:339–345, 1974.

68. Gazzard BD, Portmann B, Murray-Lyon IM, et al. Causes of death in fulminant hepatic failure and relationship to quantitative histologic assessments of parenchymal damage. Q J Med 44:615–626, 1975.

69. Ware AJ, D'Agostino A, Combes B. Cerebral edema: A major complication of massive hepatic necrosis. Gastroenterology 61:877–884, 1971.

70. Hanid MA, MacKenzie RL, Jenner RE, et al. Intracranial pressure in pigs with surgically induced acute liver failure. Gastroenterology 76:123–131, 1979.

71. Lee WM. Acute liver failure. N Engl J Med 1862–1872, 1993.

72. Traber PG, Dal Canto M, Ganger DR, et al. Electron microscopic evaluation of brain edema in rabbits with galactosamine-induced fulminant hepatic failure: Ultrastructure and integrity of the blood-brain barrier. Hepatology 7:1272–1277, 1987.

73. McClung HJ, Sloan HR, Powers P, et al. Early changes in the permeability of the blood-brain produced by toxins associated with liver failure. Pediatr Res 15:227–231, 1992.

74. Kato M, Hughes RD, Keays RT, et al. Electron microscopic study of brain capillaries in cerebral edema from fulminant hepatic failure. Hepatology 15:1060–1066, 1992.

75. Ede RJ, Williams RW. Hepatic encephalopathy and cerebral edema. Sem Liver Dis 6:107–118, 1986.

76. Blei AT. Cerebral edema and intracranial hypertension in acute liver failure: Distinct aspects of the same problem. Hepatology 13:376–379, 1991.

77. Murray-Lyon IM, Portmann B, Gazzard BC, et al. Analysis of the causes of death in the treatment failures. In: Williams R, Murray-Lyon IM (eds) Artifical Liver Support. Pitman Medical, Tunbridge Wells, England; 242, 1975.

78. Bernardi M, Wilkinson SP, Poston L, et al. The renin-angiotensin-aldosterone system in fulminant hepatic failure. Digestion 16:350 (abstract), 1977.

79. Bernardi M, Wilkinson SP, Wernze H, et al. The renin-angiotensin-aldosterone system in fulminant hepatic failure. Scand J Gastroenterol 18:369–375, 1983.

80. Trewby P, Bennett A, Murray-Lyon IM, et al. Plasma prostaglandins in fulminant hepatic failure. Br Med J 4:442, 1975.

81. Trewby PN, Chase R, Davis M, et al. The role of false neurotransmitter octopamine in the hypotension of fulminant hepatic failure. Clin Sci Mol Med 52:305–310, 1977.

82. Bihari DJ, Gimson AES, Williams R. Cardiovascular, pulmonary and renal complications of fulminant hepatic failure. In: Williams R (ed) Seminars in Liver Disease, Vol. 6. Thieme, New York, 119–128, 1986.

83. Trewby PN, Warren R, Contini S, et al. Incidence and pathophysiology of pulmonary edema in fulminant hepatic failure. Gastroenterology 74:859–865, 1978.

84. Dawson DJ, Babbs C, Warnes TW. Hypophosphataemia in acute liver failure. Brit Med J 295:1312–1313, 1987.

85. Forrester SD, Moreland KJ. Hypophosphatemia: Causes and clinical consequences. J Vet Int Med 3:149–159, 1989.

86. Bihari D, Wendon J. Tissue hypoxia in fulminant hepatic failure. In: Williams R, Hughes RD (eds) Acute Liver Failure: Improved Understanding and Better Therapy. Miter Press, London, 42–44, 1991.

87. Williams A, Trewby P, Williams RM, et al. Structural alterations to the pulmonary circulation in fulminant hepatic failure. Thorax 34:447–453, 1979.

88. Bihari D, Gimson AE, Lindridge J, et al. Lactic acidosis in fulminant hepatic failure. Some aspects of pathogenesis and prognosis. J Hepatol 1:405–416, 1985.

89. Stanley NN, Salisbury BG, McHenry LC, Jr, et al. Effect of liver failure on the response of ventilation and cerebral circulation to carbon dioxide in man and in the goat. Clin Sci Mol Med 49:157–169, 1975.

90. Stanley NN, Cherniak NS. Effect of liver failure on the cerebral circulatory and metabolic responses to hypoxia in the goat. Clin Sci Mol Med 50:15–24, 1976.

91. Stanley NN, Kelsen SG, Cherniack NS. Effect of liver failure on the ventilatory response to hypoxia in man and in the goat. Clin Sci Mol Med 50:25–35, 1976.

92. Record CO, Iles RA, Cohen RD, et al. Acid-base and metabolic disturbances in fulminant hepatic failure. Gut 16:144–149, 1975.

93. Kosaka Y, Tanaka K, Sawa H, et al. Acid-base disturbance in patients with fulminant hepatic failure. Gastroenterol Jpn 14:24–30, 1979.

94. Moore K, Taylor G, Ward P, et al. Aetiology and mangement of renal failure in acute liver failure. In: Williams R, Hughes RD (eds) Acute Liver Failure: Improved Understanding and Better Therapy. Miter Press, London, 47–53, 1991.

95. Wilkinson SP, Portmann B, Hurst D, et al. Pathogenesis of renal failure in cirrhosis and fulminant hepatic failure. Postgrad Med J 51:503–505, 1975.

96. Wilkinson SP, Hurst D, Day DW, et al. Spectrum of renal tubular damage in renal failure secondary to cirrhosis and fulminant hepatic failure. J Clin Pathol 31:101–107, 1978.

97. Wyke RJ, Yousif-Kadaru AG, Rajkoviz IA, et al. Serum stimulatory activity and polymorphonuclear leukocyte movement in patients with fulminant hepatic failure. Clin Exp Immuno 50:442–449, 1982.

98. Wyke RJ, Canalese JC, Gimson AE, et al. Bacteremia in patients with fulminant hepatic failure. Liver 2:45–52, 1982.

99. Bailey RJ, Woolf IL, Cullens H, et al. Metabolic inhibition of polymorphonuclear leucocytes in fulminant hepatic failure. Lancet 1:1162–1163, 1976.

100. Sewell RB, Hughes RD, Postin L, et al. Effects of serum from patients with fulminant hepatic failure on leucocyte sodium transport. Con Sci 63:237–242, 1982.

101. Altin M, Rajkovic IA, Hughes RD, et al. Neutrophil adherence in chronic liver disease and fulminant hepatic failure. Gut 24:746–750, 1983.

102. Larcher VF, Wyke RJ, Mowat AP, et al. Bacterial and fungal infection in children with fulminant hepatic failure: Possible role of opsonization and complement deficiency. Gut 23:1037–1043, 1982.

103. Larcher VF, Wyke RJ, Vergani D, et al. Yeast opsonization and complement in children with liver diseases. Analysis of 69 cases. Pediatr Res 17:296–300, 1983.

104. Imawari M, Hughes RD, Gove CD, et al. Fibronectin and Kupffer cell function in fulminant hepatic failure. Dig Dis Sci 30:1028–1033, 1985.

105. Gonzalez-Calvin J, Scully MF, Sanger Y, et al. Fibronectin in fulminant hepatic failure. Br Med J 285:1231–1232, 1982.

106. Wyke RJ, Raajkovic IA, Eddleston ALWF, et al. Defective opsonization and complement deficiency in serum from patients with fulminant hepatic failure. Gut 21:643–649, 1980.

107. Weinbren K. Experimental aspects of regeneration. In: Williams R, Murray-Lyon IM (eds) Artificial Liver Support. Pitman Medical, Tunbridge Wells, England, 255, 1975.

108. Gohda E, Tsubouchi H, Nakayama H, et al. Purification and partial characterization of hepatocyte growth factor from plasma of a patient with fulminant hepatic failure. J Clin Invest 81:414–419, 1988.

109. Gohda E, Tsubouchi H, Nakayama H, et al. Human hepatocyte growth factor in blood of patients with fulminant hepatic failure: Basic aspects. Dig Dis Sci 36:785–790, 1991.

110. Gove CD, Hughes RD, Williams R. Rapid inhibition of DNA synthesis in hepatocytes from regenerating rat liver by serum from patients with fulminant hepatic failure. Br J Exp Pathol 63:547–553, 1982.

111. Haas T, Holloway CJ, Osterthun V, et al. Hepatotoxic effects of serum from patients with fulminant hepatitis B on isolated rat hepatocytes in culture. J Clin Chem Clin Biochem 19:283–286, 1981.

112. Ohkawa M, Hayashi H, Chaudry IH, et al. Effects of regenerating liver cytosol on drug-induced hepatic failure. Surgery 97:455–462, 1985.

113. Francavilla A, Dileo A, Polimeno L, et al. The effect of hepatic stimulatory substance, isolated from regenerating hepatic cytosol and 50,000 and 300,000 subfractions in enhancing survival in experimental acute hepatic failure in rats treated with D-galactosamine. Hepatology 6:1346–1351, 1986.

114. Tashiro K, Hagiya M, Nishizawa R, et al. Deduced primary structure of rat hepatocyte growth factor and expression of the mRNA in rat tissues. Proc Natl Acad Sci USA 87:3200–3204, 1990.

115. Darle N, Lim RC. Effect of low molecular dextran on total liver blood flow in hemorrhagic shock. Eur Surg Res 8:132–139, 1976.

116. Hanid MA, Silk DB, Williams R. Prognostic value of the oculovestibular reflex in fulminant hepatic failure. Br Med J 1:1029, 1978.

117. Davenport A, Will EJ, Davison AM. Effect of posture on intracranial pressure and cerebral perfusion pressure in patients with fulminant hepatic and renal failure after acetaminophen self-poisoning. Crit Care Med 18:286–289, 1990.

118. Jones EA, Rosenoer VM. Corticosteroid therapy in acute and chronic hepatitis. In: Rosenoer VM, Rothschild M (eds) Controversies in Clinical Care. Sp Medical and Scientific Book Publications, New York, 79, 1981.

119. Canalese J, Gimson AES, Davis C, et al. Controlled trial of dexamethasone and mannitol for the cerebral oedema of fulminant hepatic failure. Gut 23:625–629, 1982.

120. Ede RJ, Gimson AES, Bihari D, et al. Controlled hyperventilation in the prevention of cerebral oedema in fulminant hepatic failure. J Hepatology 2:43–51, 1986.

121. Hanid MA, Davies M, Mellon PJ, et al. Clinical monitoring of intracranial pressure in fulminant hepatic failure. Gut 21:866–869, 1980.

122. Williams R, Gimson AES. Intensive liver care and management of acute hepatic failure. Dig Dis Sci 36:820–826, 1991.

123. Pollay M, Fullenwider C, Roberts A, et al. Effect of mannitol and furosemide on blood-brain osmotic gradient and intracranial pressure. J Neuro Surg 59:945–950, 1983.

124. Gazzard BG, Henderson JM, Williams R. Early changes in coagulation following a paracetamol overdose and controlled trial of fresh frozen plasma therapy. Gut 16:617–620, 1975.

125. Friedel HA, Goa KL, Benfield P. S-adenosyl-L-methionine: A review of its pharmacological and therapeutic potential in liver dysfunction and affective disorders in relation to its physiological role in cell metabolism. Drugs 38:389–416, 1989.

126. Horowitz JH, Rypins EB, Henderson JM, et al. Evidence for impairment of transsulfuration pathway in cirrhosis. Gastroenterology 81:668–675, 1981.

127. Chawla RK, Lewis FW, Kutner MH, et al. Plasma cysteine, cystine, and glutathione in cirrhosis. Gastroenterology 87:770–776, 1984.

128. Lauterburg BH, Velez ME. Glutathione deficiency in alcoholics: Risk factor for paracetamol hepatotoxicity. Gut 29:1153–1157, 1988.

129. Poulsen HE, Ranek L, Andreasen PB. The hepatic glutathione content in liver disease. Scand J Clin Lab Invest 41:573–576, 1981.

130. Sieger CP, Bossen KH, Younes M, et al. Glutathione and glutathione-S-transferases in the normal and diseased human liver. Pharmacol Res Commun 14:61–72, 1982.

131. Videla LA, Iturriaga H, Pino ME, et al. Content of hepatic reduced glutathione in chronic alcoholic patients: Influence of the length of abstinence and liver necrosis. Clin Sci 66:283–290, 1984.

132. Jewell SA, Di Monte D, Gentile A, et al. Decreased hepatic glutathione in chronic alcoholic patients. J Hepatol 3:1–6, 1986.

133. Speisky H, Kera Y, Penltila KE, et al. Depletion of hepatic glutathione by ethanol occurs independently of ethanol metabolism. Alcohol Clin Exp Res 8:65–88, 1988.

134. Duce AM, Ortiz P, Cabrero C, et al. S-adenosyl-L-methionine synthetase and phospholipid methyltransferase are inhibited in human cirrhosis. Hepatology 8:65–68, 1988.

135. Cabrero C, Martin Duce Q, Ortiz P, et al. Specific loss of the high-molecular-weight form of S-adenosyl-L-methionine synthetase in human liver cirrhosis. Heptology 8:1530–1534, 1988.

136. Vendemiale G, Altomare E, Tizio T, et al. Effects of oral S-adenosyl-L-methionine on hepatic glutathione in patients with liver disease. Scand J Gastroenterol 24:407–415, 1989.

137. Adachi Y, Nanno T, Kanbe A, et al. The effects of S-adenosylmethionine on intrahepatic cholestasis. Jpn Arch Int Med 33:185–192, 1986.

138. Frezza M, Di Padova C. The Italian Study Group for SAMe in Liver Disease. Multicenter placebo controlled clinical trial of intravenous and oral S-adenosylmethionine (SAMe) in cholestatic patients with liver disease. Hepatology 7:1105 (abstract), 1987.

139. Lieber CS, De Carli IM, Kim C, et al. S-adenosylmethionine (SAMe) attenuates alcohol-induced mitochondrial injury in the baboon. Hepatology 8:1412, 1988.

140. Meister A. New developments in glutathione metabolism and their potential application in therapy. Hepatology 4:739–742, 1984.

141. Bray GP, Tredger JM, William R. S-adenosylmethionine protects against acetaminophen hepatotoxicity in two mouse models. Hepatology 15:297–301, 1992.
142. Harrison PM, Keays R, Bray GP, et al. Improved outcome in paracetamol-induced fulminant hepatic failure following late administration of acetylcysteine. Lancet 335:1572–1573, 1990.
143. Keays RT, Gove C, Forbes A, et al. Use of late N-acetyl cysteine in severe paracetamol overdose. Gut 30:A1512 (abstract), 1989.
144. Bihari D, Sithies M, Gimson A, et al. The effects of vasodilation with prostacyclin on oxygen delivery and uptake in critically ill patients. N Engl J Med 317:397–403, 1987.
145. Harrison PM, Wendon JA, Gimson AES, et al. Improvement by acetylcysteine of hemodynamics and oxygen transport in fulminant hepatic failure. N Engl J Med 324:1852–1857, 1991.
146. Lucht WD, English DK, Bernard GR, et al. Prevention of release of granulocyte aggregants into sheep lung lymph following endotoxemia by N-acetylcysteine. Am J Med Sci 294:161–167, 1987.
147. Kharazmi A, Nielsen H, Schiotz PO. N-acetylcysteine inhibits human neutrophil and monocyte chemotaxis and oxidative metabolism. Int J Immunopharmacol 10:39–46, 1988.
148. Jensen T, Kharazmi A, Schiotz PO, et al. Effect of oral N-acetylcysteine administration on human blood neutrophil and monocyte function. APMIS 96:62–67, 1988.
149. Jaeschke H, Farhood A, Smith CW. Neutrophils contribute to ishemic reperfusion injury in rat liver in vivo. FASEB J 4:3355–3359, 1990.
150. Mitchell JR. Acetominophen toxicity. N Engl J Med 319:1601–1602, 1988.
151. Ohhori I, Yabushita IK, Watanabe T, et al. Prevention of liver damage by using free radical scavengers and changes in plasma PG levels during liver ischemia. Transplant Proc 21:1309–1311, 1989.
152. Marotto ME, Thurman RG, Lemasters JJ. Early midzonal cell death during low-flow hypoxia in the isolated, perfused rat liver: Protection by allopurinol. Hepatology 8:585–590, 1988.
153. Nordstrom G, Torsten S, Hasselgren PO. Beneficial effect of allopurinol in liver ischemia. Surgery 97:679–683, 1985.
154. Metzger J, Lauterburg BH. Increased generation of glutathione disulfide (GSS G) in reperfused ischemic liver: Prevention of oxidant stress and functional improvement by allopurinol. Gastroenterology 88:1678 (abstract), 1985.
155. Jaeschke H. Glutathione disulfide formation and oxidant stress during acetaminophen-induced hepatotoxicity in mice in vivo: The protective effect of allopurinol. J Pharmacol Exp Ther 255:935–941, 1990.
156. Yoshikawa T, Furukawa Y, Murakami M, et al. Effects of vitamin E on D-galactosamine induced or carbon tetrachloride induced hepatotoxicity. Digestion 25:222–229, 1982.
157. Skaare JU, Nafstad I. Interaction of vitamin E and selenium with the hepatotoxic agent dimethylnitrosamine. Acta Pharamacol Toxicol 43:119–128, 1978.
158. Bieri JG, Corash L, Hubbard VS. Medical uses of vitamin E. N Engl J Med 308:1063–1071, 1983.
159. Fariss MW, Merson MH, O'Hara TM. α-tocopheryl succinate protects hepatocytes from chemical-induced toxicity under physiological calcium conditions. Toxicol Let 47:61–75, 1989.
160. Sanan S, Sharma G, Malhotra R, et al. Protection by desferrioxamine against histopathological changes of the liver in the post-oligaemic phase of clinical haemorrhagic shock in dogs: Correlation with improved survival rate after recovery. Free Rad Res Comms 6:29–38, 1988.
161. Janoff A, Zweifach BW, Shapiro L. Levels of plasma bound iron in experimental shock in the rabbit and dog. Am J Physiol 198:1161–1165, 1960.
162. Bucher ML, Swaffield MN. Regulation of hepatic regeneration in rats by synergistic action of insulin and glucagon. Proc Natl Acad Sci USA 72:1154–1156, 1975.
163. Feher J, Cornides A, Romany A, et al. A prospective multicenter study of insulin and glucagon infusion therapy in acute alcoholic hepatitis. J Hepatology 5:224–231, 1987.
164. Farivar M, Wands JR, Isselbacher KJ, et al. Effect of insulin and glucagon on fulminant murine hepatitis. N Engl J Med 295:1517–1519, 1976.
165. Masaki N, Yamada S, Ogata I, et al. Enhancement of carbon tetrachloride-induced liver injury by glucagon and insulin treatment. Res Exp Med 188:27–33, 1988.
166. Fujiwara K, Ogata I, Mishiro S, et al. Glucagon and insulin for the treatment of hepatic failure in dimethylnitrosamine-intoxicated rats. Scand J Gastroenterol 23:567–573, 1988.
167. Basset ML, Mullen KD, Skolnick P, et al. Amelioration of hepatic encephalopathy by pharmacologic antagonism of the GABAa-benzodiazepine receptor complex in a rabbit model of fulminant hepatic failure. Gastroenterology 93:1069–1077, 1987.
168. Basile AS, Jones EA, Skolnick P. The pathogenesis and treatment of hepatic encephalopathy: Evidence for the involvment of benzodiazepine receptor ligands. Pharm Rev 43:27–69, 1991.
169. Stachura J, Tarnawski A, Ivey KJ, et al. Prostaglandin protection of carbon tetrachloride-induced liver cell necrosis in the rat. Gastroenterology 81:211–217, 1981.
170. Ruwart MJ, Rush BD, Friedle NM. 16, 16-dimethyl PGE₂ partially prevents necrosis due to aflatoxin in rats (abstract). Gastroenterology 82:1167, 1982.
171. Stachura J, Rarnawski A, Szczudrawa J, et al. Cytoprotective effect of 16, 16-dimethyl prostaglandin E₂ and some drugs on an acute galactosamine induced liver damage in the rat. Folia Histochem Cytochem 9:311–318, 1980.
172. Ruwart MJ, Rush BD, Freidle NM, et al. 16,16-dimethyl-PGE₂ protection against α-napthylisothiocyanate-induced experimental cholangitis in the rat. Hepatology 4:658–660, 1984.
173. Ruwart MJ, Appelman HD, Rush BD, et al. The effect of 16, 16-dimethyl-prostaglandin E₂ on nutritional injury in rat liver. In: Proceedings of the International Symposium on Chronic Hepatitis. Elsevier Science Publishers BV, Amsterdam, 257–261, 1986.
174. Ruwart MJ, Rush BD, Snyder KF, et al. 16,16-dimethyl prostaglandin E₂ delays collagen formation in nutritional injury in rat liver. Hepatology 8:61–64, 1988.
175. Mizoguchi Y, Tsutsui H, Miyajima K, et al. The protective effects of prostaglandin E₁ in an experimental massive hepatic cell necrosis model. Hepatology 7:1184–1188, 1987.
176. Kurokawa T, Nonami T, Harada A, et al. Effects of prostaglandin E₁ on the recovery of ischemia-induced liver mitochondrial dysfunction in rats with cirrhosis. Scand J Gastroenterology 26:269–274, 1991.
177. Monden M, Fortner JG. Twenty-four and 48 hours canine liver preservation by simple hypothermia with prostacyclin. Ann Surg 196:38–42, 1982.
178. Hirasawa H, Chaudry IH, Baue AE. Improved hepatic function and survival with adenosine triphosphate-magnesium chloride after hepatic ischemia. Surgery 83:655–662, 1978.
179. Ferrero ME, Marni A, Gaja G. Possible enhancement of endothelial cell function induced by defibrotide. Biochem Soc Trans 16:540–541, 1988.
180. Ferrero ME, Marni A, Gaja G. Prevention of impaired liver metabolism due to ischemia in rats: Efficacy of defibrotide administration. J Hepatol 10:223–227, 1990.
181. Pescador R, Mantovani M, Prino G, et al. Pharmacokinetics of defibrotide and its fibrinolytic activity in the rabbit. Thromb Res 30:1–11, 1983.
182. Niada R, Mantovani M, Prino G, et al. Antithrombotic activity of a polydeoxyribonucleotide substance extracted from mammalian organs: A possible link with prostacyclin. Thromb Res 23:233–246, 1981.
183. Grodzinska L, Konig E, Schror K. Defibrotide is equipotent in stimulating arterial and venous thrombolysis. Pharmacol Res Commun 19:609–615, 1987.
183a.Pegg AE, McCann PP. Polyamine metabolism and function. Am J Physiol 243:c212–c221, 1982.
184. Luk GD, Casero RA. Polyamines in normal and cancer cells. Adv Enzyme Regul 26:91–105, 1986.
185. Nagoshi S, Fumiwara K. Putrescine as a comitogen of epidermal growth factor in rat liver. Hepatology 20:725–730, 1994.
186. Diehl AM, Abdo S, Brown N. Supplemental putrescine reverses ethanol-associated inhibition of liver regeneration. Hepatology 12:633–637, 1990.
187. Chang TMS. Experimental artificial liver support with emphasis on fulminant hepatic failure: Concepts and review. In: Williams R (ed) Seminars in Liver Disease, Vol. 6. Thieme, New York, 148–158, 1986.
188. Tomlinson J, Black A. Liver lobe torsion in a dog. J Am Vet Med Assoc 183:225–226, 1983.
189. Andrzejewska A, Dlugosz J, Kurasz S. The ultrastructure of the liver in acute experimental pancreatitis in dogs. Exp Path 28:167–176, 1985.
190. Edwards DF, Bauer MS, Walker MA, et al. Pancreatic masses in seven dogs following acute pancreatitis. J Am Anim Hosp Assoc 26:189–198, 1990.
191. Salisbury SK, Lantz GC, Nelson RW, et al. Pancreatic abscess in dogs: Six cases (1978–1986). J Am Vet Med Assoc 193:1104–1108, 1988.
192. Klein MK, Dow SW, Rosychuk RAW. Pulmonary thromboembolism associated with immune-mediated hemolytic anemia in dogs: Ten cases (1982–1987). J Am Vet Med Assoc 195:246–250, 1989.
193. Bunch SE, Metcalf MR, Crane SW, et al. Idiopathic pleural effusion and pulmonary thromboembolism in a dog with autoimmune hemolytic anemia. J Am Vet Med Assoc 195:1748–1753, 1989.
194. Vane JR, Anggard EE, Botting RM. Regulatory functions of the vascular endothelium. N Engl J Med 323:27–36, 1990.
195. Breider MA. Endothelium and inflammation. J Am Vet Med Assoc 203:300–306, 1993.
196. Thomas HC. Immunologic aspects of liver disease. In: Schiff L, Schiff ER (eds) Diseases of the Liver, 6th ed. JB Lippincott, Philadelphia, 163–187, 1987.
197. Rabin BS, Rogers S. Pathologic changes in the liver and kidney produced by immunization with intestinal antigens. Am J Path 84:201–210, 1976.
198. Cornwell HJC, Wright NG. The pathology of experimental infectious canine hepatitis in neonatal puppies. Res Vet Sci 10:156–160, 1969.
199. Greene CE. Infectious canine hepatitis and canine acidophil cell hepatitis. In: CE Greene (ed) Infectious Diseases of the Dog and Cat. WB Saunders, New York, 242–251, 1990.
200. Hamilton JM, Cornwell HJC, McCusker HB, et al. Studies on the pathogenesis of canine virus hepatitis. Br Vet J 122:225–238, 1966.

201. Parry HB, Larin NM, Platt H. Studies on the agent of canine virus hepatitis (Rubarth's disease). II. The pathology and pathogenesis of the experimental disease produced by four strains of virus. J Hyg 49:482–496, 1951.

202. Gocke DJ, Preisig R, Morris TQ, et al. Experimental viral hepatitis in the dog: Production of persistent disease in partially immune animals. J Clin Invest 46:1506–1517, 1967.

203. Morrison WI, Nash AS, Wright NG. Glomerular deposition of immune complexes in dogs following natural infection with canine adenovirus. Vet Rec, 522–524, June 14, 1975.

204. Garg SP, Moulton JE, Sekhri KK. Histochemical and electron microscopic studies of dog kidney cells in the early stages of infection with infectious canine heptitis virus. Am J Vet Res 28:725–730, 1967.

205. Beckett SD, Burns MJ, Clark CH. A study of the blood glucose, serum transaminase, and electrophoretic patterns of dogs with infectious canine hepatitis. Am J Vet Res 25:1186–1190, 1964.

206. Rakich PM, Prasse KW, Lukert PD, et al. Immunohistochemical detection of canine adenovirus in paraffin sections of liver. Vet Pathol 23:478–484, 1986.

207. Kakuk TJ, Conner GH. Experimental canine herpesvirus in the gnotobiotic dog. Lab Anim Care 20:69–79, 1970.

208. Huxsoll DL, Hemelt IE. Clinical observation of canine herpesvirus. J Am Vet Med Assoc 156:1706–1713, 1970.

209. Percy DH, Carmichael LE, Albert DM, et al. Lesions in puppies surviving infection with canine herpesvirus. Vet Pathol 8:37–53, 1971.

210. Carmichael LE. Herpesvirus canis: Aspects of pathogenesis and immune response. J Am Vet Med Assoc 156:1714–1725, 1970.

211. Carmichael LE, Greene CE. Canine herpesvirus infection. In: CE Greene (ed) Infectious Diseases of the Dog and Cat. WB Saunders, New York, 252–258, 1990.

212. Harari J, Miller D, Padgett GA, et al. Cerebellar agenesis in two canine littermates. J Am Vet Med Assoc 182:622–623, 1983.

213. Wright NG, Cornwell HJC. Further studies on experimental canine herpesvirus infection in young puppies. Res Vet Sci 11:221–226, 1970.

214. Cocker FM, Howard PE, Harbour DA. Effect of human alpha-hybrid interferon on the course of feline viral rhinotracheitis. Vet Rec 120:391–393, 1987.

215. Barlough JE, Stoddart CA. Feline infectious peritonitis. In: Scott FW (ed) Contemporary Issues in Small Animal Practice 3: Infectious Diseases. Churchill Livingstone, New York, 93–108, 1986.

216. Weiss RC, Scott FW. Pathogenesis of feline infectious peritonitis: Pathologic changes and immunofluorescence. Am J Vet Res 42:2036–2048, 1981.

217. Barlough JE, Stoddart CA. Feline coronaviral infections. In: Greene CE (ed) Infectious Diseases of the Dog and Cat. WB Saunders, New York, 300–312, 1990.

218. Hayashi T, Utsumi F, Takahashi R, et al. Pathology of non-effusive type feline infectious peritonitis and experimental transmission. Jpn J Vet Sci 42:197–210, 1980.

219. Lee JF, Block GE. The changing clinical pattern of hepatic abscesses. Arch Surg 194:465–470, 1972.

220. Bertel CK, van Heerden JA, Sheedy PF. Treatment of pygenic hepatic abscesses. Arch Surg 121:554–558, 1986.

221. McDonald MI, Corey GR, Gallis HA, et al. Single and multiple pyogenic liver abscesses. Natural history, diagnosis and treatment with percutaneous drainage. Medicine 63:291–302, 1984.

222. Sabbaj J, Sutter VL, Finegold SM. Anaerobic pyogenic liver abscess. Ann Int Med 77:629–638, 1972.

223. Hirsch DC, Jang SS, Biberstein EL. Blood culture of the canine patient. J Am Vet Med Assoc 184:175–178, 1984.

224. Calvert CA, Greene CE, Hardie EM. Cardiovascular infections in dogs: Epizootiology, clinical manifestations and prognosis. J Am Vet Med Assoc 187:612–616, 1985.

225. Dow SW, Curtis CR, Jones RL, et al. Results of blood culture from critically ill dogs and cats: 100 cases (1985–1987). J Am Vet Med Assoc 195:113–117, 1989.

230. Dow SW, Jones RL. Anaerobic infections. Part I. Pathogenesis and clinical significance. Comp Contin Edu 9:711–720, 1987.

268. Weiss RC, Dodds WJ, Scott FW. Disseminated intravascular coagulation in experimentally induced feline infectious peritonitis. Am J Vet Res 41:663–671, 1980.

226. Hirsch DC, Biberstein EL, Jang SS. Obligate anaerobes in clinical veterinary practice. J Clin Microbiol 10:188–191, 1979.

227. Hirsch DC, Indiveri MC, Jaang SS, et al. Changes in prevalence and susceptibility of obligate anaerobes in clinical veterinary practice. J Am Vet Med Assoc 186:1086–1089, 1985.

228. Prescott JF. Identification of some anaerobic bacteria in nonspecific anaerobic infections in animals. Can J Com Ped 43:194–199, 1979.

229. Dow SW, Jones RL, Adney WF. Anaerobic bacterial infections and response to treatment in dogs and cats: Review of 36 cases (1983–1985). J Am Vet Med Assoc 189:930–934, 1986.

231. Dow SW, Jones RL. Anaerobic infections. Part II. Diagnosis and treatment. Comp Contin Edu 9:827–840, 1987.

232. Styrt B, Gorbach SL. Recent developments in the understanding of the pathogenesis and treatment of anaerobic infections. Parts I and 2. New Engl J Med 321:240–246, 1989.

233. Sanford JP, Gilbert DN, Gerberding JL, et al. The Sanford Guide to Antimicrobial Therapy. Antimicrobial Therapy Inc. Dallas, TX, 1994.

234. Ganaway JR, McReynolds RX, Sllen AM. Tyzzer's disease in free-living cottontail rabbits (Sylvilagus floridanus) in Maryland. J Wildl Dis 12:545–549, 1976.

235. Takagaki Y, Ito M, Naiki M, et al. Experimental Tyzzer's disease in different species of laboratory animals. Jpn J Exp Med 36:519–534, 1966.

236. Boschert KR, Allison N, Allen TLC, et al. Tyzzer's disease in an adult dog. J Am Vet Med Assoc 791–792, 1988.

237. Myerslough N. Tyzzer's disease in puppies. Vet Rec 122:238, 1988.

238. Schneck G. Tyzzer's disease in an adult cat. VM SAC 70:155–156, 1975.

239. Wilkie JSN, Barker IK. Colitis due to Bacillus piliformis in two kittens. Vet Pathol 22:649–652, 1985.

240. Meads EB, Maxie MG, Baker B. Tyzzer's disease in a puppy. Can Vet J 25:134, 1984.

241. Qureshi SR, Carlton WW, Olander HJ. Tyzzer's disease in a dog. J Am Vet Med Assoc 168:602–604, 1976.

242. Waggie KS, Hansen CT, Ganaway JR, et al. A study of mouse strain susceptibility to Bacillus piliformis (Tyzzer's disease): The association of B-cell function and resistance. Lab Anim Sci 31:139–142, 1981.

243. Nii A, Nakayama H, Fujiwara K. Effect of partial hepatectomy on Tyzzer's disease of mice. Jpn J Vet Sci 48:227–235, 1986.

244. Nakayama H, Nii A, Oguihara S, et al. Effect of reticuloendothelial system blocking on Tyzzer's disease of mice. Jpn J Vet Sci 48:211–217, 1986.

245. Poonacha KB, Smith HL. Naturally occurring Tyzzer's disease as a complication of distemper and mycotic pneumonia in a dog. J Am Vet Med Assoc 169:419–420, 1976.

246. Kubokawa K, Kubo M, Takasaki Y, et al. Two cases of feline Tyzzer's disease. Jpn J Exp Med 43:413–421, 1973.

247. Webb DM, Harrington DD, Boehm PN. Bacillus piliformis infection (Tyzzer's disease) in a calf. J Am Vet Med Assoc 191:431–434, 1987.

248. Bennett AM, Huxtable CR, Lover DN. Tyzzer's disease in cats experimentally infected with feline leukaemia virus. Vet Microbiol 2:49–56, 1977.

249. Bonney CH, Schmidt RE. A mixed infection: Chaga's and Tyzzer's disease in a lesser panda. J Zoo Anim Med 6:4–7, 1975.

250. Jones BR, Johnstone AC, Hancock WS. Tyzzer's disease in kittens with familial primary hyperlipoproteinaemia. J Sm Anim Pract 26:411–419, 1985.

251. Hunter B. Eradication of Tyzzer's disease in a colony of barrier-maintained mice. Lab Anim 5:271–276, 1971.

252. Shoenbaum M, Kariv N. An outbreak of Tyzzer's disease in a commercial rabbitry in Israel. Refu Vet 33:26–30, 1976.

253. Greene CE. Salmonellosis. In: Greene CE (ed) Infectious Diseases of the Dog and Cat. WB Saunders, New York, 542–549, 1990.

254. Nation PN. Salmonella dublin septicemia in two puppies. Can Vet J 25:324–326, 1986.

255. Timbs DV, Durham PJK, Barnsley DGC. Chronic cholecystitis in a dog infected with Salmonella typhimurium. N Z Vet J 22:100–102, 1975.

256. Walker RI, French JE, Walden DA, et al. Protection of dogs from lethal consequences of endotoxemia with plasma transfusion. Circ Shock 6:190, 1979.

257. Davies ME, Skulski G. A study of beta-hemolytic streptococci in the fading puppy in relation to canine virus hepatitis infection in the dam. Br Vet J 112:404–410, 1956.

258. Kornblatt AN, Adams RL, Barthold SE, et al. Canine neonatal deaths associated with group B streptococcal septicemia. J Am Vet Med Assoc 183:700–701, 1983.

259. Dow SW, Jones RL, Thomas TN, et al. Groups B streptococcal infection in cats. J Am Vet Med Assoc 190:71–72, 1987.

260. Greene CE. Streptococcal and other gram-positive bacterial infections. In: Greene CE (ed) Infectious Diseases of the Dog and Cat. WB Saunders, New York, 599–610, 1990.

261. Blanchard PC. Wilson DW. Group G streptococcal infections in cats. In: Greene CE (ed.) Infectious Diseases of the Dog and Cat. WB Saunders, New York, 603–605, 1990.

262. Swindle MM, Narayan O, Luzarrage M, et al. Contagious streptococcal lymphadenitis in cats. J Am Vet Med Assoc. 177:829–830, 1980.

263. Swindle MM, Narayan O, Luzarraga M, et al. Pathogenesis of contagious streptococcal lymphadenitis in cats. J Am Vet Med Assoc 179:1208–1210, 1981.

264. Tillman PC, Dodson ND, Indiveri M. Group G streptococcal epizootic in a closed cat colony. J Clin Microbiol 16:1057–1060, 1982.

265. Goldman PM, Moore TD. Spontaneous Lancefield group G streptococcal infection in a random source cat colony. Lab Anim Sci 23:565–566, 1973.

266. Blanchard PC. Group G streptococcal infections in kittens: Pathogenesis, immunity and maternal carrier state. PhD thesis, University of California, Davis, 1987.

267. Turner T. A case of Listeria monocytogenes in the cat. Vet Rec 74:778, 1962.

268. Decker RA, Rogers JJ, Lesar S. Listeriosis in a young cat. J Am Vet Med Assoc 168:1025, 1976.

269. Svabic-Vlahovic M, Pantic D, Pavicic M, et al. Transmission of Listeria

monocytogenes from mother's milk to her baby and to puppies. Lancet 2:1201, 1988.

270. Greene CE. Listeriosis. In: Greene CE (ed.) Infectious Diseases of the Dog and Cat. WB Saunders, New York, 607–608, 1990.

271. Snider WR. Tuberculosis in canine and feline populations: Review of the literature. Am J Respir Dis 104:877–887, 1971.

272. Buergelt CD, Fowler JL, Wright PS. Disseminated avian tuberculosis in a cat. Calif Vet 10:13–15, 1982.

273. Shackelford CC, Reed WM. Disseminated *Mycobacterium avium* infection in a dog. J Vet Diagn Invest 1:273–275, 1989.

274. Carpenter JL, Myers AM, Conner MW, et al. Tuberculosis in five basset hounds. J Am Vet Med Assoc 192:1563–1568, 1988.

275. Grossman A. Mycobacterial hepatitis associated with long-term steroid therapy. Fel Pract 13:37–41, 1984.

276. Frolet R. Disseminated tuberculosis caused by *Mycobacterium avium* in a cat. J Am Vet Med Assoc 189:1336–1337, 1986.

277. Walsh KM, Losco PE. Canine mycobacteriosis: A case report. J Am Anim Hosp Assoc 20:295–299, 1984.

278. Monroe WE, Chickering WR. Atypical mycobacterial infections in cats. Compend Contin Educ Pract Vet 10:1044–1048, 1988.

279. Felsburg PJ, Jezyk PF, Haskins ME. A canine model for variable combined immunodeficiency. Clin Res 30:347A (abstract), 1982.

280. Greene CE, Kunkel GA. Mycobacterial infections, feline leprosy. Atypical mycobacterial infections. In: Greene CE (ed.) Infectious Diseases of the Dog and Cat. WB Saunders, New York, 558–572, 1990.

281. Liu SK, Weitzman I, Johnson GG. Canine tuberculosis. J Am Vet Med Assoc 177:164–167, 1980.

282. Studdert VP, Hughes KL. Treatment of opportunistic mycobacterial infections with enrofloxacin in cats. J Am Vet Med Assoc 201:1388–1390, 1992.

283. Fox LE, Kunkel GA, Homer BL, et al. Disseminated subcutaneous *Mycobacterium fortuitum* infection in a dog. J Am Vet Med Assoc 206:53–55, 1995.

284. Tvedten HW, Walker RD, DiPinto NM. Mycobacterium bacteremia in a dog: Diagnosis of septicemia by microscopical evaluation of blood. J Am Anim Hosp Assoc 26:359–363, 1990.

285. Ferber JA, Scherzo CS. Tuberculosis in a dog. J Am Vet Med Assoc 183:117, 1983.

286. Wallace RJ, Jr. The clinical presentation, diagnosis, and therapy of cutaneous and pulmonary infections due to the rapidly growing mycobacteria, M. fortuitum and M. chelonae. Clin Ches Med 10:419–429, 1989.

287. Wallace RJ, Swenson JM, Silcox VA, et al. Spectrum of disease due to rapidly growing mycobacteria. Rev Infec Dis 5:657–679, 1983.

288. Goble M, Iseman MD, Madsen LA, et al. Treatment of 171 patients with pulmonary tuberculosis resistant to isoniazid and rifampin. N Engl J Med 328:527–532, 1993.

289. Iseman MD. Treatment of multidrug-resistant tuberculosis. N Eng J Med 329:784–791, 1993.

290. Frieden TR, Sterling T, Pablos-Mendez A, et al. The emergence of drug-resistant tuberculosis in New York City. N Engl J Med 328:521–526, 1993.

291. Swenson JM, Wallace RJ, Silcox VA, et al. Antimicrobial susceptibility of 5 subgroups of *Mycobacterium fortuitum* and *Mycobacterium chelonae*. Antimicrob Agents Chemother 28:807–811, 1985.

292. Green CE, Shotts EB. Leptospirosis. In: CE Greene (ed) Infectious Diseases of the Dog and Cat. WB Saunders, New York, 498–507, 1990.

293. Rentko VT, Clark N, Ross LA, et al. Canine leptospirosis. A retrospective study of 17 cases. J Vet Int Med 6:235–244, 1992.

294. Barr S. Personal communication. College of Veterinary Medicine, Cornell University, Ithaca, NY.

295. Bishop L, Strandberg JD, Adams RJ, et al. Chronic active hepatitis in dogs associated with leptospires. Am J Vet Res 40:839–844, 1979.

296. Keenan KP, Alexander AD, Montgomery CA. Pathogenesis of experimental *Leptospira interrogans*, serovar *bataviae*, infection in the dog: Microbiological, clinical, hematologic, and biochemical studies. Am J Vet Res 39:449–454, 1978.

297. Fessler JF, Morter RL. Experimental feline leptospirosis. Cornell Vet 54:176–190, 1964.

298. Low DG, Hiatt CW, Gleiser CA, et al. Experimental canine leptospirosis I. *Leptospira icterohemorrhagiae* infections in immature dogs. J Infect Dis 98:249–259, 1956.

299. Navarro CEK, Kociba GJ. Hemostatic changes in dogs with experimental *Leptospira interrogans* serovar *icteroheamorrhagiae* infection. Am J Vet Res 43:904–906, 1982.

300. Munnich D, Lakatos M. Treatment of human *Leptospira* infections with ampicillin or amoxicillin. Chemother 22:372, 1976.

301. McClain JB, Ballau WR, Harrison SM, et al. Doxycycline therapy for leptospirosis. Ann Intern Med 100:696–698, 1984.

302. Takafuji ET, Kirkpatrick JJ, Miller RN. Prophylaxis against leptospirosis with doxycycline. N Engl J Med 311:54, 1984.

303. Takafuji ET, Kirkpatrick JW, Miller RN, et al. An efficacy trial of doxycycline chemoprophylaxis against leptospirosis. N Engl J Med 310:497–500, 1984.

304. Shalit I, Barnea A, Shahar A. Efficacy of ciprofloxacin against *Leptospira interrogans* serogroup *icterohaemorrhagiae*. Antimicrob Agents Chemother 33:788–789, 1989.

305. Rohrbach BW. Tularemia. J Am Vet Med Assoc 193:428–432, 1988.

306. Boyce JM. Recent trends in the epidemiology of tularemia in the United States. J Inf Dis 131:197–199, 1975.

307. Hopla CE. The ecology of tularemia. Adv Vet Sci Comp Med 18:25–53, 1974.

308. Baldwin CJ, Panciera RJ, Morton RJ, et al. Acute tularemia in three domestic cats. J Am Vet Med Assoc 199:1602–1605, 1991.

309. Rhyan JC, Gahagan R, Fales WH. Tularemia in a cat. J Vet Diag Invet 2:239–241, 1990.

310. Johnson HN. Natural occurrence of tularemia in dogs used as a source of canine distemper virus. J Lab Clin Med 29:906–915, 1944.

311. Troy GC, Forrester SD. Canine ehrlichiosis. In: Greene CE (ed) Infectious Diseases of the Dog and Cat. WB Saunders, New York, 404–418, 1990.

312. Reardon MJ, Pierce KR. Acute experimental canine ehrlichiosis. I. Sequential reaction of the hemic and lymphoreticular systems. Vet Pathol 18:48–61, 1981.

313. Hribernik T. Canine ehrlichiosis. Comp Contin Educ 3:997–1002, 1981.

314. Walker DH. Pathology and pathogenesis of the vasculotropic rickettsioses. In: Walker DH (ed) Biology of Rickettsial Diseases, Vol. I. CRC Press, Boca Raton, FL, 115–138, 1988.

315. Kakoma I, Carson CA, Ristic M. Direct and indirect lymphocyte participation in the immunity and immunopathology of tropical canine pancytopenia—a review. Comp Immuno Microbiol Infect Dis 3:291–298, 1980.

316. Hibler SC, Hoskins JD, Greene CE. Rickettsial infections in dogs. II. Ehrlichiosis and infectious cyclic thrombocytopenia. Compend Cont Educ Pract Vet 8:106–115, 1986.

317. Bouloy RP, Lappin MR, Holland CH, et al. Clinical ehrlichiosis in a cat. J Am Vet Med Assoc 204:1475–1478, 1994.

318. Greene CE, Breitschwerdt EB. Rocky Mountain spotted fever and Q fever. In: Greene CE (ed) Infectious Disease of the Dog and Cat. WB Saunders, New York, 419–433, 1990.

319. Walker DH, Firth WT, Edgell CJ. Human endothelial cell culture plaques induced by *Rickettsia rickettsii*. Infect Immun 37:301–306, 1982.

320. Silverman DJ, Bond SB. Infection of human vascular endothelial cells infected by *Rickettsia rickettsii*. J Infect Dis 149:201–206, 1984.

321. Davidson MG, Breitschwerdt EB, Walker DH, et al. Vascular permeability and coagulation during *Rickettsia rickettsii* infection in dogs. Am J Vet Res 165–170, 1990.

322. Weiser IB, Green CE. Dermal necrosis associated with Rocky Mountain spotted fever in four dogs. J Am Vet Med Assoc 195:1756–1758, 1989.

323. Rutgers C, Kowalski J, Cole CR, et al. Severe Rocky Mountain spotted fever in five dogs. J Am Anim Hosp Assoc 21:361–369, 1985.

324. Greene CE, Marks MA, Lappin MR, et al. Comparison of latex agglutination, indirect immunofluorescent antibody, and enzyme immunoassay methods for serodiagnosis of Rocky Mountain spotted fever in dogs. Am J Vet Res 54:20–28, 1993.

325. Dubey JP, Greene CE, Lappin MR. Toxoplasmosis and neosporosis, enteric coccidiosis. In: Greene CE (ed) Infectious Diseases of the Dog and Cat. WB Saunders, New York, 818–846, 1990.

326. Lappin MR, Greene CE, Prestwood AK, et al. Enzyme-linked immunosorbent assay for the detection of circulating antigens of *Toxoplasma gondii* in the serum of cats. Am J Vet Res 50:1586–1590, 1989.

327. Dubey JP, Zajac A, Osofsky SA, et al. Acute primary toxoplasmic hepatitis in an adult cat shedding *Toxoplasma gondii* oocysts. J Am Vet Med Assoc 197:1616–1618, 1990.

328. Rhyan J, Dubey JP. Toxoplasmosis in an adult dog with hepatic necrosis and associated tissue cysts and tachyzoites. Canine Pract 17:6–10, 1992.

329. Dubey JP, Johnstone I. Fatal neonatal toxoplasmosis in cats. J Am Anim Hosp Assoc 18:461–467, 1982.

330. Dubey JP, Thulliex PH. Serologic diagnosis of toxoplasmosis in cats fed *Toxoplasma gondii* tissue cysts. J Am Vet Med Assoc 194:1297–1299, 1989.

331. Lappin MR, Greene CE, Prestwood AK, et al. Diagnosis of *Toxoplasma gondii* infection utilizing an enzyme-linked immunosorbent assay for immunoglobulin M. Am J Vet Res 50:1580–1585, 1989.

332. Lappin MR, Powell CC. Comparison of latex agglutination, indirect hemagglutination, and ELISA techniques for the detection of *Toxoplasma gondii*–specific antibodies in the serum of cats. J Vet Int Med 5:299–301, 1991.

333. Lappin MR, Greene CE, Winston S, et al. Clinical feline toxoplasmosis: Serologic diagnosis and therapeutic management of 15 cases. J Vet Int Med 3:139–143, 1989.

334. Greene CE, Mahaffey EA. Clindamycin for treatment of *Toxoplasma* polymyositis in a dog. J Am Vet Med Assoc 187:631–634, 1985.

335. Dubey JP. *Neospora caninum*: A look at a new *Toxoplasma*-like parasite of dogs and other animals. Compend Cont Ed Sm Anim Pract 12:653–663, 1990.

336. Dubey JP, Lindsay DS. Fatal *Neospora caninum* infection in kittens. J Parasitol 75:148–151, 1988.

337. Dubey JP, Lindsay DS, Lipscomb TP. Neosporosis in cats. Vet Pathol 27:335–339, 1990.

338. Dubey JP, Carpenter JL, Speer CA, et al. Newly recognized fatal protozoan disease of dogs. J Am Vet Med Assoc 192:1269–1285, 1988.

339. Dubey JP, Hattel AL, Lindsay DS, et al. Neonatal *Neospora caninum* infection in dogs: Isolation of the causative agent and experimental transmission. J Am Vet Med Assoc 193:1259–1263, 1988.

340. Lindsay DS, Dubey JP. Immunohistochemical diagnosis of *Neospora caninum* in tissue sections. Am J Vet Res 50:1981–1983, 1989.

341. Dubey JP, Koestner A, Piper RC. Repeated transplacental transmission of *Neospora caninum* in dogs. J Am Vet Med Assoc 197:857–860, 1990.

342. Dubey JP, Lindsay DS. Transplacental *Neospora caninum* infection in cats. J Parasitol 75:765–771, 1989.

343. McGlennon NJ, Jefferies AR, Casas C. Polyradiculoneuritis and polymyositis due to a *Toxoplasma*-like protozoan: Diagnosis and treatment. J Sm Anim Pract 31:102–104, 1990.

344. Mayhew IG, Smith KC, Dubey JP, et al. Treatment of encephalomyelitis due to *Neospora caninum* in a litter of puppies. J Sm Anim Pract 32:609–612, 1991.

345. Hay WH, Shell LG, Lindsay DS, et al. Diagnosis and treatment of *Neospora caninum* infection in a dog. J Am Vet Med Assoc 197:87–89, 1990.

346. Lindsay DS, Dubey JP. Effects of sulfadiazine and amprolium on *Neospora caninum* (Protozoa: Apicomplexa) infections in mice. J Parasitol 76:177–179, 1990.

347. Lipscomb TP, Pletcher JM, Dubey JP, et al. Intrahepatic biliary coccidiosis in a dog. Vet Pathol 26:343–345, 1989.

348. Slappendel RJ, Greene CE. Leishmaniasis. In: Greene CE (ed) Infectious Diseases of the Dog and Cat. WB Saunders, New York, 769–777, 1990.

349. Tryphonas L, Zawidzka Z, Bernand MA, et al. Visceral leishmaniasis in a dog: Clinical, hematological, and pathological observations. Can J Comp Med 41:1–12, 1977.

350. Keenan CM, Hendricks LD, Lightner L, et al. Visceral leishmaniasis in the German shepherd dog. I. Infection, clinical disease, and clinical pathology. Vet Pathol 21:74–79, 1984.

351. Anderson DC, Buckner RG, Glenn BL, et al. Endemic canine leishmaniasis. Vet Pathol 17:94–96, 1980.

352. Swenson CL, Silverman J, Stromberg PC, et al. Visceral leishmaniasis in an English foxhound from an Ohio research colony. J Am Vet Med Assoc 193:1089–1092, 1988.

353. Sellon RK, Menard MM, Meuten DJ, et al. Endemic visceral leishmaniasis in a dog from Texas. J Vet Int Med 7:16–19, 1993.

354. Sinton JA. The successful transmission of cutaneous leishmaniasis by inoculation to man from a natural lesion occurring on a dog in India. Indian J Med Res 25:787, 1983.

355. Ferrer L, Rabanal R, Fondevila D, et al. Skin lesions in canine leishmaniasis. J Sm Anim Pract 29:381–388, 1988.

356. Font A, Closa JM, Mascort J. Monoclonal gammopathy in a dog with visceral leishmaniasis. J Vet Int Med 8:233–235, 1994.

357. Slappendel RJ. Canine leishmaniasis: A review based on 95 cases in the Netherlands. Vet Q 35:1100–1102, 1988.

358. Huss BT, Ettinger SJ. Visceral leishmaniasis, Rocky Mountain spotted fever, and von Willebrand's disease in a giant schnauzer. J Am Anim Hosp Assoc 28:221–225, 1992.

359. Gonzalez JL, Rollan E, Novoa C, et al. Structural and ultrastructural hepatic changes in experimental canine leishmaniasis. Histol Histopath 3:323–329, 1988.

360. Corbeil LB, Wright-George J, Shively JN, et al. Canine visceral leishmaniasis with amyloidosis: An immunopathological case study. Clin Immunol Immunopathol 6:165–173, 1976.

361. Bungener W, Mehlitz D. Atypisch verlaufende *Leishmania donovani* infektion bei hunden. Histopathologische befunde. Topenmed Paraasit 28:175–180, 1977.

362. Ferrer L, Rabanal R, Domingo M, et al. Identification of leishmania amastigotes in canine tissues by immunoperoxidase staining. Res Vet Sci 44:194–196, 1988.

363. Harith AE, Slappendel RJ, Reiter I, et al. Application of direct agglutination test for detection of specific anti-*Leishmania* antibodies to the canine reservoir. J Clin Microbiol 27:2252–2257, 1989.

364. Jaffe CL, Zalis M. Use of purified parasite proteins from *Leishmania donovani* for the rapid serodiagnosis of visceral leishmaniasis. J Infect Dis 157:1212–1220, 1988.

365. Blouin EF, Kocan AA, Glenn BL, et al. Transmission of *Cytauxzoon felis* from bobcats, *Felis rufus*, to domestic cats by *Demacenter variabilis*. J Wildl Dis 20:241–242, 1984.

366. Simpson CF, Harvey JW, Lawman MJP, et al. Ultrastructure of schizonts in the liver of cats with experimentally induced cytauxzoonosis. Am J Vet Res 46:384–390, 1985.

367. Simpson CF, Harvey JW, Carlisle JW. Ultrastructure of the intraerythrocytic stage of *Cytauxzoon felis*. Am J Vet Res 46:1178–1180, 1985.

368. Kier AB. Cytauxzoonosis. In: Greene CE (ed) *Infectious Diseases of the Dog and Cat*. WB Saunders, New York, 792–795, 1990.

369. Franks PT, Harvey JW, Shields RP, et al. Hematological findings in experimental feline cytauxzoonosis. J Am Anim Hosp Assoc 24:395–401, 1988.

370. Wagner JE. A fatal cytauxzoonosis-like disease in cats. J Am Vet Med Assoc 168:585–588, 1976.

371. Malek EA, Ash LR, Lee HF, et al. *Heterobilharzia* infection in the dog and other mammals in Louisiana. J Parasitol 47:619–623, 1961.

372. Thrasher JP. Canine schistosomiasis. J Am Vet Med Assoc 144:1119–1126, 1964.

373. Pierce KR. *Heterobilharzia americana* infection in a dog. J Am Vet Med Assoc 143:496–499, 1963.

374. Slaughter JB, Billups LH. Canine heterobilharziasis. Comp Contin Educ 10:606–612, 1988.

375. Ronald RC, Craig TM. Fenbendazole for the treatment of *Heterobilharzia americana* infection in dogs. J Am Vet Med Assoc 182:172, 1983.

376. Troy GC, Forrester D, Cockburn C, et al. *Heterobilharzia americana* infection and hypercalcemia in a dog: A case report. J Am Anim Hosp Assoc 23:35–40, 1987.

377. Parsons JC, Bowman DD, Grieve RB. Pathological and haematological responses of cats experimentally infected with *Toxocara canis* larva. Int J Parasitol 19:479–488, 1989.

378. Dillon AR, Teer PA, Powers RD, et al. Canine abdominal histoplasmosis: A report of four cases. J Am Anim Hosp Assoc 18:497–502, 1982.

379. Shelton GD, Stockham SL, Carrig CB, et al. Disseminated histoplasmosis with bone lesions in a dog. J Am Anim Hosp Assoc 18:143–146, 1982.

380. Wolf AM, Belden MN. Feline histoplasmosis: A literature review and retrospective study of 20 new cases. J Am Anim Hosp Assoc 20:996–998, 1984.

381. Clinkenbeard KD, Wolf AM, Cowell RL, et al. Canine disseminated histoplasmosis. Comp Contin Educ 11:1347–1357, 1989.

382. Clinkenbeard KD, Wolf AM, Cowell RL, et al. Feline disseminated histoplasmosis. Comp Contin Educ 11:1223–1233, 1989.

383. Clinkenbeard KD, Cowell RL, Tyler RD. Disseminated histoplasmosis in dogs: 12 cases (1981–1986). J Am Vet Med Assoc 193:1443–1447, 1988.

384. Breitschwerdt EB, Halliwell WH, Burk RL, et al. Feline histoplasmosis. J Am Anim Hosp Assoc 13:216–222, 1977.

385. Clinkenbeard KD, Cowell RL, Tyler RD. Disseminated histoplasmosis in cats: 12 cases (1981–1986). J Am Vet Med Assoc 190:1445–1448, 1987.

386. Dillon AR, Teer PA, Powers RD, et al. Canine abdominal histoplasmosis: A report of four cases. J Am Anim Hosp Assoc 18:498–502, 1982.

387. Stickle JE, Hribernik TN. Clinicopathological observations in disseminated histoplasmosis in dogs. J Am Anim Hosp Assoc 14:105–110, 1978.

388. Hugenholtz PG, Reed RE, Maddy KT, et al. Experimental coccidioidomycosis in dogs. Am J Vet Res 19:433–439, 1958.

389. Maddy KT. Disseminated coccidioidomycosis of the dog. J Am Vet Med Assoc 132:483–489, 1958.

390. Armstrong PJ, DiBartola SP. Canine coccidioidomycosis: A literature review and report of eight cases. J Am Anim Hosp Assoc 19:938–946, 1983.

391. Barsanti JA, Jeffery KL. Coccidioidomycosis. In: Greene CE, (ed) Infectious Diseases of the Dog and Cat. WB Saunders, New York, 696–706, 1990.

392. Legendre AM. Blastomycosis. In: Greene CE (ed) Infectious Diseases of the Dog and Cat. WB Saunders, New York, 669–678, 1990.

393. Wolf AM. Histoplasmosis. In: Greene CE, (ed) Infectious Diseases of the Dog and Cat. WB Saunders, New York, 679–695, 1990.

394. Day MJ. Canine disseminated aspergillosis. In: Greene CE, (ed) Infectious Diseases of the Dog and Cat. WB Saunders, New York, 719–721, 1990.

395. Foil CS. Miscellaneous fungal infections. In: Greene CE, (ed) Infectious Diseases of the Dog and Cat. WB Saunders, New York, 731–741, 1990.

396. Patterson JM, Rosendal S, Humphrey J, et al. A case of disseminated paecilomycosis in the dog. J Am Anim Hosp Assoc 19:569–574, 1983.

397. Jang SS, Biberstein EL, Slauson DO, et al. Paecilomycosis in a dog. J Am Vet Med Assoc 159:1775–1779, 1971.

398. Patnaik JAK, Liu SK, Wilkins RJ, et al. Paecilomycosis in a dog. J Am Vet Med Assoc 161:806–813, 1972.

399. Elliott GS, Whitney MS, Reed WM, et al. Antemortem diagnosis of paecilomycosis in a cat. J Am Vet Med Assoc 184:93–94, 1984.

400. Littmann MP, Goldschmidt MH. Systemic paecilomycosis in a dog. J Am Vet Med Assoc 191:445–447, 1987.

401. Kurtz HJ, Finco DR, Perman V. Maduromycosis (*Allescheria boydii*) in a dog. J Am Vet Med Assoc 157:917–921, 1970.

402. Jang SS, Popp JA. Eumycotic mycetoma in a dog caused by *Allescheria boydii*. J Am Vet Med Assoc 157:1071–1076, 1970.

403. Rippon JW. Medical mycology. WB Saunders, Philadelphia, 79–114, 595–614, 1982.

404. Rhyan JC, Stackhouse LL, Davis EG. Disseminated geotrichosis in two dogs. J Am Vet Med Assoc 197:358–360, 1990.

405. Lincoln SD, Adcock JL. Disseminated geotrichosis in a dog. Pathol Vet 5:282–289, 1968.

406. Brodey RS, Schryver HF, Deubler MJ, et al. Mycetoma in a dog. J Am Vet Med Assoc 151:442–451, 1967.

407. Coyle V, Isaacs JP, O'Boyle DA. Canine mycetoma: A case report and review of the literature. J Sm Anim Pract 25:261–268, 1984.

408. Mezza LE, Harvey HJ. Osteomyelitis associated with maduromycotic mycetoma in the foot of a dog. J Am Anim Hosp Assoc 21:215–218, 1985.

409. Greene CE, Chandler FW. Candidiasis. In: Greene CE, (ed) Infectious Diseases of the Dog and Cat. WB Saunders, New York, 723–727, 1990.
410. Ehrensaft DV, Epstein RB, Sarpel S, et al. Disseminated candidiasis in leukopenic dogs. Proc Soc Exp Biol Med 160:6–10, 1979.
411. Chow HS, Sarpel SC, Epstein RB. Experimental candidiasis in neutropenic dogs: Tissue burden of infection and granulocyte transfusion effects. Blood 59:328–333, 1982.
412. Andersonn PG, Pidgeon G. Candidiasis in a dog with parvoviral enteritis. J Am Anim Hosp Assoc 23:27–30, 1987.
413. Lorenzini R, DeBernardis F. Antemortem diagnosis of an apparent case of feline candidiasis. Mycopathologica 93:13–14, 1986.
414. Holoymoen JI, Bjerkas I, Olberg IH, et al. Disseminated candidiasis (moniliasis) in a dog. A case report. Nord Vet Med 34:362–367, 1982.
415. McCaw D, Franklin R, Fales W, et al. Pyothorax caused by *Candida albicans* in a cat. J Am Vet Med Assoc 185:311–312, 1984.
416. Pichler ME, Gross TL, Kroll WR. Cutaneous and mucocutaneous candidiasis in a dog. Comp Contin Ed 7:225–230, 1985.
417. Haron E, Feld R, Tuffenell P, et al. Hepatic candidiasis: An increasing problem in immunocompromised patients. Am J Med 83:17–26, 1987.
418. Lopez-Berestein G, Bodey GP. Treatment of hepatosplenic candidiasis in cancer patients with liposomal amphotericin B (abstract). Proc Am Soc Clin Oncol 5:259, 1986.
419. Mehta R, Lopez-Berestein G, Fainstein V, et al. Liposomal amphotericin-B for the treatment of systemic fungal infections in patients with cancer: A preliminary study. J Infect Dis 151:704–710, 1985.
420. Ader PL. Phycomycosis in fifteen dogs and two cats. J Am Vet Med Assoc 174:1216–1223, 1979.
421. Pavletic MM, Miller RI, Turnwald GH. Intestinal infarction associated with canine phycomycosis. J Am Anim Hosp Assoc 19:913–916, 1983.
422. Migaki G, Font RL, Sauer RM, et al. Canine prototheocosis: Review of the literature and report of an additional case. J Am Vet Med Assoc 181:794–797, 1982.
423. Cook JR, Tyler DE, Coulter DB, et al. Disseminated prototheocosis causing acute blindness and deafness in a dog. J Am Vet Med Assoc 184:1266–1272, 1984.
424. Pegram PS, Kerns FT, Wasilauskas BL, et al. Successful ketoconazole treatment of prototheocosis with ketoconazole associated hepatotoxicity. Arch Intern Med 143:1802–1805, 1983.
425. Coloe PJ, Allison JF. Prototheocosis in a cat. J Am Vet Med Assoc 180:78–79, 1982.
426. Finnie JW, Coloe PJ. Cutaneous prototheocosis in a cat. Aust Vet J 57:307–308, 1981.
427. Kaplan W, Chandler FW, Holzinger EZ, et al. Prototheocosis in a cat: First recorded case. Sabouraudia 14:281–286, 1976.
428. Dillberger JE, Homer B, Daubert D, et al. Prototheocosis in two cats. J Am Vet Med Assoc 192:1557–1559, 1988.
429. Van Kruiningen HJ. Prototheocal enterocolitis in a dog. J Am Vet Med Assoc 157:56–63, 1970.
430. Van Kruiningen HJ, Garner FM, Schiefer B. Prototheocosis in a dog. Vet Path 6:348–354, 1969.
431. Holscher MA, Shasteen WJ, Powell HS, et al. Disseminated canine prototheocosis: A case report. J Am Anim Hosp Assoc 12:49–52, 1976.
432. Caunt SD, McGrath RK, Cox HU. Disseminated prototheocosis in a dog. J Am Vet Med Assoc 185:906–907, 1984.
433. Moore FM, Schmidt GM, Desae D, et al. Unsuccessful treatment of disseminated prototheocosis in a dog. J Am Vet Med Assoc 186:705–708, 1985.
434. Tyler DE. Prototheocosis. In: Greene CE, (ed) Infectious Diseases of the Dog and Cat. WB Saunders, New York, 742–749, 1990.
435. Merideth RE, Gwin RM, Samuelson DA, et al. Systemic prototheocosis with ocular manifestations in a dog. J Am Anim Hosp Assoc 20:153–156, 1984.
436. Cook JR, Tyler DE, Coulter DB, et al. Disseminated prototheocosis causing acute blindness and deafness in a dog. J Am Vet Med Assoc 184:1266–1272, 1984.
437. De Camargo ZP, Fischman O, Silva MRRR. Experimental prototheocosis in laboratory animals. Sabouraudia 18:237–240, 1980.
438. Sudman MS. Prototheocosis: A critical review. Am J Clin Path 61:10–19, 1974.
439. Wolfe ID, Sacks HG, Samorodin CS, et al. Cutaneous prototheocosis in a patient receiving immunosuppressive therapy. Arch Dermatol 112:829–832, 1976.
440. Papich MG, Davis LE. Drugs and the liver. Vet Clin N Am 15:77–95, 1985.
441. Bunch SE, Castleman WL, Baldwin BH, et al. Effects of long-term primidone and phenytoin administration on canine hepatic function and morphology. Am J Vet Res 46:105–115, 1985.
442. Dayrell-Hart B, Steinberg SA, VanWinkle TJ, et al. Hepatotoxicity of phenobarbital in dogs: 18 cases (1985–1989). J Am Vet Med Assoc 199:1060–1066, 1991.
443. Faraj BA, Ali FM, Fulenwider JT, et al. Hepatorenal failure induced by tetracycline in dogs with portacaval shunt. J Pharm Exp Ther 221:558–563, 1982.
444. Rowland PH, Center SA, Dougherty SA. Presumptive trimethoprim-sulfadiazine-related hepatotoxicosis in a dog. J Am Vet Med Assoc 200:348–350, 1992.
445. Colucci DF, Cicero ML. Hepatic necrosis and trimethoprim-sulfamethoxazole. JAMA 233:952–953, 1975.
446. Polzin DJ, Stowe CM, O'Leary TP, et al. Acute hepatic necrosis associated with the administration of mebendazole to dogs. J Am Vet Med Assoc 179:1013–1016, 1981.
447. McEvoy GK (ed), APHIS Formulary, American Society of Hospital Pharmacists, American Hospital Formulary Service, Bethesda, MD, 1994.
448. Cowell AK, Cowell RL, Tyler RD, et al. Severe systemic reactions to *Hymenoptera* stings in three dogs. J Am Vet Med Assoc 198:1014–1016, 1991.
449. Meerdink GL. Bites and stings of venomous animals. In: Kifk RW (ed) Current Veterinary Therapy VIII: Small Animal Practice. WB Saunders Philadelphia, 155–159, 1983.
450. Glaser M. A fatal case after hornet stings and benadril medication. Harefuah 50:175–176, 1956.
451. Jonas W, Sugar M. Severe hepatic and renal damage following wasp stings. Dapim Refuim (Folia Medica) 22:L353–L356, 1963.
452. Neuman MG, Ishay JS, Eshchar J. Hornet (*Vespa orientalis*) venum sac extract causes hepatic injury in cats. Comp Biochem Physiol 74C:469–472, 1983.
453. Mayhall CG, Miller CW, Eisen AZ, et al. Cutaneous protothecosis. Successful treatment with amphotericin B. Arch Dermatol 112:1749–1752, 1976.
454. Venezio FR, Lavoo E, Williams JE, et al. Progressive cutaneous protothecosis. Am J Clin Pathol 77:485–493, 1982.
455. McDonald JS, Richard JL, Anderson AJ. Antimicrobial susceptibility of *Prototheca zopfii* isolated from bovine intramammary infections. Am J Vet Res 45:1079–1080, 1984.
456. Neuman MG, Eshchar J, Cotariu D, et al. Hepatotoxicity of hornet's venom sac extract, after repeated in vivo and in vitro envenomation. Acta Pharmacol Toxicol 53:314–319, 1983.
457. Rosenburg P, Ishay J, Gitter S. Phospholipases A and B activities of the oriental hornet (*Vespa orientalis*) venom and venom apparatus. Toxicology 15:141–156, 1977.
458. Edery H, Ishay J, Gitter S, et al. Venoms of Vespidae. In Antropod's Venom Handbook of Experimental Pharmacology. Springer, Berlin, 48:691–771, 1978.
459. Mitchell JR, Jollow DJ, Potter WZ, et al. Acetaminophen induced hepatic necrosis. I. Role of drug metabolism. J Pharmacol Exp Ther 187:185–194, 1973.
460. Smolarek RA, Higgins CV, Amacher DE. Metabolism and cytotoxicity of acetaminophen in hepatocyte cultures from rat, rabbit, dog, and monkey. Drug Metab Dispos 18:659–663, 1990.
461. Davis DC, Potter WZ, Jollow DJ, et al. Species differences in hepatic glutathione depletion, covalent binding and hepatic necrosis after acetaminophen. Life Sci 14:2099–2109, 1974.
462. Wendel A, Jaeschke H, Gloger M. Drug-induced lipid peroxidation in mice. II. Protection against paracetamol-induced liver necrosis by intravenous liposomally entrapped glutathione. Biochem Pharmacol 31:3601–3605, 1982.
463. Prescott LF. Paracetamol overdosage: Pharmacological considerations and clinical management. Drugs 25:290–314, 1983.
464. Welch RM, Conney AH, Burns JJ. The metabolism of acetophenetidin and N-acetyl-p-aminophenol in the cat. Biochem Pharmacol 15:521–531, 1966.
465. Hjelle JJ, Grauer GF. Acetaminophen-induced toxicosis in dogs and cats. J Am Vet Med Assoc 188:742–746, 1986.
466. Savides MC, Oehme FW, Nash SL, et al. The toxicity and biotransformation of single doses of acetaminophen in dogs and cats. Toxicol Appl Pharmacol 74:26–34, 1984.
467. Eder H. Chronic toxicity studies on phenacetin, N-acetyl-p-aminophenol (NAPA) and acetylsalicylic acid on cats. Acta Pharmacol et Toxicol 21:197–204, 1964.
468. Cullison RF. Acetaminophen toxicosis in small animals: Clinical signs, mode of action, and treatment. Comp Contin Educ Pract Vet 6:315–321, 1984.
469. Gaunt SD, Baker DC, Green RA. Clinicopathologic evaluation of N-acetylcysteine therapy in acetaminophen toxicosis in the cat. J Am Vet Med Assoc 42:1982–1984, 1981.
469a. Harvey JW, French TW, Senior DF. Hematologic abnormalities associated with chronic acetaminophen administration in a dog. J Am Vet Med Assoc 189:1334–1335, 1986.
470. Welsh RM, Conney AH, Burns JJ. The metabolism of acetophenetidin and N-acetyl-p-aminophenol in the cat. Biochem Pharmacol 15–521:531, 1966.
471. Bonanomi L, Gazzaniga A. Toxicological pharmacokinetic and metabolic studies on acetylcysteine. Eur J Respir Dis 61:45–51, 1980.
472. Lake BG, Harris RA, Phillips JC, et al. Studies on the effects of L-ascorbic acid on acetaminophen-induced hepatotoxicity. Toxicol Appl Pharmacol 60:229–240, 1981.
473. Nimmo J, Dixon MF, Prescott LF. Effects of mepyramine, promethazine, and hydrocortisone on paracetamol-induced hepatic necrosis in the rat. Clin Toxicol 6:75–81, 1973.
474. Rollins DE, Buckpit AR. Liver cytosol catalyzed conjugation of reduced

glutathione with a reactive metabolite of acetaminophen. Toxicol Appl Pharmacol 47:331–339, 1979.

475. Davis M. Protective agents for acetaminophen overdose. In: Williams R (ed) Seminars in Liver Disease, Vol. 6, Thieme, New York, 138–147, 1986.

476. Finco DR, Duncan JR, Schall WD, et al. Acetaminophen toxicosis in the cat. J Am Vet Med Assoc 166:469–472, 1975.

477. Schechter RD, Schalm OW, Kaneko JJ. Heinz body hemolytic anemia associated with the use of urinary antiseptics containing methylene blue in the cat. J Am Vet Med Assoc 162:34–44, 1973.

478. Panella C, Makowka L, Barone M, et al. Effect of ranitidine on acetaminophen-induced hepatotoxicity in dogs. Dig Dis Sci 35:385–391, 1990.

479. Denning DW. Aflatoxin and human disease. Adv Drug React Acute Poisoning Rev 4:175–209, 1987.

480. Wilson BJ, Teer PA, Barney GH, et al. Relationship of aflatoxin to epizootics of toxic hepatitis among animals in southern United States. Am J Vet Res 28:1217–1230, 1967.

481. Bastianello SS, Nesbit JW, Williams MC, et al. Pathological findings in a natural outbreak of aflatoxicosis in dogs. Onderstepoort J Vet Res 54:635–640, 1987.

482. Armbrecht BH, Geleta JN, Shalkop WT, et al. A subacute exposure of beagle dogs to aflatoxin. Tox Appl Pharm 18:579–585, 1971.

483. Chaffee VW, Edds GT, Himes JA, et al. Aflatoxicosis in dogs. Am J Vet Res 30:1737–1749, 1969.

484. Newberne JW, Bailey WS, Seibold HR. Notes on a recent outbreak and experimental reproduction of hepatitis X in dogs. J Am Vet Med Assoc 127:59–62, 1955.

485. Newberne PM, Russo R, Wogan GN. Acute toxicity of aflatoxin B_1 in the dog. Pathologia Veterinaria 3:331–340, 1966.

486. Newberne PM. Chronic aflatoxicosis. J Am Vet Med Assoc 163:1262–1267, 1973.

487. Seibold HR, Bailey WS. An epizootic of hepatitis in the dog. J Am Vet Med Assoc 121:201–206, 1952.

488. Liggett AD, Colvin BM, Beaver RW, et al. Canine aflatoxicosis: A continuing problem. Vet Hum Toxicol 28:428–429, 1986.

489. Ketterer PJ, Williams ES, Blaney BJ, et al. Canine aflatoxicosis. Aust Vet J 51:355–357, 1975.

490. Krishnamachari KAVR, Bhat RV, Nagarajan V, et al. Hepatitis due to aflatoxin. An outbreak in western India. Lancet 1:1061–1063, 1975.

491. Clark JD, Jain AV, Hatch RC. Effects of various treatments on induced chronic aflatoxicosis in rabbits. Am J Vet Res 106:110, 1982.

492. Clark JD, Harch RC, Jain AV, et al. Effect of enzyme inducers and inhibitors and glutathione precursor and depleter on induced acute aflatoxicosis in rabbits. Am J Vet Res 43:1027–1033, 1982.

493. Newberne PM, Butler WH. Acute and chronic effects of aflatoxin on the liver of domestic and laboratory animals: A review. Cancer Res 29:236–250, 1969.

494. Greene CE, Barsanti JA, Jones BD. Disseminated intravascular coagulation complicating aflatoxicosis in dogs. Cornell Vet 67:29–49, 1977.

495. Arp LH, Richard JL. Intoxication of dogs with mycotoxin penitrem A. J Am Vet Med Assoc 175:565–566, 1979.

496. Hayes AW, Presley DB, Neville JA. Acute toxicity of penitrem A in dogs. Toxicol Apopl Pharmacol 35:311–320, 1976.

497. Wilson BJ, Harbison RD. Rubratoxins. J Am Vet Med Assoc 163:1274–1276, 1973.

498. Hayes AW, Wilson BJ. Effects of rubratoxin B on liver composition and metabolism in the mouse. Toxicol & Appl Pharmacol 17:481–493, 1970.

499. Munro IC, Scott PM, Moodie CA, et al. Ochratoxin A—occurrence and toxicity. J Am Vet Med Assoc 163:1268–1270, 1973.

500. Lincoff G, Mitchell DH. Introduction. In: Williams WK (ed) Toxic and Hallucinogenic Mushroom Poisoning. Van Nostrand Reinhold New York, 1–14, 1977.

501. Liggett AD, Weiss R. Liver necrosis caused by mushroom poisoning in dogs. J Vet Diagn Invest 1:267–269, 1989.

502. Kallet A, Sousa C, Spahngler W. Mushroom (*Amanita phalloides*) toxicity in dogs. Calif Vet, 47, Jan./Feb. 9–11, 1988.

503. Hunt RS, Funk A. Mushrooms fatal to dogs. Mycologia 69:432–433, 1977.

504. Bernard MA. Mushroom poisoning in the dog. Can Vet J 20:82–83, 1979.

505. Wieland T. Poisonous principles of mushrooms of the genus *Amanita*. Science 159:946–952, 1968.

506. Faulstich H. New aspects of *Amanita* poisoning. Klin Wochenschr 57:1143–1152, 1979.

507. Gitlin N. Clinical aspects of liver diseases caused by industrial and environmental toxins. In: Zakim D, Boyer TD (eds) Hepatology: A Textbook of Liver Disease. WB Saunders, New York, 791–821, 1990.

508. Falustrich H. Structure of poisonous components of *Amanita phalloides*. Curr Prob Clin Biochem 71, 1988.

509. Fiume L. Pathogenesis of the cellular lesions produced by α-amanitin. In: Farber E, (ed) The Biochemistry of Disease. Dekker, New York, 105–122, 1972.

510. Hanrahan JP, Gordon MA. Mushroom poisoning. Case reports and a review of therapy. JAMA 251:1057–1061, 1984.

511. Parish RC, Doering PL. Treatment of *Amanita* mushroom poisoning: A review. Vet Hum Toxicol 28:318–322, 1986.

512. Barnes JM, Magee PN. Some toxic properties of dimethylnitrosamine. Brit J Industr Med 11:167, 1954.

513. Cotler S, Gustafson JH, Colburn WA. Pharmacokinetics of diazepam and nordiazepam in the cat. J Pharm Sci 73:348–351, 1984.

514. Decker K, Keppler D. Galactosamine induced liver injury. In: Popper H, Schaffner F (eds) *Progress in Liver Disease*, Vol. 4. Grune & Stratton, New York, 183–199, 1972.

515. Decker K, Keppler D, Rudigier J, et al. Cell damage by trapping of biosynthetic intermediates. The role of uracil nucleotides in experimental hepatitis. Hoppe Seylers Z Physiol Chem 352:412–418, 1971.

516. Decker K, Keppler D. Galactosamine hepatitis: Key role for the nucleotide deficiency period in the pathogenesis of cell injury and cell death. Rev Physiolo Biochem Pharmacol 71:78–106, 1974.

517. Sabesin SM, Koff RS. D-galactosamine hepatotoxicity. IV. Further studies of the pathogenesis of fatty liver. Exp Mol Path 24:424–434, 1976.

518. Chojkier M, Fierer J. D-galactosamine hepatotoxicity is associated with endotoxin sensitivity and mediated by lymphoreticular cells in mice. Gastroenterology 88:115–121, 1985.

519. Jonker AM, Dijkhuis FWJ, Droese FGM, et al. Immunopathology of acute galactosamine hepatitis in rats. Hepatology 11:622–627, 1990.

520. Eisen TF, Lacouture PG, Lovejoy FH. Iron. In: Haddad LM, Winchester JF (eds) Clinical Management of Poisoning and Drug Overdose, 2nd ed. WB Saunders, Philadelphia, 1010–1017, 1990.

521. Yonkers J, Banner W, Picchionie A. Absorption characteristics of deferoxamine onto charcoal. Vet Human Toxicol 22:361 (abstract), 1980.

522. Whitten CF. Deferoxamine as a chelating agent. Clin Toxicol 4:597–602, 1977.

523. Arena JM, Drew RH. Poisoning, 5th ed. Charles C Thomas, Springfield, IL, 597–585, 1986.

33

Chronic Hepatitis, Cirrhosis, Breed-Specific Hepatopathies, Copper Storage Hepatopathy, Suppurative Hepatitis, Granulomatous Hepatitis, and Idiopathic Hepatic Fibrosis

SHARON A. CENTER

INTRODUCTION

Chronic hepatitis in dogs and cats has been classified into many different necroinflammatory entities based on morphologic criteria (Table 33–1). This classification has confused our understanding of hepatic disease because too many specific characteristics have overshadowed the commonalities among lesions. The definition of chronic hepatitis in humans is applied to any chronic necroinflammatory hepatocellular disorder that continues without improvement for longer than 6 months.[1,2] The lymphocyte is the dominant inflammatory cell. Idiopathic disease or liver disease associated with viral or bacterial infection, drug reactions, toxicities, or autoimmune phenomenon are included, and disorders in which components of the biliary tree are the primary disease targets are excluded. The natural history of disease and its response to therapy have been used to differentiate the biologic behavior of particular syndromes. Thus, classification of chronic hepatitis is made according to etiologies and behavior rather than morphologic appearance, which is vastly different from the state of veterinary hepatology.[3–9]

In humans, the term *chronic persistent hepatitis* is used for disorders that are clinically mild and histologically nonprogressive. It is not known if a similar category of disease exists in the dog and cat. The term *chronic active hepatitis* (CAH) is evolving in its application. This lesion is characterized by clinical features indicative of a likely progression to cirrhosis. Initially, use of this nomenclature required the presence of piecemeal necrosis and/or bridging necrosis. Piecemeal necrosis indicates involvement of the hepatocytes adjacent to the portal triad; this area is considered the "limiting plate." Bridging necrosis indicates the presence of tracts of necrosis extending across the hepatic acinus from portal area to portal area or from portal area to hepatic veins. Diseases associated with this lesion are often partially responsive to glucocorticoids or other anti-inflammatory or antifibrotic drugs. Currently, the definition of CAH is not inexorably linked to limiting plate destruction, serologic markers of autoimmune phenomenon, or a particular etiology. It does not have a sex-

ual predisposition and is associated with a wide array of etiopathogenic variables. Etiologic categories considered to evolve into CAH in humans include viral and drug-related hepatopathies; autoimmune injury; immunologic disorders; metabolic disorders including copper storage hepatopathy, α-1-antitrypsin deficiency, and hemochromatosis; biliary tract disease and pancreatitis-related hepatopathies; and inflammatory bowel disease. Some of these categories also are recognized in animals. In this chapter, *chronic hepatitis* is used rather than the term *CAH*. Chronic hepatitis should not be mistaken for "reactive hepatitis," a change characterized by mild mononuclear infiltrates in the periportal area, minor foci of liver cell necrosis associated with small infiltrates of leukocytes, and increased numbers of Kupffer cells and mild hepatocellular vacuolar change. This is a common morphologic hepatic reaction seen with clinically significant extrahepatic disease processes, particularly disorders of the gastrointestinal tract.[10]

Table 33–1

TERMINOLOGY APPLIED TO HEPATITIS

Inflammatory Hepatopathies	Noninflammatory Hepatopathies/ Idiopathic Hepatic Fibrosis
Acute hepatitis	
Nonspecific reactive hepatitis	Lobular dissecting hepatitis
Chronic persistent hepatitis	Perivenular fibrosis
Chronic active hepatitis	Veno-occlusive disease
Chronic aggressive hepatitis	Perisinusoidal fibrosis
Chronic hepatitis	Idiopathic hepatoportal fibrosis
Chronic cholangiohepatitis	Idiopathic periportal fibrosis
Chronic lobular hepatitis	
Cholangitis	
Drug-induced hepatitis	
Toxic hepatitis/hepatopathy	
Biliary cirrhosis	
Micronodular cirrhosis	
Macronodular cirrhosis	
Suppurative hepatitis	
Nonsuppurative hepatitis	

In most animals with chronic hepatitis the disease is not recognized until it is advanced. Anicteric disease is more common in the dog than in the cat. The dog is more able to eliminate bilirubin in the urine and is more commonly affected with chronic parenchymal destruction that does not lead to early compromise of bilirubin processing or excretion. The cat is more commonly afflicted with disorders causing canalicular collapse or portal triad targeted injury, classic examples including hepatic lipidosis and the cholangitis/cholangiohepatitis syndrome.

This chapter describes chronic hepatitis and its sequelae; cirrhosis, including its pathogenesis, clinical presentation, diagnostic features, and therapeutic considerations; breed-specific chronic inflammatory hepatopathies; and disorders recognized in young dogs associated with fibrosis but lacking an active inflammatory component.

NONSUPPURATIVE CHRONIC HEPATITIS

Clinical Synopsis

Diagnostic Features

- Several breed predispositions: Dobermans, Cockers, Skye terriers
- Depression, anorexia, vomiting common
- Ascites, icterus, CNS signs in later stages
- Serum ALT, AST, ALP increased
- Bilirubin often elevated; hypoalbuminemia frequent
- Liver function tests usually abnormal
- Hepatic biopsy reveals inflammation and provides pathological classification of hepatitis

Standard Management

- Attend to any identifiable cause
- Restricted to normal protein, low residue, balanced diet fed in small amounts frequently; supplemental zinc useful
- Use dairy or soy protein souece
- Prednisone 2.2 mg/kg/day 2–4 weeks, followed by 1.1 mg/kg/day for 2 weeks, followed by 0.6 mg/kg/day dose titrated to maintain remission
- Management of hepatic encephalopathy (neomycin 20 mg/kg PO q 6 to 12 h; lactulose 0.25–2 mL/kg PO q 6–12 h; saline and retention enemas)
- Management of infection: clavulanic acid-amoxicillin 11 mg/kg PO q 12/h
- Management of ascites: Sodium restriction, judicious use of spironolactone (1–2 mg/kg q 12 h PO) and furosemide; paracentesis
- Miscellaneous strategies of importance in some cases include fluid therapy; zinc therapy; copper chelation; H_2 blockers; antiemetics; vitamin K; azathioprine; ursodeoxycholic acid; colchicine (see text)

Chronic hepatitis can be responsive to treatment when recognized early. Prompt recognition is aided by use of screening chemistry profiles that reveal persistent unexplained increased liver enzyme activity. Use of total serum bile acid measurement will often prompt pursuit of a liver biopsy relatively early compared to the procrastination encouraged by sequential evaluation of abnormal enzymes. Recognition of increased serum bile acid values in the presence of unexplained significant elevations of liver enzymes indicates a high likelihood of serious active hepatic disease. Hepatitis is only diagnosed definitively through liver biopsy. The propriety of liver biopsy collection is ascertained by consideration of clinical and laboratory information and procedural risks. These are discussed in detail in Chapter 8.

Etiopathogenesis

Hepatitis can be primary or secondary to disease in other organ systems. Primary hepatitis is caused by viral and microbial infections, exposure to drugs, toxins, and endotoxins delivered through the portal circulation, and immune responses. Unfortunately, in many cases, the underlying cause is never established. Secondary hepatitis occurs with systemic infections, disseminated neoplasia, or pathology in other major organ systems (cardiovascular, gastrointestinal, urogenital, and endocrine systems, and the pancreas).

Viral infections are a well-documented cause of hepatitis in humans and animals. In humans, viral infections are so common that serologic investigation for specific etiologic agents and their antibodies have become routine clinical tests. In dogs, the canine infectious hepatitis virus (canine adenovirus I: CAV I) is a well-established cause of acute hepatitis. Experimental infection of dogs partially immune to the virus can lead to chronic hepatitis.[11] In a more recent study, immunohistochemical staining of liver tissue from dogs with various types of liver disease demonstrated the presence of the canine adenovirus antigen; a relationship between latent virus and hepatic disease was proposed.[12] A transmissible agent described in Great Britain[13,14] was shown to induce acute hepatitis, chronic hepatitis, and cirrhosis in infected dogs. The index cases were recognized in a region with an exceptionally high incidence of hepatocellular carcinoma in dogs. The suggested name was "acidophil cell hepatitis" based on consistent findings of a strongly acidophilic cytoplasm in hepatocytes of infected dogs. An infectious etiology was proposed but has not yet been proven. Anecdotal reports of viral particles found on ultrastructural examination of liver tissue suggest that other viruses are probably also involved with hepatitis in dogs. In cats, the feline infectious peritonitis virus is a well-documented cause of hepatitis. This coronavirus damages liver tissue through host immune response against the virus.[15] The feline immunodeficiency virus (FIV) or FeLV have not been specifically linked to liver-directed injury other than as a result of patient immunosuppression and propensity for infection and neoplasia. Dogs and other animals have been shown to have serum antibodies against hepatitis B, a deadly human hepatitis virus.[16] A nonpathologic, short-lived infection was postulated by one author, but little is known about this specific phenomenon.

Bacterial infections can also lead to chronic hepatitis. Chronic hepatitis has been experimentally produced by infection with leptospires in dogs.[17] Clinical cases of leptospirosis-associated chronic hepatitis are rarely documented. Certain strains of leptospirosis seem to be more pathologic for the liver in spontaneous infection; these include *icterohaemorrhagiae* and *canicola*.

Mycotic infections can lead to chronic granulomatous hepatitis. These are usually seen in dogs with systemic infection where the reticuloendothelial system of the liver is invaded. A similar reaction is seen with disseminated mycobacterial infection.

Many different drugs, metals, and chemicals can cause acute and chronic hepatitis. Hepatoinjurious agents and their pathophysiologic mechanisms are discussed in Chapters 30 and 32. When an adverse reaction is first recognized, withdrawal of the offensive agent may result in complete resolution of liver injury. If injury has damaged the structural support of the acinar unit, regenerative nodules and residual fibrosis will permanently distort the hepatic architecture, and in some cases, a self-sustaining inflammatory reaction may become established.

Immune mechanisms are central to the etiopathogenesis of chronic hepatitis.[18–33] The predominant inflammatory cells involved are the lymphocyte and plasma cell. The presence of these cells supports the contention that continued tissue inflammation has an immune-mediated pathogenesis as depicted in Figure 33–1.[18,19,21] These immunocytes can produce cells that are (1) directly cytotoxic for hepatocytes or biliary epithelium, (2) mount an antibody-mediated cytotoxic response, (3) produce antibodies enabling formation of complement-fixing antigen-antibody complexes, and (4) release cytokines that are injurious or recruit other inflammatory cells to the area. Early experimental work demonstrated that immunocytes infiltrating the liver can synthesize antibodies directed against liver-specific antigens.[19] Large numbers of lymphocytes and plasma cells found in biopsies from patients with chronic hepatitis may reflect in situ formation of antibodies against liver-specific antigens or activity of cytotoxic lymphocytes.[19,23,24–26]

Antiorganelle immune responses are well described in humans with chronic liver disorders, and in some cases serve as important criterion of disease classification. Abnormal immunoreactivity has been shown to be related to impaired suppressor cell activity.[34] Development of antibodies against smooth muscle, nuclear histones, DNA, or mitochondria do not perpetuate injury to hepatocytes because these antigens are hidden within the confines of the cell membrane. Rather, these are nonspecific markers of immune response to cellular

components released during tissue injury. These are associated with injury to a large number of tissues and have been found among a breadth of animal species. Chronic hepatitis in dogs has been seen in association with immune-mediated disorders such as hemolytic anemia, glomerulonephritis, systemic lupus erythematosis, polyarthritis, and inflammatory bowel disease, suggesting that some immunoinjurious conditions exist in which abnormal responses become more generalized. Immunoinjury precipitated by disturbed patient immunoreactivity was described in one dog treated with a biologic response modifier (*Corynebacterium parvum* immunotherapy) that developed glomerulonephritis, chronic hepatitis, and hepatic cirrhosis.[35] Remission of active injury was seen upon discontinuation of the immunoadjuvant. This example, a large amount of experimental evidence, and clinical studies of human patients suggest that restoring normalcy to the immune system has therapeutic value in the patient with chronic hepatitis.

Immunologic reactions against liver-specific surface antigens are believed to be integral in the perpetuation of liver injury in chronic hepatitis. This can result from exposure of normally hidden antigens within the hepatocyte membrane, alteration of normal surface antigens, or from an abnormal immune response. Involved antigenic moieties are controversial. A liver-specific lipoprotein (LSP) on the hepatocyte surface and liver membrane antigens (LMA) are believed to be involved in chronic active hepatitis in humans and in some animal models.[24,27,30] Antibodies from affected individuals have been shown to bind to the surface of intact hepatocytes in vitro. The antigenic complexity of membrane substrates is great and believed to generate a heterogenous immune response. This has led to contradictive findings among studies. Nevertheless, the pathogenetic mechanism of immunoinjury targeted to liver membrane antigens is well accepted as

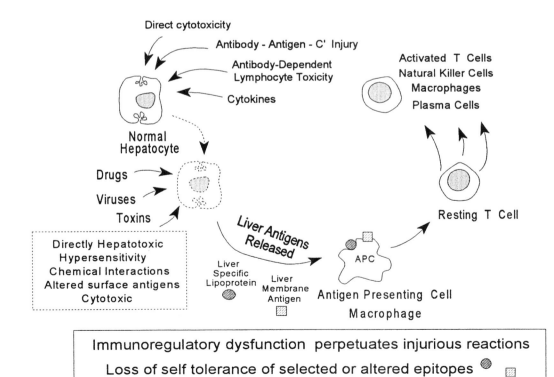

FIGURE 33–1. Diagrammatic representation of the etiopathogenic events involved with the initiation and perpetuation of chronic hepatitis.

Table 33–2

ABNORMAL IMMUNE FACTORS ASSOCIATED WITH CHRONIC HEPATITIS AND CIRRHOSIS IN HUMANS

Abnormal Response to Infectious Agents	Abnormal Ratio Helper to Suppressor T Cells	
↓ Leukocyte chemotaxis	Insufficient regulation of B cells	
↓ Phagocytosis	Polyclonal hyperglobulinemia	
↓ Complement	↑ antibody titers to infectious agents	
↓ Opsonization	Familial tendency (heritable predisposition)	
↓ Bactericidal activity against *E. coli*	Autoantibody formation:	
	ANA	Liver-Specific Lipoprotein (LSP)
	Double-stranded DNA	membrane antigen
	Antimicrosomal	not species specific protein,
	Antithyroid	lecithin sphingomyelin, fatty acids,
	Anti-smooth muscle (actin)	and cholesterol
	Bowel antigens	Liver Membrane Antigen (LMA)
	Fecal antigens	determinants differ from LSP

the basis for perpetuation of nonsuppurative chronic hepatic inflammation. A multitude of abnormalities in immune response have been shown in humans with different types of chronic hepatitis (Table 33–2). These may be causal to the hepatic injury or may be epiphenomena. Autoimmmune responses develop as a result of either a primary defect in the regulatory apparatus of the immune system or a change in tissue antigenicity. Altered tissue antigenicity may develop as a consequence of inflammation. This is associated with expression of histocompatibility proteins on epithelial cells, in this case, hepatocytes or biliary epithelium. Impairing the expression of the histocompatibility proteins can suppress the host's inflammatory response and is the basis for use of ursodeoxy-

cholic acid and anti-inflammatory drugs in control of hepatic inflammation as discussed in the therapeutic section.

A retrospective survey of conditions associated with chronic hepatitis in the dog and cat shows that nearly 66% of canine cases are idiopathic, whereas nearly 75% of feline cases are associated with major disease in another organ system (Table 33–3). This information is biased in favor of more complete systemic evaluation of cats because more definitive diagnoses were attained at necropsy; necropsies were done in 75% of cats and only 33% of dogs. It is interesting that evidence of chronic renal disease is found in a substantial number of animals, perhaps reflecting another organ response to immunoinjury or infection.

Table 33–3

DISORDERS ASSOCIATED WITH HEPATITIS IN THE DOG AND CAT

CANINE HEPATITIS

Histomorphology		Definitive Organ System Disorders					
	Idiopathic	Infectious	Neoplasia	Renal	GI	Steroid	Misc
Granulomatous	9	7	2	2	—	—	—
Periportal mild to moderate	27	1	2	6	4	5	—
Periportal severe	32	3	—	2	1	1	2
Chronic	21	9	—	1	3	—	1
Chronic active	32	—	1	1	3	—	—
Mild	12	4	2	6	2	1	2
Multifocal	9	2	2	2	1	—	2
Multifocal: acute to subacute	18	9	2	—	6	1	—
Cholangiohepatitis	12	—	—	—	4	—	—
Totals	172	35	11	20	24	8	7
% of cases	63%	13%	4%	7%	9%	3%	3%

FELINE HEPATITIS

Histomorphology		Definitive Organ System Disorders					
	Idiopathic	Infectious	Neoplasia	Renal	GI	FIP	Misc
Granulomatous	5	—	—	1	1	3	—
Periportal mild to moderate	14	5	5	8	7	—	1
Periportal severe	4	1	2	2	2	—	—
Chronic	2	—	1	—	1	—	—
Diffuse: mild to moderate	—	3	1	2	1	1	—
Multifocal: acute to subacute	1	5	5	4	1	3	1
Multifocal: acute to severe	—	5	—	—	2	—	—
Cholangiohepatitis	7	—	3	9	7	—	—
Totals	33	19	17	26	22	7	3
% of cases	26%	15%	13%	20%	17%	6%	2%

Courtesy of Small Animal Clinic, College of Veterinary Medicine, University of California at Davis, Davis, CA.

Signs consistent with inflammatory bowel disease and/or pancreatitis are frequently recognized in patients with secondary chronic hepatitis and moderate to severe involvement of the portal triad. Experimentally, immunization with intestinal antigens has been shown to cause inflammatory changes throughout the portal tracts.[26,36–38] In humans with inflammatory bowel disease the frequency of hepatic involvement ranges from 10% up to 83% depending on the type of histologic change recorded.[26] As would be expected, increased serum enzyme activity is more common than significant changes in liver function and histomorphology. The association of inflammatory bowel disease and cholangiohepatitis lesions is discussed in detail in Chapter 37.

Hepatic injury following bile duct obstruction is initially characterized by mixed suppurative/nonsuppurative inflammation focused within the biliary system.[39,40] Inflammation initially involves the biliary epithelium and adjacent periductal tissues. With chronicity (4 to 6 weeks) it is difficult to distinguish the primary cause of the portal triad inflammation and associated fibrosis. Tissue injury is believed to develop as a result of (1) increased pressure in the biliary tree, (2) retention of noxious bile acids that injure cellular membranes, and (3) ascending or hematogenously disseminated infection that biliary obstruction seems to potentiate.[41,42]

Multifocal hepatitis is usually found associated with systemic infections or disease in other organ systems; referring to Table 33–3 this was shown in nearly 50% of dogs and in 26 of 27 cats. It is suspected that upon closer scrutiny, a similar high association with other problems would be found in dogs. Finding multifocal hepatitis on hepatic biopsy should initiate a search for systemic infection or diseases in other organ systems.

Progression of Initial Injury to Chronic Hepatitis

Initial injury to hepatocytes or biliary epithelium results in the production of cytokines and mediators that recruit inflammatory cells. These are responsible for the necrosis and fibrosis in chronic hepatitis.[43,44] In most cases, the portal area is involved first. Destruction of hepatocytes permits movement of inflammatory cells and diffusion of their cytokines and mediators into an expanding area (Figure 33–2) Inflammatory cell invasion precedes or accompanies cell necrosis; hepatocyte dropout due to necrosis creates a new space for invasion by inflammatory cells. If the space created by cellular injury collapses, it distorts acinar architecture. If the architectural framework of the acinus is preserved, regeneration is possible that will have some resemblance to a normal lobule. If the framework is destroyed, regeneration may not occur or will be so haphazard that sinusoidal circulation is irreparably altered. This can be predicted by histologic evaluation after acute necrosis by application of a reticulin stain. Inflammation causes necrosis of the hepatocytes, forming a "plate" adjacent to the portal triads (Figure 33–3). Necrosis of limiting plates signifies that portal inflammation is destroying hepatocytes.

The liver responds to necrosis by regenerating hepatocytes and bile duct epithelium. There is a great capacity for hepatic regeneration. Isolated cells may be replaced or lost portions of the acinus may be repaired by regenerative nodule formation (Figure 33–4). Regenerative nodules are often encircled by obvious fibrous septa (Figures 33–4 to 33–6). In some cases, the extent of fibrosis is not obvious on routine hematoxylin and eosin (H&E) staining, and special staining of connective tissue (Masson trichrome stain) is used to specifically mark the

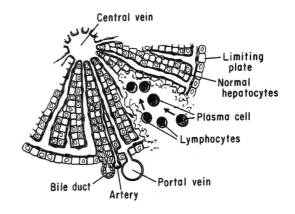

CHRONIC ACTIVE HEPATITIS

PATHOLOGY

INITIAL INSULT
↓
INFLAMMATORY CELL INFILTRATION
PORTAL AREA
↓
PLASMA CELLS AND LYMPHOCYTES
CAUSE NECROSIS OF LIMITING PLATE
↓
INFLAMMATORY PROCESS EXTENDS INTO PARENCHYMA

FIGURE 33–2. Pathology of chronic hepatitis produced by plasma cells and lymphocytes that destroy the limiting plate of hepatocytes and enter the interior of the hepatic acinus.

location of deposited collagen. Reticulin stain can also show distortion of the hepatic acinus that may not be apparent on routine staining (Figure 33–7). Initial regenerative responses in portal triad injury include proliferation of bile ductules. These are derived from specialized hepatocytes in the periportal area. Newly formed bile ductules seemingly offer another avenue for inflammatory cells to enter previously uninvolved portions of the acinus. Sometimes, bile duct proliferation is the major reparative response to hepatic injury. This results in extension of newly grown bile ducts between portal triads and, sometimes, adjacent to hepatic venules.

The pattern of necrosis establishes the histologic extension of inflammation and pattern of eventual fibrosis. Bridging portal fibrosis develops in many cases of chronic hepatitis in the dog and cat as a result of bridging necrosis and extension of inflammation from one portal triad to another. Bridging fibrosis can also extend from portal areas to the hepatic veins (zone 1 to zone 3 bridging). When associated with regenerative nodule formation and permanent distortion of the hepatic architecture, development of bridging fibrosis is classified as *cirrhosis* (Figure 33–8). *Micronodular cirrhosis* forms when fibrous septa transect acinar zones. The fibrosis may be greater in one zone than in others. Newly formed blood vessels develop in the septa, but these do not or only poorly perfuse sinusoidal channels. Blood that perfuses sinusoidal pathways is prohibited from optimal exchange with hepatocytes because of transformation of the sinusoidal endothelial cells to more closely resemble the less porous systemic capillaries. This is termed capillarization of the sinusoids and leads to intrahepatic microvascular portosystemic shunting. *Macronodular cirrhosis* develops when fibrous septa divide the liver

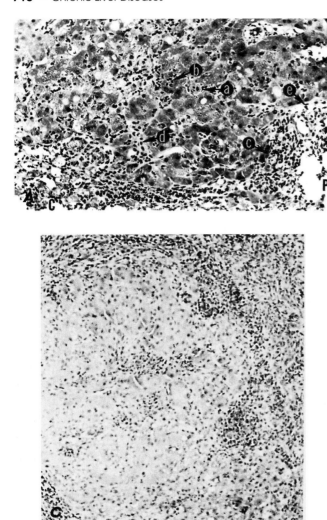

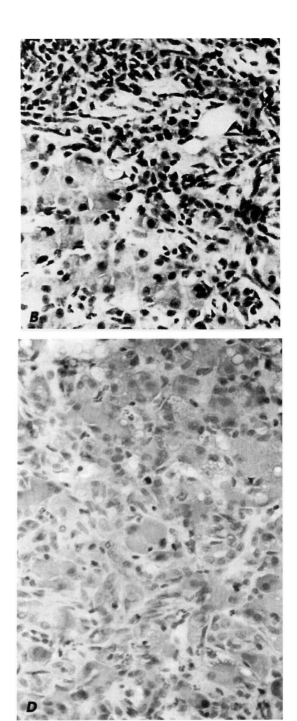

FIGURE 33–3. Photomicrographs of biopsy specimens from liver of dogs with chronic hepatitis. In (*A*), changes include necrosis of hepatocytes (a), foci of inflammation within lobule (b), and at periphery (c), and fibrosis within lobule (d) and at periphery (e). P = portal area; C = hepatic vein area (central vein). In (*B*) and (*C*), most of the inflammatory changes remain confined to the periphery of the lobule, causing so-called piecemeal necrosis of hepatocytes. In (*D*), inflammation and fibrosis are diffuse throughout the liver so that normal architecture has been lost.

into groups or clusters of acini. More than one portal tract is found within each nodule. Blood vessels in the septa surrounding nodules shunt blood away from sinusoids. In humans, micronodular cirrhosis is found in association with liver injury attributed to drug toxicity, chronic obstruction, or inflammation of the biliary tree, or impaired hepatic venous outflow. Macronodular cirrhosis is most often associated with chronic viral hepatitis and autoimmune forms of hepatitis. Regeneration of hepatocytes expands the size of regenerative nodules, compresses adjacent cell plates, and further distorts normal circulation. These events contribute to continued hepatocyte injury within nodules, and are the basis by which

macronodules evolve within micronodules. These factors promote a worsening of the liver injury even though the original insult is no longer present. Fibrosis and inflammation leading to cirrhosis can be restricted to the bile ducts and surrounding tissues. This is referred to as biliary cirrhosis (Figure 33–9), and may be initiated by periportal hepatitis resulting from a variety of insults and by chronic bile duct occlusion. Infection, drug toxicity, toxic hepatopathy, parasites, and immune-mediated injury are proposed specific causes. Advanced biliary cirrhosis may be difficult to distinguish from chronic hepatitis, especially when inflammation has extended into the interior of the hepatic lobules.

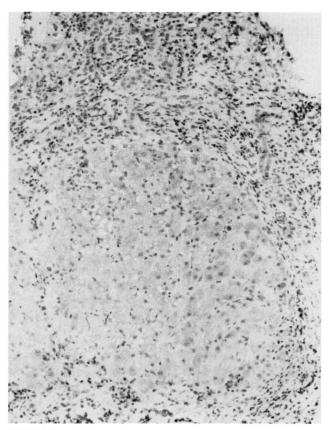

FIGURE 33-4. Photomicrograph of a biopsy specimen from a dog showing nodule of hepatocytes surrounded by inflammatory cells and fibrosis.

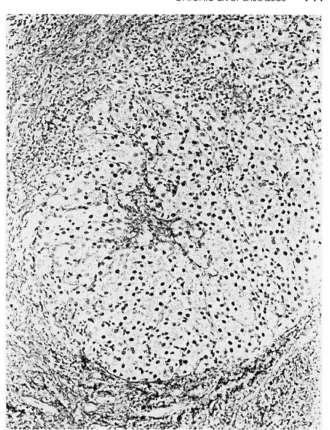

FIGURE 33-5. Photomicrograph of reticulin stain of biopsy specimen shown in Figure 33–4. The reticulin stain demonstrates the anatomic distortion and constraints imposed by encircling fibrous tissue on hepatocyte regeneration.

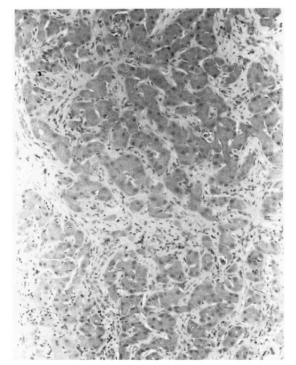

FIGURE 33-6. Photomicrograph of a biopsy specimen from a dog showing marked fibrosis that is widespread and has caused marked obvious change in the hepatic architecture. In this case, changes are easily identified on routine hematoxylin and eosin staining.

Pathophysiologic Mechanisms of Hepatic Fibrosis and Cirrhosis

The development of hepatic fibrosis is a dynamic and complex process.[45-53] It involves numerous mediators and cellular constituents and results in modification and excessive production of extracellular matrix (ECM). Extensive tissue remodeling occurs as fibrosis progresses to cirrhosis. Although the architectural changes that develop in hepatic cirrhosis have been described in detail, the pathophysiologic mechanisms leading to cirrhosis are poorly understood. This is an active area of research because elucidation of this process will permit identification of susceptible sites for effective therapeutic intervention. An overview of the interactions involved in the genesis of hepatic fibrosis is summarized in Figure 33–10.

The ECM is that conglomeration of insoluble proteins which constitutes the "ground substance" of the mesenchyme and the basement membrane of epithelia and blood vessels. In tissue sections, the ECM appears as a thin acellular layer. In health, the ECM is produced by hepatocytes and nonparenchymal cells; in hepatic fibrosis, the nonparenchymal cells dominate.[43,45,54] The ECM wields a profound influence on the cells it surrounds and supports. It is an active participant in the determination of hepatocellular function through influence on cells that abut it in the perisinusoidal space. The ECM components, laminin, fibronectin, and integrins, play important roles in cell matrix interactions. Cells

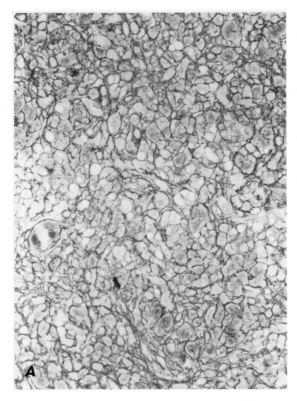

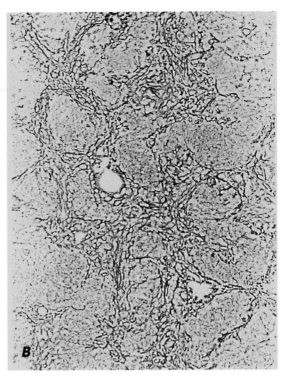

FIGURE 33-7. Photomicrographs of biopsy specimens with reticulin stains from dogs with diffuse fibrosis and sinusoidal distortion. In (*A*), the fibrosis was not apparent from routine tissue stains. Reticulin-stained preparation elucidates the sinusoidal involvement. In this specimen, the normal linear alignment of the sinusoids has been lost and interposing reticulin fibers are seen between hepatocytes. In (*B*) and (*C*), lower power magnification provides an overview perspective of the extent of lobule separation by fibrous tissue.

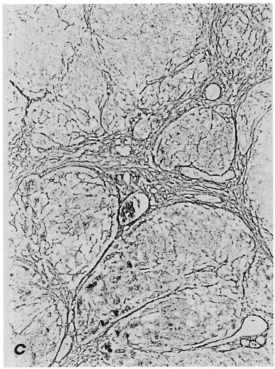

that abut the ECM sense matrix components by surface receptors. When the ECM becomes modified by disease, the phenotypic expression of its associated cells also changes.

There are three major components of the ECM: collagens, proteoglycans, and noncollagenous glycoproteins. Different tissues have different matrix components that determine form, tensile strength, and cell interactions.

Collagens are the major structural components in all tissues. A heterogenous group has been characterized including 13 distinct forms.[45,46,55] Each type of collagen is immunologically and chemically unique and can be identified using immunohistologic and molecular biologic techniques.[56–58] Collagens are comprised of subunit polypeptide chains, some with differing amino acid sequences. Most have repetitious sequences wound into a triple helix that contributes tensile strength. Collagens type I and III are common in the liver and increase in hepatic fibrosis. Intervention in collagen synthesis, secretion, or digestion are general approaches in control of fibrogenesis.

Proteoglycans are a heterogenous group of large molecules comprised of a protein core covalently bound to glycosaminoglycan side chains and oligosaccharides.[59–61] They commonly bind to hyaluronic acid and in the normal liver, heparan sulfate is the most abundant moiety. Proteoglycans are found in all connective tissues where they participate with collagens and elastin in determining matrix biomechanics. Cell surface–associated proteoglycans are believed to function in transmembrane signaling, cell adhesion, and in regulation of cell growth and differentiation. Their role in hepatic fibrosis is currently poorly understood.

Many different ECM glycoproteins have been characterized. These interact with other ECM components and bind to cell surface receptors. Fibronectin is the best known ECM gly-

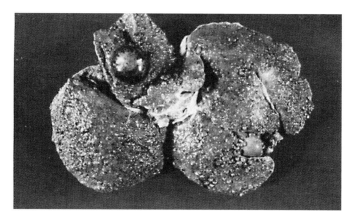

FIGURE 33-8. Gross photograph of the appearance of a cirrhotic liver as a result of chronic hepatitis.

coprotein. It is plentiful in the space of Disse in the normal liver and is believed to be derived from plasma fibronectin and fibronectin synthesized by Ito cells and sinusoidal endothelium. Fibronectin and laminin, another glycoprotein, play important roles in promoting hepatocyte regeneration. These molecules form strong bonds between cells and ECM components and are involved in the architectural changes that develop in hepatic fibrosis and cirrhosis. Fibronectin and laminin accumulate in the fibrotic liver as a result of increased production. Hepatocellular damage associated with sinusoidal capillarization is one change that stimulates laminin synthesis. Laminin is chemoattractive to neutrophils that deliver injurious enzymes. Fibronectin imparts a fibrogenic influence on hepatocytes, and a chemotactic influence on fibroblasts, smooth muscle cells, and endothelial cells.[46,49,62-64] Myofibroblasts, which synthesize and deposit collagen, may differentiate from either Ito cells or central (hepatic) vein endothelium under the influence of several different soluble mediators.

In both immune reponses and tissue wound repair, the stimulus to fibrogenesis is indirect, arising from the inflammatory infiltrate. Major constituents in progression and perpetuation of the inflammatory processes involve the local release of cytokines. The biochemical cascades involved with stimulation and release of interleukins, lymphokines, and eicosinoids are summarized in Figure 33–11; see also Chapter 3 where these mediators are discussed in relation to the gastrointestinal immune system.

Inflammatory infiltrates comprised of neutrophils and macrophages are associated with most forms of liver injury, irrespective of inititating circumstances. In some forms of injury, immune complex deposition precedes tissue damage. The ECM between parenchymal cells can serve as a depot of inflammatory mediators and immune complexes and can in this way sustain an active inflammatory condition long after the initiating event has resolved. Leukocytes migrating into an area of inflammation release lysosomal proteases and reactive radicals that disrupt the normal hepatic ECM and cellular membranes. This liberates not only prostaglandins, prostacyclin, thromboxane, and leukotrienes but also biologically active peptides that function as chemoattractants for collagen-producing cells. Transforming growth factor (TGF-beta) is the best known of a family of low molecular weight soluble factors that stimulate collagen deposition by Ito cells.[64-71] TGF-beta is produced by many cells, including Kupffer cells, lymphocytes, macrophages, and platelets. It has several additional adverse effects. It impairs hepatocyte DNA synthesis, necessary for cell repair and normal metabolism. It

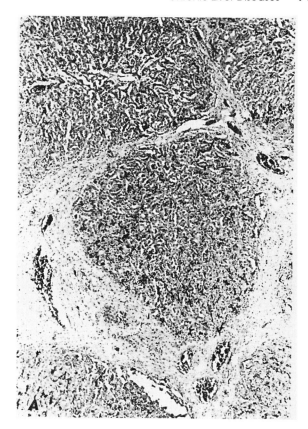

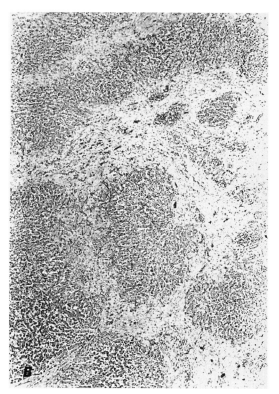

FIGURE 33-9. Photomicrograph of a liver biopsy from (*A*) a dog with diffuse biliary cirrhosis H&E and (*B*) a cat with chronic cholangitis/cholangiohepatitis that progressed to biliary cirrhosis. Large amounts of connect tissue bridge between regenerative nodules (H&E, 35× magnification).

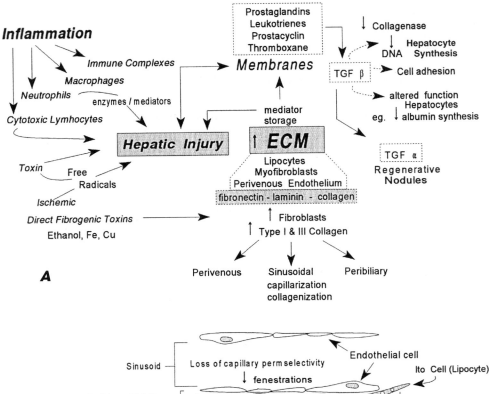

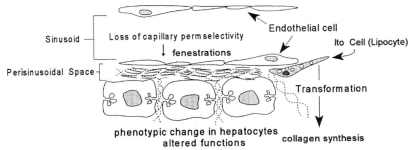

Influence of Fibrosis on the Sinusoids

B

FIGURE 33-10. Overview of the interactions involved in the generation of hepatic fibrosis in (*A*). In (*B*), the effect on the sinusoid is illustrated.

also up-regulates receptors for cell matrix adhesion and cell to cell adhesion, thus promoting development of a fibrotic network and an architecturally deranged acinus. Transformation of the lipocyte to a collagen-producing cell involves an increase in the cell's protein-synthesizing capacity, expression of receptors for platelet-derived growth factor (PDGF), and release of its normal retinoid stores. It is projected that biologic inhibition of this transformation would be beneficial for control of hepatic fibrogenesis.

As hepatic fibrosis evolves, the ECM undergoes remodeling. In early fibrosis, both collagen synthesis and collagenase activity are increased so that the processes simultaneously proceed but in separated areas. Collagenase degradation of ECM protein may promote the extension of inflammatory injury be removal of the ECM that was "holding" mediators. Degradation of ECM occurs through action of specific proteinases, the largest group being metalloproteinases.[46] As fibrosis progresses, collagen synthesis exceeds degradation; this accompanies a transition from predominantly type III collagen to type I collagen. TGF-beta seems to retard collagen degradation; this, along with its stimulatory influence on fibrogenesis, disturbs the balance between ECM synthesis and degradation, favoring collagen accumulation.

Some hepatoinjurious agents have a direct fibrogenic

effect. Examples include ethanol and excessive stores of iron and copper. In general, the role of direct fibrogenic influences is not understood and is thought to play only a minor role relative to inflammation and the cascade of events just described.

ECM in the Cirrhotic/Fibrotic Liver

In the normal liver, type I and III collagen exist in approximately equal amounts. In fibrosis, the amounts of collagen increase but the increase in type I exceeds that of type III.[46] A four- to sevenfold increase in total collagen and glycosaminoglycans occurs in the cirrhotic liver compared to normal.[72,73] Assays for detection of enzymes, metabolites, and mediators of connective tissue metabolism have been developed for assessing the activity of collagen biosynthesis in fibrogenic disorders.[74–77] Some of the enzymes and metabolites involved with fibrogenesis spill into the systemic circulation in liver disease and can be used to reflect the activity of collagen metabolism. These include serum activities of enzymes important in collagen synthesis (lysyl oxidase and prolyl hydroxylase), and concentrations of laminin, type III procollagen amino propeptide, and TGF-beta. Their use in the small animal

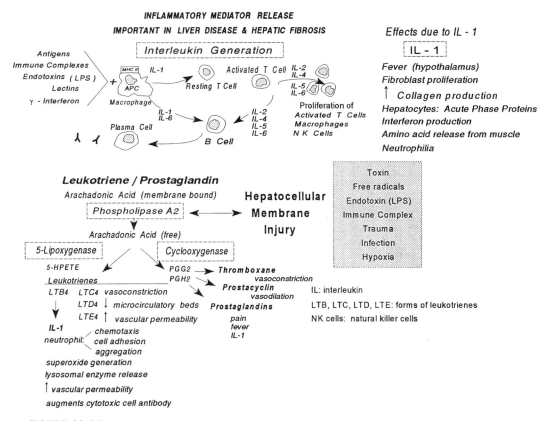

INFLAMMATORY MEDIATOR RELEASE
IMPORTANT IN LIVER DISEASE & HEPATIC FIBROSIS

Interleukin Generation

Antigens
Immune Complexes
Endotoxins (LPS)
Lectins
γ - Interferon

MHC II
APC
Macrophage
IL-1
Resting T Cell
Activated T Cell
IL-2
IL-4
IL-5
IL-6

Proliferation of
Activated T Cells
Macrophages
N K Cells

IL-1
IL-6
Plasma Cell
B Cell
IL-2
IL-4
IL-5
IL-6

Effects due to IL - 1

IL - 1

Fever (hypothalamus)
Fibroblast proliferation
↑ Collagen production
Hepatocytes: Acute Phase Proteins
Interferon production
Amino acid release from muscle
Neutrophilia

Leukotriene / Prostaglandin

Arachadonic Acid (membrane bound)

Phospholipase A2 ◄──► **Hepatocellular Membrane Injury**

Arachadonic Acid (free)

5-Lipoxygenase   Cyclooxygenase

5-HPETE   PGG2 ──► **Thromboxane**
Leukotrienes   PGH2   vasoconstriction
LTB4 LTC4 vasoconstriction   **Prostacyclin**
       LTD4 ↓ microcirculatory beds   vasodilation
       LTE4 ↑ vascular permeability **Prostaglandins**
IL-1   pain
neutrophil: chemotaxis   fever
         cell adhesion   IL-1
         aggregation
superoxide generation
lysosomal enzyme release
↑ vascular permeability
augments cytotoxic cell antibody

Toxin
Free radicals
Endotoxin (LPS)
Immune Complex
Trauma
Infection
Hypoxia

IL: interleukin
LTB, LTC, LTD, LTE: forms of leukotrienes
NK cells: natural killer cells

FIGURE 33–11. Biochemical cascades involved with stimulation and release of lymphokines, interleukins, and eicosinoids, and their interactions.

patient has not yet been well investigated. A radioimmunoassay kit for detection of type III procollagen peptide in humans was shown not to be valid in the dog.[78]

As the ECM is modified, the functional capabilities of the hepatocyte changes. For example, hepatocytes grown on type I or IV collagen lose the ability to produce albumin. This change in hepatocyte function may be reflected in clinicopathologic parameters used to appraise liver health or function. As cirrhosis develops, changes in the blood vessels, sinusoidal continuity, and phenotypic behavior of parenchymal and perisinusoidal cells occur simultaneously. The development of regenerative nodules is encouraged by TGF-beta, and these impair parenchymal cell sinusoidal orientation and perfusion. As fibrosis progresses, large bundles of collagen fibers accumulate and limit the distensibility of vascular pathways in sinusoids, portal veins, or hepatic veins and cause resistance to blood flow (Figure 33–12). Increase in fibrillar collagen beneath hepatocytes may also impair sinusoidal blood flow. Elastin increases in the walls of arteries, creating a barrier and occupying space. Alteration in the permselectivity of the specialized sinusoidal endothelial fenestrae also develops. This alteration makes the sinusoids function more like

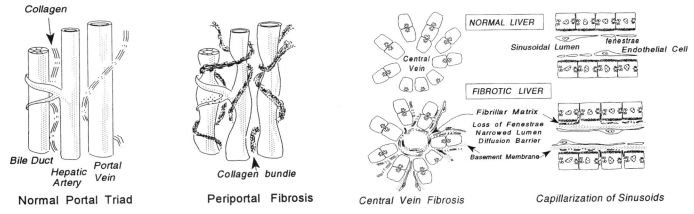

Collagen

Bile Duct
Hepatic Artery
Portal Vein
Normal Portal Triad

Collagen bundle
Periportal Fibrosis

Central Vein
Central Vein Fibrosis

NORMAL LIVER
Sinusoidal Lumen   fenestrae
Endothelial Cell

FIBROTIC LIVER
Fibrillar Matrix
Loss of Fenestrae
Narrowed Lumen
Diffusion Barrier
Basement Membrane
Capillarization of Sinusoids

FIGURE 33–12. Diagrammatic representation of the direct mechanisms impairing normal hepatic perfusion in the patient with extensive hepatic fibrosis and cirrhosis. Adapted from reference 46.

typical systemic capillaries and is termed *capillarization*,[79-81] and it markedly alters the availability of oxygen and nutrients to hepatocytes and impairs metabolite exchange with sinusoidal blood. Oxygen consumption is reduced in cirrhosis as is effective delivery of oxygen to hepatocytes.[82-84] This may be critical for some patients because even a small reduction in hepatic oxygen delivery can impair elimination of substances metabolized by enzyme systems that directly use oxygen.[85-94] Lack of oxygen has far-reaching consequences and should be considered when formulating a therapeutic plan for the critically ill patient with hepatic cirrhosis that for some reason has undergone acute decompensation.

Chronology of Hepatic Fibrosis and Its Potential for Resolution

The length of time it takes to develop substantial fibrosis is widely variable depending on the causal event or agent; reported intervals for various pathogenic mechanisms are given in Table 33–4.[40,95-105] The noxious effect of toxins reliant on bioactivation to yield a reactive metabolite or toxic moiety can be augmented by activation of the mixed function oxidases. For example, rats given carbon tetrachloride develop an irreversible condition with a four- to fivefold increase in collagen within 20 weeks and pretreatment with phenobarbital accelerates the process twofold.[95]

In experimental models, removal of an injurious agent at a critical interval can result in resolution of hepatic fibrosis.[95,104] For example, the hepatic fibrosis caused by administration of carbon tetrachloride to rats for 14 weeks can completely resolve over 3 months.[95] Regression of periportal fibrosis after resolution of neonatal and acquired extrahepatic bile duct occlusion has been occasionally reported in humans.[106-108] Resolution of true cirrhosis is rare however.[43]

One of the major reasons cirrhosis is unresolvable is that the predominant type of collagen which accumulates is type I. This type of collagen is not as susceptible to in vitro collagenase activity as type III collagen, which is more prevalent in early fibrosis. In addition, once cirrhosis is well established, the inherent production of tissue collagenase declines.[109,110]

Severe hepatic necrosis that is acute and self-limiting, up to the extent of massive necrosis, rarely leads to cirrhosis.[94] Early diagnosis and provision of supportive care can permit regeneration and preservation of nearly normal structure.

Clinical Features

Hepatitis is an insidious malady because the associated clinical signs often do not draw attention to the hepatobiliary system until a diffuse and well-established pathologic process has developed. The following discussion of hepatitis in the dog and cat is distinct from the descriptions for the cirrhotic patient that follow and the discussion of the feline cholangitis/cholangiohepatitis syndrome presented in Chapter 37.

The average age of presentation of dogs with chronic hepatitis ranges between 4 to 7 years.[3,5,9,111,112] Particular breeds of dogs seem to have an increased incidence of chronic hepatitis (see Table 33–5). The primary clinical signs of chronic hepatitis in both dogs and cats include lethargy, anorexia, and vomiting. The estimated frequency of signs demonstrated by dogs is shown in Table 33–6. A small number of dogs with chronic hepatitis show no clinical signs. That is often true in cats, where jaundice often appears following only intermittent anorexia or vomiting. Some cats with chronic cholangiohepatitis may become polyphagic, which may be related to malassimilation.

Palpation of the abdomen of a dog with chronic hepatitis is usually unremarkable. A small liver may exist but will not be detected by physical assessment. Compared to dogs, cats with liver disease usually have an easily palpable liver. The differential diagnosis for alterations in hepatic size are provided in Table 8–3. When chronic hepatitis is not recognized early, the number of patients presented with the primary complaint of ascites increases. In these animals ascites may be initially detected by ballottement of an abdominal fluid wave or is discovered during abdominal radiography or ultrasonography.

Table 33–4

TIME OF DEVELOPMENT OF HEPATIC FIBROSIS/CIRRHOSIS IN DIFFERENT SPECIES

MECHANISMS	SPECIES	LESION	FIBROSIS	CIRRHOSIS
Toxin				
CCl₄	Rats	Zone 3[a]	> 6 weeks	> 12 weeks
		Bridging zone 1 to zone 3		
CCl₄ and phenobarbital	Rats	same	> 1–2 weeks	> 4 weeks
Dimethylnitrosamine	Dogs	Bridging zone 3 to zone 1[b]	> 3–4 weeks	> 13 weeks
Immunologic				
Heterologous serum	Rats	Periportal[c]	> 5 weeks	> 10 weeks
Bacterial cell wall	Rats	Periportal[d]	> 6 weeks	—
		Bridging zone 3 to zone 1		
Murine schistosomiasis	Mice	Periportal[e]		
		granulomatous	> 6 weeks	—
Endotoxin	Mice	Rabbits[f]	—	> 9 days
Biliary Obstruction				
Mechanical ligation	Dogs	Periportal	> 4 weeks	> 12 weeks
	Cats	Periportal	> 5 weeks	> 5 weeks
Spontaneous	Humans	Periportal	—	> 12 weeks

[a] 0.1–0.2 mL/100 g body weight twice weekly, or inhalation twice weekly.
[b] 2.0–2.5 mg/kg twice weekly, PO.
[c] Swine sera given intraperitoneally 150–200 mg/g twice weekly.
[d] Single intraperitoneal injection 20 mg/g body weight.
[e] 50 cercariae given subcutaneously.
[f] *E. coli* into portal vein, then 24 hours later systemically IV, 0.1 mg total.
Data derived from reference 105 and others.

Table 33–5

BREEDS OF DOGS WITH INCREASED INCIDENCE
OF CHRONIC HEPATITIS

Doberman pinscher	Beagle
Cocker spaniel	Labrador retriever
Bedlington terrier	German shepherd dog
West Highland white terrier	Standard poodle

Table 33–6

FREQUENCY OF CLINICAL SIGNS IN DOGS
WITH CHRONIC HEPATITIS

Lethargy	>50%	Seizures	10–20%
Vomiting	40–50%	Polydipsia	10–15%
Weight loss	30–40%	Fever	10–15%
Weakness	20–30%	Bleeding	10–15%
Diarrhea	20–30%	CNS signs	5–10%
Ascites	15–25%	No signs	5–10%
Icterus	15–25%		

Ascites formation is rare in the cat with chronic hepatitis and usually indicates a grave prognosis. The abdominal effusion of dogs with ascites may fluctuate in severity for months to years.

Clinicopathologic Features of Hepatitis

Clinicopathologic features of hepatitis vary with the severity of tissue involvement and the histologic region of organ injury. Considering the broad range of histologic injuries, the most sensitive test during active disease is determination of the serum enzyme activities. The mean values and ranges for clinicopathologic tests in dogs and cats with chronic hepatitis are shown in Figure 33–13.

In dogs with chronic hepatitis, serum ALT, AST, and ALP activities are almost always increased. Mean ALT activities increase from 5 to 18 times the upper limit of normal; ALT is abnormal in more than 90% of affected dogs. In cats with chronic hepatitis, plasma ALT, AST, and/or gamma-GT are almost always increased. The mean ALP activities are increased from two- to fivefold the upper limit of normal in more than 85% of affected dogs. The serum ALP activity may not increase in cats with hepatitis unless there is substantial biliary or periportal inflammation.

Other clinicopathologic abnormalities in dogs with chronic hepatitis include hypoalbuminemia in approximately 40% and hypergammaglobulinemia in 25%. Evaluation of the coagulation status shows an abnormally pro-

longed prothrombin time in 36% and a prolonged partial thromboplastin time in approximately 60%. A prolonged prothrombin time has been shown to predict early death in affected dogs.[112] In cats, approximately 40% develop hypoalbuminemia and more than 50% become hyperglobulinemic. There are no dependable trends in the total serum cholesterol concentration in either species unless chronic hepatitis is severe. In the circumstance of hepatic failure, hypocholesterolemia may develop in both dogs and cats. Abnormalities of the blood glucose concentration are not reliable indicators of chronic hepatitis unless end-stage liver disease or portosystemic shunting has developed. In that circumstance, hypoglycemia may develop in dogs, but is relatively rare in cats. Dogs that present with hypoglycemia have a poor prognosis; a recent report characterized this clinicopathologic feature with failure to survive the first week after diagnosis.[112]

Jaundice develops in animals early when the primary lesion is focused on the portal triad. This is often the case in dogs and cats with cholangiohepatitis. Experimentally, dogs with necrotic lesions confined to the periportal hepatocytes readily become icteric[113] whereas necrosis of other parts of the lobule must be extensive before jaundice appears. Periportal inflammation causes cholestasis by obstruction of bile flow in bile ductules entering the portal area and also causes canalicular injury.

Clinicopathologic Features of Chronic Hepatitis

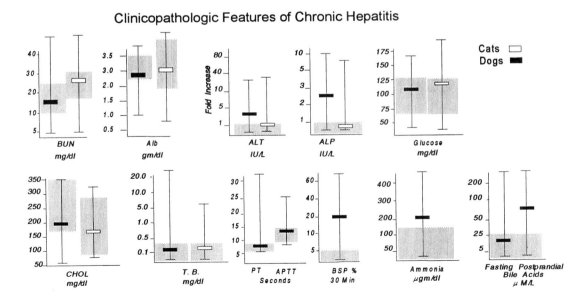

FIGURE 33–13. Clinicopathologic features of dogs and cats with chronic hepatitis, showing median, mean, and ranges. Data derived from the College of Veterinary Medicine, University of California, Davis, CA.

Estimation of liver function should be done when an animal is not overtly jaundiced and the severity of the hepatobiliary disorder is in question. Mean sulfobromophthalein (BSP) retention percentage is increased in approximately 95% of dogs with chronic hepatitis.

Baseline hyperammonemia has been detected in 54% of unfed dogs with chronic hepatitis. Ammonia intolerance is demonstrable in more than 90% when an ammonia chloride tolerance test is performed. The presence of ammonia intolerance cannot be used to predict a prognosis.[112]

Total fasting and/or postprandial bile acid concentrations are usually abnormal in dogs with chronic hepatitis. In a recent study of chronic hepatic disease in dogs intoxicated with dinitrosamines, the serum bile acids and ammonia tolerance became abnormal at the same stage of morphologic injury as did the plasma BSP retention. The serum bilirubin concentration lagged behind these function tests, becoming abnormal only with more advanced injury.[114] The sensitivity of combined pre- and post-prandial bile acids in dogs with chronic hepatitis is nearly 89%, but it has not yet been adequately evaluated in cats due to the high frequency of jaundice and the clinical lack of a need for serum bile acid analysis. The sensitivity of serum bile acids compared to other clinicopathologic tests used in the detection of chronic hepatitis in the dog and cat is shown in Figure 33–14.

Diagnosis

Diagnosis of chronic hepatitis requires acquisition of an hepatic biopsy. Polymorphonuclear leukocytes are usually not abundant and when present usually reflect the extent of necrosis. Macrophages are seen in small numbers and in proportion to the amount of necrosis. Nodular regeneration is common. Semiquantitative copper staining may subjectively disclose the presence of increased copper stores in hepatocytes. If this is suspected, tissue should be submitted for quantitative copper analysis in order to determine whether copper storage is a contributing factor to the hepatic disease. In Doberman pinschers and some other dogs, increased Kupffer cell iron stores may be seen and quantitative iron determination will reveal high values. The significance of the finding of Kupffer cell iron stores and its relation to the etiopathogenesis of chronic hepatitis is not understood. It likely is merely an epiphenomenon of the inflammation.

Hepatic fibrosis increases with chronicity and intensity of the inflammatory lesions. The severity of fibrosis and necrosis has been shown to correlate with a poor survival prognosis.[112] Cirrhosis is diagnosed when the lobular architecture is irreparably altered with bridging fibrosis and regenerative nodule formation has distorted the normal hepatic anatomy. Lesions suggestive of a glucocorticoid or vacuolar hepatopathy may be seen in the chronically ill dog and is expected in dogs treated with glucocorticoids.

Cytologic evaluation of a biopsy specimen should always be done. Impression smears of the tissue are stained with a modified Wright's Giemsa for rapid evaluation; a Diff Quik stain is adequate. Observing large numbers of neutrophils or bacterial organisms should initiate submission of aerobic and anerobic bacterial cultures. The patient should be immediately started on bactericidal antimicrobials if sepsis is possible. A specimen of liver should be reserved for metal analysis (copper and iron) and for special stains should they be indicated. See Chapter 8 for a discussion of optimal utilization of a liver biopsy.

Management

Treatment of primary chronic hepatitis is directed at arresting inflammation, correcting metabolic derangements, and resolving fibrosis. Management of secondary hepatitis is directed at the primary problem with the expectation the hepatitis will resolve once the initiating illness is under control. However, this is usually not the case and so supportive care is offered appropriate for the extent of hepatic dysfunction. No therapy for chronic hepatitis in animals has been rigidly evaluated for effectiveness.

It is currently believed that affected animals will benefit from nutritional modifications and interventional drug therapy aimed at resolution of inflammation and ongoing collagen deposition. This is based on the extensive collective information available from human studies and of dogs as experimental models of liver disease. The benefits and risks of treatment with glucocorticoids and other immunomodulatory and antifibrotic agents are addressed in the treatment section that follows discussion of hepatic cirrhosis. Such treatment is only offered once a diagnosis of chronic hepatitis has been confirmed by tissue biopsy examination. It is important to differentiate between patients with acute and chronic hepatitis. Only the latter group should receive anti-inflammatory drugs to modulate their disease, and their nutritional management can be quite different (see Chapter 32) to that of patients with acute disease.

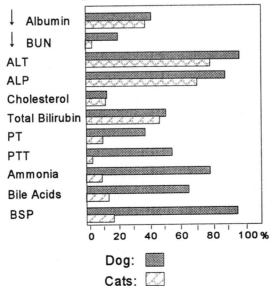

Sensitivity of Clinical Tests in Diagnosis of Chronic Hepatitis

Dog:
Cats:

FIGURE 33–14. Sensitivity of different clinicopathologic tests in the diagnosis of chronic hepatitis in the dog and cat.

CIRRHOSIS

Cirrhosis is the end result of many different chronic liver disorders. Although it is considered irreversible, eradication or control of etiopathogenic mechanisms may the limit its progression. The consequences of cirrhosis include a diversity of abnormalities. Vascular disturbances may impair portal venous inflow, hepatic venous outflow, or cause intrahepatic portosystemic shunting. *Collagenization* and *capillarization* of the hepatic sinusoids impair the vital exchange of metabolites, nutrients, and toxins between blood and hepatocytes. Portal venous hypertension may develop due to presinusoidal, sinusoidal, or postsinusoidal alterations in intrahepatic circulation. Extrahepatic portosystemic collaterals open, providing new hepatofugal pathways for the splanchnic circulation. Ascites may develop when hypertension, hypoalbuminemia, and impaired sodium and water regulation coexist. Impaired synthetic, regulatory, storage, and detoxification functions of the liver lead to the development of many different constitutional signs and clinicopathologic abnormalities.

HISTOLOGIC DEFINITION. Cirrhosis is defined as a diffuse process characterized by both fibrosis and the conversion of normal architecture into structurally abnormal nodules (regenerative nodules).[115] The mere presence of excessive fibrous tissue is not sufficient for a diagnosis of hepatic cirrhosis. As discussed later in this chapter, there are disorders of the liver associated with excessive fibrosis in the absence of cirrhosis. Cirrhosis is difficult to confirm by needle biopsy unless multiple samples are acquired to demonstrate that the characteristic lesions are widespread. For this reason in human medicine, there is general consensus that a biopsy sample should be at least 2 cm in length to optimize histologic interpretation. In addition, clinicopathologic manifestations and/or ultrasonographic imaging usually assist in determining that a process is diffuse (Figures 33–15 and 33–16). Ultrasonography may disclose the presence of nodular areas and an irregular liver margin. Gross inspection of the liver during laparotomy or laparoscopy permits direct appraisal.

A diagnosis of cirrhosis implies an abnormality in blood flow within the liver. Histopathologic examination demonstrates architectural changes that impair normal acinar perfusion. Direct and indirect mechanisms whereby hepatic fibrosis impairs normal circulation and promotes portal hypertension have been identified. Direct mechanisms include (1) compression of portal vessels by fibrous bands, (2) excessive deposition of extracellular matrix (ECM) in the space of Disse, and (3) perivenous fibrosis. These changes are diagrammatically illustrated in Figure 33–12.[46] Indirect mechanisms include the influence of expanding regenerative nodules against liver tissue that has become less malleable owing to collagen deposition and the effect of hepatocellular swelling within a space limited by fibrous septa and confined by a nondistensible hepatic capsule.

Clinical Features

The clinical features displayed by the cirrhotic animal depend on the underlying cause of the liver injury, whether it persists or not, and the presence or absence of portal hypertension and hepatocellular failure. Some animals are presented in the acute stage of cirrhosis, others present with occult cirrhosis; or after they have undergone an acute decompensation and are in fulminant hepatic failure.

Clinical signs associated with hepatic cirrhosis are highly variable; those seen in dogs are summarized in Table 33–7. Compared to dogs with chronic hepatitis, there usually are tangible signs of illness when cirrhosis develops. Nevertheless, animals are vaguely ill and a wide differential diagnostic list is considered possible initially.

The clinicopathologic features of dogs with cirrhosis presenting with portal hypertension and abdominal effusion are summarized in Figure 33–17. Most dogs have a normal hematocrit but approximately 50% have microcytic erythrocytes. The WBC is often in the normal range and a stress leukogram

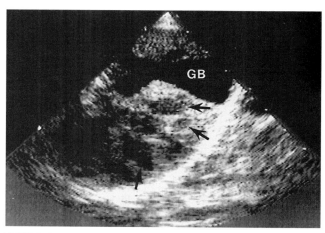

FIGURE 33–15. Ultrasonogram showing the nodular appearance (arrows) of the liver of a dog with macronodular cirrhosis. Regenerative nodules (arrows) are hypoechoic compared to the general hyperechogenicity of the hepatic parenchyma. The nodules are less than 1 cm in diameter. Gallbladder = GB. (Courtesy Dr. A. Yeager, Section of Radiology, Department of Clinical Sciences, Cornell University)

is common. A neutrophilic leukocytosis develops in some dogs with infections or inflammatory processes in other organ systems that have contributed to their clinical decompensation. Despite the common complaints of polyuria and polydipsia, few dogs present with hyposthenuric urine typical of water diuresis. Many present with minimally concentrated urine considering their dehydrated status. Few dogs demonstrate ammonium biurate crystalluria on initial urine sediment examination. In the patient with ascites, a subnormal BUN is less common than in the cirrhotic patient without ascites. This may be related to compromised renal perfusion due to the shift in Starling forces and perhaps is a manifestation of the hepatorenal syndrome in some dogs. The hepatorenal syndrome is a unique complication of cirrhosis identified in humans and is only seen in patients with ascites. Many of these dogs demonstrate melena or hematemesis; gastroenteric bleeding may have increased their BUN concentration disproportionate to their serum creatinine. Of interest is the very low creatinine seen in approximately 28% of dogs. This may be related to a combination effect of reduced muscle mass and diuresis. As expected in this subset of dogs, 75% have a subnormal albumin concentration. Of interest is an observed

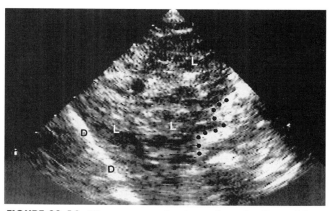

FIGURE 33–16. Ultrasonogram showing an irregular "bumpy" border on the caudal margin of the liver (black dots delineate the irregular margin) in a dog with hepatic cirrhosis. L = liver, D = diaphragm. (Courtesy Dr. A. Yeager, Section of Radiology, Department of Clinical Sciences, Cornell University)

Table 33–7

CLINICAL SIGNS SHOWN BY DOGS
WITH CIRRHOSIS

Lethargy	Ascites with abdominal distension
Anorexia	Edema (rare)
Vomiting	Hepatic encephalopathy
Weight loss	Ammonium biurates:
Polydipsia/polyuria	crystalluria
Poor hair coat	hematuria
Jaundice	pollakiuria
Weakness	obstructive uropathy
Melena	Drug intolerances:
Fever	barbiturates phenothiazines
Bleeding tendencies	aminophylline benzodiazepines
Microhepatica	narcotics anticonvulsants
Splenomegaly	antihistamines

tendency for low globulin concentrations considering the immunogenic stimuli assumed to be present in these dogs. Low globulins may reflect protein-losing enteropathy associated with portal hypertension or synthetic failure of hepatic origin acute-phase proteins. Sequestration of globulins within the ascitic fluid is unlikely because most dogs have a pure transudate. The activity of serum enzymes cannot be relied on to indicate the presence of serious liver disease in these patients. Some dogs have only minor enzyme activity and some have quiescent disease. Increased enzyme activity indicates the presence of active inflammation and adequate surviving hepatocytes to provide a source of enzyme for release. Approximately 50% of dogs with ascites and cirrhosis have very low serum cholesterol concentrations. This finding coupled with microcytosis should markedly increase the clinical suspicion of hepatoportal shunting. The low cholesterol is considered to be due to synthetic failure as well as possible fat malabsorption due to portal hypertension and altered enteric microcirculation. Up to 20% of dogs with cirrhosis and ascites have a normal bilirubin concentration. Many of these dogs have normal or slightly increased liver enzyme activities and may be in a compensated quiescent stage of disease. Evaluation of the coagulation status reveals an increased APTT more commonly than an abnormal PT. The most common abnormality is hypofibrinogenemia. Only 30% have moderately increased FDP values. A substantial number of these dogs are thrombocytopenic. Consideration of all abnormalities together suggests the presence of DIC. However, few dogs have schistocytes or acanthocytes on peripheral blood smears. The low fibrinogen could be due to synthetic failure rather than a consumptive coagulopathy and this may contribute to the low FDPs. Approximately 25% of affected dogs have splenomegaly. It is unknown if this contributes to the low platelets as has been shown in humans with cirrhosis and portal hypertension. Most dogs in which a BSP retention test has been done have abnormal values. Serum bile acids measured after a 12 hour fast may be normal. Two hours after a meal they are usually profoundly abnormal and often display a "shunting" pattern.

Compared to the dog with chronic liver disease, cirrhosis in the cat is relatively uncommon. Affected cats may have a normal or large liver whereas most dogs develop microhepatica. Weight loss due to intermittent anorexia is common. Diarrhea and constipation are frequent complicating problems and may reflect the underlying primary health problem that led to cirrhosis, namely, inflammatory bowel disease or chronic absorption of colonic toxins. Jaundice is more common in the cirrhotic cat than in the dog. In contrast, development of ascites seems more common in the dog than in the cat, although at least 50% of the dogs with cirrhosis do not initially present with ascites. Systemic disorders and hepatic diseases leading to cirrhosis in the dog and cat are provided in Table 33–8. Hepatic disorders evolving into cirrhosis in the cat are focused on the portal areas, specifically the bile ducts. Comparatively, hepatic disorders in the dog are more diverse in anatomic orientation.

The prognosis of the patient with cirrhosis varies with the intensity of the clinical effort in providing supportive care. The presence of jaundice or ascites does not indicate a hopeless response to therapeutic intervention.

In selecting management strategies for an animal with cirrhosis, general categories of hepatobiliary and metabolic support are first considered. This is followed by individual tailor-

Clinicopathologic Features of Canine Cirrhosis

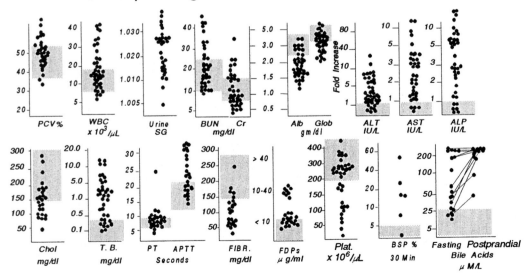

FIGURE 33–17. Scattergram showing the clinicopathologic features observed in dogs with hepatic cirrhosis associated with portal hypertension and ascites. Data derived from the College of Veterinary Medicine, Cornell University, Ithaca, NY.

Table 33–8

EXTRAHEPATIC AND HEPATIC DISORDERS ASSOCIATED WITH CHRONIC HEPATITIS

Systemic Disorders
  Recurrent pancreatitis
  Inflammatory bowel disease
    Small-bowel inflammation
    Lymphangiestasia
    Colitis
  Chronic renal disease
    Glomerulonephritis
    Chronic interstitial nephritis
  Chronic infection: systemic
    Bacterial: leptospirosis, campylobacter, *E. coli* endotoxin,
      mycobacteria
    Mycoses: histoplasmosis
  Immune-mediated diseases:
    SLE
    Vasculitis
    Polyarthritis
    Thyroiditis
  Endocarditis
  Chronic passive congestion
    Cardiac disease
    Pericardial disease
    Kinked vena cava
    Cor triatrium dextor
    Budd-Chiari syndrome
    Hepatic veno-occlusive disease
Hepatic Disorders
  Chronic bile duct obstruction (many causes)
  Liver fluke infestation (cat)
  Chronic cholangitis
  Chronic cholangiohepatitis
  Chronic active hepatitis
  Copper storage hepatopathy
  Hepatic iron toxicosis: hemochromatosis
  Chronic toxin ingestion: e.g., aflatoxicosis, CCl_4,
    dimethylnitrosamine; certain drugs: consult Chapter 30

ing of therapy to the particular needs of the patient and inhibition of active ongoing necroinflammatory injury and continued hepatic collagen deposition.

THERAPEUTICS FOR THE PATIENT WITH HEPATIC INSUFFICIENCY: CHRONIC HEPATITIS AND CIRRHOSIS

CATEGORIES OF THERAPEUTIC CONCERN. The categories of therapeutic support for patients with diffuse liver disease and hepatic insufficiency are presented in an algorithm in Figure 33–18. These include (1) nutritional modifications (caloric intake, carbohydrate supplementation, protein quantity and quality, fat quantity and quality, sodium restriction and potassium supplementation); (2) vitamin (water soluble, fat soluble) and micronutrient supplementation; (3) management of hepatic encephalopathy; (4) modification of gastroenteric ammonia and toxin production; (5) prophylactic antibiotic therapy; (6) management of gastroenteric complications; (7) management of coagulopathies; (8) antifibrotic/anti-inflammatory drugs; (9) minimization of ischemia and endotoxin-induced injury; (10) modification of endogenous bile acid milieu; (11) management of ascites/edema; (12) acid-base and electrolyte disturbances; and (13) consideration of altered drug metabolism (see Chapter 30).

Nutritional Modifications

CALORIC INTAKE. The nutritional management of the patient with hepatic insufficiency is the cornerstone of therapy. See Chapter 39 for general nutritional recommendations for the patient with hepatic disease. Without adequate caloric intake a catabolic state is unavoidable. Cirrhosis is by definition a catabolic disease.[117] The caloric and nitrogen balance of patients with chronic hepatitis with or without hepatic insufficiency is disrupted by the anorexia associated with liver disease and some well-intentioned attempts to alter their food for clinical benefit. Catabolism results in increased mobilization and metabolism of nitrogenous products such as amino acids from muscle. This leads to reduced strength and vigor and loss of an important site of ammonia detoxification and can increase a patient's proclivity for HE. The caloric needs of dogs and cats with different liver diseases are undetermined. In humans, patients with different types of liver injury are suspected to have differences in metabolic rates and thus in maintenance caloric needs.[118–121] Those with severe hepatic necrosis undergoing active tissue repair may require higher caloric and protein intake than those with relatively quiet disease. The metabolism of the cirrhotic human is similar to that during starvation where a large proportion of energy is derived from fat oxidation. A general approach to the dog and cat with serious liver disease including cirrhosis is to provide 1.25 to 1.5 times the normal, healthy animal's maintenance caloric energy requirement (MER). The ratio of nonprotein to protein calories is important from the standpoint that an increased calorie to nitrogen ratio increases the utilization of dietary protein.[122] This also tends to reduce plasma glucagon levels that, when high, are associated with increased blood ammonia concentrations.[123,124]

CARBOHYDRATE SUPPLEMENTATION. The carbohydrate component of the diet should be increased, especially in patients shown to be episodically hypoglycemic or hyperammonemic. Frequent feedings of foodstuffs high in simple and complex carbohydrates benefit these patients. Carbohydrate sources useful in any patient with significant liver disease include boiled whole white rice, pasta, and vegetables. An increase in complex carbohydrates in the form of soluble vegetable fiber is advantageous for two reasons. First, it reduces the availability and production of noxious nitrogenous wastes in the alimentary canal.[117,125] Although low-residue diets were previously advocated for patients with liver disease in an effort to maximize digestion and absorption and to reduce colonic residues considered the major source of encephalopathic toxins, this is now not recommended. Vegetable fiber encourages nitrogen fixation by enteric bacteria, resulting in smaller amounts of nitrogenous materials for alimentary absorption. Fiber is also useful in maintaining euglycemia. In addition, insoluble fiber is beneficial in binding toxic substances such as endotoxins, other bacterial products, and noxious bile acids such as lithocholic acid, which reduces their enteric absorption. Sources of beneficial vegetable fiber include bran, canned pumpkin, amaranth, squash, beans, and psyllium. For patients demonstrating signs of hypoglycemia, oral supplementation with glucose, Karo syrup, or honey is advised as emergency supportive care. For humans, the carbohydrate component of the diet should provide 50% to 60% of the total kcal ingested and this seems beneficial also for dogs with hepatic insufficiency.[117,126]

PROTEIN QUANTITY AND QUALITY. The protein component of the diet should be modified in quantity only when it is apparent that protein intolerance is causing a problem. Patients undergoing hepatic regeneration require adequate protein intake to remain anabolic; protein plays the leading

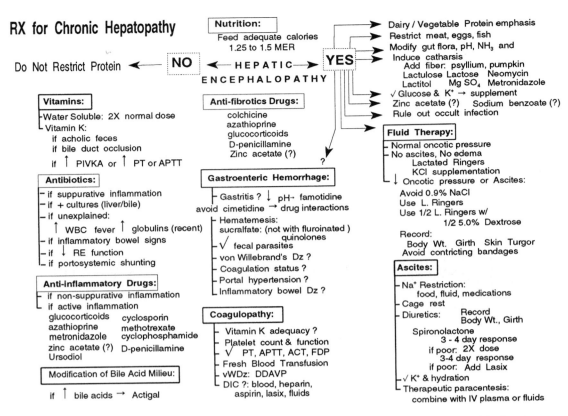

FIGURE 33-18. Algorithm summarizing the categories of therapeutic concern in the patient with chronic hepatitis and cirrhosis.

role in hepatic regeneration.[117-123] Humans with hepatic necrosis, inflammatory hepatopathies, and cirrhosis have been suggested to have increased protein requirements as compared to healthy individuals.[117,127] Although restriction of certain protein sources is advantageous in the circumstance of HE,[128] a negative protein balance leads to depletion of liver protein stores, breakdown of body protein and RNA, and conversion of polysomes to free ribosomes. Protein synthesis is curtailed and reflected in reduced albumin synthesis. The variables influencing the serum albumin concentration can delay the appearance of this reduced synthetic capacity. General protein restriction as a therapy for all patients with hepatic disease or increased serum enzyme activity is inappropriate. A study of the apparent dietary protein requirements of dogs with surgically created portosystemic shunts indicated that a low-protein intake of 1.62 g of crude protein/kg/day was inadequate to maintain normal protein stores. A diet containing at least 2.1 g of crude protein per kg body weight per day of 80% or better digestibility was recommended.[129] An interesting finding in that study was that branched chain amino acid supplementation did not appear to be beneficial when compared to an aromatic amino acid–supplemented diet. The importance of dietary amino acid balance in patients with hepatic insufficiency remains controversial. Management of a positive nitrogen balance is important in patients with portosystemic shunting as improved nitrogen balance in rats with portosystemic shunts appears to reduce plasma and brain concentrations of the hepatoencephalopathic aromatic amino acids.[129] Humans with cirrhosis undergo an improvement in their physical and mental condition when protein intake is adjusted to maintain a positive nitrogen balance.[130,131]

The clinician should look for signs of protein intolerance before deciding that a restricted protein diet is necessary. Clinicopathologic signs of protein intolerance include irrefutable signs of HE (linked to protein ingestion or gastroenteric hemorrhage), hyperammonemia documented by determination of high blood ammonia concentration or by demonstration of ammonium biurate crystalluria or biurate uroliths, or by the presence of a disproportionately low BUN compared to the creatinine in a patient on a normal maintenance (not a protein-restricted) diet. The latter sign should be carefully scrutinized because some patients with severe liver disease become polydipsic and polyuric. In these patients a low BUN may be due to the rapid water turnover that prohibits renal tubular urea absorption. Protein restriction should be instituted if signs of intolerance are identified. It was recently shown that protein-deficient diets can result in increased liver enzyme activity and minor increases in the postprandial serum bile acid concentrations.[132]

There are no definitive measures of protein adequacy and positive nitrogen balance that are appropriate for clinical use. Estimates are made using the patient's body weight (muscle mass) and serum albumin concentration. These are sequentially followed if the patient is placed on a protein-restricted diet. A continued decline in strength, vigor, muscle mass, and the concentration of serum albumin may indicate that the patient has a greater need for protein than is being supplied. See Chapter 30 for a discussion of the complexities regarding protein metabolism and albumin regulation.

When protein restriction is necessary and when hepatic insufficiency is firmly established, the quality of protein should also be altered. High biologic value proteins are not necessarily the best choice. Diets formulated for patients with renal insufficiency based on an egg and meat origin protein base may not be optimal for the patient with hepatic insufficiency. Meat- and fish-derived protein has been shown to be the least appropriate and most encephalopathic source of protein in humans with cirrhosis. The type of proteins that seem best for the patient with hepatic insufficiency are of dairy and vegetable origin.[117,123,125,133–137]

The possible benefits of a vegetable-protein diet include (1) lower concentrations of encephalopathic components and (2) alteration in enteric microbial flora. As mentioned above, vegetable fiber is beneficial in reducing intestinal ammonia generation and provides a cathartic effect that mechanically cleanses the bowel.[117] Certain forms of vegetable fiber also bind endotoxins and noxious bile acids that can be detrimental in the patient with hepatic insufficiency and portosystemic shunting.[138] Psyllium, pectin, and guar fibers are fermented in the colon where they acidify the luminal contents.[138,139] In humans with cirrhosis placed on a high vegetable-protein source diet (high-fiber diet), use of neomycin and/or lactulose may be discontinued without causing patient deterioration.[117] In these patients, fiber has now been shown to increase their tolerance of dietary protein and to induce a reduction in BUN and, presumably, the blood ammonia concentration. This occurs by an increase in the fecal elimination of nitrogen and without a change in the plasma amino acid pattern.[117,140,141] Studies in which a vegetable-protein diet with amino acid profile similar to that of meat have been fed to humans with cirrhosis have been done with *Amaranthus hypochondrium* as the vegetable fiber source. The dried seeds of amaranth contain 5% to 7% hemicellulose as nonsoluble fiber and 70% starch as soluble fiber.[117,142] This grain was one of the staples of the Aztec populations in Mexico and is still used as a food source. It provides a favorable protein and fiber source in these patients.

Diets containing a soy protein base are beneficial in dogs with experimentally induced hepatic insufficiency and in clinical patients.[126,129,143] These are described in Chapter 35. The only problem with soy protein (tofu) based diets is palatability. Some of the commercially available reduced calorie fiber-supplemented dry foods made for older dogs have worked well in dogs with chronic hepatitis and cirrhosis in the author's experience.

FAT QUANTITY AND QUALITY. The fat content of the diet is proportional to the diet's caloric density and increases palatability. Patients with portal hypertension may develop a minor degree of fat malabsorption due to overwhelmed lymphatic capacity and deranged intestinal microcirculation.[144] A minor reduction in fat digestibility was shown in dogs with experimentally created portosystemic shunts.[129] If steatorrhea is recognized, the animal should be evaluated for adequacy of pancreatic function with a TLI determination. If this is normal, the fat content of the diet should be reduced, but pancreatic enzyme therapy is inappropriate. Some clinicians advocate inclusion of medium chain triglycerides in the diet of patients developing steatorrhea to ensure that caloric needs are met. Choleretic bile acid ursodeoxycholic (Actigall; Ciba Geigy) but not dehydrocholic acid (Decholin) provides some micelle-forming properties. Medium chain triglycerides have greater digestibility than long chain triglycerides but should not be used as lipid supplements in cats because they may promote hepatic lipid vacuolation of hepatocytes.[145]

Certain free fatty acids are believed by some to be involved in the pathogenesis of HE by direct neuroencephalopathic effects or by changing the protein binding of other neurotoxic substances.[146,147] However, increases in the medium chain fatty acids by threefold had no effect on brain function in humans with cirrhosis.[148] The short chain fatty acids, which are believed to be synergistic neurotoxins, are derived by colonic fermentation of a variety of substrates including amino acids, albumin, blood, and dietary polysaccharides (fiber).[149–151] These are considered beneficial to the colonic epithelium.[150–152] In consideration of this information, there is no global recommendation to alter or restrict the fat content of most diets in the absence of malabsorption.

SODIUM RESTRICTION AND POTASSIUM SUPPLEMENTATION. Dietary sodium restriction is necessary in animals with ascites and in those with portal hypertension and/or significant hypoalbuminemia (albumin <1.5 g/dl). Sodium restriction as recommended for patients with renal and cardiac insufficiency is appropriate. Potassium supplementation is important in cats with chronic liver injury and in any patient receiving a loop diuretic for management of ascites. Cats should receive at least 7 mEq per day orally of available potassium supplement along with their food. Potassium gluconate is commercially marketed for this purpose (Tumil K).

Vitamin and Micronutrient Supplementation

All patients with hepatic insufficiency should receive a doubled dose of *water soluble vitamins* each day. The dog has a particular need for ascorbic acid.[126] It has been estimated that some humans with hepatic insufficiency have demonstrated a need of up to a 10-fold increase in some of the water soluble vitamins; these patients had other nutritional deficiencies induced by alcoholism.[153] When selecting a vitamin source, the need to avoid copper must be considered in patients with copper-associated hepatopathies. The need for supplementation of the *fat soluble vitamins* (except vitamin K) is less well established than the need for water soluble vitamins. Supplementation with vitamin D can lead to toxic side effects of hypercalcemia, renal injury, and soft tissue mineralization if the dose is not carefully monitored. Supplementation with too much vitamin A can lead to hepatotoxicity. Supplementation with vitamin E is advocated as a free radical scavenger.

A micronutrient of particular concern to the patient with hepatic insufficiency is *zinc*. The proposed benefits of zinc supplementation in patients with hepatic insufficiency are summarized in Figure 33–19 and are discussed in Chapter 30. Zinc supplementation may be appropriate in any patient with hepatic insufficiency, hepatic fibrosis, or severe inflammation. The dose of zinc used is based on experience in dogs with hepatic copper storage disease and in humans with Wilson's disease; see the anti-inflammatory/antifibrotic section of this chapter.[154] Generally, a dose of 50 to 100 mg elemental zinc is given once daily to medium- and large-sized dogs. The serum zinc concentration is sequentially measured at several week intervals over the first 2 months of treatment to guard against inadvertent zinc toxicity that can lead to hemolytic anemia and gastrointestinal signs. The availability of elemental zinc from several different zinc sources is shown in Table 33–9.

Iron supplementation may be necessary in the patient experiencing repeated gastrointestinal hemorrhage due to portal hypertension and hepatic insufficiency. This also may become necessary in the circumstance of an iron-deficient diet. The need for iron supplementation should be decided on the basis of a serum iron panel and red blood cell morphology. Microcytosis can develop in patients with portosystemic shunting despite adequate iron stores.[155–158] Iron supplementation

Benefits of Zinc Supplementation

replenishes Zn deficits

may rectify aberrant immune responses

↑ impedes copper enteric uptake

↑ metallothionein Cu binding

↑ urea cycle function

↑ neurologic status in humans with HE

↓ free radical reactions

protects against iron initiated injury

↓ collagen accumulation in experimental hepatic necrosis

FIGURE 33–19. Proposed benefits of zinc therapy in the patient with hepatic insufficiency.

is indicated when low serum iron concentration is reported, when hypochromia is recognized, and if gastroenteric bleeding or other source of chronic blood loss is recognized. It is unclear yet whether iron deficiency is induced by chronic therapeutic use of zinc; until this is known it should be considered a possible complication. The best measure of the adequacy of body iron stores is determination of a serum ferritin concentration, but this assay is not yet widely available. When iron supplements are necessary, the clinician must consider the amount of available iron in a particular product (see Table 33–9). Hepatocyte and Kupffer cell iron loading has been recognized in some animals with inflammatory liver diseases. When iron storage is copious, supplementation may be contraindicated.

Management of Hepatic Encephalopathy

A variety of clinical conditions and diagnostic or treatment complications promote development of HE (see Table 33–10). The most obvious detrimental effect is the increased toxin production that occurs following ingestion of a high-quantity meat-quality protein meal. A similar complication occurs as a result of the increased alimentary protein load following gastrointestinal hemorrhage. In humans, the most severe HE is precipitated by gastrointestinal bleeding.[117] The presence of endoparasitism should be avoided by frequent stool evaluations and judicious use of anthelmintics. Oxibendazole should be avoided. Development of a coagulopathy should be considered if unexplained gastroenteric bleeding

Table 33–9

MEDICAL SOURCES OF IRON AND ZINC

SOURCE	AVAILABLE ELEMENTAL
Ferrous sulfate	20%
Ferrous sulfate exsiccated	30%
Ferrous gluconate	12%
Iron dextran	varies with product
Whole blood transfusion (45% PCV)	0.5 mg/mL iron
Zinc gluconate	14%
Zinc sulfate	23%
Zinc acetate	31%

For each 100 mg × % is the mg elemental availability.

Table 33–10

CLINICAL CONDITIONS KNOWN TO PRECIPITATE HEPATIC ENCEPHALOPATHY

Dehydration
Increased dietary protein intake
Gastrointestinal hemorrhage and inflammation
Blood transfusion: especially stored blood or plasma
Alkalosis
Hypokalemia
Hypoglycemia
Infections: fever, ↑ catabolism
Azotemia: prerenal, renal, postrenal
Uremia: azotemia, ↑ toxins, altered neuroreceptors
Constipation: anaerobic colonic flora: major source of toxins
Drugs: diuretics (those inducing alkalosis, hypokalemia)
    tranquilizers (acepromazine)
    anesthetics (deranged neurotransmitters and neuroreceptors)
    benzodiazepines (diazepam)
    methionine, choline (lipotropic agents metabolized to toxins in GI tract)
    tetracyclines

is recognized. Vitamin K_1 should be administered while coagulation tests are pending. If coagulation tests are normal and fecal examinations are negative, a gastroduodenal vasculopathy or ulcer associated with portal hypertension should be considered (see Chapter 30). In this circumstance, modification of the portal hypertension might be beneficial. This may be accomplished by use of low doses of propranolol and/or the oral administration of neomycin.[159,160] There is no experience in veterinary clinical patients with portal hypertension and propranolol, although this is a common therapeutic intervention for portal hypertension and critical varicocele bleeding in humans. Neomycin has been shown to reduce the hyperdynamic nature of the splanchnic circulation in animals with cirrhosis induced by chronic bile duct occlusion.[160] There have been no clinical studies of its efficacy in this regard in veterinary patients. Relieving abdominal pressure due to tense ascites might also be beneficial in alleviating microcirculatory collapse that could contribute to the gastrointestinal insult. Use of sucralfate and an H_2 blocker would be indicated if a gastric lesion is suspected as the source of bleeding.

Dehydration is particularly contraindicated in these patients in that it generates azotemia and contracture alkalosis. Azotemia increases the blood ammonia concentration as a result of diffusion of increased amounts of urea into the gut where it is transformed into ammonia. Contracture alkalosis is dangerous because alkalemia promotes the formation of the soluble form of ammonia (NH_3), which easily passes across the blood-brain barrier.

Hypoglycemia is problematic because associated neuroglycopenia results in encephalopathic signs and because hypoglycemia potentiates both the activity and production of other neurotoxins. Constipation is detrimental because many of the purported HE toxins are produced and absorbed in the lower bowel. The development of inflammatory bowel disease may promote transmural passage of enteric toxins and endotoxin into the portal circulation and, consequently, into the systemic circulation. This can result in increased hepatic injury and a multitude of adverse systemic consequences. Hypokalemia promotes the development of metabolic alkalosis and encephalopathy as a result of increased renal loss of H^+ and absorption of ammonia. Severe hypokalemia may also impair renal concentration capabilities and induce diuresis, which can lead to dehydration if fluid intake does not keep pace. Hypokalemic animals are weakened and anorexic and more susceptible to dehydration.

Use of certain drugs and catabolic conditions can contribute to HE. Cachexia, starvation, and glucocorticoid administration can increase protein catabolism and production of nitrogenous wastes that contribute ammonia and other toxic substances. Antianabolic effects of certain drugs, for example tetracyclines, also increase production of waste products that contribute toxigenic substances. Adverse reactions to a variety of drugs that interact with the GABA/barbiturate/benzodiazepine receptor can directly produce hepatoencephalopathic signs.

INTERVENTION AT THE GABA-BENZODIAZEPINE RECEPTOR. GABA and its receptor are implicated in the pathogenesis of HE (see Chapter 30).[193] Intervention with the benzodiazepine antagonist *flumazenil* has been shown to be of benefit in some humans in deep HE coma. Initial reports were quite favorable, but well-controlled clinical trials have not been as enthusiastic in patients with intractable encephalopathic signs.[194]

In humans, flumazenil is used at a dose of 0.25 mg/hour after an initial 1.0 mg dose given intravenously. It has a short-term effect and thus needs slow intravenous infusion or repeated bolus administration. It has best effect in patients with acute onset of HE. Studies in dogs or cats with hepatic insufficiency have not been done.

Modification of Gastroenteric Ammonia and Toxin Production

A summary of methods used to modify gut flora responsible for ammonia generation and formation of other toxins is presented in Table 33–11.

Patients showing evidence of protein intolerance, hyperammonemia, or ammonium biurate crystalluria benefit from therapy aimed at modifying enteric ammonia production and absorption. This is accomplished by reducing the quantitative intake of dietary protein, qualitatively changing the type of dietary protein (excluding meat source and egg source protein and including dairy and vegetable source protein), the inclusion of dietary vegetable fiber, minimizing urease-producing enteric flora, and acidification of colonic pH, which impairs production of ammonia and its mucosal absorption.

A reduction in protein intake should initially be no lower than the minimum requirement established for healthy dogs and cats. This is 1.3 to 1.5 g/kg/day for dogs and 3.3 to 3.5 g/kg/day for cats.[161] The minimal amount of protein required by animals with different liver disorders has not been determined. Based on studies done in humans with cirrhosis, patients probably require a greater intake than the minimal amount of protein designated for healthy animals and patients with renal insufficiency. If the serum albumin concentration shows sequential decline or if clinically obvious catabolism (weight loss, poor hair coat, reduced vitality) occurs following dietary protein restriction, the protein content of the diet should be titrated upward to achieve an optimum for that individual. Generally, changes in dietary protein should be made in increments of 0.5 mg/kg body weight, with the effects appraised at 14 day intervals. If an increase in dietary protein generates HE signs, hyperammonemia, or biurate crystalluria, the maximal tolerated level of protein has been determined, and a reduction to the prior presumably "balanced" level of protein intake that did not produce adverse side effects is recommended. Complicating

Table 33–11

METHODS USED TO MODIFY ENTERIC PRODUCTION AND ABSORPTION OF TOXINS

Dietary Modifications
↓ Protein quantity

Modify protein quality: dairy and vegetable preferred
↑ Dietary soluble fiber
↑ Carbohydrate dietary component to 50% to 60%

Modification of Enteric Microbial Population
Acidify colonic pH: lactose, lactulose, lactitol, fiber

Antimicrobials:
neomycin	22 mg/kg PO BID–TID
metronidazole	7.5 mg/kg PO BID–TID
amoxicillin	11 mg/kg PO BID

Modify enteric substrates: dietary, nonabsorbable disaccharides, fiber
Lactulose	0.25–0.5 mg/kg PO BID–TID
Lactitol	0.5–0.75 g/kg PO SID/BID
Lactose	slightly sweet solution, BID; dairy products
Fiber	Metamucil, psyllium, dietary vegetable matter

These are used to effect, attaining several soft stools per day.

Modify bacterial population directly with additional beneficial substrates
Lactobacilli:	live yogurt culture
	dairy protein, lactose, and organisms

Direct Elimination of Microorganisms, Substrates, and Products
Cleansing enemas:	5–10 mL/kg, repeat until clear
	use warm polyionic fluids

Retention enemas:	as necessary, respect total systemic drug dose
neomycin:	15–20 mL 1% solution BID/TID
lactulose:	5–15 mg diluted 1:3 with water BID/TID
lactitol:	0.5–0.75 g/kg/diluted with water BID/TID
metronidazole:	7.5 mg/kg (systemic dose) with water, BID
betadine:	dilute 1:10 with water; flush out within 10 minutes
activated charcoal:	administered and retained in crisis situation
diluted vinegar:	1:4 dilution: reduces pH via acetic acid

factors must be carefully considered during these nutritional trials, such as gastroenteric hemorrhage, dehydration, or side effects induced by other therapeutic or diagnostic measures.

Modification of enteric flora to reduce the quantity of toxin-producing microorganisms can be accomplished through dietary alterations (see above), use of absorbable and nonabsorbable antibiotics, and administration of nonabsorbable disaccharides. An experimental method has included the immunization of animals with urease or urease-producing bacteria, resulting in some reduction of colonic urease activity.[162] Other efforts include treatment with substances that augment utilization of ammonia into nontoxic products. Any substance supporting and promoting urea cycle activity can do this, including administration of glucose (reduces the need for gluconeogenesis from amino acids), arginine (which directly augments substrates and enzymes in the urea cycle), and alpha-keto acids (which can be aminated to form amino acids and, in the process, consume ammonia).[163] Outside of treatment with glucose, the latter two modalities are of dubious benefit.

Oral administration of a nonabsorbable antibiotic, such as *neomycin*, has been used in large numbers of clinical patients to beneficially modify gut flora. Neomycin given orally is minimally absorbed in the normal intestine and attains high concentrations in the colon. Neomycin given at 200 mg/kg (a dose too high for clinical use) combined with polymyxin B at 20 mg/kg, divided and given in two doses orally, reduces fecal gram negative bacteria to almost zero within 9 days in dogs.[166] The dose of neomycin used in clinical patients is much lower than this dose. Using 22 mg/kg PO BID has produced clinical response in encephalopathic dogs and cats without recognized toxic side effects. Neomycin may be effective for reasons other than reducing bacterial populations. For example, it also reduces the intestinal production of ammonia from glutamine metabolism, similar to the effect shown for lactulose. In patients with inflammatory bowel disease, systemic absorption of neomycin may occur and cause toxicity.[167] The most notable problems in humans are ototoxicity and malabsorption. Chronic administration of neomycin can also lead to enteric bacterial overgrowth and gut malabsorption. These effects should be watched for if chronic treatment is advised. Frequently, neomycin is used for HE crises intervention, and then discontinued. Owners are advised to reinstate therapy if dietary indiscretions or other situations occur. Combination of neomycin with lactulose or with sorbital can provide synergistic effects; this is discussed more fully later.[168,169] Neomycin can be used as an oral agent or can be employed as a retention enema during HE crisis.

Lactobacillus organisms are safe and may be advantageous in the patient with hepatic insufficiency. These organisms are not urease producers. Whether a benefit is gained from orally administered lactobacilli, other than those due to its combination with dairy products, is controversial. Some clinicians believe they act synergistically with other measures used to modify gut flora. However, many experimental studies have shown that it is difficult to alter bacterial populations in the colon. There are no clinical studies of lactobacilli supplementation in dogs or cats with liver disease and it remains controversial.

Use of synthetic disaccharides is a popular measure for modifying gut ammonia production. These products, *lactulose* and *lactitol*, are not digested by mammalian enzymes. Rather, they are digested and fermented by enteric organisms producing a large quantity of organic acids that provide a variety of benefits (shown in Figure 33–20). Lactulose is primarily converted to acetate.[149] These molecules provide a variety of benefits including (1) reduction of colonic luminal pH, (2) reduction of urease-producing organisms, (3) reduction in the activity of urease, (4) provision of a cathartic effect, and (5) encouragement of bacterial nitrogen fixation. Acidification of the colon encourages NH_3 conversion to the poorly

absorbed NH_4^+ (ammonium) ion.[169–179] The low luminal pH is inhospitable to urease producers, which reduces their population. It also is the wrong pH for optimal urease activity necessary for conversion of urea to ammonia. Fermentation of lactulose to organic acids invokes a cathartic influence through an osmotic effect, which encourages passage of several soft stools per day. This directly cleanses the colon of toxigenic substrates, products, endotoxins, and urease-producing organisms. Lactulose is also proposed to provide an antiendotoxin effect.[180]

Lactulose is the most frequently used synthetic disaccharide in veterinary practice. It is sweet and well accepted by most patients. In humans, 20% to 30% complain of nausea when placed on lactulose. An alternative product, lactitol, is less sweet and preferred by many humans.[174,178,181,182] The starting dose of lactulose is 0.25 to 0.5 mL/kg PO BID to TID and for lactitol is 0.5 to 0.75 g per kg BID. The desirable therapeutic dose of either product is based on stool consistency and frequency of bowel movements; two or three soft stools (consistency comparable to pudding) per day are optimal. Documentation of fecal pH adjustment can be used to monitor whether the dose is adequate; an optimal pH is less than 6. Overdosage with lactulose can produce flatulence, bloating, dehydration, and, rarely, metabolic acidemia. Steatorrhea has been shown in healthy humans treated with lactulose.[183] If lactose is used, powder can be dissolved in water to make a slightly sweet solution. A lactose tolerance test is used in humans to predict who will respond to this therapy. Magnesium sulfate has been used as a method of inducing chronic catharsis in some human patients with recurrent HE.[117] This approach has not been used in veterinary patients.

Although lactulose activity relies on enteric organisms for its fermentation, concurrent use with neomycin has synergistic effects. Studies conducted on humans with cirrhosis and HE have evaluated various combinations of lactulose and neomycin therapy.[167–169] Like neomycin, lactulose, lactitol, and lactose can be administered rectally (following cleansing enemas) in addition to the oral route.[177]

Enemas may be used as an emergency therapy for patients with profound HE signs. Warm isotonic saline, lactated Ringer's, or pure water cleansing enemas are first advised. Cold solutions should be avoided; the fluids should be warmed to body temperature or slightly warmer especially in the petite collapsed patient. If the patient has ascites or circumstances that warn against sodium loading, hypertonic saline solutions should be avoided because the absorptive capability of the colonic mucosa is considerable. Also worthy of consideration in a small dehydrated patient is water intoxication, which can result from retention of large-volume pure water enemas. After colonic cleansing, administration of neomycin or lactulose, singly or in combination, provides a direct therapeutic effect. Enemas can be repeated on a TID basis as necessary. Betadine diluted in water is an alternative method of direct bowel flora modification. Betadine can be toxic to cells, and iodination can result in cats and small dogs in which the enema solution dwells too long. Betadine solution *must* be removed after 10 to 15 minutes. This is not the optimal enema supplement but can be used in an emergency situation. Alternatively, a dilute solution of vinegar can also be used to modify colonic pH.

A novel approach to ammonia trapping involves use of *sodium benzoate*, which has been used in children with urea cycle enzyme deficiencies.[184–186] Sodium benzoate is used to "bypass" the urea cycle, diverting nitrogen from urea to other waste products. The involved biochemistry concerns utilization of glycine, which is in equilibrium with blood ammonia

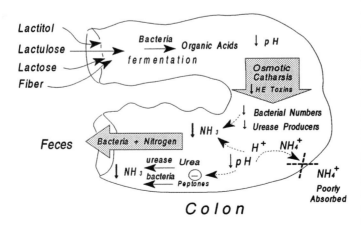

Mechanism of Action of Lactulose

FIGURE 33-20. Diagram showing the effect of lactulose on enteric nitrogen absorption and elimination and ammonia production. A similar mechanism is realized with lactitol, lactose (in the lactase-deficient patient), and soluble dietary fiber.

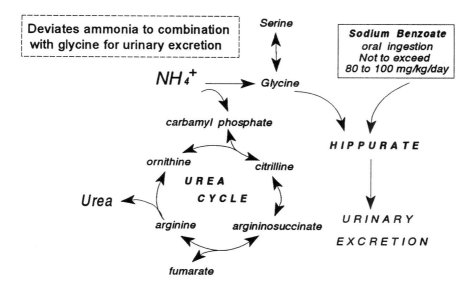

FIGURE 33-21. Diagrammatic representation of the benefits of sodium benzoate in elimination of ammonia in patients with insufficient urea cycle function.

(Figure 33–21). Because glycine is rapidly replenished, this pathway for nitrogen "deviation" remains continually operative as long as benzoate is supplied. A dose of 10 g sodium benzoate per day has been used in adult humans with HE. Clinical trials in humans where sodium benzoate has been compared to lactulose have shown it to be equivalent or better. However, this approach cannot be recommended without some concern. Very large doses of sodium benzoate (500 mg/kg) given to mice intoxicated with ammonium has a paradoxical effect.[187,188] Subsequent to that report, the dose in humans is recommended to not exceed 6 to 10 g per day or 80 to 100 mg/kg per day.[186]

The use of *L-carnitine* in experimentally induced ammonia toxicity has shown that it provides protection against hyperammonemia and neurologic signs. This is believed to be due to the multiplicity of metabolic functions attributed to L-carnitine.[189–192] In part, this is due to stimulation of urea synthesis. A preliminary trial of carnitine supplementation in human cirrhotics with HE showed an improvement in their mental function, but not in their blood ammonia concentrations, after an ammonium chloride challenge.[190]

Prophylactic Antibiotic Therapy

Prophylactic use of antibiotics has been advocated in patients with hepatic insufficiency and portosystemic shunting and in patients in acute hepatic failure.[195,196] Humans with cirrhosis have been shown to have impaired leukocyte chemotaxis, impaired cell-mediated immunity, low levels of complement, defective opsonization, and reduced bactericidal activity against *E. coli*. In addition, these patients have reduced availability and function of Kupffer cells and hepatofugal blood flow that deprives normal sinusoidal circulation. In health, enteric microorganisms and their toxins routinely gain entrance to the portal circulation or lymphatics through mural transfer and within macrophages entering the portal or lymphatic circulations.[197] Larger particles enter through the mesenteric lymphatics and smaller ones through the portal vessels. Hepatic phagocytes normally render intestinal-derived antigens nonimmunogenic, whereas the spleen and lymph node–associated macrophages enhance immunogenicity.[197–199] Development of gastrointestinal ulceration or inflammation in the patient with hepatic insufficiency is relatively common, and it further increases the animal's susceptibility to gut-derived bacterial infections.[200] Endotoxemia has been repeatedly documented in humans and animal models with chronic hepatic insufficiency, although it was not detected in dogs with congenital portosystemic vascular anomalies undergoing medical management.[201,202] The adverse consequences of endotoxemia are discussed later in this chapter. Septicemia, septic endocarditis, urinary tract infections, and spontaneous bacterial peritonitis are complications reported in humans with hepatic insufficiency, acquired portosystemic shunting, and ascites. The frequency of similar disorders in dogs and cats is undetermined. Some animals with chronic hepatitis are suspected to have an infection-linked etiology. Patients demonstrating unexplained fever, leukocystosis with or without a left shift, and rising globulin concentrations should be suspected of having an infection. Without culture of blood, urine, or ascitic fluid, diagnosis can be difficult. Infectious organisms are rarely observed on histologic sections of a liver biopsy; rather, they are identified on cytologic imprints of the tissue or examination of bile, ascitic fluid, or tissue aspirates. The clinician should remain vigilant in his or her inspection for infectious sequellae in these patients. Iatrogenically impaired immune responses due to therapeutic use of anti-inflammatory and immunosuppressive drugs makes these patients more susceptible to infections as does the common association of gastroenteric ulceration as a side effect of glucocorticoids, antimetabolites or immunosuppressives, and the presence of portal hypertension. In addition, inherently abnormal immunoregulation may underlie chronic hepatic disease in some patients, making them more susceptible to infection. Septicemia severely aggravates hyperammonemia and HE, and antibiotic therapy seems to minimize this complication.[42]

Bacterial cell products and toxins have been shown to act synergistically with other hepatotoxic events.[196–201,203–211] Treatment against coliforms and other gram negative enteric organisms is advisable considering the association between endotoxins, periportal hepatitis, and veno-occlusive lesions related to gram negative organisms.[26,36,37,209] Coadministration of *E. coli* with antibacterial lipopolysaccharide (LPS) sera to dogs induces narrowed and thickened peripheral portal veins associated with fibrosis and various degrees of aberrant vasculature in and around portal triad areas. Dogs become splenomegalic and develop a hyperdynamic splanchnic circulation typical of that seen with naturally developing cirrhosis.

Absorbable antibiotics such as amoxicillin, cephalosporins, and metronidazole have been used to modify gut flora in an attempt to reduce urease-producing organisms. Although evidence suggests that permanent modification of the gut flora is not possible, such treatment has shown clinical benefit in dogs and cats with congenital portosystemic shunts. In some cases, treatment is continued for prolonged intervals and seems effective in protecting against septicemia, endotoxemia, and HE. Such treatment is empiric, based on our understanding of the pathophysiologic mechanisms associated with HE, the impaired Kupffer cell function, and endotoxemia suspected in these patients. There have been no rigorous evaluations of its benefit in veterinary patients. Providing it does not cause symptomatic bacterial overgrowth or vitamin K deficiency, it has no recognized adverse side effects. Superinfection with resistant organisms is always a concern when chronic antibiotic therapy is used and thus the clinician must remain alert for this eventuality. Prophylactic use of antibiotics may be of particular value in patients with hepatic failure and in those with ascites. A prospective study of bacterial infection in humans with acute liver failure demonstrated a high incidence of infection early in the course of the illness.[196] The author concluded that prophylactic therapy was justified in this subset of patients. Antibiotic therapy is also initially indicated in the patient with bile duct occlusion, cholangiohepatitis, or cholangitis, especially when surgical intervention becomes necessary. A high risk of infection is associated with biliary diversion or biliary tree repair in humans.[212–214]

Antibiotics that are biotransformed or eliminated through the hepatobiliary system should be avoided unless specific therapy is directed by bacterial culture. Antibiotics deemed appropriate and inappropriate for use in the presence of compromised hepatic function are shown in Tables 33–12 to 33–14. Designation as a nondesirable antibiotic is determined on the basis of (1) reliance on hepatic biotransformation for activation or elimination, (2) impairment of mixed function oxidase activity that creates polypharmaceutic complications (chloramphenicol enrofloxacin with theophylline), or (3) consistent or idiosyncratic hepatic toxicity. Tetracycline is not used because it promotes hepatic lipidosis and, in high doses, can be toxic to dogs with portosystemic shunts.[215]

Management of Gastroenteric Complications

Clinical signs of vomiting, diarrhea, anorexia, and gastrointestinal hemorrhage are relatively common in patients with hepatic insufficiency associated with portal hypertension.

Table 33–12

ANTIMICROBIALS CONSIDERED APPROPRIATE FOR USE IN CHRONIC HEPATITIS/CIRRHOSIS

Indications:	Suspected hepatobiliary infection
	Suspected systemic infection
	↓Kupffer cell surveillance, phagocytosis
	Prophylaxis: after liver biopsy
	during gastroenteritis
	inflammatory bowel disease

Preferences:	Systemic antimicrobials achieving therapeutic concentrations in liver, bile, and other tissues, and undergoing renal elimination
Ampicillin	22 mg/kg	PO, SQ, IV	TID
Amoxicillin	11 mg/kg	PO	BID
Cephalexin	15 mg/kg	PO, SQ, IV	BID
Enrofloxacin	2.5 mg/kg	PO	BID
Metronidazole	7.5 mg/kg	PO or Rectal	BID–TID
Chloramphenicol:	11 mg/kg	PO, SQ, IV	BID

Chloramphenicol dose empirically reduced; undergoes enterohepatic circulation; associated with hematopoietic toxicity in humans; may cause anorexia and lethargy. Causes profound P-450 cytochrome oxidase inhibition and consequent drug interactions. Used *only* based on culture/sensitivity.

Nausea and vomiting can result from HE toxins and may resolve following aggressive supportive care centered on diet modification and reduced enteric ammonia production. In some cases gastric vasculopathy is the source of the problem and requires management with gastric cytoprotectants. Sucralfate is an appropriate therapeutic medication with a multitude of beneficial effects.[216] H_2 blocking drugs may be valuable in the presence of gastric erosions. When an H_2 receptor blocking drug is deemed necessary, cimetidine

Table 33–13

ANTIMICROBIALS ACHIEVING THERAPEUTIC BILIARY CONCENTRATIONS

ANTIMICROBIAL	BILE:SERUM CONCENTRATION
Aminoglycosides	
amikacin	0.3
gentamicin	0.3–0.6
kanamycin	1
streptomycin	0.4–3.0
Cephalosporins	
cefazollin	0.7–3.0
defoxitin	2.8
cephalothin	0.4–0.8
ceftriaxone	10
Penicillins	
ampicillin	1.0–2.0
penicillin G	0.5
oxacillin	0.2–0.4
mezlocillin	10
nafecillin	40
Tetracyclines	
tetracycline	5–10
doxycycline	10–20
Miscellaneous	
chloramphenicol	0.2
clindamycin	2.5–3
ciprofloxacin	2.0
erythromycin	8–25
metronidazole	1
trimethoprim/sulfa	1–2/0.4–0.7

From Sanford JP. Guide to Antimicrobial Therapy. 1993. Antimicrobial Therapy Inc., 5910 North Central Expressway, Suite 1955, Dallas, TX 75206.

Table 33–14

ANTIBIOTICS TO AVOID AS FIRST-CHOICE
ANTIMICROBIALS IN HEPATOBILIARY DISEASES
ASSOCIATED WITH HEPATIC INSUFFICIENCY

Chloramphenicol	Hetacillin
Chlortetracycline	Streptomycin
Oxytetracycline	Sulfonamides
Lincomycin	Trimethoprim-Sulfa combinations (especially
Erythromycin	Dobermans, Samoyeds)

These drugs are either *inactivated* by the liver, require *hepatic metabolism*, or are capable of causing *hepatic injury* that will complicate the interpretation of clinical response to therapy.

should not be chosen because of its powerful P-450 microsomal enzyme inhibition. Cimetidine causes numerous and complex drug interactions and these complications should be avoided. Ranitidine causes similar, albeit, fewer complications. The most commonly used alternative H$_2$ receptor blocker is famotidine (Pepcid), which is 15 to 20 times more potent than cimetidine and only needs oral administration once daily or intravenous administration twice daily.[217]

If nausea and vomiting persist, metoclopramide can be used orally, subcutaneously, or by a slow steady rate intravenous infusion. This drug acts directly on the chemoreceptive trigger zone and is effective in some patients in which vomiting is a manifestation of HE. Unfortunately, metoclopramide is a dopamine antagonist that stimulates aldosterone production; this may blunt the action of spironolactotone to mobilize ascitic fluid.[218] The patient with ascites that displays persistent vomiting and nausea should be aggressively treated for HE. If ascitic fluid accumulation causes a tautly distended abdomen, it should be relieved as discussed later, and metoclopramide avoided.

Fluid Therapy

Fluid therapy in the patient with chronic hepatitis can be problematic. The clinician must consider the individual's propensity to retain sodium and water. If biochemical indicators and clinical evaluations suggest hypoalbuminemia and portal hypertension, then 0.9% sodium chloride should be avoided. Use of solutions with a lower concentration of sodium and chloride, such as lactated Ringer's or Ringer's diluted 50% with 5% dextrose in water, is preferred. Lactated Ringer's should not pose a problem with lactate metabolism because clinical evidence in humans suggests this is one of the last biochemical pathways to be significantly impaired in hepatic failure. The volume of fluid to be administered should be carefully calculated and the patient's response to fluid therapy must be reassessed several times each day. Recording the patient's weight, measuring abdominal girth circumference, and estimating hydration by skin turgidity and tarsal fold thickness provides objective information relevant to water and sodium retention. Use of central venous pressure measurements are ill advised owing to the potential for subclinical bleeding tendencies. No vessel should be catheterized that cannot have hemostasis ensured by application of topical pressure. Arterial punctures for blood gas analysis should be avoided. Jugular veins should not be invaded. Attention must be given to dressings applied to secure catheters to maintain sterility. Occlusive bandages should be avoided in these patients because of their tendency to form edema.

If a patient with ascites and/or edema is dehydrated, administration of plasma is recommended during initial volume expansion. This will supply valuable oncotic pressure. Dextrans have been used in humans with cirrhosis and ascites and seem safe. These provide a relatively inexpensive method for increasing plasma oncotic pressure. Plasma is theoretically preferred because these patients would likely benefit from its coagulation proteins, antithrombin III, and transport proteins. Fresh plasma should be used because stored plasma can contain noxious amounts of ammonia.[219]

Management of Coagulopathies

The patient with chronic hepatitis may have occult bleeding tendencies. In human patients with liver disease, bleeding occurs mostly after invasive medical procedures rather than as a spontaneous event. All jaundiced patients should be given therapeutic doses of vitamin K$_1$ at least 24 hours before invasive procedures. The dose of vitamin K$_1$ recommended is variable and ranges between 0.5 and 2 mg/kg. The author customarily gives cats and small dogs 5 mg, medium-sized dogs 10 to 15 mg, and large dogs 15 to 20 mg, total dose given subcutaneously or intramuscularly. Vitamin K$_1$ is not given intravenously because it has produced signs of anaphylactic shock when so administered. Oral administration is not used in a jaundiced patient until it is determined that bile duct occlusion is not a problem. The absence of bile acids in the enteric canal will impair fat soluble vitamin absorption. Physical examination for petechial hemorrhages, fundic examination, and fresh fecal evaluation for signs of bleeding should be routinely completed. Bench tests of coagulation and a mucosal bleeding time should be done before invasive diagnostic or therapeutic endeavors. If tests indicate a coagulopathy despite the lack of observed spontaneous bleeding, a blood transfusion should be given before invasive procedures.

The author has biopsied a considerable number of dogs with hepatic insufficiency and abnormal coagulation profiles. Management with a blood transfusion before the procedure is effective in more than 90% of the cases in avoiding hemorrhagic complications.

The patient with chronic liver disease may be vitamin K deficient or not be able to rejuvenate vitamin K$_1$ to its active form (see Chapter 30). Evaluation of a PIVKA assay (consult Chapter 8) will indicate whether the patient is responsive to vitamin K administration. If vitamin K inadequacy is surmised, vitamin K may become part of that patient's chronic management. In most cases, chronic treatment requires dosing at 7 to 14 day intervals and can be given orally. Too much vitamin K should be avoided because it can lead to Heinz body hemolytic anemia and can be expensive.

In some patients with active hepatitis or decompensated hepatic insufficiency, DIC can become the major clinical problem. Treatment with fresh whole blood transfusions, mini-dose aspirin (0.5 mg/kg PO BID), and low-dose heparin (50 to 75 μ/kg SQ TID) has been successful in some cases. If aspirin is used, it should be combined with low-dose furosemide to provide renal protection. It has been shown experimentally that loss of autoregulatory renal prostaglandins is associated with the hepatorenal syndrome and that furosemide provides a protective influence.[220] In addition to supportive care for the coagulation system, the patient must be fully evaluated for the precipitating cause of DIC. If such can be identified and eliminated, there is hope for patient survival.

Therapeutic Intervention Against Hepatic Fibrogenesis: Antifibrotic/Anti-inflammatory/Immunosuppressant Therapy

The development of hepatic fibrosis is the result of multilevel regulation of extracellular matrix (ECM) composition and turnover (see earlier discussion). New information regarding the process of fibrogenesis is opening wider avenues for therapeutic interventions in the patient with chronic hepatitis and cirrhosis. Of primary importance in learning to use anti-inflammatory and antifibrotic agents in the patient with liver disease is an understanding of the process of collagen synthesis, cellular assembly, cell secretion, and degradation; these are schematically depicted in Figure 33–22. Collagen deposition in the liver is either the result of (1) increased collagen production or (2) reduced collagen degradation. Therapeutic intervention in this process can take a number of appoaches. Theoretically, inhibition could be directed at any of the different steps of collagen biosynthesis.[43,44,221–224] Ideally, such agents would act only in the liver, be nontoxic, and be specific for collagen or related ECM components. At the present time, only a limited number of therapeutic agents are available that intervene in these processes, although there are a considerable number of agents under experimental investigation. Drugs targeted at promotion of collagenase activity would also curtail accumulation of excessive collagen. Concurrent inhibition of collagen synthesis and induction of collagenase activity would be optimal. Colchicine is one therapeutic agent that seems to accomplish both effects, although the physiologically realized benefit of its collagenase influence remains controversial. Polyunsaturated lecithin is suggested to increase collagenase activity from lipocytes in an experimental model of hepatic fibrosis.[225] It is also possible that it reduces the activity of lipocytes and therefore lowers collagen synthesis.[225–228] A summary of agents that intervene in collagen production or invoke collagenase activity is presented in Table 33–15, which complements Figure 33–22.[43–45,52,229–233]

Interventions directed at control of the inflammatory process either initiating or perpetuating liver injury is one major method of disease intervention. Therapeutic agents used for this purpose and their dosages are listed in Table 33–16, the mechanisms of action as anti-inflammatory agents are shown in Figures 33–23 and 33–24.

Glucocorticoids have received the most attention in the human and veterinary medical literature for the management of chronic hepatitis.[5,8,9,112,114,234] Although glucocorticoids have a favorable effect on mortality during the first year of use and for many years thereafter, it has still not been established that they retard progression to cirrhosis in human patients with chronic hepatitis.[235–237] Glucocorticoids provide several benefits in the patient with chronic nonsuppurative hepatitis, including (1) reduced lymphocyte replication, circulation, and involvement in inflammation, (2) reduced macrophage receptors for immunoglobulin, which impairs their participation in inflammation, (3) stabilization of lysosomal membranes, which reduces tissue injury, (4) inhibition of neutrophil chemotaxis, which reduces their participation in inflammatory tissue injury, (5) inhibition of prostaglandin and leukotrine production, (6) impaired fibrogenesis, and (7) provision of a choleretic effect.[238–244] These are summarized along with their adverse effects in Figure 33–23. In high doses, glucocorticoids also have been shown to decrease antibody production.[244]

The most common drugs used are prednisolone and prednisone. Although prednisone must be activated in the liver to prednisolone, a number of pharmacokinetic variables that become altered in the patient with hepatic insufficiency result in adequate therapeutic prednisolone concentrations.[239,245,246] A recommended daily dose of prednisone is 2.2 mg/kg given for 2 to 4 weeks. This is tapered to 1.1 mg/kg for another 14 days, and followed by gradual adjustment to the assessed "lowest effective dose," which often approximates 0.6 mg/kg/day. It is controversial whether alternate-day therapy is advisable. In humans, glucocorticoid-responsive diseases seem to be controlled better with a daily regimen; unfortunately, this causes more side effects.[244,247] It is unclear if humans with chronic hepatitis do better on a daily rather than an alternate-day regimen,[236] although it has been shown that some patients have an exquisite sensitivity to a particular drug threshold during dose titration.[248] Dose adjustments are coordinated with clinical patient assessment, as described later. It is not known whether dividing the daily dose of prednisone into two treatments makes a difference in the clinical response.

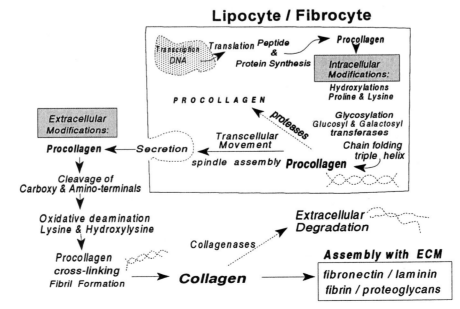

FIGURE 33–22. Diagrammatic representation of the process of collagen formation.

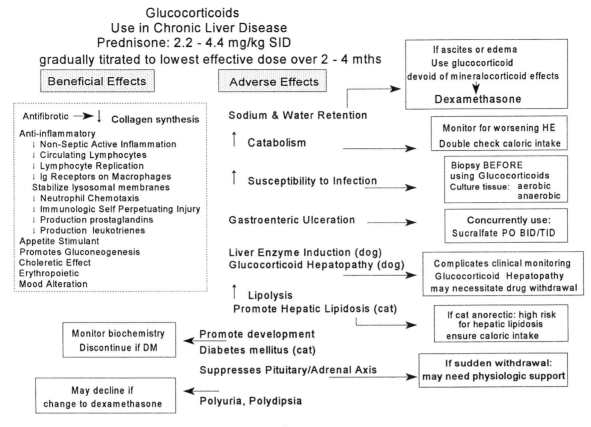

FIGURE 33-23. Beneficial and adverse effects of glucocorticoids in the patient with hepatic fibrosis/insufficiency.

The adverse consequences of chronic glucocorticoid administration are well established (Figure 33–23).[249] Intolerable side effects necessitate dose reduction and use of alternative immunosuppressive agents, usually used in combination with the reduced dose of the glucocorticoid. Combined use with azathioprine is common and has been shown to be effective in humans.[236,250] This approach reduces the detrimental side effects of each drug by permitting a lowered dose. Each animal should be evaluated as an individual and therapy tailored to its particular needs.

The initiating dose of prednisolone for cats with chronic liver disease associated with lymphoplasmacytic inflammation is twofold greater than for dogs: 4 mg/kg. Cats are less prone to displaying signs of hypercortisolism as compared to the dog, although they similarly developed a suppressed pituitary adrenal axis upon high-dose treatment.

In humans with active cirrhosis and ascites, prednisone has been shown to have a negative effect on survival.[237] In some animals with portal hypertension, ascites, and those with tenuously compensated hepatic failure, treatment with prednisone may produce side effects that hasten death. Worsening of ascites, edema, gastroenteric bleeding, and development of HE may occur. Patients with portal hypertension and/or ascites should be preferentially treated with dexamethasone, a synthetic glucocorticoid lacking the mineralocorticoid effects inherent with prednisone (prednisolone). Dexamethasone has a long half-life in the circulation (> 48 hrs) and does not lend itself to alternate-day therapy for preservation of the pituitary adrenal axis. Dogs are started on a dose of 0.2 to 0.4 mg/kg body weight. This may be titrated to every other or every third day to minimize adverse effects.

In comparison to prednisone, dexamethasone seems to produce less polydipsia and polyuria. It must be emphasized that dexamethasone is not the appropriate glucocorticoid to use in modulation of immune disease as a first-line choice. It is used only when there are extenuating circumstances and a need to avoid mineralocorticoid-associated problems.

The potential for gastroenteric hemorrhage is high in patients with hepatic disease that are treated with glucocorticoids. Sucralfate may reduce this risk, although this remains unproven. A BID or TID dose of 0.25 g is given to animals weighing up to 15 lbs, 0.5 g to animals weighing from 15 to 50 lbs, and 1 g to animals weighing more than 50 lbs. The only adverse effect of sucralfate in animals with liver disease is constipation, which can be problematic in the patient prone to HE. Concurrent treatment with lactulose and a high-fiber diet seems to obviate this problem. It should be remembered that sucralfate impairs absorption of tetracyclines and fluoroquinolones. If gastric irritation develops and persists despite sucralfate administration, an H_2 blocking drug may be helpful.

In humans, it has been recommended that glucocorticoid therapy be continued for 6 months after secure clinical remission. Only then is chronic therapy suspended. A relapse rate of 50% was shown when withdrawal occurred within the 6 month window of observation, whereas the relapse rate fell to 8% after that interval.[236,251] Knowing when a good clinical remission has been achieved is difficult without reevaluation of a liver biopsy. The histologic response in dogs with chronic hepatitis to treatment with glucocorticoids is shown in Figure 33–25 and 33–26.

If a follow-up tissue biopsy is not available, treatment response may be gauged on the basis of clinical response

Table 33–15

SUMMARY OF AGENTS THAT INTERVENE IN COLLAGEN PRODUCTION OR INVOKE COLLAGENASE ACTIVITY

SYNTHESIS REGULATORS	MECHANISM	SOURCE
Tumor necrosis factor alpha	↓ Collagen synthesis	Fibroblasts
	↑ Interstitial collagenase	
Interleukin-1	↑ Collagen synthesis	Macrophages
	↑ Collagenase	
Transforming growth factor beta	↑ ECM/Collagen synthesis	Kupffer cells
	↓ Collagenase	
Platelet-derived growth factor	↑ Collagenase	Platelets
Glucocorticoids	↓ Inflammation → ↓ cytokine release → ↓ collagen synthesis	Exogenous
	↓ Collagen synthesis	Exogenous
	↓ Collagenase	
Retinoids	↓ Collagen synthesis	Exogenous
	↓ Collagenase	
Azathioprine	↓ Inflammation → ↓ cytokine release → ↓ collagen synthesis	Exogenous
Cyclosporine	↓ Inflammation → ↓ cytokine release → ↓ collagen synthesis	Exogenous
Methotrexate	↓ Inflammation → ↓ cytokine release → ↓ collagen synthesis	Exogenous
Colchicine	↓ Collagen synthesis	Exogenous
	↑ Collagenase	
D-penicillamine	↓ Collagen synthesis	Exogenous
Zinc	↓ Collagen synthesis	Exogenous
Gamma-interferon	↓ Collagen synthesis	Exogenous
Inhibitors of proline and lysine hydroxylation in collagen*	↓ Collagen synthesis	Exogenous
Drugs ↑ intracellular cyclic AMP†	↓ Collagen synthesis (intracellular before secretion)	Exogenous
Ursodeoxycholic acid	Improves bile acid membranocytotoxicity Anti-inflammatory (↓ MHC expression)	Exogenous

*Zinc, pyridine 2,4-dicarboxylate, 3,4-dihydroxybenzoate, 3,4-dehydroproline, cis-r-hydroxyproline, L-azetidine-2-carboxylate, corticosteroids.
†Prostaglandin E_1, theophylline, epinephrine.
Information derived from references 44, 45, 46, 52, 229, 233.

including (1) improved parameters on biochemical screening profiles, (2) improved liver function on specific function tests, (3) increased patient weight not related to ascites or edema, and (4) owners' impression of their pet's vitality. Examination of the biochemical screening profile is complicated in the dog by the enzyme induction due to glucocorticoid therapy. In some dogs with steroid responsive hepatitis, the transaminases will become relatively quiescent as the disease is brought under control; steroid-related induction of ALP activity renders this enzyme useless as a monitoring parameter. Nuances suggesting improved hepatic function should be looked for on the screening profile; these include (1) an increased albumin concentration in the absence of dehydration, (2) normalized fibrinogen concentration, (3) increased cholesterol concentration in a patient with a previously low cholesterol, (4) reduced retention of bilirubin pigments, and (5) maintenance of euglycemia. Recognition of an increasing BUN disproportionate to the creatinine concentration indicates either tissue catabolism, feeding of a high-protein diet, or gastroenteric bleeding. These patients must be scrutinized for fecal blood loss because gastroenteric bleeding is a major cause of HE. Evaluation of liver function using specific tests such as bile acids, ammonia tolerance, or organic anion dye elimination may be used to document improvement. Unfortunately, development of steroid hepatopathy in the dog will compromise hepatic function.

Treatment with glucocorticoids was shown to improve long-term survival time in dogs with chronic hepatitis that survived at least 1 week after they were presented for diagnosis. This data is presented in Table 33–17 and Figure 33–27.

Dogs were treated with an initial dose of 2.2 mg/kg body weight per day for 7 to 10 days, followed by 1.1 mg/kg/day for another 7 to 10 days, and then 0.6 mg/kg/day until the disease was judged to be in remission. Treatment of dogs with glucocorticoids did not significantly influence overall survival; approximately 38% of dogs in the treated and 33% in the nontreated group survived. However, treated dogs that survived had a significantly longer mean survival interval averaging 33 months, almost three times longer than in nontreated dogs. The findings in this study are mixed and need to be challenged with a well-planned prospective study. Other studies report varied responses to glucocorticoid therapy. The success of treatment of Doberman pinschers seems to vary with the stage of disease at which therapy is begun.[114,252] There may be a difference between the glucocorticoid-responsiveness of certain breed-related hepatopathies and the more general category of chronic hepatitis. Similar problems of determining the benefit of glucocorticoid treatment exists in human medicine where efficacy is still in question in patients with chronic nonviral hepatitis.[253,254]

Azathioprine is often used in combination with glucocorticoids when objectionable side effects to cortisone develop. It is not believed to be efficacious when used alone in humans for chronic active hepatitis or primary biliary cirrhosis. This drug is an antimetabolite that is transformed in the liver to 6-mercaptopurine via xanthine oxidase and metabolites excreted in urine. Concurrent use of allopurinol, which inhibits xanthine oxidase activity, will cause drug toxicity. If such combined therapy is necessary, the dose of azathioprine should be reduced to one-third or one-fourth.[255] Azathio-

Table 33–16

TREATMENT REGIMEN FOR ANTI-INFLAMMATORY/ANTIFIBROTIC MEDICATIONS USED TO CONTROL INFLAMMATION LEADING TO HEPATIC FIBROSIS

DRUG	DOSE	FREQUENCY		COMMENTS
Glucocorticoids:				
prednisolone	2.2 mg/kg	SID	dog	Used if lymphocytic, plasmacytic inflammation, no infection. Initial dose given for at least 14 to 28 days. Serial biochemistry profiles are used to monitor enzymes and bilirubin. In many cases enzymes will be reduced despite induction phenomenon in the dog. Titrate dose of prednisolone to 0.6 mg/kg PO SID and then, if continued improvement, to the lowest effective dose. Dexamethasone is only used for patients that cannot tolerate mineralocorticoids; this may eventually be titrated to every third day if response is good. It remains controversial whether alternate-day glucocorticoids will maintain chronic hepatitis in remission.
prednisone	2.2–4.4 mg/kg	SID	cat	
dexamethasone	0.2 to 0.4 mg/kg SID reserved for animals with ascites, no mineralocorticoids			
Azathioprine	1.0 mg/kg 0.3 mg/kg	SID EOD	dog cat	Used in conjunction with glucocorticoids; allows a lower dose of each drug. Monitor CBC 7 to 14 days initially to avoid hematopoietic toxicity. If leukopenic, neutropenic, withdraw drug, reinstate at a 25% reduction upon recovery. If chronic therapy, monitor CBC intermittently to watch for marrow aplasia.
Methotrexate	0.1 mg/kg total dose per dog 0.4 mg total dose per cat in 3 bolus injections over 24 hours repeat q 2 weeks? *investigational*			Trial therapy for cats with cholangiohepatitis not responding to conventional glucocorticoid treatment. Used if biliary ductule destruction is recognized or if suspected lymphosarcoma.
Colchicine	0.3 mg/kg PO	SID	dog	Colchicine is indicated when active fibroplasia is observed and the histomorphologic diagnosis is consistent with chronic hepatitis. Avoid drug combined with probenicid. Too high a dose will induce hemorrhagic diarrhea. Colchicine has several mechanisms of action. Is of unproven efficacy although clinical experience is encouraging. No experience in cats.
D-Penicillamine	10–15 mg/kg PO	BID	dog	If induces gastric upset, give medication with a small piece of meat. No experience in cats.
Zinc acetate	50–100 mg elemental zinc 7 mg elemental	SID SID	dog cat	Monitor serum zinc concentration to avoid zinc toxicity; values 200 to 400 μg/dl advised. Do not permit serum zinc concentrations to approach 1000 μg/dl → hemolysis.
Metronidazole	7.5 mg/kg PO	BID–TID	dog/cat	Cell-mediated immune modulator used in conjunction with glucocorticoids especially in animals with inflammatory bowel disease and chronic hepatitis. Neurotoxicity if dose too high: vestibular signs, ataxia, nystagmus. Discontinue drug, reinstitute at lower dose if recovery complete. Inappetance and vomiting; some patients cannot tolerate metronidazole.
Ursodeoxycholic acid	10–15 mg/kg PO	SID	dog/cat	Adjunctive therapy, anti-inflammatory, alters hepatobiliary cell participation in ongoing inflammation, beneficially alters the serum bile acid milieu.
Polyunsaturated phosphatidylcholine	45 mg/lb per day (rats); 3 g/day (humans)			Restores membrane health; may modify immune injury. Reduces fibrosis in model of alcoholic liver disease in rats. Do not use pure lecithin for supplementation; choline content may not be well tolerated by patients with hepatic insufficiency.

prine seems more effective in modifying T-lymphocyte function than B-lymphocyte function, and has been shown to impair cell-mediated immunity and T-lymphocyte-dependent antibody synthesis. Azathioprine is well tolerated in dogs and is suggested to be more effective than cyclophosphamide in treatment of immune-mediated disorders because of its T cell suppressive effects.[256] The dose of azathioprine in dogs is 1 to 2 mg/kg body weight given SID daily or on alternate days. In cats, a reduced dose is recommended, no greater than 0.3 mg/kg per day or on alternate days. If long-term response seems good, the azathioprine dose may be reduced by 50%. Toxicity is usually related to the gastrointestinal tract and bone marrow; vomiting, diarrhea, inappetance, and pancytopenia may develop. Hematologic response should be carefully monitored during the first month of therapy; the nadir occurs between day 7 and 14. A CBC and a biochemical profile should be done every 2 weeks for the first 2 months of use and then monthly or every other month thereafter. If hematopoietic toxicity occurs (leukopenia, thrombocytopenia), the drug should be temporarily discontinued and reinstituted at a 25% dose reduction when the marrow has recovered. In some cases, the patient does not tolerate long-term treatment without hematopoietic toxicity at any dose. Pancreatitis, dermatologic reactions, and cholestatic hepatotoxicity are other reported complications, but these are rare in small animal patients. Good disease control has been achieved in dogs treated with azathioprine and glucocorticoids by the author.

D-penicillamine has been used as an immunosuppressant, immunomodulator, inhibitor of fibrillar collagen deposition, stimulator of collagenase activity, to improve function of the RE system, and for copper chelation.[257–269] Extensive studies in humans with chronic liver disease have shown inconsistent response. It may be more effective than glucocorticoids in delaying or reversing hepatic fibrosis, but this remains highly controversial.[266–270] D-penicillamine is associated with a myriad of side effects in humans, and in dogs, persistent vomiting can be problematic. This may be obviated by splitting the daily dose and administering the drug at mealtime. A dose of 10 to 15 mg/kg PO BID has been recommended for copper chelation therapy, discussed later. This drug has not been used in cats.

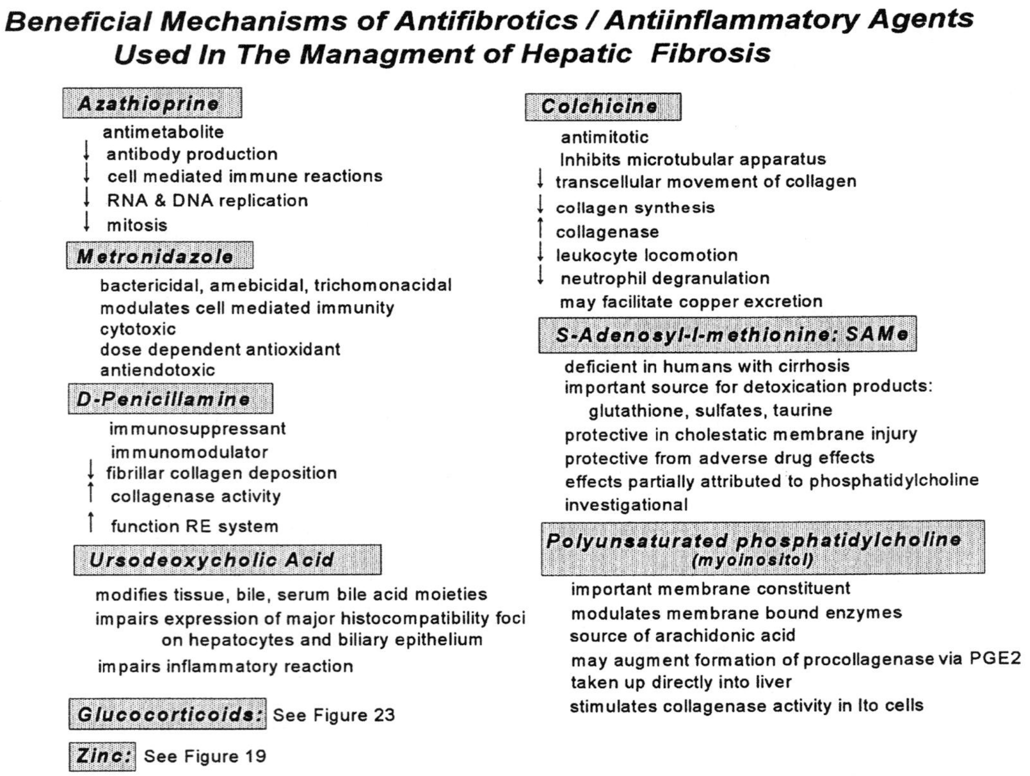

Beneficial Mechanisms of Antifibrotics / Antiinflammatory Agents Used In The Managment of Hepatic Fibrosis

Azathioprine

antimetabolite
↓ antibody production
↓ cell mediated immune reactions
↓ RNA & DNA replication
↓ mitosis

Metronidazole

bactericidal, amebicidal, trichomonacidal
modulates cell mediated immunity
cytotoxic
dose dependent antioxidant
antiendotoxic

D-Penicillamine

immunosuppressant
immunomodulator
↓ fibrillar collagen deposition
↑ collagenase activity
↑ function RE system

Ursodeoxycholic Acid

modifies tissue, bile, serum bile acid moieties
impairs expression of major histocompatibility foci
    on hepatocytes and biliary epithelium
impairs inflammatory reaction

Glucocorticoids: See Figure 23

Zinc: See Figure 19

Colchicine

antimitotic
Inhibits microtubular apparatus
↓ transcellular movement of collagen
↓ collagen synthesis
↑ collagenase
↓ leukocyte locomotion
↓ neutrophil degranulation
may facilitate copper excretion

S-Adenosyl-l-methionine: SAMe

deficient in humans with cirrhosis
important source for detoxication products:
    glutathione, sulfates, taurine
protective in cholestatic membrane injury
protective from adverse drug effects
effects partially attributed to phosphatidylcholine
investigational

Polyunsaturated phosphatidylcholine (myoinositol)

important membrane constituent
modulates membrane bound enzymes
source of arachidonic acid
may augment formation of procollagenase via PGE2
taken up directly into liver
stimulates collagenase activity in Ito cells

FIGURE 33-24. Beneficial effects of selected anti-inflammatory/antifibrotic agents used to treat chronic hepatitis leading to hepatic fibrosis and/or cirrhosis.

Colchicine has been used for the control of hepatic fibrosis in humans with cirrhosis and primary biliary cirrhosis and has shown variable success.[270-278] This is an antimitotic agent that acts by inhibiting the microtubular apparatus. It has been used to arrest and resolve hepatic fibrosis in experimental models of liver disease by its ability to interfere with the transcellular movement of procollagen or the synthesis of collagen.[279] It also may act as an antifibrotic by inducing the production of collagenase.[280] It alters leukocyte locomotion during inflammation, degranulation of polymorphonuclear cells, and has been shown to increase interleukin-1 in mononuclear cells, to inhibit fibroblast proliferation and fibronectin expression.[281] Recently, it has also been suggested to facilitate copper excretion. Several studies in humans with cirrhosis have shown that chronic treatment with colchicine results in improvement in ascites, hyperbilirubinemia, HE, and survival rate. Side effects have included hemorrhagic gastroenteritis, bone marrow suppression, renal injury, and neuromyopathies.[282] The liver is the primary site of drug elimination. Studies in rats have shown that bile duct ligation, intrahepatic cholestasis, and severe hepatocellular necrosis significantly decrease drug elimination.[283]

The use of colchicine in dogs with hepatic fibrosis with or without associated active inflammation has not been well documented. Only three clinical papers report the use of colchicine in a few dogs.[284,285] Nevertheless, it has been used in many clinical patients with chronic hepatitis not included in documented case studies, where it has provided an apparent clinical (but unproven) benefit. Clinical experience of the author is that there is limited toxicity if a dose no greater than 0.03 mg/kg PO SID is used in the dog. Colchicine is available in two forms: colchicine combined with probenicid, which delays its renal excretion, or colchicine alone. Use of the combination product in dogs has been associated with

intolerance. The drug has not been used in the cat to the author's knowledge and there is no information regarding pharmacology of colchicine in the cat.

Cyclophosphamide (Cytoxan) is an alkalating agent and cytotoxic drug used in cancer chemotherapy and for the management of immune-mediated disorders.[286,287] Cytoxan has also been evaluated along with prednisone in humans with chronic active hepatitis.[288] In that study, cytoxan did not produce a consistently good response. This drug should be considered a "last resort measure" in the patient with liver disease. In dogs and cats the dose used for the patient with hepatic disease is 0.5 to 1 mg/kg PO for 4 days on and 3 days off, or given on alternate days. In severe hepatic insufficiency a lower dose may be appropriate and is titrated by evaluation of serial CBCs or signs of toxicity.

Chlorambucil, another alkalating agent, is a less potent drug compared to cyclophosphamide. Use of chlorambucil in humans with primary biliary cirrhosis leads to improved biochemical parameters, IgM concentrations, and some histologic features. Unfortunately it has been associated with unacceptable side effects (bone marrow toxicity) that necessitated drug withdrawal.[289] This drug should be used as an alternative agent if other therapeutic measures have failed or resulted in unacceptable toxicity.

Methotrexate is an antimetabolite that inhibits dihydrofolate reductase; this reduces the availability of tetrahydrofolate, the active form of folic acid. Insufficient intracellular folic acid interferes with nucleic acid synthesis. Methotrexate has recently received increased attention as an anti-inflammatory-immunomodulator in a variety of immune-mediated disorders in humans, including primary biliary cirrhosis and sclerosing cholangitis.[290-293] Its mechanism as an immunomodulatory/anti-inflammatory agent remains undetermined, although it is speculated to interact with lymphocytes. It has been used in one clini-

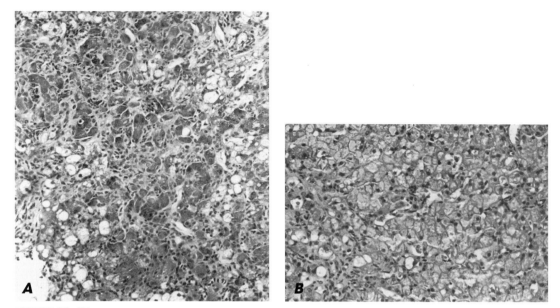

FIGURE 33–25. Photomicrograph of liver tissue from a dog with chronic hepatitis before (*A*) and 16 weeks after (*B*) treatment with glucocorticoids. Improvement includes reduction in both inflammation and fibrosis. The vacuolar change in hepatocytes is associated with use of glucocorticoids. (H&E)

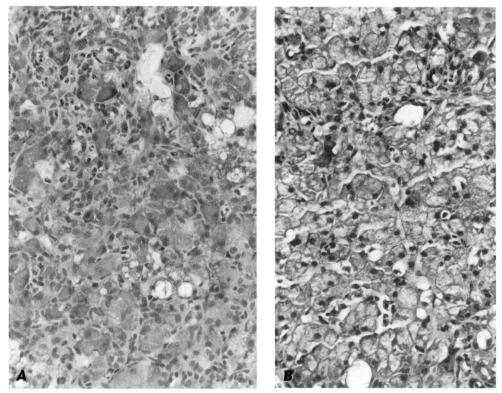

FIGURE 33–26. Photomicrograph of liver tissue from a different dog than in Figure 33–25 that also had chronic hepatitis. Biopsies are taken before (*A*) and 16 weeks after (*B*) treatment with glucocorticoids. Improvement includes reduction in both inflammation and fibrosis. (H&E)

cal trial of chronic hepatitis in humans in which it improved biochemical parameters and liver function but showed variable histologic benefit.

Methotrexate is concentrated in bile and undergoes an active enterohepatic circulation. It has thus received attention for use in immune-mediated disorders involving the bil-

iary tree and is currently undergoing clinical evaluation in humans with such immune-mediated liver disorders.[290–292] The value of methotrexate in chronic hepatitis of dogs and cats is unknown. There is one report of hepatotoxicity in a dog given 5 mg/m² 4 days a week for 12 weeks.[294]

Cyclosporin A has been used extensively in transplantation

Table 33–17

EFFECTS OF CORTICOSTEROID TREATMENT ON SURVIVAL TIME
OF DOGS WITH CHRONIC HEPATITIS

STATUS	SURVIVAL (MONTHS)*	NO. OF DOGS	SURVIVAL (MONTHS)	NO. OF DOGS
Alive	33.1 ± 5.5	14 (24%)	19.3 ± 3.9	10 (26%)
Alive: no follow-up	22.1 ± 4.7	8	4.3 ± 1.8	3
Died of hepatic disease	18.2 ± 3.2	23 (49%)	5.5 ± 1.4	23 (59%)
Died of nonhepatic disease	22.5 ± 9.3	13 (22%)	20.3 ± 9.8	3 (8%)
Total		58		39

*P < 0.005 significantly different from untreated group.
Data are expressed as mean ± SE.
Courtesy College of Veterinary Medicine, University of California at Davis, Davis, CA.

medicine and as an immunomodulator in a large variety of pathologic conditions in humans including chronic hepatitis.[295,296] It reversibly inhibits T cell–mediated immune and autoimmune responses, particularly lymphokine production, but spares suppressor T cell activity. It reduces interleukin-2 synthesis and synthesis of gamma-interferon, the lymphokine that activates macrophages and monocytes involved in antigen presentation. Cyclosporin spares most T cell independent, antibody-mediated immunity.[297–300] Cyclosporin can result in cholestatic hepatotoxicity in humans with renal transplants. It alters calcium fluxes across the hepatocyte cell membranes, increases serum bile acids, and impedes bile flow. However, use in dogs with an end-to-side portacaval shunt (Eck fistula) has shown it has a profound hepatotrophic influence, as have other studies.[301–305] A dose-related choleresis without any change in bile salt secretion has also been shown in dogs.[305] Erratic gastroenteric absorption of the oral formulation requires that trough levels of the plasma drug concentration be monitored to guard against toxicity and to ensure that therapeutic levels of the drug have been attained.[306] This is too inconvenient and cost prohibitive for most clients. Studies in dogs with 70% hepatectomy and complete bile duct ligation have shown that serious hepatic dysfunction significantly influences the pharmacokinetics of cyclosporin.[307] Dose adjustment is therefore of special concern when this drug is used in the presence of hepatic disease.[307] The dose and administration regimen for animals with hepatic disease has not been established. Furthermore, the taste of the liquid oral preparation is objectionable to many animals. This drug has interesting potential

in the patient with chronic hepatitis if the problems associated with dosing and toxicity can be monitored.

Metronidazole is bactericidal, amebicidal, trichomonacidal, and cytotoxic.[308–310] It has also been shown to have immunosuppressive activity, specifically against cell-mediated immune responses, and a dose-dependent antioxidant effect.[309] It may provide a good response combined with glucocorticoids, particularly when immune-mediated inflammatory bowel disease is a concurrent problem.[311] Drug elimination relies partially on hepatic metabolism (30% to 60%), and on renal and fecal elimination. An empirical dose reduction has been recommended for patients with compromised hepatic function, on the basis of experience in human beings where a 50% reduction in drug dosage has been recommended. A dose of 7.5 mg/kg PO BID to TID has been used in clinical patients (dogs and cats) with hepatic insufficiency without toxicity. The author has treated some dogs and cats with an apparent metronidazole intolerance indicated by intractable vomiting whenever the drug is given. Owing to its low protein binding, metronidazole achieves good concentration in bile, bone, body cavity effusions, CSF, and hepatic abscesses. It is readily absorbed across the colonic mucosa and may be administered in this way in patients that cannot tolerate oral dosing.[312]

Zinc acetate or *gluconate* also may provide benefit in the patient with chronic hepatitis and hepatic fibrosis. The functions of zinc and its influence on hepatic disease are described in Chapter 30. A summary of the beneficial effects of zinc therapy in the patient with chronic hepatitis and hepatic insufficiency is provided in Figure 33–19.

Currently, the dose of zinc used in these patients is based on preliminary work done on a small number of dogs with copper storage hepatopathies.[154] An initial dose of 50 to 200 mg of elemental zinc is given in divided doses BID (separated by 1 hour from food ingestion) to dogs weighing 25 pounds or more. This is tailored on the basis of plasma zinc concentrations measured at 7 to 14 day intervals, with a goal of 200 to 400 µg/dl (2 ppm). Zinc concentrations approaching 1000 µg/dl are associated with red cell hemolysis and must be avoided. There is no scientific evidence that zinc therapy is beneficial or harmful in animals with chronic hepatitis and/or cirrhosis other than the information available regarding its use in dogs with copper storage hepatopathy.[154] Treatment is based on experience in humans and animal models described here. The author has been using this adjunctive therapy routinely for the past 3 years in dogs. A more conservative dose has been used in cats, 7 mg elemental zinc per day. No animal has developed signs of zinc toxicity, iron deficiency, or copper deficiency that was clinically apparent. Dogs are supplemented with zinc acetate preferably because this form of zinc is best tolerated. Alternatively, zinc gluconate or sulfate can be used, although they are more commonly asso-

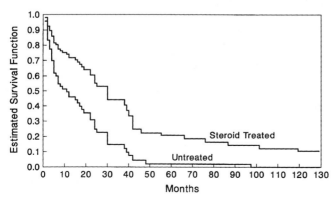

FIGURE 33–27. Graph showing differential survival in months of dogs that were treated with glucocorticoids compared to dogs that were not treated. Data derived from the College of Veterinary Medicine, University of California, Davis, CA.

Table 33–18

MICRONUTRIENT AND THERAPEUTIC ANTIOXI-
DANT SUBSTANCES PROVIDING CELLULAR AND
MEMBRANE PROTECTION FOR CONSIDERATION
IN THE PATIENT WITH ONGOING
HEPATOCELLULAR INJURY

Copper	Constituent of superoxide dismutase Constituent of ceruloplasmin (a scavenger) (contraindicated if copper storage hepatopathy, cholestasis)
Iron	Constituent of catalase (contraindicated if iron status adequate)
Selenium	Constituent of glutathione peroxidase
Zinc	Constituent of cytosolic superoxide dismutase
Manganese	Constituent of mitochondrial superoxide dismutase
Vitamin C (ascorbic acid)	Cytosolic antioxidant
Vitamin E (alpha-tochoperol)	Membrane lipid antioxidant (cell membrane)
Vitamin A (beta-carotene, retinoids)	Membrane lipid antioxidant
Allopurinol	Inhibits xanthine oxidase, a major cause of cell free radical production
Prostaglandin E_2	Prevents cytokine-mediated cell injury, pre- serves circulation, maintains cellular ATP, stabilizes lysosomes
Deferroxamine	Chelates free iron involved in tissue injury; used in acute reperfusion injuries and iron toxicity
Glucocorticoids	Stabilizes membranes; reduces arachidonic acid metabolism to injurious prosta- glandins and leukotrienes

ciated with gastroenteric irritation. When using zinc supplements, the clinician must pay attention to the quantity of available zinc in a particular source so the correct dose of elemental zinc is provided; see Table 33–9.

Polyunsaturated phosphatidylcholine has been used experimentally in humans with chronic active hepatitis and with alcoholic cirrhosis.[225–228] Myo-inositol, a component of phosphatidylcholine, is classified in the group of B vitamins. This is a lipotropic compound, important membrane constituent, and lipoprotein component.[313] Phosphatidylinositol has diverse activities. It modulates the activity of several membrane-bound enzymes including sodium-potassium ATPase, mediates transmembrane signaling processes through effects on protein kinase C, and influences intracellular calcium and protein phosphorylations.

Phosphatidylcholine production can be reduced in liver disease. In humans with chronic active hepatitis, it is suggested that it may modify immune injury.[228] It is possible that this is linked to restored membrane function or signaling. In humans, it has been used in combination with glucocorticoids and azathioprine.[228] A dose of 3 g per day was given to humans, 100 mg/kg to rats, and 4.1 mg/kcal diet in baboons in a model of alcoholic liver disease.[225–228] S-adenosylmethionine supplementation is being used in experimental studies in patients with cholestatic liver disease.[313] It is believed to protect them from cholestatic-associated membrane injury and adverse drug effects and to provide them with important antioxidant protection. Part of its beneficial effect is believed to rest in generation of phosphatidylcholine; consult Figure

32–9. This drug is not yet available in the United States and has not been used in dogs or cats with liver disease to the author's knowledge.

Ursodeoxycholic acid also has potential as an anti-inflammatory drug. Two studies have suggested a cytoprotective effect.[314,315] The expression of HLA foci in liver is induced by cholestasis, and this is reduced by treatment with ursodiol.[316,317] This effect may be suppressing the target of cytotoxic T cells that initiate destruction of bile ducts and periportal tissue in chronic hepatitis. It is possible that this modulates or prevents immune-mediated periportal and lobular necrosis. This drug is discussed extensively in the following section regarding modification of the endogenous serum and tissue bile acid profile in patients with hepatic insufficiency.

Protection Against Ongoing Ischemia/ Eicosinoid/Endotoxin/and Reperfusion-Related Tissue Injury

The damaging effects of hepatic ischemia associated with reperfusion injury also warrants consideration in the context of chronic hepatic inflammation because it can perpetuate the hepatic fibrosis.[318,319] Oxygen-derived free radicals enhance inflammation by perpetuating cellular injury and liberation of cytokines that nourish the inflammatory process.

The natural protective mechanisms against oxygen radical injury include glutathione, superoxide dismutase, catalases, and peroxidases. The hepatic content of glutathione may be reduced in patients with chronic liver disease, cirrhosis, and severe diffuse necrosis.[320–322] When hepatocytes are injured, smaller amounts of catalase and peroxidase are available. Other antioxidants are listed in Table 33–18. Some of these have been suggested for use as interventional therapies for reperfusion injury, and some may be advantageous in the management of hepatic fibrogenesis. However, it is unknown which of these drugs may provide the best effect with minimal side effects. Commonly used interventional approaches that modify this component of the pathobiology of hepatic fibrosis include the use of vitamin E, vitamin C, glucocorticoids, and in some exceptional cases low-dose aspirin.

Delivery of endotoxin to the liver from the alimentary canal may also contribute to hepatic parenchymal injury. In health, endotoxin is continuously delivered to the liver from the portal system and removed by the Kupffer cell population. In patients with hepatic fibrosis or cirrhosis, the Kupffer cells are unable to detoxify sufficient endotoxin. The deleterious effects of endotoxemia are related and interactive with the interleukin, cytokine, and eicosinoid cascades, summarized in Figures 33–11 and 33–28. Therapy targeted at modifying the effects of endotoxin and gram negative portal bacteremia should be considered in the patient with chronic hepatitis or cirrhosis, particularly if portosystemic shunting has developed. Cholestyramine and activated charcoal have been shown to attenuate the production and absorption of intestinal endotoxin; these are used as emergency treatments. Cholestyramine, an ion exchange resin, also appears to have a direct bacteriostatic effect and impairs the production of toxic bile acids in the alimentary canal.[323] Hepatic cytoprotection afforded by prostaglandin E_1, E_2, and I_2 has been shown in endotoxin-initiated hepatic necrosis as well as a variety of models of liver injury.[324–330] The benefit is believed to be associated with impaired release of cytotoxic factors, stabilization of lysosomal membranes, increased cellular ATP, and vasodilation.

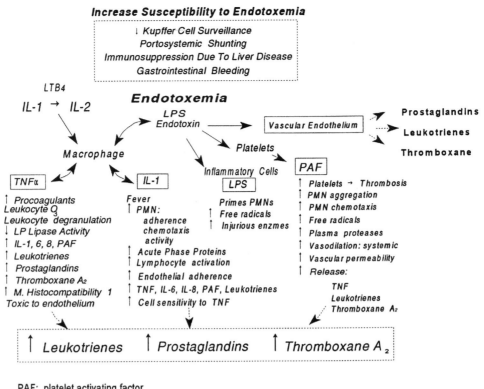

FIGURE 33–28. The effects of endotexemia and its interaction with other inflammatory mediators. See also Figure 33–11.

Modification of Altered Bile Acid Metabolism

Ursodeoxycholic acid has been found to be an effective treatment in certain forms of chronic liver disease in humans.[314,315,331–342] Initially marketed as a medical treatment for gallstone dissolution because of its choleretic action, it was discovered to produce clinical improvement in patients with serious hepatobiliary disease.[331] Numerous clinical trials have shown remarkable improvements in serum biochemical parameters, patient well-being, and resolution of jaundice in humans with chronic active hepatitis, primary biliary cirrhosis, sclerosing cholangitis, and cirrhosis. It has also been shown to improve the transplant potential of children with biliary atresia and to benefit patients with cystic fibrosis that have cholestatic liver injury.[338,340–342] Despite the many testimonials for its clinical benefit, a consistent improvement in histologic lesions has not been shown. The mechanism(s) of action are poorly understood. Before its benefit in human patients was realized, experimental studies of ursodiol showed that it could reduce the bile ductular proliferation and portal inflammation in bile duct–ligated animals and reduce the hepatotoxicity of lithocholic acid.[343,344]

As hepatic fibrogenesis progresses, the ability of hepatocytes to process bile acids becomes altered. The normal balance between the trihydroxy and dihydroxy bile acids in liver tissue, bile, and sera changes as disease progresses, resulting in an increased concentration of lipophilic and cytotoxic dihydroxy bile acids.[345–350] Cytotoxicity of a bile acid is inversely related to its degree of hydroxylation and to the ori-

entation of hydroxyl groups. Cytotoxic bile acids increase cell and organelle membrane permeability and cause injury.[351–355] This permits release of lysosomal enzymes that damage cell structure and promote inflammation, cytokine generation, and an ECM-favoring fibrogenesis. Beneficial modification of the bile acid balance was shown in early studies of ursodeoxycholic acid in which it reduced the concentration of toxic membranocytolytic bile acid moieties by up to 70% in healthy individuals.[356–358] This work was consistent with in vitro and in vivo studies which showed that ursodiol could mitigate the hepatotoxicity of lithocholic acid, the most toxic of all known bile acids.[344] The mechanism of ursodiol protection was linked to a competitively reduced ileal absorption of toxic bile acids.[359–362] Recently, contradictive evidence has been shown for this mechanism in patients with cholestatic liver injury.[340] Rather than alteration of endogenous bile acid moieties, a direct cytoprotective effect on hepatocytes is proposed.[314–317] Consistent with this hypothesis is the fact that patients demonstrate clinical improvement before they develop bile enriched with ursodeoxycholic acid. This is currently an area of intense study because ursodiol has shown promise as an adjunctive therapy in chronic liver disease of any etiology.

Currently, it is believed that ursodeoxycholic acid has an anti-inflammatory influence because of its ability to inhibit expression of cell surface histocompatibility antigens, an essential component of tissue participation in inflammation. This would curtail continued inflammation dependent on hepatobiliary tissue targeting and thus impair continued production and release of interleukins and other cytokines. It is also possible that other cytoprotective influences are responsible.

The clinician should remember that if an underlying primary disturbance can be identified as a cause of liver damage, its elimination will assist in arresting further tissue injury and fibrogenesis. Ursodeoxycholic acid is adjunctive therapy used with other measures aimed at control of disease pathogenesis. This drug is an inappropriate medical intervention for extrahepatic bile duct occlusion; definitive treatment in that circumstance is biliary decompression or diversion. The dose of ursodeoxycholic acid currently used in dogs and cats is 10 to 15 mg/kg PO SID, an empiric dose based on studies in human beings. The drug is prohibitively expensive for large dogs at this dose because it is marketed in 300 mg capsules. A dose range of 4 to 15 mg/kg of ursodiol has been recommended for humans with chronic liver disease. Ursodeoxycholic acid is toxic to rhesus monkeys, baboons, and rabbits, but it is not toxic to normal dogs even in very high doses. A preliminary study of its safety in healthy cats showed that a 15 mg/kg dose is not toxic.[363] Use in dogs and cats with cholestatic liver disease has not shown any sign of toxicity. The author has routinely used this drug as adjunctive therapy in clinical patients for the past 7 years; the clinical impression is that it is beneficial. There has been no controlled study of its efficacy in veterinary patients.

Ascites

The pathophysiologic mechanisms involved with ascites formation in the patient with chronic hepatic disease are discussed in Chapter 30. The physical signs of ascites are variable, ranging from obvious abdominal distension and dyspnea due to restricted diaphragm movement to a vague indistinction of visceral boundaries on abdominal palpation. A fluid wave can be detected when enough ascites has accumulated to allow this physical maneuver. Abdominal ultrasonography is an excellent method of fluid documentation and for differentiating between free fluid, loculated fluid, and normal and abnormal fluid-filled structures (see Chapter 8). Paracentesis should be performed and the physicochemical characteristics of the abdominal effusion determined to verify that no other process has caused or contributed to fluid accumulation.

The evaluation of ascitic fluid should include protein determination, specific gravity, and cytology.[364] A small portion should be retained for culture should the cytology indicate this need. In humans, it has been advocated that ascitic fluid be placed immediately in broth blood culture tubes to optimize organism retrieval.[364] In most dogs with ascites due to liver disease, the fluid is characterized as a pure transudate. The total protein concentration is less than 2.5 g/dl, the specific gravity is usually in the range of 1.010 to 1.015, and the cytology discloses a relative acellularity showing few reactive mesothelial cells and neutrophils. If neutrophils are present in high enough quantity to be estimated as moderate, the fluid should be cultured. In the jaundiced patient, the fluid will be yellow stained and bilirubin crystals may be visualized on microscopic evaluation. Evaluation of the GGT activity may indicate a value above the normal serum range. Comparison of the concentration of albumin in the serum to that in the abdominal effusion permits calculation of a serum to ascites protein ratio. In humans, a value more than 1.1 is associated with portal hypertension as a major cause of the fluid accumulation. Patients with a low gradient (< 1.1 g/dl) have other factors involved with their fluid accumulation.

Application of this ratio to animals has not yet been closely scrutinized.

TREATMENT.   Management of factors contributing to ascites formation is important in the cirrhotic patient. In humans, the presence of ascites worsens the patient's overall prognosis and these patients feel ill and inappetant. This appears true for the cat but may not apply to the dog. Many dogs with cirrhosis have "transient" recurrent ascites that can be successfully managed with little obvious impact on the well-being of the patient. Many complications are associated with the presence, evaluation, and management of ascites. Complications associated with ascites in humans include spontaneous bacterial peritonitis, pleural effusions, and the hepatorenal syndrome. The latter condition is a complication of hepatic insufficiency exclusive to patients with ascites; this disorder is discussed in Chapter 30. The presence of ascites can increase intra-abdominal pressure, which increases portal venous pressure. This can lead to gastroenteric hemorrhage, protein-losing enteropathy, mild steatorrhea, and azotemia. Tense ascites has significant negative hemodynamic effects on cardiac function; it impedes venous return and decreases cardiac output.[365–367] Studies of patients before and after fluid removal have shown a progressive increase in cardiac output, stroke volume, and ejection rate of both ventricles.[365–368] Tense ascites also can seriously impair ventilation. Iatrogenic problems related to paracentesis and induced diureses can lead to serious hydration and electrolyte derangements.

The approach for treatment of ascites is summarized in Figure 33–29. The first consideration is to restrict patient mobility and sodium intake. Enforced rest increases renal perfusion and reduces renin, which stimulates aldosterone liberation. Theoretically, patient rest increases the opportunity for sodium excretion. Usually this does not make a great deal of difference in the patient response. Gradual sodium restriction from the excessive amount in most commercial foods, 0.5% (dry foods), 0.7% (semimoist food), and 1.0% (canned food), to a range between 0.1% to 0.3% has been established as safe. This can be accomplished by feeding one of a variety of prescription or homemade diets. In humans, dietary salt restriction is usually inadequate when used alone for the management of ascites. Dietary sodium restriction is not risk free. In some patients, sodium restriction results in hypovolemia, renal hypoperfusion, and compensatory polydipsia, which results in worsening hyponatremia. During initial salt restriction, patients should be monitored for complications of azotemia and hyponatremia.

Use of diuretics will markedly increase fluid and sodium excretion in most patients (90%), although in some ascites will appear refractory.[369–371] A safe loss of 0.5% to 1.0% body weight per day has been suggested for humans. A lower margin of weight loss may be prudent in some patients, given the threat diuresis poses to the circulating plasma volume. When ascites has been mobilized adequately, intermittent use of the diuretic is advised. Intermittent therapy is guided by fluid reaccumulation. In most cases, administration of a diuretic two or three times per week will sustain control of fluid accumulation. Determining when ascites has been adequately mobilized may be difficult in some patients and is determined by abdominal palpation, measurement of abdominal girth and body weight, or use of abdominal radiographs or ultrasonography.

Considering the mechanisms underlying ascites formation, an aldosterone-blocking diuretic is most logical as a first-choice drug.[365,371,372] Spironolactone competes with aldosterone for its intracellular receptor sites, thus promoting sodium excretion and potassium retention in the renal tubule. This is beneficial for the patient with ascites because,

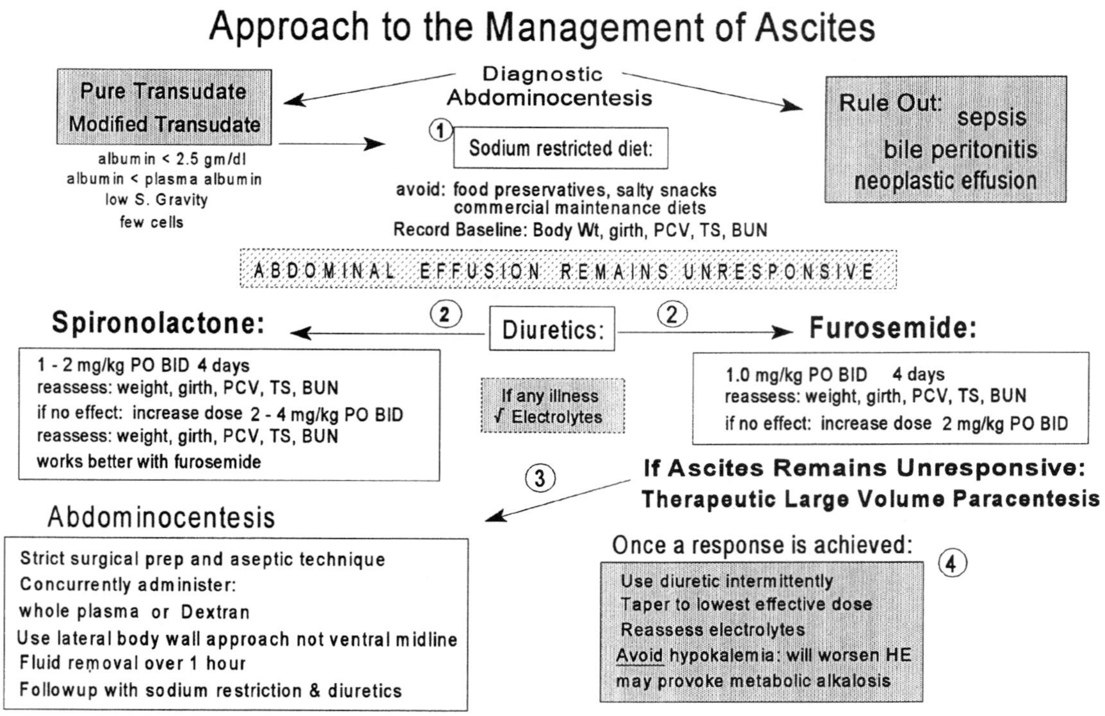

Approach to the Management of Ascites

Diagnostic Abdominocentesis

Pure Transudate
Modified Transudate

albumin < 2.5 gm/dl
albumin < plasma albumin
low S. Gravity
few cells

① Sodium restricted diet:

avoid: food preservatives, salty snacks
commercial maintenance diets
Record Baseline: Body Wt, girth, PCV, TS, BUN

Rule Out: sepsis
bile peritonitis
neoplastic effusion

ABDOMINAL EFFUSION REMAINS UNRESPONSIVE

Spironolactone: ② Diuretics: ② **Furosemide:**

1 - 2 mg/kg PO BID 4 days
reassess: weight, girth, PCV, TS, BUN
if no effect: increase dose 2 - 4 mg/kg PO BID
reassess: weight, girth, PCV, TS, BUN
works better with furosemide

If any illness
√ Electrolytes

1.0 mg/kg PO BID 4 days
reassess: weight, girth, PCV, TS, BUN
if no effect: increase dose 2 mg/kg PO BID

If Ascites Remains Unresponsive:
③ **Therapeutic Large Volume Paracentesis**

Abdominocentesis

Strict surgical prep and aseptic technique
Concurrently administer:
whole plasma or Dextran
Use lateral body wall approach not ventral midline
Fluid removal over 1 hour
Followup with sodium restriction & diuretics

Once a response is achieved: ④

Use diuretic intermittently
Taper to lowest effective dose
Reassess electrolytes
Avoid hypokalemia: will worsen HE
may provoke metabolic alkalosis

FIGURE 33-29. Therapeutic strategies for the management of ascites.

irrespective of the measured serum electrolyte concentrations, total body water sodium stores are increased and potassium stores are reduced. Total body potassium can be reduced by 10% to 30% in humans with cirrhosis. Hypokalemia is dangerous because it may precipitate HE. Administration of large potassium supplements combined with spironolactone in humans does not easily restore normal body potassium stores; in some patients, potassium deficits require weeks to correct. In others, potassium toxicity occurs. Therefore, when spironolactone is used, serum electrolyte concentrations should be measured to determine the patient's electrolyte status in order to use potassium supplement judiciously. Some patients with cirrhosis have reduced serum sodium concentrations due to impaired water excretion; these develop dilutional hyponatremia. This has been seen in dogs. Treatment is focused on water restriction, a clinical maneuver not to be considered without careful monitoring. These patients also require discontinuation of any diuretics. Prerenal azotemia induced by dehydration must be avoided because it can lead to hepatoencephalopathic signs. Compared to the loop diuretics, spironolactone is less potent in mobilizing fluid so it is unlikely that rapid dehydration will occur. Hyperchloremic metabolic acidosis has developed in humans with cirrhosis treated with spironolactone but has not been seen in dogs.[373]

In most cases, furosemide is used in conjunction with spironolactone. Spironolactone has a slow onset of activity; it may take up to 14 days to invoke diuresis in humans. When combined with furosemide it seems safe and is effective. This combination has been used safely in dogs. Furosemide is used alone in cats. As a loop diuretic, furosemide causes as much as 25% of the filtered sodium to be excreted. Loop diuretics inhibit sodium and chloride transport in the ascending limb of Henle's loop, and thus impair the maximal ability of the kidneys to dilute or concentrate urine. They increase urinary potassium loss by increasing urine flow within the nephron segments regulating potassium excretion. A vigorous diuresis with loop diuretics can lead to dehydration and a contraction metabolic alkalosis. Furosemide has been shown to precipitate more complications when used alone than when used with spironolactone in humans with ascites.[374,375] In a prospective study of furosemide-induced adverse effects in people, 51% of 172 cirrhotic patients developed complications with either electrolyte derangements (23%), volume contraction (14%), or HE (12%).[376] One benefit of furosemide is that it protects renal prostaglandins from the adverse effects of nonsteroidal anti-inflammatory agents, should they be purposely or accidentally given to a cirrhotic patient.[220]

The best approach for ascites mobilization is detailed in Figure 33-29. Spironolactone is used initially in conjunction with furosemide. The dose of each is progressively titrated from 1 to 2 mg/kg per day to 2 to 4 mg/kg BID. Onset of action is delayed for 2 to 4 days and so dose adjustments should respect this treatment interval. If there is no response to a doubled dose, it may be followed by a third incremental increase. However, large-volume paracentesis is a preferable method of initiating fluid mobilization. Spironolactone used alone effects diuresis in from 50% to 95% of humans; similar data have not been evaluated for dogs.[371,372,374,377] Combination of potassium-sparing and potassium-wasting diuretics may obviate the acid-base and electrolyte derangements induced by use of either as single diuretic agents. Monitoring a patient with sequential body weight, girth measurements, PCV, total solids, BUN, and serum electrolytes is optimal. At-home monitoring with weight and girth measurement is advised. Marking a spot on the abdomen with nonerasable ink for abdominal girth assessment and using a consistent operator and measuring tape will optimize the information recorded. Body weight reductions approaching 5% per day are dangerous and indicate a need for veterinary examination. Diuretic dosage must be reduced or discontinued if dehydration, too rapid weight loss, electrolyte abnormalities, prerenal azotemia, or HE occur.

Amiloride has been substituted in humans for spironolactone because it has a faster onset of action.[364] There is no experience yet in cirrhotic dogs with this drug. A new diuretic being evaluated in humans with ascites, ibopamine, is a dopamine agonist that improves renal blood flow, glomerular filtration rate, and reduces plasma ADH concentrations. There is no information regarding use of this drug in veterinary patients with liver disease.

In some animals, diuresis and natriuresis is promoted by expansion of the plasma compartment. This maneuver increases the effective plasma volume and promotes release of atrial natriuretic factor, which stimulates sodium excretion. Plasma volume can be expanded with plasma or albumin transfusion, dextrans, or the patient's ascitic fluid. The most practical solution is use of fresh plasma. Plasma should be used instead of whole blood because of the potential for protein loading and hyperammonemia should donor cells be incompatible. Reuse of ascitic fluid is dangerous because it can induce sepsis.

In some patients, diuretics fail to mobilize ascites. In these, large-volume paracentesis is used to initiate a response.[374] Paracentesis as a therapeutic technique for management of ascites is controversial. The old theory was that removal of a large volume of ascites was dangerous and could precipitate hemodynamic crisis, renal failure, and HE. Furthermore, studies in humans indicated that following removal of from 2 to 10 L, approximately 60% of the removed volume reaccumulated within 4 days.[378] A major adverse consequence of repeated large-volume paracentesis is depletion of the circulating albumin and complement concentrations. Patients with cirrhosis are known to have low complement and often are already maximally synthesizing albumin. However, fluid removal has the beneficial effect of improving cardiac function and stimulating diuresis. These effects are due to reduction of intra-abdominal pressure, which compromises venous return and possibly by modulation of sympathetic and angiotensin moderated influences. Recent studies have shown that removal of ascites coupled with the concurrent administration of dextrans or albumin is a safe, convenient, expedient, and affordable treatment option for humans.[365,374,377–382] Fluid removal is done over a 30 to 60 minute interval. This approach has not been studied in large numbers of veterinary patients, but the author has used it in both dogs and cats without ill effects. Initiating ascites mobilization with large-volume paracentesis results in a notable improvement in diuresis in most cases. Sodium restriction and continuation of diuretics must also be used in conjunction with this approach.

In humans with intractable ascites, peritoneovenous shunts and surgically created portosystemic shunts are occasionally used to relieve the ascites.[365,383,384] The use of these treatments is relatively unexplored in practical veterinary medicine. Development of a portosystemic shunt can lead to devastating clinical and clinicopathologic consequences similar to the problems well documented in animals with congenital portosystemic shunts.

Spontaneous bacterial peritonitis is a serious complication of ascites in human patients with cirrhosis.[385–387] Affected patients may be asymptomatic or may display signs of septic peritonitis. Some asymptomatic patients are discovered serendipitously during routine clinical evaluation. The etiopathogenesis of this disorder remains uncertain. Proposed routes of abdominal contamination include (1) transmural passage of microorganisms across the gastrointestinal border, (2) transmission from lymphatics draining the alimentary canal, (3) hematogenous entry, (4) the reproductive tract (in females), and (5) from diagnostic or therapeutic abdominocentesis. Most organisms cultured from affected patients are normal aerobic flora of the gut.[387] Management is focused on use of nontoxic antibiotics that are easily distributed into ascites; amoxicillin-clavulanic acid, third-generation cephalosporins, fluorinated quinolones, and penicillins are reasonable choices. Short-term (4 day) treatment cycles are recommended because the lack of tissue involvement allows rapid organism clearance. Discontinuation of an antibiotic is based on the elimination of white blood cells in the effusion (< 250 cell/mm^3). The occurrence of this complication in ascitic veterinary patients is rare.

The development of hydrothorax as a complication of ascites is relatively rare in veterinary patients with cirrhosis.[388] Pleurodesis with tetracycline has been done in humans and in one dog with this complication, but this is an aggressive and dangerous form of treatment even in a patient in otherwise good health.[389] In experimental models of portosystemic shunts where dogs have been used to study HE, high doses of tetracycline have been lethal.

Electrolyte and Acid-Base Disturbances

Acid-base disturbances occur frequently in human patients with cirrhosis.[390] The most common disturbance is hyperventilation-induced respiratory alkalosis. A metabolic alkalosis may also develop due to vomiting, dehydration, or as a complication of certain diuretics. In dogs with hepatic insufficiency, acid-base disturbances are not consistent, although respiratory alkalosis and metabolic acidemia are most common. Respiratory alkalosis is usually attributed to HE. Contraction metabolic alkalosis can be induced by the potassium-wasting diuretics such as furosemide or fluid losses associated with vomiting or diarrhea. Contraction alkalosis is treated with fluid volume replacement, and potassium deficiency is judiciously corrected using the sliding potassium scale. Inhibition of distal renal tubular hydrogen ion secretion by the potassium-sparing diuretics may induce a metabolic acidosis and hyperammonemia.[373] Administration of glucose-containing fluids may promote renal potassium loss and stimulate the intracellular movement of potassium that will aggravate preexisting hypokalemia. Magnesium may also be depleted along with potassium in patients with liver disease, and supplementation may be required. Little is known about magnesium deficiency in small animal patients because this ion is rarely measured.

Water balance may be disrupted in animals with hepatic disease. In compensated cirrhosis, water excretion may be normal. In those with ascites, either impaired or increased water excretion may occur. Polyuria and polydipsia are occasionally the major problem for which an affected animal is presented. Although these animals may respond partially to water deprivation, this is ill advised, considering their other metabolic and physiologic handicaps. Primary psychogenic polydipsia may develop as a manifestation of HE. Other causes include potassium depletion or alterations in osmoreceptors in the portal vein.[391] A renal concentrating defect is also probable in many patients due to loss of the renal medullary solute gradient created by the low urea concentration, potassium depletion, or increased glucocorticoids associated with hepatic insufficiency or treatment.[392,393] Dilutional hyponatremia may develop when water intake exceeds urinary water excretion. If these patients are receiving diuretics, treatment should be temporarily discontinued. Water restriction may be attempted to achieve a mild to moderate negative water balance. Careful monitoring for dehydration is essential to avert HE crisis.

CHRONIC HEPATITIS IN THE DOBERMAN PINSCHER

Clinical Synopsis

Diagnostic Features

- Middle-aged female Dobermans predisposed
- Usually present with signs of advanced liver failure
- Bleeding tendencies are common and may be exacerbated by von Willebrand's disease
- ALT elevated proportionately more than SAP
- Hypoalbuminemia and hyperbilirubinemia are common
- Biopsy reveals varying degrees of periportal hepatocellular degeneration and necrosis often with copper and iron accumulation

Standard Management

- As for chronic hepatitis (see clinical synopsis on p. 706) with particular attention to immunosuppressive therapy (prednisone/azathioprine) and measures to reduce hepatic copper content (zinc, prednisone)

Middle-aged female Doberman pinschers seem to be extraordinarily susceptible to an aggressive form of chronic hepatitis.[114,252,394,395] Our current understanding of this disorder is based on two detailed retrospective studies that characterized the clinical and pathologic features of affected dogs.[114,252] Information derived from these reports and extracted from case records of the author's hospital are detailed in Figure 33–30; information presented indicates initial evaluations. Of

52 dogs, 46 were females and 6 were males. In each data source, the representation of affected females far surpasses that of males. Affected dogs may present in fulminant hepatic failure as the first sign of disease or may be detected early on the basis of serum enzyme activity on a routine screening biochemical profile. Dogs with advanced liver disease present for weight loss, anorexia, polyuria/polydipsia, icterus, ascites, bleeding tendencies, severe depression, or signs of HE. These animals generally have a short and fulminant clinical course. Despite intensive therapeutic efforts they usually die within 1 week of presentation. Dogs presenting in reasonable condition on first examination (bright, responsive, without overt weight loss or ascites) survive longer. However, these may decompensate rapidly and in some this appears to be accelerated by invasive diagnostic efforts. Dogs detected serendipitously via routine screening health profiles have lived for years when given interventional therapy, discussed later. Earlier diagnosis of this condition seemingly has made a difference in survival, although we remain naive about the biologic behavior of the disorder because only dogs with advanced liver disease have been well characterized.

The typical hematologic features include a normal to high hematocrit and normal red cell indices. If the dog is chronically ill, a microcytosis may develop. A neutrophilic leukocytosis develops in some dogs, particularly those undergoing massive hepatic necrosis associated with a suppurative response. Many dogs have presented with polyuria and polydipsia. The BUN and creatinine concentrations are disproportionate in dogs presenting in acute fulminant hepatic failure. Low blood urea concentration occurs concurrent with hyperammonemia. Some dogs develop acute renal failure terminally, possibly an expression of the hepatorenal syndrome. Serum albumin concentrations have been within the normal range for at least 50% of affected dogs. Those with hypoalbuminemia were dogs with fulminant hepatic failure. Serum transaminase activity is increased in all dogs. In most, ALT activities are at least twofold above the normal range. Values

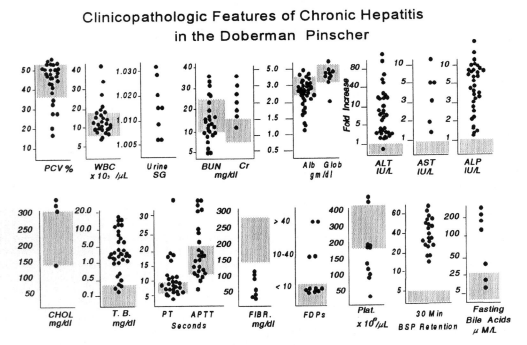

FIGURE 33–30. Scattergram showing the clinicopathologic features of chronic hepatitis in the Doberman pinscher. Data derived from references 114, 252, and the College of Veterinary Medicine, Cornell University, Ithaca, NY.

up to 90-fold normal have been documented in dogs undergoing massive necrosis. Serum ALP activity is less markedly increased compared to the transaminases in many dogs. This reflects the necroinflammatory nature of the diffuse fulminant disease. Most dogs are hyperbilirubinemic and many are jaundiced at initial presentation. The presence of jaundice does not indicate prognosis because some dogs that have responded to corticosteroid therapy underwent normalization of their serum bilirubin concentration. Evaluation of the coagulation status has revealed prolonged PT or APTT in between 40% to 55% of dogs tested. Low serum fibrinogen concentrations seem consistent and may reflect consumption coagulopathy or synthetic failure. Not all of these dogs have increased FDPs but many are thrombocytopenic. The high incidence of von Willebrand's disease in this breed puts them at high risk for pathologic hemorrhage during liver biopsy considering their deranged coagulation tests. Pretreatment with DDAVP of patient and blood donor is prudent in this circumstance to maximize availability of von Willebrand's factor. This prophylactic measure must be carefully orchestrated to temporally coincide with the biopsy procedure because it provides only a few hours of benefit. Immediately before the procedure, DDAVP (1-desamino-8-D-arginine vasopressin, Desmopressin acetate; USV Laboratories, Tarrytown, NY) is administered to the patient at a dose of 1 to 5 μg/kg diluted in 10 to 20 mL of saline given IV slowly (over 10 minutes) or given subcutaneously.[544] If a blood transfusion is deemed appropriate, only fresh blood should be administered. If possible, the donor should be pretreated with DDAVP. Using fresh blood optimizes platelet function, coagulation factor delivery, and reduced concentrations of ammonia as compared to previously stored blood. Optimally, the patient should be cross-matched to the donors; this requires anticipation of potential transfusion before the biopsy procedure is performed.

Remarkably increased BSP percentage retention is not surprising in this disorder considering the hyperbilirubinemia in most dogs. Bile acids have been evaluated only in the fasting condition, and in some, these have been normal. Bile acid values have been determined only in dogs that were not overtly jaundiced. Physicochemical evaluation of abdominal effusion in dogs with ascites shows a pure or modified transudate.

Histomorphologic features of chronic hepatitis in the Doberman pinscher include variable degrees of degeneration and necrosis of periportal hepatocytes (Figure 33–31 and 33–32). Many biopsies also show necrosis and fibrosis of perivenular (zone 3) hepatocytes and bridging tracts crossing the lobule.[252] Mixed inflammatory cell infiltrates develop in periportal areas. Areas of acute hepatocellular necrosis are infiltrated with neutrophils and macrophages. Bile ductule proliferation may also develop, but the large bile ducts appear uninvolved. Portal fibrosis may be mild or severe and bridging. Hepatic cirrhosis occurs in severely affected dogs. Accumulation of copper predominates in periportal hepatocytes, particularly in areas of degeneration and necrosis (Figure 33–31 and 33–32).[252] In severely affected dogs, a multifocal distribution of copper-laden cells occurs. Lipogranulomas may occur in the periportal area and some of these areas stain positively for iron. Iron accumulates in Kupffer cells and macrophages rather than hepatocytes. Extramedullary hematopoiesis has been seen in liver tissue from some animals. Ultrastructural studies have failed to recognize viral agents in liver tissue.

Quantitative copper and iron determinations have been completed in some dogs (see Figure 33–33). Moderately increased copper and notably increased iron concentrations have been shown in affected dogs. The role of copper in this

disease is not understood but is believed to be an epiphenomenon due to the cholestatic nature of the disorder. Accumulated iron is probably associated with the hepatic parenchymal necrosis, hemorrhage, and inflammation. Pathophysiologically, accumulation of either of these metals could aggravate ongoing local inflammation if excessive stores accumulate.

Definitive treatment of affected dogs is not well established. Complete medical management requires consideration of the various factors described in the therapeutic section of this chapter. Specific anti-inflammatory treatment with prednisone is believed to be beneficial in dogs diagnosed early. An immunosuppressive dose of prednisone is gradually tapered to achieve a daily total dose between 10 and 20 mg. In some dogs, an eventual titration to alternate-day treatment has been successful. If treatment is successful, sequential evaluations usually show a gradual reduction in transaminase activity.[114] Hepatic copper values were reduced to less than 400 μg/g dry tissue after 3 to 12 months of treatment in one dog sequentially biopsied.

It is important that Doberman pinschers with liver disease have tissue biopsy and careful review of their case record before breed-related chronic hepatitis is assumed. This breed has an increased tendency for trimethoprim-sulfa, oxibendazole, and perhaps other drug hepatotoxicities. If any medication has temporal association with newly recognized liver disease or with recrudescence of an older problem, that drug must be discontinued. It is advisable that routine screening profiles be evaluated on Doberman pinschers as a method of early disease detection.

COPPER STORAGE HEPATOPATHY IN THE BEDLINGTON TERRIER

Clinical Synopsis

Diagnostic Features

- Young adult to middle-aged Bedlington terriers
- Clinical signs of acute or chronic anorexia, vomiting, and/or diarrhea are common
- Jaundice, ascites, and hepatic encephalopathy occur in chronically affected dogs
- Acute hemolytic crises occur in some dogs
- Elevated ALT common
- Four histologic classifications: copper staining only, focal hepatitis, chronic hepatitis, or cirrhosis
- Liver copper concentration greater than 850 μg/g dry weight

Standard Management

- Low copper diets and zinc supplementation (100 mg PO BID for 3 months followed by 50 mg PO BID)
- Keep plasma zinc concentration below 1 mg/dl
- Copper chelation with D-penicillamine (10–15 mg/kg PO BID), 2,2,2 tetramine (10–15 mg/kg PO) or 2,3,3 tetramine (15 mg/kg PO BID) initially
- Prednisone (0.5–1.0 mg/kg PO if hemolytic crisis)

The first report of chronic progressive hepatitis in Bedlington terriers was published in 1975 by Hardy et al.[396] Since then, the disorder has been linked to pathologic copper retention in hepatocytes, determined to be an inherited autosomal recessive defect, and found to have a pathogenesis simi-

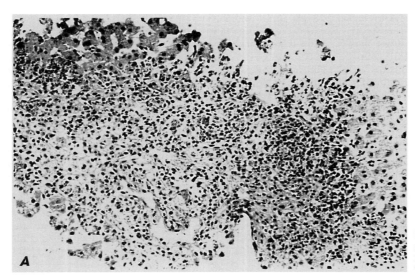

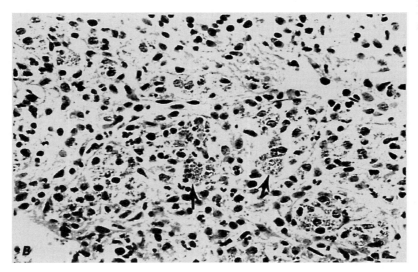

FIGURE 33–31. Photomicrograph of liver tissue from a Doberman pinscher with chronic hepatitis. In (*A*), low-power magnification of a needle biopsy specimen. There is marked periportal inflammation, sinusoidal disarray, and developing fibrosis. In (*B*), a higher power magnification is shown (140×: magnification) that illustrates the increased fibrous tissue, segmentation of the sinusoids, and a granular appearance to hepatocytes.

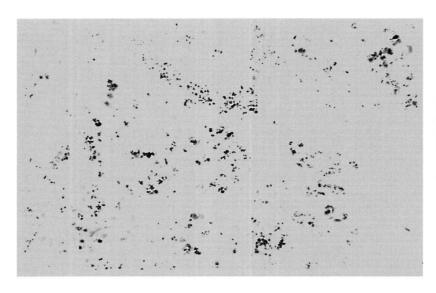

FIGURE 33–32. Photomicrograph of liver tissue from the dog in Figure 33–31, stained with rubeanic acid. The granules stain positive for copper. This photomicrograph should be compared to Figure 33–35 in which the copper deposition in a Bedlington terrier is shown. Quantitative copper was 2500 µg/g dry weight liver tissue.

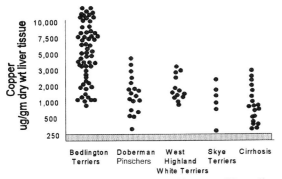

Dogs with histologic evidence of liver disease

FIGURE 33-33. Hepatic copper concentrations expressed on a dry weight basis in different types of chronic liver disease in the dog and certain pure breed dogs.

lar to Wilson's disease in humans.[397–402] In health, copper acquired from the diet is circulated to the liver where it is temporarily stored bound to hepatic cytosolic proteins. If not used, copper is sequestered in hepatic lysosomes and eventually excreted in bile and eliminated in feces; see Chapter 30 for a more detailed discussion of copper metabolism. The genetic defect in the Bedlington terrier causes expression of an abnormal hepatic metallothionein. This results in reduced biliary excretion of copper.[400,403] Excessive copper becomes sequestered in hepatocellular lysosomes where it is best detected using copper-specific stains. It can also be detected on light microscopy as red/brown granules with routine H&E staining[403–406] (Figures 33–34 and 33–35). Special stains such as rubeanic acid, rhodanine, or Timms are used to identify copper-laden lysosomes definitively (Figure 33–34). Estimation of hepatic copper content can be made with these stains. Staining differentiates copper granules from granules associated with iron, lipofuscin, or bile pigments. Quantitative copper determinations confirm a copper storage hepatopathy and in the Bedlington have shown pathologically increased hepatic copper concentrations in all affected dogs. An increasing hepatic copper concentration correlates with the severity of tissue injury and progressively accumulates as the dog ages (Figure 33–36).[397] Once a critical burden of copper accumulates, acute hepatic necrosis develops with only slight provocation. Crises occur after stressful events or in the preterminal stages of hepatic failure. When excess copper is released into the systemic circulation it invokes red cell hemolysis and abrupt development of severe anemia, acute renal failure, and DIC.

The clinical and morphologic features of copper toxicosis in the Bedlington terrier has been well described.[396,397,407,408] One large survey[397] identified 68 affected dogs on the basis of hepatic biopsy and quantitative determination of tissue copper concentration. Only 5 of 63 (12.6%) had palpable organomegaly. Clinical signs were displayed by only 19 of these dogs and were classified into three distinct syndromes. In 5 dogs less than 6 years old, signs consisted of acute episodes of anorexia, vomiting, weakness, lethargy, and dehydration. These dogs had biochemical evidence of active liver disease (increased ALT activity) and morphologic abnormalities on tissue examination. Each recovered from bouts of illness with provision of only supportive care. In 13 dogs, ages ranging between 5 and 12 years, a more insidious illness was characterized. These dogs lost condition due to anorexia, intermittent vomiting, and diarrhea. Clinical signs were recognized weeks to months before development of overt liver failure. Jaundice, ascites, cachexia, HE, and death ultimately

occurred in dogs of this group. Four dogs developed an abrupt episode of hemolytic anemia, jaundice, and marked increases in their ALT activities. One dog had a hemolytic crisis following whelping and the others were insidiously ill and had hemolytic crises preterminally. Dogs with clinical signs had variable abnormalities in liver function, but almost all had increased serum ALT activity. Of all 68 dogs with morphologic hepatic lesions or excessive copper storage, 22 (32%) had abnormally increased serum ALT activity. Histologic staging of the liver injury allowed the authors to evaluate the association between clinicopathologic features and the extent of tissue damage. The association between tissue injury and the frequency of increased ALT activity is shown in Figure 33–37.[397] It was deduced that abnormal enzyme activity occurs rather late in the disorder and reflects the stage of morphologic injury rather than the earlier stage of uncomplicated copper accumulation. Dogs with advanced disease developed other clinicopathologic features of hepatic injury including increased ALP activity, hyperbilirubinemia, prolonged prothrombin time, and reduced serum albumin concentration.

Determinations of serum or plasma copper concentration were not different between affected and unaffected dogs: 54 ± 10 μg/dl in affected dogs (n = 15), 56 ± 10μg/dl (n = 7), and 49 ± 5 μg/dl in mixed-breed dogs (n = 7).[397] The plasma

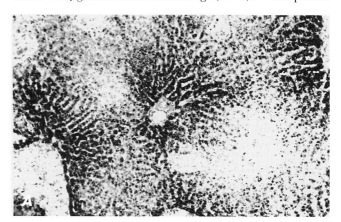

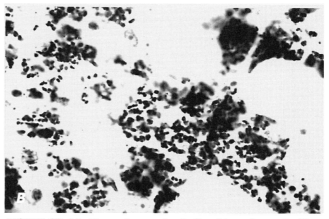

FIGURE 33-34. Photomicrograph of a liver biopsy from a Bedlington terrier with copper storage hepatopathy. In *A*, the tissue copper deposition is well displayed on low-power magnification of the biopsy specimen stained with rubeanic acid, as a copper-specific stain. This dog had severe copper deposition and was clinically ill. Quantitative copper determination was 8000 μg/g dry weight liver tissue (normal <400 μg/g). In *B*, a high-power view of the copper granules is provided. Background hepatocyte nuclei are seen for size comparison.

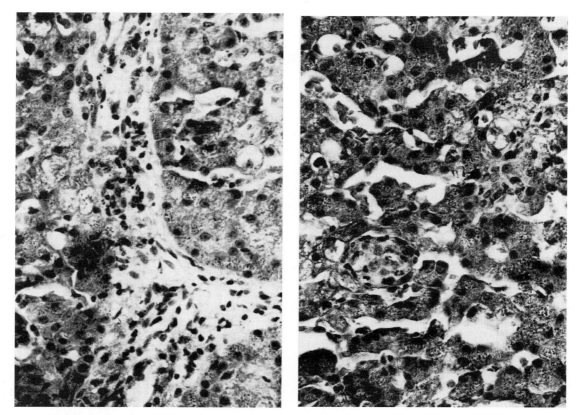

FIGURE 33–35. Photomicrograph showing copper granules as they appear with routine H&E staining in a Bedlington terrier with no clinical evidence of liver disease except an ALT activity 10 times normal. Copper content of the liver was 1723 µg/g wet weight (normal = 40 µg/g). Plasma copper was 91 µg/dl and ceruloplasmin was 27 mg/dl, both in the normal range. Histology shows infiltration of portal areas with inflammatory cells, focal necrosis with macrophages, and hepatocyte changes that include granules and lipidosis.

concentration of ceruloplasmin (a copper transport protein) is not diagnostic, unlike the situation in Wilson's disease in humans. Definitive diagnosis requires tissue biopsy examination, staining copper with specific stains, and quantitative tissue copper determination. Hepatic tissue copper concentrations become profoundly increased in affected dogs and reach maximal values in dogs ranging in age between 2 and 10 years. Tissue copper concentrations have ranged between 850 and 10,600 µg/g dry weight. Affected dogs older than 10 years of age have had significantly lower tissue copper concentrations than dogs between 4 and 6 years of age. It is possible that this occurs beacause of the earlier death of severely affected dogs, a reduction in tissue copper due to connective tissue displacement of hepatic parenchyma, and a lower concentration of copper in regenerative nodules. Hepatic concentrations of iron also increase with copper toxicosis in the

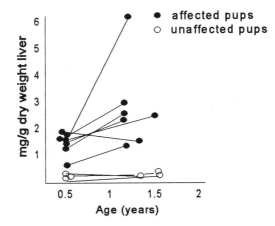

FIGURE 33–36. Association between hepatic copper content and increasing age of young Bedlington terriers affected with a copper storage hepatopathy. Data adapted from reference 397, with permission.

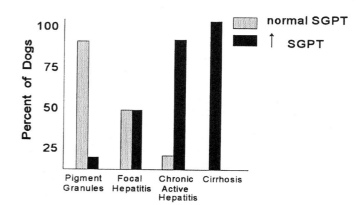

FIGURE 33–37. The association between tissue injury and the frequency of increased ALT activity in the Bedlington with copper storage hepatopathy. Data adapted from reference 397, with permission.

Bedlington terrier. Quantitation of iron in the liver has shown a fourfold increase compared to normal dogs. It is possible that this is related to red cell hemolysis or parenchymal cell necrosis and inflammation.

The histologic lesions in Bedlington terriers with copper storage hepatopathy have been categorized into four groups: (1) pigment granules only, (2) focal hepatitis, (3) chronic hepatitis, and (4) cirrhosis.[397,404] The first group was comprised of biopsies from 11 of 68 dogs that did not show signs of liver injury. In young dogs in this group the copper granules were predominantly perivenular (zone 3). Group 2 was comprised of 25 of 68 specimens characterized by randomly distributed focal hepatitis; foci involved Kupffer cell hyperplasia and infiltrates of neutrophils and macrophages. Fibrosis extending from the portal triads was observed in some areas. Copper-laden granules were more plentiful than in group 1 and were diffusely distributed throughout the hepatic acinus. Group 3 included 21 of 68 specimens typified as chronic hepatitis; these had infiltrates of lymphocytes, plasma cells, and neutrophils extending mainly from the portal triads. Bridging necrosis was occasionally seen. Kupffer cells were prominent and contained pigmented inclusions. Fibrosis was variable and in some was characterized as bridging between portal areas and in others as extending from portal areas into the lobules. Copper-laden granules were diffuse and evident in most hepatocytes. Group 4 was comprised of 11 of 68 specimens from dogs with micro- or macronodular cirrhosis; these had ongoing tissue injury, diffusely distributed copper granules, and occasional dilated lymphatics. Extramedullary hematopoiesis was a common observation. Grossly, the livers of dogs with severe liver injury were normal or slightly decreased in size. The relationship between the histomorphologic lesion and the age of the dog is shown in Figure 33–38.

It has been suggested that a presumptive diagnosis of copper toxicosis can be made in a Bedlington terrier if persistently increased and unexplainable ALT activity is recognized. At one time up to two-thirds of dogs of this breed were considered affected. The frequency of disease occurrence has been reduced by selective breeding. Combination of tests permits recognition of the disorder in dogs as young as 6 months. A study of heterozygotes of this trait showed they could develop transiently increased tissue copper concentrations during the first 2 years of life. Biopsy between 5 and 7 months and again after 14 to 15 months was recommended. The dog free of this trait will have normal tissue copper concentrations on each biopsy, the homozygote will have increasing concentrations, and the heterozygote will have an early rise but subsequent normalization of its tissue copper concentrations.[408]

Management of Bedlington terriers with copper storage hepatopathy is initially focused on avoiding excessive copper ingestion and absorption in the young affected dog. This is accomplished by assuring that excessive dietary or water sources of copper are eliminated and by using zinc to block enteric copper absorption and excess hepatic copper storage.[409–412] Once excessive copper storage has developed (tissue copper > 2000 µg/g dry weight), initial treatment with a copper chelator is advised. Subsequently, treatment with zinc is continued as lifelong therapy. Coadministration of zinc and a chelator is not recommended at the present time, although they may share a common mechanism of action in induction of metallothionein.[413]

If serious hepatic injury has not yet developed, avoidance of an intake of excessive copper is paramount. Preparation of a copper-free diet is impossible and not believed to be necessary if chelation and zinc therapy are used as indicated. Foodstuffs or water containing high concentrations of copper should obviously be avoided (Table 33–19).[262] The dietary copper level rec-

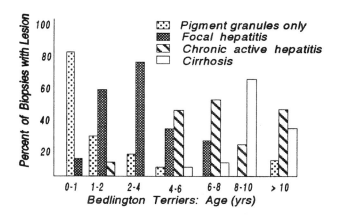

FIGURE 33–38. The relationship between the histomorphologic hepatic lesion and the age of an affected Bedlington terrier with copper storage hepatopathy. Data adapted from reference 397, with permission.

ommended by the National Research Council equates to 0.8 mg of copper per 1000 kcal of metabolizable energy, believed by some nutritionists to be excessive supplementation.[462] The allowed dietary intake of humans with Wilson's disease is 1.0 mg/day.[262] The Wilson's patient on zinc therapy absorbs far less copper than this. Most commercial dog foods contain copper concentrations in excess of 7 mg/kg diet on a dry weight basis. Commercial human enteral diets are also often high in copper and should be avoided.[262] Mineral supplements, vitamins, or treats containing copper should also be avoided.

Feeding copper-restricted diets slows hepatic copper accumulation but does not facilitate removal of preexistent copper stores. Although chelation therapy is currently believed to be necessary when excessive hepatic copper concentrations have already accumulated, preliminary studies in humans with Wilson's disease suggest zinc therapy may be beneficial in halting hepatic injury even before copper chelation.[262] When chelation therapy is used, copper is bound by the chelating agent either in the circulation or tissues and is then mobilized for renal excretion. Chelation removal of copper takes months to years to mobilize a significant amount from the liver. The most commonly used drug has been *D-penicillamine* (Cuprimine, 250 mg capsules; Merck Sharp & Dohme; or Depen, 250 mg tablets; Wallace). This is a potent chelator and an average loss of 900 µg of copper per gram of dry weight liver per year from affected Bedlingtons given penicillamine has been reported.[414] It would thus take

Table 33–19

FOODS RICH IN ZINC AND COPPER

Foods Rich in Zinc	Foods Rich in Copper
Red meat	Shellfish*
Milk	Liver*
Gelatin	Kidney
Egg yolks	Heart
Shellfish	Meat
Beans	Nuts
Peas	Mushrooms
Liver	Cereals
Whole grains	Cocoa
Lentils	Legumes
Rice	Soft water (copper pipes)
Potatoes	

*Very high.

several years to decopper a liver containing 5000 μg/g, a concentration commonly found in affected middle-aged Bedlington terriers. The recommended dose for D-penicillamine is 10 to 15 mg/kg given PO BID on an empty stomach because food interferes with drug absorption. Some dogs vomit when treated and this may be alleviated by reducing the dose and giving it more frequently. Side effects associated with D-penicillamine are uncommon in dogs but include reversible renal disease, proteinuria, cutaneous eruptions, and vomiting.[414] In humans experiencing side effects of penicillamine, the drug is withdrawn and then reinstituted at a lower dose. If problems continue, prednisone is given concurrently.[414,415] If this is unsuccessful, treatment is switched to an alternative chelator. Humans receiving chronic D-penicillamine therapy develop pyridoxine deficiency.[250] Although this has not been identified in dogs, it is recommended they be supplemented with B vitamins to avoid this potential problem. Bedlingtons on long-term therapy with D-penicillamine do not develop hepatic failure despite continued increased copper levels and apparent ongoing hepatic injury.[416]

An alternative chelator that is less toxic then D-penicillamine is *2,2,2 tetramine* (Trientine, Cuprid, 250 mg capsules; Merck Sharp & Dohme).[417-418] A clinical trial with tetramine in healthy and affected dogs demonstrated it was free of objectionable side effects.[418] At a dose of 10 to 15 mg/kg PO BID, chelation effects were comparable to D-penicillamine. A urinary loss of approximately 0.5 mg copper per day was reported. Studies in the dog have shown that 2,2,2 tetramine does not have a significant effect on zinc or iron concentrations. Experimental work suggests that tetramine may prove beneficial for treating dogs in acute hemolytic crises due to high serum copper concentrations; D-penicillamine is not useful in this circumstance.[418]

Modification of 2,2,2 tetramine to *2,3,2 tetramine* produces a four- to nine-fold increase in potency as a copper chelator. Use in affected Bedlington terriers (n = 5) showed that it reduced liver copper concentrations by a mean of 3282 μg/g dry weight after 200 days of treatment at a dose of 15 mg/kg.[419] This produced an approximate daily loss of 2 mg copper in the urine. It also was effective in one dog undergoing acute hepatic necrosis and hemolysis. This drug is not commercially available. It can be obtained from chemical supply companies in the form of N,N'-bis(2-aminoethyl-)-1,3-propanediamine and then prepared as a salt to be given orally.[419]

Another important approach to the management of copper storage hepatopathy is reducing intestinal copper absorption. This is done by avoiding excess copper intake in food or water, by ingesting ascorbic acid with meals, using glucocorticoids, and ingesting oral zinc at least 1 hour before or after meals. *Ascorbic acid* is believed to reduce enteric copper absorption as well as to facilitate urinary copper elimination. However, its efficacy in this function is poorly documented. The recommended dose for these effects is 500 to 1000 mg/day.[154,262,410-412,420,421] The mechanisms of action of *glucocorticoids* is through their effect on metallothionein induction, similar to the effect described for zinc. Glucocorticoids thereby reduce enteric copper absorption and increase the storage potential in the nontoxic cytosolic copper storage pool. A dose of 0.5 to 1.0 mg/kg has been recommended to stabilize lysosomes against rupture in dogs undergoing hemolytic crises.[422,423] Glucocorticoids are reserved only for this purpose.

Zinc therapy has shown success in the management of humans with chronic Wilson's disease and in Bedlington terriers with copper toxicosis.[154,262,415-420,424-427] The physiologic benefits of zinc therapy in the patient with hepatic insufficiency have been discussed in Chapter 30 and previously in this chap-

ter (see Figure 33-19).[428,429] The major benefit of zinc therapy in the patient with copper hepatotoxicosis is through its induction of intestinal metallothionein that covalently binds copper, blocking its absorption. This has been accomplished in humans with doses as small as 25 mg PO TID.[410] A pilot study in dogs, three Bedlington terriers with copper hepatotoxicity and three West Highland white terriers with an ill-defined tendency for hepatic copper storage, reported the efficacy of zinc acetate in the management of hepatic copper accumulation.[154] Of note in this study was that it took 3 to 6 months to obtain a therapeutic plasma zinc response and suppression of enteric copper absorption in the dogs studied. Loading with 100 mg elemental zinc PO BID for 3 months was recommended. Thereafter, the dosage of elemental zinc was reduced to 50 mg PO BID to maintain adequate control within a safe plasma zinc concentration. Plasma zinc concentrations should be monitored periodically, every 2 to 3 months, to assure that therapeutic and nontoxic levels of zinc are attained. Plasma zinc concentrations of 1000 μg/dl or above are avoided because they can be associated with red cell hemolysis.

An abbreviated algorithm for current recommendations for treatment of biopsy-confirmed hepatic copper toxicosis is provided in Figure 33-39. Zinc acetate is better tolerated than zinc sulfate or gluconate. It is best administered in gel capsules and must be separated by at least 1 hour from food ingestion.

Hepatic Copper Concentrations in Liver Disorders

The association between an increased hepatic copper concentration and its relationship to tissue injury is controversial in breeds other than the Bedlington terrier. Because biliary excretion is the major mechanism regulating body copper homeostasis, hepatic diseases associated with cholestasis cause abnormal hepatic copper retention.[400,422-426,430,431] There is also concern that limited synthesis of transport proteins, such as ceruloplasmin, may promote hepatocyte copper sequestration. There have been a number of reports showing that Doberman pinschers, West Highland white terriers, and other breeds have increased hepatic copper concentrations when they develop substantial liver disease.[114,252,395,427,432-436] The West Highland white terrier may have an inborn propensity to accumulate copper in the liver, but this has not been shown to be inexorably linked to liver disease.[433,434] Experimental creation of major bile duct occlusion is associated with an increased uptake of radio-labeled copper and a reduced biliary elimination of copper.[400] The Bedlington terrier defect simulates biliary obstruction in its influence on copper.[400] The hepatic tissue copper concentrations in cats with major bile duct occlusion have also been shown to be increased, although not to the same magnitude as in dogs.[436] Chronic hepatitis, chronic cholestasis, and cirrhosis have been shown to lead to increased tissue copper concentrations in dogs; these values are compared graphically in Figure 33-33. This phenomenon has also been shown in humans where it is clearly established that hepatic copper concentrations increase in the majority of patients with primary biliary cirrhosis, prolonged extrahepatic bile duct obstruction, or chronic liver disease to the extent that they can overlap with values reported for humans with Wilson's disease.[422-426,430,431] It is probable that in many dogs with liver disease, an increased tissue copper concentration develops as an epiphenomenon of cholestasis or other aspects of reduced hepatic function. The increased copper, however, could contribute to tissue injury if hepatocellular lysosomes become over-

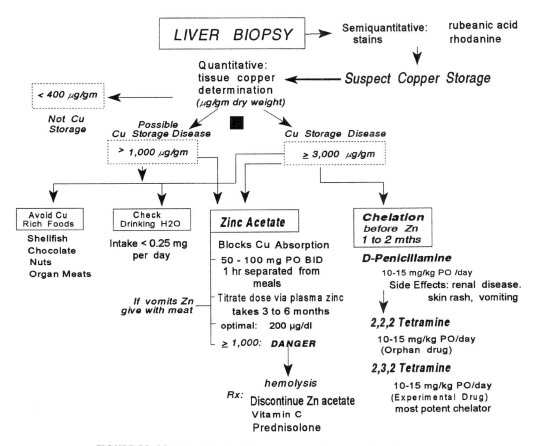

FIGURE 33–39. Algorithm for the treatment of copper toxicosis in the dog.

whelmed and toxic copper is released into the cytosol. It is interesting to note that the normal adult dog has a 10-fold greater hepatic concentration of copper than a normal adult human. The canine liver is amazingly well adapted for storing copper compared to other species.[437] This high concentration may be due to the high copper content of commercial dog foods, which contribute more copper per pound of body weight for the dog than a person consumes with a well-balanced diet. One author proposed a plausible scenario of this difference. The concentration of copper in hepatic tissue in dogs has progressively increased from 6.8 µg/g dry weight in 1929, 44 µg/g dry weight in 1932, up to 200 µg/g dry weight in 1982.[400] This corresponds to the change in customs of feeding pet dogs commercially prepared pet foods that are excessively fortified with copper. A concentration less than 400 µg/g dry weight is considered normal. The liver copper concentration is greater in neonates than in adults, and can approach 600 µg/g dry weight in the puppy.

WEST HIGHLAND WHITE TERRIERS AND HEPATIC COPPER RETENTION

Clinical Synopsis

Diagnostic Features

- Young adult to middle-aged West Highland white terriers
- Clinical and biochemical evidence of chronic hepatitis
- Increased serum ALT is earliest abnormality

- Four histologic categories: normal liver, copper staining only, multifocal hepatitis, or cirrhosis
- No clear relationship between severity of hepatitis and hepatic copper level

Standard Management

- As for chronic hepatitis (see clinical synopsis on p. 706)

A detailed report of West Highland white terriers described the histologic distribution and quantitative measurements of hepatic copper.[433] Liver tissue from 71 dogs was studied; samples were derived from biopsy and necropsy acquisitions in a diagnostic laboratory and a prospective study of a kindred of dogs suspected to be affected with inheritable liver disease. Not all dogs were showing signs of liver disease, and there was no indication that biochemical screening profiles were done in each dog. A subsequent report indicates that increased serum ALT activity is the earliest biochemical abnormality.[434] With advanced disease, clinicopathologic features include increased liver enzyme activity, hyperbilirubinemia, increased serum bile acid concentrations and BSP retention, hyperammonemia and hypoalbuminemia. Hemolytic anemia has not been recognized.

Upon retrospective evaluation of 71 dogs, four different histomorphologic categories were characterized: normal liver without excessive copper staining, normal liver with excessive copper staining, multifocal hepatitis with excessive copper staining, and cirrhosis with excessive copper staining. Quantitative copper measurements were taken from a small number of dogs in each group; see Figure 33–40. Comparison of age

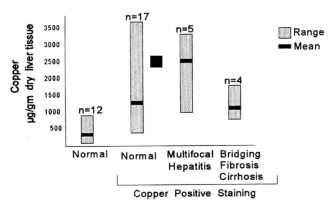

FIGURE 33-40. Association between histomorphologic lesions, quantitative hepatic copper measurements, and qualitative copper detection with a copper-specific stain in West Highland white terrier dogs with suspected copper storage hepatopathy. Adapted from reference 433.

with quantitative hepatic copper concentration showed no relationship. This is contrary to the circumstance in Bedlington terriers where there is a progressive increase in tissue copper accumulation until 8 years of age. There also was no consistent association between abnormal histomorphology and quantitative tissue copper content. This too is contrary to the circumstance in Bedlington terriers where hepatic injury shows a positive association with tissue copper concentration, until the development of cirrhosis.

Early copper retention appeared in the perivenular (zone 3) region of the acinus, similar to the Bedlington terrier. Foci of hepatitis were characterized by focal hepatocellular necrosis, pigment-filled phagocytes, and a few lymphocytes, plasma cells, and neutrophils. These foci were associated with the largest and most numerous copper-containing granules. Phagocytic cells in the foci contained iron and copper. Dogs with cirrhosis had bridging fibrosis between portal regions and between hepatic vein and portal areas. These dogs also developed biliary hyperplasia. Copper-containing hepatocytes were evident bordering fibrous septa and in some, diffusely throughout regenerative nodules.

The copper concentration attained in dogs with obvious hepatic disease did not exceed 3500 μg/g dry weight liver. In contrast, affected Bedlington terriers commonly have values of 5000 μg/g dry weight liver or greater. Values as high as 10,000 have been reported.

The relationship between copper toxicosis and liver disease in the West Highland white terrier is not understood. In a demographic study done in Sweden, West Highland white terriers were found to have an increased incidence of chronic hepatitis, but copper accumulation was not a consistent feature.[111] Some dogs with high copper concentrations have no sign of liver injury as we know it in the Bedlington terrier. The genetics of this defect may be an incomplete expression of a simple Mendelian trait or a polygenic abnormality with variable expression as this mode of genetic transmission would produce the confusing characteristics so far described. It is also possible that this is an epiphenomenon of some other predisposition to liver disease. Long-term study of dogs with high hepatic copper concentrations will clarify whether or not the copper storage precedes serious liver disease and whether chelation or zinc acetate treatments are appropriate in this breed.

LIVER DISEASE IN SKYE TERRIERS

A liver disease of Skye terriers was reported in 1984 and was recently more fully characterized.[438–440] In the detailed report, nine related Skye terriers ranging between the ages of 18 months and 15 years were included. Seven (78%) of these dogs had preterminal clinical signs of progressive liver disease including anorexia, vomiting, ascites, and jaundice. Three dogs that either died from or were euthanized because of their liver disease had variable increases in serum ALP activity. Two dogs were asymptomatic and one of these had an increased serum ALP activity and high globulins. The last dog was found to have cirrhosis on necropsy after euthanasia for old-age-related problems.

Liver histomorphology and copper content allowed categorization of the tissue into three groups. It was felt these groups most accurately described disease chronicity rather than severity. In the first group (n = 2), liver architecture was normal. Perivenular hepatocytes appeared swollen, there was evidence of retained biliary debris, and inflammatory changes were mild and limited to a few neutrophils, monocytes, and occasional plasma cells in periportal and perivenular areas. Copper was not evident on histochemical staining and quantitative copper was within the normal range in one dog. In the second group (n = 5), liver tissue was architecturally disrupted by parenchymal nodules separated by wide bands of connective tissue containing hyperplastic bile ductules, capillaries, and many pigment-containing macrophages and inflammatory cells. Regional variation in tissue injury was notable but active degenerative/necrotizing processes seemed to originate in the perivenular (zone 3) area. Modest accumulation of copper-positive pigment was shown in the involved hepatocytes. Inflammatory changes were moderate and were comprised of neutrophils, macrophages, and a few plasma cells and lymphocytes. Copper-positive pigmentation was minimal to moderate in zone 3 and in regions adjacent to fibrous bands. Mean copper concentration was 926 μg/g dry weight liver. The third group (n = 2) was characterized by advanced macronodular cirrhosis. There was severe intracanalicular cholestasis and considerable zonal variation in the extent of tissue injury. Periacinar zonal necrosis was marked in the less fibrotic areas. Marked copper deposition was observed in hepatocytes extending from zone 3 into zone 2 and adjacent to fibrous tracts. The mean copper concentration was 1860 μg/g dry weight liver.

Hepatic copper accumulation is inconsistent in these dogs. It was not shown to accompany initial injury and did not appear to decline with severity of injury as it does in the Bedlington terrier. Intracanalicular cholestasis was felt to be a distinguishing difference between this disorder and those described for Bedlington terriers and West Highland white terriers. Copper accumulation in the Skye terrier appears to be in the perivenular (zone 3) area, which is inconsistent with other disorders associated with cholestasis and subsequent tissue copper retention. Cholestasis in the Doberman pinscher, cholestatic liver injury and primary biliary cirrhosis in humans, and copper loading in experimental animals result in periportal copper accumulation. Intrahepatic canalicular cholestasis was proposed as the mechanism of copper accumulation in zone 3. An inheritable metabolic defect was suggested but has not been clarified.

COCKER SPANIEL HEPATOPATHY

A preliminary report of hepatic disease in Cocker spaniels (n = 16) detailed an increased incidence in males (n = 14).[441]

Clinical illness was short lived; most dogs were ill for only 2 weeks or less prior to presentation for diagnostic evaluations. In two dogs, liver disease was discovered on the basis of biochemical screening profiles done for other purposes. The most common clinical problem and obvious physical abnormality was acute abdominal distension due to ascites (n = 11). Other vague signs common to hepatic disease were also present, including anorexia, lethargy, vomiting, diarrhea, polydipsia/polyuria, weight loss, and melena. In addition to ascites (n = 12), other physical abnormalities included depression (n = 7), icterus (n = 4), melena (n = 2), dehydration (n = 2), subcutaneous edema (n = 1), and coma (n = 1).

Clinicopathologic features included a borderline anemia in 50% of the dogs and a mature neutrophilia in 86%. Half of the dogs had isosthenuric urine and all were bilirubinuric. Evaluation of ascitic fluid yielded a pure or modified transudate. The biochemical profile detailed ongoing hepatic injury by virtue of increased transaminase and ALP activity. Hyperbilirubinemia was present in less than 50% of the dogs; mean bilirubin concentration was 1.4 mg/dl. Serum bile acid concentrations were abnormal in 6 of 8 dogs (fasting or portprandial was unspecified), fasting ammonia concentrations were abnormal in 3 dogs, a low BUN developed in 8 of 14 dogs, and a prolonged activated clotting time developed in 9 of 16 dogs. Prediction of liver size varied depending on the method of assessment (radiography vs. ultrasonography). At necropsy, livers were small, firm, and had many small regenerative nodules.

All biopsies showed moderate to severe portal hepatitis with variable degrees of portal fibrosis. Periportal inflammation was comprised predominantly of lymphocytes, plasma cells, and fewer numbers of neutrophils. Portal to portal bridging fibrosis and biliary hyperplasia were observed in most biopsies. Pathologic diagnoses included micronodular cirrhosis, macronodular cirrhosis, chronic hepatitis, and chronic periportal inflammation. Some dogs showed moderate to "abundant" copper on rhodanine stain; quantitative copper determination on one dog was 623 μg/g dry weight liver tissue.

Six dogs died within one week of presentation for diagnostic evaluation and six others died within a month. Of the longest surviving dogs (265 days and 395 days), one was treated with D-penicillamine and one was treated with prednisone. The later dog had "less mature" histologic lesions compared to the group in general. The two oldest dogs in the study also were under the influence of cortisone, which may have promoted long-term survival; one was hyperadrenocorticoid and the other on long-term prednisone therapy (10 mg PO every other day for 8 years). Treatment of other Cocker spaniels with chronic hepatitis using glucocorticoids, dietary modifications, ursodeoxycholic acid, and measures to manage ascites has permitted long-term survival in some for 12 months.

CHOLESTATIC LIVER DISEASE ASSOCIATED WITH EXTRAHEPATIC SEPSIS, PYOGENIC ABSCESS, AND SUPPURATIVE HEPATITIS

Bacterial organisms causing cholestatic injury without hepatic tissue colonization are shown in Table 33–20.[442–449] In humans, infants are more commonly affected than adults. The urinary tract is the usual site of primary infection and *E. coli* the most common pathogen.[449] Nonhepatic soft tissue abscesses, pneumonia, inflammatory bowel disease, pyelonephritis, prostatitis, endocarditis, and generalized bacteremia have been sources of infections in humans and in dogs.[442,444,448,450–452] Parvoviral infection can lead to this form of cholestatic jaundice in the dog due to coliform septicemia.[450] The etiopathogenesis of jaundice associated with extrahepatic sepsis, in the absence of direct hepatic colonization, involves bacterial toxins and inflammatory reactants, fever, malnutrition, and hypoxia. Endotoxin, teichoic acid (a lipopolysaccharide component of the cell wall of *Staphylococcus* spp.), and exotoxins have each been implicated as cholestatic toxins.[443,445,451–454] Endotoxin produces a dose-dependent reduction in the bile salt-dependent and independent bile flow. Acute-phase reactants associated with sepsis and inflammation have been shown to interfere with the transport of bile acids into canaliculi.[454] Despite the development of jaundice, the alteration in liver function and structure that develops in systemic infection is rarely severe enough to cause significant illness or death. Morbidity and mortality are attributed to the effects of septicemia rather than liver dysfunction. Clinicopathologic features may include a hemogram reflective of the systemic infectious process, and a disproportionate increase in bilirubin compared to the increases in liver enzyme activities.[444,446,449] Total bilirubin concentrations of up to 30 mg/dl have been seen in dogs.[446] The histologic lesions are often mild and nonspecific. Those most commonly linked to cholestasis associated with extrahepatic sepsis include perivenular canalicular stasis, the absence of hepatocellular necrosis, and mild accumulations of inflammatory cells in the portal areas.[443] If necrosis is seen, it is usually perivenular (zone 3). Ultrastructural lesions include canalicular dilatation and flattening of the canalicular microvilli, which reflect the cholestatic injury.[442]

Pyogenic Hepatic Abscess

Clinical Synopsis

Diagnostic Features

- Signs may relate more to underlying condition
- Fever, lethargy, and vomiting common
- Cranial abdominal pain may be present
- Neutrophilia common
- Increased ALT, ALP, globulins and bilirubin may occur
- Radiographs may show gas-filled hepatic lesion
- Ultrasonography usually detects a cystic or complex mass

Standard Management

- Antibiotics for 2–3 months
- Choice guided by culture results but amoxicillin, metron-

Table 33–20

BACTERIAL SEPSIS ASSOCIATED WITH INTRAHEPATIC CHOLESTASIS AND JAUNDICE

Bacteriodes*	Proteus
Enterobacter*	Pseudomonas
*Escherichia coli**	Salmonella
Hemophilus	Shigella
Klebsiella	Staphylococci*
Legionella	Streptococcus
Listeria	

*Most common.

idazole, cephalosporins, and short courses of aminoglycosides are suitable
- Needle or surgical drainage speeds resolution
- Lobectomy may be indicated

Pyogenic abscesses of the liver, occurring without evidence of a primary site of infection elsewhere in the body, is a relatively uncommon antemortem diagnosis in dogs and cats. Likely origins of infection are occult omphalitis in neonates and portal bacteremia in older animals. In adult animals, hepatic abscesses are more commonly associated with extrahepatic infection or regional hepatic parenchymal injury. Hematogenous spread from other sites of infection may occur; examples include prostatitis, pyometritis, pancreatitis, or pyelonephritis. Endocarditis and hepatic abscessation commonly occur together. It is unclear if one system becomes infected first or if infection becomes established during the same hematogenous shower of organisms.

In cats, the biliary system seems to be a more important route of infection than in the dog. In the cat, cholangitis associated with stagnant bile flow due to major bile duct occlusion, duodenitis, or pancreatitis seems to initiate retrograde infection that seeds a cholangiolar and periportal septic inflammation. Experimentally an intravenous injection of *Bacteroides fragilis* can lead to hepatobiliary sepsis if biliary tract obstruction coexists.[214] The portal vein is considered to be a more important route of infection compared to the lymphatic or the systemic circulatory routes.[213] A preexistent or concurrent ischemic insult is also believed to predispose the liver to infection.[455] Neoplastic conditions impinging on sinusoidal blood flow can make a focal area more susceptible to infection.[455] Necrosis of the interior of regenerative nodules or tumors can also predispose to infection.

The clinical signs of pyogenic hepatic abscesses are often nonspecific. Fever, lethargy, anorexia, and vomiting are common, and splenomegaly has been observed in affected dogs and cats. Weight loss develops if the problem is chronic. Physical assessment may reveal a tender cranial abdomen or evidence of diseases that increase susceptibility to infection; examples include hyperadrenocorticism, poorly controlled diabetes mellitus, and lymphosarcoma. The signs of hepatic disease may be minimal compared to the clinical signs of a primary underlying condition. Recognition of a recently developed cardiac murmur may signal the presence of endocarditis related to the hepatic abscess. If an abscess has ruptured, a septic exudative abdominal effusion may accumulate causing peritonitis, abdominal distension, and ileus.

Clinicopathologic features may include a neutrophilic leukocytosis with or without a left shift, increased liver enzyme activities (ALP and transaminases), hyperglobulinemia, and, in some cases, hyperbilirubinemia. However, liver enzymes may only be intermittently increased. In some animals, a neutropenia and degenerative left leukocyte shift develop due to overwhelming sepsis.

Hepatic abscessation may be detected on abdominal radiography if a gas-producing organism is involved or if the abscess has become mineralized (Figure 33–41). If an abscess has ruptured, free or loculated abdominal fluid may be observed. Ultrasonography is a more reliable investigative method. The reported sensitivity ranges between 80% to 100% for ultrasonographic detection of hepatic abscesses in humans.[456] Figure 33–42 shows the ultrasonographic appearance of an hepatic abscess. An ultrasound examination can determine whether a lesion is cystic, complex, or solid. When the index of suspicion for abscess is high, a cystic or complex mass is strongly suggestive. Abscesses containing a large amount of lipid content and those with gas may be hypere-

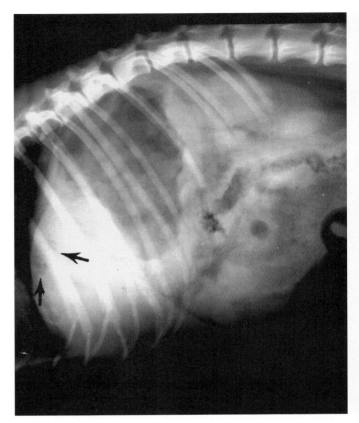

FIGURE 33–41. Abdominal radiograph showing free gas (arrows) within the hepatic parenchyma adjacent to the diaphragm. This dog had a septic cholangiohepatitis. (Courtesy Dr. N. Dykes, Section of Radiology, Department of Clinical Sciences, Cornell University)

choic and overlooked.[456] More sensitive imaging procedures include the use of ^{99m}Tc sulfur colloid scans, computed axial tomography (CT) scans, and magnetic resonance imaging (MRI). A biopsy of the lesion should always be submitted because cystic malformations (acquired or congenital) or neoplasia may become secondarily infected.

At laparotomy, there may be no gross evidence of an hepatic abscess by direct visualization. Palpation may reveal a change in tissue consistency. Needle aspiration may be

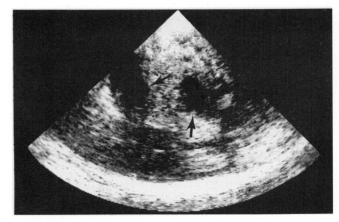

FIGURE 33–42. Ultrasonogram showing a two-cavitated hepatic abscess (arrows) in a dog with recurrent fever, neutrophilic leukocytosis, and anorexia. (Courtesy Dr. A. Yeager, Section of Radiology, Department of Clinical Sciences, Cornell University)

needed to localize the involved area. A percutaneous needle aspirate or biopsy of a suspected hepatic abscess should be directed by ultrasonographic guidance. If this is not done, a representative sample may not be collected. Needle biopsy may lead to complications of abdominal contamination and bacteremia.

Multiple small abscesses are more difficult to diagnose than large abscesses. These are found on routine examination of a tissue biopsy. Sepsis is more easily discerned on cytologic evaluation of tissue imprints rather than on histopathologic evaluation. Frequently, organisms can be cultured and observed on cytologic preparation when the histomorphology only describes suppurative inflammation. For this reason, liver imprints should always be made of the biopsy specimen. Sterile tissue sections should be reserved for aerobic and anaerobic bacterial culture and submitted after review of the tissue cytology. Organisms commonly cultured from hepatic abscesses in veterinary patients are shown in Table 33–21. In humans, if strict anaerobic techniques are adhered to, 50% of abscesses have an anerobic component.[455,457,458] Gram staining of the cytologic preparation will permit selection of initial antimicrobials. If one type of organism is seen, an antibiotic that has a high likelihood of efficacy should be chosen based on the gram stain. If two or more types of organisms are observed, combination antibiotic therapy is recommended, including metronidazole or clindamycin, and ampicillin or amoxicillin and an aminoglycoside or second- or third-generation cephalosporin.[457–459] Antibiotic therapy is more specifically targeted when culture and sensitivity results become available. Antibiotics should be given for at least 2 to 3 months; during the first week parenteral treatment is recommended.[457] Repeat ultrasonography and evaluation of the serum biochemical profile will assist in evaluating the response to treatment. Abscess drainage by needle, catheter, or surgical methods is usually done, although there is evidence that some patients may do well given only appropriate antibiotics.[460–462] In patients with single large abscesses, surgical removal of the involved liver lobe may be most efficient if the patient's condition will withstand the anesthetic and surgical risks.

Suppurative Hepatitis

Suppurative hepatitis may develop in association with infection or as a response to a regional hepatocellular necrosis. Regional injury can occur due to trauma, hypoxia, thromboembolism, copper toxicity, or neoplasia. Devitalized hepatic tissue is less able to remove the normal onslaught of microorganisms from the portal circulation. This tissue is thus more likely to become infected. Hepatic artery ligation in the dog often leads to hepatic necrosis and infection unless large doses of neomycin are orally administered preoperatively.[212]

Severe inflammatory bowel disease is an important cause of acute suppurative hepatitis in veterinary patients. These animals rarely undergo early liver biopsy because of initial diagnostic focus on the primary disease process. Later on when a chronic hepatopathy is recognized, nonsuppurative periportal inflammation is often found.

Tyzzer's disease, caused by a gram negative spore-forming bacteria (*Bacillus pilliformis*), is an uncommon but well-documented cause of multifocal hepatic necrosis and suppurative hepatitis in dogs and cats.[463] It is discussed in Chapter 32.

When suppurative hepatitis or a mixed inflammatory reaction (features of suppurative and nonsuppurative inflammation) are diagnosed, infection should be assumed although it

Table 33–21

BACTERIA CULTURED FROM PYOGENIC LIVER ABSCESSES IN DOGS AND CATS

Aerobic	Anaerobic
Bacillus piliformis	Actinomyces
Corynebacterium	Bacteroides
Enterobacter	*Clostridium perfringens*
Enterococcus	Fusobacterium
Escherichia coli	Proprionobacterium
Francisella tularensis	Anaerobic streptococci
Listeria monocytogenes	
Proteus	
Pseudomonas	
Salmonella	
Streptococcus	
Staphylococcus	

is not always present. Antimicrobial coverage should be directed at the most likely pathogens, which include the anaerobic enteric flora. Chronic treatment of liver inflammation may become necessary because a suppurative inflammatory reaction is thought to transform into a nonsuppurative self-perpetuating process.

GRANULOMATOUS HEPATITIS

Clinical Synopsis

Diagnostic Features

- Signs often relate to underlying condition
- Clinical and laboratory evidence of chronic hepatitis
- Liver biopsy shows granulomatous inflammation
- Special stains and titers for infectious or parasitic agents are indicated

Standard Management

- Treatment directed at underlying cause if identified
- Empirical antibiotic and/or glucocorticoid therapy may be valuable in idiopathic cases

Granulomatous hepatitis is characterized by small collections of histiocytes (or macrophages) often associated with lymphocytes and plasma cells, and occasionally with neutrophils and/or eosinophils.[464–472] Often this is a biopsy or postmortem finding that reflects a systemic disease process that incites granuloma formation. The sensitizing agent can be a foreign substance, immune complex, infectious agent, neoplastic cell, or an autoimmune phenomenon. A typical granulomatous foci from the liver of a dog with granulomatous hepatitis is shown in Figure 33–43. The cause of granulomatous hepatitis remains unknown in many animals. There are many potential etiologies (see Table 33–22).[470–487] Important differential diagnoses include neoplasia,[471] feline infectious peritonitis, and mycobacterial infection.[479]

Parasite migration has been cited as a cause in colonies of beagle dogs.[465–474] Coccidioidomycosis and histoplasmosis cause granulomatous hepatitis in dogs living in endemic areas.[482,483] Affected dogs are systemically infected. In the absence of an identifiable infectious cause, concurrent drug therapy should be considered as a possible cause because there are a considerable number of drugs that can produce this response in humans (see Chapter 30). Drug toxicity

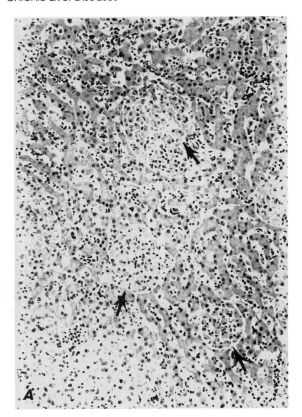

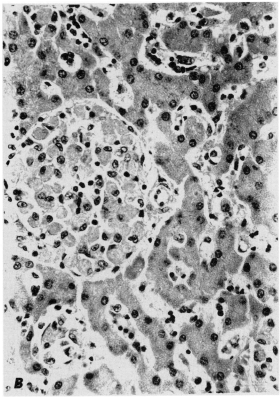

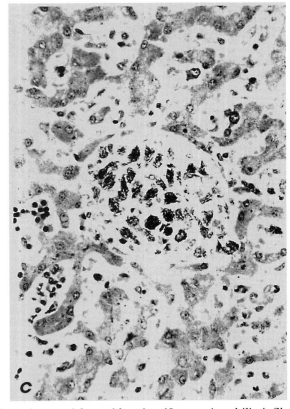

FIGURE 33–43. Photomicrograph of the liver from a dog with a granulomatous hepatitis. In (*A*), arrows indicate a large granuloma containing histiocytes and giant cells (140×: magnification). In (*B*) a higher magnification 350×:) does not disclose any infectious organisms H&E. In (*C*), the section is stained with Ziehl- Neelsen stain, which clearly demonstrates the presence of mycobacterial organisms; *Mycobacterium fortuitum* was later cultured.

should receive special consideration if an eosinophilic infiltrate is associated with granulomas.[468]

Clinical signs common in dogs with granulomatous hepatitis include lethargy, hepatomegaly, episodic or persistent fever, anorexia, and weight loss. Ascites, polydipsia, vomiting and/or diarrhea, icterus, abdominal pain, and peripheral lymphadenopathy are less consistent.

A diagnosis of granulomatous hepatitis warrants special staining of liver tissue for mycotic and microbial agents and serum testing for brucellosis, borreliosis, dirofilarrosis, and the common systemic fungal pathogen. Tissue for aerobic and anaerobic bacterial culture and for fungal culture should also be submitted. If peripheral lymphadenopathy is recognized, lymph node aspirates or Tru-cut biopsies should be collected for cytologic and histopathologic examination. This may confirm the presence of a neoplastic cell population. If a definitive cause is not recognized after liver biopsy and lymph node aspirates, cytologic evaluation and culture of aspirates of bone marrow and spleen should be performed. If a mycobacterial organism is involved, growth is slow in culture and will not guide therapy. Mycobacterial and fungal organisms should be looked for with special stains in all tissues submitted. Unfortunately, reports of retrospective studies in humans with granulomatous hepatitis have indicated that a cause cannot be found in up to 50% of patients even after extensive investigation.[465,466]

Treatment of granulomatous hepatitis involves therapy directed at the specific etiologic agent if such is identified. In some cases, improvement with empiric use of broad-spectrum antibiotics has been realized. Use of glucocorticoids to modulate the immune response involved with granuloma formation has been successful concurrent with antimicrobial therapy when an underlying etiology has not been established. Care must be given that all reasonable diagnostic evaluations have been completed before immunosuppression is contemplated. Frequent reevaluations including physical, hematologic, and biochemical assessments should be scheduled for the first several months of treatment if empirical glucocorticoid therapy is undertaken. If a positive response to glucocorticoids occurs, slow careful titration of the dose to alternate-day therapy and combination with azathioprine has been successful for long-term management in dogs believed to have immune-mediated disease.

IDIOPATHIC HEPATIC FIBROSIS IN YOUNG DOGS

Hepatic fibrosis in the absence of marked inflammation or some other underlying acquired hepatobiliary disorder has been recognized as a clinical syndrome in young to middle-aged dogs. Several different histomorphologic lesions have been characterized in groups of dogs: (1) periportal fibrosis (idiopathic hepatoportal fibrosis), (2) central perivenular fibrosis, and (3) perisinusoidal (pericellular) fibrosis, also termed reticulofibrosis. A lesion associated with random sinusoidal inflammation and fibrosis has been termed *lobular dissecting hepatitis*.[488–491]

The historical features and clinical signs at presentation include mild to marked ascites, lethargy, weight loss associated with variable gastrointestinal signs leading to poor body condition (vomiting, diarrhea, and anorexia), polyuria and polydipsia, and neurobehavioral changes compatible with HE. The clinicopathologic features of these dogs are shown in Table 33–23; the dogs with lobular dissecting hepatitis have been segregated from those with a noninflammatory lesion. Histopathologically, dogs have liver lesions characterized by differing degrees and severities of fibrosis. There is no evidence of pathologic copper retention and usually little to mild evidence of cholestasis. The clinical signs and clinicopathologic features seem independent of the histologic classification and are predominantly due to portal hypertension and acquired portosystemic shunting. The only other disorder in the dog with similar clinical signs is hepatic arteriovenous fistula, which can be distinguished by ultrasonography, angiography of hepatic artery, and liver biopsy.

Lobular Dissecting Hepatitis

As a distinct histologic lesion, lobular dissecting hepatitis was described in a small number of dogs that presented with ascites and acquired portosystemic shunts.[490] A mixed inflammatory infiltrate and dissection of lobular parenchyma by reticulin and fine collagen fibers characterizes the lesion (Figure 33–44). Portal inflammation is inconstant and usually a minor feature. Periportal fibrosis was minimal in the initial report and there was little bile duct proliferation. Dilated vascular channels presumed to be derived from sinusoids and portal venous radicles were prominent in most biopsies. Dilated lymphatics but no evidence of hepatic vein obstruction were also observed. All dogs presented for ascites and inappetance, and some were polydipsic. The report did not

Table 33–22

CAUSES OF GRANULOMATOUS HEPATITIS

Infectious Disorders	Noninfectious Disorders
Bacterial	**Primary Liver Disease**
Actinomyces	Biliary obstruction
Borrelia	Acute/chronic pericholangitis
Brucella	Chronic hepatitis
Norcardia	Postnecrotic cirrhosis
Tularemia	Copper hepatopathy
Yersinia	**Collagen/Vascular Diseases**
Mycotic	SLE
Aspergilla Histoplasma	Rheumatoid arthritis
Blastomyces Paecilomycosis	Polyarthritis
Cryptococcus Sporotrichosis	**Immunodeficiency**
Coccidiodes	Predisposition to infections
Parasitic	**Neoplasia**
Capillaria	Lymphoreticular cancer
Lungworms	Malignant histocytosis
Dirofilaria	Systemic histocytosis
Schistosomiasis	Other: poorly differentiated
Hepatozoonosis	**Other Diseases**
Trematodes	Inflammatory bowel disease: lymphangiectasia
Larval migration	Ulcerative colitis
ascariasis	**Drug Toxicity**
ancylostoma	Consult Chapter 30, Table 30–22
stronglyoides	**Idiopathic Granulomatous Hepatitis**
Protozoal	
Amebiasis	
Protothecosis	
Toxoplasmosis	
Viral	
FIP	

Table 33–23

CLINICOPATHOLOGIC FEATURES OF DOGS WITH
IDIOPATHIC HEPATIC FIBROSIS[489,491] AND
LOBULAR DISSECTING HEPATITIS[490,491]

Test Parameter	Idiopathic Fibrosis: Perivenous, Periportal, and Sinusoidal Categories	Lobular Dissecting Hepatitis
RBC microcytosis	12/15*	—
Leukocytosis	5/15	0/6
↓ Total protein	13/18	6/6
↓ Albumin	7/18	6/6
↓ Globulins	6/15	0/6
↑ Liver enzymes:		
ALP	15/18	N–↑
Gamma-GT	2/3	—
ALT	10/18	N–↑
AST	2/3	—
↑ Total bilirubin	8/18	—
↓ Total cholesterol	5/15	—
↑ BSP% retention	8/8	6/6
↑ Total fasting serum bile acids	5/7	—
↑ Fasting NH_3 or ↓ NH_3 tolerance	11/12	4/4
Microhepatica	18/18	6/6
Obvious ascites	15/18	6/6

*Data expressed as number abnormal/number evaluated.

detail the presence of jaundice, and total bilirubin measurements were not provided. The clinical cases of lobular dissecting hepatitis in the dog seen by the author have had variable bilirubin concentrations and not all dogs have had ascites on initial presentation. Three unrelated male black standard poodles were included in the initial report of this disorder. In dogs of that report, the gross appearance of the liver usually resembled micronodular cirrhosis. Liver copper levels in three dogs were within normal limits.

Idiopathic Hepatoportal Fibrosis

Idiopathic hepatoportal fibrosis associated with portal atresia was first described in dogs by Ewing and Suter.[488] It was recently clarified as a distinct entity in four dogs: (3 dogs, 6 months of age or less).[489–491] Hematologic findings included a normal hematocrit or mild nonregenerative anemia. Microcytosis consistent with portosystemic shunting was verified in one dog. Serum biochemistry findings included hypoproteinemia and hypoalbuminemia but normal globulin concentrations. Increased activities of serum ALP and ALT developed in all dogs and hyperbilirubinemia was evident in two dogs. A subnormal or low normal BUN was consistent with impaired urea cycle ammonia detoxification or reduced renal tubular urea absorption. The serum cholesterol concentration was low in the only dog for which it was reported, consistent with portosystemic shunting or hepatic parenchymal insufficiency. Baseline ammonia and ammonia tolerance tests were abnormal and increased fasting serum bile acids and prolonged BSP retention were documented in one dog tested. One dog was shown to have increased fecal quantities of fatty acids, indicating reduced fat absorption.

Livers were small and congested with a slightly irregular surface. Two had obvious hyperplastic nodules. All three dogs had splenomegaly. Variable occurrence of thoracic effusion, pericardial effusion, subcutaneous edema, and edema of the submucosa of stomach and small and large intestines were recognized. Histologic evaluation of liver revealed prominent portal fibrosis with portoportal bridging and focal disruption of the "limiting plate" (hepatocytes bordering the portal triad). An increased number of arteriolar cross sections, bile ductular proliferation, and a minor infiltration of mononuclear cells were found in fibrotic areas. There were few small venules or capillaries in the portal area. Dilated lymphatics were described around the sublobular hepatic veins and in large portal areas. There were minimal inflammatory changes in the hepatic parenchyma.

Portal hypertension was proposed to be due to hepatoportal fibrosis and concurrent atresia or hypoplasia of the terminal branches of the portal veins. This condition was likened to specific disorders described in humans (see Table 33–24). Survival of 30 months occurred in one dog treated with colchicine, metronidazole, lactulose, multivitamins, furosemide, and a protein-restricted diet. During treatment, the serum albumin declined, and dietary protein supplementation was provided to avert worsening hypoalbuminemia. This dog succumbed to renal infarction associated with multiple thromboemboli. The other dogs for which hepatoportal fibrosis has been well described were euthanized shortly after diagnosis.

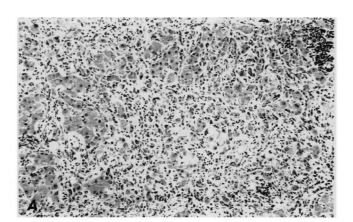 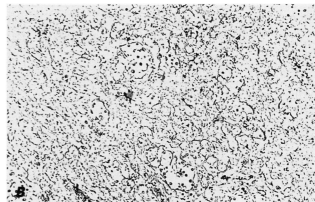

FIGURE 33–44. Photomicrograph of liver tissue from a dog with lobular dissecting hepatitis. In (*A*), the hepatic sinusoids are in disarray and hepatocytes are abnormally separated by fine reticulin fibers (H&E). In (*B*), Reticulin stain of the biopsy shown in (*A*) demonstrating the fine reticulin fiber dissection throughout the hepatic parenchyma.

Table 33–24

HEPATIC DISORDERS ASSOCIATED WITH IMPAIRED INTRAHEPATIC PORTAL PERFUSION IN HUMANS

SYNDROME	HISTOLOGIC LESION/DISEASE MECHANISM
Idiopathic hepatoportal sclerosis, portal hypertension, congenital hepatic fibrosis (infants)	Congenital hypoplasia or atresia of terminal portal vein branches
Toxins: copper sulfate, arsenic, vinyl chloride, methotrexate	Medium and large portal vein branches obliterated
Idiopathic portal hypertension (adults) (Banti's disease)	Medium and large portal vein branches obliterated
Schistosomiasis	Granulomas around portal venules
Wilson's disease (copper storage hepatopathy)	Peribiliary fibrosis associated with copper deposition
Cystic fibrosis	Peribiliary fibrosis due to obstructed bile ducts (inspissated mucus)
Chronic active hepatitis	Immune-mediated chronic hepatopathy focused in the portal triad; round cell infiltration
Primary biliary cirrhosis	Immune-mediated chronic hepatopathy focused on small bile ducts leading to periportal fibrosis

Idiopathic Sinusoidal (Pericellular) Fibrosis

Subsequent to the initial report of lobular dissecting hepatitis, a second paper describes a similar pattern of fibrosis in the absence of a marked inflammatory component.[491] This lesion is denoted as idiopathic pericellular (sinusoidal) fibrosis and was described in nine dogs. Affected dogs ranged in age from 4 months to 7 years. Four of these dogs were German shepherds. One dog was euthanized at diagnosis, one dog died shortly thereafter of renal failure, four dogs were euthanized within 1 month of diagnosis for failure to respond to therapy, and two dogs were lost to follow-up. One dog survived more than 4 years.

The diffuse parenchymal involvement in these dogs correlates with a severe clinical disease course compared to dogs with idiopathic periportal or perivenular fibrosis. Although a poorer prognosis was proposed by the authors for these dogs compared to dogs in the other "idiopathic fibrosis" categories, significant numbers of dogs have not been studied.

Idiopathic Perivenous Fibrosis (Idiopathic Veno-Occlusive Disease)

Idiopathic perivenous fibrosis has been described in five young dogs.[491] Four of these dogs were young German shepherds and one was a young Rottweiler. One of these dogs was euthanized at diagnosis, two dogs survived more than 4 years, one dog was being monitored and had not been followed for longer than 6 months, and one dog was lost to follow-up. Of the dogs that survived for longer than 4 years, one was treated only with dietary protein restriction and one was treated with prednisolone for 3 years. Liver biopsy shows a diffuse fibrosis surrounding the hepatic veins and a lack of inflammatory components. Specific staining for reticulin and connective tissue discloses considerable fibrous tissue peripheral to the intima of the vein. A two-year follow-up liver biopsy in the dog treated with glucocorticoids revealed an increase in the luminal diameter of central veins. One dog undergoing treatment with colchicine was doing well on the basis of clinical signs after 6 months. Figure 33–45 shows the hepatic lesions in a young German shepherd with this syndrome.

Nodular Hyperplasia

Nodular hyperplasia of the liver is a well-recognized age-related condition in the dog and lacks a breed or sex predilection. It is a common finding on postmortem examination of dogs over 8 years of age. No underlying disease condition has been recognized. This is contrary to findings in humans where they may represent a preneoplastic development. Nodular hyperplasia should be differentiated from regenerative nodules associated with liver cell injury and neoplasia. Regenerative nodules are usually associated with fibrosis, whereas nodular hyperplasia is not. Lipogranulomata, foci of macrophages, Ito cells, and ceroid pigment occur with increased frequency in dogs with nodular hyperplasia. The association among these phenomena remains undetermined.[492]

Mild increases in the serum ALP and ALT activities have been seen in conjunction with nodular hyperplasia in the dog. Hepatocytes in hyperplastic nodules are somewhat larger than normal adjacent hepatocytes and are variably vacuolated either with triglyceride or glycogen. There may be focal areas of sinusoidal dilation and accumulations of hematopoietic cells. When nodules enlarge, they can lead to compression and atrophy of surrounding hepatic

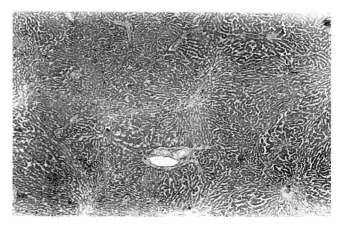

FIGURE 33–45. Photomicrograph of liver tissue from a young German shepherd dog with noninflammatory dissecting fibrosis. This dog presented with ascites.

parenchyma; this is likely the source of the increased serum enzyme activity. Ultrasonography may disclose homogenous hypoechoic masses or mixed hypoechoic to hyperechoic lesions.[493] Some lesions are invisible; they have similar echogenicity as the surrounding normal tissue. When visualized, ultrasound evaluation cannot differentiate these benign nodules from primary or secondary neoplasia. Histologic evaluation is augmented by collection of a wedge rather than a needle biopsy. Needle specimens of nodular hyperplasia can be difficult to differentiate from hepatocellular adenoma or adenocarcinoma because of the very small size of the collected tissue. Rarely, hyperplastic nodules may become large and clinically appear similar to hepatoacellular adenoma. These may develop necrotic centers.

REFERENCES

1. Boyer JL, Miller DJ. Chronic hepatitis. In: Schiff L, Schiff ER (eds) Diseases of the Liver. JB Lippincott, Philadelphia, 687–723, 1987.
2. MacSween RNM, Anthony P, Scheuer PJ. Pathology of the Liver. Churchill Livingstone, New York, 1987.
3. Strombeck DR, Gribble D. Chronic active hepatitis in the dog. J Am Vet Med Assoc 173:380–386, 1978.
4. Strombeck DR, Rogers W, Gribble D. Chronic active hepatic disease in a dog. J Am Vet Med Assoc 169:802–804, 1976.
5. Doige CE, Lester S. Chronic active hepatitis in dogs—a review of 14 cases. J Am Anim Hosp Assoc 17:725–730, 1981.
6. Doige CE, Furneaux RW. Liver disease and intrahepatic portal hypertension in the dog. Can Vet J 16:209–214, 1975.
7. Hardy RM. Chronic hepatitis: An emerging syndrome in dogs. Vet Clin N Am: Sm Anim Pract 15:135–150, 1985.
8. Hardy RM. Chronic hepatitis in dogs: A syndrome. Comp Cont Ed 8:904–914, 1986.
9. Rutgers HC, Haywood S. Chronic hepatitis in the dog. J Sm Anim Pract 29:679–690, 1988.
10. Dillon AR. The liver in systemic disease. Vet Clin N Am: Sm Anim Pract 15:97–117, 1985.
11. Gocke DF, Morris TQ, Bradley SE. Chronic hepatitis in the dog: The role of immune factors. J Am Vet Med Assoc 156:1700–1705, 19??.
12. Rakich PM, Rogers KW, Lukert PD, et al. Immunohistochemical detection of canine adenovirus in paraffin sections of liver. Vet Pathol 23:478–484, 1986.
13. Jarrett WFH, O'Neil BW. A new transmissible agent causing acute hepatitis, chronic hepatitis and cirrhosis in dogs. Vet Record 116:629–635, 1985.
14. Jarrett WFH, O'Neil BW, Lindholm I. Persistent hepatitis and chronic fibrosis induced by canine acidophil cell hepatitis virus. Vet Rec 120:234–235, 1987.
15. Weiss RC, Scott FW. Pathogenesis of feline infectious peritonitis: Pathologic changes and immunofluorescence. Am J Vet Res 42:2036–2048, 1981.
16. Robinson WS. Why do animals have antibodies to hepatitis B surface antigen? Gastroenterology 84:1614–1615, 1983.
17. Bishop L, Strandberg JD, Adams RJ, et al. Chronic active hepatitis in dogs associated with leptospires. Am J Vet Res 40:839–844, 19??.
18. Frazer IH, Mackay IR, Bell J, et al. The cellular infiltrate in the liver in auto-immune chronic active hepatitis: Analysis with monoclonal antibodies. Liver 5:162–167, 1985.
19. Hopf U, Meyer zum Buschenfelde KH. Studies on the pathogenesis of experimental chronic active hepatitis in rabbits. II. Demonstration of immunoglobulin on isolated hepatocytes. Brit J Exp Path 55:509–513, 1974.
20. Hopf U, Meyer zum Buschenfelde KH. Diagnosis of autoimmune chronic active hepatitis: A method for the detection of liver membrane autoantibodies (LMA). Zeit Gastroenterologie 16:261–264, 1978.
21. Onji M, Kumohn I, Miyaoka H, et al. Identification of intrahepatic lymphocyte subpopulations in patients with drug-induced allergic hepatitis. J Gastroenterol Hepatol 2:407–412, 1987.
22. Zum Buschenfelde KHM, Hopf U. Studies on the pathogenesis of experimental chronic active hepatitis in rabbits. I. Induction of the disease and protective effect of allogeneic liver specific proteins. Br J Exp Pathol 55:498–508, 1974.
23. Kawanishi H. In vitro morphological studies on antibody-dependent non-immune lymphocyte-mediated cytotoxicity in chronic active liver disease. Am J Dig Dis 23:97–109, 1978.
24. Meyer zum Buschenfelde KH, Manns M, Hutterroth TH, et al. LM-Ag and LSP—two different target antigens involved in the immunopatho-

genesis of chronic active hepatitis. Clin Exp Immuno 37:205–212, 1979.
25. Montano L, Aranguibel F, Boffill M, et al. An analysis of the composition of the inflammatory infiltrate in autoimmune and hepatitis B virus induced chronic liver disease. Hepatology 3:292–296, 1984.
26. Vierling JM. Hepatobiliary complications of ulcerative colitis and Crohn's disease. In: Zakim D, Boyer TD (eds) Hepatology, a Textbook of Liver Disease. WB Saunders, Philadelphia, 1126–1158, 1990.
27. Krawitt EL, Kilby AE, Albertini RJ, et al. Immunogenetic studies of autoimmune chronic active hepatitis: HLA, immunoglobulin allotypes and autoantibodies. Hepatology 7:13??–1310, 1987.
28. Maddrey WC. Subdivisions of idiopathic autoimmune chronic active hepatitis. Hepatology 1372–1375, 1987.
29. Mackay IR. Induction by drugs of hepatitis and autoantibodies to cell organelles: Significance and interpretation. Hepatology 5:904–906, 1985.
30. Thomas HC. Immunologic mechanisms in chronic liver disease. In: Zakim D, Boyer TD (eds) Hepatology, a Textbook of Liver Disease. WB Saunders, Philadelphia, 1114–1126, 1990.
31. Worman HJ, Courvalin J-C. Autoantibodies against nuclear envelope proteins in liver disease. Hepatology 14:1269–1279, 1991.
32. Lohse AW, Manns M, Dienes H-P, et al. Experimental autoimmune hepatitis: Disease induction, time course and T-cell reactivity. Hepatology 11:24–30, 1990.
33. Bassedine MF, Yeaman SJ. Serological markers of primary biliary cirrhosis: Diagnosis, prognosis and subsets. Hepatology 15:545–547, 1992.
34. Krawitt EL, Kilby AE, Albertini RJ, et al. An immunogenetic study of suppressor cell activity in autoimmune chronic active hepatitis. Clin Immunol Immunopath 46:249–257, 1988.
35. Leifer CE, Page RL, Matus RE, et al. Proliferative glomerulonephritis and chronic active hepatitis with cirrhosis associated with *Corynebacterium parvum* immunotherapy in a dog. J Am Vet Med Assoc 190:78–80, 1987.
36. Schrumpf E, Fausa O, Elgjo K, et al. Hepatobiliary complications of inflammatory bowel disease. Sem Liver Dis 8:201–209, 1988.
37. Dew MJ, Thompson H, Allan RN. The spectrum of hepatic dysfunction in inflammatory bowel disease. Q J Med, New Series 48:113–135, 1979.
38. Rabin BS, Rogers S. Pathologic changes in the liver and kidney produced by immunization with intestinal antigens. Am J Pathol 84:201–207, 1976.
39. Ohlsson EG, Rutherford RB, Boitnott JK, et al. Changes in portal circulation after biliary obstruction in dogs. Am J Surg 120:16–22, 1970.
40. Center SA, Castleman W, Roth L, et al. Light microscopic and electron microsocopic changes in the livers of cats with extrahepatic bile duct obstruction. Am J Vet Res 47:1278–1282, 1986.
41. Dooley JS, Hamilton-Miller JMT, Brumfitt W, et al. Antibiotics in the treatment of biliary infection. Gut 25:988–998, 1984.
42. Wyke RJ. Problems of bacterial infection in patients with liver disease. Gut 28:623–641, 1987.
43. Rojkind M, Dunn MA. Hepatic fibrosis. Gastroenterology 76:849–863, 1979.
44. Chojkier M, Brenner DA. Therapeutic strategies for hepatic fibrosis. Hepatology 8:176–182, 1988.
45. Bissell DM, Friedman SL, Maher JJ, et al. Connective tissue biology and hepatic fibrosis: Report of a conference. Hepatology 11:488–498, 1990.
46. Bissell DM, Roll J. Connective tissue metabolism and hepatic fibrosis. In: Zakim D, Boyer TD (eds) Hepatology; a Textbook of Liver Disease, 2nd ed. WB Saunders, Philadelphia, 424–444, 1990.
47. Sherlock S. Hepatic cirrhosis. In: Sherlock S (ed) Diseases of the Liver and Biliary System, 8th ed. Blackwell Scientific, Oxford, England, 410–424, 1989.
48. Conn HO, Atterbury CE. Cirrhosis. In: Schiff L, Schiff ER (eds) Diseases of the Liver. JB Lippincott, Philadelphia, 725–864, 1987.
49. Rojkind M, Greenwel P. The liver as a bioecological system. In: Arias IM, Jakoby WB, Popper H, et al. (eds) The Liver: Biology and Pathobiology, 2nd ed. Raven Press, New York, 1269–1285, 1988.
50. Friedman SL. Cellular sources of collagen and regulation of collagen production in liver. Sem Liver Dis 10:20–29, 1990.
51. Schuppan D. Structure of the extracellular matrix in normal and fibrotic liver: Collagens and glycoproteins. Sem Liver Dis 10:1–9, 1990.
52. Bissell M. Cell matrix interactions and hepatic fibrosis. In: Popper H, Schaffner F (eds) Progress in Liver Diseases, Vol. 9. WB Saunders, Philadelphia, 143–155, 1990.
53. Biagini G, Ballardini G. Liver fibrosis and extracellular matrix. J Hepatol 8:115–124, 1989.
54. Martin GR, Kleinman HK. The extracellular matrix in development and in disease. Sem Liv Dis 5:147–156, 1985.
55. Burgeson RE. New collagens, new concepts. Annu Rev Cell Biol 4:551–577, 1988.
56. Grimaud J-A, Druguet M, Peyrol S, et al. Collagen immunotyping in human liver. J Histochem Cytochem 28:1145–1156, 1980.
57. Clement B, Grimaud J-A, Campion J-P, et al. Cell types involved in collagen and fibronectin production in normal and fibrotic human liver. Hepatology 66:225–234, 1986.

58. Zern MA, Czaja MJ, Weiner FR. The use of molecular hybridization techniques as tools to evaluate hepatic fibrogenesis. In: Rojkind M (ed) Connective Tissue in Health and Disease. CRC Press, Boca Raton, FL, 99–122, 1990.

59. Hassell JR, Kimura JH, Hascall VC. Proteoglyan core protein families. Annu Rev Biochem 55:539–567, 1986.

60. Poole AR. Proteoglycans in health and disease: Structures and functions. Biochem J 236:1–14, 1986.

61. Gallagher JT, Lyon M, Steward WP. Structure and function of heparan sulphate proteoglycans. Biochem J 236:313–325, 1986.

62. Weiner FR, Giambrone MA, Czaja MJ, et al. Ito-cell gene expression and collagen regulation. Hepatology 11:111–117, 1990.

63. Maher JJ, McGuire RF. Extracellular matrix gene expression increases preferentially in rat lipocytes and sinusoidal endothelial cells during hepatic fibrosis in vivo. J Clin Invest 86:1641–1648, 1990.

64. Matsuoka M, Tsukamoto H. Stimulation of hepatic lipocyte collagen production by Kupffer cell-derived transforming growth factor β: Implication for pathogenetic role in alcoholic liver fibrogenesis. Hepatology 11:599–605, 1990.

65. Castilla A, Prieto J, Fausto N. Transforming growth factors β1 and α in chronic liver disease: Effects of interferon α therapy. N Engl J Med 324:933–940, 1991.

66. Braun L, Mead JE, Panzica M, et al. Transforming growth factor β mRNA increases during liver regeneration: A possible paracrine mechanism of growth regulation. Proc Natl Acad Sci USA 85:1539–1543, 1988.

67. Fausto N, Mead JE. Regulation of liver growth: Protooncogenes and transforming growth factors. Lab Invest 60:4–13, 1989.

68. Czaja MJ, Weiner FR, Flanders KC, et al. In vitro and in vivo association of transforming growth factoer-β1 with hepatic fibrosis. J Cell Biol 108:2477–2482, 1989.

69. Roberts AB, Sporn MB, Assoian RK, et al. Transforming growth factor type β: Rapid induction of fibrosis and angiogenesis in vivo and stimulation of collagen formation in vitro. Proc Natl Acad Sci USA 83:4167–4171, 1986.

70. Roberts AB, Sporn MB. The transforming growth factor-βs. In: Sporn MB, Roberts AB (eds) Peptide Growth Factors and Their Receptors I. Vol. 95 of Handbook of Experimental Pharmacology. Springer-Verlag, Berlin, Germany, 419–472, 1989.

71. Nakatsukasa H, Naguy P, Everts RO, et al. Cellular distribution of transforming growth factor-β1 and procollagen types I, III and IV transcripts in carbon tetrachloride-induced rat liver fibrosis. J Clin Invest 85:1833–1843, 1990.

72. Rojkind M, Giambrone M-A, Biempica L. Collagen types in normal and cirrhotic liver. Gastroenterology 76:710–719, 1979.

73. Seyer JM, Hutcheson ET, Kang AH. Collagen polymorphism in normal and cirrhotic human liver. J Clin Invest 59:241–248, 1977.

74. Murawaki Y, Kusakabe Y, Hirayama C. Serum lysyl oxidase activity in chronic liver disease in comparison with serum levels of prolyl hydroxylase and laminin. Hepatology 14:1167–1173, 1991.

75. Risteli L, Risteli J. Noninvasive methods for detection of organ fibrosis. In: Rojkind M (ed) Connective Tissue in Health and Disease. CRC Press, Boca Raton, FL, 61–98, 1990.

76. Hahn EG. Blood analysis for liver fibrosis. J Hepatol 1:67–73, 1984.

77. Kivirikko KI, Savolainen E-R. Serum markers of hepatic collagen metabolism. Acta Hepatol Jpn 26:1421–1425, 1985.

78. Dimski D, Brooks CL, Johnson SE. Evaluation of a radioimmunoassay for Type III procollagen peptide in the dog. Vet Clin Pathol 19:40–44, 1990.

79. Henriksen JH, Horn T, Christoffersen P. The blood-lymph barrier in the liver: A review based on morphological and functional concepts of normal and cirrhotic liver. Liver 4:221–223, 1984.

80. Horn T, Christoffersen P, Henriksen JH. Alcoholic liver injury: Defenestration in noncirrhotic livers—a scanning electron microscopic study. Hepatology 7:77–82, 1987.

81. Villeneuve JP, Huet PM. Microcirculatory abnormalities in liver disease. Hepatology 7:186–187, 1987.

82. Kamada T, Hayashi N, Sato N, et al. Estimated hepatic oxygen consumption in patients with chronic liver diseases as assessed by organ reflectance spectrophotometry. Dig Dis Sci 31:119–124, 1986.

83. Miyamoto K, French SW. Hepatic adenine nucleotide metabolism measured in vivo in rats fed ethanol and a high fat-low protein diet. Hepatology 8:53–60, 1988.

84. Lieber CS, Baraona E, Hernandez-Munoz R, et al. Impaired oxygen utilization: A new mechanism for the hepatotoxicity of ethanol in subhuman primates. J Clin Invest 83:1662–1690, 1989.

85. Morgan DJ, McLean AJ. Therapeutic implications of impaired hepatic oxygen diffusion in chronic liver disease. Hepatology 14:1280–1282, 1991.

86. Wilkinson GR. Clearance approaches in pharmacology. Pharmacol Rev 39:1–47, 1987.

87. Wilkinson GR. Influence of hepatic disease on pharmacokinetics. In: Evans WE, Schentag JJ, Jusko WJ (eds) Applied Pharmacokinetics: Principles of Therapeutic Drug Monitoring, 2nd ed. Applied Therapeutics, Spokane, 116–138, 1986.

88. Secor JW, Schenker S. Drug metabolism in patients with liver disease. In: Stollerman GH (ed) Advances in Internal Medicine, Vol. 32. Year Book Medical Publishers, Chicago, 379–406, 1987.

89. McLean AJ, Morgan DJ. Clinical pharmacokinetics in patients with liver disease: 1990. Clin Pharmacokinet 21:42–69, 1991.

90. Angus PW, Mihaly GW, Morgan DJ, et al. Oxygen dependence of omperazole clearance and sulfone and sulfide metabolite formation in the isolated perfused rat liver. J Pharmacol Exp Therap 250:1043–1047, 1989.

91. Angus PW, Mihaly GW, Morgan DJ, et al. Oxygen dependence of salbutamol elimination by the isolated perfused rat liver. Biochem Pharmacol 38:1443–1449, 1989.

92. Reichen J, Egger B, Ohara N, et al. Determinants of hepatic function in liver cirrhosis in the rat: Multivariate analysis. J Clin Invest 82:2069–2076, 1988.

93. Reichen J, Hirlinger A, Ha HR, et al. Chronic verapamil administration lowers portal pressure and improves hepatic function in rats with liver cirrhosis. J Hepatol 3:49–58, 1986.

94. Reichen J, Le M. Verapamil favourably influences hepatic microvascular exchange and function in rats with cirrhosis of the liver. J Clin Invest 78:448–455, 1986.

95. Cameron GR, Karunaratne WAE. Carbon tetrachloride cirrhosis in relation to liver regeneration. J Pathol Bacteriol 42:1–21, 1936.

96. Scobie BA, Summerskill WHJ. Hepatic cirrhosis secondary to obstruction of the biliary system. Am J Dig Dis 10:135–146, 1965.

97. Unikowsky B, Wexler MJ, Levey M. Dogs with experimental cirrhosis of the liver but without intrahepatic hypertension do not retain sodium or form ascites. J Clin Invest 1594–1604, 1983.

98. Bosch J, Enriquez R, Groszmann RJ, et al. Chronic bile duct ligation in the dog: Hemodynamic characterization of a portal hypertensive model. Hepatology 3:1002–1007, 1983.

99. McLean EK, McLean AEM, Sutton PM. An improved method for producing cirrhosis of the liver in rats by simultaneous administration of carbon tetrachloride and phenobarbitone. Br J Exp Pathol 50:502–506, 1969.

100. Proctor E, Chatamra K. High yield micronodular cirrhosis in the rat. Gastroenterology 83:1183–1190, 1982.

101. Madden JW, Gertmen PM, Peacock EE, Jr. Dimethylnitrosamine-induced hepatic cirrhosis: A new canine model of an ancient human disease. Surgery 68:260–268, 1970.

102. Levy M. Sodium retention and ascites formation in dogs with experimental portal cirrhosis. Am J Physiol 233:572–585, 1977.

103. Levy M, Wexler MJ. Renal sodium retention and ascites formation in dogs with experimental cirrhosis but without portal hypertension or increased splanchnic vascular capacity. J Lab Clin Med 91:520–536, 1978.

104. Morcos SH, Khayyal MT, Mansour MM, et al. Reversal of hepatic fibrosis after praziquantel therapy of murine schistosomiasis. Am J Trop Med Hyg 34:314–321, 1985.

105. Tsukamoto H, Matsuoka M, French SW. Experimental models of hepatic fibrosis: A review. Sem Liver Dis 10:56–65, 1990.

106. Leevy CM, Dvorshak CK, Gnassi AM. The liver in extrahepatic biliary obstruction. Am J Med Sci 227:272–278, 1954.

107. Cameron R, Bunton GL. Congenital biliary atresia. Brit Med J 2:1253–1257, 1960.

108. Thaler MM, Gellis SS. Studies in neonatal hepatitis and biliary atresia. III. Progression and regression of cirrhosis in biliary atresia. Am J Dis Child 116:271–279, 1968.

109. Okazaki I, Maruyamo K. Collagenase activity in experimental hepatic fibrosis. Nature 252:49–50, 1974.

110. Montfort I, Perez-Tamayo R. Collagenase in experimental carbon tetrachloride cirrhosis of the liver. Am J Pathol 92:411–420, 1978.

111. Andersson M, Sevelius E. Breed, sex and age distribution in dogs with chronic liver disease: A demographic study. J Sm Anim Pract 32:1–5, 1991.

112. Strombeck DR, Miller LM, Harrold D. Effects of corticosteroids on survival time in dogs with chronic hepatitis: 151 cases (1977–1985). J Am Vet Med Assoc 193:1109–1113, 1988.

113. Gopinath C, Ford EJH. Location of liver injury and extent of bilirubinaemia in experimental liver lesions. Vet Pathol 9:99–108, 1972.

114. Crawford MA, Schall WD, Jensen RK, et al. Chronic active hepatitis in 26 Doberman pinschers. J Am Vet Med Assoc 187:1343–1350, 1985.

115. Anthony PP, Ishak KG, Nayak NC, et al. The morphology of cirrhosis: Definition, nomenclature and classification. Bulletin of the World Health Organization 55:521–540, 1977.

116. Schlichting P, Holund B, Poulsen H. Liver biopsy in chronic aggressive hepatitis. Diagnostic reproducibility in relation to size of specimen. Scand J Gastroenterol 18:27–32, 1983.

117. Uribe M. Treatment of portal systemic encephalopathy: The old and new treatments. In: Grisolia S, et al. (eds) Cirrhosis, Hepatic Encephalopathy, and Ammonium Toxicity. Plenum Press, New York, 235–253, 1990.

118. Schneeweiss B, Graninger W, Ferenci P, et al. Energy metabolism in liver disease. Hepatology 11:387–393, 1990.

119. Heymesfield ST, Waki M, Reinus J. Are patients with chronic liver disease hypermetabolic? Hepatology 11:502–504, 1990.

120. Schneeweiss B, Graninger W, Ferenci P, et al. Energy metabolism in patients with acute and chronic liver disease. Hepatology 11:387–393, 1990.

121. Fiaccadori F, Ghinelli F, Pedretti G, et al. Negative nitrogen balance in cirrhotics. La Ricerca Clin Lab 11:259–268, 1981.

122. Plough IC, Iber FL, Shipman ME, et al. The effects of supplementary calories on nitrogen storage at high intakes or protein in patients with chronic liver disease. Am J Clin Nutr 4:224–230, 1956.

123. Mullen KD, Weber FL. Role of nutrition in hepatic encephalopathy. Sem Liver Dis 11:292–304, 1991.

124. Strombeck DR, Harrold D, Rogers Q, et al. Plasma amino acid, glucagon, and insulin concentrations in dogs with nitrosamine-induced hepatic disease. Am J Vet Res 44:2028–2036, 1983.

125. Greenberger NJ, Carley J, Schenker S, et al. Effect of vegetable and animal protein diets in chronic hepatic encephalopathy. Am J Dig Dis 22:845–855, 1977.

126. Strombeck DR, Schaeffer MC, Rogers QR. Dietary therapy for dogs with chronic hepatic insufficiency. In: Kirk RW (ed) Current Veterinary Therapy VIII. WB Saunders, Philadelphia, 817–821, 1983.

127. Kondrup J, Nielsen K, Hamberg O. Nutritional therapy in patients with liver cirrhosis. Eur J Clin Nutr 46:239–246, 1992.

128. Rosen HM, Soeters PM, James JH, et al. Influences of exogenous intake and nitrogen balance on plasma and brain amino acid concentrations. Metabolism 27:393–404, 1987.

129. Laflamme DP, Allen SW, Huber TL. Apparent dietary protein requirement of dogs with portosystemic shunt. Am J Vet Res 54:719–723, 1993.

130. Swart GR, van den Berg JWO, Wattimena JLD, et al. Elevated protein requirements in cirrhosis of the liver investigated by whole body protein turnover studies. Clin Sci 75:101–107, 1988.

131. Swart GR, van den Berg JWO, van Vuure JK, et al. Minimum protein requirements in liver cirrhosis determined by nitrogen balance measurements at three levels of protein intake. Clin Nutr 8:329–336, 1989.

132. Davenport DJ, Mostardi RA, Gross KL. Effect of a protein-deficient diet on serum proteins, urea nitrogen, hepatic enzymes and bile acids in dogs. Proc Waltham Symposium on the Nutrition of Companion Animals, Adelaide (abstract), 69, 1993.

133. Bianchi GP, Marchesini G, Fabbri A, et al. Vegetable versus animal protein diet in cirrhotic patients with chronic encephalopathy. A randomized cross-over comparison. J Int Med 233:385–392, 1993.

134. Keshavarsian A, Meek J, Sutton C, et al. Dietary protein supplementation from vegetable sources in the management of chronic portal systemic encephalopathy. Am J Gastroenterol 79:945–949, 1984.

135. Shaw S, Worner MT, Lieber CS. Comparison of animal and vegetable protein sources in the dietary management of hepatic encephalopathy. Clin Nutr 38:59–63, 1983.

136. Uribe M, Dibildox M, Malpica S, et al. Beneficial effect of vegetable protein diet supplemented with psyllium plantago in patients with hepatic encephalopathy and diabetes mellitus. Gastroenterology 88:901–907, 1985.

137. Uribe M, Marquez MA, Ramos GG, et al. Treatment of chronic portal-systemic encephalopathy with vegetable and animal protein diets: A controlled crossover study. Dig Dis Sci 27:1109–1116, 1982.

138. Pomare EW, Branch WJ, Cummings JM. Carbohydrate fermentation in the human colon and its relation to acetate concentration in venous blood. J Clin Invest 74:1448–1454, 1985.

139. Lupton J, Codei D, Jacobs L. Long term effects of fermentable fibers on rat colonic pH and epithelial cell cycle. J Nutr 118:840–845, 1988.

140. Weber FL, Jr, Minco D, Fresard KM, et al. Effects of vegetable diets on nitrogen metabolism in cirrhotic subjects. Gastroenterology 89:538–544, 1985.

141. Weber FL, Jr, Stephen AM, Karagiannis EN. Effects of dietary fiber on nitrogen metabolism in cirrhotic patients. Gastroenterology 88:1704, 1985.

142. Max JL. Amaranthus, a comeback for the food of the Aztecs. Science 98:4312, 1977.

143. Schaeffer MC, Rogers QR, Buffington CA, et al. Long-term biochemical and physiologic effects of surgically placed portacaval shunts in dogs. Am J Vet Res 47:346–355, 1986.

144. Linscher WG, Patterson JF, Moore EW, et al. Medium and long chain fat absorption in patients with cirrhosis. J Clin Invest 45:1317–1325, 1966.

145. MacDonald ML, Anderson BC, Rogers QR, et al. Essential fatty acid requirements of cats: Pathology of essential fatty acid deficiency. Am J Vet Res 45:1310–1317, 1984.

146. Sampson FE, Jr, Dahl N, Dahl DR. A study on the narcosis action of short chain fatty acids. J Clin Invest 35:1291–1298, 1956.

147. Muto YI. Clinical study on the relationship of short chain fatty acids and hepatic encephalopathy. Jpn J Gastroenterol 63:19–32, 1966.

148. Morgan MH, Bolton CH, Morris JS, et al. Medium chain triglycerides and hepatic encephalopathy. Gut 15:180–188, 1974.

149. Mortensen PB, Holtug K, Bonnen H, et al. The degradation of amino acids, proteins, and blood to short-chain fatty acids in colon is prevented by lactulose. Gastroenterology 98:353–360, 1990.

150. Mortensen PB, Holtug K, Bonnen H, et al. Effect of lactulose on the metabolism of short-chain fatty acids. Gastroenterology 98:353–360, 1990.

151. Cummings JH. Fermentation in the human large intestine: Evidence on implication for health. Lancet 1:1206–1209, 1983.

152. Royall D, Wolever TMS, Jeejeebhoy KN. Clinical significance of colonic fermentation. Am J Gastroenterol 85:1210–1312, 1990.

153. Russell RM. Vitamin and mineral supplements in the management of liver disease. Med Clin N Am 63:537–544, 1979.

154. Brewer GJ, Dick RD, Schall W, et al. Use of zinc acetate to treat copper toxicosis in dogs. J Am Vet Med Assoc 201:564–568, 1992.

155. Griffiths GL, Lumsden JH, Valli VEO. Hematologic and biochemical changes in dogs with portosystemic shunts. J Am Anim Hosp Assoc 17:705–710, 1981.

156. Laflamme D, Mahaffey E, Allen S, et al. Microcytosis in dogs with portocaval shunt. Proc 8th ACVIM Forum (abstract), 113, 1990.

157. Bunch SE, Jordan HL, Sellon RK, et al. Iron status in 12 dogs with congenital portosystemic shunts. Proc 10th ACVIM Forum (abstract), 809, 1992.

158. Meyer DJ, Harvey JW. Hematologic changes associated with serum and hepatic iron alterations in dogs with congenital portosystemic vascular anomalies. J Vet Int Med 8:55–56, 1994.

159. Bichet DG, Van Putten VJ, Schrier RW. Potential role of increased sympathetic activity in impaired sodium and water excretion in cirrhosis. N Engl J Med 307:1552–1557, 1982.

160. Blei AT, Gottstein J, Ganger D. Oral neomycin normalizes hyperdynamic features of awake portal hypertensive rats (abstract). Hepatology 8:1253, 1988.

161. Plozin DJ, Osborne CA. Update-conservative medical management of chronic renal failure. In: Kirk RW (ed) Current Veterinary Therapy IX. WB Saunders, Philadelphia, 1167–1173, 1986.

162. Moreau MC, Ducluzeau R, Raibaud P. Hydrolysis of urea in the gastrointestinal tract of "monoxenic" rats: Effect of immunization with strains of ureolytic bacteria. Infect Immun 13:9–15, 1976.

163. Maddrey WC, Weber FL, Coulter AW, et al. Effects of keto analogues of essential amino acids in portal-systemic encephalopathy. Gastroenterology 71:190–195, 1976.

164. Stephen AM, Cumming JH. Mechanism of action of dietary fibre in the human colon. Nature 284:283–284, 1980.

165. Herrmann R, Shakoor T, Weber FL, Jr. Beneficial effects of pectin in chronic hepatic encephalopathy (abstract). Gastroenterology 92:1795, 1987.

166. Hirsch DW. Infectious complications of cancer. In: Kirk RW (ed) Current Veterinary Therapy IX. WB Saunders, Philadelphia, 1167–1173, 1986.

167. Conn HO, Leevy CM, Vlahcevic ZR, et al. Comparison of lactulose and neomycin in the treatment of chronic portal-systemic encephalopathy. Gastroenterology 72:573–583, 1977.

168. Atterbury CE, Maddrey WC, Conn HO. Neomycin-sorbitol and lactulose in the treatment of acute portal-systemic encephalopathy. A controlled, double-blind clinical trial. Dig Dis 53:398–406, 1978.

169. Weber FL, Banwell JG, Fresard KM, et al. Nitrogen in fecal bacterial, fiber, and soluble fractions of patients with cirrhosis: Effects of lactulose and lactulose plus neomycin. J Lab Clin Med 110:259–263, 1987.

170. Vince A, Killingley M, Wrong OM. Effect of lactulose on ammonia production in a fecal incubation system. Gastroenterology 74:544–549, 1978.

171. Bircher J, Haemmerli UP, Trabert E, et al. The mechanism of action of lactulose in portal-systemic encephalopathy. Non-ionic diffusion of ammonia in the canine colon. Rev Europ Etudes Clin Et Biol 16:352–357, 1971.

172. Zeegen R, Dringwater J, Fenton J, et al. Some observations on the effects of treatment with lactulose on patients with chronic hepatic encephalopathy. Q J Med, New Series XXXIX; 34:245–263, 1970.

173. Agostini L, Down PF, Murison J, et al. Faecal ammonia and pH during lactulose administration in man: Comparison with other cathartics. Gut 13:859–866, 1972.

174. Morgan MY, Hawley KE. Lactitol vs. lactulose in the treatment of acute hepatic encephalopathy in cirrhotic patients: A double-blind randomized trial. Hepatology 7:1278–1284, 1987.

175. Mason VC. An explanation of effect of lactulose in treatment of hepatic encephalopathy. Gastroenterology 66:1271, 1974.

176. Leber G, Luginbuhl M. In: Conn HO, Bircher J (eds) Hepatic Encephalopathy: Management with Lactulose and Related Carbohydrates. Medi-Ed Press, East Lansing, 271–281, 1988.

177. Uribe M, Berthier JM, Lewis H, et al. Lactose enemas plus placebo tablets vs. neomycin tablets plus starch enemas in acute portal systemic encephalopathy. A double-blind randomized controlled study. Gastroenterology 81:101–106, 1981.

178. Blanc P, Daures J-P, Rouillon JM, et al. Lactitol or lactulose in the treatment of chronic hepatic encephalopathy: Results of a meta-analysis. Hepatology 15:222–228, 1992.

179. Elkington SG, Floch MH, Conn HO. Lactulose in the treatment of chronic portal-systemic encephalopathy. A double-blind clinical trial. N Engl J Med 281:408–412, 1969.

180. Liehr H, Englisch G, Rasenack U. Lactulose—a drug with anti-endotoxin effect. Hepatogastroenterology 27:356–360, 1980.

181. Riggio O, Balducci G, Ariosto F, et al. Lactitol in prevention of recurrent episodes of hepatic encephalopathy in cirrhotic patients with portal-systemic shunt. Dig Dis Sci 34:823–829, 1989.

182. Uribe M, Toledo H, Perez F, et al. Lactitol, a second-generation disaccharide for treatment of chronic portal-systemic encephalopathy. A double-blind, crossover, randomized clinical trial. Dig Dis Sci 32:1345–1353, 1987.

183. Holgate AM, Read NW. Relationship between small bowel transit time and absorption of a solid meal. Influence of metoclopramide, magnesium sulfate, and lactulose. Dig Dis Sci 28:812–819, 1983.

184. Bathshaw ML, Brusilow S, Lewis MD, et al. Treatment of inborn errors of urea synthesis. N Eng J Med 306:1387–1392, 1982.

185. Mendenhall CL, Rouster S, Marshall L. A new therapy for portal systemic encephalopathy. Am J Gastroenterology 81:540–543, 1986.

186. Uribe M, Poo JL, Bosques F. Hyperammonemia hepatic encephalopathy treated with sodium benzoate. Final report of a double blind evaluation. Presented at annual AASLD, November 1989.

187. O'Connor JE, Ribelles M, Grisolia S. Potentiation of hyperammonemia by sodium benzoate in animals: A note of caution. Eur J Pediatr 138:186–187, 1982.

188. O'Connor JE, Costell M, Grisolia S. The potentiation of ammonia toxicity by sodium benzoate is prevented by L-carnitine. Biochem Biophys Res Comm 145:817–824, 1987.

189. Ohtsuka Y, Clark DJ, Griffith OW. Metabolic effects of carnitine and carnitine analogs. In: Grisolia S (ed) Cirrhosis, Hepatic Encephalopathy, and Ammonium Toxicity. Plenum Press, New York, 159–174, 1990.

190. del Olmo JA, Castillo M, Rodrigo JM, et al. Effect of L-carnitine upon ammonia tolerance test in cirrhotic patients. In: Grisolia S (ed) Cirrhosis, Hepatic Encephalopathy, and Ammonium Toxicity. Plenum Press, New York, 197–208, 1990.

191. Silliprandi N, Di Lisa F, Menabo R. Clinical use of carnitine past, present and future. In: Grisolia S (ed) Cirrhosis, Hepatic Encephalopathy, and Ammonium Toxicity. Plenum Press, New York, 175–181, 1990.

192. O'Connor JE, Costell M. New roles of carnitine metabolism in ammonia cytotoxicity. In: Grisolia S (ed) Cirrhosis, Hepatic Encephalopathy, and Ammonium Toxicity. Plenum Press, New York, 183–195, 1990.

193. Brogden RN, Goa KL. Flumazenil: A reappraisal of its pharmacological properties and therapeutic efficacy as a benzodiazepine antagonist. Drugs 42:1061–1089, 1991.

194. Van der Rijt CCD, Schalm SW, Meulstee J, et al. Flumazenil therapy for hepatic encephalopathy: A double blind crossover study. Hepatology 10:590, 1989.

195. Wright TL, Boyer TD. Diagnosis and management of cirrhotic ascites. In: Zakim D, Boyer TD (eds) Hepatology, a Textbook of Liver Disease. WB Saunders, Philadelphia, 616–634, 1990.

196. Rolando N, Harvey F, Brahm J. Prospective study of bacterial infection in acute liver failure: An analysis of fifty patients. Hepatology 11:49–53, 1990.

197. Rimola A, Soto R, Bory F, et al. Reticuloendothelial system phagocytic activity in cirrhosis and its relation to bacterial infections and prognosis. Hepatology 4:53–58, 1984.

198. Wells CL, Maddaus MA, Simmons RL. Role of the macrophage in the translocation of intestinal bacteria. Arch Surg 122:48–53, 1987.

199. Thomas HC, McSween RNM, White RG. The role of the liver in controlling the immunogenicity of commensal bacteria in the gut. Lancet 1:1288–1291, 1973.

200. Murray M, Robinson PB, McKeating FJ, et al. Peptic ulceration in the dog: A clinico-pathological study. Vet Rec 91:441–447, 1972.

201. Grun HL, Thiel H, Brunswig D, et al. Endotoxin-induced liver necrosis and intravascular coagulation in rats enhanced by portacaval collateral circulation. Gut 16:429–436, 1975.

202. Peterson SL, Koblik PD, Whiting PG, et al. Endotoxin concentrations measured by a chromogenic assay in portal and peripheral venous blood in ten dogs with portosystemic shunts. J Vet Int Med 5:71–74, 1991.

203. Nolan JP. The role of endotoxin in liver injury. Gastroenterology 69:1346–1356, 1975.

204. Tiegs G, Niehorster M, Wendel A. Leukocyte alterations do not account for hepatitis induced by or TNFα in galactosamine-sensitized mice. Biochem Pharm 40:1317–1322, 1990.

205. Campbell LV, Gilbert EF. Experimental giant cell transformation in the liver induced by E. coli endotoxin. Am J Pathol 51:855–868, 1967.

206. Simjee AE, Hamilton-Miller JMT, Thomas HC, et al. Antibodies to Escherichia coli in chronic liver diseases. Gut 16:871–875, 1975.

207. Thomas HC, McSween RNM, White RG. The role of the liver in controlling the immunogenicity of commensal bacteria in the gut. Lancet 1:1288–1291, 1973.

208. Rutenburg AM, Sonnenblick E, Koven I, et al. The role of intestinal bacteria in the development of dietary cirrhosis in rats. J Exp Med 106:1–13, 1987.

209. Levy E, Slusser RJ, Reubner BH. Hepatic changes produced by a single dose of endotoxin in the mouse by electron microscopy. Am J Pathol 52:477–502, 1968.

210. Leach BE, Fobes JC. Sulfonamide drugs as protective agents against carbon tetrachloride poisoning. Proc Soc Exp Biol Med 48:361–363, 1941.

211. Sugita S, Ohnishi K, Saito M, et al. Splanchnic hemodynamics in portal hypertensive dogs with portal fibrosis. Am J Physiol 252:G748–G754, 1987.

212. Schatten WE. The role of intestinal bacteria in liver necrosis following experimental excision of the hepatic arterial supply. Surgery 36:256–269, 1954.

213. Dineen P. The importance of the route of infection in experimental biliary tract obstruction. Surg Gyn Obstet 1001–1008, 1964.

214. Lykkegaard NM, Asaes S, Justesen T. Susceptibility of the liver and biliary tract to anaerobic infection in extrahepatic biliary tract obstruction. III. Possible synergistic effect between anaerobic and aerobic bacteria. Scand J Gastroenterol 11:263–272, 1976.

215. Faraj BA, Ali FM, Fulenwider JT, et al. Hepatorenal failure induced by tetracycline in dogs with portacaval shunt. J Pharm Exp Ther 221:558–563, 1982.

216. McCarthy DM. Sucralfate. N Engl J Med 325:1017–1025, 1991.

217. Feldman M, Burton ME. Histamine₂-receptor antagonists. N Engl J Med 323:1672–1680, 1990.

218. D'Arinenzo A, Ambrogio G, Di Siervi P, et al. A randomized comparison of metoclopramide and domperidone on plasma aldosterone concentration and on spironolactone-induced diuresis in ascitic cirrhotic patients. Hepatology 5:854–857, 1985.

219. Prytz B, Grossi CE, Rousselot LM. In vitro formation of ammonia in blood of dog and man. Clin Chem 16:277–278, 1970.

220. Planas R, Arroyo V, Rimola A, et al. Acetylsalicylic acid suppresses the renal hemodynamic effect and reduces the diuretic action of furosemide in cirrhosis with ascites. Gastroenterology 84:247–252, 1983.

221. Uitto J, Ryhanen L, Tan EML, et al. Pharmacological inhibition of excessive collagen deposition in fibrotic diseases. Fed Proc 43:2815–2820, 1984.

222. Brenner DA, Alcorn JM. Therapy for hepatic fibrosis. Sem Liver Dis 10:1–9, 1990.

223. Arthur MJ. Matrix degradation in liver disease. Sem Liver Dis 10:47–55, 1990.

224. Kivirikko KI, Savolaine ER. Hepatic collagen metabolism. In: Testa B (ed) Liver Drugs: Experimental Pharmacology to Therapeutic Application. CRC Press, Boca Raton, FL, 42–53, 1989.

225. Li J, Kim C-I, Leo MA, et al. Polyunsaturated lecithin prevents acetaldehyde-mediated hepatic collagen accumulation by stimulating collagenase activity in cultured lipocytes. Hepatology 15:373–381, 1992.

226. Friedman SL. "Cuts both ways": Collagenases, lipocyte activation and polyunsaturated lecithin. Hepatology 15:549–551, 1992.

227. Lieber CS, DeCarli LM, Mak KM, et al. Attenuation of alcohol-induced hepatic fibrosis by polyunsaturated lecithin. Hepatology 12:1390–1398, 1990.

228. Jenkins PJ, Portmann BP, Eddleston ALWF, et al. Use of polyunsaturated phosphatidyl choline in HBsAg negative chronic active hepatitis: Results of prospective double-blind controlled trial. Liver 2:77–81, 1982.

229. Millward-Sadler GH, Hahn EG, Wright R. Cirrhosis: An appraisal. In: Wright R, et al. (eds) Liver and Biliary Disease: Pathophysiology, Diagnosis, Management. Bailliere Tindall, WB Saunders, Philadelphia, 821–860, 1985.

230. Rojkind M. Inhibition of liver fibrosis by L-azetidine-2-carboxylic acid in rats treated with carbon tetrachloride. J Clin Invest 52:2451–2454, 1973.

231. Uitto J, Tan EL, Ryhanen L. Inhibition of collagen accumulation in fibrotic processes: Review of pharmacologic agents and new approaches with amino acids and their analogues. J Invest Dermatol 79:113s–120s, 1982.

232. Kivirikko KL, Majamaha K. Synthesis of collagen: Chemical regulation of post-translational events. In: Ciba Foundation Symposium on Fibrosis. Pitman, London, 34–59, 1985.

233. Leveille CR, Arias IM. Pathophysiology and pharmacologic modulation of hepatic fibrosis. J Vet Int Med 7:73–84, 1993.

234. Dalton JRF, Hill FWG, Kelly DF. Intrahepatic cholestasis in a dog: A clinicopathological study. Vet Rec 97:383–386, 1975.

235. Tygstrop N. Use of corticosteroids in liver disease. In: Testa B (ed) Liver Drugs: Experimental Pharmacology to Therapeutic Application. CRC Press Boca Raton, FL, 162–173, 1989.

236. Summerskill WHJ, Korman MG, Ammon HV, et al. Prednisone for chronic active liver disease: Dose titration, standard dose, and combination with azathioprine compared. Gut 16:876–883, 1975.

237. Copenhagen Study Group for Liver Diseases. Effect of prednisone on the survival of patients with cirrhosis of the liver. Lancet 1:119–121, 1969.

238. Weiner FR, Czaja MJ, Ciambrone MA, et al. Transcriptional and posttranscriptional effects of dexamethasone on albumin and procollagen

messenger RNAs in murine schistosomiasis. Biochemistry 26:1557–1562, 1986.

239. Tanner A, Powel L. Corticosteroids in liver disease: Possible mechanisms of action, pharmacology, and rational use. Gut 20:1109–1124, 1979.

240. Weiner FR, Czaja MJ, Jefferson DM, et al. The effects of dexamethasone on in vitro collagen gene expression. J Biol Chem 262:6955–6958, 1987.

241. Ikeda T, Uchihara M, Daiguji Y, et al. Immunological mechanisms of corticosteroid therapy in chronic active hepatitis: Analysis of peripheral blood suppressor T-cell and interleukin 2 activities. Clin Imm Immunopath 48:371–379, 1988.

242. Nouri-Aria KT, Hegarty JE, Alexander GJM, et al. Effect of corticosteroids on suppressor-cell activity in "autoimmune" and viral chronic active hepatitis. N Engl J Med 307:1301–1304, 1982.

243. Gans JH, McEntee K. Comparative effects of prednisolone and thyroid hormone on bile secretion in the dog. Am J Physiol 201:577–581, 1961.

244. Miller E. Immunosuppressive therapy in the treatment of immune-mediated disease. J Vet Int Med 6:206–213, 1992.

245. Uribe M, Summerskill WHJ, Go VLW. Comparative serum prednisone and prednisolone concentration following administration to patients with chronic active liver disease. Clin Pharmacokinet 7:452–459, 1982.

246. Schalm SW, Summerskill WHJ, Go VLW. Prednisone for chronic active liver disease: Pharmacokinetics including conversion to prednisolone. Gastoenterology 72:910–913, 1977.

247. Hegarty JE, Nouri AKT, Portmann B, et al. Relapse following treatment withdrawal in patients with autoimmune chronic active hepatitis. Hepatology 3:685–689, 1983.

248. Runyon BA. Exquisite sensitivity to small decrements in corticosteroid dose in autoimmune chronic active hepatitis. J Clin Gastroenterol 9:541–542, 1987.

249. Uribe M, Wolf AM, Summerskill WMJ. Steroid side effects during therapy of chronic active liver disease (CALD). What to expect. Gastroenterology 71:932, 1976.

250. Murray-Lyon IM, Stern RB, Williams R. Controlled trial of prednisone and azathioprine in active chronic hepatitis. Lancet 735–737, 1973.

251. Summerskill WHJ. Chronic active liver disease re-examined: Prognosis hopeful. Gastroenterology 66:450–464, 1974.

252. Johnson GF, Zawie DA, Gilberston SR, et al. Chronic active hepatitis in Doberman pinschers. J Am Vet Med Assoc 180:1438–1442, 1982.

253. Czaja AJ, Ludwig J, Baggenstoss AH, et al. Corticosteroid-treated chronic active hepatitis in remission-uncertain prognosis of chronic persistent hepatitis. N Engl J Med 304:5–9, 1981.

254. Combes B. The initial morphologic lesion in chronic hepatitis, important or unimportant? Hepatology 6:518–522, 1986.

255. Beale KM. Azathioprine for treatment of immune-mediated disease of dogs and cats. J Am Vet Med Assoc 192:1316–1318, 1988.

256. Ogilvie GK, Felsburg PJ, Harris CW. Short-term effect of cyclophosphamide and azathioprine on selected aspects of the canine blastogenic response. Vet Imm Immunopath 18:119–127, 1988.

257. Nimni ME. A defect in the intramolecular and intermolecular cross-linking of collagen caused by penicillamine. J Biol Chem 243:1457–1466, 1968.

258. Mezey E, Potter JJ, Iber FL, et al. Hepatic collagen proline hydroxylase activity in alcoholic hepatitis: Effect of D-penicillamine. J Lab Clin Med 93:92–100, 1979.

259. Bodenheimer HC, Charland C, Thayer WR, et al. Effects of penicillamine on serum immunoglobulins and immune complex-reactive material in primary biliary cirrhosis. Gastroenterology 88:412–417, 1985.

260. Bodenheimer HC, Jr, Schaffner F, Sternlieb I, et al. A prospective clinical trial of D-penicillamine in the treatment of primary biliary cirrhosis. Hepatology 5:1139–1142, 1985.

261. Lipsky PE, Ziff M. Inhibition of human helper T cell function in vitro by D-penicillamine and CuSO$_4$. J Clin Invest 65:1069–1076, 1980.

262. Brewer GJ, Yuzbasiyan-Gurkan V. Wilson's disease: An update with emphasis on new approaches to treatment. Dig Dis 7:178–193, 1989.

263. Binderup L, Bramm E, Arrigoni-Martelli E. Effect of D-penicillamine in vitro and in vivo on macrophage phagocytosis. Biochem Pharmacol 29:2273–2278, 1980.

264. Dickson ER, Fleming CR, Geall MG, et al. A double-blind controlled study using D-penicillamine in chronic cholangiolitic hepatitis (primary biliary cirrhosis) (abstract). Gastroenterology 72:1049, 1977.

265. Fleming CR, Ludwig J, Dickson ER. Asymptomatic primary biliary cirrhosis: Presentation, histology, and results with D-penicillamine. Mayo Clin Proc 53:587–593, 1978.

266. Dickson ER, Gleming RT, Wiesner RH, et al. Trial of penicillamine in advanced primary biliary cirrhosis. N Engl J Med 312:1011–1015, 1985.

267. James OFW. D-penicillamine for primary biliary cirrhosis. Gut 26:109–113, 1985.

268. Maddrey WC. Chronic hepatitis. In: Zakim D, Boyer TD (eds) Hepatology, a Textbook of Liver Disease. WB Saunders, Philadelphia, 1025–1061, 1990.

269. Kershenobich D, Uribe M, Suarez GI, et al. Treatment of cirrhosis with colchicine: A double-blind randomized trial. Gastroenterology 77:532–536, 1979.

270. Kerschenobich D, Vargas F, Garcia-Tsao G, et al. Colchicine in the treatment of cirrhosis of the liver. N Engl J Med 318:1709–1713, 1988.

271. Floridi A, Fini C, Palmerini CA, et al. Experimental liver cirrhosis: Effects of low and high doses of colchicine (abstract). Gastroenterology 84:1371, 1983.

272. Ilfeld D, Kuperman O. Correction of a suppressor cell deficiency in four patients with familial Mediterranean fever by in vitro or in vivo colchicine. Clin Exp Immunol 50:99–105, 1982.

273. Bodenheimer H, Schaffner F, Pezzullo J. Evaluation of colchicine therapy in primary biliary cirrhosis. Gastroenterology 95:124–129, 1988.

274. Warnes TW, Smith A, Lee FI, et al. A controlled trial of colchicine in primary biliary cirrhosis. J Hepatol 5:1–7, 1987.

275. Kaplan MM. Medical treatment of primary biliary cirrhosis. Sem Liver Dis 9:138–142, 1989.

276. Zifroni A, Schaffner F. Long-term follow-up of patients with primary biliary cirrhosis on colchicine therapy. Hepatology 14:990–993, 1991.

277. Rojkind M, Kershenobich D. Effect of colchicine on collagen, albumin and transferrin synthesis by cirrhotic rat liver slices. Biochem Biophys Acta 378:415–423, 1975.

278. Gorden S, Werb Z. Secretion of macrophage neutral proteinase is enhanced by colchicine. Proc Natl Acad Sci USA 73:872–876, 1976.

279. Rennard SI, Bitterman PB, Ozaki T, et al. Colchicine suppresses the release of fibroblast growth factors from alveolar macrophages in vitro. Am Rev Respir Dis 137:181–185, 1988.

280. Kuncl RW, Duncan G, Watson D, et al. Colchicine myopathy and neuropathy. N Engl J Med 316:1562–1568, 1987.

281. Liu YK, Hymowitz R, Carrol MG. Marrow aplasia induced by colchicine: A case report. Arthritis Rheum 21:731–735, 1978.

282. Freeman DL. Frequent doses of intravenous colchicine can be lethal. N Engl J Med 309:310, 1983.

283. Leighton JA, Bay MK, Maldonado AL, et al. The effect of liver dysfunction on colchicine pharmacokinetics in the rat. Hepatology 11:210–215, 1990.

284. Boer HH, Nelson RW, Long GG. Colchicine therapy for hepatic fibrosis in a dog. J Am Vet Med Assoc 185:303–305, 1984.

285. Rutgers HC, Haywood S, Batt RM. Colchicine treatment in a dog with hepatoportal fibrosis. J Sm Anim Pract 31:97–101, 1990.

286. Meischer PA, Beris P. Immunosuppressive therapy in the treatment of autoimmune diseases. Springer Sem Immunopath 7:69–90, 1984.

287. Stanton M, Legendre AM. Effects of cyclophosphamide in dogs and cats. J Am Vet Med Assoc 188:1319–1322, 1986.

288. Meischer PA, Beris P. Immunosuppressive therapy in the treatment of autoimmune diseases. Springer Sem Immunopath 7:69–90, 1984.

289. Hoofnagle JH, Davis GL, Schafer DF, et al. Randomized trial of chlorambucil for primary biliary cirrhosis. Gastroenterology 91:1327–1334, 1986.

290. Kaplan MM, Knox TA, Arora S. Primary biliary cirrhosis treated with low-dose oral pulse methotrexate. Ann Int Med 109:429–431, 1988.

291. Kaplan MM, Knox TA, Arora S. Low-dose oral pulse methotrexate in the treatment of primary biliary cirrhosis (PBC): Resolution of symptoms and improvement in biochemical tests of liver function (abstract). Gastroenterology 94:A552, 1988.

292. Kaplan MM, Arora S, Pincus SH. Primary sclerosing cholangitis and low-dose oral pulse methotrexate therapy. Ann Int Med 106:231–235, 1987.

293. Bertino JR, Dicker AP. On the mechanism of methotrexate action in rheumatoid arthritis. In: Wilke WS (ed) Methotrexate Therapy in Rheumatic Disease. Marcel Dekker, New York, 129–144, 1989.

294. Pond EC, Morrow D. Heptotoxicity associated with methotrexate therapy in the dog. J Sm Anim Pract 23:659–666, 1982.

295. Minuk G, Bohme C, Burgess E, et al. A prospective, double-blind, randomized, controlled trial of cyclosporin A in primary biliary cirrhosis (abstract). Hepatology 7:1119, 1987.

296. Wiesner RH, Dickson ER, Lindor KE, et al. A controlled clinical trial evaluating cyclosporin in the treatment of primary biliary cirrhosis. A preliminary report (abstract). Hepatology 7:1025, 1987.

297. Fathman CG, Myers BD. Cyclosporine therapy for autoimmune disease. N Engl J Med 326:1693–1696, 1992.

298. Hess AD, Esa AH, Colombani PM. Mechanisms of action of cyclosporine: Effect on cells of the immune system and on subcellular events in T cell activation. Transplant Proc 20:29–40, 1988.

299. Kahan BD. Cyclosporin. N Engl J Med 321:1726–1738, 1989.

300. Yocum DE, Allen JB, Wahl SM, et al. Inhibition by cyclosporin A of streptococcal cell wall-induced arthritis and hepatic granulomas in rats. Arthrit Rheum 29:262–272, 1986.

301. Mazzaferro V, Porter KA, Scotti-Foglieni CL, et al. The hepatotropic influence of cyclosporin. Surgery 107:533–539, 1990.

302. Makowka L, Svanas G, Esquivel CO, et al. Effect of cyclosporin on hepatic regeneration. Surg Forum 37:352–354, 1986.

303. Kim YI, Salvini P, Auxilia F, et al. Effect of cyclosporin A on hepatocyte proliferation after partial hepatectomy in rats: Comparison with standard immunosuppressive agent. Am J Surg 155:245–249, 1988.

304. Kim YI, Calne RY, Nagasue N. Cyclosporin A stimulates proliferation of the liver cells after partial hepatectomy in rats. Surg Gynecol Obstet 166:317–322, 1988.

305. Sutherland FR, Preshaw RM, Shaffer EA. The effect of cyclosporin A on bile secretion in dogs. Can J Physiol Pharmacol 68:136–138, 1990.

306. Gregory CR. Cyclosporine. In: Kirk RW (ed) Current Veterinary Therapy X. WB Saunders, Philadelphia, 513–514, 1989.

307. Takaya S, Iwatsuki S, Noguchi T, et al. The influence of liver dysfunction on cyclosporin pharmacokinetics—a comparison between 70 per cent hepatectomy and complete bile duct ligation in dogs. Jap J Surg 19:49–56, 1989.

308. Lau AH, Lam NP, Piscitelli SC, et al. Clinical pharmacokinetics of metronidazole and other nitroimidazole anti-infectives. Clin Pharmakinet 23:328–364, 1992.

309. Grove DI, Mahmoud AAAF, Warren KS. Suppression of cell-mediated immunity by metronidazole. Int Arch Allergy Appl Imm 54:422–427, 1977.

310. Goldman P. Metronidazole. N Engl J Med 303:1212–1218, 1980.

311. Sutherland L, Singleton J, Sessions J, et al. Double blind, placebo controlled trial of metronidazole in Crohn's disease. Gut 32:1071–1075, 1991.

312. Ioannides L, Somogyi A, Spicer J, et al. Rectal administration of metronidazole provides therapeutic plasma levels in postoperative patients. N Engl J Med 305:1569–1570, 1981.

313. Friedel HA, Goa KL, Benfield P. S-adenosyl-l-methionine: A review of its pharmacological properties and therapeutic potential in liver dysfunction and affective disorders in relation to its physiological role in cell metabolism. Drugs 38:389–416, 1989.

314. Hoffman AF. Bile acid hepatotoxicity and the rationale of UDCA therapy in chronic cholestatic liver disease: Some hypotheses. In: Paumgartner G, Stiehl A, Barbar L, et al. (eds) Strategies for the Treatment of Hepatobiliary Diseases. Kluwer Academic, Dordrecht, the Netherlands, 13–33, 1990.

315. Kitani K. Hepatoprotective effect of ursodeoxycholate in experimental animals. In: Paumgartner G, Stiehl A, Barbar L, et al. (eds) Strategies for the Treatment of Hepatobiliary Diseases. Kluwer Academic, Dordrecht, the Netherlands, 43–56, 1990.

316. Calmus Y, Gane P, Rouger P, et al. Hepatic expression of class I and class II major histocompatibility complex molecules in primary biliary cirrhosis: Effect of ursodeoxycholic acid. Hepatology 11:12–15, 1990.

317. Leuschner U, Dienes HP, Guldutuna S, et al. Ursodeoxycholic acid (UDCA) influences immune parameters in patients with primary biliary cirrhosis (PBC) (abstract). Hepatology 12:957, 1990.

318. Silver EH, Szabo S. Role of lipid peroxidation in tissue injury after hepatic ischemia. Exp Mol Pathol 38:69–76, 1983.

319. Tribble DL, Aw TY, Jones DP. The pathophysiological significance of lipid peroxidation in oxidative cell injury. Hepatology 7:377–387, 1987.

320. Chawla RK, Lewis FW, Kutner MH, et al. Plasma cysteine, cystine, and glutathione in cirrhosis. Gastroenterology 87:770–776, 1984.

321. Burk RF, Lane JM, Patel K. Relationship of oxygen and glutathione in protection against carbon-tetrachloride-induced hepatic microsomal lipid peroxidation and covalent binding in the rat. Rational for the use of hyperbaric oxygen to treat carbon tetrachloride ingestion. J Clin Invest 74:1996–2001, 1984.

322. Horowitz JH, Rypins EB, Henderson JM, et al. Evidence for impairment of transulfuration pathway in cirrhosis. Gastroenterology 81:668–675, 1981.

323. De Heer K, Sauer H-D, Werner B, et al. Protective effects of cholestyramine on liver cirrhosis induced by carbon tetrachloride in the rat. Gut 21:860–865, 1980.

324. Ueda Y, Matsuo K, Kamei T, et al. Protective effect of prostaglandin E1 (PGE1) on energy metabolism and reticuloendothelial function in the ischemically damaged canine liver. Liver 9:6–13, 1989.

325. Ohhori I, Izumi R, Yabushita K, et al. Prevention of liver damage by using free radical scavengers and changes in plasma PG levels during liver ischemia. Transplant Proc 21:1309–1311, 1989.

326. Ruwart MJ, Rush BD, Snyder KF, et al. 16, 16-dimethyl prostaglandin E$_2$ delays collagen formation in nutritional injury in rat liver. Hepatology 8:61–64, 1988.

327. Ruwart MJ, Rush BD, Friedle NM, et al. 16,16-dimethyl prostaglandin E$_2$ protection agains α-naphthylisothiocyanate-induced experimental cholangitis in the rat. Hepatology 4:658–660, 1984.

328. Stachura J, Tarnawski A, Ivey KJ, et al. Prostaglandin protection in carbon-tetrachloride-induced liver cell necrosis in the rat. Gastroenterology 81:211–217, 1981.

329. Stachura J, Tarnawski A, Szczudrawa J, et al. Cytoprotective effect of 16, 16' dimethyl prostaglandin E$_2$ and some drugs on an acute galactosamine induced liver damage in rat. Folia Histochem, Cytochem 18:311–318, 1980.

330. Mizoguchi Y, Tsutsui H, Miyajima K, et al. The protective effects of prostaglandin E$_1$ in an experimental massive hepatic necrosis model. Hepatology 7:1184–1188, 1987.

331. Leuschner U, Leusschcner M, Sieratzki J, et al. Gallstone dissolution with ursodeoxycholic acid in patients with chronic active hepatitis and two years follow-up. A pilot study. Dig Dis Sci 30:642–649, 1985.

332. Podda M, Ghezzi C, Battezzati PM, et al. Ursodeoxycholic acid for chronic liver diseases. J Clin Gastroenterol 10(suppl. 2):S25–S31, 1988.

333. Bateson MC. Ursodeoxycholic acid therapy in chronic active hepatitis. Postgrad Med J 66:781–783, 1990.

334. Batta AK, Salen G, Shefer S, et al. Effect of ursodeoxycholic acid on bile acid metabolism in primary biliary cirrhosis. Hepatology 10:414–419, 1989.

335. Poupon RE, Balkau B, Eschwege E, et al. A multicenter, controlled trial of ursodiol for the treatment of primary biliary cirrhosis. N Engl J Med 324:1548–1554, 1991.

336. Poupon R, Poupon RE, Calmus Y, et al. Is ursodeoxycholic acid an effective treatment for primary biliary cirrhosis? Lancet, 834–836, 1987.

337. Stiehl A, Raedsch R, Kommerell B. The effect of ursodeoxycholic acid (URSO) in primary sclerosing cholangitis. A comparison to primary biliary cirrhosis (abstract). Gastroenterology 98:A595, 1988.

338. Senior JR, O'Brien CB, Wiesner RH. Ursodiol therapy of primary sclerosing cholangitis reduces the predicted mortality risk (abstract). Gastroenterology A630, 1988.

339. Ullrich D, Tating D, Schroter W, et al. Treatment with ursodeoxycholic acid renders children with biliary atresia suitable for liver transplantation. Lancet, 1324, 1987.

340. Beuers U, Spengler U, Zwiebel FM, et al. Effect of ursodeoxycholic acid on the kinetics of the major hydrophobic bile acids in healthy and in chronic cholestatic liver disease. Hepatology 15:603–608, 1992.

341. Colombo C, Setchell KDR, Podda M, et al. Effects of ursodeoxycholic acid therapy for liver disease associated with cystic fibrosis. J Pediatr 117:482–489, 1990.

342. Nakagawa M, Colombo C, Setchell KDR. Comprehensive study of the biliary bile acid composition of patients with cystic fibrosis and associated liver disease before and after UDCA administration. Hepatology 12:322–334, 1990.

343. Krol T, Kitamura T, Miyai K, et al. Tauroursodeoxycholate reduced ductular proliferation and portal inflammation in bile duct–ligated hamsters. Hepatology 80:881, 1983.

344. Miyai K, Toyota N, Jones HM, et al. Protective effect of ursodeoxycholic acid against cholestatic and heptotoxic effects of lithocholic acid (abstract). Hepatology 2:705, 1982.

345. Struthers JE, Mehta SJ, Kaye DM, et al. Relative concentrations of individual nonsulfated bile acids in the serum and bile of patients with cirrhosis. Dig Dis 22:861–865, 1977.

346. Vlahcevic ZR, Juttijudata P, Bell CC, et al. Bile acid metabolism in patients with cirrhosis. II. Cholic and chenodeoxycholic acid metabolism. Gastroenterology 62:1174–1183, 1972.

347. Akashi Y, Miyazaki H, Yanagisawa J, et al. Bile acid metabolism in cirrhotic liver tissue-altered synthesis and impaired hepatic secretion. Clin Chimica Acta 199–206, 1987.

348. Yoshida T, McCormick WC, Swell L, et al. Bile acid metabolism in cirrhosis. IV Characterization of the abnormality in deoxycholic acid metabolism. Gastroenterology 68:335–341, 1975.

349. Patteson TE, Vlahcevic ZR, Schwartz CC, et al. Bile acid metabolism in cirrhosis. VI. Sites of blockage in the bile acid pathways to primary bile acids. Gastroenterology 79:620–628, 1980.

350. Poupon RY, Poupon RE, Lebrec D, et al. Mechanisms for reduced hepatic clearance and elevated plasma levels of bile acids in cirrhosis. Gastroenterology 80:1438–1444, 1981.

351. Miyazaki K, Nakayama F, Koga A, et al. Effects of chenodeoxycholic and ursodeoxycholic acids on isolated adult human hepatocytes. Dig Dis Sci 4:661–666, 1984.

352. Schubert R, Jaroni H, Scholmerich J, et al. Studies on the mechanism of bile salt-induced liposomial membrane damage. Digestion 28:181–190, 1983.

353. Salvioli G, Lugli R, Pradell JM. In: Calandra S, Carulli N, Salvioli G (eds) Effects of Bile Salts on Membranes. Elsevier, New York; 163–185, 1984.

354. Lillemoe KD, Kidder GwW, Harmon JW, et al. Tauroursodeoxycholic acid is less damaging than ursochenodeoxycholic acid on the gastric and esophageal mucosa. Dig Dis Sci 28:359–364, 1983.

355. Gaetti E, Salvioli GF, Gualdi GL, Lugli R. Effect of bile salts on red blood cell membrane: A method to evaluate their membrane-damaging effect (abstract). International Meeting on Pathochemistry, Pathophysiology and Pathomechanics of the Biliary System: New Strategies for the Treatment of Biliary Tract Disease, Bologna, Italy, March 14–16, 1988.

356. Lee D, Bonorris G, Cohen H, et al. Effect of ursodeoxycholic acid on bile acid kinetics and hepatic lipid secretion. Hepatology 1:526, 1981.

357. Roda E, Roda A, Sama C, et al. Effect of ursodeoxycholic acid administration on biliary lipid composition and bile acid kinetics in cholesterol gallstone patients. Am J Dig Dis 24:123–128, 1979.

358. Von Bergmann K, Epple-Gutsfeld M, Leiss O. Differences in the effects of chenodeoxycholic and ursodeoxycholic acid on biliary lipid secretion and bile acid synthesis in patients with gallstones. Gastroenterology 87:136–143, 1984.

359. Marteau P, Chazouilleres O, Myara A, et al. Effect of chronic administration of ursodeoxycholic acid on the ileal absorption of endogenous bile acids in man. Hepatology 12:1206–1208, 1990.

360. Batta AK, Arora R, Salen G, et al. Characterization of serum and urinary bile acids in patients with primary biliary cirrhosis by gas-liquid chro-

360. matography-mass spectrometry: Effect of ursodeoxycholic acid treatment. J Lipid Res 30:1953–1962, 1989.

361. Stiehl A, Raedsch R, Rudolph G. Acute effects of ursodeoxycholic and chenodeoxycholic acid on the small intestinal absorption of bile acids. Gastroenterology 98:424–428, 1990.

362. Eusufzai S, Ericsson S, Cederlund T, et al. Effect of ursodeoxycholic acid treatment on ileal absorption of bile acids in man as determined by the SeHCAT test. Gut 32:1044–1048, 1991.

363. Nicholson BT, Center SA, Rowland PJ, et al. Evaluation of the safety of ursodeoxycholic acid in healthy cats (abstract). Proc 11th ACVIM Forum, 949, 1993.

364. Runyon BA. Current concepts: Care of patients with ascites. N Engl J Med 330:337–342, 1994.

365. Stassen WN, McCullough AJ. Management of ascites. Sem Liver Dis 5:291–307, 1985.

366. Guazzi M, Polese A, Magrini F, et al. Negative influences of ascites on the cardiac function of cirrhotic patients. Am J Med 59:165–170, 1975.

367. Panos MA, Moore K, Vlavianos P, et al. Single, total paracentesis for tense ascites: Sequential hemodynamic changes and right atrial size. Hepatology 11:662–667, 1990.

368. Knauer CM, Lowe HM. Hemodynamics in the cirrhotic patient during paracentesis. N Engl J Med 276;491–496, 1967.

369. Sherlock S. Ascites. In: Sherlock S (ed) Diseases of the Liver and Biliary System, 6th ed. Blackwell Scientific, Oxford, 116–133, 1981.

370. Boyer TD, Warnock DG. Use of diuretics in the treatment of cirrhotic ascites. Gastroenterology 84:1051–1055, 1983.

371. Campra JL, Reynolds TB. Effectiveness of high dose spironolactone therapy in patients with chronic liver disease and relatively refractory ascites. Dig Dis Sci 23:1025–1030, 1978.

372. Eggert RC. Spironolactone diuresis in patients with cirrhosis and ascites. Br Med J 4:401–403, 1970.

373. Gabow PA, Moore S, Schrier RW. Spironolactone-induced hyperchloremic acidosis in cirrhosis. Ann Intern Med 90:338–340, 1979.

374. Perez-Ayuso RM, Arroyo V, Plana SR, et al. Randomized comparative study of efficacy of furosemide versus spironolactone in non-azotemic cirrhosis with ascites. Relationship between the diuretic response and the activity of the renin-aldosterone system. Gastroenterology 84:961–968, 1983.

375. Gines P, Arroyo V, Quintero E, et al. Comparison of paracentesis and diuretics in the treatment of cirrhotics with tense ascites. Gastroenterology 93:234–241, 1987.

376. Naranjo CA, Pontigo E, Valdenegro C, et al. Furosemide induced adverse reactions in cirrhosis of the liver. Clinic Pharmacol Ther 25:154–160, 1979.

377. Descos L, Gauthier A, Levy VG, et al. Comparison of six treatments of ascites in patients with liver cirrhosis. A clinical trial. Hepatogastroenterology 30:15–20, 1983.

378. Shear L, Ching S, Gabuzda GJ. Compartmentalization of ascites and edema in patients with hepatic cirrhosis. N Engl J Med 282:1391–1396, 1970.

379. Kao HW, Rakov NRE, Reynolds TB. The effect of large volume paracentesis on plasma volume. A cause of hypovolemia? Gastroenterology 84:1202A, 1983.

380. Cabrera J, Inglada L, Quintero E, et al. Large-volume paracentesis and intravenous saline: Effects on the renin-angiotensin system. Hepatology 14:1025–1028, 1991.

381. Reynolds TB. Therapeutic paracentesis. Gastroenterology 93:386–388, 1987.

382. Schiff ER. Paracentesis: A safe and effective form of therapy. Hepatology 7:591–592, 1987.

383. LeVeen HH, Christoudias G, Ip M, et al. Peritoneo-venous shunting for ascites. Ann Surg 180:580–591, 1974.

384. Furneaux RW, Mero KN. End-to-side portocaval anastomosis for the correction of ascites in a terrier dog. J Am Anim Hosp Assoc 9:562–566, 1973.

385. Pinzello G, Simonetti R, Craxi A, et al. Spontaneous bacterial peritonitis: A prospective investigation in predominantly non-alcoholic cirrhotic patients. Hepatology 3:545–549, 1983.

386. Tito L, Rimola A, Gines P, et al. Recurrence of spontaneous bacterial peritonitis in cirrhosis: Frequency and predictive factors. Hepatology 8:27–31, 1988.

387. Hoefs JC, Canawati HN, Sapico FL, et al. Spontaneous bacterial peritonitis. Hepatology 2:399–407, 1982.

388. Steyn PF, Wittum TE. Radiographic, epidemiologic, and clinical aspects of simultaneous pleural and peritoneal effusions in dogs and cats: 48 cases (1982–1991). J Am Vet Med Assoc 202:307–312, 1993.

389. Falchuk KR, Jacoby I, Colucci WS, et al. Tetracycline-induced pleural symphysis for recurrent hydrothorax complicating cirrhosis. A new approach to treatment. Gastroenterology 72:319–321, 1977.

390. Mulhasen R, Eichenholz A, Blumentals A. Acid-base disturbances in patients with cirrhosis of the liver. Medicine (Baltimore) 46:185–189, 1967.

391. Kozlowski S, Drzewiecki K. The role of osmoreceptors in portal circulation in control of water intake in dogs. Acta Physiol Polonica 24:325–330, 1973.

392. Whang R, Papper S. The possible relationship of renal cortical hypoperfusion and diminished renal concentrating ability in Laennec's cirrhosis. J Chron Dis 27:263–265, 1974.

393. Vaamonde CA, Vaamonde LS, Morosi HJ, et al. Renal concentrating ability in cirrhosis. I. Changes associated with the clinical status and course of the disease. J Lab Clin Med 70:179–194, 1967.

394. Franklin JE, Saunders GK. Chronic active hepatitis in Doberman pinschers. Comp Cont Ed 10:1247–1255, 1988.

395. Thornburg LP, Rottinghaus G, Koch J, et al. High liver copper levels in two Doberman pinschers with subacute hepatitis. J Am Anim Hosp Assoc 20:1003–1005, 1984.

396. Hardy RM, Stevens JB, Stowe CM. Chronic progressive hepatitis in Bedlington terriers associated with elevated liver copper concentrations. Minn Vet 15:13–20, 1975.

397. Twedt DC, Sternlieb I, Gilbertson SR. Clinical, morphologic, and chemical studies on copper toxicosis of Bedlington terriers. J Am Vet Med Assoc 175:269–275, 1979.

398. Johnson GF, Sternlieb I, Twedt DC, et al. Inheritance of copper toxicosis in Bedlington terriers. Am J Vet Res 41:1865–1866, 1980.

399. Herrtage ME, Seymour CA, White RAS, et al. Inherited copper toxicosis in the Bedlington terrier: The prevalence in asymptomatic dogs. J Sm Anim Pract 28:1141–1151, 1987.

400. Su L-C, Owen CA, Zollman PE, et al. A defect of biliary excretion of copper in copper-laden Bedlington terriers. Am J Physiol 243:G231–G236, 1982.

401. Su L-C, Ravanshad S, Owen CA, et al. A comparison of copper-loading disease in Bedlington terriers and Wilson's disease in humans. Am J Physiol 243:G226–G230, 1982.

402. Owen CA, McCall JT. Identification of the carrier of the Bedlington terrier copper disease. Am J Vet Res 44:694–696, 1983.

403. Lerch K, Hohnson GF, Grushoff PS, et al. Canine hepatic lysosomal copper protein: Identification as metallothionein. Arch Biochem Biophys 243:108–114, 1985.

404. Johnson GF, Gilbertson SR, Goldfischer S, et al. Cytochemical detection of inherited copper toxicosis of Bedlington terriers. Vet Pathol 21:57–60, 1984.

405. Johnson GF, Morell AG, Stockert RJ, et al. Hepatic lysosomal copper protein in dogs with an inherited copper toxicosis. Hepatology 3:243–248, 1981.

406. Thornburg LP, Beissenherz M, Dolan M, et al. Histochemical demonstration of copper and copper-associated protein in the canine liver. Vet Pathol 22:327–332, 1985.

407. Robertson HM, Studdert VP, Reuter RE. Inherited copper toxicosis in Bedlington terriers. Aust Vet J 60:235–238, 1983.

408. Ludwig J, Owen CA, Barham SS, et al. The liver in the inherited copper disease of Bedlington terriers. Lab Invest 43:82–87, 1980.

409. Oelshlegel FJ, Jr, Brewer GJ. Absorption of pharmacologic doses of zinc. In: Brewer GJ, Prasad AS (eds) Zinc Metabolism: Current Aspects in Health and Disease. Alan R. Liss, New York, 14:29–36, 1977.

410. Hill GM, Brewer GJ, Prasad AS, et al. Treatment of Wilson's disease with zinc. I. Oral zinc therapy regimens. Hepatology 7:522–528, 1987.

411. Schilsky M, Blank R, Stockert R, et al. Copper hepatotoxicity attenuated by zinc. Hepatology 8:2240, 1988.

412. Lee D-Y, Brewer GJ, Wang Y. Treatment of Wilson's disease with zinc. VII. Protection of the liver from copper toxicity by zinc-induced metallothionein in a rat model. J Lab Clin Med 114:639–646, 1989.

413. Heilmaier HE, Jiang JL, Griem H, et al. D-penicillamine induces rat hepatic metallothionein. Toxicology 42:23–31, 1986.

414. Twedt DC, Whitney EL. Management of hepatic copper toxicosis in dogs. In: Kirk RW (ed) Current Veterinary Therapy X. WB Saunders, Philadelphia, 891–893, 1989.

415. Hardy RM. Copper-associated hepatitis in Bedlington terriers. In: Kirk RW (ed) Current Veterinary Therapy. VIII. Small Animal Practice. WB Saunders, Philadelphia, 834–836, 1983.

416. Twedt DC. Copper chelator therapy. Proc 10th ACVIM Forum, San Diego, CA, 53–55, May 1992.

417. Scheinberg IH, Jaffe ME, Sternlieb I. The use of trientine in preventing the effects of interrupting penicillamine therapy in Wilson's disease. N Engl J Med 317:209–213, 1987.

418. Allen KGD, Hunsaker HA, Twedt DC. Tetramine cupruretic agents: A comparison in dogs. Am J Vet Res 48:28–30, 1987.

419. Twedt DC, Hunsaker MS, Alleid KGD. Use of 2,3,2 tetramine as a hepatic copper chelating agent for the treatment of copper hepatotoxicosis in Bedlington terriers. J Am Vet Med Assoc 192:52–56, 1988.

420. Hoogenraad TU, Van Den Hamer CJA, Koevoet R, et al. Oral zinc in Wilson's disease. Lancet 2:1262–1269, 1978.

421. Lipsky MA, Gollan JL. Treatment of Wilson's disease: In D-penicillamine we trust—what about zinc? Hepatology 7:593–595, 1987.

422. LaRusso NR, Summerskill WHJ, McCall JT. Abnormalities of chemical tests for copper metabolism in chronic active liver disease. Gastroenterology 70:653–655, 1976.

423. Owen CA. Copper metabolism after biliary fistula, obstruction or sham operation in rats. Mayo Clin Proc 50:412–418, 1975.

424. Fleming CR, Dickson ER, Baggenstoss AH, et al. Copper and primary biliary cirrhosis. Gastroenterology 67:1182–1187, 1974.

425. Ritland S, Steinnes E, Skrede S. Hepatic copper content, urinary copper excretion, and serum ceruloplasmin in liver disease. Scand J Gastroenterol 12:81–88, 1977.

426. Hunt AH, Parr RM, Taylor DM, et al. Relation between cirrhosis and trace metal content of liver with special reference to primary biliary cirrhosis and copper. Br Med J 2:1498–1501, 1963.

427. Thornburg LP, Rottinghaus G. What is the significance of hepatic copper values in dogs with cirrhosis? Vet Med 80:50–54, 1985.

428. Sullivan JF, Burch RE. Potential role of zinc in liver disease. In: Prasad AS (ed) Trace Elements in Human Health and Disease. Academic, New York, 67–85, 1976.

429. Prasad AS. Clinical, biochemical and pharmacological role of zinc. Ann Rev Pharmacol Toxicol 20:393–426, 1979.

430. Smallwood RA, Williams HA, Rosenoer VM, et al. Liver copper levels in liver disease: Studies using neutron activation analysis. Lancet 2:1310–1313, 1968.

431. Fleming CR, Dickson ER, Baggenstoss AH, et al. Copper and primary biliary cirrhosis. Gastroenterology 67:1182–1187, 1974.

432. Thornburg LP, Polley D, Dimmitt R. The diagnosis and treatment of copper toxicosis in dogs. Canine Practice 11:36–39, 1984.

433. Thornburg LP, Shaw D, Dolan M, et al. Hereditary copper toxicosis in West Highland white terriers. Vet Pathol 23:148–154, 1986.

434. Thornburg LP. Copper metabolism defect in West Highland white terriers. In: Kirk RW (ed) Current Veterinary Therapy: Small Animal Practice X. WB Saunders, Philadelphia, 889–890, 1989.

435. Thornburg LP, Rottinghaus G, Gage H. Chronic liver disease associated with high hepatic copper concentration in a dog. J Am Vet Med Assoc 188:1190–1191, 1986.

436. Center SA, Baldwin BH, King JM, et al. Hematologic and biochemical abnormalities associated with induced extrahepatic bile duct obsturction in the cat. Am J Vet Res 44:1822–1829, 1983.

437. Keen CL, Lonnerdal B, Fisher GL. Age-related variations in hepatic iron, copper, zinc, and selenium concentration in beagles. Am J Vet Res 42:1884–1887, 1981.

438. Christian MK. Liver disease in Skye terriers. Vet Rec 114:127, 1984.

439. Haywood S, Rutgers HC, Christian MK. Hepatitis and copper accumulation in Skye terriers. Vet Pathol 25:408–414, 1988.

440. Thornburg LP, Moxley RA, Jones BD. An unusual case of chronic hepatitis in a Kerry blue. Vet Med/Sm Anim Clin 76:363–364, 1981.

441. Hardy RM. Chronic hepatitis in cocker spaniels—another syndrome? Proc 11th ACVIM Forum, 256–258, 1993.

442. Brandborg LL, Goldman IS. Bacterial and miscellaneous infections of the liver. In: Zakim D, Boyer TD (eds) Hepatology: a Textbook of Liver Disease, 2nd ed. WB Saunders, Philadelphia, 1086–1114, 1990.

443. Zimmerman HJ, Fang M, Utili R, et al. Jaundice due to bacterial infection. Gastroenterology 77:362–374, 1979.

444. Miller DJ, Keёton GR, Webber RL, et al. Jaundice in severe bacterial infection. Gastroenterology 71:94–97, 1976.

445. Rose HD, Lentino JR, Mavrelis PG, et al. Jaundice associated with non-hepatic *Staphylococcus aureus* infection. Does teichoic acid have a role in pathogenesis? Dig Dis Sci 27:1046–1050, 1982.

446. Toboada J, Meyer DJ. Cholestasis associated with extrahepatic bacterial infection in five dogs. J Vet Int Med 216–221, 1989.

447. Seeler RA, Hahn K. Jaundice in urinary tract infection in infancy. Am J Dis Child 118:553–558, 1969.

448. Agrez MV, House AK, Quinlan MF. Jaundice may herald an appendiceal abscess. Aust NZ J Surg 56:511–513, 1986.

449. Franson TR, Hierholzer WJ, LaBrecque DR. Frequency and characteristics of hyperbilirubinemia associated with bacteremia. Rev Infect Dis 7:1–9, 1985.

450. Turk J, Miller M, Brown R, et al. Coliform septicemia and pulmonary disease associated with canine parvoviral enteritis: 88 cases (1987–1988). J Am Vet Med Assoc 196:771–773, 1990.

451. Utili R, Abernathy CO, Zimmerman HJ. Cholestatic effects of *Escherichia coli* endotoxin on the isolated perfused rat liver. Gastroenterology 70:248–253, 1976.

452. Utili R, Abernathy CO, Zimmerman HJ. Studies on the effects of E. coli on canalicular bile formation in the isolated perfused rat liver. J Lab Clin Med 89:471–482, 1977.

453. Utili R, Abernathy CO, Zimmerman HJ. Inhibition of Na^+, K^+, adenosine triphosphatase by endotoxin: A possible mechanism for endotoxin induced cholestasis. J Infect Dis 136:583–587, 1977.

454. Oelberg DG, Lester R. Cellular mechanisms of cholestasis. Annu Rev Med 37:297–317, 1986.

455. Lee FS, Block GE. The changing clinical patterns of hepatic abscesses. Arch Surg 104:465–470, 1972.

456. Rubinson HA, Isikoff MB, Hill MC. Diagnostic imaging of hepatic abscesses: A retrospective analysis. Am J Roentgenol 135:735–740, 1980.

457. Barnes PF, DeCock KM, Reynolds TN, et al. A comparison of amoebic and pyogenic abscess of the liver. Medicine 66:472–483, 1987.

458. Sabbaj J, Sutter VL, Finegold SM. Anaerobic pyogenic liver abscess. Ann Intern Med 77:629–638, 1972.

459. McDonald MI, Corey GR, Gallis HA, et al. Single and multiple pyogenic liver abscesses; natural history, diagnosis and treatment with emphasis on percutaneous drainage. Medicine 63:291–302, 1984.

460. Gerzof SG, Johnson WC, Robbins AH, et al. Intrahepatic pyogenic abscesses: Treatment by percutaneous drainage. Am J Surg 149:487–494, 1985.

461. Bertel CK, VanHeerden JA, Sheedy PF. Treatment of pyogenic hepatic abscesses; Surgical vs. percutaneous drainage. Arch Surg 121:554–563, 1986.

462. Maher JA Jr, Reynolds TB, Yellin A. Successful medical treatment of pyogenic liver abscess. Gastroenterology 77:618–622, 1979.

463. Greene CE, Jones BR. Tyzzer's disease. In: Greene CE (ed) Infectious Diseases of the Dog and Cat. WB Saunders, Philadelphia, 552–553, 1990.

464. Guckian JC, Perry JE. Granulomatous hepatitis. An analysis of 63 cases and review of the literature. Ann Int Med 65:1081–1100, 1966.

465. Sartin JS, Walker RC. Granulomatous hepatitis: A retrospective review of 88 cases at the Mayo Clinic. Mayo Clin Proc 66:914–918, 1991.

466. Anderson CS, Nicholls IJ, Rowland R, et al. Hepatic granulomas: A 15 year experience in the Royal Adelaide Hospital. Med J Aust 148:71–74, 1988.

467. Wyler DJ, Wolff SM. Granulomatous liver disease. In: Schiff L, Schiff ER (eds) Diseases of the Liver, 6th ed. JB Lippincott, Philadelphia, 1438–1442, 1988.

468. McMaster KR, Hennigar GR. Drug induced granulomatous hepatitis. Lab Invest 44:61–73, 1981.

469. Chapman BL, Hendrick MJ, Washabau RJ. Granulomatous hepatitis in dogs: Nine cases (1987–1990). J Am Vet Med Assoc 203:680–684, 1993.

470. Chavanet P, Pillon D, Lancon JP, et al. Granulomatous hepatitis associated with Lyme disease. Lancet 623–624, 1987.

471. Aderka D, Kraus M, Avidor E, et al. Hodgkin's and non-Hodgkin's lymphomas masquerading as "idiopathic" liver granulomas. Am J Gastroenterol 79:642–644, 1984.

472. Hottendorf GH, Hirth RS. Lesions of spontaneous subclinical disease in beagle dogs. Vet Pathol 11:240–258, 1974.

473. Barron CN, Saunders LS. Visceral larva migrans in the dog. Vet Pathol 3:315–330, 1966.

474. Hirth RS, Hottendorf GH. Lesions produced by a new lungworm in beagle dogs. Vet Pathol 10:385–407, 1973.

475. Thrasher JP. Canine schistosomiasis. J Am Vet Med Assoc 144:1119–1126, 1964.

476. Tyler DE. Protothecosis. In: Greene CE (ed) Clinical Microbiology and Infectious Diseases of the Dog and Cat. WB Saunders, Philadelphia, 747–756, 1984.

477. Craig TM. Hepatoozoonosis. In: Greene CE (ed) Clinical Microbiology and Infectious Diseases of the Dog and Cat. WB Saunders, Philadelphia, 771–780, 1984.

478. Hardie EM. Actinomycosis and nocardiosis. In: Greene CE (ed) Clinical Microbiology and Infectious Diseases of the Dog and Cat. WB Saunders, Philadelphia, 663–674, 1984.

479. Carpenter JL, Myers AM, Conner MW, et al. Tuberculosis in five basset hounds. J Am Vet Med Assoc 192:1563–1568, 1988.

480. Grossman A. Mycobacterial hepatitis associated with long-term steroid therapy. Feline Pract 13:37–41, 1983.

481. Barasanti JA. Sporotrichosis. In: Greene CE (ed) Clinical Microbiology and Infectious Diseases of the Dog and Cat. WB Saunders, Philadelphia, 722–727, 1984.

482. Barsanti JA, Jeffery KL. Coccidioidomycosis. In: Greene CE (ed) Clinical Microbiology and Infectious Diseases of the Dog and Cat. WB Saunders, Philadelphia, 710–721, 1984.

483. Clinkenbeard KD, Cowell RL, Tyler RD. Disseminated histoplasmosis in dogs: 12 cases (1981–1986). J Am Vet Med Assoc 193:1443–1447, 1988.

484. Jang SS, Biberstein EL, Slauson DO, et al. Paecilomycosis in a dog. J Am Vet Med Assoc 159:1775–1779, 1971.

485. Stampley AR, Barsanti JA. Disseminated cryptococcosis in a dog. J Am Anim Hosp Assoc 24:17–24, 1988.

486. Jang SS, Dorr TE, Biberstein EL, et al. *Aspergillus deflectus* infection in four dogs. J Med Vet Mycol 24:95–104, 1986.

487. Day MJ, Penhale WJ, Eger CE, et al. Disseminated aspergillosis in dogs. Aust Vet J 63:55–59, 1986.

488. Ewing GO, Suter PF, Bailey CS. Hepatic insufficiency associated with congenital anomalies of the portal vein in dogs. JAAHA 10:463–476, 1974.

489. den Ingh TSGAM, Rothuizen J. Hepatoportal fibrosis in three young dogs. Vet Rec 110:575–577, 1982.

490. Bennett AM, Davies JD, Gaskell CJ, et al. Lobular dissecting hepatitis in the dog. Vet Pathol 20:179–188, 1983.

491. Rutgers HC, Haywood S, Kelly DF. Idiopathic hepatic fibrosis in 15 dogs. Vet Rec 133:115–118, 1993.

492. Bergaman JR. Nodular hyperplasia in the liver of the dog: An association with changes in the Ito cell population. Vet Pathol 22:427–438, 1985.

493. Stowater JL, et al. Ultrasonographic features of canine hepatic nodular hyperplasia. Vet Radiol 31:268–272, 1990.

34

Hepatic Lipidosis, Glucocorticoid Hepatopathy, Vacuolar Hepatopathy, Storage Disorders, Amyloidosis, and Iron Toxicity

SHARON A. CENTER

INTRODUCTION

There are a number of disorders in the dog and cat in which the hepatocytes become distended with vacuoles of endogenous products. These syndromes are usually associated with hepatomegaly and clinicopathologic features of intrahepatic cholestasis. In most cases, clinicopathologic evidence of the disorder is marked by increased liver enzyme activity, particularly ALP. Later, as hepatocytes become more severely distended, intrahepatic cholestasis associated with canalicular compression and microtubular disruption is marked by high serum bile acid concentrations. In cats with lipidosis, overt jaundice develops when the hepatocellular cytosol is at least 50% displaced by triglyceride (TG). Dogs with glucocorticoid and vacuolar hepatopathies rarely become jaundiced. These disorders are more closely associated with profound increases in the serum enzyme activity (ALP), which prompts diagnostic evaluation. Some dogs with glucocorticoid hepatopathies develop this lesion due to endogenous or iatrogenic hyperadrenocorticism. However, glucocorticoid and vacuolar hepatopathies are fairly common in dogs without endogenous hyperadrenocorticism or a history of therapeutic exposure to corticosteroid medications. In these, some other underlying systemic disease process is often found and thus clinical signs are highly variable.

A rare cause of hepatocellular injury due to extracellular deposition of an endogenous product is amyloidosis. In this disorder, hepatomegaly develops as a result of diffuse deposition of amyloid in the space of Disse, which leads to sinusoidal congestion and hepatocellular compression. Affected animals display a spectrum of clinical signs related to the diverse causes of immune dysregulation associated with amyloid formation and deposition.

The least common cause of storage hepatopathies in the dog and cat are inborn errors of metabolism leading to the inability to degrade or utilize a metabolic substrate or product. These are the lysosomal storage disorders, some of which lead to profound increases in organ size, including hepatomegaly. These disorders usually manifest at a young age and lead to progressive debilitation.

HEPATIC LIPIDOSIS

Clinical Synopsis

Diagnostic Features

- Obese, anorectic female cats predisposed
- Substantial weight loss usually precedes the disorder
- Anorexia, vomiting, and diarrhea are common
- Hepatomegaly and jaundice are frequently detected
- Signs of hepatic encephalopathy are unusual
- ALP usually elevated to a greater extent than GGT and often ALT
- Hyperbilirubinemia and hypokalemia common
- Serum globulin level is usually normal

Standard Treatment

- Fluid therapy with 0.9% NaCl and 20 mEq/L of KCl
- Protein-replete diet fed by gastrostomy tube sufficient to meet daily caloric requirements
- Supplementation with arginine (1 g/day) and taurine (250–500 mg BID/day), L-carnitine (250–500 mg/day), thiamine (50–100 mg/day), zinc (7–10 mg of elemental zinc/day), vitamin E (20–100 mg/day) and vitamin K_1 (5 mg BID for 1 day, repeated SID every 3–5 days) may be valuable during first 2 to 3 weeks of treatment

The syndrome of feline hepatic lipidosis (HL) is one of the most common severe hepatobiliary disorders affecting the domestic cat in North America. It is an uncommon diagnosis in the dog. Mistaken diagnosis of HL in the dog sometimes occurs in animals with a vacuolar hepatopathy in which the vacuoles become distended with glycogen or the cytoplasm assumes a frothy appearance. Specific histologic staining of tissue processed to preserve vacuolar contents can be performed to confirm the presence of cytosolic lipid. Otherwise, the diagnosis is based on a pathologist's subjective impression of vacuole morphology.

Hepatic lipidosis in the cat is a serious acquired syndrome that mimics the clinicopathologic features of other feline cholestatic disorders. It is most commonly diagnosed in obese female cats that have become anorectic. Correct diagnosis requires examination of liver tissue either by cytologic or histologic evaluation. In health, approximately 5% of the normal liver is lipid. Feline HL is characterized by the massive accumulation of TG in greater than 50% of the liver parenchymal cells. This extensive vacuolation compromises hepatocellular function to the extent that affected cats become systemically ill and untreated cats die.

Hepatic lipidosis as a disease entity has been reported in human beings, cows, horses, dogs, and cats as a spontaneous or reactive hepatobiliary disorder.[1–27] Many causal factors have been incriminated, as discussed in Chapter 30. Accumulation of TG in hepatocytes is not directly noxious to the cell, but is a common response to a variety of metabolic aberrations or underlying liver disorders. Physiologically, lipid accumulation is benign and a potentially reversible process. Compared to other species, feline hepatocytes appear to have a propensity for lipid vacuole formation. Cats with a variety of systemic abnormalities develop hepatic lipid vacuolation.[20] Consequently, mild to moderate hepatic lipidosis is a fairly common histologic observation in this species and should not be confused with the pathologic lipidosis syndrome.[20] Diffuse involvement of greater than 50% of the hepatocytes is required before a diagnosis of HL syndrome is made (Figure 34–1A and B).

In addition to their tendency to develop extensive hepatic lipid vacuolation, the cat also seems uniquely susceptible to hepatocellular dysfunction when diffuse lipidosis develops. Whether the lipid accumulation causes the hepatic dysfunction or vice versa has not been clarified. Currently, the HL syndrome in the cat is believed to be multifactorial in its etiopathogenesis. There is no question that it is related to starvation, but it appears cats have variable susceptibility to the syndrome. Analysis of adipose and hepatic vacuolar fat from affected cats has revealed similarities; hepatic vacuolar fat is comprised mainly of TGs and has a fatty acid content similar to that of adipose tissue.[28] This supports the contention that increased mobilization of peripheral fat stores during starvation serves as the source of hepatic TGs. The following discussion addresses some of the possible reasons for individual variation in development of the HL syndrome.

Etiopathogenesis

Triglycerides may accumulate in the liver as a result of a variety of imbalances in normal fat metabolism. Figures 30–3, 30–4, and 34–2 present a simplified overview of lipid metabolism and abnormalities in metabolism that may be involved in the feline HL syndrome. It is believed the feline HL syndrome is multifactorial in origin, even though it appears to be related to obesity and anorexia. In health, a balance is maintained between the hepatic (1) uptake of fatty acids, (2) use of fatty acids for energy (production of ketone and fatty

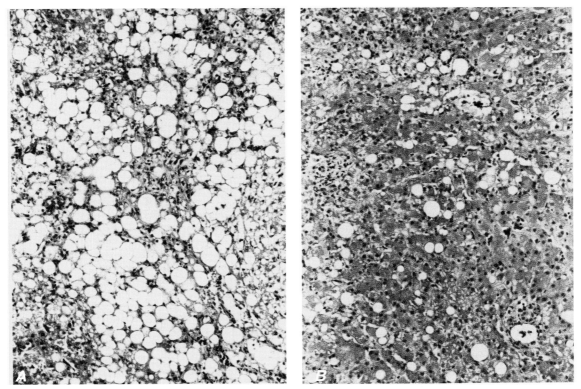

FIGURE 34–1. Photomicrographs showing (*A*), severe diffuse hepatic lipidosis and (*B*), mild hepatic lipid vacuole formation. A diffuse lesion such as that in (*A*) is associated with the feline hepatic lipidosis syndrome. A mild lesion such as that in (*B*) is common in feline liver biopsies and is not indicative of the hepatic lipidosis syndrome. Hepatocytes containing lipid appear empty with an inconspicuous nucleus when processed routinely with formalin fixation, paraffin embedment, and H&E stain. Paraffin embedment results in vacuolar fat extraction.

Possible Abnormalities in Hepatic Lipidosis

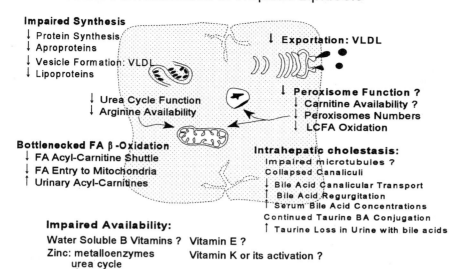

Impaired Synthesis
↓ Protein Synthesis
↓ Aproproteins
↓ Vesicle Formation: VLDL
↓ Lipoproteins

↓ Exportation: VLDL

↓ Urea Cycle Function
↓ Arginine Availability

↓ Peroxisome Function ?
↓ Carnitine Availability ?
↓ Peroxisomes Numbers
↓ LCFA Oxidation

Bottlenecked FA β -Oxidation
↓ FA Acyl-Carnitine Shuttle
↓ FA Entry to Mitochondria
↑ Urinary Acyl-Carnitines

Intrahepatic cholestasis:
Impaired microtubules ?
Collapsed Canaliculi
↓ Bile Acid Canalicular Transport
↑ Bile Acid Regurgitation
↑ Serum Bile Acid Concentrations
Continued Taurine BA Conjugation
↑ Taurine Loss in Urine with bile acids

Impaired Availability:
Water Soluble B Vitamins ?   Vitamin E ?
Zinc: metalloenzymes
    urea cycle   Vitamin K or its activation ?
    free radical scavanger

FIGURE 34-2. Simplified overview of abnormalities in hepatocellular metabolism involved in the feline hepatic lipidosis syndrome.

acid α-oxidation), (3) production and dispersal of lipoproteins, which are essential for distribution of fat to other body systems, and (4) de novo synthesis of TGs. Adipose tissue is an important fat and energy store. Lipolysis and esterification of fatty acids into TG in adipose occur simultaneously, the net outcome depending on their relative rates. In health, mobilization of adipose fat for energy is regulated by the blood glucose concentration and a complex balance of hormonal, neural, and nutritional mechanisms.

The activities of lipoprotein lipase (LPL) and hormone sensitive lipase (HSL) govern the rate of adipocyte fat uptake and lipolysis. LPL activity varies in different metabolic states. In the well-fed animal, LPL activity promotes adipocyte fat uptake and storage. During starvation, LPL activity is downregulated and HSL activity prevails. This results in hydrolysis of adipocyte TG and release of free fatty acids (FFA) into the systemic circulation. HSL is stimulated by norepinephrine, epinephrine, growth hormone, corticosteroids, glucagon, and thyroxine and is inhibited by insulin. The stress associated with illness and starvation may shift the hormonal milieu in favor of increased HSL activity. Insulin is an important regulator of HSL. An absence or insensitivity to insulin impairs HSL suppression, permitting continued lipolysis of adipocyte fat and mobilization of FFA to the liver. Poorly controlled diabetes mellitus is associated with hepatic lipidosis.

Many metabolic conditions, nutritional factors, drugs, and toxins can facilitate the accumulation of excessive hepatic fat (see in Table 34–1). The conditions of concern in the cat with the HL syndrome include obesity, anorexia, nutritional management with poorly balanced rations (i.e., IV glucose infusion in the anoretic, euglycemic cat or forced nutritional support with high fat restricted protein diet), inflammatory bowel disease or development of small intestinal bacterial overgrowth, diabetes mellitus, acquired abnormalities in peroxisomal or mitochondrial function, inadequate carnitine availability, and the accumulation of lipogenic hepatic toxins.

OBESITY. Constant overnutrition with foods high in fat or simply just excessive caloric intake each lead to hepatic TG accumulation. Obesity results in excessive mobilization of FFA from adipose, release of FFA increasing proportionately with the extent of obesity. This alone can lead to excessive hepatic lipid accumulation because up to one-third of the

mobilized FFA may be taken up by the liver.[1] The normal liver is capable of extracting FFA and reesterifying them into TG at a rate that exceeds its capacity for their use in energy or lipoprotein dispersal. This underlying tendency favoring greater ingress than egress sets the stage for TG accumulation should excess fat uptake occur. In obesity, derangements in carbohydrate metabolism lead to mild hyperglycemia. Under normal circumstances this situation would permit insulin to suppress FFA mobilization from adipocytes through its effect on HSL. However, in the presence of marked obesity, the ability of insulin to suppress lipolysis is overwhelmed. Obese cats are believed to have an increased risk of developing the HL syndrome when they become anorectic for any reason. Complicating medical conditions may facilitate the process as can the feeding of poorly balanced high-fat diets.

ANOREXIA OR RAPID WEIGHT REDUCTION. Starvation for 2 weeks or chronic undernutrition lead to hepatic TG accumulation. Adipocyte lipolysis is promoted due to reduced glucose availability, decreased insulin concentrations, increased concentration of growth hormone and glucocorticoids, and heightened sympathetic tone.[1-3] Increased fat turnover increases the serum FFA. Upon uptake into the liver these are either oxidized to ketone bodies or reesterified to TG. Dispersed ketone bodies are used for energy by the CNS, and the TG are exported as VLDL for systemic distribution. The limited hepatic capacity for fatty acid oxidation and ketone formation creates a metabolic blockade favoring fatty acid reesterification into TG. When starvation reduces the availability of proteins, choline, and possibly other important lipotropes for synthesis of apoproteins and lipoproteins, storage of hepatic TG rather than lipoprotein synthesis is favored. Experimentally, administration of choline to animals with HL associated with long-term starvation assists in hepatic metabolic recovery if coadministered with a nutritionally replete diet. Other causes of HL will not respond to this therapy. During absolute starvation, adaptation to fat metabolism is nearly complete; muscle and brain rely on fatty acids or ketones for 95% of their energy requirements. This metabolic adaptation conserves glucose, reduces the need for using amino acids in gluconeogenesis, and results in only a low level of hepatic TG accumulation. However, several factors modulate the development of lipidosis in the circum-

Table 34-1

FACTORS PROMOTING DEVELOPMENT OF HEPATIC LIPIDOSIS

Nutritional Conditions	Proposed Mechanisms
Starvation	
2 weeks or longer	↑ mobilization of FFA from adipose
	↓ protein, ↓ choline: ↓ synthesis of apoproteins and lipoproteins
	↓ synthesis of apoproteins and lipoproteins
Chronic undernutrition	↓ availability of carnitine, ↓ export VLDL
	impaired export of VLDL from liver
	impaired adaptation to efficient beta-oxidation
Protein depletion	↓ synthesis of apoproteins and lipoproteins
	impaired export of VLDL from liver
	↑ susceptibility to peroxidation and free radical injuries
	↓ enzyme activity
Depletion of choline, methionine,	↓ synthesis of apoproteins and lipoproteins
myoinositol:	impaired export of VLDL from liver
Chronic parenteral nutrition	excessive calorie:protein nitrogen ratio
	deficiency of essential fatty acids
	↑ de novo hepatic fatty acid synthesis
	↓ hepatic VLDL formation, acquired carnitine deficiency
	hepatotoxic products: tryptophan breakdown moieties, ↑ enteric production endotoxins, toxic bile acids
Medium chain TG	experimental evidence in cats that this leads to lipidosis
	mechanism unknown
Miscellaneous	
Intestinal bacterial overgrowth	formation of toxic bile acids, endotoxins, dietary inadequacies
Diabetes mellitus	↑ adipose lipolysis
Carnitine deficiency	impaired preprocessing of FA for beta-oxidation
Peroxisome dysfunction	impaired preprocessing of FA for beta-oxidation, oxidation of long chain FA
Mitochondrial dysfunction	↓ beta-oxidation of FA
Congenital ↓ LPL	hypertriglyceridemia, ↑ hepatic fat accumulation
Pregnancy	impaired mitochondrial beta-oxidation
Hepatic hypoxia	↓ FFA oxidation or exportation, ↓ energy used for maintenance of euglycemia
Hepatic regeneration	metabolism deviated to reparative processes
Toxins	
Inflammatory bowel	altered intestinal flora endotoxins, noxious bile acids
Chronic alcohol ingestion	direct hepatic injury, metabolite-mediated injury
	altered nutrient metabolism
	↑ TG deposition
CCl_4	metabolites produced by P-450 microsomes: toxic free radicals, lipid peroxidation ↓ cell protein synthesis, ↓ synthesis and export lipoproteins
Ethionine, phosphorus	↓ apolipoprotein synthesis → ↓ lipoprotein exportation
Puromycin	ethionine: ↓ ATP in hepatocyte
Hypoglycin (Akee tree)	impairs fatty acid beta-oxidation and metabolism by conversion to nonmetabolizable CoA and carnitine derivatives
Aflatoxins	inhibit RNA synthesis and thus synthesis of proteins and enzymes, suppressed glucose metabolism. Protein depletion increases susceptibly
Orotic acid	impaired assembly or exportation of VLDL from the liver
Bacterial toxins and endotoxins	impaired fatty acid oxidation, ↓ apoprotein synthesis
Drugs	
Tetracycline	↓ apoprotein production, impaired VLDL exportation
Valproic acid	impaired fatty acid oxidation and decreased availability of coenzyme A and carnitine
Amiodarone	lysosomal phospholipidosis is due to accumulated drug metabolites
Methotrexate	mechanism undetermined, suspected ↓ lipotrope availability (↓ folate metabolism)
Glucocorticoids	↑ peripheral lipolysis → ↑ FFA mobilization to the liver

stance of starvation, including the completeness of starvation, the extent of protein deficiency, and the adaptive capabilities of the hepatocyte for VLDL dispersal. With less than absolute starvation this efficient adaptation to fatty acid metabolism is lost. This is relevant to the feline patient with HL because ingestion or IV administration of dextrose or forced feeding of some but insufficient calories may disrupt the efficient adaptation to fatty acid metabolism.[29] This results in augmented hepatic TG accumulation because fats are not efficiently oxidized and not expediently exported as VLDL due to relative apoprotein deficiencies or inefficient lipoprotein synthesis.[30] Low-level glucose infusions should be avoided in anorectic obese cats because they may facilitate the development or worsening of hepatic TG storage. Feeding of a diet replete with calories and protein appears to facilitate recovery from the HL syndrome. This is of particular importance for the cat, considering its status as a pure carnivore and its limited ability to adapt to a restricted protein diet.[31,32]

Characterization of the serum lipoprotein concentrations in normal and obese cats undergoing weight reduction but not developing HL has shown no significant alterations that would explain the feline propensity for hepatic lipid accumulation.[33]

IMBALANCED NUTRITION. Nutritional factors essential for normal hepatic fat metabolism include precursors necessary for lipoprotein synthesis (lipotropic agents). These include choline, methionine, myo-inositol, and vitamin B_{12}. Methionine is a choline precursor, and methionine and cysteine can replace choline. Choline is important for hepatic lipoprotein synthesis and dispersal.[34,35] In rats, increased hepatic lipid deposition can be shown within hours after feeding a choline deficient diet. Myo-inositol is lipotropic by virtue of its incorporation in the phospholipid phosphatidylinositol, an important membrane and lipoprotein component.[36] Phosphatidylinositol has diverse activities that can influence the health and activity of the hepatocyte including modulation of several membrane-bound enzymes, intercellular communications, and intracellular calcium and protein phosphorylations.[36–38] Deficiency can lead to a variety of abnormalities of lipid metabolism.[37,38] Provision of additional inositol to animals with fatty livers has no beneficial effect unless its deficiency was involved in its etiopathogenesis. However, the administration of choline-sparing substances such as B_{12}, folic acid, and inositol may assist in protecting a liver from the consequences of choline deficiency.[39–41] Vitamin B_{12} is involved in the methylation of certain lipotropic amino acids and other intermediary metabolites, such as choline and methionine.[35] Choline and inositol deficiencies are unlikely as spontaneous disorders in pet cats because commercial foods contain adequate quantities. However, choline deficiency may develop due to intestinal malabsorption or maldigestion; this also may lead to B_{12} deficiency. An acquired and a congenital deficiency of cobalamin (with suspected B_{12} deficiency), each associated with HL and in the later case with methylmalonic acidemia, have been described in cats.[42,43] It is unknown if these abnormalities are common in cats with the HL syndrome.

A fatty liver can develop from protein-deficient diets. Protein deficiency is the cause of HL in Kwashiorkor, an important cause of hepatic failure in children. Initial injury in these patients is believed to be derived from exposure to endotoxins, infections, or aflatoxin. These initiate cellular injury through production of free radicals and this injury is promoted by the deficiency in cellular antioxidants and inadequate reparative capabilities due to protein deficiency and hepatic dysfunction associated with HL.[44] Hepatic lipid accumulates due to deficient synthesis of VLDL. It is possible that similar mechanisms to these initiate HL in some cats.

Hepatic lipidosis may develop in association with imbalances in the relative amounts of carbohydrates and lipids consumed, such as when the primary source of calories is fat. In this circumstance, diet supplementation with choline, vitamins, protein, and micronutrients protects against hepatic TG deposition. Considering that the feeding of rations with an excessive lipid and insufficient protein content can promote lipidosis, use of protein-restricted diets supplemented with additional fat to increase the caloric content of the diet may be detrimental in cats already affected with the lipidosis syndrome. Careful attention must be paid to the nutritional balance of the recovering cat. Supplementation with adequate protein is essential. Chronic parenteral alimentation has been associated with hepatic lipidosis in human beings.[45,46] Moderate hepatic lipid accumulation has also been shown in short-term parenteral alimentation in healthy cats.[45] Proposed causes are numerous and include excessive calorie-to-protein nitrogen ratio, essential fatty acid deficiency, enhanced de novo hepatic synthesis of fatty acids,

reduced hepatic VLDL formation, hepatotoxicity derived from tryptophan metabolites, acquired carnitine deficiency, or alimentary production of hepatotoxic endotoxins and bile acids.

DIABETES MELLITUS. Fatty liver is associated with diabetes mellitus in humans, dogs, and cats. An absolute or relative insulin deficiency promotes fasting hyperglycemia, glucose intolerance, and increased adipocyte lipolysis due to failure to suppress HSL activity and the perceived physiologic need for continued lipolysis. These influences encourage hepatic lipid accumulation. In humans, there is no apparent association between the degree of glycemic control or the duration of diabetes with the extent or severity of hepatic fat infiltration. Rather, hepatic lipid accumulation seems more related to the degree of patient obesity. Overt diabetes is an uncommon underlying cause of the HL syndrome in cats.[25] However, diabetic animals have not undergone rigorous evaluation for this disorder.

TOXINS. A number of toxins have been associated with HL in human beings and experimental animals. Most of these are listed in Table 34–1 and reviewed in Chapter 30. Many drugs, chemicals, and plant toxins may produce lipidosis if chronic exposure to small quantities occurs. However, acute severe intoxications are usually associated with hepatic necrosis or inflammation, which is inconsistent with the histomorphologic lesion seen in the feline HL syndrome. Because lipid vacuolation is one of the few morphologic responses of the hepatocyte to metabolic injury, different toxins, with different injurious effects, can produce this same morphologic response. Few toxins have been specifically identified that can induce clinical HL in the cat. In one study, a diet composed of safflower seed oil (5%), chicken fat (5%), and hydrogenated coconut oil (15%) produced lipidosis.[47] It was assumed the coconut oil medium chain TGs were responsible. These substances are now considered contraindicated for nutritional support of cats.

Orotic acid has been shown to induce hepatic lipidosis in rats[48] and has been suggested to be involved in the genesis of the feline HL syndrome.[16,19,49] This toxin accumulates when entrance of nitrogenous wastes into the urea cycle is blocked and they are deviated to the pyrimidine synthetic pathway.[50] Entrance to the urea cycle can become compromised when a deficiency of urea cycle substrate intermediates such as arginine develops (Figure 34–3). When orotic acid accumulates, it interferes with the formation and exportation of hepatic lipoproteins.

However, the relevancy of orotic acid toxicity to the feline HL syndrome remains speculative and is waning in popularity as a causal factor. A recent preliminary investigation of orotic acid toxicity in overfed obese cats failed to induce hepatic lipid vacuolation consistent with the HL syndrome.[51,52] High concentrations of orotic acid in serum or urine of cats with spontaneous clinical HL or in cats with experimentally induced HL have not been found.[22,53]

Loading of cats with HL with large concentrations of dietary citrulline was proposed as a treatment for this syndrome.[21] It is theorized that provision of citrulline would ensure arginine repletion in the urea cycle and reduce the production of orotic acid (Figure 34–3). Experimentally it has been shown that large concentrations of ornithine can block the development of hyperammonemia in cats fed an arginine-depleted high-protein elemental diet. Citrulline has been suggested to be superior to ornithine in ensuring adequate concentrations of arginine in kittens.[54] As of yet no evidence indicates that citrulline or ornithine loading would be superior to the feeding of an arginine-replete balanced feline diet.

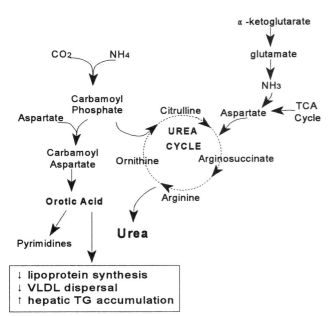

FIGURE 34–3. Diagrammatic representation of the urea cycle and its association with orotic acid generation. If urea cycle function is impaired, ammonia is directed to the pyrimidine synthetic pathway and formation of orotic acid. Orotic acid can impair VLDL synthesis and dispersal. It has been implicated as a cause of hepatic lipidosis in the rat but has not been shown to be involved with the feline syndrome.

Toxic substances produced by intestinal bacteria have been suggested to induce hepatic lipid vacuolation in humans and cats. Endotoxin has received the most attention. Bacterial overgrowth in the small bowel, as occurs with the stagnant loop syndrome or with maldigestion/malabsorption problems, can also induce hepatocellular vacuolation in humans. Proposed mechanisms include formation of bacterial toxins and toxic bile salts, or development of nutrient inadequacies. Certain bacterial toxins impair fatty acid oxidation and decrease apoprotein synthesis. Overgrowth of intestinal anaerobes is believed to generate lipidosis-inducing toxins in some humans with severe HL. Reportedly, hepatic fat deposition can be reversed by eliminating anaerobic overgrowth.[6]

Tetracycline has been associated with diffuse HL in cats, humans, and experimental animals.[29,54–60] Microvesicular lipid vacuolation of hepatocytes develops in humans within 3 to 12 days after treatment initiation.[29] One cat with suspected hepatic toxicity due to tetracycline administration developed markedly increased serum ALT activity and a mild degree of HL.

SYSTEMIC OR LOCAL HEPATIC CARNITINE INSUFFICIENCY. It is possible that an acquired carnitine deficiency may be related to the development of the feline HL syndrome. Carnitine is primarily synthesized in the liver and essential for enzyme-mediated uptake of fatty acids into mitochondria[61,62] (Figure 34–4). Carnitine also facilitates the export of short chain acyls from the intra- to the extramitochondrial space. It is also found in peroxisomes where it is associated with the oxidation of long chain fatty acids.[62–64] Under normal circumstances, hepatic lipid accumulation stimulates liver carnitine synthesis to meet increased metabolic demands for fatty acid mitochondrial transport.[65,66] During a fast, humans initially develop reduced serum and urine-free carnitine concentrations. However, the serum concentration and urinary excretion of acyl-carnitines thereafter increase as small acyl-carnitine moieties are refluxed into the systemic circulation from the liver (see Figure 34–4).[67]

Congenital (primary) and acquired (secondary) carnitine deficiency in human beings is associated with severe lipid accumulation in the liver and other tissues. The hepatic lipid accumulation can be associated with hepatic dysfunction similar to that in cats with the HL syndrome. A deficiency of carnitine is detrimental in regard to its role in transporting fatty acids into the mitochondria. Carnitine deficiency is also thought to impair normal ammonia detoxification through effects on the urea cycle and to augment the neurotoxic effects of ammonia.[68,69] In addition, carnitine deficiency is believed to promote the accumulation of toxic intramitochrondrial concentrations of acetyl CoA.

Several different congenital enzyme deficiencies are suspected in human beings to cause primary defects in carnitine metabolism or utilization; these include disorders of transcellular carnitine transport, deranged carnitine biosynthesis, abnormal renal conservation of carnitine, altered cellular uptake or release mechanisms, excessive carnitine degradation, or defective intestinal absorption.[61,70–72] Affected individuals episodically accumulate excessive hepatic lipid. "Attacks" are precipitated by caloric deprivation and increased depen-

FIGURE 34–4. Diagrammatic representation of carnitine participation in fatty acid oxidation and of the proposed theory for "regional" carnitine inadequacy in cats with severe hepatic lipidosis. Increased delivery of long chain free fatty acids in the vicinity of the mitochondria requires available carnitine for transport across the organelle wall. Beta-oxidation in mitochondria and peroxisomes may be inadequate for processing of increased amounts of acyl-CoA moieties formed. Consequently, increased amounts of acyl-carnitines accumulate and diffuse out of the hepatocyte into the perisinusoidal space (space of Disse) from which they are swept away into the peripheral circulation. Ultimately, these undergo renal excretion. The clinical impression that carnitine hastens recovery from the feline hepatic lipidosis syndrome supports some degree of carnitine inadequacy.

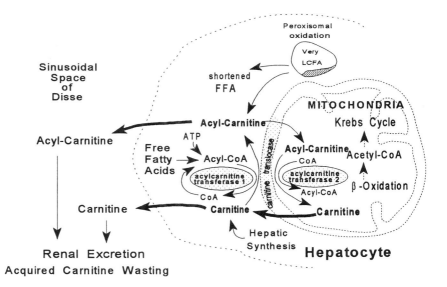

dency on fatty acid–derived energy. No congenital enzymatic defects influencing carnitine availability or function have been recognized in cats, but the presence of such defects has not been rigorously evaluated.

It may be that this species is predisposed to development of acquired carnitine deficiencies. Conditions associated with acquired carnitine deficiencies in humans include chronic parenteral hyperalimentation, prematurity, myopathies, cirrhosis associated with cachexia, Fanconi syndrome, Kwashiorkor, hypothyroidism, hypopituitarism, hypoadrenocorticism, pregnancy, starvation, and inborn errors of fatty acid oxidation.[61,66,67,73]

Plasma, liver tissue, and urine concentrations of free- and acyl-carnitine moieties in cats with severe hepatic lipidosis are increased compared to normal, short-term fasted cats.[22,74] This is similar to findings in studies of lean and obese mice and humans subjected to starvation but differs from findings in some obese rats.[67,73,75–77] In starvation, both lean and obese rats conserve hepatic carnitine for the essential purpose of fatty acid oxidation.[73] In cats, the higher concentrations of carnitine moieties in blood and urine as compared to control animals likely reflects increased mobilization and urinary loss of acyl-carnitines due to regurgitation from hepatocytes where they have accumulated. The normal hepatic capabilities for uptake of FFA exceeds the capabilities for fatty acid β-oxidation or export of VLDL. This natural tendency to sequester TG in the liver becomes profoundly imbalanced in the cat with the HL syndrome. The continued cytosolic egress of acyl-carnitine moieties either awaiting β-oxidation or accumulating in the mitochondria after partial oxidation may lead to a relative carnitine deficiency inside the cell where its availability is essential. If this circumstance is realized, carnitine availability could become a rate-limiting factor in fatty acid utilization.

Carnitine supplementation for humans with acquired carnitine deficiency states has been shown to be therapeutically beneficial based on subjective and objective evaluations.[78] A preliminary study of carnitine supplementation for obese cats undergoing weight loss suggests it may be beneficial; conclusions from that study were difficult owing to the finding of lipid vacuolation in control specimens taken before weight loss was initiated.[79] Clinical use of carnitine supplementation in cats with spontaneous HL seems to hasten their recovery; however, this observation has not been evaluated in a controlled study.

ABNORMAL MITOCHONDRIAL OR PEROXISOMAL FUNCTION. Peroxisomes are small organelles distributed throughout mammalian cells (see Figure 29–20). They are particularly populous in hepatocytes. Peroxisomes participate in a large number of diverse functions including respiration, gluconeogenesis and β-oxidation.[80–82] They are known to collaborate with mitochondria in some of their essential metabolic functions, such as fatty acid β-oxidation.

Inherited enzyme disorders that impair normal fatty acid oxidation and peroxisome availability or function can also lead to extensive hepatic lipid accumulation. These disorders have been characterized in humans and rodents and do not exclusively involve the liver. They have not been documented in dogs or cats. When defects in fatty acid oxidation occur, organic acids that undergo chain shortening at the point of the metabolic defect become abnormally elevated. These end-point products can be detected to determine the exact metabolic site of the enzyme defect. Evaluation of organic acids in urine of affected cats has failed to reveal the presence of dicarboxylic acids, products of β-oxidation that indicate a specific focal enzymatic abnormality impairing normal fatty acid oxidation in the cat with HL.[22]

An acquired mitochondrial or peroxisomal dysfunction could possibly underlie the HL syndrome in the cat. Ultrastructural study of hepatocytes from cats with spontaneous disease compared to healthy cats and cats with mechanical cholestasis (extrahepatic bile duct obstruction) has revealed several distinct features; these are summarized in Table 34–2 and illustrated in Figure 34–5A and 5B.[83] The most intriguing finding that may have etiopathogenic significance is that reduced numbers of peroxisomes, as expressed per cell view and per number of mitochondria, were detected.

Peroxisomal enzyme activity for fatty acid oxidation has been shown to be suppressed as a nonspecific host response to inflammation.[84,85] It is possible that this could contribute to the accumulation of hepatocellular TG in cats that develop HL secondary to a primary inflammatory or septic disease process. It is also possible that some cats or cats in general fail to increase peroxisomal number and/or function appropriately upon uptake of an excessive amount of FFA in the liver. An acquired peroxisomal dysfunction would augment cytosolic retention of TG.

INBORN ERRORS OF METABOLISM. A variety of inheritable metabolic defects have been identified in humans with hepatic lipidosis. Only a few lipid storage disorders have been recognized in the cat that can result in retention of fatty material in visceral organs, reticuloendothelial cells, or the central nervous system. These include an acquired disorder of ceroid-lipidosis, a sphingomyelin storage abnormality, and a cholesterol ester storage disease.[86] These disorders do not present with the clinical or histologic features typical of the feline HL syndrome.

A congenital deficiency of LPL has also been characterized in cats.[87–89] Affected animals develop hypertriglyceridemia and large numbers of lipid vacuoles in hepatocytes. The disorder is obvious because affected animals are severely hyperlipidemic. Cats with the HL syndrome are usually not hyperlipidemic unless they concurrently have diabetes mellitus.

Diseases Associated with the Feline Hepatic Lipidosis Syndrome

Many different pathologic disorders have been associated with the HL syndrome in cats (see Table 34–3). Cats are considered to have idiopathic HL if no underlying medical condition is detected after a thorough diagnostic investigation. Approximately 50% of affected cats have idiopathic disease. Investigation for an underlying disorder is of utmost impor-

Table 34–2

ULTRASTRUCTURAL FEATURES OF HEPATOCYTES IN CATS WITH HEPATIC LIPIDOSIS AS COMPARED TO CATS WITH EXTRAHEPATIC BILE DUCT OBSTRUCTION AND HEALTHY CATS

Mitochodrial	reduced numbers, abnormal shapes, appearance of megamitochondria blunted cristae, ↑ electron density
Peroxisomes	reduced numbers per cell altered morphology
Golgi apparatus	reduced numbers per cell
Endoplasmic reticulum	reduced numbers per cell
Lysosomes	reduced numbers per cell
Canaliculi	blunted, short villi; collapsed lumen
Glycogen	reduced quantity

Data derived from reference 83.

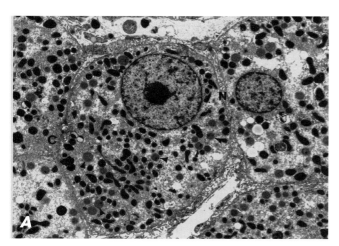 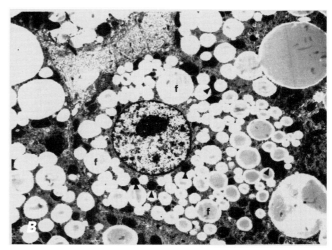

FIGURE 34-5. *(A),* Transmission electron micrograph showing hepatocytes from a healthy cat. Peroxisomes are indicated by black arrowheads, nucleus (N), canaliculus (C to left of canaliculus), and numerous mitochondria.[83] *(B),* Transmission electron micrograph showing hepatocytes from a cat with severe hepatic lipidosis. Notice the paucity of cytosolic space for organelles and the small number of visible organelles. Pale fat inclusions (f) and mitochondria (arrowheads) are evident.[83]

tance in order to alleviate the clinical condition causing the cat to remain anorectic or undernourished.

Signalment and Clinical Signs

The feline HL syndrome occurs twice as often in females as compared to males. There is no predilection for pure bred animals; the syndrome is most commonly seen in domestic shorthair cats. Most affected cats are middle aged, although cats of any age may be affected. The majority of cats weigh 4.0 kg or more and are considered overweight by their owners. A common historical feature is for an owner to recognize a substantial weight loss, often exceeding 25% of the cat's usual body weight, before presentation for veterinary care.

Common presenting complaints in addition to weight loss include a protracted course of anorexia (usually 2 weeks duration or longer but sometimes as brief as 24 hours), vomiting, lethargy, or weakness. Diarrhea and constipation occur in more than 50% of affected cats. Commonly detected physical features include jaundice, hepatomegaly, and dehydration. Ptyalism or other signs typical of hepatic encephalopathy are uncommon. There is no recognized association between FeLV or FIV infection and this disorder.

Clinicopathologic Features

Certain clinicopathologic abnormalities associated with the feline HL syndrome are consistent enough to strongly increase clinical suspicion prior to biopsy inspection. Nevertheless, this disorder is only definitively confirmed upon tissue evaluation. The clinicopathologic features of severe HL in 77 afflicted cats is illustrated in Figure 34–6. Urinalysis will disclose the presence of hyperbilirubinemia before jaundice becomes clinically evident. Bilirubinuria is always abnormal in the cat and, when detected consistently, indicates hyperbilirubinemia. In some cats, marked lipiduria is observed upon examination of urine sediment. A fatty layer may develop on the surface of urine. The origin of the lipiduria has not been determined but is suspected to be related to

fatty vacuolation in the renal tubules or abnormal amounts of circulating lipid moieties. Renal tubule vacuolation presumably with fat has been commonly observed upon necropsy of affected cats.

The hemogram often reveals a borderline anemia. Depending on the underlying primary medical disorder, the anemia may be regenerative or nonregenerative. The development of poikilocytes (erythrocytes with unusual shapes) is common in cats with the HL syndrome (Figure 34–7). Poikilocytes are not pathognomonic for the syndrome; they also

Table 34–3

DISORDERS ASSOCIATED WITH THE FELINE HEPATIC LIPIDOSIS SYNDROME IN DESCENDING ORDER OF PREVALENCE

Other Liver Disorders
  Cholangiohepatitis
  Choledochitis extrahepatic bile duct obstruction
  Chronic suppurative hepatitis
  Bile duct adenocarcinoma
  Hepatic lymphosarcoma
Neoplasia (nonhepatic)
  Urinary bladder transitional cell carcinoma
  Metastatic carcinoma
  Intestinal lymphosarcoma
  Intestinal adenocarcinoma
Pancreatitis
Diabetes mellitus
Small Intestinal Diseases
  Eosinophilic enteritis
  Lymphocytic/plasmacytic enteritis
  Chronic bowel obstruction
  Salmonella enteritis
Renal Disorders
  Chronic FUS
  Chronic interstitial nephritis
  Pyelonephritis
Hyperthyroidism
Severe Anemia
Pyometra
Cardiomyopathy
Central Neurologic Disease

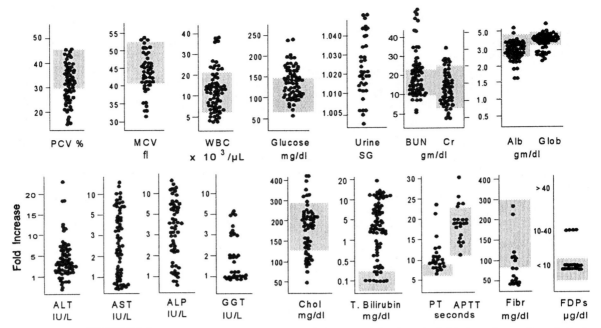

FIGURE 34-6. The clinicopathologic features of the severe feline hepatic lipidosis syndrome. Data derived from the College of Veterinary Medicine, Cornell University.

develop in association with other severe hepatobiliary disorders in the cat.[25,90] Microcytosis develops in approximately 20% of affected cats. Investigation as to the cause of microcytosis has not been completed; an association with deranged iron metabolism or iron deficiency or the abnormal red cell shape remains possible. The leukogram generally reflects the underlying medical disorder with which the lipidosis syndrome is associated. An inflammatory leukogram is not expected in idiopathic lipidosis because the hepatic histomorphology is typically free of inflammation or cell necrosis.

The biochemical profile usually reveals more specific abnormalities than the hemogram. Approximately 80% of cats develop a twofold or more and 55% a fivefold or more increase in the serum ALP activity. Comparatively, the serum GGT activity is unimpressive. Only 16% of cats develop an increased serum GGT activity. In no case of idiopathic lipidosis has the fold increase in GGT activity equaled or exceeded

the fold increase in ALP activity in the author's practice. Increased GGT activity has been seen in cats with secondary HL when other underlying conditions produce increased GGT activity (pancreatitis, cholangiohepatitis, bile duct obstruction). The normal GGT activity or its minor increase in most cats with HL contrasts to the substantial increases in GGT activity that develop in other forms of acquired feline liver disorders (see Figure 8–10).[91] In many cats with HL, the fold increase in ALP activity also exceeds the fold increase in serum ALT or AST activities. In some cats, abnormal serum enzyme activity is detected before derangements in the total bilirubin concentration. This is consistent with observations in the experimental induction of the HL syndrome in cats.[26] The discrepant increases in ALP compared to serum GGT activity has led to early diagnosis in affected cats.

Most cats are hyperbilirubinemic when presented for clinical evaluation. The author has occasionally examined cats

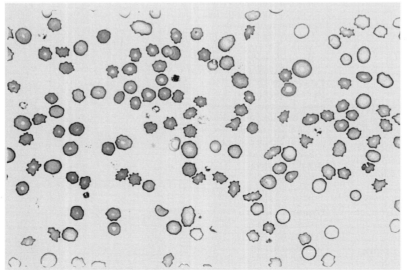

FIGURE 34-7. Photomicrograph showing the typical appearance of poikilocytes, abnormally shaped erythrocytes, associated with the feline hepatic lipidosis syndrome and other severe hepatobiliary disorders in the cat.

that were not overtly jaundiced and in these animals, the HL syndrome was serendipitously discovered in a seemingly early stage of development. These cats were being evaluated for other primary disease processes.

Hypoproteinemia and hypoalbuminemia are relatively uncommon in this disorder. Approximately 12% of cats become hypoproteinemic and 18% become hypoalbuminemic. Serum globulin concentrations tend to remain within the normal range. This is another feature that helps to distinguish this hepatobiliary disorder from other acquired feline cholestatic diseases because the latter disorders are commonly associated with increased serum globulin concentrations. Mild to moderate hyperglycemia occurs in 38% of cats; of 77 cats studied, approximately 20% of hyperglycemic animals were diabetics.

The serum cholesterol concentration is increased in approximately 30% of cats. The variable expression of hypercholesterolemia in cats with severe HL may reflect differences in the metabolic condition of the liver, a major determinant of the rate of cholesterol synthesis.[92,93] It is also possible that the extent of patient anorexia also influences the serum cholesterol concentration. In the rat, fasting is associated with the lowest rate of cholesterol biosynthesis.[93] A prior study of rapid weight loss in obese cats demonstrated a transient reduction in the total serum cholesterol concentration during initial short-term starvation.[42] It is possible that fasting and a reduced hepatocellular metabolic rate curtails the development of hypercholesterolemia. Gross hyperlipidemia is rarely encountered in cats with the HL syndrome.

A subnormal BUN develops in approximately 50% of affected cats. This usually occurs in combination with a normal serum creatinine concentration and minimally concentrated urine. The subnormal BUN in cats with the HL syndrome may be related to their chronic anorexia or compromised urea cycle function. Arginine, an important urea cycle substrate, has been shown to be reduced in the serum of cats with the severe HL syndrome.[22] This is compatible with what is known about the dependency of the cat on ingested sources of arginine for normal urea cycle function. Unfortunately, it is not known if these cats are concurrently hyperammonemic, as would be expected if the low BUN is related to reduced urea cycle function and insufficient arginine concentrations.

Results of coagulation profiles are abnormal in one or more tests in 45% of cats tested. The most common abnormalities are a prolonged prothrombin time in 40% of cats and an increased activated partial thromboplastin time in 35% of cats. The serum fibrinogen concentration is reduced in 13% of cats. The FDPs have been increased in nearly 30% of cats tested. Despite evidence of deranged coagulation balance, of 77 cats with severe HL, only three animals demonstrated clinical signs of bleeding. The discrepancy between laboratory test results and the demonstration of bleeding tendencies is not unusual in the patient with hepatic disease. Abnormal coagulation tests may reflect hepatic synthetic failure, vitamin K deficiency, or a consumptive coagulopathy (see Chapter 30). Because cats affected with the HL syndrome are chronically anorectic and frequently have received empiric antibiotic treatment before the syndrome is suspected, iatrogenic vitamin K deficiency remains possible. It is also possible that malabsorption of vitamin K could develop as a result of enterocyte atrophy due to starvation or restricted enterohepatic circulation of bile acids. Reduced formation of secondary bile acids, products of enteric bacterial dehydroxylation reactions, has been shown in cats with the HL syndrome.[94]

Severe HL is unlike other acquired hepatic disorders in the cat because hyperglobulinemia is not a typical feature.

Stimuli capable of inducing an acute-phase response leading to hyperglobulinemia include inflammation and cell necrosis, which are lacking in cats with the idiopathic form of this syndrome. Hypofibrinogenemia in this disorder is possibly due to hepatic synthetic failure and/or a consumptive coagulopathy. Synthetic failure is likely considering the remarkable displacement and elimination of hepatocellular organelles observed upon ultrastructural examination of affected hepatocytes.[83] A redesignation of hepatocyte and Kupffer cell functions rather than synthetic failure could also explain the low serum fibrinogen and the normal globulin concentrations. Low serum fibrinogen concentrations are not thought to be due to DIC. Although increased FDPs have been found in a few cats, other evidence of a consumptive coagulopathy such as schistocytes, thrombocytopenia, thromboembolic complications, or petechiation have not been observed. An additional observation has been that hypofibrinogenemia is not significantly related to failure to survive, which would be suspected if DIC was a related phenomenon.

Serum electrolyte concentrations are highly variable. The most significant derangements are in serum potassium and phosphorus concentrations. Approximately 30% of cats are hypokalemic, which is significantly related to failure to survive. Marked hypophosphatemia associated with hemolytic anemia was reported in one cat with severe HL, but overall is relatively rare in cats with severe HL.[22,24]

Total serum bile acid concentrations are increased in most cats, particularly at the 2 hour postprandial interval. Because the HL syndrome causes intrahepatic cholestasis, the serum bile acid concentrations become demonstrably abnormal before hyperbilirubinemia develops. In the anicteric patient, the postprandial serum bile acid concentration may provide evidence of hepatic dysfunction, which permits early definitive diagnosis and therapeutic intervention. Fractionation of serum and urine bile acids in cats with the HL syndrome has shown similarities to the bile acid profiles associated with extrahepatic bile duct occlusion.[94] This suggests that the enterohepatic circulation of bile acids is severely disrupted in the affected cat. This study revealed that substantial amounts of taurine conjugated bile acids are eliminated in urine. Despite development of low plasma taurine concentrations, cats with the HL syndrome continue to conjugate bile acids with taurine and to eliminate the taurine conjugates in urine. This is not unique to the HL syndrome but suggests that the HL cat should be supplemented therapeutically, at least initially, with taurine.

Retrospective evaluation of clinicopathologic features of cats with severe HL has shown that survivors are younger and have a higher PCV and serum potassium concentration than nonsurvivors. Those with idiopathic HL have a better survival than cats with secondary HL. Aggressive early intervention results in a 60% or higher survival rate. However, it is important that any primary underlying medical problems be identified and alleviated.

Abdominal Radiography and Ultrasonography

Abdominal radiography rarely provides information important in the evaluation of the cat with the HL syndrome. Hepatomegaly is common and usually recognized during the initial physical examination. Lateral abdominal radiographs will confirm this feature. On occasion, radiographic details will permit identification of an underlying disease process that has initiated anorexia and, subsequently, the HL syndrome.

Abdominal ultrasonography has been shown to have high sensitivity, specificity, and predictive value for the diagnosis of HL.[95] In the hands of an experienced ultrasonographer, HL can be differentiated (provisionally) from extrahepatic bile duct occlusion, cholangiohepatitis, and metastatic neoplasia. These disorders may each produce physical features and clinicopathologic abnormalities similar to the HL syndrome. The ultrasonographic features of HL include a diffuse homogeneous parenchymal hyperechogenicity, hepatomegaly, and an absence of bile duct wall thickening, lumenal distension, or gallbladder abnormalities. The gallbladder usually appears large due to anorexia, but the wall appears normal. There may be some degree of bile sludge, a feature commonly observed in anorectic animals. Liver echogenicity is usually described relative to that of the normal renal cortex. However, in the cat with lipidosis, comparison of the liver and kidney will not permit discrimination of hyperechogenicity. Cats with hepatic lipidosis also accumulate considerable fat within the renal tubular epithelium, which makes their kidneys also appear hyperechoic. Comparison of hepatic parenchymal echogenicity with falciform fat has been more useful (Figure 34–8). In HL, the liver takes on the hyperechoic appearance of the falciform fat. The ultrasonographic features of diffuse lipidosis, considered along with the typically disproportionate increase in the serum ALP relative to the serum GGT activity in a jaundiced cat, provides enough diagnostic information to pursue aspiration or biopsy of the liver under ultrasonographic guidance. This can be accomplished during the initial ultrasonographic evaluation if prophylactic vitamin K_1 was given at least 12 hours previously.

Hepatic Biopsy

Definitive diagnosis of the HL syndrome requires histopathologic or cytologic evaluation of liver tissue. Histologic evaluation is more accurate than cytology in ruling out other underlying hepatobiliary disorders. The coagulation status of the patient must be appraised before liver biopsy or aspiration, especially if the patient is jaundiced (see Chapter 30). If coagulation tests are abnormal, blood transfusion is necessary. Nevertheless, even if a prebiopsy blood transfusion is not indicated, the clinician should ensure that compatible fresh blood is available before embarking on the biopsy procedure. Vitamin K_1 3 to 5 mg total dose per cat is given IM BID the first day, then SID every 3 to 5 consecutive days. The first dose of vitamin K_1 should be administered at least 12 hours prior to the biopsy/aspiration procedure.

Because hepatomegaly is common, a variety of biopsy techniques may be used safely. Procedures used successfully include percutaneous blind needle aspirate or biopsy, keyhole needle or pinch biopsy, pinch biopsy via laparoscopy, and laparotomy for wedge biopsy. These techniques are described in detail in Chapter 8.

Irrespective of the biopsy technique employed, enough tissue should be obtained to permit imprint cytology, culture, and histopathology. A portion of the biopsy tissue should be fixed in buffered formalin. Liver tissue heavily laden with TG will usually float in formalin. The tissue fixed in formalin should be subdivided for two separate staining procedures: (1) routine hematoxylin and eosin, and (2) specific staining for fat on a cryostat cut section. Routine processing requires paraffin embedment of tissue, which results in fat extraction. Empty cytoplasmic vacuoles are subsequently observed on microscopic examination. The only way to be sure that fat has occupied these vacuoles is to apply a specific fat stain such as oil red-O or Sudan black to a tissue specimen in which the fat

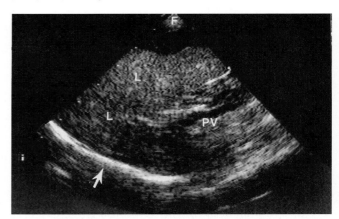

FIGURE 34–8. Ultrasonogram showing the diffuse hepatic parenchymal hyperechogenicity (L) as determined by comparison to falciform fat (F). Portal vein (PV), diaphragm (arrow). (Courtesy Dr. A. Yeager, Section of Radiology, Department of Clinical Sciences, College of Veterinary Medicine, Cornell University.)

has not been extracted. To ensure proper sample processing, the clinician should alert the pathologist that HL is a highly considered differential diagnosis.

Cytologic and Histopathologic Features of Hepatic Lipidosis

The typical gross appearance of the liver in the cat with severe HL is pale, yellow, friable, greasy, and enlarged. Cytologic evaluation of a modified Wright's-Giemsa stained specimen will adequately distinguish the vacuolar distortion of hepatocytes typical of the HL syndrome (Figure 34–9). The tissue imprints may appear greasy. Cytologic evaluation readily reveals the multivacuolated nature of the hepatic parenchymal cells. The vacuoles may be few and large (macrovesicular) or multiple and small (microvesicular). The patient with severe diffuse HL will have very few normal-appearing hepatocytes. Because lipid vacuolation is common in feline hepatocytes, the number of vacuolated hepatocytes should be estimated. At least 50% of the hepatocytes observed on an aspirate or imprint cytology specimen should be vacuolated before a diagnosis of the HL syndrome is considered plausible. Careful cytologic evaluation for inflammatory cells should be undertaken. The cholangitis/cholangiohepatitis syndrome can be associated with HL in some cats. If inflammatory cells are identified on the cytology specimen, another concurrent acquired hepatobiliary disorder should be considered. Hepatic lipidosis is a nonreactive hepatopathy. It is *not* associated with tissue necrosis, infection, or inflammation unless an underlying or associated malady coexists.

The histologic evaluation of liver tissue for HL is fairly straightforward. In normal liver, fat is not readily evident in hepatocytes on routine histologic examination. Only small lipid droplets may be observed on tissue specifically stained for fat with oil red-O or Sudan black. An occasional Ito cell filled with lipid is normal. In a fatty liver, vacuoles are obvious in hepatocytes even without application of a fat-specific stain (Figure 34–10). Care must be taken to estimate the degree of hepatocyte vacuolation. Focal or zonal involvement of less than 50% of the parenchyma is not consistent with the HL syndrome (Figure 34–1*B*). Unfortunately, some pathology reports suggest the lipidosis syndrome as a differential diagnosis whenever lipid vacuoles are observed. An oil red-

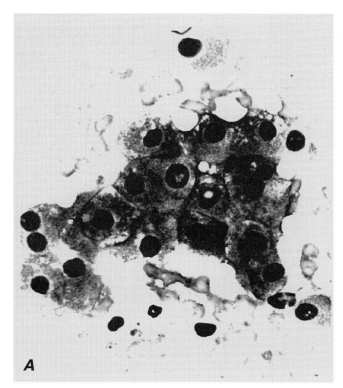

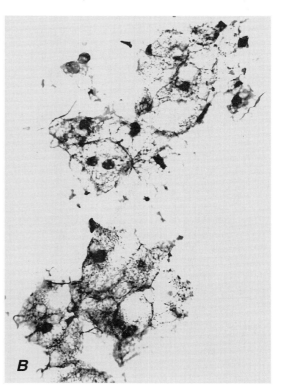

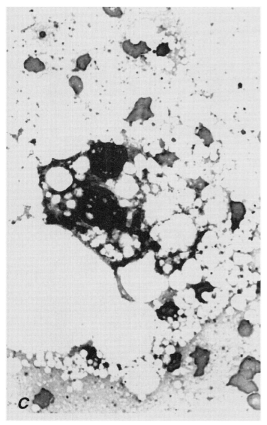

FIGURE 34-9. Photomicrographs showing cytologic features of hepatocytes from a healthy cat and from cats with severe hepatic lipidosis. In (*A*), hepatocytes from a healthy cat have a homogeneous cyptoplasm and minimal fatty vacuolation (modified Wrights-Giemsa stain, 450X magnification). In (*B*), hepatocytes are devoid of normal cytoplasm because they are filled with microvesicular fatty vacuolation. There was no cytologic evidence of inflammation and no normal-appearing hepatocytes on the preparation. Hepatocellular nuclei have remained central in position (modified Wright's-Giemsa stain, 600× magnification). In (*C*), large amounts of globular-appearing lipid surround hepatocytes showing macrovesicular vacuolation. The preparation appeared greasy on gross inspection. There was no cytologic evidence of inflammation (modified Wright's-Giemsa stain, 875× magnification).

microvesicular. Most cats with severe HL have large single vacuoles that displace cytoplasm, organelles, and nucleus to the cell margin. The fat is deposited in a large liposome globule that fills the cell, causing the hepatocyte to resemble an adipocyte. This type of vacuolation is termed macrovesicular. The second less common form of fat dispersal involves fat distribution in small discrete fat droplets; this is termed a microvesicular pattern. These small vacuoles may be dispersed throughout the cytoplasm with only minimal disruption of the normal organelle or nuclear position; Figure 34–9 shows cytology from cats with the microvesicular and macrovesicular form of vacuolation. In humans, it has been suggested that the microvesicular form of vacuolation is the precursor to the large vacuole formation. It has also been suggested that the microvesicular form reflects a more serious disturbance of hepatocyte metabolism. It is unknown if this holds true for the cat.

O–stained liver biopsy taken from a cat with severe HL is shown in Figure 34–11; this preparation verifies the nature of the vacuolar contents as neural fat.

Lipid vacuolation in hepatocytes may be macrovesicular or

Treatment

For effective treatment, recognition of the HL syndrome requires a careful inspection for underlying primary disease.

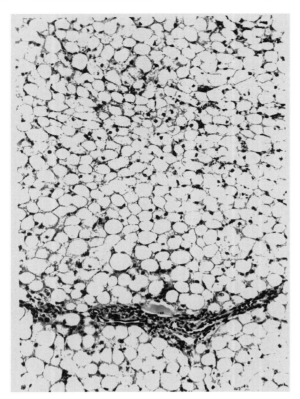

FIGURE 34-10. Photomicrograph of liver biopsy from a cat with severe hepatic lipidosis. Liver tissue was fixed and stained routinely. Large macrovesicular empty vacuoles occupy the majority of the hepatocyte cytoplasm (H&E, 140×).

Identification and elimination or effective management of an underlying condition, along with provision of thorough supportive care, will permit a cure in more than 60% of cases. Idiopathic lipidosis can be more difficult to manage in some cats because there is no underlying disorder to eliminate. Nevertheless, aggressive treatment of these cats also results in a more than 60% survival rate. A general overview of treatment is provided in Table 34–4.

FLUID THERAPY. Rehydration is essential to avoid prerenal azotemia that could precipitate hyperammonemia and encephalopathic signs. Maintenance fluid requirements are estimated as 66 to 88 mL/kg per day. Initially, fluids are administered intravenously, but once nutritional support is implemented, fluid intake is combined with feedings. During the initial stages of treatment, continued reappraisal of hydration status is imperative. Polyionic isotonic fluids should be used. Lactated Ringer's may not be the best choice because increased urine lactic acid has been detected in severely affected cats, implying an inability to metabolize lactate.[22] Although cats with HL have increased circulating ketone concentrations compared to normal cats, serious acidosis requiring intervention with bicarbonate is uncommon. It is inappropriate to supplement cats with the HL syndrome with dextrose-containing fluids because most cats are euglycemic to moderately hyperglycemic. Carbohydrate infusions could stimulate de novo synthesis of TG in the liver and block efficient conversion to β-oxidation of fat for energy production. Furthermore, diuresis with a dextrose-enriched solution could promote the development of hypokalemia, which worsens the prognosis for survival.

Potassium supplementation should be provided on the basis of the serum electrolyte concentration and use of the sliding scale commonly used in veterinary practice (Table 34–4). Maintenance potassium chloride is commonly given at 5 mEq/250 mL of fluid volume if the serum potassium status cannot be repeatedly determined. It is important to avoid potassium supplementation at a rate exceeding 0.5 mEq/kg/hour because this rate is cardiotoxic.

If severe hypophosphatemia is recognized (serum phosphorus < 2.1 mg/dl), the intravenous administration of potassium phosphate is recommended; appropriate dosage[24] is provided in Table 34–4. Severe hypophosphatemia should be treated because it can cause hemolysis, weakness, and vague neurologic signs (Table 32–5).[24]

NUTRITIONAL CONSIDERATIONS. Dedication on the part of the owner and clinician toward aggressive nutritional management is the most important factor determining a positive outcome. The feeding program should be aimed at getting the cat home where nutritional support may be provided with a minimum of stress.

Caloric Intake. Provision of adequate calories for maintenance support with additional calories added for the heightened maintenance requirement of the ill stressed cat is the cornerstone of successful medical management. A target caloric intake between 65 and 90 kcal/kg per day has been used with good clinical outcome in the author's hospital. The goal is to provide adequate calories to inhibit peripheral lipolysis yet to avoid overnutrition, which will promote hepatic TG accumulation. The exact caloric needs of these patients have not been determined. Targeting a high caloric intake usually ensures that adequate calories are fed. Feeding too few calories is detrimental because it will lead to continued lipolysis and hepatic fatty acid uptake.

Route of Alimentation. Because most cats with lipidosis are

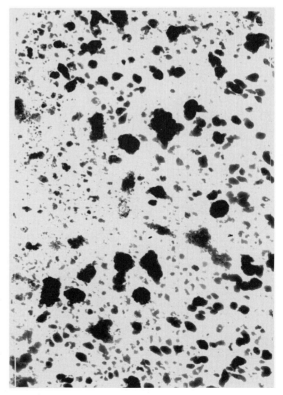

FIGURE 34-11. Photomicrograph of liver tissue from a cat with severe hepatic lipidosis. This tissue was unextracted and stained with oil red-O, demonstrating the neutral fat content of the hepatic vacuoles which appear as the darkened areas (140× magnification).

Table 34–4

RX: FELINE HEPATIC LIPIDOSIS

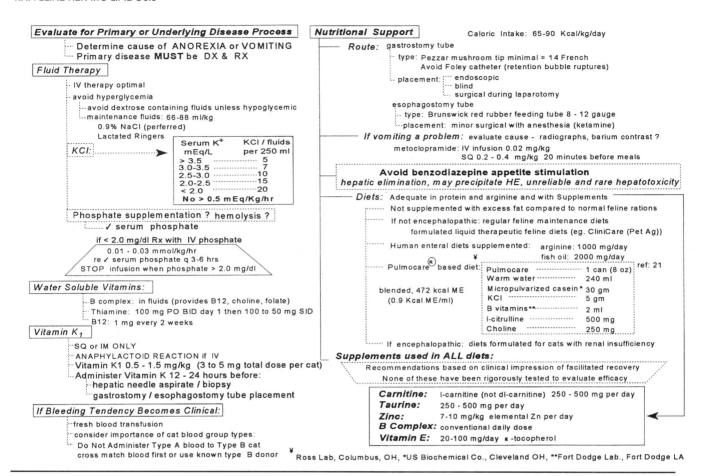

anorectic, they must be force-fed. Administration of benzodiazepines (diazepam, oxazepam) or cyproheptadine increases appetite momentarily but is unreliable in ensuring adequate caloric intake. Furthermore, benzodiazepines are contraindicated in patients with severely reduced hepatic function, particularly if they have or are showing signs of hepatic encephalopathy.

Force feeding by the oral route with a liquified diet is successful in some cats where a dedicated owner has the time and patience to provide the necessary nursing care. Feeding of a liquified baby food diet (beef or chicken with additional supplements as shown in Table 34–4) or a liquified commercial feline diet (CliniCare Maintenance; Pet Ag Inc., Hampshire, IL) has been successful in some cats. Force feeding by nasogastric intubation or gastrostomy tube is the most reliable and efficient method of assuring adequate alimentation. Nasogastric tubes are best used as a temporary feeding route during stabilization of the patient. The nasal and pharyngeal discomfort associated with nasogastric tubes and their propensity to block make them less suitable than gastrostomy tubes for long-term alimentation. Recently, esophagostomy tubes have also been used by some clinicians.[96] Pharyngostomy tubes are not tolerated well by most cats and should be avoided.

Gastrostomy tube alimentation is vastly preferred by many clinicians as the best alternative for long-term alimentation. A reinforced mushroom tip self-retaining 14 to 20 French catheter (Bardex self-retaining catheter; Pizzer, Bard Urological Division, CR Bard, Inc., Murray Hill, NJ) is usually used. The large diameter of a gastrostomy tube permits feeding of a variety of alternative diets and provides an easy access for fluid supplementation and medication administration. Tube displacement is uncommon in comparison to the problems experienced with nasogastric tubes. Tube insertion, maintenance, and removal are manageable in most practices and owners can successfully feed their pet using the gastrostomy tube without the stress and discomfort associated with forced oral or nasogastric feeding. A soft body bandage holds the tube in proper position and the owner is instructed to change this wrap at 3 to 5 day intervals after the initial 10 days of healing. It is not necessary for most cats to wear an Elizabethan collar when a gastrostomy tube is used. Recommended procedures for gastrostomy tube insertion are described elsewhere in this text and in other publications.[97] Gastrostomy tubes have been maintained in many cats with HL for 16 weeks. In a few cases, a longer term treatment interval and reinsertion of a different tube has been necessary. This can usually be done merely with manual restraint.

Initial feeding through a gastrostomy tube begins 36

hours after insertion. A small volume of water (5 mL/kg) is first administered. If there is no sign of nausea or vomiting, small volumes of water are repeated at 2 to 4 hour intervals. If there are no problems, a small volume of food is administered within 12 to 24 hours. Initially, feedings are divided into 4 to 6 meals per day. An initial 20 mL total volume per feeding is used for the first day and then is progressively increased until the necessary volume of food can be delivered in a reasonable number of feedings. Total meal volume per feeding usually does not exceed 20 mL/kg body weight per meal. Before administration of a meal, the gastrostomy tube is aspirated to assess the degree of ingesta retention. If 10 mL or more of food or water can be aspirated into the syringe after a reasonable interdigestive interval, delayed gastric emptying is suspected. Metoclopramide is used to control vomiting and to facilitate gastric emptying if these problems occur after a gastrostomy tube is placed. In rare cases cats will not tolerate the position of a gastrostomy tube and it must be removed.

When a cat begins to recover from HL, it will demonstrate an interest in food. Gastrostomy or esophagostomy tubes do not interfere with this desired outcome. Nasogastric tubes often discourage the patient's interest in sniffing or tasting offered food because of the facial, nasal, and pharyngeal discomfort associated with the feeding apparatus. When a cat begins to consume food voluntarily, the gastrostomy tube should be kept patent by periodic flushes of small volumes of warm water, and eventually removed after it is clear the patient will consume adequate calories and is well on its way to full recovery.

Diet Formulations. Because most cats with the HL syndrome do not demonstrate overt signs of hepatic encephalopathy, a well-balanced maintenance feline ration is a suitable diet. A commercially prepared feline diet is recommended over home-prepared diets to ensure provision of essential amino acids and fatty acids.

Cats require almost twice the dietary protein of dogs and cannot adapt to a lower protein intake because of an inherent high activity of hepatic enzymes that deaminate and transaminate amino acids.[31,98] Consequently, a fixed amount of protein is always catabolized for energy. Insufficient protein intake rapidly induces tissue catabolism. A study of rapid weight loss in obese cats indicates that dietary support with a protein rather than a carbohydrate- or lipid-enriched diet protects against HL.[53] This is consistent with clinical results observed in cats with HL fed feline maintenance diets.

Feline diets should not be supplemented with medium chain triglycerides because this is believed to have produced HL experimentally in cats.[47] Similarly, use of certain commercially available elemental diets for humans are not appropriate because their fat sources heavily depend on coconut oil, which is high in medium chain triglycerides (e.g., Isocal; Mead Johnson). It is unknown whether a diet relatively restricted in fat is beneficial for cats with the HL syndrome.

Dietary Supplements. A number of dietary supplements have been used in cats with the HL syndrome, but no scientific evidence confirms these treatments are necessary or beneficial. Their use is based on experience in clinical cases where survival rates have appeared to improve and recovery has been seemingly hastened. Most of these are routinely used in the author's hospital.

Arginine. Cats develop hepatic encephalopathy if fed a diet deficient in arginine.[99] Because animal origin protein is generally rich in arginine, most balanced commercial feline diets are well fortified with this amino acid. The cat with severe HL is catabolic and thus is mobilizing peripheral protein stores, such as muscle, to provide essential amino acids.

A constant, albeit restricted endogenous supply of arginine is made available via this mechanism. Determinations of serum arginine concentrations have verified that affected cats have low serum arginine concentrations.[22] Arginine supplementation should be offered to cats demonstrating encephalopathic signs and to any patient being fed a home-formulated diet or human enteral diet in which the arginine concentration has not been clearly defined. Arginine supplementation at a rate of 1 g/day has been previously recommended[49] and used by the author without ill effects. It is possible that supplementation of arginine benefits the cat with HL by provision of an essential protein for apoprotein synthesis. Arginine is essential for the formation of certain important apoproteins in humans. Presently, the composition of feline apoproteins is ill defined and so it remains speculative whether this would help a cat.

Taurine. Taurine is an essential amino acid for the cat. Signs of taurine deficiency do not occur in cats with HL given the relatively short duration of this clinical disorder. However, because of the cholestatic nature of the lipidosis syndrome and obligate conjugation of bile acids with taurine, a considerable amount of taurine is localized in the bile acid pool in ill cats. Evaluation of serum and urine bile acid profiles has documented the high degree of taurine conjugated bile acids both in the peripheral circulation and in urine, and the relative absence of the glycine conjugated moieties.[94] A continued loss of taurine in urine and deviation of available taurine for use in bile acid conjugation suggests that other body systems requiring taurine for normal function may become compromised. Supplementation with "extra" taurine may therefore provide a protective function during initial recovery from the HL syndrome. It is also possible that taurine supplementation may assist in detoxification and/or urinary elimination of cytotoxic bile acids. Amino acid conjugation of bile acids increases their water solubility and their potential for renal excretion. Routine supplementation of cats with HL with taurine (250 to 500 mg PO BID) through the first 3 to 4 weeks of nutritional support has been used clinically by the author with apparent good success, but this is a subjective assessment. If the maintenance diet is known to contain adequate taurine, then supplementation is thereafter discontinued. If a cat is showing signs of hepatic encephalopathy, taurine supplementation should be undertaken with caution to avoid oversupplementation because it is a recognized hepatoencephalopathic toxin.

Carnitine. Carnitine supplementation is recommended on the assumption that it may assist in optimizing fatty acid β-oxidation and ensure carnitine repletion within the hepatocellular cytosol, mitochondria, and peroxisomes. There is scanty clinical and experimental work to support or refute the presence of an acquired deficiency of carnitine in the cat with HL. Because a relative carnitine insufficiency remains possible and therapy with L-carnitine (but *not* D-carnitine or DL-carnitine) is not harmful, HL cats are routinely supplemented with L-carnitine in the author's hospital. A dose ranging between 250 to 500 mg L-carnitine per cat/day, given orally, is used. Clinically, supplemented cats appear to have an accelerated rate of recovery but this has not been verified with controlled clinical evaluations. Analytic grade L-carnitine (99.4%; Ajinomoto Co. Inc., Tokyo, Japan) has been routinely used.

Vitamins. Considering that many of the water soluble vitamins are essential for intermediary metabolism and hepatic activation is necessary for some of these, daily provision of a well-balanced vitamin supplement is recommended. Thiamine (B_1) is of major importance because cats are easily depleted of this vitamin unless it is regularly replenished. The signs of thiamine deficiency are easily confused with those of hepatic encephalopathy and hypokalemia. Thiamine deficiency is associated with dilated unresponsive pupils, apparent blindness, head and neck ventroflexion, ataxia, stupor, and weakness. Treatment during the early stages of deficiency results in complete resolution of clinical signs. Thiamine deficiency is treated or easily avoided by supplementation with 50 to 100 mg of thiamine hydrochloride, given BID by oral, subcutaneous, or intramuscular routes.

Vitamin K_1 is routinely administered to all cats with the severe HL syndrome because of the frequency with which abnormal coagulation test results have been observed. To circumvent the problems associated with delayed hepatic activation of vitamin K or gut malabsorption, supplementation is initially provided at 12 hour intervals for two or three treatments of 3 to 5 mg per dose per cat. Thereafter, vitamin K_1 is provided every 3 to 5 days either by injection or mixed with food, until it is clear that clinical recovery is occurring. Overdosage with vitamin K must be avoided because it results in hemolytic anemia associated with Heinz body formation in the cat.

Use of lipotropes cannot be specifically recommended in this disorder other than provision of water soluble vitamins and a well-balanced feline ration. If these are administered, adequate quantities of choline, methionine, and inositol will be ingested. Specific supplementation with methionine should be avoided due to the potential for metabolism in the gut to an encephalotoxigenic substance.

Supplementation with vitamin E is recommended on the basis that this vitamin provides important antioxidant function and reduced peroxisomal numbers develop experimentally on vitamin E deficient diets. The therapeutic dose is undetermined but dose recommendations for clinical use in vitamin E–deficient states include 20 to 100 mg per day of β tocopheral acetate per os in addition to maintenance vitamin E levels in the diet.[100,101]

In humans with hepatic insufficiency due to a variety of different disease processes, low serum and liver tissue zinc concentrations have been well documented.[102,103] Low zinc concentrations are believed to augment the expression of hepatic encephalopathy as a result of influence on neuroreceptors and neurotransmitters as well as on impairment of urea cycle enzyme activity, which promotes hyperammonemia.[103,104] Accordingly, a daily zinc supplement is advised for cats with the HL syndrome until full recovery is realized. A dose of 7 to 10 mg of elemental zinc is recommended. Care must be taken to avoid zinc oversupplementation because hemolysis may develop.

ANTIBIOTICS. Prophylactic administration of antibiotics to cats with the HL syndrome is common. Antibiotic treatment is given because it is surmised that hepatic sinusoidal circulation and Kupffer cell function are compromised. Additional reasons for antibiotic administration are that gastrointestinal lesions may be sustained during gastrostomy tube insertion or may be related to the primary underlying disease process that initially induced the anorexia and HL syndrome. Experimentally, endotoxemia derived from gut microorganisms is thought to potentiate the development of hepatic lipidosis after toxic hepatic injury.

If antibiotics are used, those reliant on hepatic biotransformation or excretion are avoided as are those known to diminish appetite or have other debilitating effects. Tetracyclines should be avoided because of their causal association with hepatic lipidosis. Ampicillin, amoxicillin, Clavamox, cephalexin, cephalothin, and metronidazole (reduced dose by 50%) have each been used without ill effects.

MEDICATIONS TO AVOID. In addition to tetracyclines, other antibiotics that should be avoided include chloramphenicol (nausea, inappetance, impaired drug metabolism) and trimethoprim-sulfa combinations (immune reactions, idiosyncratic hepatopathy). If an H_2 blocker is desired, cimetidine should be avoided due to its adverse influence on drug-metabolizing enzymes. Anabolic steroids should not be used because they have a propensity to cause a cholestatic hepatopathy.

Glucocorticoids should be avoided whenever possible because they are lipolytic. Although the cat does not develop a steroid hepatopathy similar to the dog, the catabolic and lipolytic effects of glucocorticoids promote FFA mobilization to the liver. The metabolic effects of glucocorticoids, coupled with obesity and intrinsic defects of hepatic TG dispersal and FA oxidation, would promote hepatic lipid accumulation.

The use of benzodiazepines as an appetite stimulant or sedative should be avoided. Benzodiazepines require hepatic biotransformation and excretion and may produce substantial sedation. In addition, the benzodiazepine neuroreceptor is recognized to be involved in the genesis of hepatic encephalopathy.

Lipotropic compounds containing choline or methionine are not necessary if cats are fed a balanced feline ration. Excessive methionine can produce hepatoencephalopathic signs if administered by the oral route in patients with compromised hepatic function, even though its importance as a major hepatoencephalopathic toxin is controversial. Supplementation with B complex vitamins will usually provide optimal choline and B_{12}, an important consideration because two separate reports have detailed an association between B_{12} deficiency and HL in cats.[42,43]

INSULIN THERAPY. It has been suggested that the HL syndrome in the cat is linked with an absolute or relative deficiency of insulin or insulin resistance. It seems unlikely that insulin therapy would correct the underlying metabolic imbalances associated with this syndrome, especially considering that glucose intolerance in the obese cat may be insulin resistant. However, some authors have previously suggested that conservative doses of regular insulin be used to treat this disorder. It is not clear that a clinical benefit is realized from this treatment, and considering the inherent dangers of insulin administration to an animal that may not need it, this form of therapy is ill advised.

HEPATIC ENCEPHALOPATHY. The few cats with HL that demonstrate overt encephalopathic signs should be treated with medications and dietary adjustments aimed at reducing the production and absorption of alimentary-derived toxins (see chapters 30 and 33). They should be carefully examined for evidence of gastroenteric bleeding or inflammation, systemic infection, azotemia, and constipation. Each of these conditions can precipitate the expression of encephalopathic signs. Animals presented in encephalopathic crisis should be treated with warm saline cleansing enemas to evacuate the colon. Retention enemas containing lactulose (5 to 10 mL diluted 1:3 with water, three or four times daily) or neomycin (15 to 20 mL of a 1% solution, TID or QID) may be used to retard absorption and production of colonic toxins. The acid-base status should be monitored and alkalemia avoided. Hypokalemia must be recognized and corrected. Fluid therapy is selected on the basis of the acid-base status, serum electrolytes, and blood glucose concentration. If severe hepatic insufficiency is suspected, lactated Ringer's solution should not be selected as a first-choice fluid therapy because of the potentially limited capacity for hepatic lactate metabolism in these cats. This is the only form of hepatic insufficiency in animals where an impaired metabolism of lactate is currently suspected.

Following appropriate management of an encephalopathic crisis, dietary modification, including a restricted protein diet and the daily administration of lactulose and/or neomycin or metronidazole, is recommended. The commercially available diet formulated for cats with renal insufficiency seems adequate. If a home-cooked diet is used, care must be given to the sufficiency of arginine and taurine in the recipe. It is safer to supplement additional amino acids than to fail to provide optimal amounts.

Hepatic Lipidosis in Toy Breed Dogs

A tendency for the puppies of toy breeds to develop hepatic lipidosis has been described. The Yorkshire terrier was the predominant breed affected.[13] Major clinical signs were anorexia, vomiting, diarrhea, and neurologic signs. Prolonged fasting of three pups aged 9 weeks old resulted in hypoglycemia associated with ketonemia and hepatic lipidosis; two of these pups died.[14] Blood insulin concentrations decreased while glucagon and cortisol concentrations increased. An expansive retrospective study of liver biopsy results in pediatric patients revealed lipidosis to be common among puppies when ill for a variety of reasons. However, the clinical spectrum of clinicopathologic features has not been described. Liver biopsies show considerable macrovesicular fatty vacuolation but not as severe as that in cats with HL. The fact that a large number of these dogs were Yorkshire terriers is a concern that microvascular portal dysplasia or portosystemic vascular anomalies may be associated with this lesion; see Chapter 35. Liver function tests have not been reported in affected pups.

VACUOLAR HEPATOPATHY/GLUCOCORTICOID HEPATOPATHY

Clinical Synopsis

Diagnostic Features

- Clinical signs pertain to hypercortisolemia or other underlying disease rather than hepatopathy
- Hepatomegaly common
- Cats are rarely affected
- ALP and GGT are usually markedly increased
- Biopsy of liver reveals vacuoles containing glycogen or unidentified material

Standard Treatment

- Directed at underlying cause of the hepatopathy (if identified)

The development of a vacuolar hepatopathy, having either a multifocal or diffuse zonal distribution, is common in the dog. Hepatocytes become enlarged and distended as a result of cytosolic formation of microvesicular or macrovesicular vacuoles; vacuoles contain either glycogen, intracellular edema, or lipid. The contents of the vacuoles determine the classification of the hepatopathy. Like lipid, glycogen may be lost during routine tissue processing, resulting in the formation of a cytosolic void. Special fixation and staining of tissues not subjected to the leaching effects of routine processing are necessary to verify vacuolar contents. Some confusion exists between the differentiation of vacuole formation and the development of hydropic degeneration. *Hydropic degeneration*

describes the histologic appearance of hepatocytes distended due to enlargement of cytoplasmic membranous or organelle compartments. This term has been applied to liver lesions typical of a glucocorticoid hepatopathy as well as to conditions in which the vacuolar appearance is the earliest sign of impending hepatocyte degeneration or necrosis. Insults such as hypoxia, damage by a variety of toxins including endotoxin, and overload by bile pigments can each produce hydropic degeneration and lead to hepatocellular death.

A diagnosis of vacuolar hepatopathy is proposed when contents of the hepatocellular vacuoles are neither lipid nor glycogen or definitive identification of the vacuolar contents has not been completed and preterminal hydropic degeneration is not suspected. A glucocorticoid hepatopathy in the dog is typified by cytosolic distension with vacuoles containing glycogen. This is a common histologic diagnosis in chronically ill dogs, dogs receiving exogenous glucocorticoids, or dogs with hyperadrenocorticism. Unfortunately, the distinction that vacuoles are filled with glycogen is not clear cut without special processing. Many pathologists continue to denote the general lesion of a vacuolar hepatopathy as a glucocorticoid hepatopathy. A variety of illnesses or conditions have been observed in association with a vacuolar or glucocorticoid hepatopathy in the dog (see Table 34–5).

Development of vacuolar hepatopathies usually is linked with marked increases in the serum ALP activity. Several different ALP isoenzymes exist in the dog and cat;[106–119] a unique glucocorticoid isoenzyme has been characterized in the dog.[120–127] When the liver lesion is chronic, a large component of the serum ALP activity is usually comprised of the glucocorticoid-induced isoenzyme (G-ALP).[105–107] A variety of different methods of estimating the ALP isoenzymes have been described. A recently developed quantitative technique (levamisole-inhibition assay) has been adapted for use on automated analyzers.[127] This method is more accurate than determination of G-ALP as a percentage of total ALP activity. Using this methodology, the association between increased serum ALP activity and the glucocorticoid-induced isoenzyme has been clarified in dogs with (1) spontaneous hyperadrenocorticism, (2) iatrogenic hyperadrenocorticism, and (3) a number of different chronic disease conditions.[128–130] With the levamisole-inhibition assay, determination of the G-ALP activity can be used as a crude screening test to decide whether further diagnostic evaluations for hyperadrenocorticism are warranted because these dogs usually have markedly increased G-ALP activity. Unfortunately, many false positive test results occur in clinically ill dogs. This has been attributed to induction of the G-ALP isoenzyme as a result of stress-induced endogenous glucocorticoid release stimulated by a chronic underlying disease.[128,131–133] These dogs often have a vacuolar hepatopathy. A liver biopsy demonstrating a vacuolar hepatopathy, therefore, *cannot* be used to confirm a diagnosis of hyperadrenocorticism, although its absence in a dog with hyperadrenocorticism is unusual.

Induction of a Glucocorticoid Hepatopathy

The hepatic response to treatment with glucocorticoids varies considerably among species. The dog and rabbit liver are most sensitive; in the dog, exogenous glucocorticoids have long been known to have an effect on liver histomorphology.[134,135] The sensitivity of the dog to glucocorticoids is manifested by the ease with which the serum ALP activity is increased; a rise in ALP from 50- to 100-fold normal is common following prolonged high-dose glucocorticoid treatment. There is a high degree of variation to this influence

Table 34-5

CONDITIONS ASSOCIATED WITH VACUOLAR
HEPATOPATHY IN THE DOG

Hyperadrenocorticism
Treatment with glucocorticoids
   oral, parenteral, topical: skin, eye, ear
Chronic Stress: other diseases (ill > 4 weeks)
   Severe dental disease
   Chronic infections
   Chronic inflammation
   Pyelonephritis
   Inflammatory bowel disease
   Neoplasia
      lymphosarcoma
      other
Disorders of lipid metabolism
   Diabetes mellitus
   Schnauzer hyperlipidemia
   Shetland sheepdog hyperlipidemia
Pancreatitis
Hepatocutaneous syndrome
Severe hypothyroidism

determined by the animal's inherent sensitivity, drug dosage, the particular glucocorticoid administered, and the route of administration.

The adverse influence of a variety of different therapeutic glucocorticoids on the liver of the dog has been chronicled.[105,134–137] The initial clinical report of dogs (n = 22) with a glucocorticoid hepatopathy described clinical signs that included hepatomegaly, increased serum enzyme activity, and increased BSP 30 minute percentage retention.[138] The hepatopathy was reversible if exposure to exogenous or endogenous glucocorticoids was eliminated. One of the first experimental studies of the effects of glucocorticoids on the liver of dogs demonstrated that daily SQ administration of cortisone acetate (5 mg/kg for 3 to 4 weeks) caused severe vacuolar lesions, marked hepatomegaly due to hepatocellular distension, and a twofold increase in the hepatic glycogen content.[135]

Subsequent studies have shown that dogs given glucocorticoids (prednisolone) daily in large doses (4 mg/kg body weight) develop liver lesions within 2 or 3 days, before biochemical abnormalities are well developed.[105] Glucocorticoids given at high doses by injection cause the earliest and most severe changes. Clinical experience verifies great individual variation in the development of this hepatopathy in response to small single doses of glucocorticoids as well as to large repeatedly given doses.[138–142] Hepatic and adrenal changes have been shown to develop following application of steroids topically to the eye, ear, and skin.[139–141,143,144] A glucocorticoid hepatopathy developed in dogs receiving ocular treatment after 8 to 16 weeks and only partially resolved in dogs biopsied 60 days after cessation of glucocorticoid treatment. After initiation of topical otic treatment, liver enzyme activities increased within 1 week and peaked at 3 weeks. Enzyme activity seemed higher in dogs receiving topical dexamethasone compared to prednisone or triamcinolone.[141] Although development of a glucocorticoid hepatopathy has not been inexorably linked to a suppressed pituitary adrenal axis, it is likely that the two conditions coexist.

Recently, use of oral prednisone at an anti-inflammatory dose (1.1 mg/kg body weight PO per day) was shown to be free of marked enzyme induction even after 35 days of drug administration.[142] Although a single intramuscular injection of 2.2 mg/kg prednisone (Metacortin) does not cause a sup-

pressed pituitary-adrenal axis at 1 week posttreatment,[145] a single intramuscular 2.5 mg/kg dose of methylprednisolone acetate (Depo-medrol) or 0.22 mg/kg triamcinolone acetonide (Vetalog) has been reported to alter canine adrenocortical function for at least 5 weeks.[145,146] Repeated parenteral treatment with depot-injectable forms of glucocorticoids, such as that used to control signs of seasonal allergic dermatitis, commonly leads to liver enzyme induction and suppression of the pituitary-adrenal axis. It is assumed that dogs with a suppressed pituitary-adrenal axis and clinicopathologic markers of a glucocorticoid hepatopathy concurrently develop the hepatic histomorphologic lesions, although most of these patients do not undergo liver biopsy. This is based on a study of the effects of dexamethasone where increased serum ALP, with or without increased ALT, develops after 5 days of dexamethasone given at a dose of 2.2 mg/kg SQ BID.[137] Histomorphologic hepatic lesions preceded the marked increases in serum ALP activity. In another study, a dose of 2 mg/kg dexamethasone per day, given in two divided doses for 7 to 28 consecutive days, resulted in histologic changes after only 3 days of treatment. The initial diffuse hepatocellular vacuolation changed to a periportal (zone 1) distribution with chronicity.

The initial increase in ALP activity is due to the liver isoenzyme rather than the G-ALP isoenzyme.[125,136] With chronicity, the activity of the G-ALP progressively increases. This explains why the levamisole-inhibition assay has high sensitivity in selecting for dogs with hyperadrenocorticism; this subset of dogs has chronic exposure to supraphysiologic quantities of glucocorticoids and G-ALP induction.

Cats differ in their response to glucocorticoids compared to the dog. An early study of cats (n = 4) given methylprednisolone acetate (Depo-Medrol), 20 mg SQ once weekly for 4 weeks, showed an increase in the serum total protein, albumin, cholesterol, and glucose concentrations and the activities of amylase and lactate dehydrogenase.[147] Serum activities of ALT, AST, and ALP remained normal in 3 of 4 cats; one cat developed 4-fold increases in AST activity and 10-fold increases in ALT activity. Each cat demonstrated suppression of its pituitary-adrenal axis when evaluated using an ACTH response test. Another study of the effects of glucocorticoids in the cat evaluated prednisolone given at a dose of 2 mg/kg/day PO for 1 week and at 4 mg/kg/day PO for a second week.[148] In this study the response of cats to prednisolone was comparison to megestrol acetate (5 mg/cat/day). In only 5 circumstances (5 of 340 estimations) up to threefold increases in enzyme concentrations were found. It was not specified which enzymes were abnormal or which group the affected cats represented. Diffuse hepatocyte swelling and pallor were detected on day 8 in two cats given megestrol acetate and in one cat given prednisolone. Two of these cats became glycosuric. It was speculated that vacuoles contained glycogen. These findings were partially coroborated by results of another study where healthy cats were given prednisolone acetate at a dose of 2 mg/kg IM or 8 mg/kg IM for 14 days.[149] Some cats developed increased serum ALT activity and a vacuolar hepatopathy. The most spectacular changes occurred in cats receiving 8 mg/kg, in which the ALT activity increased from 3- to 10-fold normal on day 14. Although enzyme activity declined by day 28, the ALT activity remained significantly increased. All cats developed an hepatocellular vacuolar change by the third day of treatment. Normal cats receiving 5 mg/kg methylprednisolone acetate (Depo-Medrol) SQ once weekly for 4 weeks do not develop increased liver enzyme activity.[147] However, if treatment is extended to 9 weeks, progressive hyperglycemia and increases in serum transaminases develop (but no change in ALP activity).[150] In one cat treated for 13 weeks, a moderate centrilobular vacuolation with glycogen was described. Clinical experience with cats on high-dose glucocorticoid therapy suggests it is unusual for cats to develop substantial liver changes or serum enzyme activities consistent with steroid hepatopathy as it is known in the dog, unless very large doses are given for several months. Rather, it is more common for cats to accumulate hepatic lipid vacuoles, particularly if they become anorectic. It appears that the cat requires higher doses of glucocorticoids, as compared to the dog, to develop hepatic lesions.

Histology

As can be gleaned from the preceding discussion, the dog treated with glucocorticoids may develop histologic liver lesions within a few days of initial drug administration, before overt biochemical abnormalities have developed. Hepatocyte vacuolation is associated with cellular swelling and a fine reticulum that encloses multiple vacuole-like areas (Figure 34–12). Ballooned hepatocytes ranging from 2 to 20 times normal size are usually interspersed among enlarged hepatocytes. In severely distended cells, the nucleus and organelles become displaced to the cell periphery, resembling hepatocytes filled with lipid in the feline HL syndrome. Hepatocyte swelling compresses and reduces the size of sinusoids and results in marked organ enlargement.

Variables influencing the severity of the morphologic features are the same ones that influence the induction of the glucocorticoid ALP isoenzyme. These include (1) the amount of steroid given, (2) the chronicity of drug administration, (3) the individual susceptibility of the patient, and (4) the type of drug and its route of administration. A parallel ultrastructural, histochemical, and quantitative analytical study of the vacuolar contents in dogs with a glucocorticoid hepatopathy has shown that hepatocellular enlargement is due predominantly to hepatic glycogen and that there is no appreciable increase in hepatic lipid or water content.[151] Hepatocellular glycogen was best preserved for histologic demonstration when tissues were fixed in absolute alcohol rather than buffered formalin or Bouin's solutions.[151] With uninterrupted cortisone administration, the hepatic glycogen content gradually increased, reaching a maximum after 2 weeks and thereafter declined. Early changes were diffuse and evolved into a midzonal (zone 2) or centrolobular (zone 3) distribution as the lesion progressed. Variation in zonal distribution of the hepatic vacuolation has been described by different investigators seemingly because of the evolving pattern of tissue involvement. Differences in zonal distribution of the vacuolation among studies is consistent with the high variation in histomorphometry seen in clinical cases (Figure 34–13).

Along with vacuolar change, single cell dropout, minor focal necrosis, and multifocal accumulations of small aggregates of polymorphonuclear cells are commonly observed in clinical patients with a severe glucocorticoid or vacuolar hepatopathy (Figure 34–13A). Areas of cell necrosis are typically very small

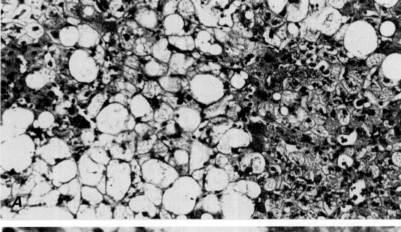

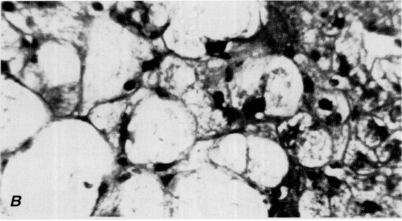

FIGURE 34–12. Photomicrograph of a liver biopsy from a dog with a glucocorticoid hepatopathy associated with spontaneous hyperadrenocorticism. In (A), vacuolar changes vary from mild to severe. In (B), a higher power magnification of (A), the reticulation or cytoplasmic strands extending between vacuoles is evident. This contrasts to the macrovesicular form of hepatic lipidosis where the vacuole is empty and cytoplasmic strands are not seen (H&E stain).

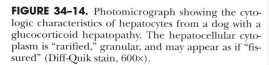

FIGURE 34-13. Photomicrograph of a liver biopsy from a dog with a glucocorticoid hepatopathy showing the variation in tissue involvement. In (*A*), diffuse severe vacuolation and a small foci of cell dropout and neutrophil infiltration are seen. In (*B*), a multifocal and random involvement was observed (H&E stain).

and are randomly distributed. This can lead to stromal collapse and development of a nodular appearance in the absence of extensive fibrosis. In some dogs, extramedullary hematopoiesis is observed in the absence of anemia.

Cytologic characteristics of hepatocytes typical of a glucocorticoid or vacuolar hepatopathy in the dog are shown in Figure 34–14. Because of the common finding of this cytologic change in dogs with chronic illness, cytologic evaluation is not clinically useful. This change may coexist with other clinically significant hepatobiliary disorders.

Clinical Signs

Clinical signs in dogs with a glucocorticoid hepatopathy are primarily related to the hypercortisolism rather than liver disease per se. The signs are variable depending on the cause and route of the glucocorticoid exposure. In dogs with spontaneous hyperadrenocorticism, typical signs variably include polyuria, polydipsia, polyphagia, a pot-bellied appearance, bilaterally symmetric alopecia, cutaneous hyperpigmentation, comedomes, thin skin, excessive panting, muscle wasting and

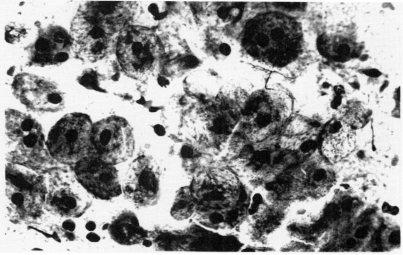

FIGURE 34-14. Photomicrograph showing the cytologic characteristics of hepatocytes from a dog with a glucocorticoid hepatopathy. The hepatocellular cytoplasm is "rarified," granular, and may appear as if "fissured" (Diff-Quik stain, 600×).

weakness, increased susceptibility to infections, hepatomegaly, and in rare cases, a myopathy. These signs may also develop in dogs receiving excessive exogenous glucocorticoids for several weeks or longer. Dogs with underlying medical conditions that can lead to chronic stress and high basal glucocorticoid concentrations usually show only the increased liver enzyme activity on biochemical screening profiles and hepatomegaly. In some cases, polyuria, polydipsia, and equivocal cutaneous changes also develop.

Clinicopathologic Features

In most dogs with a glucocorticoid hepatopathy, the clinical signs are nonspecific and the increased liver enzyme activity initiates diagnostic concern. In dogs that have hyperadrenocorticism, either endogenous or iatrogenic, a relative polycythemia, stress leukogram, and thrombocytosis are also recognized. The plasma may be lipemic. The urine specific gravity is usually in the isosthenuric or hyposthenuric range but may be in the zone of minimal urine concentration. A significant increase in the serum albumin and total protein concentration may develop due to enhanced protein synthesis by glucocorticoids.[152,153] This has been recognized in both dogs and cats receiving large doses of glucocorticoids chronically.

The biochemical abnormalities found on screening profiles usually include modestly increased ALT and AST activities, and marked increases of ALP and GGT. The presence of the G-ALP does not always correspond to the presence of a vacuolar or glucocorticoid hepatopathy as the single hepatic lesion; many other primary hepatic conditions can be associated with induction of this isoenzyme, as shown in Table 34–6.

As previously discussed, in healthy dogs, glucocorticoid administration causes striking biochemical abnormalities after 5 days of drug administration.[105,136,137,151,154,155] Although there is great variability, plasma ALP activity continues to increase and peaks at 20 to 30-fold normal at 3 weeks in dogs given high doses of prednisone daily for 2 weeks. A similar pattern is seen for plasma ALT activity with mean peak values of 10- to 15-fold normal. Mean plasma GGT activity increases to peak at three- to fourfold normal at 4 weeks. Serum enzyme activities return to normal ranges slowly after drug discontinuation, but may remain increased beyond 40 days; Figure 34–15 shows the fold increases in serum enzyme activities that developed in healthy dogs given high doses of glucocorticoids.[105]

The G-ALP isoenzyme accounts for less than 15% of the total ALP activity in the serum of healthy dogs.[125] In dogs with hyperadrenocorticism, this isoenzyme may comprise more than 85% of the total ALP activity. In dogs treated with 4 mg/kg of prednisone IM SID (Meticorten) for 32 consecutive days, the initial increase in ALP was attributed to the liver

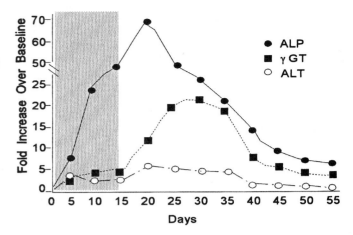

FIGURE 34–15. Fold increase over baseline of mean serum enzyme activities in dogs (n = 6) given daily IM injections of prednisone (4.4 mg/kg; Metacortin) for 14 consecutive days (shaded area). (ALP = alkaline phosphatase, GGT = gamma-glutamyl transpeptidase, ALT = alanine aminotransferase). Data adapted from reference 105, with permission.

isoenzyme. The glucocorticoid isoenzyme progressively increased from day 5 through day 24 (Figure 34–16).[125]

The G-ALP isoenzyme is derived from the hepatocyte membranes, which comprise the bile canaliculi.[126] Exposure to supraphysiologic concentrations of glucocorticoids is required to induce the G-ALP to the extent it becomes the predominant ALP isoenzyme in serum. It is proposed that the marked initial increases in total ALP and G-ALP isoenzyme may develop due to the severe hepatocellular swelling caused by cytosolic distension with glycogen. Accumulation of bile acids as a result of cholestasis can solubilize ALP in the area of the canalicular membrane, releasing it to the peripheral circulation.[156] In some animals, ALP cannot be histochemically localized to the area of the canalicular membranes. It is postulated that this occurs as a result of the marked cell distension which causes membrane devitalization and loss of canalicular microvilli, similar to changes shown in

Table 34–6

CANINE LIVER DISEASES ASSOCIATED WITH INCREASED GLUCOCORTICOID ALP ISOENZYME IN THE ABSENCE OF A DOMINANT VACUOLAR OR GLUCOCORTICOID HEPATOPATHY

Septic necrotizing hepatitis
Hepatic neoplasia
    Lymphosarcoma
    Hepatocellular carcinoma
    Hepatoma
Extrahepatic bile duct obstruction
Cholangitis / cholangiohepatitis
Chronic active hepatitis

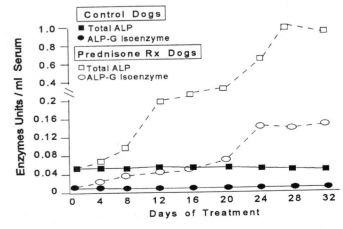

FIGURE 34–16. The total mean serum alkaline phosphatase (ALP) activity and the total mean activity of the glucocorticoid isoenzyme of alkaline phosphatase (ALP-G) in prednisone-treated dogs (n = 4; 4 mg/kg SID for 32 days) and control dogs (n = 3). Isoenzyme was determined by levamisole inhibition assay. Data adapted from reference 125, with permission.

livers from bile duct–ligated rats.[157] In vitro studies have not been able to demonstrate that increased protein synthesis is directly involved in the increased production of the G-ALP as it is with the liver isoenzyme.[158]

Experimentally, serum arginase activity has also been shown to increase up to 16-fold normal in dogs after 11 days of treatment with dexamethasone (3 mg/kg IV).[154] Hypercholesterolemia also is common in dogs with a glucocorticoid hepatopathy.

Development of a glucocorticoid hepatopathy can impair hepatic function. It is believed this is due to impaired sinusoidal perfusion and diminished perisinusoidal space related to the cellular distension. A cholestatic effect may be realized from compression and injury of the canaliculi and displacement or impaired function of cellular microtubules. Daily dexamethasone treatment caused mean serum bile acid concentrations to increase from a normal of 1.0 μg/dl to 19.2 μg/dl within 12 days in dogs.[154] The sulfobromophthalein (BSP) 30 minute retention doubled in these dogs. Serum bile acid concentrations are often modestly increased in both the fasting and postprandial intervals in clinical patients with a glucocorticoid hepatopathy, consistent with an intrahepatic cholestatic pattern.[159] Only rarely does an increased total bilirubin concentration develop.

Functional compromise can be used to recognize which dogs with enzyme induction have significant morphologic hepatic change. Short-term treatment with low-dose glucocorticoids will induce serum enzymes but will not significantly alter liver function tests unless diffuse morphologic lesions

develop.[159] The ammonia tolerance test remained normal in one study of dogs where prednisone administration induced abnormal bile acid values and impaired BSP clearance.[154] The findings suggested a cholestatic effect before sinusoidal perfusion becomes impaired.

A glucagon tolerance test has been evaluated in dogs treated with prednisolone.[160] An abnormal response consistent with glucose intolerance was suggested to be an indicator of hepatic glycogen accumulation. This has not been found to be useful in clinical patients for differential diagnoses.

Abdominal radiographs may suggest the presence of hepatomegaly. Abdominal ultrasonography reveals either a diffuse or multifocal hyperechoic appearance of the hepatic parenchyma. In some animals, discrete nodular lesions are identified. These correspond to large focal areas of severe vacuolation. The echogenicity of the hepatic parenchyma cannot be differentiated from hepatic lipid accumulation or diffuse fibrosis.

Treatment

When a vacuolar or glucocorticoid hepatopathy is discovered, diagnostic efforts should be directed to identifying an underlying endocrine, metabolic, infectious, or inflammatory condition. The appropriate diagnostic appraisals are summarized in Figure 34–17. Initial steps are to rule out exposure to

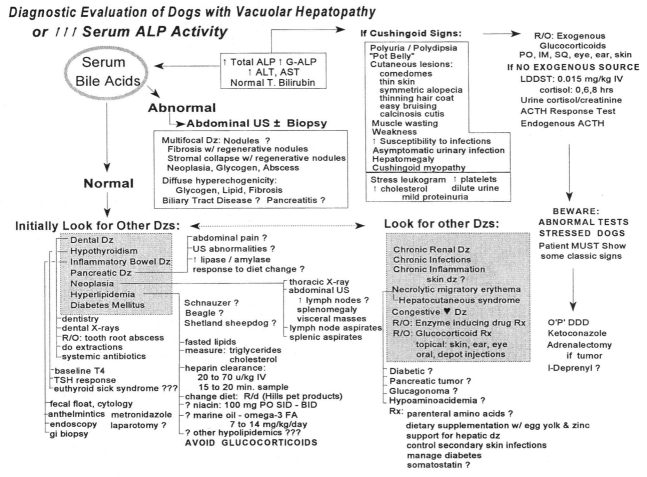

FIGURE 34–17. Diagnostic appraisals appropriate for the dog with marked increases in the serum activity of total alkaline phosphatase, serum glucocorticoid isoenzyme activity, or in which a glucocorticoid or vacuolar hepatopathy has been diagnosed.

exogenous glucocorticoids or the presence of endogenous hyperadrenocorticism. Tests used for the diagnosis of hyperadrenocorticism must be interpreted with caution. Chronically stressed dogs may develop abnormal low-dose dexamethasone suppression, ACTH response, and urine cortisol to creatinine ratios. These animals may also develop hyperplastic adrenal glands that may be considered as enlarged on abdominal ultrasonography. Accordingly, if abnormal test results support a diagnosis of hyperadrenocorticism, the animal should be carefully evaluated for other causes of stress. This is of particular importance in the animal demonstrating few of the classic clinical signs of Cushing syndrome. Evaluation of the patient for severe dental disease, inflammatory bowel disease, pancreatitis, neoplasia, other underlying endocrinopathies, and inherent problems in lipid metabolism should be undertaken, as each may be responsible for vacuolar hepatopathy.

If the underlying problem is hyperadrenocorticism or exogenous glucocorticoid administration, appropriate treatment will permit resolution of the vacuolar hepatopathy over several months. In some dogs with Cushing disease, sufficient control to allow complete resolution of the hepatopathy is never obtained.

SCHNAUZER HYPERLIPIDEMIA-ASSOCIATED VACUOLAR HEPATOPATHY

Clinical Synopsis

Diagnostic Features

- Intermittent signs include abdominal pain, vomiting, and pancreatitis
- Hepatomegaly is common
- Fasting lipemia often recognized
- Increased plasma cholesterol and ALP activity
- Liver biopsy reveals severe vacuolation
- May develop sludged bile and choleliths requiring surgical management

Standard Treatment

- Low-fat diets
- Avoidance of glucocorticoids

An inborn error of lipoprotein metabolism has been characterized in miniature schnauzer dogs and briards.[161-165] Abnormalities of lipoprotein metabolism also exist in Shetland sheepdogs and beagles. Schnauzers and Shetland sheep dogs with hyperlipidemia develop this hepatic lesion.

Clinical Signs

Based on a number of dogs seen by the author and clinical reports of affected schnauzers, associated clinical signs include recurrent lethargy, abdominal pain, inappetance, vomiting, hepatomegaly, episodic grand mal seizure activity, pancreatitis, and, in some dogs, eventual development of diabetes mellitus.

Clinicopathologic Features

Affected dogs have had moderate to marked increases in their serum ALP activity. When the glucocorticoid-induced isoenzyme (G-ALP) has been measured, it has been markedly increased but does not account for the total ALP activity.

Most dogs have increased plasma concentrations of total cholesterol, TGs, and phospholipids.[161,162,165] Fasting lipemia is common. Hyperchylomicronemia is apparent by formation of a cream layer in plasma upon sample refrigeration. In some dogs, IV injection of heparin at a dose of 20 to 70 IU/kg body weight has been used to stimulate lipoprotein lipase (LPL) activity and has resulted in a transient reduction of the circulating hyperlipidemia. This suggests that the metabolic defect causing this disorder is not related to the absence or dysfunction of LPL.

Recently, the ultracentrifugal and electrophoretic characteristics of the plasma lipoproteins in affected schnauzers have been clarified.[164] An increased concentration of very low density lipoproteins (VLDL) and a lack of lipoproteins with characteristics of normal low density lipoproteins (LDL) were found. Screening tests have ruled out underlying primary metabolic or endocrine disorders leading to the lipoprotein abnormality. It is proposed that there is delayed clearance of triglyceride-rich lipoproteins from the circulation. However, some dogs have been able to clear their lipemia during a protracted fast. It is possible that the primary defect is removal of VLDL from the circulation. The clearance mechanism for VLDL is shared by chylomicrons; thus, competition for clearance of VLDL can impede clearance of chylomicrons and lead to chylomicronemia.[165,166] Disorders that increase production of VLDL (obesity, diabetes mellitus) can compound the problem, causing increased VLDL and chylomicron concentrations.[165,167] It is possible that a primary underlying defect of VLDL clearance sets the stage for development of hyperchylomicronemia under the influence of a high-fat meal. This may lead to induction of pancreatitis during bouts of hyperchylomicronemia and, eventually, to diabetes mellitus, as has been reported in humans.[168-170]

Hepatic Histopathology

Some schnauzers with hyperlipoproteinemia have developed hepatic insufficiency as a result of hepatic injury attributed to a severe vacuolar hepatopathy. These animals develop a macroscopically nodular liver due to stromal collapse and regenerative nodule formation. The microscopic features are shown in Figure 34–18. Vacuolated hepatocytes are severely distended with the cytosol containing either a few large clear vacuoles or frothy microvesicles. Specific staining of unextracted hepatic tissue for glycogen and triglyceride has confirmed their presence (Figure 34–19). In most cases, inflammation is rare and hepatocellular necrosis is only detected in small focal areas or is absent. The bile ducts may appear prominent as a result of collapse of surrounding parenchyma. Thin strands of reticulin fibers bridge between portal triads. Masson's trichrome staining for connective tissue shows very little collagen deposition. Dogs may develop choleliths that are green and gelatinous on gross inspection or severely sludged bile. Some dogs also have had concurrently recognized cystic and renal calculi that are believed to be unassociated with the lipid metabolism defect.

Treatment

The most important therapeutic intervention in an affected dog is to limit its intake of dietary fat and to avoid treatment with glucocorticoids. Dietary management is focused on fat restriction and fiber supplementation. A prescription diet R/d (Hill's Pet Products) usually results in marked improvement in clinical signs. Care should also be

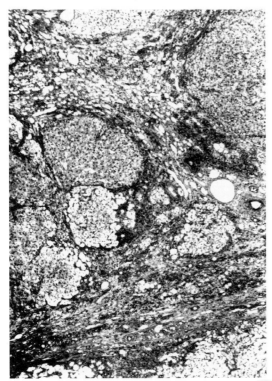

FIGURE 34–18. Photomicrograph of a liver biopsy from a schnauzer with hyperlipoproteinemia, and episodic abdominal pain that eventually developed diabetes mellitus 5 years after the liver biopsy was collected. The vacuolar hepatopathy progressed to cause hepatic insufficiency. Notice the absence of large amount of connective tissue and inflammation. Although this liver was macroscopically nodular, it is not cirrhotic (H&E stain, 87X).

taken to avoid addition of any "fatty" supplements. Administration of capsules containing eicosinoids and vitamin E have produced signs of abdominal pain and pancreatitis in some dogs. Once dietary modification is optimized and the client strictly adheres to the nutritional recommendations, complete resolution of clinical signs can be expected. Dogs that have become diabetic will require continued insulin therapy. Circulating lipoprotein abnormalities will not resolve, but their absolute concentrations will improve toward normal.

Although many efficacious hypolipidemic agents have been developed, none is effective in all lipoprotein disorders, and all have associated side effects. Nicotinic acid generally decreases levels of plasma triglyceride and VLDL cholesterol by 30% to 40% in hyperlipidemic humans. It appears to reduce the synthesis of VLDL. Anecdotal reports of its use in schnauzers suggests that a dose of 100 mg PO SID to BID provides some benefit. Nicotinic acid can be hepatotoxic in humans and may increase the activity of liver enzymes and glucose concentration. It is contraindicated in humans with underlying liver disease. Limited information is available about the toxicity of nicotinic acid in dogs. *LOPID*

Fibric acid derivatives (clofibrate, gemfibrozil) are believed to increase the activity of lipoprotein lipase. These agents also are potent peroxisiome inducers. Clofibrate is contraindicated in patients with liver disease and does not seem a logical choice for use in the schnauzer disease. Gemfibrozil is similar to clofibrate and shares its side effects. There is no experience with either clofibrate or gemfibrozil in affected schnauzers.

Neomycin has been effective in lowering plasma cholesterol levels in humans and is a comparatively safe, well-tolerated, and efficacious agent for controlling certain hyper-

lipoproteinemia disorders in humans. To the author's knowledge, this has not been tried in affected schnauzers.

Marine oils rich in omega-3 fatty acids have been shown to reduce plasma triglycerides by 60% and cholesterol by 27% in humans with hypertriglyceridemia.[171] Use of marine oils in humans with hypertriglyceridemia has also reduced the concentration of circulating chylomicrons after ingestion of a fatty meal. It is possible that this may benefit dogs with hyperlipidemia. One author has suggested a dose of 6.8 to 13.6 mg/kg per day in dogs and has used this without adverse consequence.[172] The dose used in humans is 20 to 30 g per day.[171] It is proposed that the omega-3 fatty acids reduce VLDL concentrations by suppressing hepatic VLDL and fatty acid synthesis or via increased clearance of VLDL by the liver or peripheral tissues. Reduction in the plasma cholesterol concentrations may be related to increased fecal steroid excretion.[171]

Drugs that competitively inhibit 3-hydroxy-3-methylglutaryl-coenzyme A reductase (HMG-CoA reductase), the rate-controlling enzyme in cholesterol synthesis, have been effective in lowering cholesterol levels in humans with some forms of hypercholesterolemia.[173] Lovastatin (Mevacor) is known to produce cataracts in dogs when used at very high doses.[174] It also has (rarely) been associated with a myopathy and increased hepatic enzymes. There is no experience with this drug as a therapeutic agent in clinical patients.

Avoidance of treatment with glucocorticoids is an important aspect of long-term management. It is prudent to avoid treatment with glucocorticoids because of their effect on fat metabolism and inducing effects on G-ALP, pancreatitis, and vacuolar hepatopathy. Treatment of affected dogs with ursodeoxycholic acid is recommended if a sludged bile syndrome is suspected or verified. A dose of 4 to 15 mg/kg per day is recommended

NECROLYTIC MIGRATORY ERYTHEMA OR HEPATOCUTANEOUS SYNDROME

Clinical Synopsis

Diagnostic Features

- Crusting and/or erosive lesions of the pads, mucocutaneous junctions, and pressure points
- Skin biopsies show diffuse parakeratosis and intercellular edema in upper half of the epidermis
- Elevated serum ALP, ALT; bile acids are common
- Hyperglycemia due to diabetes mellitus is common
- Plasma amino acids 30% to 50% of normal
- Liver biopsy shows moderate to severe vacuolation with fat

Standard Treatment

- Symptomatic management of skin (cleansing, antibiotics, ketaconazole)
- High-protein, egg-yolk–supplemented diets (1 yolk per 4.5 kg/day)
- Supplemental B complex vitamins and zinc (1.5 mg/kg zinc gluconate divided BID)

A unique dermatologic lesion characterized by epidermal parakeratosis and laminar intracellular edema has been recognized in dogs and likened to a disorder in humans termed necrolytic migratory erythema. The canine counterpart was originally referred to as superficial necrolytic dermatitis.[175–179] In humans, this disorder has been linked to the presence of hyperglucagonemia secondary to glucagon-secreting pancre-

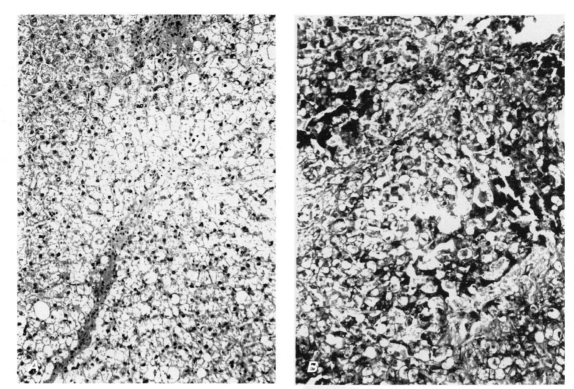

FIGURE 34-19. Photomicrographs of a liver biopsy from a schnauzer with hyperlipoproteinemia and a vacuolar hepatopathy. This dog was evaluated extensively for hyperadrenocorticism that could not be documented. In (A), a diffuse vacuolar hepatopathy is shown (H&E, 140×). In (B), staining with periodic acid–Schiff (PAS) stain after treatment with diastase confirmed the presence of glycogen, which appears in this photograph as very dark globular areas that impair visualization of the underlying hepatocytes (140×). Application of Oil-Red-O to this tissue also documented increased neural fat stores within vacuolated hepatocytes.

atic neoplasia, although there have been cases reported in which no pancreatic endocrine tumors could be identified. Some of these patients have hepatic insufficiency.[180] The initial report of this dermatologic disorder in the dog characterized four dogs, of which one dog was definitively proven to have hepatic insufficiency associated with a macronodular cirrhosis.[175] Subsequent reports have shown a minority of dogs to have endocrine pancreatic tumors and a majority of dogs to have substantial hepatic insufficiency.[176-179] Many, but not all, dogs develop diabetes mellitus. None have been shown to have hyperadrenocorticism.

Clinical Signs

Initial diagnosis of this disorder is based on clinical and skin biopsy findings. Most dogs present for painful crusting lesions of the pads. Most develop bilaterally symmetric lesions characterized by erythema, erosion, ulceration, and crusting of the oral, ocular, anal, and/or genital mucocutaneous junctions, ears, and pressure points (especially the elbows). Some intact male dogs have developed lesions involving the scrotum. Some dogs have developed paronychia and deformed nails. Rarely, stomatitis also develops. Most dogs have recently lost weight.

Multiple skin biopsies should be examined. The classic lesions involve a moderate to severe diffuse parakeratotic hyperkeratosis associated with marked intracellular and intercellular edema in the upper one-half of the epidermis. The edema leads to formation of intraepidermal clefts and vesi-

cles.[177] Skin biopsies taken from old or traumatized areas may fail to distinguish the typical epidermal edema that is characteristic of the necrolytic-migratory-erythema lesion.[177]

Clinicopathologic Features

A mild normocytic normochromic nonregenerative anemia is usually found. Erythrocytic morphologic abnormalities consistent with severe liver disease are common and include poikilocyte and target cell formation.

Approximately 50% of reported cases have developed diabetes. These dogs become hyperglycemic late in the course of the disease after cutaneous lesions and hepatic insufficiency are well established. However, in a few dogs, cutaneous lesions have developed after the dog developed diabetes mellitus. Insulin concentrations have been increased in 8 of 11 dogs tested, indicating that insulinopenia is not the cause of the glucose intolerance.

All dogs with this disorder develop marked increases in their serum ALP activities. Most dogs also develop increased ALT and AST activities. Some dogs become jaundiced. Signs consistent with pancreatitis have developed in a few dogs. Hypoalbuminemia develops in approximately 30% of dogs. In all dogs tested, abnormal bile acid concentrations have been shown. As expected, the postprandial values are most profoundly increased.

In eight dogs, severe reductions in the concentrations of most plasma amino acids were found in the range of 30% to 50% of normal.[179] Some amino acids were reduced even further, most notably hydroxyproline, threonine, glutamine, proline, alanine, citrulline, and arginine. Some amino acids are normal or mildly increased, most notably glutamic acid, α-amino-n-butyric acid, cystathionine, phenylalanine, ornithine, and 3-methylhistidine. Plasma glucagon values were not increased in five dogs in one report,[179] but were increased in a total of five dogs in two other reports.[175,177] The discordant findings in measured glucagon concentrations may reflect different glucagon or glucagon-like moieties measured by different techniques as well as deterioration of the hormone stored in plasma.

Hepatic Histopathology

The liver may be small, normal, or slightly enlarged. The surface is nodular due to the presence of regenerative nodule formation. An end-stage lesion demonstrating the severity of nodular regeneration is shown in Figure 34–20. The microscopic lesion is characterized by a moderate to severe vacuolation of hepatocytes, parenchymal collapse, and the presence of large hyperplastic nodules.[179] In most dogs, vacuolated hepatocytes are severely ballooned. The cytosol contains either a few large clear vacuoles with discrete borders or is frothy with a microvesicular appearance. In most cases, inflammation is rare and hepatocellular necrosis is absent. The bile ducts may appear prominent as a result of collapse of surrounding parenchyma. Strands of reticulin fibers bridge between portal triads. Specific staining of the vacuole is consistent with an increased fat content. Masson's trichrome staining reveals only a small increase in connective tissue in most cases.

In most dogs, pancreatic tissue appears grossly normal. Microscopically, some dogs have evidence of mild to moderate pancreatitis. In some dogs, interstitial pancreatic fibrosis has been notable and has been associated with atrophy and mild infiltration with lymphocytes and macrophages.[179] Rarely, a pancreatic tumor is identified.

Pathogenesis

The underlying cause of this disorder remains undetermined. A severe hypoaminoacidemia characterizes the human counterpart of necrolytic migratory erythema.[181–183] In the few dogs tested, amino acid profiles are consistent with a general trend toward hypoaminoacidemia.[179] In humans, the association between hyperglucagonemia and this syndrome has been related to the hypoaminoacidemia. Persistent hyperglucagonemia may reduce plasma amino acids as a result of unremitting gluconeogenesis. Reversal of the cutaneous lesions has been shown in humans given intravenous amino acid infusions.[181,184] A marked improvement in the cutaneous lesions in six dogs was observed when egg yolks were used as a dietary supplement.[179] Because egg yolks are a concentrated source of protein, it was proposed that a similar pathogenic connection between hypoaminoacidemia and the cutaneous lesions exists in the dog. The consumption of high-protein diets by humans with inoperable glucagonoma has reportedly reduced the severity of their cutaneous lesions.[185] The association between the low plasma amino acid concentrations and the skin lesions is believed to be due to protein depletion in the epidermis that curtails its ability to replicate. A relationship between low amino acid concentrations and abnormal zinc metabolism has also been proposed as a result of the similarity between the cutaneous lesions induced by each deficiency.

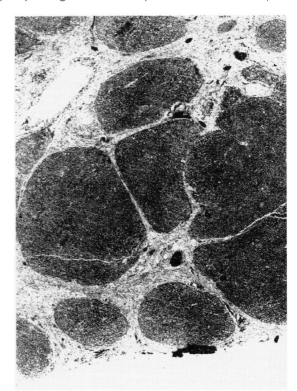

FIGURE 34–20. Photomicrograph of a liver biopsy from a dog with necrolytic migratory erythema (hepatocutaneous syndrome). This low-power photomicrograph demonstrates severe nodule formation typical of this disorder. This dog had no evidence of active inflammation. Clinicopathologic evaluations indicated hepatic insufficiency (H&E, 14× magnification).

Primary severe vacuolar liver disease does not explain the hypoaminoacidemia. Experimentally induced liver disease can be associated with reduced concentrations of amino acids in dogs, but not to the severity shown in these patients. Increased glucagon values have been shown in humans with cirrhosis and in animal models of hepatic insufficiency.[186–188] It remains possible that hyperglucagonemia is a major etiopathogenic factor in this disorder. The increased plasma insulin concentrations demonstrated in dogs with glucose intolerance supports this consideration. Determination of plasma glucagon concentrations have produced conflicting results, partly because of assay difficulties but also because glucagon levels in peripheral blood may not reflect those in portal blood, which signals hepatic gluconeogenesis.[179,189–192]

Treatment

Treatment of affected dogs involves management of their cutaneous lesions with a focus on keeping them clean and free of secondary infectious agents. Bacterial and fungal infections have been found in skin lesions of some dogs. Ketaconazole transiently improved the cutaneous lesions in one dog.[175] A broad-spectrum bactericidal antibiotic effective against *Staphylococcus intermedius* should be used. The diabetes should be managed appropriately with insulin therapy and a high-fiber diet. The use of hypoglycemic agents has not been evaluated. It is inappropriate to feed these patients a high-fat and protein-restricted diet, such as that used for management of severe hepatic insufficiency. Dogs treated with egg yolk as a protein supplementation have shown improvement in their cutaneous lesions and survival. Egg yolk is used as a dietary supplement in long-term management at a dose of 1 yolk per 4.5 kg body weight per day. An alternative source of amino acid supplementation is Amino Pro-Mod (Ross Labs) at a dose of 10g/7kg body weight SID. It is reported that one dog has remained relatively well controlled on egg yolk supplementation for at least one year. In dogs presented in a debilitated condition, hyperalimentation with a nutritionally balanced amino acid–enriched solution seems prudent. Cutaneous lesions have improved in humans treated with parenteral amino acid infusions.

Treatment with prednisone has been used in enough cases to indicate that such therapy is overall ineffective, although it modulates the inflammation, pain, and severity of the cutaneous lesions.

Addition of water soluble vitamins and zinc to the diet is also recommended. Water soluble vitamins are important for intermediary metabolism and some of these are activated in the liver. Zinc supplementation is prudent considering the importance of zinc in several essential metalloenzymes involved in intermediary metabolism, the urea cycle, and because of the known deficiencies that develop in humans with hepatic insufficiency. Furthermore, the parakeratotic lesions associated with zinc deficiency share similarities with the cutaneous lesions of this syndrome. Thus far there has been limited experience with zinc supplementation in these patients. A dose of 1.5 mg per kg body weight of zinc gluconate has been suggested.

It is possible that a recently marketed recombinant form of somatostatin may be useful in managing this disorder. Somatostatin might curtail pathologic release of glucagon that may be important in etiopathogenesis of this syndrome. Use of the long-acting somatostatin analogue (Octreotide, Sandostatin; Sandoz) has been described in dogs with acromegaly, insulinomas, and other APUDomas.[193]

FELINE HYPERLIPOPROTEINEMIA

Clinical Signs and Clinicopathologic Features

An inherited lipoprotein lipase deficiency has been described in cats.[87–89,194–196] Affected animals have fasting hyperlipemia, hyperchylomicronemia, hypertriglyceridemia, hypercholesterolemia, and a slight increase in VLDL. Lipemia retinalis and peripheral neuropathies due to compression of nerves by lipid granulomata have been reported. Nerve compression is attributed to trauma and resulting granuloma formation. Pressure point cutaneous xanthomatosis has been recognized in some cats. Fat-specific stains demonstrate lipid droplets within foamy macrophages associated with xanthomas. In some cats, intra-abdominal viscera-associated fatty granulomas may be palpable but are nonpainful.

The metabolic defect in this disorder is characterized as production of an aberrant form of LPL.[195,196] The protein is amply produced but is unable to bind to the vascular endothelium and to interact with heparin.[195] This inheritable defect is believed to be due to a point mutation in the LPL gene.

Hepatic Histopathology

Examination of hepatic tissue from affected cats by light and electron microscopy has shown large numbers of lipid-containing cytoplasmic vacuoles ranging from small to very large and, in some cases, occupying the majority of the cell cytoplasm. Kupffer cells also appear vacuolated with lipid. Chylomicrons are observed in the space of Disse. Hepatocytes and macrophages also contain ceroid inclusions. Ceroid is formed by the intracellular oxidation and polymerization of lipid at the periphery of a lipid droplet. Ceroid accumulates as a nonsoluble residual body (secondary lysosome).

These animals do not develop signs of liver disease, although in some older animals hepatomegaly has been detected.

There is no known treatment for this condition and morbidity due to liver disease has not been reported. Only slight clearance of chylomicronemia occurs in response to intravenous heparin.[196]

STORAGE DISORDERS: LYSOSOMAL AND GLYCOGEN STORAGE DISORDERS

A variety of lysosomal storage disorders have been described in humans, dogs, and cats.[89,197] These diseases include most of the lipid, mucopolysaccharidoses, glycoprotein, and mucolipid storage disorders. These usually are inherited defects that become apparent when the animal demonstrates a growth or developmental deficit. Most affected animals are normal at birth. Target organs affected by pathologic product storage are the usual sites of degradation for the involved macromolecules (Figure 34–21). Hepatomegaly develops in disorders in which the lysosomes of hepatocytes or Kupffer cells serve as an important site of product degradation. Examples of storage disorders in dogs and/or cats associated with hepatomegaly and abnormal hepatic or Kupffer cell lysosomal inclusions include type I α-mannosidosis in cats, GM$_1$ gangliosidosis in dogs and cats, mucopolysaccharidosis in dogs and cats, ceroid lipofuscinosis in dogs and cats, α-glucosidase deficiency in dogs, and acid lipase deficiency (cholesteryl ester storage disease) in cats. These disorders are uncommon. Many are associated with neurologic signs in young animals and are progressive. Hepatic signs are minor and organ involvement is obvious upon necropsy evaluation. Histologic evaluation of liver tissue reveals cytoplasmic distension due to storage of the involved macromolecules.

Glycogen storage diseases are inherited disorders involving a deficiency of specific enzymes necessary for normal glycogen metabolism. Enzyme deficiency results in impaired glycogen mobilization and subsequent accumulation of visceral glycogen. Impaired hepatic glycogen catabolism is usually associated with fasting hypoglycemia. In certain disorders, glycogen accumulation in the liver causes massive hepatomegaly. In humans eight types of glycogen storage disorders are described. Three of these are suspected to occur in dogs: type 1 (von Gierke's disease), type II (Pompe's disease), and type III (Cori's disease). Types II and III have been confirmed in dogs with specific enzymatic assays.

Type II glycogenosis is caused by deficiency of lysosomal α-1,4-glucosidase. This has been described in Lapland dogs; an autosomal recessive inheritance is suspected.[198] The type II disease is a variant from the typical manifestations of a glycogen storage disorder because it is not associated with fasting hypoglycemia or hepatic glycogen accumulation. Clinical signs are related to cardiac and skeletal muscle glycogenosis and include regurgitation due to megaesophagus, systemic muscle weakness, and cardiac dysfunction. The prognosis is poor; affected dogs died by 1.5 years of age.

The type III glycogenosis is caused by a deficiency of debranching amyloclastic enzyme (amylo-1,6-glucosidase). This has been described in related female German shepherd dogs.[199,200] Clinical signs include weakness, failure to grow,

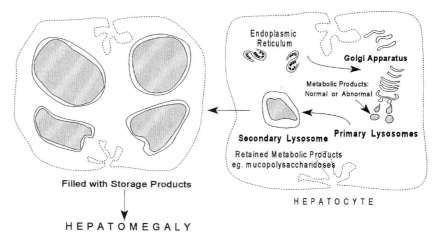

FIGURE 34–21. Diagrammatic representation of the hepatopathy that develops with lysosomal storage disorders. The absence of an essential lysosomal enzyme limits degradation and excretion of an endogenous product or substrate. With no alternative for disposal, the substance accumulates within the hepatocyte. This results in hepatocellular enlargement and progressive hepatomegaly, depending on the metabolic defect.

and massive hepatomegaly causing abdominal distension. Mild hypoglycemia was documented in one dog as was a suboptimal glycemic response to epinephrine administration. At necropsy, glycogen infiltration was found in visceral organs, skeletal muscle, and CNS. The hepatic activity of amylo-1,6-glucosidase ranged from 0% to 7% of normal.

These disorders are rare but should be considered in young animals with persistent or recurrent fasting hypoglycemia. They must be differentiated from all other causes of hypoglycemia in the young dog, particularly portosystemic vascular anomalies. Abnormal response to glucagon has been shown in dogs with vascular anomalies. Demonstration of massive hepatic glycogen deposition should increase the index of suspicion of type I and III storage disorders. However, definitive diagnosis requires tissue biopsy for enzyme analysis on freshly frozen tissue. Treatment for these metabolic errors is unavailable other than frequent feedings of simple carbohydrates and intravenous dextrose in the event of neuroglycopenia.

AMYLOIDOSIS

Clinical Synopsis

Diagnostic Features

- Shar Pei dogs and Abyssinian cats are predisposed
- Most animals are presented because of renal dysfunction
- Liver involvement manifests as hepatomegaly and raised liver enzymes
- Shar Peis also show recurrent pyrexia, nonspecific pain, swollen joints, and vague gastrointestinal upsets
- Proteinuria, nephrotic syndrome, and/or azotemia are common
- Renal and/or liver biopsy reveals amyloid deposits

Standard Treatment

- Treat any underlying cause
- Supportive therapy for renal or liver failure
- Colchicine 0.03 mg/kg SID has improved some dogs
- DMSO (80 mg/kg SQ three times per week or 125 mg/kg PO BID) remains investigational

Amyloidosis is not a single disease entity, but rather a pathologic response to inflammatory or lymphoproliferative disorders.[201] The syndrome of amyloidosis results from the extracellular deposition of an insoluble fibrillar protein (amy-

loid). The amyloid protein is produced as an acute-phase reactant or as a product from a neoplastic clone of cells. There are several different types of amyloid proteins. Although they have widely different amino acid sequences, all amyloid substance has an antiparallel β-pleated sheet structure that makes it poorly antigenic, resistant to enzymatic digestion, and poorly soluble. Its unique β-pleated sheet configuration permits unique staining reactions and birefringence with polarized light.

The patient with amyloidosis develops illness as a result of impaired organ function due to extracellular deposition of the inert amyloid fibrils.[201–203] Fibril deposition leads to pressure atrophy of adjacent cells and tissue injury due to impaired microcirculation, exchange of metabolic products, and nutrients. Normal function of affected vital organs becomes irreparably compromised and eventually leads to death. Amyloidosis is now classified into the following descriptive categories. Immunocyte-dyscrasia related amyloidosis (type AL protein with characteristics similar to light chains) refers to acquired amyloidosis not associated with infectious, inflammatory, or nonimmunocyte neoplastic conditions.[201] Reactive systemic amyloidosis refers to amyloid deposition (AA protein) associated with recognized recurrent acute or chronic inflammatory, infectious, or other debilitating disorders.[201] The amyloid protein usually found in dogs and cats is believed to be reactive or AA amyloid; the protein subunits are believed to be originally derived from the liver and behave as acute-phase reactants. Amyloidosis develops when the acute-phase reactant is synthesized at a rate that exceeds the systemic capacity for its degradation. It is postulated that acute-phase reactants undergo proteolytic cleavage by macrophage or neutrophil proteinases, forming amyloid AA protein which is deposited in the extracellular space within target organs.[201] It is not known why certain organs or tissues are targeted or what determines the pattern of deposition within a particular organ. In some humans, resolution and degradation of amyloid substance has been observed after eradication of the infectious or inflammatory condition that stimulated formation and release of the acute-phase reactants. The variety of conditions associated with systemic amyloidosis in the dog and cat are listed in Table 34–7.[202–206] Unfortunately, a large number of animals have no recognized underlying condition. This is similar to the situation in human beings and places these patients in an idiopathic disease category.

When densely deposited in tissues, routine H&E staining shows amyloid as a homogeneous pink amorphous extracellular material. With Congo red staining and evaluation under polarized light, amyloid appears birefringent and apple

Table 34-7

DISORDERS ASSOCIATED WITH AMYLOIDOSIS
IN DOGS AND CATS
(PATIENTS WITH RENAL AMYLOIDOSIS

Chronic Infections
   nocardiosis
   tuberculosis
   blastomycosis
   coccidioidomycosis
   dirofilariasis
Chronic Suppurative Inflammation
   chronic prostatitis
   chronic pancreatitis
   chronic gastroenteritis
   cholangitis
   biliary cirrhosis
   endometritis
   bronchopneumonia
   peritonitis
   pleuritis
   stomatitis, gingivitis
Hypothyroidism
Hereditary Cyclic Neutropenia (gray collie syndrome)
Systemic Lupus Erythematosus
Polyarthritis
Neoplasia
   lymphosarcoma
   lymphocytic leukemia
   squamous cell carcinoma
   thyroid carcinoma
   adrenal carcinoma
   hepatocellular carcinoma
   splenic hemangioma
   mammary tumors
Idiopathic: no underlying conditions

---

green. When viewed under ultraviolet light after staining with Thioflavin T, amyloid shows a yellow-green fluorescence. Amyloid in cats seems to stain more reliably with Thioflavin T. Amyloid AA fibrils are sensitive to oxidative treatment by permanganate.[201,207-209] Comparison of tissues stained with Congo red before and after such treatment permits identification of the AA fibril type.

Although the liver can be a major site of amyloid deposition, this is an uncommon primary site in the dog or cat. In the dog, renal amyloidosis is more common and causes proteinuria. Amyloidosis is uncommon in the cat. When it occurs it may affect multiple organs, often the liver and kidneys.[209-216] In the cat, it has been best described in the Abyssinian as a familial disorder.[213,214] Most of these animals are presented for veterinary attention because of renal dysfunction.

Abyssinian cats and Shar Pei dogs appear to have a predisposition for systemic amyloid formation.[215,216] In the sharpei, kindreds of dogs have been affected with recurrent disease resembling the human disorder of familial Mediterranean fever.[217-219] Hepatic amyloid can be a complication in these dogs. In both the Shar Pei dog and Abyssinian cat, the deposits are composed of amyloid protein AA.

Clinical Signs

The clinical signs of amyloidosis reflect the functional disturbances due to its deposition in organs or tissues. Involvement of the liver is indicated by marked hepatomegaly, increased liver enzyme activity, jaundice, and ascites. Rarely,

an animal will present for spontaneous liver lobe hemorrhage causing hypovolemic shock or death.[219a,241a,b] Liver lobe bleeding is believed to be associated with increased tissue fragility attributed to vascular deposition of amyloid. It is unknown if an aquired coagulopathy coexists.

Cats with amyloidosis usually present for evaluation of inappetence, weight loss, polyuria, polydipsia, and poor hair coat. Physical examination may reveal the presence of normal- to small-sized kidneys with an irregular surface contour.

Dogs with renal amyloidosis usually present for evaluation of polyuria, polydipsia, and weight loss. Later in the course of their disease, azotemia and signs of uremia become apparent. Shar Pei dogs with systemic amyloidosis usually present for recurrent severe pyrexia, nonspecific pain, swollen joints, vague gastrointestinal distress, diarrhea, polyuria, and polydipsia. Breeders refer to this syndrome as "Shar Pei fever" and it has been estimated that as many as 18% of Shar Peis are affected. Typically, fevers range between 104° to 107° and last from 12 to 36 hours. During this time the dog is lethargic, painful, and reluctant to move.[218,219] Some dogs have episodes of fever only in their youth; most dogs initially become symptomatic during the first year of life. Dogs with severe hepatic involvement or the nephrotic syndrome may present with ascites and/or edema. Hepatomegaly may be noted when hepatic involvement is marked. In some dogs, other inflammatory liver disorders and a glucocorticoid or vacuolar hepatopathy have been coexistent and contribute to hepatomegaly and clinical signs.

Clinicopathologic Features

In cats with systemic amyloidosis, clinicopathologic tests indicate the presence of impaired renal function. Cats with hepatic involvement may show mild increases in liver enzymes, and when deposition is severe, become hyperbilirubinemic.

Most dogs develop pathologic proteinuria. The urinalysis may or may not reveal active sediment (hyaline, granular or waxy casts, and increased WBCs and RBCs). The urine protein:creatinine ratio is markedly increased and may be more than 10. As the renal disorder progresses, hypoalbuminemia, hypercholesterolemia, and third space fluid sequestration may become apparent and the magnitude of the urine protein loss increases. Thromboembolism and renal insufficiency develop later in the course of the disease.

Microcytosis is frequent in affected Shar Peis but is also common in Shar Peis with other disorders; approximately 60% to 70% of Shar Peis seen by the author for a variety of disorders have been microcytic. An inflammatory leukogram is present in many dogs with systemic amyloidosis. Some dogs have a left-shifted leukogram associated with a high fever, suggesting the presence of infection. However, it appears that some of these dogs are merely responding to inflammatory mediators or cytokines associated with their immunoreactive disorder. Some Shar Pei dogs only develop a medullary interstitial renal deposition of amyloid.

Marked hepatomegaly may develop in the presence of minimal alterations in liver function. Initially the hepatic deposition of amyloid produces little injury and so the liver enzymes and total bilirubin concentration may remain within the normal range. With increasing severity of deposition, sinusoidal flow becomes impaired. Abdominal radiography may disclose the presence of hepatomegaly. Abdominal ultrasonography reveals a diffuse homogeneous hypoechogenic parenchyma.

In dogs with systemic amyloidosis, it has been suggested

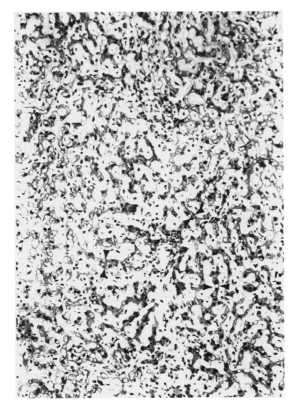

FIGURE 34-22. Photomicrograph showing the distribution of amyloid in the liver of a Shar Pei with relapsing fevers and joint pain. Amyloid is distributed diffusely in the space of Disse and appears as a pale gray amorphous material that virtually fills the sinusoid. Small nuclei seen within the sinusoidal space represent blood cells traversing the narrowed channel. Arrowheads indicate the location of three cords of hepatic cells for orientation. This dog had massive hepatomegaly (H&E, 140× magnification).

that colonic pinch biopsy or bone marrow aspiration may disclose the presence of amyloid deposition as it can in humans with systemic reactive amyloidosis.[220,221] In this circumstance, the deduction of hepatic involvement may be possible on the basis of other clinicopathologic and physical signs. In humans, amyloid can be diagnosed with fine needle aspirate of abdominal fat (in systemic amyloidosis) and liver tissue.[222,223] Efforts to duplicate these findings in Shar Pei dogs have not been successful.

Hepatic Histopathology

A liver diffusely infiltrated with amyloid is usually large, firm, and has a normal or pale color. Distribution occurs in two general lobular areas: (1) involvement of blood vessels in the portal triads, and (2) diffuse deposition in the perisinusoidal space of Disse. A liver severely infiltrated with diffuse amyloidosis in a Shar Pei dog is shown in Figure 34–22. In humans, there is no stepwise gradation from one hepatic pattern of deposition to another. Either distribution may appear independently. Massive intralobular amyloid distribution causes sinusoidal obstruction and compression of adjacent hepatocytes. Hepatic cords may undergo atrophy and individual hepatocytes may drop out (see Figure 34–22).

Hepatic amyloid deposition in the Abyssinian cat usually involves vessels within the portal triads, the area around the central veins, and extension into the space of Disse along sinusoids. In some cats, a mild periportal infiltration with lymphocytes and plasma cells and a mild multifocal hepatocellular necrosis also develops. A specific predisposing inflammatory disease has been found in some but not all affected cats.

Shar Pei dogs may develop hepatic amyloidosis involving the vessels of the portal triads as well as distribution in the space of Disse. Other tissues also are involved. Unlike other dogs with amyloidosis, Shar Peis with renal amyloidosis usually develop medullary involvement similar to the Abyssinian cat, although some dogs also develop typical canine glomerular involvement.

Treatment

The treatment of amyloidosis should focus on three approaches, including (1) supportive care for the organ dysfunction resulting from amyloid deposition; (2) efforts to control or eradicate any primary underlying infectious, inflammatory, or neoplastic conditions; and (3) attempts to block further amyloid deposition and to mobilize already established amyloid protein. Despite these considerations and the discussion that follows, the prognosis for animals with diffuse hepatic involvement is dismal because there is no reliable medical therapy for systemic or hepatic amyloidosis.[224]

Supportive care for hepatic insufficiency should be tailored to the individual patient and should follow the principles outlined in Chapter 33. Administration of prophylactic antimicrobials may be necessary if the patient shows signs of inflammatory bowel disease, a leukogram indicating possible sepsis, or recurrent pyrexia. Unfortunately, fevers commonly will cycle in association with the immune dysregulation underlying the amyloid formation and may not reflect infection.

A thorough diagnostic evaluation should be undertaken to discover any underlying primary disease process that may be amenable to treatment. If occult neoplasia is suspected, thoracic radiographs, lymph node aspirates, abdominal ultrasonography, and bone marrow aspirate should be evaluated. If an infectious disease seems possible, specific tests for antibody titers or antigenemia should be undertaken. Evaluation of joints for effusion or pain may indicate the presence of polyarthropathy. If such is suspected, arthrocentesis should be done and synovial fluid cultured and cytologically evaluated. Tests for autoimmunity, such as an antinuclear antibody, rheumatoid factor, and thyroid antibodies, should be submitted if no other disease process is defined. If hyperglobulinemia is detected, a cellulose acetate electrophoresis may disclose the presence of a monoclonal gammopathy suggestive of a globulin-producing plasmacytic or lymphoplasmacytic neoplasia.

Treatments aimed at limiting the deposition of amyloid have not been routinely successful in humans or in animal models of systemic or reactive amyloidosis. Immunosuppressive therapy and chemotherapy have been used with occasional benefit in humans with AL amyloid. In a few cases, treatment of primary underlying inflammatory disorders or suppression of an inflammatory process has led to curtailed amyloid deposition and resorption in patients with reactive amyloidosis.[225,226]

Colchicine has shown benefit in the treatment of humans with familial Mediterranean fever and in a murine model of amyloidosis.[201,224,227] Use of colchicine should most benefit animals with familial amyloidosis early in the disease process. However, later use might also control further amyloid deposition. Controlled trials in veterinary patients have not yet been completed with colchicine. A daily dose of no greater than 0.03 mg/kg body weight is recommended for the dog; the author has used this dose without adverse effects in dogs with developing hepatic fibrosis/cirrhosis. Overdosage results in gastroenteric toxicity typified by hemorrhagic diarrhea and vomiting. There is no experience with colchicine in the cat.

Some therapeutic trials of dimethylsulfoxide (DMSO) in laboratory animals with systemic reactive amyloidosis have produced encouraging results.[228–235] Use of large doses of DMSO has caused partial or total disappearance of amyloid deposits in the murine casein-induced amyloid model and a reduced incidence and degree of amyloidosis in a mouse model of spontaneous amyloidosis.[229,231,232] Experimental work with DMSO has shown that it can split amyloid fibrils in vitro and in vivo.[228] DMSO has not been consistently impressive as a therapeutic agent in clinical trials in humans.[234–236] Anecdotally, some dogs treated with DMSO for management of renal amyloidosis (80 mg/kg SQ three times weekly; 125 mg/kg PO BID) have survived for several years when the disease was diagnosed before azotemia was established.[237,238] However, considerable doubt remains regarding the many clinical reports that suggest a beneficial response to DMSO in experimental animals and clinical patients with renal amyloidosis.[239]

Use of glucocorticoids in the treatment of amyloidosis is controversial. One experimental study showed that glucocorticoids accelerate amyloid deposition in a model of reactive amyloidosis.[201] A similar effect was suggested in humans.[201,240] However, if an underlying disease is considered responsive to glucocorticoids, a trial course of therapy should be considered.

If an associated immunocyte dyscrasia is documented, use of glucocorticoids and cytotoxic drugs such as the alkylating agent melphalen should be used as appropriate.[201] Cytotoxic agents have also been used to treat amyloid associated with collagen vascular disorders in humans.

HEMOSIDEROSIS

Clinical Synopsis

Diagnostic Features

- Signs usually relate to underlying hepatic or hematologic condition
- Liver dysfunction usually subclinical, but mildly elevated liver enzymes and hypoalbuminemia may occur in extreme cases
- Liver biopsy reveals excessive hemosiderin and minimal inflammation
- Cirrhosis can develop in experimental models of the disease

Standard Treatment

- Attend to primary cause of underlying hepatic or hematologic disease
- In severe cases, phlebotomy or deferoxamine (40 mg/kg IM TID for 7 days) can be used

The liver is the major organ that stores iron. In normal dogs, the mean hepatic iron content approximates 1000 µg/g dry weight tissue (range 311–1579).[241] Most of the nonheme iron is stored in the form of ferritin, the soluble form of iron located in hepatocytes. This iron is mainly derived from circulating iron bound to transferrin. Ferritin functions as a readily available iron depot that makes iron continuously available for reutilization. Heme iron, derived from effete erythrocytes and hemolysis, tends to be stored in Kupffer cells as hemosiderin, an insoluble aggregate form of iron. Iron mobilized from senescent erythrocytes is stored in the liver until reused for hemoglobin synthesis. In the storage pool, iron is kept in balance with utilization needs. If erythrogenesis is not balanced with hepatic iron deposition, iron tends to accumulate. (See Chapter 30 for a detailed review of iron metabolism.)

Hemosiderosis refers to the deposition of visible iron pigments in tissue. The accumulation of hepatic hemosiderin can occur as a primary or secondary phenomenon. Primary hemosiderosis results from excessive iron uptake or administration. Secondary hemosiderosis is usually related to hepatic inflammation, hemolysis, or repeated blood transfusions.

Primary hemosiderosis from chronic low-dose parenteral iron loading (injection of iron dextran or iron sorbital over 1 to 2 years) in dogs and baboons leads to hepatic fibrosis or cirrhosis.[242,243] Portal fibrosis and cirrhosis develops with only slight inflammation. The severity of fibrosis is proportional to the concentration of iron in the liver. Excessive iron accumulates in the hepatic parenchyma in this model. Iron accumulating within hepatocytes is more noxious than that deposited in Kupffer cells.

An important cause of primary hemosiderosis in humans is the inherited disorder of hemochromatosis. This is a unique disease for which there is no recognized animal counterpart. In this disorder, an excessive inappropriate absorption of dietary iron results in the progressive accumulation of storage iron in hepatocytes which eventually results in severe liver damage.

Secondary hemosiderosis is usually associated with increased Kupffer cell iron. Inflammatory hepatic disorders in which hemorrhage and inflammation result in focal areas of erythrocyte stagnation and injury can result in the accumulation of hemosiderin in lipogranulomata and adjacent to active inflammation. In Bedlington terriers with copper storage hepatopathy, the mean hepatic iron concentration is fourfold normal at 4000 µg/g dry weight (range 2197–6792). The hepatic iron concentration is also increased in Doberman pinschers with chronic active hepatitis. Small foci of lipogranulomata are also observed in animals with portosystemic shunts.

Tissue iron (hemosiderin) can be stained with Prussian blue for a crude estimation of hepatic iron storage. However, the relation between histochemical grading of tissue iron content and the quantitative hepatic iron content is not linear. A slight siderosis (iron storage) is common in normal canine and feline liver. Although animals with secondary iron "overload" accumulate iron predominantly in Kupffer cells, with progressive accumulation, hepatocellular iron accumulation also occurs.

The specific pathophysiologic mechanisms for hepatocyte iron toxicity and hepatic fibrosis are not known. However, two proposed theories explain its toxicity.[241,244] One theory focuses on the role of hemosiderin as a toxin destabilizing hepatocellular lysosomes. As iron accumulates, it is stored as hemosiderin in lysosomes.[245,246] When in excess, iron is released into the acidic intraorganelle compartment, lysosomal membranes are injured, and hydrolytic enzymes released into the cytosol. The alternative theory suggests a more general role for iron in causing peroxidative injury to fatty acids of membrane phospholipids. According to this theory, intracellular membrane damage initiates lysosomal instability and damage to cell organelles. It is proposed that a toxic threshold exists beyond which initiating injury occurs.

Iron Complex	Elemental Iron
Ferrous carbonate	48%
Ferric phosphate	37%
Ferrous sulfate (dry)	37%
Ferrous fumarate	33%
Ferrous sulfate (hydrate)	20%
Ferroglycine sulfate	16%
Peptonized iron	16%
Ferrous gluconate	12%

FIGURE 34-23. Amount of elemental iron provided by common iron salts.

Clinical Signs

Clinical signs of secondary hepatic hemosiderosis are related to the underlying hepatic or hematologic conditions.

Dogs given chronic parenteral iron causing experimental hemochromatosis develop small increases in their serum transaminase activities and hypoalbuminemia after 1 to 2 years of iron administration.[242] Once iron administration ceases, clinical signs do not progress.

Treatment

Treatment of animals with increased hepatic iron stores should include management of underlying conditions and avoidance of supplemental parenteral or oral iron products. Effective treatment of chronic active hepatitis in the Doberman pinscher has been associated with a diminution of hepatic iron stores. If iron stores are excessive, phlebotomy has been used as one method to remove iron. Feeding of a nutritionally replete diet with adequate vitamin supplementation is important. Dietary levels of iron are reduced to a minimum. In extreme cases, deferoxamine could be used, as recommended for persons with hemochromatosis.

ACUTE IRON TOXICITY

Acute toxicity with iron can occur when a massive dose of iron is given orally.[247] Doses of iron less than 20 mg/kg body weight are considered nontoxic, 20 to 60 mg/kg may cause mild to moderate toxicosis, and quantities exceeding 60 mg/kg are toxic. Dosages of more than 200 mg/kg are potentially lethal. Under normal circumstances, the rate-limiting factor for iron uptake is the saturable, carrier-mediated uptake of iron across the enterocyte. With massive overdosage, a passive, concentration-dependent absorption occurs. This results in increased circulatory concentrations of free or unbound iron. Acute iron toxicity leads to vomiting, diarrhea, depression, bloody stools, tremors, shock, and death. Clinical signs are related to hemorrhagic gastroenteritis, hepatic failure, metabolic acidemia, coagulation defects, and cardiovascular collapse. These effects are attributable to direct gastroenteric toxicity and to the presence of large amounts of unbound iron in the circulation. The most profound effects of acute iron toxicity are on the cardiovascular

system where it increases capillary permeability related to augmented release of serotonin and histamine. This leads to vascular stasis, reduced cardiac output, and compromised microcirculation. Hepatic necrosis and hepatocellular swelling are believed to be due to mitochondrial and microsomal injury. Coagulation defects have been attributed to an inhibition of thrombin generation and to hepatic injury. A severe metabolic acidosis is related to the microcirculatory collapse and to the conversion of ferrous to the ferric form of iron.

Diagnosis of acute iron toxicity is made on the basis of history, physical signs, and determination of the serum iron concentration. The amount of elemental iron provided by iron salts varies considerably (Figure 34–23). Dogs remaining asymptomatic for 6 hours after iron ingestion are considered free of toxicity. Measurement of serum iron that estimates the amount of iron bound to transferrin can be used to indicate the necessity for chelation. Values exceeding 500 µg/dl (normal 84 to 243 µg/dl), 4 to 6 hours after ingestion, are proposed to require chelation. Determination of the total iron-binding capacity has not been consistently reliable in the diagnosis of toxicosis. Abdominal radiographs may indicate the presence of large amounts of unabsorbed iron. In humans, hyperglycemia and leukocytosis commonly accompany increased serum iron concentrations.

Treatment of acute iron toxicity is directed to (1) stabilize the patient's vital signs, (2) decontaminate the gastrointestinal tract, and (3) remove excessive circulating iron by chelation. Activated charcoal does not effectively bind iron. Chelation with deferoxamine (Desferal; Ciba Giegy) has been recommended. In the severely poisoned dog, a continuous IV infusion of 15 mg/kg per hour has been recommended.[247] Care must be exercised to avoid more rapid administration because it may cause cardiac arrhythmias and aggravation of preexistent hypotension. Alternatively, deferoxamine can be given IM at 40 mg/kg every 4 to 8 hours. Chelation is continued until the patient's serum iron concentration is less than 350 µg/dl. This may require 2 to 3 days of treatment.

REFERENCES

1. Hoyumpa AM, Greene HL, Dunn GD, et al. Fatty liver: Biochemical and clinical considerations. Digest Dis 20:1142–1170, 1975.
2. Cello JP, Grendell JH. The liver in systemic conditions. In: Zakim D, Boyer TD (eds) Hepatology, a Textbook of Liver Disease. WB Saunders, Philadelphia, 1411–1437, 1990.
3. Holdstock G, Millward-Sadler GH, Wright R. Hepatic changes in systemic disease. In: Wright R, et al. (eds). Liver and Biliary Disease, 2nd ed. WB Saunders, Philadelphia, 1033–1076, 1985.
4. Smuckler EA. Patterns of reaction of the liver to injury. In: Zakim D, Boyer TD (eds). Hepatology, a Textbook of Liver Disease. WB Saunders, Philadelphia, 681–692, 1982.
5. Vierling JM. Hepatobiliary complications of ulcerative colitis and Crohn's disease. In: Zakim D, Boyer TD (eds) Hepatology, a Textbook of Liver Disease. WB Saunders, Philadelphia, 797–824, 1982.
6. Drenick EJ, Fisler J, Johnson D. Hepatic steatosis after intestinal bypass: Prevention and reversal by metronidazole, irrespective of protein calorie malnutrition. Gastroenterology 82:535–548, 1982.
7. Quigley EMM, Zetterman RK. Hepatobiliary complications of malabsorption and malnutrition. Sem Liver Dis 8:218–228, 1988.
8. Klein S, Nealon WH. Hepatobiliary abnormalities associated with total parenteral nutrition. Sem Liver Dis 8:237–246, 1988.
9. Gerloff BJ, Herdt TH. Hepatic lipidosis from dietary restriction in nonlactating cows. J Am Vet Med Assoc 185:223–224, 1984.
10. Herdt TH, Gerloff BJ. Hepatic lipidosis and liver function in 49 cows with displaced abomasums. Proc XIIth World Congress on Diseases of Cattle, the Netherlands, Vol. I, 522–526, 1982.
11. Gerloff BJ, Herdt TH, Emery RS, et al. Inositol as a lipotropic agent in dairy cattle diets. J Anim Sci 59:806–812, 1984.
12. Murray M. Hepatic lipidosis in a post parturient mare. Equine Vet J 17:68–69, 1985.
13. van der Linde-Sipman JS, van den Ingh TSGAM, van Toor AJ. Fatty liver syndrome in puppies. Am Anim Hosp Assoc 26:91–12, 1990.
14. van Toor AJ, van der Linde-Sipman, van der Ingh TSGAM, et al. Experi-

mental induction of fasting hypoglycaemia and fatty liver syndrome in three Yorkshire terrier pups. Vet Q 13:16–23, 1991.

15. Barsanti JA, Jones BD, Spano JS, et al. Prolonged anorexia associated with hepatic lipidosis in three cats. Fel Pract, 52–57, May 1977.

16. Burrows CF, Chiapella AM, Jezyk P. Idiopathic feline hepatic lipidosis: The syndrome and speculations on its pathogenesis. Florida Vet J, 18–20, Winter 1981.

17. Thornburg LP, Simpson S, Digilio K. Fatty liver syndrome in cats. J Am Anim Hosp Assoc 18:397–400, 1982.

18. Pritchard DH, Jolly RD, Howell LJ, et al. Ceroid-lipidosis: An acquired storage-type disease of liver and hepatic lymph node. Vet Pathol 20:242–244, 1983.

19. Zawie D, Garvey MS. Feline hepatic disease. Vet Clin N Am 14:1201–1230, 1984.

20. Center SA. Hepatic lipidosis in the cat. Proc 4th ACVIM Forum 13:71–79, 1986.

21. Biourge V, MacDonald MJ, King L. Case report feline hepatic lipidosis: Pathogenesis and nutritional management. Comp Cont Educ Pract Vet 12:1244–1258, 1990.

22. Center SA, Thompson M, Wood PA, et al. Hepatic ultrastructural and metabolic derangements in cats with severe hepatic lipidosis. Proc 9th ACVIM Forum, 193–196, 1991.

23. Hubbard BS, Vulgamott JC. Feline hepatic lipidosis. Comp Contin Ed 14:459–463, 1992.

24. Adams LG, Hardy RM, Weiss DJ, et al. Hypophosphatemia and hemolytic anemia associated with diabetes mellitus and hepatic lipidosis in cats. J Vet Int Med 7:266–271, 1993.

25. Center SA, Crawford MA, Guida L, et al. A retrospective study of cats (n = 77) with severe hepatic lipidosis: 1975–1990. J Vet Int Med 7:349–359, 1993.

26. Biourge V, Pion P, Lewis J, et al. Spontaneous occurrence of hepatic lipidosis in a group of laboratory cats. J Vet Int Med 7:194–197, 1993.

27. Akol KG, Washabau RJ, Saunders HM, et al. Acute pancreatitis in cats with hepatic lipidosis. J Vet Int Med 7:205–209, 1993.

28. Hall JA, Barstad LA, Voller BE, et al. Lipid composition of liver and adipose tissues from normal cats and cats with hepatic lipidosis (abstract). Proc 10th ACVIM Forum, 810, 1992.

29. Read AE. The liver and drugs. In: Wright R, et al. (eds) Liver and Biliary Disease, 2nd ed. WB Saunders, Philadelphia, 1003–1032, 1985.

30. Cooper AD. Hepatic lipoprotein and cholesterol metabolism. In: Zakim D, Boyer TD (eds) Hepatology, a Textbook of Liver Disease. WB Saunders, Philadelphia, 109–138, 1982.

31. Rogers QR, Morris JF, Freedland RA. Lack of hepatic enzymatic adaptation to low and high levels of dietary protein in the adult cat. Enzyme 22:348–356, 1977.

32. MacDonald ML, Rogers QR, Morris JG. Nutrition of the domestic cat, a mammalian carnivore. Ann Rev Nutr 4:521–562, 1984.

33. Dimski DS, Buffington CA, Johnson SE, et al. Serum lipoprotein concentrations and hepatic lesions in obese cats undergoing weight loss. Am J Vet Res 53:1259–1262, 1992.

34. Lombardi B, Oler A. Choline deficiency fatty liver, protein synthesis and release. Lab Invest 17:308–321, 1967.

35. Lombardi B, Pant P, Schlunk FF. Choline-deficiency fatty liver: Impaired release of hepatic triglycerides. J Lipid Res 9:437–446, 1968.

36. Holub BJ. The nutritional importance of inositol and the phosphoinositides. N Engl J Med 326:1285–1288, 1992.

37. Holub BJ. The nutritional significance, metabolism and function of myoinositol and phosphatidylinositol in health and disease. In: Draper HH (ed) Advances in Nutrition Research, Vol. 4. Plenum, New York, 107–141, 1982.

38. Wells WW, Burton LE. Requirement for dietary myo-inositol in the lactating rat. In: Wells WW, Eisenberg F, Jr (eds) Cyclitrols and Phosphoinositides. Academic Press, New York, 471–485, 1978.

39. McHenry EW, Patterson JM. Lipotropic factors. Physiol Rev 24:128, 1944.

40. Drill VA. Lipotropic effects of vitamin B$_{12}$ and other factors. Ann NY Acad Sci 57:654–663, 1954.

41. Van Lancker JL. Molecular and cellular mechanisms in disease. Springer-Verlag, Berlin-Heidelberg, 284–293, 1976.

42. Frank A, Feinstein RE. Hepatic lipidosis associated with severe vitamin B$_{12}$ deficiency recognized by liver cobalt status in three cats. Fel Pract 19:16–20, 1991.

43. Vaden SL, Wood PA, Ledley FD, et al. Cobalamin deficiency associated with methylmalonic acidemia in a cat. J Am Vet Med Assoc 200:1101–1103, 1992.

44. Golden MHN, Ramdath D. Free radicals in the pathogenesis of kwashiorkor. Proc Nutr Soc 46:53–68, 1987.

45. Lippert AC, Faulkner JE, Evans TA, et al. Total parenteral nutrition in clinically sound cats. J Am Vet Med Assoc 194:669–676, 1989.

46. Alpers D H, Isselbacher KJ. Fatty liver: Biochemical and clinical aspects. In: Schiff L (ed) Diseases of the Liver, 5th ed. JG Lippincott, Philadelphia, 815–832, 1975.

47. MacDonald ML, Anderson BC, Rogers QR, et al. Essential fatty acid requirements of cats: Pathology of essential fatty acid deficiency. Am J Vet Res 45:1310–1317, 1984.

48. Windmueller HG, Levy RI. Total inhibition of hepatic β-lipoprotein production in the rat by orotic acid. J Biol Chem 242:2246–2254, 1967.

49. Bauer JE. Feline lipid metabolism and hepatic lipidosis. Feline Medicine. Proc 12th Ann Kal Kan Symposium for Treatment of Small Animal Diseases, 75–78, 1988.

50. Milner JA, Prior RL, Visnek WJ. Arginine deficiency and orotic aciduria in mammals. Proc Soc Exp Biol Med 150:282–288, 1975.

51. Dimski DS, Toboada J, Taylor HW, et al. Preliminary study of orotic acid induction of hepatic lipidosis in cats (abstract). Proc 9th ACVIM Forum, 886, 1991.

52. Dimski DS. Idiopathic hepatic lipidosis: A research update. Proc 11th ACVIM Forum, 198–201, 1993.

53. Biourge V, Groff JM, Kirk CA, et al. Induction of hepatic lipidosis in cats by voluntary fasting. Proc 11th ACVIM Forum, 948, 1993.

54. Dow SW, LeCouteur RA, Poss ML, et al. Central nervous system toxicosis associated with metronidazole treatment of dogs: Five cases (1984–1987). J Am Vet Med Assoc 195:365–368, 1989.

55. Kaufman AC, Greene CE. Increased alanine transaminase activity associated with tetracycline administration in a cat. J Am Vet Med Assoc 202:628–630, 1993.

56. Freneaux E, Gilles L, Letteron P, et al. Inhibition of the mitochondrial oxidation of fatty acids by tetracycline in mice and man: Possible role in microvesicular steatosis induced by this antibiotic. Hepatology 8:1056–1062, 1988.

57. Breen KJ, Schenker S, Heimberg M. Effect of tetracycline on the metabolism of (1-^{14}C) oleate by the liver. Biochem Pharmacol 28:197–200, 1979.

58. Gwee MCE. Can tetracycline-induced fatty liver in pregnancy be attributed to choline deficiency? Med Hypotheses 9:157–162, 1982.

59. Hansen CH, Pearson LH, Schenker S, et al. Impaired secretion of triglycerides by the liver: A cause of tetracycline-induced fatty liver. Proc Soc Exp Biol Med 128:143–146, 1968.

60. Romert P, Matthiessen ME. Tetracycline-induced changes in hepatocytes of mini-pigs and mini-pig foetuses as revealed by electron microscopy. Acta Pathol Microbiol Immunol Scand 94:125–131, 1986.

61. Rebouche CJ, Engel AG. Carnitine metabolism and deficiency syndromes. Mayo Clin Proc 58:533–540, 1983.

62. Bremer J. Carnitine metabolism and its functions. Physiol Rev 63:1420–1480, 1983.

63. Buechler KF, Lowenstein JM. The involvement of carnitine intermediates in peroxisomal fatty acid oxidation: A study with 2-bromofatty acids. Arch Biochem and Biophys 281:233–238, 1990.

64. Van Hoof F, Vamecq J, Draye J-P, et al. The catabolism of medium- and long-chain dicarboxylic acids. Biochem Soc Trans 16:423–424, 1988.

65. Snoswell AM, Henderson GD. Carnitine metabolism in ruminant animals. In: Frenkel RA, McGarry JK (eds) Carnitine Biosynthesis, Metabolism and Functions. Academic Press, New York, 191–205, 1980.

66. Mitchell ME. Carnitine metabolism in human subjects. III. Metabolism in disease. Am J Clin Nutr 31:645–659, 1978.

67. Frohlich J, Seccombe DW, Hahn P, et al. Effect of fasting on free and esterified carnitine levels in humans' serum and urine: Correlation with serum levels of free fatty acids and β-hydroxybutyrate. Metabolism 27:555–561, 1978.

68. Siliprnadi N, Lisa FC, Menabo R. Clinical use of carnitine: Past, present and future. In: Grisolia S, et al. (eds) Cirrhosis, Hepatic Encephalopathy, and Ammonium Toxicity. Plenum Press, New York, 175–181, 1990.

69. O'Conneer JE, Costell M. New roles of carnitine metabolism in ammonia cytotoxicity. In: Grisolia S, et al. (eds) Cirrhosis, Hepatic Encephalopathy, and ammonium toxicity. Plenum Press, New York, 183–195, 1990.

70. Engel AG, Rebouche CJ. Carnitine metabolism and inborn errors. J Inher Metab Dis 7(suppl) 1:38–43, 1984.

71. Chapoy PR, Angelini C, Broren WJ, et al. Systemic carnitine deficiency: A treatable inherited lipid-storage disease presenting as Reye's syndrome. N Engl J Med 303:1389, 1980.

72. Treem WR, Stanley CA, Finegold DN, et al. Primary carnitine deficiency due to a failure of carnitine transport in kidney, muscle and fibroblasts. N Engl J Med 319:1331–1336, 1988.

73. Hahn P, Skala JP. The effect of starvation on obese mice. Can J Physiol Pharmacol 59:355–357, 1981.

74. Jacobs G, Cornelius L, Keene B, et al. Comparison of plasma, liver and skeletal muscle carnitine concentrations in cats with idiopathic hepatic lipidosis and in healthy cats. Am J Vet Res 51:1349–1351, 1990.

75. Hoppel CL, Genuth SM. Carnitine metabolism in normal weight and obese human subjects with fasting. Am J Physiol 238:E409–E415, 1980.

76. Brass EP, Hoppel CL. Carnitine metabolism in the fasting rat. J Biol Chem 253:2688–2693, 1978.

77. Brady LJ, Brady PS, Albers L, et al. Carnitine metabolism in lean and obese Zucker rats during starvation. J Nutr 116:668–674, 1986.

78. Goa KL, Brogden RN. L-carnitine: A preliminary review of its pharmacokinetics and its therapeutic use in ischemic cardiac disease and primary and secondary carnitine deficiencies in relationship to its role in fatty acid metabolism. Drugs 34:1–24, 1987.

79. Armstrong PJ, Hardie EM, Cullen JM, et al. L-carnitine reduces hepatic fat accumulation during rapid weight reduction in cats (abstract). Proc 10th ACVIM Forum, 810, 1992.

80. Mannaerts GP, van Veldhoven PP. The peroxisome: Functional properties in health and disease. Biochem Soc Trans 18:87–89, 1990.

81. Mannaerts GP, Debeer IJ. Mitochondrial and peroxisomal β-oxidation of fatty acids in rat liver. In: Kindl H, Lazarow PB (eds) Peroxisomes and Glyoxysomes. Annals of the New York Academy of Sciences, New York, 30–38, 1982.

82. Buechler KF, Lowenstein JM. The involvement of carnitine intermediates in peroxisomal fatty acid oxidation: A study with 2-bromofatty acids. Arch Biochem Biophys 281:233–238, 1990.

83. Center SA, Guida L, Zanelli MJ, et al. Ultrastructural hepatocellular features associated with severe hepatic lipidosis in cats. Am J Vet Res 54:724–731, 1993.

84. Canonico PG, Rill W, Ayala E. Effects of inflammation on peroxisomal enzyme activities, catalase synthesis and lipid metabolism. Lab Invest 37:479–486, 1977.

85. Goldfisher S, Reddy JK. Peroxisomes (microbodies) in cell pathology. Int Rev Exp Pathol 26:45–84, 1984.

86. Thrall MA, Mitchell T, Lappin M, et al. Cholesteryl ester storage disease in two cats. In: Proc 42nd Annual Meeting ACVP, 17, 1991.

87. Thompson JC, Johnstone AC, Jones BR, et al. The ultrastructural pathology of five lipoprotein lipase-deficient cats. J Comp Pathol 101:251–262, 1989.

88. Jones BR, Johnstone AC, Hancock WS. Inherited hyperchylomicronaemia in the cat. Vet Ann 26:330–340, 1986.

89. Jones BR, Johnstone AC, Cahill JI, et al. Peripheral neuropathy in cats with inherited primary hyperchylomicronaemia. Vet Rec 119:268–272, 1986.

90. Christopher MM, Lee SE. Red cell morphologic alterations in cats with hepatic disease. Vet Clin Pathol 23:7–12, 1994.

91. Center SA, Dillingham S, Baldwin BH, et al. Serum gamma glutamyl transferase and alkaline phosphatase in cats with hepatobiliary disease. J Am Vet Med Assoc 188:507–510, 1986.

92. Back P, Hamprecht B, Lynen F. Regulation of cholesterol biosynthesis in rat liver: Diurnal changes of activity and influence of bile acids. Arch Biochem Biophys 133:11–21, 1969.

93. Weis HJ, Dietschy JM. The interaction of various control mechanisms in determining the rate of cholesterogenesis in the rat. Biochim Biophys Acta 398:315–324, 1975.

94. Center SA, Thompson M, Guida L. 3 α-hydroxylated bile acid profiles in clinically normal cats, cats with severe hepatic lipidosis, and cats with complete extrahepatic bile duct occlusion. Am J Vet Res 54:681–688, 1993.

95. Yeager AE, Mohammed HO. Accuracy of ultrasonography in the detection of severe hepatic lipidosis in cats. Am J Vet Res 53:597–599, 1992.

96. Crowe DT. Nutritional support for the hospitalized patient: An introduction to tube feeding. Compend Cont Ed Pract Vet 12:1711–1720, 1990.

97. Bright RM. Percutaneous tube gastrostomy. In: Bojrab MJ. (ed.) Current Techniques in Small Animal Surgery, 3rd ed. Lea & Febiger, Philadelphia, 221–224, 1990.

98. Morris AR, Rogers QR. Nutritional implications of some metabolic anomalies of the cat. Proc Amer Anim Hosp Assoc, 325–332, 1983.

99. Stewart PM, Batshaw M, Valle D, et al. Effects of arginine-free meals on ureagenesis in cats. Am J Physiol 241:E310–E315, 1981.

100. Lewis LD, Morris ML, Hand MS. Small Animal Clinical Nutrition III. Mark Morris Associates, Topeka, 1-3–1-25, 4-1–4-12, 12-1–12-15, 1987.

101. Buffington CAT. Nutritional diseases and nutritional therapy. In: Sherding RG (ed.) The Cat: Diseases and Clinical Management, 2nd ed. Churchill Livingstone, New York, 161–190, 1994.

102. Bode JC, Hanisch P, Henning H, et al. Hepatic zinc content in patients with various stages of alcoholic liver disease and in patients with chronic active and chronic persistent hepatitis. Hepatology 8:1605–1609, 1988.

103. Kahn AM, Helwig HL, Redeker AG, et al. Urine and serum zinc abnormalities in disease of the liver. Am J Clin Pathol 44:426–435, 1965.

104. Cossack ZT, Prasad AS. Hyperammonemia in zinc deficiency: Activities of urea cycle related enzymes. Nutr Res 7:1161–1167, 1987.

105. Badylak SF, Van Vleet JF. Sequential morphologic and clinicopathologic alterations in dogs with experimentally induced glucocorticoid hepatopathy. Am J Vet Res 42:1310–1318, 1981.

106. Dorner JL, Hoffmann WE, Long GB. Corticosteroid induction of an isoenzyme of alkaline phosphatase in the dog. Am J Vet Res 35:1457–1458, 1974.

107. Eckersall PD, Nash AS. Isoenzymes of canine plasma alkaline phosphatase: An investigation using isoelectric focusing and related diagnosis. Res Vet Sci 34:310–314, 1983.

108. Bengmark S, Olsson R. Elimination of alkaline phosphatases from serum in dog after intravenous injection of canine phosphatases from bone and intestine. Acta Chir Scand 140:1–6, 1974.

109. Hoffmann WE, Dorner JL. A comparison of canine normal hepatic alkaline phosphatase and variant alkaline phosphatase of serum and liver. Clin Chim Acta 62:137–142, 1975.

110. Hoffmann WE, Dorner JL. Separation of isoenzymes of canine alkaline phosphatase by cellulose acetate electrophoresis. J Am Anim Hosp Assoc 11:283–285, 1975.

111. Hoffmann WE. Diagnostic value of canine serum alkaline phosphatase

112. Hoffman WE, Dorner JL. Disappearance rate of intravenous injected canine alkaline phosphatase isoenzymes. Am J Vet Res 38:1553–1555, 1977.

113. Everett RM, Duncan JR, Prasse KW. Alkaline phosphatase in tissues and sera of cats. Am J Vet Res 38:1533–1538, 1977.

114. Hoffman WE, Renegar WE, Dorner JL. Alkaline phosphatase and alkaline phospatase isoenzymes in the cat. Vet Clin Pathol 6:21–24, 1977.

115. Hoffman WE, Dorner JL. Serum half-life of intravenously injected intestinal and hepatic alkaline phosphatase isoenzymes in the cat. Am J Vet Res 38:1637–1639, 1977.

116. Saini PK, Peavy GM, Hauser DE, et al. Diagnostic evaluation of canine serum alkaline phosphatase by immunochemical means and interpretation of results. Am J Vet Res 39:1514–1518, 1978.

117. McLain DL, Nagode LA, Wilson GP, et al. Alkaline phosphatase and its isoenzymes in normal cats and in cats with biliary obstruction. JAAHA 14:94–99, 1978.

118. Saini PK, Saini SK. Origin of serum alkaline phosphatase in the dog. Am J Vet Res 39:1510–1513, 1978.

119. Amacher DE, Smith DJ, Martz LK, et al. Characterization of alkaline phosphatase in canine serum. Enzyme 37:141–149, 1987.

120. Dorner JL, Hoffmann WE, Long GB. Corticosteroid induction of an isoenzyme of alkaline phosphatase in the dog. Am J Vet Res 35:1457–1458, 1974.

121. Wellman ML, Hoffmann WE, Dorner JL, et al. Comparison of the steroid-induced, intestinal, and hepatic isoenzymes of alkaline phosphatase in the dog. Am J Vet Res 43:1204–1207, 1982.

122. Wellman ML, Hoffmann WE, Dorner JL, et al. Immunoassay for the steroid-induced isoenzyme of alkaline phosphatase in the dog. Am J Vet Res 43:1200–1203, 1982.

123. Oluju MP, Eckersall PD, Douglas TA. Simple quantitative assay for canine steroid-induced alkaline phosphatase. Vet Rec 115:17–18, 1984.

124. Eckersall PD, Nash AS, Marshall GM, et al. The measurement of canine steroid-induced alkaline phosphatase by L-phenylalanine inhibition. J Sm Anim Pract 27:411–418, 1986.

125. Sanecki RK, Hoffman WE, Gelberg HB, et al. Subcellular location of corticosteroid-induced alkaline phosphatase in canine hepatocytes. Vet Pathol 24:296–301, 1987.

126. Sanecki RK, Hoffmann WE, Dorner JL, et al. Purification and comparison of corticosteroid-induced and intestinal isoenzymes of alkaline phosphatase in dogs. Am J Vet Res 51:1964–1968, 1990.

127. Hoffman WE, Sanecki RK, Dorner JL. A technique for automated quantification of canine glucocorticoid-induced isoenzyme of alkaline phosphatase. Vet Clin Pathol 66–70, 1991.

128. Solter PF, Hoffmann WE, Hungerford LL, et al. Assessment of corticosteroid-induced alkaline phosphatase isoenzyme as a screening test for hyperadrenocorticism in dogs. J Am Vet Med Assoc 203:534–538, 1993.

129. Teske E, Rothuizen J, de Bruijne JJ, et al. Corticosteroid-induced alkaline phosphatase isoenzyme in the diagnosis of canine hyperadrenocorticism. Vet Rec 125:12–14, 1989.

130. Wilson SM, Feldman EC. Diagnostic value of the steroid-induced isoenzyme of alkaline phosphatase in the dog. Am Anim Hosp Assoc 28:245–250, 1992.

131. Chastain CB, Franklin RT, Ganjam VK, et al. Evaluation of the hypothalamic pituitary-adrenal axis in clinically stressed dogs. J Am Anim Hosp Assoc 22:435–442, 1986.

132. Stephens DB. Stress and its measurement in domestic animals: A review of behavioral and physiological studies under field and laboratory situations. Adv Vet Sci Comp Med 24:179–210, 1980.

133. Schmidt RE, Booker JL. Effects of different surgical stresses on hematologic and blood chemistry values in dogs. J Am Anim Hosp Assoc 191:1212–1215, 1982.

134. Fielder FG, Hoff EJ, Thomas GB. A study of the subacute toxicity of prednisolone, methylprednisolone, and triamcinalone in dogs. Toxicol Appl Pharmacol 1:305–314, 1959.

135. Thompson SW, Sparano BM, Diener RM. Vacuoles in the hepatocytes of cortisone-treated dogs. Am J Pathol 63:135–148, 1971.

136. Dillon AR, Spano JS, Powers RD. Prednisolone induced hematologic, biochemical and histologic changes in the dog. J Am Anim Hosp Assoc 16:831–836, 1980.

137. Dillon AR, Sorjonen DC, Powers RD, et al. Effects of dexamethasone and surgical hypotension on hepatic morphologic features and enzymes in dogs. Am J Vet Res 44:1996–1999, 1983.

138. Rogers WA, Ruebner BH. A retrospective study of probable glucocorticoid-induced hepatopathy in dogs. J Am Vet Med Assoc 170:603–606, 1977.

139. Roberts SM, Lavach JD, Macy DW, et al. Effect of ophthalmic prednisolone acetate on the canine adrenal gland and hepatic function. Am J Vet Res 45:1711–1714, 1984.

140. Glaze MB, Crawford MA, Nachreiner RF, et al. Ophthalmic corticosteroid therapy: Systemic effects in the dog. J Am Vet Med Assoc 192:73–75, 1988.

141. Meyer DJ, Moriello KA, Feder BM, et al. Effect of otic medications containing glucocorticoids on liver function test results in healthy dogs. J Am Vet Med Assoc 196:743–744, 1990.

142. Moore GE, Mahaffey EA, Hoenig M. Hematologic and serum biochemical effects of long-term administration of anti-inflammatory doses of prednisone in dogs. Am J Vet Res 53:1033–1037, 1992.

143. Moriello KA, Fehrer-Sawyer SL, Meyer DJ, et al. Adrenocortical suppression associated with topical otic administration of glucocorticoids in dogs. J Am Vet Med Assoc 193:329–331, 1988.

144. Zenoble RD, Kemppainen RJ. Adrenocortical suppression by topically applied corticosteroids in healthy dogs. J Am Vet Med Assoc 191:685–688, 1987.

145. Kemppainen RJ, Lorenz MD, Thompson FN. Adrenocortical suppression in the dog after a single dose of methylprednisolone acetate. Am J Vet Res 42:822–824, 1981.

146. Kemppainen RJ, Lorenz MD, Thompson FN. Adrenocortical suppression in the dog given a single intramuscular dose of prednisone or triamcinolone acetonide. Am J Vet Res 42:204–206, 1982.

147. Scott DW, Kirk RW, Bentinck-Smith J. Some effects of short-term methylprednisolone therapy in normal cats. Cornell Vet 69:104–115, 1979.

148. Middleton DJ, Watson ADJ, Howe CJ, et al. Suppression of cortisol reponses to exogenous adrenocorticotrophic hormone, and the occurrence of side effects attributable to glucocorticoid excess, in cats during therapy with megestrol acetate and prednisolone. Can J Vet Res 51:60–65, 1987.

149. Fulton R, Thrall MA, Weiser MG, et al. Steroid hepatopathy in cats (platform presentation). Proc Am Soc Vet Clin Pathol, 23, 1988.

150. Scott DW, Manning TO, Reimers TJ. Iatrogenic Cushing's syndrome in the cat. Feline Pract 12:30–36, 1982.

151. Fittschen C, Bellamy JEC. Prednisone-induced morphologic and chemical changes in the liver of dogs. Vet Pathol 21:399–406, 1984.

152. Rothschild MA, Schreiber SS, Oratz M, et al. The effects of adrenocortical hormones on albumin metabolism studied with albumin-I[131]. J Clin Invest 37:1229–1235, 1958.

153. Bancroft FC, Levine L, Tashjian AH, Jr. Serum albumin production by hepatoma cells in culture: Direct evidence for stimulation by hydrocortisone. Biochem Biophys Res Commun 37:1028–1035, 1969.

154. DeNovo RC, Prasse KW. Comparison of serum biochemical and hepatic functional alterations in dogs treated with corticosteroids and hepatic duct ligation. Am J Vet Res 44:1703–1709, 1983.

155. Badylak SF, Van Vleet JF. Tissue γ-glutamyl transpeptidase activity and hepatic ultrastructural alterations in dogs with experimentally induced glucocorticoid hepatopathy. Am J Vet Res 43:649–655, 1982.

156. Hatoff DE, Hardison WGM. Bile acid–dependent secretion of alkaline phosphatase in rat bile. Hepatology 2:433–439, 1982.

157. Kako M, Toda G, Torii M, et al. Electron microscopic studies on hepatic alkaline phosphatase in experimentally induced biliary obstruction of the rat. Clin Sci 15:600–605, 1980.

158. Hadley SP, Hoffman WE, Kuhlenschmidt MS, et al. Effect of glucocorticoids on ALP, ALT and GGT in cultured dog hepatocytes. Enzyme 43:89–90, 1990.

159. Center SA, ManWarren T, Slater MR, et al. Evaluation of twelve-hour preprandial and two-hour postprandial serum bile acids concentrations for diagnosis of hepatobiliary disease in dogs. J Am Vet Med Assoc 199:217–226, 1991.

160. Roberts SM, Lavach JD, Macy DW, et al. Effect of ophthalmic prednisolone acetate on the canine adrenal gland and hepatic function. Am J Vet Res 45:1711–1714, 1984.

161. Rogers WA, Donovan EF, Kociba GJ. Idiopathic hyperlipoproteinemia in dogs. J Am Vet Med Assoc 166:1087–1091, 1975.

162. Rogers WA, Donovan EF, Kociba GJ. Lipids and lipoproteins in normal dogs and in dogs with secondary hyperlipoproteinemia. J Am Vet Med Assoc 166:1092–1100, 1975.

163. Bodkin K. Seizures associated with hyperlipoproteinemia in a miniature schnauzer. Canine Pract 17:11–15, 1992.

164. Whitney MS, Boon GD, Rebar AH, et al. Ultracentrifugal and electrophoretic characteristics of the plasma lipoproteins of miniature schnauzer dogs with idiopathic hyperlipoproteinemia. J Vet Int Med 7:253–260, 1993.

165. Watson P, Avella M, Simpson K, et al. Characterization of plasma apolipoproteins of briards with idiopathic hypercholestrolemia (abstract). Proc 11th ACVIM Forum, 948, 1994.

166. Havel RJ, Goldstein JL, Brown MS. Lipoproteins and lipid transport. In: Bondy PK, Rosenberg LE, (eds) Metabolic Control and Disease, 8th ed. WB Saunders, Philadelphia; 393–494, 1980.

167. Brunzell JD, Bierman EL. Chylomicronemia syndrome. Interaction of genetic and acquired hypertriglyceridemia. Med Clin N Am 66:455–468, 1982.

168. Schaefer EJ, Levy RI. Pathogenesis and management of lipoprotein disorders. N Engl J Med 312:1300–1310, 1985.

169. Brunzell JD, Miller NE, Alaupovic P, et al. Familial chylomicronemia due to a circulating inhibitor of lipoprotein lipase activity. J Lipid Res 24:12–19, 1983.

170. Nikkila EA. Familial lipoprotein lipase deficiency and related disorders of chylomicron metabolism. In: Stanbury JB, Wyngaarden JB, Frederickson DS, et al. (eds) The Metabolic Basis of Inherited Disease, 5th ed. McGraw-Hill, St. Louis, 622–642, 1983.

171. Phillipson BE, Rothrock DW, Connor WE, et al. Reduction of plasma lipids, lipoproteins, and apoproteins by dietary fish oils in patients with hypertriglyceridemia. N Engl J Med 312:1210–1216, 1985.

172. Mandelker L. New treatment for hyperlipidemia: Important steps to consider. Vet Forum, 46–47, July 1993.

173. Oates JA, Wood AJJ, Grundy SM. HMG-CoA reductase inhibitors for treatment of hypercholesterolemia. N Engl J Med 319:24–33, 1988.

174. Garg A, Grundy SM. Lovastatin for lowering cholesterol levels in non-insulin-dependent diabetes mellitus. N Engl J Med 318:81–86, 1988.

175. Walton DK, Center SA, Scott DW, et al. Ulcerative dermatosis associated with diabetes mellitus in the dog: A report of four cases. J Am Anim Hosp Assoc 22:79–88, 1986.

176. Turnwald GH, Foil CS, Solfsheimer KJ, et al. Failure to document hyperglucagonemia in a dog with diabetic dermatopathy resembling necrolytic migratory erythema. J Am Anim Hosp Assoc 25:363–369, 1989.

177. Miller WH, Scott DW, Buerger RG, et al. Necrolytic migratory erythema in dogs: A hepatocutaneous syndrome. J Am Anim Hosp Assoc 26:573–581, 1990.

178. Gross TL, O'Brien RD, Davis AP, et al. Glucagon-producing pancreatic endocrine tumors in two dogs with superficial necrolytic dermatitis. J Am Vet Med Assoc 197:1619–1622, 1990.

179. Gross TL, Song MD, Havel PJ, et al. Superficial necrolytic dermatitis (necrolytic migratory erythema) in dogs. Vet Pathol 30:75–81, 1993.

180. Doyle JA, Schroeter AL, Rogers RS. Hyperglucagonaemia and necrolytic migratory erythema in cirrhosis—possible pseudoglucagonoma syndrome. Br J Dermatol 100:581–587, 1979.

181. Boden G. Insulinoma and glucagonoma. Semin Oncol 14:253–262, 1987.

182. Goodenberger DM, Lawley TJ, Strober W, et al. Necrolytic migratory erythema without glucagonoma. Arch Dermatol 115:1429–1432, 1979.

183. Miller SJ. Nutritional deficiency and the skin. J Am Acad Dermatol 21:1–30, 1989.

184. Bhathena SJ, Higgins GA, Recant L. Glucagonoma and glucagnonoma syndrome. In: Unger RH, Orci L (eds) Glucagon: Physiology, Pathophysiology, and Morphology of the Pancreatic A-Cells. Elsevier, New York, 413–438, 1981.

185. Bloom SR, Polak JM. Glucogonoma syndrome. Am J Med 82:25–36, 1987.

186. Jaspan JB, Huen A, Morley CG, et al. The role of the liver in glucagon metabolism. J Clin Invest 60:421–428, 1977.

187. Johnson DG, Alberti KGMM. The liver and the endocrine system. In: Wright R, Millward-Sadler GH, Alberti KGMM, et al. (eds) Liver and Biliary Disease, 2nd ed. London: Bailliere Tindall, 161–188, 1985.

188. Van Thiel DA. The liver and the endocrine system. In: Arias IM, Jakoby WB, Popper H, et al. (eds) The Liver: Biology and Pathobiology, 2nd ed. Raven Press, New York, 1007–1032, 1988.

189. Valverde I, Dobbs R, Unger RH. Heterogeneity of plasma glucagon immunoreactivity in normal, depancreatized and alloxan-diagetic dogs. Metabolism 24:1021–1028, 1975.

190. Jaspan JB, Huen A, Morley CG, et al. The role of the liver in glucagon metabolism. J Clin Invest 60:421–428, 1977.

191. Conlon MJ. Molecular forms of the glucagon-like polypeptides (IRG and GLI) in tissues and plasma. In: Unger RH, Orci L (eds) Glucagon: Physiology, Pathophysiology, and Morphology of the Pancreatic A-Cells. Elsevier, New York, 55–75, 1981.

192. Kelly CP, Johnston CF, Nolan N, et al. Necrolytic migratory erythema with elevated plasma enteroglucagon in celiac disease. Gastroenterology 96:1350–1353, 1989.

193. Lothrop C, Jr. Medical treatment of neuroendocrine tumors of the gastroenteropancreatic system with somatostatin. In: Kirk RW (ed) Current Veterinary Therapy X. WB Saunders, Philadelphia, 1020–1024, 1989.

194. Johnstone AC, Jones BR, Thompson JC: The pathology of inherited hyperlipoproteinaemia of cats. J Comp Pathol 102:125–137, 1990.

195. Peritz LN, Brunzell JD, Harvey-Clarke C, et al. Characterization of a lipoprotein lipase class III type defect in hypertriglyceridemic cats. Clin Invest Med 13:259–263, 1990.

196. Jones BR, Wallace A, Harding DRK, et al. Occurrence of idiopathic, familial hyperchylomicronaemia in a cat. Vet Record 112:543–547, 1983.

197. Braund KG. Diseases of the nervous system: Degenerative and developmental diseases. In: Oliver JE, Hoerlein BF, Mayhew IG (eds) Veterinary Neurology. WB Saunders, Philadelphia, 185–187, 1987.

198. Walvoort HC, Dormans JA, van den Ingh TS. Comparative pathology of the canine model of glycogen storage disease Type III (Pompes disease). J Inherit Metab Dis 8:38–46, 1985.

199. Ceh L, Hauge JG, Svenkerud R, et al. Glycogenosis type III in the dog. Acta Vet Scand 17:210–222, 1976.

200. Rafiquzzaman M, Svenkerud R, Strande A, et al. Glycogenosis in the dog. Acta Vet Scand 17:196–209, 1976.

201. Glenner GG. Amyloid deposits and amyloidosis: The β-fibrilloses. N Engl J Med 302:1283–1292, 1333–1343, 1980.

202. Slauson DO, Gribble DH, Russel SW. A clinicopathological study of renal amyloidosis in dogs. J Comp Path 80:335–343, 1979.

203. Dibartola SP, Tarr MJ, Parker AT, et al. Clinicopathologic findings in dogs

with renal amyloidosis: 59 cases (1976–1986). J Am Vet Med Assoc 195:358–364, 1989.

204. Osborne CA, Johnson KH, Perman V, et al. Renal amyloidosis in the dog. J Am Vet Med Assoc 153:660–688, 1968.

205. Sherwood BF, Lemay JC, Castellanos RA. Blastomycosis with secondary amyloidosis in the dog. J Am Vet Med Assoc 150:1377–1381, 1967.

206. Thornburg LP, Moody GM. Hepatic amyloidosis in a dog. J Am Anim Hosp Assoc 17:721–723, 1981.

207. Van Rijswijk MH, Van Heudsen CWGJ. The potassium permanganate method: A reliable method for differentiating amyloid AA from other forms of amyloid in routine laboratory practice. Am J Pathol 97:43–58, 1979.

208. Chopra S, Rubinow A, Kopf RS, et al. Hepatic amyloidosis: A histopathologic analysis of primary (AL) and secondary (AA) forms. Am J Pathol 115:186–193, 1984.

209. Boyce JT, DiBartola SP, Chew DJ, et al. Familial renal amyloidosis in Abyssinian cats. Vet Pathol 21:33–38, 1984.

210. Crowell WA, Goldston RT, Schall WD, et al. Generalized amyloidosis in a cat. J Am Vet Med Assoc 161:1127–1133, 1972.

211. Nakamatsu M, Goto M, Morita M. A case of generalized amyloidosis in the cat. Jpn J Vet Sci 28:259–265, 1966.

212. Clark L, Seawright AA. Generalized amyloidosis in seven cats. Pathol Vet 6:117–134, 1969.

213. Chew DJ, DiBartola SP, Boyce JT, et al. Renal amyloidosis in related Abyssinian cats. J Am Vet Med Assoc 181:139–142, 1982.

214. DiBartola SP, Tarr MJ, Benson MD. Tissue distribution of amyloid deposits in Abyssinian cats with familial amyloidosis. J Comp Pathol 96:387–398, 1986.

214a. Zuber RM: Systemic amyloidosis in Oriental and Siamese cats. Aust Vet Practit 23:66–70, 1993.

214b. Blunden AS, Smith KC: Generalised amyloidosis and acute liver haemorrhage in four cats. J Sm Anim Pract 33:566–570, 1992.

215. DiBartola SP, Hill RL, Fechheimer NS, et al. Pedigree analysis of Abyssinian cats with familial amyloidosis. J Am Vet Med Assoc 47:2666–2668, 1986.

216. DiBartola SP, Tarr MJ, Webb DM, et al. Familial renal amyloidosis in Chinese Shar Pei dogs. J Am Vet Med Assoc 197:483–487, 1990.

217. Sohar E, Gafni J, Pras M, et al. Familial Mediterranean fever: A survey of 470 cases and review of the literature. Am J Med 43:227–253, 1967.

218. Tintle LJM. Amyloidosis: Familial reactive systemic amyloidosis of Chinese shar-pei. The Shar-Pei Magazine, 52–58, 1990.

219. Tintle L. Familial shar-pei fever, swollen hock syndrome, and secondary systemic amyloidosis. The Barker, 98–100, Jan./Feb. 1992.

219a. Loeven KO: Spontaneous hepatic rupture secondary to amyloidosis in a Chinese Shar Pei. J Am Anim Hosp Assoc 30:577–579.

220. Kyle RA, Spencer RJ, Dahlin DC. Value of rectal biopsy in the diagnosis of primary systemic amyloidosis. Am J Med Sci 251:501–506, 1966.

221. Kyle RA, Pease GL, Richmond H, et al. Bone marrow aspiration in the antemortem diagnosis of primary systemic amyloidosis. Am J Clin Pathol 45:252–257, 1966.

222. Libbey CA, Skinner M, Cohen AS. Use of abdominal fat tissue aspirate in the diagnosis of systemic amyloidosis. Arch Intern Med 143:1549–1552, 1983.

223. Yerba M, Albarran F, Durantez A, et al. Diagnosis of hepatic amyloidosis by fine neeedle aspiration biopsy (letter). Am J Med 82:1275–1276, 1987.

224. Wegelius O. The resolution of amyloid substance. Acta Med Scand 212:273–275, 1982.

225. Fitchen JH. Amyloidosis and granulomatous ileocolilitis: Regression after surgical removal of the involved bowel. N Engl J Med 292:352–353, 1975.

226. Lowenstein J, Gallo G. Remission of the nephrotic syndrome in renal amyloidosis. N Engl J Med 282:128–132, 1970.

227. Kisilevsky R, Boudreau L, Foster D. Kinetics of amyloid deposition. II. The effects of dimethylsulfoxide and colchicine therapy. Lab Invest 48:60–67, 1983.

228. Hanai N, Ishihara T, Uchino F, et al. Effects of dimethylsulfoxide and colchicine on the resorption of experimental amyloid. Virchows Arch (Pathol Anat) 384:45–52, 1979.

229. Kedar I, Greenwald M, Ravid M. Treatment of experimental murine amyloidosis with dimethyl sulfoxide. Eur J Clin Invest 7:149–150, 1977.

230. Greenwald M, Kedar I, Sohar E. The effect of colchicine and dimethylsulfoxide (DMSO) on the genetic amyloidosis of the white Peking duckt. In: Glenner GG, Costa PP, de Freitas F, (eds). Amyloid and Amyloidosis. Excerpta Medica, Amsterdam, 584–586, 1980.

231. Isobe T, Osserman EF. Effects of dimethyl sulfoxide (DMSO) on Bence Jones proteins, amyloid fibrils and casein induced amyloidosis. In: Wegelius O, Pasternack A (eds) Amyloidosis. Academic Press, New York, 247–257, 1976.

232. Eisenbud LE, Lerner CP, Chai CK. The effect of dimethyl sulfoxide (DMSO) upon spontaneous amyloidosis in mice. Proc Soc Exp Biol Med 168:172–174, 1981.

233. Ravid M, Keizman IK, Sohar E. Effect of a single dose of dimethyl sulphoxide on renal amyloidosis. Lancet 1:730–731, 1977.

234. Falck HM, Tornroth T, Skrifvars B, et al. Resolution of renal amyloidosis secondary to rheumatoid arthritis. Acta Med Scan 205:651–656, 1979.

235. van Rijswijk MH, Ruinen L, Donker AJM. Dimethyl sulfoxide in the treatment of AA amyloidosis. Ann NY Acad Sci, 67–83, 1983.

236. Osserman EF, Sherman WH, Kyle A. Further studies of therapy of amyloidosis with dimethyl sulfoxide (DMSO). In: Glenner GG, Costa PP, Freitas F, (eds) Amyloid and Amyloidosis. Excerpta Medica, Amsterdam; Proceedings of the Third Symposium on Amyloidosis, Povoa de Varzim, Portugal, 563, 1980.

237. Spyridakis L, Brown S, Barsanti J, et al. Amyloidosis in a dog: Treatment wiht dimethylsulfoxide. J Am Vet Med Assoc 189:690–691, 1986.

238. Cowgill LD. Diseases of the kidney. In: Ettinger SJ (ed) Textbook of Veterinary Internal Medicine, 2nd ed. WB Saunders, Philadelphia, 1843, 1983.

239. Gruys E, Sijens RJ, Biewenga WJ. Dubious effect of dimethylsulphoxide (DMSO) therapy on amyloid deposits and amyloidosis. Vet Res Com 5:21–32, 1981.

240. Hardt F. Acceleration of casein induced amyloidosis in mice by immunosuppressive agents. Acta Path Microbiol Scand, Sec. A 79:61–64, 1971.

241. Ludwig J, Owen CA, Barham SS, et al. The liver in the inherited copper disease of Bedlington terriers. Lab Invest 43:82–87, 1980.

242. Lisboa PE. Experimental hepatic cirrhosis in dogs caused by chronic iron overload. Gut 12:363–368, 1971.

243. Brissot P, Campion JP, Guillozo A, et al. Experimental hepatic iron overload in the baboon: Results of a two-year study. Evolution of biological and morphologic hepatic parameters of iron overload. Dig Dis Sci 28:616–624, 1983.

244. Falck H, Skrifvars B, Wegelius O. Treatment of amyloidosis secondary to rheumatoid arthritis with cyclophosphamide. In: Glenner GG, Costa PP, Freitas F (eds) Amyloid and Amyloidosis. Proceedings of the Third Symposium on Amyloidosis, Povoa de Varzim, Portugal. Excerpta Medica, Amsterdam, 592, 1980.

245. Gollan JL. Diagnosis of hemochromatosis. Gastroenterology 84:418–431, 1983.

246. Bothwell TH, Charlton RW. Hemochromatosis in the liver. In: Schiff L, Schiff ER (eds) Diseases of the Liver. JB Lippincott, Philadelphia, 1001–1035, 1987.

247. Greentree WF, Miller J, Buck WB. Diagnosis and management of acute iron toxicosis. Can Pract 18:20–23, 1993.

35 Hepatic Vascular Diseases

SHARON A. CENTER

INTRODUCTION

In health, the liver receives 25% of the cardiac output, the portal vein supplying approximately two-thirds and the hepatic artery the remainder. Hepatic tissue oxygenation is provided by both circulatory beds, and important hepatotrophic factors are derived from the portal circulation. The portal venous circulation is a valveless, low-pressure system. In health, portal pressure approximates 6 to 10 cm water (to convert to mm Hg, divide by 1.36). Portal circulation follows the path of least resistance, pressure gradients between the abdominal visceral arteries and the right atrium determining its flow. Conditions altering blood flow through the caudal portion of the thoracic vena cava, hepatic veins, hepatic artery, and portal vein have differing effects on hepatic histology and function. Chronic passive congestion results in hepatic venous congestion, sinusoidal distension, hepatomegaly, impaired parenchymal perfusion, zone 3 necrosis, formation of ascites, and portal hypertension. Portal venous hypertension can result in collateral portosystemic shunting when interconnecting venous beds provide an alternate low-resistance pathway. The circulatory bed recruited depends on the cause of hepatic venous congestion. Acute or chronic occlusion of the portal venous circulation results in a compensatory increase in the hepatic arterial blood flow. Loss of portal circulation leads to hepatocyte atrophy, collapse of intrahepatic portal veins, and augmentation of the hepatic arterial vasculature. A reciprocal circulatory compensation does not occur in the event of acute or chronic loss of the hepatic arterial circulation. In fact, abrupt loss of the hepatic arterial perfusion can lead to fatal hepatic necrosis. Acute occlusion of the main portion of the portal vein in an individual without open functioning portosystemic communications results in severe portal hypertension, splanchnic congestion, mesenteric and intestinal hypoxia, ascites, endotoxemia, and death within hours to a few days. Within 3 weeks of partial obstruction of portal blood flow, sustained portal hypertension results in development of multiple portosystemic collaterals. These collateral vessels develop from nonfunctional vascular structures. Portosystemic shunting, whether associated with congenital portal venous malformations or acquired portal hypertension, leads to marked derangements in hepatic function and clinical signs of hepatic encephalopathy (HE).

Important relationships among portal blood flow, hepatic function, and overall homeostasis were first recognized a century ago by Eck.[1,2] In the 1930s and 1940s it was experimentally demonstrated that liver function was significantly reduced in animals with an Eck fistula, a surgically created communication between the portal vein and the vena cava that deviates portal flow to the caudal vena cava. After creation of an Eck fistula, the liver receives circulation only from the hepatic artery. Intolerance to orally administered amino acids, evidence of progressive deterioration of hepatic function, HE, and impaired regeneration of liver tissue were reported in these early studies.[2,3] These studies also indicated that the quality, and not the quantity, of blood flowing to the liver determines its size. It was subsequently discovered that the portal venous blood is an important determinant of hepatic size because of its delivery of hepatotrophic factors derived from the gastrointestinal tract and pancreas.[4] Hepatotrophic factors consist of nutrients and hormones that influence the size of individual hepatocytes. Reduced portal blood flow and deprivation of hepatotrophic substances results in hepatocyte atrophy, loss of glycogen stores, hepatocellular vacuolation, and a marked reduction in liver size.

Portosystemic shunting or hepatofugal blood flow can develop as a result of congenital malformations of the hepatic microcirculation or portal vein or be an acquired response to impaired portal blood flow. Portosystemic vascular anomalies (PSVA) have been recognized in humans, rats, dogs, cats, foals, calves, and miniature pigs.[5-58] Generally, these are not associated with portal hypertension. They have most commonly been recognized in small animals.[15-58] Animals with portosystemic shunting can demonstrate a variety of neurobehavioral and clinical laboratory abnormalities. Medical management aimed at palliation of metabolic derangements caused by hepatofugal circulation benefits all affected animals. Surgical ligation of PSVA usually results in remarkable clinical improvement. In rare cases, PSVAs are associated with portal hypertension. This occurs when PSVAs are linked with severe microvascular portal dysplasia (portal vein atresia). Severe portal hypertension also develops in animals with congenital or acquired hepatic arteriovenous fistulas. Intrahepatic anastomosis between a branch of the hepatic artery and hepatic portal vein results in arterialization of the portal venous circulatory system. This causes portal hypertension, acquired portosystemic shunting, and marked changes in hepatic microvasculature.

Acquired portosystemic shunting is always associated with

portal hypertension related to one of the following conditions: (1) increased resistance to sinusoidal blood flow due to obstructed blood flow in the thoracic portion of the caudal vena cava, hepatic veins, sinusoids, or severe microvascular portal dysplasia, (2) prehepatic compression, stricture, or thromboembolism of the abdominal portion of the portal vein, or (3) arterialization of the portal venous system. Treatment of acquired portosystemic shunts focuses on the underlying hepatic or vascular disease causing portal hypertension. In most cases, surgical extirpation of acquired portosystemic shunts is ill advised if the underlying pathologic condition cannot be resolved.

PORTOSYSTEMIC VASCULAR ANOMALIES (PSVA)

Clinical Synopsis

Diagnostic Features

- Episodic neurobehavioral signs common (dullness, circling, disorientation, blindness, ataxia, seizures, stupor)
- Poor growth and gastroenteric upsets common
- Cats often show seizures, hypersalivation, and copper iris color
- Large-breed dogs usually have intrahepatic shunts
- Small-breed dogs usually have extrahepatic shunts
- Microhepatica and renomegaly usual
- Mild nonregenerative anemia with microcytosis and poikilocytes common
- ALT and ALP only mildly elevated; bilirubin usually normal
- Low BUN, cholesterol, glucose, and globulin frequent
- Ammonium biurate crystalluria and urate calculi are common
- Abnormal ammonia tolerance and postprandial bile acid tests

Standard Treatment

- Diet based on dairy or vegetable proteins in restricted quantities with supplemental fermentable fiber and water soluble vitamins and taurine (cats)
- For hepatoencephalopathic crisis: Cleansing enemas followed by retention enema (5–10 mL/kg) with added antibiotics or lactulose
- Lactulose (0.25–1.0 mL/kg PO TID-QID to effect)
- Neomycin (22 mg/kg BID PO) and/or metronidazole (7.5 mg/kg BID PO)
- Surgical attenuation of shunt if possible

The first naturally occurring PSVA was described in 1949 by Hickman.[15] This dog had a normal hepatic arterial supply, but the portal vein was absent and a portoazygos shunt was identified. Clinical signs of disease were not described. The clinical entity caused by portal vein anomalies was not recognized until reports by Ewing et al. and Audell et al. in 1974.[16,17] Since then, multiple reports of single cases and case series have reiterated the characteristics of affected animals.[18–58] This is a well-characterized disorder of the dog and cat, although it is relatively uncommon in routine veterinary practice. An incidence of 0.02% to 0.6% in dogs and from 0.02% to 0.1% in cats in a referral-based hospital has been estimated.[59] A retrospective survey of 30 North American veterinary teaching hospitals over a 20 year period from 1964 to 1985 yielded over 700 cases of PSVA in the dog.[60] The frequency of this diagnosis seems to be increasing as the clinical characteristics have become widely recognized and serum bile acid testing has become routine.

Embryology

Consideration of the hepatic vascular embryology assists in understanding how PSVAs develop (Figure 35–1). The liver develops from endoderm of the ventral portion of the foregut destined to become the duodenum.[61–63] The hepatic parenchyma and biliary system develop from the hepatic diverticulum. This diverticulum grows into the mesoderm of the septum transversum (destined to become the diaphragm) and forms two outgrowths: (1) the pars hepatica, which becomes the hepatic parenchymal cells, and (2) the pars cystica, which becomes the gallbladder (biliary structures).

The intrahepatic venous structures, including the portal veins, hepatic sinusoids, and hepatic veins, develop from mesoderm of the septum transversum and from the vitelline (omphalomesenteric vein) and umbilical veins.[64,65] The abdominal extrahepatic veins are derived from the umbilical, vitelline, and caudal cardinal veins. The portal vein and all its tributaries are derived from the vitelline and umbilical veins and the nonportal abdominal veins, including the renal and gonadal veins, from the cardinal veins.[64,65] The vena cava forms from a fusion between the cardinal veins and the right vitelline vein. No normal *functional* communications develop between the cardinal veins and the umbilical or vitelline veins caudal to the liver. However, there are many *nonfunctional* portocaval and portoazygos communications that may become functional should portal hypertension develop.[66]

The paired vitelline veins originate from the yolk sac and join the sinus venosus (Figure 35–1A). Three communications develop between these two veins. The ductus venosus develops between the cranial anastomosis of the vitelline veins and the left umbilical vein. This provides a direct route for blood from the placental circulation to the developing heart (Figure 35–1B and C). The liver develops between the cranial and middle vitelline vein anastomoses. The left proximal portion of the vitelline vein atrophies and the right proximal portion forms the hepatic segment of the caudal vena cava. The middle portion of the vitelline veins becomes subdivided and participates in formation of the developing hepatic sinusoids. The remaining portion of the cranial anastomosis becomes the left hepatic vein. Degeneration of the right distal vitelline vein, caudal anastomosis of the vitelline veins, and the cranial extrahepatic portion of the left middle vitelline vein occurs before or concurrent with the leftward rotation of the developing stomach.[63] The portal vein is entirely derived from the vitelline system: (1) caudal portion of the left vitelline vein, (2) the middle anastomosis of the vitelline vein, and (3) the distal portion of the right middle vitelline vein. The cranial mesenteric and splenic veins are derived from the distal segments of the vitelline veins and empty into the left distal vitelline vein being transformed into the portal vein (Figure 35–1C).

The paired umbilical veins lie lateral and parallel to the vitelline veins. As the liver develops, the umbilical veins form anastomoses with the hepatic sinusoids. These communications permit umbilical venous blood to flow through developing sinusoids. Preferential flow to the left side from the placenta causes this segment to enlarge as the right side

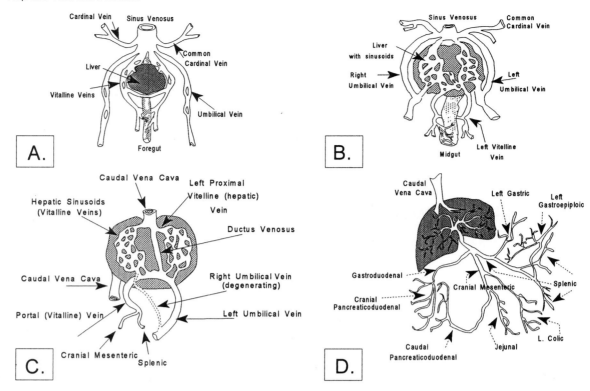

FIGURE 35-1. Diagrammatic representation of the embryologic development of the portal vein and hepatic sinusoids and the final mature tributaries of the portal vein. Adapted from references 60 and 63.

atrophies. The cranial umbilical veins degenerate as blood flow deviates into the sinusoids. The communication between the left umbilical vein and portal vein caudal to the ductus venosus is the umbilical-portal sinus, which becomes the left branch of the portal vein when umbilical flow terminates.[67] This is the only segment of the portal vein not derived from the vitelline structures.

The paired cardinal veins develop into the caudal vena cava and the azygos vein. The only normal functional anastomosis of the cardinal and vitelline systems occurs where they form the caudal vena cava at the level of the liver.[64,67]

Anatomy of the Mature Hepatic Circulation

The vascular network of the liver is comprised of the portal veins, hepatic artery, and hepatic veins. Portal circulation derives blood from the gastrointestinal tract, pancreas, and spleen. The major contributors to the portal vein include the cranial and caudal mesenteric veins, the splenic vein, the gastroduodenal vein, and the left gastric vein[67,68] (Figure 35–1D). The portal vein is relatively constant in its distribution to the liver (Figure 35–2). The liver lobes are designated as hepatic divisions based on their blood supply.[63] The left division includes the papillary process of the caudate lobe and the left lateral and medial lobes. The right division includes the caudate process of the caudate lobe and the right lateral lobe, and the central division includes the right medial and quadrate lobes. There are two main hepatic branches of the portal vein; the left branch supplies the left and central divisions and the right branch the right hepatic divisions. The blood in the right branch reaches the liver before blood in the left branch; this may be observed during contrast portography.

The hepatic artery originates from the celiac artery, a direct branch of the aorta located proximal to the cranial mesenteric artery. The celiac artery lies dorsal to the portal vein and common bile duct within the hepatoduodenal ligament.[68] It completes an arch before terminating as the right gastric and gastroduodenal arteries. Usually, two or three arterial branches derived from this arch supply the liver; each hepatic division having a separate arterial supply.[67]

The hepatic veins are variable in number and location, but each enters the vena cava before it crosses the diaphragm. Usually there are between six to eight major veins.[67] The largest and most consistent is the left hepatic vein, which is the most cranial segment. This vessel is derived from the left branch of the cranial anastomosis of the embryonal vitelline

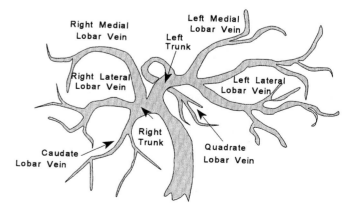

FIGURE 35-2. Diagrammatic representation of the normal intrahepatic distribution of the portal vein as observed on radiographic portal venography.

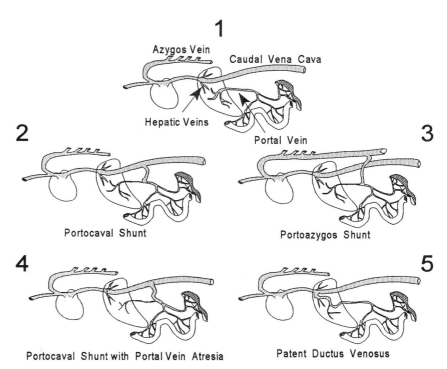

FIGURE 35-3. Diagrammatic representation of the most common portosystemic vascular anomalies in the dog and cat.

veins and always drains the left hepatic division and may partially drain the central hepatic division.[63,67,68]

Developmental Anomalies

Congenital portosystemic vascular anomalies can be either intrahepatic or extrahepatic. Extrahepatic PSVA are more common than intrahepatic malformations. The types of PSVA described most often in dogs and cats are shown in Figure 35–3. The estimated prevalence of different types of anomalies are shown in Table 35–1.

The development of extrahepatic shunts is different from that of intrahepatic shunts. All extrahepatic shunts represent aberrant communications between the vitelline and cardinal venous systems,[63–65] the extrahepatic portal vessels representing the vitelline system and the extrahepatic caudal vena cava and azygos veins the cardinal system. The majority of extrahepatic PSVA involve an anomalous vessel or vessels arising from a major tributary of the portal veins. Most PSVA arise from the main trunk of the portal vein or from the left gastric or splenic veins. Fewer have been described that involve the gastroduodenal and mesenteric vessels. All of these vessels originate from the most caudal vitelline system and typically empty directly into the caudal vena cava cranial to the phrenicoabdominal veins.[39,54,63] Thus, extrahepatic PSVA rec-

Table 35-1

PREVALENCE OF DIFFERENT TYPES OF PSVA IN DOGS AND CATS

TYPE OF VASCULAR ANOMALY	NUMBER	MEDIAN AGE (MONTHS)	RANGE
Dogs			
Portocaval	39	9	1–144
Ductus venosus	18	4	2–11
Left gastric	11	17	2–60
Portal atresia	5	24	6–72
Portoazygos	4	14.5	2–60
Arteriovenous fistula			
Cats			
Left gastric	23	9	4–50
Portocaval	13	24	3–48
Ductus venosus	7	6	3.5–36
Portal atresia	4	10	6–17
Portoazygos	2	11	NA
Gastrosplenic	3	3	7–36

Data acquired from the College of Veterinary Medicine, Cornell University (dogs and cats) and cats from many references.[24,29,33,34,37,40,43,46,49]

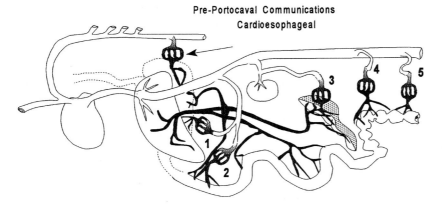

Pre-Portocaval Communications
Cardioesophageal

FIGURE 35-4. Diagrammatic representation of the most common portosystemic vascular shunts associated with acquired liver disease and portal hypertension. These represent normally present but nonfunctional portosystemic communications that become functional in response to portal hypertension.

Post-Portocaval Communications
1. Gastrophrenic
2. Duodenal
3. Velaromental
4. Left Colic
5. Cranial Rectal

ognized in dogs and cats represent developmental errors between two embryonic vascular systems.[60] These aberrant vascular structures are discrete from the normally present but nonfunctional portosystemic communications that only become functional in response to portal hypertension (Figures 35–3 and 35–4). Portoazygos shunts are the second most common type of PSVAs. These arise from the portal vein or a normal portal tributary and empty into the azygos vein. These also represent anomalous fusions between the vitelline and cardinal venous systems.

The least common type of extrahepatic PSVAs are complicated malformations involving multiple vessels and, in some cases, severe microvascular portal dysplasia and portal vein atresia. In the circumstance of severe portal venous atresia, portal hypertension leads to the development of multiple acquired shunts and hepatofugal portal flow to the caudal vena cava. The anomaly of portal atresia is relatively rare but may be more common in cats than in dogs. Affected patients present at an older age compared to animals with single uncomplicated PSVA.

An intrahepatic PSVA represents a patent ductus venosus.[63] Although these are most common in large-breed dogs, they also occur in small dogs and in cats. Most of these malformations involve the left hepatic division, which makes them consistent with the normal embryonic position of the ductus venosus. Right hepatic divisional shunts usually directly enter the caudal vena cava and are difficult to correct surgically because there is little if any vascular segment amenable to ligature placement.

In the normal dog, the ductus venosus functionally closes within 3 days after birth.[69,70] Closure is initiated by cessation of umbilical flow and is related to active closure of a sphincter at the proximal end of the vessel. Thromboxane A_2 released from the vascular endothelium or liver is believed to initiate closure of this sphincter.[71] By 15 to 18 days of age, structural closure of the ductus is established in the dog.[67] Histologically, closure begins in the connective tissue at the junction of the ductus and umbilical-portal sinus. This tissue proliferates and expands from the sinus to the termination of the ductus at the left hepatic vein.[69] A patent ductus venosus results from failure of the initiation or progression of this closure process. Prostaglandin I_2 has been shown to cause sphincter relaxation, but it is not known whether this response is causally related to failed closure.

Clinical Signs

Dogs with experimentally created Eck fistula have been shown to remain clinically normal for 8 years or more when fed an adequate diet.[1] It is thus not surprising that some dogs with PSVA remain clinically normal for long periods prior to diagnosis. A variety of conditions and medical problems may predispose the dog or cat with PSVA to HE. These conditions become the focus of medical management in these patients and are discussed in the treatment section of this chapter.

Portosystemic vascular anomalies are most commonly diagnosed in purebred dogs and domestic shorthair cats. There is no sex predisposition in dogs, but a predisposition for male cats has been observed. A list of dog breeds and the frequency of occurrence of PSVA seen in the author's hospital and reported in large case series over the past 18 years is given in Table 35–2. Portosystemic vascular anomalies and microvascular portal dysplasia have been observed in kindreds of Irish wolfhounds, Yorkshire terriers, and Cairn terriers.[72,73] Purebred littermates with PSVA have been seen in several breeds, including miniature schnauzers, old English sheepdogs, Yorkshire terriers, Irish wolfhounds, and boxers. Dogs with porto-azygos or porto-hemiazygos shunts have generally been older than dogs with other PSVAs, suggesting that the type of shunt influences the age of onset and the severity of clinical manifestations.[24] One dog with situs inversus associated with PSVA has been described; combination of PSVA and visceral malposition has also been reported in humans.[16] Large dogs are more likely to have intrahepatic shunts (60% to 70%) whereas small- to medium-sized dogs are more likely to have single extrahepatic shunts (90%). Although half of the male dogs in one study (n = 20) were cryptorchid,[41] this finding has not been consistently reported.

Most animals with PSVAs demonstrate neurobehavioral signs at a young age and are presented for veterinary examination before 1 year. Many present between 4 and 6 months of age because they are unable to manage normal high-protein growth foods. Some cats have not been presented until 4 years of age and some dogs not until 10 years of age. Clinical signs may remain vague, with some animals merely demonstrating an unusually quiet or dull disposition or apparent learning disabilities. Recognition of neurobehavioral abnormalities may be difficult for the owner inexperienced in ani-

Table 35–2

PREVALENCE OF DIFFERENT DOG BREEDS
AFFECTED WITH PSVA*

BREED OF DOGS	NUMBER
Yorkshire terrier	26
Miniature schnauzer	21
Mixed breed	14
Cairn terrier	9
German shepherd	7
Poodle	7
Shih Tzu	6
Irish wolfhound	6
Old English sheepdog	6
Golden retriever	6
Doberman pinscher	6
Collie	6
Pug	5
Lhasa apso	4
Labrador retriever	4
Siberian husky	3
Samoyed	3
Dachshund	3
Bernese mountain dog	3
Beagle	3
Brittany spaniel	3
Cocker spaniel	3
Irish setter	2
Akita	3
Shetland sheepdog	2
Bouvier	2
Newfoundland	2
Pomeranian	2
Komondor	2
West Highland white terrier	2

*If two or more affected individuals.
Data acquired from the College of Veterinary Medicine, Cornell University (1978–1994) and large published case series. A total of 190 cases were surveyed.

mal husbandry. In humans with PSVA, diagnosis is commonly not confirmed until the fourth or fifth decade owing to the vague signs and subtle histologic hepatic lesions.

Neurobehavioral manifestations of HE include a variety of abnormal responses; these are detailed in Table 35–3. Signs are episodic and often are temporally associated with food ingestion or a gastrointestinal disturbance causing hemorrhage, inflammation, or constipation. Signs usually develop gradually and abate over several hours to days. Some animals display propulsive circling or pacing and head press. Some develop amaurotic blindness (sudden onset of transient unexplained blindness). Others display ataxia consistent with a transverse myelopathy. Personality changes may be remarkable; many cats become intractably aggressive and some dogs become hyperactive and bark manically. Severe signs of stupor and coma develop in some animals that may resolve within 12 hours following institution of aggressive supportive care. In some cases, grand mal seizure activity is the only reported clinical sign. On closer investigation, seizures usually are related to other neurobehavioral abnormalities having slow onset and resolution, which distinguishes them from typical idiopathic epilepsy. Cats with PSVA are more commonly afflicted with grand mal seizure activity than dogs in the author's experience. Neurologic signs in some animals have been precipitated by administration of psychotropic medications: tranquilizers, antihistamines, anesthetics, and barbiturates. In some dogs (especially toy breeds, e.g., Yorkshire terriers), neurologic signs may indicate the presence of neuroglycopenia.

Nonspecific gastroenteric signs may be another reason for owner concern. In some animals, recurrent vomiting is the major clinical abnormality. Others have demonstrated anorexia, polyphagia and pica, or diarrhea. Some dogs have repeatedly ingested foreign objects necessitating enterotomy. Delayed recovery from anesthesia may prompt consideration of PSVA in these. Most cats and some dogs demonstrate ptyalism (hypersalivation). The cause of this phenomenon remains undetermined but may be related to nausea. The author has seen two dogs with severe recurrent gastroenteric hemorrhage necessitating blood transfusion. This problem resolved upon surgical correction of the PSVA.

Some dogs and cats have presented for signs related to urolithiasis, recurrent urinary tract infection or inflammation.[40,44,49,52,74] Hematuria is common in animals having ammonium biurate calculi. Renal, obstructing ureteral, cystic, and obstructing urethral calculi have each been documented in these patients. Cystic and renal calculi are most common. Calculi are far more common than was previously considered;

Table 35–3

CLINICAL SIGNS DISPLAYED BY DOGS AND CATS
WITH PSVA

Personality changes:
   aggression in cats
   manic barking in dogs
Neurologic signs:
Chronologically related:
   meals, gastrointestinal hemorrhage, infection, fever
Lethargy
Unresponsiveness
Difficulty training
Aimless wandering
Pacing / circling
Head pressing
Hallucinations
Head down posture
Amaurotic blindness
Ataxia / weakness
Collapse
Stupor
Seizures
Coma
Physical signs:
Small body size
Weight loss
Small liver
Prominent kidneys
Copper-colored iris: cats
Ptyalism: cats especially
Vomiting
Diarrhea
Constipation: worsens HE
Anorexia
Polyphagia: foreign body ingestion
Polydipsia / polyuria
Fever: intermittent
Ammonium biurate crystalluria
   hematuria   pollakiuria
   urinary calculi→   urethral obstruction
   nephrolithiasis→   ureteral obstruction
Drug intolerance
   barbiturates
   narcotics
   benzodiazepines
   metronidazole
   tetracycline
   anesthetics
   phenothiazines
   antihistamines
   methionine

more than 50% of PSVA patients have uroliths detected during abdominal ultrasonographic assessment. Cystic calculi are usually removed at the time of surgical ligation of the PSVA.

Physical Abnormalities

The typical patient with a PSVA has a small body stature. In most animals the liver is smaller than normal, but in some, the liver size is close to normal. More cats than dogs have what appears to be a nearly normal hepatic size. The presence of prominent kidneys is fairly common.[16,17,75] An increase in kidney size is believed to be related to increased work demands on the renal tissue, perhaps the delivery of trophic factors, and an increased renal circulation. There is evidence that exposure of renal cells to high concentrations of ammonia results in hypertrophy. Renal gluconeogenesis is also associated with renal hypertrophy. Increased renal gluconeogenesis could occur as an adaptation to systemic hypoglycemia resulting from impaired hepatic gluconeogenesis and glycogenolysis. Renal gluconeogenesis also increases upon renal exposure and production of increased concentrations of ammonia.[74] Kidney enlargement may also be associated with an increased GFR as has been shown with rats with experimentally created portosystemic communications.

A unique golden-copper color of the iris has been observed in most affected cats seen by the author. The exceptions have been in Siamese and Himalayan cats. This unique iris color in PSVA cats is similar to that naturally occurring in the Persian breed. Heart murmurs have been detected in some cats with PSVA. In one cat, a truncus arteriosus cardiac malformation was confirmed. A few dogs with PSVA have been intensely pruritic on initial presentation. Atopy has been diagnosed in these dogs rather than bile salt related pruritus as is seen in humans with liver diseases associated with increased serum bile acid concentrations. Ascites is rare in the patient with a typical PSVA before surgical intervention. However, after surgical attenuation of a PSVA, transient ascites may develop for 7 to 14 days. This usually resolves without complication. When ascites is detected on initial veterinary examination, the presence of portal hypertension is inferred and suggests that either an arteriovenous fistula, severe microvascular portal dysplasia, or acquired liver disease are underlying factors.

Clinicopathologic Features

The metabolic abnormalities associated with portosystemic shunting have been well characterized. A study of dogs with surgically created portosystemic shunts has detailed the chronologic appearance of most abnormalities recognized in clinical patients (Figure 35–5).[76] The clinicopathologic fea-

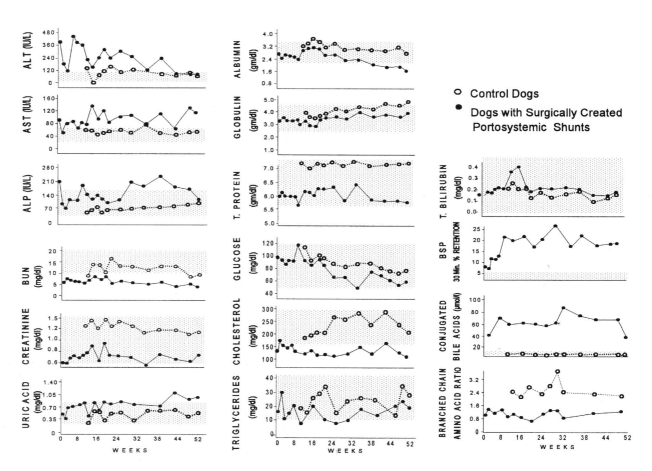

FIGURE 35–5. Chronology of clinicopathologic aberrations associated with surgically created portosystemic vascular anomalies in the dog.[76]

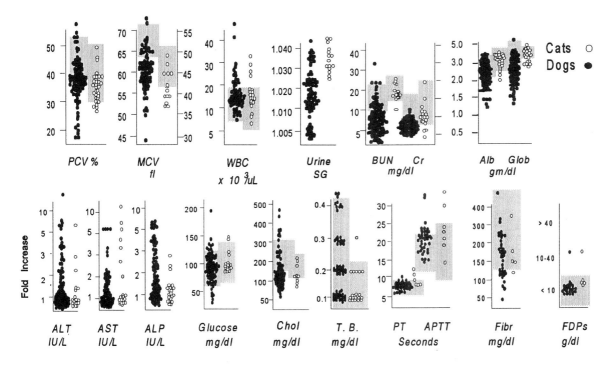

Cats ○
Dogs ●

FIGURE 35-6. Clinicopathologic features associated with congenital portosystemic vascular anomalies in the dog and cat. Data derived from the College of Veterinary Medicine, Cornell University.

tures from dogs (n = 100) and cats (n = 33) with PSVA are summarized in Figure 35–6. Detailed discussion of possible underlying causes of these laboratory abnormalities can be found in Chapter 30.

Hematology

Many animals with PSVA have microcytic normochromic erythrocytes and red blood cell conformational changes.[13,52,77] A nonregenerative anemia develops in approximately 50% of dogs and 15% to 20% of cats. Postulated causes include deficient utilization of marrow iron, chronic gastroenteric blood loss, iron deficiency, decreased red cell survival, subnormal nutritional status, decreased serum erythropoietin levels, and abnormal cholesterol and lipid metabolism leading to poor erythrocyte membrane stability. Microcytosis in documented case series ranges between 29% to 65% of dogs and 54% of cats. Nearly 80% of dogs seen by the author have had microcytosis. Microcytosis is not uniquely associated with PSVA; it has also been reported in dogs that are hepatoencephalopathic due to acquired liver disease.[77] An association between microcytosis and hepatoportal shunting is apparent. Although microcytosis is likely related to iron metabolism, evaluation of serum iron binding capacity, serum iron total binding capacity (TBC), protoporphyrin, serum ferritin, and bone marrow staining with Prussian blue have not revealed consistent abnormalities.[52,78–80]

Target cells and poikilocytes (acanthocytes) are common in patients with PSVA. Target cells are most commonly identified in dogs. Poikilocytes have been observed in blood smears from many cats and in some dogs with PSVA (see Figure 8–2). Although not pathognomonic for PSVA, especially in the cat, poikilocytosis prompts consideration of serious hepa-

tobiliary disease. Although the cause of these RBC conformational changes is unproven, it is speculated they are associated with abnormal lipid metabolism or retention of bile acids.[81]

The white blood cell count is usually in the normal range or only slightly increased. When leukocytosis occurs, a mature neutrophilia is most common. The peripheral dispersal of enteric toxins and microorganisms or increased concentration of cortisol resulting from impaired hepatic biotransformation and elimination of steroid hormones may be underlying causes.

Serum Biochemistry

LIVER ENZYMES. Normal or only mild increases in serum ALT, AST, and ALP activities are most common in dogs and cats with PSVA and surgically created portosystemic shunts (Figures 35–5 and 35–6). It is speculated that reduced hepatic perfusion leads to hypoxic cellular damage and enzyme leakage. This concept is consistent with the hepatocellular degeneration and vacuolation observed microscopically. Because animals with PSVA are usually seen when they are very young and growing, and considering that cholestasis is not a pathologic feature of this disorder, the two- to threefold increase in serum ALP activity frquently seen in dogs with PSVA may be related to increased production and release of the bone isoenzyme. However, subcellular fractionation and study of hepatocellular enzymes in dogs with PSVA have disclosed a prominent change in the activity and distribution of ALP in the absence of other membrane-related enzyme changes.[82] Increased ALP activity was found in the biliary canalicular region. This was suggested to be due to increased biosynthesis and/or decreased enzyme release.[82–84]

Synthesis of ALP might be increased in response to the high bile acid concentrations that develop with portosystemic shunting. Bile acids have been shown to induce hepatic synthesis of ALP from hepatocytes in vitro and after biliary tract obstruction.[82,83] It is also postulated that the membrane solubilizing effects of bile acids may elute membrane-bound enzymes.[82,84] It is not known whether increased hepatocellular ALP is related to the elevated serum ALP enzyme activity.

Some animals with PSVA develop chronic progressive hepatic fibrosis. This is particularly common in Yorkshire terriers and Maltese. At some point in the progression of this disorder, animals develop increased serum enzyme activities. Histologically, periportal fibrosis is associated with mild to moderate inflammation. Dogs subjected to the experimental creation of an Eck fistula develop mild, moderate to extensive hepatic fibrosis associated with variable increases in liver enzyme activities over time (Figure 35–5).[76]

TOTAL BILIRUBIN. In most animals with PSVA, the serum total bilirubin concentration is within the normal range. Mild hyperbilirubinemia has been seen in a few cases. When hyperbilirubinemia is detected, investigation for some other hepatobiliary or hemolytic process should be undertaken because PSVA is not a cholestatic disorder.

CHOLESTEROL. Very low serum cholesterol concentrations are found in most animals with PSVA: approximately 70% of dogs and between 60% to 70% of cats. Most others have cholesterol concentrations within the low normal range. Hypocholesterolemia is a consistent clinicopathologic feature developing after the surgical creation of portocaval shunts in humans, dogs, and rats.[76,85–90] The underlying pathogenetic mechanisms may involve (1) reduced intestinal absorption of cholesterol, (2) reduced hepatic synthesis of cholesterol, lipoproteins, or triglycerides, or (3) a change in the distribution of cholesterol among its various pools. There is evidence that certain bile acids directly inhibit cholesterol synthesis. The high bile acid concentrations invariably associated with hypocholesterolemia of PSVA make this hypothesis appealing.

SERUM PROTEINS. Between 30% to 50% of dogs and approximately 15% of cats with PSVA develop mild to moderate hypoalbuminemia. Suspected causes include (1) reduced hepatic synthesis because of insufficient hepatic mass, (2) down-regulation of synthesis due to anorexia, feeding of a diet containing insufficient protein, or patient immaturity, (3) intestinal loss due to bowel inflammation or endoparasitism, and (4) blood volume expansion due to sodium and water retention. At least one report has shown that total body water increases in dogs having an Eck fistula.[91] In some clinical cases, hypoalbuminemia has been iatrogenically aggravated by aggressive fluid therapy.

Hyperglobulinemia is relatively uncommon in dogs and cats with PSVA, unlike many other liver diseases. In contrast, almost 50% of dogs and 30% to 40% of cats are hypoglobulinemic. Hypoglobulinemia likely reflects either reduced hepatic globulin synthesis or expansion of the circulating blood volume. Lower globulins, as compared to sham-operated controls, developed also in dogs with experimentally created portosystemic shunts (Figure 35–5).[76]

BLOOD UREA NITROGEN AND CREATININE. The BUN concentration is often in the low normal or subnormal range; approximately 60% to 80% of dogs and 10% to 20% of cats have a low BUN. A subnormal BUN in a patient with hepatic insufficiency may reflect a number of variables including (1) insufficient hepatic urea synthesis from ammonia, (2) fluid diuresis subsequent to fluid therapy, primary polydipsia, or primary polyuria, (3) ingestion of a protein-restricted diet, or (4) simply individual variation. Approximately 75% of dogs

having a low BUN also have a subnormal serum creatinine concentration. Only 10% to 15% of cats are so affected. Dogs with experimentally created portosystemic shunts also developed low creatinine concentrations when compared to sham-operated controls (Figure 35–5).[76] The development of a low urine specific gravity, low BUN, and a low creatinine concentration suggests that fluid diuresis plays an important role in their genesis. Altered renal perfusion or changes in osmoreceptors associated with the portal circulation may promote reduced urine concentration and polydipsia.[92,93] The small muscle mass in very young dogs and toy breeds may permit only a very limited creatinine turnover, which would augment development of a low serum creatinine concentration. Additionally, the small muscle mass may also reduce the quantity of ammonia produced. Rats with surgically created portosystemic shunts develop increased renal creatinine and inulin clearances associated with reduced urine concentration.[94] This suggests an increased GFR and polyuria. It is probable that this also occurs in the dog. The cat's reliance on higher nutritional protein intake and its inability to down-regulate amino acid transamination may make this species relatively more resistant to development of a low BUN.

BLOOD GLUCOSE. Approximately 30% to 40% of dogs with PSVA are hypoglycemic, whereas hypoglycemia is rare in affected cats. Fasting hypoglycemia associated with PSVA is most common in toy breeds, pediatric patients and animals that develop complicating medical conditions, such as severe diarrhea, endoparasitism, or systemic infection. Symptomatic hypoglycemia complicates the recognition of HE. Less than 20% of dogs with PSVA seen in the author's hospital have developed clinical signs attributable to neuroglycopenia (hypoglycemia causing neuroencephalopathic signs). There are many postulated causes of hypoglycemia in the PSVA patient: (1) insufficient hepatic mass for gluconeogenesis, (2) insufficient hepatic glycogen storage, (3) slow or insufficient response to glucagon, (4) hyperglucagonemia, (5) impaired insulin metabolism, or (6) abnormally balanced counterregulatory hormones (cortisol and epinephrine). Additional problems in very young animals include the presence of immature hepatic gluconeogenic enzyme systems, insufficient peripheral stores of gluconeogenic amino acids, and suboptimal function of feedback and counterregulatory mechanisms. Animals with PSVA show decreased responsiveness to exogenously administered glucagon, which may reflect a number of factors, including (1) reduced glucagon delivery to the liver, (2) decreased hepatic glycogen storage, or (3) abnormal function of glucagon receptors.[95] In liver biopsies taken from animals with Eck fistulas and those with PSVA, hepatic glycogen stores have inconsistently been depleted.

Neonatal animals have difficulty recovering from either hypoglycemia or hyperglycemia. Care must be taken when regulating their blood glucose concentrations with intravenous dextrose because their glycemic response varies widely.

COAGULATION TESTS. Abnormal coagulation tests are unusual in the patient with PSVA. Increased partial thromboplastin times occur in approximately 30% of dogs and 25% of cats. The prothrombin time is normal in most dogs but was abnormal in 3 of 6 cats tested in the author's clinic. Hypofibrinogenemia develops in approximately 30% of dogs and is rare in cats. In only a few situations has clinical bleeding been realized. Prophylactic use of blood transfusions before surgery for portography or shunt ligation is not advocated unless there is clinical evidence of a hemorrhagic tendency. Judicious use of blood transfusion requires consideration of the dangers inherent with the administration of an exogenous protein challenge. Incompatibility of blood components or aged poorly viable erythrocytes may induce signs of HE. Hemolysis generates a nitrogen/protein challenge similar to that associated with a meat meal, gastroenteric hemorrhage, or an ammonia tolerance test. Day-old stored human blood has been shown to contain 170 μg ammonia per deciliter. Although canine blood has been shown to be less ammoniogenic than human blood,[96] if a blood transfusion seems necessary, only freshly collected blood should be given. If possible, cross-match compatibility should be verified.

SERUM ELECTROLYTES. There are no consistent electrolyte aberrations in animals with PSVA. Mild hypernatremia develops in approximately 12% of dogs, mild asymptomatic hypokalemia develops in 28% of dogs, and mild hyperchloremia in 35% of dogs. In cats, hypokalemia may develop as a result of anorexia, vomiting, or diarrhea or as a complication associated with fluid diuresis or use of loop diuretics. As a result of hypokalemia, renal ammonia production increases and a metabolic alkalosis is promoted.[97] A metabolic alkalosis has the potential to facilitate the transfer of unionized ammonia across the blood-brain barrier. Fluid supplementation with potassium chloride is recommended to avoid this complication, provided the potassium balance is monitored with serial electrolyte determinations. It is important to remember that serum potassium measurement may not reflect body potassium stores because acid-base changes shift potassium between intracellular and extracellular compartments.

Hyponatremia that is relatively resistant to fluid therapy has been reported in a small number of dogs that have developed status epilepticus following PSVA ligation. A causal association was not demonstrated between the electrolyte aberration and seizures. Although reduced sodium excretion and increased fluid retention are known to occur in humans with hepatic insufficiency, their occurrence in small animal patients with PSVA remains speculative. Only one study suggested water and sodium retention in dogs with an Eck fistula.[91] This phenomenon is difficult to study because serum sodium measurements do not accurately reflect sodium retention as fluid is retained proportionally.

Urinalysis

Although polydipsia and polyuria have been repeatedly described as routine findings in dogs and cats with PSVA, this is a highly variable observation. Routine urinalysis may disclose isosthenuria, hyposthenuria, or hypersthenuria. More dogs than cats are polyuric. Approximately 88% of cats and 20% of dogs have urine with a specific gravity equal to or

more than 1.030. Isosthenuric or hyposthenuric urine has been detected in 44% of dogs, 18% with a urine specific gravity less than 1.008.

Animals presenting with polyuria and polydipsia usually show at least a partial response to water deprivation, and concentrating defects typically resolve following successful shunt ligation. In the initial report of PSVA by Ewing, abrupt water restriction in 11 dogs resulted in only 5 of 11 being able to concentrate their urine.[16] Another study of 5 polydipsic dogs concluded that 3 of 5 were able to produce concentrated urine upon abrupt water restriction.[45] The formation of concentrated urine following water deprivation supports the presence of primary polydipsia and maintenance of an adequate renal medullary solute gradient. Dogs unable to concentrate their urine either had renal medullary washout or primary polyuria. It was interesting that two dogs in the later report were miniature schnauzers, a breed of dog previously shown to be afflicted with deranged osmostat function.[98]

Ammonium urate or biurate crystals and calculi develop in the urinary tracts of animals with experimentally created Eck fistula and in both humans and animals with PSVA.[14,16,21,74,99,100] Urate calculi usually are green, smooth, fairly small, and typically have obvious concentric laminations. They may be mixed with struvite or oxalate components. High serum concentrations of uric acid have not been documented in large numbers of clinical patients with PSVA because this test is seldom performed. However, in dogs with experimentally created portosystemic shunts, uric acid concentrations consistently exceeded those of sham-operated controls and were above the normal range after 40 weeks (Figure 35–5). High serum uric acid concentrations have also been shown in other studies of rats and dogs with experimentally created portosystemic shunts.[99,101] The hyperuricemia leads to elevated urinary uric acid concentrations, which in combination with elevated urinary ammonia levels leads to the precipitation of ammonium urates.

Ammonium biurate crystalluria is detected in a fresh urine sediment (Figure 35–7). Crystal precipitation does not appear to be associated with urine concentration or pH. In some animals with PSVA, ammonium urate crystals are repeatedly observed; in others, they are never observed. Some animals with nondemonstrable ammonium urate crystalluria have ammonium urate uroliths. Depending on reports, between 40% to 74% of dogs and approximately 13% of cats have had ammonium urate crystalluria. The overall frequency of urolith development in animals with PSVA is unknown but is suspected to be very high. Two-dimensional ultrasonography commonly reveals what are presumed to be uroliths in the renal pelvis or bladder in more than 50% of dogs and cats with PSVA. Rare obstructing ureteral and ure-

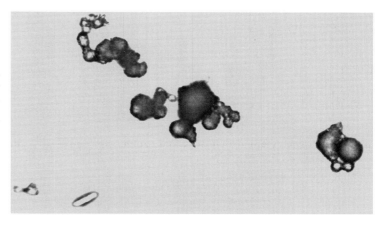

FIGURE 35–7. Photomicrograph showing ammonium biurate crystals in the urine of a cat with a portosystemic vascular anomaly. The condenser of the microscope is moved to a lower position than is conventionally used to view slides. Increased refractility of the crystals and examination under 400× magnification increases the ability to identify them.

thral calculi have also been recognized. The recognition of urate calculi or ammonium biurate crystalluria in any non-Dalmatian dog should raise suspicion of hepatic disease and warrants evaluation of fasting and postprandial serum bile acids. If the animal is young and acquired liver disease is considered unlikely, a PSVA should be highly suspected.

Hematuria, pyuria, and proteinuria may also be detected in animals with PSVA. These are usually associated with ammonium urate crystalluria or uroliths. In the author's experience, nearly 40% of dogs and 80% of cats have proteinuria and/or hematuria on initial urinalysis.

Liver Function Tests

PLASMA BSP AND ICG RETENTIONS. The numerous variables interfering with the use of BSP and ICG are reviewed in Chapter 8. Test values for dogs and cats with PSVA are shown in Figure 35–8. As a result of the inadequacies associated with the use of organic anions for estimation of liver function, some dogs and cats with PSVA have had normal BSP 30 minute percentage retentions. These are artifactual and either due to hypoalbuminemia or dosing errors.

AMMONIA TOLERANCE TESTING. Animals with PSVA do not dependably demonstrate fasting hyperammonemia. Fasting blood ammonia values may be normal in up to 21% of dogs and in 10% of cats. After administration of ammonium chloride, increases of 300% to 400% usually develop. Abnormal values are determined by comparison with normal ranges established by the laboratory analyzing the sample and the control ammonia sample. The ATT is reliable in detecting hepatic insufficiency in PSVA when the test is properly done. Using a meal to simulate an ATT does not reliably challenge a patient's ammonia detoxification capabilities. The plasma ammonia concentrations in dogs and cats with PSVA before and after the oral administration of ammonium chloride are shown in Figure 35–8. Ammonia intolerance is clearly demonstrated in each patient.

SERUM BILE ACIDS. Serum bile acid (SBA) concentrations are good indicators of portosystemic shunting, no matter what the cause (Figure 35–9).[102–114] Intrahepatic as well as extrahepatic shunting are reflected by abnormal values. The postprandial SBA concentration is the most dependable diagnostic test for detection of PSVA in routine practice.[102–110]

The SBA concentrations cannot distinguish between liver disorders because there is a wide overlap of abnormal values.[103,108–111,113,114] Combination with other diagnostic tests, however, may yield useful patterns that predict the type of hepatobiliary disease. In animals with PSVA, the patient signalment, the presence of erythrocyte microcytosis, low serum cholesterol, normal or mildly increased serum enzyme activity, and neurobehavioral signs along with markedly increased SBA concentrations usually provides strong indication of the disorder. The presence of a "shunting" pattern to the bile acid values is a strong indication of a perfusion abnormality. The shunting pattern is typified by normal or moderately increased fasting bile acid concentrations and a profoundly increased postprandial serum bile acid concentration (Figure 35–8) (for a review of the patterns of bile acid with various diseases see Figure 8–35). Not all animals with PSVA show this pattern; some have remarkably increased fasting and postprandial SBA values, similar to the pattern seen in cholestatic disorders. The duration of the fast prior to testing determines how low the fasting SBA concentrations may become. As with baseline ammonia concentrations, prolonged fasting may provide enough time for the hepatic arterial circulation to "cleanse" the systemic blood. The postprandial SBA concentrations provide the best diagnostic indicator of hepatic perfusion abnormalities in animals with PSVA.[104,109,110] A random fasting SBA value, as a single test, should not be used to diagnose this disorder.

Diagnostic Imaging of Portosystemic Shunts

Radiographic contrast imaging of the portal venous system is the gold standard for documentation and anatomic localization of congenital and acquired portocaval shunts.[16,75,115–121] The patient must be under general anesthesia for each of the procedures used. It has been suggested that intrahepatic and extrahepatic shunts can be differentiated radiographically using portography.[121] If a shunting vessel is located cranial to the T_{13} vertebra, it is probably intrahepatic, and if any part is caudal to this vertebra, it is most likely extrahepatic.[121]

CRANIAL MESENTERIC ARTERIAL PORTOGRAPHY. This procedure requires prior experience with selective mesenteric catheterization and availability of fluoroscopy. Contrast medium is directly injected into the cranial mesenteric artery. Catheterization is accomplished through the femoral artery

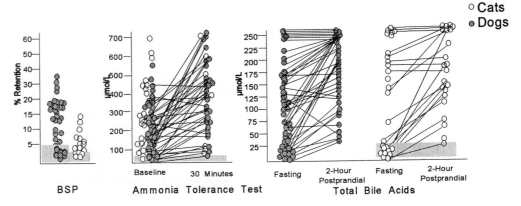

FIGURE 35–8. Results of liver function tests (BSP 30 minute percentage retention, ammonia tolerance tests, and 12 hour fasting and 2 hour postprandial serum bile acid determinations) on dogs and cats with congenital portosystemic vascular anomalies. Data derived from the College of Veterinary Medicine, Cornell University.

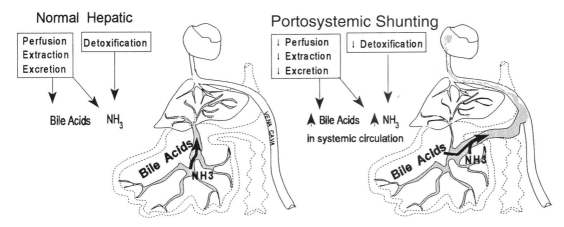

FIGURE 35-9. The effect of portosystemic shunting on hepatic extraction of bile acids and ammonia.

by use of a long radiopaque "pigtailed" catheter. The catheter is inserted into the femoral artery and under fluoroscopic observation is moved into the aorta to the level of the first lumbar vertebra. The catheter tip is rotated and moved until it enters the cranial mesenteric artery. This is ascertained by test injection of contrast under fluoroscopic visualization. Mistaken passage of the catheter into the celiac artery will result in an arteriogram yielding a nondiagnostic study in dogs with typical PSVA. Selective celiac artery catheterization is used as the diagnostic procedure of choice for documentation of an hepatic arteriovenous fistula, discussed later in this chapter. With the catheter in position, water soluble contrast media such as Conray 400 (Mallinckrodt Medical, Inc.; St. Louis, MO) or Renographin 76 (ER Squibb Co.; Atlanta, GA) is injected at a dose of 1.5 to 3.0 mL/kg body weight using 150 to 300 psi via an automatic injector.[75,115–119] The automatic high-pressure injector rather than hand injection delivers contrast in a rapid bolus that permits dense vessel opacification. Use of a high-pressure injector requires that a catheter with an adequate lumen be used to avoid disconnection of injector lines and catheter at its hub as a result of catheter-related flow resistance. From 3 to 6 radiographs are made during the 4 to 10 second arterial phase.[75] Eight to 10 radiographs are made during the 6 to 14 second venous phase.[75] A rapid film changer permits exposure of numerous films in rapid succession. This imaging technique is the least invasive of all described radiographic procedures for PSVA identification. The disadvantages include (1) delayed and blunted shunt visualization due to the fact that the venous phase follows contrast dilution in the arterial and capillary phases, (2) catheter movement resulting in a nonselective aortogram, (3) expense of the necessary support equipment, (4) a possibility of induced arterial spasm and thromboembolism as a result of contrast media, injection pressure irritation, or catheter-related mechanical trauma, and (5) the need for an experienced radiologist. Examples of anterior mesenteric portography are shown in Figures 35–10, 35–11, and 35–12. A photographic subtraction technique can be used to improve shunt visualization by removing images of overlying abdominal structures.[120]

SPLENOPORTOGRAPHY. This can be a minimally invasive technique in the best circumstance, but it usually requires laparotomy. Splenic pulp portography involves direct contrast medium injection into the splenic parenchyma. It is hoped that contrast will rapidly move into the splenic vein and subsequently into the portal circulation. The venous drainage of the spleen originates as sinuses delineated by reticular fibers.

Collagenous trabeculae coalesce to form the splenic venules that emerge at its hilus. Many venules exiting the hilus of the spleen converge to form the splenic vein, which accepts major tributaries (the left gastric, gastroepiploic, and pancreatic veins) as it courses toward the portal vein (Figure 35–1D). This procedure can be done using percutaneous, keyhole, or laparotomy approaches. An 18 to 20 gauge intravenous catheter is inserted obliquely into the spleen with the intent of positioning the tip as close to the hilus as possible. Venous backflow is realized if positioning is correct.[75,118] A test injection of contrast is done and is observed either fluoroscopically or on a single survey film taken at 2 to 4 seconds after contrast injection. If the contrast appears to be flowing appropriately, from 5 to 15 mL of contrast medium is injected by hand. Optimally, 6 to 10 radiographs are made at 1 second intervals after an initial 2 to 4 second delay. Adequate studies can be made without a rapid film changer and fluoroscopy. Two or three radiographs taken over a 4 to 6 second interval have been diagnostic using this technique.[118] A small tunnel built to support the patient above the radiographic cassettes can permit rapid hand advancement of several films to attain multiple sequential exposures.

Successful splenoportography delineates the portion of the portal vein cranial to the splenic vein. Usually, good opacification of the vessels occurs because there is minimal dilution of contrast medium. Portosystemic collateral vessels from the

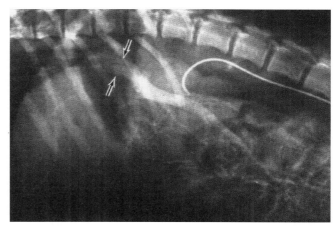

FIGURE 35-10. Anterior mesenteric artery portogram showing a large portosystemic anastomosis between the portal vein and azygos vein (arrows). This shunt could only be partially closed.

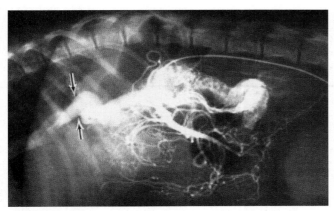

FIGURE 35–11. Anterior mesenteric artery portogram in a dog with a patent ductus venosus (arrows). This study is unusual because most of the contrast entered the portal vein without dilution in the arterial and capillary circulation.

splenic vein but not from the anterior mesenteric vein are well visualized. Thus, some PSVA will be completely missed using this procedure. Complications associated with this procedure include (1) splenic laceration, (2) splenic infarction, (3) loss of catheter position resulting in a poor study and peritoneal contamination with contrast, and (4) postoperative splenic abscessation. This technique, however, can be performed by most veterinary practitioners.

Operative catheterization of a major splenic vein with a through-the-needle catheter has been described as an alternative method for portography.[122] The parietal surface of the spleen is punctured with a 14 to 16 gauge needle opposite the venule selected for catheterization. An 18 gauge needle is suggested for petite patients. The needle is manipulated into position and the catheter is carefully advanced into the venule. Digital manipulation directs placement of the catheter within the splenic vein. The operator has the option of positioning the catheter at various levels within the splenic-portal vasculature. The catheter is secured against the parietal surface of the spleen so as to ensure that gentle traction will not dislodge it, the abdomen is closed, and portography completed. It has been suggested that the catheter can be removed uneventfully by simply pulling it out, without reopening the abdomen. This requires proper tautness and positioning of the securing suture and knots.[122] Tearing of the splenic capsule, surface hemorrhage, splenic abscessa-

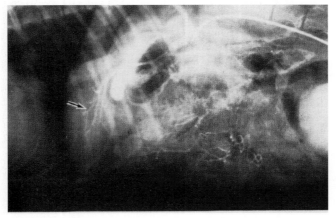

FIGURE 35–12. Anterior mesenteric artery portogram in a dog with a portosystemic shunt demonstrating a small intrahepatic portal system (arrow) and a large shunting vessel.

tion, and splenic vein thromboembolism are potential complications. Pre- and postligation portal pressures can be estimated with a water manometer using this technique.

MESENTERIC PORTOGRAPHY. The best and most complete studies of the portal venous system are usually attained with this procedure. This is one of the most invasive of the diagnostic radiographic techniques for PSVA visualization. A loop of jejunum is isolated and a jejunal vein is selected that may be catheterized without jeopardizing intestinal arcade perfusion.[50] Two ligatures are placed around a selected jejunal vein and an over-the-needle 18 to 20 gauge (22 to 24 gauge in cats) intravenous catheter is introduced and ligated in position with 4-0 silk suture.[39] The abdomen is temporarily closed and the animal is moved to the radiographic equipment. A 1 to 2 mL/kg bolus of contrast medium is injected by hand into the mesenteric catheter.[115,118] One or more radiographs are made as the final volume of contrast medium is injected. An optimal study results when 4 to 6 radiographs are made over 6 to 10 seconds.[75,115,118] Good quality studies can result from single radiographic exposures using this method. Both lateral and ventrodorsal views should be made, requiring at least two separate injections. These studies provide high-quality detail because the contrast medium is directly injected into the portal vein, minimizing circulatory dilution. An example of mesenteric portography in a cat with a left gastric vein PSVA is shown in Figure 35–13. No special equipment other than that used for routine radiography is required, making this technique useful to most small animal practices. Drawbacks to this procedure include (1) the need for laparotomy, (2) prolonged anesthetic time, (3) potential dislodgement of mesenteric catheter during transport from surgical suite to radiography equipment, (4) risk of peritonitis resulting from failure to maintain aseptic conditions, and (5) potential jejunal loop infarction from iatrogenic vascular injury to the mesenteric arcade (uncommon problem for the experienced surgeon). After the study is complete, the patient is returned to surgery and the abdomen is reopened. If the animal's condition is stable, the PSVA is ligated and the liver is biopsied. The jejunal catheter is used to pre- and post-PSVA attenuation portal venous pressures using a water manometer. Afterward, the jejunal catheter is removed and the access vein is ligated.

ABDOMINAL ULTRASONOGRAPHY. Hepatic ultrasonography can assist in identifying the presence of a PSVA but the high dependence on operator skill gives this diagnostic modality highly variable sensitivity and specificity.[123–126] The use of equipment augmented with Doppler capabilities improves the diagnostic performance of ultrasonography for PSVA identification. The liver of the patient with a PSVA is usually small, but this is a subjective ultrasonographic assessment. In most patients, few hepatic or portal veins are visualized. Unfortunately, these structures may also be difficult to visualize in a healthy individual.[123] Often the ultrasonographer is left with an impression that the hepatic portal vasculature is diminished, but this finding does not carry much diagnostic significance. The small hepatic size may substantially hinder a thorough evaluation for a PSVA. Overlying ribs, lungs, and gastrointestinal tract may impede thorough inspection of hepatic and vascular structures.[123,125,126] The use of general anesthesia and positive pressure ventilation can improve conditions for ultrasonographic visualization of a portosystemic shunt. Increased ventilatory pressure pushes the diaphragm and liver caudally, away from the overlying ribs and lungs. This also results in expansion of the abdominal vena cava and intrahepatic veins and may assist in their identification.

Intrahepatic shunts are easier to visualize than extrahepatic shunts. Communications between the intrahepatic cau-

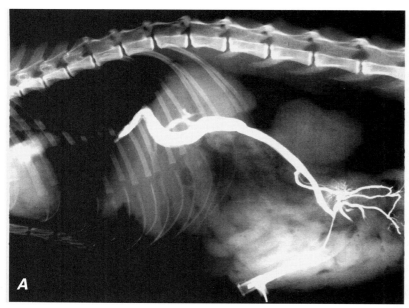

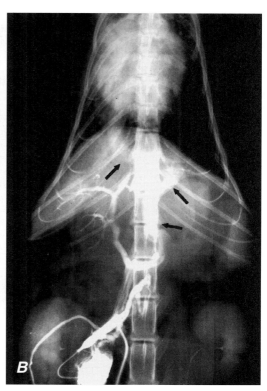

FIGURE 35-13. Mesenteric portogram in a cat with a left gastric vein portosystemic vascular anomaly. In (A) the lateral view clearly defines the shunting vessel. In (B) the right division of the portal vein is perfusing the liver with contrast and the very large anomalous shunting vessel (arrows). (Courtesy Dr. N. Dykes, Section of Radiology, Department of Clinical Sciences, Cornell University.)

dal vena cava and the portal vein may be directly seen or only the turbulence associated with dilated venous structures may be identified (similar to the findings associated with an intrahepatic arteriovenous fistula).[123,124] Intraoperative use of ultrasound can locate intrahepatic shunts if surgical inspection is unable to localize the vascular anomaly.[32] Transducers may be placed inside sterile surgical gloves for intraoperative use and saline used as an acoustic coupling agent.[32,118]

Extrahepatic shunts may be directly visualized by a diligent operator following a tedious systematic evaluation of portal tributaries and the caudal vena cava using Doppler (Figure 35-14). Identification of turbulent blood flow within the vena cava usually signifies the entrance of a shunting vessel. Visualization of an extrahepatic shunt can be impaired by overlying bowel gas. Of all the extrahepatic shunts commonly diagnosed, the portoazygos shunts are the most difficult to visualize.[127] When a shunting vessel cannot be visualized ultrasonographically, the presence of an extrahepatic PSVA remains probable in the face of the following findings: (1) high clinical index of suspicion based on signalment, routine clinicopathologic testing, and high serum bile acids, (2) subjective evaluation that the liver appears small, (3) the lack of visualization of an intrahepatic shunt, and (4) the presence of minimally dilated intrahepatic portal veins and a small extrahepatic portal vein. There is danger in putting full confidence in this assumption because some animals fulfilling these criteria do not have extrahepatic portosystemic shunts but have a newly described entity of microvascular portal dysplasia, an aberration of the hepatic circulatory system restricted to the microvasculature.

Pulsed-wave Doppler ultrasound can be used as a noninvasive method of estimating portal blood flow. This is a tedious procedure that requires the patient's full cooperation. Estimations of portal blood flow in normal dogs and dogs with experimentally induced biliary cirrhosis have been reported.[128,129] There is operator-induced error inherent in these estimations. Currently, detection of abnormal portal blood flow unique to PSVA has not been shown to be a useful diagnostic parameter using this technology.

COLORECTAL SCINTIGRAPHY. Scintigraphic study of the liver involves the administration of a radioisotope that is circulated to the liver and taken up into the organ. The most commonly used scintigraphic procedures on PSVA patients require minimal restraint because the images are collected over a very short time span following isotope administration. If sedation is necessary, intravenous butorphanol at a dose of 0.05 mg/kg has been successfully used without causing serious long-term sedation or neurologic signs.

Early studies of hepatic function used technetium (^{99m}Tc) sulfur colloid. Following intravenous injection, radiocolloid particles circulated to the liver whereupon they were

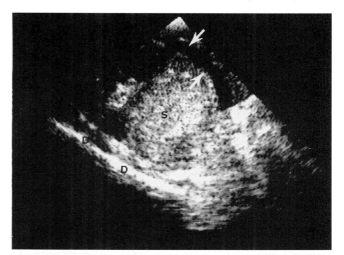

FIGURE 35-14. Combination of two separate ultrasonographic images of the left gastric shunt shown in Figure 35-13 to demonstrate the ability to follow the anomalous shunting vessel around the structure of the stomach. The PSVA is indicated by arrows, the stomach = S, diaphragm = D. (Courtesy Dr. A. Yeager, Section of Radiology, Department of Clinical Sciences, Cornell University.)

extracted by the hepatic reticuloendothelial cells. These also were taken up by the spleen. Estimation of the rate and quantity of isotope taken into the liver provides an estimation of hepatic blood flow and function of the hepatic reticuloendothelial system. Circulation of radioactive colloid during initial hepatic arterial and portal venous transit can be used to estimate the relative blood flow through each circulatory bed. A time-activity curve can be constructed from this information that graphically depicts the arterial and portal venous phase. The slope of the extraction curve is calculated and provides an hepatic perfusion index (HPI). The HPI expresses the relationship between the arterial phase slope and the portal venous phase slope and thus the relative perfusion from each system.[130-132] Initial studies using radiocolloid techniques showed significant differences in HPI between normal dogs and dogs with PSVA.[130] Scintigraphic studies of cats using 99mTc sulfur colloid were difficult to analyze due to the small size of the patient. In these, isotope uptake into pulmonary tissue interfered with imaging of the hepatic arterial and portal venous systems.

Scintigraphy using an 99mTc-labeled imidoacetic acid analogue, used primarily for hepatocholescintigraphy, has yielded HPI indices in animals with PSVA similar to those in normal dogs.[133] Further evaluation of the application of the HPI using different imaging agents in dogs with PSVA has shown a substantial number of false positive and indeterminant results.[134] Subsequently another imaging substance (N-isopropyl-p-(123I) iodoamphetamine (IMP), used primarily for brain imaging, was evaluated. This substance has optimal characteristics for use in the estimation of hepatic blood flow; it has rapid colonic absorption into the portal circulation and high first-pass hepatic extraction (Figure 35–15). After intracolonic administration, IMP can be followed as it traverses the portal circulatory system. Estimation of cardiopulmonary and hepatic parenchymal activity provides an approximation of the percentage of portal blood flow effectively bypassing the liver.[134,135] The fraction of mesenteric blood flow that bypasses the liver is determined from data acquired on a computer-linked scanner. Two studies have shown significantly higher shunt fractions for dogs with PSVA than for normal dogs.[113,114] This radiopharmaceutic has a long half-life permitting convenient storage, but it has limited availability and is expensive.

Use of 99mTechnetium pertechnetate (99mTcO4-) is an inexpensive alternative to the more costly imaging isotopes.[136,137] It too has rapid colonic absorption; approximately 14% of a delivered dose enters the portal circulation with an absorption half-time of 1.41 ± 0.57 minutes.[138] Recording a dynamic image over 1 to 5 minutes following colonic instillation produces a nuclear venogram of the portal circulation.[139] A small dose of isotope, between 5 to 20 mCI, is administered in a small volume of fluid (1.5 to 2 mL) to minimize colonic retention of tracer.[137] This very small dose is flushed through a soft blunt-ended rubber feeding tube, shortened to minimize dead space and yet permit dose deposition between 10 and 20 cm into the descending colon. Air rather than saline or water is used to ensure dose delivery; 10 to 15 mL of air is usually used but this is determined by the size of the instillation apparatus. Dilution of the isotope dose with a fluid flush results in an inferior portal image. It is recommended that a cleansing enema be given 6 to 12 hours before dose administration to ensure rapid contact between isotope and colonic mucosa which will optimize isotope absorption. It is important to avoid the complication caused by residual enema fluid retention because that dilutes the isotope, resulting in a poor quality study. Animals are imaged in right lateral recumbency to maintain consistency with conventional positioning on radiographic studies. A large field of view gamma camera is used and initial imaging started a few seconds before isotope

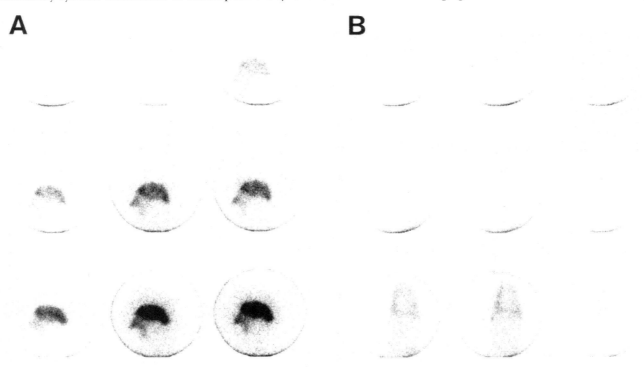

A

B

FIGURE 35–15. Transcolonic 123I-iodoamphetamine studies performed on a normal dog (*A*) and a dog with a PSVA (*B*). The sequential series of 1 minute ventral microdot images demonstrate exclusive uptake of the tracer by the liver in the normal dog, whereas the dog with the shunt has obvious pulmonary uptake. A ratio of lung counts to lung counts plus liver counts provides an estimate of the relative shunt flow. (From Koblik PD, Yed C-K, Hornof WJ, et al. Use of transcolonic 123I-iodoamphetamine to diagnose spontaneous portosystemic shunts in 18 dogs. Vet Radiol 30:67–73, 1989.)

administration. Approximately one image every 4 seconds is recorded.[137] In a normal animal, the portal vein is visualized between 10 to 22 seconds after isotope instillation. The isotope is first delivered to the liver and subsequently to the heart and lungs. In animals with a PSVA, the isotope is first delivered to the heart and lungs or simultaneously to the liver, heart, and lungs (Figure 35–16). Sometimes the isotope never obviously marks the hepatic circulation as a result of systemic circulatory dispersal. There is sufficient definition on some studies to distinguish large-diameter shunting ves-

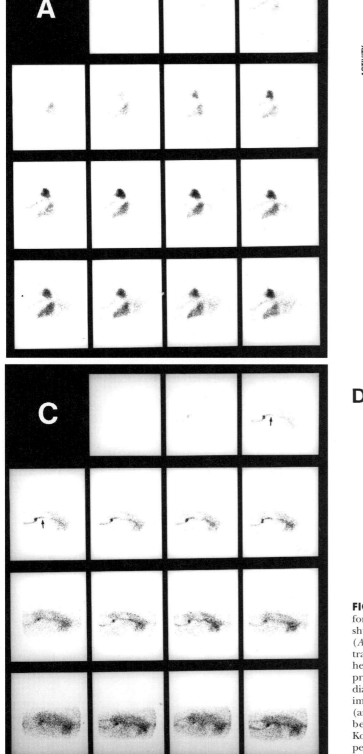

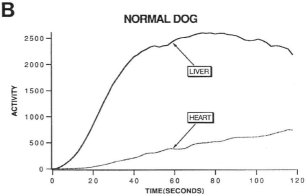

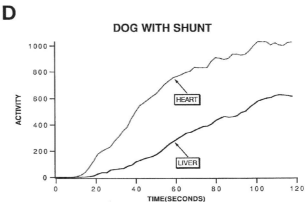

FIGURE 35-16. Transcolonic [99m]-Tc pertechnetate studies performed on a normal dog (*A, B*) and on a dog with a portosystemic shunt (*C, D*). The sequential 5 second right lateral microdot images (*A*) and accompanying time activity curves (*B*) demonstrate the tracer arrives in the liver several seconds before it arrives in the heart. In the dog with a PSVA (*C, D*), the tracer arrives in the heart prior to its arrival in the liver. The reversal of temporal events is diagnostic for portosystemic shunting. In this instance, the microdot images indicate a single and probably intrahepatic shunt vessel (arrow). Analysis of the areas under the liver and heart curves can be used to estimate relative shunt flow. (From Koblik PD, Komtebedde J, Yen C-K, et al. Use of transcolonic [99m]technectium-pertechnetate as a screening test for portosystemic shunts in dogs. J Am Vet Med Assoc 196:925–930, 1990.)

sels. However, as a rule, nuclear images provide less anatomic information than that afforded by radiographic venography. Colorectal scintigraphy has high diagnostic specificity for detection of portosystemic shunting without requiring general anesthesia and invasive catheterization procedures. Results using ^{99m}Tc pertechnetate are usually so obvious that they can be interpreted without computer processing. Because ^{99m}Tc pertechnetate is not extracted by the heart or lungs, quantification of an HPI is not possible. Instead, a shunt index is computed based on the ratio of integrated heart to liver counts collected over an operator-defined interval and area following initial isotope appearance at either one of the targets. The shunt index is used to express the severity of the shunt. The percentage of blood that shunts past the liver is calculated by dividing the summed counts in the heart by the summed counts in the heart and liver. In normal dogs, the shunt index is less than 15%.[137] For dogs and cats with PSVA, the shunt index ranges between 22% to 89%.[114] This procedure can be used to estimate the extent of surgical correction of a PSVA in the immediate postoperative period. Whether or not this provides prognostic information has not been determined. Follow-up of some dogs with PSVA only partially ligated has shown a decremental reduction in shunt index over time.[140] Immediate postoperative scintigraphy of some dogs that have had their PSVA completely ligated, according to the surgeon performing the procedure, has shown residual shunting. This either is due to the presence of more than one shunting vessel or incomplete attenuation of the anomalous vessel. Dogs with microvascular portal dysplasia without a PSVA usually have a normal to slightly increased shunt index ranging up to 30%.[140] One shortcoming of colorectal scintigraphy is the underestimation of shunting when a gastrosplenic vessel is involved. This occurs because portal blood from the colon does not normally circulate through this area. This may complicate use of the test in cats where left gastric vein shunts are one of the most common types of PSVA.

Hepatic Histology Associated with PSVA

A liver biopsy should always be collected in animals with PSVA to ascertain the presence or absence of hepatic fibrosis and acquired hepatobiliary disease. In addition, hepatic biopsy is the only diagnostic test that confirms the presence of microvascular portal dysplasia. The histologic features of PSVA and microvascular portal dysplasia are similar to those developing after creation of an Eck fistula.[141–147] Histologic changes in dogs after surgical creation of a portosystemic shunt have been well characterized.[142]

Representative photomicrographs detailing liver lesions in dogs with PSVA are shown in Figures 35–17 and 35–18. Lesions are subtle and, consequently, many early studies of animals with PSVA failed to describe the classic features that are now acknowledged. In humans with PSVA, hepatic lesions were not identified until autopsy in several cases. Antemortem liver biopsies were called normal. Histologic changes in all species in which PSVA have been recognized are similar, although not every animal displays each of the so-called classic features. Sinusoids surrounding the portal triad (zone 1) are narrowed and sinusoids surrounding the hepatic vein (zone 3) may be widened. Fatty vacuole formation or vacuolation is common in hepatocytes in zone 3 as is deposition of small amounts of connective tissue around the hepatic vein. Hepatic arterioles are obvious in the portal triad and portal veins may be small or indistinguishable. Small- to medium-sized arteries in the portal triad have distended lumens and

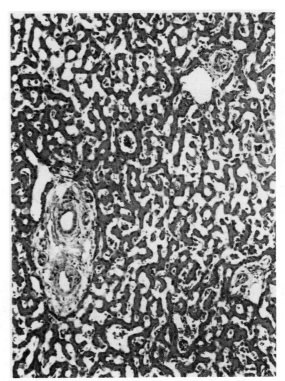

FIGURE 35–17. Photomicrograph of a liver biopsy from a dog with a portosystemic vascular anomaly. Hepatic changes included sinusoidal distension, parenchymal atrophy, and relatively few branches of portal veins in portal triads. The number of portal triad branches is excessive for the magnification shown.

thickened walls. An increase in the number of small- and large-caliber vascular structures in the periportal area, presumably capillaries or possibly lymphatics, are observed in many patients. An increased number of bile ducts has been notable in some portal triads. Inconsistently, hyperplastic foci

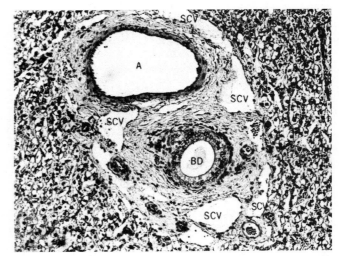

FIGURE 35–18. Photomicrograph of a liver biopsy from a dog with a portosystemic vascular anomaly. This close-up view of a portal triad demonstrates the increased numbers of small caliber vessels (SCV) and absence of convincing portal veins. The hepatocytes are atrophied. The caliber of the hepatic artery (A) is large because of the compensatory increase in blood flow. BD = bile duct. (From Breznock EM. Surgical manipulation of portosystemic shunts in dogs. JAVMA 174:819–826, 1979.)

of hepatocytes may be seen in zone 1. In some animals, an increased deposition of iron in hepatic Kupffer cells and within lipogranulomatous foci have been observed. Similar "hemosiderosis" has been related to portosystemic shunting since early investigations.[148]

Hyperplastic changes of hepatic arterioles represents either a response to an increased arterial flow or a compensatory change to accommodate a greater flow. Increased numbers of vascular channels presumably communicating with the hepatic arterioles, portal veins, and sinusoids suggests that arteriovenous and arteriosinusoidal shunting permits a compensatory increase in hepatic arterial flow. The fibroplasia around central veins and altered appearance of the sinusoids reflects the deranged hepatic blood flow. Stasis of RBC movement through sinusoids may be associated with increased release of iron, focal inflammation, and subsequent storage of iron in Kupffer cells. Deposition of iron in hepatic Kupffer cells, and with chronicity, in hepatocytes, has been shown in dogs and rats with portocaval anastomoses.[142,146] Progressive fibrosis seen in some animals remains unexplained but seems to be associated with progressive worsening of the hepatic insufficiency.

The lesions just described are also seen in animals with microvascular portal dysplasia lacking PSVA or acquired portosystemic shunting. These animals have abnormal liver function tests and may or may not display other clinicopathologic features typical of PSVA. In severe cases, secondary or acquired portosystemic shunting develops due to portal venous atresia and hypertension. Severely affected animals develop multiple portosystemic collaterals. The most severe form of microvascular portal dysplasia is denoted as portal venous atresia, diagnosed when an atretic portal vein is recognized at the time of surgery. It is probable that all animals with PSVA have some degree of permanent microvascular anatomic malformation. This explains the lack of normalization of liver function after complete surgical attenuation of a single PSVA. Comparisons of hepatic histology before and months after complete PSVA ligation have shown persistent hepatic lesions in some dogs and cats (Figure 35–19). Although residual vascular abnormalities are usually evident, hepatocyte atrophy seemingly resolves.

In health, the high-pressure arteriolar circulation joins the low-pressure portal circulation during sinusoidal admixture and through direct arteriovenular anastomoses that are regulated by sphincters.[149,150] Arteriosinusoidal and arterioportal communications regulate the mixture of blood perfusing the hepatic sinusoids. Shunting through these regions increases after portacaval anastomosis.[149,150] Arterioportal communications also are associated with the intrahepatic shunting that occurs in patients with hepatic cirrhosis.[151–154] The portal venous/hepatic artery admixture has been evaluated by use of radioisotope-labeled colloids in normal rats and in rats in which the portal vein and hepatic artery have been variably ligated.[155,156] This work verifies that arterial flow is the predominant component of the afferent hepatic circulation and that the high-pressure arterial blood mixes with the portal system before the sinusoidal level. Increased blood flow through the liver was shown when the portal vein was ligated. Autoregulatory response of the hepatic artery compensates for loss of portal perfusion. Faster flow of blood through the sinusoids and exposure of periportal vasculature to higher pressures is assumed.

The normal hepatic microcirculation has been evaluated in a number of different studies.[149–151,156–160] In health, the hepatic arterial blood enters the majority of the sinusoids from the portal venule so that flow is generally through the sinusoidal bed toward the central venule. The sinusoidal blood fed by arteriosinus twigs (branches of the hepatic

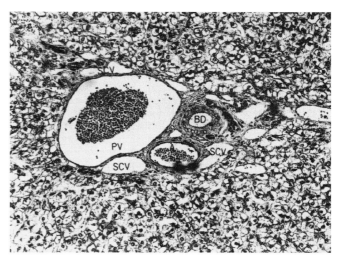

FIGURE 35–19. Photomicrograph of a liver biopsy from the same dog as in Figure 35–18, after ligation of the anomalous shunting portal vessel. Portal triads still retain small caliber vessels (SCV). There is now a large portal vein (PV). The hepatic artery (A) is less prominent in size compared to the entire portal triad. These changes may only be ascertained after review of many portal triads in a specimen. BD = bile duct. (From Breznock EM. Surgical manipulation of portosystemic shunts in dogs. JAVMA 174:819–826, 1979.)

artery terminating in zone 1) flows toward both the central venules and through short separate segments of the sinusoids into portal venules. Normally the arteriosinusoidal twigs contain little flow. In rats with an Eck fistula, flow in these vessels is remarkably increased. The lack of normal portal perfusion likely leads to focal necrosis in sinusoidal areas not supplied by an arteriosinus twig. This could be pathogenically associated with the areas of multifocal vacuolar transformation commonly observed in hepatic biopsies from PSVA patients. Upon creation of an Eck fistula, hepatic sinusoids in zone 3 become dilated and lose their normal parallel organization. Scattered islands of thickened plates of hepatic cells bounded by narrowed sinusoids also are often observed. These areas are speculated to have rapid blood flow that would impair the ability of hepatocytes to extract nutrients and metabolites; this results in a "shunting effect." Sinusoidal walls are likely damaged by the high pressure in the now "arterialized" system.[157,158] This leads to a transformation of the vascular pathways in zone 1 into poorly fenestrated capillaries. These changes could explain the abnormal portal triads lacking portal veins and containing marginal small caliber vascular structures. The small-caliber vessels may provide a reservoir for blood from the now "arterialized" system. Light microscopy and transmission electron microscopy of liver from rats with PSVA suggest that sinusoidal capillarization is an adaptive response to the lack of normal portal venous perfusion.[14] Ultrastructurally, sinusoids adjacent to the portal triad develop a thickened endothelial barrier lacking the normal complement of hepatic endothelial fenestrae. These resemble nonfenestrated "true" or systemic capillaries. It was pointed out that these structures could easily be misinterpreted as abnormal portal tracts .

Hepatic atrophy is microscopically and grossly evident in most animals with PSVA. It is grossly more obvious in the dog than in the cat. Similar atrophy has been shown in animals with Eck fistulas.[161,162] Histologically and cytologically, hepatocytes appear smaller than normal. Regeneration has been shown to be slowed when portal circulation is deviated.

Surgical Management

Surgical attenuation of a PSVA is the treatment of choice. Surgical therapy may not result in complete cure even though clinical signs are vastly improved or eliminated. A normal life expectancy can be achieved after ligation of a PSVA if medical management is adjunctively used as necessary. A large number of dogs and cats that have had complete surgical ligation of a PSVA *never* normalize their liver function.

In some patients, surgical attenuation of the shunting vessel is not done during the same anesthetic interval as portography. Survival has improved in the author's hospital if hypothermia and procedures longer than 3 hours are avoided. This has been particularly true for pediatric and petite patients (especially cats and Yorkshire terriers). We have staged surgical ligations as early as 3 days from diagnostic portography. Obviously this approach requires owner preparation for repeated anesthetic and surgical intervention. Previously reported mortality rates for animals undergoing surgical ligation of a PSVA have been approximated as 14% and 21%. This has improved with increasing experience of clinicians managing these cases. In the author's hospital, the mortality rate within the past 8 years is less than 10% .

Understanding the normal anatomy of the portal and azygos venous systems is essential for correct identification of aberrant shunting vessels. This is not a surgical procedure that should be undertaken by an inexperienced surgeon or individual not fully familiar with the normal portal and splenic vasculature. Many surgeons use radiographic portography to confirm the presence and position of shunting vessels. Without portography, misidentification of the PSVA and failure to locate and ligate multiple shunting vessels is possible. Most extrahepatic portocaval shunts are prominent or tortuous on visual inspection and the portal vein is smaller than normal.[23,30,39,53,54] The most common extrahepatic portocaval shunts enter the caudal vena cava cranial to the phrenicoabdominal veins. A systematic evaluation of normal venous structures is necessary in order to conclusively identify an anomalous vessel. The portal vein, caudal vena cava, and renal veins are first identified.[48,51] The paired phrenicoabdominal veins are located entering the caudal vena cava immediately cranial to the renal veins after coursing across the adjacent adrenal gland.[50] Any vein entering the caudal vena cava in front of the phrenicoabdominal veins may be considered anomalous.[53] If a shunt is not visualized, further inspection requires cranial retraction of the stomach, a right and ventral retraction of the duodenum, and a caudal retraction of the left pancreatic lobe.[53] This permits visualization of the left gastric vein, splenic vein, and other portal vein branches and portoazygos shunts.[53] Portoazygos shunts are distinguished by careful identification of normal portal tributaries and tracing their route to the liver. These shunts usually are large and tortuous and originate from a portal venous tributary that deviates to the azygos or hemiazygos vein dorsal to the stomach near the crus of the diaphragm.[63] Identification and surgical correction of a patent ductus venosus is the most challenging of all portosystemic vascular communications. Most of these are located in the left or central hepatic divisions and empty into the left hepatic vein before entering the caudal vena cava.[41,53,63] These may be ligated by left hepatic vein attenuation, intracaval techniques, or intraparenchymal dissection.[3,30,39,54,58] Surgical approaches and procedures for attenuating intrahepatic PSVA are complicated and have been well reviewed in recently published surgical textbooks.[39,54] Some dogs and cats have PSVA and portal vein atresia associated with multiple peripheral portosystemic shunts.[16,28,75] An example of a portogram from a cat with this collection of abnormalities, before and 8 months after surgery, is shown in Figure 35–20A and B. These patients often cannot be corrected by shunt attenuation, although some authors have suggested vena caval banding procedures.

The degree of attenuation of a PSVA depends on the response of the individual patient's portal circulation to the applied ligature. Temporary attenuation is done with the surgeon observing the abdominal viscera. Subtle and acceptable signs of portal hypertension include a slight pallor or blanching of the duodenum and jejunum followed by obvious distension and pulsation of jejunal arteries.[47] The motility of the small intestine may become vigorous and the pancreas may become slightly congested.[47] Visceral cyanosis should not develop. Cyanosis warrants immediate loosening of the ligature around the PSVA. The viscera are grossly observed for 15 minutes and if no further changes indicative of continuing portal hypertension are noted, the ligatures are permanently set. Many surgeons also measure the portal pressure and use this parameter to determine if acceptable shunt attenuation has been accomplished. Normal values for portal pressure have been reported to range between 3 and 26 cm H_2O and between 8 to 10 mm Hg.[16,39,161–164] Most authors report a range between 6 and 13 cm H_2O. Fewer values are published for cats, but a similar range to that of dogs has been reported.

When attenuating a PSVA, different authors have recommended that either or both the gradient of change and the final portal pressure be considered. A general recommendation is that the portal pressure should not rise 10 cm H_2O greater than the preattenuation pressure[35] or greater than 23 cm H_2O.[30,35,39] A retrospective study evaluating the reliability and safety of determining the degree of shunt attenuation on the basis of visually estimated and H_2O manometer–determined portal pressures indicates a wide variation in postattenuation portal pressure in dogs successfully ligated and no consistent parameter that consistently indicates when a safe end point of attenuation is reached.[47] Absolute values of portal pressure appeared of little use.[47] Approximate doubling of the preattenuation value appeared to be safe and effective and coincided with the gross estimations of the degree of portal hypertension judged to be safe. The major conclusion that most surgeons seem to agree on is that relative changes in portal pressure are more important than absolute measurements.

Surgical complications of shunt ligation include (1) portal hypertension due to an inability to accommodate increased hepatic portal flow, which can lead to transient ascites, bowel ischemia, or portal thromboembolism; (2) mesenteric venous hemorrhage from the site of jejunal or splenic vein catheterization; and (3) septic peritonitis due to contamination during surgical and/or radiographic procedures. Excessive manipulation of the abdominal viscera and circulation and deep anesthesia may compromise the ability of a surgeon to judge the suitability of ligature tautness. The visceral response to manipulation is increased vascular resistance, which reduces splanchnic blood flow.[140] Both halothane and enflurane decrease hepatic arterial, portal venous, and total liver blood flow.[165,166] These variations may lead to excessive shunt attenuation and subsequent postoperative complications.

Immediate Postoperative Recovery

Postoperative management of animals with PSVA is outlined in Figure 35–21. The surgical ligation of a PSVA has appropriately been labeled "a dynamic event."[47] The hemodynamic adjustments to shunt attenuation are established over several postoperative days. Ascites may form and resolve and

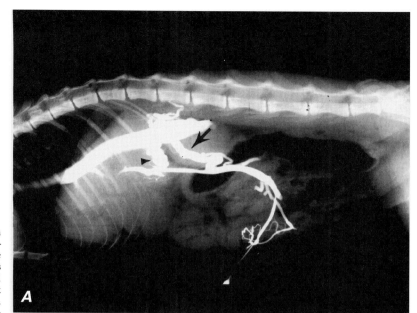

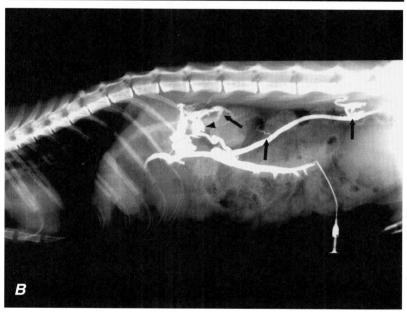

FIGURE 35–20. Mesenteric portogram of a cat with severe microvascular portal dysplasia and a portosystemic shunt. In (*A*), completed before surgery, a large shunting vessel is shown (arrow). Accompanying this vessel is a tortuous acquired portosystemic collateral (arrowhead). Liver biopsy revealed features consistent with PSVA and no evidence of acquired liver disease. In (*B*), completed 8 months after initial surgery, the location of shunt ligation is marked by surgical clip (arrowhead). Notice the development of other acquired portosystemic collaterals (arrows), lack of intrahepatic portal circulation, and microhepatica. Despite medical management, this cat was showing profound hepatoencephalopathic signs.

the gut undergoes a short interval of postoperative ileus. During the immediate postoperative interval, attention must be directed to avoidance and correction of hypothermia and hypoglycemia as each of these can slow recovery. Hypothermia is a particular problem in toy breeds of dogs and in cats. During the first several postoperative hours, the patient should be closely assessed for development of abdominal hemorrhage and intestinal ischemia. Rapid development of abdominal distension, concurrent with ileus, diffuse intestinal distension with gas, hemorrhagic diarrhea, tachycardia, and impending shock, indicate a need for emergency surgical intervention for ligature removal. Abdominal ultrasound may assist in patient assessment.[167]

Fever ranging up to 103.8 °F is common during the first 48 hours after surgery. Abdominal pain should be modulated with narcotics. Oxymorphone or butorphanol are commonly used and titrated to the animal's ability to metabolize the sedative effects of either drug (each drug is metabolized/excreted by the liver). Oxymorphone and

butorphanol cannot be used together because they have competitive antagonistic effects. A dose at the low end of the normally prescribed range for analgesia is initially used and modified according to patient response. Butorphanol is given at a dose of 0.1 to 0.2 mg/kg and oxymorphone is given at a dose of 0.05 to 0.1 mg/kg. Oxymorphone is preferred because it has a stronger analgesic effect. Some cats develop agitation and bizarre reactions to opiates; if this occurs, use of the drug is suspended. If hepatoencephalopathic stupor or coma are evident, opiates should be avoided because they can increase intracranial pressure. Laparotomy incisions are painful and pain increases sympathetic tone and splanchnic vascular resistance, which can adversely influence mesenteric perfusion. Postoperatively, animals should not be so uncomfortable that they stand in their cage or remain restless. The clinician should not be afraid to modulate pain in these animals. Acepromazine should not be given because it may cause depression and stupor and has no analgesic effect. If the animal is agitated or uncomfortable, pain modulation and treatment

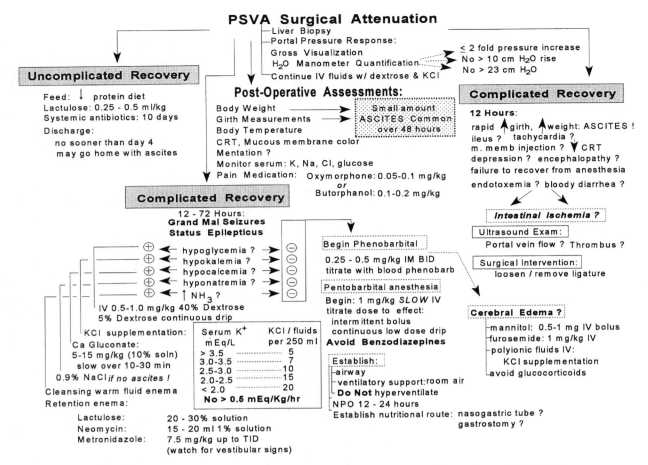

FIGURE 35–21. Treatment algorithm for the postoperative management of dogs and cats with PSVA. Treatment is specified for uncomplicated and complicated recoveries.

of HE is more appropriate. Intravenous fluids containing dextrose are continued until the patient is able to eat and drink. Serious hypoglycemia can develop during recovery from anesthesia and may be overlooked unless blood glucose concentrations are monitored.

Monitoring of vital signs includes initial hourly assessments of pulse quality and rate, mucous membrane color and capillary refill, blood glucose, urine production, and measurement of body weight and abdominal girth. Body weight and girth determinations will allow early recognition of ascitic fluid accumulation.

A gradual accumulation of abdominal effusion is common within the first 48 hours and will usually resolve within 7 to 10 days. In normal dogs in which moderate portal hypertension is created by portal venous banding, shunting through portosystemic collaterals is well developed within 3 weeks. Patients unable to accommodate surgically induced portal hypertension following PSVA ligation develop multiple portosystemic collaterals within a similar time interval.[66,168,169] When modest and reversible portal hypertension develops, fluid is characterized as a modified transudate and the abdomen usually does not become tautly distended. Because the presence of abdominal effusion signals the presence of portal hypertension, fluid therapy with 0.9% saline should be avoided. Rather, sodium-restricted fluids should be given if continued parenteral fluid support is required. Most animals can be discharged for at-home owner care before complete resolution of their effusion. The sudden development of

abdominal distension associated with worsening depression and/or failure to fully recover from anesthesia should prompt consideration of obstructed portal venous blood flow associated with thromboembolism. This complication is rare but can be confirmed by ultrasonographic imaging. Portovenography can also be done, but less invasive diagnostic evaluations are preferred.[167]

In patients undergoing uncomplicated recovery, feeding is usually resumed within 36 to 48 hours of surgery. Continued use of lactulose and a restricted protein diet is recommended until the success of surgical therapy can be appraised. This usually is not evaluated for several weeks. Systemic antibiotics are continued for 10 days as a prophylactic measure; amoxicillin or cephalexin are often used. If a neutrophilic leukocytosis, toxic neutrophils, and/or a left shift develop, antibiotics should be changed to a broader spectrum and consideration be given to surgical complications.

Postoperative Seizures

A rare postoperative complication is the development of grand mal seizures within 12 hours to 3 days after uneventful and successful ligation of PSVA. There is no predictive variable associated with this complication other than a seemingly greater occurrence in animals older than 18 months of age, dogs of small breeds, and a greater occurrence in Maltese.[47,170,171] In the author's hospital, cats with PSVA have more commonly demonstrated pre- and postoperative seizure activity than dogs. The cause of sudden onset seizure activity remains unexplained. Hypoglycemia, hyperammonemia, thromboembolism, cerebral infarction, and encephalitis have been ruled out as etiologic factors based on blood chemistry, CSF analysis, and necropsy findings. Some animals have had subnormal serum concentrations of potassium and calcium, but clinical signs persist when these abnormalities are rectified. Hyponatremia has been recognized in some dogs that resists correction with fluid therapy.[171] Treatment with fluids, oral and rectal lactulose, neomycin, or metronidazole is ineffective in ameliorating seizure activity. Because the cause of the seizure activity remains unclarified, the recommended treatment is supportive and symptomatic. An appropriate approach is detailed in Figure 35–21.

At first onset of seizure activity the patient's glucose and electrolyte status (calcium, potassium, sodium) should be evaluated. An intravenous bolus of a concentrated dextrose solution should be given if hypoglycemia is detected and an infusion of a dextrose-enriched solution continued. Symptomatic neuroglycopenia is usually rapidly responsive to dextrose infusion, although in some animals that have experienced severe persistent hypoglycemia, a seizure focus may become established. Hypokalemia can promote ammonia toxicity in the central nervous system and so this problem must be corrected as rapidly as is safe. Infusion of potassium is given according to the conventional sliding scale for potassium supplementation with care given to avoid a dose exceeding 0.5 mEq/kg/hour (Figure 35–21). Serial determinations of the serum potassium concentration are used to guide potassium supplementation. If hypocalcemia is recognized, consideration of the influence of total protein and albumin binding on the total calcium determination is essential in the dog. If spurious hypocalcemia is discounted, a slow infusion of 10% calcium gluconate is provided as the patient's neurologic condition and vital signs are monitored. Development of bradycardia indicates a too rapid infusion of calcium. If HE is considered likely, intravenous fluid therapy and cleansing warm enemas should be given. Fluid therapy will guard against development of prerenal azotemia, which will promote hyperammonemia. The colon should be evacuated to eliminate a source of continued release of hepatoencephalopathic toxins. Once the colon is evacuated, a retention enema containing lactulose, neomycin, and/or metronidazole is used to modify further gut toxin formation.

Initially, these patients should be kept off oral food and water. Because most patients suffering postoperative seizures do not rapidly recover from their neurologic impairment, it may be necessary to establish a method of nutritional support. Gastrostomy or nasogastric tubes have worked well in these patients, but sometimes hand feeding of a slurried or liquified diet mixture is successful. If cerebral edema is considered possible on the basis of clinical signs (increased muscle tone in extremities, hyperventilation, and slowed pupillary light reflexes), mannitol has been recommended at a dose of 0.5 to 1.0 g/kg given by rapid intravenous bolus.[171,172] Because nonosmotic loop diuretics like furosemide have been reported to inhibit the secretion of CSF by the choroid plexus, these may be synergistic when used with mannitol to reduce intracranial pressure.[173] Care must be taken to monitor serum electrolytes when mannitol and/or furosemide are administered because either drug may induce diuresis that can lead to electrolyte depletions. Use of glucocorticoids cannot be advocated in these patients. Although some forms of cerebral edema are responsive to glucocorticoids, this has not been shown in patients with HE associated with fulminant hepatic failure.[172] Furthermore, glucocorticoids promote catabolism, gastroenteric bleeding, and polyuria, side effects that may worsen a patient's clinical status and tendency to develop HE. The use of barbiturates (pentobarbital and phenobarbital) for seizure control offers a benefit in protection against cerebral edema. Barbiturates have been shown to lower cerebral metabolic rate and blood flow.[174] Ventilatory support may become necessary if a patient is anesthetized. This may require use of a mechanical ventilator. Ventilation with room air is appropriate. Hyperventilation is not recommended on the basis of work in humans with HE where it has not been effective in protecting against development of cerebral edema.[174,175] Hyperventilation may prove detrimental via induction of respiratory alkalosis, which can promote CNS ammonia toxicity.

Postoperative seizures in patients with PSVA are usually poorly responsive to anticonvulsants. Consequently, general anesthesia with pentobarbital is usually used for immediate control. A wide-ranging dose between 1 and 14 mg/kg has been required to anesthetize affected dogs. Initial anesthesia should be accomplished with very small doses given at intervals of 5 to 10 minutes to avoid inadvertent overdosage. It is prudent to be conservative at first because of the severe derangement of the GABA neuroreceptors and neutrotransmitters in the patient with HE and because of the PSVA patient's impaired hepatic drug metabolism.[176–179] Use of benzodiazepines has been ineffectual. This is not surprising considering the role that benzodiazepines are believed to serve in the etiopathogenesis of HE. Initiation of phenobarbital at a 0.25 mg/kg to 0.5 mg/kg dose and subsequent dose titration based on the serum phenobarbital concentrations has been used for chronic seizure control in surviving animals. Phenobarbital is usually begun concurrent with initial pentobarbital anesthesia. Approximately 25% of phenobarbital is eliminated by the kidneys, which permits its use in patients with compromised hepatic function. Treatment with potassium bromide has been successful for long-term seizure control in some dogs with PSVA that suffer recurrent seizure activity and have residual hepatic insufficiency. The majority of dogs reported in the literature and approximately 50% of dogs and cats treated in the author's hospital for postoperative seizure activity have died or been euthanized. In the few patients that recover, recurrent seizure activity may or may not become an intermittent medical problem. Recovery from neurologic impairments is usually slow and often is incomplete. The best responses have been observed in animals managed by vigilant dedicated owners. One severely impaired cat that developed postoperative seizures underwent nearly full recovery only after 12 months of at-home nursing care.

Histologic Brain Lesions

Animals with PSVA that have chronic recurrent HE develop histologic lesions in the brain. Some of these lesions are reversible. Described abnormalities include bilateral symmetric polymicrocavitation of the brain stem and the cerebellar nuclei and an Alzheimer type II reaction and polymicrocavitation in the cerebral cortex and adjoining white matter.[27,180,181]

Long-Term Response to Surgical Management of PSVA

Portosystemic vascular anomalies should be considered amenable to surgical palliation. For animals showing signs of

HE, clinical signs nearly always improve. A good clinical response is achieved in most cases. However, a considerable number of dogs and cats never regain normal liver function tests, either BSP, ammonia tolerance test, serum bile acid concentrations, or hepatic scintigraphy.[23,30–32,36,44,48,49,56] Estimation of shunt fraction using ^{99m}Tc pertechnetate colorectal scintigraphy has shown that even animals with completely ligated PSVA have residual shunting.[137] Failure to eliminate portal systemic shunting and to normalize liver function in a patient that has undergone what is believed to be complete surgical ligation of a PSVA has been attributed to a variety of possibilities including (1) failure to identify and ligate all contributory shunting vessels, (2) ligation of the wrong vessel, (3) induced portal hypertension and development of acquired portosystemic shunts, (4) incomplete PSVA ligation, and (5) the presence of nonresolvable microvascular portal malformations (microvascular portal dysplasia). Although ligation of PSVA usually results in improved clinical status, the persistence of abnormal liver function tests is extremely common and has been perplexing to clinicians managing these cases. In one reported case, residual shunting through what was erroneously believed to be a completely ligated shunt was shown by a photographic subtraction procedure applied to a routinely done portogram.[120] The residual shunting was not recognized on routinely evaluated portography.

Short-term prognosis for good clinical outcome was recently evaluated retrospectively for partial or complete PSVA ligation in dogs (n = 20).[56] Short-term postoperative clinical response (reduction of clinical signs) was the same for partial and total occlusion of a PSVA. Progressive reduction in shunting as estimated by colorectal scintigraphy has been shown in some dogs with partial PSVA ligation.[140] One retrospective study of 7 cats, however, has suggested that incomplete ligation of a PSVA does not produce a good long-term outcome.[49] In cats with PSVA unable to be completely attenuated, some temporarily improve and some continue to demonstrate clinical signs severe enough to warrant routine continuous medical intervention. Repeat laparotomy and complete shunt attenuation after 2 to 6 months has improved some of these patients. However, some cats have had severe microvascular portal dysplasia and cannot tolerate further shunt occlusion (Figure 35–20) because they develop multiple acquired portosystemic communications. In dogs and cats, clinical results and whether a shunt can be partially or totally occluded at surgery cannot be predicted from preoperative serum bile acid values, portograms, colorectal scintigraphy, or liver biopsy. The inability to observe hepatic portal vasculature in a portogram performed preoperatively cannot be used to deduce that the intrahepatic vasculature is lacking (Figure 35–22). It does seem that younger animals do better than older animals. One study concluded that dogs younger than 12 months of age can be given a better prognosis than those older than 2 years at the time of surgery.[56]

There is ample evidence that dogs with PSVA have more derangement in liver function than can be explained by simple extrahepatic shunting. Work with kindreds of Cairn terriers, Yorkshire terriers, and individuals of other pure breeds has described a microvascular portal dysplasia lesion that likely thwarts full recovery.[73,182]

Medical Management

Adjunctive medical management of PSVA should precede and accompany surgical intervention. Chronic medical management becomes necessary when surgical therapy does not fully alleviate clinical signs, when severe microvascular portal dysplasia exists, or in the patient who develops portal hypertension and acquired portosystemic shunting following PSVA attenuation. Medical therapy is also essential for the acute management of HE that often precedes definitive diagnosis of a PSVA.

Medical management of portosystemic encephalopathy is focused on avoidance of conditions known to precipitate HE (Table 35–4). Therapy is aimed at alleviating encephalopathic signs and/or ammonium biurate urolithiasis. The impaired hepatic ability to biotransform, conjugate, and eliminate certain drugs is considered before prescribing medications used routinely in other patients. Decreased mixed function oxidase activity has been shown following experimental creation of portosystemic shunts in rats.[176–179] This phenomenon as well as the perfusion alterations may underlie or worsen drug intolerance in these patients.

Medical management of dogs and cats with PSVA usually is not a successful long-term treatment. Liver dysfunction seems to progress over time and in some cases appears to culminate in hepatic fibrosis and portal hypertension. Clinical signs of HE episodically relapse despite optimal dietary management in most patients denied surgical intervention.

Chronic management is individually tailored to include the fewest number of therapeutic agents that achieve the very best control of clinical signs. The treatment regimen for each patient must be individualized. The lowest dose of medications that achieves a beneficial effect should be sought to conserve expenses and to avoid drug interactions.

Management of HE

The medical management of HE for the patient with PSVA is outlined in Figure 35–23 and has been discussed elsewhere in this text. When an animal presents with obvious encephalopathic signs, the initial step is to stop food ingestion for 12 to 48 hours. If neurologic signs are severe, the colon should be evaluated, cleansed, and a retention enema given to directly curtail further production of enteric toxins. When the patient recovers to the extent that per os medication is possible, lactulose, neomycin, and a protein-restricted diet are initiated. It is essential that a thorough investigation be made for medical conditions known to precipitate encephalopathic crises.

Dietary Therapy

Patients with portosystemic encephalopathy must be kept in positive nitrogen and calorie balance to avoid tissue catabolism that generates ammonia. The first important nutritional concern is to keep the patient eating.

Total caloric intake may be more important or at least as important as the protein intake in determining outcome in the Eck fistula dog.[183] It is not precisely known what level of caloric intake the patient with PSVA requires. General formulas for calculation of caloric needs have been empirically used in these animals.[184]

Suitable protein sources include cottage cheese, yogurt, and tofu. When diets restricted to these protein sources and containing the bulk of calories from carbohydrates and fat were evaluated in dogs with experimentally created portosystemic shunts, animals remained free of clinical signs, maintained body weight and protein reserves, and survived uneventfully for months when fed adequate calories.[183,185,186] When compared to dogs fed conventional diets, hepatic atro-

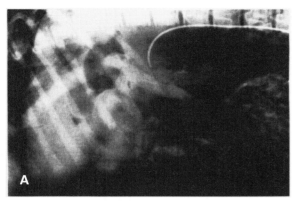

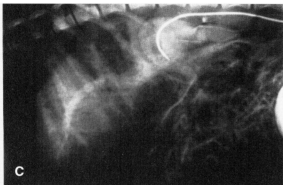

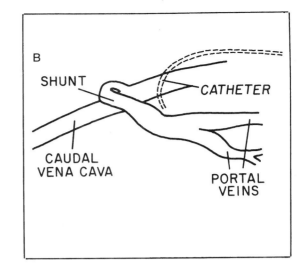

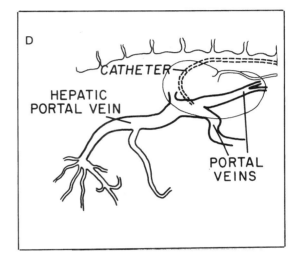

FIGURE 35–22. Angiogram of venous phase after injection of contrast medium through cranial mesenteric artery. Before surgery (*A*), the portosystemic shunt is filled with contrast medium because it provides the route of least resistance for the portal circulation. In (*B*), a diagrammatic representation of the anatomic structures is depicted. In (*C*), after surgical ligation of the portosystemic shunt, the venous phase of the angiogram shows no contrast medium entering the caudal vena cava directly. In (*D*), a diagrammatic representation of the anatomic structures is depicted. Before surgery, an hepatic portal circulatory system could not be seen, whereas after surgery, a normal system was defined.

phy occurred irrespective of the diet fed, but degenerative hepatic changes were more severe in animals ingesting insufficient calories and conventional canine diets. In spite of their high biological value, meat and egg proteins are considered detrimental to patients with HE.

The amount of protein the PSVA patient requires has been roughly estimated from a nutritional study in dogs with surgically created portosystemic shunts. This study showed that ingestion of 2.11 g/kg/day crude protein with an 80% or greater bioavailability is adequate to maintain body protein reserves without producing HE.[185] It is important to individually titrate a given patient to their optimal protein intake.[187] If the serum albumin concentration shows sequential decline or if clinically obvious catabolism (weight loss, poor hair coat, reduced vitality) occurs following dietary protein restriction, the protein content of the diet should be titrated upward to provide an optimal protein level for that individual. Changes in dietary protein are made in increments of 0.5 mg/kg body weight, with the effects appraised at 14 day intervals. If an increase in dietary protein generates HE signs, hyperammonemia, or biurate crystalluria, the maximal tolerated level of protein has been determined. Resumption of the previous protein intake that did not produce adverse side effects is recommended.

Use of prescription diets formulated for animals with renal insufficiency has commonly been recommended for management of portosystemic encephalopathy in both the dog and cat. Diets that are moderately protein restricted have been used successfully (Hills Prescription Diet k/d; Waltham Low Protein diet), although subjectively, these patients seem to do better on home-formulated diets or home modifications of the prescription renal diets (Table 35–5 and 35–6).

Abnormalities of branched chain to aromatic amino acid ratios have been documented in dogs with portosystemic shunting (Figure 35–5). However, a causal relationship between a deranged BCAA to AAA ratio and HE remains unproven (see Chapter 30). The deranged BCAA to AAA ratio associated with portosystemic shunting correlates better with the severity of shunting and hepatic insufficiency than with the presence or absence of HE.[188–190] Although formulating diets to minimize development of this adverse ratio has long been recommended, it is not clear this provides a related benefit.[185,188] Milk protein and soybean protein have similar amounts of adverse amino acids as meat proteins and most commercial maintenance dog foods. However, milk and soy protein are more effective in eliminating clinical signs of HE despite their association with a low BCAA to AAA ratio.

Provision of adequate usable nutrients in a moderately

Table 35-4

CONDITIONS ASSOCIATED WITH DEVELOPMENT OF HEPATIC ENCEPHALOPATHY

Dehydration:	prerenal azotemia
	renal azotemia
Azotemia:	↑ NH_3
Alkalemia:	↑ CNS NH_3 toxicity
Hypokalemia:	↑ NH_3
	↑ alkalemia
	polyuria
	anorexia
Hypoglycemia:	neuroglycopenia
Catabolism:	↑ protein turnover
Infection:	↑ protein turnover
	urease producers → urea → ↑ NH_3 = urease producers→urea→↑NH_3
Polydipsia/polyuria:	↓ K^+
	inappetence
Anorexia:	catabolism
	↓ K^+, ↓ zinc
	dehydration
	hypoglycemia
Constipation:	↑ toxin production
	↑ toxin absorption
Hemolysis:	↑ RBC breakdown → ↑ protein
Blood transfusion:	↑ RBC breakdown → ↑ protein
GI Hemorrhage:	RBC digestion→ ↑ protein
	inflammation ↑ protein
	parasitism ↑ protein
High dietary protein:	
(animal, fish, eggs)	↑ protein load
	↑ many other toxins
Drugs:	
benzodiazepines: diazepam, oxazepam	
antihistamines: Atarax®	
barbiturates: phenobarbital, pentobarbital	
metronidazole	
tetracyclines	
methionine	
organophosphates	
anesthetics	
diuretic overdosage: furosemide	

restricted protein diet, rather than focusing on provision of a theoretically optimal amino acid balance, has now been shown to prevent weight loss and development of neurologic signs in dogs with portosystemic shunts.[76,185,187] Study of dogs with surgically created shunts demonstrated that feeding protein-restricted diets high in BCAA versus a similar diet supplemented with AAA did not produce the expected benefits or side effects.[185] Surprisingly, feeding a moderately protein-restricted diet supplemented with BCAA produced neuroencephalopathic signs. Energy and diet digestibility were discounted as factors influencing the development of signs in these dogs. These findings contest previously published information suggesting that dietary restriction of AAA or supplementation with BCAA is neurologically protective.[191-200] Other investigators have also shown that dietary use of BCAA does not always benefit in prevention or reversal of HE in Eck fistula dogs.[188,194]

Another theoretical concern in diet preparation for the patient with HE has been to minimize patient exposure to methionine. It is incontestible that when fed in high amounts (25 g per dog) to animals with experimentally created portosystemic shunts, in one cat given methionine as a urinary acidifier and one dog reported in the literature, that methionine precipitates encephalopathic signs.[201-203] Despite these concerns, it has been shown that foodstuffs containing equivalent

quantities of methionine do not generate encephalopathic effects proportional to their methionine concentrations. Therefore, focus on preparation of a methionine-restricted diet is considered inappropriate, although excess supplementation should be avoided.

The importance of the source of dietary protein has been studied in humans in which HE is incapacitating. Provision of vegetable and dairy quality protein has clearly produced the best results in maintaining a positive protein balance with minimal encephalopathic effects.[204-207] The difference between the amino acid composition of meat and vegetable protein diets is not significant and so other dietary components are considered to be neuroprotective. The carbohydrate component of the dairy and vegetable protein diets is now recognized as the pivotal ingredient. Inclusion of fermentable, poorly absorbed disaccharides (such as lactose in the lactase deficient patient) and fiber (pectin and psyllium) has been shown to influence metabolism of nitrogenous and other encephalopathic toxins.[204,205,208,209] Fermentable carbohydrates induce increased microbial nitrogen fixation and subsequently fecal elimination.[209-211] They also reduce ammonia production and absorption and act as cathartics that assist in evacuation of encephalopathic colonic toxins.

It is interesting that soybean meal has been used as the protein source in several experimental studies in dogs with portosystemic shunts where neuroencephalopathic signs were averted.[76,183,185] One recently reported effect of soy protein is in reduction of enteric absorption of bile acids, which could moderate changes in cell membrane permeability; it is theoretically possible that this could favorably influence permeability of the blood-brain barrier.[212]

Feeding a diet with a high carbohydrate to protein component is advantageous in dogs and rats with an Eck fistula and humans with cirrhosis.[210] It appears that provision of at least 50% of the dietary calories in the form of easily digested and assimilated carbohydrates successfully averts encephalopathic signs.[76,183,185,204,206,210] This has been attributed to a lowered need for peripheral gluconeogenesis, which promotes protein anabolism rather than ammoniogenic protein catabolism.[204,213] Beneficial dietary carbohydrate sources include cornstarch, sucrose, pasta (wheat based, not egg noodles), and rice (polished). Each of these carbohydrate sources are palatable, easily digested, and simple to prepare.

Fat is an important source of calories and essential fatty acids, augments absorption of fat soluble vitamins, and enhances diet palatability. However, the role of fat in the diet of patients with hepatic insufficiency has not been determined. In humans with portal hypertension associated with cirrhosis, fat malabsorption may become a problem.[214] Only a minor decrease in the digestibility of dietary fat (from 92% to 85%) was shown in dogs with experimentally created portosystemic shunts.[185] A number of studies of the Eck fistula dog has shown that they do well on diets containing 20% to 25% fat.[76,198,210,215] Animal fat is commonly used in diets for animals with PSVA; vegetable oil and seed oil are also added for additional caloric and essential fatty acid supplementation. Although short chain fatty acids were previously considered to be important encephalopathic toxins, this is now contested.

Use of diets rich in carbohydrates, high in soluble fiber, supplemented with animal fat, and protein derived from dairy and vegetable sources have proven to be effective in the management of canine patients with hepatic insufficiency and PSVA. Soy protein in the form of tofu has worked well but takes some imagination to flavor so that it is well accepted. Soy sauce should not be used because uncooked sauce has recently been shown to contain high concentra-

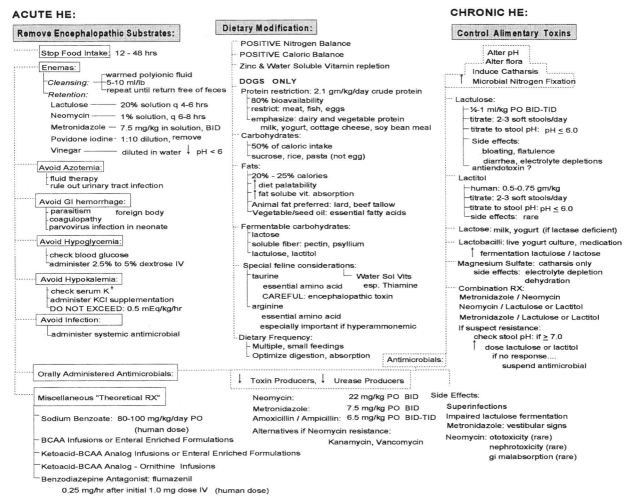

FIGURE 35-23. Treatment algorithm for the management of hepatic encephalopathy in dogs and cats with congenital PSVA. Consult Table 35–7 for drug dosages and side effects.

tions of ammonia.[216] A number of diets that have worked well in dogs with PSVA are provided in Table 35–6. It is useful to remember that lactose functions much like lactulose when some degree of lactase deficiency exists. Dairy products containing lactose (not cottage cheese) therefore provide good quality supplemental protein as well as beneficial fermentable carbohydrates.

Cats require a relatively high-protein diet in comparison to dogs. Protein should account for 14% to 20% of their caloric needs, which is approximately twice that needed by dogs.[184] There is little information on feeding cats with hepatic insufficiency. It is expected that they are like other mammals with hepatic insufficiency in that feeding high meat diets exacerbates encephalopathic signs. If milk and vegetable protein diets are used in cats it is essential that taurine and arginine be supplemented. At least 50 mg of taurine per day is recommended for the adult cat. Use of taurine should be individually tailored to each patient because taurine has been implicated as an encephalopathic toxin. A dose of 150 to 250 mg of taurine per day per cat has not produced adverse effects. Protein-restricted diets formulated for cats with renal insufficiency have been successfully used for long-term management of cats with HE due to PSVA (Table 35–5).

In order to optimize diet digestion and absorption and to minimize catabolic intervals, food should be fed in several small meals over the day or as free choice. Dietary supplementation with vegetable fiber may even out the assimilation of nutrients throughout the day. This minimizes the risk of hypoglycemia, ammoniogenesis promoted by gluconeogenesis, and increased free fatty acid mobilization related to lipolysis. Protracted fasting should be avoided. High-carbohydrate snacks should be fed to dogs and cats with PSVA. Some cats like caramels, cantaloupe, canned creamed corn, and vanilla pudding bottled for infants. Many dogs enjoy buttered popcorn and high carbohydrate cookies. Foods containing large numbers of preservatives should be avoided, especially foods containing MSG (monosodium glutamate).

Supplementation of water soluble vitamins is recommended for most patients. This becomes particularly important if home-prepared diets are used for chronic management or if an animal becomes anorectic. Water soluble vitamin supplementation also is important in patients that are polydipsic and polyuric where increased urinary losses are anticipated. Anorectic cats may require additional B complex vitamins to ensure adequate thiamine intake. Water soluble vitamin supplementation ranging from two to eightfold more than dogs receive has been suggested for cats.[217] A balanced commercial pet vitamin supplement is usually an adequate

Table 35–5

DIETS FOR CATS WITH PSVA AND HEPATIC ENCEPHALOPATHY	
K/D DRY HILLS PRESCRIPTION DIET	**RESTRICTED PROTEIN/PHOSPHORUS DIET[184]**
Nutrient g/100 g dry weight	
Protein 28.1%	¼ lb (115 g) liver (diced and braised, retain fat)
Poultry by-product meal	½ cup creamed cottage cheese
Dried whole egg	2 cups (350 g) cooked rice without salt
Dired poultry digest	1 T (15 g) vegetable oil
Fat: 27.4%	1 T (15 g) chicken fat
Animal fat	1 t (5 g) calcium carbonate
Carbohydrates: 38.3%	Balanced vitamin supplement
Brewer's rice	½ cup 2% milk
Cornmeal	Taurine 50 to 100 mg per day
Calories: 544/kcal cup (4.3 oz)	1 t pectin
Calorie derivation:	Calories: 635 kcal/lb
protein: 22%, fat: 48.2%, carbohydrates: 29.8%	Protein: 21%, carbohydrate: 35%, fat: 44%
	Calorie derivation:
	protein: 13.6%, fat: 63.9%, carbohydrates: 22.6%

vitamin source. Extra supplementation with fat soluble vitamins or lipotrophic substances containing methionine is not appropriate and may prove hazardous.

In summary, the important issues in nutritional management for these patients centers around (1) provision of adequate calories; (2) provision of a positive nitrogen balance to maintain body mass and protein reserves, (3) for the dog at least, avoidance or minimization of meat, egg, and fish origin protein and provision of vegetable and/or dairy quality protein, (4) supplementation of soluble fiber such as pectin or psyllium, (5) provision of adequate trace minerals, water soluble vitamins, and (6) adequate arginine and taurine for the cat.

Nondietary Strategies

CONTROLLING ALIMENTARY TOXINS. Modification of the alimentary environment is possible through use of medications that alter the microbial flora, enteric pH, and the absorption of toxic substances. Simple provision of enteric catharsis is also beneficial. The dosage and adverse side effects for a variety of therapeutic interventions are provided in Table 35–7.

LACTULOSE, LACTITOL, LACTOSE. Lactulose is a synthetic disaccharide that cannot be digested by mammalian enzymes. It is fermented in the lower bowel to organic acids by bacterial organisms. The fermentation products—lactic, acetic, and formic acids—acidify the lumenal pH, which discourages proliferation of urease-producing organisms and the catalytic activity of urease.[218–224] Lactulose also augments the uptake and incorporation of nitrogen into bacterial organisms, thereby promoting the fecal elimination of ammoniagenic products.[204] This activity is similar to the influence of carbohydrates in optimizing nitrogen fixation in ruminants. With proper dosing, fermentation of lactulose also serves as a gentle cathartic that encourages colonic evacuation. This beneficial effect protects against development of constipation, a recognized cause of encephalopathic crises. It is also possible that lactulose provides an antiendotoxic effect, useful in patients with compromised portal circulation and Kupffer cell surveillance.[225] The activity of lactulose is illustrated in Figure 33–20. Lactulose is sweet tasting and most animals take it willingly. Overdosage can result in bloating, abdominal

cramping, diarrhea, metabolic acidosis, dehydration, and electrolyte aberrations; these side effects are uncommon. Rarely, an animal will vomit after drug administration. Side effects are easily avoided by starting treatment with a low dose and having the owner gradually increase the amount given to achieve passage of several "pudding" consistency stools per day.

Lactitol is a newer generation synthetic disaccharide similar to lactulose that is marketed in a crystalline form. Its mechanism of action mimics that of lactulose. It is less sweet tasting than lactulose and has been evaluated in several clinical trials in humans.[226–229] It is not clear that it offers a substantial benefit over lactulose. It is claimed to be associated with fewer adverse side effects in humans (bloating, diarrhea) and has a more dependable and rapid cathartic effect. A dose of 0.5 to 0.75 g/kg body weight is recommended for humans.[229]

Lactose, when not optimally digested, provides a clinical effect similar to lactulose and lactitol.[151] This is an inexpensive and easy way to modify the gut environment in some PSVA patients. Lactose can be administered as a powder dissolved in water (to make a slightly sweet solution) or via ingestion of milk or yogurt. Provision of milk as necessary to produce a loose stool has been used in some clinical patients with success. Cottage cheese contains relatively little lactose. Yogurt with live lactobacillus culture has been successfully used as supplemental therapy in some PSVA patients. Whether the dairy quality protein, lactobacilli organisms, or residual lactose are beneficial is unresolved.

ANTIMICROBIALS. A number of different antimicrobials have been advocated for use in patients with portosystemic encephalopathy. The goal of such therapy is modification of the enteric flora such that toxin-producing organisms are reduced. Most drugs effective in this regard are inhibitory to urease-producing bacteria believed to be largely comprised of gram negative anaerobic organisms.[220] Anaerobic bacteria are most numerous in the large intestine and terminal ileum.[230,231] It is important to realize that some bacteria become resistant to antibiotics within 24 to 48 hours and suppression of sensitive strains can allow resistant ones to multiply. Thus, use of antibiotics may not be effective for longer than a few days in directly modifying the enteric microbial flora. However, there are probably other beneficial effects of antimicrobial administration related to impaired production of other encephalopathic toxins. Examples include interference in production of noxious products from methionine, endotoxins from bacteria, and volatile fatty acids from polysaccharide fermentation.

Certain antibiotics should be avoided. Tetracyclines should not be used because they have led to portosystemic encephalopathy in dogs with surgically created portosystemic shunts.[197] Tetracylines are also implicated as a cause of hepatic lipidosis. Consult Chapter 33 if use of a different antibiotic than those discussed is anticipated in the PSVA patient.

Amoxicillin/Ampicillin. Administration of oral amoxicillin or oral or parenteral ampicillin appears to provide short-term clinical benefit in both dogs and cats with acute HE associated with PSVA. These antibiotics are especially useful when systemic infection is a coexistent problem. Both drugs have been used independently as alternatives for neomycin and metronidazole, the more traditionally used enteric antimicrobials. Penicillin derivatives are advised over aminoglycoside products when renal insufficiency is suspected or when a patient initially presents dehydrated. Ampicillin has been shown to have efficacy comparable to that of neomycin in reducing gastric ammonia concentration in azotemic patients.[232] Cats demonstrating ptyalism as a sign of HE appear particularly responsive to amoxicillin, fluid therapy, and food withdrawal.

Neomycin. Oral treatment with neomycin is the standard for control of toxin-producing enteric microorganisms because it is effective against urease-producing organisms and is poorly absorbed from the gastrointestinal tract.[233–236] Even though neomycin is not known to have a wide efficacy against anaerobes, it produces good short-term clinical response in most encephalopathic patients. Although an aminoglycoside, the risk of toxicity with neomycin is low because less than 3% of an administered dose is absorbed.[235] Alternative aminoglycosides useful when intractable encephalopathy is thought to be associated with neomycin-resistant organisms include orally administered kanamycin and vancomycin. Toxic side effects associated with chronic oral administration of high-dose neomycin can occur. Chronic use can impart toxic effects to the intestinal mucosa, leading to epithelial atrophy and malabsorption.[237] Rarely, chronic neomycin use leads to bacterial or mycotic superinfections. Side effects associated with routine maintenance use of neomycin have been rare in dogs and cats with PSVA. However, animals with inflammatory bowel disease may absorb a larger proportion of an administered dose leading to ototoxicity and nephrotoxicity

Metronidazole. Metronidazole has broad-spectrum activity against enteric anaerobes such as *Bacteroides* spp. that are believed to metabolize nitrogenous dietary substrates. In one study, metronidazole was as effective as neomycin in the management of chronic portosystemic encephalopathy in humans.[238] In that study, an adjunctive benefit was detected when both medications were co-administered. If the oral route of administration cannot be used, rectal administration can provide therapeutic concentrations.[239] The dose of metronidazole must be restricted in patients with hepatic insufficiency because of drug dependence on hepatic biotransformation and elimination. In humans, a 50% dose reduction is recommended.[238] This is equivalent to an empiric dose reduction to 7.5 mg/kg PO BID for animals. This dose has not been verified to achieve therapeutic plasma concentrations in animals but seems clinically effective. Toxic neurologic side effects (vestibular signs) reported in animals[240] and humans with conventional doses have not developed with this dose in patients with hepatic insufficiency.

Combination Therapy: Lactulose and Antimicrobials. Combined treatment with lactulose and an antimicrobial may be effective in ameliorating encephalopathic signs when individual therapy is unsuccessful. In severely affected patients, a combination of an antimicrobial and lactulose are initiated early. Although lactulose and neomycin have been shown to act synergistically[241] one study suggests that neomycin can inhibit the organisms necessary for lactulose fermentation.[242] It is speculated that this is an uncommon complication because of the resistance of *Bacteriodes* spp. to neomycin, *Bacteriodes* being one of the strong lactulose fermenters. Whenever lactulose is used in combination with an antibiotic, its fermentation to organic acids can be monitored by assessing fecal pH using a urine dipstick pH pad. After 1 to 2 weeks of lactulose administration, a fecal pH of more than 7.0 indicates inadequate fermentation. In most cases, this is rectified by withdrawal of the concurrently administered antimicrobial, although in some patients an increase in the dose of lactulose identifies that a suboptimal dosage was being used. Coadministration of metronidazole and lactulose also has been effective clinically in severe HE. Although in theory metronidazole inhibition of *Bacteroides* should impair lactulose fermentation, this has not been realized.

Removal of Encephalopathogenic Substrates and Organisms

Osmotic Catharsis. Daily administration of magnesium sulfate has been used in humans with moderate portosystemic encephalopathy to cleanse the colon of encephalogenic toxins.[205] Chronic administration of lactulose, lactitol, lactose (if it is poorly digested), and soluble fiber (pectin, psyllium) provide a less dangerous method of catharsis for the small animal patient.

Cleansing Enemas and Retention Enemas. Cleansing enemas are used to directly eliminate retained colonic debris that serves as a source of encephalogenic toxins. Mechanical cleansing of the colon is important in the patient showing severe encephalopathic signs. Warmed polyionic fluids are initially used to avoid induction of hypothermia and water intoxication, concerns of particular importance in the petite or pediatric patient. The enema volume should be adequate to fill the colon but not be excessive so as to cause vomiting. These patients may lack conscious control of laryngeal reflexes and are thus subject to aspiration. Small-volume enemas intended to fill the colon and lower portion of the small bowel are repeated until the fluid return is relatively fecal free. A volume of approximately 10 to 25 mL per kg body weight is safely used. If the patient is constipated, dioctyl sodium succinate is mixed with the enema solution with the intent of softening the stool. Following complete evacuation of colonic contents, a retention enema is administered.

Retention Enemas

Retention enemas are given to provide immediate active modification of the colonic environment. These are small-volume enemas (5 to 10 mL per kg body weight) that remain within the colon and modify the lumenal environment by either influencing pH, microbial proliferation, microbial enzyme production, or enzyme activity. Diluted solutions of lactulose, lactitol, lactose, neomycin, metronidazole, vinegar, or povidone iodine are slowly injected into the bowel. Acidifying enemas comprised of 20% lactulose, lactitol, or lactose have been shown to reduce the blood ammonia concentration in humans.[205] Single or combination use of lactulose,

Table 35–6

Diets for Dogs with PSVA and Hepatic Encephalopathy: These diets are protein restricted. The protein is derived from dairy products and vegetables (soy). Restricted protein diets are suitable for the patient showing encephalopathic signs but *not* if the PSVA has been successfully managed with surgery. Gradual transition to higher protein diet is appropriate if clinical response to surgical shunt ligation appears good. Transition is made slowly and titrated to the quantity of protein the animal can tolerate without adverse signs. Dietary therapy is combined with other treatments used to control hepatoencephalopathy; consult Table 35–7 and Figure 35–23. Soluble fiber should be added to these diets: Pectin or Metamucil can be used. Approximate amounts are 1 Tablespoon pectin or Metamucil per 15 to 20 pound body weight per day.

STROMBECK/ROGERS DIET FOR DOGS WITH SEVERE LIVER DISEASE:[215]

Canine Diet 1

3 C	Instant nonfat dry milk fortified with vitamins A and D
⅖ C	Blackstrap molasses
1 C + 2 T	Raw wheat germ, ground
⅕ C	Bonemeal (sterilized for PO use)
½ C	Safflower oil
½ C	Animal fat
1½ t	Table salt (NaCl), iodized
3 C	Cornstarch
Vitamin C:	10 mg/lb/day
Choline:	250 mg per day if ≤ 33 lb 500 mg per day if > 33 lb (choline chloride or bitartrate)

Nutrient	*g/100 g dry weight*
Protein	11.1%
Fat	21.2%
Carbohydrate	55.2%

Calories: 4.6 kcal/g dry weight.
Calorie derivation: Protein: 9.6%, Fat 42.0%, Carbohydrate: 48.4%

Mix wheat germ and cold safflower oil with an electric mixer. Cut tallow or lard with scissors into small portions. Raise temperature to facilitate mixing with other components. Mix salt, bonemeal, and cornstarch separately and add to above ingredients. Add dry instant milk and molasses and mix. Diet resembles granola in appearance. A small amount of water may be added to improve palatability. Do not add water to diet intended for storage. Stored portions are refrigerated or frozen. If diarrhea develops, reduce quantity of diet fed per day for several days. If diarrhea persists, change to Diet 2 because lactose intolerance may be complicating use of Diet 1. Palatability may be enhanced by the addition of garlic powder, tomato sauce (fresh, no preservatives), or other inducements.

Canine Diet 2

2 lb	Low-fat cottage cheese
½ lb	Animal fat
¼ C	Safflower oil
1 lb + 3 T	Sugar
1 lb + 5 T	Cornstarch
1⅓ oz	Bonemeal
3¼ t	Salt substitute (KCl), iodized
	Not lite salt: NaCl + KCl
2 t	Table salt (NaCl), iodized
Vitamin C:	10 mg/lb/day
Choline	250 mg per day if ≤ 33 lb 500 mg per day if > 33 lb (choline chloride or bitartrate)
	High potency multivitamin / multimineral supplement

Nutrient	*g/100 g dry weight*
Protein	10.3%
Fat	19.0%
Carbohydrate	65.5%

Calories: 4.7 kcal/g dry weight
Calorie derivation: Protein: 8.7%, Fat: 36.1%, Carbohydrates: 55.3%

Mix sugar, cornstarch, bonemeal, and salt. Cut up lard or beef tallow as for Diet 1. Bring animal fat to room temperature prior to mixing with other ingredients. Mix the cottage cheese and safflower oil and blend with other ingredients. Palatability may be enhanced by addition of garlic powder, tomato sauce (fresh, no preservatives), or other craved foodstuffs in small quantities.

Quantities to Feed of Diets 1 and 2

Body Wt (lbs)	Maintenance Adult Energy	Diet 1		Diet 2	
		g	oz	g	oz
10	410	89	3.2	128	4.5
20	692	150	5.3	216	7.6
30	935	203	7.2	292	10.2
35	1051	228	8.1	328	11.6
45	1267	275	9.7	396	14.0
55	1476	321	11.3	461	16.3
80	1956	425	15.0	611	21.6

(Continued)

(Table 35–6 *continued)*

Canine Diet 3: General Liver Formula[215]

Nutrient	g/100 g dry weight
Casein	9.0%
Animal fat	20.0%
Sucrose	32.35%
Cornstarch	32.35%
Vitamin mix	1.0%
Mineral mix	5.0%
Choline chloride	0.3%

Calorie derivation:
    Protein: 7.5%, Fat: 38%, Carbohydrates: 54.5%

Mineral Mix: United States Biochemical Corp., Cleveland, OH
Vitamin Mix: Total Vitamin Supplement, United States Biochemical Corp., Cleveland, OH. To 1 kg of vitamin mix, 1 g of 0.1% vitamin B_{12} in gelatin.

Canine Diet 4[76]

Nutrient	g/100 g dry weight
Soy protein	18.0%
Chicken fat	25.0%
Sucrose	25.2%
Cornstarch	25.2%
Vitamin mix	1.0%
Mineral mix	5.0%
Choline chloride	0.3%
L-Methionine	0.3%

Calorie derivation:
    Protein: 14.4%, Fat: 45.1%, Carbohydrates: 40.4%

Canine Diet 5[183]

Nutrient	g/100 g dry weight
Isocal (Mead-Johnson)	
Enteric nutritional supplement	
Protein	13%
Caseinate (sodium, calcium)	
Soy protein	
Fat:	37%
Soy oil	
Medium chain triglycerides	
Carbohydrates:	
Maltodextrin	
Calories: 1 kcal/ml	

Calorie derivation:
    Protein: 8%, Fat: 57%, Carbohydrates: 34%

Canine Diet 6: Dry Canine k/d[184]

Nutrient	g/100 g dry weight
Protein	14.6%
Corn	
Dried whole egg	
Dried whey	
Fat:	19.5%
Animal fat	
Carbohydrates:	61.3%
Corn	
Brewers rice	
Calories: 362/cup (2.9 oz)	

Calorie derivation:
    Protein: 12%, Fat: 37.5%, Carbohydrates: 51%

Canine Diets 1 and 2 have been repeatedly used in clinical patients developing intermittent severe hepatoencephalopathic signs with excellent success.
Canine Diet 3 is a general formulation from which Diets 1 and 2 were derived.
Canine Diet 4 is an experimentally used diet derived from the Diet 3 recipe. This was used in a long-term study of dogs with surgically created portosystemic shunts and maintained dogs in good body condition without neuroencephalopathic signs for more than 40 weeks.
Canine Diet 5 was used for management of dogs with surgically created portosystemic shunts that maintained body weight without developing encephalopathic signs for 4 months. Dogs were given 85 kcal/kg body weight per day. This diet requires vitamin and fiber supplementation. Adequacy of protein repletion must be closely monitored.
Canine Diet 6 is commercially marketed for animals with renal insufficiency. This diet differs from the other diets in the origin of protein. It is a convenient alternative to home-cooked meals.

neomycin, and metronidazole has been used successfully in small animal patients. Because metronidazole is well absorbed from the intestines, rectal administration will not only influence the alimentary canal but will also provide a systemic antimicrobial effect. A dose no greater than the 7.5 mg/kg BID to TID oral dose is recommended, considering that hepatic metabolism of metronidazole is likely impaired. If lactulose, lactitol, neomycin, or metronidazole is not available, a dilute solution of povidone iodine and water (1:3) or vinegar (acetic acid) and water may be used. Iodine-containing solutions directly alter the viability of colonic organisms and should be removed after 10 minutes in young animals and cats especially, to avoid toxicity and mucosal irritation. Enema solution containing diluted vinegar can reduce the colonic lumenal pH, making it inhospitable to enteric ammonia producers and urease activity.

Retention enemas are repeated at 4 to 6 hour intervals, or more frequently if evacuation is frequent and complete. Care should be taken to avoid overdosing neomycin or metronidazole with repeated dosing. Retention enemas are continued while an animal displays obvious hepatoencephalopathic signs. Chronic use at home is not advised, but owners are taught to administer enemas in the event of acute encephalopathic decompensation. It is important that enema administration be done carefully so enteric inflammation and hemorrhage are not induced. These complications add potential toxigenic materials to the bowel.

MISCELLANEOUS TREATMENTS. Over the past 20 years, a number of treatments have been devised to target specific encephalopathic toxins. Most of these treatments do not provide a consistent response because of the multifactorial nature of HE and the fact that different factors may be operant within an individual at different times.

Sodium benzoate and sodium phenylacetate have been used in the management of hyperammonemia in children that have inborn errors of urea cycle enzymes.[243-245] This metabolic scheme is presented in Figure 33–21. There have been only a few clinical trials of sodium benzoate in humans with portosystemic encephalopathy.[205,245] Although improvement in clinical status and reduction of blood ammonia has been shown, a paradoxical side effect of hyperammonemia in an animal model was reported by one group.[246,247]

Intravenous infusions of BCAA or their keto-analogues have also been evaluated as therapeutic interventions. Study of dogs with experimentally created portosystemic shunts has shown that emphasis on attaining a high BCAA to AAA ratio vía an oral route does not improve condition or neurologic status.[185] This area of therapy is controversial and ongoing.

The administration of L-dopamine has been investigated in effort to normalize neurotransmission in humans and ani-

Table 35–7

MEDICATIONS USED FOR MODIFYING ENTERIC PRODUCTION OF ENCEPHALOPATHOGENIC TOXINS

Modifications of pH, Urease Activity, Toxin Generation, Microbe Population and Nitrogen Fixation

Lactulose:	0.25 to 1.0 mL/kg PO BID-TID per 4 kg body weight	Toxicity: with overdosage, flatulence, abdominal distension, diarrhea and metabolic acidemia. Dose titrated on the basis of stool character and frequency. Several soft stools with pH < 6.0 per day are desirable.
Lactitol:	0.5 to 0.75 g/kg PO BID	Less sweet than lactulose, may be more reliable in production of catharsis Minimal toxicity: flatulence, abdominal distension, diarrhea.
Lactose:	Milk or dry powder 10 to 50 g dissolved in water	Advantageous in lactose intolerant animals where lactose is digested/fermented similar to lactulose. Prepare a slightly sweet solution.
Dietary fiber:	soluble fiber pectin, Metamucil to diet 1 T per 7–10 kg body weight	Improves bacterial nitrogen utilization, reduces toxin production, and provides a mild cathartic effect. Pectin and Metamucil (unflavored) are advised. Dose is unknown, humans consume 10 to 20 g/day.
Lactobacilli:	live yogurt culture rather than pure culture	Continued oral administration can modify GI flora only temporarily with lactulose fermenting, nonurease-producing organisms.

Modification of Enteric Microbial Population, Toxin Generation

Neomycin:	22 mg/kg PO BID	Not absorbed well across the bowel wall. Chronic use in humans has been associated with ototoxicity, atrophy of enterocytes and malabsorption, and rarely, nephrotoxicity. Toxicity is uncommon in animals on chronic therapy. Antiendotoxic and synergistic with lactulose. Rarely, neomycin may impair lactulose fermentation. This is deduced by examining fecal pH for acidity.
Metronidazole:	7.5 mg/kg PO BID	Minor protein binding permits wide tissue distribution. Is efficacious against anaerobes. Modulates cell-mediated immune reactions, believed to have antiendotoxic properties, may be synergistic with lactulose. Rectal administration can be effectively used. Care must be given to avoid overdosage because metronidazole is reliant on hepatic metabolism and elimination. Toxicity: vestibular signs, nausea, and inappetence.
Amoxicillin:	5 mg/kg PO BID	Good systemic protection, can modify GI flora in some animals. Can be used in cats with PSVA to modulate encephalopathic signs.

Osmotic Catharsis

Magnesium sulfate:		Rarely used, can precipitate dehydration and electrolyte aberrations.

Lactulose, lactose, dairy products, soluble fiber: as described elsewhere in this table.

Cleansing and Retention Enemas

Warm saline cleansing enemas: 5–25 mL/kg	Isotonic polyionic, warmed fluids to avoid hypothermia and water intoxication. Enemas are given until fecal material is eliminated.
Retention Enemas	Dwell time imparts beneficial modifications within colonic lumen
lactulose:	5 to 15 mL of a 1:3 dilution
neomycin:	15 to 20 mL of a 1% solution
metronidazole:	systemic dose dissolved in water and administered per rectum
povidone iodine:	1:10 in water, remove after 10 to 15 minutes
diluted vinegar:	1:10 in water, ↓ pH of colonic lumen
lactose:	20 to 40 g in water

Avoidance or Elimination of Complicating Disorders

hypoglycemia: dextrose-enriched fluids	gastroenteric bleeding: famotidine, sucralfate
dehydration / azotemia → hyperammonemia	endoparasitism: fecal evaluation, anthelmintics
hypokalemia: KCl in fluids	infections: systemic antibiotics
alkalemia: avoid HCO_3 influsions	constipation

Avoid vitamin (B_1 in cats) and minerals (zinc) deficiency
Avoid animal and egg protein, focus on dairy and vegetable protein, high carbohydrate and ample fat diet.

Miscellaneous

Benzodiazepine antagonist: flumazenil	Initial 1.0 mg IV by slow bolus, followed by 0.25 mg/h (flumazenil) has been used in humans in deep encephalopathic coma. Seems to perform best in acute HE.
Sodium benzoate: 80–100 mg/kg/day	Do not exceed this dose because it may be toxic and/or lethal.
BCAA and/or BCAA keto-analogues:	Controversial, may be used in parenteral nutrition

mal models with severe portosystemic encephalopathy. Despite initial encouraging results, controlled studies have failed to confirm a beneficial effect.[205,248] Similarly, treatment with bromocriptine, a dopamine agonist, has not produced a consistently positive response.[249,250] More recent studies have

been unable to relate impaired dopaminergic neural transmission to HE.[248]

Animals and humans with unresponsive HE have been reported to improve following administration of a benzodiazepine antagonist (flumazenil). Unfortunately, recent clinical trials in humans have failed to substantiate a benefit in all patients.[251-253] It seems probable that acute encephalopathy is more responsive to flumazenil than is chronic encephalopathy. There have been no reports of flumazenil use in dogs and cats with spontaneous portosystemic encephalopathy.

MANAGEMENT OF AMMONIUM URATE CALCULI. Urate calculi seen in young non-Dalmatian dogs and cats are usually associated with PSVA. Medical management of urate calculi is especially important when (1) a PSVA is not amenable to surgical ligation, (2) surgical attenuation fails to correct portosystemic encephalopathy, or (3) surgical therapy is refused. If surgical ligation is planned, the urinary system should be thoroughly evaluated by ultrasonography to determine whether a cystotomy should be done at the time of laparotomy. Surgical removal of uroliths is often accomplished at the time of portography or shunt attenuation.

Medical management of ammonium urate calculi focuses on reducing factors known to favor crystal and urolith precipitation. These include (1) the formation of urine supersaturated with uric acid and ammonium, (2) stagnation of bladder urine, and (3) the presence of a urinary tract infection that can promote stone precipitation and aggravate preexisting hyperammonuria. Control of the blood ammonia concentration is the first goal to consider. Hyperammonemia can be partially controlled, through dietary modifications and use of lactulose and enteric antimicrobials. Although feeding a low-protein high-sodium diet is theoretically appropriate, the PSVA patient may lose condition and become catabolic on the ultra-low protein diet conventionally used to dissolve other types of urinary calculi (s/d prescription diet, Hills Pet Products). A restricted protein diet devised for control of HE containing vegetable and dairy quality proteins, is beneficial in control of ammonium biurate crystalluria/calculi because it reduces the enteric production and absorption of ammonia and restricts exposure to uric acid precursors (which are rich in meat- and egg-derived proteins). Maintenance of a low urine specific gravity is recommended as a prophylactic treatment for all types of uroliths; many patients with PSVA are polydipsic and polyuric and already are undergoing diuresis. The feeding of a high-salt diet, as recommended for dissolution of other types of uroliths, may be detrimental to some of these patients. Salt loading may promote development of ascites and may augment preexisting portal hypertension. These side effects are more common and serious in animals with acquired hepatic insufficiency associated with portal hypertension but can develop in some patients with PSVA postoperatively. Modification of urine pH to optimize solubility of ammonium urate uroliths may not be possible because ammonium urate calculi are theoretically more soluble in alkalinized urine. In animals with an inborn error of uric acid metabolism (such as Dalmatians), urine alkalinization inhibits renal tubular production of ammonium, which limits formation of ammonium urate colloids. In patients with PSVA, systemic hyperammonemia provides a ready source of ammonia for glomerular filtration. Without amelioration of recurrent hyperammonemia, ammonium biurate crystalluria remains uncontrolled. Alkalinization of urine with sodium bicarbonate may endanger the PSVA patient's neurologic status as a result of systemic alkalemia and preservation of ammonia in the nonionized and readily diffusable state. Chronic administration of sodium bicarbonate also can deleteriously load these patients with sodium. Retrospective evaluation of the urine characteristics in patients with PSVA demonstrating ammonium urate crystals has not clearly indicated a trend for a specific pH that augments their precipitation.

Dogs proven to have a concurrent urinary tract infection should receive chronic treatment with an antibiotic that does not rely on hepatic metabolism for biotransformation or elimination. Urease-producing organisms are particularly problematic because they will hydrolyze urea to ammonia. As long as urinary calculi are retained, infection can persist or become a relapsing problem.

Although anecdotal recommendations for the use of allopurinol in patients with PSVA have been given, such treatment has not been critically evaluated. Allopurinol is commonly used in Dalmatians to control formation of uric acid uroliths. Allopurinol undergoes hepatic metabolism to oxypurinol; both moieties are competitive and noncompetitive inhibitors of xanthine oxidase, the enzyme that transforms xanthine and hypoxanthine to uric acid. In humans, oxypurinol has a longer half-life than allopurinol. Because allopurinol is metabolized in the liver, compromised hepatic function or portosystemic shunting likely extends the plasma concentration of both parent drug and its derivative. Side effects of allopurinol in humans with normal hepatic function include inhibition of hepatic drug metabolizing enzymes and an infrequently reported idiosyncratic hepatotoxicity. Interference with drug metabolism would be particularly troublesome in the PSVA patient already burdened with deranged drug metabolism (P-450 cytochrome suppression) and hepatic insufficiency. In Dalmatians, chronic excessive dosing of allopurinol results in hyperxanthemia and subsequent formation of xanthine calculi.[254] The currently recommended treatment protocol suggests evaluation of urine uric acid clearance to estimate whether an effective and safe dose of allopurinol is being administered. In Dalmatians, approximately 300 mg of urate per 24 hours is considered optimal and avoids further precipitation of uric acid calculi and iatrogenic xanthine calculi.[254,255] The guidelines for similar titration of uric acid in the urine of the PSVA are not established. If allopurinol is used for chronic management, the owner should be cautioned that such use is investigational in these patients and that xanthine calculi may become a future complication.[255]

Feeding a low-protein diet (k/d, Hills Pet Products; primarily corn-derived protein) was associated with stone dissolution in dogs in one report.[256] It is probable these animals also received other treatments aimed at correcting clinical signs of portosystemic encephalopathy that concurrently controlled or reduced their blood ammonia concentration.

MICROVASCULAR PORTAL DYSPLASIA

Clinical Synopsis

Diagnostic Features

- Young Cairn or Yorkshire terriers are predisposed
- Usually subclinical but signs similar to PSVA may be seen
- Postprandial serum bile acids abnormal
- Colorectal scintigraphy normal to marginally abnormal
- Radiographic portography reveals diminution of tertiary branches of intrahepatic portal veins
- Hepatic biopsy reveals malformation of portal vascular axis similar to that seen with PSVA

Standard Treatment

- If clinically affected, treat as for PSVA

Microvascular portal dysplasia is a nonreversible congenital malformation of the intrahepatic portal vascular axis. This

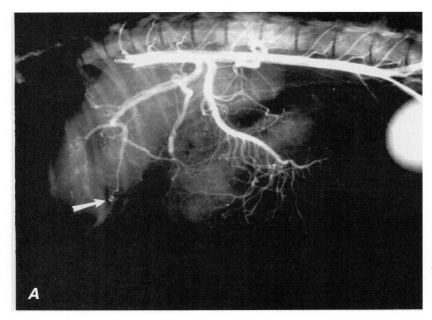

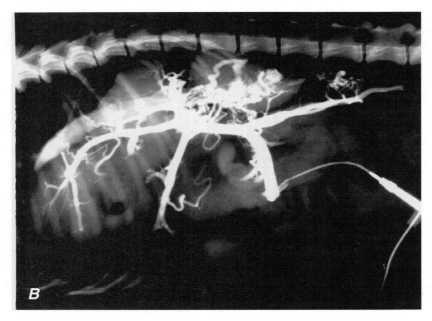

FIGURE 35-24. Nonselective arteriogram (*A*) made by injecting contrast into the aorta cranial to the celiac artery. This patient was too small to permit selective catheterization of the celiac artery. In (*B*) a jejunal venogram is shown. In (*A*), a tortuosity of the intrahepatic arterioles is demonstrated. In some terminal areas (arrow) contrast ballooned into what appeared to be small arteriovenous fistulas. Histologically, vascular malformations were consistent with the presence of an hepatic arteriovenous fistula. The arteriography was done because this dog presented with ascites and clinical signs and laboratory evidence of portosystemic shunting. A common PSVA was not anticipated. In (*B*), the portal hypertension associated with the vascular malformations in this dog has led to the opening of many portosystemic collateral communications. There was no surgical therapy that could assist this patient.

disorder is characterized by hepatic histology identical to that considered pathognomonic for PSVA. The commonality of the hepatic lesions suggests that PSVA and microvascular portal dysplasia are varying expressions of a more general portal vascular malformation. All dogs with PSVA have microvascular portal dysplasia, and there is evidence that these lesions do not fully resolve upon surgical ligation of the shunting vessel. This disorder has been extensively studied in kindreds of Cairn terriers and in individual Yorkshire terriers and other small purebred dogs.[73,182] Cairn terriers with this disorder have abnormal bile acids, impaired ICG clearances, reduced hepatic portal vascularity on ultrasonographic evaluation, and a normal to mildly increased shunt index on colonic scintigraphy. Mesenteric portography and surgical exploration fail to disclose large shunting vessels. Liver biopsy reveals varying degrees of vascular malformation among liver lobes. Serial sections cut from one biopsy suggest a merging of vascular structures with the central vein. An impression of diminished small distributing portal vessels may be apparent in individual liver lobes on mesenteric portography. Studies of the inheritance of this disorder in Cairn terriers suggest it is transmitted as a polygenic trait.[73] In this breed, clinically asymptomatic microscopic portovascular dysplasia is far more common than PSVA. Expression of this disorder appears to be most severe in the Yorkshire terrier, a breed already known to have a high incidence of PSVA. In its most severe form, microvascular portal dysplasia has been termed "portal venous atresia" and is associated with multiple acquired portosystemic communications, clinical signs of HE, progressive hepatic fibrosis, and clinicopathologic features of PSVA.

Dogs with the milder form of microvascular portal dysplasia, lacking PSVA or acquired shunts, receive veterinary attention when abnormal liver function tests (bile acid concentrations) are serendipitously recognized. They do not present with clinical signs of hepatic insufficiency. In the mild form of expression, there may be no other clinicopathologic abnormalities. When these animals become ill from nonhepatic disorders, abnormal liver function is recognized and pursued as if it were the etiologic factor in the animal's current illness. The disorder is diagnosed when a shunt is not documented, but hepatic histology details classic PSVA lesions. One of the most common features is the presence of multiple small-caliber vascular components in the portal triad. It is undocumented if the milder form of this congenital abnormality progresses to clinical disease or acquired hepatic lesions because aged affected dogs have not yet been rigorously evaluated. However, it is a clinical impression that this does not occur in Cairn terriers but may occur in Yorkshire terriers.

HEPATIC ARTERIOVENOUS FISTULA

Clinical Synopsis

Diagnostic Features

- Clinical and laboratory findings as for PSVA
- Liver enzyme activity tends to be higher than in PSVA
- Ascites more common than in PSVA
- Ultrasound or celiac arteriogram confirms arteriovenous shunt
- Histologic lesions are distinct showing marked increase in arteriolarized portal vessels throughout the liver

Standard Management

- Medical support as for PSVA
- Resection of affected lobe(s)

Intrahepatic arteriovenous (A–V) fistulas are rare congenital malformations of hepatic vasculature that have been recognized in dogs and cats.[258–262] Fistulas between a branch of the hepatic artery and portal venous radicals can also develop secondary to trauma, iatrogenic injury during diagnostic or surgical procedures, as a result of neoplastic erosion of a branch of the hepatic artery, or rupture of an hepatic arterial aneurysm.[262–264] Because arteries and veins develop from a common embryologic capillary plexus, the congenital malformations are believed to be the result of failure of the common embryologic anlage to differentiate. Intrahepatic arterioportal fistulas are associated with portal hypertension and shunting through multiple portosystemic collaterals. Increased pressure in the portal vein, hepatic vein, and hepatic sinusoids is caused by arterialization of the portal circulation. Arteriovenous fistulas located elsewhere in the body increase cardiac output and lead to high-output cardiac failure associated with a hyperdynamic circulation. The interposition of the hepatic sinusoids between the heart and fistula cushions the heart from the typical hemodynamic effects of an A–V fistula, the sinusoidal capacitance and resistance providing cardioprotection.

Animals with congenital intrahepatic A–V fistulas have clinical presentations and clinicopathologic features analogous to animals with PSVA. Most animals are less than 6 months of age and have become acutely ill prior to presentation for veterinary care. Vomiting, diarrhea, and HE are common. Liver enzyme activity has a tendency to be higher and albumin to be lower than in animals with typical PSVA. The patient with an intrahepatic A–V fistula develops multiple portosystemic shunts and usually also has ascites due to the portal hypertension caused by arterialization of the normally low-pressure portal circulation.

Survey radiographs usually are not helpful because a ground glass appearance of the abdomen due to abdominal effusion that obscures visceral detail. Abdominal ultrasonography reveals anechoic, tortuous, irregular cystic (blood-filled) lesions in the area of the fistula.[265] Doppler-assisted ultrasonography reveals areas with unidirectional fluid flow and areas of turbulent flow in apparent cystic regions. The hepatic artery and portal vein branches may appear dilated and tortuous. Hepatofugal blood flow (flow through portosystemic collaterals) may be notable, especially in the area of the kidneys. The affected liver lobe is larger than the other liver lobes, which may be subjectively appraised as small. Increased blood pressure and flow in the tissue region of the A-V fistula results in distension of the involved liver lobe.

Definitive diagnosis is accomplished via selective catheterization of the celiac artery. Routine procedures used for portography in animals with PSVA, such as jejunal vein portography or splenoportography, cannot confirm the presence of an intrahepatic A-V fistula. These procedures will only document the existence of multiple portosystemic collaterals. Contrast medium must be injected into the hepatic artery to detail the A-V interconnection; consult Figure 35–24.

Surgical correction of an intrahepatic A-V fistula can be more difficult than attenuation of a PSVA. At surgery, the affected liver lobe is usually quite obvious due to the presence of a pulsating vascular structure.[266] Palpation of this area may reveal a thrill.[257] Surgical treatment is completed by resection of affected liver lobes, ligation of involved vessels, and/or establishment of normal circulatory communications by vascular anastomosis. Although resection of the aberrant circulation may be successful, it is probable that residual vascular lesions persist in the microcirculatory bed. Residual hepatic dysfunction and progressive hepatic fibrosis has been shown in some dogs.

The histologic features of intrahepatic A-V fistula include (1) increased numbers of hepatic arterioles and capillaries, (2) arteriolar proliferation in hepatic tissue distant to the fistula location, (3) multiple arterioportal communications in affected lobes, (4) hepatic parenchymal atrophy, (5) relative collapse of distributing portal veins, and (6) bile duct proliferation (Figure 35–25).[262] Some of these features are similar to lesions associated with PSVA. Arteriolar intimal smooth muscle hyperplasia, to the extent of causing lumenal occlusion, is marked in vessels directly involved with the fistula. Branches of the portal vein in the region of the fistula appear "arterialized" with apparent mural smooth muscle hyperplasia and increased elastin. These veins may become widely distended. The adjacent hepatic sinusoids become congested. Manifestations of prior portal vein thrombosis and recanalization are frequently found.

PORTAL VEIN OCCLUSION/THROMBOSIS

Clinical Synopsis

Diagnostic Features

- Abdominal pain and distension (effusion)
- Dysentery and adynamic ileus
- Schistocytes
- Ultrasonography discloses diminution of intrahepatic portal vasculature or presence of thrombi
- Portography shows portal obstruction

Standard Management

- Treat underlying cause if identified

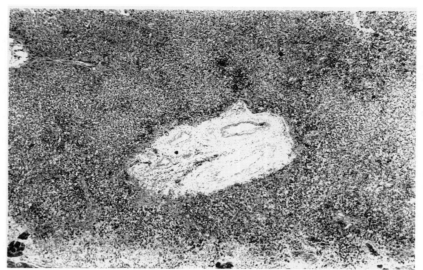

FIGURE 35–25. Photomicrograph of liver tissue from a dog with an hepatic arteriovenous fistula. Large vascular structures were commonly seen throughout this liver. Three large vascular structures are shown that have characteristics of arteries (smooth muscle hyperplasia in the wall and increased elastin fibers). There were few vessels resembling venous structures in portal triads and hepatocytes were atrophied. A large single A-V fistula was identified and surgically resected. Liver dysfunction persisted.

- Aspirin (0.5 mg/kg PO BID)
- Heparin (50–75 IU/kg SQ TID)
- Surgical embolectomy may be required
- Long-term coumadin therapy may be necessary in some animals (consult text)

Portal vein thrombosis is a relatively uncommon occurrence in the dog and has not been described in the cat to the author's knowledge.[267–273] Acute obstruction of the portal circulation is compensated by an increase in hepatic arterial blood flow and improved efficiency of hepatocellular oxygen extraction. In the acute stage of obstruction, cardiac output declines and ischemic endomyocardial effects occur in dogs.[274,275] If the acute stage is survived, recanalization of obstructing thrombi and/or development of hepatofugal circulation through portosystemic collaterals develops within 3 to 5 weeks. In humans, portal vein thrombosis is a well-recognized cause of portal hypertension.[276–285] Conditions causally associated with portal thromboembolism involve one or more of the following procoagulative changes (1) stasis of flow, (2) damage to the portal vascular endothelium, or (3) hypercoagulability. In infants, umbilical infection and congenital malformation of the portal vein are common predisposing conditions.[277] A number of different conditions lead to portal thromboembolism in adults, including abdominal trauma; neoplastic invasion, compression, or entrapment of the portal vein; inflammation and/or entrapment of the portal vein as a result of pancreatitis; and hypercoagulable conditions. Portal vein thrombosis can occur as sequelae to other causes of portal hypertension.[281] For example, it is estimated that as many as 10% to 20% of humans with cirrhosis and portal hypertension develop portal thrombosis.[284,285] An underlying cause is not determined in 50% of cases reported in adult humans.[276] A list of conditions associated with portal venous thromboembolism in the dog is provided in Table 35–8.

Clinical features displayed by dogs with portal venous thromboembolism include tachycardia, abdominal pain and distension, ileus, bloody diarrhea, and an acute accumulation of an abdominal effusion having a total protein content of more than 2.5 g/dl. Microvascular disease is usually evidenced by the presence of schistocytes in the peripheral blood. Liver enzyme activity may be normal if the portal venous obstruction is extrahepatic, or markedly increased if small intrahepatic portal radicals are involved in the thrombotic process. Abdominal radiographs may disclose a diffuse gaseous or fluid distension of the intestines consistent with ileus. Ultrasonographic evaluation will disclose a diminution of the intrahepatic portal vasculature or the presence of thrombi in vessels (Figure 35–26). Portal venous blood flow in the area of the thrombus will be absent or greatly diminished.[286] Portal vein collaterals and enlargement of the thrombosed segment of the vein may also be recognized.

Therapy should be directed toward determined causal factors and control of thrombotic tendencies. Obstruction due to neoplasia is difficult to resolve if the tumor has invaded the portal vein. Lymphosarcoma causing compression of the portal venous system may be palliated with chemotherapy. Vasculitis and DIC require mini-dose aspirin (0.5 mg/kg PO BID) and whole blood or plasma transfusion to provide antithrombin III. In most cases mini-dose heparin is used (50 to 75 IU/kg SQ TID) in acute management. Repeated infusions of whole blood or fresh plasma may be necessary to replenish antithrombin III in the presence of a consumptive coagulopathy, protein-losing enteropathy, or protein-losing nephropathy to ensure heparin efficacy. When heparin is dis-

Table 35–8

CONDITIONS ASSOCIATED WITH PORTAL VENOUS THROMBOEMBOLISM IN THE DOG

Pancreatitis
Frostbite
Neoplasia
   lymphosarcoma
   adenocarcinoma
   myeloproliferative disease
Immune-mediated hemolytic anemia
Systemic lupus erythematosus
Vasculitis
Hyperadrenocorticism
Chronic glucocorticoid treatment
Protein-losing enteropathy
Protein-losing nephropathy
   amyloidosis
   glomerulonephritis
Postoperative complication
   PSVA ligation
Splenic torsion
Gastric dilatation–volvulus
Cirrhosis and portal hypertension

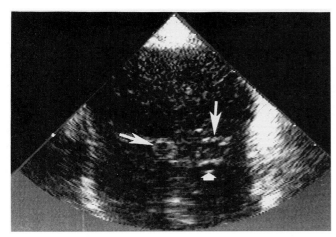

FIGURE 35–26. Ultrasonogram of the liver of a dog with diffuse portal vascular thromboembolism caused by metastatic adenocarcinoma. The portal vein with occluding thrombi are indicated by arrows. The hepatic vein is indicated by an arrowhead. (Courtesy Dr. A. Yeager, Section of Radiology, Department of Clinical Sciences, Cornell University)

continued, it is slowly tapered over 48 hours to avoid rebound hypercoagulation. Treatment with coumadin may also be necessary. Coumadin therapy permits chronic "at home" anticoagulation if a thrombotic tendency persists. In some cases this is manifest by recognition of persistent subnormal PT or APTT clotting times. A dose of coumadin approximating 0.22 mg/kg SID is given for 3 to 5 days. The maintenance dose of coumadin is carefully titrated on the basis of the PT; the goal is 1.5- to 2-fold increase in the PT without overt hemorrhage. There is great individual variation in response to this drug. Some animals need more and some need less. Because coumadin is highly protein bound, use of medications that compete for albumin-binding sites will cause a dangerous drug interaction. In this circumstance, the dose of coumadin is titrated while the competitor drug is being consistently administered. This avoids inadvertent overdosage of coumadin and disastrous hemorrhagic consequences. When coumadin is used with aspirin therapy (aspirin is highly protein bound) for long-term management of vasculitis, consistent administration of each drug is necessary to sustain steady anticoagulation. In some patients, the maintenance dose of coumadin is difficult to stabilize and is best achieved when the drug is given once every 2 or 3 days or by alternate-day dose adjustments (e.g., 2.5 mg one day and 0.5 mg the next). Long-term survival in dogs with portal venous thrombosis is possible if aggressive medical and/or surgical therapy is initially provided.

There are several reports of humans with portal thrombosis surviving with only conservative medical management consisting of heparin, coumadin, and blood transfusion.[283,284,287] The use of thrombolytic agents, such as tissue plasminogen activating factor (TPA), to resolve portal venous thromboembolism, has not been evaluated in animals. It should be remembered that spontaneous lysis of a formed clot and recanalization of residual emboli occurs over a 3 to 5 week interval if the patient can be kept alive through the acute episode and if thromboembolism is restricted.

Management may require surgical embolectomy, a complicated and high-risk procedure. Resection of ischemic bowel may also be necessary. Accurate diagnosis and localization of thrombi in the portal venous system is essential if embolectomy is pursued. This requires preoperative mesenteric portography to display the venous involvement; Figures 35–27 and 35–28 demonstrate portograms used to locate portal thrombi that were successfully removed. Performance of portal venography may aggravate thrombotic tendencies as a result of vascular irritation resulting from radiographic contrast medium and catheter placement. Postoperative portography should be evaluated to determine the extent of residual thrombi and hepatopetal portal flow. Portal venous embolectomy is a complicated procedure that should be attempted only by a well-experienced surgeon having the proper equipment.

CHRONIC PASSIVE CONGESTION, BUDD-CHIARI SYNDROME, AND VENO-OCCLUSIVE DISEASE

Anything that obstructs hepatic venous outflow causes severe congestive changes in the perivenular area (zone 3). This leads to pressure atrophy and ischemic necrosis of

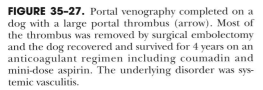

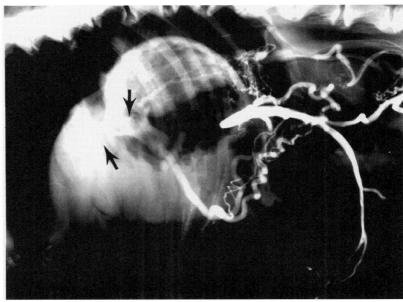

FIGURE 35–27. Portal venography completed on a dog with a large portal thrombus (arrow). Most of the thrombus was removed by surgical embolectomy and the dog recovered and survived for 4 years on an anticoagulant regimen including coumadin and mini-dose aspirin. The underlying disorder was systemic vasculitis.

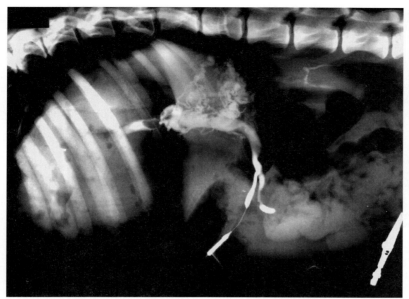

FIGURE 35-28. Intraoperative portal venography completed in a dog with a portal thrombus (arrow) secondary to frostbite injury to the feet. This lesion has been chronic because there are numerous secondary portosystemic collaterals that have developed to ameliorate portal hypertension. This study was done after partial embolectomy was completed. The remainder of the clot was resected and the dog recovered. Portal thromboembolism recurred within 4 months.

perivenular hepatocytes. Chronic obstruction of the hepatic venous outflow leads to perivenular fibrosis, and eventually this extends toward the portal tracts, which may become involved.[288-291] Causes include anything that increases central venous pressure: the Budd-Chiari syndrome, a general term applied to a variety of noncirrhotic pathologic processes that cause an outflow block from the sinusoidal bed of the liver; and veno-occlusive disease, a disorder affecting small terminal hepatic venous radicles.[292] Extravasation and trapping of erythrocytes in the space of Disse has been described as pathognomonic of the Budd-Chiari syndrome and hepatic veno-occlusive disease. Similar changes are seen in severe right heart failure and with left ventricular failure in the absence of right ventricular failure in humans.

Chronic Passive Congestion

Clinical Synopsis

Diagnostic Features

- Clinical signs usually of cardiac not hepatic disease
- Hepatomegaly and ascites are common
- ALP and ALT usually two-to fourfold normal
- BSP or ICG plasma clearance abnormal
- Bile acid and ammonia tolerance tests are usually normal
- Hepatic ultrasound may reveal diffuse hyperechogenicity
- Biopsy reveals sinusoidal congestion, hepatocellular atrophy, and fibrosis and hemosiderosis about central veins

Standard Management

- Treat underlying cause of hepatic congestion

The animal with chronic passive congestion associated with cardiac disease typically has a relative or absolute polycythemia resulting from impaired cardiac function and an inability to optimally oxygenate tissues. Increased liver enzyme activity is common; both transaminases and ALP are increased by magnitudes of two- to fourfold normal. Evaluation of liver function by BSP or ICG clearance demonstrates impaired hepatic perfusion. Evaluation of liver function with serum bile acids or ammonia tolerance testing will not indicate impaired hepatic function until morphologic hepatic lesions have developed. A summary of the sensitivity of different tests in dogs and cats with hepatic congestion is shown in Figure 35–29. The clinicopathologic features of hepatic congestion in dogs and cats are shown in Figure 35–30.

Hepatomegaly is usually obvious on physical examination. Ascites develops when the central venous pressure increases and hepatic venous outflow becomes severely compromised. Chronic passive congestion develops as a result of (1) congenital or acquired cardiac disease (right or left sided), (2) pericardial disease (pericardial tamponade, restrictive or constrictive pericarditis), (3) mass lesions impairing right atrial filling, (4) severe heartworm disease with or without development of the vena cava syndrome, (5) obstructed flow through the caudal vena cava cranial to the diaphragm, or (6) obstructed flow through the pulmonary circulation. Signs of the underlying medical condition may be difficult to detect on initial physical examination, except in the circumstance of acquired cardiac dysfunction and certain congenital cardiac malformations.

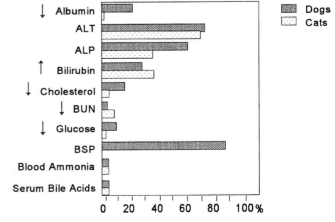

FIGURE 35-29. Comparison of the sensitivities for different tests in dogs and cats with hepatic congestion.

Clinicopathologic Features of Hepatic Congestion

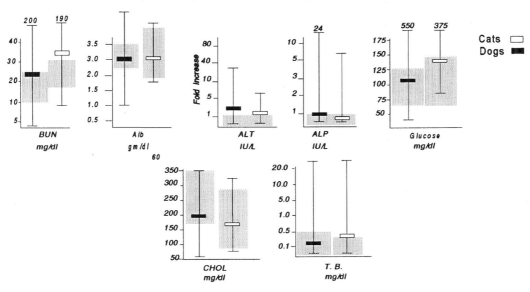

FIGURE 35–30. The clinicopathologic features in dogs and cats with hepatic congestion. Numbers in selected columns represent outliers of the expressed range. (Data derived from the College of Veterinary Medicine, University of California.)

Thoracic radiographs may increase the index of suspicion for cardiac or pulmonary disorders or dirofilariasis. A lateral thoracic radiograph may also reveal an abnormally small or misshapen caudal vena cava just cranial to the diaphragm in the circumstance of a constricted or "kinked" caudal vena cava.

Abdominal ultrasonography will often detail a subjectively large liver. Subtle dilation of hepatic veins may be detected upon careful examination where they merge with the vena cava (Figure 35–31). Doppler evaluation usually reveals an exaggerated reverse flow of blood into the hepatic veins if passive congestion is associated with an abnormality at the level of the heart.[125] A diffuse hepatic parenchymal hyperechogenicity is typical.[125]

The classic hepatic lesions associated with chronic passive congestion are disappearance of hepatocytes from zone 3 as the sinusoids become engorged with blood and the amount of perivenular collagen increases.[288–291] Increased hydrostatic pressure, cellular anoxia, and impaired nutrition are believed to underlie hepatocellular necrosis and atrophy. When necessary, hepatocytes have the ability to increase their efficiency of oxygen extraction. With reduced cardiac output, it is believed hepatic perfusion drops below a critical threshold that impairs this compensatory response. Cells in zone 1 are maintained in relative good health while cells in zone 3 are perfused with blood that does not contain sufficient oxygen to meet cellular requirements.[293] Impedance of hepatic venous outflow leads to increased sinusoidal hydrostatic pressure and increased formation and flow of hepatic lymph. Enlargement of the periportal hepatic lymphatics reflects a compensatory effort to transport this increased volume of lymph. When the quantity of lymph exceeds the capacity of the intrahepatic lymphatic system, a protein-rich fluid weeps from the surface of the liver into the abdominal cavity. With chronicity, a sclerotic thickening of the walls of the hepatic veins develops and perivenular scars extend into the lobular parenchyma.[293] Perivenular and midzonal necrosis may develop in some animals and contrasts with the preserved periportal architecture. Increased accumulation of ceroid pigment and hemosiderin is observed in Kupffer cells in zone

3, presumably as a result of vascular stasis, erythrocyte phagocytosis, and cellular anoxia.

Budd-Chiari Syndrome

Clinical Synopsis

Diagnostic Features

- Signs of HE may develop
- Ascites and hepatomegaly usually overt

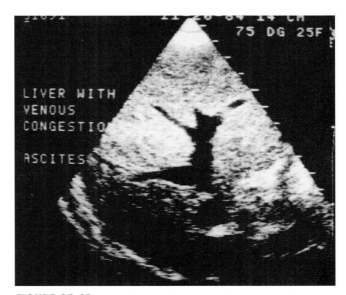

FIGURE 35–31. Ultrasonogram of the liver of a dog with severe congestive heart failure. The hepatic veins are markedly distended. (Courtesy Dr. A. Yeager, Section of Radiology, Department of Clinical Sciences, Cornell University.)

- Mildly elevated liver enzymes
- Serum bile acid and ammonia tolerance tests abnormal
- Hepatic biopsy findings as for passive congestion
- Venograms may reveal portosystemic shunting or evidence of posthepatic or hepatic venous obstruction

Standard Management

- Treat underlying cause of venous obstruction
- Symptomatic management of HE

The initial definition of the Budd-Chiari syndrome limited application to a very specific pathologic entity of "endophlebitis obliterans" of the small hepatic veins.[292] Today, the term is diffusely applied to the clinical signs and pathologic changes developing in response to postsinusoidal obstruction of hepatic venous flow at any site between the liver and the right atrium. A multitude of different conditions can produce this hemodynamically generated lesion, including (1) obstructed blood flow due to tumors or abscesses located in the liver or the inferior vena cava, (2) hepatic venous or vena caval thrombosis, (3) a congenital web, kink, or acquired stricture occluding the lumen of the hepatic veins or vena cava, or (4) cardiac malformations impairing right atrial function or filling. In humans, the Budd-Chiari syndrome develops from hepatic vein thrombosis related to a variety of disorders, but in approximately two-thirds of patients an underlying cause is never substantiated.[294] Conditions similar to the Budd-Chiari syndrome have been infrequently reported in dogs and are extremely rare in the cat.[295-307]

Clinical signs of the Budd-Chiari syndrome invariably include the development of ascites and hepatomegaly. Increased sinusoidal hydrostatic pressure results in formation of lymph exceeding the capacity of the hepatic lymphatic vasculature. Subsequently, protein-rich interstitial fluid weeps from the hepatic surface through the capsule into the peritoneal cavity. Hepatic vein obstruction forces the portal vein to become the route of egress for the hepatic circulation. Portosystemic collaterals open and the patient is susceptible to all the ramifications of deviated portal blood flow. The portosystemic collaterals open between the portal vein and azygos vein and other venous pathways separate from the caudal vena cava.

A variety of different conditions have been associated with the Budd-Chiari syndrome in dogs. Occlusion of the caudal vena cava cranial to the diaphragm by extrinsic compression (tumor, diaphragmatic hernia), an intraluminal congenital membranous web, or a "kink" causing vessel stricture have been well described.[298-300] A kink in the caudal vena cava is usually related to prior trauma. Web and kink lesions can be surgically corrected. Impaired cardiac filling or outflow due to right atrial tumors or cor triatrium dextor have also been well documented.[295-297,301-303] Cor triatrium dextor is a congenital malformation in which the atrium is partitioned by an obstructing fibrous membrane. Obstructive pulmonary lesions or vena caval syndrome caused by dirofilariasis have also been described in dogs showing signs of the Budd-Chiari syndrome.[306,307] Intrahepatic postsinusoidal venous obstruction was described in a Basenji dog in which the lesion was speculated to be a congenital malformation.[304]

The hallmark of obstructed postsinusoidal venous flow is formation of ascites characterized as a modified transudate. The clinical features vary depending on the underlying disorder. Typically, liver enzymes are only mildly increased and the serum albumin is only marginally subnormal. Signs of HE are uncommon. Serum bile acids and ammonia tolerance testing reflect hepatic insufficiency after acquired portosystemic shunting has developed. Dilated intestinal lymphatics and protein-losing enteropathies have developed in some dogs.

Venograms done by contrast injection into a lateral saphenous vein in dogs with a kinked intrathoracic caudal vena cava have revealed hepatofugal blood flow through systemic venous collaterals involving the azygous, phrenicoabdominal, lumbar and intercostal veins, and the vertebral venous sinuses.[299] Hepatic ultrasonography details the same lesions as described for chronic passive congestion, except that portosystemic collateral circulation may be observed in some cases. Depending on the anatomic area of vena caval obstruction, radiographic and/or ultrasonographic evaluations may disclose the abnormality. Vena caval malformation (kinking) or stricture cranial to the diaphragm may be initially suspected on evaluation of a lateral thoracic radiograph disclosing an inappropriately narrowed or misshapened malpositioned vessel. In some cases, the vena caval lesion can be seen during ultrasonographic evaluation. Ultimately, selective contrast injection is required to detail the extent, nature, and localization of the obstructive lesion. Dogs with cor triatrium dextor have their lesion initially recognized on the basis of echocardiography. Follow-up cardiac contrast studies assist in definitively identifying the anatomic defect. Selective catheterization of the thoracic portion of the caudal vena cava has revealed vascular stricture, kinks, or membranes in some patients.

Hepatic histologic lesions are characterized by distension of the hepatic veins, perivenous sinusoidal congestion, and with chronicity, increased perivenous connective tissue, typical of chronic passive congestion. In the acute stage of postsinusoidal obstruction, hepatomegaly due to increased blood storage and edema can be observed. With chronicity, the liver may become reduced in size. The hepatic histologic lesions associated with cor triatrium dextor in a young dog are shown in Figure 35–32. This dog had tense ascites but liver function remained normal.

The clinical outcome of patients with the Budd-Chiari syndrome depends on the underlying causal factors and the ability to resolve them. When underlying factors cannot be eliminated, a slow progression to hepatic cirrhosis usually occurs. In some cases, where thromboembolism develops, hepatic necrosis and a short illness precedes death. Use of diuretics to resolve or control the ascites usually has limited effect. Institution of a sodium-restricted diet is recommended. When hepatic insufficiency or portosystemic shunting result in HE, a protein-restricted diet and other interventional therapies, as appropriate for the patient with PSVA, are initiated. The development of protein-losing enteropathies and reduced nutrient assimilation as a result of the portal and lymphatic hypertension and intestinal wall edema complicate the delivery of adequate nutrition. Optimal management of this condition requires surgical resolution of the obstructing lesion. In the case of the vena caval syndrome associated with heartworm disease, this involves manual removal of obstructing parasites and follow-up adulticidal therapy. A kinked or obstructed intrathoracic caudal vena cava is treated either by membranotomy (resection of a "weblike lesion") or resection of the malformed section of the vessel. Cor triatrium dextor is amenable to surgical membrane obliteration. Creation of a portosystemic shunt is a possible option if intrahepatic venous thrombosis is identified as the underlying cause. Resolution of the histologic lesions associated with obstructed venous outflow has been shown experimentally in dogs following creation of a decompressive shunt.[308]

Veno-Occlusive Disease

Hepatic veno-occlusive disease in humans is a major differential diagnosis for the Budd-Chiari syndrome. This disorder

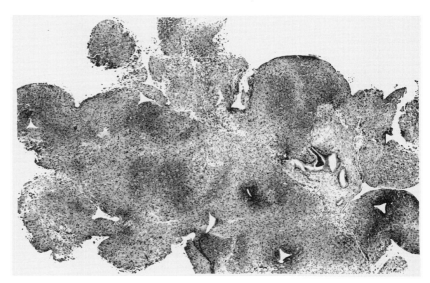

FIGURE 35-32. Photomicrograph of the liver biopsy from a young dog with cor triatrium dextor. This dog had tense ascites. The most obvious hepatic abnormalities were the enlarged and slightly thickened hepatic veins, which appear triangular in shape. There is no evidence of nonreversible hepatic parenchymal changes (H & E, 35× magnification).

is characterized as the nonthrombotic fibrous obliteration of sublobular veins and terminal hepatic venules. This leads to portal hypertension, hepatomegaly, ascites, and abdominal pain. The veno-occlusive lesion is proposed to develop from damaged sinusoidal endothelium, resulting in an accumulation of erythrocytes and fibrin in the space of Disse. This leads to subintimal fibroplasia and collagen deposition and a progressive obliteration of hepatic veins.[309–311]

In humans, veno-occlusive disease has been associated with many disorders, including pyrrolizidine alkaloids and aflatoxin toxicity, radiation injury to the liver, administration of certain antimetabolites, alkylating agents, oral progestational agents, vitamin A toxicity, and SLE.[311–327] The histologic findings of veno-occlusive disease may be subtle, and it is proposed that this lesion is underdiagnosed in humans with serious liver disease.[327] Histologic lesions of veno-occlusive disease have been created in dogs fed dimethylnitrosamines for the intent of modeling chronic hepatic fibrosis.[328–330] A portal veno-occlusive lesion has also been produced by chronic injection of *E. coli* and *E. coli* antisera into the portal vein of dogs.[331] A veno-occlusive lesion has been described in captive cheetahs and snow leopards in North America.[332–334] The exact cause remains unproven.

IDIOPATHIC VENO-OCCLUSIVE DISEASE IN COCKER SPANIELS. A report of four related female American cocker spaniels between 10 and 19 months of age detailed what was proposed as a "functional" hepatic vein occlusion associated with portal hypertension.[335] Each dog developed multiple acquired portosystemic shunts. This lesion seemingly progressed to perivenular fibrosis and veno-occlusion. Initially, affected dogs presented for severe diarrhea and weight loss; one dog presented for ascites of 24 hours duration and one dog presented for signs of HE. Clinicopathologic features of these dogs included a panhypoproteinemia, variable liver enzyme activity, and ammonia intolerance.[335]

Initial histologic lesions included multiple prominent smooth muscle "sphincters" in terminal and interlobular hepatic veins observed in cut sections longitudinally. In some sections, the vascular lumen appeared to be occluded by sphincters. Large vascular channels were seen traversing acini from portal tracts to terminal hepatic veins; these were confirmed on serially sectioned tissues. Both portal and terminal hepatic veins were dilated and surrounded by distended lymphatics. Portal triads contained a normal complement of hepatic arterioles and portal veins. There was mild hepatic

atrophy but no evidence of acute or previous hepatocellular injury or fibroplasia. Intestinal biopsies revealed submucosal edema and marked lymphangiectasia in one dog. Repeat biopsies in the index case at 21 months following initial biopsy (and 19 months after ligation of large shunting vessels until portal pressure was increased) revealed moderate periacinal fatty degeneration and hemosiderosis, extensive cholangiolar proliferation, hepatic atrophy, and early regenerative nodule formation. Walls of portal veins were thickened and distended and there was extensive smooth muscle hyperplasia and fibrosis in walls of terminal and interlobular hepatic veins. Several hepatic veins were seen to be obliterated. Liver biopsies from two other dogs also demonstrated occlusive venous sphincters, mild to moderate perivenular fibrosis, widely dilated vascular channels between portal triads and central interlobular veins (one dog), and mild cholangiolar proliferation (one dog). It was proposed that this was a genetically linked lesion that developed into a veno-occlusive disorder over time. Further reports of affected dogs have not been made.

REFERENCES

1. Whipple GH, Robscheit Robbins FS, Hawkins WB. Eck fistula liver subnormal in producing hemoglobin and plasma proteins on diets rich in liver and iron. J Exp Med 81:171–191, 1945.
2. Bollman JL. The animal with Eck fistula. Physiol Rev 41:607–621, 1961.
3. Silen W, Mawdsley DL, Weirich WL, et al. Studies of hepatic function in dogs with Eck fistula or portacaval transposition. AMA Arch Surg 74:964–973, 1957.
4. Starzl TE, Porter KA, Watanube K, et al. Effects of insulin, glucagon, and insulin/glucagon infusions on liver morphology and cell division after complete portacaval shunt in dogs. Lancet 1:821–825, 1976.
5. Raskin NH, Price JB, Fishman RA. Portal-systemic encephalopathy due to congenital intrahepatic shunts. N Engl J Med 270:225–229, 1964.
6. Barsky MR, Rankin RN, Wall WJ, et al. Patent ductus venosus: problems in assessment and management. Can J Surg 32:203–216, 1989.
7. Raskin NH, Bredesen D, Ehrenfield WK, et al. Periodic confusion caused by congenital extrahepatic portacaval shunt. Neurology 34:666–669, 1984.
8. Piccone VA, Lentino W, LeVeen HH. Radiological demonstration of patent ductus venosus in an adult. Gastroenterology 52:263–266, 1967.
9. Marois D, Van Heerden JA, Carpenter HA, et al. Congenital absence of the portal vein. Mayo Clin Proc 54:55–59, 1979.
10. Olling S, Olsson R. Congenital absence of portal venous system in a fifty year old woman. Acta Med Scand 196:343–345, 1974.
11. Hellweg JG. Congenital absence of intrahepatic portal venous system simulating Eck fistula. Report of a case with necropsy findings. AMA Arch Pathol 57:425–430, 1954.
12. Abernethy J. Account of two instances of uncommon formation in the

viscera of the human body. Phil Trans R Soc Long (Biol) 83:59–66, 1973.

13. Vonnahme F-J, Dubuisson L, Kubale R, et al. Ultrastructural characteristics of hyperplastic alterations in the liver of congenital portocaval-shunt rats. Br J Exp Path 65:585–596, 1984.

14. Bioulac-Sagae P, Saric J, Boussarie L, et al. Congenital portacaval shunt in rats: Liver adaptation to lack of portal vein—a light and electron microscopic study. Hepatology 5:1183–1189, 1985.

15. Hickman J, Edwards JE, Mann F. Portal venous anomalies in a dog. I. Absence of the portal vein. II. Continuity of lower part of inferior vena cava with azygos vein. Anat Rec 104:137–146, 1949.

16. Ewing GO, Suter PF, Bailey CS. Hepatic insufficiency associated with congenital anomalies of the portal vein in dogs. J Am Anim Hosp Assoc 10:463–476, 1974.

17. Audell L, Jonson L, Lannak B. Congenital portacaval shunt in the dog. Zbl Vet Med 1:797–805, 1974.

18. Simpson ST, Hribernik TN. Portosystemic shunt in the dog. Two case reports. J Sm Anim Pract 17:163–170, 1976.

19. Lohse CL, Selcer RR, Suter PF. Hepatoencephalopathy associated with situs inversus of abdominal organs and vascular anomalies in a dog. J Am Vet Med Assoc 168:681–688, 1976.

20. Cornelius LM, Thrall DE, Halliwell WH, et al. Anomalous portosystemic anastomoses associated with chronic hepatic insufficiency in six young dogs. J Am Vet Med Assoc 167:220–228, 1975.

21. Barrett RE, DeLahunta A, Renick WJ, et al. Four cases of congenital portacaval shunt in the dog. J Sm Anim Pract 17:71–85, 1976.

22. Gofton N. Surgical ligation of congenital portosystemic venous shunts in the dog: A report of three cases. Am Anim Hosp Assoc 14:728–733, 1978.

23. Breznock EM. Surgical manipulation of portosystemic shunts in dogs. J Am Vet Med Assoc 174:819–826, 1979.

24. Vulgamott JC, Turnwald GH, King GK, et al. Congenital portacaval anomalies in the cat: Two case reports. J Am Anim Hosp Assoc 16:916–919, 1980.

25. Campbell TM, Lording PM, Wrigley JRH, et al. Portal vein anomaly and hepatic encephalopathy in three dogs. Aust Vet J 56:593–598, 1980.

26. Maddison JE. Portosystemic encephalopathy in two young dogs: Some additional diagnostic and therapeutic considerations. J Sm Anim Pract 22:731–739, 1981.

27. Rothuizen J, van den Ingh SGAM, Voorhout G, et al. Congenital portosystemic shunts in sixteen dogs and three cats. J Sm Anim Pract 23:67–81, 1982.

28. van den Ingh TSGAM, Rothuizen J. Hepatoportal fibrosis in three young dogs. Vet Rec 110:575–577, 1982.

29. Levesque DC, Oliver JE, Cornelius LM, et al. Congenital portacaval shunts in two cats: Diagnosis and surgical correction. J Am Vet Med Assoc 181:143–145, 1982.

30. Breznock EB, Berger B, Pendray D, et al. Surgical manipulation of intrahepatic portacaval shunts in dogs. J Am Vet Med Assoc 182:798–805, 1983.

31. Rawlings CA, Wilson SA. Intracaval repair of a persistent ductus venosus in a dog. Vet Surg 12:155–159, 1983.

32. Wrigley RH, Macy DW, Wykes PM. Ligation of ductus venosus in a dog using ultrasonographic guidance. J Am Vet Med Assoc 183:1461–1464, 1983.

33. Gandolfi RC. Hepatoencephalopathy associated with patent ductus venosus in a cat. J Am Vet Med Assoc 185:301–302, 1984.

34. Hawe RS, Mullen HS. An unusual portocaval anomaly as a cause of hepatic encephalopathy in a cat. J Am Anim Hosp Assoc 20:987–993, 1984.

35. Birchard SJ. Surgical management of portosystemic shunts in dogs and cats. Compend Contin Educ Pract Vet 6:795–801, 1984.

36. Carr SH, Thornburg LP. Congenital portacaval shunt in two kittens. Fel Pract 14:43–45, 1984.

37. Gandolfi RC. Hepatoencephalopathy associated with patent ductus venosus in a cat. J Am Vet Med Assoc 185:301–302, 1984.

38. Vulgamott JC. Portosystemic shunts. Vet Clin N Am [Sm Anim Pract] 15:229–242, 1985.

39. Breznock EM, Whiting PG. Portacaval shunts and anaomalies. In: Slatter DH (ed.) Textbook of Small Animal Surgery, Vol 1. WB Saunders, Philadelphia, 1156–1173, 1985.

40. Ware WA, Montavon P, DiBartola SP, et al. Atypical portosystemic shunt in a cat. J Am Vet Med Assoc 188:187–188, 1986.

41. Martin RA, August JR, Barber DL, et al. Left hepatic vein attenuation for treatment of patent ductus venosus in a dog. J Am Vet Med Assoc 189:1465–1468, 1986.

42. Scavelli TD, Hornbuckle WE, Roth L, et al. Portosystemic shunts in cats: Seven cases (1976–1984). J Am Vet Med Assoc 189:317–325, 1986.

43. Berger B, Whiting PG, Breznock EM, et al. Congenital feline portosystemic shunts. J Am Vet Med Assoc 188:517–521, 1986.

44. Johnson CA, Armstrong PJ, Hauptman JG. Congenital portosystemic shunts in dogs: 46 cases (1979–1986). J Am Vet Med Assoc 191:1478–1483, 1987.

45. Grauer GF, Pitts RP. Primary polydipsia in three dogs with portosystemic shunts. J Am Anim Hosp Assoc 23:197–200, 1987.

46. Blaxter AC, Holt PE, Pearson GR, et al. Congenital portosystemic shunts in the cat: A report of nine cases. J Sm Anim Pract 29:631–645, 1988.

47. Mathews K, Gofton N. Congenital extrahepatic portosystemic shunt occlusion in the dog: Gross observations during surgical correction. J Am Anim Hosp Assoc 24:387–394, 1988.

48. Johnson SE, Crisp SM, Smeak DD, et al. Hepatic encephalopathy in two aged dogs secondary to a presumed congenital portosystemic shunt. J Am Anim Hosp Assoc 25:129–137, 1989.

49. VanGundy TE, Boothe HW, Wolf A. Results of surgical management of feline portosystemic shunts. J Am Anim Hosp Assoc 26:55–62, 1990.

50. Butler LM, Fossum TW, Boothe HW. Surgical management of extrahepatic portosystemic shunts in the dog and cat. Sem Vet Med Surg (Sm Anim) 5:127–133, 1990.

51. Swalec KM, Smeak DD. Partial versus complete attenuation of single portosystemic shunts. Vet Surg 19:406–411, 1990.

52. Center SA, Magne M. Historical, physical examination, and clinicopathologic features of portosystemic vascular anomalies in the dog and cat. Sem Vet Med Surg(Sm Anim) 5:83–93, 1990.

53. Martin RA, Payne JT. Angiographic results of intrahepatic portocaval shunt attenuation in three dogs. Sem Vet Med Surg (Sm Anim) 5:134–141, 1990.

54. Whiting PG, Breznock EM. Portosystemic shunts. In: Bojrab MJ (ed) Current Techniques in Small Animal Surgery, 3rd ed. Lea & Febiger, Philadelphia, 295–299, 1990.

55. Cape L, Panciera DL, Partington B, et al. Glomerulonephritis and a congenital portocaval shunt in a seven-year old dog. Am Anim Hosp Assoc 28:419–424, 1992.

56. Lawrence D, Bellah JR, Diaz R. Results of surgical management of portosystemic shunts in dogs: 20 cases (1985–1990). J Am Vet Med Assoc 201:1750–1753, 1992.

57. Birchard SJ, Sherding RG. Feline portosystemic shunts. Comp Continu Ed 114:1295–1300, 1992.

58. Partington BP, Partington CR, Biller DS, et al. Transvenous coil embolization for treatment of patent ductus venosus in a dog. J Am Vet Med Assoc 202:281–284, 1993.

59. Strombeck DR, Guilford G. Small Animal Gastroenterology, 2nd ed. Stonegate, Davis, CA, 1990.

60. Whiting PG, Breznock EM. Unpublished information.

61. Noden DM, deLahunta A. Digestive System in the Embryology of Domestic Animals. Williams & Wilkins, Baltimore, 293–311, 1985.

62. Latshaw WK. The Digestive System in Veterinary Developmental Anatomy. Dekker, New York, 1987.

63. Payne JT, Martin RA, Constantinscu GM. The anatomy and embryology of portosystemic shunts in dogs and cats. Sem Vet Med Surg (Sm Anim) 5:76–82, 1990.

64. Noden DM, de Lahunta A. Cardiovascular System III. Venous System and Lymphatics in the Embryology of Domestic Animals. Williams & Wilkins, Baltimore, 257–269, 1985.

65. Latshaw WK. Blood Vascular System in Veterinary Developmental Anatomy. Dekker, New York, 1987.

66. Vitums A. Portosystemic communications in the dog. Acta Anat 39:271–299, 1959.

67. Sleight DR, Thomford NR. Gross anatomy of the blood supply and biliary drainage of the canine liver. Anat Rec 166:153–160, 1970.

68. Evans HE, Christensen GC (eds.). Miller's Anatomy of the Dog 2nd ed. Saunders, Philadelphia, 1979.

69. Edelstone DI. Regulation of blood flow through the ductus venosus. J Dev Physiol 2:219–238, 1980.

70. Lohse CL, Suter PF. Functional closure of the ductus venosus during early postnatal life in the dog. Am J Vet Res 38:839–844, 1977.

71. Adeagbo ASO, Bishera I, Lees J, et al. Evidence for a role of prostaglandin I_2 and thromboxane A_2 in the ductus venosus of the lamb. Can J Physiol Pharmacol 63:1601–1605, 1985.

72. Meyer HP, Rothuizen J. Congenital portosystemic shunts (PSS) in dogs are a genetic disorder. Tijdschrift voor diergeneeskunde 116:809–810, 1991.

73. Schermerhorn T, Center SA, Rowland PJ, et al. Characterization of inherited portovascular dysplasia in Cairn terriers (abstract). Proc 11th ACVIM Forum, 949, 1993.

74. Marretta SM, Pask AJ, Greene RW, et al. Urinary calculi associated with portosystemic shunts in six dogs. J Am Vet Med Assoc 178:133–137, 1981.

75. Suter PF. Portal vein anomalies in the dog: Their angiographic diagnosis. Vet Radiol 16:84–97, 1975.

76. Schaeffer MC, Rogers QR, Buffington CA, et al. Long-term biochemical and physiologic effects of surgically placed portacaval shunts in dogs. Am J Vet Res 47:346–355, 1986.

77. Griffiths GL, Lumsden JH, Valli VEO. Hematologic and biochemical changes in dogs with portosystemic shunts. J Am Anim Hosp Assoc 17:705–710, 1981.

78. Laflamme D, Mahaffey E, Allen S, et al. Microcytosis in dogs with portocaval shunt (abstract). Proc 8th ACVIM Forum, 113, 1990.

79. Bunch SE, Jordan HL, Sellon RK, et al. Iron status in 12 dogs with congenital portosystemic shunts (abstract). Proc 10th ACVIM Forum, 809, 1992.

80. Meyer DJ, Harvey JW. Hematologic changes associated with serum and hepatic iron alterations in dogs with congenital portosystemic vascular anomalies. J Vet Intern Med 8:55–56, 1994.

81. Cooper RA, Jandl JH. Destruction of erythrocytes. In: Williams WJ (ed) Hematology, 3rd ed. New McGraw-Hill, New York, 377, 1983.

81a. Doll DC. Spur cells. N Engl J Med 333:1183, 1995.

82. Rutgers HC, Batt RM, Haywood S, et al. Hepatic organelle pathology in dogs with congenital portosystemic shunts. J Vet Int Med 5:351–356, 1991.

83. Hatoff DE, Hardison WG. Bile acids modify alkaline phosphatase induction and bile secretion pressure after bile duct obstruction in the rat. Gastroenterology 80:666–672, 1981.

84. Low MG, Ferguson MAJ, Futerman AH, et al. Covalently attached phosphatidylinositol as a hydrophobic anchor for membrane proteins. Trends Biochem Sci 11:212–215, 1986.

85. Beher WT, Toledo-Pereyra LH. Effect of caval shunts on lipid metabolism. Prog Lipid Res 18:165–177, 1980.

86. Francavilla A, Jones AF, Benichou J, et al. The effect of portacaval shunt upon hepatic cholesterol synthesis and cyclic AMP in dogs and baboons. J Surg Res 28:1–7, 1980.

87. Coyle JJ, Schwarz MZ, Marubbio AT, et al. The effect of portacaval shunt on plasma lipids and tissue cholesterol synthesis in the dog. Surgery 80:54–60, 1976.

88. Coyle JJ, Guzman IJ, Varco RL, et al. Cholesterol pool sizes and turnover following portacaval shunt in the dog. Surg Gynecol Obstet 148:723–727, 1979.

89. Castellanos J, Toledo-Pereyra LH, Mittal VK, et al. Prolonged hypocholesterolemic effects of portacaval transposition in dogs: An experimental study. Eur Surg Res 13:438–443, 1981.

90. Proia JA, McNamara DJ, Edwards KDG, et al. Cholesterol homeostasis in the rat with a portacaval anastomosis. Proc Natl Acad Sci USA 148:723–727, 1979.

91. Riveron E, Kukral JC, Henegar GC. Blood volume, water and electrolyte spaces in human beings with cirrhosis and in dogs with Eck's fistula. Surg Forum 17:365–366, 1966.

92. Whang R, Papper S. The possible relationship of renal cortical hypoperfusion and diminished renal concentrating ability in Laennec's cirrhosis. J Chron Dis 27:263–265, 1974.

93. Kozlowski S, Drzewiecki K. The role of osmoreceptors in portal circulation in control of water intake in dogs. Acta Physiol Polonica 24:325–330, 1973.

94. Lauterburg B, Bircher J. Defective renal handling of water in the rat with a portacaval shunt. Eur J Clin Invest 6:439–444, 1976.

95. Magne ML, Macy DW. Intravenous glucagon challenge test in the diagnosis and assessment of therapeutic efficacy in dogs with congenital portosystemic shunts (abstract). ACVIM Scientific Proc, 36, 1984.

96. Schenker S, Breen KJ, Hoyumpa AM. Hepatic encephalopathy: Current status. Gastroenterology 66:121–151, 1974.

97. Gabuzda GJ, Hall PW. Relation of potassium depletion to renal ammonia metabolism and hepatic coma. Medicine 45:481–490, 1966.

98. Crawford MA, Kittleson MD, Fink GD. Hypernatremia and adipsia in a dog. J Am Vet Med Assoc 184:3818–3821, 1984.

99. Lauterburg B, Sautter V, Herz R, et al. The defect of uric acid metabolism in Eck-fistula rats. J Lab Clin Med 90:92–100, 1977.

100. Herz R, Sautter V, Bircher J. Fortuitous discovery of urate nephrolithiasis in rats subjected to portacaval anastomosis. Experientia 28:27–28, 1972.

101. Condon RE. Effect of dietary protein on symptoms and survival in dogs with an Eck fistula. Am J Surg 121:107–114, 1971.

102. Horak W, Gangi A, Funovics J, et al. Effect of portacaval shunt and arterialization of the liver on bile acid metabolism. Gastroenterology 69:338–341, 1975.

103. Center SA, Baldwin BH, Erb N, et al. Bile acid concentrations in the diagnosis of hepatobiliary disease in the dog. J Am Vet Med Assoc 187:935–940, 1985.

104. Center SA, Baldwin BH, de Lahunta A, et al. Evaluation of serum bile acid concentrations for the diagnosis of portosystemic venous anomalies in the dog and cat. J Am Vet Med Assoc 186:1090–1094, 1986.

105. Meyer DJ. Liver function tests in dogs with portosystemic shunts: Measurement of serum bile acid concentration. J Am Vet Med Assoc 188:168–169, 1986.

106. Center SA. Serum bile acids in companion animal medicine. Vet Clin N Amer [Sm Animal Practice] 23:625–657, 1993.

107. Center SA. Liver function tests in the diagnosis of portosystemic vascular anomalies. Sem Vet Med and Surg (Sm Anim) 5:94–99, 1990.

108. Center SA, Baldwin BH, Erb H, et al. Bile acid concentrations in the diagnosis of hepatobiliary disease in the cat. J Am Vet Med Assoc 189:891–896, 1986.

109. Center SA, Slatter M, ManWarren T, et al. Evaluation of twelve-hour preprandial and two-hour postprandial serum bile acids concentrations for diagnosis of hepatobiliary disease in dogs. J Am Vet Med Assoc 199:217–226, 1991.

110. Center SA, Joseph SA, Erb HN. Measurement of twelve hour fasting and two-hour postprandial serum bile acids for the diagnosis of hepatobiliary disease in cats. J Am Vet Med Assoc, in press.

111. Herz R, Paumgartner G, Preisig R. Bile salt metabolism and bile formation in the rat with a portacaval shunt. Eur J Clin Invest 4:223–228, 1974.

112. Center SA, Leveille CR, Baldwin BH, et al. Direct spectometric determination of serum bile acids in the dog and cat. Am J Vet Res 45:2043–2050, 1984.

113. Johnson SE, Rogers WA, Bonagura JD, et al. Determination of serum bile acids in fasting dogs with hepatobiliary disease. Am J Vet Res 46:2048–2053, 1985.

114. Hauge JG, Abdelkader SV. Serum bile acids as an indicator of liver disease in dogs. Acta Vet Scand 25:495–503, 1984.

115. Schmidt S, Suter PF. Angiography of the hepatic and portal venous system in the dog and cat: An investigative method. Vet Radiol 21:57–77, 1980.

116. Schmidt S, Lohse CL, Suter PF. Branching patterns of the hepatic artery in the dog: Arteriographic and anatomic study. Am J Vet Res 41:1090–1097, 1980.

117. Enge IR, Flatmark A. Selective coeliac and hepatic artery angiography in the dog. Can J Gastroenterol 7:361–368, 1972.

118. Moon ML. Diagnostic imaging of portosystemic shunts. Sem Vet Med Surg (Sm Anim) 5:120–126, 1990.

119. Gomez JA, Lawson TL, Korobkin M, et al. Selective abdominal angiography in the dog. Am Vet Radiol Soc J 14:72–80, 1973.

120. Wrigley RH, Park RD, Konde LJ, et al. Subtraction portal venography. Vet Radiol 28:208–212, 1987.

121. Birchard SJ, Biller DS, Johnson SE. Differentiation of intrahepatic versus extrahepatic portosystemic shunts in dogs using positive-contrast portography. Am Anim Hosp Assoc 25:13–17, 1989.

122. Schulz KS, Martin RA, Henderson RA. Trans-splenic portal catheterization: Surgical technique and use in two dogs with portosystemic shunts. Vet Surg 22:363–369, 1993.

123. Wrigley RH, Konde LJ, Park RD, et al. Ultrasonographic diagnosis of portocaval shunts in young dogs. J Am Vet Med Assoc 191:421–424, 1987.

124. Bailey MQ, Willard MD, McLoughlin MA, et al. Ultrasonographic findings associated with congenital hepatic arteriovenous fistula in three dogs. J Am Vet Med Assoc 192:1099–1101, 1988.

125. Nyland TG, Park RD. Hepatic ultrasonography in the dog. Vet Radiol 24:74–84, 1983.

126. Nyland TG, Hager DA. Sonography of the liver, gallbladder, and spleen. Vet Clin N Am (Sm Anim Pract) 15:1123–1148, 1985.

127. Yeager A. Department of Clinical Sciences, Section of Radiology, College of Veterinary Medicine, Cornell University, personal communication.

128. Kantrowitz BM, Nyland TG, Fisher P. Estimation of portal blood flow using duplex real-time and pulsed Doppler ultrasound imaging in the dog. Vet Radiol 30:222–226, 1989.

129. Lamb DR. Doppler ultrasonography of portosystemic shunts in dogs: Work in progress. 1933 Annual Scientific Meeting, American College of Veterinary Radiology.

130. Koblik PD, Hornof WJ, Breznock EM. Quantitative hepatic scintigraphy in the dog. Vet Radiol 24:226–231, 1983.

131. Koblik PD, Hornof WJ, Breznock EM. Use of quantitative hepatic scintigraphy to evaluate spontaneous portosystemic shunts in 12 dogs. Vet Radiol 24:232–236, 1983.

132. Hornof WJ, Koblik PD, Breznock EM. Radiocolloid scintigraphy as an aid to the diagnosis of congenital portacaval anomalies in the dog. J Am Vet Med Assoc 182:44–46, 1983.

133. Kerr LY, Hornof WJ. Quantitative hepatobiliary scintigraphy using 99mTc-DISIDA in the dog. Vet Radiol 27:173–177, 1986.

134. Koblik PD, Yed C-K, Hornof WJ, et al. Use of transcolonic 123-I-iodoamphetamine to diagnose spontaneous portosystemic shunts in 18 dogs. Vet Radiol 30:67–73, 1989.

135. Yen C-K, Koblik P, Breznock B, et al. Portosystemic shunt fraction quantification using transrectal administration of iodine-123 iodoamphetamine in dogs with chronic bile duct ligation and after propranolol administration. J Nucl Med 30:1701–1702, 1989.

136. Koblik PD, Komtebedde J, Yen C-K, et al. Use of transcolonic 99mtechnectium-pertechnate as a screening test for portosystemic shunts in dogs. J Am Vet Med Assoc 196:925–930, 1990.

137. Daniel GB, Bright R, Ollis P, et al. Per rectal portal scintigraphy using 99mTechnectium pertechnetate to diagnose portosystemic shunts in dogs and cats. J Vet Int Med 5:23–27, 1991.

138. Caride VJ. Rectal absorption of 99mTc-pertechnetate in the dog. Concise communication. J Nucl Med 14:600–603, 1973.

139. Shiomi S, Kuroki T, Kurai O, et al. Portal circulation by Technectium-99m pertechnetate per rectal portal scintigraphy. J Nucl Med 29:460–465, 1988.

140. Dykes NL. Department of Clinical Sciences, Section of Radiology, College of Veterinary Medicine, Cornell University, personal communication.

141. McCuskey RS, Vonnahme FJ, Grun M. In vivo and electron microscopic observation of the hepatic microvasculature in the rat following portacaval anastomosis. Hepatology 3:96–104, 1983.

142. Lanier VC, Buchanan RD, Foster JH. Hepatic morphologic changes following end-to-side portacaval shunt in dogs. Am Surg 34:185–195, 1968.

143. McCusky RS, Vonnahme R-J, Crun M. In vivo and electron microscopic observations of the hepatic microvasculature in the rat following portacaval anastomosis. Hepatology 3:96–104, 1983.

144. Rubin F, Gevirth NRT, Cohan P, et al. Liver cell damage by portacaval shunts. Proc Soc Exp Biol Med 59:111–115, 1965.

145. Weinbren K, Stirling GA, Washington SLA. The development of a proliferative response in liver parenchyma deprived of portal blood flow. Br J Exp Path 53:54–58, 1972.

146. Kyu MH, Cavanagh JP. Some effects of porto-caval anastomosis in the male rat. Br J Exp Pathol 51:217–227, 1970.

147. Meyers OL, Hicckman R, Keraan M, et al. Acute biochemical and histological effects of portacaval shunt in the normal rat. S Afr J Lab Clin Med 49:1048–1050, 1975.

148. Doberneck RC, Kline DG, Morse AS, et al. Relationship of hemosiderosis to portocaval shunting. Surgery 54:912–920, 1963.

149. Rappaport AM. Hepatic blood flow: Morphologic aspects and physiologic regulation. In: Javitt NB (ed.) Liver and Biliary Tract Physiology. University Park Press, Baltimore, 1–63, 1980.

150. McCuskey RS. A dynamic and static study of hepatic arterioles and hepatic sphincters. Am J Anat 119:455–478, 1966.

151. Huet P-M, Goresky CA, Villeneuve J-P, et al. Assessment of liver microcirculation in human cirrhosis. J Clin Invest 70:1234–1244, 1982.

152. Rector WG, Hoefs JC, Hossack KF, et al. Hepatofugal portal flow in cirrhosis: Observations on hepatic hemodynamics and the nature of the arterioportal communications. Hepatology 8:16–20, 1988.

153. Schaffner F, Popper H. Capillarization of hepatic sinusoids. Gastroenterology 44:239–242, 1963.

154. Villeneuve J-P, Huet P-M. Microcirculatory abnormalities in liver diseases. Hepatology 7:186–187, 1987.

155. Rabinovici N, Shapira?. The intrahepatic distribution of portal venous and arterial blood. J Surg Res 6:74–79, 19??.

156. Hanson KM, Johnson PC. Local control of hepatic arterial and portal venous flow in the dog. Am J Physiol 211:712–720, 1966.

157. Fraser R, Bowler LM, Day WA, et al. High pressure perfusion damages the sieving ability of the sinusoidal endothelium in rat liver. Br J Exp Pathol 61:222–223, 1980.

158. Raffucci MD. The effects of temporary occlusion of the afferent hepatic circulation in dogs. Surgery 33:342–351, 1953.

159. Fraser D, Rappaport AM, Vuylsteke CA, et al. Effects of ligation of the hepatic artery in dogs. Surgery 30:624–641, 1951.

160. Drapanas T, Becker DR, Alfano GS, et al. Some effects of interrupting hepatic blood flow. Ann Surg 142:831–835, 1955.

161. Fisher B, Lee S, Fisher ER, et al. Liver regeneration following portacaval shunt. Surgery 52:88–102, 1962.

162. Grun M, Liehr H, Heine WD, et al. Liver hyperegeneration after end-to-side portacaval anastomosis as a consequence of lack of cell differentiation control by factors originating from the upper intestinal tract. In: Lie TS (ed), Microsurgery. Excerpta Medica, Amsterdam, 1980.

163. Schmidt S, Suter PF. Indirect and direct determination of the portal vein pressure in normal and abnormal dogs and normal cats. Vet Rad Soc 21:246–259, 1980.

164. Doige CE, Furneaux RW. Liver disease and intrahepatic portal hypertension in the dog. Can Vet J 16:209–216, 1975.

165. Ahlgren I, Aronsen KF, Ericsson B, et al. Hepatic blood flow during different depths of halothane anesthesia in the dog. Acta Anaesth Scand 11:91–96, 1967.

166. Boettner RB, Ankeney JL, Middleton H. Effect of halothane on splanchnic and peripheral flow in dogs. Anesth Analg 44:214–219, 1965.

167. Merritt CRB. Ultrasonographic demonstration of portal vein thrombosis. Radiology 133:425–427, 1979.

168. Volwiler W, Grindlay JH, Bollman JL. The relationship of portal vein pressure to the formation of ascites—an experimental study. Gastroenterology 14:40–55, 1980.

169. Wiles CE, Schenk WG, Lindenberg J. The experimental production of portal hypertension. Ann Surg 136:811–817, 1952.

170. Matushek KJ, Bjorling D, Mathews K. Generalized motor seizures after portosystmic shunt ligation in dogs: Five cases (1981–1988). J Am Vet Med Assoc 196:2013–2014, 1990.

171. Hardie EM, Hornegay JN, Cullen JM. Status epilepticus after ligation of portosystemic shunts. Vet Surg 19:412–417, 1990.

172. Canalese J, Gimson AES, Davis C, et al. Controlled trial of dexamethasone and mannitol for the cerebral oedema of fulminant hepatic failure. Gut 23:625–629, 1982.

173. Munoz SJ, Maddrey WC. Major complications of acute and chronic liver disease. Gastroenterol Clin N Am 17:265–287, 1988.

174. Ede RJ, Williams R. Hepatic encephalopathy and cerebral edema. Sem Liver Dis 6:107–118, 1986.

175. Ede RJ, Gimson AES, Bihari D, et al. Controlled hyperventilation in the prevention of cerebral oedema in fulminant hepatic failure. J Hepatol 2:43–51, 1986.

176. Prioa AD, Edwards DG, McNamara DJ, et al. Dietary influences on the hepatic mixed-function oxidase system in the rat after portacaval anastomosis. Gastroenterology 86:618–626, 1984.

177. Ossenberg FW, Pointard L, Benhamou JP. Effect of portacaval shunt on hepatic cytochrome P-450 in rats. Rev Eur Etudes Clin et Biol 17:791–793, 1972.

178. Pector JC, Ossenberg FW, Peignoux M, et al. The effect of portacaval transposition on hepatic cytochrome P-450 in the rat. Biomedicine 23:160–162, 1975.

179. Rubin E, Hutterer F, Ohshiro T, et al. Effect of experimental portacaval shunt on hepatic drug metabolizing enzymes. Proc Soc Exp Biol Med 127:444–447, 1968.

180. Nance FC, Kline DG. Eck's fistula encephalopathy in germfree dogs. Ann Surg 174:856–862, 1971.

181. Hooper PT. Spongy degeneration in the central nervous system of domestic animals. III. Occurrence and pathogenesis-hepatocerebral disease caused by hyperammonaemia. Acta Neuropath (Berl) 31:343–351, 1975.

182. Phillips L, Tappe J, Lyman. Hepatic microvascular dysplasia without demonstrable macroscopic shunts. Proc 11th ACVIM Forum, 438–439, 1993.

183. Thompson JS, Schafer DF, Haun J, et al. Adequate diet prevents hepatic coma in dogs with Eck fistulas. Surg Gynecol Obstet 162:126–130, 1986.

184. Lewis LD, Morris ML, Jr, Hand MS. Small Animal Clinical Nutrition III. Mark Morris Associates, Topeka, KS, 1987.

185. Laflamme DP, Allen SW, Huber TL. Apparent dietary protein requirement of dogs with portosystemic shunt. Am J Vet Res 54:719–723, 1993.

186. Smith AR, Rossi-Fanelli F, Freund H, et al. Sulfur-containing amino acids in experimental hepatic coma in the dog and the monkey. Surg 85:677–683, 1979.

187. Gabuzda GJ, Shear L. Metabolism of dietary protein in hepatic cirrhosis. Nutritional and clinical considerations. Am J Clin Nutr 23:479–487, 1970.

188. Eriksson LS, Conn HO. Branched-chain amino acids in the management of hepatic encephalopathy: An analysis of variants. Hepatology 10:228–246, 1989.

189. Eriksson LS, Persson A, Wahren J. Branched-chain amino acids in the treatment of chronic hepatic encephalopathy. Gut 23:801–806, 1982.

190. Maddison JE. Hepatic encephalopathy: Current concepts of the pathogenesis. J Vet Int Med 6:341–353, 1992.

191. Swart GR, van den Berg FW, Wattimena JL, et al. Elevated protein requirements in cirrhosis of the liver investigated by whole body protein turnover studies. Clin Sci 75:101–107, 1988.

192. Swart GR, van den Berg FW, van Vuure FK. Minimum protein requirements in liver cirrhosis determined by nitrogen balance measurements at three levels of protein intake. Clin Nutr 8:329–336, 1989.

193. Young VR, Marchini JS. Mechanisms and nutritional significance of metabolic responses to altered intakes of protein and amino acids, with reference to nutritional adaptation in humans. Am J Clin Nutr 51:270–289, 1990.

194. Aguirre A, Yoshimura N, Westman T, et al. Plasma amino acids in dogs with two experimental forms of liver damage. J Surg Res 16:339–345, 1974.

195. Soeters PB, Weir G, Ebeid AM, et al. Insulin, glucagon, portal systemic shunting, and hepatic failure in the dog. J Surg Res 23:183–188, 1979.

196. Smith AR, Rossi-Fanelli F, Ziparo V, et al. Alterations in plasma and CSF amino acids, amines and metabolites in hepatic coma. Ann Surg 187:343–350, 1978.

197. Faraj BA, Farouk MA, Fulenwider JT, et al. Hepatorenal failure induced by tetracycline in dogs with portocaval shunt. J Pharmacol Exp Ther 22:558–563, 1982.

198. Thompson JS, Schafer DF, Schafer GJ, et al. Gamma-amino butyric acid plasma levels and brain binding in Eck fistula dogs. J Surg Res 38:143–148, 1985.

199. Okamoto H, Fujimura T. Normalization of abnormal eletroencephalograms in beagles with portacaval anastomosis by infusion of solutions rich in branched-chain amino acids. J Parenter Nutr 10:34–39, 1986.

200. Sato S, Tateishi K, Kato A, et al. Marked depression of brain cholecystokinin and vasoactive intestinal polypeptide levels in Eck fistula dogs. Regul Pept 25:111–121, 1989.

201. Merino GE, Jetzer T, Dorzaki WFD, et al. Methionine induced hepatic coma in dogs. Am J Surg 130:41–46, 1975.

202. Phear EA, Tuebner B, Sherlock S, et al. Methionine toxicity in liver disease and its prevention by chlortetracycline. Clin Sci 15:93–117, 1956.

203. Branam JE. Suspected methionine toxicosis associated with a portacaval shunt in a dog. J Am Vet Med Assoc 181:929–931, 1982.

204. Mullen KD, Weber FL. Role of nutrition in hepatic encephalopathy. Sem Liv Dis 11:292–304, 1991.

205. Uribe M. Treatment of portal systemic encephalopathy: The old and new treatments. In: Grisolia S (ed) Cirrhosis, Hepatic Encephalopathy, and Ammonium Toxicity. Plenum Press, New York, 235–253, 1990.

206. Bianchi GP, Marchesini G, Fabbri A, et al. Vegetable versus animal pro-

tein diet in cirrhotic patients with chronic encephalopathy. A randomized cross-over comparison. J Int Med 233:385–392, 1993.

207. Weber FL, Minco D, Fresard KM, et al. Effects of vegetable diets on nitrogen metabolism in cirrhotic subjects. Gastroenterology 89:538–544, 1985.

208. Uribe M. Nutrition, diet and hepatic encephalopathy. In: Butterworth RF, Pomier Layrargues G (eds) Hepatic Encephalopathy. Humana Press, Clifton, NJ, 529–548, 1989.

209. Uribe M, Dibildox M, Mapica S, et al. Beneficial effect of vegetable protein diet supplemented with psyllium plantago in patients with hepatic encephalopathy and diabetes mellitus. Gastroenterology 88:901–907, 1985.

210. Zieve L, Zieve FJ. The dietary prevention of hepatic coma in Eck fistula dogs: Ammonia and the carbohydrate to protein ratio. Hepatology 7:196–198, 1987.

211. Stephen AM, Cummings JH. Mechanism of action of dietary fiber in the human colon. Nature 284:283–284, 1980.

212. Iwami K, Kitagawa M, Nagasaki T, et al. Comparison of intestinal taurocholate uptake in rats given soy protein- or casein-based diet. Nut Res 10:547–554, 1990.

213. Strombeck DR, Harrold D, Rogers Q, et al. Plasma amino acid, glucagon, and insulin concentrations in dogs with nitrosamine-induced hepatic disease. 44:2028–2036, 1983.

214. Linscheer WG. Malabsorption in cirrhosis. A J Clin Nutr 23:488–492, 1970.

215. Strombeck DR, Schaeffer MC, Rogers QR. Dietary therapy for dogs with chronic hepatic insufficiency. In: Kirk RW (ed.) Current Veterinary Therapy. VIII. Small Animal Practice. WB Saunders, Philadelphia, 817–821, 1983.

216. Yokoyama M, Fukumoto S, Shimada Y. Determination of NH3-N content in foods and seasonings and low NH3-N diets in the treatment of hepatic encephalopathy. J Jap Soc Nutr Food Sci 44:351–356, 1991.

217. Kronfeld DS. Feeding cats and feline nutrition. Compend Contin Educ Pract Vet 5:419–424, 1983.

218. Castell DO, Moore EW. Ammonia absorption from the human colon. The role of non-ionic diffusion. Gastroenterology 60:33–42, 1971.

219. Vince A, Killingley M, Wrong OM. Effect of lactulose on ammonia production in a fecal incubation system. Gastroenterology 74:544–549, 1978.

220. Vince AJ, Burridge SM. Ammonia production by intestinal bacteria: The effects of lactose, lactulose, and glucose. J Med Microbiol 13:177–191, 1980.

221. Bircher J, Haemmerli UP, Trabert E, et al. The mechanism of action of lactulose in portal-systemic encephalopathy. Non ionic diffusion of ammonia in the canine colon. Rev Eur Etud Clin Biol 16:352–357, 1971.

222. Down PF, Agostini L, Murison J, et al. The interrelations of faecal ammonia pH and bicarbonate: Evidence of colonic absorption of ammonia by non-ionic diffusion. Clin Sci 43:101–114, 1972.

223. Agostini L, Down PF, Murison J, et al. Fecal ammonia and pH during lactulose administration in man: Comparison with other cathartics. Gut 13:859–866, 1972.

224. Leber G, Luginbuhl M. Effect of lactitol and lactulose on human intestinal flora in portal-systemic encephalopthy. In: Conn HO, Bircher J (eds.) Hepatic Encepahlopathy: Management with Lactulose and Related Carbohydrates. Medi-Ed Press, East Lansing, 271–281, 1988.

225. Liehr H, Englisch G, Rasenaek U. Lactulose—a drug with antiendotoxin effect. Hepatogastroenterology 27:356–360, 1980.

226. Riggio O, Balducci G, Ariosto F, et al. Lactitol in prevention of recurrent episodes of hepatic encephalopathy in cirrhotic patients with portal-systemic shunt. Dig Dis Sci 34:823–829, 1989.

227. Patil DH, Westaby D, Mahida YR, et al. Comparative modes of action of lactitol and lactulose in the treatment of hepatic encephalopathy. Gut 28:255–259, 1987.

228. Lanthier PL, Morgan MY. Lactitol in the treatment of chronic hepatic encephalopathy: An open comparison with lactulose. Gut 26:415–420, 1985.

229. Uribe M, Toledo H, Perez F, et al. Lactitol, a second generation disaccharide for treatment of chronic portal systemic encephalopathy. A double blind crossover randomized clinical trial. Dig Dis Sci 32:1345–1353, 1987.

230. Brown CL, Hill MJ, Richards P. Bacterial ureases in uraemic men. Lancet 2:406–409, 1971.

231. Drasar BS, Hill MJ. Human Intestinal Flora. Academic Press, London, 90–94, 1974.

232. Myers S, Lievber CS. Reduction of gastric ammonia by ampicillin in normal and azotemic sugjects. Gastroenterology 70:244–247, 1976.

233. Faloon WW, Fisher CJ. Clinical experience with the use of neomycin in hepatic coma. Arch Intern Med 105:43–49, 1959.

234. Dawson AM, McClaren J, Sherlock S. Neomycin in the treatment of hepatic coma. Lancet 2:1263–1268, 1957.

235. Hoyumpa AM, Desmond PV, Avant GR, et al. Hepatic encephalopathy. Gastroenterology 76:184–195, 1979.

236. Wolpert E, Phillips SF, Summerskill WHJ. Ammonia production in the human colon. Effects of cleansing, neomycin and acetohydroxamic acid. N Engl J Med 283:159–164, 1970.

237. Jacobsen ED, Prior JT, Faloon WW. Malabsorptive syndrome induced by neomycin: Morphologic alterations in the jejunal mucosa. Lab Clin Med 56:245–250, 1960.

238. Morgan MH, Read AE, Speller DCE. Treatment of hepatic encephalopathy with metronidazole. Gut 23:1–7, 1982.

239. Ioannides L, Somogyi A, Spicer J, et al. Rectal administration of metronidazole provides therapeutic plasma levels in postoperative patients. N Engl J Med 1569–1570, 1981.

240. Dow SW, LeCouteur RA, Poss ML, et al. Central nervous system toxicosis associated with metronidazole treatment of dogs: Five cases (1984–1987). J Am Vet Med Assoc 195:365–368, 1989.

241. Pirotte J, Guffens JM, Devos J. Comparative study of basal arterial ammonemia and of orally-induced hyperammonemia in chronic portal systemic encephalopathy, treated with neomycin and lactulose. Digestion 10:435–444, 1974.

242. Orlandi F, Freddara U, Candelaresi MT, et al. Comparison between neomycin and lactulose in 173 patients with hepatic encephalopathy: A randomized clinical study. Dig Dis Sci 26:498–506, 1981.

243. Batshaw ML, Brusilow S, Waber L, et al. Treatment of inborn errors of urea synthesis: Activation of alternative pathways of waste nitrogen synthesis and excretion. N Engl J Med 306:1387–1392, 1982.

244. Brusilow SW, Danney M, Waber LJ, et al. Treatment of episodic hyperammonemia in children with inborn errors of urea synthesis. N Engl J Med 310:1630–1634, 1984.

245. Mendenhall CL, Rouster S, Marshall L, et al. A new therapy for portal systemic encephalopathy. Am J Gastroenterology 81:540–543, 1986.

246. O'Conner JE, Ribelles M, Grisolila S. Potentiation of hyperammonemia by sodium benzoate in animals: A note of caution. Eur J Pediatr 138:186–187, 1982.

247. O'Conner JE, Costell M, Grisolia S. The potentiation of ammonia toxicity by sodium benzoate is prevented by L-carnitine. Biochem Biphys Res Comm 145:817–824, 1987.

248. Jones EA, Schafer DF. Hepatic encephalopathy: A neurochemical disorder. In: Popper H, Schaffner F (eds) Progress in Liver Disease 57:525–540, 1986.

249. Uribe M, Farca A, Marquez MA, et al. Treatment of chronic portal systemic encephalopathy with bromocriptine. A double blind controlled trial. Gastroenterology 76:1347–1351, 1979.

250. Uribe M, Garcia Ramos G, Ramos MH, et al. Standard and higher doses of bromocriptine for severe chronic portal systemic encephalopathy. Am J Gastroenterology 78:517–522, 1983.

251. Van der Rijt CCD, Schalm SW, Meulstee J, et al. Flumazenil therapy for hepatic encephalopathy: A double blind crossover study. Hepatology 10:590, 1989.

252. Zieve L, Ferenci P, Rzepczynski D, et al. A benzodiazepine antagonist does not alter the course of hepatic encephalopathy or neural GABA binding. Metab Brain Dis 2:201–205, 1987.

253. Sutherland LR, Minuk RY. Ro 151788 and hepatic failure. Ann Intern Med 108:158, 1988.

254. Ling GV, Ruby AL, Harrold DR, et al. Xanthine-containing urinary calculi in dogs given allopurinol. J Am Vet Med Assoc 198:1935–1940, 1991.

255. Sorenson JL, Ling GV. Diagnosis, prevention and treatment of urate urolithiasis in Dalmations. J Am Vet Med Assoc 203:863–869, 1993.

256. Osborne CA, Kruger JM, Plolzin DJ. Dissolution of canine ammonium urate uroliths. Vet Clin N Am (Sm Anim Pract) 16:375–388, 1986.

257. van den Ingh TSGAM, Rothuizen J. Hepatoportal fibrosis in three young dogs. Vet Rec 110:575–577, 1982.

258. Easley JC, Carpenter JL. Hepatic arteriovenous fistula in two Saint Bernard pups. J Am Vet Med Assoc 166:167–171, 1975.

259. Legendre AM, Krahwinkel DJ, Carrig CB, et al. Ascites associated with intrahepatic arteriovenous fistula in the cat. J Am Vet Med Assoc 168:589–590, 1976.

260. Rogers WA, Suter PF, Breznock EM, et al. Intrahepatic arteriovenous fistulae in a dog resulting in portal hypertension, portacaval shunts, and reversal of portal blood flow. J Am Anim Hosp Assoc 13:470–475, 1977.

261. McGavin MD, Henry J. Canine vascular hamartoma associated with ascites. J Am Vet Med Assoc 160:864–866, 1970.

262. Moore PF, Whiting PG. Hepatic lesions associated with intrahepatic arterioportal fistulae in dogs. Vet Path 23:57–62, 1986.

263. Foley WJ, Turcotte JG, Hoskins PA, et al. Intrahepatic arteriovenous fistulas between the hepatic artery and portal vein. Ann Surg 174:849–855, 1971.

264. Gomes MMR, Bernatz PE. Arteriovenous fistulas: A review and ten-year experience at the Mayo Clinic. 45:81–102, 1970.

265. Bailey MQ, Willard MD, McLoughlin MA, et al. Ultrasonographic findings associated with congenital hepatic arteriovenous fistula in three dogs. J Am Vet Med Assoc 192:1099–1101, 1988.

266. Whiting PG, Breznock EM, Moore P, et al. Portal hepatectomy witih temporary hepatic vascular occlusion in dogs with hepatic arteriovenous fistulas. Vet Surg 15:171–180, 1986.

267. Owen LN, Hall LW. Ascites in a dog due to a metastasis from an adenocarcinoma of the ovary. Vet Rec 74:220–223, 1962.

268. Hoskins JD, Ochoa R, Hawkins BJ. Portal vein thrombosis in a dog: A case report. J Am Anim Hosp Assoc 15:497–500, 1979.

269. Willard MD, Bailey MQ, Hauptman J, et al. Obstructed portal venous flow and portal vein thrombus in a dog. J Am Vet Med Assoc 194:1449–1451, 1989.

270. Thornburg LP. Diseases of the liver in the dog and cat. Compend Contin Educ Pract Vet 4:538–546, 1982.

271. Roy RG, Post GS, Waters DJ, et al. Portal vein thrombosis as a complication of portosystemic shunt ligation in two dogs. J Am Anim Hosp Assoc 28:53–58, 1992.

272. Willard MD, Bailey MQ, Hauptman J, et al. Obstructed portal venous flow and portal vein thrombus in a dog. J Am Vet Med Assoc 194:1449–1451, 1989.

273. Van Winkle TJ, Bruce E. Thrombosis of the portal vein in eleven dogs. Vet Pathol 30:28–35, 1993.

274. Tanturi C, Mejia RH, Canepa JF, et al. Electrocardiographic and humoral changes in transient occlusion of the portal vein in the dog. Surg Gynecol Obstet 537–540, 1960.

275. Hanna SS, Maheshwari Y. Effect of portal vein occlusion on liver blood flow in normal and cirrhotic dogs. J Surg Res 41:293–300, 1986.

276. Sherlock S. Extrahepatic portal venous hypertension in adults. Clin Gastroenterol 14:1–18, 1985.

277. Orozco H, Guraieb E, Takahashi T, et al. Deficiency of protein C in patients with portal vein thrombosis. Hepatology 8:1110–1111, 1988.

278. Webb LJ, Sherlock AS. The aetiology, presentation and natural history of extra-hepatic portal venous obstruction. Q J Med 48:627–639, 1979.

279. Scully RE, Mark EJ, McNeely WF, et al. Weekly clinicopathological exercises. N Engl J Med 329:301–310, 1989.

280. Brown KM, Kaplan MM, Donowitz M. Extrahepatic portal venous thrombosis: Frequent recognition of associated diseases. J Clin Gastroenterol 7:153–159, 1985.

281. Ohnishi K, Saito M, Terabayashi H, et al. Development of portal vein thrombosis complicating idiopathic portal hypertension. A case report. Gastroenterology 88:1034–1040, 1985.

282. Belli L, Romani F, Sansalone CV, et al. Portal thrombosis in cirrhotics: A retrospective analysis. Ann Surg 203:286–291, 1986.

283. Burke GW, III, Ascher NL, Hunter D, et al. Orthotopic liver tranplantation: Nonoperative management of early, acute portal vein thrombosis. Surgery 104:924–928, 1988.

284. Triger DR. Extrahepatic portal venous obstruction. Gut 28:1193–1197, 1987.

285. Sack J, Aldrete JS. Primary mesenteric venous thrombosis. Surg Gynecol Obstet 154:205–208, 1982.

286. Van Gansbeke D, Avni EF, Delcour C, et al. Sonographic features of portal vein thrombosis. A J R 144:749–752, 1985.

287. Verbanck JJ, Rutgeerts LJ, Haerens MH, et al. Parital splenoportal and superior mesenteric venous thrombosis: Early sonographic diagnosis and successful conservative management. Gastroenterology 86:949–952, 1984.

288. Safran AP, Schaffner F. Chronic passive congestion of the liver in man. Am J Path 50:447–463, 1967.

289. Drapanas T, Schenk WG, Pollack EL, et al. Hepatic hemodynamics in experimental ascites. Ann Surg 152:705–715, 1961.

290. Lefkowitch JH, Mendez L. Morphologic features of hepatic injury in cardiac disease and shock. J Hepatology 2:313–327, 1986.

291. Armstrong CD, Richards V. Results of long term experimental constriction of hepatic veins in dogs. Arch Surg 48:472–481, 1944.

292. McDermott WV, Stone MD, Bothe A, et al. Budd-Chiari syndrome: Historical and clinical review with an analysis of surgical corrective procedures. Am J Surg 147:463–467, 1984.

293. Ware AJ. The liver when the heart fails. Gastroenterology 74:627–628, 1978.

294. Murphy FB, Steinberg HV, Shires GT, et al. The Budd-Chiari syndrome: A review. A J R 147:9–15, 1986.

295. Linde-Sipman JS, Stokhof AA. Triple atria in a pup. J Am Vet Med Assoc 165:536–541, 1974.

296. Edwards DF, Bahr RJ, Suter PF, et al. Portal hypertension secondary to a right atrial tumor in a dog. J Am Vet Med Assoc 173:750–755, 1978.

297. Lombard CW, Goldschmidt MH. Primary fibroma in the right atrium of a dog. J Sm Anim Pract 21:439–448, 1980.

298. Kolata RJ, Cornelius LM, Bjorling DE, et al. Correction of an obstructive lesion of the caudal vena cava in a dog using a temporary intraluminal shunt. Vet Surg 11:100–104, 1982.

299. Crowe DT, Lorenz MD, Hardie EM, et al. Chronic peritoneal effusion due to partial caudal vena cava obstruction following blunt trauma: Diagnosis and successful surgical treatment. J Am Anim Hosp Assoc 20:231–238, 1984.

300. Cornelius L, Mahaffey M. Kinking of the intrathoracic caudal vena cava in five dogs. J Sm Anim Pract 26:67–80, 1985.

301. Stern A, Fallon RK, Aronson E, et al. Cor triatrium dexter in a dog. Comp Cont Ed Pract Vet 8:401–413, 1986.

302. Miller MW, Bonagura JD, DiBartola SP, et al. Budd-Chiari-like syndrome in two dogs. J Am Anim Hosp Assoc 25:277–283, 1989.

303. Otto CM, Mahaffey M, Jacobs C, et al. Cor triatrium dexter with Budd-Chiari syndrome and a review of ascites in young dogs. J Sm Anim Pract 31:385–389, 1990.

304. Cohn LA, Spaulding KA, Cullen JA, et al. Intrahepatic postsinusoidal venous obstruction in a dog. J Vet Int Med 5:317–321, 1991.

305. Mallik R, Hunt GV, Chard RB, et al. Congenital obstruction of the caudal vena cava in a dog. J Am Vet Med Assoc 197:880–882, 1990.

306. von Lictenberg, Jackson RF, Otto FG. Hepatic lesions in dogs with dirofilariasis. J Am Vet Med Assoc 141:121–128, 1962.

307. Jackson RF, von Lictenberg F, Otto GF. Occurrence of adult heartworms in the venae cavae of dogs. J Am Vet Med Assoc 141:117–128, 1962.

307a. Macintire DK, Henderson RH, Banfield C, et al. Budd-Chiari syndrome in a kitten caused by membranous obstruction of the caudal vena cava. J Am Anim Hosp Assoc 31:484–491, 1995.

308. Orloff MJ, Johansen KH. Treatment of Budd-Chiari syndrome by side-to-side portacaval shunt: Experimental and clinical results. Ann Surg 188:494–512, 1978.

309. Brooks SEH, Miller CG, McKenzie K, et al. Acute veno-occlusive disease of the liver. Arch Pathol 89:507–520, 1970.

310. Leopold JG, Parry TE, Storring FK. A change in the sinusoid-trabecular structure of the liver with hepatic venous outflow block. J Pathol 100:87–98, 1970.

311. Fajardo LF, Colby TV. Pathogenesis of veno-occlusive liver disease after radiation. Arch Pathol Lab Med 104:584–588, 1980.

312. Bras G, Jellife DNB, Stuart KL. Veno-occlusive disease of the liver with non-portal types of cirrhosis occurring in Jamaica. AMA Arch Pathol 57:285–300, 1954.

313. Stillman A, Huxtable R, Consroe P, et al. Hepatic veno-occlusive disease due to pyrrolizidine (Senecio) poisoning in Arizona. Gastroenterology 73:349–352, 1977.

314. Mohabbat P, Younos MS, Merzad AA, et al. An outbreak of hepatic veno-occlusive disease in northwestern Afghanistan. Lancet 2:269–271, 1976.

315. Tandon BN, Tandon HD, Tandon RK, et al. An epidemic of veno-occlusive disease of the liver in central India. Lancet 2:271–272, 1976.

316. Feigen M. Fatal veno-occlusive disease of the liver associated with herbal tea consumption and radiation. Aust NZ J Med 14:61–62, 1984.

317. Reed GB, Cox AJ. The human liver after radiation injury, a form of veno-occlusive disease. Am J Pathol 48:597–612, 1966.

318. Brodsky I, Johnson H, Killman SA, et al. Fibrosis of central and hepatic veins and perisinusoidal spaces of the liver following prolonged administration of urethane. Am J Med 30:976–980, 1961.

319. Griner PF, Elbodawi A, Packman CH. Veno-occlusive disease of the liver after chemotherapy of acute leukemia. Report of two cases. Ann Intern Med 85:579–582, 1976.

320. Asbury RF, Rosenthal SN, Descalzi ME, et al. Hepatic veno-occlusive disease due to DTIC. Cancer 45:2670–2674, 1980.

321. Menard DB, Gisselbrecht MM, Marty M, et al. Antineoplastic agents and the liver. Gastroenterology 78:142–164, 1980.

322. Girardin MFSM, Zafrani ES, Prigent A, et al. Unilobular small hepatic vein obstruction: Possible role of progestogen. Gastroenterology 84:630–635, 1983.

323. Zafrani ES, Pimaudeau Y, Dhumeaux D. Drug induced vascular lesions of the liver. Arch Intern Med 143:495–502, 1983.

324. Goodman ZA, Ishak KG. Occlusive venous lesions in alcoholic liver disease. Gastroenterology 83:786–796, 1982.

325. Mellis C, Bale PM. Familial hepatic veno-occlusive disease in a patient with probable immune deficiency. J Pediatr 88:236–242, 1976.

326. Pappas SC, Malone DB, Rabin L, et al. Hepatic veno-occlusive disease in a patient with systemic lupus erythematosus. Arthritis Rheum 27:104–108, 1984.

327. Katzka DA, Saul SH, Jorkasky D, et al. Azathioprine and hepatic venocclusive disease in renal transplant patients. Gastroenterology 90:446–454, 1986.

328. Madden JW, Gertmen PM, Peacock EE Jr. Dimethylnitrosamine-induced hepatic cirrhosis: A new canine model of an ancient human disease. Surgery 68:260–268, 1970.

329. Strombeck DR, Harrold D, Rogers Q, et al. Plasma amino acid, glucagon, and insulin concentrations in dogs with nitrosamine-induced hepatic disease. Am J Vet Res 44:2028–2036, 1983.

330. Boothe DM, Jenkins WL, Green RA, et al. Dimethylnitrosamine induced hepatotoxicosis in dogs as a model of progressive canine hepatic disease. Am J Vet Res 53:411–420, 1992.

331. Sugita S, Ohnishi K, Saito M, et al. Splanchnic hemodynamics in portal hypertensive dogs with portal fibrosis. Am J Physiol 252:G748–G754, 1987.

332. Setchell KDR, Gosselin SJ, Welsh MB, et al. Dietary estrogens—a probable cause of infertility and liver disease in captive cheetahs. Gastroenterology 93:225–233, 1987.

333. Munson L, Worley MB. Veno-occlusive disease in snow leopards (Panthera uncia) from zoological parks. Vet Pathol 28:37–45, 1991.

334. Gosselin SJ, Loudy DL, Tarr MJ, et al. Veno-occlusive disease of the liver in captive cheetah. Vet Pathol 25:48–57, 1988.

335. Rand JS, Best SJ, Mathews KA. Portosystemic vascular shunts in a family of American cocker spaniels. J Am Anim Hosp Assoc 24:266–272, 1988.

36 Hepatic Neoplasms

DONALD R. STROMBECK AND W. GRANT GUILFORD

INTRODUCTION

The liver can be the site of primary and metastatic neoplastic disease. The prevalence of primary hepatic tumors in necropsied dogs ranges from 0.6% to 0.8%. Primary hepatobiliary neoplasms account for 1.2% of all tumors seen in dogs. The most common primary neoplasms in dogs are hepatocellular carcinomas and adenomas (i.e., neoplasms that arise from hepatocytes).[1] Bile duct carcinomas are seen less frequently. Fibromas, fibrosarcomas, hemangiomas, and hemangiosarcomas are uncommon primary hepatic neoplasms accounting for approximately 13% of all primary hepatic neoplasms.

Metastatic tumors are approximately three times more common than primary liver tumors in dogs.[2] The liver is the organ most commonly affected by tumor metastasis. It is involved in 31% to 37% of all cases in comparison to the lungs, which are involved in 24% of cases. Metastases can invade the liver from many different tissues in addition to the abdominal viscera (Table 36–1).

In cats, hepatic neoplasms are reported to represent 1.5% to 2.3% of all neoplastic disease.[3,4,5] The majority (approximately 75%) is accounted for by malignant lymphoma, which can be multicentric or in some cases restricted to the liver. Myeloproliferative disorders and mast cell neoplasia also frequently involve the liver in cats. Primary hepatic neoplasms are unusual in cats but include bile duct adenomas, bile duct carcinomas, hepatocellular adenomas, hepatocellular carcinomas, and myelolipomas.

NODULAR HYPERPLASIA

Nodular hyperplasia refers to a benign nodular regeneration of hepatocellular tissue that is most common in older dogs (Figure 36–1A). The regenerative process is unable to restore the normal architecture and forms nodules of normal or near-normal-appearing hepatocytes without their typical arrangements with the vasculature. Vacuolation of the regenerating cells is common and their communication with the afferent portal and arterial blood supply or the efferent blood flow in the central vein is often abnormal. Bile canaliculi also regenerate within the nodule, but often without connections to bile ducts so that secreted bile is unable to leave the liver. The exchange of substances between hepatocytes and circulation is impaired because regenerated parenchymal cells reform in thicker than usual plates. The nodules may or may not be encapsulated by a thin layer of fibrous tissue. In humans, evidence has been accumulating that regenerative nodules can be preneoplastic.[6] There is as yet no evidence that the same is true in dogs.

Nodular hyperplasia is usually not responsible for clinical signs but is sometimes associated with mild elevations in the activity of serum liver enzymes. From a clinical perspective, the primary importance of nodular hyperplasia is that it can be difficult to differentiate from liver neoplasia. The ultrasonographic findings in nodular hyperplasia often resemble those seen in primary or metastatic neoplasia.[7] Gross examination of a liver affected by nodular hyperplasia reveals tan to pink nodules up to a few centimeters in size that can easily be confused with adenomas or adenocarcinomas. Even on histologic examination the difficulties can continue, particularly when the pathologist is provided with a needle biopsy rather than a large surgical biopsy specimen.

HEPATOCELLULAR ADENOMAS

Hepatocellular adenomas are commonly seen in dogs but are less frequently reported in cats. Affected dogs are usually over 10 years of age. Grossly and histologically, adenomas can be difficult to distinguish from nodular hyperplasia or even

Table 36–1

CANINE METASTATIC LIVER DISEASE			
TUMOR TYPE		**PRIMARY SITE**	
Hemangiosarcoma	29%	Generalized	27%
Lymphosarcoma	23%	Unknown	14%
Adenocarcinoma	13%	Spleen	12%
Carcinoma	13%	Heart	8%
Leiomyosarcoma	6%	GI	7%
Sarcoma	6%	Pancreas	6%
Myeloma	3%	Islet Cell	5%
Osteosarcoma	2%	Bone	3%
Miscellaneous	5%	Oral Cavity	3%
		Adrenal	3%
		Renal	3%
		Lung	2%
		Other	7%

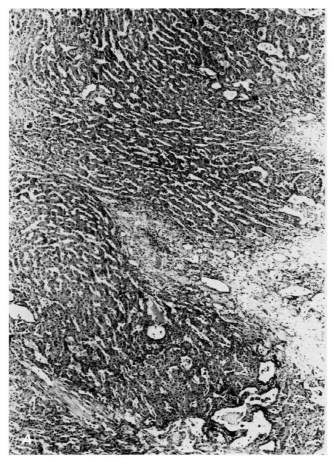

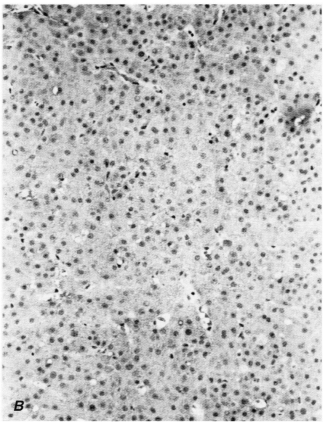

FIGURE 36-1. (*A*) Nodules of regenerating hepatocytes as shown in this photo are often mistaken for hepatic tumors during gross postmortem examination. Biopsy shows the nodules to contain normal hepatocytes, which are usually replicating in a manner that does not restore hepatic architecture. (*B*) Hepatic regeneration and adenomas. Photomicrograph of biopsy specimen shows normal-appearing well-differentiated hepatocytes, no recognizable portal areas or central veins, and no evidence for rapid cell multiplication. This photo does not differentiate hepatic regeneration from adenomas. When adenomas are diffuse and not capsulated, a definitive diagnosis is not possible. Hepatic regeneration can progress to hepatocellular carcinoma; see text on pathogenesis.

normal liver tissue. They usually appear as a well-circumscribed single nodule less than 10 cm in diameter but occasionally will be larger (up to 20 cm in diameter) or multiple. Grossly they are yellow-brown and often relatively soft and friable. They are usually of little clinical significance but, because of their friable nature, can sometimes rupture, resulting in abdominal hemorrhage. Hemorrhage is more likely from larger adenomas. Microscopically they have a well-defined trabecular pattern and the tumor cells resemble normal hepatocytes (Figure 36–1*B*). They show compression of adjacent hepatic parenchyma and are not necessarily encapsulated. Mitotic figures are infrequently seen. Affected liver cells tend to be larger and clearer than normal. Adenomas consist solely of liver cells. There are no portal tracts, and they show a normal reticulin pattern that aids in their differentiation from regenerative nodules and hepatocellular carcinomas.

Diagnosis of hepatocellular adenomas is made by biopsy. Treatment is by surgical excision.

HEPATOCELLULAR CARCINOMAS

Hepatocellular carcinomas are the most common primary hepatic malignancy reported in dogs, accounting for more than 50% of the total number.[1,2,8,9] Greater than 80% of affected dogs are older than 10 years. More males than females have been reported to develop the disease. In contrast to dogs, hepatocellular carcinomas are less common than bile duct neoplasms in cats.[10]

Etiology and Pathogenesis[11,12]

Most current information suggests that environmental factors play an important role in the pathogenesis of hepatocellular carcinomas. Incrimination of environmental factors is based on experimental studies showing that primary hepatic tumors can be induced by toxins. Carcinogens can be naturally occurring substances, such as aflatoxins, produced by toxigenic strains of the fungus *Aspergillus flavus*. This organism is widespread in nature and under appropriate conditions it multiplies and produces the toxin. Of particular concern is the spoilage of prepared animal foods during storage. Aflatoxins can produce acute hepatic lesions as well as causing hepatic neoplasms in experimental animals. The relationship of aflatoxins in animal feeds to naturally occurring hepatic tumors is not known. A number of other hepatic carcinogens are found in nature, although they are not normally available to small animals. They include pyrrolizidine alkaloids, cycasin, and safrole, all of which are found in plants.

Nitrosamines are able to cause hepatic necrosis and primary neoplastic disease in experimental animals. Nitrosamines are produced from nitrites and secondary amines. Nitrites are an important food additive used in meat products. Secondary amines are ubiquitous in nature, being found in both plants and animals. Nitrosamines are easily formed from those two types of chemicals either outside the body or inside the gastrointestinal tract.

A variety of other chemicals and some drugs can be carcinogenic. They include carbon tetrachloride, polycyclic hydrocarbons, aromatic amines, azo dyes, organochloride pesticides, polychlorinated biphenyls, griseofulvin, and tannic acid. Most chemicals are not carcinogenic in their native form; they must first be metabolized by the liver to an active agent. Metabolic conversion is by cytochrome enzymes of the endoplasmic reticulum. They catalyze aromatic ring oxidation, aliphatic hydroxylation, oxidative demethylation, and N-hydroxylation, which results, in most cases, in the formation of highly reactive epoxides. The nucleic acids readily react with these carcinogens. Cell proteins and polysaccharides also form chemical bonds with the carcinogens. The net effect is alteration of cell macromolecules, resulting in injury to cell organelles and structural membranes. The persistence of carcinogens makes repair impossible, and the host responds to the overall loss of hepatic function by cell proliferation. Inhibition of microsomal enzyme activity can prevent primary hepatic neoplasms despite the presence of high levels of carcinogen precursors. Conversely, stimulation of cytochrome enzyme activity, such as by phenobarbital, can increase the risk for other chemicals to be converted to carcinogens.

Other factors influencing the carcinogenic potential of a drug or chemical include state of nutrition and rate of hepatocyte turnover. The exposure of regenerating hepatocytes to a carcinogen is more likely to result in carcinoma than exposure of nonregenerating liver to the same carcinogen.

The development of hepatic neoplasms has been associated with viruses in humans and some animal species. However, it is unknown whether the viruses that cause liver damage in dogs and cats (see Chapter 32) can also induce hepatic neoplasia.

Clinical and Laboratory Findings[2,9,13]

The clinical signs of primary hepatocellular carcinoma are nonspecific and characteristic of hepatic disease in general. The most consistent signs—depression, weakness, anorexia, weight loss, polydipsia, diarrhea, and vomiting—usually do not appear until the disease is advanced. Hepatomegaly is a consistent feature, and clinical signs are often subtle until marked hepatomegaly develops. Abdominal hemorrhage occasionally occurs. Increased bleeding tendency, icterus, and signs of hepatic encephalopathy are seen infrequently. Clinical signs frequently do not become apparent until the core of the tumor becomes necrotic or the tumor encroaches on adjacent organs.

Hematologic changes are inconsistent and nonspecific but can include leukocytosis and anemia. Coagulation profiles are sometimes abnormal (Figure 36–2). Biochemical evaluation of animals with primary hepatocellular carcinomas reveals a pathologic process more severe than suggested by the clinical signs (Figure 36–2). Plasma alanine aminotransferase (ALT) activity increases in about 80% of affected dogs. The mean activity is 4 to 7 times the upper limit of normal. This is in contrast to the slight elevation, if any, of plasma ALT activity that occurs as a result of metastatic hepatic neoplasms (Figure 36–3). The increase in plasma ALT activity that accompanies hepatic carcinoma is most likely due to an increased rate of release of ALT by hepatic carcinoma cells and, in later stages, ischemic necrosis of the tumor core and pressure necrosis of adjacent normal hepatocytes.

Plasma alkaline phosphatase (ALP) activity also increases as a result of hepatocellular carcinoma in dogs. The usual ALP activity in affected dogs ranges from 400 to 800 IU/L,

although increases up to 9500 IU/L can occur. The increased ALP activity found in dogs with hepatocellular carcinomas is most likely due to increased hepatic synthesis and release of alkaline phosphatase by proliferating biliary epithelium. In some dogs, cholestasis may contribute to the increased ALP activity. Alternatively, the marked increases in some dogs may represent the excessive production of abnormal ALP isoenzyme. Such "atypical" alkaline phosphatase is found in some humans with hepatocellular carcinoma.[14]

Plasma albumin concentration usually decreases with hepatocellular carcinoma. The cause for the hypoalbuminemia is uncertain. There is no evidence that hepatic carcinomas reduce hepatic function sufficiently to reduce albumin synthesis. Nor is there evidence for increased loss of albumin through the gastrointestinal tract or kidneys. It is possible that the albumin produced by the neoplastic liver is abnormal, resulting in a shorter half-life.

Increased plasma globulin concentrations have been found in dogs with primary hepatocellular carcinoma.[9] Eighty percent of the globulins in these dogs were gamma-globulins, which are not produced by the liver. The basis for the hypergammaglobulinemia is unknown. Abnormal globulins have been detected in humans with hepatic carcinoma (Table 36–2).[14]

Hypoglycemia in adult dogs is most often caused by insulinoma, but hepatic carcinoma is an important differential diagnosis. Hypoglycemia has been associated with hepatic tumors in humans as well as animals.[13,15–17] The hypoglycemia has been attributed to the tumor's increased utilization of glucose, or to the tumor's production and release of insulin-like activity or other hormones that affect the maintenance of normal blood glucose concentrations. Plasma insulin concentrations are low normal in affected animals. One reported case of hypoglycemia with a hepatoma in a dog showed a normal mobilization of hepatic glycogen following the administration of glucagon.[16] Blood sugar levels remained elevated abnormally long, however, and there was not the normal response of insulin release to cause blood glucose to return to normal. Plasma insulin concentrations during fasting and hyperglycemia were abnormally low. Fasting hypoglycemia associated with normal hepatic glycogen stores indicated that glucagon or other glycogen-mobilizing hormones were not being released. There was evidence for inhibition of the release of both insulin and glucagon in this dog. A possible cause is the release of a somatostatin-like hormone by anaplastic carcinoma cells. In addition, some hypoglycemia-

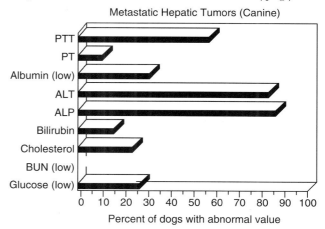

FIGURE 36–2. Comparison of sensitivities for different tests in dogs with hepatocellular carcinoma. Following graphs show distribution of clinical pathology values in dogs with hepatocellular carcinoma. Points on graphs represent 0%, 25%, 50%, 75%, and 100% medians. Normal range is in shaded area. *Figure continued on following page*

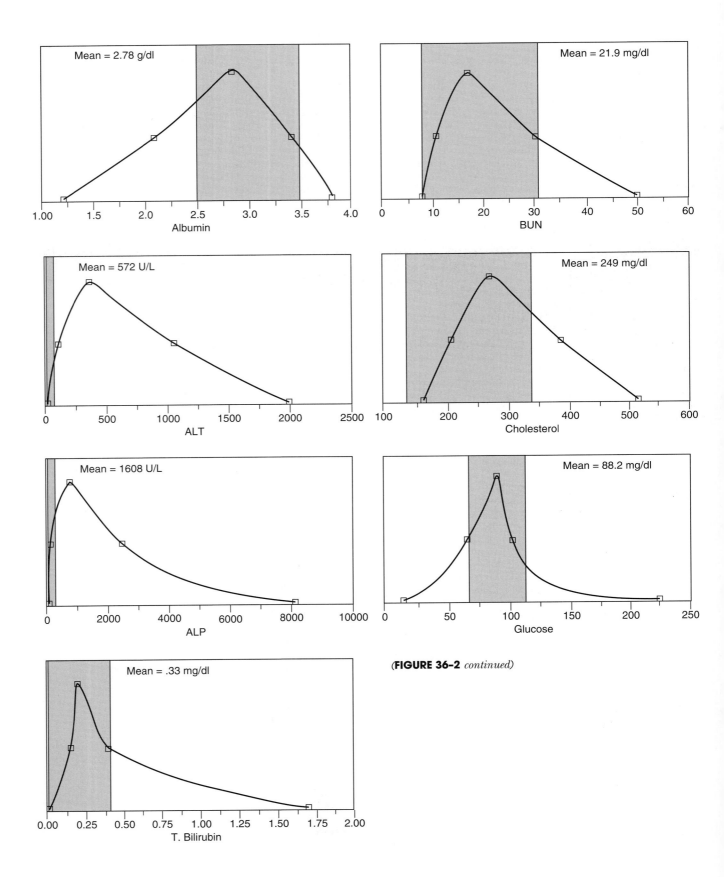

Mean = 2.78 g/dl — Albumin

Mean = 21.9 mg/dl — BUN

Mean = 572 U/L — ALT

Mean = 249 mg/dl — Cholesterol

Mean = 1608 U/L — ALP

Mean = 88.2 mg/dl — Glucose

Mean = .33 mg/dl — T. Bilirubin

(**FIGURE 36–2** *continued*)

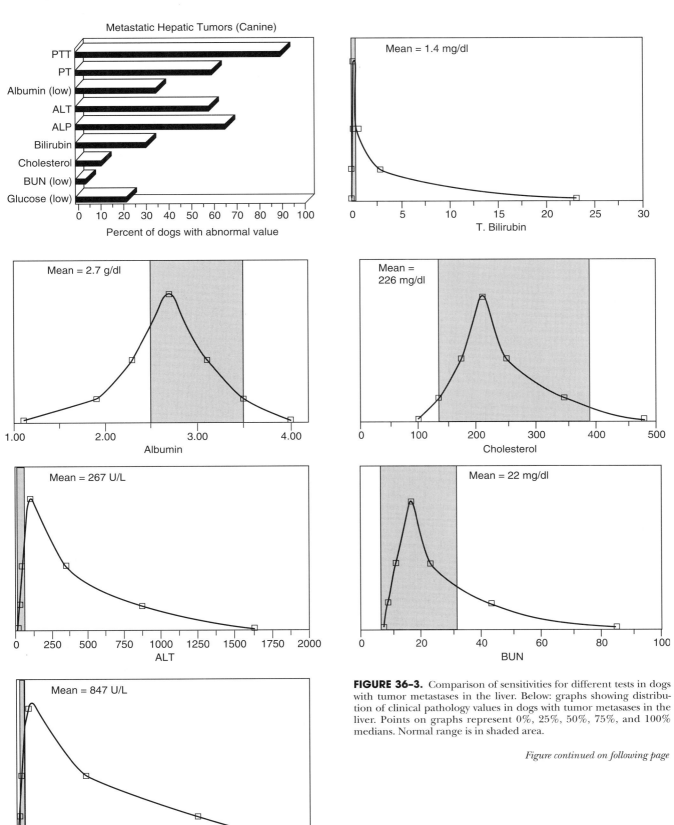

FIGURE 36–3. Comparison of sensitivities for different tests in dogs with tumor metastases in the liver. Below: graphs showing distribution of clinical pathology values in dogs with tumor metasases in the liver. Points on graphs represent 0%, 25%, 50%, 75%, and 100% medians. Normal range is in shaded area.

Figure continued on following page

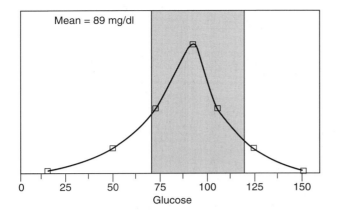

Mean = 89 mg/dl

Glucose

(FIGURE 36–3 *continued)*

inducing liver tumors, previously reported as hepatocellular carcinomas, may have actually been hepatic carcinoids (see later). The latter are able to produce a variety of hormones capable of causing hypoglycemia, such as somatostatin.[14]

Hypercholesterolemia and mild hyperbilirubinemia are found in a few dogs with hepatocellular carcinoma. Liver function tests, such as serum bile acid analysis, are not consistently abnormal in hepatic neoplasia, probably a reflection of the large areas of normal liver tissue that are present in all but advanced neoplasia.

Alpha-fetoprotein is a major plasma protein in the developing fetus. Its function in the fetus is unknown. The protein does not appear in adults unless there is a reversion of hepatocytes to the primitive fetal form. Plasma alpha-fetoprotein levels increase during the development of primary hepatic neoplasms in a variety of species including dogs[18] and measurement of alpha-fetoprotein levels have been used to screen for hepatic cancer in humans. Unfortunately, elevations of total plasma alpha-fetoprotein levels are not specific for cancer and can occur in some human patients with cirrhosis and biliary tract obstruction.[19] Cell injury resulting in regeneration is the common denominator signifying its appearance. High levels of alpha-fetoprotein (> 250 ng/mL) were found in a small number of dogs with hepatocellular carcinoma and cholangiocarcinoma in one study.[18] Although the sensitivity and specificity of total alpha-fetoprotein levels for the diagnosis of these tumors in dogs remains to be determined, this study suggests that detection of high alpha-fetoprotein levels in a dog along with other indicators of liver cancer (e.g., ultrasonographic evidence of a mass in the liver) is strongly suggestive of liver cancer. In humans, the specificity of the diagnosis of hepatic carcinoma can be improved by the measurement of more specific molecular variants of alpha-fetoprotein.[6] The role of these alpha-fetoprotein variants in the diagnosis of hepatic neoplasia in dogs and cats has yet to be examined.

Diagnostic Imaging Findings

Survey radiographs are only abnormal once hepatic carcinoma is advanced. Radiographs can reveal an asymmetrically enlarged liver, an irregular hepatic border, or caudal and lateral displacement of the stomach. Ultrasonography can detect hepatic carcinoma at an earlier stage than radiography, but the changes in echogenicity observed are not pathognomonic for carcinoma and the diagnosis ultimately depends on biopsy.

Diagnosis

Diagnosis of liver cancer can be made only by liver biopsy. Asymmetric enlargements of the liver detected on physical examination or radiography should not be assumed to be neoplastic until granulomas, hematomas, and hepatic cysts have been ruled out. Similarly, laboratory evaluation does not distinguish hepatocellular carcinoma from hepatic necrosis, chronic hepatitis, or any of the many other hepatic problems that can cause abnormal serum biochemical findings.

Pathology Findings

Hepatocellular carcinoma may develop as a discrete mass (61%) or as multiple nodules (29%) (Figure 36–4). Alternatively, the carcinoma may diffusely infiltrate the liver (10%).[13] The massive form of the disease has the lowest rate of metastasis. Metastasis of hepatocellular carcinoma usually occurs to other liver lobes, hepatic lymph nodes, lung, and peritoneum. Neoplastic hepatic tissue varies in color from almost white to the color of normal liver. Large carcinomas are readily identifiable at neocropsy. They frequently develop a necrotic core because they outdistance their blood supply. The nodular form of the disease is easily confused with regenerative nodules on gross examination. Diffuse hepatocellular carcinoma causes hepatomegaly, and the neoplastic process is not identified until the tissue is examined microscopically.

The histologic appearance of hepatocellular carcinomas ranges from well-differentiated cells that closely resemble normal hepatocytes to those that are so anaplastic they are barely recognizable as being of hepatocellular origin (Figure 36–4). On occasion, well-differentiated hepatocellular carcinoma cells develop vacuolation and are referred to as "clear

Table 36–2

METABOLIC ABNORMALITIES IN HUMANS WITH HEPATOCELLULAR CARCINOMA

Serum Protein Abnormalities
 Fetoprotein
 Abnormal globulin
 Increased hepatoglobin
 Increased ceruloplasmin
 Increased alpha-1-antitrypsin
 Aberrant alkaline phosphatase
 Abnormal isoferritins
 Increased levels of chorionic gonadotrophins
 Increased levels of chorionic somatotrophins
Hematologic Abnormalities
 Dysfibrinogenemias, cryofibrinogenemia
 Antifibrinolysis
 Plasmacytosis
 Hemolytic processes
 Erythrocytosis
Lipid Abnormalities
 Hypercholesterolemia
 Hypertriglyceridemia
Other Abnormal Serum Factors
 Porphyria
 Cystathioninuria
 Ethanolaminuria
Functional and Hormone-like Abnormalities
 Hypoglycemia
 Pseudohyperparathyroidism
 Precocious Puberty
 Gynecomastia
 Hypertrophic pulmonary osteoarthropathy

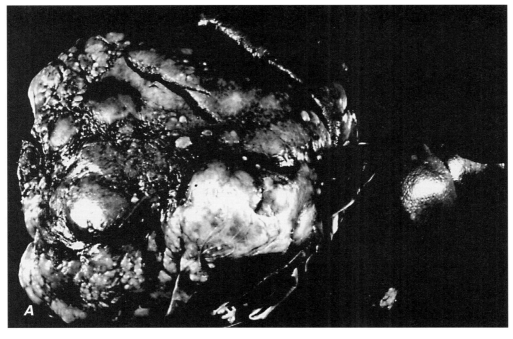

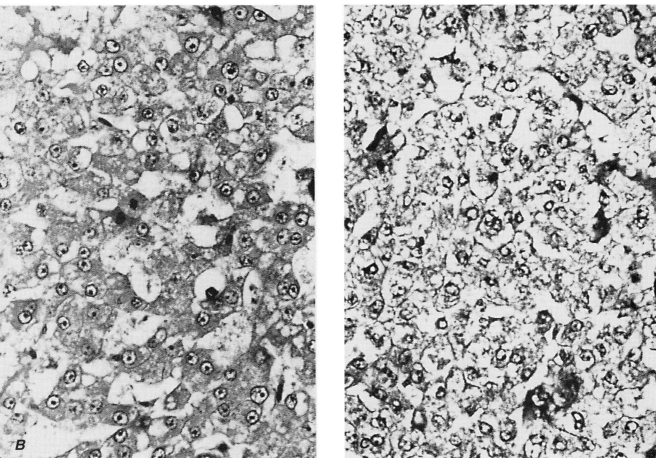

FIGURE 36–4. (*A*) Gross pathologic specimen of hepatocellular carcinoma in a dog. Note the marked thickening of the affected lobe. (*B*) Hepatocellular carcinoma. Mitotic figure is seen in center of photo. Increased rate of cell division is also suggested by many large nuclei (in hepatocytes) that contain dark-staining chromatin. (*C*) Hepatocellular carcinoma. Hepatocytes are well differentiated and show many clear cells, suggesting glycogen or lipid accumulation. Normal architecture is noticeably absent. Mitotic figures are not seen. (*D*) Hepatocellular carcinoma. Hepatocytes are less well differentiated than in (*C*). Cells are pleomorphic with more basophilic-staining cytoplasm and dark-staining nuclei (suggesting greater activity). (*E*) Hepatocellular carcinoma. Poorly differentiated cells often make it difficult to identify their origin. (*F*) Hepatocellular carcinoma. Well-differentiated cells are arranged predominantly in an acinar pattern. Excessive fibrous tissue was seen in other sections of this biopsy. (*G*) Hepatocellular carcinoma. Well-differentiated cells are arranged in a trabecular pattern in this biopsy specimen.

Figure continued on following page

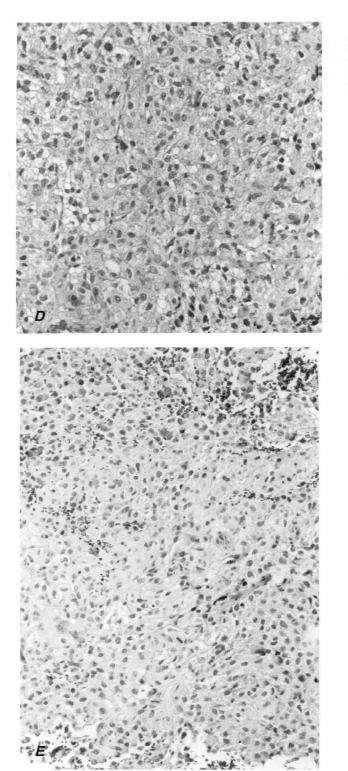

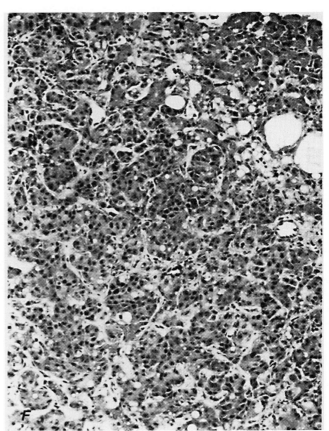

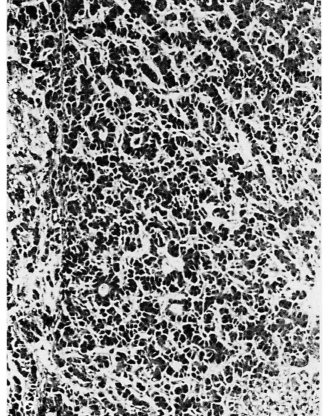

(**FIGURE 36-4** *continued*)

cells" (Figure 36-4). In humans, monoclonal antibodies have been developed that give reasonably specific staining of malignant liver tissue.[20] These are useful when the identification of the tumor is difficult by regular histologic procedures.

Hepatocellular carcinoma cells can form a number of different histologic patterns. In one pattern, the hepatocytes form trabeculi comprised of well-differentiated carcinoma cells. The trabeculi appear normal with the exception that they are several cells thick in contrast to the single cell thickness of normal trabeculi. In addition, Kupffer cells are not seen and sinusoids may not be evident because of compression from the thickened plates. In a second histologic pattern, the carcinoma cells are arranged into acinus-like or gland-like structures. The acinus lumen usually contains protein-like material that may stain PAS positive. In a third pattern, the carcinoma appears to be compact, solid, or scirrhous, growing in solid sheets without any sinusoids or fibrous tissue evident. In some cases, metastatic carcinoma can be difficult to differentiate from primary hepatocellular carcinoma. In addition, hepatic carcinoids can be difficult to differentiate from hepatocellular carcinoma unless silver stains are used.

Management

Most hepatocellular carcinomas are not recognized until they have reached an advanced stage, whereupon clinical signs begin to appear and metastasis is common. In one case study, less than 30% of surgically explored dogs with hepatocellular adenomas and carcinomas had resectable tumors.[21] If a single lobe of the liver is involved, surgical removal is possible and often results in survival times of several years or more.[21]

When the neoplastic involvement is diffuse and extensive, little can be done to remove the diseased tissue and the prognosis is poor. In this situation, hepatic dearterialization may provide a degree of palliation because hepatic neoplasms derive most of the blood supply from the hepatic arterial supply rather than the portal venous system. Hepatic dearterialization has been reported to be well tolerated in dogs.[22] As yet, chemotherapy has little documented value in hepatocellular carcinoma in animals. Human experience suggests that best results are obtained with arterial infusion of chemotherapeutics rather than intravenous administration.[6] Percutaneous ethanol injection is an alternative to multiple lobectomy for the treatment of diffuse nodular neoplastic disease of the liver. Small quantities of ethanol are injected in and around the nodules.[6] The technique has been used successfully in humans.

HEPATIC CARCINOIDS

Hepatic carcinoids are neoplasms originating from amine precursor uptake and decarboxylation (APUD) cells.[23] Tumors derived from these cells produce and release a number of biogenic amines and peptide hormones normally found in the gastrointestinal tract, such as somatostatin.[14] Hepatic carcinoids closely resemble hepatocellular carcinoma but can be differentiated with special stains.[23] Until recently, carcinoids were believed to be rare, but one survey showed they account for 14% of primary hepatic neoplasms in dogs.[23] They were found most often in dogs less than 10 years of age with a mean of 8 years. They are highly malignant and spread rapidly to the hepatic lymph nodes and peritoneum. Hepatic carcinoids are rare in cats, but one report has been recently published.[24]

BILE DUCT ADENOMAS AND ADENOCARCINOMAS

Bile duct adenocarcinomas account for 22% to 35% of all primary hepatic neoplasms in dogs.[1,2,25] Although bile duct adenocarcinomas are less common than hepatocellular carcinomas in dogs, they are more malignant and show a higher frequency of metastasis (88%). In cats, bile duct adenomas are the most common nonhematopoietic hepatic neoplasm followed by bile duct adenocarcinomas.[10,24] Collectively, bile duct adenomas and adenocarcinomas account for approximately 75% of nonhematopoietic hepatic neoplasms in cats.[10] Tumors may originate from any area of the biliary tract including intrahepatic biliary ducts, extrahepatic biliary ducts, and gall bladder.

In both dogs and cats, most bile duct adenocarcinomas are seen in animals over 10 years of age. The predominant clinical signs of the disease are anorexia, lethargy, weight loss, vomiting, depression, ascites, and dyspnea. Hepatomegaly and icterus are seen in a few animals. The clinical pathology for dogs with bile duct adenocarcinoma is similar to that for hepatocellular carcinoma. The most consistent abnormalities are increased activities of ALP (69%) and ALT (54%), decreased albumin, and increased bilirubin (31%). In cats with bile duct neoplasia, the most frequent laboratory abnormalities are uremia and hyperbilirubinemia.[10]

In an analogous manner to hepatocellular carcinomas, intrahepatic bile duct adenocarcinomas are classified as massive, nodular, or diffuse lesions (Figure 36–5). Histologically, intrahepatic bile duct adenocarcinomas can be tubular carcinomas or bile cystadenocarcinomas (Figure 36–5). The tubular or cholangiocarcinomas consist of many tubular structures lined with cuboidal or columnar cells and dissected by diffuse fibrous stroma. Bile duct adencarcinomas are different from primary hepatocellular carcinomas in that they result in the formation of more fibrous stroma. When the fine structure of these tumors is examined, the finding of microvilli on the luminal border of the cells clearly indicates their origin. Mucus secretion may be evident in some. Some carcinoma cells may be poorly differentiated. Cystadencarcinomas are characterized by many cysts lined with single or multiple layers of epithelial cells. In some, papillary structures lined with cuboidal or columnar epithelium, arranged as in an acinus with papillary infolding, fill the cystic spaces. Metastatic adenocarcinomas and carcinoids may be difficult to differentiate from bile duct adenocarcinomas.

No attempt has been made to treat bile duct adenocarcinomas. Affected patients usually die shortly after diagnosis.

HEPATIC HEMANGIOSARCOMA

Hemangiosarcomas often metastasize to the liver from primary sites in other organs such as the heart and spleen. Occasionally the tumor is reported to originate in the liver.[3] Often affected animals have no clinical signs until the tumor ruptures and causes massive abdominal hemorrhage. Because blood can be readily absorbed from the abdomen, affected dogs may show only transient evidence of weakness before recovering. Clinical pathologic abnormalities are few (Figure 36–6). The most consistent finding is reduced hematocrit from the bleeding. The tumor usually diffusely infiltrates the liver, and no successful treatment is currently available.

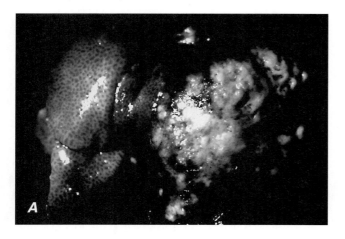

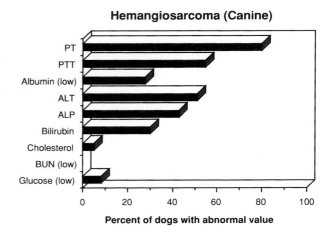

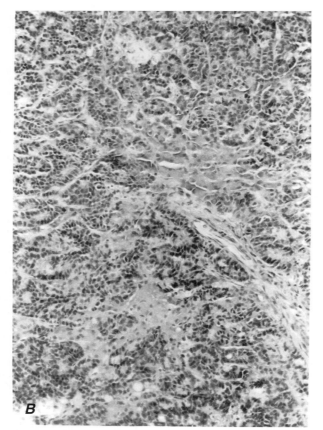

FIGURE 36-5. (*A*) Gross specimen of bile duct carcinoma in a cat. (*B*) Cholangiocarcinoma. Acini are formed but are not well defined, making the tumor moderately differentiated. Carcinoma involves most of this biopsy specimen, leaving only a few recognizable cords of hepatocytes.

FIGURE 36-6. Comparison of sensitivities for different tests in dogs with hemangiosarcoma in the liver. Following graphs show distribution of clinical pathology values in dogs with hemangiosarcoma in the liver. Points on graphs represent 0%, 25%, 50%, 75%, and 100% medians. Normal range is in shaded area.

HEPATIC LYMPHOSARCOMA

Hepatic lymphosarcoma may occur as a component of multicentric lymphoma or as an apparently primary hepatic disease (Figure 36–7). The disorder occurs in both cats and dogs but is most common in cats. The clinical signs are those of hepatic dysfunction. Hepatomegaly is usually present and is often symmetric. The ultrasonographic appearance of the disease is variable and ranges from mild general-ized hyperechogenicity or hypoechogenicity to multifocal hypoechogenicity. Diagnosis is usually made by needle aspiration or biopsy of the liver. The chemotherapy protocols used for multicentric lymphoma usually produce a short period of remission of hepatic lymphoma. The prognosis is guarded.

METASTATIC NEOPLASIA[8,9,26]

Necropsies of dogs and cats indicate that the liver is frequently invaded by metastatic neoplasia (31% to 37% of all

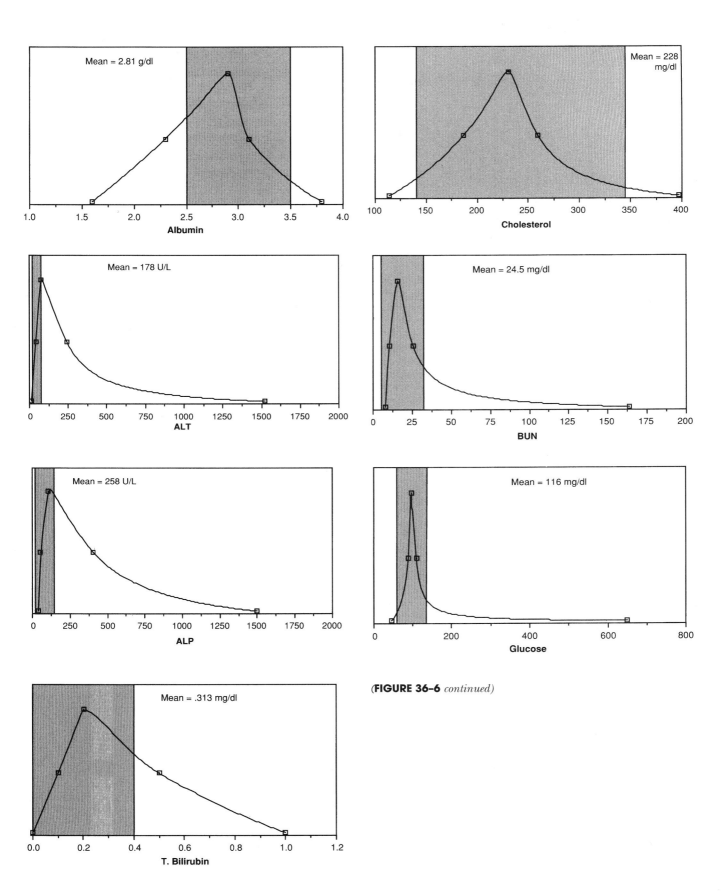

(**FIGURE 36–6** *continued*)

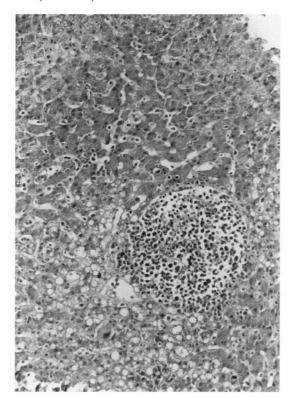

FIGURE 36-7. Hepatic lymphosarcoma. Biopsy of dog's liver showing abnormal clusters of lymphocytes.

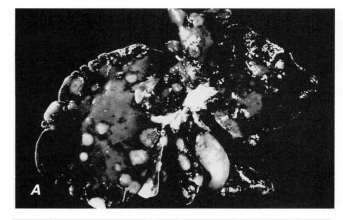

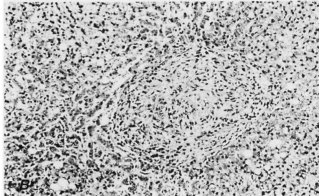

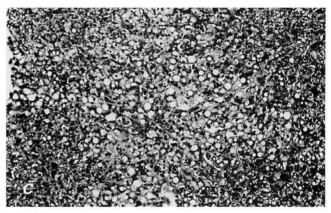

FIGURE 36-8. (*A*) Fibrosarcoma metastases in the liver of a dog. (*B*) Metastasis of gastric carcinoma to the liver is shown by large cluster of neoplastic cells in center of biopsy specimen. Such lesions are focal and can be missed on blind needle biopsy. (*C*) Hepatic changes with myeloproliferative disease. Biopsy shows fatty changes, atrophy of hepatic cords, and extramedullary hematopoiesis.

malignancies have metastases in the liver). The liver can be involved diffusely without developing the changes consistently seen in animals with primary hepatocellular carcinomas (Figure 36–8). The clinical signs seen are frequently nonspecific and include polydipsia, anorexia, weight loss, and vomiting. Hepatomegaly is a variable finding that is reported in some dogs with lymphosarcoma (37%), leukemias (44%), pancreatic carcinomas (57%), hemangiosarcomas (8%), and other carcinomas or sarcomas (20%).[2] Abdominal pain is reported in fewer than one-third of all dogs.

Metastatic neoplasia less frequently causes serum biochemical abnormalities than do primary hepatic tumors (Figure 36–3). Plasma ALT activities are usually normal to mildly elevated (see section on hepatic carcinoma). Plasma ALP activities are usually normal or mildly to moderately elevated, similar to the increases seen with hepatocellular carcinomas. Hyperbilirubinemia is infrequently seen.

Ultrasonographic examination of the liver has greatly facilitated the diagnosis of hepatic metastatic neoplasia.[27] Focal variations in echogenicity are suggestive of multifocal neoplastic disease but must be carefully differentiated from nodular hyperplasia. Diffuse hyperechogenicity has been reported as a feature of hepatic lymphosarcoma.[28] Blind biopsy or fine needle aspiration of the liver is a poorly sensitive technique for diagnosing multifocal hepatic cancer. With the advent of ultrasound-guided biopsy or fine needle aspiration, tissue samples from even small focal lesions can now be readily and safely obtained. In the absence of ultrasound examination, diagnosis of metastatic hepatic neoplasia may require surgical biopsy of the liver (Figure 36–8).

HAMARTOMAS

Angiomatous hamartomas are congenital malformations characterized by vascular proliferations that resemble hemangiomas grossly and microscopically. They are considered to be a tumor-like lesion. Hamartomas appear in very young animals and cause clinical signs similar to those seen in older animals with hepatic masses.[29]

REFERENCES

1. Patnaik AK, Hurvitz AI, Lieberman PH. Canine hepatic neoplasms: A clinicopathologic study. Vet Pathol 17:553–564, 1980.
2. Trigo FJ, Thompson H, Breeze RG, et al. The pathology of liver tumors in the dog. J Comp Path 92:21–39, 1982.
3. Theilen GH, Madewell BR. Veterinary Cancer Medicine. Lea and Febiger, Philadelphia, 34, 1987.
4. Engle GC, Brodey RS. A retrospective study of 395 feline neoplasms. J Am Anim Hosp Assoc 5:21–31, 1969.
5. Schmidt RE, Langham RF. A survey of feline neoplasms. J Am Vet Med Assoc 151:1325–1328, 1967.
6. Franco D, Vons C. Primary and secondary liver tumors. C Opin G 10:337–343, 1994.
7. Stowater JL, Lamb CR, Schelling SH. Ultrasonographic features of canine hepatic nodular hyperplasia. Vet Radiol 31:268–272, 1990.
8. Magne ML, Withrow SJ. Hepatic neoplasia. Vet Clin N Am Sm Anim Pract 15:243–256, 1985.
9. Strombeck DR. Clinicopathologic features of primary and metastatic neoplastic disease of the liver in dogs. J Am Med Assoc 173:267–269, 1978.
10. Post G, Patnaik AK. Nonhematopoietic hepatic neoplasms cats: 21 cases (1983–1988). J Am Vet Med Assoc 201:1080–1082, 1992.
11. Farber E, Sarma DSR, Rajalakshimi S, et al. Liver carcinogenesis: A unifying hypothesis. In: Becker FF (ed) The Liver: Normal and Abnormal Function. Part B. The Biochemistry of Disease. Vol. 5. Marcel Dekker, New York, 755–771, 1975.
12. MacSween RNM, Anthony PP, Scheuer PJ. Tumours and tumour-like lesions of the liver and biliary tract. In: Pathology of the Liver. Churchill Livingstone, New York, 574–637, 1987.
13. Patnaik AK, Hurvitz AI, Liebermann PH, et al. Canine hepatocellular carcinoma. Vet Pathol 18:427–438, 1981.
14. Edmundson HA, Craig JR. Neoplasms of the liver. In: Schiff L, Schiff ER (eds) Diseases of the Liver. JB Lippincott, Philadelphia, 1109–1158, 1987.
15. Marks IJ, Steinke J, Podolsky S, et al. Hypoglycemia associated with neoplasia. Am NY Acad Sci 230:147–160, 1974.
16. Strombeck DR, Krum S, Meyer D, et al. Hypoglycemia and hypoinsulinemia associated with hepatoma in a dog. J Am Vet Med Assoc 169:811–812, 1976.
17. Leifer CE, Peterson ME, Matus RE, et al. Hypoglycemia associated with nonislet cell tumor in 13 dogs. J Am Vet Med Assoc 186:53–55, 1985.
18. Lowseth LA, Gillet NA, Chong IY, et al. Detection of serum alpha-fetoprotein in dogs with hepatic tumors. J Am Vet Med Assoc 199:735–741, 1991.
19. Bloomer JR, Waldman RA, McIntire KR, et al. Alpha-fetoprotein in nonneoplastic hepatic disorders. J Am Med Assoc 233:38–41, 1975.
20. Lefkowitch JH. Pathology of the liver. C Opin G 10:249–256, 1994.
21. Kosovsky JE, Manfra-Marretta S, Matthiesen DT, et al. Results of partial hepatectomy in 18 dogs with hepatocellular carcinoma. J Am Anim Hosp Assoc 25:203–206, 1989.
22. Gunn C, Gourley IM, Koblik PD. Hepatic dearterialization in the dog. Am J Vet Res 47:170–175, 1986.
23. Patnaik AK, Liebermann PH, Hurvitz AI, et al. Canine hepatic carcinoids. Vet Pathol 18:445–453, 1981.
24. Patnaik AK. A morphologic and immunocytochemical study of hepatic neoplasms in cats. Vet Pathol 29:405–415, 1992.
25. Patnaik AK, Hurvitz AL, Lieberman PH, et al. Canine bile duct carcinoma. Vet Pathol 18:439–444, 1981.
26. McConnell MF, Lumsden JH. Biochemical evaluation of metastatic liver disease in the dog. J Am Anim Hosp Assoc 19:173–178, 1983.
27. Cartee RE. Diagnostic real time ultrasonography of the liver of the dog and cat. J Am Anim Hosp Assoc 17:731–737, 1981.
28. Voros K, Vrabely T, Papp L, et al. Correlation of ultrasonographic and pathomorphological findings in canine diseases. J Anim Pract 32:627–634, 1991.
29. Castellano MC, Idiart JR, Ortega CF, et al. Multiple hepatic angiomatous hamartomas in a puppy. Canine Pract 13:30–33, 1986.

37 Diseases of the Gallbladder and Biliary Tree

SHARON A. CENTER

INTRODUCTION

Patients are evaluated for disease of the biliary system when hyperbilirubinemia or overt jaundice are recognized and when enzyme changes suggest a primarily cholestatic lesion. The incidence of disorders restricted to the gallbladder and biliary tree is low compared to the many parenchymal hepatic conditions. Although cholelithiasis has been amply reported in the dog and cat, until recently it was considered an uncommon diagnosis. This disease is now being diagnosed more frequently due to use of abdominal ultrasonography as a routine investigative procedure in clinical practice. Extrahepatic bile duct obstruction is a well-recognized condition because of its association with pancreatitis or biliary tract neoplasia. The syndrome of cholangitis/cholangiohepatitis is one of the most common diffuse hepatobiliary disorders seen in the cat; in three large referral-based hospital populations, this syndrome has been responsible for 20% to 30% of jaundice in cats.

FUNCTIONAL ANATOMY OF THE BILIARY SYSTEM

The biliary system is comprised of gallbladder, cystic duct, common bile duct, hepatic ducts, segmental, septal, and interlobular bile ducts, bile ductules, and hepatic canaliculi, as illustrated in Figure 29–10. Bile ductules are a synonym for cholangioles, the smallest branches of the biliary system lined by bile duct epithelium and having a basement membrane. These lack an individual capillary supply and conduct bile received from canaliculi. They terminate at the (interlobular) bile ducts, which are the smallest branches of the intrahepatic biliary tree. These are accompanied by branches of the hepatic artery and portal vein and are lined by cuboidal epithelium. Septal bile ducts are the small branches of the intrahepatic biliary system that begin with the union of two or more interlobular bile ducts. These eventually fuse into segmental bile ducts, which are medium-sized branches of the intrahepatic biliary system located at the main drainage areas of the liver lobes. These are distinguished only on the basis of their anatomic location. Segmental bile ducts transport bile to the hepatic bile ducts. In the dog, hepatic ducts enter the cystic duct and common bile duct separately. The cystic duct extends from the neck of the gallbladder to its junction with

the first hepatic duct. Distal to this, it continues to the duodenum, still receiving hepatic ducts as it becomes the common bile duct. Communication of the common bile duct with the duodenum is anatomically unique in the dog and cat. In a medium-sized dog, the common bile duct is approximately 5 cm long and 2.5 mm in diameter.[1] It empties into the duodenum 1.5 to 6.0 cm distal to the pylorus at the major duodenal papilla after coursing intramurally for approximately 2 cm.[1] In the dog, the common bile duct opens near the smaller of two pancreatic ducts (the pancreatic duct). The larger duct is the accessory pancreatic duct; this opens into the duodenum a few centimeters caudal to the common bile duct on the minor duodenal papilla. In the cat, the common bile duct and the pancreatic duct are usually fused prior to entrance in the duodenal papilla (Figure 37–1). In some cats the major pancreatic duct opens separately but immediately adjacent to the common bile duct. Approximately 2 cm caudal to the major duodenal papilla, the accessory pancreatic duct enters the duodenum at the minor duodenal papilla. This duct is sometimes absent in the cat. Although the pancreas in dogs and cats is almost always drained by two ducts, a great deal of variation occurs. Pancreatic and biliary disease (extrahepatic and intrahepatic) are commonly associated in the cat, seemingly as a result of the anatomic fusion of the pancreatic and common bile ducts. Despite the separation of these systems in the dog, acute and chronic pancreatitis also commonly initiate biliary tract disease. This is usually associated with extra-

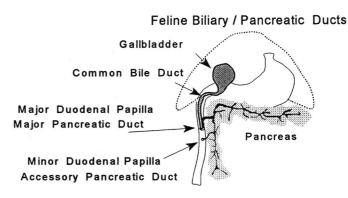

FIGURE 37-1. Normal anatomy of the common bile duct and pancreatic duct in the cat.

hepatic biliary obstruction (partial or complete) as a result of regional inflammation and duodenitis.

The circulation to the gallbladder and common bile ducts is derived from the left branch of the proper hepatic artery.[1] This circulation must be preserved when decompressive biliary surgery is performed. Injury to this vessel can result in necrotizing cholecystitis and bile peritonitis within 48 to 72 hours.

The gallbladder is positioned between the quadrate and right medial lobes of the liver on its visceral surface. It may not be readily apparent on gross inspection unless distended, as it normally lies deep between liver lobes. The location of the gallbladder can be appreciated by review of radiographs of animals with gallbladders containing gas or mineralized opacities (see Figure 8–41). The gallbladder provides four distinct functions: reservoir, absorptive, secretory, and motor.[2] It serves as a bile reservoir and under neuroendocrine influence synchronizes its contraction and bile ejection with the digestive interval. The gallbladder modifies bile through reabsorption of isotonic fluid (water absorption is coupled to active transport of sodium and chloride across the gallbladder mucosa) and secretion of glycoproteins and H^+ ions. In dogs, bile has a pH more than 6.0; acidification is accomplished through H^+ secretion rather than HCO_3^- reabsorption.[3] More than 90% of the biliary solids are comprised of bile acids. In concentrated bile, total bile salt concentration may exceed 300 mM/L, 10^5-fold greater than the serum bile acid concentrations. The bile salts are kept in solution by incorporation into micelles. These maintain a biliary isosmotic balance with plasma. The gallbladder resorbs more than 50% of the calcium in bile. This maintains free Ca^+ at a relatively low concentration and protects against cholelith precipitation. Lipid solubility is the major determinant of absorption of organic compounds in the gallbladder. Conjugation of bilirubin, steroid hormones, biliary contrast media, and bile acids increases their water solubility, thereby inhibiting their absorption by the gallbladder epithelium.[4] Consequently, concentrated gallbladder bile contains large amounts of conjugated bile acids and bilirubin and lesser quantities of lipid soluble cholesterol. Increased absorption of conjugated bile acids and cholecystographic contrast agents can occur in the presence of gallbladder inflammation or sepsis as a result of deconjugation reactions. This leads to greater bile saturation with cholesterol and greater bile lithogenicity. This also contributes to the inability to visualize the inflamed and/or infected gallbladder during cholecystography.

Filling of the gallbladder with bile occurs continuously. Bile flow in the biliary tree is driven by hepatic secretion and gallbladder contraction. This is a low-pressure, low-flow system. The distribution of bile within the common and cystic bile ducts is determined by the relative resistances of the cystic duct and the sphincter of Oddi. The sphincter of Oddi is the functional sphincter located at the terminal portion of the common bile duct. The resistance in the cystic duct and sphincter have both active and passive components. The sphincter of Oddi exhibits both tonic and rhythmic contractions. The rhythmic contractions regulate duodenal bile flow into spurts rather than a continuous stream. The sphincter functions as a one-way valve and can regulate pressure within the biliary system. It provides resistance against retrograde passage of duodenal contents or pancreatic secretions into the biliary tree. During fasting, 75% of hepatic bile enters the gallbladder; the remainder flows into the common bile duct and episodically enters the duodenum. After a meal, a sustained gallbladder contraction empties 50% or more of its bile within 30 minutes.[5] Emptying of the gallbladder is slow and has been estimated at 2% per minute. Consequently, only small-pressure gradients develop within the ductal sys-

tem. Large-pressure changes, such as those resulting from mechanical distension and inflammation of the extrahepatic biliary tree, can each stimulate mechanoreceptors and pain receptors causing right cranial abdominal pain or ill-defined discomfort. In humans, abdominal discomfort can occur with sphincter dysmotility disturbances, cholelithiasis, septic or nonseptic inflammation, and certain drugs (e.g., meperidine given IV). Hyperkinesia or hypokinesia of the gallbladder in response to cholecystokinin, and sphincter of Oddi stenosis, spasm, dyskinesia, and paradoxical response to cholecystokinin have been defined as clinical problems in humans with chronic intermittent epigastric pain. These disorders have not been characterized in dogs or cats. In humans, biliary pain is severe and can be difficult to distinguish from esophageal pain and anginal pain due to coronary artery spasm.[5] We remain unaware of such discomfort in veterinary patients, although occasionally animals with choleliths are examined because of episodic abdominal discomfort, vomiting, and anorexia.

Cholecystokinin, a hormone secreted by the duodenal mucosa, is the principal hormone that stimulates gallbladder contraction.[6] It is one of the most potent cholagogues recognized. Cholagogues are substances that stimulate bile flow from the biliary system into the duodenum. Its choleretic effects are due in part to stimulation of release of glucagon and insulin.[7] It also is known to inhibit the phasic contractions of the sphincter of Oddi, an effect favoring discharge of bile into the duodenum. Other substances, such as motilin, and the cholinergic pathways also appear to be important in stimulation of gallbladder evacuation. As expected, atropine and somatostatin decrease gallbladder evacuation.

In health, cholecystokinin release is stimulated by ingestion of food containing fat and protein; this subsequently invokes gallbladder contraction and the alimentary provision of bile acids for digestive purposes. Cholecystectomy, ileal resection, and administration of cholestyramine (an anion exchange resin that binds enteric bile acids) each increases cholecystokinin release.[8]

Spontaneous contraction of the gallbladder is known to occur in the interdigestive interval and at night.[9–12] This results in a continued but variable availability of bile acids within the alimentary canal during the fasting interval. This spontaneous gallbladder contraction is the reason that serum bile acid values may be higher after a 12 hour fast than during a 2 hour postprandial interval.

EVALUATION OF THE PATIENT WITH BILIARY TRACT DISEASE

A general diagnostic approach for disorders of the biliary tree is presented in Figure 37–2. Initial evaluation of these patients is usually pursued due to the presence of jaundice or hyperbilirubinemia. If a septic process is involved, fever and a neutrophilic leukocytosis with a left shift is often found. Target cells and poikilocytes are common, as with other hepatobiliary disorders. Animals with complete bile duct occlusion, necrotizing cholecystitis, and septic bile peritonitis are the most symptomatic. Patients with extrahepatic bile duct obstruction are overtly jaundiced, have lost weight, and are vaguely ill. Patients with necrotizing cholecystitis or septic bile peritonitis may present with fever, anorexia, diffuse abdominal pain, and/or shock. Clinical signs most common for each disease entity are discussed separately in this chapter.

Serum biochemical profiles usually indicate cholestasis: increased serum transaminases, ALP and GGT activities, and

Diagnostic Evaluation of Biliary Tract Disorders

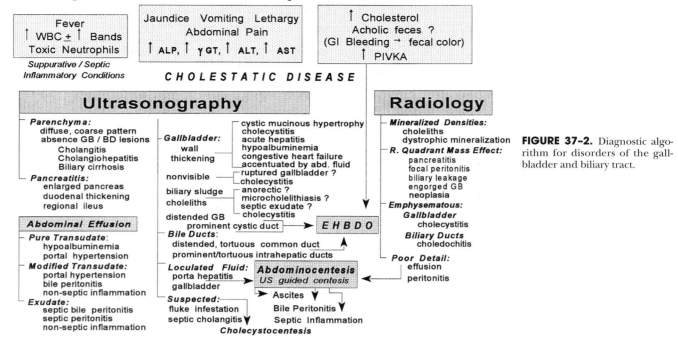

FIGURE 37-2. Diagnostic algorithm for disorders of the gallbladder and biliary tract.

hyperbilirubinemia. Animals with an obstructed bile duct usually become hypercholesterolemic. The detection of acholic stools in an overtly jaundiced animal indicates a high likelihood of extrahepatic bile duct occlusion. Abdominal pain associated with peritoneal effusion containing a disproportionately high bilirubin concentration suggests a ruptured biliary tree often associated with cholecystitis or choledochitis. If abdominal fluid is detected, abdominocentesis and fluid evaluation should be promptly completed. Bile peritonitis with or without sepsis requires immediate surgical attention. Blood cultures may expedite confirmation of associated septicemia.

Radiography

Abdominal radiographs are usually of limited assistance in these patients. Occasionally information having diagnostic value is disclosed. Mineralized densities within the biliary structures can be associated with chronic cholangiohepatitis (dystrophic mineralization) or cholelithiasis (Figures 8–41, 37–3, and 37–4A and B). Approximately 50% of choleliths in dogs and cats are mineralized and thus can be detected by survey radiography. A mass in the region of the gallbladder in patients with major bile duct obstruction may represent an engorged gallbladder, pancreatitis, neoplasia, or focal peritonitis associated with ruptured biliary structures. An appearance of diffuse abdominal effusion could lead to rapid diagnosis of bile peritonitis. Gas within the biliary structures or hepatic parenchyma indicates the presence of emphysematous cholecystitis, choledochitis, or an abscess and warrants prompt surgical and antimicrobial therapy (Figure 37–5).

Cholecystography

Contrast radiographic imaging of the biliary tree is not commonly done in small animals because abdominal ultrasonography usually provides more diagnostic information. A number of studies with different contrast agents have been conducted in dogs and cats. Successful dosages and time intervals for proper exposure of radiographs are provided in Table 37–1.[12–19] Cholecystography can be done with iodinated contrast agents given either by mouth or intravenously. These studies are influenced by the numerous variables. At its best, cholecystography can disclose stones, polyps, or sludge in the gallbladder.

Abdominal Ultrasonography

Ultrasonography is a better method for appraisal of the extrahepatic biliary structures than survey or contrast radiography. The distension and wall thickness of components of the biliary system can be defined. The gallbladder is easily

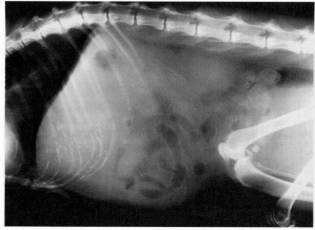

FIGURE 37-3. Radiographic appearance of microlithiasis in a cat with chronic cholangiohepatitis.

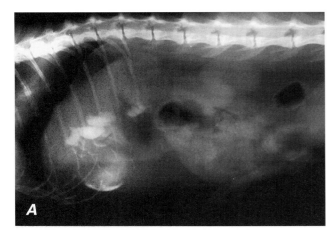

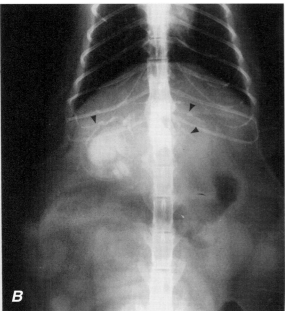

FIGURE 37-4. (*A*) Lateral abdominal radiograph showing radio-dense choleliths and a "porcelain" gallbladder in a cat that intermittently showed signs consistent with epigastric pain and pancreatitis. Serum biochemical parameters suggested cholangitis/cholangiohepatitis. (Courtesy Dr. Ann Chiapella): (*B*) Dorsoventral abdominal radiograph in a different cat from that in (*A*), showing radiopaque densities in the gallbladder and outlining the segmental and lobar bile ducts (arrows). (Courtesy Dr. N. Freeborough)

identified as an oval anechoic structure between the quadrate and right medial liver lobes.[20-22] When healthy, the wall of the gallbladder is poorly visualized. The common bile duct, cystic duct, hepatic ducts, and intrahepatic biliary system can also be difficult to visualize.

When thickening of the gallbladder wall is observed, consideration of several diverse conditions is necessary. These include a partially empty gallbladder with a relaxed wall, the presence of cholecystitis or hepatitis, or wall edema due to portal hypertension, hypoalbuminemia, or congestive heart failure[20] (Figure 37-6). The presence of ascites may also make the gallbladder wall become more apparent (spurious wall thickening). The size of the gallbladder varies depending on whether the patient has recently eaten. Animals that are anorectic can have a remarkably distended gallbladder. Biliary sediment or sludge is commonly visualized in the gall-

bladder in its dependent portion. Sludge does not produce postacoustic shadowing.[2] In humans, echogenic sludged material is comprised of cholesterol crystals and calcium bilirubinate granules suspended in a mucin gel matrix.[2] The cholesterol crystals are the reported source of acoustic echoes.

Common bile duct enlargement can be recognized within 24 to 48 hours of acute complete bile duct obstruction[23,24] (Figure 37-7). Intrahepatic biliary duct dilation is not apparent until 5 to 7 days of acute obstruction. These are differentiated from portal vessels by their irregular branching patterns and tortuosity.[24] Absolute measurement of bile duct diameter varies among dogs and cannot be used as a determinant of the duration of obstruction.

Cholelithiasis and choledocholithiasis may be diagnosed by abdominal ultrasonography as shown in Figure 37-6 and in Figure 8-46. Both radiodense and radiopaque stones can be imaged. Stones within the gallbladder are easiest to see, and these produce strong acoustic shadowing when of sufficient size and density. Calculi are differentiated from lesions attached to the wall of the gallbladder by demonstration of their gravitational mobility. Calculi in the common or cystic duct may be difficult to visualize because of adjacent bowel gas and because they are not surrounded by anechoic bile.[20-22]

Sessile or polypoid lesions can be seen on the gallbladder wall in dogs with cystic hyperplasia of the gallbladder. Adenomas or adenocarcinomas are less common and usually produce an irregular and focal wall involvement. Cats with polycystic liver disease may have biliary cysts visible in the porta hepatis. Choledochal cysts and cystadenomas have also been visualized in this area.

The association of pancreatitis or pancreatic neoplasia with biliary tract disease can also be appraised using ultrasonography. Pancreatic enlargement or masses, focal steatitis due to fat necrosis, and enlarged lymph nodes may be disclosed; Figure 37-8 shows pancreatic enlargement in a dog with pancreatitis associated with major bile duct occlusion. The accumulation of small quantities of fluid associated with focal peritonitis, thickening of the duodenal wall, and lack of normal duodenal motility suggestive of duodenitis and focal ileus may also be detected.

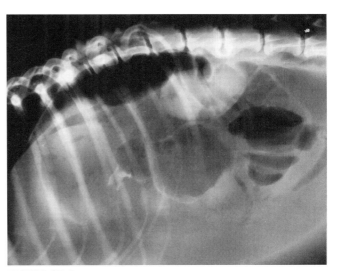

FIGURE 37-5. Radiograph of a dog with septic bile peritonitis. Linear gas densities within the biliary tree indicate the presence of a gas-producing organism. This animal had a septic abdominal effusion and free gas within the abdominal cavity. Campylobacter was subsequently cultured.

Table 37-1

CHOLECYSTOGRAPHIC AGENTS

AGENT	SPECIES	DOSE (MG/KG)	ROUTE	EXPOSURE TIME INTERVAL
Iodipamide	dog	0.5 mg/kg	IV	1 hour
Iobenzamic acid	dog	2–3 g/10–15 kg 5—150 mg/kg	PO	12 hour
Meglumine iotrixinate	dog	0.5–1.0 mg/kg	IV slow	30 minutes
Ipodate calcium	dog	150–450 mg/kg	PO	12 hours
	cat	150–500 mg/kg	PO	12 hours
Ipodate sodium	cat	150–500 mg/kg	PO	12 hours
Iodipamide meglumine	cat	0.5–1.5 mL/kg	IV slow	3–5 hours
Cholecystokinin	cat	5 μ/cat	IV	
		(aided gallbladder contraction without side effects)		

Ultrasonography can be used to visualize small quantities of fluid loculated by fibrinous adhesions in the area of the gallbladder and porta hepatis. Bile peritonitis may be diagnosed by ultrasonographically guided needle aspirate of small fluid pools when bile duct rupture is suspected. In some cases this has afforded rapid diagnoses permitting prompt surgical intervention. In the presence of a ruptured biliary tree, the gallbladder may be extremely difficult to image, a phenomenon that strengthens an index of suspicion for the diagnosis.

For patients with suspected cholangitis or cats with the cholangitis/cholangiohepatitis syndrome, ultrasonography allows diagnostic decision making. If suppurative cholangitis is suspected and the biliary tree is not "pathologically" distended, cholecystocentesis can be done to sample bile for cytology and culture. In cats from climates where hepatic flukes are endemic, a bile sample may disclose the presence of operculated eggs. The likelihood of hepatic lipidosis versus a diffuse parenchymal cholangitis may be predicted by combination use of the clinical biochemical profile and ultrasonographic features. High ALP and minimal change in GGT associated with a diffuse hyperechogenic hepatic parenchyma suggests lipidosis. High ALP and GGT with multifocal hyperechogenicity and thickened biliary structures suggests cholangiohepatitis. This information can assist in deciding whether a laparotomy or ultrasound-guided needle aspirate or biopsy is most appropriate. Lipidosis can be confirmed on aspirate; cholangiohepatitis cannot be confirmed without biopsy. Unfortunately, both disorders may coexist so a clear-cut diagnostic strategy cannot be dogmatically followed.

Hepatic Scintigraphy

Alternative methods for imaging the biliary tree are available at some referral practices. These involve use of short-lived radioisotopes, such as technetium (^{99m}TC) used as labels on a new class of organic anions, the iminodiacetic (IDA) analogues[25] (see Chapter 8). Hepatic scintigraphy using ^{99m}TC-IDA agents in humans can achieve early diagnosis of common bile duct occlusion, acute and chronic cholecystitis, segmental biliary tree obstruction, and problems associated with gallbladder or sphincter of Oddi function.[25] Scintigraphy also provides a noninvasive method of documenting small-volume bile leakage into the peritoneal cavity (Figure 37–9).

Few reports of the use of these analogues in veterinary patients have been published relevant to clinical practice. Two studies have demonstrated their utility in dogs with spontaneous cholestatic disease.[26,27]

Cholecystocentesis

Percutaneous ultrasound-guided cholecystocentesis has been described in humans, dogs, swine, and cattle.[28–33] Risks associated with this procedure are low and complications seem infrequent. Aspiration of the gallbladder can be accomplished from a direct transpercutaneous/transperitoneal route or transhepatically. The transhepatic approach is considered the safest percutaneous method of bile aspiration. A 22 gauge spinal needle is used for this method in both dogs and cats. The safest procedures are completed using an ultrasound biopsy guide. The patient must be heavily sedated or preferably anesthetized to avoid serious iatrogenic injury. The transhepatic approach is done by inserting the needle into the hepatic tissue adjacent to the gallbladder and then puncturing the wall of the gallbladder from this vantage point. This method permits the juxtaposed hepatic parenchyma to assist hemostasis and entrap escaped bile by virtue of the tissue pressure over the puncture site and entrapment of escaped bile. Liver tissue effectively seals off the area of gallbladder puncture and minimizes the risk of peritonitis due to bile leakage. Liver fluke infestation in cattle and cats can be detected using this procedure. Needle puncture of a distended, friable, or

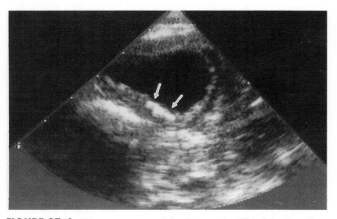

FIGURE 37-6. Ultrasonogram of the liver and gallbladder in a dog with a thickened gallbladder wall due to cholecystitis. Three small (2 mm sized) choleliths (arrows) are visualized in the gallbladder. (Courtesy Dr. A. Yeager, Section of Radiology, Department of Clinical Sciences, College of Veterinary Medicine, Cornell University)

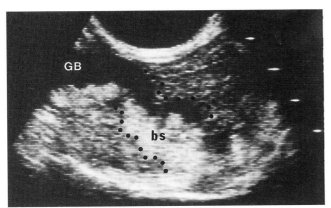

FIGURE 37-7. Ultrasonogram of the liver and gallbladder (GB) in a dog with extrahepatic bile duct obstruction. The gallbladder was distended. There is a large amount of biliary sludge (bs) and a tortuous cystic duct (dotted black line). Liver tissue is observed to the right and left of the cystic duct. (Courtesy Dr. A. Yeager, Section of Radiology, Department of Clinical Sciences, College of Veterinary Medicine, Cornell University)

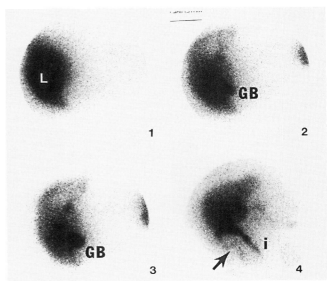

FIGURE 37-9. Scintigram showing bile leakage into the peritoneal cavity in a dog with bile peritonitis subsequent to reconstructive biliary tract surgery following trauma. An intravenously administered technetium-labeled iminodiacetic analogue was used. Scintigrams were recorded sequentially for 3 hours. This study shows rapid accumulation of radionuclide in the liver and slower accumulation in the area of the gallbladder. Between 2 and 3 hours, there is progressive accumulation of radionuclide in a loop of intestine that likely comprises the cholecystojejunostomy that had been surgically constructed. A less well-defined serpentine area of increased activity extends from the area of the gallbladder. This is consistent with leakage of bile from the surgical site. Liver (L), Gallbladder (GB), Intestine (i), bile leakage (arrow); sector 1 = 30 minutes, 2 = 48 minutes, 3 = 75 minutes, and 4 = 180 minutes. (Courtesy Dr. B. Nicholson and Dr. N. Dykes, Section of Radiology, Department of Clinical Sciences, College of Veterinary Medicine, Cornell University)

diseased gallbladder wall carries more risk than cholecystocentesis of a normal gallbladder. Hemorrhagic tendencies must be considered before the procedure is undertaken and appropriate preparations should be made for intervention of possible complications. The patient should be observed for 24 hours following this procedure to monitor for signs of peritonitis, particularly if a septic exudate is collected. In humans, severe vagal complications, which have progressed to cardiac arrest, have been described in patients with acute cholecystitis undergoing vigorous diagnostic or therapeutic manipulations of the gallbladder.[33] Similar problems have not been seen in dogs or cats undergoing simple gallbladder aspiration.

DISEASES OF THE GALLBLADDER

Cystic Mucinous Hypertrophy of the Gallbladder

This lesion has been described in elderly dogs and dogs treated with progestational compounds. It is not associated with obstruction of the cystic duct or any clinical symptoma-

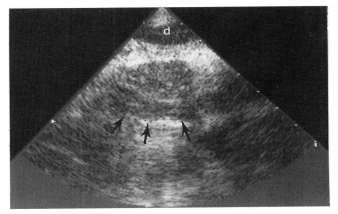

FIGURE 37-8. Ultrasonogram of a dog with pancreatitis showing an enlarged pancreas (arrows) adjacent to the duodenum (d). (Courtesy Dr. A. Yeager, Section of Radiology, Department of Clinical Sciences, College of Veterinary Medicine, Cornell University)

tology.[34,35] The clinician should be aware of this "lesion" because it may be detected on ultrasonographic evaluation of the biliary tree. On gross inspection of an affected gallbladder, the normally white mucosa is grossly thickened and proliferative. The lumen is often filled with thick, viscous, green mucus. Histologically, the surface epithelium is intact and normal and a distinct lamina propria can be identified. There is no evidence of inflammation and the serosal, muscular, and vascular structures appear intact and normal. The mucosal surface is irregular and comprised of a polypoid cystic lining. Ultrasonographically, a thickened and slightly irregular gallbladder wall is imaged. Biliary sludge is usually observed. Review of the patient's record fails to detail symptomatology suggestive of cholecystitis or cholestasis.

Cholecystitis

Clinical Synopsis

Diagnostic Features

- Abdominal pain, fever, vomiting, and jaundice
- Leukocytosis with toxic neutrophils common
- Elevated bilirubin and liver enzymes
- Abdominal radiology may suggest peritonitis, gas in biliary tree, or a mass in right cranial quadrant

Standard Treatment

- Fluid therapy (colloids may be required)

- Broad spectrum antibiotic coverage (e.g., ampicillin/gentamicin) tailored specifically to cultured organisms
- Vitamin K_1
- Surgical exploration, cholecystectomy, or biliary diversion

Cholecystitis, or inflammation of the gallbladder, is an uncommon diagnosis in the dog and cat. If not diagnosed and treated promptly, it can be lethal.

PATHOGENESIS. The genesis of cholecystitis has been explored with a large number of experimental animal models. Cholecystitis can be induced by ligating the cystic duct and allowing inflammation to develop from bile stasis. Inflammation is seemingly accelerated by implantation of a mechanical irritant.[36–38] Inflammation contributes to the formation of cholesterol choleliths.[36,37,39–41] After obstruction of the cystic duct, the gallbladder wall thickens and the organ decreases in diameter. Hydrops, or gallbladder distension with a clear or white viscid mucoid bile (bile lacking bilirubin pigments), is often seen if there are no complications. In the presence of septic inflammation, cystic duct obstruction results in empyema and acute septic cholecystitis.[36] Alternatively, choleliths can mechanically incite inflammation. Increased gallbladder volume to the point of causing taut distension of the wall occurs with common bile duct obstruction. This has been shown to impair mural circulation and to predispose to necrosis and perforation of the gallbladder.

In dogs and humans, cholecystitis and cholelithiasis can be induced by creation of a wide opening between the common bile duct and the intestine.[42] This is related to retrograde invasion by enteric flora. Reflux of pancreatic enzymes into the biliary tree has also been implicated in some cases of cholecystitis.[43] A pathogenic role for lysolecithin has also been proposed.[38,40,44] Lecithin in normal bile can be converted to lysolecithin by phospholipase A released from the inflamed gallbladder epithelium. Lysolecithin is cytotoxic and increases the permeability of the gallbladder wall. Prolonged exposure of the gallbladder mucosa to high concentrations of cholesterol or bile salts may also result in inflammation that progresses to acute cholecystitis. Impaired gallbladder circulation by cystic artery occlusion, primary bacterial infection, or cystic duct obstruction due to cholelithiasis, neoplasia, or an adjacent inflammatory process can each induce acute cholecystitis. In most clinical cases of acute cholecystitis, combination of surface irritants and impaired cystic duct flow are thought to coexist.

The most severe forms of cholecystitis are associated with necrosis of the gall bladder wall (necrotizing cholecystitis and emphysematous septic inflammation (emphysematous cholecystitis or choledochitis).

NECROTIZING CHOLECYSTITIS. Necrotizing cholecystitis has been reported infrequently in the dog.[45–52] In the largest case series, the clinical findings in 23 dogs were provided.[45] There was no breed or sex predilection, mean age was 9.5 years, and 8 dogs presented in shock. Three types of cholecystitis were recognized: (1) necrotizing cholecystitis without gallbladder rupture (5/23), (2) acute cholecystitis with gallbladder perforation and peritonitis (13/23), and (3) chronic cholecystitis with cholecystic, omental, and hepatic adhesions and with fistulas to other abdominal structures (5/23). Of these dogs 18 of 23 had a ruptured gallbladder, 12 of 23 had obstruction of the common bile duct, and 14 of 23 had cholelithiasis. Histologic lesions in the liver were defined as chronic active cholangiohepatitis (n = 4), hepatic necrosis (n = 3), hepatic fibrosis (n = 2), and hepatic degeneration (n = 2). Nearly 80% of these dogs had a ruptured gallbladder, seemingly due to acute exacerbation of chronic cholecystitis associated with

common bile duct obstruction. Biliary cultures were positive in 13 of 16 dogs: *E. coli* (9/13), *Klebsiella* (2/13), *Clostridia* (1/13), and *Pseudomonas* (1/13). Three dogs with emphysematous cholecystitis had an *E. coli* infection. This study demonstrated that prompt diagnosis and surgical treatment is essential for a positive outcome.

EMPHYSEMATOUS CHOLECYSTITIS OR CHOLEDOCHITIS. Emphysematous cholecystitis is an uncommon condition that has been associated with diabetes mellitus, acute cholecystitis with or without cholecystolithiasis, and traumatic ischemia of the gallbladder.[53–55] Recognition of gas within the gallbladder and/or biliary tree, in the absence of a surgically created cholecystoenterostomy, indicates serious septic inflammation, likely associated with gangrene. Ischemia is believed to be important in the pathogenesis of emphysematous cholecystitis, especially when anaerobic organisms are involved. Clostridial organisms and *E. coli* have been cultured from the biliary tree of affected dogs. Because gangrene is a common feature of the pathologic process of emphysematous cholecystitis, a cholecystectomy is mandatory.

CLINICAL SIGNS. Clinical manifestations of acute cholecystitis include abdominal pain, fever, vomiting, ileus, and mild to moderate jaundice. A mass effect may be recognized in the right cranial abdomen. Some animals present in endotoxic shock. A variable leukocytosis is associated with toxic neutrophils but inconsistently with a left shift. Hyperbilirubinemia may be modest or overt, depending on chronicity, involvement of the extrahepatic biliary tree, and the presence or absence of bile duct occlusion. Hepatic transaminases and ALP activity are usually moderately increased. Rupture of the gallbladder may occur as a result of gangrenous changes in the wall. This may result in formation of a pericholecystic abscess localized by the omentum or development of generalized peritonitis. Finding free bile within the abdominal cavity is diagnostic for a ruptured biliary tree and bile peritonitis.

Abdominal radiology may reveal evidence of focal peritonitis characterized by indistinct detail in the cranial abdomen and a sentinel loop indicating a focal ileus. A sentinel loop signifies an ileus in a focal segment of gut and indicates the likelihood of an adjacent inflammatory lesion. In exceptional cases, the wall of the gallbladder may become radiodense due to dystrophic mineralization. In some animals choleliths will be easily identified. Gas accumulation within the biliary tree and/or gallbladder heralds the presence of emphysematous cholecystitis. This is always associated with sepsis and indicates an urgent need for antibiotics and cholecystectomy. An example of the radiographic features observed in an animal with acute necrotizing cholecystitis is shown in Figure 37–10. Abdominal ultrasonography may detect small pockets of fluid adjacent to the gallbladder and liver. This may be sampled with ultrasonographic guidance disclosing the presence of infection or bile leakage.

TREATMENT OF CHOLECYSTITIS. Medical and surgical management must focus on restoring the patient's fluid and electrolyte status, providing broad-spectrum antibiotics effective against enteric organisms, and prompt surgical intervention. Some of these patients will need administration of colloids or a plasma transfusion. Hypoalbuminemia results from protein sequestration in an inflammatory abdominal effusion. If jaundice has been notable for several weeks and major bile duct occlusion is considered possible, Vitamin K_1 should be administered intramuscularly 12 to 24 hours prior to surgical intervention. If this time lag is not advisable considering the patient's condition, provision of a fresh whole blood transfusion may be necessary to avert hemorrhagic complications. Some animals present in shock due to bile peritonitis; appropriate treatment for this sequela is described later in this

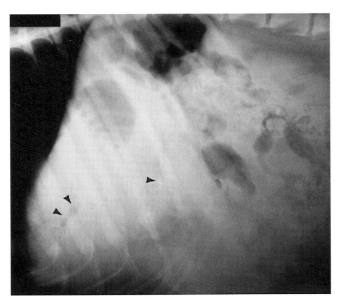

FIGURE 37-10. Lateral abdominal radiograph of a dog with acute necrotizing cholecystitis. This radiograph demonstrates the lack of cranial abdominal detail due to free fluid and peritoneal inflammation, the presence of choleliths (single arrow), and gas within the biliary tree (double arrowheads). This patient developed endotoxic shock subsequent to septic bile peritonitis.

chapter. Considering the underlying factors associated with cholecystitis and choledochitis, surgical exploration of the biliary tree is necessary. At surgery, the patency of the cystic and common bile duct must be appraised as well as an assessment of the viability of the gallbladder. The surgeon should be prepared to perform a cholecystectomy and/or biliary-enteric anastomosis. The procedures for biliary enteric anastomosis, cholecystectomy, and utilization of T-tubes for temporary extracorporeal bile drainage are provided in several current surgical textbooks.[56,57] Bile, gallbladder wall, choleliths, and liver tissue should be submitted for aerobic and anaerobic cultures. Cytologic evaluation of tissue imprints and bile should always be completed, which will assist in optimal selection of the initial antimicrobial therapy. A combination of an aminoglycoside, metronidazole or clindamycin, and ampicillin or a fluorinated quinolone is often used in the initial postoperative interval. This provides broad protection against enteric opportunists that are most commonly isolated. If the gallbladder is the only necrotic tissue, a simple cholecystectomy may be curative. If the common bile duct, cystic bile duct, or hepatic ducts are involved, a more guarded prognosis is warranted.

CHOLECYSTECTOMY. There are few side effects of removal of a functional gallbladder.[58,59] Cholecystectomy results in the loss of the absorptive and pressure-regulating function of the gallbladder and the fasting reservoir where bile acids are concentrated.[60,61] After gallbladder removal, bile increases in volume due to increased output of sodium, the size of the bile acid pool diminishes, and the enterohepatic circulation of bile acids becomes a continuous process.[60–63] A decrease in the bile acid pool by more than 80% was shown in cats cholecystectomized for 6 to 8 weeks.[58] A shift in the composition of the bile acid pool to an increase in the secondary (dihydroxy) bile acids occurs due to their increased formation by gut bacterial dehydroxylation. The greater exposure of bile acids to the enteric flora permits this change.[58,64,65] The concentration of bile acids in hepatic bile increases as a result of a decreased rate of bile acid–independent bile flow. The bile

duct epithelium appears to compensate somewhat for the loss of the absorptive function of the gallbladder. The common bile duct appears to enlarge after cholecystectomy and this change may be appreciated on subsequent ultrasonographic evaluations.

Cholelithiasis

Clinical Synopsis

Diagnostic Features

- Often asymptomatic
- May lead to episodic abdominal pain, vomiting, fever, and jaundice
- Laboratory evidence of cholestasis common
- Radiographs may reveal radiopaque calculi
- Diagnosis usually made by ultrasonography

Standard Treatment

- Ursodeoxycholic acid (10–15 mg/kg/day PO)
- Antibiotics (e.g., fluoroquinilones, ampicillin/gentamicin)
- Surgical removal if symptomatic

Cholelithiasis has been amply reported in the veterinary literature despite the fact that it is a rather uncommon clinical diagnosis.[66–80] As a clinical problem, cholelithiasis seems most common in small dogs, the miniature schnauzer and poodle having a higher incidence. The popular use of abdominal ultrasonography in evaluation of veterinary patients has increased the recognition of cholelithiasis in small animals.

PATHOGENESIS. Gallstones are a common malady of human beings where they often lead to cholecystitis and cholecystectomy. Stone formation is known to depend on a number of biliary variables including bile saturation with cholesterol and biliary pigments, and the type and proportion of bile acids, protein, and mucin in bile. High biliary protein and lipid concentrations are risk factors for gallstone formation in humans. It is believed that high cholesterol concentrations in bile lead to local inflammation and can provide a nucleation nidus for subsequent cholelith precipitation.[81,82]

Cholelith composition in the dog and cat has not been well characterized. It appears that canine choleliths are not particularly rich in cholesterol.[50,52,66–73,80,83] Their primary constituents usually are mucin, calcium, and bilirubin. Compared to humans, canine bile has higher quantities of total solids, lipids, bile acids, and phospholipids and lower quantities of bilirubin, cholesterol, and monoglycerides.[83] Canine bile has a very low lithogenic index; in fact, human cholesterol gallstones dissolve when placed in the gallbladder of dogs. This low lithogenic index is attributed to the low concentrations of cholesterol and free Ca^+. The low calcium concentration is maintained by the efficient resorption of calcium by the canine gallbladder.[84] Although recurrent choleliths removed from one cat were found to be 86% cholesterol, other feline choleliths have not been rich in cholesterol. The calcium concentration of many choleliths in dogs and cats is low enough that they remain radiolucent. However, in a recent retrospective study of cholelithiasis in the dog, 50% of 27 dogs had choleliths that were radiodense.[80] It is probable that this study overrepresents the proportion of choleliths that are radiodense in dogs.

Diet can induce cholelithiasis in several laboratory animals.

Gallstones have been produced in dogs fed a diet comprised of purified casein (10%), sucrose (50%), cornstarch (26%), lard (5%), cholesterol (1%), and other minor components.[85,86] Gelatinous, rubbery to firm choleliths began forming within 1 week. Choleliths were dark brown or black and were qualitatively analyzed. Components included protein, cholesterol, bilirubin, carbonate, fat, calcium, phosphorus, lecithin, and bile acids. The lithogenic mechanisms of this low-protein, low-taurine diet is not understood.

Gallbladder sludge is commonly identified during abdominal ultrasonography in dogs and cats, particularly if they have been anoretic. This is considered a nonpathologic phenomenon unless the clinical history typifies recurrent abdominal distress and vomiting and a serum biochemical profile details episodic or persistent evidence of cholestasis.

Gallbladder stasis is believed to favor cholelith precipitation. Upon ligation of the cystic duct, dogs develop pigment sludge, increased mucin production, and increased biliary cholesterol concentrations.[87,88] The gallbladder sludge contains solid particles ranging between 1 and 4 mm in diameter. Mucin-bilirubin complexes form first, but as the mucin content increases, sludge particles coalesce and precipitate as gravel and stones. Increased bile lithogenicity impairs gallbladder evacuation leading to biliary stasis and gallbladder distension. Distension stimulates mucin production, which may lead to occlusion of the cystic duct and futher promotion of sludge formation. Theoretically, impaired gallbladder motility contributes to gallstone precipitation. However, this may only be circumstantial because stasis usually coexists with other conditions causally linked to increased bile lithogenicity. Cholecystitis is lithogenic by virtue of its collective associations with prostaglandin-mediated inflammation, increased mucin production, hemorrhage, bacterial enzymes, and bile stagnation. Clearly, diseases of the gallbladder and major bile ducts can lead to cholelithiasis as surely as cholelithiasis can injure these structures.

CLINICAL FEATURES. Most humans with gallstones have no clinical signs. It is suspected this also is true for animals. Episodic right upper quadrant pain or epigastric distress are most common. This scenario is difficult to recognize in small animals. In a few dogs, this symptomatology has been recognized in the presence of cholelithiasis detected during routine abdominal ultrasonography. Similar to humans, some dogs with cholelithiasis remain asymptomatic until they present with acute cholecystitis. Severe abdominal pain, nausea, vomiting, fever, leukocytosis, and mild jaundice are usually displayed. Bile duct obstruction and bile infection commonly coexist in these patients. In a recent retrospective study of canine cholelithiasis, 14 of 20 aerobic and 8 of 18 anaerobic bile cultures were positive.[80] The most common isolates were *E. coli*, *Enterococcus*, and *Klebsiella*. Other single isolates were *Proteus*, *Clostridia*, *Citrobacter*, *Serratia*, *Fusobacteria*, *Bacillus*, and *Eubacterium* spp.

In humans, passage of common bile duct stones can induce acute pancreatitis due to transient obstruction of the main pancreatic duct.[89-94] Cholecystectomy or therapy with ursodeoxycholic acid reduces the incidence of relapsing pancreatitis in some of these patients. Considering the anatomic similarity of the feline and human bile duct/pancreatic duct union and the recognition that cholangitis can be associated with pancreatitis in the cat, a similar phenomenon is suspected.

DIAGNOSIS OF CHOLELITHIASIS. Diagnosis of gallstones is usually made by abdominal ultrasonography because many stones are not detected on survey abdominal radiographs. Ultrasonography can detect stones 2 mm or more in diameter when located in the gallbladder. Stone identification is aided by demonstration of their mobility. It is much more difficult to visualize choleliths in the common duct because of adjacent bowel gas and the absence of an anechoic (fluid) interface. During ultrasonographic evaluation of the biliary system, structural information regarding the gallbladder, including the presence of wall thickening or common duct occlusion, should be obtained. A thickening of the gallbladder wall suggests inflammation but also may be due to circulatory congestion, hypoalbuminemia, inflammatory hepatopathies, portal hypertension, or enhanced wall visibility due to the presence of an abdominal effusion. Most animals with cholelithiasis reported before the common clinical use of ultrasound were symptomatic and had serum biochemical features suggestive of obstructive biliary tract disease. The clinical presentation of this disorder is evolving in veterinary medicine as the ultrasonographic recognition of asymptomatic cholelithiasis becomes more common. Currently, most affected dogs and cats are being recognized before onset of obstructive biliary tract disease, necrotizing cholecystitis, and severe jaundice.

TREATMENT. Gallstones should not be surgically removed unless a patient is symptomatic, either clinically or biochemically, for related disease. Stone removal along with cholecystectomy is usually done if cholecystitis or obstructed biliary flow is recognized. Stones in the common duct require urgent removal. An attempt to "dissolve" gallstones with ursodeoxycholic acid is advised for patients not showing acute or relapsing clinical signs. Stones rich in calcium are reported to be poorly soluble and do not regress with medical therapy. In humans where gallstone dissolution has been intensely studied, stones dissolve no faster than approximately 1 mm (stone diameter) per month and recurrence has been shown in 43% after 4 years.[95,96] Other means of gallstone dissolution or removal have been investigated in humans because of the high incidence of this disorder. These include contact dissolution with methyl tert-butyl ether and n-propyl acetate, extracorporeal biliary lithotripsy, endoscopic retrograde retrieval from the common duct, and laparoscopic cholecystectomy. These are not appropriate for use in veterinary patients for a variety of reasons.

The common association of cholithiasis with biliary tract infection requires that broad-spectrum antibiotic therapy be provided. In a recent review of canine cholelithiasis, more than 80% of biliary isolates were susceptible to aminoglycosides. Fluorinated quinolones also are suspected to be efficacious considering their activity against many gram negative organisms and their good penetration into bile. The clinician must remember that cholestasis associated with common bile duct obstruction must be rectified to achieve adequate antibiotic penetration in bile. Antibiotics that achieve good penetration in bile are listed in Table 33-14.

Surgical removal of choleliths is the treatment of choice for calculi causing clinical signs. If the gallbladder appears inflamed and infected, a cholecystectomy is usually done. Dogs in which a cholecystectomy is done seem to have better survival.[80] Most dogs have multiple stones and so exploration of the biliary tree is important at the time of surgery. Patency of the cystic and common bile ducts can be ascertained by passage of a soft flexible catheter. Injection of sterile saline into the tube permits assessment of flow resistance. A liver biopsy should be collected to assess the extent of hepatic injury due to mechanical cholestasis, biliary tract inflammation, and infection. Cholecystotomy is done if cholecystectomy is appraised as too dangerous considering the condition of the bile ducts and if the patient's condition contraindicates a lengthy surgical procedure.

BILE PERITONITIS

Clinical Synopsis

Diagnostic Features

- Low-grade abdominal pain (if nonseptic peritonitis)
- Malaise, weight loss, and abdominal effusion
- Septicemia and septic peritonitis may develop
- Liver enzymes mildly to moderately elevated
- Abdominocentesis discloses inflammatory cells and bilirubin crystals in a turbid golden-brown or green fluid

Standard Treatment

- Fluid therapy (colloids often required)
- Abdominal lavage and surgical repair of leakage
- Antibiotics and open abdominal drainage if septic peritonitis

Rupture of the extrahepatic biliary tree has been well documented in the veterinary literature.[47,66,67,97–115] In the dog, the most common sites of rupture are the common bile duct and gallbladder. Etiologic factors include blunt or penetrating abdominal trauma, biliary tree sepsis, necrotizing cholecystitis, and cholelithiasis (Table 37–2). Iatrogenic injury of the biliary tree during hepatic percutaneous needle biopsy or other surgical manipulations may also occur. Needle biopsy of a patient with an obstructed extrahepatic biliary tree or severe choledochitis, especially when done as a blind or unguided procedure, carries the greatest risk of iatrogenic injury and subsequent bile peritonitis. Perforation of the gallbladder may be either immediate or delayed after blunt trauma or iatrogenic injury.

Leakage of bile into the peritoneal cavity can be associated with vague clinical signs. Because biliary tract tissue is invariably injured or inflamed, the serum transaminase, ALP, and GGT activities are increased. Jaundice may or may not occur depending on the underlying cause and the chronicity of the biliary tract rupture. In the absence of infection, bile leakage

Table 37–2

CAUSES OF BILIARY TRACT RUPTURE IN 60 DOGS	
SITE OF RUPTURE	**DOGS**
Bile Duct Rupture:	36
recent blunt abdominal trauma	32
penetrating abdominal injury	3
choledocholith	
Gallbladder Rupture:	27
cholelithiasis	17
necrotizing cholecystitis	8
recent blunt abdominal trauma	2

into the abdomen results in a variable peritoneal reaction. In many dogs, cytology discloses the presence of numerous neutrophils, macrophages, and few to moderate free bilirubin crystals. Large volumes of fluid may accumulate with relatively few overt adverse effects. Studies in germ-free dogs have shown survival for more than 2 weeks with few ill effects other than large-volume abdominal effusion (several liters in medium-sized dogs).[116] As a result, definitive diagnosis may be delayed until the animal displays signs of illness. Bile peritonitis is a potentially life threatening condition and should be diagnosed and definitively treated as soon as possible.

Escape of small amounts of sterile bile into the peritoneal cavity during surgery or subsequent to cholecystocentesis is usually uneventful. However, when large amounts of bile accumulate, sepsis may soon follow and this transforms bile peritonitis into a lethal condition (Figure 37–11). Unconjugated bile salts are cytotoxic and induce tissue inflammation. Although virtually all bile acids derived from the biliary tree are conjugated, the presence of a bacterial infection within the biliary tree or a low pH will result in bile acid deconjugation. Unconjugated bile acids alter the permeability of vascular structures within the peritoneal membranes. Transudation of fluid and transmural migration of enteric organisms into

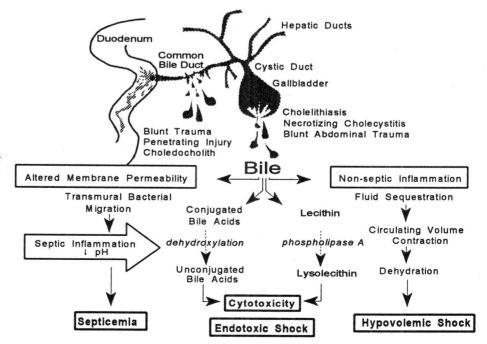

FIGURE 37–11. Pathophysiology of bile peritonitis leading to sepsis and endotoxemia.

the peritoneal cavity follows. Systemic hypovolemia and absorption of bacteria and their toxins leads to septicemia and endotoxic and hypovolemic shock. Abdominal palpation usually reveals vague pain and an obvious fluid wave. Patients usually are febrile, lethargic, jaundiced, anorectic, and may have pale or acholic stools. An interval ranging between 3 days and 3 weeks before presentation has been reported.[98]

In some animals, a focal bile peritonitis occurs due to omental entrapment of spilled biliary material. An intense local inflammatory reaction leads to formation of fibrinous adhesions at the site of biliary tree rupture, which serves to contain the process. Abdominal pain may be notable on palpation and a focal reaction associated with radiographic evidence of right cranial quadrant peritonitis. Abdominal ultrasonography usually reveals a pocket of fluid and "deranged" local anatomy. The gallbladder may not be well visualized if it is ruptured.

Diagnosis of diffuse bile peritonitis is usually easily accomplished upon cytologic evaluation of the abdominal effusion. An inflammatory reaction is apparent as well as many particles of bile both free and engulfed in macrophages and neutrophils (Figure 37–12). Sepsis is easily recognized. Grossly, the effusion is turbid and golden-brown or golden-green in color. Determination of bilirubin concentrations in fluid and serum usually discloses a disproportionate increase in the abdominal effusion. This, however, is usually a redundant diagnostic effort.

In some animals, for example the jaundiced patient that has recently undergone biliary tree surgery, substantiation of bile peritonitis is difficult. Use of abdominal lavage may assist in detecting spilled bile. A sensitive method of demonstrating bile spillage into the abdomen is by use of nuclear scintigraphy done with an organic anion labeled with an isotope (see Figure 37–9). Radiographic cholecystography is less definitive for a variety of reasons.

TREATMENT.   Successful treatment requires prompt diagnosis and surgical correction of bile leakage. Treatment for endotoxic and hypovolemic shock may be necessary. At surgery, the abdomen should be lavaged until it is grossly free of bile-stained fluid. Attention must be given to the fluid and electrolyte status of the patient and to the provision of colloid if hypoalbuminemia has developed. Effusion should be collected adjacent to the area of bile leakage and a cytologic preparation and gram stain immediately examined to assist in initial selection of antimicrobials. Adequate postoperative

abdominal drainage should be provided. If necrotizing cholecystitis is recognized, a cholecystectomy is mandatory. Unless the inflammation or injury is restricted to the gallbladder, this problem carries with it a poor prognosis. The presence of necrotizing choledochitis along with cholecystitis makes diversion of the biliary tree a difficult task. Utilization of extracorporeal T-tube drainage and later creation of a biliary enteric fistula are the only recourse. If substantial delay in surgical therapy is anticipated, the abdomen should be lavaged to remove as much bile as possible. Care must be taken to avoid inadvertent bacterial infection during paracentesis and lavage.

EXTRAHEPATIC BILE DUCT OBSTRUCTION

Clinical Synopsis

Diagnostic Features

- Jaundice and hepatomegaly
- Intermittent fever, vomiting, and acholic feces
- Neutrophilia, nonregenerative anemia, and elevated liver enzymes, bilirubin, and cholesterol common
- Absence of urobilinogen sometimes seen
- Ultrasonography reveals obstructed biliary structures

Standard Treatment

- Fluid therapy
- Surgical exploration and biliary decompression
- Cholecystoenterostomy
- Broad-spectrum antibiotics may be required
- Sucralfate and/or famotidine

Obstruction of the extrahepatic bile duct is associated with a number of diverse conditions shown in Table 37–3. Cholestasis resulting from occlusion of the major bile ducts leads to serious hepatobiliary injury within just a few

Table 37–3

CAUSES OF BILE DUCT OBSTRUCTION

Cholelithiasis
Choledochitis
Neoplasia
    Bile duct adenocarcinoma
    Pancreatic adenocarcinoma
    Lymphosarcoma
    Local tumor invasion
    Biliary cystadenomas
Malformation
    Choledochal cysts
    Polycystic liver disease
Parasitic
    Trematode infestation
Extrinsic Compression
    Lymph nodes
    Pancreatic mass
    Entrapment in diaphragmatic hernia
Fibrosis
    Blunt trauma
    Peritonitis
    Pancreatitis
Stricture
    Blunt trauma
    Iatrogenic: surgical

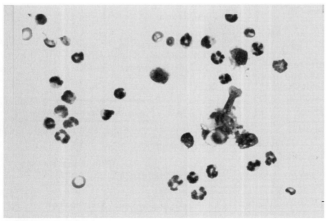

FIGURE 37–12. Cytologic preparation made from the abdominal effusion from a dog with nonseptic bile peritonitis. Many neutrophils, macrophages, and moderate numbers of bilirubin crystals were observed (Wright's-Giemsa stain; 480× magnification).

weeks.[117-125] Following complete obstruction, hepatomegaly and dilated intrahepatic bile ducts promptly follow. Obstructed bile flow leads to cell membrane and organelle injury as a result of stagnation of bile acids, lysolecithin, and possibly copper. Biliary injury is associated with eicosinoid-mediated inflammation and free radical injury-which inevitably involves other mediators. Biliary epithelial hyperplasia and bile ductule proliferation are early histologic features. Distension of the biliary structures, devitalization of the biliary epithelium, necrotic debris and suppurative inflammation within the bile duct lumen, periportal accumulations of neutrophils, lymphocytes, and plasma cells, periportal edema, and multifocal parenchymal necrosis are classic histologic changes of major duct occlusion of several weeks or longer (Figure 37–13). With chronicity, irreparable distension of the major bile ducts develops. Periportal fibrosis usually is obvious within 2 weeks and evolves into an "onion skin" appearance around the bile ducts. If obstruction is alleviated within the first several weeks, the periductal fibrosis and bile duct distension may completely resolve. If obstruction persists beyond 6 weeks, biliary cirrhosis predictably develops.

In the presence of complete bile duct obstruction, bile may become colorless (white bile) due to the reduced secretion of bilirubin pigments and an increased production of mucin.[126]

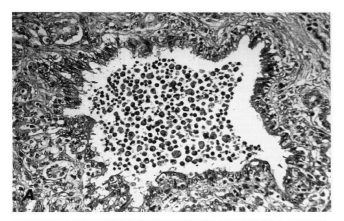

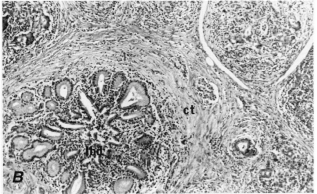

FIGURE 37-13. *(A)* Photomicrograph of the liver from a cat with extrahepatic bile duct occlusion of several weeks duration. A suppurative exudate has formed within the lumen of a distended large bile duct. Peribiliary inflammation and edema also were observed (H&E stain). *(B)* Photomicrograph of the liver from a cat with extrahepatic bile duct occlusion of several weeks duration. There is an accumulation of inflammatory cells (mainly neutrophils) within the large bile duct, (lbd), evidence of bile duct proliferation surrounding the large duct, and periportal connective tissue deposition (ct). A mixed suppurative/nonsuppurative inflammatory infiltrate has accumulated in the portal area (H&E stain).

Bacterial colonization of the gallbladder may develop due to either biliary reflux of intestinal bacteria or their hematogenous or lymphatic dissemination. Risk factors associated with the development of biliary bacteria in humans include advanced age, recent episodes of cholangitis, acute cholecystitis, choledocholithiasis, cholecystitis, and obstructive jaundice of any cause.[127] It is important to remember that treatment of biliary tract sepsis without biliary decompression will be ineffective because no antibiotic will achieve adequate levels in the biliary tree in the presence of extrahepatic obstructive jaundice.

CLINICAL SIGNS. Following bile duct obstruction, animals become lethargic, have intermittent fevers, and become markedly jaundiced within a few days. Increased serum concentrations of bilirubin are demonstrable within 4 hours. Some animals are intermittently inappetent but others may become polyphagic, possibly associated with fat malabsorption. Vomiting may be episodic. Hepatomegaly, acholic feces, and the absence of urine urobilinogen may develop within the first week. Bleeding tendencies may be notable within 3 weeks and seem to be more common in cats. Gastroenteric ulceration at the pyloric-duodenal junction is common and can lead to substantial blood loss. With intestinal bleeding, bilirubin pigments gain access to the bowel and formation of urobilinogen and fecal stercobilin may follow. Feces may resultantly become brown and urobilinogen may appear in urine. Patients with obstructive jaundice have a tendency to become hypotensive and are more susceptible to shock during surgery and anesthesia.[128-132]

DIAGNOSTIC FEATURES. The major clinicopathologic features of extrahepatic bile duct obstruction are shown in Figure 37–14. The chronologic changes in serum enzyme activities, cholesterol, and total bilirubin concentrations are shown in Figure 37–15.

The CBC may show a neutrophilic leukocytosis, and with increased chronicity of bile duct occlusion, a nonregenerative anemia may develop. A strongly regenerative anemia has been seen in some animals with persistent severe gastrointestinal hemorrhage. Usually, the hematocrit is within the normal range and microcytosis is uncommon. As bile stagnates in the liver and the biliary pressure increases, hepatic transaminases are released due to altered cell membrane permeability and cell necrosis. Induction of ALP and GGT occurs within 8 to 12 hours and causes a substantial increase in the serum enzyme activities within a few days.[123,133-137] The cholestatic enzymes are induced and released from the periportal canaliculi and the biliary duct epithelium.[138] As parenchymal necrosis and periportal inflammation proceed, both transaminases and cholestatic enzymes remain markedly increased. The magnitude of increase in ALP activity in the cat is less dramatic than in the dog (Figures 37–14 and 37–15). The activity of the serum AST mitochondrial isoenzyme has been proposed to be a useful marker of hepatic injury following obstructive jaundice in the dog.[139] After decompression of the biliary obstruction, this isoenzyme has been shown to reflect resolution or continuation of the hepatic injury. Persistent high mitochondrial AST activity reflects ongoing hepatocellular damage. After 4 to 6 weeks of continued biliary tree obstruction, serum transaminases and bilirubin values may slowly decline but usually not to within normal ranges. Hypercholesterolemia develops within 2 weeks of bile duct obstruction as a result of impaired cholesterol elimination and increased hepatic cholesterol biosynthesis. With chronic obstruction and development of biliary cirrhosis, the serum cholesterol concentration may normalize or become subnormal. This occurs because of impaired hepatic cholesterol synthesis and development of portosystemic shunting. Coagulopathies associated with vitamin K

Clinicopathologic Features of Extrahepatic Bile Duct Obstruction

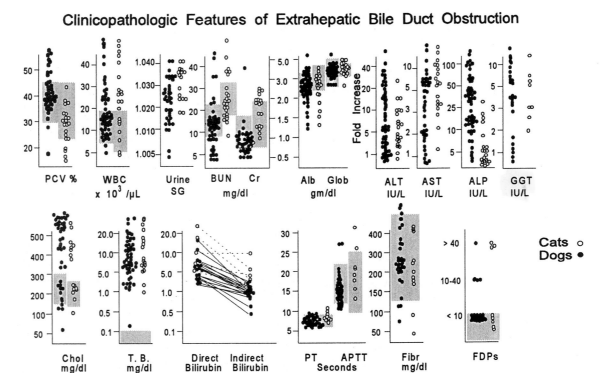

FIGURE 37–14. Scattergrams showing the clinicopathologic features associated with extrahepatic bile duct obstruction in the dog and cat (data derived from the College of Veterinary Medicine, Cornell University, Ithaca, NY, 1980–1993).

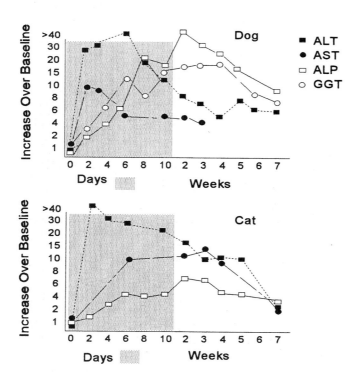

FIGURE 37–15. Chronologic change of serum enzyme activities (ALP: alkaline phosphatase, GGT: gamma glutamyl transferase, AST: aspartate aminotransferase, ALT: alanine aminotransferase) and serum total bilirubin and cholesterol in dogs and cats after acute complete extrahepatic bile duct obstruction.

deficiency may develop within 21 days and can be detected best with a PIVKA assay (Proteins Induced by Vitamin K Absence), which is more sensitive than the PT or APTT for this problem. PIVKAs are discussed in more depth in Chapter 8. In clinical patients, demonstrable abnormalities in the routinely used coagulation tests are uncommon (Figure 37–14), possibly because they are presented early in the course of biliary tree obstruction.

Diagnosis of major bile duct occlusion is confirmed on ultrasonographic evaluation or exploratory surgery. Survey radiography or cholecystography are not useful. Cholecystographic agents will not opacify biliary structures in the presence of overt jaundice, significant hepatocellular disease, intrahepatic cholestasis, or extrahepatic biliary obstruction. In the absence of ultrasonography, surgical exploration of the abdomen is necessary for definitive diagnosis. Ultrasonographic features of bile duct occlusion include a distended and tortuous common bile duct, large gallbladder, and prominent, tortuous intrahepatic bile ducts (Figure 37–7). These findings are obvious by 5 to 7 days postobstruction to an experienced ultrasonographer. The actual cause of biliary obstruction may be difficult to determine during an ultrasonographic evaluation. In humans, early diagnosis of major bile duct occlusion can be facilitated by feeding a fatty meal and watching for dimensional changes in duct size.[140–142] An unobstructed duct should become smaller in width. A duct that does not change in size after feeding cannot be used alone as a diagnostic indicator of obstruction. Unfortunately, once the elasticity of the bile ducts is irreparably damaged, a floppy duct will be persistent and may lead to inaccurate assessments.

Biliary scintigraphy is a sensitive method of detecting biliary tree obstruction when combined with ultrasonography. Impaired excretion of isotope into the biliary tract coupled with the ultrasonographic features of duct distension can make a diagnosis within the first few days.

TREATMENT. Whenever an obstructed biliary tree is a considered cause of jaundice, an exploratory laparotomy rather than a percutaneous needle biopsy or laparoscopy should be done. Confirmation of the diagnosis and management of extrahepatic bile duct obstruction requires surgical exploration of the abdomen and inspection of the biliary structures. Gross inspection of the gallbladder and common bile duct usually reveals the site and cause of the obstruction. Palpation of the ducts may reveal an intramural mass. Gentle compression on the gallbladder may be needed to verify obstruction in some animals, especially in the early stages of duct occlusion. Later on, grossly distended and tortuous bile ducts make the diagnosis apparent. The most difficult obstructive lesions to identify are those involving the biliary tree proximal to the cystic duct. In some animals, performing a duodenotomy, cholecystotomy, or choledochotomy may be necessary for passage of a flexible catheter into the common bile duct to verify its patency and for removal of inspissated biliary sludge.

A common cause of bile duct occlusion in the dog and cat is pancreatitis due to periductal fibrosis and duct stricture.[48,143–146] Deciding on whether or not surgical intervention is appropriate for these patients can be difficult. The first indication for biliary decompression by surgical treatment is a steadily climbing or plateaued hyperbilirubinemia (> 7 mg/dl or a 15- to 20-fold increase over normal) transpiring over a 7 day interval. This combined with one or more of the following criteria should promote surgical intervention: (1) a palpable mass in the right cranial abdominal quadrant, (2) radiographic suggestion of a mass or focal peritonitis in the area of the body of the pancreas and proximal duodenum, or (3) ultrasonographic evidence of pancreatitis and bile duct obstruction. Sequential monitoring of serum transaminases, cholestatic enzymes, or pancreatic enzymes *cannot* be used to verify the need for surgical intervention because enzyme activities will invariably be increased with serious pancreatitis or bile duct inflammation in the absence of biliary tree obstruction. In addition, the magnitude of serum enzyme elevation has no correlation with the degree of hepatobiliary injury or obstruction.

Prompt surgical management of biliary tract obstruction by creation of a cholecystoduodenostomy or cholecystojejunostomy can have a high rate of success. Treated animals can have a good quality long-term survival. Prior to surgical intervention, Vitamin K_1 should be given for 12 to 48 hours to allow for activation of the dependent clotting factors. Cholecystoduodenostomy is more physiologic than cholecystojejunostomy considering that ingested materials will mix with pancreatic secretions in a nearly normal manner.[147] Unfortunately, some animals with pancreatitis have focal peritonitis, which complicates surgical manipulation of the duodenum. Cholecystojejunostomy has been successful in the author's clinic even without creation of a Roux-en-Y anastomosis. The long-term clinical course of dogs and cats (> 7 year survival) in the author's hospital has been quite satisfactory following this procedure.

The most critical factor in creation of a biliary enteric anastomosis is provision of a large enough opening to permit drainage of refluxed intestinal contents from the biliary tract.[148] An opening of at least 2.5 cm is advised. Bacterial growth in the biliary tract is expected during the initial postoperative period; however, clinical cholangitis usually does not develop unless the biliary tree becomes obstructed.[149–151] When cholecystoduodenostomies and cholecystojejunostomies were done in healthy dogs, variable histologic lesions

were seen in the liver over a 6 month interval.[152] These included bile duct proliferation, portal fibrosis, and periportal infiltration by lymphocytes and plasma cells. The severity of these lesions varied markedly between animals. Lesions worsened in severity with an increasing postoperative interval.

Follow-up abdominal radiographs in animals with cholecystoenterostomies may detail gas within the gallbladder or large extrahepatic bile ducts (Figure 37–16). Subsequent contrast studies of the lower gastrointestinal tract may demonstrate the free reflux of enteric contents into the biliary structures (Figure 37–17).

The decision to perform a biliary enteric anastomosis in

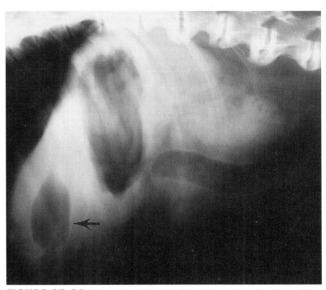

FIGURE 37-16. Lateral abdominal radiograph of a dog with a cholecystojejunostomy done to relieve extrahepatic bile duct obstruction due to fibrosing pancreatitis. Gas derived from the alimentary canal fills the gallbladder (arrow). There was no evidence of symptomatic cholangitis or cholecystitis in this patient.

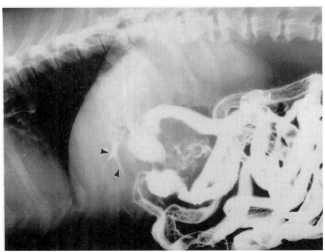

FIGURE 37-17. Lateral abdominal radiograph taken during a barium contrast study of the lower gastrointestinal tract in a dog with a cholecystoduodenostomy that was done to relieve extrahepatic bile duct obstruction due to fibrosing pancreatitis. A retrograde cholangiogram resulted from reflux of barium contrast into dilated hepatic or segmental ducts (arrowheads). There was no evidence of symptomatic cholangitis or cholecystitis in this patient.

animals with neoplasia obstructing the common bile duct can be an ethical dilemma. Adenocarcinomas of the bile duct are common in elderly cats presenting with extrahepatic bile duct occlusion. Thoracic radiographs should be reviewed before surgery to detect obvious metastasis. If metastases are seen, surgical decompression of the biliary tree will not assist in prolonging survival. In the absence of overt metastasis, tumor resection and biliary diversion should be pursued. Some of these tumors are very slow growing and cats can survive for 6 months or longer if a biliary diversion is created. They have a better quality of life if the cholestasis is palliated. If judged to be surgically resectable, the tumor should be removed. A biliary enteric anastomosis should still be done owing to the likelihood of tumor recurrence and postoperative bile duct scarring.

During and following biliary tree decompression, the patient should be maintained on intravenous fluids to ensure adequate volume expansion for blood pressure support and for the choleresis that will follow. Broad-spectrum antibiotics should be administered. This is of special importance for animals receiving a biliary-enteric anastomosis. Cultures of bile and tissue should be submitted to rule out a complicating infectious process. Biopsy of the liver and biliary tract in the area of obstruction is essential. Liver histology will predict future hepatobiliary compromise based on the degree of portal triad and bile ductule injury, periductal fibrosis, and cellular necrosis. Biopsy of duct tissue will permit diagnosis of benign or malignant neoplasia or inflammation. Sequential evaluation of a biochemical profile will indicate resolution of the cholestasis, hepatocellular inflammation, and necrosis. Serum bilirubin concentrations decline rapidly over 3 to 6 days but may not completely normalize for several weeks. A CBC should be appraised every few days to monitor for infection associated with surgery; these patients are predisposed to postoperative biliary tract infection. The clinician must remain alert for the development of bile peritonitis. Administration of sucralfate and famotidine are indicated initially due to the high incidence of gastroenteric ulceration in animals with bile duct obstruction. Sucralfate administration is probably a good idea in patients with biliary-enteric anastomosis considering the development of intestinal inflammation associated with the newly established bile drainage. This treatment has not been tested for efficacy. It is important to remember that fluorinated quinolones cannot be used concurrently with sucralfate due to their incompatibility.

In the patient with a cholecystojejunostomy, trial therapy with exocrine pancreatic enzymes can be considered if the patient appears to lose weight and condition, despite a good appetite, after recovery from surgery. Experimental study of dogs with choledochoduodenostomies and choledochojejunostomies showed that only the latter dogs lost weight.[153] Although not proven, this is presumed to be associated with maldigestion. The diet should be tailored to the animal's weight gain and tolerance of fat by observation of the fecal character.

CHOLANGITIS/CHOLANGIOHEPATITIS COMPLEX

Cholangitis and cholangiohepatitis are more common in the cat than in the dog. The anatomic difference in the biliary duct/pancreatic duct anatomy has long been considered an important predisposing factor for this species difference.[154-161] Suppurative and nonsuppurative cholangitis arise from similar causative factors; a list of associated disorders in the cat is provided in Table 37–4. The clinicopathologic fea-

Table 37–4

DISORDERS ASSOCIATED WITH CHOLANGITIS/CHOLANGIOHEPATITIS IN THE CAT	
SUPPURATIVE	**NONSUPPURATIVE**
Primary bacterial infection	Inflammatory bowel disease
Septicemia	Primary cholangitis
Chronic bacterial infections	Pancreatitis
sinusitis	Extrahepatic bile duct obstruction
splenic abscess	Cholelithiasis
pyelonephritis	Cholecystitis
Cholecystitis	Neoplasia
Cholelithiasis	Gallbladder adenocarcinoma
Pancreatitis	Bile duct cystadenoma
Inflammatory bowel disease	Malformation: choledochal cyst
Extrahepatic bile duct	Chronic trematode infestation
obstruction	Chronic bacterial infection
Acute trematode infestation	
Toxoplasmosis	

tures of the cholangitis/cholangiohepatitis syndrome in cats are shown in Figure 37–18.

Suppurative Cholangitis/Cholangiohepatitis

Clinical Synopsis

Diagnostic Features

- Male cats predisposed
- Duration of illness usually short (<5 days)
- Jaundice and fever common
- Liver enzymes mildly to moderately elevated
- Left-shifted leukogram occasionally seen
- Liver biopsy shows periductal suppurative inflammation

Standard Treatment

- Broad-spectrum antibiotics (ampicillin/gentamicin/metronidazole) initially followed by 3–6 months of an antibiotic dictated by sensitivity pattern
- Ursodeoxycholic acid (10–15 mg/kg PO, SID) for 3–6 months
- Rapid surgical biliary diversion needed in some cats

Compared to nonsuppurative cholangitis, suppurative cholangitis has more severe clinical manifestations, usually a shorter duration before diagnosis is made, and is associated with purulent exudate within the biliary tract. Acute suppurative cholangitis has a high degree of association with complete or partial obstruction of the biliary tract.[162-165] In the absence of biliary obstruction, bacterial contamination of bile is asymptomatic. Other conditions conducive to biliary tract infections include septicemia concurrent with biliary tract inflammation or obstruction, surgical biliary reconstruction, abnormalities of gallbladder structure or function, or preexisting cholecystitis, choledochitis, acute pancreatitis, inflammatory bowel disease, and immunodeficiencies.[163-166] The presence of biliary tract disease allows the enterohepatic-biliary bacterial cycle to become pathologic.[166-169] Gallbladder ischemia encourages growth of enteric anaerobes inadequately cleared from the biliary tract. In humans, infections of the biliary tree usually begin in the gallbladder and spread into the biliary system rather than ascending from the gut through the bile ducts into an obstructed biliary system. In suppurative cholangitis associated with complete bile duct obstruction, duct pressure increases rapidly as bacteria prolif-

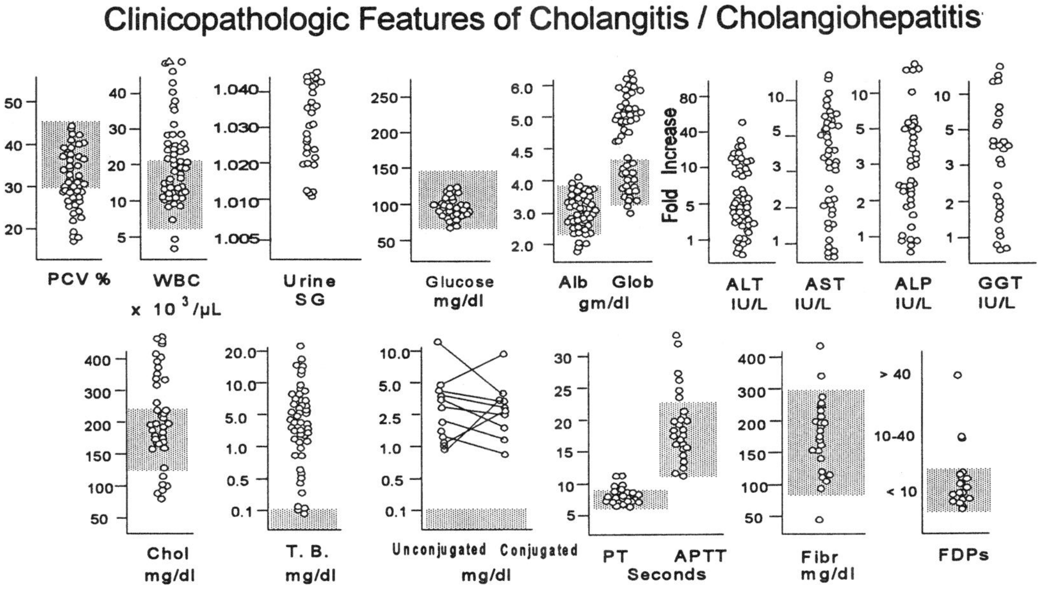

Clinicopathologic Features of Cholangitis / Cholangiohepatitis

FIGURE 37-18. Scattergrams showing the clinicopathologic features associated with the cholangitis/cholangiohepatitis syndrome in cats (data derived from the College of Veterinary Medicine, Cornell University, Ithaca, NY, 1980–1993).

erate. When ductal pressure reaches a critical threshold, exceeding the secretory biliary pressure generated by the liver, bacteria and their toxic products gain entrance into the systemic circulation via the hepatic sinusoids.[167-169] This leads to fulminant bacteremia and endotoxic shock. The most commonly isolated organisms in cats with acute suppurative cholangitis are consistent with an enteric origin: *E. coli, Enterobacter*, alpha-hemolytic *Streptococcus, Klebsiella, Actinomyces, Clostridia*, and *Bacteroides*.

Many other organisms have also been associated with suppurative cholangitis and cholangiohepatitis. Toxoplasmosis in the cat has been associated with suppurative cholangiohepatitis, but usually this organism does not show a particular tropism for the biliary tree.[170] *Campylobacter jejuni* was associated with suppurative cholangitis and cholecystitis in a dog that subsequently died of this infection in the author's hospital; an abdominal radiograph of this dog is shown in Figure 37-5. In the acute stages, leptospirosis can also be associated with suppurative portal tract inflammation. Severe chronic suppurative cholangiohepatitis was reported in a dog that had intrahepatic biliary coccidiosis associated with intermittent diarrhea of 4 weeks duration.[171] Chronic cholecystitis and cholangiohepatitis has also been observed in dogs infected with Salmonella.[172]

Suppurative cholangitis/cholangiohepatitis has been reported in a small number of cats as a distinct syndrome.[159,160] A retrospective study of cats with suppurative cholangitis in the author's hospital has helped to clarify the features of this condition.[173] Cats with suppurative cholangitis/cholangiohepatitis ranged in age between 3 months and 16 years; most cats were middle aged or younger. Significantly more males than females were affected. Most cats had a short duration of clinical illness (<5 days). Less than 50% had hepatomegaly, and most were jaundiced, febrile, lethargic, and dehydrated on initial presentation. Abdominal pain was commonly detected during initial physical examination. Vomiting or diarrhea was reported in 50%.

Similar to the situation in humans with suppurative cholangitis/cholangiohepatitis, most cats have underlying disorders of the biliary system leading to bile duct obstruction that would augment development of a septic process. Acute or short-term inflammatory bowel disease, pancreatitis, or acute extrahepatic bile duct obstruction were predisposing conditions in 75%. Two cats developed hepatic lipidosis as a result of illness attributed to suppurative cholangitis. Some cats have had histologically confirmed cholecystitis.

The clinicopathologic features of cats with all forms of cholangitis/cholangiohepatitis are shown in Figure 37-18. Most cats with suppurative inflammation have moderate increases in activities of ALT, AST, and GGT and a mild increase in ALP activity. Approximately 30% have a left-shifted leukogram and toxic neutrophils, with or without leukocytosis.

Severe ascending cholangitis is associated with thickening of the extrahepatic biliary system. This may be evident on ultrasonographic evaluation (Figure 37-19). Histologic lesions include dilation of the intrahepatic bile ducts, periportal edema, periductular suppurative inflammation, and an accumulation of suppurative exudate within the biliary lumen (Figure 37-20). Depending on chronicity, varying degrees of periductal fibrosis can be found associated with the bile duct proliferation and biliary hyperplasia (Figure 37-21). Associated cholecystitis and obvious exudation within the gallbladder and common bile duct may also occur. Associated pancreatic lesions include interstitial fibrosis, periductal fibrosis, and intraductal suppurative inflammation. Pancreatitis has previously been documented in cats with suppurative cholangitis and is supported by findings in our retrospective study.[159,160,173]

Cholelithiasis is found in some cats with suppurative cholangitis/cholangiohepatitis. These cats display intermittent or persistent fever, anorexia, and vomiting. Most have recently lost weight and are overtly jaundiced. Hemogram and biochemistry features are not different from other cats with suppurative cholangitis/cholangiohepatitis. Some calculi are radiodense and easily visualized. Some appear as miliary densities throughout the biliary tree (Figure 37-3). As previously discussed, ultrasonography is the most sensitive and specific method of cholelith diagnosis.

Early use of biliary diversion is vital in the prevention or control of septicemia in aggressive acute obstructive suppurative cholangitis. Survival reflects the speed of definitive treatment and biliary decompression. Following creation of a biliary to intestinal diversion, bacterial cholangitis should be anticipated as a complicating problem.

When suppurative cholangitis is suspected, cultures for aerobic and anaerobic bacteria should be requested from one or more of the following specimens: biliary secretions,

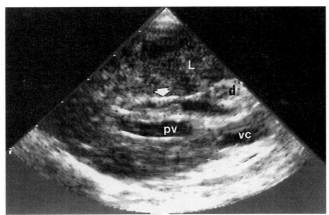

FIGURE 37-19. Ultrasonogram showing an area of the porta hepatis in a cat with suppurative cholangitis/cholangiohepatitis. A thickened wall of the common bile duct (arrow) and the presence of biliary sludge or an exudate in the lumen is visualized. The hepatic parenchymal echogenicity is coarse (L) and the liver margins were rounded. Landmarks include the duodenum (d), portal vein (pv), and vena cava (vc). (Courtesy Dr. A. Yeager, Section of Radiology, Department of Clinical Sciences, College of Veterinary Medicine, Cornell University)

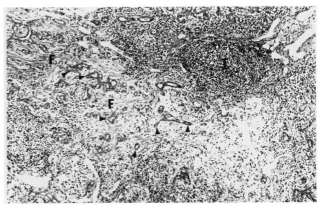

FIGURE 37-21. Photomicrograph of a liver biopsy from a cat with chronic suppurative cholangiohepatitis. Biliary ductule proliferation (arrowheads), fibrosis (F), and focal accumulation of a mixed inflammatory infiltrate (I) are seen (H&E stain). (Courtesy Dr. P. Rowland, Department of Pathology, College of Veterinary Medicine, Cornell University)

gallbladder wall, choleliths, and liver tissue. Cytologic evaluation of biliary secretions and liver imprints should be done as soon as possible. If bacteria are observed, a gram stain will facilitate optimal selection of antibiotics during the initial postoperative interval. Bacterial organisms are more easily visualized on cytologic preparations as compared to histopathologic sections (Figure 37-22). Prior treatment with

antibiotics may result in negative cultures despite cytologic visualization of bacteria.

Treatment with an appropriate antibiotic, cholelith removal, biliary tree decompression as indicated, maintenance of normal fluid and electrolyte balance, and use of ursodeoxycholic acid as a choleretic are advised for patients with suppurative cholangitis/cholangiohepatitis. Ursodeoxycholic acid is given at a dose of 10 to 15 mg/kg PO SID and is used preferentially over dehydrocholic acid (Decholin). This therapy is *only* given when bile duct obstruction has been eliminated. Initial antibiotic therapy should cover the broad

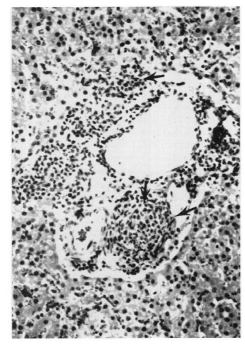

FIGURE 37-20. Photomicrograph of a liver biopsy from a cat with suppurative cholangiohepatitis showing a portal triad and surrounding hepatocytes. The bile ducts (arrows) are surrounded and filled with neutrophils. Suppurative inflammation is extending out of the portal triad and into the surrounding hepatic parenchyma (H&E stain). (Courtesy Dr. P. Rowland, Department of Pathology, College of Veterinary Medicine, Cornell University)

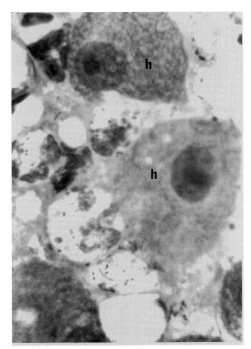

FIGURE 37-22. Photomicrograph of an impression smear made from the hepatic biopsy from a cat with suppurative cholangiohepatitis. Hepatocytes (h) are shown with adjacent neutrophils containing bacterial organisms. Culture was positive for *E. coli* and *Actinomyces*. Histopathology did not disclose the presence of microorganisms (modified Wright's-Giemsa, 900×).

spectrum of enteric organisms that may be involved. Combination therapy with an aminoglycoside, penicillin, and metronidazole or clindamycin is recommended as initial therapy. Recently, vancomycin was reported to be successful in treatment of a cat with suppurative cholangitis associated with *Enterobacter*.[174] Antimicrobial therapy should be ultimately tailored on the basis of organisms identified on culture. Prognosis is usually good if the animal survives the immediate postoperative interval (48 hours). Normalization of biochemical abnormalities may occur within 4 weeks. Treatment with antibiotics for several months (3 to 6 months) is advised. If no underlying cause for cholelithiasis is identified, chronic treatment with ursodeoxycholic acid is recommended for its hydrocholeretic influence. If liver enzyme activity remains increased, and especially if an inflammatory leukogram persists, continued suppurative inflammation should be suspected. Ultrasound-guided cholecystocentesis can be used for sampling bile for cytology and repeat bacterial culture (consult section on cholecystocentesis). It is suspected, but has not been proven, that septic inflammation evolves into a chronic lymphocytic or lymphoplasmacytic inflammatory process. If nonsuppurative inflammation is verified, treatment with anti-inflammatory drugs is appropriate. In some cats with suppurative cholangitis, an abscess in another organ, such as the spleen, has been an underlying problem. In these cases, the source of chronic infection must be vigorously treated.

Nonsuppurative Cholangitis/Cholangiohepatitis

Clinical Synopsis

Diagnostic Features

- Cats predisposed
- Duration of illness usually long (>2 weeks)
- Jaundice, hepatomegaly, vomiting, and diarrhea common
- High-protein abdominal effusion occasionally seen
- Liver enzymes mildly to moderately increased
- Lymphocytosis and hyperglobulinemia occasional in lymphocytic form
- Biopsy reveals lymphocytic or mixed lympho-plasmacytic periductal infiltration

Standard Treatment

- Attend to any underlying cause (e.g., IBD, pancreatitis)
- Glucocorticoids (2–4 mg/kg/day decreasing over 3 months to lowest dose needed for remission)
- Metronidazole (7.5 mg/kg PO, BID) for 2–4 weeks or indefinitely
- Ursodeoxycholic acid (10–15 mg/kg PO, SID) for 2–3 months or indefinitely
- High-fiber diet

Animals with nonsuppurative cholangitis/cholangiohepatitis have either a mixed lymphoplasmacytic inflammatory infiltrate or a pure lymphocytic infiltrate. There have been several reports that have characterized nonsuppurative cholangitis in the cat and one case series including 21 cats.[161,175–177] These in combination with 60 cats reviewed in the author's hospital have characterized the disorder.[173]

Lymphoplasmacytic Cholangitis/Cholangiohepatitis

Cats with lymphoplasmacytic cholangitis/cholangiohepatitis range in age between 2 and 17 years. Most are middle aged and have been ill 3 weeks or longer. Infection with FeLV is uncommon. There is no sex or breed predisposition. Hepatomegaly occurs in 50% and most are jaundiced. Although diarrhea and/or vomiting are clinical signs displayed by 60%, these cats generally are not profoundly lethargic and some have remarkably good appetites. Hyperthyroidism has been discounted in these cats on the basis of baseline T_4 concentrations. In the author's hospital very few cats have developed abdominal effusion.

Common concurrent disorders in cats include cholecystitis, pancreatitis, extrahepatic bile duct obstruction, and inflammatory bowel disease. In some cats, cholangitis has been the only disease process identified.

Cats in this group tend to have greater magnitudes of increased ALT, AST, ALP, and GGT than cats with pure lymphocytic cholangitis. Some have concurrent bacterial infection of the biliary tree. Cytologic impression smears of liver tissue or bile cannot definitively diagnose mixed nonsuppurative cholangitis/cholangiohepatitis. Rather, it is useful in ruling out a major suppurative and septic component.

Ultrasonographic evaluation of these cats often discloses diffuse or blotchy hepatic hyperechogenicity and sometimes thickening of the walls of biliary structures.

Hepatic histology details a mixed lymphoplasmacytic inflammatory infiltrate surrounding and invading portal triads (Figure 37–23). Bile duct epithelium is focally invaded by inflammatory cells. In some bile ducts, epithelial cell vacuolation and dropout is observed leading to a generalized reduction in the number of the medium- and small-sized bile ductules (Figure 37–24). With severe and apparently chronic inflammation, bridging portal fibrosis develops and progresses to biliary cirrhosis, although cirrhosis is an uncommon occurrence.

Lymphocytic Cholangitis/Cholangiohepatitis

Cats with lymphocytic cholangitis/cholangiohepatitis range in age between 1 and 16 years although most are older

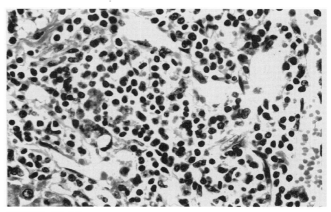

FIGURE 37-23. Photomicrograph of a liver biopsy from a cat with nonsuppurative lymphoplasmacytic cholangiohepatitis. This high-power view shows the mixed infiltrate in a portal triad (H&E stain). (Courtesy Dr. P. Rowland, Department of Pathology, College of Veterinary Medicine, Cornell University)

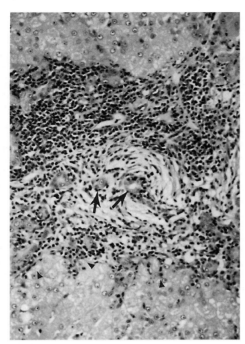

FIGURE 37-24. Photomicrograph of a liver biopsy from the same cat as shown in Figure 37-23. Portal infiltration with inflammatory cells, periductal edema, and duct epithelial dropout (arrows) are shown. Invasion of the surrounding hepatic parenchyma with inflammatory cells is obvious (small arrowheads). This cat had a subjective paucity of medium-sized bile ducts on review of its entire biopsy specimen (H&E eosin stain). (Courtesy Dr. P. Rowland, Department of Pathology, College of Veterinary Medicine, Cornell University)

than 9 years of age. Duration of illness ranges between 2 weeks and several years; most are ill 2 months or more. None have been FeLV infected. Hepatomegaly, jaundice, vomiting, and/or diarrhea develop in 70%. In the author's hospital, very few of these cats have developed abdominal effusion. In a prior report, ascites was one of the most common presenting signs seen in 11 of 21 cats.[175] That report also described generalized lymph node enlargement in 5 of 21 cats. Ascitic fluid had a high total protein concentration attributable largely to globulins.

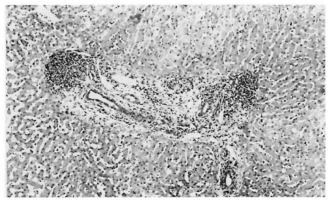

FIGURE 37-25. Photomicrograph of a liver biopsy from a cat with lymphocytic cholangiohepatitis showing a portal triad structure. Lymphoid follicles and a moderate diffuse periductular infiltration with lymphocytes are seen. An impression of increased connective tissue deposition was confirmed by application of a trichrome stain. There is minimal infiltration of inflammatory cells into the adjacent

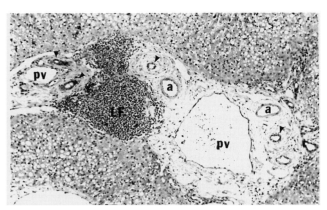

FIGURE 37-26. Photomicrograph of a liver biopsy from a cat with lymphocytic cholangiohepatitis showing a lymphoid follicle (LF) in a portal triad. There is periductal fibrosis and a suggestion of ductopenia with minimal residual periductal inflammation (hepatic artery (a), portal vein (pv), bile ducts (arrowheads). The portal triad has an increased deposition of connective tissue. A moderate diffuse hepatic vacuolation with lipid is also present. Application of an immunoperoxidase stain for biliary cytokeratins confirmed the minimal residual biliary epithelial structures (H&E stain). (Courtesy Dr. P. Rowland, Department of Pathology, College of Veterinary Medicine, Cornell University)

Cats with lymphocytic inflammation have variable WBC counts, but some of these have had the highest WBC counts seen in cats with the cholangitis/cholangiohepatitis syndrome. Some cats have had a remarkable lymphocytosis (> 14,000/μL); lymphocyte morphology and bone marrow evaluations could not confirm lymphosarcoma in these. Cats in this group comparatively have the most modest increases in hepatic transaminase and GGT activities. Approximately 50% are hyperglobulinemic. In a prior report, serum protein electrophoresis showed a prominent gamma globulin peak in 5 of 7 cats.[175] IgG was shown to be the principal globulin detected. Testing for serologic markers of autoimmunity (ANA, and antibodies to mitochondria, smooth muscle, thyroid, and parietal cells) was negative except for one weak positive ANA.[175] Cats with lymphocytic inflammation are the only cats observed to develop symptomatic coagulopathies.[173]

Common concurrent disorders include inflammatory bowel disease, chronic pancreatitis, cholecystitis, and extrahepatic bile duct occlusion. Some cats have had chronic bacterial infections or inflammatory conditions centered elsewhere in their bodies.

Hepatic histology is characterized by a periportal lymphocytic infiltrate associated with bile duct hypertrophy and hyperplasia (Figure 37-25). Lymphocytes are small and do not have morphology consistent with lymphoma. Deposition of connective tissue around and bridging between portal triads is obvious when the condition becomes chronic (Figure 37-26). In some cats, small bile ducts diminish in number, and in some, residual lipogranulomatous foci remain (Figures 37-26 and 37-27). A variable involvement of portal triads is observed. Some areas demonstrate active ongoing injury and others lack active inflammation and demonstrate the residual tissue injury (ductopenia). Application of a cytokeratin stain specific for biliary epithelium has confirmed the absence of bile duct epithelium in the midst of periportal lymphocytic infiltrates in some cats. Portal hypertension has been detected on abdominal ultrasound in some cats due to venous congestion caused by impaired flow at the level of the porta hepatis. Some have had portal hypertension associated with biliary cirrhosis and ascites. Organisms have been

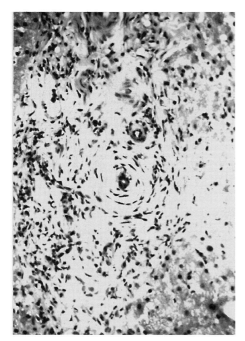

FIGURE 37-27. Photomicrograph of a liver biopsy from a cat with lymphocytic cholangiohepatitis showing the consequent ductopenia that develops in some cats. These bile ducts are representative of the small- and medium-sized biliary ductules in this cat. An inflammatory component is absent; the ductopenia is believed to represent the residual tissue injury. Other areas of the biopsy specimen revealed active ongoing periductal inflammation (H&E stain). (Courtesy Dr. P. Rowland, Department of Pathology, College of Veterinary Medicine, Cornell University)

isolated from tissue and bile cultures in very few of these cats. Cytologic evaluation of liver and bile is rarely diagnostic.

Pathogenesis of Nonsuppurative Cholangitis/Cholangiohepatitis Syndrome

Lymphocytic and lymphoplasmacytic cholangitis represents tissue response to chronic, nonseptic injury. The most common historical complaints in cats affected with this syndrome are vomiting and/or diarrhea. Most cats are insidiously and chronically ill. Although evaluation for inflammatory bowel disease and pancreatitis has not been thorough in every cat reported to date, they appear to be common associated conditions. Pyogranulomatous cholangiohepatitis was reported in one cat that had immune-complex glomerulonephritis. This case links immune disturbances in other systems with biliary tree injury.[178] Recently, a form of primary hepatic lymphosarcoma has been described in humans in which small lymphocytes are the predominant infiltrate.[179-183] Immunocytologic characterization indicates that these are usually T cell–rich B cell lymphomas.[183] It is undetermined whether some cats with lymphocytic cholangitis have a similar syndrome.

INFLAMMATORY BOWEL DISEASE. An association between inflammatory bowel disease and liver disease is well established in humans.[184-186] The most common lesions include pericholangitis (small duct sclerosing cholangitis), primary sclerosing cholangitis, and development of cirrhosis and cholangiocarcinoma. The pericholangitis observed in cats with nonsuppurative cholangitis/cholangiohepatitis appears similar to the portal triaditis seen in humans with inflammatory bowel disease.

In humans, liver lesions can precede or follow recognition of inflammatory bowel symptomatology. Lesions seem to be independent of the severity of bowel disease. Their pathogenesis has not been clearly defined. Proposed mechanisms include low-grade portal bacteremia, iatrogenic drug injury, and genetic and/or immunologic factors. The clinical, clinicopathologic, and pathologic characteristics of the human disease are quite similar to the findings in cats with nonsuppurative cholangiohepatitis.

PANCREATITIS. Pancreatitis is also seemingly associated with this syndrome. In dogs with experimental and spontaneous chronic pancreatitis, lymphoid "portal triaditis" is common.[187] The etiologic factors associated with pancreatitis in cats have not been clearly defined. Pancreatitis could occur by retrograde passage of duodenal organisms into the pancreatic duct. Inflammatory bowel disease could be associated with pancreatitis as a result of transient pancreatic duct occlusion, hematogenous or transmural dissemination of inflammatory mediators into the pancreatic microcirculation, or retrograde passage of infectious or inflammatory substances up the pancreatic duct. Obstruction of the distal portion of the common bile duct, such as by a gallstone, can induce pancreatitis by occluding the pancreatic duct at the time of maximal pancreatic secretion. Obstruction of the distal portion of the common bile duct also could promote bile reflux into the pancreas. Although choleliths are uncommonly recognized in cats, sludged or inspissated bile is not, and so this relationship remains possible although speculative. Pancreatic lesions and cholangitis in the cat have also been reported with infectious disorders including trematode and protozoal infections (toxoplasmosis).[188-192]

INFECTIOUS DISORDERS. Infection with toxoplasmosis, a coccidia-like organism (possibly this was toxoplasmosis), *Hepatozoan*, cytauxzoonosis, Tyzzer's disease, and feline immunodeficiency virus have been described in cats with cholangiohepatitis.[188-194] Cholangiohepatitis has also been recognized in association with bacterial infections in dogs including Campylobacter, Salmonellosis, and Leptospirosis. Liver flukes in cats also can produce cholangitis and major bile duct inflammation and obstruction. The clinical manifestations of liver fluke infestation are described separately in the next section of this chapter.

EXTRAHEPATIC BILE DUCT OBSTRUCTION, CHOLECYSTITIS, AND CHOLELITHIASIS. Bile duct obstruction, cholelithiasis, and cholecystitis are also associated with the cholangitis/cholangiohepatitis complex. It is possible that initial injury of the biliary tree transforms into an immune-mediated inflammatory process. It is also possible that an immune-mediated cholangitis could progress to involve the major bile ducts and gallbladder. Immunologic reactions are well recognized to be involved in almost all types of chronic inflammatory liver disease in humans, although whether they are causal or an epiphenomenon has not been definitively established in all instances.[195] See Chapter 33 for a discussion of the immunoregulatory disturbances associated with chronic hepatobiliary disorders.

VANISHING BILE DUCT SYNDROMES. A number of disorders characterized in humans share the histologic feature of vanishing bile ducts. These syndromes are classified into developmental, immunologic, infectious, vascular, or chemical origins and according to the size of the involved ducts (Table 37–5).[196,197] A subset of cats with nonsuppurative cholangitis/cholangiohepatitis have been found to have disappearing small-to medium-sized bile ducts.[173,176,177] Several of these cats have had lymphocytic inflammation in their pancreas.

Three types of vanishing bile duct syndromes in dogs have been reported.[198-200] Spontaneous loss of bile ducts in the small portal triads was characterized in 7 dogs seen as clinical

Table 37–5

CLASSIFICATION OF BILE DUCT DISEASE IN HUMANS BY SIZE AND MECHANISM[196]

CONDITION	BILE DUCTS INJURED	MECHANISM
Primary biliary cirrhosis	Small ducts	Immunologic
Graft-versus-host	Small ducts	Immunologic
Hepatic transplant rejection	Small ducts	Immunologic
Sarcoidosis	Small ducts	Immunologic
Idiopathic inflantile ductopenia	Small ducts	Genetic/infectious ?
Idiopathic adult ductopenia	Small ducts	Infections/immunologic ?
Idiosyncratic drug induced	Small ducts	Idiosyncratic/immunologic
Vascular cholangitis	Small or large ducts	Ischemic
Primary sclerosing cholangitis	Small or large ducts	Immunologic/infection
Extrahepatic bile duct obstruction	Largel ducts	Mechanical
Bacterial cholangitis	Small and large ducts	Infection

patients.[198] There was minimal inflammation associated with this lesion. Dogs ranged in age from 2 to 11 years (median 6 years) and the duration of clinical signs ranged between 2 weeks to 4 months (median 5 weeks). Common clinical signs included anorexia, lethargy, weight loss, and jaundice. Acholic feces were observed in 4 of 7, vomiting in 3 of 7, and polydipsia in 2 of 7. Hematologic findings were variable. All dogs had increased transaminase and cholestatic enzyme activities. The authors speculated that lesions resembled those seen with adverse drug reactions, such as phenothiazines. Only two dogs had recently received medication; one had been given trimethoprim-sulfa for 1 week before onset of clinical signs and the other had been given diphenylsulphon (Dapsone) 9 weeks before clinical signs.

Vascular injury to radicals of the hepatic artery supplying bile ducts can induce destructive cholangitis. This leads to necrosis of bile duct epithelium. Protracted hepatic arterial infusions of floxuridine, a chemotherapy agent, administered through an implanted drug delivery system causes such lesions in humans and in dogs.[199] Four to 6 weeks after initiation of drug infusion in dogs, focal strictures involving central bile ducts and diffuse attenuation of the intrahepatic ducts develops.

Among the many and diverse disorders associated with vanishing bile ducts in humans are several that are known or are speculated to involve immune-mediated mechanisms. Granulomatous destruction of small bile ducts is a hallmark of sarcoidosis, an autoimmune disease of humans. The liver is only one of many tissues that may be involved.

An immune-mediated hepatic disorder of humans that shares some features with the nonsuppurative cholangitis/cholangiohepatitis syndrome in cats is primary biliary cirrhosis.[177] This is a chronic, progressive, and usually fatal cholestatic liver disorder affecting middle-aged women. In the early stages of primary biliary cirrhosis, there is an obvious symmetric destruction of septal and interlobular bile ducts. Damaged ducts are usually densely surrounded by lymphocytes. Granulomas develop in the portal triads. With chronicity, the number of normal bile ducts in portal triads declines and many remaining bile ducts appear deformed. Eventually, bridging fibrosis progresses to biliary cirrhosis. An absence of bile ducts in portal triads in a cirrhotic liver suggests this disease. There are a large number of immunologic abnormalities in these patients but no direct proof of an autoimmune or immune-mediated disease mechanism.

Idiosyncratic (drug-induced) destructive cholangitis has been associated with administration of acetaminophen, chlorpromazine, cromolyn sodium, haloperidol, imipramine, methyltestosterone, phenylbutazone, and tolbutamide. Some of these drug reactions are immunologically mediated.

Other types of ductal injury are also recognized, although the mechanism of injury is not always fully understood. Bacterial cholangitis can lead to bile duct damage as a result of neutrophilic infiltration, enzyme release, and epithelial destruction. Ultimately the bile duct is replaced by fibrous tissue which resembles that of primary sclerosing cholangitis. Fluke infestation can cause similar lesions. Biliary atresia in infants (idiopathic infantile ductopenia) is believed to be a congenital disorder in some cases and acquired in others. The ductopenia is believed to be a postinflammatory condition. Some cases are genetically linked and others are thought to be associated with cytopathic viruses that have a tropism for immature bile duct epithelium. Idiopathic adulthood ductopenia is an unusual disorder associated with a history and laboratory profile of chronic cholestatic liver disease, histologic evidence of ductopenia, and normal cholangiography. These patients may have an atypical form of sclerosing cholangitis.

ATYPICAL PRIMARY HEPATIC LYMPHOMA. Recently, recognition of non-Hodgkins lymphoma presenting as a primary tumor of the liver has been described in humans.[179–183] Although many of these patients have solitary tumor masses in the liver, some have small-cell lymphoma that has been initially diagnosed as nonspecific inflammation, primary biliary cirrhosis, or chronic active hepatitis. Some of these patients have diffuse lymphocytic infiltrates surrounding and invading the portal triads. In a few cases, bone marrow evaluation has disclosed the presence of neoplastic cells. On the basis of immunocytologic staining of liver tissue, T cell–rich B cell lymphoma has been shown. The neoplastic B cells are few in number and have been suggested to elaborate cytokines that have stimulatory effects on T cells.[183] Combination chemotherapy for lymphoma has been used to attain remission in some patients. Specific immunocytologic markers for differentiating lymphocytes in cats have not yet been evaluated in cats with severe lymphocytic cholangitis. The possibility of lymphoma should be considered when there is an absence of fibroplasia and bile duct destruction on histopathologic evaluation of liver biopsy showing dense periportal lymphocytic infiltration (Figures 37–28 and 37–29). The suspicion of an underlying neoplastic condition is increased when conventional therapy fails to improve a cat's condition or clinicopathologic markers of disease. Combination chemotherapy is appropriate for cats with confirmed lymphoma but also may be useful in cats with lymphocytic cholangiohepatitis if conventional therapy fails. This treat-

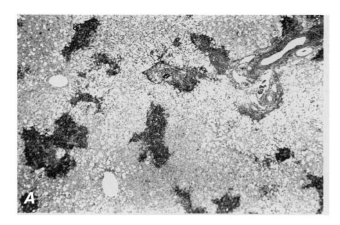

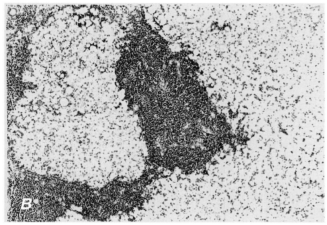

FIGURE 37-28. Photomicrographs of a liver biopsy from a cat with hepatic lymphosarcoma. *(A)* a lower power and *(B)* a higher power perspective is presented. A dense mantle of lymphocytes is observed around portal triads. Bile duct hyperplasia was moderate. In this case, the monomorphic appearance of the lymphocytes (Figure 37–29) and documentation of bone marrow involvement confirmed the diagnoses. (Courtesy Dr. P. Rowland, Department of Pathology, College of Veterinary Medicine, Cornell University)

ment alternative may produce remission due to non-neoplastic immunoinjury but should be considered as a last resort until further studies of its efficacy are evaluated.

Treatment for Nonsuppurative Cholangitis/Cholangiohepatitis

Considering the underlying or associated disorders, any cat with nonsuppurative cholangitis should be evaluated for extrahepatic bile duct obstruction, cholelithiasis, pancreatitis, inflammatory bowel disease, and other nonhepatic sites of chronic bacterial infection. In dogs, chronic pancreatic disease and inflammatory bowel disease seem most commonly associated with both suppurative and nonsuppurative portal triaditis. Both septicemia and infectious gastroenteritis can cause acute periportal inflammation. These relationships should be fully explored and therapeutically managed.

The histologic lesions of nonsuppurative inflammation indicate cell-mediated immunoinjury. The following discussion of therapeutic options focuses on disease in the cat, which is far more common than in the dog. Similar therapeutic considerations would apply to the dog.

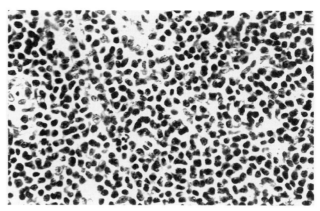

FIGURE 37-29. A photomicrograph of a high-power magnification of the lymphocytic infiltrate in the cat shown in Figure 37–26. Lymphosarcoma was confirmed in this case. (Courtesy Dr. P. Rowland, Department of Pathology, College of Veterinary Medicine, Cornell University)

Intervention with an immunosuppressive dose of glucocorticoids (4 mg/kg/day for cats, 2mg/kg/day for dogs) has resulted in solid remission in very few instances. Glucocorticoids provide some degree of choleresis and also may be beneficial in managing a coexistent inflammatory bowel disease. Concurrent treatment with metronidazole, at an empirically reduced dose to avoid toxicity due to impaired hepatic metabolism (7.5 mg/kg PO BID), has been used in combination with glucocorticoids. Metronidazole is selected in an attempt to modulate cell-mediated immune mechanisms involved with the chronic inflammation. This may benefit both the cholangitis and an associated inflammatory bowel disorder.

Ursodeoxycholic acid is added to the treatment regimen to modulate the accumulated "noxious" bile acids, to produce a choleresis, and to provide an anti-inflammatory influence. Ursodeoxycholic acid has been shown to reduce expression of the class 2 histocompatibility foci on the surface of hepatocytes/bile duct epithelium, considered essential for continued self-perpetuating immunoinjury. Actigal capsules (Ciba Geigy; 300 mg capsules) may be compounded into 30 mg gel capsules for once a day administration to cats. A dose ranging between 10 to 15 mg/kg is prescribed. Actigal has not been associated with any adverse effects in dogs or cats with liver disease. It is imperative that extrahepatic bile duct obstruction is rectified or ruled out before Actigal is prescribed.

If hyperbilirubinemia is severe and the cat is passing acholic feces, injectable vitamin K_1 is given intramuscularly every 14 to 21 days at a dose of 1.5 to 5 mg. This is done over concern for fat soluble vitamin malabsorption. Oral vitamin K may not be well absorbed in the absence of adequate enteric bile salts. Malabsorption of fat soluble vitamins has been documented in humans with sclerosing cholangitis and biliary cirrhosis. Care must be taken to avoid overdosing an animal with vitamin K because it can cause hemolytic anemia associated with formation of heinz bodies. Supplementary water soluble vitamins are also given on a daily basis. Nutritional intake is modified to a diet supplemented with soluble and insoluble fiber. This benefits not only the liver disease but may also assist in management of inflammatory bowel disease and avoidance of recurrent pancreatitis.

A restricted protein diet as formulated for renal insufficiency is not appropriate for these cats, especially if they have inflammatory bowel disease or pancreatitis as associated conditions. Signs of hepatic encephalopathy are extremely rare in these patients and thus a protein-restricted diet is not advocated. Protein restriction may impair regenerative capabilities and make a cat more susceptible to development of hepatic lipidosis. If hepatic cytology or histology reveals vacuolated hepatocytes consistent with hepatic lipidosis, supplemental taurine (250 to 500 mg PO per day) and L-carnitine (250 mg PO per day) are usually given for the first several weeks along with strict attention that the cat consumes an adequate caloric intake.

Antibiotics are usually continued until it is clear there is no bacterial infection requiring continued treatment. If inflammatory bowel disease is an ongoing problem, antibiotics may be necessary to provide protection against portal bacteremia and biliary sepsis.

Only a few cats attain full remission on glucocorticoid therapy. Rarely, a cat may be able to be weaned completely off immunosuppressive therapy. The poor control of this syndrome with glucocorticoids has led to the investigation of other immunomodulatory drug regimens. Many different modes of treatment have been tried in clinical trials of humans with sclerosing cholangitis and primary biliary cirrhosis. These have included studies of systemic glucocorticoids, high-dose pulse methylprednisolone, nasobiliary administered glucocorticoids, D-penicillamine, cyclosporine, methotrexate, azathioprine, and glucocorticoids in combination with colchicine and ursodeoxycholic acid. Experience with azathioprine has not been very rewarding because cats become inappetant and can develop leukopenia with very small doses (0.3 mg/kg PO SID) given on every other or every third day. Low-dose weekly pulse methotrexate has recently been reported to result in improved biochemical parameters, stabilization of bile duct injury, and to markedly improve liver histology in small numbers of humans with sclerosing cholangitis and primary biliary cirrhosis. Clinical trials of high-dose pulse methylprednisolone and low-dose pulse methotrexate (total dose of 0.4 mg divided into three treatments over 24 hours; e.g., 0, 12, 24 hours) are in process in cats that have failed to substantially improve on glucocorticoids and metronidazole. Methotrexate use is not without some risk; it has been associated with hepatotoxicity in human beings treated daily for a variety of immune-mediated disorders (rheumatoid arthritis, inflammatory bowel disease, psoriasis). Use of methotrexate in these cats is not recommended for initial management and if used, must be accompanied by an explanation to the owner that it is an investigational form of therapy.

It will probably be a long time before an effective form of treatment for this feline syndrome is firmly established. The biologic behavior of the nonsuppurative cholangitis/cholangiohepatitis syndrome has a fluctuating nature and the lesions appear to be very slowly progressive. Survival is widely variable without treatment, some cats surviving for 6 years or more with fluctuating liver enzyme activity and minimal clinical signs.

LIVER FLUKES

Clinical Synopsis

Diagnostic Features

- Travel of cats to tropical areas (Florida)
- Jaundice, hepatomegaly, and abdominal distension may be seen
- Fluke eggs in feces

- Eosinophilia and clinicopathologic evidence of cholestasis common

Standard Treatment

- Treatment is ill defined
- Albendazole (50 mg/kg/day) until fluke eggs disappear from feces may be valuable

Several different digenetic trematodes have been found in domestic cats in the United States that can cause biliary tree injury. The trematode species that have been reported are shown in Table 37–6.[189,201–213] Infection in the pancreatic ducts has also been observed.

Platynosomum concinnum has been reported to cause hepatic disease in domesticated cats. This parasite is primarily found in tropical areas, although it has been reported in cats from the continental United States. A land snail is the first intermediate host. Subsequent development occurs in either a reptile or amphibian. Following ingestion by a cat, the infective stage of the fluke migrates up the common bile duct into the gallbladder and bile ducts where it matures into the adult fluke in 8 to 12 weeks. Embryonated eggs are passed in bile into the alimentary canal and can be detected in feces (Figure 37–30). Progressive clinical signs in cats with naturally acquired platynosomiasis have included weight loss, anorexia, vomiting, mucoid diarrhea, jaundice, hepatomegaly, emaciation, and abdominal distension. Severely affected cats die as a result of chronic fluke infestation. Some animals, however, are asymptomatic. The 21 month clinical course of small (125 flukes per cat) and large (1000 flukes per cat) dose infection of healthy cats with *Platynosomum concinnum* has been studied.[201] Clinical signs attributable to fluke infection were observed in 5 of 8 cats given high-but not low-dose infection. Observed signs were first notable between 7 to 16 weeks after infection and included anorexia, lethargy, weight loss, and abdominal tenderness. All symptomatic cats returned to normal clinical health by 24 weeks postinfection. Three of 8 cats did not develop obvious clinical signs. None of the cats became febrile, and none displayed vomiting or diarrhea. Fluke ova were detected in feces from several cats as early as 8 weeks after infection. All infected cats passed fluke ova by 12 weeks postinfestation at which time embryonated ova appeared. The number of recoverable ova in feces gradually decreased

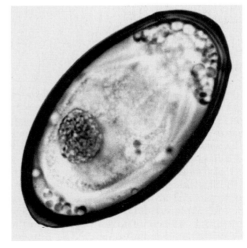

FIGURE 37–30. Photomicrograph showing the characteristics of a trematode egg harvested from stool. These can also be found in bile; see Figure 37–31.

after 4 months of infection. Hematologic changes included an increase in the circulating eosinophils 3 weeks after infection. In some male cats given small doses of flukes, eosinophilia was not apparent until 14 weeks of infection. A circulating eosinophilia was maintained throughout the following 9 month interval. Increased serum activity of ALT and AST developed in large-dose cats between 3 to 10 weeks postinfection. Only a small increase in ALT and AST activity developed in cats given small doses of flukes; these normalized within 3 months. The serum activity of ALP remained within the normal range throughout the study. Hyperbilirubinemia developed in cats in the high-dose group at 7 to 16 weeks of infection.

Hepatobiliary lesions were not discernible until 3 weeks of infection. Initial changes occurred in the biliary epithelium, which assumed a columnar rather than normal cuboidal appearance. At 6 weeks of infection, inflammation and distension of the proximal bile ducts was obvious. A neutrophilic and eosinophilic infiltrate characterized the inflammatory changes. With chronicity, bile ducts throughout the liver were affected in both the low- and high-dose infected cats. Severe adenomatous hyperplasia of bile duct epithelium and periductal inflammation was present by 4 months of infection. By 6 months, extensive fibrous connective tissue encircled bile ducts. The liver parenchyma remained unaffected in low- and high-dose affected cats, except for one cat that developed some degree of lipidosis. Enlarged mesenteric and hepatic lymph nodes developed in some cats. Flukes were recovered from bile ducts and gallbladder of all infected cats. In clinical cases, chronic fluke infection is associated with bile duct fibrosis and distension and biliary epithelial hyperplasia (Figure 37–31). Biliary cirrhosis occurs with chronicity and is associated with a periductal infiltrate comprised of histiocytes, plasma cells, and lymphocytes. Small numbers of neutrophils and eosinophils may also be seen. Occasionally, adult flukes and fluke eggs are visualized (Figure 37–31). The experimental work has shown a correlation between the developmental stages of the parasite in the liver and the clinical manifestations. Bile duct distension increases with growth of adult flukes. Upon sexual maturation of the flukes, bile ducts containing parasites become fibrotic and the serum transaminase activities normalize.

Given the absence of clinical signs in some infected cats, diagnosis of fluke infestation may be difficult. Fecal examination may fail to detect the parasite for several reasons, including (1) passage of only a small number of eggs daily, (2) passage of eggs with variable morphology (immature and mature eggs), (3) the small size of the eggs, and (4) the inefficiency of detecting eggs through direct smears and routine fecal screening procedures. Cholecystocentesis has been used to document the presence of fluke eggs in cats where the index of suspicion for fluke infestation was high (signs of cholestatic liver injury, travel history to Florida or another tropical climate, and an opportunity to hunt the intermediate host).

Treatment of platynosomiasis is ill defined. Praziquantel and nitroscanate catrodifene resulted in an initial increase in egg passage but was followed by a reduced and then sporadic egg production. The efficacy of albendazole and fenbendazole remains unclear. Albendazole has been used at a dose of 50 mg/kg/day to clear *Paragonimus* pulmonary infections from cats. The drug is administered until fluke eggs disappear from feces. Treated cats should be observed for albendazole-associated bone marrow toxicity when doses of 50 mg/kg PO, SID are administered for more than 5 consecutive days.

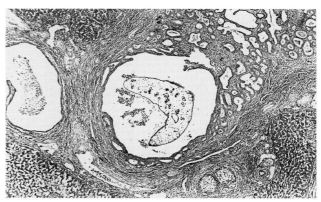

FIGURE 37–31. Photomicrograph of a liver biopsy from a cat with liver disease attributed to a fluke infestation. A fluke is shown within a distended bile duct that has hyperplastic epithelium. Adenomatous hyperplasia of the biliary structures and peribiliary fibrosis was extensive. Eggs can be seen in the bile duct with the fluke. Eggs would have been seen in a sample of bile from this cat (H&E stain). (Courtesy Dr. P. Rowland, Department of Pathology, College of Veterinary Medicine, Cornell University)

BILIARY CIRRHOSIS

Biliary cirrhosis is the end-stage liver lesion that can evolve from any disorder causing protracted inflammation of the intrahepatic biliary tree (Figures 37–32 and 37–33). It can develop in dogs and cats subjected to extrahepatic bile duct occlusion of 6 weeks or longer and is usually associated with hepatomegaly, which is surprising considering the extent of tissue injury that has occurred. Dogs develop portal hypertension and portosystemic collaterals within 6 to 10 weeks following acute complete bile duct occlusion. Cats with the cholangitis/cholangiohepatitis syndrome are uncommonly seen with well-developed cirrhosis. These animals seem to succumb to their disease before cirrhosis is florid. Synthetic failure, hepatic encephalopathy, and formation of ascites seem uncommon in cats compared to dogs with cirrhosis.

No matter the cause, once biliary cirrhosis is established, the lobular architecture and hepatic microcirculation is permanently altered. Recognition and arrest of biliary tract disease can avert progression to biliary cirrhosis. Biliary tract enteric diversion is one means to palliate obstructive common duct disease to avoid this sequela.

CYSTIC HEPATOBILIARY DISORDERS

Congenital and acquired hepatic cysts derived from ductular epithelium have been seen in both dogs and cats.[214–222] It is thought that most hepatic cysts are of ductular origin, arising from one or more primitive bile ducts lacking a connection with the biliary tract. These subsequently develop into retention cysts. Cysts may be either solitary or multiple (polycystic). The polycystic condition may be associated with cystic lesions in other organs, most notably the kidneys. Cysts vary in size from a few millimeters to several centimeters (Figure 37–34). Most are asymptomatic, although symptoms may develop owing to encroachment of cystic structures on normal tissues or organs. Rarely, fluid may accumulate in the peritoneal cavity as a consequence of cyst rupture or portal hypertension resulting from impingement of the portal vasculature. Cyst contents are usually clear but sometimes may contain bile or blood. Cysts containing blood or bile-contami-

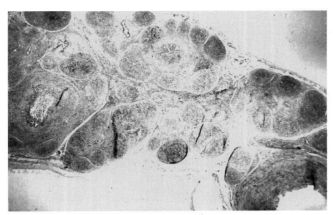

FIGURE 37–32. Low-power magnification of the liver of a cat with chronic lymphocytic cholangitis/cholangiohepatitis that has progressed to cirrhosis. Bridging fibrosis and nodular regeneration have replaced the normal hepatic architecture. The dark nuclei are foci of lymphocytes involved with ongoing inflammation. This cat had demonstrated clinical signs for more than 5 years (H&E stain). (Courtesy Dr. P. Rowland, Department of Pathology, College of Veterinary Medicine, Cornell University)

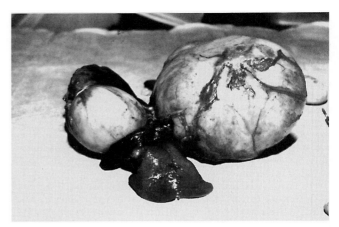

FIGURE 37–34. Photograph of large biliary cysts that developed in a cat. (Courtesy Dr. H. A. Miller)

nated fluid may be acquired lesions resulting from trauma, inflammation, or neoplasia. Acquired cysts are usually solitary, whereas congenital or developmental cysts are commonly multiple.

Occasionally, hepatic cysts become apparent when they cause a palpable abdominal mass. Hepatic insufficiency rarely develops because there usually is sufficient reserve tissue that remains unaffected. Confusion may exist in differentiating these masses from neoplasia unless abdominal ultrasonography or mass aspiration is performed.

Survey abdominal radiographs may reveal an irregular hepatic margin or focal densities if a few large cysts are present (Figure 37–35). Ultrasonographic evaluation readily demonstrates the cystic nature of these lesions and the extent of parenchymal or biliary tract involvement.

Treatment of biliary cysts is restricted until clinical signs are related to their presence. If a large cyst causes abdominal discomfort, impairs diaphragmatic motion, or appears to be causing pressure injury on normal tissues, the cyst should be aspirated. If fluid rapidly reaccumulates, repeated centesis or surgical removal of the cyst will be necessary. In some animals, this requires resection of a lobe of liver. If biliary cysts seem to be impinging on bile flow at the extrahepatic ducts, surgical excision or a biliary diversion should be done. Some cats have multiple biliary cysts within the common and hepatic bile ducts. This causes extrahepatic bile duct obstruction that cannot be corrected. Biliary cirrhosis gradually develops. Rarely, when large cysts cannot be surgically removed, creation of communication with the abdominal cavity may allow fluid efflux into the peritoneal cavity, relieving pressure on essential hepatic structures. However, if the cystic structure is producing a biliary type secretion, this is contraindicated.

Polycystic malformations in the kidney and liver have been documented as congenital or developmental abnormalities in Cairn terrier dogs and Persian cats during the first few months of life.[216,217] In severely affected animals, clinical features include abdominal enlargement due to organomegaly and insufficient renal function. When clinical signs develop during the first several months of life, the condition is usually lethal. In some Persian cats, the polycystic disorder is mild, does not cause overt symptoms, and is recognized as an incidental finding later in life. The polycystic disorder appears to

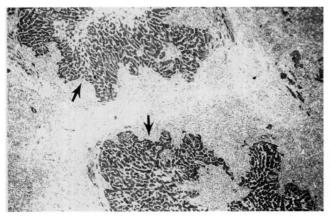

FIGURE 37–33. Low-power photomicrograph of liver tissue showing extensive loss of viable hepatocytes and massive connective tissue deposition. Only small islands of viable hepatocytes (arrows) remain. This cat had clinicopathologic features of cholangitis/cholangiohepatitis for more than 7 years (Masson's trichrome stain). (Courtesy Dr. P. Rowland, Department of Pathology, College of Veterinary Medicine, Cornell University)

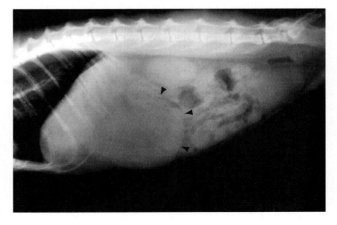

FIGURE 37–35. Radiograph of a cat with the large biliary cyst shown in Figure 37–34. The cyst extends caudal to the surface of the liver into the mid-abdominal region. Caudal margins of the cyst are marked by arrowheads. This cyst was managed with repeated centesis. (Courtesy Dr. H. A. Miller)

dental finding later in life. The polycystic disorder appears to be inheritable and runs a benign course in many affected animals.

REFERENCES

1. Evans HE, Christensen GC. Miller's Anatomy of the Dog. WB Saunders, Philadelphia, 1979.
2. Hueman DM, Moore EW, Vlahcevic ZR. Pathogenesis and dissolution of gallstones. In: Zakim D, Boyer TD (eds) Hepatology, a Textbook of Liver Disease. WB Saunders, Philadelphia, 1480–1516, 1990.
3. Rege RV, Moore EW. Evidence for H+ secretion by the canine gallbladder. Gastroenterology 92:281–289, 1987.
4. Scharschmidt BF. Bile formation and cholestasis. In: Zakim D, Boyer TD (eds) Hepatology, a Textbook of Liver Disease. WB Saunders, Philadelphia, 303–340, 1990.
5. Hogan WJ, Geenen JE, Dodds WJ. Dysmotility disturbances of the biliary tract: Classification, diagnosis, and treatment. Sem Liver Dis 7:302–310, 1987.
6. Shiratori K, Watanabe S, Chey WY. Endogenous cholecystokinin drives gallbladder emptying in dogs. Am J Physiol 251 (Gastro Intest Liver Physiol 14):G553–G558, 1986.
7. Westfall SG, Deshpande YG, Kaminski DL. Role of glucagon and insulin in canine bile flow stimulated by endogenous cholecystokinin release. Am J Surg 157:130–136, 1989.
8. Janes JO, Dietschy JM, Berk RN, et al. Determinants of the rate of intestinal absorption of oral cholecystographic contrast agents in the dog jejunum. Gastroenterology 76:970–977, 1979.
9. Nally CV, McMullin LJ, Clanachan AS, et al. Periodic gallbladder contraction maintains bile acid circulation during the fasting period: A canine study. Br J Surg 74:1134–1138, 1987.
10. Itoh A, Takahashi I. Periodic contractions of the canine gallbladder during the interdigestive state. Am J Physiol 240:G183–G189, 1981.
11. Traynor OJ, Dozois RR, DiMagno EP. Canine interdigestive and postprandial gallbladder motility and emptying. Am J Physiol 246:G426–G432, 1984.
12. Scott RB, Strasberg SM, El-Sharkawy TY, et al. Regulation of the fasting enterohepatic circulation of bile acids by the migrating myoelectric complex in dogs. J Clin Invest 71:644–654, 1983.
13. Carlisle CH. A comparison of technics for cholecystography in the cat. Am Vet Rad Soc 18:173–176, 1977.
14. Carlisle CH. Radiographic anatomy of the cat gallbladder. JAVRS 18:170–176, 1977.
15. van der Linden W, Kempi V, Edlund G. Function of the liver, gallbladder and sphincter of Oddi after major surgery studied by computer assisted cholescintigraphy and real time ultrasonography. Br J Surg 70:497–501, 1983.
16. Singh SS, Kumar R, Sobti VK. Oral cholecystography in dogs. Can Pract 11:30–38, 1984.
17. Allan GS, Dixon RT. Cholecystography in the dog: Assessment of radiographic positioning and the use of double-contrast examination by visual and densitometric methods. JAVRS 18:177–180, 1977.
18. Allan GS, Dixon RT. Cholecystography in the dog. The choice of contrast media and optimum dose rates. JAVRS 16:98–104, 1975.
19. Ibrahim IM, Abdel-Hamid MA, Ahmed AS, et al. Intravenous cholecystography in dogs. Comp Anim Pract 2:31–33, 1988.
20. Nyland TG, Hager DA, Herring DS. Sonography of the liver, gallbladder, and spleen. Sem Vet Med Surg 4:13–31, 1989.
21. Shlaer WJ, Leopold GR, Scheible FW. Sonography of the thickened gallbladder wall: A nonspecific finding. Am J Roentenol 136:337–339, 1981.
22. Cooperberg PL, Gibney RG. Imaging of the gallbladder. Radiology 163:605–613, 1987.
23. Zeman RK, Raylor KJW, Rosenfield AT, et al. Acute experimental biliary obstruction in the dog: Sonographic findings and clinical implications. AJR 136:965–967, 1981.
24. Nyland TG, Gillett NA. Sonographic evaluation of experimental bile duct ligation in the dog. Vet Radiol 13:252–260, 1982.
25. Krishnamurthy S, Krishnamurthy GT. Technetium-99m-iminodiacetic acid organic anions: Review of biokinetics and clinical application in hepatology. Hepatology 9:139–153, 1989.
26. Rothuizen J, van den Brom. Quantitative hepatobiliary scintigraphy as a measure of bile flow in dogs with cholestatic disease. Am J Vet Res 51:253–256, 1990.
27. Boothe HW, Boothe DM, Komkov A, et al. Use of hepatobiliary scintigraphy in the diagnosis of extrahepatic biliary obstruction in dogs and cats: 25 cases (1982–1989). J Am Vet Med Assoc 201:134–141, 1992.
28. Braun U, Gerber D. Percutaneous ultrasound-guided cholecystocentesis in cows. Am J Vet Res 53:1079–1084, 1992.
29. McGahan JP, Walter JP. Diagnostic percutaneous aspiration of the gallbladder. Radiology 155:619–622, 1985.
30. Klapdor R, Scherer K, Sepehr H, et al. The ultrasonically guided puncture of the gallbladder in animals: A new methodological procedure for a simple and non-surgical collection of gallbladder bile. Endoscopy 9:166–169, 1977.
31. Hogan MT, Watne A, Mossburg W, et al. Direct injection into the gallbladder in dogs, using ultrasonic guidance. Arch Surg 111:564–565, 1976.
32. McGahan JP, Phillips HE, Nyland T, et al. Sonographically guided percutaneous cholecystostomy performed in dogs and pigs. Radiology 149:841–843, 1983.
33. van Sonnenberg E, Wittich GR, Casola G, et al. Diagnostic and therapeutic percutaneous gallbladder procedures. Radiology 160:23–26, 1986.
34. Kovatch RM, Hilderbrandt PK, Marcus LC. Cystic mucinous hypertrophy of the mucosa of the gallbladder in the dog. Pathol Vet 2:574–574, 1965.
35. Mawdesley Thomas LE, Noel PRB. Cystic hyperplasia of the gallbladder in the beagle associated with administration of progestational compounds. Vet Rec 80:658–659, 1967.
36. Svanvik J, Pellegrini CA, Allen B, et al. Transport of fluid and biliary lipids in the canine gallbladder in experimental cholecystitis. J Surg Res 41:425–431, 1986.
37. Svanvik J, Thornell E, Zettergren L. Gallbladder function in experimental cholecystitis: Reversal of the inflammaorty net fluid "secretion" into the gallbladder by indomethacin. Surgery 89:500–506, 1981.
38. Neiderhiser DH. Animal model of human disease: Acute acalculous cholecystitis induced by lysophosphatidylcholine. Am J Pathol 124:559–563, 1986.
39. Kaminski DL, Daneshmand H, Dean P, et al. Prostanoids and leukotrienes in experimental feline cholecystitis. Hepatology 11:1003–1009, 1990.
40. LaMorte WW, Lamont JT, Habe W, et al. Gallbladder prostaglandins and lysophospholipids as mediators of mucin secretion during cholelithiasis. Am J Physiol 251:G701–G709, 1986.
41. Lamont JT, Turner BS, Dibenedetto D, et al. Arachidonic acid stimulates mucin secretion in prairie dog gallbladder. Am J Physiol 245:G92–G698, 1983.
42. Large AM. Regurgitation cholecystitis and cholelithiasis. Ann Surg 146:607–612, 1957.
43. Anderson MC, Hauman RL, Suriyapa C, et al. Pancreatic enzyme levels in bile of patients with extrahepatic biliary tract disease. Am J Surg 137:301–306, 1979.
44. Sjodahl R, Tagesson C. The prerequisites for local lysolecithin formation in the human gallbladder. Scand J Gastroenterol 10:459–463, 1975.
45. Church EM, Matthieson DT. Surgical treatment of 23 dogs with necrotizing cholecystitis. J Am Anim Hosp Assoc 24:305–310, 1988.
46. Lipowitz AJ, Poffenbarger E. Gallbladder perforation in a dog. J Am Vet Med Assoc 184:838–839, 1984.
47. Hunt CA, Gofton N. Primary repair of a transected bile duct. J Am Anim Hosp Assoc 20:57–64, 1984.
48. Martin RA, MacCoy DM, Harvey HJ. Surgical management of extrahepatic biliary tract disease: A report of eleven cases. J Am Anim Hosp Assoc 22:301–307, 1986.
49. Scott DW, Hoffer RE, Amand WB, et al. Cholelithiasis in a dog. J Am Vet Med Assoc 163:254–256, 1973.
50. Harari J, Ettinger S, Lippincott CL. Extrahepatic bile duct obstruction due to cholecystitis and choledocholithiasis: Case report. J Am Anim Hosp Assoc 18:347–349, 1982.
51. Matthiesen DT, Lammerding J. Gallbladder rupture and bile peritonitis secondary to cholelithiasis and cholecystitis in a dog. J Am Vet Med Assoc 184:1282–1283, 1984.
52. Cosenza SF. Cholelithiasis and choledocholithiasis in a dog. J Am Vet Med Assoc 184:87–88, 1984.
53. Burk RL, Johnson GF. Emphysematous cholecystitis in the nondiabetic dog: Three case histories. Vet Radiol 21:242–245, 1980.
54. Lord PF, Wilkins RJ. Emphysema of the gallbladder in a diabetic dog. J Am Vet Rad Soc 13:49–52, 1972.
55. Mentzer RM, Golden GT, Chandler JG, et al. A comparative appraisal of emphysematous cholecystitis. Am J Surg 129:10–15, 1975.
56. Tangner CH. Biliary surgery. In: Bojrab JM, Birchard SJ, Tomlinson JL, Jr (eds) Current Techniques in Small Animal Surgery, 3rd ed. Lea & Febiger, Philadelphia, 299–303, 1990.
57. Walshaw R. Liver and biliary system surgical diseases. In: Slatter DH (ed) Textbook of Small Animal Surgery. WB Saunders, Philadelphia, 798–827, 1985.
58. Friman S, Radberg G, Bosaeus I, et al. Hepatobiliary compensation for the loss of gallbladder function after cholecystectomy—an experimental study in the cat. Scand J Gastroenterol 25:307–314, 1990.
59. Mahour GH, Wakim KG, Soule EH, et al. Effects of cholecystectomy on the biliary ducts in the dog. Arch Surg 97:570–574, 1968.
60. Pomare EW, Heaton KW. The effect of cholecystectomy on bile salt metabolism. Gut 14:753–762, 1973.
61. Simmons F, Ross APJ, Bouchier IAD. Alterations in hepatic bile composition after cholecystectomy. Gastroenterology 63:466–471, 1972.
62. Roda E, Aldini R, Mazzela G, et al. Enterohepatic circulation of bile acids after cholecystectomy. Gut 19:640–649, 1978.

63. Nahrwold DL, Rose RC. Changes in hepatic bile secretion following cholecystectomy. Surgery 80:178–182, 1976.
64. Hepner GW, Hofmann AF, Malagelada JR, et al. Increased bacterial degradation of bile acids in cholecystectomized patients. Gastroenterology 66:556–564, 1974.
65. Breuer NF, Jaekel S, Dommes P, et al. Fecal bile acid excretion pattern in cholecystectomized patients. Dig Dis Sci 31:953–960, 1986.
66. Mullowney PC, Tennant BC. Choledocholithiasis in the dog: A review and a report of a case with rupture of the common bile duct. J Sm Anim Pract 23:631–638, 1982.
67. Schall WD, Chapman WL, Finco DR et al. Cholelithiasis in dogs. J Am Vet Med Assoc 163:469–472, 1973.
68. Prowse EA. Cholecystolithiasis and cholecystectomy in a dog. Can Vet J 25:201–000, 1984.
69. Binns RM. Cholelithiasis causing obstructive jaundice in a boxer dog. Vet Rec 76:239–243, 1964.
70. Cantwell HD, Blevins WE, Hanika-Rebar C, et al. Radiopaque hepatic and lobar duct choleliths in a dog. J Am Anim Hosp Assoc 19:373–375, 1983.
71. Doster-Virtue ME, Virtue RW. Gallstones in a dog. J Am Vet Med Assoc 101:197, 1962.
72. Harris SJ, Simpson JW, Thoday KL. Obstructive cholelithiasis and gall bladder rupture in a dog. J Sm Anim Pract 25:661–667, 1984.
73. Jorgensen LS, Pentlarge VW, Flanders JA, et al. Recurrent choleithiasis in a cat. Comp Contin Educ 9:265–270, 1987.
74. O'brien RT, Mitchum GD. Cholelithiasis in a cat. J Am Vet Med Assoc 156:1015–1017, 1970.
75. Heidner GL, Cambell KL. Cholelithiasis in a cat. J Am Vet Med Assoc 186:176–177, 1985.
76. Wolf AM. Obstructive jaundice in a cat resulting from choledocholithiasis. J Am Vet Med Assoc 185:85–87, 1984.
77. Naus MJA, Jones BR. Cholelithiasis and choledocholithiasis in a cat. NZ Vet J 26:160–161, 1978.
78. Gibson KS. Cholelithiasis and choledocholithiasis in a cat. J Am Vet Med Assoc 121:288–289, 1952.
79. Joseph RJ, Matthiesen DT. What's your diagnosis. J Am Vet Med Assoc 188:879–880, 1986.
80. Kirpensteijn J, Fingland RB, Ulrich T, et al. Cholelithiasis in dogs: 29 cases (1980–1990). J Am Vet Med Assoc 202:1137–1142, 1993.
81. Borgman RF, Haselden FH. Ear lesions produced in rabbits by sterol injections. Am J Vet Res 33:2309–2315, 1972.
82. Netsky MG, Clarkson TB. Response of arterial wall to intramural cholesterol. Proc Soc Exp Biol Med 98:773–775, 1958.
83. Nakayama F. Composition of gallstone and bile: Species difference. J Lab Clin Med 73:623–630, 1969.
84. Rege RV, Nahrwold DI, Moore EW. Absorption of biliary calcium from the canine gallbladder: Protection against the formation of calcium-containing gallstones. J Lab Clin Med 110:381–386, 1987.
85. Englert E, Harman CG, Wales EE. Gallstones induced by normal foodstuffs in dogs. Nature 224:280–281, 1969.
86. Englert E, Harmon CG, Freston JW, et al. Studies on the pathogenesis of diet-induced dog gallstones. Dig Dis Sci 22:305–313, 1977.
87. Soloway RD, Powell KM, Senior JR, et al. Interrelationships of bile salts, phospholipids, and cholesterol in bile during manipulation of the enterohepatic circulation in the conscious dog. Gastroenterology 64:1156–1162, 1973.
88. Bernhoft RA, Pellegrini CA, Broderick WC, et al. Pigment sludge and stone formation in the acutely ligated dog gallbladder. Gastroenterology 85:1166–1171, 1983.
89. Lee SP, Nicholls JF, Park HZ. Biliary sludge as a cause of acute pancreatitis. N Engl J Med 326:589–593, 1992.
90. Ros E, Navarro S, Bru C, et al. Occult microlithiasis in 'idiopathic' acute pancreatitis: Prevention of relapses by cholecystectomy or ursodeoxycholic acid therapy. Gastroenterology 101:1701–1709, 1991.
91. Acosta JM, Ledesma CL. Gallstone migration as a cause of acute pancreatitis. N Engl J Med 290:484–487, 1974.
92. Acosta JM, Pellegrini CA, Skinner DB. Etiology and pathogenesis of acute biliary pancreatitis. Surgery 88:118–125, 1980.
93. Kelley TR. Gallstone pancreatitis. Arch Surg 109:294–297, 1974.
94. Kelley TR. Gallstone pancreatitis: Pathophysiology. Surgery 80:488–492, 1976.
95. Senior JR, Johnson MF, DeTurck DM, et al. In vivo kinetics of radiolucent gallstone dissolution by oral dihydroxy bile acids. Gastroenterology 99:243–251, 1990.
96. O'Donnell LDJ, Heaton KW. Recurrence and re-recurrence of gall stones after medical dissolution: A longterm follow up. Gut 29:655–658, 1988.
97. Suter PF, Olsson SE. The diagnosis of injuries to the intestines, gallbladder, and bile ducts in the dog. J Sm Anim Pract 11:575–584, 1970.
98. Watkins PE, Pearson H, Denny HR. Traumatic rupture of the bile duct in the dog: A report of seven cases. J Sm Anim Pract 24:731–740, 1983.
99. Bellenger CR. Surgery for bile duct rupture and obstruction in the dog. Aust Vet J 49:298–306, 1973.
100. Berzon JL. Surgical repair of traumatic injuries of the biliary system: Case report and discussion. J Am Anim Hosp Assoc 17:421–426, 1981.
101. Matthiesen DT, Lammerding J. Gallbladder rupture and bile peritonitis secondary to cholelithiasis and cholecystitis. J Am Vet Med Assoc 184:1282–1283, 1984.
102. Kipnis RM. Cholelithiasis, gallbladder perforation, and bile peritonitis in a dog. Canine Pract 13:15–27, 1986.
103. Robins G, Thornton J, Mills J. Bile peritonitis and pleuritis in a dog. J Am Anim Hosp Assoc 13:55–60, 1977.
104. Slappendel RJ, Rijnberk A. Traumatic bile duct rupture in dogs and its surgical treatment. Tijdschr Diergeneesk 95:392–399, 1970.
105. O'Brien JA, Shields DR, Berg P, et al. Traumatic pleural biliary fistula in a dog. J Am Vet Med Assoc 146:1054–1058, 1965.
106. Bieritz WG, Brasmer TH. Traumatic rupture of the cystic duct. J Am Anim Hosp Assoc 2:35–39, 1966.
107. Jeffrey KL. A technique for repair of ruptured common bile duct: A case report. VM/SAC 64:1061–1064, 1969.
108. Hoffer RE, Niemeyer KH, Patton M. Common bile duct repair utilizing the gallbladder and t-tube. VM/SAC 66:889–894, 1971.
109. Watson ADJ, Porges WL. Ruptured bile duct in a dog. Aust Vet J 47:340–342, 1971.
110. Parker GW. Rupture of the common bile duct: A case report. J Am Anim Hosp Assoc 8:328–329, 1979.
111. Borthwick R, Mackenzie CP, Lewis ND, et al. Rupture of the bile duct in a dog. Vet Rec 92:356–359, 1973.
112. Long RD. Rupture of the common bile duct in a dog. A case report. Vet Rec 92:370, 1973.
113. Richardson F, Hobson HP, Morris EL. Rupture of the gallbladder in the canine and its surgical correction: Case report. Southwest Vet 28:251–254, 1975.
114. Kelch WT, Rabaut SM. Traumatic rupture of the bile duct in a dog. VM/SAC 73:732–734, 1978.
115. Parchman MB, Flanders JA. Extrahepatic biliary tract rupture: Evaluation of the relationship between the site of rupture and the cause of rupture in 15 dogs. Cornell Vet 80:267–272, 1990.
116. Cain JL, Labat JA, Cohn I. Bile peritonitis in germ-free dogs. Gastroenterology 53:600–603, 1967.
117. Stewart HL, Lieber MM. Ligation of the common bile duct in the cat. Arch Pathol 34–46, 1935.
118. Cameron GR, Hasan SM. Disturbances of structure and function in the liver as the result of biliary obstruction. J Path Bact 75:333–347, 1958.
119. Center SA, Castleman W, Roth L, et al. Light microscopic and electron microscopic changes in the livers of cats with extrahepatic bile duct obstruction. Am J Vet Res 47:1278–1282, 1986.
120. Trams EG, Symeonidis A. Morphologic and functional changes in the livers of rats after ligation or excision of the common bile duct. Am J Pathol 33:13–27, 1957.
121. Steiner JW, Carruthers JS. Experimental extrahepatic biliary obstruction. Am J Pathol 40:253–270, 1962.
122. Stewart HL, Cantarow A. Decompression of the obstructed biliary system of the cat. Am J Dig Dis Nutr 2:101–108, 1935.
123. Van Vleet JF, Alberts JO. Evaluation of liver function tests and liver biopsy in experimental carbon tetrachloride intoxication and extrahepatic bile duct obstruction in the dog. J Am Vet Med Assoc 29:2119–2131, 1968.
124. Gliedman ML, Carrol HJ, Popowitz L, et al. An experimental hepatorenal syndrome. Surg Gynecol Obstet 10:519–523, 1970.
125. Ohlsson EG. The effect of biliary obstruction on the distribution of the hepatic flow and reticuloendothelial system in dogs. Acta Clin Scand 138:159–164, 1972.
126. Tavoloni N. Role of ductular bile water reabsorption in canine bile secretion. J Lab Clin Med 106:154–156, 1985.
127. Pitt HA, Postier RG, Cameron JL. Biliary bacteria: Significance and alterations after antibiotic therapy. Arch Surg 117:445–449, 1982.
128. Saito H. Clinical and experimental studies on the hyperdynamic states in obstructive jaundice. J Jap Surg Soc 82:483–497, 1981.
129. Sasha SM, Better OS, Chaimovitz C, et al. Hemodynamic studies in dogs with chronic bile duct ligation. Clin Sci Mol Med 50:533–537, 1976.
130. Fineberg JPM, Syrop HA, Better OS. Blunted pressor response to angiotensin and sympathomimetic amines in the bile duct ligated dogs. Clin Sci 61:535–539, 1981.
131. Binah O, Bomzon A, Blendis LM, et al. Obstructive jaundice blunts myocardial contractile response to isoproterenol in the dog: A clue to the susceptibility of jaundiced patients to shock. Clin Sci 69:647–653, 1985.
132. Bomzon A, Rosenberg M, Gali D, et al. Systemic hypotension and decreased pressor response in dogs with chronic bile duct ligation. Hepatology 6:595–600, 1986.
133. Center SA, Baldwin BH, King JM, et al. Hematologic and biochemical abnormalities associated with induced extrahepatic bile duct obstruction in the cat. Am J Vet Res 44:1822–1829, 1983.
134. Carlstein A, Edlund Y, Thulesois P. Bilirubin, alkaline phosphatase and transaminases in blood and lymph during biliary obstruction in the cat. Acta Physiol Scand 53:58–67, 1961.
135. Guelfi JF, Braun JP, Benard P, et al. Value of so-called cholestasis markers in the dog: An experimental study. Res Vet Sci 33:309–312, 1982.

136. Stein TA, Burns GP, Wise L. Diagnostic value of liver function tests in bile duct obstruction. J Surg Res 46:226–229, 1989.
137. Kryszewski AJ, Neale G, Whitfield JB, et al. Enzyme changes in experimental biliary obstruction. Clin Chim Acta 47:175–183, 1973.
138. Hagerstrand I. Enzyme histochemistry of the liver in extrahepatic biliary obstruction. Acta Pathol Microbiol Scand 81:737–750, 1973.
139. Sada E, Tashiro S, Morino Y. The significance of serum mitochondrial aspartate aminotransferase activity in obstructive jaundice: Experimental and clinical studies. Jap J Surg 20:392–405, 1990.
140. Willson SA, Gosink BB, van Sonnenberg E. Unchanged size of a dilated common bile duct after a fatty meal: Results and significance. Radiology 160:29–31, 1986.
141. Simeone JF, Mueller PR, Ferrucci JT, et al. Sonography of the bile ducts after a fatty meal: An aid in detection of obstruction. Radiology 143:211–215, 1982.
142. Simeone JF, Butch RJ, Mueller PR, et al. The bile ducts after a fatty meal: Further sonographic observations. Radiology 154:763–768, 1985.
143. Cribb AE, Burgener DC, Reimann KA. Bile duct obstruction secondary to chronic pancreatitis in seven dogs. Can Vet J 29:654–657, 1988.
144. Edwards DF, Bauer MS, Walker MA, et al. Pancreatic masses in seven dogs following acute pancreatitis. J Am Anim Hosp Assoc 26:189–198, 1990.
145. Salisbury SK, Lantz GC, Nelson RW. Pancreatic abscessation in the dog. In: ACVIM Proc 5th Ann Vet Med Forum. Madison, WI: Omnipress, 905, 1987.
146. Matthiesen DT, Rosin E. Common bile duct obstruction secondary to chronic fibrosing pancreatitis: Treatment by use of cholecystoduodenostomy in the dog. J Am Vet Med Assoc 189:1443–1446, 1986.
147. Kajiwara T, Suzuki T. Effect of biliary diversion on exocrine pancreas. Surg Gynecol Obstet 147:343–349, 1978.
148. Johnson AG, Stevens AE. Importance of the size of the stoma in choledochoduodenostomy. Gut 10:68–70, 1969.
149. Tangner CH. Cholecystoduodenostomy in the dog: Comparison of two techniques. Vet Surg 13:126–134, 1984.
150. Boey JH, Way LW. Acute cholangitis. Ann Surg 141:254–270, 1980.
151. Large A, Musgrove JE, Grindlay JH, et al. Intestinal biliary reflux after anastomosis of common duct to duodenum or jejunum: An experimental study. Arch Surg 64:579–589, 1952.
152. Martin RA, Walsh KM, Zimmer JF, et al. Effects of intestinal reflux into the hepatobiliary ducts following biliary enteric anastomosis in the dog (abstract). Vet Surg 14:59–60, 1985.
153. Breen JJ, Molina E, Ritchie WP, Jr. Effect of common bile duct transplantation on gastric acid secretion in the dog. Brit J Surg 55:282–284, 1968.
154. Duffell SJ. Some aspects of pancreatic disease in the cat. J Sm Anim Pract 16:365–375, 1975.
155. Williams RD. Effects of partial and complete biliary tract obstruction. Oklahoma State Med Assoc 60:390–394, 1966.
156. Wilkins RJ, Hurvitz AI. Chemical profiles in the cat. J Am Vet Med Assoc 159:1142–1145, 1971.
157. Twedt D, Gilberton S. Icteric cats: A survey of 47 necropsied cats. Anim Med Ctr Lab Newsletter 48, 1977.
158. Owens JM, Drazner FH, Gilbertson SR. Pancreatic disease in the cat. J Am Anim Hosp Assoc 83–89, 1975.
159. Kelly DF, Baggot DG, Gaskell CJ. Jaundice in the cat associated with inflammation of the biliary tract and pancreas. J Sm Anim Pract 16:163–175, 1975.
160. Hirsch VM, Doige CE. Suppurative cholangitis in cats. J Am Vet Med Assoc 182:1223–1226, 1983.
161. Prasse KW, Mahaffey EA, DeNovo R, et al. Chronic lymphocytic cholangitis in three cats. Vet Pathol 19:99–108, 1982.
162. Chock E, Wolfe BM, Matolo NM. Acute suppurative cholangitis. Surg Clin N Am 61:885–892, 1981.
163. Scott AJ. Bacteria and disease of the biliary tract. Gut 12:487–492, 1971.
164. Scott AJ, Khan GA. Origin of bacteria in bile duct bile. Lancet 2:790–792, 1967.
165. Hancke E, Marklein G, Helpap B. Keimbesiedlung der Gallenwege, experimentelle hinweise auf einen entero-hepatico-biliaren bakterienreislauf. Langenbecks Arch Chir 353:121–127, 1980.
166. Sung JY, Shaffer EA, Olson ME, et al. Bacterial invasion of biliary system by way of the portal venous system. Hepatology 14:313–317, 1991.
167. Cardoso V, Pimenta A, Correa da Fonseca J, et al. The effect of cholestasis on hepatic clearance of bacteria. World J Surg 6:330–334, 1982.
168. Huang R, Bass JA, Williams RD. The significance of biliary pressure in cholangitis. Arch Surg 98:629–632, 1969.
169. Jacobsson B, Kjellander J, Rosengren B. Cholangiovenous reflux. Acta Chir Scand 123:316–321, 1962.
170. Dubey JP, Zajac A, Osofsky SA, et al. Acute primary toxoplasmic hepatitis in an adult cat shedding Toxoplasma gondii oocysts. J Am Vet Med Assoc 197:1616–1618, 1990.
171. Lipscomb TP, Dubey JP, Pletcher JM, et al. Intrahepatic biliary coccidiosis in a dog. Vet Pathol 26:343–345, 1989.
172. Timbs DV, Durham PJK, Barnsley DGG. Chronic cholecystitis in a dog infected with Salmonella typhimurium. NZ Vet J 22:100–102, 1974.
173. Center SA, Rowland P, Corbett J, et al. Suppurative and non-suppurative cholangitis in the cat, a retrospective study. Submitted for publication.
174. Jackson MW, Panciera DL, Hartmann F. Administration of vancomycin for treatment of ascending bacterial cholangiohepatitis in a cat. J Am Vet Med Assoc 204:602–605, 1994.
175. Lucke VM, Davies JD. Progressive lymphocytic cholangitis in the cat. J Sm Anim Pract 25:249–260, 1984.
176. Edwards DF, McCracken MD, Richardson DC, et al. Sclerosing cholangitis in a cat. J Am Vet Med Assoc 182:710–712, 1983.
177. Nakayama H, Uchida K, Lee S-K, et al. Three cases of feline sclerosing lymphocytic cholangitis. J Vet Med Sci 54:769–771, 1992.
178. Johnson ME, DiBartola SP, Gelberg HG. Nephrotic syndrome and pericholangiohepatitis in a cat. J Am Anim Hosp Assoc 19:191–196, 1983.
179. Antony PP, Sarsfield P, Clarke T. Primary lymphoma of the liver: Clinical and pathological features of 10 patients. J Clin Pathol 43:1007–1013, 1990.
180. DeMent SH, Mann RB, Staal SP, et al. Primary lymphomas of the liver: Report of six cases and review of the literature. Am J Clin Pathol 88:255–263, 1987.
181. Scoazec J-Y, Degott C, Brousse N, et al. Non-Hodgkin's lymphoma presenting as primary tumor of the liver: Presentation, diagnosis and outcome in eight patients. Hepatology 13:870–875, 1991.
182. Ryan J, Straus DJ, Lange C, et al. Primary lymphoma of the liver. Cancer 61:370–375, 1988.
183. Khan SM, Cottrell BJ, Millward-Sadler GH, et al. T cell-rich B cell lymphoma presenting as liver disease. Histopathology 21:217–224, 1993.
184. Schrumpf E, Fausa O, Elgjo K, et al. Hepatobiliary complications of inflammatory bowel disease. Sem Liver Dis 8:201–209, 1988.
185. Dew MJ, Thompson H, Allan RN. The spectrum of hepatic dysfunction in inflammatory bowel disease. Q J Med, New Series 58:113–135, 1979.
186. Schrumpf E, Elgjo K, Fausa O, et al. Sclerosing cholangitis in ulcerative colitis. Scand J Gastroenterol 15:689–697, 1980.
187. Tuzhilin SA, Podolsky AE, Dreiling DA. Hepatic lesions in pancreatitis. Clinicoexperimental data. Am J Gastroenterol 64:108–114, 1975.
188. Smart ME, Downey RS, Stockdale PHG. Toxoplasmosis in a cat associated with cholangitis and progressive pancreatitis. Can Vet J 14:313–316, 1973.
189. Rothenbacher H, Lindquist WD. Liver cirrhosis and pancreatitis in a cat infected with Amphimerus pseudofelineus. J Am Vet Med Assoc 143:1099–1102, 1963.
190. Ewing GO. Granulomatous cholangiohepatitis in a cat due to a protozoan parasite resembling Hepatozoon canis. Feline Pract 7:37–40, 1977.
191. Neufeld JL, Brandt RW. Cholangiohepatitis in a cat associated with a coccidia-like organism. Can Vet J 15:156–159, 1974.
192. Wagner JE. A fatal cytauxzoonosis-like disease in cats. J Am Vet Med Assoc 168:585–588, 1976.
193. Kovatch RM, Zebarth G. Naturally-occurring Tyzzer's disease in a cat. J Am Vet Med Assoc 162:136–138, 1973.
194. Callanan JJ, Thompson H, Toth SR, et al. Clinical and pathological findings in feline immunodeficiency virus experimental infection. Vet Imm Immnopath 35:3–13, 1992.
195. Meyer zum Buschenfelde KH, Manns M, Gerken G. Immunological aspects of chronic hepatitis. J Gastroenterol Hepatol 3:177–185, 1988.
196. Sherlock S. The syndrome of disappearing intrahepatic bile ducts. Lancet 2:493–496, 1987.
197. Ludwig J. New concepts in biliary cirrhosis. Sem Liver Dis 7:293–301, 1987.
198. van den Ingh TSGAM, Rothuizen J, van Zinnicq Bergman HMS. Destructive cholangiolitis in seven dogs. Vet Q 10:240–245, 1988.
199. Andrews JC, Knol J, Wollner I, et al. Floxuridine-associated sclerosing cholangitis—a dog model. Invest Radiol 24:47–51, 1989.
200. Uchida H, Tomikawa S, Nishimura Y, et al. Vanishing bile duct syndrome in canine liver allotransplants. Transpl Proc 21:404–406, 1989.
201. Taylor D, Perri SF. Experimental infection of cats with the liver fluke Platynosomum concinnum. Am J Vet Res 38:51–54, 1977.
202. Palumbo NE, Perri SF, Loo B, et al. Cat liver fluke, Platynosomum concinnum, in Hawaii. Am J Vet Res 35:1455, 1974.
203. Retnasabapathy A, Prathap K. The liver fluke Platynosomum fastosum in domestic cats. Vet Rec 88:62–65, 1971.
204. Greve JH, Leonard PO. Hepatic flukes (Platynosomum concinnum) in a cat from Illinois. J Am Vet Med Assoc 149:418–420, 1966.
205. Learn G, Walker IE. The occurrence of Platynosomum fastosum in domestic cats in the Bahamas. Vet Rec 75:46–47, 1963.
206. Barriga OO, Caputo CA, Weisbrode SE. Liver flukes (Platynosomum concinnum) in an Ohio cat. J Am Vet Med Assoc 179:901–903, 1981.
207. Bielsa LM, Greiner EC. Liver flukes (Platynosomum concinnum) in cats. J Am Anim Hosp Assoc 21:269–274, 1985.
208. Hitt HE. Liver fluke infection in South Florida cats. Feline Pract 11:26–29, 1981.
209. Levine ND, Beamer PD. Platynosomum fastosum in an Illinois cat. J Parasitol 43(suppl):29–30, 1957.
210. Essex HE, Ballman JL. Parasitic cirrhosis of the liver in a cat infected with Opisthorchis pseudofelineus and Metorchis complexus. Am J Trop Med 10:65–70, 1930.

211. Oppong ENW, Rommel W. *Platynosomum concinnum* infection in cats in West Africa. Vet Rec 90:462, 1972.

212. Robinson VB, Ehrenford FA. Hepatic lesions associated with liver fluke (*Platynosomum fastosum*) infection in a cat. Am J Vet Res 23:1300–1303, 1962.

213. Palumbo NE, Taylor D, Perri SF. Evaluation of fecal techniques for the diagnosis of cat liver fluke infection. Lab Anim Sci 26:490–493, 1976.

214. Black M. Solitary congenital hepatic cyst in a cat. Aust Vet Pract 13:166–168, 1983.

215. Crowell WA, Hubbell JJ, Riley JC. Polycystic renal disease in related cats. J Am Vet Med Assoc 175:286–294, 1979.

216. Biller DS, Chew DJ, DiBartola SP. Polycystic kidney disease in a family of Persian cats. J Am Vet Med Assoc 196:1288–1290, 1990.

217. McKenna SC, Carpenter JL. Polycystic disease of the kidney and liver in the Cairn terrier. Vet Pathol 17:436–442, 1980.

218. Mendham JH, Roszel JF, Bovee KC. Clinical-pathologic conference. J Am Vet Med Assoc 154:935–944, 1969.

219. Scherzo CS. Cystic liver and persistent urachus in a cat. J Am Vet Med Assoc 151:1329–1330, 1967.

220. Reid JS, Frank RJ. Liver cyst in a cat (a case report). Vet Med/ Sm Anim Clin 68:1127–1130, 1973.

221. Van den Ingh TS, Rothuizen J. Congenital cystic disease of the liver in seven dogs. J Comp Pathol 95(3):405–414, 1985.

222. Stebbins KE. Polycystic disease of the kidney and liver in an adult Persian cat. J Comp Pathol 100:327–300, 1989.

38 Nutritional Management of Gastrointestinal Diseases

W. GRANT GUILFORD

INTRODUCTION

Most gastrointestinal diseases are treated by a combination of pharmacologic and nutritional management. Unfortunately, pharmaceutical agents are often given inappropriate precedence. Drug therapy without appropriate nutritional management is likely to result in, at best, incomplete or delayed resolution of signs and, at worst, exacerbation of the disorder. Many gastrointestinal diseases can be (and should be) managed by dietary therapy only. Dietary modification provides the clinician with a powerful tool for the treatment of gastrointestinal diseases because of the numerous effects of nutrients on the bowel (Table 38–1 and Figure 38–1).

This chapter provides practical recommendations on the nutritional management of selected gastrointestinal problems. The discussion is prefaced by a description of the influence of deficiency or excess of important macronutrients and micronutrients on gastrointestinal system structure and function and, conversely, the nutritional consequences to the animal of gastrointestinal disease. Prepared with this knowledge, the clinician will be in a position to rationally formulate diets for any alimentary problem encountered in clinical practice.

INFLUENCE OF NUTRIENTS AND NUTRITIONAL STATUS ON THE GASTROINTESTINAL TRACT

Protein meals increase gastroesophageal sphincter pressure, perhaps because dietary protein is a potent stimulus for gastrin and gastric acid release. Dietary protein is also a strong stimulant of pancreatic secretion.[1] The type of protein in the diet influences gastric emptying rate and small-bowel transit time.[2] Food proteins comprise the majority of antigens and allergens in the diet.

Malabsorbed protein is an important source of ammonia, which in excess is toxic to the large-bowel mucosa and can result in encephalopathy, if inadequately metabolized by the liver. Malabsorbed protein is energetically costly to replace but does not appear to be a major stimulus for diarrhea in comparison to malabsorbed carbohydrate and fat. Thus, in spite of significant protein loss into the bowel, dogs with lymphangiectasia sometimes do not have diarrhea.

Protein deficiency can occur in association with carbohydrate deficiency resulting in protein-calorie malnutrition. The systemic manifestations of protein-calorie malnutrition

Table 38–1

INFLUENCE OF DIET ON THE GI TRACT

Diet May Contain
  Toxic food additives
  Allergenic proteins
  Antigenic proteins
Diet May Correct
  Nutritional deficiencies
Diet May Alter
  Cell renewal rate
  Motility
  Absorption
  Secretion of mucus, acid, and enzymes
  Bacterial flora
  Luminal ammonia content
  Colonic volatile fatty acid content

include poor hair coat, weight loss, weakness, inactivity, poor healing, and susceptibility to infections. The predominant effects of malnutrition on the bowel are mucosal atrophy, delayed gastric emptying of fluid and food, impaired absorption of nutrients, decreased gastric, pancreatic, and biliary secretions, and diarrhea.[3–6] Mucin secretion is decreased, bacterial overgrowth is common, and susceptibility to enteric

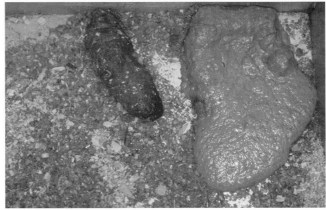

FIGURE 38–1. The litter tray of a cat with chronic diarrhea. The diarrhea resolved within 12 hours of the cat's diet being changed to a high-quality, selected-protein, restricted-fat product.

pathogens is increased.[4,5] Dysphagia due to functional decline in somatic and visceral muscle can occur.[7] Adequate dietary protein is required to maintain serum albumin levels and allow mucosal turnover and repair. Protein-deficient diets result in mildly increased serum alkaline phosphatase levels and abnormal postprandial serum bile acid concentrations in dogs.[8]

Glutamine

Glutamine is the most abundant amino acid in plasma. It is involved in a number of physiologic processes and is the principal fuel for rapidly dividing cells such as those in the small intestinal mucosa.[9–11] Glutamine plays a prominent role in the maintenance of intestinal metabolism, structure, and function, and is an important respiratory fuel for the pancreas.[11] The importance of glutamine to the gastrointestinal tract was demonstrated by experiments in which plasma glutamine levels were reduced by infusion of glutaminase, resulting in mild villous atrophy, mucosal ulceration, intestinal necrosis, and diarrhea.[12]

Intestinal mucosal cells derive glutamine from the intestinal lumen during feeding and from the bloodstream during fasting. In dogs, the principal sources of plasma glutamine are muscle and, during starvation, the liver.[13] Catabolic states (other than septicemia) reduce the supply of glutamine by muscle and increase uptake by the small intestine.[9,11] As a result, glutamine supply can become limiting, and glutamine may be considered a conditionally essential amino acid during certain catabolic states such as starvation, advanced malignancy, and operative stress.[11] Interestingly, glucocorticoid administration markedly increases gut extraction of circulating glutamine but decreases luminal uptake of glutamine.[11]

The administration of glutamine has been beneficial in a number of experimental models. Provision of glutamine-enriched diets reduces bacterial translocation through the bowel of burned rats[14] and improves survival in a rat model of experimentally induced peritonitis.[15] Glutamine stimulates sodium and chloride absorption in pig rotavirus enteritis.[16] Glutamine supplementation of TPN solution reduces the gastric, small intestinal, and colonic mucosal atrophy associated with standard TPN solutions.[11,17] Glutamine has also been reported to enhance mucosal hyperplasia after small-bowel resection in dogs and to improve small-bowel cellularity after toxic injury.[18,19] Glutamine may also be necessary for normal gut-associated lymphoid tissue function.[11] Other studies have suggested that the provision of glutamine-supplemented nutritional support reduces the severity of intestinal mucosal injury from chemotherapeutic agents and radiation.[11]

Carbohydrate

Carbohydrate is a major component of most pet foods, even though an obligate requirement for carbohydrate in dogs and cats has not been demonstrated. The predominant carbohydrate in pet foods is starch. The digestibility of starch is determined by its plant origin and the degree and type of processing (Table 38–2). Some starch, such as that in rice, wheat, and cooked maize, is well digested by healthy cats and dogs, but considerable amounts of other starches such as potato and tapioca can escape assimilation particularly if they are poorly cooked.[20–23] It is perhaps surprising that cats can efficiently digest carbohydrate considering the low carbohydrate content of their ancestral diet. Footprints of this

Table 38–2

FACTORS AFFECTING STARCH DIGESTIBILITY

FOOD FORM	FIBER (TYPE)
Particle size	Antinutrients
Starch source	Phytate
Amylose content	Lectins
Amylopectin content	Tannins
Degree of gelatinization	Saponins
Cooking process	Enzyme inhibitors
Degree of hydration	
Starch-nutrient interactions	

carnivorous past can be detected, however. The amylase activity in the pancreas and small intestinal chyme of cats is low in comparison to dogs (Table 38–3).[25] Furthermore, unlike omnivorous animals, inductive effects of dietary carbohydrate on pancreatic amylase activity and intestinal sugar transporters are small.[24,25] These observations support the suspicions of some clinicians that cats suffering from gastrointestinal disease are less tolerant of carbohydrate than dogs with the same disorders.[26,27] It is possible, however, that malabsorbed carbohydrate has fewer adverse consequences to cats than other species because cats have limited capacity for microbial fermentation of carbohydrate.[25] The reduced ability to ferment carbohydrate may be due to the relatively low activity of microbial amylases in cats and the low fecal water percentage.[25]

LACTOSE. Sugars such as lactose are included in the diet of many pets. Brush-border lactase levels show individual variation in dogs and cats but are normally low (Table 38–4)[28] and are reduced further when the bowel is diseased. Lactose is poorly tolerated by most dogs and cats, resulting in soft feces or liquid diarrhea.[23,29] In contrast, sucrose is well tolerated in healthy dogs and cats.[23,29,30] Healthy dogs can tolerate dietary lactose of 1 g/kg/day without clinical evidence of diarrhea. However, increased intake of lactose to more than 1.5 g/kg/day results in severe osmotic diarrhea in many dogs. These figures have practical relevance because as little as 1 cup of whole milk (244 g) provides 11 g of lactose.[31] Any more milk than 1 cup per 7 kg body weight would be likely to result in diarrhea in the dog. Lactose has a dose-related effect on fecal consistency (decrease in dry matter), pH (decrease), osmolality (increase), and lactic acid concentration (increase).[32] These changes are observable even at dietary levels of lactose insufficient to produce clinical evidence of diarrhea. Intolerance of lactose in milk can be prevented by prior enzymatic digestion of the lactose with commercially available beta galactosidase.[32] The lactose contents of various foods are shown in Table 38–5.

CARBOHYDRATE MALASSIMILATION. Carbohydrate malassimilation contributes to the pathophysiology of a number of different diseases including exocrine pancreatic insufficiency, dumping syndromes, short-bowel syndrome, and mucosal dis-

Table 38–3

ACTIVITY OF AMYLASE IN PANCREAS AND SMALL INTESTINAL CHYME

	PANCREAS	SMALL INTESTINE
	U/g wet weight	
Cat	70	20–50
Dog	3000	50–600

From Kienzle E (1993).[25]

Table 38–4

ACTIVITY OF BRUSH BORDER DISACCHARIDASES
IN THE DOG

	LACTASE	SUCRASE	MALTASE
	(μ moles/g wet mucosa/minute)		
Duodenum	3.1	6.7	29.0
Jejunum	3.5	7.8	38.1
Ileum	0.7	4.6	27.7

From Hill FWG, Kelly DF (1974).[28]

eases of the small intestine. The consequences of carbohydrate malassimilation include osmotic diarrhea, loss of water and electrolytes (especially potassium), intestinal gaseousness, bacterial overgrowth of the small intestine, reduced small intestinal protein assimilation, acidification of colonic content, and alteration of the composition of intestinal flora.[27,33–36] For these reasons, carbohydrates included in therapeutic diets must be highly digestible.

Fat

The ingestion of a fatty meal decreases gastroesophageal tone, slows gastric emptying, and is a potent stimulus for pancreatic secretion.[3,5,37,38] Fat-induced delay of gastric emptying is less pronounced in humans adapted to high-fat diets, emphasizing the importance of recent dietary history when evaluating the effects of nutrients on the gastrointestinal tract.[39] The quantity and type of fat included in the diet are important considerations when treating gastrointestinal disease.

MEDIUM CHAIN TRIGLYCERIDES (MCTs). Medium chain triglycerides (carbon chain lengths less than 12) have theoretical advantages over long chain triglycerides (LCTs) for the treatment of gastrointestinal disease.[40] In contrast to LCTs, considerable amounts of MCTs are directly absorbed without the need for hydrolysis or formation of micelles. The MCT that is hydrolyzed by pancreatic lipase is hydrolyzed more completely than LCT. The medium chain fatty acids produced by hydrolysis are minimally reesterified in the enterocyte. Instead, they are absorbed directly into the portal circulation. The small quantity of MCT that is reesterified is incorporated into chylomicrons in the same manner as LCT. The amount of MCT incorporated into chylomicrons increases when the diet is high in MCTs or when MCTs are fed for prolonged periods.[41] Thus, feeding of MCT oil, particularly in large quantities, is likely to increase lymph flow but not to the same degree as LCT.

Medium chain triglycerides are most commonly used in dogs and cats to increase the energy intake of animals with

Table 38–5

AMOUNT OF LACTOSE IN VARIOUS FOODS*

	LACTOSE (g)	PROTEIN (g)	CALORIES (cal)
Whole milk	11	8	157
Yogurt	11	8	139
Cottage cheese	6	31	200
Cheddar cheese	5	57	800

*Per 8 oz cup.

lymphangiectasia. Unfortunately, the ability to supply significant quantities of calories by MCTs is hampered by their potential to cause osmotic diarrhea and inappetence. MCT oils are ketogenic and should not be given to patients with ketosis or acidosis. They are poorly metabolized in hepatic cirrhosis and may accumulate in plasma.

OMEGA-3 POLYUNSATURATED FATTY ACIDS. Omega-3 polyunsaturated fatty acids such as eicosapentaenoic acid (20:5 omega-3) and docosahexaenoic acid (C22:6 omega-3), are found in high concentrations in fish oils. The addition of omega-3 fatty acids to the diet has been shown to alter the fatty acid and eicosanoid profiles of the gastrointestinal mucosa[42,43] and to reduce the degree of inflammation in experimental models of colitis.[42] Furthermore, dietary supplementation with omega-3 fatty acids has a favorable impact on endotoxemia and allergic processes.[40]

ESSENTIAL FATTY ACIDS. Essential fatty acid deficiency impairs the recovery of damaged intestinal mucosa in rats.[44] A polyunsaturated fat-supplemented diet (40% of calories as corn oil) improves water and electrolyte absorption from the small intestine of rats.[45]

FAT MALASSIMILATION. Most fats are almost entirely digested (85% to 99%) in healthy cats and dogs.[46] In comparison to other macronutrients, the assimilation of fat is a relatively complex process, however, and it is comparatively easy to disrupt during gastrointestinal disease. The consequences of fat malassimilation include fatty acid, bile salt, vitamin, and mineral malabsorption. Malabsorbed fatty acid and bile acids are hydroxylated and deconjugated, respectively, by colonic bacteria to produce potent secretagogues (Figure 38–2). The deconjugated bile acids and hydroxylated fatty acids are toxic to the colonic mucosa, inducing morphologic changes, increased mucosal permeability, altered motility, and secretory diarrhea (Figure 38–1).[47]

Fiber

DEFINITION. Fiber is plant material resistant to digestion by enzymes of monogastrics. Fiber is the predominant nutrient entering the colon and has considerable therapeutic value for disorders of the large bowel. Insufficient ingestion of fiber has been incriminated as causing a variety of bowel disorders including irritable bowel disease and colon cancer. In veterinary medicine, there is a tendency to treat fiber as a single entity and to label fiber-responsive diarrhea as a single disease process: "irritable bowel syndrome." In reality, there are several hundred types of fiber each with different biologic effects, many different fiber-responsive diseases, and a large

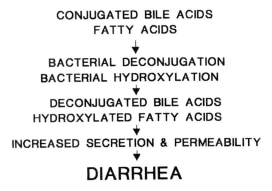

FIGURE 38–2. Consequences of malabsorbed fat.

variety of ways in which fiber influences the gastrointestinal tract in addition to its effects on motility. Major constituents of fiber include nonstarch polysaccharides (cellulose, hemicellulose, and pectins) and noncarbohydrate components such as lignin and waxy materials. The amount of these constituents varies considerably in fibers of different origins.

SOLUBLE VERSUS INSOLUBLE FIBERS. There are a number of methods for classifying fibers.[48] One system divides fibers into soluble and insoluble fractions. Traditionally, division into these groups has reflected the solubility of a fiber in hot buffer with thermostable amylase.[49] The nutritional relevance of such nonphysiologic methods has been challenged,[49,50] and Monro (1993) has suggested a new technique for estimating soluble and insoluble fiber contents that more accurately reflects solubility of fiber in the upper gastrointestinal tract.[49] It is probable that this more physiologic method will improve the clinical relevance of the soluble/insoluble classification of fibers. The solubility of dietary fiber largely depends on the chemical structure of the fiber. In general, fibers with high lignin content as insoluble. Other factors that influence the solubility of a fiber in vivo include particle size, other meal constituents, and meal volume.[49] Because the chemical structure of fibers is diverse, many fibers will share properties of both soluble and insoluble fibers.

The physiologic properties of the different types of fibers are somewhat predictable by the soluble/insoluble classifica-tion. As a general rule, soluble fibers attract water, form gels, delay gastric emptying, inhibit the absorption of cholesterol, are poor bulking agents, are highly fermentable in the colon by bacteria, increase the numbers of colonic bacteria, form colonic short chain fatty acids (SCFA), lower colonic pH, and stimulate colonic cell proliferation. In contrast, insoluble fibers do not form gels, do not delay gastric emptying, and have only mild effects on macronutrient absorption. Insoluble fibers are usually poorly fermentable, and are good bulk-forming agents particularly if their water-holding capacity is high.

Foods high in soluble fiber include psyllium husks, pectins, oats, barley, and certain fruits and legumes.[48,49] Soluble fibers of importance are guar gum, pectin, and psyllium. In contrast, wheat and rye fibers and most cereal brans have relatively high contents of insoluble fiber such as cellulose.[48]

EFFECTS OF FIBER ON UPPER GASTROINTESTINAL FUNCTION. Although fiber predominantly influences the large bowel, many effects on gastric, small intestinal, and pancreatic structure and function have been observed (Figure 38–3).[51] Prolonged intake of fiber is thought to increase the number of goblet cells and the secretion of mucus in the intestine.[51] It also influences villus morphology, intestinal IgA secretion, and intestinal hormone responses.[51–53] Water soluble gel-forming fibers such as psyllium, guar gum, pectins, and hydroxypropylmethylcellulose slow gastric emptying and

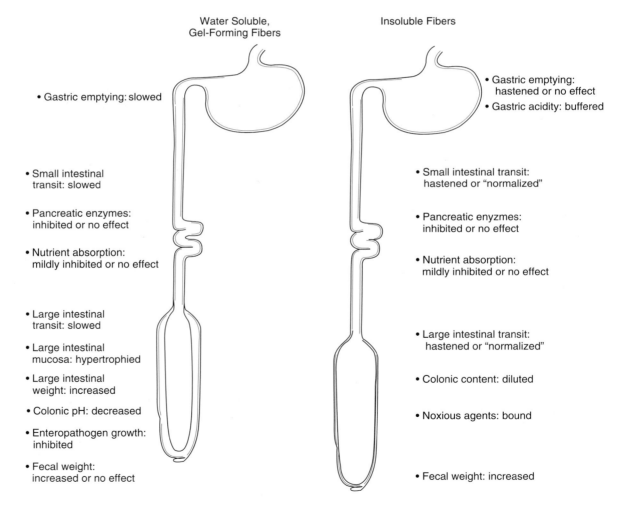

FIGURE 38–3. Effect of fiber on the gastrointestinal tract.

small intestinal transit in dogs, whereas certain insoluble fibers may actually hasten gastric emptying and small intestinal transit.[50,54-56] Cellulose decreases mouth-to-anus transit time in dogs[57] as does pectin.[58] The more rapid mouth-to-anus transit of pectin-containing diets is difficult to reconcile with the delay in gastric emptying caused by pectin unless transit through the large bowel is accelerated. "Normalization" of transit time was observed in some dogs fed a cellulose-containing diet; slow transit became faster and rapid transit was slowed.[57] The primary mechanism by which gel-forming fibers slow gastrointestinal transit is the hydrodynamic effects of increased intraluminal viscosity, and not marked alteration in neuromuscular function.[54,55]

Insoluble fibers modestly buffer gastric acid, and various fibers inhibit pancreatic enzyme activity.[51] For instance, wheat bran decreases pancreatic lipase secretion in dogs,[59] and pectin is known to markedly inhibit lipase activity in pigs and humans. Some fibers reduce brush border enzyme activity.[51] Soluble fibers may increase the viscosity of the unstirred water layer of the small intestinal mucosa, thus decreasing the absorption of some nutrients.[50] Fecal fat is increased by some fibers, perhaps via the effects on bile acid metabolism and pancreatic enzyme activity.[51,60] In one study, the apparent digestibility of protein and fat in dogs was found to be slightly decreased by the addition of cellulose to the diet.[57] Other studies in dogs, however, have not been able to detect a detrimental effect of fiber on digestibility of macronutrients.[35,58] It has been suggested that antinutrients associated with fibers (such as pectins, saponins, phytates, tannins, and enzyme inhibitors) may partly explain the mild detrimental effects of fibers on digestion and absorption of micronutrients and macronutrients observed in some studies.[48]

EFFECTS OF FIBER ON LARGE-BOWEL FUNCTION. Fiber influences the large bowel through a number of mechanisms (Figures 38–3 and 38–4).[48] Insoluble fibers bind various materials and dilute colonic content by their bulking activity.[50] This has the potential to reduce mucosal injury caused by noxious agents such as bile acids, ammonia, and toxic metals in the bowel lumen.[48,51] The gel-forming fibers and the lignins appear to be the most effective bile acid binding agents. The binding appears to be primarily an adsorption phenomenon and it is influenced by pH, osmolality, bile acid structure, and the form of the fiber.[51] Some fibers also bind fatty acids. In contrast to insoluble fibers, some soluble fibers increase colonic ammonia concentration. The increase in ammonia may be due to the trapping of ammonium ion in the colon by low colonic pH resulting from fermentation of soluble fiber. Alternatively, the increase may be due to mildly decreased protein absorption in the small intestine, providing increased substrate for colonic ammonia generation. Ammonia is toxic to the colonic mucosa, stimulates epithelial turnover, and increases tumorigenesis.

Colonic transit time is variably affected by different fibers

and is not necessarily predictable based on their solubility or insolubility. Some residue is necessary to stimulate normal colonic segmentation so that transit rates are normal. Colonic morphology is also affected by variations in dietary fiber.

Short chain fatty acids from fermented fiber markedly influence large-bowel structure and function. The quantity, composition, and site of production of SCFA varies considerably with species, microflora, and chemical composition of the fiber.[61,63,64] Fermentation of most soluble fibers generates large quantities of SCFA including acetate, propionate, and butyrate. Locus bean gum, corn grits, and pectin fibers are good sources of butyrate, at least in the cat.[64] Because of rapid fermentation in the upper large bowel, highly soluble fibers may actually produce less SCFA in the rectum than their poorly soluble counterparts that survive passage to the rectum in greater quantity.[61]

The salvage of fluid and electrolytes by the colon is closely associated with the absorption of SCFA,[65] perhaps via SCFA-bicarbonate and sodium-hydrogen exchange mechanisms.[50] Butyrate and, to a lesser extent, other SCFA are the principal energy sources of colonocytes.[65] These SCFA have a trophic effect on the large-bowel mucosa.[62] Butyrate enemas are effective therapy for diversion colitis and distal ulcerative colitis in humans.[67] Dogs fed a poorly fermentable fiber (cellulose) have colons that are significantly lighter in weight per kg body weight, and have a lower surface area to mucosal mass ratio than dogs fed fermentable fibers.[66] These changes are due to colonic mucosal hypertrophy in the dogs fed fermentable fiber. Also of interest is that the accumulation of inflammatory cells and/or necrotic crypt enterocytes (cryptitis) is higher in dogs fed a cellulose-based diet compared to dogs fed a diet containing beet pulp, a moderately fermentable fiber.[66]

Short chain fatty acids lower pH in the colon. Acidification of colonic content is associated with increased cell proliferation and, potentially, tumorigenesis.[68] Fortunately, however, butyrate appears to directly inhibit tumor formation in the large bowel.[61] Lowered luminal pH in the large bowel supports increased numbers of anaerobic flora and discourages the growth of pathogens including *Clostridium perfringens, Salmonella,* and pathogenic *E. coli.*[69,70] Furthermore, the secretion of colonic IgA can be increased or decreased by different types of dietary fiber.[51]

Mean fecal weight of dogs increases linearly with the addition of cellulose to the diet.[57] In contrast, low-residue diets such as cottage cheese and rice reduce the fecal volume of dogs by up to 85%, and also reduce the frequency of defecation. Fiber increases fecal bulk by two mechanisms. First, indigestible fiber acts as a sponge for water, increasing the weight and water content of the stool. Second, fiber that can be metabolized by bacteria provides substrate for bacterial growth and increases fecal bulk by elevating fecal bacterial numbers.[50,71] Psyllium (6 g q 8 hours) has been shown to improve fecal consistency and viscosity in humans with secretory diarrhea to a much greater extent than wheat bran. This property may be due to the gel-forming properties of psyllium.[72]

SUMMARY OF FIBER. In conclusion, it has been recommended that diets for small intestinal diseases be low in residue to avoid physical trauma to the inflamed gastrointestinal tract and to minimize the presumed negative effects of fiber on small intestinal assimilation of nutrients. This recommendation is in need of reexamination because there is little evidence to support the concept that fiber causes harmful physical abrasion to the intestinal tract, and accumulating evidence indicates that many fibers (in nutritionally practical amounts) cause very little interference with digestion of

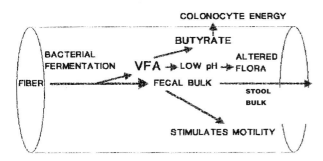

FIGURE 38–4. Effect of fiber on the large bowel.

macronutrients. Futhermore, on theoretical grounds, the binding and gelling properties of fiber may be beneficial in some small intestinal diseases.

The ability of fiber to markedly influence large-bowel physiology supports its continued use in the treatment of large-bowel diseases. What requires further definition, however, is which types of fiber are suitable for different large-bowel disorders and to which mechanism their beneficial effects can be attributed. These questions are particularly important because it appears fiber can have both detrimental and beneficial effects on large-bowel function.

Vitamins and Minerals

Deficiencies and excesses of vitamins and minerals have a series of well-recognized systemic effects,[73] but their influence on the bowel is less well studied. Deficiencies of vitamins and minerals are not uncommon in chronic gastrointestinal diseases. Thiamin deficiency may cause anorexia and vomiting in addition to its more classic CNS signs (Figure 38–5).[74] Pantothenic acid and riboflavin deficiency cause fatty liver. In cats, pantothenic acid deficiency causes gastrointestinal mucosal damage.[73] In dogs, niacin deficiency results in fatty liver, hemorrhagic diarrhea, and ulceration of the mucous membranes of the mouth and tongue (black tongue). In cats, the signs of niacin deficiency include diarrhea and emaciation.[74] Biotin deficiency can produce bloody diarrhea, and choline deficiency can result in a fatty liver. Vitamin A deficiency results in a significant reduction in the numbers of intestinal goblet cells and abnormalities in intestinal mucus.[75] Vitamin D or choline toxicity can result in diarrhea. Potassium deficiency can cause adynamic ileus, and zinc deficiency has been associated with vomiting.[74] Copper deficiency causes diarrhea, anemia, and depigmentation. Selenium deficiency has been associated with esophageal cancer in humans. Excess dietary iron is irritating to the mucosa and will induce diarrhea.

NUTRITIONAL DEFICIENCIES RESULTING FROM GASTROINTESTINAL DISEASE

The principal nutritional consequences of gastrointestinal disease are protein-calorie malnutrition and vitamin and mineral deficiencies.[76] The protein-calorie malnutrition usually results from a combination of decreased food intake and increased energy and protein requirements due to the disease process, malassimilation, and increased direct loss of protein into the gastrointestinal tract. Correction of protein-calorie malnutrition is hampered in some animals by recommendations to feed controlled diets of low palatability and caloric density.

Deficiencies of sodium, potassium, chloride, and bicarbonate are common with intestinal disease, and are discussed in Chapter 39. The demand for potassium and phosphorus is greatly increased by the anabolism that accompanies the resumption of appropriate nutrition. Increased loss of divalent cations such as magnesium, zinc, and calcium are known to occur in human gastrointestinal diseases. Chronic intestinal hemorrhage is a common cause of iron deficiency.

Vitamin B deficiencies can result from prolonged periods of anorexia and diarrhea.[73] Serum concentrations of cobalamin will decrease in some dogs with bacterial overgrowth or exocrine pancreatic insufficiency, and serum folate levels will be low in some severe small intestinal diseases.[77,78] Fat soluble vitamin deficiencies can occur with prolonged steatorrhea. A

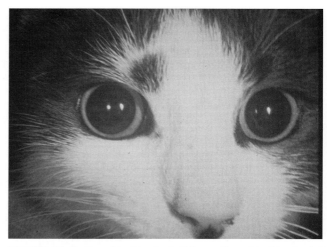

FIGURE 38–5. Cat with thiamin deficiency. Cats with thiamin deficiency are usually anorexic and can vomit, in addition to showing neurologic signs such as dilated pupils and postural abnormalities.

vitamin K-responsive coagulopathy has been noted in cats with lymphocytic-plasmacytic enteritis.[79]

PRINCIPLES IN FORMULATING DIETS

To undertake successful nutritional management of gastrointestinal disorders, the clinician must be able to assess the protein-calorie status of the patient, formulate a balanced diet that fulfills its energy and protein demands, and be familiar with which nutrients and which routes of nutrient administration are appropriate in particular gastrointestinal disorders. The nutrient contents of some commonly used ingredients for homemade diets are listed in Table 38–6. Unfortunately, most homemade diets recommended by veterinarians are unbalanced.[80]

Assessment of Protein-Calorie Status

An accurate assessment of the caloric and protein needs of a patient is important to successful nutritional management. Unfortunately, there is as yet no simple and accurate means of assessment that is both diagnostic of nutritional deficit and predictive of a favorable response to nutritional intervention.[81] In dogs and cats, the best approximation of caloric status comes from a combination of dietary history, physical examination, and patient's body weight.

DIET HISTORY. The dietary history helps determine the severity of deprivation. The calorie and protein content of the patient's present diet is estimated, and the duration if its nutrient restriction determined. The relative severity of the protein-calorie deficit can then be assessed by comparing the estimated intake with the calculated requirements of the animal. Where possible it is preferably to base the calculated requirements on the premorbid body weight.

PHYSICAL EXAMINATION. Assessment of coat condition, mental state, muscle and adipose mass, muscle strength, and body weight greatly assists determination of nutritional status. Nutritional deprivation results in a dull coat, mild to moderately depressed mentation, muscle weakness, and loss of muscle and adipose mass. Reduced protein mass can often be discerned by comparison of muscle mass with an adjacent bony prominence such as the sagittal crest of the cranium or the

Table 38–6

COMPOSITION OF VARIOUS FOODS*

	CHO (g)	ENERGY (kcal)	WATER (g)	PROTEIN (g)	FAT (g)
Meat, fatty	——	350	50	20	30
Meat, medium	——	275	56	24	20
Meat, lean	——	200	63	27	10
Heart	1	105	78	17	4
Milk, whole	4.7	67	87	3.5	3.8
skim	5.1	35	90	3.5	0.1
Casein powder	——	370	6	90	2.0
Cottage cheese (2% low fat)	3.6	90	79	14	2.0
Eggs, whole	0.7	163	74	13	12
Liver, beef	6	136	70	20	3
Liver, chicken	3	141	70	22	4
Kidney, beef	1	141	75	15	8
Tuna, in water	——	130	69	30	0.5
Brewer's yeast	34	330	13	42	2
Soybean meal	36	330	13	44	1
Oatmeal	56	360	13	16	8
Barley, pearl	78	353	11	8	1
Farina	76	357	11	11	1
Rice, brown	78	355	12	7	1.7
white	80	350	12	7	0.3
Tapioca	86	350	12	1	0.2
Pasta	70	385	10	14	5
Bread, white	52	270	35	8	3
whole wheat	49	260	37	9	3

*Per 100 g serving; uncooked.

spine of the scapula. Body weight is particularly valuable if it can be compared to the patient's usual body weight. In humans, recent weight loss as little as 2% to 6% per month has been used to predict significant calorie-protein malnutrition.[82] Acute weight loss of 10% of body mass will result in measurable decreases in muscle performance.[82] Fasted healthy dogs lose 1% to 3% of body weight daily.[83] More chronic weight loss in humans of 10% to 20% of ideal body weight is considered indicative of mild protein-calorie malnutrition. Reduction of ideal body weight of 20% to 30% is considered moderate deficiency and greater than 30% is considered severe.[76] An obvious confounding factor is that weight can fluctuate markedly as a result of fluid loss or gain due to dehydration, ascites, or edema.

BIOCHEMICAL PARAMETERS. Biochemical measures have been utilized in human medicine as a guide to nutritional status. Albumin is the most commonly used parameter, although it is considered by some to be of little value.[85] The serum concentration of albumin is affected by many factors other than nutritional status.[85] Furthermore, it has a relatively long serum half-life so there is a considerable lag time before serum albumin concentration reflects nutritional deprivation. For these reasons, serum albumin is a poor indicator of the nutritional status of a newly admitted patient. Serial serum albumin levels may, however, be of some value in monitoring the response to nutritional therapy, provided the clinician is cognizant of the confounding factors. Recently, plasma insulin-like growth

factor has been shown in humans to have many of the attributes of a reliable nutritional marker.[81]

Stress versus Simple Starvation

When deciding the patient's nutritional requirements, it is important to differentiate "simple starvation" from "stress starvation." Simple starvation refers to ingestion of insufficient calories in a healthy adult animal. Stress starvation refers to inadequate nutritional intake in an animal that is stressed by intercurrent disease or some energetically demanding process such as growth or lactation. These processes force the patient into an obligatory hypermetabolic state that utilizes fat and protein stores simultaneously. The hypermetabolic state resulting from disease is mediated by the release of cytokines such as interleukin-1, interleukin-6, and tumor necrosis factor. In contrast, simple starvation is a carefully controlled process in which metabolic rate declines and there is a shift to ketogenesis with the result that fat provides the majority of energy, and protein stores are spared. The clinical significance of this differentiation is that animals with stress starvation will rapidly develop complications of malnutrition whereas those subjected to simple starvation can survive weeks without significant complications.[86] Therefore, nutritional intervention is required much earlier in patients with stress starvation.

Calculation of Energy Requirements

Estimation of a patient's energy and protein requirements can be difficult because demand varies according to weight, age, activity level, and physiologic state.[74,87–89] For an in-depth discussion of the calculation of energy requirements, see recent publications on the subject.[74,83,89] For purposes of this discussion, you should be familiar with the term *basal energy expenditure* (basal metabolic rate). Basal energy expenditure is the energy expended by an animal to maintain life while it is resting quietly in the postabsorptive state in a thermoneutral environment. The basal energy expenditure (BEE) for dogs and cats is provided in Table 38–7. By using the table, and the following adjustments factors, the energy requirements for different physiologic and pathologic states may be calculated. Thus, maintenance energy requirements for a caged animal are approximately $1.25 \times BEE$ (maintenance energy expenditure is greater than that required for BEE because of the energy demands made by the small amount of movement of a caged animal and the energy lost in the digestion of food). Energy requirements for normal canine activity are approximately 1.75 to $2.0 \times BEE$, and for normal feline activity approximately $1.4 \times BEE$. Energy requirements during major infections or inflammatory diseases have been estimated to range from 1.25 to $2.0 \times BEE$. Recent studies on the metabolic requirements of humans have found that the energy requirements of such patients rarely, if ever, exceed $1.5 \times BEE$,[82] suggesting the estimated energy requirements for severe illness in the dog should be reexamined. Extreme physical activity can raise energy requirements to 3 to $4 \times BEE$. Growth raises energy requirements to 2 to $3 \times BEE$, and lactation raises energy requirements to 4 to $6 \times BEE$.

The principal energy sources in diets are usually carbohydrate and fat. The relative proportion of energy provided as carbohydrate or fat depends on a number of factors. Fat has more caloric density than carbohydrates but it is also more difficult to assimilate when the gastrointestinal tract is compromised. The

Table 38–7

ENERGY REQUIREMENTS FOR DOGS AND CATS*

BODY WEIGHT (kg)	ESTIMATED BASAL ENERGY EXPENDITURE[a] (kcal/day)	ESTIMATED AVERAGE ENERGY EXPENDITURE[b] (kcal/day)
1	70	105
1.5	95	142
2	118	177
2.5	139	209
3	160	239
3.5	179	269
4	198	297
4.5	216	324
5	234	351
6	268	403
7	301	452
8	333	499
9	364	546
10	394	590
11	423	634
12	451	677
13	479	719
14	507	760
15	534	800
16	560	840
17	586	879
18	612	918
19	637	956
20	662	993
21	687	1030
22	711	1067
23	735	1103
24	759	1139
25	783	1174
26	806	1209
27	829	1244
28	852	1278
29	875	1312
30	897	1346
35	1107	1511
40	1113	1670
45	1216	1824
50	1316	1974
60	1509	2264
70	1694	2541
80	1872	2809
90	2045	3068
100	2214	3320

[a]$70 \times BW \text{ kg } 0.75$
*Average energy requirements for the critically ill patient; calculated as $1.5 \times BEE$. Caged animals with minimal activity and minor disease stress perhaps would be more closely approximated by $1.25 \times BEE$. Normal canine activity or very severe disease stress in either the dog or cat perhaps would be more accurately approximated by 1.75 or $2.0 \times BEE$. Lactation, late-stage pregnancy, and heavy exercise may increase energy requirements 4 to $6 \times BEE$.
[b]Average energy requirements of a dog with normal activity.
Courtesy of Dr. S.C. Haskins, Department of Surgery, School of Veterinary Medicine, University of California, Davis, CA.

caloric density of long chain triglycerides is approximately 9 kcal per g whereas that of carbohydrate is approximately 4 kcal per g. The advantage of high caloric density is that it reduces dietary volume which can be a major concern in an inappetent patient. Medium chain triglycerides are better assimilated than long chain triglycerides and provide approximately 8.3 kcal per g. Unfortunately they are at times poorly tolerated by the patient. The amount of dietary fat given to animals with small-bowel-type diarrhea is usually severely limited by the adverse consequences of malassimilated lipid on digestive function. As a general rule, fat in the diet of animals with diarrhea is limited to less than 15% of the diet on a dry matter basis.

Calculation of Protein Requirements

Careful attention must be paid to the level of protein being fed. The dysfunction resulting from protein deficiency is most obvious in growing animals because growth potential will not be satisfied. Adults are also affected, however. Initially, the dysfunction is subclinical, and includes such phenomena as impaired immunity and decreased physical and mental activity. As protein loss continues decreased muscle mass becomes obvious, the immune response becomes more severely comprised, wound healing is impaired, organ dysfunction occurs (such as cardiomypathy), and skeletal muscle weakness (including that of the diaphragm) becomes obvious. If excess protein is ingested, it is not stored as a protein reserve but is metabolized to provide energy. This is an inefficient way to feed an animal because protein is an expensive component of the diet. Furthermore, excess protein has been incriminated as a contributor to hepatic encephalopathy in patients with pre-existing liver disease.

Arbitrary requirements for protein are provided in Tables 38–8 and 38–9. Protein requirements can increase considerably with intestinal diseases. In healthy animals, large amounts of protein (approximately 1 g per kg per day) enter the gastrointestinal tract in pancreatic and intestinal secretions and from desquamated mucosal cells. The majority of this is reabsorbed (approximately 90%). Any disease that speeds transit time, increases the mucosal cell turnover rate, or promotes mucus secretion is likely to increase protein requirements. Another obvious example is the syndrome of protein-losing enteropathy. In humans, fecal protein loss in protein-losing enteropathies can amount to as much as 0.5 g/kg/day. Unfortunately, there is no practical way to estimate the increased protein requirements for a patient with protein-losing enteropathy, and requirements are usually determined by trial and error using clinical condition and plasma albumin concentration as a guide. It has been determined in humans that, with the exception of major fractures and burns, protein requirements during diseases (including intestinal diseases) are rarely more than double basal requirements.[82] As a rule of thumb, it has been recommended that patients with mild diseases receive dietary protein to provide 130% of basal daily requirements, and patients with moderate and severe disease receive 160% and 200% of daily basal requirements, respectively.[82]

Conversely, the protein fed to an animal may have to be reduced because of diseases such as liver disease. In these circumstances the amount of protein provided is selected to minimize clinical signs of encephalopathy but with consideration of the minimum protein requirements for that species (dog, 1.3–1.5 g/kg/day; cat, 3.3–3.5 g/kg/day).[90] For instance, it has been recommended that dogs with portosystemic shunts receive a minimum of 2.11 g of crude protein (> 80% digestibility) per kg of body weight per day.[91]

Calculation of Other Nutritional Requirements

The vitamin and mineral requirements of dogs and cats are listed in Tables 38–8 and 38–9. As with protein and energy, the requirements for micronutrients vary with the life stage

Table 38–8

NUTRIENT ALLOWANCES OF NORMAL DOGS*

NUTRIENT	UNITS DM BASIS	GROWTH AND REPRODUCTIVE MINIMUM	ADULT MAINTENANCE MINIMUM	MAXIMUM
Protein	%	22.0	18.0	
Arginine	%	0.62	0.51	
Histidine	%	0.22	0.18	
Isoleucine	%	0.45	0.37	
Leucine	%	0.72	0.59	
Lysine	%	0.77	0.63	
Methionine/cystine	%	0.53	0.43	
Phenylal/tyrosine	%	0.89	0.73	
Threonine	%	0.58	0.48	
Tryptophan	%	0.20	0.16	
Valine	%	0.48	0.39	
Fat	%	8.0	5.0	
Linoleic acid	%	1.0	1.0	
Minerals				
Calcium	%	1.0	0.6	2.5
Phosphorus	%	0.8	0.5	1.6
Ca:P ratio	—	1:1	1:1	2:1
Potassium	%	0.6	0.6	
Sodium	%	0.3	0.06	
Chloride	%	0.45	0.09	
Magnesium	%	0.04	0.04	0.3
Iron	mg/kg	80	80	3000
Copper	mg/kg	7.3	7.3	250
Manganese	mg/kg	5.0	5.0	
Zinc	mg/kg	120	120	1000
Iodine	mg/kg	1.5	1.5	50
Selenium	mg/kg	0.11	0.11	2
Vitamins				
Vitamin A	IU/kg	5000	5000	50,000
Vitamin D	IU/kg	500	500	5,000
Vitamin E	IU/kg	50	50	1,000
Thiamin	mg/kg	1.0	1.0	
Riboflavin	mg/kg	2.2	2.2	
Pantothenate	mg/kg	10.0	10.0	
Niacin	mg/kg	11.4	11.4	
Pyridoxine	mg/kg	1.0	1.0	
Folic acid	mg/kg	0.18	0.18	
Vitamin B_{12}	mg/kg	0.022	0.022	
Choline	mg/kg	1200	1200	

*This table is derived from the recommendations of the Canine Nutrition Expert Committee of the American Association of Feed Control Officials. The recommendations assume the food eaten has an energy density of approximately 3.5 kcal ME/g DM. Dogs eating diets of significantly higher energy density (> 4.0 kcal/g) should have their intakes of protein, vitamins, and minerals increased proportionately to the percentage increase in energy density. Many of the values listed exceed NRC (1985) recommended minimums because allowance has been made for predicted processing losses and the limited digestibility of the ingredients commonly used in pet foods. Animals receiving intravenous nutrition solutions, enteral diets, and some homemade diets may not require the full allowance recommended in these tables because of the greater availability of some of the nutrients in these diets in comparison to commercial foods.

and physiologic condition of the animal. For instance, the requirements for B vitamins are increased during accelerated metabolism, and the requirements for fat soluble vitamins increase in proportion to the severity of steatorrhea. As discussed earlier, the ideal fiber percentage of the diet also varies with the clinical condition.

Summary

In summary, the first step in the formulation of a diet for a patient with a digestive system disorder is the calculation of energy needs, which determines the quantity of food to be fed. The energy requirement is based on estimates of the protein-calorie status of the patient, the basal energy expendi-

ture for an animal of that size, and the increased energy requirements due to the particular disease. The next consideration is the protein requirement of the patient, which is calculated in an analogous manner to the energy requirement. Decisions are then made on dietary levels of fat and fiber, based on a knowledge of the influence of these nutrients on gastrointestinal function. Finally, it must be decided whether adequate nutrients can be provided by the oral route or if nutritional support by other means is required.

It is important to emphasize that the calculations made in the formulation of a diet make a number of arbitrary assumptions, and the potential for significant error is high. Therefore, it is essential that the condition of the patient be carefully monitored and the diet subsequently modified according to patient response.

Table 38–9

NUTRIENT ALLOWANCES OF NORMAL CATS*

NUTRIENT	UNITS DM BASIS	GROWTH AND REPRODUCTIVE MINIMUM	ADULT MAINTENANCE MINIMUM	MAXIMUM
Protein	%	30.0	26.0	
Arginine	%	1.25	1.04	
Histidine	%	0.31	0.31	
Isoleucine	%	0.52	0.52	
Leucine	%	1.25	1.25	
Lysine	%	1.20	0.83	
Methionine/cystine	%	1.10	1.10	
Methionine	%	0.62	0.62	1.5
Phenylal/tyrosine	%	0.88	0.88	
Phenylalanine	%	0.42	0.42	
Taurine (extruded)	%	0.10	0.10	
Taurine (canned)	%	0.20	0.20	
Threonine	%	0.73	0.73	
Tryptophan	%	0.25	0.16	
Valine	%	0.62	0.62	
Fat	%	9.0	9.0	
Linoleic acid	%	0.5	0.5	
Arachidonic acid	%	0.02	0.02	
Minerals				
Calcium	%	1.0	0.6	
Phosphorus	%	0.8	0.5	
Ca:P ratio	—	1:1	1:1	
Potassium	%	0.6	0.6	
Sodium	%	0.2	0.2	
Chloride	%	0.3	0.3	
Magnesium	%	0.08	0.04	
Iron	mg/kg	80.0	80.0	
Copper	mg/kg	5.0	5.0	
Iodine	mg/kg	0.35	0.35	
Zinc	mg/kg	75.0	75.0	2000
Manganese	mg/kg	7.5	7.5	
Selenium	mg/kg	0.1	0.1	
Vitamins				
Vitamin A	IU/kg	5000	5000	750,000
Vitamin D	IU/kg	500	500	10,000
Vitamin E	IU/kg	30	30	
Vitamin K†	mg/kg	0.1	0.1	
Thiamin	mg/kg	5.0	5.0	
Riboflavin	mg/kg	4.0	4.0	
Pyridoxine	mg/kg	4.0	4.0	
Niacin	mg/kg	60.0	60.0	
Pantothenate	mg/kg	5.0	5.0	
Folic acid	mg/kg	0.8	0.8	
Vitamin B_{12}	mg/kg	0.02	0.02	
Choline	mg/kg	2400	2400	

*This table is derived from the recommendations of the Feline Nutrition Expert Committee of the American Association of Feed Control Officials. The recommendations assume the food eaten has an energy density of approximately 4.0 kcal ME/g DM. Cats eating diets of significantly higher energy density (> 4.5 kcal/g) should have their intakes of protein, vitamins, and minerals increased proportionately to the percentage increase in energy density. Many of the values listed exceed NRC (1986) recommended minimums because allowance has been made for predicted processing losses and the limited digestibility of the ingredients commonly used in pet foods. Animals receiving intravenous nutrition solutions, enteral diets, and some homemade diets may not require the full allowance recommended in these tables because of the greater availability of some of the nutrients in these diets in comparison to commercial foods.
†Supplementary vitamin K is needed in fish-based diets only.

NUTRITIONAL THERAPY OF GASTROINTESTINAL PROBLEMS

Controlled diets are helpful in the management of most gastrointestinal diseases.[92] The term *controlled diet* refers to a diet in which a veterinarian has control over the ingredients. There have been few studies to determine the nutritional requirements of dogs and cats with gastrointestinal disorders. The recommendations provided here are based predominantly on clinical experience and pathophysiologic theory and must be regarded as tentative.

Dysphagia, Aversion, Anorexia, and Polyphagia

PHYSIOLOGY OF INTAKE. Food intake is controlled by a complex interaction of many factors. In the healthy animal, food intake is programmed to maintain body weight with remarkable consistency in spite of marked fluctuations of energy requirements on a day-to-day and week-to-week basis. The ebb and flow of appetite and satiety results from various gastrointestinal, environmental, and CNS phenomena. The gastrointestinal phenomena include gastric distention, rate of gastric emptying, the release of gastric hormones (in particular CCK and bombesin), and the absorption of nutrients such as glucose, fatty acids, and amino acids.[93,94] The gut hormones have effects both locally on the gastrointestinal tract and centrally on the thalamic centers that control feeding behavior. An important example is CCK, which decreases appetite by inhibiting gastric emptying and by inhibiting the CNS feeding "center." The inhibitory influence of absorbed nutrients on intake has been proposed to operate through "glucostats," "lipostats," "aminostats," and "purinostats," although the importance, location, structure, and function of these "appetostats" remains poorly elucidated.

Feeding behavior is ultimately under control of the CNS feeding centers. Threatening environmental factors operating through these centers will reduce food intake. In addition to the gastrointestinal and environmental phenomena already mentioned, the CNS can be directly influenced by the diet. The ingestion of a protein meal results in the absorption of amino acids that cross the blood-brain barrier and directly alter the concentration of neurotransmitters in the CNS. Furthermore, some of the absorbed nutrients may alter the responsiveness of CNS receptors.

Neurotransmitters of importance in the control of intake include catecholamines operating through beta adrenergic receptors (inhibitory) and alpha adrenergic receptors (stimulatory); dopamine (inhibitory); serotonin (inhibitory); opioids operating through kappa receptors and mu receptors; and gamma aminobutyric acid (GABA). Naloxone, binding to opioid receptors, is inhibitory to food intake, whereas butorphanol stimulates feeding. Benzodiazepines operate in conjunction with GABA to increase appetite, and inhibit the serotonergic satiety system. Glucocorticoids increase intake, partly by a direct effect on CNS inhibitors of appetite, such as serotonin, and partly by an anti-inflammatory effect.

PALATABILITY, ACCEPTABILITY, AND FOOD AVERSION. Diets of poor palatability result in poor acceptability of a food so the amount of food consumed may not satisfy caloric requirements. The animal is not anorectic per se, in that a more palatable food is readily consumed. Properties of a food that influence palatability include smell, taste, texture, temperature, pH, and even appearance. High fat content and moderate levels of protein are generally preferred by cats and dogs. Nucleotides, monosodium glutamate, and animal digests encourage palatability in cats.[95] Cats also prefer their food warm (30°–40° C) and with a low pH (3 to 5).[95,96] Palatability enhancers for dogs include animal digests, certain amino acids (such as L-lysine), nucleotides, and monosodium glutamate.[95] Dogs also prefer their food warm (20°–40° C).[95] Rancidity negatively affects palatability in both cats and dogs. Learned food aversion occurs when the ingestion of a food is associated with nausea or vomiting. Dogs and cats will also become averse to diets of imbalanced amino acid composition. Poor dietary palatability and food aversion result in a capricious intake in dogs and often complete refusal to eat in cats.

PATHOPHYSIOLOGY OF INTAKE. Prolonged, inappropriate satiety is termed *anorexia* or *inappetence*. The causes of anorexia are legion. Threatening environments, including veterinary clinics and boarding establishments, inhibit appetite. Inflammatory, infectious, or neoplastic diseases can cause inappetence, probably as a result of the release of a variety of chemical mediators such as cachectin and interleukin-1. Painful oropharyngeal lesions can cause reluctance to eat or dysphagia. Diseases that cause nausea or delay gastric emptying result in inappetence, perhaps partly through gastric distension. Anorexia is not the only cause of decreased food intake. Others include dysphagia, poor dietary acceptability, and food aversion.

A prolonged and inappropriately excessive appetite is termed *polyphagia*. Most causes of polyphagia are due to endocrine disorders such as diabetes mellitus, hyperthyroidism, and hyperadrenocorticism. Occasionally, gastrointestinal diseases such as pancreatic insufficiency or malabsorption will cause polyphagia. Some dogs and cats appear to eat to excess for indeterminate reasons. One consequence of polyphagia is obesity, which in turn increases the likelihood of joint, skin, and respiratory problems. Gastrointestinal causes of polyphagia do not result in obesity.

MANAGEMENT OF ANOREXIA AND POOR DIETARY ACCEPTABILITY. The management of anorexia begins with attention to the primary cause if identifiable. Symptomatic therapy includes attention to fluid and electrolyte derangements, reduction of environmental stressors, and modification of the diet to improve palatability. Reduction in stress is best attained by careful and considerate handling. With reassurance, some frightened animals can be coaxed to eat.

Palatability of the diet can be improved by adding flavored toppings such as chicken or beef broths, seasoning with condiments such as garlic powder, increasing the fat or protein content, varying the texture and appearance of the food, and heating the food to improve its aroma and temperature (no more than body temperature).

If such manipulations fail, and the patient is capable of ingesting food, drug therapy can be tried prior to offering the food. Benzodiazepine derivatives such as diazepam (0.1 mg/kg IV) and oxazepam (0.5 mg/kg PO q 12–24 hours) will produce an increase in appetite in most cats and some dogs. Butorphanol (0.2 mg/kg SC) may also be useful, particularly if analgesia is also required. Cyproheptadine, an antihistamine with antiserotonergic properties, has been used as an appetite stimulant in cats and dogs (0.2–0.5 mg/kg PO q 12 hours) with mixed success. Metoclopramide (0.2–0.4 mg/kg SC, PO) is useful if anorexia is associated with delayed gastric emptying or ileus and may also have a central influence by way of its antidopaminergic-antiemetic effects. If these efforts fail, or if nutritional support greater than several days duration is required, enteral feeding techniques should be considered.

NUTRITIONAL MANAGEMENT OF DYSPHAGIA. The symptomatic management of dysphagia includes altering the texture of the diet and feeding from an elevated receptacle. Abnormal motility of the pharynx and/or esophagus sometimes causes great difficulty in swallowing solid boluses of food although the swallowing of liquid or gruels is little affected. Occasionally, solids are swallowed better than liquids, perhaps because the solid food bolus provides sufficient sensory stimulus to initiate the swallowing reflex in those animals with a vagal sensory deficit. Nutritional management is thus largely directed by trial and error, although dogs with megaesophagus generally fare better with liquid diets. Many dysphagic patients must be fed via gastrostomy tubes.

Acute Gastroenteritis

Standard dietary recommendations for dogs and cats with acute gastroenteritis include fasting for 12 to 48 hours, followed by small quantities of a "bland" diet fed 3 to 4 times per day for 3 to 7 days. These dietary recommendations have stood the test of time but are based more on common sense than scientific investigations.

Fasting the animal for a short period provides so-called bowel rest. This is traditionally considered of prime importance in the treatment of most gastrointestinal problems, although it has been recently challenged in the treatment of diarrhea (see later). In acute problems, bowel rest is accomplished by completely restricting the oral intake of food. The advantage of small frequent feedings might be to limit the duration of acid secretion at each meal. A moment's introspection confirms that small volumes of food provoke less nausea during acute gastritis.

"Bland" diets are diets without coarse and spicy foods. Most commercial pet food could, therefore, be thought of as bland. One theoretical justification for *not* feeding a vomiting dog or cat its usual diet is the observation in humans that acquired food allergies to proteins eaten during acute gastroenteritis can delay recovery.[97,98] There is clinical and gastroscopic food sensitivity testing evidence to suggest that the same phenomenon also occurs in the cat and dog. Acquired food allergies to novel protein sources temporarily introduced into a vomiting animal's diet (such as chicken or cottage cheese) are not as problematic as an acquired allergy to a dietary staple such as beef.

Gastric Diseases

Little information is available on suitable diets for inflammatory or ulcerative gastric diseases. Most authorities recommend a bland diet.[99,100] Milk, which was recommended in the past as a buffering/coating agent, fell from favor because of concern about the stimulatory effects on gastric acid secretion of calcium and protein in milk.[99,100] However, interest in milk feeding is now undergoing a resurgence because of evidence that intragastric administration of lipid emulsions improves the hydrophobicity of the gastric mucosal barrier.[101] Frequent small feeding may provide symptomatic relief but have not been shown to hasten healing.[100] Liquidizing the diet will hasten gastric emptying, reducing gastric acid secretion. Minimizing the protein content of the food may also reduce gastric acid secretion. The buffering action of insoluble fiber and its acceleration of gastric emptying may one day be proven valuable for the treatment of gastric diseases. A suitable commercial diet is i/d (Hill's Pet Products), and suitable homemade diets are the cottage cheese or chicken and rice diets given in Tables 38–10 and 38–11.

Nutritional management of delayed gastric emptying has limited effectiveness. Fluids and solids empty differently from the stomach, which suggests that altering the consistency of the diet may help some patients. Vagotomy accelerates the emptying of fluids but decreases the emptying of solids, implying that emptying disorders resulting from neuropathies (such as dysautonomia or diabetic neuropathy) may be ameliorated by use of liquid diets. Emptying is delayed by the use of hyperosmolar and high-fat foods. Therefore, in the first few days of therapy the liquid diet should be diluted to iso-osmolarity and should contain little fat. Unfortunately, such foods are often without sufficient caloric density to maintain animals for prolonged periods.

Gastric dumping disorders result from the accelerated emptying of hyperosmolar chyme into the duodenum. Diets with a high soluble fiber content (such as 3% w/v psyllium) slow gastric emptying in dogs[55] and may therefore be useful

Table 38–10

CONTROLLED DIET FOR VOMITING AND/OR DIARRHEA IN DOGS*

1. 8 ounces of cooked white rice
2. 4 ounces of low-fat cottage cheese†
3. 1 teaspoon of vegetable oil‡
4. 1 teaspoon of dicalcium phosphate‡
5. 0.75 teaspoons of iodized "lite" salt (KCl)‡
6. Multivitamin and mineral supplement to fulfill recommended daily allowances‡§
7. Consider 1 to 6 teaspoons Metamucil per meal if suspect large-bowel diarrhea

*Diet contains 19%–20% DM protein; 7.3% DM fat; and provides approximately 400 kcal.
†For elimination diets, the cottage cheese can be substituted with another protein source such as tofu, cooked lamb, or skinned and cooked chicken.
‡If using this diet as an elimination diet, these ingredients can be omitted for the first 1–2 weeks of therapy.
§Especially vitamin A, B vitamins, iron, copper, and zinc.

in the management of dumping.[48] Small frequent feedings and avoidance of diets high in simple carbohydrates have been recommended in humans.[100] Feeding dry food and avoiding drinking fluids with the meal may also slow gastric emptying.[102]

Acute "Small-Bowel" Diarrhea

The traditional dietary therapy of acute diarrhea is similar to that described for acute gastroenteritis. Dogs and cats with acute diarrhea are usually fasted for 12 to 48 hours and then offered a bland, low-fat diet fed frequently and in small quantities for 3 to 7 days. Dietary fat is kept to a minimum because fat undergoes a complex digestion and absorption process that is easily disrupted by gastroenteritis. Furthermore, malabsorbed fatty acids and bile acids promote secretory diarrhea in the large bowel.

Recently, the long-held belief in the value of bowel rest for the treatment of diarrhea has been challenged by the concepts of food-based oral rehydration therapy and feeding-through-diarrhea. Food-based oral rehydration therapy differs from feeding-through-diarrhea primarily in the amount of nutrients provided.

Oral rehydration therapy, using inorganic salts, dextrose, and amino acids, has been successfully practiced for many years in humans, production animals, and dogs (see Chapter

Table 38–11

CONTROLLED DIET FOR VOMITING AND/OR DIARRHEA IN CATS*

1. 5 ounces rice cereal powder cooked in chicken soup or broth
2. 5 ounces of finely chopped poultry
3. 1 teaspoon vegetable oil‡
4. 1 teaspoon of dicalcium phosphate‡
5. 0.5 teaspoons of iodized "lite" salt (KCl)‡
6. Multivitamin and mineral supplement to fulfill recommended daily allowances§‡
7. Add small quantities of liver (0.5 oz) if required for palatability‡

*Modified from Kronfeld DS (1983).[162]
†Diet contains 40% DM protein; 11% DM fat; and provides approximately 400 kcal.
‡If using this diet as an elimination diet, these ingredients can be omitted for the first 1–2 weeks of therapy.
§Especially B vitamins, iron, copper, and zinc.

39). It has recently become apparent that the addition of small quantities of cereals, such as rice, to the solution enhances salt and water absorption, and provides slightly more calories than standard oral rehydration solutions.[103] The glucose and peptides in rice furnish organic substrates for fluid and electrolyte pumps without markedly increasing dietary osmolality.[104-107] Furthermore, at least in some studies, food-based oral rehydration solutions reduce stool volume and shorten the course of diarrhea in comparison to glucose-based solutions.[103,108,109] One such riced-based rehydration solution used in humans is shown in Table 39–4. It is possible similar solutions, fed through nasogastric tubes or per os, may be of value in the short-term symptomatic treatment of cats and dogs with acute diarrhea.

Feeding-through-diarrhea (with sufficient solid or semi-solid food to satisfy the approximate caloric requirements) has recently proven beneficial in humans with acute diarrhea. Feeding-through-diarrhea maintains greater mucosal barrier integrity and helps minimize malnutrition, usually without prolonging the duration of diarrhea.[103,110] At first sight these observations might encourage veterinary clinicians to feed their diarrhea patients. Caution is required, however, before the tried-and-true "no food per os" recommendation is abandoned in dogs and cats with diarrhea. Most of the studies showing beneficial effects of feeding-through-diarrhea were performed in children affected by secretory diarrhea due to toxigenic organisms such as cholera.[103] Feeding-through was less successful in children with severe diarrhea or those with rotavirus infection,[103] which produces an osmotic diarrhea. Osmotic diarrhea due to viral infections (parvovirus, corona-virus, rotavirus, etc.) and dietary indiscretions are more common in dogs and cats than are secretory diarrheas. Furthermore, daily stooling frequency was increased in several studies of humans fed during diarrhea.[103] This may not be of major consequence to humans (provided duration of the diarrhea is not extended) but can be disastrous to the owner of a pet defecating in the house. Consequently, feeding-through-diarrhea is likely to be less successful in veterinary practice than current recommendations of "no food per os."

Chronic "Small-Bowel" Diarrhea

The ideal diet for chronic small-bowel-type diarrhea is based on a highly digestible protein and carbohydrate source, is gluten free, low in lactose and fat, hypoallergenic, isotonic, and contains generous overages of potassium and water soluble and fat soluble vitamins. Good palatability, nutritional balance, and convenience are also required. The diet should incorporate the fewest ingredients possible, so the influence of each ingredient on the patient's bowel function can be assessed. Strict adherence to a controlled diet depends on the effectiveness of client education. Owners often incorrectly believe that minor dietary alterations are of no consequence. Suitable diets for dogs and cats with small-bowel diarrhea are provided in Tables 38–10 and 38–11.

DIGESTIBILITY. High digestibility results in more complete absorption in the cranial small intestine, permitting the remainder of the bowel to rest. Highly digestible diets reduce the likelihood of gaseousness and osmotic diarrhea due to malabsorption. Highly digestible protein is less antigenic because little dietary protein is absorbed intact into the mucosa. Furthermore, less protein will enter the colon, preventing excessive colonic ammonia generation. Diets needing minimal digestion stimulate pancreatic, biliary, and intestinal secretion less than do regular diets.

The diet is known to have an important effect on the num-

ber and type of enteric bacteria.[33,111] The rate of bacterial growth is directly related to nutrient availability. Total intestinal bacterial counts decline with the feeding of highly digestible diets such as elemental diets. These diets are virtually completely absorbed in the proximal small intestine. Thus, the bacterial flora is "starved," and its total population is reduced. By reducing the total number of bacteria, the number of potential invaders, the amount of enterotoxin produced, and the total antigenic load in the intestinal tract is limited.

PROTEIN SOURCES. Protein used in the treatment of small-bowel diarrhea should be derived from one food source and, as described earlier, should be highly digestible to limit antigenicity. A protein source not commonly included in the animal's usual diet is advantageous because it reduces the likelihood of feeding a protein to which the animal is allergic. Furthermore, acquired allergy (resulting from gastrointestinal inflammation; see Chapter 24) to an infrequently fed protein is less problematical than acquired allergy to a dietary staple. Suitable protein sources for dogs include cottage cheese, tofu, eggs, chicken, venison, lamb (except Australasia), and rabbit, but any other highly digestible meat not commonly included in the animal's diet is also likely to be well tolerated. Cottage cheese is advantageous because it contains less lipid than eggs and meat (Table 38–6). Cottage cheese is less palatable to cats than dogs, but chicken, turkey, fish, and liver (provided liver is not fed continuously) are readily accepted alternatives.

The amount of protein used in the initial diet should comfortably meet the animal's protein requirements. Excess protein should be avoided to minimize dietary antigenicity and to limit the amount of protein in the ileal effluent.

CARBOHYDRATE SOURCES. An ideal carbohydrate source for dogs and cats with small-bowel diarrhea is rice. White rice is highly digestible and does not induce gluten enteropathy. Furthermore, there are few reported allergies to rice proteins in dogs or cats. Boiled white rice is suitable for dogs and baby rice cereals for cats. Other carbohydrates that can be used include corn, potatoes, or tapioca. These are all gluten free. Potato and tapioca starches are less digestible than rice starch, however.[20] Corn starch is very well digested[20] but, because corn is widely used in pet foods, the prevalence of allergies to corn proteins is likely to be higher than that of rice. Pasta is another alternative but is not gluten free.

The advisability of including carbohydrate in the diet of cats with diarrhea has been questioned[26,27] because of concern about the palatability and digestibility of carbohydrate in cats. For the first few weeks of treatment, there is no compelling reason to include carbohydrate in the diet of cats with diarrhea. In the long term, however, it is sensible from the economic point of view (and perhaps also for renal health) to "dilute" the protein with carbohydrate. The palatability of rice baby cereals to cats can be enhanced by cooking the cereal with chicken soup or broth.

Sudden change of an animal to a high carbohydrate diet should be avoided. Large quantities of newly introduced carbohydrate in the diet may initially be inadequately digested and absorbed, until pancreatic enzyme and brush border enzyme levels increase to meet the changed digestive requirements.[3,112,113] This problem is minimized by feeding small meals frequently.

LACTOSE AND GLUTEN CONTENT. Disaccharides, especially lactose, should be avoided because the brush border disaccharidases (lactose, maltase, isomaltose, and sucrase) are temporarily reduced following diarrhea due to any cause. Diets for the treatment of small-bowel diarrhea are preferably gluten free (see Chapter 24) in case the diarrhea is due to gluten enteropathy.

FAT CONTENT. Restriction of fat is usually necessary because fat malassimilation commonly complicates small-bowel diarrhea. Fat restriction is not necessary in all motility disorders or in many cases of chronic colitis. It has been suggested that cats with diarrhea tolerate high-fat diets better than high-carbohydrate diets. This suggestion needs further investigation before widespread application. Low-fat foods include vegetables, bread, cereals, low-fat milk products, most fish, and lean meats such as boiled poultry (without skin). MCT oil can be used to supplement the dietary fat (see earlier).

HYPOALLERGENICITY. Hypoallergenicity minimizes the risks of acquired gastrointestinal allergies secondary to mucosal barrier dysfunction. The principles of hypoallergenic diets are discussed in Chapters 24 and 25. The allergenicity of a diet is reduced by decreasing the amount of protein fed, and choosing highly digestible proteins. The protein source fed should be one to which the animal has had little exposure.

OSMOLALITY. The ideal diet has a restricted osmolality to prevent excessive extracellular fluid moving into the intestine and to minimize the damage to the mucosa that can occur with such diets. High osmolality is one stimulus for gastrointestinal inflammation, and can also disrupt tight junction structure.[115] Furthermore, if the constituents of the hyperosmolar diet are not readily absorbed, osmotic diarrhea will develop. Hyperosmolarity is most often of concern when feeding excessive amounts of hyperosmolar liquid elemental diets.

VITAMIN AND MINERAL CONTENT. Increased loss of water soluble vitamins and electrolytes, such as sodium and potassium, occurs with diarrhea. Steatorrhea results in increased loss of fat soluble vitamins. For these reasons, diets used for the treatment of diarrhea should be adequately supplemented with vitamins and minerals.[73] This is particularly important in cats, a species in which thiamin and potassium depletion are not infrequently seen. Thiamin deficiency can develop in as little as 3 to 4 days in cats with watery diarrhea in which the combination of poor body stores, decreased intake from anorexia, and increased loss of thiamin in diarrhea lead to rapid depletion (Figure 38–5). Most diets contain more than adequate amounts of sodium, but conservative increases in the content of dietary potassium may be advantageous in animals with diarrhea because the potassium content of some commercial foods may not be high enough to meet the increased losses induced by diarrhea.

In general, no controlled diet should be used for greater than 2 to 3 weeks without adequate vitamin and mineral supplementation. These micronutrients are best supplied by way of fractionated doses from a multivitamin and mineral capsule that fulfills all human recommended daily allowances. Using a human vitamin and mineral capsule avoids accidental inclusion in the diet of the potentially allergenic proteins contained in "palatable" or "chewable" veterinary vitamin and mineral supplements. In addition to the multivitamin and mineral capsule, it is usually necessary to provide supplementary calcium, phosphorus, potassium (usually as "lite" salt), and essential fatty acids (like vegetable or corn oil).

Most patients can be adequately supported with oral mineral supplements but, in the presence of severe malabsorption, parenteral administration of vitamins is sometimes required. If administered parenterally, B vitamins are usually included in intravenous fluids or given every 2 to 3 days subcutaneously, and fat soluble vitamins are given intramuscularly every week. If oral supplementation is used in the face of malabsorptive diseases, the daily dose of vitamins and minerals provided is often arbitrarily doubled to compensate for decreased absorption. The adequacy or necessity of such adjustments has not been examined in the dog or cat.

FIBER CONTENT. As discussed earlier it is traditional to use low-fiber diets in the treatment of small-bowel diarrhea. This practice is in need of revaluation, however, because fiber potentially has beneficial effects on small-bowel function.

YOGURT FOR TREATMENT OF DIARRHEA. Yogurt is sometimes used for therapy of chronic diarrhea in the mistaken belief that the bacteria contained in the yogurt (*Lactobacillus acidophilus* or *Lactobacillus bulgaricus*) will colonize the bowel and displace unfavorable microorganisms. Yogurt has bactericidal properties in vitro but not in vivo. Orally administered bacteria in yogurt do not displace resident or pathogenic bacterial populations in normal or diseased intestines of a variety of species.[115-117] The bacteria in yogurt are generally acid labile, limiting the numbers surviving passage through the stomach.

Yogurt and milk have approximately twice the lactose content of cottage cheese per calorie (Table 38–5).[31] Thus, cottage cheese is the preferred milk-based substrate for the treatment of diarrhea. Interestingly, however lactose in yogurt has greater digestibility than lactose in milk, perhaps because of the presence of bacterial-derived beta-galactosidase (lactase) that assists digestion of lactose in yogurt.[118]

EVALUATION OF THE DIET. The success of a controlled diet for the treatment of diarrhea is determined primarily by changes in the character of the feces, but additional signs such as halitosis, bloating, borborygmus, flatulence, and the frequency of vomiting are also monitored. If the bowel has suffered little morphologic damage, improvement in clinical signs resulting from appropriate nutritional management can occur as quickly as 1 to 3 days and is usually apparent within 7 days even after extended periods of diarrhea. In contrast, if morphologic changes such as villus atrophy are present, feeding the correct therapeutic diet may not result in clinically evident benefit for 3 to 4 weeks or more.

WEANING OFF THE CONTROLLED DIET. Controlled diets are often impractical for long-term use because of expense, inconvenience, or lack of dietary balance. Therefore, it is common practice to attempt to wean the animal back to a complete and balanced commercial diet. If the controlled diet results in complete remission, it is subsequently modified by introducing one new dietary ingredient every 1 to 2 weeks. The animal is closely observed for adverse effects due to the new ingredient. If there is any evidence of diarrhea or flatulence (an early sign of malabsorption), the new ingredient is eliminated from the diet. With time, a number of dietary ingredients are identified that are well tolerated, and others may be recognized that provoke clinical signs. Eventually a commercial food free of the poorly tolerated ingredients can usually be chosen.

COMMERCIAL DIETS FOR SMALL-BOWEL DIARRHEA. A number of different commercial diets are available to manage small animals with chronic gastrointestinal problems. These include Prescription diet i/d (Hill's Pet Products), Eukanuba (Iams Co), Waltham Selected Protein Diet (Kal Kan Foods, Inc.), Waltham Low Fat Diet (Kal Kan Foods Inc.), and the CNM (Provisions) and Innovative Veterinary Diets ranges. These foods vary considerably in their ingredients and proximate analyses. The commercial diet to feed in an individual animal is determined by the animal's dietary history and the elimination-challenge trials described earlier. As a general rule, the most successful commercial diets for the treatment of chronic diarrhea are based on ingredients not commonly found in pet foods and contain highly digestible carbohydrates and protein derived from single rather than multiple foodstuffs.

Protein-Losing Enteropathies

The diet of patients with protein-losing enteropathy should include additional high-quality protein to make up for increased fecal loss. Fat is usually restricted in protein-losing enteropathies because of the likelihood of increasing lymph flow (lymphangiectasia) or difficult assimilation (e.g., inflammatory bowel disease). In spite of the reduced dietary fat content, daily caloric intake must be sufficient to provide additional energy to support the formation of replacement protein.

As discussed earlier, there is as yet no practical way to assess the amount of protein lost in the feces. As a rule of thumb, in patients with clinical evidence of debilitation from protein-losing enteropathy, protein requirements should be considered to be a minimum of 150% of basal requirements and probably nearer 200%. Tuna packed in water, skinned poultry, and low-fat cottage cheese are convenient low-fat protein sources (Table 38–6). The diet provided in Table 38–10 is suitable for the management of protein-losing enteropathy provided sufficient protein is added to cover suspected additional protein losses. In my opinion, the use of commercial weight-reducing diets for the treatment of lymphangiectasia (as has been recommended) is contraindicated. These diets are too calorie restricted to support the increased protein and energy requirements of these usually malnourished and often inappetent patients.

Inflammatory Bowel Disease

The dietary therapy of inflammatory bowel disease (IBD) is similar to that recommended for chronic small-bowel diarrhea. Immunosuppressive drugs (e.g., prednisone) are also usually required in the therapy of IBD. In my experience, acquired food allergies are particularly important in this disorder. To avoid recurrence of clinical signs due to acquired allergy the dietary protein source can be changed after the first 6 weeks of therapy. This diet change is made just prior to the lowering of the prednisone dose from the immunosuppressive to the anti-inflammatory range. The dietary management of IBD is discussed in more detail in Chapter 24.

Large-Bowel Disease

As described earlier, fiber has a variety of influences on the bowel, and the type of fiber used markedly influences the nature of these effects. Fecal incontinence is best treated with low-fiber diets whereas constipation can be prevented (but not treated) by high-fiber diets. As discussed in Chapter 24, dietary recommendations for the management of colitis are controversial. Low-residue diets such as Prescription Diet i/d (Hill's Pet Products),[119] lamb and rice, and cottage cheese and rice have been successfully used as the sole management in many dogs. Others have recommended the use of fiber, with some finding success with soluble fibers such as psyllium (hemicellulose) and others preferring insoluble fibers such as bran.[120] I recommend a diet containing moderate amounts of a highly digestible protein that is not included in the animal's usual diet (reduced colonic ammonia generation and low dietary allergenicity) in association with the addition of a fermentable fiber such as psyllium, oat bran, or soy fiber. The beneficial effect of the soluble fibers probably relates to the generation of volatile fatty acids that nourish the colonic epithelium and discourage growth of bacterial pathogens. A suggested diet for colitis is provided in Table 38–10.

Borborygmus and Flatulence

Gastrointestinal fat is produced by aerophagia or bacterial degradation of unabsorbed nutrients. Excessive gas usually results from dietary indiscretions but, on occasion, can herald more serious gastrointestinal disease such as malassimilation. In human beings, diets high in soybeans, whole wheat products, bran, lactose, and fats can cause gaseousness. Similar associations appear to occur in some dogs and cats. Spoiled diets and diets high in protein or fat are particularly likely to yield odoriferous gases. Milk products can cause gaseousness in animals with lactase deficiency.

The management of these problems begins with a change to a highly digestible, low-fiber diet of moderate fat and protein content. Suitable commercial products are available. Alternatively, the owner can prepare a homemade diet comprised of highly digestible protein and carbohydrate sources (such as cottage cheese and rice) appropriately balanced with vitamins and minerals. In the rare event that dietary manipulation is not successful, consider investigation of the patient for malassimilation.

Pancreatic Disease

The nutritional management of pancreatic diseases is discussed in Chapter 20. Traditionally, low-fat, highly digestible diets are recommended for the treatment of exocrine pancreatic insufficiency and for the prevention of recurrence of acute pancreatitis. The need for low-fat (low-calorie) diets in exocrine pancreatic insufficiency is currently under question, given the availability of modern high potency pancreatic enzyme supplements. In severe cases of acute pancreatitis, total parenteral nutrition and enteral administration of high-carbohydrate, low-fat diets with amino acids stimulate pancreatic secretion less than high-fat diets containing unhydrolyzed protein.[121] Avoiding duodenal distention and the sight and smell of food may also be important in reducing pancreatic secretion. Total parenteral nutrition is the best method of supporting animals in which pancreatitis is complicated by paralytic ileus. Fat emulsions can form part of the intravenous formula. Fat emulsions do not exacerbate acute pancreatitis in humans[121] and have been used safely in dogs with acute pancreatitis at the University of California, Davis, VMTH.

Liver Disease

The nutritional management of liver diseases is discussed in Chapters 33 through 36, and additional information is available elsewhere.[91,122,123] Protein in the diet of a patient with liver disease should be highly digestible and should be moderately restricted in quantity if the animal shows signs of hepatic encephalopathy (even early signs such as depression). Milk or vegetable proteins are well tolerated but red meats are best avoided.[123,124] The debate over the value of diets rich in branched chain amino acids continues.[125,126] Low-fat diets are usually not necessary unless fat malabsorption due to biliary obstruction is diagnosed. Two suitable diets for patients with hepatic insufficiency are provided in Table 38–12. A parenteral nutritional formula suitable for support of patients with liver failure is given in Table 38–13. Commercial diets of value for dogs with liver disease include Prescription diets k/d or i/d (Hill's Pet Products) and Waltham low-protein diet (Kal Kan Foods, Inc.). If ascites occurs, canine h/d can be use-

Table 38–12

DIETARY THERAPY FOR DOGS WITH CHRONIC HEPATIC INSUFFICIENCY

INGREDIENT	OUNCES
Diet 1*	
Instant nonfat dry milk fortified with vitamins A and D	7.4
Blackstrap molasses	4.75
Wheat germ (raw ground)	4.0
Bonemeal	1.0
Safflower oil	3.5
Animal fat	3.5
Cornstarch	14.2
Table salt (iodized)†	1 tsp
Vitamin C	20 mg/kg/day
Choline	250 mg/day for dogs < 15 kg
	500 mg/day for dogs > 15 kg
B-complex supplement to fulfill recommended daily allowances	

*Mixing directions: Mix wheat germ and cold safflower oil with an electric mixer if possible. If beef tallow is used as the source of animal fat, allow it to come to room temperature before mixing. Add animal fat and mix. Mix salt, bonemeal, and cornstarch separately and then add mixture to above ingredients. Add dry instant milk and molasses and mix. Refrigerate. Add a small amount of water at feeding to improve palatability. Calories provided are 4.6 kcal/g DM. Provides 13% protein DM.

†If ascites is present, salt can be reduced, but identify another source of iodine if the diet is going to be used for a prolonged period.

Diet 2*	
Low-fat cottage cheese	2 lb
Animal fat	1/2 lb
Safflower oil	1/4 cup
Sugar	1 lb & 3 tbsp
Cornstarch	1 lb & 5 tbsp
Bonemeal	1.3 Oz
Salt substitute KCl (iodized)	3.5 tsp
Table salt (iodized)	1.0 tsp
Vitamin C	20 mg/kg/day
Choline	As for diet 1
Multivitamin and mineral supplement to fulfill recommended daily allowances	

*Mixing instructions: Mix the sugar, cornstarch, bonemeal, and salt. If beef tallow used, allow to come to room temperature before mixing. Blend animal fat with sugar mixture. Mix the cottage cheese and safflower oil and blend in with other ingredients. Keep refrigerated. Contains 4.7 kcal/g DM. Provides 11% protein DM.

Modified from Strombeck DR et al. (1983).[123]

ful. If encephalopathy develops, canine k/d or u/d can be used. For cats, feline k/d is a useful diet for liver disease.

Vitamin supplementation is appropriate in hepatobiliary disease because of decreased absorption due to steatorrhea and because reduction in liver size decreases the vitamin storage capacity of the body.[73,124] Furthermore, plasma levels of vitamin C are low in dogs with liver disease.[123]

INTENSIVE NUTRITIONAL SUPPORT

Intensive nutritional support is indicated in animals unwilling or unable to eat or in those patients in which deranged gastrointestinal function prevents adequate assimilation of food.[83,128–132] The decision whether to institute intensive therapy is guided by the nutritional status of the patient and the nature and expected longevity of its disease process. Methods of assessment of protein-calorie status, and energy and protein requirements of dogs and cats have been described. As a general rule, dogs and cats with debilitating disease condi-

tions (stress starvation) should not be allowed to go without food for longer than 3 to 5 days.

Selection of Nutrition Technique

Nutritional support may be achieved by enteral or parenteral alimentation. The route of administration of nutrients is determined by the site of gastrointestinal dysfunction, expense of administration, and availability of intensive care facilities. In general, enteral administration is preferred unless prevented by marked gastrointestinal dysfunction. Enteral nutrition is more physiologic, preserves gastrointestinal mucosal architecture, decreases the potential for bacterial and endotoxin translation, and is cheaper, safer, and easier to administer than total parenteral nutrition.

Enteral alimentation may be provided by a number of different techniques including forced oral feeding and nasogastric, pharyngostomy, gastrostomy, and jejunostomy tubes.[83,133] Forced oral feeding is usually too stressful for animals (and staff) to be continued for more than a few days. Nasogastric, pharyngostomy, or gastrostomy tubes can be utilized for nutritional support of animals with anorexia or dysphagia. These methods are not appropriate if the patient is persistently vomiting. In general, gastrostomy tubes are the preferred technique for the long-term nutritional support of animals. Gastrostomy tubes are preferable to pharyngostomy or nasogastric tubes because they are more comfortable for the patient, and completely bypass the esophagus with no risk of compromising the lower esophageal sphincter. An additional disadvantage of pharyngostomy tubes is the risk of interfering with laryngeal function if incorrectly placed. Gastrostomy tubes allow the administration of blended dog or cat foods, unlike nasogastric tubes whose fine diameter necessitates use of enteral formula. The primary advantage of nasogastric

Table 38–13

STANDARDIZED INTRAVENOUS NUTRITION FORMULAS

Dogs
500 mL 50% dextrose
500 mL 8.5% Travasol with electrolytes
250 mL 20% Intralipid
1 mL B-complex vitamins
20 mEq potassium phosphate

Provides 1.06 nonprotein kcal/mL; 40 mEq potassium per liter; 3.15 g protein per 100 nonprotein kcal

Cats
250 mL 50% dextrose
500 mL 8.5% Travasol with electrolytes
250 mL 20% Intralipid
1 mL B-complex vitamins
10 mEq potassium phosphate

Provides 0.92 nonprotein kcal/mL; 40 mEq potassium per liter; 4.6 g protein per 100 nonprotein kcal

Dogs with Liver Failure
500 mL 50% dextrose
250 mL 8.5% Travasol with electrolytes
500 mL 20% Intralipid
1 mL B-complex vitamins
36 mEq potassium phosphate

Provides 1.44 nonprotein kcal/mL; 40 mEq potassium per liter; 1.15 g protein per 100 nonprotein kcal

Courtesy Dr. SC Haskins, UCD VMTH.

tubes is that they do not require general anesthesia to place. They are therefore convenient for the short-term maintenance of critical patients.

The placement of jejunostomy tubes is indicated for gastrointestinal diseases in which gastric dysfunction is prominent. Jejunostomy tubes are less desirable than gastrostomy tubes because they are more difficult to place, usually require the use of elemental diets, and are complicated by a high incidence of iatrogenic osmotic diarrhea.

Total parenteral nutrition (TPN) is usually reserved for severely debilitated patients that cannot take enteral sustenance and require a short period of intensive nutritional support. It is particularly useful in the management of patients with persistent ileus or acute pancreatitis, or if the intestinal tract is unable to absorb nutrients. One advantage in comparison to gastrostomy tubes is that anesthesia is not required. Disadvantages include the limited duration for which TPN can be used, the expense of the procedure, the requirement for intensive monitoring of the patient, and the risk of sepsis. Moreover, the bowel undergoes significant mucosal atrophy during total parenteral nutrition with currently available TPN formulations.

Enteral Nutrition Techniques

FORCED ORAL FEEDING. Patients may be force fed by a number of different techniques including the use of modified syringes and orogastric intubation. The syringe technique involves the removal of the distal fifth of the syringe barrel of a 5 to 10 mL syringe to create a plunger system that can be used to introduce canned food into the pharynx and proximal esophagus. The technique is described more fully elsewhere.[74] Stomach tubing is an effective way to feed neonates but otherwise has limited application because of attendant stress, time-consuming nature, and the risk of tracheal administration.

NASOGASTRIC INTUBATION. Nasogastric intubation is the technique of choice for the short-term support of critical patients with adequately functioning gastrointestinal tracts. The technique has been described in detail by others.[74,132,133,163] Nasogastric tubes should be soft, flexible, and of appropriate diameter (usually 5–8 Fr) and length (sufficient to reach the distal esophagus). Pediatric polyurethane nasogastric tubes (NCC Div; Argyle, NY) are suitable. The tube is marked to allow judgment of the length inserted and is then lubricated and gently passed into the ventral nasal meatus after the instillation of a few drops of local anesthetic. Once the tube has been successfully maneuvered to the distal esophagus or stomach and its position verified, it is sutured or glued in place at the nasal meatus and its free end passed to behind the animal's head where it is secured. Verification of the position of the tube may be made by aspiration or radiography. The initiation of coughing, failure to pass the tube to its full length, or aspiration of copious amounts of free air raises the likelihood of tracheal intubation.

PHARYNGOSTOMY TUBES. With the advent of percutaneous placement of gastrostomy tubes, the indications for pharyngostomy are now few and far between. In practices that do not utilize endoscopy, pharyngostomy tubes have a place in the long-term nutritional support of patients. The technique of placement is described elsewhere.[133,135,136] To minimize the risk of interference with the epiglottis the tube should enter the pharynx caudal to the hyoid apparatus and immediately rostral to the upper esophageal sphincter. A major disadvantage of pharyngostomy tubes is that they can be uncomfortable for the patient.

ESOPHAGOSTOMY TUBES. Esophagostomy tubes have been recommended for use in cats and dogs.[133] The tubes are easy to insert under light general anesthesia and are well tolerated with minimal complications.[133] To date, esophageal strictures resulting from the technique have not been described. The technique is described elsewhere.[133]

GASTROSTOMY TUBES. Gastrostomy tube placement is the technique of choice for long-term enteral support. The primary advantages of gastrostomy tubes are that they are well tolerated, produce minimal discomfort, allow the feeding of regular dog or cat foods, and can be easily managed at home by owners. Gastrostomy tubes are very useful for the support of patients with swallowing disorders. They do not cause pharyngitis, and do not interfere with function of the larynx, pharynx, or lower esophageal sphincter. Patients are able to eat normally with the tube in place, thus facilitating weaning the animal back to oral feeding. The major disadvantage of gastrostomy tubes is the need for general anesthesia (or heavy sedation and local block of the abdomen) and the risk of peritonitis. The latter complication is very rare. Gastrostomy tubes can be placed endoscopically, blindly, or surgically. Endoscopic placement of gastrostomy tubes is the preferred technique and is described in Chapter 7 and elsewhere.[74,137–140]

The blind placement of gastrostomy tubes is performed with the aid of a stomach tube and a length of guide wire.[141] The patient is anaesthetized and placed in right lateral recumbency. The left flank is clipped and surgically prepared. A stomach tube is passed per os into the stomach and manipulated until the gastric end of the tube displaces the lateral abdominal wall beyond the 13th rib. The operator grasps the tip of the stomach tube and positions the tip 2 to 3 cm caudal to the end of the 13th rib. A stab incision is made over the tip and a large-bore catheter is inserted through the incision, abdominal muscles, and stomach wall into the lumen of the stomach tube. A guide wire is inserted through the catheter and into the stomach tube. The wire is threaded up the stomach tube until the end of the wire exits the stomach tube at the mouth of the animal. The stomach tube is then removed and the guide wire tied to a gastrostomy tube prepared in the same manner as described for endoscopically placed gastrostomy tubes (Chapter 7). The guide wire is now grasped at the flank of the animal and pulled steadily to draw the gastrostomy tube through the animal's mouth, esophagus, stomach, and flank. The gastrostomy tube is then secured in position as described in Chapter 7.

The surgical placement of gastrostomy tubes has been described.[142,143] Briefly, a celiotomy is performed and the lateral or caudal aspect of the greater curvature of the stomach is isolated. Two purse-string sutures are placed concentrically about the site of the intended incision in the stomach. A small incision is made just ventral to the 13th rib on the left side, and the catheter inserted through the body wall and into the stomach. The purse-string sutures are tightened about the gastrostomy tube and the stomach is sutured to the abdominal wall. The abdominal incision is closed, and the tube secured by abdominal bandages. Suitable tubes for surgical gastrostomy are 14 to 24 Fr mushroom-tipped (Bardex) or balloon-tipped (Foley) catheters. Gastric motility derangements have been demonstrated in dogs with surgically placed gastrostomy tubes[144] but these rarely cause clinically significant problems. Any debilitated and anorexic animal that undergoes celiotomy for diagnostic or therapeutic reasons should be considered a prime candidate for the placement of a gastrostomy tube at the time of the celiotomy. Such forward thinking greatly facilitates the nutritional support of the patient in the postoperative period.

When the need for a gastrostomy tube has finished, the tube is carefully pulled from the stomach through the abdominal wall. If the gastrostomy tube cannot be removed in this manner, the tube should be cut flush with the abdominal wall. The tip of the tube will pass uneventually in most animals but can be retrieved endoscopically if preferred. The stoma is allowed to heal by secondary intention.

JEJUNOSTOMY TUBES. Jejunal feeding is indicated whenever the upper gastrointestinal tract must be rested. This need may arise in a persistently vomiting animal or in a patient undergoing surgery of the upper gastrointestinal tract. Furthermore, jejunal feeding minimizes the stimulation of pancreatic secretion, and can be of value in the treatment of intractable acute pancreatitis. In dogs and cats, jejunostomy tubes are usually placed via the abdominal wall (needle catheter jejunostomy). These techniques have been previously described.[133,145,146] Jejunal tubes can also be threaded through a gastrostomy tube and into the jejunum via the pylorus (gastrojejunal tubes). Gastrojejunal tubes have undergone preliminary investigation in dogs.[147] Unfortunately, standard gastrojejunal tubes designed for human enteral feeding are unreliable in dogs because of frequent reflux of the jejunal portion of the tube back into the upper gastrointestinal tract.[147] Osmotic diarrhea is a common complication of jejunal feeding.

Products Available for Enteral Nutrition

Products useful for enteral alimentation include blenderized pet foods and various elemental or polymeric enteral feeding solutions.[83,143] Elemental diets consist of carbohydrates and lipids in forms requiring little or no digestion, and nitrogen in the form of amino acids and di- or tripeptides. Polymeric diets contain large peptides or whole proteins and a mixture of coarse starch hydrolysates and long chain triglycerides. Nutrient additives, otherwise known as "feeding modules," are also available. Theses are sources of one nutrient, such as protein, and are used to supplement diets.

BLENDERIZED PET FOODS. Blenderized pet foods are inexpensive balanced diets but cannot be used through fine bore feeding tubes because of clogging. The pet food used should be highly digestible and contain animal-based protein sources. Blenderizing the food with an enteral diet, oral rehydration solution, or small quantities of vegetable oil minimizes the decreases in caloric density resulting from blenderizing with water.

ELEMENTAL DIETS. Elemental diets have a number of theoretical advantages for the treatment of intestinal problems. They have a low fat content, need little or no digestion, and minimize gastric, pancreatic, and biliary secretions. They are hypoallergenic and reduce bacterial microflora numbers. In recent years, however, there has been a move away from elemental solutions to diets with less hydrolyzed constituents. Elemental diets are associated with a higher incidence of diarrhea and abdominal cramping (due to higher osmolality) and have not been shown to provide significant clinical benefit over polymeric diets for nutritional support of humans in spite of their theoretical promise.[84,149,150] Elemental diets are probably still the enteral solution of choice in short bowel syndrome, however, and an enteral diet containing partially hydrolyzed proteins has recently been shown to compare favorably to a polymeric diet in humans undergoing abdominal surgery.[151] Elemental diets have been recommended for short-term use in dogs when initiating feeding following acute pancreatitis or severe gastrointestinal disease such as parvoviral enteritis.[83] Higher protein elemental diets, such as

Vivonex T.E.N. (Norwich Eaton) and Criticare H.N. (Mead Johnson), are the elemental diets favored by the author for use in dogs. The protein content of these products (15% of calories as protein) is too low for long-term use in cats.

POLYMERIC ENTERAL DIETS. A wide variety of polymeric diets designed for humans is available. Many have marginal or inadequate arginine, protein, and thiamine for prolonged use in cats. In addition, most are deficient in arachidonic acid and taurine and have insufficient calcium and phosphorus. For chronic use in cats, human enteral formulas should be supplemented with protein (e.g., 15–30 g casein powder per 8 fl oz can), B complex vitamins (2 mL per can), taurine (250 mg per can), and a calcium/phosphorus source (e.g., 0.25 teaspoons bone meal). Dogs receiving human enteral solutions for long periods may require supplemental B vitamins (especially niacin) and calcium and phosphorus.

The most suitable human enteral products for use in dogs and cats are the higher protein, more energy dense formulas, such as Pulmocare (Ross) and Traumacal (Mead Johnson). Jevity (Ross Labs) and Enrich (Ross Labs) are examples of new generation enteral feeds that contains small quantities of fiber to maintain large-bowel health and help prevent diarrhea and constipation. These products are gaining favor in humans[152] and we have used them successfully in dogs and cats (supplemented as previously described) at Massey University. Recently, a human enteral formula containing supplemental arginine and added RNA and fish oil (Impact, Sandoz Nutrition) has received favorable reports.[153,154] A dietary source of nucleotides is thought to be important in maintaining optimal growth and function of lymphocytes, macrophages, and enterocytes.[154]

Polymeric products specially formulated for use in dogs and cats (Prescription diet a/d, Hill's; Canine and Feline Clinicare, Pet-Ag) are now available. These products are reputed to cause less diarrhea than polymeric diets designed for humans and are better suited for the nutritional requirements of the dog and cat.[133]

NUTRIENT MODULES. Protein modules are regularly used to fortify enteral solutions for use in dogs and cats (see earlier). Suitable protein modules include ProMagic (American Nutritional Labs), ProMod (Ross Labs), and casein powder. The protein contents of a number of commonly used protein supplements are listed in Table 38–6. Fat modules are occasionally required to increase the energy density of the food and to supplement linoleic acid. Corn or MCT oil are the most commonly used fat modules. Fiber, such as psyllium, oat bran, or wheat bran, are occasionally required for large-bowel disorders.

Enteral Feeding Plans

Vomiting and diarrhea often complicate enteral feeding of dogs and cats. These signs usually result from rapid administration of large volumes of enteral formula. Even when carefully used, many products still cause mild diarrhea. The clinical significance of mild diarrhea is probably negligible. In fact, stool weights of humans with enteral-feeding associated "diarrhea" are often normal.[135] Moderate or severe osmotic diarrhea in hospitalized dogs and cats is of concern, however. Diarrhea and gastric atony is thought to be more prevalent in hypoalbuminemic patients, but this belief has recently been challenged.[156]

Initial feeding volumes should be conservative and not exceed 3 to 5 mL per kg body weight per feed, or infusion rates of 1 to 3 mL per kg body weight per hour[86] until approximately one-half of the calculated daily requirements are provided.[133] Intermittent feedings are initially administered every 2 hours. Prior to each feeding, the feeding tube should be aspirated to ensure the previous instillation has emptied from the stomach. If more than 50% of the feeding solution is still recoverable, then no additional feedings should be performed until the stomach has emptied.[86] If the majority of the enteral solution has not left the stomach within 4 to 6 hours, the gastrointestinal tract should be considered currently unsuitable for nutritional support because of ileus. Reversal of ileus can sometimes be achieved with prokinetic drugs and parenteral potassium supplementation.

If the enteral food is well tolerated, and the stomach empties normally, subsequent feedings can be increased in volume over the ensuing 2 days until the patient's requirements are met in 3 to 6 daily feeds. Tubes should be flushed with water between feedings, and then capped. When feeding hyperosmolar diets, additional water must be provided via the tube if the animal is unable to drink.

If the patient demonstrates signs of dietary intolerance such as nausea, abdominal pain, vomiting, or diarrhea, the volume of food should be reduced, the enteral diet diluted, or the interval of feeding increased until the signs resolve. An infusion pump can be used for constant delivery of diet, a procedure that may minimize the adverse effects of enteral solutions. Feeding by gravity drip is acceptable if the rate is carefully controlled.

Parenteral Nutrition

Some patients with gastrointestinal problems cannot be fed enterally, and it is necessary to maintain nutritional homeostasis with parenteral nutrition. Specific indications include severe malabsorption or prolonged ileus or pancreatitis. Parenteral nutrition may be used to provide partial nutritional requirements or total nutritional requirements (TPN).

PARTIAL PARENTERAL NUTRITION. Partial parenteral nutrition endeavors to minimize the loss of body protein that occurs during stress starvation. A protein-sparing effect may be achieved by the infusion of small amounts of dextrose or amino acids. Intravenous infusion of dextrose can reduce nitrogen losses by as much as one-half even though it does not meet total energy requirements.[157] Similarly, intravenous administration of 3% amino acid solution with electrolytes has a protein-sparing-effect.[33] The addition of 3% glycerine to 3% amino acids (ProcalAmine, Kendall McGraw) appears even more effective.[133] One of the major advantages of these solutions is that they can be administered by peripheral veins. Partial parental nutrition is also considerably less expensive than TPN and potentially has wide application in small animal practice.

ROUTES OF ADMINISTRATION OF TPN. Parenteral nutrition solutions are usually hypertonic, and must be infused into a central vein to avoid phlebitis and thrombosis. Veins of choice are the jugular veins, and in the cat the medial saphenous vein through which a catheter can be threaded to reach the caudal vena cava. The catheter for delivery of the TPN solution must be dedicated to TPN alone and never be used for other purposes, otherwise sepsis will result. An antibiotic-antifungal cream should be placed at the catheter insertion site and the catheter inspected and rebandaged every 24 hours. Central vein catheters, carefully cared for, can last a week or more.

FORMULATION OF TPN SOLUTIONS. The energy and protein requirements of the patient are calculated as described earlier. Energy should be supplied by both fat and carbohydrate (Table 38–13). Clinical trials in humans have shown that there is a limit to the protein-sparing effect of glucose, and if glucose is provided as the sole calorie source protein repletion cannot be achieved.[158] Furthermore, fat solutions may reduce the thrombogenicity of TPN solutions,[159] provide a source of essential fatty acids, and lower the osmolality of the parenteral solution because of their high caloric density. Intralipid (Cutter) has been administered to dogs at a rate as high as 9 g of fat/kg body weight/day for a month with no undesirable effects.

Use of standardized mixtures of nutrients simplify TPN. The mixtures in Table 38–13 are adequate to supply the nutritional requirements of the majority of dogs and cats. These mixtures should be mixed in as sterile manner as possible. The "All-in-One" mixing bags (Baxter) greatly facilitate this procedure. To ensure the stability of the mixture, the order of addition to the all-in-one bag should be dextrose solution, amino acid solution, and then lipid solution. The bag can be hung at room temperature for several days (as long as they are agitated regularly), after which time any remaining solution should be discarded.

ADDITIONAL NUTRIENT AND FLUID REQUIREMENTS DURING TPN. Cats have dietary requirements for protein, arachidonate, and taurine that are difficult to meet with parenteral solutions. However, positive nitrogen balance can be achieved in cats receiving standard amino acid mixtures.[160] Oral supplementation of these nutrients should be provided if prolonged nutritional support is envisioned. Taurine is best supplied as taurine tablets (250 mg).

Small animals require about 40 to 60 mL water/kg body weight per day. Parenteral nutrition solutions, provided in sufficient amounts to meet an animal's daily caloric requirements, usually also meet the daily water requirements unless there is some reason for increased water loss (such as hyperglycemia or diarrhea). Unless specifically contraindicated by the patient's condition it is advisable to allow animals receiving TPN to have free access to water, to avoid dehydration.

Potassium requirements double when parenteral nutrition solutions are infused.[161] The high potassium requirements are necessary for protein accretion and to match the urinary excretion of potassium. Protein accretion also results in a high demand for phosphorus. Phosphate-free parenteral nutrition solutions rapidly reduce serum phosphorus levels. The complications of hypophosphatemia in dogs include weakness, seizures, hemolytic anemia, and, without correction, death within 5 to 6 days. For these reasons, the addition of potassium phosphate to TPN solutions is recommended (Table 38–13).

ADMINISTRATION RATE OF TPN SOLUTIONS AND MONITORING. The volume of solution required to meet nutritional requirements can be calculated from the caloric content of the TPN solution (provided in Table 38–13) and the estimated requirements of the patient. The nutritional solutions is initially administered slowly (50% of the calculated rate necessary to maintain the patient) and after 4 hours the blood glucose is checked. If the glucose remains below 250 mg/dl, the infusion rate is increased to full ration in a step-wise fashion over the ensuing 8 hours. If the patient's blood glucose reaches 250 to 300 mg/dl, the rate is maintained constant until the patient develops a tolerance for the glucose (serum concentration decreases) whereupon the rate can be increased. If the serum glucose concentration exceeds 300 mg/dl, the rate should be temporarily reduced.[86] Monitoring should include observation for persistent lipemia, and a blood ammonia level should be determined after the first day of therapy to ensure protein administration is not excessive. PCV, total protein, and serum glucose and electrolyte concen-

Table 38–14

COMPLICATIONS OF TOTAL PARENTERAL NUTRITION

WITH GLUCOSE-BASED SOLUTIONS	WITH ALL TYPES OF SOLUTIONS
Hyperosmolarity	Peptide hypersensitivity
Osmotic dehydration	Potassium depletion
Glucosuria	Phosphate depletion
Metabolic acidosis	Fluid overload
Fluid overload	Hyperammonemia
Phlebitis	Infection

tration should be followed closely. Close observation for evidence of acidosis, fluid overload or dehydration, and evidence of sepsis is essential.

COMPLICATIONS OF TPN. The most important complication of parenteral nutrition is sepsis (Table 38–14). The frequency can be particularly high if care is not taken during the mixing of the solutions and if correct catheter protocol is not observed. Other important complications include phlebitis and thrombosis.[159] This can be particularly catastrophic if a central vein is involved. Hyperglycemia and fluid and electrolyte imbalances are relatively common, with hypernatremia, hypokalemia, and hypophosphatemia being particularly frequent. In cats, 2 weeks of total parenteral nutrition has been associated with vomiting, lethargy, lingual ulcers, mild to moderate anemia, mild to severe thrombocytopenia, metabolic acidosis, villus atrophy, and a reversible fatty liver.[160]

REFERENCES

1. Liddle RA, Green GM, Conrad CK et al. Proteins but not amino acids, carbohydrates or fats stimulate cholecystokinin secretion in the rat. Am J Physiol 251:G243–G248, 1986.
2. Hara H, Nishikawa H, Kiriyama S. Different effects of casein and soybean protein on gastric emptying of protein and small intestinal transit after spontaneous feeding of diet in rats. Br J Nutr 68:59–66. 1992.
3. Greenberg GR. The exocrine pancreas: Nutrient interactions with function and structure. In: Shils ME, Young VR (eds) Modern Nutrition in Health and Disease, 7th ed. Lea & Febiger, Philadelphia, 1108–1113, 1988.
4. Torun B, Viteri FE. Protein-energy malnutrition. In: Shils ME, Young VR (eds) Modern Nutrition in Health and Disease, 7th ed. Lea & Febiger, Philadelphia, 746–773, 1988.
5. Wilson PC, Greene HL. The gastrointestinal tract: Portal to nutrient utilization. In: Shils ME, Young VR (eds) Modern Nutrition in Health and Disease, 7th ed. Lea & Febiger, Philadelphia, 481–499, 1988.
6. Desai AJ, Moyer LL, Deveney CW, et al. Malnutrition significantly prolongs the delay in gastric emptying in rats. Nutr Res 13:715–722, 1993.
7. Veldee MS, Peth LD. Can protein-calorie malnutrition cause dysphagia? Dysphagia 7:86–101, 1992.
8. Davenport DJ, Mostardi RA, Gross KL. Effect of a protein-deficient diet on serum proteins, urea nitrogen, hepatic enzymes, and bile acids in dogs. Proc Waltham Symposium on the Nutrition of Companion Animals, Adelaide (abstract), 69, 1993.
9. Klein S. Glutamine: An essential nonessential amino acid for the gut. Gastroenterology 99:279–281, 1990.
10. Souba WW, Herskowitz K, Salloum RM, et al. Gut glutamine metabolism. J Parenter Enteral Nutr 14:45S–55S, 1990.
11. Souba WW. Glutamine: A key substrate for the splanchnic bed. Ann Rev Nutr 11:285–308, 1991.
12. Baskerville A, Hambleton P, Benbough JE. Pathologic features of glutaminase toxicity. Br J Exp Pathol 61:132–138, 1980.
13. Abumrad NN, Yazigi N, Cersosimo E, et al. Glutamine metabolism during starvation. J Parenter Enteral Nutr 14:71S–76S, 1990.
14. Alexander JW. Nutrition and translocation. J Parenter Enteral Nutr 14:170S–174S, 1990.
15. Inoue Y, Grant JP, Snyder PJ. Effect of glutamine-supplemented intravenous nutrition on survival after Escherichia coli–induced peritonitis. J Parenter Enteral Nutr 17:41–46, 1993.
16. Rhoads JM, Keku EO, Quinn J, et al. L-glutamine stimulates sodium and chloride absorption in pig rotavirus enteritis. Gastroenterology 100:683–691, 1991.
17. O'Dwyer ST, Smith RJ, Huang TL, et al. Maintenance of small bowel mucosa with glutamine-enriched parenteral nutrition. J Parenter Enteral Nutr 13:579–585, 1989.
18. Gouttebel MC, Astre C, Briand D, et al. Influence of N-acetylglutamine or glutamine infusion on plasma amino acid concentrations during the early phase of small-bowel adaptation in the dog. J Parenter Enteral Nutr 16:117–120, 1992.
19. Penn D, Lebenthal E. Intestinal mucosal energy metabolism—a new approach to therapy of gastrointestinal disease. J Parenter Gastroenterol Nutr 10:1–4, 1990.
20. Schunemann C, Muhlum A, Junker S, et al. Prececal and postileal digestibility of various starches, and pH values and organic acid content of digesta and faeces. Advs Anim Physiol Anim Nutr 19:44–58, 1989.
21. Baker DH, Czarnecki-Maulden GL. Comparative nutrition of cats and dogs. Ann Rev Nutr 11:239–263, 1991.
22. Kienzle, E. Carbohydrate metabolism of the cat. 2. Digestion of starch. J Anim Physiol Anim Nutr 69:102–114, 1993.
23. Morris JG, Trudell J, Pencovic T. Carbohydrate digestion by the domestic cat (Felis catus). Br J Nutr 37:365–373, 1977.
24. Buddington RK, Chen JW, Diamond JM. Dietary regulation of intestinal brush-border sugar and amino acid transport in carnivores. Am J Physiol 261:R793–R801, 1991.
25. Kienzle E. Carbohydrate metabolism of the cat. 1. Activity of amylase in the gastrointestinal tract of the cat. J Anim Physiol Anim Nutr 69:92–101, 1993.
26. Sherding RG. Diseases of the intestines. In: The Cat: Diseases and Clinical Management. Churchill Livingston, New York, 955–1006, 1989.
27. Washabau RJ, Buffington CA, Strombeck DR. Evaluation and management of carbohydrate malassimilation. In: Kirk RW (ed) Current Veterinary Therapy IX. WB Saunders, Philadelphia, 889–892, 1986.
28. Hill FWG, Kelley DF. Naturally occurring intestinal malabsorption in the dog. Am J Dig Dis 19:649–665, 1974.
29. Muhlum A, Ingwersen M, Schunemann C, et al. Prececal and postileal digestion of sucrose, lactose, stachyose and raffinose. Advs Anim Physiol Anim Nutr 19:31–43, 1989.
30. Kienzle E. Carbohydrate metabolism of the cat. 3. Digestion of sugars. J Anim Physiol Anim Nutr 69:203–210, 1993.
31. Pennington JAT. Food Values of Portions Commonly Used, 15th ed. JB Lippincott, Philadelphia, 1989.
32. Mundt HC, Meyer H. Pathogenesis of lactose-induced diarrhea and its prevention by enzymatic splitting of lactose. In: Burger IH, Rivers JPW (eds) Nutrition of the Dog and Cat. Cambridge University Press, Cambridge, 267–274, 1989.
33. Amtsberg G, Stock V, Treschnak, E., et al. Composition of intestinal microorganisms in the dog in relation to diet and decontamination of the intestinal tract with various antibacterial substances. Advs Anim Physiol Anim Nutr 19:120–130, 1989.
34. Muhlum A, Ingwersen M, Schunemann C, et al. Prececal and postileal digestion of sucrose, lactose, stachyose and raffinose. Advs Anim Physiol Anim Nutr 19:31–43, 1989.
35. Meyer H, Arndt J, Behfeld T, et al. Prececal and postileal digestibility of various proteins. Advs Anim Physiol Anim Nutr 19:59–77, 1989.
36. Meyer H, Behfeld T, Schunemann C, et al. Intestinal water, sodium and potassium metabolism. Advs Anim Physiol Anim Nutr 19:109–119, 1989.
37. Roman C, Gonella J. Extrinsic control of digestive tract motility. In: Johnson LR (ed) Physiology of the Gastrointestinal Tract, 2nd ed. Raven Press, New York, 595–612, 1987.
38. Christensen J. Motor functions of the pharynx and esophagus. In: Johnson LR (ed) Physiology of the Gastrointestinal Tract, 2nd ed. Raven Press, New York, 595–612, 1978.
39. Cunningham KM, Daly J, Horowitz M, et al. Gastrointestinal adaptation to diets of differing fat composition in human volunteers. Gut 32:482–486, 1991.
40. Maliakkal RJ, Hendra KP, Mascioli EA. Recent advances in medium-chain triglycerides and fish oil. Curr Opin G 8:314–325, 1992.
41. Swift LL, Hill JO, Peters JC, et al. Medium chain fatty acids: Evidence for incorporation into chylomicron triglyceride in humans. Am J Clin Nutr 52:834–836, 1990.
42. Vilaseca J, Salas A, Guarner F, et al. Dietary fish oil reduces progression of chronic inflammatory lesions in a rat model of granulomatous colitis. Gut 31:539–544, 1990.
43. Hillier K, Jewell R, Dorrell L, et al. Incorporation of fatty acids from fish oil and olive oil into colonic mucosal lipids and effects upon eicosanoid synthesis in inflammatory bowel disease.
44. Vanderhoof JA, Park JHY, Mohammadpour H, et al. Effects of dietary lipids on recovery from mucosal injury. Gastroenterology 98:1226–1231, 1990.
45. Sagher FA, Didge JA, Moore R, et al. Modulation of fluid absorption and

the secretory response of rat jejunum to cholera toxin by dietary fat. Gut 312:1256–1261, 1990.

46. Meyer H. Fat in dog and cat nutrition. Effen-Forschung-fur-Heimtier-nahrung-Report 28:1–13, 1989.

47. Binder HJ, Sandle GI. Electrolyte absorption and secretion in the mammalian colon. In: Johnson LR (ed) Physiology of the Gastrointestinal Tract, 2nd ed. Raven Press, New York, 1389–1418, 1987.

48. Jenkins DJA. Carbohydrates. In: Shils ME, Young VR (eds) Modern Nutrition in Health and Disease, 7th ed. Lea & Febiger, Philadelphia, 52–71, 1988.

49. Monro JA. A nutritionally valid procedure for measuring soluble dietary fibre. Food Chem 47:187–193, 1993.

50. Eastwood MA. The physiological effect of dietary fiber: An update. Ann Rev Nutr 12:19–35, 1992.

51. Vahouny GV. Effects of dietary fiber on digestion and absorption. In: Johnson LR (ed) Physiology of the Gastrointestinal Tract. Raven Press, New York. 1623–1648, 1987.

52. Kritchevsky D. Dietary fiber. Ann Rev Nutr 8:301–328, 1988.

53. Urban E. A feast of fiber. Gastroenterology 88:211–212, 1985.

54. Reppas C, Meyer JH, Sirois PJ, et al. Effect of hydroxypropylcellulose on gastrointestinal transit and luminal viscosity in dogs. Gastroenterology 100:1217–1223, 1991.

55. Russell J, Bass P. Canine gastric emptying of fiber meals: Influence of meal viscosity and antroduodenal motility. Am J Physiol 249:G662–G67, 1985.

56. Jenkins DJA, Jenkins AL, Wolever TMS, et al. Simple and complex carbohydrates. Nutr Rev 44:44–49, 1986.

57. Burrows CF, Kronfeld DS, Banta CA, et al. Effects of fiber on digestibility and transit time in dogs. J Nutr 112:1726–1732, 1982.

58. Lewis LD, Morris ML, Mitchell EE, et al. Dietary fiber effect on canine stools, intestinal function, and nutrient digestibility. Proc Waltham Symposium on the Nutrition of Companion Animals, Adelaide (abstract), 91, 1993.

59. Stock-Damge C, Aprahamian M, Raul F, et al. Effects of wheat bran on the exocrine pancreas and the small intestinal mucosa in the dog. J Nutr 114:1076–1082, 1984.

60. Isaksson G, Asp NG, Ihse I. Effects of dietary fiber on pancreatic enzyme activities of ileostomy evacuates and on excretion of fat and nitrogen in the rat. Gastroenterology 18:417–423, 1983.

61. McIntyre A, Gibson PR, Young GP. Butyrate production from dietary fibre and protection against large bowel cancer in a rat model. Gut 34:386–391, 1993.

62. Sakata T. Stimulatory effect of short-chain fatty acid on epithelial cell proliferation in rat intestine: A possible explanation for trophic effects of fermentable fibre, gut microbes and luminal tropic factors. Br J Nutr 58:95–103, 1987.

63. Sunvold GD, Fahey GC, Merchen NR, et al. Fermentability of selected fibrous substrates by dog fecal microflora as influenced by diet. Proc Waltham Symposium on the Nutrition of Companion Animals, Adelaide (abstract), 95, 1993.

64. Sunvold GD, Titgemeyer EC, Bourquin LD, et al. Fermentability of selected fibrous substrates by cat fecal microflora. Proc Waltham Symposium on the Nutrition of Companion Animals, Adelaide (abstract), 97, 1993.

65. Reinhart D, Lebenthal E. Intestinal mucosal energy metabolism—a new approach to therapy of gastrointestinal disease. J Pediatr Gastroenterol Nutr 10:1–4, 1990.

66. Reinhart GA, Moxley RA, Clemens ET. Dietary fiber source and its effects on colonic microstructure and histopathology of Beagle dogs. Proc Waltham Symposium on the Nutrition of Companion Animals, Adelaide (abstract), 79, 1993.

67. Scheppach W, Sommer H, Kirchner T, et al. Effect of butyrate enemas on the colonic mucosa in distal ulcerative colitis. Gastroenterology 103:51–56, 1992.

68. Lupton JR, Kurtz PP. Relationship of colonic luminal short-chain fatty acids and pH to in vivo cell proliferation in rats. J Nutr 123:1522–1530, 1993.

69. Brockett M, Tanner GW. Dietary influence on microbial activities in the cecum of mice. Can J Microbiol 28:493–499, 1982.

70. Twedt DC. Dietary Fiber in Gastrointestinal Disease. Proc 11th ACVIM Forum, Washington, DC, 225–229, 1993.

71. Stephen AM, Cummings JH. The microbial contribution to human fecal mass. J Med Microbiol 13:45–49, 1980.

72. Eherer AJ, Santa Ana CA, Porter J, et al. Effect of psyllium, calcium polycarbophil, and wheat bran on secretory diarrhea induced by phenolphthalein. Gastroenterology 104:1007–1012, 1993.

73. Buffington CA. Therapeutic use of vitamins in companion animals. In: Kirk RW (ed) Current Veterinary Therapy IX. WB Saunders, Philadelphia. 40-47, 1986.

74. Lewis LD, Morris ML, Hand NS. Small Animal Clinical Nutrition, Mark Morris Associates, Topeka, 1987.

75. De Luca L, Maestri N, Bonanni F, et al. Maintenance of epithelial cell differentiation; The mode of action of vitamin A. Cancer 30:1326–1331, 1972.

76. Rosenberg IH, Alpers DH. Nutritional deficiency in gastrointestinal disease. In: Sleisenger MH, Fordtran JS (eds) Gastrointestinal Disease. Pathophysiology, Diagnosis, Management, 4th ed. WB Saunders, Philadelphia, 1983–1994, 1989.

77. Batt RM, Morgan JO. Role of serum folate and vitamin B_{12} concentrations in the differentiation of small intestinal abnormalities in the dog. Res Vet Sci 32:17:22, 1982.

78. Batt RM, Horadagoda NU, Simpson KW. Role of the pancreas in the absorption and malabsorption of cobalamin (vitamin B-12) in dogs. J Nutr 121:11S, S75–S76, 1991.

79. Edwards DF, Russell RG. Probable-vitamin K deficient bleeding in two cats with malabsorption syndrome secondary to lymphocytic-plasmacytic enteritis. J Vet Int Med 1:97–101, 1987.

80. Roudebush P, Cowell CS. Results of a hypoallergenic diet survey of veterinarians in North America with a nutritional evaluation of homemade diet prescriptions. Vet Dermatol 3:23–28, 1992.

81. Lipman TO. Nutritional assessment. Curr Opin G 7:271–276, 1991.

82. Alpers DH, Rosenberg IH. Eating behavior and nutrient requirements. In: Sleisenger MH, Fordtran JS (eds) Gastrointestinal Disease. Pathophysiology, Diagnosis, Management, 4th ed. WB Saunders, Philadelphia, 1971–1983, 1989.

83. Donoghue S. Nutritional support of hospitalized patients. Vet Clin N Am 19:475–495, 1989.

84. Clouse RE, Rosenberg IH. Intensive nutritional support. In: Sleisenger MH, Fordtran JS (eds) Gastrointestinal Disease. Pathophysiology, Diagnosis, Management, 4th ed. WB Saunders, Philadelphia. 2007–2027, 1989.

85. Klein S. The myth of serum albumin as a measure of nutritional status. Gastroenterology 99:1845–1846, 1990.

86. Haskins SC. Personal communication, 1989.

87. Rogers QR, Baker DH, Hayes KC, et al. Nutrient Requirements of Cats. National Academy Press, Washington, DC, 1986.

88. Sheffey BE, Hayes KC, Knapka JJ, et al. Nutrient Requirements of Dogs. National Academy Press, Washington, DC, 1986.

89. Rivers JPW, Burger IH. Allometric considerations in the nutrition of dogs. In: Burger IH, Rivers JPW (eds) Nutrition of the Dog and Cat. Cambridge University Press, Cambridge, 67–112, 1989.

90. Polzin DJ, Osborne CA. Update—conservative medical management of chronic renal failure. In: Kirk RW (ed) Current Veterinary Therapy IX. WB Saunders, Philadelphia, 1167–1173, 1986.

91. Leflamme DP. Dietary management of canine hepatic encephalopathy. Comp Contin Ed Pract Vet 10:1259–1263, 1988.

92. Zimmer JF. Nutritional management of gastrointestinal diseases. In: Kirk RW (ed) Current Veterinary Therapy IX. WB Saunders, Philadelphia. 909–916, 1986.

93. Pappas TN, Melendez RL, Debas HT. Gastric distension is a physiologic satiety signal in the dog. Dig Dis Sci 34:1489–1493, 1989.

94. Durrans D, Taylor TV, Holt S. Intragastric device for weight loss: Effect on energy intake in dogs. Dig Dis Sci 36:893–896, 1991.

95. Allen TA. Food preference and palatability. Proc 9th ACVIM Forum, 239–242, 1991.

96. Stein BS. Feeding the anorectic cat. Tijdschrift-voor-Diergeneeskunde 116:71S–76S, 1991.

97. Iyngkaran N, Robinson MJ, Sumithran E, et al. Cow's milk protein sensitive enteropathy: An important factor prolonging diarrhea of acute infectious enteritis in early infancy. Arch Dis Ch 53:150–153, 1978.

98. Gryboski JD. Gastrointestinal aspects of cow's mild protein intolerence and allergy. Immunol Allergy Clin N Am 11:733–797, 1991.

99. Desai MB, Jeejeebhoy KN. Diet and peptic ulcer disease. In: Shils ME, Young VR (eds) Modern Nutrition in Health and Disease, 7th ed. Lea & Febiger, Philadelphia. 1099–1102, 1988.

100. Pemberton CM, Moxness KE, German MJ, et al. Mayo Clinic Diet Manual. BC Decker, Toronto, 168–170, 1988.

101. Lichtenberger LM. Mechanisms of gastric mucosal protection. Proc ACVIM Forum, Washington, DC, 74–79, 1993.

102. Desai MB, Jeejeehoy KN, Nutritional support of patients with short bowel syndrome and malabsorption, In: Shils ME, Young VR (eds) Modern Nutrition in Health and Disease, 7th ed. Lea & Febiger, Philadelphia, 1114–1150, 1988.

103. Snyder JD, Molla AM, Cash RA. Home-based therapy for diarrhea. J Pediatr Gastroent Nutr 11:438–447, 1990.

104. Armstrong WM. Cellular mechanisms of ion transport in the small intestine. In: Johnson LR (ed) Physiology of the Gastrointestinal Tract, 2nd ed. Raven Press, New York, 1251–1265, 1987.

105. Carpenter CCI, Greenough WB, Pierce NF. Oral-rehydration therapy—the role of polymeric substrates. New Eng J Med 319:1346–1348, 1988.

106. Patra FC, Mahalanabis D, Jalan KM, et al. Is oral rice electrolyte solution superior to glucose electrolyte solution in the infantile diarrhea? Arch Dis Ch 57:910–912, 1982.

107. Powell DW. Intestinal water and electrolyte transport. In: Johnson LR (ed) Physiology of the Gastrointestinal Tract, 2nd ed. Raven Press, New York, 1267–1305, 1987.

108. Molla AM, Molla A, Rhode J, et al. Turning off the diarrhea, the role of food and ORS. J Pediatr Gastroenterol Nutr 8:81–84, 1989.

109. Lebenthal E. Rice as a carbohydrate substrate in oral rehydration solutions (ORS). J Pediatr Gastroenterol Nutr 11:293–300, 1990.

110. Isolauri E, Juntunen M, Wiren S. Intestinal permeability changes in acute gastroenteritis: Effects of clinical factors and nutritional management. J Pediatr Gastroenterol Nutr 8:466-473, 1989.

111. William REO, Drasar BS. Alterations in gut bacterial flora in disease. In: Badenoch J, Brooke BN (eds) Recent Advances in Gastroenterology. Churchill and Livingston, London, 31–53, 1972.

112. Deren JJ, Broitman SA, Zamcheck N. Effect of diet upon intestinal disaccharidases and disaccharide absorption. J Clin Invest 46:186–195, 1967.

113. Grossman MI, Greenard H, Ivy AC. The effect of dietary composition on pancreatic enzymes. Am J Physiol 138:676–682, 1942–43.

114. Madara JL, Trier JS. Functional morphology of the mucosa of the small intestine. In: Johnson LR (ed) Physiology of the Gastrointestinal Tract. Raven Press, New York, 1209–1249, 1987.

115. Kotz CM, Peterson LR, Moody JA, et al. Effect of yogurt on clindamycin-induced *Clostridium difficile* colitis in hamsters. Dig Dis Sci 37:129–132, 1992.

116. Gotteland M, Pochart P, Dabbech M, et al. In vivo effect of yogurt on excretion of enteropathogen *Escherichia coli* RDEC–1 during acute diarrhea in the just-weaned rabbit. J Pediatr Gastroenterol Nutr 14:264–267, 1992.

117. Goldin BR, Gorbach SL, Saxelin M, et al. Survival of *Lactobacillus* species (strain GG) in human gastrointestinal tract. Dig Dis Sci 37:121–128, 1992.

118. Boudraa G, Touhami M, Pochart P, et al. Effect of feeding yogurt versus milk in children with persistent diarrhea. J Pediatr Gastroenterol Nutr 11:509–512, 1993.

119. Nelson RW, Stookey LJ, Kazacos E. Nutritional management of idiopathic chronic colitis in the dog. J Vet Int Med 2:133–137, 1988.

120. Simpson JW. Role of nutrition in aetiology and treatment of diarrhea. J Sm Anim Pract 33:167–171, 1992.

121. Russell RI. Nutritional support of patients with pancreatic diseases. In: Shils ME, Young VR (eds) Modern Nutrition in Health and Disease, 7th ed. Lea & Febiger, Philadelphia, 1115–1123, 1988.

122. Bauer JE, Schenck PA. Dietary therapy for hepatic disease. Vet Clin N Am 19:515–526, 1989.

123. Strombeck DR, Schaeffer MC, Rogers QR. Dietary therapy for dogs with chronic hepatic insufficiency. In: Kirk RW (ed) Current Veterinary Therapy VIII. WB Saunders, Philadelphia, 817–821, 1983.

124. Blendis LM, Jenkins DJA. Nutritional support in liver disease. In: Shils ME, Young VR (eds) Modern Nutrition in Health and Disease, 9th ed. Lea & Febiger, Philadelphia, 1182–1200, 1988.

125. Naylor CD, O'Rourke K, Detsky AS, et al. Parenteral nutrition with branched-chain acids in hepatic encephalopathy. A meta analysis. Gastroenterology 97:1033–1042, 1989.

126. Blackburn GL, O'Keefe SJD. Nutrition in liver failure. Gastroenterology 97:1049–1051, 1989./

127. Strombeck DR, Harold D, Rogers QR, et al. Plasma amino acid, glucagon, and insulin concentrations in dogs with nitrosamine-induced hepatic disease. Am J Vet Res 44:2028, 1983.

128. Armstrong J, Lippert AC. Selected aspects of enteral and parenteral nutritional support. Sem Vet Surg 3:216–226, 1988.

129. Crowe DT. Enteral nutrition for critically ill or injured patients, part 1. Comp Contin Ed Pract Vet 8:603–612, 1986.

130. Crowe DT. Enteral nutrition for critically ill or injured patients, part II. Comp Contin Ed Pract Vet 8:719–732, 1986.

131. Crowe DT. Nutrition in critical patients: Administering the support therapies. Vet Med 84:152–180, 1989.

132. Crowe DT. Clinical use of an indwelling nasogastric tube for enteral nutrition and fluid therapy in the dog and cat. J Am Anim Hosp Assoc 22:675–679, 1986.

133. Crowe DT. Nutritional support for the hospitalized patient: An introduction to tube feeding. Comp Contin Ed Pract Vet 12:1711–1721, 1990.

134. Crowe DT, Downs MO. Pharyngostomy complications in dogs and cats and recommended technical modifications: Experimental and clinical investigations. J Am Anim Hosp Assoc 22:493–498, 1986.

135. Fox SM. Placing a pharyngostomy tube for enteral feeding. Vet Med 82:903–906, 1987.

136. Lantz GC. Pharyngostomy tube placement. In: Bojorab MJ (ed) Current

137. Mathews KA, Binnington AG. Percutaneous incision-less placement of a gastrostomy tube utilizing a gastroscope: Preliminary observations. J Am Vet Med Assoc 202:601– 610, 1986.

138. Debowes LJ, Coyne B, Layton CE. Comparison of French-Pezzar and Malecot catheters for percutaneously placed gastrostomy tubes in cats. J Am Vet Med Assoc 202:1963–1965, 1993.

139. Armstrong PJ, Hardie EM. Percutaneous endoscopic gastrostomy: A retrospective study of 54 clinical cases in dogs and cats. J Vet Intern Med 4:202–206, 1990.

140. Bright RM. Percutaneous endoscopic gastrostomy. Vet Clin N Am 23:531–545, 1993.

141. Fulton RB, Dennis JS. Blind percutaneous placement of a gastrostomy tube for nutritional support in dogs and cats. J Am Vet Med Assoc 201:6967–700, 1992.

142. Crane SW. Placement and maintenance of a temporary feeding tube gastrostomy in the dog and cat. Comp Contin Ed Pract Vet 2:770–776, 1980.

143. Williams JM, White RAS. Tube gastrostomy in dogs. J Sm Anim Pract 34:50–64, 1993.

144. Sampley AR, Burrows CF, Ellison GW, et al. Gastric myoelectric activity after experimental gastric dilatation-volvulus and tube gastrostomy in dogs. Vet Surg 21:10–14, 1992.

145. Orton EC. Enteral hyperalimentation administered via needle catheter jejunostomy as an adjunct to cranial abdominal surgery in dogs and cats. J Am Vet Med Assoc 188:1406–1411, 1986.

146. Orton EC. Needle catheter jejunostomy. In: Bojorab MJ (ed) Current Techniques in Small Animal Surgery, 3rd ed. Lea & Febiger, Philadelphia, 257–259, 1990.

147. Hardie EM, Armstrong J. Development of a gastro-jejunal tube for the dog. J Nutr 121:11S, S154, 1991.

148. Bury KD. Elemental diets. In: Fischer JE (ed) Total Parenteral Nutrition. Little, Brown, Boston, 395–411. 1976.

149. Rigaud D, Cosnes J, Le Quintrec Y, et al. Controlled trial comparing two types of enteral nutrition in treatment of active Crohn's disease: Elemental vs. polymeric diet. Gut 32:1492–1497, 1991.

150. Raouf AH, Hildrey V, Daniel J, et al. Enteral feeding as sole treatment for Crohn's disease: Controlled trial of whole protein v amino based feed and a case study of dietary challenge. Gut 32:702–707, 1991.

151. Ziegler F, Olivier JM, Cynober L, et al. Efficiency of enteral nitrogen support in surgical patients: Small peptides v non-degraded proteins. Gut 31:1277–1283, 1990.

152. Silk DBA, Grimble GK, Payne-James JJ. Enteral nutrition. Curr Opin G 8:290–295, 1992.

153. Cerra FB, Lehman S, Konstantinides N, et al. Effect of enteral nutrition on in vivo tests of immune function in ICU patients: A preliminary report. Nutrition 6:84–87, 1990.

154. Baumgartner TG, Cerda JJ. Enteral nutrition. Curr Opin G 9:284–291, 1993.

155. Benya R, Layden TJ, Mobarhan S. Diarrhea associated with tube feeding: The importance of using objective criteria. J Clin Gastroenterol 13:167–172, 1991.

156. Patterson ML, Dominguez JM, Lyman B, et al. Enteral feeding in the hypoalbuminemic patient. J Parenter Enteral Nutr 14:362–365, 1990.

157. Rydberg U. Alcohol metabolism. In: Ghadimi H (ed) Total Parenteral Nutrition. John Wiley, New York, 47–56, 1975.

158. Macfis J, Smith RC, Hill GL. Glucose or fat as a non-protein energy source? A controlled clinical trial in patients requiring intravenous nutrition. Gastroenterology 80:103–108, 1981.

159. Wakefield A, Cohen Z, Craig M, et al. Thrombogenicity of total parenteral nutrition solutions: I. Effect on induction of monocyte/macrophage procoagulant activity. Gastroenterology 97:1210–1219, 1989.

160. Lippert AC, Faulkner JE, Evans AT, et al. Total parenteral nutrition in clinically normal cats. J Am Vet Med Assoc 194:669–676, 1989.

161. Giovanoni R. The manufacturing pharmacy solutions and incompatibilities. In: Fischer JE (ed) Total Parenteral Nutrition. Little, Brown, Boston, 27–53, 1976.

162. Kronfeld DS. Feeding cats and feline nutrition. Comp Contin Ed Pract Vet 5:419–423, 1983.

163. Abood SK, Buffington CA. Enteral feeding of dogs and cats: 51 cases (1989–1991). J Am Vet Med Assoc 201:619–622, 1992.

39 Fluid Therapy of Gastrointestinal Disease

W. GRANT GUILFORD AND DONALD R. STROMBECK

INTRODUCTION

Gastrointestinal diseases are the most common cause of fluid and electrolyte disturbances in small animal patients. Many of the clinical signs of gastrointestinal disorders are due to fluid and electrolyte imbalances, and correction of these imbalances is the single most important treatment in many gastrointestinal diseases. Effective management of fluid and electrolyte imbalances requires a thorough knowledge of the physiology and pathophysiology of body fluids. The reader is referred to readily available authoritative texts and articles on this subject.[1-10] This chapter is concerned less with the theory of fluid and electrolyte homeostasis and more with the practicalities of fluid use in gastrointestinal diseases.

Appropriate fluid and electrolyte therapy is determined by synthesizing information acquired from the patient's history, physical examination, and laboratory evaluation. Clinical findings or laboratory tests used in isolation of one another do not allow optimal correction of imbalances. Clinical findings dictate the fluid volume required to correct dehydration, and indicate the preferred rate and route of administration. In contrast, laboratory tests provide the most accurate assessment of the required composition of the replacement fluid. A good understanding of fluid and electrolyte pathophysiology allows clinicians to estimate the electrolyte and acid-base derangements likely to accompany a particular gastrointestinal problem. This knowledge assists suitable fluid therapy when laboratory evaluations of electrolyte and acid-base balance are not available. In addition, discordance between expected electrolyte and acid-base derangements and the actual electrolyte and acid-base results provided by the laboratory helps lead the clinician to undiagnosed problems or to laboratory error, both of which may result in inappropriate therapy.

FLUID, ELECTROLYTE, AND ACID-BASE DERANGEMENTS FROM VOMITING AND DIARRHEA

Loss of body fluid with the same composition as extracellular fluid results in dehydration without major changes in body electrolyte composition. Gastric and intestinal secretions differ from extracellular fluids in electrolyte composition (Table 39-1), and their loss results in electrolyte and acid-base abnormalities.

Vomiting

Gastric secretions contain less sodium and higher concentrations of both potassium and chloride than extracellular fluid. The secretion is iso-osmotic with respect to body fluids, and the total number of anions and cations is approximately equivalent. When acid is secreted at a high rate, the gastric juices contain a high concentration of hydrochloric acid and a low concentration of sodium. Conversely, when acid secretion is low, the hydrogen ion concentration is low and that of sodium is high, approaching that of extracellular fluid. The gastric mucosa is a semipermeable membrane, and small amounts of acid secreted in the stomach soon equilibrate with the extracellular fluid.

Water is lost in excess of sodium during vomiting, producing hypernatremia. If vomiting patients are allowed to drink water, however, dilution of their plasma electrolytes by the absorbed water will result in hyponatremia.

Alkalosis is to be expected if the vomiting patient loses gastric hydrogen and chloride ions in excess of gastric, intestinal, and pancreatic sodium and bicarbonate. This is most likely to occur as a result of pyloric or upper duodenal intestinal obstruction. The hypochloremia perpetuates the alkalosis by increasing renal bicarbonate absorption. The alkalosis is

Table 39-1

COMPOSITIONS OF NORMAL PLASMA ELECTROLYTES, GASTRIC SECRETIONS, AND INTESTINAL SECRETIONS*

| | CONCENTRATIONS (mEq/L) | | |
	Plasma	Gastric Juice	Intestinal Secretions
Na	140-148	20-100	126-152
K	4.4-5.6	7-20	4-20
Cl	100-105	120-173	65-153
HCO$_3$	24	trace	5-60

*Compilation of data from a number of different sources including Biological Handbook of Federation of American Societies for Experimental Biology, 402-419, 1961.

particularly profound if concomitant hypokalemia and mild to moderate hypovolemia are present. Through a variety of mechanisms, hypokalemia is a potent stimulus for renal hydrogen secretion and bicarbonate reabsorption.[7] The result is paradoxical aciduria causing further loss of hydrogen ions in the urine and exacerbation of the alkalosis.[7] Alkalosis can also be caused by, or perpetuated by, mild to moderate hypovolemia. In this case the pathophysiology relates to a strong drive for the resorption of sodium and to "contraction alkalosis."

The composition of fluids secreted in the cranial small intestine is similar to the extracellular fluid, except for the chloride and bicarbonate concentrations (Table 39–1). Upper intestinal secretion has a pH of about 6.0 to 6.5. Because of its slightly acidic nature, excessive loss of upper intestinal secretions produces metabolic alkalosis, similar to that which can occur with loss of gastric juices. Alkalosis from the loss of upper gastrointestinal secretions occurs most frequently with duodenal obstruction. The alkalosis develops whether or not the obstruction is above or below the pancreatic and duodenal papilla, suggesting that the development of alkalosis does not depend on the exclusion of pancreatic and biliary secretions from the stomach, as is often suggested.

Acidemia can also occur in vomiting patients. This is particularly likely if the vomited gastric fluid is of relatively low hydrogen and chloride ion content (e.g., during fasting), if there is concurrent loss of intestinal sodium and bicarbonate, or if the animal becomes markedly hypovolemic. Loss of intestinal fluid via gastroduodenal reflux frequently occurs during vomiting and produces an acidosis because sodium (and bicarbonate) are lost in excess of chloride. Hypovolemia occurs as a result of loss of body water and sodium in the vomitus, producing contraction of the extracellular fluid volume and reduced blood volume. When the volume contracture is marked, tissue perfusion becomes inadequate and anaerobic metabolism ensues, generating lactic acid and a metabolic acidosis.

Diarrhea

Fluid secreted in the caudal small intestine and large intestine contains concentrations of bicarbonate higher than in plasma fluid and sodium in excess of chloride ion. The forfeiture of this fluid in diarrhea results in acidosis via loss of bicarbonate and, perhaps more importantly, a decrease in the strong ion difference. The acidosis can be compounded by the development of hypovolemia and accumulation of lactic acid. The sodium concentration of intestinal secretions is similar to that of plasma. As a result, loss of intestinal fluid causes a contraction of the extracellular fluid volume with little alteration of plasma sodium concentration unless continued water consumption occurs, diluting plasma sodium and producing hyponatremia.

Changes in Potassium

The potassium concentration of both gastric and intestinal secretions is high (Table 39–1) in relation to plasma. Thus, total body depletion of potassium is a predictable consequence of gastrointestinal disease. Hypokalemia may not be present, however, even in the face of significant total body potassium depletion because potassium is primarily an intracellular ion. Alteration of the proportionate distribution of potassium in the intracellular and extracellular spaces due to

acidosis can also affect the plasma potassium concentration, although this effect seems most marked with inorganic rather than organic acids. Hypokalemia in association with gastrointestinal disease will be particularly profound if the high daily losses of potassium are not matched by sufficient intake of potassium in food.

Prevalence of Fluid and Electrolyte Disorders in Vomiting and/or Diarrhea

Dogs and cats with vomiting and diarrhea may have any of the following fluid and electrolyte abnormalities: dehydration; low, normal, or high serum sodium, potassium, and chloride; and acidosis or alkalosis. The derangement that predominates in a particular animal depends on the severity of the disease and the influence of such factors as site of lesion, nutritional status, and amount of water consumed. Which of these fluid and electrolyte derangements are most prevalent in dogs and cats with vomiting and diarrhea has not been adequately determined.

The most common abnormalities seen in dogs with parvoviral enteritis have been reported to be alkalemia, hypochloremia, and hyponatremia.[11] The alkalemia and hyponatremia were primarily associated with vomiting. In this small series of cases hypokalemia or acidemia were not seen. In the authors' experience, *profound* alkalemia is more often a result of vomiting due to upper gastrointestinal obstruction rather than gastroenteritis. In another study, 34% of vomiting dogs had normal acid-base balance, 34% had metabolic acidosis, and 20% had metabolic alkalosis.[12] Fifty percent of the small number of dogs in the same study with diarrhea or a combination of diarrhea and vomiting had a primary metabolic acidosis. Metabolic acidosis is frequent in dogs with dehydration. Normal acid-base balance is usual in dogs with liver disease.[12] Of the electrolyte abnormalities associated with vomiting and diarrhea, mild hypokalemia, hyponatremia, hypernatremia, and hypochloremia appear to be the most common. Occasionally, vomiting and diarrhea from a variety of causes will produce hyponatremia in association with hyperkalemia, and may lead to an erroneous diagnosis of hypoadrenocorticism.[13]

In summary, whereas the spectrum of electrolytes depleted from the body during vomiting and diarrhea is predictable, the magnitude of the electrolyte loss and the resultant blood concentration of the electrolytes is highly variable. For these reasons, blood electrolyte and acid-base assessments are helpful in tailoring the fluid therapy of vomiting patients. Laboratory evaluation is not necessary, however, to choose the basic constituents of that fluid.

CHOICE OF FLUID COMPOSITION TO ADMINISTER

Replacement Fluids: Composition for Patients with Vomiting and Diarrhea

As already discussed, every patient with vomiting or diarrhea can be considered depleted, to a greater or lesser extent, of sodium, potassium, chloride, and water. Therefore, every vomiting or diarrheal patient whose clinical condition is sufficiently severe to warrant fluid therapy should receive fluid containing these electrolytes (Table 39–2). Thus, the fluid of choice for the initial therapy of vomiting or diarrhea

Table 39-2

RECOMMENDED FLUIDS FOR THE THERAPY OF GASTROINTESTINAL PROBLEMS

Maintenance of patients with anorexia-adypsia
First choice: Normosol-M or Plasmalyte 56 with 5% dextrose
Second choice: 1 part lactated Ringer's solution mixed with 1 to 2 parts 5% dextrose and spiked with 10 to 20 mEq/L of KCl

Initial volume replacement of patients with vomiting or diarrhea*
First choice: Lactated Ringer's solution with additional 5 to 10 mEq/L of KCl
Second choice: 0.9% NaCl spiked with 10 to 15 mEq/L of KCl

Maintenance of patients with uncomplicated vomiting or diarrhea
First choice: Lactated Ringer's solution spiked with 10 to 20 mEq/L of KCl
Second choice: 0.9% NaCl spiked with 15 to 20 mEq/L of KCl

Rehydration or maintenance of patients with vomiting or diarrhea complicated by hypokalemia†
First choice: Lactated Ringer's solution spiked with 15 to 75 mEq/L of KCl
Second choice: 0.9% NaCl spiked with 20 to 80 mEq/L of KCl

Treatment of patients with lactic acidosis and a blood pH < 7.2
First choice: 0.9% NaCl spiked with 10 to 15 mEq/L of KCl and sufficient $NaHCO_3$ to replace 0.25% of the total body deficit of bicarbonate
Second choice: None

Treatment of patients with metabolic alkalosis and a blood pH > 7.6
Nonedematous: 0.9% NaCl spiked with 15 to 20 mEq/L of KCl
Edematous (e.g., hepatic failure): acetazolamide 10 mg/kg q 6 hours PO; HCl if required; avoid sodium-containing fluids

*If serum electrolyte analysis subsequently rules out hyperkalemia, potassium concentration of the volume replacement fluids may be judiciously increased as required. Maintenance potassium requirements in an anoretic patient are approximately 0.03 to 0.05 mEq/kg/hour; maximum rate is 0.5 mEq/kg/hour.
†See text for precautions regarding KCl therapy.

is a balanced polyionic electrolyte solution such as lactated Ringer's solution (LRS). The primary properties of this fluid are that it is not acidifying (nor is it alkalinizing), and it provides small amounts of potassium and large quantities of sodium chloride. To this fluid may be added additional constituents as dictated by the results of electrolyte analysis. The additive most commonly required is potassium. This is added as potassium chloride (KCl) in amounts guided by the serum potassium level of the patient at admission (Table 39–3).

In contrast to LRS, normal saline is an acidifying fluid and it contains no potassium. It should only be used for the rehydration of vomiting patients that are alkalotic. It should never be used without the addition of supplemental potassium

Table 39-3

POTASSIUM REPLACEMENT GUIDELINES

SERUM POTASSIUM (mEq/L)	mEq KCL TO ADD TO 500 mL OF FLUID*	MAXIMUM INFUSION RATE† (mL/kg/HOUR)
< 2.0	40	6
2.1 to 2.5	30	8
2.6 to 3.0	20	12
3.1 to 3.5	14	16

*Assuming potassium-free fluid. If using LRS reduce potassium added by 5 mEq/L.
†Do not exceed 0.5 mEq/kg/hour.
Modified from Bell FW, Osborne CA. Maintenance fluid therapy. In: Kirk RW (ed) Current Veterinary Therapy X. WB Saunders, Philadelphia, 37–43, 1989.

(Table 39–2). As mentioned earlier, most patients with vomiting or diarrhea have significant total body potassium depletion, and many are hypokalemic. The rapid administration of a potassium-free fluid exacerbates the hypokalemia (by dilution) and does not counteract ongoing losses of potassium. The result can be a rapid onset of profound hypokalemia with disastrous consequences. A minor advantage for KCl-spiked normal saline over LRS in the treatment of the vomiting animal is that it contains slightly higher concentrations of sodium. An additional advantage of this fluid is that it is more compatible with sodium bicarbonate should alkalinization of the patient prove necessary.

It is important to reiterate that both LRS and normal saline fluids require modification to constitute ideally tailored volume replacement solutions for individual patients. The addition of more potassium over and above "physiologic" levels is particularly likely to be required. A major problem for the private practitioner is that rapid access to blood gas and electrolyte analysis may not be available. Without these analyses it is very difficult to determine the precise fluid and electrolyte requirements of the patient, particularly if the animal has been vomiting or has had diarrhea for prolonged periods whereupon fluid and electrolyte derangements can be considerable. The marked variations in the electrolyte concentration and acid-base abnormalities that accompany gastrointestinal disease, in particular vomiting (see earlier), make it difficult to provide standard recipes suitable to all patients. Therefore, it is suggested that until electrolyte results become available, the patient with vomiting and diarrhea is rehydrated with a fluid that is unlikely to exacerbate any potential preexisting metabolic derangements such as hypokalemia, hyperkalemia, acidosis, or alkalosis. A suitable fluid is LRS to which has been added conservative amounts of KCl (5–10 mEq per liter). This is sufficient KCl to meet and slightly exceed maintenance requirements when the fluid is administered at the rapid rates required to replace typical fluid deficits over a 6 to 12 hour period. This additional potassium should only be added to the replacement fluids of patients that have no evidence of renal azotemia (as judged by a reagent stick analysis of BUN and by the urine specific gravity) or hyperkalemia (bradycardia). In our opinion, it is best not to *rehydrate* patients empirically with solutions containing greater amounts of potassium than 15 mEq/L until the patient's blood potassium level is known. Use of fluids containing very high concentrations of potassium during resuscitation would be regretted if the patient had a hyperkalemia from, for instance, hypoadrenocorticism or concomitant renal disease. Furthermore, some dogs with primary gastrointestinal disease have serum potassium concentrations as high as 9.6 mEq/L.[13] Moreover, the use of high-concentration potassium-containing fluids significantly restricts the rapidity with which fluid can be administered during volume replacement of patients with shock.

Maintenance Fluids: Composition for Patients with Vomiting and Diarrhea

Neither LRS nor 0.9% sodium chloride are suitable maintenance fluids. LRS contains enough potassium (4 mEq/L), so that it will not exacerbate hypokalemia by dilution, but it does not contain sufficient to match maintenance losses of potassium in normal patients, let alone the exaggerated losses of this electrolyte that occur in animals with gastroenteritis. When used as a maintenance fluid, LRS must be routinely "spiked" with an additional 10 to 15 mEq/L of KCl to raise its potassium concentration to at least match that being lost in the urine and feces. Very often patients with gastrointestinal disease are depleted of total body potassium and may have ongoing losses of potassium in vomiting or diarrhea. Therefore, these patients often require greater than maintenance levels of potassium to replace their losses and maintain their serum potassium concentration. Once again, the amount of additional potassium provided is best guided by the results of a serum electrolyte analysis (Table 39–3). If electrolyte analysis is not available, a reasonably safe empirical dose is to add to LRS (used at maintenance rates) an additional 20 to 30 mEq/L of KCl for 2 to 3 days until the patient's vomiting and diarrhea abates and it begins to eat. Once again, it is essential to ensure there is no concomitant renal disease before adding high doses of potassium to the fluids.

As mentioned earlier, 0.9% sodium chloride is an acidifying fluid, and if used for several days will result in significant acidosis. This phenomenon occurs because of the high concentration of chloride ion (relative to sodium) in normal saline, and because the bicarbonate-free sodium chloride dilutes plasma bicarbonate and results in reduced reabsorption of urinary bicarbonate. Therefore, 0.9% sodium chloride should not be used as a maintenance fluid.

Both normal saline and LRS contain greater amounts of sodium than is required to replace maintenance losses in the normal animal. This may seem paradoxical because the sodium concentration of both these fluids, and the potassium concentration of LRS, closely approximate the serum concentrations of these electrolytes. However, for purposes of maintenance, the ideal fluid should match the concentration of electrolytes that are lost in the urine and stool, not the concentration of electrolytes in plasma (e.g., a healthy 4 kg cat loses approximately 6.6 mEq of potassium and 7.5 mEq of sodium per day[14]). In general, the potassium concentration of both urine and feces is higher than the concentration of potassium in the plasma, and the concentration of sodium is lower in these fluids than in plasma. The use of fluids with high sodium concentrations for maintenance of animals with vomiting and diarrhea is appropriate because losses of this ion are greater than normal. However, if continued fluid therapy is required in a patient whose vomiting and diarrhea have ceased, the patient should be switched to purpose-designed maintenance fluids, such as Normosol-M (CEVA Labs), which have a lower concentration of sodium and a higher concentration of potassium. Alternatively, a "home-made" maintenance fluid can be made by mixing 1 part LRS solution with 1 to 2 parts 5% dextrose.[3] Potassium chloride (10–20 mEq/L) is then added to the mixed solutions.

An example of a situation in which a maintenance fluid, such as Normosol-M, is indicated is a normovolemic animal whose vomiting and diarrhea have resolved but which remains anorexic and adypsic. If such an animal is maintained on LRS alone it will become hypernatremic and hypokalemic. If it is switched to a maintenance fluid, serum electrolytes are more likely to stay in the normal range provided there are no ongoing occult excessive losses of electrolytes. If there is any suggestion that the patient's diarrhea or vomiting have not completely resolved, these low-sodium fluids should not be used because the patient will become rapidly hyponatremic.

If the patient's disease process is complicated by significant hypokalemia, hypernatremia, acidemia, hypoalbuminemia, anemia, or various other abnormalities, modifications of the composition of these basic recipes will be required. These modifications are discussed, according to the particular derangement, in subsequent sections of this chapter.

CHOICE OF FLUID VOLUME TO ADMINISTER

Determination of Fluid Volume Required for Rehydration

The severity of the dehydration is a major determinant of the initial volume of fluid to be administered. The detection of dehydration and the estimation of the degree of fluid deficit is an inexact process. Laboratory results such as the presence of a high total protein, a high PCV, and especially a high serum albumin or sodium concentration should make a clinician suspicious of dehydration. These results can be misleading, however, and they cannot be used to judge the volume of fluid deficit. Instead, evaluation of hydration status most often relies on clinical assessment of skin turgor, dryness of mucous membranes, capillary refill time, mental attitude, and character and rate of pulse. Certain clinical findings have been associated with different degrees of dehydration. These findings have been tabulated, and allow the clinician to arrive at a crude estimation of the percentage of body water the patient has lost (Table 39–4). Certain circumstances can mislead clinicians in to wrongly estimating the percentage dehydration. For instance, panting can dry the oral mucous membranes, and obesity results in a tight skin that will not "tent" even in the face of dehydration. Conversely, weight loss and malnutrition can result in a baggy, poorly inelastic skin that tents excessively even though hydration is adequate.

Once the percentage of dehydration has been estimated, the volume of fluid required to replace that deficit (liters) is calculated by multiplying the percentage of dehydration by the body weight (kg). Thus, a 10 kg dog that has lost 10% of its body weight through dehydration requires $10/100 \times 10 = 1$ L of fluid to replace the deficit.

Additional fluid will be required to match ongoing obligatory fluid loss particularly from breath, feces, and urine. Charts relating obligatory (maintenance) fluid requirements to body weight (or surface area) are available. A rule of thumb is that daily maintenance fluid requirements of normal dogs and cats will range from 40 to 60 mL/kg/day. Smaller animals require higher volumes of fluids for maintenance than do larger animals. The daily fluid requirements of animals with vomiting or diarrhea are greatly increased over those of normal animals because of the large volumes of fluid that are lost in vomitus or diarrhea. These so-called contemporary or ongoing losses are estimated as best as possible, and added to the obligatory daily fluid requirement of the

Table 39–4

ESTIMATION OF THE SEVERITY OF DEHYDRATION

PERCENTAGE DEHYDRATION	CLINICAL SIGN
< 5	No detectable abnormalities
5–6	Slight loss of skin turgor
6–8	Skin tents momentarily but slowly flattens to normal, mucous membranes slightly dry, capillary refill time is normal to slightly prolonged, moderate depression but still alert
9–10	Skin remains tented, mucous membranes are dry and tacky, eyes are sunken into orbits, capillary refill is prolonged, tachycardia, weak pulse, markedly depressed, dull
>12	Profound shock, moribund

patient. Thus, in summary, the amount of fluid initially required to rehydrate and maintain the patient is calculated by the addition of the estimated volume of initial fluid deficit, the volume of fluid known to be necessary to maintain a normal animal, and the estimated additional volume of fluid lost in the patient's diarrhea or vomitus.

Measuring central venous pressure (CVP) is an objective way of estimating the volume of fluid required for rehydration. It is particularly useful in situations where rapid fluid administration is considered necessary because of evidence of hypovolemic shock, and has been used to monitor fluid administration in dogs with parvovirus enteritis.[15] Fluid is administered quickly until the patient's CVP begins to rise rapidly. An increase of 2 cm of water within 15 to 30 minutes is an indication to decrease the rate of fluid administration to maintenance rates. Because of reflex venoconstriction during hypovolemia, some dehydrated patients will have a normal or elevated CVP.[16] The usual response to fluid administration in these patients is an initial fall in central venous pressure because of relaxation of the venoconstriction. The CVP will begin to rise again once fluid replacement has been adequate. Normal CVP is usually 0 to 5 cm of water, but this is markedly influenced by the position of the transducer or water column. Because of this, and the previously mentioned phenomenon of reflex venoconstriction, it is better to estimate fluid requirements by dynamic changes in CVP rather than by using standardized "normal" values. Arterial blood pressure cannot be used in an analogous way to CVP to estimate dehydration because arterial blood pressure does not change until the patient becomes severely dehydrated or overhydrated. Thus, a weak pulse in a dehydrated patient is suggestive of severe fluid and electrolyte deficits or coexisting cardiac disease. More sophisticated means to evaluate water balance are seldom used. They involve the administration and subsequent measurement of tracers that distribute to total body water.

Determining Fluid Volume Required for Maintenance

Once fluid deficits have been replenished, the volume of fluid administered is reduced to match the estimated maintenance requirements of the patient. Because the estimation of both the obligatory losses and the contemporary (ongoing) losses is somewhat arbitrary, it is critical that the adequacy of maintenance fluid therapy be closely monitored to avoid overhydration or, more commonly, underhydration. This is best achieved by repeated daily physical examination, weighing the patient, estimation of urine output, and evaluation of the PCV, total protein, and urine specific gravity. Assessing these parameters not only determines the adequacy of fluid therapy but also may detect concomitant disease processes such as gastrointestinal bleeding and oliguric renal failure.

Clinical signs of overhydration include an increase in body weight, serous nasal discharge, restlessness, soft cough, late inspiratory crackles in the dependent portions of the lungs (pulmonary edema), polyuria, and diarrhea. In overhydrated patients, PCV and total protein will decline and the urine specific gravity will become hyposthenuric (in animals with normal renal function).

Signs of dehydration were described earlier. Fasted healthy dogs lose 1% to 3% of their body weight per day due to tissue catabolism. A fasted adult cat will lose approximately 0.1 kg/day. Greater daily weight loss in fasting animals should be attributed to dehydration.

CHOICE OF FLUID ADMINISTRATION ROUTE

Fluid supplementation may be provided by a variety of routes, including oral, intravenous, subcutaneous, and intramedullary. The route chosen largely depends on the severity of the patient's condition and the volume and composition of fluid to be replaced.

Oral Rehydration Solutions

Oral fluid therapy is ideally reserved for patients with minor fluid deficits or to supply maintenance fluid requirements. The oral route is not desirable if the patient is vomiting, but oral rehydration fluids can still be successfully administered to vomiting patents provided the vomiting is not persistent or severe. A major advantage of oral rehydration solutions (ORS) in comparison to intravenous fluids is reduced cost. A recent description of oral rehydration in small animals is available.[17]

The best ORS contain glucose (monomeric or polymeric) and amino acids in addition to water and electrolytes to take advantage of the cotransport pathways for the absorption of electrolytes and organic molecules.[18-20] During acute diarrheal diseases (especially secretory diarrheas but including rotaviral diarrhea), such sodium-coupled organic solute absorption remains largely intact.[21] Glucose increases the absorption of sodium in the jejunum by a factor of four and the absorption of water as much as sixfold. The correct concentrations of sodium and glucose are critical for optimal efficiency and safety.[18] Glucose-stimulated absorption plateaus at glucose concentrations of 50 mM.[20] Interestingly, this is the maximum glucose concentration found in the intestine of animals following ingestion of normal meals.[22] Glucose-containing ORS that result in intestinal glucose concentrations significantly in excess of 50 mM are likely to exacerbate diarrhea. There is evidence in humans that sucrose can be successfully used in homemade ORS.[19] This may also be true in dogs and cats; it is known that healthy dogs and cats can comfortably assimilate small quantities of sucrose.

Multiple cotransporters are involved in the absorption of different amino acids resulting in cumulative increases in sodium resorption when the small bowel is exposed to mixes of different amino acids. This additive effect of amino acids means that a mixture of amino acids can increase the rate of sodium absorption fivefold over that achieved by glucose/sodium cotransport.[20,23] A glucose and amino acid based, proprietary ORS for dogs and cats is now available (Enterolyte; Beecham).

It is very important that ORS are approximately isosmolar (300–350 mOsm); otherwise, iatrogenic osmotic diarrhea could exacerbate the diarrheal disease of the patient.[19] The desire to provide more organic substrate (and hence greater fluid and electrolyte absorption) but not exceed osmolality limits has led to the recent usage of ORS containing synthetic glucose polymers or glucose and amino acid polymers derived from foods ("food-based ORS").[19,24,25] Cooked cereal powders (especially rice) have proved suitable for this purpose. The glucose and amino acids in the cereal are slowly released during digestion, avoiding a deleterious osmotic load. It has been demonstrated in humans that the starches (and to a minor extent peptides) in rice are effective substrates for use in ORS, and can reduce the severity and duration of diarrhea.[19,24,26] Table 39–5 shows the composition of a rice-based ORS that has been successfully used in humans.[18] This solution may prove to have application in dogs and cats.

Table 39–5

COMPOSITION OF A RICE-BASED ORAL
REHYDRATION SOLUTION USED IN HUMANS

COMPONENT	g/L
Rice powder	50–80
Sodium chloride	3.5
Sodium bicarbonate	2.5
Potassium chloride	1.5

Concern has been expressed by some,[19] but not by others,[27] that food-based ORS may be inappropriate in neonates because of immature starch digestive processes.[19] It is also important to remember that food-based ORS contain insufficient calories to maintain an animal.

Bicarbonate or citrate are commonly incorporated in ORS to power further sodium resorption and provide alkalinization.[19] For practical purposes (such as shelf life) citrate is generally preferred to bicarbonate.[28] Others, however, have questioned the need for base or base precursors in ORS, pointing out that acidosis due to diarrhea usually corrects spontaneously with rehydration, and that bicarbonate may actually have a detrimental effect on sodium absorption in the face of enterotoxins.[29]

Potassium is necessary in ORS to address potassium losses in the diarrhea. Volatile fatty acids, such as lactate, pyruvate, and propionate, stimulate sodium and water absorption two- to sixfold in the colon of mammals.[20] These may also prove useful additions to ORS.

Intravenous Route

Intravenous administration is required for the rapid replacement of significant fluid deficits. Catheterization of a cephalic vein is suitable for the administration of fluids in most situations. The medial saphenous vein is also very useful in cats, and the lateral saphenous can be used in dogs. The jugular vein is preferred if large volumes of fluid need to be administered rapidly. An advantage of the jugular route in critically ill patients is that it allows assessment of CVP. The jugular vein is also preferred for the administration of hypertonic solutions. The caudal vena cava can be accessed through the medial saphenous of most cats and can also be used for the administration of hypertonic fluids.

Intramedullary Route

In hypovolemic animals in which percutaneous venous access can not be gained, a surgical cut-down on a vein is indicated. Alternatively, fluids may be administered directly into the medullary cavity of a long bone.[30] The intraosseous technique is particularly useful in pediatric patients because of the difficulty in catheterizing such animals. The femur is usually used because of convenient access. To minimize the risk of osteomyelitis, the area over the trochanteric fossa is surgically prepared. Local anesthetic (0.5–1.0 mL) is infiltrated under the skin and into the periosteum of the trochanteric fossa. A 20 gauge spinal needle is advanced into the femur via the trochanteric fossa. Bone marrow is aspirated to confirm placement, and the point of entry is protected with antiseptic cream and a light dressing. Fluids can be run into the marrow cavity at quite rapid rates.

Subcutaneous Route

The subcutaneous route is a convenient route for the administration of small volumes of fluids required for maintenance. It is not an ideal route for replacing large fluid deficits because fluid is absorbed slowly and unpredictably from the subcutaneous tissues of hypovolemic animals. Furthermore, the administration of large volumes of fluid subcutaneously is uncomfortable and, if excessive, can lead to skin necrosis. Subcutaneous administration is particularly useful for intractable patients and for correction of minor dehydration in animals treated as outpatients. Only isotonic fluids can be administered subcutaneously. The volume injected at one site should be determined by the degree of patient discomfort but, in small patients, should not exceed 100 to 150 mL per site. After administration, the fluid should be massaged in a ventral direction away from the needle puncture; otherwise, considerable loss of fluid will occur through the puncture site.

Intraperitoneal Route

This neglected route of administration can be very effective in neonates. Blood, electrolytes, and dextrose can be given by this route and appear to be rapidly absorbed. Solutions used intraperitoneally should be approximately isotonic and nonirritating. They must be administered in a sterile manner.

CHOICE OF FLUID ADMINISTRATION RATE

The rapidity of administration depends on the patient's hydration status, its ongoing fluid losses, and the presence or absence of concomitant medical conditions such as heart failure or renal disease.

During shock, fluids can be administered to cats or dogs as rapidly as 70–90 mL/kg/hour, respectively (preferably with CVP monitoring). In dehydrated patients that are not in shock, fluid volume deficits are usually replaced over a 6 to 24 hour period as dictated by the patient's medical condition. Overly rapid infusion is avoided so that the administered fluid and electrolytes have time to equilibrate with the tissues rather than cause vascular volume overload and excessive diuresis. Most volume deficits in patients with uncomplicated gastrointestinal disease can be safely replenished in 6 to 8 hours. Volume replacement must be slow and carefully monitored in patients with renal, pulmonary, or heart disease. If fluid administration can only be observed for part of the day, it is usually better to provide the majority of the patient's deficit and daily needs during the period of observation.

CAUSE, RECOGNITION, AND THERAPY OF HOMEOSTATIC DERANGEMENTS COMMON IN GASTROINTESTINAL DISEASE

Hypokalemia

CAUSE. Common causes of hypokalemia include vomiting, diarrhea, secondary hyperaldosteronemia due to dehydration or liver disease, and rapid correction of acidosis by the administration of bicarbonate.[31–33] Additional causes of hypokalemia are provided in Table 39–6.

Table 39–6

CAUSES OF POTASSIUM DEPLETION

Gastrointestinal losses
Vomiting
Diarrhea

Renal losses
Anorexia
Hyperaldosteronism (hypovolemia, liver disease)
Metabolic alkalosis
Renal disease
Drugs (diuretics, nephrotoxic drugs)

"Third" spaces
Gastric dilatation-volvulus
Subcutaneous administration of potassium-free fluid

Intracellular shifts
Insulin administration
Bicarbonate administration

CLINICAL SIGNS. Mild hypokalemia is subclinical. Clinical manifestations of severe hypokalemia include weakness, anorexia, vomiting, constipation, adynamic ileus, variable ECG changes (especially prolonged QT interval, small T-wave, and arrhythmias), polyuria, and neurologic signs (Table 39–7). In cats, hypokalemia is associated with head and neck ventroflexion, myalgia, and polymyopathy. Hypokalemia may produce glucose intolerance because of impaired insulin release, and polyuria may develop due to deficient renal concentrating ability. Plasma concentrations of other ions frequently change with that of potassium, and can exaggerate the clinical signs of hypokalemia.

TREATMENT. It is important to reiterate that plasma potassium concentrations do not accurately reflect the total body stores of potassium because potassium is largely an intracellular ion. As a result, if clinical signs consistent with low body potassium are noted, consideration should be given to supplemental potassium therapy even in the presence of a normal serum potassium level. An example of where such an approach has proved useful is in the treatment of arrhythmias associated with gastric-dilatation volvulus. Supplemental potassium is also indicated during adynamic ileus associated with vomiting or diarrhea because there is high probability that the ileus is compounded by potassium depletion.

Potassium can be replaced by means of parenteral fluids, oral supplements, or conventional diets. In order to replace large deficits of potassium, KCl should be added to the intravenous fluid solution to bring the potassium concentration to 30 to 80 mEq/L. The amount of KCl added depends on the severity of the potassium deficit; a guideline is provided in Table 39–3. In animals with normal renal function, potassium may be supplemented as rapidly as 0.5 mEq/kg/hour. Careful monitoring of serum potassium levels during therapy is advisable. Alternatively, the electrocardiogram can be monitored.

Potassium can also be added to subcutaneous fluids. The concentration of potassium in subcutaneous fluids should not exceed 30 mEq/L. Oral potassium replacement is best achieved with elixirs such as potassium gluconate (Kaon Elixir; Adria). Potassium tablets are a recognized cause of esophageal perforation in people, and must be used with care in animals. The elixir is usually administered at doses of 2 to 3 mEq/kg once to three times per day. Higher rates may be used if required, provided potassium concentrations can be monitored. Oral forms are as potentially hazardous as the parenteral solutions because potassium given orally is rapidly and completely absorbed from the small intestine.

Potassium deficits are often not readily replaced until food intake is resumed, and even then potassium losses sometimes exceed intake. The approximate potassium content of some common foods is as follows: beef (6.5 mEq/100 g), chicken (9.5 mEq/100 g), and potatoes (10.5 mEq/100 g). Foods containing high amounts of potassium include halibut (14 mEq/100 g), banana (11.3 mEq per medium-sized banana), and tomato (7.7 mEq per medium-sized tomato).

Potassium-depleted patients should not be administered potassium-free fluids. The consequences of potassium-free solutions are more severe when the fluids used contain glucose or bicarbonate. Both of these substances promote the transfer of potassium from the extracellular fluid to intracellular stores, worsening the hypokalemia.

Hyperkalemia

Hyperkalemia is not usually associated with gastrointestinal diseases. Some exceptions do occur, however. Concomitant renal disease, hypoadrenocorticism, and inadvertent oversupplementation with KCl can produce hyperkalemia.[34] Furthermore, as mentioned earlier, some dogs with primary gastrointestinal diseases can develop significantly elevated potassium concentrations in association with hyponatremia (electrolyte changes that mimic hypoadrenocorticism).[13] The hyponatremia in these dogs has been attributed to gastrointestinal loss, and the hyperkalemia to acidosis-induced translocation of potassium from the intracellular to the extracellular compartment.[13] Decreased glomerular filtration rate may have also contributed to the hyperkalemia. Hyperkalemia resulting from primary gastrointestinal causes is usually mild and can be treated by the administration of potassium-free fluids such as saline or 5% dextrose.

Table 39–7

NEUROLOGIC MANIFESTATIONS OF ELECTROLYTE DISTURBANCES

DISTURBANCE	LISTLESSNESS CONFUSION, COMA	SEIZURES	MUSCLE WEAKNESS	PARALYSIS	TETANY
Hypernatremia	+	+	+	–	–
Hyponatremia	+	+	+	–	–
Hyperkalemia	–	–	+	+	–
Hypokalemia	±	±	+	+	±
Acidosis	+	±	–	–	–
Alkalosis	+	+	+	–	+

Hyponatremia

CAUSE. Hyponatremia is relatively common in gastrointestinal disease. The usual cause is the continued intake of water in the face of loss of sodium-rich gastrointestinal fluids in vomitus or diarrhea. It is also commonly associated with edematous states such as hepatic cirrhosis. Additional causes are listed in Table 39–8.

CLINICAL SIGNS. Hyponatremia can cause anorexia, lethargy, vomiting, tachycardia, shock, and a variety of neurologic signs including muscle cramping, myoclonus, seizures, and coma (Table 39–7). The appearance of clinical signs is determined by the rate at which plasma sodium concentration decreases. Rapid reductions from normal concentrations to concentrations in the vicinity of 130 mEq/L will usually result in the development of neurologic signs. In contrast, if sodium depletion is gradual, clinical signs may not be evident until a plasma sodium concentration of 110 mEq/L is reached.

TREATMENT. Mild hyponatremia in association with hypovolemia due to loss of gastrointestinal secretions is treated with sodium-containing fluids such as normal saline or LRS. Profound hyponatremia is corrected by careful intravenous administration of hypertonic salt solutions (3%). The sodium deficit is calculated by the formula 0.6 × lean body weight × sodium deficit per liter. In general, only enough sodium should be given to raise the serum sodium concentration to just above 120 to 130 mEq/L. Hypertonic saline solutions are rarely necessary in the treatment of gastrointestinal disorders. Too rapid correction of chronic hyponatremia can lead to delayed myelinolysis in dogs.[35] Signs of myelinolysis usually begin 3 to 4 days after correction of the sodium imbalance and consist of depression, weakness, and ataxia progressing to spastic episodic quadriparesis, myoclonus, and hypermetria.[35] Neurologic improvement of affected dogs can occur with time. To avoid such complications, rates of correction of chronic hyponatremia should not exceed 0.5 mEq/L/hour.

Hyponatremia due to edematous states such as cirrhosis is treated by attention to the primary cause and careful water restriction. If the hyponatremia is severe, the edematous patient can be treated by the concurrent administration of a loop diuretic and slow infusion of hypertonic saline. The diuretic induces the loss of both salt and water, but only the salt is replaced by the hypertonic saline. In these patients, administration of sodium without the loop diuretic is contraindicated because it will worsen the severity of the edema. Thiazide diuretics should not be used in this situation because they exacerbate the hyponatremia by inducing sodium and potassium loss in excess of water.[7]

Table 39–8

CAUSES OF HYPONATREMIA

Vomiting and/or diarrhea
Hypoadrenocorticism
Iatrogenic (low-salt diet; hypotonic fluids; diuretics)
Inappropriate use of maintenance (low-sodium) intravenous fluids
"Third space" loss (GDV; pancreatitis)
Edematous states (hepatic cirrhosis; hypoalbuminemia; heart disease)
Exudative fluid losses (burns; body cavity lavage)
Renal disease (renal failure; sodium-wasting nephropathy; nephrotic syndrome)
Psychogenic polydipsia
Syndrome of inappropriate ADH secretion (CNS disease; drugs; paraneoplastic)
Pseudohyponatremia (hyperlipidemia; hyperproteinemia; hyperglycemia)

Table 39–9

CAUSES OF HYPERNATREMIA

Excessive pure water loss (fever, hyperventilation, heat stroke, diabetes insipidus)
Excessive hypotonic water loss (vomiting and/or diarrhea; diabetes mellitus; renal failure; hyperadrenocorticism)
Adypsia (primary [CNS]; pharyngeal or esophageal diseases; lack of access; miscellaneous diseases)
Iatrogenic (hypertonic saline fluids; sodium bicarbonate; prolonged use of LRS or 0.9% saline; hypertonic saline enemas)
Sodium avidity (hyperadrenocorticism, hyperaldosteronemia)
Cushing's syndrome
Salt poisoning

Hypernatremia

The primary gastrointestinal cause of hypernatremia is the loss of greater amounts of water than sodium in vomitus. Other causes of hypernatremia are provided in Table 39–9.

The most common clinical signs of hypernatremia are weakness, extreme thirst, irritability, depression, ataxia, tremors, myoclonus, and coma (Table 39–7). Acute elevations of sodium to approximately 170 mEq/L are likely to cause clinical signs. More chronic elevations may be asymptomatic because of the development of idiogenic osmoles in the CNS. Diagnosis of hypernatremia is made by measuring plasma electrolytes. No consistent changes are observed on electrocardiograms.

Hypernatremia indicates intracellular dehydration as well as contraction of the extracellular fluid volume, and it is treated by attention to the primary cause and careful administration of isotonic or hypotonic fluids (e.g., 0.45% sodium or 5% dextrose solutions). The isotonic fluids are indicated when volume repletion is necessary and when the hypernatremia is not severe. Hypotonic fluids are indicated if hypernatremia is severe. They must be administered very slowly (over 2–3 days) to patients with chronic hypernatremia; otherwise, cerebral edema and death will result. Serum sodium concentration should not decrease any more rapidly than 0.5 to 1 mEq/hour.

Metabolic Acidosis

Acidosis is a process that causes acid to accumulate in the body. It tends to cause a decrease in blood pH but, because of the buffering capacity of the blood, marked abnormality in blood pH may not occur. In contrast, the term *acidemia* implies a decrease in blood pH to below normal (Table 39–10). In other words, acidosis is a process causing a tendency toward acidemia. Acidosis may result from a respiratory disease that causes carbon dioxide to accumulate in the body (respiratory acidosis) or from a metabolic process that causes a decrease in the strong ion difference (increase in chloride relative to sodium ion), an addition of strong organic acids (e.g., lactate, acetoacetate, beta-hydroxybutyrate), or the loss of alkaline reserve (bicarbonate). In gastrointestinal diseases, metabolic acidosis is of prime importance.

CAUSE. The most common gastrointestinal causes of acidosis are diarrhea and dehydration. As discussed earlier, severe diarrhea is associated with both an accelerated loss of sodium and bicarbonate-rich intestinal fluid and an accelerated production of lactic acid as a result of dehydration and

Table 39–10

VENOUS BLOOD GAS DATA IN HEALTHY DOGS AND CATS

	DOGS	**CATS**
pH	7.35 +/− 0.02	7.3 +/− 0.09
PO_2 (torr)	55.0 +/− 9.6	38.6 +/− 11.4
PCO_2 (torr)	36.6 +/− 1.2	41.8 +/− 9.1
Bicarbonate (mEq/L)	23.0 +/− 1.4	19.4 +/− 4.0
TCO_2 (mEq/L)	24.1 +/− 1.4	20.1 +/− 4.2
Base excess (mEq/L)	−1.2 +/− 1.1	−5.7 +/− 4.6

hypovolemia. Expansion of the extracellular fluid compartment with solutions containing little or no bicarbonate, such as normal saline, is another cause of acidosis (see earlier). Additional causes of acidosis are provided in Table 39–11.

Acidosis caused by decrease in strong ion difference, bicarbonate loss, or acid accumulation will all lower plasma bicarbonate concentration. These types of metabolic acidosis have different effects on plasma chloride concentrations, however. When acids are retained in extracellular fluid, plasma chloride concentrations remain normal. The retained acids replace bicarbonate and have no effect on chloride concentrations (Figure 39–1). When excessive chloride is retained or increased bicarbonate is lost, plasma chloride concentrations increase above normal. Therefore, classification of metabolic acidosis as hyperchloremic (normal anion gap) or normochloremic (high anion gap) may help identify cause.[36]

CLINICAL SIGNS AND DIAGNOSIS. Metabolic acidosis should be suspected in any animal showing evidence of diarrhea, dehydration, or hypovolemia. The clinical signs of acidosis are nonspecific and include CNS signs (Table 39–7) and hyperventilation (a means of compensation for metabolic acidosis). Urine pH is of little diagnostic value because urine can be either alkaline or acid, depending on the availability of potassium for excretion. Blood gas analysis is the only reliable means of identifying metabolic acidosis (Table 39–10). It allows differentiation of the various forms of acid-base derangements, and provides the serum pH, base excess, and bicarbonate concentration values on which therapeutic decisions are based. When blood gas analysis is unavailable, total CO_2 measurement can be used as a guide to acid-base derangements. Serum total CO_2 is usually 1 to 2 mEq higher than serum bicarbonate concentration (Table 39–10).

TREATMENT. Metabolic acidosis resulting from diarrhea

Table 39–11

CAUSES OF METABOLIC ACIDOSIS

Excess Formation and Retention of Metabolically Produced Acids
  Diabetes mellitus
  Lactic acidosis (marked volume depletion, shock)
  Advanced renal failure
  Distal renal tubular acidosis
  Ingestion of acidifying products (ethylene glycol, salicylates)
  Hyperproteinemia

Excessive Loss of Bicarbonate
  Diarrhea
  Chronic renal disease
  Proximal renal tubular acidosis
  Drugs (carbonic anhydrase inhibitors, cholestyramine)
  Expansion of extracellular fluid volume with bicarbonate-free fluids (dilutional acidosis)

seldom needs specific alkalinizing treatment. On most occasions, the condition is readily correctable by rehydration. Should pronounced acidemia be present, however, consideration may be given to the use of intravenous bicarbonate therapy. The administration of sodium bicarbonate can be associated with a number of undesirable consequences (Table 39–12). Therefore, most clinicians will not administer bicarbonate until the serum pH has decreased to a range in which patient safety is compromised. In humans, once pH drops below 7.2 cardiac function is thought to be compromised through decreased contractility and arrhythmias. Therefore, most veterinary clinicians will institute bicarbonate therapy at blood pH of 7.2 or below.

During administration, bicarbonate distributes rapidly to the extracellular space but requires 2 to 4 hours to equilibrate with the intracellular compartment. The total body bicarbonate deficit can be calculated with the following formula:

$$\text{mEq } HCO_3 \text{ needed} = \text{body weight (kg)} \times 0.6 \, [24 \text{ mEq/L} - \text{measured plasma } HCO_3 \text{ concentration}].$$

The constant "0.6" refers to the space that bicarbonate distributes to, that of total body water. Some clinicians prefer to calculate the extracellular bicarbonate deficit by using the factor 0.3 instead of 0.6. Once the decision to utilize bicarbonate is made, the bicarbonate deficit is calculated and a proportion (usually 25%) of the total body deficit is administered intravenously over a 2 to 3 hour period. Additional bicarbonate is given only after the pH is reevaluated. Titration of the bicarbonate dose in this manner minimizes the potential side effects associated with its use. If blood gas results are not available, but the clinician feels bicarbonate therapy is indicated, an alternative approach is to empirically administer bicarbonate at a dose of 1 to 4 mEq/kg depending on the suspected severity of the acidosis. Sodium bicarbonate is best administered as an infusion in 0.45% or 0.9% saline. In theory, it is not compatible with LRS because of the calcium contained in this fluid.

Unfortunately, there is considerable doubt about the efficacy of plasma bicarbonate for the treatment of lactic acidosis and heightening concern, born of experimental work in dogs, that it may actually worsen the situation by producing a transient intracellular acidosis (in an analogous manner to paradoxical cerebral acidosis).[37–39] The buffering of hydrogen ion by bicarbonate is thought to result in the accumulation of CO_2 in the tissues. This is a freely diffusible gas and rapidly enters the intracellular fluid, generating carbonic and lactic acid and further reducing intracellular pH. The relevance of the phenomenon is still disputed by some authorities, however.[40] As mentioned earlier, an additional important potential complication of bicarbonate administration is hypokalemia.

Metabolic acidosis can also be corrected with sodium lactate. Lactate is metabolized by the liver and other tissues to form bicarbonate, with 1 mEq of Na lactate forming 1 mEq of Na bicarbonate. Conversion of lactate to bicarbonate is not immediate because it depends on the rates of lactate transport into cells, on intracellular metabolism, and on bicarbonate transport into extracellular fluid. Administration of lactate offers no advantages over the administration of bicarbonate for the correction of acidosis,[7] and it is likely to be poorly efficacious for alkalinization therapy in lactic acidosis (there is evidence to suggest that lactate utilization is depressed in lactic acidosis as well as the rate of production increased).[7] As its name would suggest, LRS contains lactate, but it should not be considered a suitable fluid for alkalinization therapy during serious acidemia. There is sufficient lac-

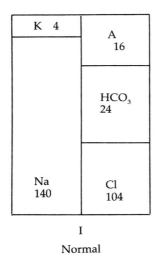 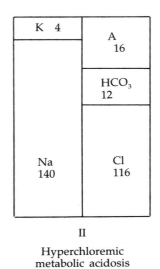 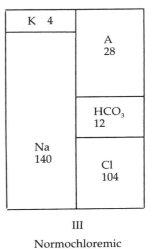

I	II	III
Normal	Hyperchloremic metabolic acidosis	Normochloremic metabolic acidosis

FIGURE 39–1. Composition of plasma fluid in the normal state and with hyperchloremic and normochloremic metabolic acidosis. A = unmeasured anions that increase with metabolic disease such as diabetes mellitus.

tate in LRS to prevent reduction of plasma bicarbonate and hence the exacerbation of a preexisting acidosis. There is not sufficient lactate in LRS to reverse an acidemia, however. These comments notwithstanding, LRS is still the fluid of choice for the treatment of acidosis and mild acidemias. Its beneficial effect in these situations comes not from an ability to "neutralize" acid but from volume replenishment and the reestablishment of adequate perfusion to previously ischemic tissues.

Metabolic Alkalosis

Alkalosis is a process that causes base to accumulate in the body. Although blood pH tends to increase when alkalosis occurs, because of the buffering capacity of blood, no abnormality in blood pH may occur.[36] In contrast, alkalemia refers to an increase in blood pH above normal. Metabolic alkalosis usually results from a loss of hydrogen and chloride ions (in

Table 39–12

COMMON CAUSES OF MORBIDITY AND MORTALITY ASSOCIATED WITH FLUID THERAPY

Underestimation of fluid requirements
Iatrogenic hypokalemia by administration of fluids too low in potassium
Cerebral edema from too rapid administration of hypoosmolar fluids to hyperosmolar patients
Cardiac arrhythmias and phlebitis from too rapid administration of KCl
Too rapid administration of sodium bicarbonate resulting in paradoxical cerebral acidosis, paradoxical intracellular acidosis, hypokalemia, decreased ionized calcium, hyperosmolality, decreased tissue oxygen delivery, and "overshoot" alkalosis
Sepsis from inadequate catheter care or poor placement technique
Thrombophlebitis from poor catheter technique or administration of hyperosmolar solutions
Pulmonary edema from too rapid administration of sodium-containing fluids to patients with congestive heart failure, pneumonitis, or renal disease

excess of sodium) from the gastrointestinal tract or from an accumulation of bicarbonate.

CAUSE. Metabolic alkalosis is most commonly due to vomiting (Table 39–13). Other causes of chloride depletion, such as diuretic administration or chloride-secreting diarrhea, will also cause metabolic alkalosis. As discussed earlier, potassium depletion and mild to moderate hypovolemia may cause or perpetuate metabolic alkalosis. Excessive administration of antacids can cause metabolic alkalosis. This is infrequent, however, occurring only in animals with renal function that is inadequate to excrete excess base. Alkalosis is likely in patients with hepatic cirrhosis. In cirrhotic patients the alkalosis most commonly develops from a combination of excessive diuretic use and a reduced effective circulating volume. The latter leads to sodium avidity and bicarbonate resorption in an analogous manner to hypovolemia.

CLINICAL SIGNS AND DIAGNOSIS. The clinical signs of alkalosis are nonspecific and usually relate to the cause of the alkalosis rather than the alkalosis itself. Alkalotic animals hypoventilate. Many problems cause respiratory depression, however, so this sign is of little diagnostic value for alkalosis. Low plasma chloride concentration associated with near normal levels of sodium and potassium are suggestive of alkalosis. Plasma bicarbonate concentration is often increased when plasma chloride is low. Suspected alkalosis is confirmed by blood gas analysis.

TREATMENT. The aim of therapy is to correct the three primary factors that perpetuate alkalemia, that is, hypochloremia, hypovolemia, and hypokalemia.[7] These aims can usually be achieved by the use of a 0.9% sodium chloride spiked with an appropriate amount of KCl. Additional therapy of value in alkalotic vomiting patients is the use of an H_2 receptor blocker such as cimetidine. Saline-resistant alkalosis is rarely encountered in patients with gastrointestinal disease. One cause is severe hypokalemia (< 2 mEq/L). In this situation, potassium supplementation will lead to saline-responsive alkalosis. In patients with hepatic cirrhosis, saline administration is not indicated because it will precipitate edema. In these patients, the drug of first choice is acetazolamide, which serves the dual purpose of increasing the renal secre-

Table 39–13

CAUSES OF METABOLIC ALKALOSIS

Vomiting (high intestinal obstruction)
Gastric dilatation-volvulus
Chloride-secreting diarrhea?
Excessive administration of bicarbonate or citrate
Hypoproteinemia
Contraction alkalosis (mild to moderate dehydration)

tion of sodium and bicarbonate.[7] If this measure fails, and the blood pH remains above 7.6, dilute hydrochloric acid (1.0 N)(1 mEq/mL) can be used at a rate of 1 mEq/minute and a dose calculated by the following formula:

$$HCl\ (mEq) = 0.3 \times body\ (kg)\ weight \times base\ excess\ (mEq/L).$$

One-third to two-thirds of the calculated deficit is given and the blood pH carefully monitored.[39] It should be noted that ammonium chloride or arginine chloride should not be used in the treatment of alkalosis due to liver failure as they may result in ammonia toxicity.[7]

Respiratory Acidosis and Alkalosis

Respiratory acidosis or alkalosis are often detected in patients with gastrointestinal disease. On most occasions, however, these processes are appropriate compensatory responses for the metabolic derangement induced by the gastrointestinal disorder. On occasion a mixed acid-base disorder will be apparent in which the alteration in pH induced by the metabolic abnormality is exacerbated by a concomitant respiratory acidosis or alkalosis. This usually reflects a secondary disease process affecting the animal or an inappropriate physiologic response. For instance, pain or distress in a vomiting animal will occasionally induce hyperventilation and respiratory alkalosis that can complicate a metabolic alkalosis from vomiting.

Hypoproteinemia and Hypoalbuminemia

Loss of albumin and globulin are common problems in gastrointestinal diseases in which mucosal permeability is increased (protein-losing enteropathies). In hepatic insufficiency, hypoalbuminemia is common because of reduced hepatic synthesis of albumin. The consequences of hypoalbuminemia are decreased oncotic pressure and reduced effective circulating volume. The result is edema and sodium avidity that compounds the edema. Hypoalbuminemic patients develop sodium avidity either as a result of their disease (e.g., liver failure) or as a result of decreased effective circulating volume (poor tissue perfusion). The sodium retention results in increased extracellular fluid and plasma volume but paradoxically need not improve effective circulating volume.

The treatment of choice for hypoalbuminemia is administration of plasma in association with the judicious use of a loop diuretic. The loop diuretic reduces the extracellular fluid volume back toward normal. The amount of plasma administered depends on the severity of the hypoalbuminemia. The aim is to return the serum albumin concentration to 1.5 to 2.0 g/dl. A suitable starting dose is 20 mL/kg. If sufficient plasma is unavailable, alternative colloidal fluids of value for short-term maintenance of oncotic pressure are dextran 70 (5 mL/kg/hour to a maximum of 20 mL/kg/day) or hetastarch 6% (10–20 mL/kg/day).

REFERENCES

1. Brobst D. Pathophysiologic and adaptive changes in acid-base disorders. J Am Vet Med Assoc 183:773–780, 1983.
2. Stewart PA. Modern quantitative acid-base chemistry. Can J Physiol Pharmacol 61:1444–1461, 1983.
3. Haskins SC. Fluid and electrolyte therapy. Comp Contin Ed Pract Vet 6:244–254, 1984.
4. Brobst D. Review of the pathophysiology of alterations in potassium homeostasis. J Am Vet Med Assoc 188:1019–1025, 1986.
5. Bell FW, Osborne CA. Maintenance fluid therapy. In: Kirk RW (ed) Current Veterinary Therapy X. WB Saunders, Philadelphia, 37–43, 1989.
6. Orsini JA. Pathophysiology, diagnosis, and treatment of clinical acid-base disorders. Comp Contin Ed Pract Vet 11:593–604, 1989.
7. Rose BD. Clinical Physiology of Acid-Base and Electrolyte Disorders, 3rd ed. McGraw-Hill, New York, 1989.
8. Leith DE. The new acid-base: Power and simplicity. Proc 9th ACVIM Forum, New Orleans, 611–617, 1991.
9. Pascoe PJ. Acid-base and blood gas abnormalities. In: Allen DG, Kruth SA, Garvey MS (eds) Small Animal Medicine. JB Lippincott, Philadelphia, 935–948, 1991.
10. de Morais HSA. Disorders of PCO_2, [SID] and [A_{TOT}]. Proc 10th ACVIM Forum, San Diego, 165–167, 1992.
11. Heald RD, Jones BD, Schmidt DA. Blood gas and electrolyte concentrations in canine parvoviral enteritis. J Am Anim Hosp Assoc 22:745–748, 1986.
12. Cornelius LM, Rawlings CA. Arterial blood gas values in dogs with various diseases and signs of disease. J Am Vet Med Assoc 178:992–995, 1981.
13. Di Bartola SP, Johnson SE, Davenport DJ, et al. Clinicopathologic findings resembling hypoadrenocorticism in dogs with primary gastrointestinal disease. J Am Vet Med Assoc 187:60–63, 1985.
14. Harrison JB, Sussman HH, Pickering DE. Fluid and electrolyte therapy in small animals. J Am Vet Med Assoc 137:637–640, 1960.
15. Horvath L, Lajos Z, Mikecz A. Study of the efficacy of fluid therapy in dogs suffering from parvovirus enteritis. Magyar-Allatorvosok-Lapja 46:93–99, 1991.
16. Wilson RF, Sibbald WJ. Editorial: A new look at an old approach to resuscitation: Early aggressive fluid administration. Circulatory Shock 2:1–3, 1975.
17. Zenger E, Willard MD. Oral rehydration therapy in companion animals. Comp Anim Pract 19:6–10, 1989.
18. Carpenter CCJ, Greenough WB, Pierce NF. Oral-rehydration therapy—the role of polymeric substrates. New Eng J Med 319:1346–1348, 1988.
19. Snyder JD, Molla AM, Cash RA. Home-based therapy for diarrhea. J Pediatr Gastroenterol Nutr 11:438–447, 1990.
20. Powell DW. Intestinal water and electrolyte transport. In: Johnson LR (ed) Physiology of the Gastrointestinal Tract, 2nd ed. Raven Press, New York, 1267–1305, 1987.
21. Rhoads JM, Keku EO, Quinn J, et al. L-glutamine stimulates sodium and chloride absorption in pig rotavirus enteritis. Gastroenterology 100:683–691, 1991.
22. Ferraris RP, Yasharpour S, Lloyd KCK, et al. Luminal glucose concentrations in the gut under normal conditions. Am J Physiol 259:G822–G837, 1990.
23. Armstrong WM. Cellular mechanisms of ion transport in the small intestine. In: Johnson LR (ed) Physiology of the Gastrointestinal Tract, 2nd ed. Raven Press, New York, 1251–1265, 1987.
24. Lebenthal E. Rice as a carbohydrate substrate in oral rehydration solutions (ORS). J Pediatr Gastroenterol Nutr 11:293–303, 1990.
25. Saunders DR, Saunders MD, Sillery JK. Beneficial effects of glucose polymer and an H_2 receptor blocker in a patient with a proximal ileostomy. Am J Gastroenterol 84:192–194, 1989.
26. Patra FC, Mahalanabis D, Jalan KN, et al. Is oral rice electrolyte solution superior to glucose electrolyte solution in the infantile diarrhea? Arch Dis Child 57:910–912, 1982.
27. Lebenthal E. Glucose polymers in diarrhea—high caloric density nutrients with low osmolality. J Pediatr Gastroenterol Nutr 11:1–6, 1990.
28. ESPGAN Working Group. Recommendations for composition of oral rehydration solutions for the children of Europe. J Pediatr Gastroenterol Nutr 14:113–115, 1992.
29. Elliot EJ, Watson AJM, Walker-Smith JA, et al. Bicarbonate and citrate in oral rehydration therapy: Studies in a model of secretory diarrhea. J Pediatr Gastroenterol Nutr 16:278–283, 1993.
30. Otto CM, Kaufman GM, Crowe DT. Intraosseous infusion of fluids and therapeutics. Comp Contin Ed Pract Vet 11:421–424, 1989.
31. Bell FW, Osborne CA. Treatment of hypokalemia. In: Kirk RW (ed) Current Veterinary Therapy IX. WB Saunders, Philadelphia, 101–107, 1986.
32. Kleeman CR: Water metabolism. In: Maxwell MH, Kleeman CR (eds) Clin-

ical Disorders of Fluid and Electrolyte Metabolism, 2nd ed. McGraw-Hill, New York, 215–295, 1972.

33. Whang R. Hyperkalemia: Diagnosis and treatment. Am J Med Sci 272:19–29, 1976.

34. Willard MD. Treatment of hyperkalemia. In: Kirk RW (ed) Current Veterinary Therapy IX. WB Saunders, Philadelphia, 94–101, 1986.

35. O'Brien D. The CNS effects of sodium imbalances. Proc 10th ACVIM Forum, San Diego, 741–744, 1992.

36. Polzin DJ, Osborne CA. Anion gap—diagnostic and therapeutic applications. In: Kirk RW (ed) Current Veterinary Therapy IX. WB Saunders, Philadelphia, 52–59, 1986.

37. Arieff AI, Park R, Leach WJ, et al. Pathophysiology of experimental lactic acidosis in dogs. Am J Physiol 239:F135–F142, 1980.

38. Arieff AI, Leach W, Park R, et al. Systemic effect of sodium bicarbonate therapy in experimental lactic acidosis in dogs. Am J Physiol 242:F586–F591, 1982.

39. Hardy RM, Robinson EP. Treatment of alkalosis. In: Kirk RW (ed) Current Veterinary Therapy IX. WB Saunders, Philadelphia, 67–75, 1986.

40. Narins RG, Cohen JJ. Bicarbonate therapy for organic acidosis: The case for its continued use. Ann Int Med 106:615–618, 1987.

40 Experimental Models of Digestive System Diseases

DENNY J. MEYER

INTRODUCTION

The purpose of this chapter is to assist medical and veterinary researchers in identifying experimental models of digestive system diseases. In general, more recent citations are given so that modifications of the models can be appreciated. The original sources are referenced to enable researchers to trace the origin of the model where necessary.

LIVER

General

Strain A. Isolated hepatocytes: Use in experimental and clinical hepatology. Gut 35:433–436, 1994.
- the recent developments and their impact on experimental and clinical hepatology pertaining to the use of isolated hepatocytes, hepatocyte couplets, and liver slices are succinctly discussed. Areas covered include artificial hepatic support, hepatocyte transplantation, and use of hepatocytes for gene therapy.

Brown DE, Thrall MA, Walkley SU, et al. Feline Niemann-Pick disease type C. Am J Pathol 144:1412–1415, 1994.
- a colony of cats is described with a neurovisceral lysosomal storage disorder similar to human Niemann-Pick disease type C; cholesterol lipidosis develops as a consequence of defective intracellular transport of unesterified cholesterol.

Adachi Y, Kobayashi H, Shouji M, et al. Functional integrity of hepatocyte canalicular membrane transport of taurocholate and bilirubin diglucuronide in Eisai hyperbilirubinuria rats. Life Sci 52:777–784, 1993.
- in this model, like the TR- rat, the biliary excretion of conjugated bilirubin, the glutathione conjugate of sulfobromophthalein, reduced glutathione, cysteinyl leukotriene C_4, lithocholic acid sulfate, and taruolithocholic acid sulfate is moderately to severely impaired while taurocholate is excreted into bile normally.

Verkade HJ, Wolters H, Gerding A, et al. Mechanism of biliary lipid secretion in the rat: A role for bile acid-independent bile flow? Hepatology 17:1074–1080, 1993.
- Groningen Yellow Wistar rats express a genetic defect in the biliary secretion of various organic anions.
- bile acid-independent flow is reduced approximately 50% probably because of the absence of glutathione in bile.

Yang L, Faris RA, Hixson DC. Long-term culture and characteristics of normal rat liver bile duct epithelial cells. Gastroenterology 104:840–852, 1993.

Tarsetti F, Lenzi R, Salvi R, et al. Liver carcinogenesis associated with feeding of ethionine in a choline-free diet: Evidence against a role of oval cells in the emergence of hepatocellular carcinoma. Hepatology 18:596–603, 1993.
- the use of a choline-free diet without or with ethionine at two concentrations affected the occurrence of oval cell proliferation, hepatocellular nodule, and hepatocellular carcinoma development.

Hosokawa S, Tagaya O, Mikami T, et al. A new rat mutant with chronic conjugated hyperbilirubinemia and renal glomerular lesions. Lab Anim Sci 42:27–30, 1992.
- a new mutant strain of inbred Sprague Dawley rats with autosomal recessive hyperbilirubinuria.

Mori M, Hattori A, Sawaki M, et al. The LEC rat: A model for human hepatitis, liver cancer and much more. Am J Pathol 144:200–204, 1994.
- See commentary on this article pertaining to the use of this model for the study of the pathogenetic mechanisms (oxidant stress) associated with copper overload–associated tissue injury, in Sokol RJ. At long last: An animal model of Wilson's disease. Hepatology 20:533–535, 1994.

Okayash T, Tochimaru T, Hyuga T, et al. Inherited copper toxicity in Long-Evans Cinnamon rats exhibiting spontaneous hepatitis: A model of Wilson's disease. Pediatr Res 31:253–257, 1992.
- fulminant hepatitis that develops in this mutant strain is controlled by a single autosomal recessive gene.
- copper accumulates in the liver, decreased ceruloplasmin in the serum, and a high concentration of copper in the urine. See also Kasai N, Miyoshi I, Osanai T, et al. Effects of sex hormones on fulminant hepatitis in LEC rats: A model of Wilson's disease. Lab Anim Sci 42:363–368, 1992.

Enomoto K, Takahashi H, Mori M. A new rat model for the study of hepatocarcinogenesis. J Gastroenterol Hepatol 7:98–104, 1992.
- a mutant rat (LEC rat) spontaneously develops hepatitis and hepatocellular carcinoma at a high incidence.
- natural history of LEC rats is described and there is a discussion on the genesis of liver cancer.

Saville BA, Gray MR, Tam YK. Models of hepatic drug elimination. Drug Metab Rev 24:49–88, 1992.

Kamada N: Animal models of hepatic allograft rejection. Sem Liver Dis 12:1–15, 1992.

Gridelli B, Batti S, Piazzini A, et al. Xenogeneic orthotopic liver transplantation from sheep to pig. Transplant Proc 24:614–616, 1992.
- the focus of rejection at the hepatic vasculature following liver transplantation was studied in allotransplant studies (pigs used as donors and recipients) and xenotransplant studies (sheep as donors and pigs as recipients).

Reimer P, Weissleder R, Nickeleit V, et al. Animal models for magnetic resonance imaging research of the liver. Inv Radiol 27:390–393, 1992.

Terblance J, Hickman R. Animal models of fulminant hepatic failure. Dig Dis Sci 36:770–774, 1991.
- examines five requirements for a satisfactory animal model.

Ray DC, Drummond GB. Halothane hepatitis. Brit J Anaest 67:84–99, 1991.
- reviews animal models for halothane hepatitis.

Tsukamoto H, Matsuoka M, French SW. Experimental models of hepatic fibrosis: A review. Sem Liver Dis 10:56–65, 1990.

Miao S, Bao-En W, Annnoni G, et al. Two rat models of hepatic fibrosis: A morphologic and molecular comparison. Lab Invest 63:467–472, 1990.
- an antigen-antibody model and a carbon tetrachloride model are compared and contrasted.

Klir P, Pravenec M. Models in experimental medicine. In: Deyl Z, Zicha J (eds) Methods in Animal Physiology. CRC Press, Boca Raton, 3–10, 1989.
- general discussion pertaining to animal "modeling" and extrapolation of experimental data.

Baudysova M. Isolated organs and explanted tissue. In: Deyl Z, Zicha J (eds) Methods in Animal Physiology. CRC Press, Boca Raton, 42–73, 1989.

Mullen KD, McCullough AJ. Problems with animal models of chronic liver disease: Suggestions for improvement in standardization. Hepatology 9:500–503, 1989.

Better OS, Bomzon A. Effects of jaundice on the renal and cardiovascular systems. In: Epstein M (ed) The Kidney in Liver Disease. Williams & Wilkins, Baltimore, 508–534, 1988.
- review of animal studies with tables comparing findings in dog, rat, rabbit, baboon.

Cornelius CE. Animal models. In: Arias IM, Jakoby WB, Popper H (eds) The Liver: Biology and Pathobiology, 2nd ed. Raven Press, New York, 1315–1336, 1988.

Methods

Bail J, Foultier M, Patrice T. Experimental model of liver metastasis: Adhesion and growth of cells on contact with endothelial or hepatocyte cell monolayer cultures. Res Exp Med 194:53–61, 1994.
- a model is discussed using rat colon carcinoma in which two cell types are selected and administered intracecally; one produced hepatic metastasis and the other both hepatic and pulmonary. A method for the study of the adhesion and growth of the carcinoma cells upon contact with hepatocytes and/or endothelial cells is also described.

Young A, Hare G, Hay J. Blood-to-lymph migration of small lymphocytes through the liver of the sheep. Hepatology 19:758–763, 1994.
- an ovine model is described for the study of lymphocyte trafficking through the liver and hepatic lymph node. The methodology facilitates investigations into the unique role of the liver in lymphocyte homing and the systemic immune response especially in hepatic diseases in which mononuclear cells predominate.

Simonsen K, Horn T, Mortensen A, et al. Liver fibrosis in heterozygous WHHL rabbits fed cholesterol and fats; a new animal model. Int Hepatol Commun 3:310–315, 1995.
- hepatic histopathology similar to that seen in humans with alcoholic liver disease was induced by a cholesterol-enriched diet plus either vegetable oil or marine oil fed for 14 weeks. The notable findings included pericellular fibrosis in a "chicken wire" pattern, bridging fibrosis, steatosis, and Mallory-like bodies.

Goldin R. Rodent models of alcoholic liver disease. Int J Exp Pathol 75:1–7, 1994.
- a concise review of rodent models of alcoholic liver disease with a focus on studies that have enhanced our understanding of its pathogenesis; confounding risk factors are also discussed.

Pietrangelo A, Gualdi R, Casalgrandi G, et al. Enhanced hepatic collagen type I mRNA expression into fat-storing cells in a rodent model of hemochromatosis. Hepatology 19:714–721, 1994.
- hepatocellular iron overload similar to that in humans with primary iron overload was induced in rats by feeding a carbonyl iron-enriched diet. Immunocytochemistry combined with in situ hybridization was used to identify the fat-storing cell (Ito cell) as the major effector of enhanced collagen type I gene activation. Northern-blot analysis on RNA extracted from purified cell isolates was used to confirm the finding.

Alpini G, Phillips JO, Vroman B, et al. Recent advances in the isolation of liver cells. Hepatology 20:494–514, 1994.
- provides a concise overview of the separation techniques for the isolation of specific cell types from the liver.

Friman S, Egestad B, Sjovall J, et al. Hepatic excretion and metabolism of polyethylene glycols and mannitol in the cat. J Hepatol 17:48–55, 1993.
- cat model to study the biliary clearances of mannitol and PEG 900.

Ikeda H, Wu GY, Wu CH. Lipocytes from fibrotic rat liver

have an impaired feedback response to procollagen propeptides. Am J Physiol 264:G157–G162, 1993.
- describes isolation and culture of Ito cells and measurement of collagen production.

Vlahcevic ZR, Pandak WM, Hylemon PB, et al. Role of newly synthesized cholesterol or its metabolites on the regulation of bile acid biosynthesis after short-term biliary diversion in the rat. Hepatology 18:660–668, 1993.
- model to study the bile acid biosynthetic pathway.

Aggerbeck M, Garlati M, Feilleux-Duche S, et al. Regulation of the cytosolic aspartate aminotransferase housekeeping gene promoter by glucocorticoids, cAMP, and insulin. Biochemistry 32:9065–9072, 1993.
- rat hepatoma clone Fao, derived from the H411EC3 line of the Reuber H35 hepatoma used to examine subcellular regulation of cytosolic enzyme.

Marin JJG, Barbero ER, Herrera MC, et al. Bile acid-induced modifications in DNA synthesis by the regenerating perfused rat liver. Hepatology 18:1182–1192, 1993.
- discusses advantages of using a modification of the isolated in situ perfused rat liver preparation following two-thirds hepatectomy to study liver regeneration.

Sokol RJ, Devereaux M, Khandwala R, et al. Evidence for involvement of oxygen free radicals in bile acid toxicity to isolated rat hepatocytes. Hepatology 17:869–881, 1993.
- discusses advantages of using an isolated hepatocyte suspension system vs. cultured hepatocytes to study bile acid toxicity.

Rogiers V, Vercruysse A. Rat hepatocyte cultures and co-cultures in biotransformation studies of xenobiotics. Toxicology 82:193–208, 1993.
- discusses properties for maintaining long-term cultures as a suitable model.

Roberts RA, Soames AR. Hepatocyte spheroids: Prolonged-hepatocyte viability for in vitro modeling of nongenotoxic carcinogenesis. Fund Appl Toxicol 21:149–158, 1993.
- three-dimensional multicellular hepatocyte spheroids prolong cell viability and are used for studying peroxisome proliferator-induced hepatocellular carcinogenesis.

Accatino L, Hono J, Koenig C, et al. Adaptive changes of hepatic bile salt transport in a model of reversible interruption of the enterohepatic circulation in the rat. J Hepatol 19:95–104, 1993.
- a model of reversible enterohepatic circulation interruption was characterized in unrestrained, free-moving rats.

Chesne C, Guyomard C, Fautrel A, et al. Viability and function in primary culture of adult hepatocytes from various animal species and human beings after cryopreservation. Hepatology 18:406–414, 1993.
- hepatocytes from human, monkey, dog, rabbit, mouse, hamster, and rat were investigated.

Berry MN, Halls HJ, Grivell MB. Techniques for pharmacological and toxicological studies with isolated hepatocyte suspensions. Life Sci 51:1–16, 1992.

Peloux AF, Federici C, Bichet N, et al. Hepatocytes in primary culture: An alternative to LD50 testing? Validation of a predictive model by multivariant analysis. Alter to Lab Anim 20:8–20, 1992.

Adachi Y, Arii S, Sasaoki T, et al. Hepatic macrophage malfunction in rats with obstructive jaundice and its biological significance. J Hepatol 16:171–176, 1992.
- labeled endotoxin used to determine phagocytic index following bile duct ligation.

Porquet D, Appel, Fournier T, et al. Evaluation of the hepatotoxicological effects of a drug in an in vivo/in vitro model. Experientia 48:257–263, 1992.

Kawamori Y, Matsui O, Kadoya M, et al. Differentiation of hepatocellular carcinomas from hyperplastic nodules induced in rat liver with ferrite-enhanced MR imaging. Radiology 183:65–72, 1992.
- evaluates a noninvasive procedure for identifying and differentiating hyperplastic from neoplastic hepatic proliferative lesions; stainable iron demonstrated in hyperplastic nodules but not carcinomas.

Kurebayashi Y, Ikeda T, Honda Y. Protective effect of 16, 16-dimethyl prostaglandin E_2 on isolated rat hepatocytes against complement-mediated immune attack. Dig Dis Sci 37:645–649, 1992.
- in vitro model of complement-mediated liver cell membrane injury utilizing an antigen-antibody reaction between the plasma membrane of isolated rat hepatocytes and a monoclonal antibody to a rat liver-specific membranous antigen.

Winter HS, Fox CH, Hendren RB, et al. Use of an animal model for the study of the role of human immunodeficiency virus 1 in the human intestine. Gastroenterology 102:834–839, 1992.
- subcutaneous transplantation of human fetal bowel into nude mice; develops into adult-appearing tissue with a lumen after 8 weeks.

Schreiber RA, Kleinman RE, Barksdale EM, Jr, et al. Rejection of murine congenic bile ducts: A model for immune-mediated bile duct disease. Gastroenterology 102:924–930, 1992.
- segments of the common bile duct from fetal, postnatal, and adult mice were grafted under the renal capsule of adult congenic mice. The immunologic and histologic changes associated with rejection were similar to the histopathology of neonatal biliary atresia or primary sclerosing cholangitis.

Kay MA, Baley P, Rothenberg S, et al. Expression of human alpha-1-antitrypsin in dogs after autologous transplantation of retroviral transduced hepatocytes. Proc Natl Acad Sci USA 89:89–93, 1992.
- retrovirus delivered gene to hepatocytes in dogs with production of alpha-1-antitrypsin up to 1 month.

Rothuizen J, van den Brom WE, Fevery J. The origins and kinetics of bilirubin in healthy dogs, in comparison with man. J Hepatol 15:25–34, 1992.
- describes labeled bilirubin studies.
- important paper contrasting the difference in bilirubin kinetics between dog and human.

Stiglmair-Herb M, Scheid R, Hanichen T. Spontaneous inclusion body hepatitis in young tamarins. I. Morphological study. Lab Anim 26:80–87, 1992.

Dieter Nagel J, Kort WJ. A new liver-tumor model in the rat. Cancer Chemother Pharmacol 30:70–72, 1992.

- single liver tumors were induced in the liver of rats by the implantation of small pieces of a colon adenocarcinoma CC531 from the subcutaneous location of growth.

Harms G, Dijkhuis FWJ, Hardonk MJ, et al. Immunopathology of alkaline phosphatase-induced granulomatous hepatitis in rats. Virchows Archiv B Cell Pathol 62:35–43, 1992.

- intravenous administration of porcine intestinal alkaline phosphatase causes hepatitis with granulomas as early as 2 weeks after injection and persists for up to 30 weeks.

Heitmeyer SA, Powers JF. Improved method for bile collection in unrestrained conscious rats. Lab Anim Sci 42:312–315, 1992.

- technique establishes near physiologic conditions postsurgery to minimize potential artifacts during bile collection.

Saville BA, Gray MR, Tam YK. Models of hepatic drug elimination. Drug Metab Rev 24:49–88, 1992.

Robinson RJ: Hepatic modeling and risk assessment: Compartmental versus tube models and interspecies scaling. Drug Metab Rev 23:601–617, 1991.

Carp NZ, Saputelli J, Halbherr TC, et al. A technique for liver biopsy performed in Pekin ducks using anesthesia with Telazol. Lab Anim Sci 41:474–475, 1991.

- Pekin ducks (*Anas domesticus platyrhynkos*) are susceptible to duck hepatitis B virus, an analogue of the human hepatitis B virus. Chemical restraint that avoids intubation and a technique for obtaining liver biopsies is described to support studies in the Pekin duck.

Faidley TD, Galloway ST, Luhman CM, et al. A surgical model for studying biliary bile acid and cholesterol metabolism in swine. Lab Anim Sci 41:447–450, 1991.

- technique to simultaneously collect and reinfuse bile in Large White x Landrace pig 10 to 12 weeks of age.

Walpole HE, Lee WM, Walle T, et al. Rabbit hepatocytes in primary culture: Preparation, viability and use in studies of propranolol metabolism. Hepatology 11:394–400, 1990.

- indicates rat and hamster show significant differences in the cytochrome P-450 complex compared to humans.
- suggests rabbit hepatocyte metabolic pathways more closely resemble human cell metabolism in the study of drug interactions.

Piasecki C, Seifalian AM. Continuous intraoperative monitoring of hepatic blood perfusion using a noninvasive surface electrode. Dig Dis Sci 35:399–405, 1990.

- used rabbit; length of portal vein in dog acceptable.
- apparently sheep swine, mini-pig, and cat not acceptable.

Yamashita Y, Kimitsuki H, Hiraki M, et al. Direct observation of the portal vein interior by intra-operative angioscopy in the dog and man. J Gastroenterol Hepatol 5:234–238, 1990.

- Olympus BF3C10 (3.5 mm) inserted through portal venotomy in dog.

Shiomi S, Kuroki T, Ueda T, et al. Portal circulation in monkeys and humans studied after ingestion of a capsule containing a radionuclide. J Gastroenterol Hepatol 5:228, 1990.

- improved method for assessing portal circulation.

Kamada N. Historical background to experimental liver transplantation. In: Experimental Liver Transplantation. CRC Press, Boca Raton, 1–35, 1988.

- discusses development of techniques in animal models.

Stone BG, Udani M, Sanghvi A, et al. Cyclosporin A-induced cholestasis: The mechanism in a rat model. Gastroenterology 93:344–350, 1987.

Sato K, Ikeda T, Katami K, et al. Preparation of monoclonal antibody to hepatocellular membranes and its application to induction of liver cell membrane damage. Acta Pathol Jpn 35:1375–1383, 1985.

In Vivo

Sirica AE, Cole SL, Williams T. A unique rat model of bile ductular hyperplasia in which liver is almost totally replaced with well-differentiated bile ducts. Am J Pathol 144:1257–1268, 1994.

- a combination of bile duct ligation with short-term chronic furan treatment causes remarkable bile duct proliferation in the rat. Approximately 70% of the total liver section area was bile ductule tissue; the homogenates contained high gamma glutamyltransferase activity.

Merton Boothe D, Cullen JM, Calvin JA, et al. Antipyrine and caffeine dispositions in clinically normal dogs and dogs with progressive liver disease. Am J Vet Res 55:254–261, 1994.

- pathology of varying severity was induced with dimethylnitrosamine.
- relates hepatic function to pathologic changes.
- serum biochemical changes in this model in Boothe DM,

Brown SA, Jenkins WL, et al. Indocyanine green disposition in healthy dogs and dogs with mild, moderate, or severe dimethylnitrosamine-induced hepatic disease. Am J Vet Res 53:382–388, 1992; and Boothe DM, Jenkins WL, Green RA, et al. Dimethylnitrosamine-induced hepatotoxicosis in dogs as a model of progressive canine hepatic disease. Am J Vet Res 53:411–420, 1992.

Schoeniger LO, Andreoni KA, Ott GR, et al. Induction of heat-shock gene expression in postischemic pig liver depends on superoxide generation. Gastroenterology 106:177–184, 1994.

- total liver ischemia model that used an active portal systemic venous bypass system to obviate gut injury from venous congestion and subsequent liver injury due to systemic factors.

Bhunchet E, Fujieda K. Capillarization and venularization of hepatic sinusoids in porcine serum-induced rat liver fibrosis: A mechanism to maintain liver blood flow. Hepatology 18:1450–1458, 1993.

- intraperitoneal administration or porcine serum over 10 weeks.

Pacot C, Petit M, Caira F, et al. Response of genetically obese Zucker rats to ciprofibrate, a hypolipidemic agent, with peroxisome proliferation activity as compared to Zucker lean and Sprague-Dawley rats. Bio Cell 77:27–35, 1993.

- genetically obese old Zucker rats have a lipoprotein metabolism closer to that of humans than Sprague-Dawley rats. The drug effects on liver morphology and parameters reflecting hepatic peroxisome proliferation and cytochrome P4504A1 induction are described and compared in these three strains of rats.

Bacon BR, O'Neill R, Britton RS. Hepatic mitochondrial energy production in rats with chronic iron overload. Gastroenterology 105:1134–1140, 1993.
- increased hepatic iron induced by feeding carbonyl iron.

Carthew, Dorman BM, Edwards RE, et al. A unique model for both the cardiotoxic and hepatotoxic effects of prolonged iron overload. Lab Invest 69:217–220, 1993.
- iron dextran administered subcutaneously to gerbils weekly for 7 weeks produced severe hepatic iron overload.

Schwartz KA, Fisher J, Adams ET. Morphologic investigations of the guinea pig model of iron overload. Tox Pathol 21:311–320, 1993.
- intraperitoneal administration of iron dextran used to increase iron in hepatic and cardiac muscle tissues.

Bjorkhem I, Andersson U, Sudjama-Sugiaman E, et al. Studies on the link between HMG-CoA reductase and cholesterol 7 alpha-hydroxylase in lymph-fistula rats: Evidence for both transcriptional and post-transcriptional mechanisms for down-regulation of the two enzymes by bile acids. J Lipid Res 34:1497–1503, 1993.
- in this model there is no transport of absorbed cholesterol to the liver; thus, the stimulatory effect of bile acids on cholesterol absorption is minimized and permits evaluation of feedback mechanisms.

Myers BM, Prendergast FG, Holman R, et al. Alterations in hepatocyte lysosomes in experimental hepatic copper overload in rats. Gastroenterology 105:1814–1823, 1993.
- to study the subcellular effects of increased hepatic copper, increased tissue concentrations were achieved by adding copper acetate to the drinking water for 6 weeks.

Xu G, Salen G, Shefer S, et al. Different feedback regulation of hepatic cholesterol and bile acid synthesis by glycodeoxycholic acid in rabbits. Gastroenterology 105:1192–1199, 1993.
- a bile fistula rabbit model with a depleted bile acid pool and up-regulated bile acid synthesis is used to study the feedback regulation of bile acid formation.

Cullen JM, Sandgren EP, Brinster RL, et al. Histologic characterization of hepatic carcinogenesis in transgenic mice expressing SV40 T-antigens. Vet Pathol 30:111–118, 1993.
- use of transgenic mice to study the carcinogenic effects of selected oncogenic genes in the whole animal and in differentiated tissues.

Suou T, Yamada S, Kobasyashi J, et al. Changes of serum 7S fragment of type IV collagen and N-terminal propeptide of type III procollagen after transcatheter arterial embolization as a model of acute liver injury. Hepatology 18:809–815, 1993.
- humans with hepatocellular carcinoma were studied following therapeutic transcatheter arterial embolization.

Gonzalez-Flecha B, Reides C, Cutrin JC, et al. Oxidative stress produced by suprahepatic occlusion and reperfusion. Hepatology 18:881–889, 1993.
- oxidative stress and cell injury produced in rat liver by occlusion and release of the suprahepatic inferior vena cava.
- spontaneous liver chemiluminescence, hydrogen peroxide, mitochondrial respiratory control, and antioxidant enzymes measured.

Ohara N, Boelkel NF, Chang S. Tissue eicosanoids and vascular permeability in rats with chronic biliary obstruction. Hepatology 18:111–118, 1993.
- "cirrhosis" induced by ligation of the bile duct.
- methods given for measurement of vascular permeability and tissue eicosanoids.

Wahler JB, Swain MG, Carson R, et al. Blood-brain barrier permeability is markedly decreased in cholestasis in the rat. Hepatology 17:1103–1108, 1993.
- two models used: bile duct ligation and alpha-naphthylisothiocyanate (ANIT).
- method for assessing blood-brain barrier described.

Arai M, Mochida S, Ohno A, et al. Sinusoidal endothelial cell damage by activated macrophages in rat liver necrosis. Gastroenterology 104:1466–1471, 1993.
- uses model from Yamada S, Ogata I, Hirata K, et al. Intravascular coagulation in the development of massive hepatic necrosis induced by *Corynebacterium parvum* and endotoxin in rats. Scand J Gastroenterol 24:293–298, 1989.
- *C. parvum* activation of macrophages followed by the administration of endotoxin results in massive hepatic necrosis.
- this study used isolated hepatic nonparenchymal cells and liver perfusion to investigate pathogenesis.

Peterson TC. Pentoxifylline prevents fibrosis in an animal model and inhibits plate-derived growth factor-driven proliferation of fibroblasts. Hepatology 17:486–493, 1993.
- extensive fibrosis in Duroc-Hampshire pigs using long-term, low-dose yellow phosphorus administration.

Gaudio E, Pannarale L, Onori P, et al. A scanning electron microscopic study of liver microcirculation disarrangement in experimental rat cirrhosis. Hepatology 17:477–485, 1993.
- chronic intragastric administration of carbon tetrachloride results in biochemical and structural features of micronodular cirrhosis.

Aller MA, Lorente L, Alonso S, et al. A model of cholestasis in the rat, using a microsurgical technique. Scand J Gastroenterol 28:10–14, 1993.
- ligation of the biliary ducts that drain each of the four lobes in proximity to the "common" bile duct.
- fewer postoperative complications reported.

Scheibner J, Fuchs M, Schiemann M, et al. Bile acid synthesis from newly synthesized vs. preformed cholesterol precursor pools in the rat. Hepatology 17:1095–1102, 1993.
- recovered rat model to study bile acid formation from cholesterol after interruption of the enterohepatic circulation.

Wang XD, Ar'Rajab A, Andersson R, et al. The influence of surgically induced acute liver failure on the intestine in the rat. Scan J Gastroenterol 28:31–40, 1993.
- 90% hepatectomy results in altered intestinal structure and function and bacterial translocation.

Kim JK, Summer SN, Howard RL, et al. Vasopressin gene expression in rats with experimental cirrhosis. Hepatology 17:143–147, 1993.

- cirrhosis induced by a combination of phenobarbital and intragastric administration of carbon tetrachloride.

Jacquemin E, Dumont M, Mallet A, et al. Ursodeoxycholic acid improves ethinyl estradiol-induced cholestasis in the rat. Eur J Clin Invest 23:794–802, 1993.
- bile flow, bile output, and composition of bile evaluated in this model.

Halsted CH, Villanueva J, Chandler CJ, et al. Centrilobular distribution of acetaldehyde and collagen in the ethanol-fed micropig. Hepatology 18:954–960, 1993.
- model of alcoholic liver disease in the Yucatan micropig that voluntarily consumes alcohol in its diet.

Sullivan MP, Cerda JJ, Robbins FL, et al. The gerbil, hamster, and guinea pig as rodent models for hyperlipidemia. Lab Anim Sci 43:575–578, 1993.
- the effects of hyperlipidemic diets evaluated.
- guinea pig suggested as the most appropriate model for studying hypercholesterolemia and the hamster as a model for studying hypertriglyceridemia.

Tsutsui H, Mizoguchi Y, Morisawa S. Importance of direct hepatocytolosis by liver macrophages in experimental fulminant hepatitis. Hepatogastroenterology 39:553–559, 1992.
- massive liver necrosis develops in mice injected with heat-killed *Propionibacterium acnes* followed by the administration of lipopolysaccharide.

Cornelius CE, Freedland RA. Fasting hyperbilirubinemia in normal squirrel monkeys. Lab Anim Sci 42:35–37, 1992.
- Bolivian squirrel monkey manifests a bilirubin paradigm for human Gilbert's syndrome type I; unconjugated hyperbilirubinemia after an overnight fast.

Gonzalez J, Fevery J. Spontaneously diabetic biobreeding rats and impairment of bile acid-independent bile flow and increased biliary bilirubin, calcium and lipid secretion. Hepatology 16:426–432, 1992.
- model of bile acid–independent cholestasis with enhanced biliary bile acid and calcium secretion and with presumably an enhanced bilirubin production.

Kabemura T, Misawa, T, Chijiiwa Y, et al. Substance P, vasoactive intestinal polypeptide, and gastrin catabolism in canine liver and kidney. Dig Dis Sci 37:1661–1665, 1992.
- model to study metabolism of gastrointestinal hormones.

Kanai M, Tanaka M, Nimura Y, et al. Mitochondrial dysfunction in the non-obstructed lobe of rat liver after selective biliary obstruction. Hepatogastroenterology 39:385–2391, 1992.
- 70% or 90% of the biliary drainage was stopped and biochemical parameters in the nonobstructed lobe studied.

Roth L, Harbison RD, James RC, et al. Cocaine hepatotoxicity: Influence of hepatic enzyme inducing and inhibiting agents on the site of necrosis. Hepatology 15:934–940, 1992.
- multiple references including discussion on variable zonation of hepatic necrosis.

Jonker AM, Dijkhuis WJ, Boes A, et al. Immunohistochemical study of extracellular matrix in acute galactosamine hepatitis in rats. Hepatology 15:423–431, 1992.
- a single intraperitoneal injection of D-galactosamine hydrochloride induces acute transient liver disease that

morphologically resembles drug-induced hepatitis in humans.

Nishimura T, Nakahara M, Kobayashi S, et al. Ischemic injury in cirrhotic livers: An experimental study of the temporary arrest of hepatic circulation. J Surg Res 53:227–233, 1992.
- intraperitoneal administration of thioacetamide used to induce macronodular cirrhosis.
- biochemical changes studied subsequent to an ischemic insult.

Nagai T, Yamakawa T. Experimental model with bilioenteric anastomosis in rats—technique and significance. Hepatogastroenterology 39:309–313, 1992.
- procedure evaluated for the study of morphologic changes of the biliary system.

Benoit JN, Grisham MB, Mesh CL. et al: Hepatic oxidant and antioxidant systems in portacaval-shunted rats. J Hepatol 14:253–258, 1992.
- describes a model and methodology to evaluate hepatic oxidant stress in disorders that are associated with decreased portal blood flow.

Sokal EM, Mostin J, Buts JP. Liver metabolic zonation in rat biliary cirrhosis: Distribution is reverse of that in toxic cirrhosis. Hepatology 15:904–908, 1992.
- common bile duct ligated in growing rats (40 days of age).

Kelly JH, Koussayer T, He D, et al. An improved model of acetaminophen-induced fulminant hepatic failure in dogs. Hepatology 15:329–335, 1992.
- hypoglycemia by 15 hours and encephalopathy by 48 hours.

Melzer E, Krepel Z, Ronen I, et al. Recovery of hepatic clearance and extraction following a release of common bile duct obstruction in the rat. Res Exp Med 192:35–40, 1992.
- ligation of cannulated common bile duct followed by reopening and implantation into the duodenum.

Zimmermann T, Gardemann A, Machnik G, et al. Metabolic and hemodynamic responses of bivascularly perfused rat liver to nerve stimulation, noradrenaline, acetylcholine and glucagon in thioacetamide-induced micronodular cirrhosis. Hepatology 15:464–470, 1992.
- model used arterially and portally perfused livers after cirrhosis developed.

Bioulac-Sage P, Dubuisson L, Bedin C, et al. Nodular regenerative hyperplasia in the rat induced by a selenium-enriched diet: Study of a model. Hepatology 16:418–425, 1992.

Ishiki Y, Ohnishi H, Muto Y, et al. Direct evidence that hepatocyte growth factor is a hepatotrophic factor for liver regeneration and has a potent antihepatitis effect in vivo. Hepatology 16:1227–1235, 1992.
- describes protocol for assessing effect of hepatocyte growth factor (HGF) on regeneration.

Cywes R, Greig PD, Morgan GR, et al. Rapid donor liver nutritional enhancement in a large animal model. Hepatology 16:1271–1279, 1992.
- describes rapid technique to replete hepatic glycogen stores in Yorkshire pig model.

Francavilla A, Starzl TE, Porter K, et al. Screening for candidate hepatic growth factors by selective portal infusion after canine Eck's fistula. Hepatology 14:665–670, 1991.

- underscores importance of using in vivo model for evaluating potential hepatic growth factors.

Kuhlenschmidt MS, Hoffmann WE, Rippy MK. Glucocorticoid hepatopathy: Effect on receptor-mediated endocytosis of asialoglycoproteins. Biochem Med Metabol Biol 46:152–168, 1991.

- glycogen-induced hepatomegaly associated with glucocorticoid administration.
- use of subcutaneous Alzet osmotic pumps plus catheter to jugular vein for constant intravenous infusion of compound for 30 days.

Andersson R, Poulsen HE, Ahren B. Effect of bile on liver function tests in experimental *E. coli* peritonitis in the rat. Hepatogastroenterology 38:388–390, 1991.

- two different experimental peritonitis models in the rat are described.

Koo A, Komatsu H, Tao G, et al. Contribution of no-reflow phenomenon to hepatic injury after ischemia-reperfusion: Evidence for a role for superoxide anion. Hepatology 15:507–514, 1991.

- describes hepatic reperfusion injury model.
- in vivo liver microcirculation assessed.

Ikeda T, Kurebayashi Y. A rat model of acute liver necrosis induced by a monoclonal antibody to liver-specific antigen and complement. Hepatology 13:1152–1157, 1991.

- acute massive hepatic injury induced by a monoclonal antibody against a rat liver-specific membrane antigen.
- marked deposition of the third component of complement was demonstrated in the necrotic area suggesting complement-mediated immune attachment on the liver cell membrane induced by the antigen-antibody reaction.

Paronetto F, Tennant BC. Woodchuck hepatitis virus infection: A model of human hepatic diseases and hepatocellular carcinoma. In: Popper H, Schaffner F (eds) Progress in Liver Diseases. W.B. Saunders, Philadelphia, 463–483, 1990.

- discusses infection of the woodchuck (*Marmota monax*) with woodchuck hepatitis virus with characteristics strikingly similar to those of human hepatitis B virus.

Azorin I, Minana MD, Felipo V, et al. A simple animal model of hyperammonemia. Hepatology 10:311–314, 1989.

- rats fed a diet supplemented with ammonium acetate.

Lopez-Novoa JM. Pathophysiological features of the carbon tetrachloride/phenobarbital model of experimental liver cirrhosis in rats. In: Epstein M (ed) The Kidney in Liver Disease. Williams & Wilkins, Baltimore, 309–327, 1988.

- discusses the main features of this model of cirrhosis including renal function, ascites formation, hemodynamic studies, fluid compartment redistribution, and hormonal studies (including the renin-angiotensin-aldosterone system, prostaglandins, atrial natriuretic peptide).

Mori T, Mori Y, Yoshida H, et al. Cell-mediated cytotoxicity of sensitized spleen cells against target liver cells—in vivo study with a mouse model of experimental autoimmune hepatitis. Hepatology 5:770–777, 1985.

- liver specific protein (LSP), used to induce a model of chronic hepatitis, is inhibited by EDTA, often included in the preparation, and may have affected results of earlier studies.

Mori Y, Mori T, Ueda S, et al. Study of cellular immunity in experimental autoimmune hepatitis in mice: transfer of spleen cells sensitized with liver proteins. Clin Exp Immunol 61:577–584, 1985.

Kountouras J, Billing BH, Scheuer PJ. Prolonged bile duct obstruction: A new experimental model for cirrhosis in the rat. Br J Exp Path 65:305–311, 1984.

- characterizes morphologic changes over multiple time points.

In Vitro

Strazzabosco M, Poci C, Spirli C, et al. Effect of ursodeoxycholic acid on intracellular pH in a bile duct epithelium-like cell line. Hepatology 19:145–154, 1994.

- SK-ChA-1 is a well-differentiated human cholangiocarcinoma cell line similar to bile duct epithelium in terms of intracellular pH regulatory mechanisms and morphologic markers.

Joplin R. Isolation and culture of biliary epithelial cells. Gut 35:875–878, 1994.

- intrahepatic biliary epithelial cells are a small (approximately 5%) component of the total cells in the liver making their isolation difficult. This paper discusses the conditions necessary for culture and study of biliary epithelial cells and defines their applicability for investigational studies.

Lamb RG, Koch JC, Snyder JW, et al. An in vitro model of ethanol-dependent liver cell injury. Hepatology 19:174–182, 1994.

Endoh K, Ueno K, Miyashita A, et al. An experimental model of acute liver injury using multicellular spheroids composed of rat parenchymal and non-parenchymal liver cells. Res Commun Chem Pathol Pharmacol 82:317–329, 1993.

- one model using a monolayer culture system and another using a spheroid culture system are described and evaluated as a possible alternative to an in vivo system.

Miller MG, Beyer J, Hall GL, et al. Predictive value of liver slices for metabolism and toxicity in vivo: Use of acetaminophen as a model hepatotoxicant. Toxicol Appl Pharmacol 122:108–116, 1993.

Edwards CM, Otal MP, Stacpoole PW. Lipoprotein-X fails to inhibit hydroxymethylglutaryl coenzyme A reductase in HepG2 cells. Metabolism 42:807–813, 1993.

- system used to evaluate effects of cholestasis on cholesterol metabolism.

Rieder H, Armbrust T, Meyer zum Buschenfelde K, et al. Contribution of sinusoidal endothelial liver cells to liver fibrosis: Expression of transforming growth factor-beta 1 receptors and modulation of plasmin-generating enzymes by transforming growth factor-beta 1. Hepatology 18:937–944, 1993.

- describes technique for separating sinusoidal endothelial cells from guinea pig liver.

Kato A, Gores GJ, LaRusso NF. Secretin stimulates exocytosis in isolated bile duct epithelial cells by a cyclic AMP-mediated mechanism. J Biol Chem 267:15523–15529, 1992.

- rat cholangiocytes isolated using enzymatic digestion and mechanical disruption followed by immunomagnetic separation using specific monoclonal antibodies.
- physiologic parameters evaluated.

PANCREAS

Measurement of Physiologic and Morphologic Parameters Without Experimentally Induced Pancreatitis

Toriumi Y, Samuel I, Wilcockson DP, et al. A new model for study of pancreatic exocrine secretion: The tethered pancreatic fistula rat. Lab Anim Sci 44:270–273, 1994.

- diversion and recirculation of bile and pancreatic juice to support studies of exocrine pancreatic secretion was accomplished in a partial restraint tethering system that accommodated four fistula catheters exiting at the nape of the neck yet allowing the animals the freedom to move, groom, and feed.

Conter RL, Washington JL, Kauffman GL, Jr. Stimulated pancreatic exocrine secretion does not require pancreatic hyperemia in rats: Potential cholinergic role. Dig Dis Sci 38:1270–1277, 1993.

- describes techniques and methods for the measurement of various parameters.

Nustede R, Schmidt WE, Kohler H, et al. The influence of bile acids on the regulation of exocrine pancreatic secretion and on the plasma concentrations of neurotensin and CCK in dogs. Int J Pancreatol 13:23–30, 1993.

- uses modified Herrera fistula in dog for the analysis of pancreatic secretions.

Larvin M, Alexander DJ, Switala SF, et al. Impaired mononuclear phagocytic function in patients with severe acute pancreatitis: Evidence from studies of plasma clearance of trypsin and monocyte phagocytosis. Dig Dis Sci 38:18–27, 1993.

- methods for the measurement of labeled trypsinclearance and monocyte phagocytosis.

Ainsworth MA, Svendsen P, Ladegaard L, et al. Relative importance of pancreatic, hepatic, and mucosal bicarbonate in duodenal neutralization of acid in anesthetized pigs. Scand J Gastroenterol 27:343–349, 1992.

- physiologic measurements in Danish Landrace pigs; digestive tract comparable to human.

Frick TW, Spycher MA, Heitz PU, et al. Ultrastructure of the guinea pig pancreas in acute hypercalcemia. Pancreas 7:287–294, 1992.

- techniques and methods for the study of pancreatic tissue ultrastructurally.

Manso MA, Gallego HA, DeDios I. Effect of acute and chronic administration of ethanol on the pancreatic exocrine response to cholecystokinin in rats fed different diets. Clin Sci 82:4343–438, 1992.

- a diet high in protein and fat content used.

Scholmerich J, Schumichen C, Lausen M, et al. Scintigraphic assessment of leukocyte infiltration in acute pancreatitis

using technetium-99m-hexamethyl propylene amine oxine as leukocyte label. Dig Dis Sci 36:65–70, 1991.

- technique used in humans.
- correlation identified between severity and leukocyte infiltration.

Layer P, Hotz J, Schmitz-Moormann HP, et al. Effects of experimental chronic hypercalcemia on feline exocrine pancreatic secretion. Gastroenterology 82:309–316, 1982.

- hypercalcemia induced by oral administration of calcium.
- variety of physiologic parameters measured.

Isaksson G, Lundquist I, Ihse I. Effects on the exocrine and endocrine pancreas of duct occlusion with two different tissue glues in the rat. Eur Surg Res 15:136–144, 1983.

- acrylate or prolamine were used to occlude the pancreatic ducts.

Sakakibara A, Okumura N, Hayakawa T, et al. Ultrastructural changes in the exocrine pancreas of experimental pancreatolithiasis in dogs. Am J Gastroenterol 77:498–506, 1982.

- major pancreatic duct partially ligated.
- severe interlobular fibrosis after 12 months.
- ultrastructure studies of the pancreas.

Pancreatitis

General

Lerch MM, Adler G. Experimental animal models of acute pancreatitis. Int J Pancreatol 15:159–170, 1994.

- reviews the models of this disease.

Frick TW, Wiegand D, Bimmler D, et al. A rat model to study hypercalcemia-induced acute pancreatitis. Int J Pancreatol 15:91–96, 1994.

- describes a model in the rat to study the effect of hypercalcemia on pancreatic acinar cell function with respect to the pathogenesis of hypercalcemia-induced acute pancreatitis.

Friess H, Weber A, Buchler M. Standards in monitoring acute experimental pancreatitis. Eur Surg Res 24 (suppl 1):1–13, 1992.

- provides overview for the different models.
- describes standard parameters for monitoring.

Nevalainen TJ, Heikki JA. Standards of morphological evaluation and histological grading in experimental acute pancreatitis. Eur Surg Res 24 (suppl 1):14–23, 1992.

- suggests criteria for grading severity of disease by assessing morphologic changes or histometric measurements.
- lists methods of inducing experimental pancreatitis.

Schoenberg MH, Buchler M, Helfen M, et al. Role of oxygen radicals in experimental acute pancreatitis. Eur Surg Res 24 (suppl 1):74–84, 1992.

- lists animal studies of scavenger treatment in acute pancreatitis.

Grendell JH. Experimental pancreatitis. Curr Opin Gastroenterol 7:702–708, 1991.

- evaluates various models of pancreatitis and factors that may be involved.

Braganza JM. Experimental pancreatitis. Curr Opin Gastroenterol 6:763–768, 1990.
- evaluates various models of pancreatitis and factors that may be involved.

Goke B. A critical appraisal of studies of the pancreas. Int J Pancreatol 6:181–188, 1990.

Steer ML. Workshop on experimental pancreatitis. Dig Dis Sci 30:575–581, 1985.
- panel of experts evaluates models.

In Vivo

Karanjia N, Widdison A, Lutrin F, et al. Dopamine in models of alcoholic acute pancreatitis. Gut 35:547–551, 1994.
- acute pancreatitis, edematous or hemorrhagic, was induced in cats using low pressure duct perfusion with 40% ethanol. Serum lipase activity and urinary trypsinogen activation peptide was measured and the histopathology was evaluated with and without dopamine treatment. The untreated model caused suppurative pancreatitis with an increase in the serum lipase activity and urinary trypsinogen-activating peptide concentration.

Onizuka S, Ito Masahiro, Sekine I, et al. Spontaneous pancreatitis in spontaneously hypertensive rats. Pancreas 9:54–61, 1994.

Foitzik T, Bassi DG, Schmidt J, et al. Intravenous contrast medium accentuates the severity of acute necrotizing pancreatitis in the rat. Gastroenterology 106:207–214, 1994.
- pancreatitis of varying severity induced by intravenous infusion of cerulein with or without retrograde infusion of glycodeoxycholic acid.

Karanjia ND, Widdison AL, Jehanli A, et al. Assay of trypsinogen activation in the cat experimental model of acute pancreatitis. Pancreas 8:189–195, 1993.
- models of acute edematous pancreatitis and hemorrhagic pancreatitis in the cat.

Lerch MM, Saluja AK, Runzi M, et al. Pancreatic duct obstruction triggers acute necrotizing pancreatitis in the opossum. Gastroenterology 104:853–861, 1993.
- the opossum has a long extrahepatic common bile duct that is joined by the pancreatic duct before it joins the duodenum.
- ligation of the biliopancreatic duct results in hemorrhagic pancreatitis.

Tangoku A, Doi R, Chowdhury P, et al. Humoral factors that induce alterations of the pancreas in rats with obstructive jaundice. Pancreas 8:103–108, 1993.
- measurement of DNA and RNA content, enzyme activity, and morphologic examination of the pancreas following ligation of the bile duct.

Arendt T. Bile-induced acute pancreatitis in cats: Roles of bile, bacteria, and pancreatic duct pressure. Dig Dis Sci 38:39–44, 1993.
- retrograde infusion of bile with or without bacteria into the pancreas.

Closa D, Rosello-Catafau J, Martratt A, et al. Changes of systemic prostacyclin and thromboxane A2 in sodium taurocholate- and cerulein-induced acute pancreatitis in rats. Dig Dis Sci 38:33–38, 1993.
- intravenous cerulein used for one model and retrograde infusion of sodium taurocholate into the pancreas for another.
- plasma activities for amylase and lipase; prestudy and during pancreatitis.

Dabrowski A, Gabryelewicz A. Oxidative stress: An early phenomenon characteristic of acute experimental pancreatitis. Int J Pancreatol 12:193–199, 1992.
- retrograde infusion of taurocholate used to induce hemorrhagic pancreatitis.
- markers of oxidative stress (malondialdehyde and sulfhydryl groups concentration, superoxide dismutase, and catalase activity) were measured in pancreatic, hepatic, and lung tissues. These markers were also determined (except catalase) in the serum and peritoneal exudate.

Shen J, Huang MK, Wu FL, et al. Effect of naloxone on the hemodynamics and the outcome of experimental acute pancreatitis in dogs. J Gastroenterol Hepatol 7:502–507, 1992.
- hemodynamics measurement.
- pancreatic blood flow measurement.
- pancreatitis model using bile and trypsin

Musa BB, Nelson AW, Gillette EL, et al. A model to study acute pancreatitis in the dog. J Surg Res 21:51–56, 1979.

Kukaszyk A, Bodzenta-Kukaszyk A, Gabryelewicz A, et al. Blood platelet function in canine acute pancreatitis with reference to treatment with nafamostat mesilate (FUT-175). Thromb Res 65:229–239, 1992.
- modification of model using incubated trypsin and bile infusion retrograde into the pancreatic duct.
- method for measuring platelet function.

Lerch MM, Saluja K, Dawra R, et al. Acute necrotizing pancreatitis in the opossum: Earliest morphological changes involve acinar cells. Gastroenterology 103:205–213, 1992.
- measurements of tissue enzyme activity and protein and DNA concentrations.
- preparation for electron microscopy.

Runkel NSF, Smith GS, Rodriguez LF, et al. Influence of shock on development of infection during acute pancreatitis in the rat. Dig Dis Sci 37:1418–1425, 1992.
- induced by ligation of biliopancreatic duct.
- method to study bacterial translocation to the pancreas.
- schematic illustrating anatomy of rat biliopancreatic duct for ligation.

Willemer S, Elsasser HP, Adler G. Hormone-induced pancreatitis. Eur Surg Res 24 (suppl 1):29–39, 1992.
- rat model useful for studying intracellular events in the early phase.

Niederau C, Luthen R, Niederau MC, et al. Acute experimental hemorrhagic-necrotizing pancreatitis induced by feeding a choline-deficient, ethionine-supplemented diet. Eur Surg Res 24 (suppl 1):40–54, 1992.
- rat model useful for studying novel therapies.

Schmidt J, Lewandrowski K, Fernandez-del Castillo C, et al. Histologic correlates of serum amylase activity in acute experimental pancreatitis. Dig Dis Sci 37:1426–1433, 1992.
- pancreatitis induced by retrograde infusion of bile salt with or without enterokinase followed by intravenous cerulein.

Elsasser HP, Haake T, Grimmig M, et al. Repetitive cerulein-induced pancreatitis and pancreatic fibrosis in the rat. Pancreas 7:385–390, 1992.
- attempt to induce pancreatic fibrosis failed.
- references on the formation of collagen in the pancreas.

Rueda JC, Ortega L, Arguello JM. Acute experimental pancreatitis in rat induced by sodium taurocholic acid: Objective quantification of pancreatic necrosis. Virch Archiv A Pathol Anat 420:117–120, 1992.
- describes morphometric technique.

Yazu T, Kimura T, Sumii T, et al. Alteration of cholecystokinin receptor binding after cerulein-induced pancreatitis in the rat. Digestion 50:142–148, 1991.
- cerulein is administered by the intraperitoneal route.

Tani S, Itoh H, Okabayashi Y, et al. New model of acute necrotizing pancreatitis induced by excessive dose of arginine in rats. Dig Dis Sci 35:367–374, 1990.
- L-arginine administered using the intraperitoneal route.

Frick TW, Hailemariam S, Heitz PU, et al. Acute hypercalcemia induces acinar cell necrosis and intraductal protein precipitates in the pancreas of cats and guinea pigs. Gastroenterology 98:1675–1681, 1990.
- calcium infusion using the splenic artery caused hemorrhagic pancreatitis in the cat.

Ebbehoj N, Borley L, Heyeraas KJ, et al. Effect of portal hypertension and duct ligation on pancreatic fluid pressures in cats. Scand J Gastroenterol 25:609–612, 1990.
- describes micropuncture technique for the study of interstitial fluid pressure in the pancreas.

Andrzejewskka A, Dlugosz J, Kurasz S. The ultrastructure of the liver in acute experimental pancreatitis in dogs. Exp Path 28:167–176, 1985.
- induced by retrograde infusion of an incubated mixture of bile and trypsin into the pancreatic duct.
- describes morphologic and ultrastructural changes in the hepatocyte.

Attix E, Strombeck DR, Wheeldon EB, et al. Effects of an anticholinergic and a corticosteroid on acute pancreatitis in experimental dogs. Am J Vet Res 42:1668–1674, 1981.
- uses retrograde infusion of oleic acid into the pancreas of dogs.

Chronic Pancreatitis

Tanaka T, Ichiba Y, Miura Y, et al. Canine model of chronic pancreatitis due to chronic ischemia. Digestion 55:86–89, 1994.
- intralobular fibrosis with inflammation and loss of parenchymal cells in the pancreas was produced by the ligation and separation of branches of splenic artery that supply the left pancreatic lobe of the dog.

Reber HA, Karanjia ND, Alvarez C, et al. Pancreatic blood flow in cats with chronic pancreatitis. Gastroenterology 103:652–659, 1992.
- used a model of partial duct ligation from Austin JL, Roberts C, Rosenholtz, MJ, et al. Effect of partial duct obstruction and drainage on pancreatic function. J Surg Res 28:426–433, 1980.
- illustrates measurement of pancreatic blood flow.

Strombeck DR, Wheeldon E, Harrold D. Model of chronic pancreatitis in the dog. Am J Vet Res 45:131–136, 1984.
- oleic acid was infused using the accessory pancreatic duct.

Lombardi B. Influence of dietary factors on the pancreatotoxicity of ethionine. Am J Pathol 84:633–648, 1976.
- acute hemorrhagic pancreatitis with fat necrosis develops in mice fed DL-ethionine with a choline-deficient diet.

Pancreatic Atrophy

Meyer JH, Elashoff JD, Dory JE, et al. Disproportionate ileal digestion on canine food consumption: A possible model for satiety in pancreatic insufficiency. Dig Dis Sci 39:1014–1024, 1994.
- dogs were prepared with pancreatic fistulas that allowed reversible switching of pancreatic juice from entry at duodenum to entry at mid-small intestine. Diversion of pancreatic juice to mid-intestine depressed food intake and reduced body weight, suggesting that stimulation of ileal satiety mechanisms may contribute to malnourishment.

Henry JP, Steinberg WH. Pancreatic function tests in the rat model of chronic pancreatic insufficiency. Pancreas 8:622–626, 1993.
- oleic acid infused into the pancreaticobiliary duct.
- variety of function tests evaluated.

Delaney CP, McGeeney KF, Dervan P, et al. Pancreatic atrophy: A new model using serial intra-peritoneal injections of L-arginine. Scand J Gastroenterol 28:1086–1090, 1993.
- rat model.
- four injections over 10 days; 90% acinar destruction by day 5; changes present at 6 months.

Nylander AG, Chen D, Ihse I, et al. Pancreatic atrophy in rats produced by the cholecystokinin-A receptor antagonist devazepide. Scand J Gastroenterol 27:743–747, 1992.

Little JM, Lauer C, Hogg J. Pancreatic duct obstruction with an acrylate glue: A new method for producing pancreatic exocrine atrophy. Surgery 81:243–249, 1977.

In Vitro

Githens S, Patke CL, Schexnayder JA. Isolation and culture of Rhesus monkey pancreatic ductules and ductule-like epithelium. Pancreas 9:20–31, 1994.

Matshushita K, Okabayashi Y, Koide M, et al. Potentiating effect of insulin on exocrine secretory function in isolated rat pancreatic acini. Gastroenterology 106:200–206, 1994.

- model from Williams JA, Korc M, Dormer RL. Action of secretagogues on a new preparation of functionally intact, isolated pancreatic acini. Am J Physiol 235:E517–E524, 1978.
- measurement of enzyme activity.
- determination of secretin binding and Na^{+-} and K^{+-} activated ATP phosphohydrolase activity.

Doi R, Inoue K, Chowdhury P, et al. Structural and functional changes of exocrine pancreas induced by FK506 in rats. Gastroenterology 104:1153–1164, 1993.
- describes preparation of isolated pancreatic acini.
- measurement of enzyme activity, CCK, and scopolamine binding to receptors.
- measurement of cytosolic free calcium concentration.

Nakagawa A, Stagher JI, Samols E. Suppressive role of the islet-acinar axis in the perfused rat pancreas. Gastroenterology 105:868–875, 1993.
- perfusion method modified from Okabayashi Y, Otsuki M, Ohki A, et al. Secretin-induced exocrine secretion in perfused pancreas isolated from diabetic rats. Diabetes 37:1173–1180, 1988.

Schonfeld JV, Muller MK, Augustin M, et al. Effect of cysteamine on insulin release and exocrine pancreatic secretion in vitro. Dig Dis Sci 38:28–32, 1993.
- technique of measuring exocrine pancreatic secretion using an isolated perfused rat pancreas.

Hall PA, Lemoine NR. Rapid acinar to ductal transdifferentiation in cultured human exocrine pancreas. J Pathol 166:97–103, 1992.

Kimura W, Meyer F, Hess D, et al. Comparison of different treatment modalities in experimental pancreatitis. Gastroenterology 103:1916–1924, 1992.
- describes preparation of isolated pancreatic acini.
- describes modified preparation of isolated perfused rat pancreas.

Mossner J, Bodeker H, Kimura W. Isolated rat pancreatic acini as a model to study the potential role of lipase in the pathogenesis of acinar cell destruction. Int J Pancreatol 12:285–296, 1992.

Sanfey H, Sarr MG, Bulkley GB, et al. Oxygen-derived free radicals and acute pancreatitis: A review. Acta Physiol Scand (suppl 548):109–118, 1986.
- describes an ex vivo perfused canine pancreas preparation as a model for studying ischemic pancreatitis.

GASTROINTESTINAL

General

Kararli TT. Comparison of the gastrointestinal anatomy, physiology, and biochemistry of humans and commonly used laboratory animals. Biopharm Drug Dispos 16:351–380,1995.
- a user friendly potpourri of comparative facts pertaining to anatomy, physiology, and biochemistry for dogs, cats, rats, rabbits, mice, ruminants, and swine. The information covers anatomical differences, gastric acid pH and secretion, gastric and intestinal bacterial counts, intestinal mucosal brush border enzyme activities and lipid composi-

tion, bile flow, and composition. A must for those who play trivial pursuit of the digestive system!

Lennernas H. Gastrointestinal absorption mechanisms: A comparison between animal and human models. Eur J Pharm Sci 2:39–43, 1994.
- discusses the predictability of animal models for in vivo absorption of drugs in humans.

Fiocchi C. Cytokines and animal models: A combined path to inflammatory bowel disease pathogenesis. Gastroenterology 104:1202–1219, 1993.

Stark ME, Szurszewski JH. Role of nitric oxide in gastrointestinal and hepatic function and disease. Gastroenterology 103:1928–1949, 1992.
- references made to animal models.

Kim HS, Berstad A. Experimental colitis in animal models. Scand J Gastroenterol 27:529–537, 1992.

Haxell SL, Eichberg JW, Lee DR, et al. Selection of the chimpanzee over the baboon as a model for *Helicobacter pylori* infection. Gastroenterology 103:848–854, 1992.

Greenberg D, Smith GP, Gibbs J. Cholecystokinin and the satiating effect of fat. Gastroenterology 102:1801–1803, 1992.
- cholecystokinin and vagal afferent mechanisms are the two mediators of fat-induced satiety. This editorial succinctly reviews the animal studies and models defining these mechanisms.

Lee A. Spiral organisms: What are they? A microbiologic introduction to *Helicobacter pylori*. Scand J Gastroenterol 26 (suppl 187):S9–S22, 1991.
- discusses use of animal models in the study of pathogenic mechanisms.

Szurszewski JH. Electrical basis for gastrointestinal motility. In: Johnson LR (ed) Physiology of the Gastrointestinal Tract, 2nd ed. Raven Press, New York, 383–422, 1987.
- refers to studies in a variety of animals.

Debas HT: The gastrointestinal tract. In: Gay WI (ed) Methods of Animal Experimentation, Vol. VII. Academic Press, San Diego, 119–155, 1986.
- a compilation of the various animal preparations used in the study of gastrointestinal physiology. The surgical techniques are described and examples of pertinent studies given.

Onderdonk AB. Experimental models for ulcerative colitis. Dig Dis Sci 30 (suppl):40S–44S, 1985.
- reviews naturally occurring and experimentally induced animal models.

Cheville NF. Criteria for development of animal models of diseases of the gastrointestinal system. Am J Pathol 101 (suppl):S67–S88, 1980.

Kent TH, Moon HW. The comparative pathogenesis of some enteric diseases. Vet Pathol 10:414–469, 1973.
- naturally occurring disease in swine, avian, snake, dog, monkey, horse, and bovine with abundant photomicrographs.
- acute intestinal radiation injury in the cat is covered.

Methods

Evans G, Flint N, Potten C. Primary cultures for studies of cell regulation and physiology in intestinal epithelium. Ann Rev Physiol 56:399–417, 1994.

- the application and limitations of primary cultures for the study of normal gut epithelium are discussed.

Chew C. Parietal cell culture: New models and directions. Ann Rev Physiol 56:445–461, 1994.

- the development of prototype primary parietal cell culture models are described; their utility, deficiency, and future direction are discussed.

Sorensen SH, Proud FJ, Adam A, et al. A novel HPLC method for the simultaneous quantification of monosaccharides and disaccharides used in tests of intestinal permeability. Clin Chim Acta 221:115–126, 1993.

Meunier LD, Kissinger JT, Marcello J, et al. A chronic access port model for direct delivery of drugs into the intestine of conscious dogs. Lab Anim Sci 43:466–470, 1993.

- a modified vascular-access port was developed and validated for use in the duodenum, jejunum, colon, and/or peritoneal cavity.

Fiorucci S, Morelli A. Motilin and erythromycin stimulate pepsinogen secretion by chief cells isolated from guinea pig stomach. Gastoenterology 104:1030–1036, 1993.

- isolated gastric chief cells were obtained from guinea pig stomach by collagenase digestion and calcium chelation with ethylene glycol-bis (B-amynomethyl ether) -N, N, N', N'-tetraacetic acid.

Schlesinger DP, Rubin SI, Papich MG, et al. Use of the breath hydrogen measurement to evaluate orocecal transit time in cats before and after treatment for hyperthyroidism. Can J Vet Res 57:89–94, 1993.

Loiselle J, Wollin A. Mucosal histamine elimination and its effect on acid secretion in rabbit gastric mucosa. Gastroenterology 104:1013–1020, 1993.

- elimination of histamine and its effect on acid secretion was examined on isolated mucosal sheets mounted in flux chambers and in dispersed mucosal cells.

Soediono P, Belai A, Burnstock G. Prevention of neuropathy in the pyloric sphincter of streptozotocin-diabetic rats by gangliosides. Gastroenterology 104:1072–1082, 1993.

- streptozotocin-induced diabetic rats develop changes in the adrenergic and peptidergic innervation in the gastrointestinal tract, delayed small intestinal transit, and megacolon.

Jacobson ED. Circulatory mechanisms of gastric mucosal damage and protection. Gastroenterology 102:1788–1800, 1992.

- discusses methods for measurement of mucosal perfusion and microcirculation.

Duncan A, Stewart MJ. Measurement of faecal ammonia. Med Lab Sci 49:133–134, 1992.

Hall JA, Willer RL, Seim HB, et al. Gastric emptying of nondigestible radiopaque markers after circumcostal gastropexy in clinically normal dogs and dogs with gastric dilatation-volvulus. Am J Vet Res 53:1961–1965, 1992.

Takahashi M, Maeda Y, Tashiro H, et al. A new simple test for evaluation of intestinal bacteria. World J Surg 14:628–635, 1990.

- the synthesis and use of a conjugate of ursodeoxycholic acid with para-aminobenzoic acid (PABA) for the diagnosis of bacterial overgrowth is described. Both in vitro studies and a stagnant loop model in the rat are used to demonstrate its usefulness.

Esophagus

Cassidy KT, Geisinger KR, Kraus BB, et al. Continuous versus intermittent acid exposure in production of esophagitis in feline model. Dig Dis Sci 37:1206–1211, 1992.

- exposure of esophagus to 0.1 N HCl shown to result in esophagitis histologically similar to human reflux esophagitis.

Richter JE, Bradley LA, DeMeester TR, et al. Normal 24-hr ambulatory esophageal pH values: Influence of study center, pH electrode, age, and gender. Dig Dis Sci 37:849–856, 1992.

- describes technique and determines values in humans.

Friesen CA, Hayes R, Hodge C, et al. Comparison of methods of assessing 24-hour intraesophageal pH recordings in children. J Pediatr Gastroenterol Nutr 14:252–255, 1992.

Gastric

Dubois A, Fiala N, Heman-Ackah L, et al. Natural gastric infection with *Helicobacter pylori* in monkeys: A novel model for spiral bacteria infection in humans. Gastroenterology 106:1405–1417, 1994.

- rhesus monkeys are naturally infected with *Helicobacter pylori;* they have gastritis similar to humans and an increase in a specific plasma IgG titer.

Szabo S, Folkman J, Vattay P, et al. Accelerated healing of duodenal ulcers by oral administration of a mutein of basic fibroblast growth factor in rats. Gastroenterology 106:1106–1111, 1994.

- modification of model using cysteamine-hydrochloric acid by intragastric lavage.

Piasecki CK, Thrasivoulou C. Spasm of gastric muscularis mucosae might play a key role in causing focal mucosal ischemia and ulceration: An experimental study in guinea pigs. Dig Dis Sci 38:1183–1189, 1993.

- suggests findings may contribute to model of gastric ulceration.

Krantis A, Harding RK, McKay AE, et al. Effects of compound U74500A in animal models of gastric and duodenal ulceration. Dig Dis Sci 38:722–729, 1993.

- models used 100% ethanol gavage for gastric ulcers and intragastric boluses of cysteamine-hydrochloric acid for duodenal ulcers in Sprague-Dawley rats.

Maruoka A, Fujishima H, Misawa T, et al. Evaluation of acetic acid-induced gastric ulcers in dogs by endoscopic evaluation. Scand J Gastroenterol 28:1055–1061, 1993.

- classification of ulcer depth using this model.

Brzozowski T, Konturek SJ, Majka J, et al. Epidermal growth

factor, polyamines, and prostaglandins in healing of stress-induced gastric lesions in rats. Dig Dis Sci 38:276–283, 1993.

- acute gastric lesions induced by restraint and immersion in 23° C water to the xyphoid level for 6 hours.
- salivary gland removed in one group—major source of epidermal growth factor.

Carriere F, Laugier R, Barrowman JA, et al. Gastric and pancreatic lipase levels during a test meal in dogs. Scand J Gastroenterol 28:443–454, 1993.

- used device to monitor throughout the digestion period the flows of gastric and pancreatic lipases in the digestive tract and to quantify their total secretions.

Stein HJ, DeMeester TR. Integrated ambulatory foregut monitoring in patients with functional foregut disorders. Surg Annu 24:161–180, 1992.

- discusses the technique and equipment to assess ambulatory 24 hour monitoring of foregut pH and motility in human beings.

Ross JS, Bui HX, del Rosario A, et al. *Helicobacter pylori:* Its role in the pathogenesis of peptic ulcer disease in a new animal model. Am J Pathol 141:721–727, 1992.

- gastric ulcers induced with 100% acetic acid in Sprague-Dawley rats followed by intragastric administration of *Helicobacter pylori.*

Scheiman JM, Draus ER, Yoshimura K, et al. Effect of sucralfate on components of mucosal barrier produced by cultured canine epithelial cells in vitro. Dig Dis Sci 37:1853–1859, 1992.

- describes preparation of primary culture of canine fundic surface epithelial cells.

Kleiman-Wexler RL, Ephgrave KS, Broadhurst KA. Effects of intragastric and intravenous glucose on restraint model of stress ulceration. Dig Dis Sci 37:1860–1865, 1992.

- cold stress protocol used.

Hodgson DS, Dunlop CI, Chapman PL, et al. Cardiopulmonary responses to experimentally induced gastric dilatation in isoflurane-anesthetized dogs. Am J Vet Res 53:938–943, 1992.

- an intragastric balloon was used to distend the stomach.

Lantz GC, Badylak SF, Hiles MC, et al. Treatment of reperfusion injury in dogs with experimentally induced gastric dilatation-volvulus. Am J Vet Res 53:1594–1598, 1992.

- model of gastric dilatation-volvulus.

Lee A, Fox JG, Otto G, et al. A small animal model of human *Helicobacter pylori* active chronic gastritis. Gastroenterology 99:1315–1323, 1990.

- *Helicobacter felis* was isolated, cultured, and given orally to Swiss Webster mice.

Small Bowel

Nagata H, Miyairi M, Sekizuka E, et al. In vivo visualization of lymphatic microvessels and lymphocyte migration through rat Peyer's patches. Gastroenterology 106:1548–1553, 1994.

- a micropuncture technique is described for the study of lymphocyte trafficking in Peyer's patches.

Tarr P. Enterocolitis associated with Shiga-like toxin production: An appropriate animal model at least? Gastroenterology 106:540–543, 1994.

- a rabbit model for human enterohemorrhagic disease is interrogated and questions are posed for future investigation relating to its pathophysiologic consequences. The model is described in Sjogren R, Neill R, Rachmilewitz D, et al. Role of Shiga-like toxin I in bacterial enteritis: Comparison between isogenic Escherichia coli strains induced in rabbits. Gastroenterology 106:306–317, 1994.

Crissinger K, Burney D, Velasquez O, et al. An animal model of necrotizing enterocolitis induced by infant formula and ischemia in developing piglets. Gastroenterology 106:1215–1222, 1994.

- luminal perfusion of 1-day-old piglet jejunoileum with predigested and bile acid-solubilized preterm infant formula combined with ischemia/reperfusion successfully produces necrotizing enterocolitis.

Slocum MM, Granger DN. Early mucosal and microvascular changes in feline intestinal transplants. Gastroenterology 105:1761–1768, 1993.

- model of small intestinal transplantation in which ileal grafts underwent 0 to 24 hours of cold ischemia before reperfusion.

Malbert CH, Ruckebusch Y. Duodenal pH dips as an index of transpyloric flow in conscious dogs. Gastroenterology 105:755–763, 1993.

- technique for simultaneous monitoring of transpyloric flow and pH in the duodenal bulb.

Ulshen MH, Dowling RH, Fuller R, et al. Enhanced growth of small bowel in transgenic mice overexpressing bovine growth hormone. Gastroenterology 104:973–980, 1993.

- transgenic mice with a bovine growth hormone gene linked to a mouse metallothionein I promoter (growth hormone transgenics) used to study growth of small-bowel mucosa.

Pothoulakis C, Kelly CP, Joshi MA, et al. *Saccharomyces boulardii* inhibits *Clostridium difficile* toxin A binding and enterotoxicity in rat ileum. Gastroenterology 104:1108–1115, 1993.

- standardized rat ileal loop model used to determine the effect of toxin on secretion, epithelial permeability, and morphology.

Hudson M, Piasecki C, Sankey EA, et al. A ferret model of acute multifocal gastrointestinal infarction. Gastroenterology 102:1591–1596, 1992.

- intra-arterial injection of styrene microspheres produced focal inflammation, necrosis, and ulceration; "summit" lesions observed (fibrinous and acute inflammatory exudate).

Hayashi M, Endoh D, Kon Y, et al. Higher sensitivity of LEC strain rat in radiation-induced acute intestinal death. J Vet Med Sci 54:269–273, 1992.

Longmire-Cook SJ, Lillienau J, Kim YS, et al. Effect of replacement therapy with cholylsarcosine on fat malabsorption associated with severe bile acid malabsorption: Studies in dogs with ileal resection. Dig Dis Sci 37:1217–1227, 1992.

- in addition to removal of the entire ileum, a Thomas cannula was inserted first into the duodenum and then into the anterior abdominal wall in order to attach the duodenum to the abdominal wall and create a permanent sampling access.

Stone WC, Bjorling DE, Southard JH, et al. Evaluation of intestinal villus height in rats after ischemia and reperfusion by administration of superoxide dismutase, and two 21-aminosteroids. Am J Vet Res 53:2153–2156, 1992.
- ischemia induced by placing bulldog vascular clamp across the cranial mesenteric artery and vein.

Cohen MB, Giannella RA. Jejunal toxin inactivation regulates susceptibility of the immature rat to STa. Gastroenterology 102:1988–1996, 1992.
- immature rat jejunum demonstrates an increased response, sensitivity, and susceptibility to heat stable enterotoxin.

D'Inca R, Hunt RH, Perdue MH. Mucosal damage during intestinal anaphylaxis in the rat: Effect of betamethasone and disodium cromoglycate. Dig Dis Sci 37:1704–1708, 1992.
- rats immunized with *Nippostrongylus brasiliensis* and challenged intravenously with whole worm antigen.

Erickson RA, Rivera N. Effect of difluoromethylornithine (DFMO) on NSAID-induced intestinal injury in rats. Dig Dis Sci 37:1833–1839, 1992.
- injury induced by intragastric gavage of indomethacin.

Isolauri E, Gotteland M, Heyman M, et al. Antigen absorption in rabbit bacterial diarrhea (RDEC-1): In vitro modifications in ileum and Peyer's patches. Dig Dis Sci 35:360–366, 1990.
- rabbits infected at weaning with the rabbit-specific *Escherichia coli strain* RDEC-1.
- within hours it adheres to microfold M cells of the intestinal Peyer's patches and causes acute inflammation.
- the second stage involves adherence to the intestinal epithelium and destruction of microvilli in a manner morphologically identical to what is observed in human pathology.

Heyman M, Crain-Denoyelle AM, Desjeux JF. Endocytosis and processing of protein by isolated villus and crypt cells of the mouse small intestine. J Pediatr Gastroenterol Nutr 9:238–245, 1989.
- describes isolation of intestinal cells.

Large Bowel

Wallace J, Le T, Carter L, et al. Hapten-induced chronic colitis in the rat: Alternatives to trinitrobenzene sulfonic acid. J Pharmacol Toxicol Meth 33:237–239, 1995.
- a single intracolonic administration of a hapten, trinitrobenzenesulfonic acid causes colonic inflammation that persists for approximately 8 weeks. Two structurally similar haptens that produce colonic inflammation for approximately 2 weeks in rats are evaluated in this paper. These haptens are apparently more economical.

Banerjee A. Hypothesis-pouchitis represents a useful clinical model of ulcerative colitis. Med Hypothesis 42:36–38, 1994.
- the use of pouchitis as an animal model for the study of ulcerative colitis in humans is interrogated. The bottom line: it represents a useful pathophysiologic and therapeutic model.

Basilisco G, Phillips SF. Ileal distention relaxes the canine colon: A model of megacolon? Gastroenterology 106:606–614, 1994.
- schematic illustrating experimental preparation.

Garrigues TM, Segura-Bono MJ, Bermejo MV, et al. Compared effects of synthetic and natural bile acid surfactant on xenobiotic absorption. II. Studies with sodium glycocholate to confirm a hypothesis. International J Pharm 101:209–217, 1994.
- effect of a bile acid on the intestinal absorption of drug-related xenobiotics investigated, on the basis of previously established absorption/partition relationships, using an in situ rat gut technique; the whole colon serves as a nonspecialized absorption membrane model.

Tsuchiya T, Ishizuka J, Sato K, et al. New experimental model of proximal and distal colon transposition in rats. Lab Anim Sci 43:454–456, 1993.

Rachmilewitz D, Stamler JS, Karmeli F, et al. Peroxynitrite-induced rat colitis—a new model of colonic inflammation. Gastroenterology 105:1681–1688, 1993.

Yamada T, Sartor RB, Marshall S, et al. Mucosal injury and inflammation in a model of chronic granulomatous colitis in rats. Gastroenterology 104:759–771, 1993.
- intramural injection of peptidoglycan-polysaccharide into the distal colon of genetically susceptible rats (specific pathogen-free Lewis rats).
- blood-to-lumen clearance of chromium labeled-ethylenediaminaetetraacetic acid, colonic myoelectrical activity, colon weight, and plasma nitrite and nitrate concentrations were determined to quantitate colonic mucosal injury, inflammation, and nitric oxide production, respectively.

Leung FW, Su KC, Yonei Y, et al. Regional differences in mucosal hemodynamics in experimental colonic injury in rats. Dig Dis Sci 38:1220–1223, 1993.
- colon injury induced by acetic acid and by dinitrochlorobenzene.

Gurbindo C, Russo P, Sabbah S, et al. Interleukin-2 activity of colonic lamina propria mononuclear cells in a rat model of experimental colitis. Gastroenterology 104:964–972, 1993.
- trinitrobenzene sulfonic acid was given by colic enema.

Grossi L, McHugh K, Collins SM. On the specificity of altered muscle function in experimental colitis in rats. Gastroenterology 104:1049–1056, 1993.
- distal colitis was induced by intrarectal administration of trinitrobenzene sulfonic, acetic acid, or *Trichinella spiralis* larvae, or by intraperitoneal injection of mitomycin C.

Yamada T, Marshall S, Specian RD, et al. A comparative analysis of two models of colitis in rats. Gastroenterology 102:1524–1534, 1992.
- models using acetic acid and trinitrobenzene sulfonic acid are compared and evaluated.

Kishimoto S, Kobayashi H, Shimizu S, et al. Changes of colonic vasoactive intestinal peptide and cholinergic activity in rats with chemical colitis. Dig Dis Sci 37:1729–1737, 1992.
- sodium salt of dextran sulfate added to water for 3 months used to induce lesion reported to resemble ulcerative colitis.

Mack DR, Lau AS, Sherman PM. Systemic tumor necrosis factor-alpha production in experimental colitis. Dig Dis Sci 37:1738–1745, 1992.

- colitis in New Zealand white rabbits by the induction of cellular immunity by sequential challenge with a chemical hapten 1-chloro-2, 4-dinitrobenzene dissolved in acetone and applied to shaved flank area. Ten days later the chemical was applied to the mucosa of the distal colon.

Kitsukawa Y, Saito H, Suzuki Y, et al. Effect of ingestion of eicosapentaenoic acid ethyl ester on carrageenan-induced colitis in guinea pigs. Gastroenterology 102:1859–1866, 1992.

Imray CHE, Minoura T, Davis A, et al. Comparability of hamster with human faecal unconjugated bile acids in a model of colorectal cancer. Anticancer Res 12:553–558, 1992.

PORTAL HYPERTENSION

Methods and Procedures

Lebrec D. Methods to evaluate portal hypertension. Gastroenterol Clin N Am 21:41–59, 1992.

- in addition to the contemporary review of methods, there is a short discussion on models of portal hypertension.
- opening chapter of this reference lists experimental models.

Dauzat M, Pomier-Layrargues G. Portal vein blood flow measurements using pulsed Doppler and electromagnetic flowmetry in dogs: A comparative study. Gastroenterology 96:913–919, 1989.

- Doppler flowmetry was not an ideal method to measure absolute portal vein blood flow values.

Bosch J, Mastai R, Kravetz D, et al. Hemodynamic evaluation of the patient with portal hypertension. Liver Dis 6:309–317, 1986.

- reviews techniques and methods used in humans.

In Vivo

Jaffe V, Alexander B, Mathie RT. Intrahepatic portal occlusion by microspheres: A new model of portal hypertension in the rat. Gut 35:815–818, 1994.

- microspheres given intraportally cause portal hypertension without distorting hepatic architecture as with the cirrhotic model and the technique avoids the use of constricting devices. However, the maximum pressure achieved is limited because, perhaps, of the existence of intrahepatic shunts in the normal rat liver which "open" in response to increased portal pressure. This serendipitous finding stimulates the possible use of a similar model for the investigation of the proposed syndrome of intrahepatic shunts in Cairn terriers (Schermerhorn T, Center S, Rowland P, et al. Characterization of inherited portovascular dysplasia in Cairn terriers (abstract). J Vet Int Med 7:136, 1993).

Um A, Nishida O, Tokubayashi M, et al. Hemodynamic changes after ligation of a major branch of the portal vein in rats: Comparison with rats with portal vein constriction. Hepatology 19:202–209, 1994.

- 80% of the total liver mass was deprived of portal blood

flow by ligation of the portal branch (illustrated) and the hemodynamic changes examined chronologically.

Garcia-Tsao G, Albillos A, Barden GE, et al. Bacterial translocation in acute and chronic hypertension. Hepatology 17:1081–1085, 1993.

- rat model using calibrated portal vein stenosis.
- procedure for handling tissues to determine bacterial growth.

Vorobioff J, Bredfeldt JE, Groszmann RJ. Hyperdynamic circulation in portal-hypertensive rat model: A primary factor for maintenance of chronic portal hypertension. Am J Physiol 244:G52–G57, 1992.

- portal vein stenosis model.
- methods and procedures for measurement of splanchnic hemodynamics.

Poo JL, Feldmann G, Erlinger S, et al. Ursodeoxycholic acid limits liver histologic alterations and portal hypertension induced by bile duct ligation in the rat. Gastroenterology 102:1752–1759, 1992.

- four weeks following bile duct ligation there is extensive fibrosis, portal hypertension, and alterations in the splanchnic and systemic circulation.

Pomier-Layrargues G, Giroux L, Rocheleau B, et al. Combined treatment of portal hypertension with ritanserin and propranolol in conscious and unrestrained cirrhotic rats. Hepatology 15:878–882, 1992.

- cirrhosis, induced by adding phenobarbital to the drinking water for 2 weeks, causes portal hypertension.

Sikuler E. Beta-adrenergic blockers for portal hypertension. J Hepatol 12:133–135, 1992.

- concise editorial reflecting on information obtained from various animal models.

GALLBLADDER

In Vivo

Fiorucci S, Scionti L, Bosso R, et al. Effect of erythromycin on gallbladder emptying in diabetic patients with and without autonomic neuropathy and high levels of motilin. Dig Dis Sci 37:1671–1677, 1992.

- ultrasound protocol for evaluating gallbladder emptying.

Diamond T, Dolan S, Rowlands BJ. An improved technique for choledochoduodenostomy in a rat model of obstructive jaundice. Lab Anim Sci 41:82–83, 1991.

Fujimoto JM. Some in vivo methods for studying sites of toxicant action in relation to bile formation. In: Plaa G, Hewitt WR (eds) Toxicology of the Liver. Raven Press, New York, 121–141, 1982.

- describes a variety of techniques and methods.
- small list of animal models.

Suda K, Miyano T, Suzuki F, et al. Clinicopathologic and experimental studies on cases of abnormal pancreatico-choledocho-ductal junction. Acta Pathol Jpn 37:1549–1562, 1987.

- long-term evaluation in dogs.
- cell kinetics in biliary tract mucosa observed by the use of monoclonal antibody against bromodeoxyuridine.

In Vitro

Auth MKH, Keitzer RA, Scholz M. Establishment and characterization of cultured human gallbladder epithelial cells. Hepatology 18:546–555, 1993.

Purdum PP, Ulissi A, Hylemon PB, et al. Cultured human gallbladder epithelia: Methods and partial characterization of a carcinoma-derived model. Lab Invest 68:345–353, 1993.
- a variety of physiologic parameters measured.
- model consistent with native gallbladder.
- suggested use for study of the pathophysiology of gallstone formation.

Liu YF, Saccone GTP, Thune A, et al. Sphincter of Oddi regulates flow by acting as a variable resistor to flow. Am J Physiol 263:G683-G689, 1992.
- two models of transsphincteric flow and a model evaluating pumping activity were established in the Australian brush-tailed possum to study the sphincter of Oddi.
- discussion includes information on the dog and cat models.

Shaffer EA. Abnormalities in gallbladder function in cholesterol gallstone disease: Bile and blood, mucosa and muscle—the list lengths. Gastroenterology 102:808–812, 1992.
- contains references for the prairie dog and ground squirrel models.

Conter RL, Washington JL, Liao CC, et al. Gallbladder mucosal blood flow increases during early cholesterol gallstone formation. Gastroenterology 102:1764–1770, 1992.
- experimental design uses prairie dog model; indicates extrahepatic biliary anatomy and biliary lipid composition similar to human counterparts.
- contains schematic showing catheter placement in model.

Myers SI. The role of eicosanoids in experimental and clinical gallbladder disease. Prostagland Leuk Essen Fatty Acids 45:167–180, 1992.
- reviews factors related to inflammation of the gallbladder and refers to a variety of animal models.

Pemsingh RS, MacPherson BR, Scott GW. Mucus hypersecretion in the gallbladder epithelium of ground squirrels fed a lithogenic diet for the induction of cholesterol gallstones. Hepatology 7:1267–1271, 1987.
- study uses Richardson ground squirrel to examine factors involved in the formation of cholesterol gallstones.

Index

ISBN 0-7216-3760-4

90038